Drug Therapy in Nursing

Drug Therapy in Nursing

EDITION 4

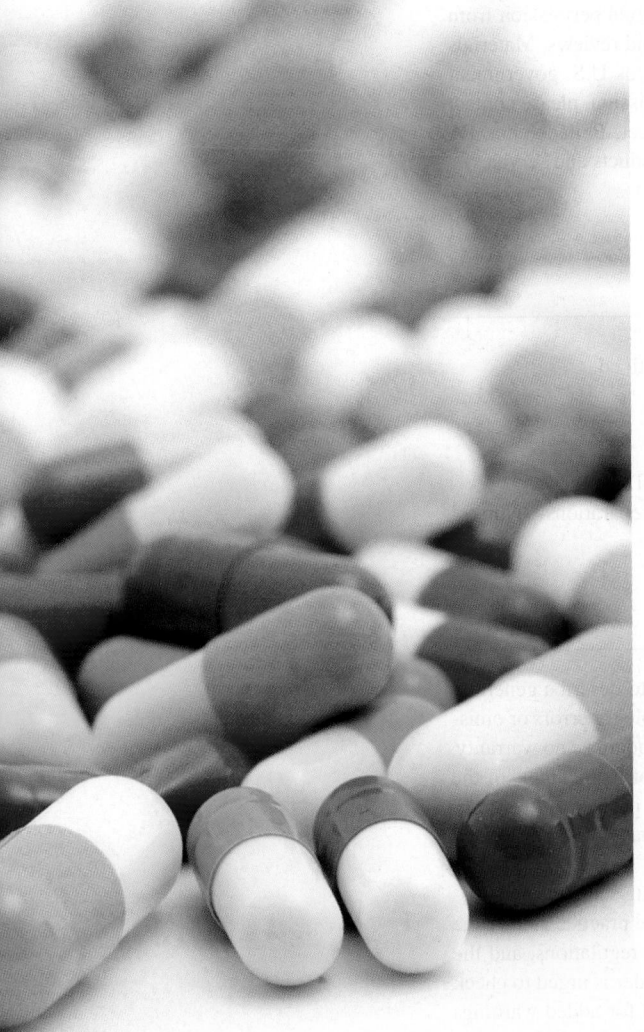

Diane S. Aschenbrenner, MS, RN
Course Coordinator
Johns Hopkins University
School of Nursing
Baltimore, Maryland

Samantha J. Venable, MS, RN, FNP, CNE
Professor
Saddleback College
Mission Viejo, California

. Wolters Kluwer | Lippincott Williams & Wilkins
Health
Philadelphia · Baltimore · New York · London
Buenos Aires · Hong Kong · Sydney · Tokyo

Acquisitions Editor: Hilarie Surrena
Product Manager: Mary Kinsella
Editorial Assistanst: Jacalyn Clay, Zachary Shapiro
Design Coordinator: Holly Reid McLaughlin
Illustration Coordinator: Brett McNaughton
Manufacturing Coordinator: Karin Duffield
Prepress Vendor: SPi Global

4th edition

Aschenbrenner, Diane S.
  Drug therapy in nursing / Diane S. Aschenbrenner, Samantha J. Venable. – 4th ed.
     p. ; cm.
  Includes bibliographical references and index.
  ISBN 978-1-60831-151-4
  1. Chemotherapy. 2. Pharmacology. 3. Nursing. I. Venable, Samantha J. II. Title.
  [DNLM: 1. Drug Therapy—Nurses' Instruction. 2. Pharmaceutical Preparations—Nurses' Instruction. 3. Pharmacology—Nurses' Instruction.   WB 330]
  RM125.N83   2011
  615.5'8—dc22
                                                                        2011013529

LWW.com

To my family for encouragement to do this again;
and to my students for all that they have taught me.

DSA

To my husband Ben who continues to support me in all
of my professional efforts, and to my students who never
cease to amaze me with their dedication and hard work.

SV

Contributors

Faye Bembry, RN, MSN, FNP-BC
Nurse Practitioner
Paradigm Health Services
University of Tennessee
School of Nursing
Milligan College
Johnson City, Tennessee

Andrew R. Benson, MS, RN, CRNA
Nurse Anesthetist
The Johns Hopkins University
School of Medicine
Baltimore, Maryland

Gerry M. deJesus, MSN
Nurse Practitioner
Health Care Agency
Santa Ana, California

Jacqueline Gilreath, ADN
Staff Nurse
Mattel's Children's Hospital
University of California
Los Angeles

Janice J. Hoffman, RN, PhD, CCRN
*Assistant Professor, Assistant Dean of the
    Baccalaureate Program*
University of Maryland
School of Nursing
Baltimore, Maryland

Barbara G. Huggins, MN, PMHCNS-BC
Professor of Nursing
Saddleback College
Mission Viejo, California

Peggy Jenkins, MS, CAS, CCRN, CNE
Professor Nursing
Hartwick College
Oneonta, New York

Mikaela Olsen, RN, MS, OCN
Oncology and Hematology Clinical Nurse Specialist
The Johns Hopkins Hospital
The Sidney Kimmel Comprehensive Cancer Center
Baltimore, Maryland

Paul L. Sacamano, BSN, RN
Clinical Nurse II
University of the Maryland, Medical Center
Department of Medicine, Division of Infectious
    Diseases
Baltimore, Maryland

Brenda K. Shelton, MS, RN, CCRN, AOCN
Clinical Nurse Specialist
The Johns Hopkins Hospital
The Sidney Kimmel Comprehensive Cancer Center
Baltimore, Maryland

Kelly A. Stauffacher, CRNA, MSN
Clinical Faculty
Duke University
School of Nursing
Durham, North Carolina

Nancy Sullivan, RN, MS
Nurse Educator
The Johns Hopkins Hospital
Adjunct Faculty
The Johns Hopkins University
School of Nursing
Baltimore, Maryland

Donna Rane-Szostak, EdD, MSN, CNE
Dean, Health Sciences & Human Services
Saddleback College
Mission Viejo, California

Joyce B. Vazzano, MS, APRN, CRNP
Instructor
The Johns Hopkins University
School of Nursing
Baltimore, Maryland

Anne B. Woods, PhD, MPH, CNM
Associate Professor
Messiah College
Department of Nursing
Grantham, Pennsylvania

Reviewers

Maureen Anthony, PhD, RN
Associate Professor
University of Detroit Mercy
McAuley School of Nursing
Detroit, Michigan

April Bigelow, PhD, ANP-BC
Clinical Assistant Professor
Adult Nurse Practitioner Program Coordinator
University of Michigan
School of Nursing
Ann Arbor, Michigan

Barbara Bostelmann, RN, BS, MS
Assistant Professor
Elmhurst College
Deicke Center for Nursing Education
Elmhurst, Illinois

Peggy Bozarth, MSN, RN, CNE
Professor of Nursing
Nursing Program Coordinator
Hopkinsville Community College
Hopkinsville, Kentucky

Marilyn Breuer, BSN, MSN
Associate Professor of Nursing
American International College
Springfield, Massachusetts

Djuana Burns, DNP, FNP-C
Assistant Professor
Troy University, School of Nursing
Troy, Alabama

Jean Cain, BSN, MSN
Nursing Faculty
Presentation College
Lakota Campus
Aberdeen, South Dakota

Joan Cawthorn, RN, BScN
Nursing Instructor
Grande Prairie Regional College
Grande Prairie, Alberta, Canada

Dominic Chan
Faculty of Nursing
University of Toronto
Ontario, Canada

Ellen Cram, PhD, RN
Assistant Dean, Undergraduate and Pre-licensure
* Programs*
Associate Professor, Clinical
University of Iowa
College of Nursing
Iowa City, Iowa

Ann Denney, RN, MSN
Associate Professor of Nursing
Thomas More College
Crestview Hills, Kentucky

Nancy W. Ebersole, RN, PhD
Associate Professor of Nursing
Salem State University
Salem, Massachusetts

Sophia Gardner, MSN, RN
Professor of Nursing
Community College of Allegheny County
Pittsburgh, Pennsylvania

Elizabeth Gephart, DNP, APRN, PNP-BC
Assistant Professor
Millikin University
Decatur, Illinois

Junell Harris, BSN, MSN/ED
Instructor
The Good Samaritan College of Nursing and
   Health Science
Cincinnati, Ohio

Barbara J. Holtrop, RN, MSN
Nursing Faculty, ADN Nursing Program
Muskegon Community College
Muskegon, Michigan

Peggy Jenkins, MS, CAS, CCRN, CNE
Professor of Nursing
Hartwick College
Oneonta, New York

James V. Jessup, PhD, RN
Associate Professor
University of Florida
Gainesville, Florida

Karen L. Joiner, MS, ARNP
Director of Nursing Programs
Lower Columbia College
Longview, Washington

J. Mari Beth Linder, PhD, RN, BC
Director & Professor of Nursing
Missouri Southern State University
Joplin, Missouri

Brenda Mason, RN, MSN, FNP-BC
Associate Professor of Nursing
Alderson Broaddus College
Philippi, West Virginia

Abigail Matos-Pagan, DNP, MS, ANPC, RN, CCA
Associate Professor
University of Puerto Rico Mayaguez
Department of Nursing
Mayaguez, Puerto Rico

Patricia McGinley, RN, MSN, FNP
Assistant Director of Nursing
El Camino College
Torrance, California

Karen Montalto, RN, PhD
BSN Chair/Associate Professor
Holy Family University
Philadelphia, Pennsylvania

Margaret Moriarty-Litz, MS, RN
Coordinator, ASN Program
St. Joseph School of Nursing
Nashua, New Hampshire

Zondra Myers
Vincennes University
Vincennes, Indiana

Linda Peake, MS, RNC, CNE
Curriculum Coordinator, Professor
St. Mary's/Marshall University
Cooperative ASN Program
Huntington, West Virginia

Karen A. Piotrowski, RNC, MSN
Associate Professor of Nursing
D'Youville College
Buffalo, New York

Lillian A. Rafeldt, MA, RN, CNE
Professor of Nursing, CT-CCNP
Three Rivers Community College
Norwich, Connecticut

Tracy Saddler, RN, APN
Union University
Jackson, Tennessee

Hana Smalley
North Island College
Courtenay, BC, Canada

Janet Thorlton, PhD, MS, RN
Assistant Professor
Purdue University School of Nursing
West Lafayette, Indiana

Diane Tomasic
Co-chair of the Nursing Department Curriculum Committee
Slippery Rock University
Slippery Rock, Pennsylvania

Maureen Tremel
Seminole Community College
Sanford, Florida

Richard Trifilo
Fitchburg State College
Fitchburg, Massachussetts

Marianne Udell, MN, RN, MSW
Retired, Formerly Assistant Professor
Santa Fe Community College
Department of Nursing
Santa Fe, New Mexico

Cecelia Vicuna-Keady, RN, BSN, MSN, DNP
Lecturer
University of Massachusetts Amherst
Amherst, Massachussetts

Melinda Wang, MSN, RN, APN, WHNP-BC
Assistant Professor
Pellissippi State College
Knoxville, Tennessee

Carol Webb, RN, MN, BSN, FPNP
Associate of Professor
The University of West Alabama
Division of Nursing
Livingston, Alabama

Teresa Wicks, MSN, RNC
Adjunct Assistant Professor
Montana State University
College of Nursing, Billings Campus
Bozeman, Montana

Preface

"How will I ever learn all of this?" and "Where do I begin?" are questions that nursing students frequently ask themselves and their faculty when beginning to study pharmacology. The subject is indeed vast for novices in the profession who lack the skills to organize drug information appropriately. Students feel overwhelmed by all of the isolated pieces of drug information they must learn. Consequently, they lose sight of "the forest for the trees."

PROTOTYPE APPROACH

For years, many pharmacology faculty have favored a prototype approach to teaching pharmacology. This method encourages identification of "the major trees" and facilitates recognition of "the forest." Use of a prototype, a drug that is representative of a class (or group) of drugs, helps students because it offers a systematic approach to grouping drug data, while beginning to recognize individual drug names. It gives students a "method" of learning and organizing large amounts of information. *Drug Therapy in Nursing, Fourth Edition,* is designed and written by faculty who themselves teach nursing pharmacology using the prototype approach. At last, nursing pharmacology faculty have a text that matches the way they teach. *Drug Therapy in Nursing, Fourth Edition,* is that text!

CLINICAL JUDGMENT AND CLINICAL APPLICATION

Drug Therapy in Nursing, Fourth Edition, is unique in that it presents a totally nursing-focused framework to support the teaching and learning of nursing pharmacology. Learning the pharmacology facts about different drug prototypes is only half of the knowledge nursing students need. Because they're learning to be nurses, they must understand how to apply this knowledge to patient care. Nurses must learn to think critically, evaluate information, and make decisions. However, this essential aspect of knowledge application has never been thoroughly addressed in nursing pharmacology texts. Frequently, students view *nursing application* of drug knowledge as less important than learning the hard drug facts. This thinking is fostered when the pharmacology textbooks they use present the nursing process after or apart from drug knowledge in a brief paragraph or chart. *Drug Therapy in Nursing, Fourth Edition,* fully integrates core drug knowledge with core patient information, appropriately stressing, as no other text does, the relationship between the two bodies of information.

As with all other factual, scientific, or medical information used by nurses, students must learn to integrate this knowledge into their practice and apply it to patient care. Applying drug information to patient care may overwhelm students because every patient is different, with different responses, positive or negative, to the same drug therapy. If the student sees each patient situation as an isolated case, learning is again hampered. This text provides a systematic framework for assessing and evaluating patient responses that change in accord with health, age, gender, lifestyle, and other factors. This important *patient focus* is strengthened by use of the nursing process framework. Pharmacologic facts are integrated into nursing, to help the student apply knowledge to practice, safely administer drugs, educate patients, and begin to make the journey from novice to expert.

USE OF A SYSTEMATIC FRAMEWORK

The authors of *Drug Therapy in Nursing, Fourth Edition,* present a systematic framework for drug therapy with every prototype drug. The framework consists of two basic areas of information: first, core drug knowledge and core patient variables; and second, actions of the nurse using this knowledge.

Core Drug Knowledge highlights the important drug facts about a prototype drug. Core drug knowledge includes pharmacotherapeutics, pharmacokinetics, pharmacodynamics, contraindications and precautions, adverse effects, and drug interactions.

Core Patient Variables identify the major topics that should be assessed in every patient to determine special considerations that need to be taken into account when administering a drug to a patient. Core patient variables include health status; life span and gender; lifestyle, diet, and habits; environment; and culture and inherited traits. The text presents the relevant variables for each particular prototype.

The nurse uses knowledge about the drug and knowledge about the patient to maximize the therapeutic effect of the drug, minimize the adverse effects of the drug, or provide patient and family education. The authors of this text call what the nurse does with knowledge about the drug and the individual patient "nursing management of drug therapy."

ORGANIZATION

Drug Therapy in Nursing, Fourth Edition, has twelve units. The first three units address the principles and process of nursing management of drug therapy, and the basics of core drug knowledge and patient-related variables. The next nine units present the nursing management of drugs affecting various body systems and disease states. Appendices are now located on the text website on thePoint.

Unit 1, Foundations for Drug Therapy in Nursing, consists of three chapters. Chapter 1 explains the framework for the text and how this framework relates to the application of drug knowledge to clinical practice. **This is a crucial chapter for students and faculty to read so that they will best understand the content in the rest of the text.** The remaining chapters address basic pharmaceutical knowledge, drug development and its related safeguards, and drug delivery, and the modes of drug administration.

Unit 2, Core Drug Knowledge, includes two chapters that present the basics of pharmacology: pharmacotherapeutics, pharmacokinetics, and pharmacodynamics; and adverse effects and drug interactions.

Unit 3, Core Patient Variables, includes seven chapters that highlight information pertinent to patient assessment relevant to drug therapy. This is not an exhaustive list of every aspect that can be considered by these variables. The topics include life-span issues (children, pregnant or breast-feeding women, and older adults); lifestyle, diet, and habits issues (substance abuse, dietary considerations, and complementary medication use); environment (influences on drug therapy); and culture and inherited traits (considerations in drug therapy). The core patient variable of health status is not presented, as this includes all physiology, pathophysiology, disease states, and their related treatments.

Units 4 through 12 present drugs affecting the various body systems and drugs used to treat diseases and their symptoms.

The Appendices, found online at **thePoint** under faculty and student resources present essential information on diagnostic imaging agents, enzymes and débridement therapy, enteral and nutritional supplements, parenteral nutrition, immunizations and immunization schedules for the United States, drugs causing photosensitivity, drugs that interact with grapefruit juice, and drugs metabolized by the P450 system. Emphasis is given in the appendices to the nursing management of these drug therapies.

PEDAGOGY

- **Chapter Learning Objectives** identify key content within the chapter to help direct student learning.
- **Key Terms** identify terms that are key to understanding each chapter's contents.
- **Pathophysiology information,** which summarizes information relevant to drug therapy, is included to assist with understanding and critical thinking.
- **Black Box warnings** from the FDA labels are included in the discussion of each prototype when applicable.
- **Separate chapters** are included on drugs affecting fungal and viral infections, with revised expanded content.
- **Chapter Summaries** highlight the most important information presented in the chapter.
- **Questions for Study and Review** encourage the student to reflect on the important aspects of the chapter. Answers are provided at the back of the book.

NEW TO THIS EDITION

- All chapters have been updated and include new drugs approved by the FDA.
  - The chapter sequence has been reorganized to promote student comprehension and learning.
  - Totally revised chapters on adrenergic and cholinergic drugs to address areas typically confusing to students
  - Separate chapter with expanded content on chemotherapy drugs that affect a specific targeted cell.
- Black Box warnings from the FDA labels have been added to the memory chips when applicable.
- NCLEX style questions have been added to many of the chapters in the Study Guide.

KEY FEATURES

- **Concept Maps** introduce the student to all drugs that will be mentioned in the chapter. Each map identifies the drug class, its prototype, and drugs in the class that are similar to or different than the prototype. Concept maps also refer the student to other chapters if related drugs are covered elsewhere.
- **Physiology Figures** illustrate physiologic processes relevant to the drug class and link drug actions to physiology.
- **Memory Chips** assist students in studying and preparing for clinical practice, providing a quick reference of key points for each prototype drug.
- **Focus on Research** boxes highlight current research in pharmacology. The implications for nursing practice are addressed for each article.
- **Community-Based Concerns** highlight nursing issues related to drug therapy carried out in patients' homes and communities.
- **Critical Thinking Scenarios** challenge students to develop critical thinking skills for applying pharmacology knowledge to patient care. Answers are provided for instructors on thePoint.
- **Drug Summary Tables** relate pharmacotherapeutics and general dosage data to pharmacokinetic parameters.
- **Drug Interaction Tables,** for every prototype drug, highlight known drug–drug and drug–food interactions. When diagnostic and laboratory test values are affected by drug use, this information is pointed out as well.

TEACHING/LEARNING PACKAGE

These excellent ancillary materials make teaching and learning even easier!

Resources for Instructors

The following tools are available upon textbook adoption to instructors on http://thePoint.lww.com/aschenbrenner4e.

- The **Test Generator** lets you generate new tests from a bank containing over 800 NCLEX-style questions to help you assess your students' understanding of the course material.

- **Lesson Plans** organize all ancillary resources by learning objective to assist in preparing your lessons.
- An **Image Bank** contains illustrations from the book in formats suitable for printing and incorporating into Power-Point presentations and Internet sites.

In addition, an extensive collection of materials is provided for each book chapter:

- **Pre-Lecture Quizzes** are quick, knowledge-based assessments that allow you to check students' reading before you begin your instruction. Answers are also provided.
- **PowerPoint Presentations** provide an easy way for you to integrate the textbook with your students' classroom experience, either via slide shows or handouts. Multiple-choice and True/False questions are integrated into the presentations to promote class participation and allow instructors to use i-clicker technology.
- **Guided Lecture Notes** walk you through the chapters, objective by objective, and provide you with corresponding PowerPoint slide numbers.
- **Discussion Topics** (and suggested answers) can be used as conversation starters or in online discussion boards.
- **Assignments** (and suggested answers) include group, written, clinical, and web assignments.
- **Case Studies** for every drug chapter in the book are provided to help your students apply their knowledge to clinical scenarios.

Valuable learning tools for students are available on Student Resources online via ThePoint include:

- **NCLEX-Style Review Questions** for every chapter feature traditional and alternative-format NCLEX-style questions.
- Appendices to support drug information found in text.
- Concepts in Action animations illustrating pharmacologic and pharmacokinetic mechanisms bring the text to life.
- Watch and Learn video clips demonstrate important concepts related to medication administration and preventing medication errors, teaching students habits for careful clinical practice.

- **Dosage Calculation Quizzes** provide review of dosage calculation concepts to further promote patient safety
- **Monographs** of the 100 most commonly prescribed drugs, a **Spanish–English Audio Glossary,** and an **NCLEX Alternate Item Format Tutorial** are also provided.

In addition to these resources, the following are also available exclusively on thePoint:

- **Drug Class Review Exercises,** based on the Concept Maps in the text, are interactive drag-and-drop exercises that allow students to place the drugs in their appropriate drug classes and hear the drug names pronounced.
- Additional animations and video clips related to physiology and pathophysiology concepts offer students additional tools for review.
- **Journal Articles,** corresponding to every book chapter, offer students access to current research available in Lippincott Williams & Wilkins journals.

Study Guide

Study Guide to Accompany Drug Therapy in Nursing, Fourth Edition, authored by Diane Aschenbrenner and Samantha Venable, has been carefully designed to complement the textbook. The study guide is unique in that the text book authors have written the study guide, which is not often the case with student study guides. The study guide truly is designed to help students master important content. Information is reviewed according to the types of knowledge presented in each textbook chapter (e.g., key terms, physiology and pathophysiology, core drug knowledge, core patient variables, and nursing management). The *Study Guide* provides students further study and learning opportunities through various techniques, such as multiple-choice questions, matching, decision trees, and case studies that encourage critical thinking and the application of knowledge. Students move through the levels of learning, beginning with knowledge of terms and acquisition of facts, and progressing to the application of knowledge in each chapter. Answers for all of the exercises are provided at the end of the study guide to assist students with independent study. This edition features additional NCLEX questions for every chapter. Visit **thePoint** for further information.

Acknowledgments

Diane Aschenbrenner would like to acknowledge the research assistance provided by Robert Caswell, Wesley Cook, Leah Hart, Anna Karuba, Jessica Klosiewicz, Erin K. Meehan, Kailee M. Rabinovitz, Paul L. Sacamano, and Christine Young

The author team would like to acknowledge the contributions of the entire Lippincott Williams & Wilkins publishing staff for their hard work on this text. Many thanks!

Contents

UNIT 1

Foundations for Drug Therapy in Nursing

Nursing Management of Drug Therapy

Learning Objectives

At the completion of this chapter the student will:

1. Identify the defining components of core drug knowledge.

2. Identify the defining components of core patient variables.

3. Define nursing management of drug therapy.

4. Describe how the prototype approach to drugs is a helpful learning tool.

5. Differentiate the three main sources of data used in assessment of core drug variables.

6. Describe how core drug knowledge and core patient variables are used in nursing management of drug therapy.

7. Explain general strategies for maximizing the therapeutic effects of drug therapy.

8. Explain general strategies for minimizing adverse effects of drug therapy.

9. Identify the importance of patient and family education in drug therapy.

10. Discuss how to evaluate drug therapy and its nursing management.

11. Describe the varied settings in which nurses use nursing management techniques to assist patients receiving drug therapy.

Key Terms

adverse effects
contraindications and precautions
core drug knowledge
core patient variables
culture and inherited traits
drug interactions

drug response
environment
health status
life span and gender
lifestyle, diet, and habits

nursing management of drug therapy
pharmacodynamics
pharmacokinetics
pharmacotherapeutics
prototype drug

Nurses have a vital role in managing drug therapy for people with medical conditions. The nurse uses knowledge about the drug (core drug knowledge) and knowledge about the individual patient (core patient variables) to maximize the therapeutic effects of the drug, to minimize the adverse effects of the drug, and to provide patient and family education. The term *patient* is used in this text to identify the person who is taking the drug. It should not be interpreted to mean that drug therapy or the nursing management involved occurs solely in an acute, inpatient setting. Most drug therapy now occurs outside of hospitals.

Nurses apply pharmacology (i.e., the scientific body of drug knowledge) to meeting the assessed care needs of the patient. The pharmacologic facts relevant to each drug, termed **core drug knowledge,** are:

- **Pharmacotherapeutics:** the desired therapeutic effect of the drug
- **Pharmacokinetics:** the changes that occur to the drug while it is inside the body
- **Pharmacodynamics:** the effects of the drug on the body
- **Contraindications and precautions:** conditions under which the drug should not be used or must be used carefully with monitoring
- **Adverse effects:** unintended and usually undesired effects that may occur with use of the drug

- **Drug interactions:** effects that may occur when the drug is given along with another drug, food, or substance

These components of core drug knowledge are discussed in more depth in Chapters 4 and 5.

In addition to knowing the pharmacologic facts about each drug that a patient receives, nurses assess the patient for factors that may or will interact with drug therapy. These areas of assessment, termed **core patient variables,** are:

- **Health status:** the presence of disease, illness, and allergy; chronic conditions causing system or organ dysfunction; diminished memory or mental capacity
- **Life span and gender:** age, physiologic development, reproductive stage, and gender
- **Lifestyle, diet, and habits:** amount of activity and exercise; sleep–wake patterns; occupation; financial resources or access to health insurance coverage to offset the cost of the drug, or both; eating preferences and patterns; use or abuse of substances (e.g., nicotine, alcohol, and illegal drugs); use of over-the-counter (OTC) drugs; use of alternative health practices (e.g., herbal medicine, folk remedies); and ability to read and write
- **Environment:** location in which the drug therapy will be administered, such as hospital, home, or long-term care facility; properties of the physical environment that may

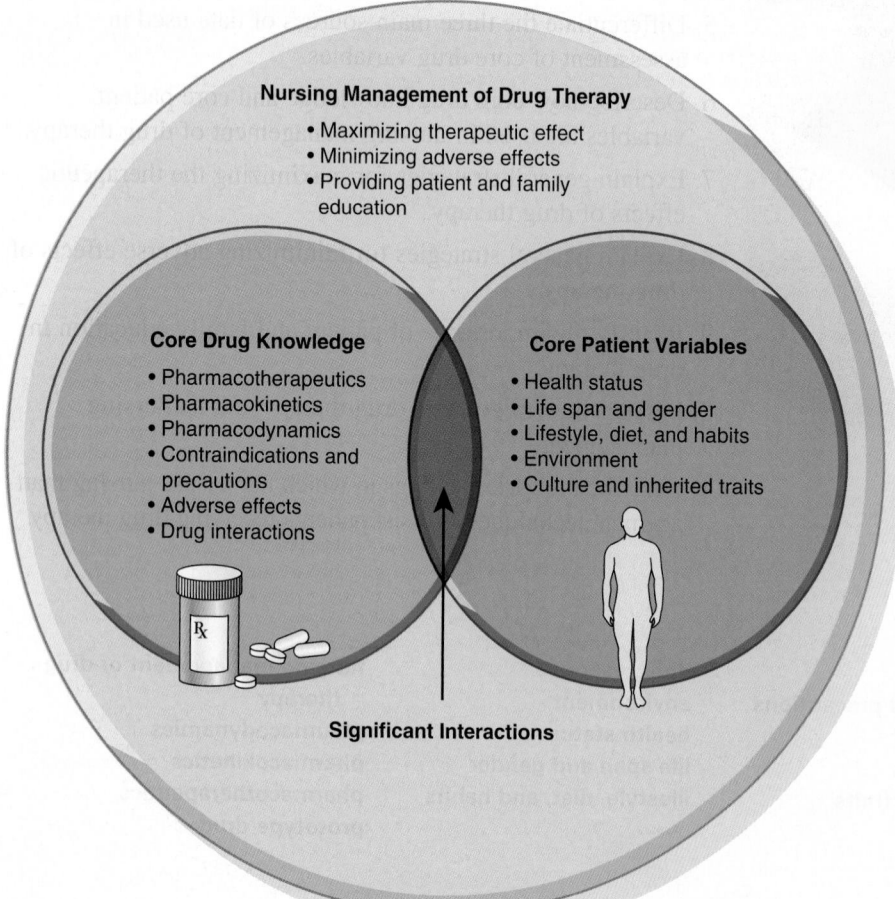

• FIGURE 1.1 Relationships among core drug knowledge, core patient variables, and nursing management of drug therapy. The nurse considers both the core drug knowledge and the core patient variables to provide appropriate nursing management of drug therapy.

alter a drug's action or effect, induce adverse effects from a drug, or set limitations on whether the drug may be administered in that setting; and exposure to potentially harmful substances, or a pathology induced from a harmful environmental substance, that requires drug therapy for treatment
- **Culture and inherited traits:** religious, social, and ethnic backgrounds that may affect the individual's receptiveness to drug therapy; also, genetic traits that affect a drug's pharmacokinetic and pharmacodynamic properties

The nurse considers the core drug knowledge and the core patient variable categories and determines potentially important interactions between them. An important interaction is an area in which key elements of the drug overlap—or potentially may overlap—with specific patient factors, thus requiring nursing management. **Nursing management of drug therapy** is the process of planning and implementing actions that will maximize the therapeutic effects and minimize the adverse effects of a drug. The nurse also considers these important interactions when planning and providing patient and family education relevant to the drug therapy. Finally, the nurse evaluates the effectiveness of both the drug therapy and the nursing interventions. Thus, the nurse applies knowledge in an individualized manner to meet the care needs of a particular patient receiving a particular drug therapy. Figure 1.1

shows how the interactions between core drug knowledge and core patient variables can be used to manage therapy.

Nursing management of drug therapy helps ensure quality and comprehensive nursing care. It occurs in all settings, including hospitals, long-term care facilities, outpatient centers and clinics, health care providers' offices, and patients' homes. Some aspects of nursing management are more relevant to a particular setting than others are; for example, considering the patient's lifestyle is more important for the nurse when drug therapy occurs in the home than when it occurs in a hospital.

MANAGING DRUG THERAPY THROUGH THE NURSING PROCESS

The nurse uses the nursing process when managing the care of a patient receiving drug therapy. The nursing process is a series of steps in which the nurse assesses and identifies a patient's response to health-related problems and then plans and implements interventions to manage the problem and promote a healthful outcome. The six steps of the nursing process are assessment, diagnosis, outcome identification, planning, intervention, and evaluation. Figure 1.2 shows how the nursing process corresponds to the phases of nursing management of drug therapy.

Nursing Process

Assessment

Nursing Diagnosis and Outcome Identification

Planning

Intervention

Evaluation

Nursing Management of Drug Therapy

Determine specific drug and identify core drug knowledge | Assess patient and identify significant core patient variables

Identify significant interactions between core drug knowledge and core patient variables

Identify actions to maximize therapeutic effects and actions to minimize adverse effects

Integrate and implement strategies to maximize therapeutic effects and minimize adverse effects

Provide patient and family education

Evaluation

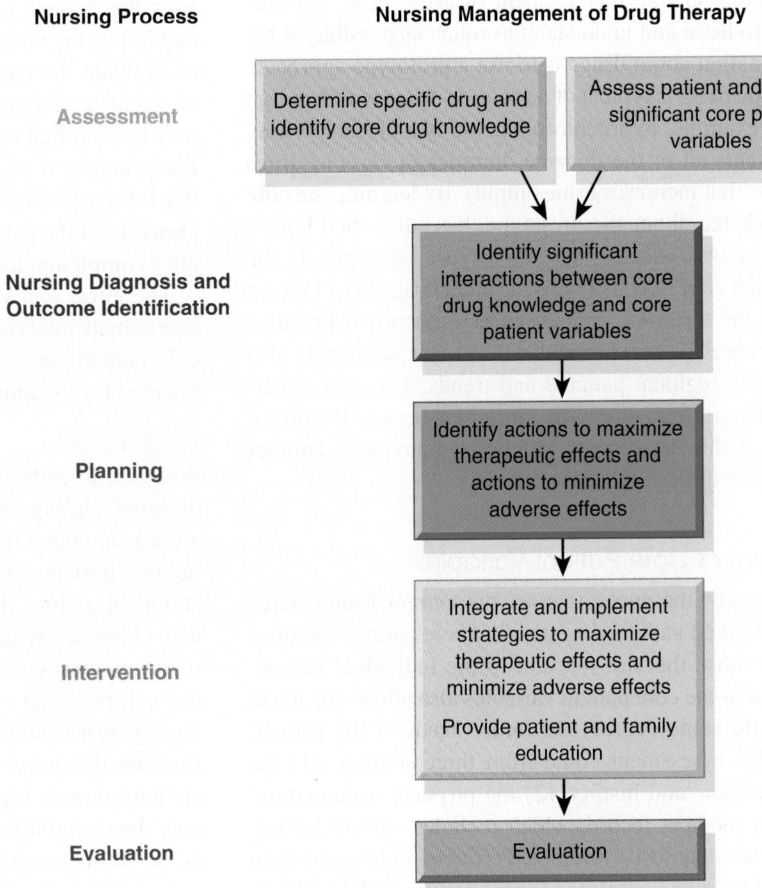

• FIGURE 1.2 Relationship of nursing management of drug therapy to the nursing process.

Assessment

Assessment of Core Drug Knowledge

Nurses need to know about all drugs a patient is taking, including prescribed and OTC drugs. In any given month, almost 45% of the U.S. population will receive one prescription drug; a little under 18% will receive three or more prescription drugs. Prescription drug use increases with each age group, with approximately 85% of adults aged 65 and older receiving one prescription and over half receiving three or more prescriptions in a month (National Center for Health Statistics, 2007).

The first step for a nurse is to identify the core drug knowledge relevant to a patient's drug therapy. The nurse needs to be familiar with every drug the patient is taking, to determine whether interactions with core patient variables are likely to occur and consider what nursing management is required. Although memorizing information on every available drug would be difficult, if not impossible, the nurse is responsible for using available, current drug references to review unfamiliar data before administering the drug or instructing the patient to self-administer the drug.

In the assessment phase, the nurse identifies the drug to be administered and its prototype. Currently there are thousands of generic and brand name prescription drugs sold in the United States. Additionally, there are numerous combination drugs, prescription and OTC, as well as brand new drugs introduced every year. The sheer volume of drug forms makes it impossible for the nurse to memorize up-to-date information regarding nursing management of every drug. An efficient way to learn and understand as much as possible of the vast information about drugs is to use a prototype approach. A **prototype drug** is typical of a group of drugs within a drug class. For example, hydrochlorothiazide is a prototype drug that represents all of the thiazide diuretics (a class of drugs in this class that increases urine output). By learning the core drug knowledge about the prototype, the nurse then knows something about related drugs. Prototypes are typically the first drug of a class. Occasionally, as other drugs in a class are developed, the "original" is not used as frequently in practice. The preference for one particular drug over another is also influenced by regional patterns and trends. This text generally uses the original, or classic, drug in a class as the prototype drug. If this drug is not widely used anymore, another representative drug of the class is used.

Assessment of Core Patient Variables

In drug therapy, the nurse assesses the current health status of the patient and gathers data on other core patient variables to identify those that are relevant to the individual patient. Assessment of the core patient variables also allows the nurse to predict (to some degree) the future needs of the patient. Data for this assessment come from three sources: (1) the patient interview and history, (2) the physical examination, and (3) the medical record, which includes current laboratory and other diagnostic findings. Pertinent findings are then assimilated to form a current, accurate picture of the patient's needs regarding drug therapy. These facts establish a baseline for the patient's treatment and care.

The Patient Interview and History

Most assessment data come from an assessment interview, in which the patient responds to questions. To be most effective, the nurse asks open-ended questions. Open-ended questions allow the patient to give details and explanations, whereas closed-ended questions require a single or particular response. Although closed-ended questions are a quick way to obtain information, they limit the depth of a response.

An example of an open-ended question is, "What kind of drug allergies do you have, if any?" An example of a closed-ended question is, "Are you allergic to penicillin?" The second question limits the patient's response to "Yes" or "No." Although this response answers the immediate question, important information can be missed. Open-ended questions may elicit the information that the patient is allergic to ampicillin. This fact is important to know because people who are allergic to ampicillin may also be allergic to penicillin (Penicillin and ampicillin are both antibiotics with similar chemical structures.). Closed-ended questions are most useful in emergency situations and when particular information must be determined quickly. An open-ended approach is preferable during the assessment interview if time and the patient's physical state permit.

Follow-up questions must be asked whenever the patient responds in a closed-ended manner. If, for example, the patient identifies an allergy to a particular drug, the nurse asks the patient to describe the allergic event. Using this technique, the nurse gains additional information with which to evaluate the patient's response. The patient may believe an event or response is a sign of an allergy, when in fact it may be a normal response to or an adverse effect of the drug. For example, if the patient describes a rash occurring on the third day of taking a drug, this may indicate a true allergy. However, if the patient describes a rash that occurred 6 weeks after completing a drug, a drug allergy is unlikely.

The nurse seeks information on several topics during the assessment interview (Box 1.1) and then determines which core patient variables are relevant to the drug therapy being planned for the individual.

Health Status

A patient's health status includes information about illnesses, diseases, chronic conditions, and allergies. This information allows the nurse to assess functioning of body systems and organs. Impaired functioning may interact with or alter the action of a drug. Pharmacotherapeutics, pharmacokinetics, and pharmacodynamics may all be affected. For example, if the patient has kidney disease, and the drug is excreted through the renal system, the drug will not be eliminated as rapidly as it would in someone with normal kidney function. Because the drug is not eliminated as quickly, the drug levels may remain higher than normally expected. The patient may then exhibit increased therapeutic effects from the drug or be at increased risk for adverse effects. Patients with impaired functioning of a body system or organ may have

Box 1.1 COMPONENTS OF THE PATIENT INTERVIEW

Health Status

- Presence of acute or chronic disease (physical or mental)
- Drug history (see Box 1.2)
- Sensory deficits (vision, hearing, speech)
- Ability to understand spoken instruction
- Cognitive or memory deficits

Life Span and Gender

- Age
- Developmental level
- Ability to read and write
- Female patients: reproductive status (e.g., pregnant or planning pregnancy, lactating), premenopausal, postmenopausal

Lifestyle, Diet, and Habits

- Occupation
- Insurance and other economic resources to pay for drug therapy
- Activity and exercise patterns
- Sleep and rest patterns
- Dietary patterns: frequency of meals and snacks, foods usually eaten, foods avoided
- Dietary supplements, including vitamins, minerals, and herbal or folk remedies
- Use of complementary medicine
- Street (illegal) drugs used: frequency and route of street drugs, last time street drugs were used
- Alcohol used: amount of alcohol consumed daily, last time alcohol consumed
- Cigarettes or other nicotine-containing products used: amount used daily, pack years of use
- Caffeine used: amount of daily caffeine consumption

Environment

- Description of home setting or living accommodations
- Location of home (city, industrial, suburban, rural)

Culture and Inherited Traits

- Religious beliefs
- Ethnic practices

Box 1.2 COMPONENTS OF A COMPLETE DRUG HISTORY

- Currently prescribed medications
- Prescribed dosages and routes of the medications
- When each medication was last taken
- Patient's description of why the medication was prescribed
- Other prescribed medications taken in the recent past but not currently
- Reason the medications were stopped
- Known drug allergies
- When allergic effect occurred
- Description of specific allergic effects that occurred
- Known food or environmental allergies
- Over-the-counter (OTC) medications used, such as cough and cold remedies, vitamins and minerals, and headache remedies
- Frequency of OTC drug use
- Last time the OTC medications were used

about recently used drugs is also important because some drugs have long-lasting effects that may interact with a newly administered drug. Finally, the patient's drug therapy may have direct bearing on the understanding and interpretation of data obtained from physical assessment and laboratory findings. The data may indicate an expected therapeutic effect, an adverse effect, or an interaction between drugs. For example, knowing that a patient regularly takes the anticoagulant warfarin (Coumadin) would explain why the patient's clotting time is prolonged. Knowing that a patient is currently taking digoxin (Lanoxin), a drug that slows the heart rate, may explain why that person is experiencing adverse drug effects, such as extreme bradycardia with nausea and weakness.

Asking a patient to describe why he or she is taking the drug provides a great deal of information about the learning needs of that patient. The nurse may find that the patient has an excellent knowledge base or, conversely, that the patient has inadequate information or misconceptions concerning drug therapy. One patient may state that the drug is a diuretic to treat hypertension; another patient may state that the drug is a fluid pill; and another patient may have no understanding of what the drug does or why it was prescribed. Patients have different learning needs that require different approaches from the nurse.

Lack of adherence to prescribed drug therapy is very important to determine. However, merely confirming lack of adherence is not enough; the nurse needs to explore the reason the patient has stopped taking drug therapy as ordered. A patient may have stopped taking a drug for a variety of reasons. The patient may no longer have a medical indication for the drug, or the patient may have had an adverse reaction. The drug may have been discontinued on the advice of the prescriber, or the patient may have discontinued it independently. People may independently stop taking a drug because they think they no longer need it, they think it is not effective, they are experiencing unpleasant adverse effects, the prescription ran out and they cannot get to the pharmacy, or they cannot afford the drug.

special educational needs for drug therapy. For example, patients with impaired vision, hearing, or dexterity or those with decreased memory or mental capacity need educational materials tailored to meet their particular needs.

A complete drug history is necessary to assess the health status of the patient adequately and to assess a patient's needs and knowledge accurately regarding current or proposed drug regimens. Components of a complete drug history are given in Box 1.2. In the drug history interview, the nurse seeks information about current drug therapy, including the drug name, dose, and time last given. Any new drugs prescribed should not interact adversely with a current drug regimen. In addition, patients who are admitted to acute or long-term care facilities must continue the drug therapy they have been taking. Information

Allergies are another aspect of the drug history that must be identified correctly and documented carefully in the medical record. Drug, food, and environmental allergies should be noted. Although allergies are an individual aspect of health status, they are usually considered part of the complete drug history and thus are discussed as part of the drug history rather than as a separate element. Health care providers need to know the patient's allergies so that they do not prescribe or administer drugs to which the individual is allergic. Ask the patient to describe the symptoms of the allergic reaction and note them in the appropriate area of the patient's record. True allergic reactions include formation of rash or hives, itching, redness, swelling, difficulty breathing, and anaphylactic shock. Nausea and vomiting, however, are adverse effects of drug therapy. In addition to drug allergies, food or environmental allergies must be identified and documented. Elements of some foods are found in some drugs; for example, iodine is an element of many contrast media used in radiologic studies. Environmental allergens, if present, may complicate the health status of the individual. The nurse also gathers data about the patient's use of OTC drugs; these preparations may interact with prescribed drugs and alter their effect or produce adverse effects.

Life Span and Gender

During assessment, the nurse determines the patient's developmental level, ability to read and write, and ability to understand directions. This information is needed to plan patient education on drug therapy, including the nurse's approach and teaching methods.

Determining the stage of the reproductive cycle of female patients is important. If a drug is extremely toxic to the fetus, women of childbearing age need to be cautioned not to become pregnant while taking the drug. If a woman is past childbearing age (postmenopausal), a drug that is toxic to the fetus may be used. Certain drugs may cross the placenta, affecting fetal growth and development and sometimes causing birth defects or teratogenic effects. Therefore, if the woman is already pregnant, alternative drug therapy is usually indicated. Additionally, assessment for breast-feeding is important because some drugs cross into breast milk and will have some effect on the infant and the mother.

Lifestyle, Diet, and Habits

The nurse asks questions about a patient's lifestyle because of its potential effect on drug therapy. For example, the patient's levels of exercise and general activity may influence drug effect. Patients who are very active and who exercise are likely to have better circulatory systems than those who are inactive. These lifestyle choices affect the distribution of drugs within the body. People who are very active may also be more likely to incur accidental injury than other, less active people. Their increased incidence of injury would put them at greater risk than their more sedentary peers for certain adverse drug effects, such as prolonged bleeding with warfarin, an anticoagulant.

Information on normal dietary intake is useful because food or food elements interact with certain drugs. For example, monoamine oxidase inhibitors (a class of antidepressants) interact with tyramine-rich foods (e.g., aged cheese, tap beers) and can induce a hypertensive crisis. Some foods affect the absorption and action of a drug; for example, milk interferes with the absorption of tetracycline, an antibiotic. Many drugs can increase or decrease appetite or alter taste sensations. The nurse needs to assess the patient for these potential effects.

Because instructions for taking many drugs include whether they should be taken with food, the nurse needs to know how frequently and regularly the patient eats. If a drug is to be taken three times a day with food and the patient eats three meals a day, the patient may be instructed to take the drug with meals. However, if the patient normally eats only one or two meals a day or eats five or six meals a day, and this pattern was not assessed, the patient will not receive the correct dosage if the instruction to take with meals is followed.

Sleep and rest patterns and occupation are important to assess because they also have a bearing on drug therapy. People who work nights and sleep during the day will need the timing of their drug dosages varied because a daytime schedule is usually recommended for taking drugs, to enable uninterrupted sleep at night. Knowledge of the patient's customary rest patterns provides a baseline to determine whether drug therapy is therapeutic (e.g., a drug given to induce sleep) or whether an adverse drug effect (e.g., insomnia) is occurring. Certain occupations may place the patient at risk for injury and consequently at risk for adverse effects from some drugs.

The patient's use of street drugs, alcohol, cigarettes, and caffeine must be determined because these substances can affect some drug actions or alter the health or physiologic functioning of the patient. For example, a cigarette smoker may have respiratory disease. Cigarette smoking also alters the pharmacokinetics of some drugs, such as theophylline, a bronchodilator.

Economic factors may determine whether the patient will adhere to prescribed drug therapy; therefore, these factors should be assessed. If the drug is very expensive and the patient cannot afford the drug or health insurance to offset or defray drug costs, the patient's inability to purchase the drug may preclude his or her adherence to therapy. A little more than $200 billion is spent yearly in the United States on prescription drugs; 12% of the amount an individual pays for health care is spent on prescription drugs and $25 billion is paid as an out-of-pocket (i.e., not covered by insurance) expense by the patient (National Center for Health Statistics, 2007).

Environment

The nurse assesses the home setting or living environment because it may give clues to the patient's adherence to the drug regimen or to potential risks from the therapy. For example, if a patient is receiving a drug that causes dizziness as an adverse effect, stairs in the house may pose a risk for falls. If the home does not have running water, a patient may be unable to adhere to instructions about handwashing before self-injection of insulin. General factors to assess include cleanliness, lighting, adequate heat, water, and refrigeration. A home visit by a visiting or home health nurse may be the most accurate way to obtain this information.

Environmental factors outside of the home may also affect drug therapy. Environmental elements or substances in the environment may predispose the patient to adverse drug effects. Direct sunlight, for example, may cause sunburn when the patient is prone to photosensitivity from tetracycline, an antibiotic.

The nurse needs to determine the environment in which the drug will be administered. Some drug therapy occurs only in certain environments or settings (e.g., general anesthetics are given only in an operating room). Other drugs, such as oral antibiotics, may be used in all health care settings, including the patient's home. The strategies selected to maximize therapeutic effect or minimize adverse effects may depend on the drug administration environment. Materials selected for patient and family teaching may also depend on the environment in which drug therapy occurs. Patients may start drug therapy in one environment and continue therapy in another—for example, the hospital and then the home—or therapy may be lifelong, as with antidiabetic agents. The patient may begin taking a drug in a hospital and continue taking it in a subacute care center or at home. Planning for discharge of a patient from an acute care setting begins the day of admission. Therefore, during assessment, the nurse must gather data that will be important in meeting the goals of drug therapy once the patient is discharged. Where the patient will go after discharge will alter the education required. If the patient will receive drug therapy at home, the nurse needs to assess the home as previously described.

Some home drug therapies, such as intravenous (IV) therapy, may require special equipment, technologies, or skills. In these cases, the nurse assesses the ability of the patient or responsible caregiver to administer drug therapy safely and effectively. Additional assessments are made about the ability to take appropriate actions if a problem occurs. For example, the nurse needs to know whether the patient or caregiver can describe the actions he or she would take if an infection occurred as a result of IV therapy. The nurse can assess this information by asking hypothetical questions about typically encountered problems and having the patient or caregiver describe how to handle the problem described.

Culture and Inherited Traits

Culture and inherited traits is the last core patient variable to include in the health history and drug assessment. This text uses the term *culture* in its broadest interpretation, which may not directly reflect the definition given by some sociologists or anthropologists. Religious restrictions or cultural practices may affect the patient's acceptance of prescribed drug therapy. Christian Scientists, for example, who believe in healing through prayer, may not accept drug therapy to manage hypertension. Patients with some ethnic backgrounds may have altered responses to particular drug therapies. African Americans, for example, exhibit a diminished therapeutic response to antihypertensive agents, such as angiotensin-converting enzyme inhibitors.

Recently, it has been determined that there may be individual variation to drug therapy. These variations are inherited but are not related to racial or ethnic backgrounds. Instead, they are caused by genetic variations. These unique genetic variations may not be evident until a patient begins therapy with a particular drug; that is, they cannot be predicted ahead of time. Many of these variations are related to the P-450 isoenzyme system. Specific knowledge about the effects of genetic variation on drug therapy is currently in its infancy. Genetic research is being conducted to identify the presence or absence of various isoenzymes in individuals. Knowing whether a patient lacks a specific isoenzyme used in metabolizing a particular drug before starting drug therapy would enable the therapy to be tailored to the patient's needs, preventing possible adverse effects.

The Physical Examination

After completing the health history interview, the nurse performs the second part of the assessment—the physical examination. The physical examination focuses on the core patient variables of health status and life span and gender and should be comprehensive. The patient's history and present complaints (the main reason for seeking health care) usually dictate which body systems require in-depth assessment.

General observation will provide some information on health status. Approximate age and, depending on the stage, pregnancy can be determined by general observation as well. Physical assessment of the systems (e.g., the respiratory system) will provide information about disease or illness.

Baseline data, such as vital signs, height, and weight, must be measured. Ideally, the height and weight are taken directly by the nurse or someone delegated by the nurse (rather than asking the patient for this information). An accurate measurement of body size is an important factor in computing the correct dose of many drugs. During emergencies, this information may be estimated.

The nurse closely inspects the skin of all patients for rashes and documents their appearance and location. Failure to do so could result in the rash being misinterpreted as a drug reaction. If IV drugs may be ordered, other areas to inspect closely are the peripheral blood vessels. If a history of IV drug abuse is reported, scarring or inflammation of the vessels may be present. In such cases, the nurse can anticipate potential problems with IVs.

The nurse must analyze all gathered data in terms of the specific current and proposed drugs, identifying any actual and potential problems related to providing drug therapy.

The Medical Record

In addition to the patient interview and history and physical examination, a review of the patient's medical record and test results provides complete assessment data for the core patient variables. The medical record provides information about the patient's health status, lifestyle, diet, habits, and environment.

Areas of the medical record that are specifically important include laboratory and other diagnostic test results. For drug therapy, pertinent findings may include blood levels of a drug or test results related to drug action. For example, blood glucose levels are pertinent findings in diabetic patients

TABLE 1.1	General Test Values: Normal Ranges Laboratory*	
System Tested	**Diagnostic Test**	**Normal Values**
Hepatic	Bilirubin (total)	0.2–1.3 mg/dL
	Direct conjugated bilirubin	0.0–0.2 mg/dL
	AST (also known as SGOT)	8–20 U/L
	ALT (also known as SGPT)	10–60 U/L
	PTT	21–35 s
	PT	11–13 s
	INR	1
Renal	BUN	7–18 mg/dL
	Serum creatinine	0.8–1.2 mg/dL
	Creatinine clearance	Women: 72–110 mL/min/1.73 m²
		Men: 94–140 mL/min/1.73 m²
Hematologic	Hct	Women: 36%–48%
		Men: 42%–52%
	Hgb	Women: 12–16 g/dL
		Men: 14–17 g/dL
	WBC count	4,500–10,500/mm³
	Platelets	140,000–400,000/mm³

*Ranges for normal laboratory test values may vary according to the health care setting, the laboratory performing the test, and the testing equipment. This information should be considered a basic guide. Nurses need to be familiar with normal ranges used in the facility or agency in which they work.

Fischbach, F. T., & Dunning, M. B. III. (2011). *Nurses' quick reference to common laboratory & diagnostic tests* (5th ed.). Philadelphia: Wolters Kluwer Health/Lippincott Williams & Wilkins.

receiving insulin to control hyperglycemia. A computed tomography scan report indicating the tumor burden of a patient receiving chemotherapy is also a relevant finding. The nurse reviews all diagnostic findings, paying special attention to those findings relevant to body systems at risk for adverse effects from currently used drugs (Table 1.1).

Past medical records may be used to verify the patient's drug history. Moreover, they may provide details relevant to the patient's current treatment. Patients may forget previous drug reactions, past illnesses, family histories, and other essential baseline information, but these data may be available in previous medical records. Review of the medical record is important regardless of whether the drug is administered in a hospital, extended care facility, outpatient center, or the patient's home. This part of the assessment can be done either before or after the interview and physical examination.

Nursing Diagnoses and Outcome Identification

Data that have been gathered throughout the patient's assessment are interpreted by the nurse according to their relevance to drug therapy. The nurse reviews the core drug knowledge and the core patient variables from which significant interactions may be generated. The nursing diagnoses and patient outcomes are names or labels given to these interactions.

Nursing diagnoses are based on classifications proposed by the North American Nursing Diagnosis Association (NANDA). The diagnosis may reflect a current, actual problem or the risk for developing a problem related to drug therapy. A patient may be receiving a drug that addresses a current problem, yet use of this drug may put the patient at risk for developing other problems. For example, a patient has a nursing diagnosis of Chronic Pain related to cancer. If the patient is taking morphine to control the pain, the diagnoses related to the drug therapy would be Risk for Injury related to sedation from narcotic drug use and Constipation related to adverse effects of morphine. Selected nursing diagnoses pertaining to drug effects are given in Box 1.3.

Box 1.3 SELECTED NURSING DIAGNOSES PERTAINING TO DRUG EFFECTS

- Constipation
- Diarrhea
- Acute Pain
- Chronic Pain
- Fatigue
- Risk for Infection
- Risk for Injury
- Disturbed Sensory Perception
- Ineffective Sexuality Patterns
- Disturbed Sleep Pattern
- Disturbed Thought Processes
- Interrupted Breast-feeding
- Acute Confusion
- Deficient Fluid Volume
- Excess Fluid Volume
- Imbalanced Nutrition: More than Body Requirements
- Imbalanced Nutrition: Less than Body Requirements
- Impaired Urinary Elimination
- Urinary Retention

IDENTIFYING CORE PATIENT VARIABLES

1. Propose questions to ask patients who tell you that they are allergic to a drug.
2. Your patient, a 75-year-old man living on a fixed income from a Social Security pension, is to be discharged on a new drug for hypertension. In assessing core drug knowledge for the patient's drug therapy, you identify adverse effects of dizziness and dry mouth. Identify the core patient variables that you would evaluate most carefully for relevance to this patient's drug therapy.

In addition to diagnoses that reflect current or potential problems from effects of drugs, many other types of drug-related diagnoses may be appropriate. The diagnosis of Deficient Knowledge may be appropriate if a new drug has been prescribed. Ineffective Therapeutic Regimen Management may be appropriate if the individual has not been taking drug therapy as prescribed because he or she has misunderstood the directions. Ineffective Coping may be a nursing diagnosis for a patient who continually forgets to take a prescribed drug for a chronic condition (e.g., insulin for diabetes). Nursing diagnoses are highly individualized and cannot be predicted from prescribed drug therapy alone. Reputable textbooks devoted specifically to nursing diagnosis contain additional information.

The next phase of the nursing process is outcome identification—that is, determining the desired results of nursing interventions. Outcomes develop from the data gained in assessment and the diagnosis selected. A plan for a patient receiving drug therapy would identify outcomes related to the patient's specific drug regimen.

Planning

Once the important interactions between the core drug knowledge and the core patient variables have been identified, the nurse devises strategies to maximize the therapeutic effects and minimize the adverse effects of the drug therapy. The nursing process step of planning is used. Planning begins with identifying interventions necessary to reach the desired outcome. Planning continues by defining what needs to be done to achieve the identified outcomes.

Maximizing Therapeutic Effects

To maximize the therapeutic effects of any given drug therapy, the nurse must know what the desired therapeutic effects are and how they are achieved. Strategies appropriate for the patient are then used to promote these effects. Although these strategies are drug specific, a few general principles exist:

• Administer the drug in a manner that will promote its absorption. A drug administered orally may be given with meals or on an empty stomach, depending on the drug. When giving a drug parenterally, use the appropriate administration technique for the desired route. A route different from that prescribed may alter absorption and the desired effect. For example, if an intramuscular injection is accidentally given subcutaneously, absorption will be slower and the onset of the therapeutic effect delayed.
• Administer the drug at the appropriate time to maintain blood levels of the drug that will promote therapeutic effects.
• Monitor laboratory values, when appropriate, to determine that the prescribed dose achieves a therapeutic drug level.

Minimizing Adverse Effects

Many of the nursing care strategies are directed at minimizing the adverse effects of drug therapy. Again, the strategies are specific to the drug, but some are common to all drug therapy:

• Before initiating drug therapy, verify that the patient is not allergic to the drug and that the drug is not contraindicated for this patient for some reason.
• Administer the drug in a manner consistent with standard safety protocols. For example, some drugs must be administered intravenously at a regular, steady rate, and the use of an IV infusion controller, or pump, is considered standard for these drugs.
• Monitor the patient and relevant laboratory findings closely for evidence of known adverse effects from drug therapy. Patients at high risk for developing a particular adverse effect should be monitored especially carefully.
• Discontinue or withhold a drug if the laboratory findings warrant doing so. Notify the prescriber of the findings and your actions.
• Report evidence of adverse effects to the prescriber as soon as possible.
• Modify administration techniques, when appropriate, to decrease the incidence of adverse effects. For example, if the drug causes the patient gastrointestinal distress on an empty stomach, administer the drug with food.
• Implement appropriate techniques for certain drugs to detect the onset of adverse effects. For example, monitor blood pressure before administering each dose of an antihypertensive drug to determine whether the blood pressure has decreased too much to administer the drug.

Intervention

The next phase of the nursing process is intervention: performing the plan. With intervention, the nurse integrates the devised strategies into the nursing care plan for the patient receiving drug therapy. These strategies are relevant to the physical act of drug administration and to patient and family education about drug therapy, an essential part of implementing any therapeutic plan. The nurse integrates the recognized interactions of the core drug knowledge and the core patient variables into this patient and family education. Thus, the education is specific to the drug therapy and specific to the patient's needs.

Core Drug Knowledge

The nurse has a crucial role in educating patients and their families about drug therapy. The goal of patient education is for the individual patient to understand the drug and its effects well enough to self-medicate safely and effectively and to monitor the **drug response** (i.e., the anticipated therapeutic and adverse effects). Basic drug therapy education should include the name of the drug, the reason the drug was prescribed (pharmacotherapeutics), the intended effect of the drug (pharmacodynamics), and important adverse effects that may occur and should be reported to the nurse or health care provider. If the patient will be taking the drug at home, he or she also needs to know when, how frequently, and for how long to take it; how to store it; and what to do if a dose is missed. In addition, the patient must be aware of any special concerns regarding other drugs or foods taken (drug interactions) and trained in any special techniques needed for self-administration of the drug to maximize therapeutic effects or minimize adverse effects. This information is obtained from the prescription and from the core drug knowledge of pharmacokinetics and pharmacodynamics.

Core Patient Variables

Any or all of the core patient variables may have a bearing on the educational needs of the patient or the family. Patient variables may affect which educational materials should be provided and the format or method of presentation.

Health Status

Education related to the core patient variable of health status includes information about those activities that must be performed while the patient receives the drug to maintain health or to detect early changes in health that are related to adverse effects of the drug. For example, there may be a need for periodic laboratory tests, such as monitoring levels of theophylline (a bronchodilator) or monitoring bleeding time in a patient receiving an anticoagulant. Periodic examination or assessment by a health care provider may also be required, for example, to monitor blood pressure when the patient is receiving antihypertensives.

The current health status of the patient must also be considered. The following are questions a nurse considers when designing a patient education program for drug therapy:

- Has any current disease or condition impaired any organ or system functioning, leaving the patient at risk for certain adverse effects? If so, information on these adverse effects should be emphasized during educational sessions.
- Does the patient have impaired vision that may prohibit reading drug labels or contribute to making errors, such as misreading the number "3" as a "5" in the instruction, "Take 3 times a day"? A vision problem may also indicate that educational material cannot be presented in written form to this patient.
- Does the patient have a hearing loss that may interfere with the comprehension of oral teaching?

- Does the patient have difficulty with small motor movements, perhaps because of arthritis in the hands? If so, difficulty in opening drug bottles may be a problem.
- Does the patient remember spoken conversations well? If not, written education may be effective. If memory loss is severe, adherence to the prescribed drug regimen may be difficult to achieve, and devices or systems developed to help the patient remember to take the correct drugs at the correct time may be indicated.
- Does the patient have the mental capacity to understand the information presented on drug therapy? If not, another person may have to be responsible for administering the drug to the patient.

Life Span and Gender

The life span variable becomes important when a drug therapy has the potential to produce adverse effects on a developing fetus. Women of childbearing age need to be educated not to become pregnant while taking certain drugs. Age is also an important consideration when determining a patient education approach. For example, drug education for a preschooler will most likely be directed to the parents, whereas education for an adolescent is directed so that the adolescent becomes an active partner in the educational process.

Lifestyle, Diet, and Habits

When planning patient education, consider lifestyle and behavioral changes the patient may need to make during drug therapy because of the action or adverse effect of the drug. For example, a patient taking narcotics for pain will be drowsy because the drug depresses the central nervous system. This patient is cautioned not to drive a car or operate potentially hazardous machinery while taking the drug. A patient receiving an antihistamine for an allergic reaction may also experience drowsiness as an adverse drug effect and should be similarly cautioned. Other lifestyle changes may be indicated, such as avoiding alcohol or cigarettes because they may alter a drug's effect. For example, cimetidine is less effective in decreasing gastric acid production in a patient who smokes cigarettes while taking this drug.

The patient's lifestyle determines the value placed on patient education. The nurse may consider the patient education information important, but if the patient does not share this view, the educational process will not be very effective. The nurse needs to determine what the patient wants to know about the drug and what the patient believes has the most significance for him or her. Ideally, the educational process begins with the nurse giving answers to the patient's questions, even if the nurse believes that other, unasked questions may be more important. Meeting the needs of the patient will increase the effectiveness of the education and promote receptivity to additional teaching at a later time.

The nurse must consider the patient's learning style when selecting an approach to patient education. Some people are visual learners, and the use of videotapes may be a better teaching medium for them than printed information. Other

---

Box 1.4 PATIENT EDUCATION GUIDELINES

When preparing educational materials for patients receiving drug therapy, the nurse includes guidelines on the following:

- Drug name: generic and trade names
- Purpose of the drug
- Contraindication to taking the drug
- When to take the drug (time, frequency)
- Duration of treatment
- How to take the drug
- What to do if a dose is forgotten
- Special instructions related to lifestyle changes while on the drug
- Hazardous activities to avoid while on the drug
- Any dietary restrictions or additions
- Drug-food interactions
- Drug-drug interactions, including those that may result from over-the-counter drugs
- Adverse effects and instructions on what to do about them
- Special storage needs if applicable
- Special directions for drug disposal
- Therapeutic monitoring needed while taking the drug
- Periodic laboratory tests needed while taking the drug
- Precautions related to pregnancy or lactation
- Health care providers who should be notified about the drug therapy (e.g., dentist, by patient taking an anticoagulant)
- Advisability of carrying or wearing a drug alert card or medical identification
- Period of time drug remains active after discontinuing therapy

---

people need to be physically involved in their learning, and role-playing or demonstration and return demonstration may be better educational techniques for them.

When using written educational materials, the nurse must consider the patient's literacy level: Can the patient read and write in the language used in those materials? Written materials are appropriate for individuals who can read. However, they must be at the patient's reading level. If appropriate, standardized drug information sheets may be used. Many health care settings distribute these sheets for patient use. Additionally, some drug references are available that are designed to be photocopied and given to patients. If a standard information sheet is unavailable, the nurse can create one or simply write down instructions for taking the drugs along with a dosage schedule (Box 1.4).

Environment

Environment is an important consideration when educating a patient and family about drug therapy. The extent of teaching will vary, depending on the environment in which the patient receives the drug. Although some education is required regardless of the setting, more information is necessary if the patient will be taking the drug at home. These patients must know about all aspects of the drug so that its administration can be safely and effectively self-managed. If another person—family member or someone else—will be responsible for the patient's drug therapy at home, that

person needs to be included in the educational process. It is also important to confirm that the patient will be able to adhere to the prescribed drug therapy in the home setting. Considerations for safe and effective home-based drug therapy are given in Box 1.5.

The physical properties of the home may also affect the patient education required; the home setup may increase the

---

Box 1.5 SAFE AND EFFECTIVE HOME-BASED DRUG THERAPY

Patient and Family Assessment

The nurse needs to assess the ability of the patient or responsible others to manage drug therapy safely at home, by considering:

- Ability to see and read labels
- Ability to remember dosage schedule
- Ability to open medication containers
- Ability to perform any special techniques required for drug administration

Home Assessment

The nurse also needs to assess the following aspects of the home environment:

- Safe storage areas for keeping medications out of the reach of small children who may live in or visit the patient's home
- Adequate refrigeration if the medication needs to be chilled
- Convenient and safe storage areas for equipment, particularly the equipment needed to administer medication (e.g., intravenous [IV] pumps and controllers, nebulizers)
- Adequate and secure disposal containers for medication or equipment

Tools Promoting Adherence and Safety

On the basis of the assessment, the nurse might provide or suggest one or more of the following to assist the patient or family in adherence to the prescribed drug therapy in a safe and effective manner:

- Clear, written instructions for medication administration
- Memory aids, such as a calendar, dosage chart with space to document that the dose was taken, setting a kitchen timer or a watch alarm to sound at the time medication is due, or a clock-faced picture with the appropriate medication doses identified at the correct times
- An organized, convenient system for accessing medication such as
  - Keeping all medication containers in a bowl, in a small box, or on a special shelf
  - Dispensing one day's medication in a pill box, a commercially available organizer, or the individual compartments of an empty egg carton
  - Numbering or color-coding drug containers if the patient has a reading or language problem
- An organized, convenient system for storing drug delivery equipment (syringes, alcohol wipes, transdermal patches, drug pumps, IV tubing, and so forth), such as a box, a plastic storage container with a snap-on lid, or clean, dry glass jars with screw tops
- An impervious, puncture-proof container with properly fitting lid for safe disposal of needles, syringes, and other equipment, such as coffee cans or plastic milk jugs

risk for injury or adverse effects from a drug. For example, if the home has scatter rugs, the patient needs to be educated about the increased risk for falls while receiving drug therapy that may cause an unsteady gait.

Culture and Inherited Traits

When educating the patient and family about drug therapy, the nurse needs to be sensitive to the patient's cultural frame of reference. A person's religious and ethnic background influences his or her beliefs about health, wellness, and the role of drug therapy in maintaining or restoring health. Cultural background may also influence communication patterns and determine the appropriate family member to be involved in educational sessions. Depending on the culture, this person may or may not be the patient. The patient's cultural background is neither right nor wrong. To provide effective education, the nurse must consider cultural issues and modify content or presentation accordingly. The nurse must adapt to meet the patient's needs. If it has been determined that the patient has a unique response to a particular drug therapy, then the patient education must also be individualized.

Evaluation

Like the nursing process, nursing management of drug therapy ends with evaluation. At the end of the established time frame for achieving an expected outcome, the nurse measures the patient's progress. Was the outcome or goal achieved? Was the nursing management effective? These two measurements are not the same. An outcome can be achieved despite an ineffective plan. For example, a patient may not have adverse effects from drug therapy despite the nurse's not thoroughly identifying actions to minimize adverse effects. Or the management may have been appropriate, although the goal was not achieved. For example, the patient may experience an adverse drug effect even though the nurse appropriately identified and implemented strategies to minimize adverse effects. In evaluating the effectiveness of drug therapy, one of the most important aspects to consider is whether the drug achieved the desired effect. For example, an antihypertensive drug is given to lower blood pressure. Did the blood pressure drop to a safe and normal range? If so, then the evaluation shows that drug therapy was effective.

If the patient does not achieve the expected outcomes, the nurse must reassess to identify the barriers to success. Perhaps the nurse missed an important interaction between the core drug knowledge and the core patient variables. Perhaps the nurse did not identify a core patient variable. Perhaps the teaching strategies used were not effective for this patient, and a different approach should be attempted. Perhaps the identified outcome is not appropriate for this patient, or the outcome may be appropriate but the time frame inadequate. Evaluation is not merely determining whether the goals were achieved or the management was effective. The evaluation must identify the reason behind any treatment failure and the steps to achieve desired results effectively.

CLINICAL PATHWAYS

Nursing management of drug therapy may be used in clinical pathways (also known as critical pathways). A clinical pathway is an interdisciplinary approach to care that establishes common protocols for patients with the same medical diagnoses. These pathways specify the responsibilities, actions, and time frame required of each discipline (e.g., nursing, medicine, physical therapy, pharmacy, respiratory therapy) to meet the objectives required to complete the care plan.

Clinical pathways provide a standard of care for all patients with the same diagnosis. The pathway accounts for the drugs ordered as a treatment for or response to a specific condition. For example, the clinical pathway for a patient with deep vein thrombosis (a blood clot) usually has drug therapy beginning with the anticoagulant heparin. After 3 to 4 days, the patient usually receives an oral anticoagulant, such as warfarin sodium, to lengthen the bleeding time and prevent blood clots from forming. When the patient's blood tests indicate that the oral anticoagulant is at a therapeutic level, heparin therapy stops. If the patient meets the requirements of the pathway in the time specified, the therapy is evaluated as effective.

Nursing management of drug therapy still occurs with the use of the clinical pathway. Clinical pathways are not substitutes for nursing assessment and judgment. Assessing core drug knowledge and core patient variables, identifying their significant interactions, developing strategies to maximize therapeutic effects and minimize adverse effects, and providing patient and family education not only form the basis of astute nursing care but also contribute to early identification of a patient at risk for "falling off" the clinical pathway. Early identification of the patient at risk alters plans of care, prevents complications, and minimizes additional inpatient days.

CHAPTER SUMMARY

- Core drug knowledge, which consists of basic pharmacologic facts about each drug, is composed of pharmacotherapeutics, pharmacokinetics, pharmacodynamics, contraindications and precautions, adverse effects, and drug interactions.
- Core patient variables are features that make a patient unique at any given time.
- The nurse determines which of the patient's core patient variables are relevant to a particular drug therapy. They include health status; life span and gender; lifestyle, diet, and habits; environment; and culture and inherited traits.
- The nurse determines which significant interactions will occur between the core drug knowledge and the core patient variables. The nurse then recommends strategies based on those interactions to maximize the therapeutic effect and minimize the adverse effects of drug therapy. The nurse integrates these strategies into a nursing plan of care. Patient and family education is also based on the interactions between core drug knowledge and core patient variables. This process is nursing management of drug therapy.

- A prototype drug is a drug that is representative of a class of drugs. Acquiring the core drug knowledge about the prototype provides the nurse with information about several other drugs in the same class as the prototype drug. Acquiring core drug knowledge organizes and simplifies learning about many different drugs.
- In providing nursing management of drug therapy, the steps of the nursing process are used. Nursing management of drug therapy occurs in all health care environments, including acute care, long-term care, and home and community settings.
- A thorough drug assessment provides the baseline information needed for effective nursing management of drug therapy. It includes the patient history, physical assessment, and examination of the medical record.
- Nursing diagnoses and outcomes are labels given to the identified interactions between core drug knowledge and core patient variables.
- Nursing diagnoses for patients receiving drug therapy reflect current or potential problems relevant to the therapy.
- Expected outcomes define the units of measure by which to gauge the effectiveness of drug therapy.
- Patient and family education is a crucial aspect of nursing management of drug therapy. Individualized education proceeds from the baseline core drug knowledge and core patient variables.
- Drug therapy is evaluated as effective if the desired effect of the drug occurs. The nurse also evaluates whether the management plan was effective. If conclusions drawn from the evaluation show that the drug effect or the management plan was not achieved, the nurse must determine why and then respond accordingly.
- An important goal of home-based drug therapy is for patients and caregivers to acquire the knowledge and skills needed to implement drug therapy safely and effectively. The nursing management of drug therapy must take the home setting into consideration. Education is structured so that patients and caregivers can assume maximal responsibility for administering and monitoring drug therapy safely and effectively.

QUESTIONS FOR STUDY AND REVIEW

1. How does the nurse assess core patient variables?
2. Why does the nurse need to assess the core drug knowledge of each drug a patient receives?
3. How does learning core drug knowledge about prototype drugs help the nurse?
4. How do the core patient variables affect the patient education that is provided?

NEED MORE HELP?

Chapter 1 of the Study Guide to Accompany *Drug Therapy in Nursing*, 4th Edition, contains NCLEX-style questions and other learning activities to reinforce your understanding of the concepts presented in this chapter. For additional information or to purchase the study guide, visit thePoint.

REFERENCES

National Center for Health Statistics. *Health, United States, 2007. Table 96: Prescription drug use in the past month by sex, age, race and Hispanic origin: United States, 1988–1994 and 1999–2002.* Retrieved from http://www.cdc.gov/nchs/data/hus/hus07.pdf#096 on March 6, 2009.

National Center for Health Statistics. *Health, United States, 2007. Figure 6: Personal health care expenditures, by source of funds and type of expenditure.* Retrieved from http://www.cdc.gov/nchs/data/hus/hus07.pdf#096 on March 6, 2009.

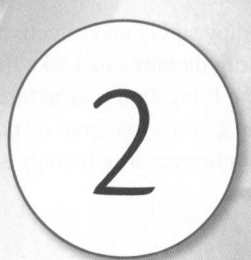

2

Pharmaceuticals: Development, Safeguards, and Delivery

Learning Objectives

At the completion of this chapter the student will:

1. Identify key concepts relevant to nursing management in pharmacotherapy.

2. Compare and contrast the four main sources of drugs and biologic products.

3. Describe the differences in the ways that drugs are named.

4. Explain the significance of drug classifications.

5. Identify sources of drug information.

6. Describe the scope of nursing responsibilities related to pharmacology.

7. Discuss the application of the nursing process related to pharmacology.

8. Describe the intent, scope, and benefits of drug standards and legislation.

9. Identify several references and resources that list standards regulating drug development, distribution, and use.

10. Explain new drug development and the role of nurses in clinical trials.

11. Differentiate between over-the-counter and legend (prescription) drugs.

12. Discuss the significance of the 1970 Controlled Substance Act and its relationship to nursing practice.

Key Terms

chemical composition	legend drugs	placebo response
chemical name	*National Formulary*	preclinical trials
clinical trials	orphan drug	therapeutic classification
controlled substance	pharmacogenetics	trade name
drug classification	pharmacogenomics	*United States Pharmacopeia*
generic name	physiologic classification	

What is a drug? By definition, a drug is any chemical that can affect living processes. Virtually all chemicals can be considered drugs because when given in large enough amounts, all chemicals will have some effect on life.

Drugs have been used throughout the ages, even in prehistoric times. The sciences of botany, physiology, quantitative chemistry, and gene mapping have enabled modern pharmacology to excel. Today, researchers examine rain forests and jungles for sources of new drugs to treat diseases. Scientists of the 21st century are able to develop new drugs through chemical synthesis, manipulation of enzymes and hormones, and genetic engineering, making pharmacology a complex science with a vast drug-manufacturing component. Highlights of advancements in pharmacology during the 20th century include the use of computer technology, which facilitates rational drug design and replaces some animal studies, and biotechnology, which permits the targeting of specific drug action and expands drug development procedures. One technique, receptor isolation, expands the potential for developing drugs with greater selectivity and reduced toxicity. Cell culture techniques permit the study of drug action at cellular and molecular levels. Immunochemistry leads to diagnosis that is more accurate and to the treatment of formerly untreatable diseases. The new drug classes that sometimes result from such advances in pharmacology provide novel means to treat and manage disease. Because pharmacotherapy is an integral piece of Western medicine, it is imperative that today's nurse understands the development, safeguards, and delivery of drugs.

SOURCES OF DRUGS

As we have learned more about drugs and how they affect the human body, pharmaceutical companies have focused on four sources of current drug products: plants, animals, synthetic chemicals, and genetically engineered chemicals.

Plants

Drug sources from the plant world date to primitive times. Common drugs from plants include digitalis (purple foxglove), morphine (opium poppy), and vincristine (periwinkle). Drugs that come from plants are classified according to their physical and chemical properties:

- *Alkaloids* (alkaline substances) react with body acids to form a salt, which is readily soluble in body fluids.
- *Glycosides* contain a carbohydrate or sugar molecule.
- *Gums* are mucilaginous secretions—usually polysaccharides—with the ability to attract and hold water.
- *Oils* are insoluble in water and are classified as volatile or fixed. Volatile oils, which are derived strictly from plants, evaporate when exposed to air. Fixed oils, also known as fatty oils, are derived from both animals and plants; their consistency varies with temperature.
- *Resins* are solid or semisolid, water insoluble, organic substances of vegetable origin that are commonly used as laxative or caustic agents.

Animals

Traditionally, drugs from animal sources include agents such as insulin, pituitary hormones, some vitamins, antibiotics, and biologic agents (such as vaccines and immune serums). Today, genetically engineered hormones (including insulin, pituitary hormone, and erythropoietin) are rapidly replacing animal-based drugs. The advantage of genetically engineered drugs is their purity. Because no foreign proteins are involved, they do not induce antibody production.

Synthetic Chemicals

Most drugs used today are either partially or wholly synthetic chemical compounds that have been produced in a laboratory. A partially synthetic agent contains a derivative of a natural substance combined with a pure chemical. An example is penicillin V, known as Pen-Vee K. The penicillin molecule, which is unstable in gastric acid, is modified so that it can be given orally. An advantage of synthetic drugs is that they are pure chemicals and, unlike drugs from a natural source, are unaffected by pharmacodynamic changes—namely, deterioration in potency and stability. Another advantage of synthetic agents is that they are usually less expensive to produce than drugs from a natural source.

Genetically Engineered Chemicals

Genetically engineered drugs are drugs developed with DNA technologies. The Human Genome Project's complete sequencing of the genetic code has ushered in a new era of "omics" technology, providing new strategies to diagnose, treat, and prevent disease. *Genomics* is the study and identification of genes and gene function. This new knowledge has enabled researchers to manipulate the chemical formulas of drugs to produce more specifically targeted drugs with fewer adverse effects. *Proteomics* is the study of protein structure and function. The term *proteome* describes the entire complement of proteins in a given biological organism or system at a given time (Wasinger et al., 1995). Proteomic technology is essential in biomarker discovery. A biomarker can be a substance that is introduced in an organism as a means to examine organ function—such as a radioactive isotope used to evaluate perfusion of heart muscle—to detect particular disease, or to indicate exposure to various environmental substances. In genetics, a biomarker is a fragment of DNA sequence that is associated with a specific disease. *Transcriptomics* is the study of the transcriptome, the complete set of RNA transcripts produced by the genome at any one time. Transcriptomics aids in understanding the development and differentiation of a cell or an organism as well as its adaptation to variable conditions. This information can be used when a single biomarker is not sufficient to differentiate between similar diseases. *Metabonomics* is the study of metabolic responses to drugs, environmental changes, and diseases. In pharmacotherapy, metabonomics can possibly predict an individual patient's response to drug treatment.

Pharmacogenomics is the application of the "omics" technology for the prediction of the sensitivity or resistance of an individual patient's disease to a specific drug or a group of drugs. **Pharmacogenetics** is the study of how genetic variables affect the pharmacodynamics of a drug in a specific patient. In the general population, 75% to 80% of people, known as extensive metabolizers, have genetic variations that do not affect drug metabolism. Ten percent to 15% of the population, referred to as poor metabolizers, have genetic variations that decrease their enzyme system's ability to metabolize certain drugs into their active form. This results in a poor response to the medication, even if the dose is increased. Ultrarapid metabolizers comprise 1% to 10% of the population. The enzyme system in these patients works rapidly, resulting in an increased concentration of the drug in the blood, which increases the potential for adverse effects.

Pharmacogenetic testing is a reality. Current testing is focused on substrates of the P-450 enzyme system. The importance of CYP enzymes in the metabolism of several antidepressant and antipsychotic drugs suggests that pharmacogenetic testing may aid in medication selection or dosing, resulting in maximal therapeutic effects and minimal adverse effects. Pharmacogenetic testing may be helpful in a variety of clinical situations, especially the management of cancer and HIV-positive patients. The future of pharmacogenetic testing will depend on economic and developmental considerations by the pharmaceutical industry.

The "omics" technologies have opened the door to the development of many drugs and treatments that had been only imagined in the past. These new technologies have the potential to identify drug targets, evaluate toxicity, classify diseases, evaluate formulations of specific drugs, assess drug response and treatments, and develop personalized medicines. The downside to drugs developed using these new technologies is the high cost of development, which is reflected in the high cost of the drug to the consumer.

DRUG NOMENCLATURE

All drugs are known by at least three names: a chemical name, a generic name (sometimes called the official name), and a trade name (Figure 2.1).

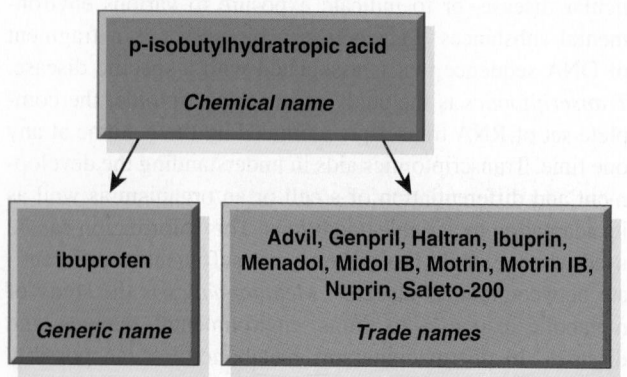

• FIGURE 2.1 A drug called by another name may still be the same drug. Nomenclature is a core feature of pharmacology. The three configurations illustrate various names for the same drug.

The **chemical name** of a drug precisely describes the drug's atomic and molecular structure, using exact chemical nomenclature (language) and terminology. The chemical name, which is usually long and complex, is not practical for everyday use but is useful to chemists and biochemists.

The **generic name** of a drug is also known as its nonproprietary name. Each drug has only one generic name, which identifies the drug's active ingredient. As a general rule, generic names are less complicated than the chemical names from which they are derived, but they are more complicated than trade names. Generic names are easily recognizable because the first letter of the name is typically not capitalized. In some cases, the prefix or suffix of the generic name may indicate the class of the drug. For example, the generic names of most beta-blocking agents end in "-olol." Similarly, the generic names of HMG-CoA reductase inhibitors have "-statin" as the suffix. The generic name of a drug also often serves as the drug's official name. The **United States Adopted Names Council** assigns an official name to each drug, as mandated by the United States government in 1962. These names are published in the *United States Pharmacopeia* and the *National Formulary*.

The **trade name**, also known as a brand or proprietary name, is given to a drug by its manufacturer. Trade names, which are usually easy to say and remember, are protected by trademark. The symbol™ or ® after the trade name indicates that the drug molecule and name are registered by the drug manufacturer, and the use of the drug and its name are restricted to the drug's manufacturer. The manufacturer receives a 17-year patent on the drug, which provides an opportunity to recover part of the costs used in research, development, and testing of the drug. The trade name is easily recognizable because the first letter is capitalized and the™ or ® symbol may be present. Unless governed by patent protection, any drug can be marketed in different formulations and by multiple drug companies. Consequently, the number of trade names a drug has can be extensive.

Implications for Nurses

Name recognition is important in drug therapy. The nurse has the responsibility of accurately transcribing drug orders, administering the drugs correctly, and documenting the patient's response. Usually, a drug is ordered by the generic name because numerous brand names may exist for the same drug. Health care practitioners and prescribers typically order drugs by generic names to avoid confusion between brand names that look and sound alike. Examples of proprietary names that may cause confusion include:

• Serzone (nefazodone) for depression and Seroquel (quetiapine) for schizophrenia
• Lamictal (lamotrigine) for epilepsy, Lamisil (terbinafine) for nail infections, Ludiomil (maprotiline) for depression, and Lomotil (diphenoxylate) for diarrhea
• Taxotere (docetaxel) and Taxol (paclitaxel), both for chemotherapy

- Zantac (ranitidine) for heartburn, Zyrtec (cetirizine) for allergies, and Zyprexa (olanzapine) for mental conditions
- Celebrex (celecoxib) for arthritis and Celexa (citalopram) for depression.

To prevent an error when administering any drug, the nurse checks the drug name at least three times—before, during, and after obtaining the drug. If the names used for the order and those on the drug label are different (e.g., trade name and generic equivalent), the nurse must verify that the two names refer to the same drug before administering the drug.

To decrease the potential for medication errors, many hospitals have implemented a pharmacy bar-code system. When entering the hospital, the patient receives a bar-coded identification wristband that can transmit information to the hospital's computer. The nurse uses a bar-code scanner to scan the patient's wristband and the medications to be given. If the patient record and the medication do not match, a warning box appears on the computer screen. Despite the use of this system, the nurse should still triple-check all drugs prior to administration.

DRUG CLASSIFICATIONS (FAMILIES)

Drugs that share similar characteristics are classified as a pharmacologic group or family. Because thousands of drugs are available today, studying them as individual agents would be an overwhelming task. Fortunately, drugs can be systematically classified into a reasonable number of drug groups known as **drug classifications** (or drug classes).

Drugs that share similar characteristics can be classified in several ways: by chemical composition, physiologic effect (on body systems), and therapeutic uses or actions (clinical indications). For example, the **chemical composition** of a drug such as morphine sulfate describes its chemical base of opium. Morphine sulfate, therefore, is classified as an opiate or opioid. The **physiologic classification** of a drug describes its effects on body systems; therefore, morphine sulfate is classified as a central nervous system depressant. The **therapeutic classification** of a drug describes the drug by its use in therapy; therefore, morphine sulfate is also known as an opioid narcotic analgesic. Thus, any one drug may belong to more than one drug class (family), depending on the classification system being used.

SOURCES OF DRUG INFORMATION

Because pharmacology is a dynamic science, new drugs are continually being developed, and new uses for existing drugs are frequently discovered. Nurses need reliable and up-to-date drug reference information. Awareness of reliable resources and the specific type of information provided in those resources enables the nurse to be efficiently and completely informed about safe drug administration and new therapeutic developments. Many drug-oriented publications help fill the need of nurses, health care providers, pharmacists, and others for current and detailed drug information. To be fully informed in a clinical situation, the nurse may have to consult several references (Table 2.1).

TABLE 2.1 Sources of Drug Information		
Resource	**Features**	**Evaluation and Commentary**
Official Pharmacopeia		
The United States Pharmacopeia (USP) and National Formulary (NF)	Drugs listed by official name Primary focus on sources, chemistry, physical properties of drugs; tests for identity, purity, and assay (measurement); and official storage requirements	• Federal Pure Food and Drug Act (1906) adopted USP and NF as official pharmacopeia • Published every 5 years with periodic supplements • Formerly listed drugs deleted and replaced by newer or better drugs, or drug listing removed after high incidence of toxicity reported • More useful as a drug reference to the pharmaceutical industry than to the nursing profession
Unofficial Compendia		
American Hospital Formulary Service (AHFS) Drug Information	Includes extensive drug information, particularly on drug classes Presents objective overviews of individual preparations of drugs available in the United States	• Published annually and updated with periodic supplements • Highly regarded drug reference
Facts and Comparisons	Provides concise but thorough monographs organized by drug class Begins each class section with a therapeutic overview, followed by additional sections organized by chemical classifications Offers comparisons of drugs (including over-the-counter [OTC] products)	• Updated monthly with supplemental entries • Available in print, online, or PDA format • Generally more usable than the Physician's Desk Reference (PDR) • Published by Facts and Comparisons, St. Louis, MO

(continued)

TABLE 2.1	Sources of Drug Information	*(continued)*
Resource	**Features**	**Evaluation and Commentary**
Unofficial Compendia		
Food and Drug Administration (FDA) Drug Bulletin	Offers recent FDA reviews of various drugs (usually common ones) and new clinical findings	• Free, quarterly newsletter • Includes a MedWatch form for reporting unusual clinical experiences with drugs to the FDA
USP Dispensing Information (USPDI)	Covers drug categories, prescribing precautions and considerations, side effects, drug actions, impact on lifestyle, dosage forms, and labeling data	• Written in nontechnical language • A major advantage is the presentation of side effect potential (rare to common) • Clearly identifies side effects to be reported to the health care provider • Highly valuable reference for nurses • Published annually and updated bimonthly
Pharmaceutical Package Inserts	Constitutes a concise compilation of specific drug information relative to clinical indications, safe dosage ranges, and unranked secondary (side) effects	• Manufacturer's leaflet enclosed with a drug product as it leaves the pharmaceutical distributor • Of limited value to the nursing process
Physician's Desk Reference (PDR)	Provides concise monograph of drug information similar to the manufacturer's package inserts	• Commonly consulted in clinical settings • Written by pharmaceutical company that manufactures the drug
PDR for Nonprescription Drugs	Besides concise monograph of OTC drug information, includes photographs of the drugs and a section on self-care of minor health problems	• Format similar to the PDR • First published in 1980 in response to the rapid growth and availability of OTC drugs and the general public's increasing health awareness and interest in managing self-care
Electronic Databases		
FDA web page, Medline, PharmInfoNet web page, Toxline, and others	Current drug-related information	• Available through the National Library of Medicine's online services
Cumulative Index to Nursing and Allied Health Literature (CINAHL)	Represents publications of major health care journals Abstracts available for many articles	• Libraries and schools have access through CD-ROM disks • Access through personal computer
IPhone, Ipod Touch, Personal Digital Assistant (PDA) Programs		
www.pdacortex.com *www.skyscape.com* *www.lexi.com* *www.unboundmedicine.com* *www.pepid.com*	Large selection of nursing-oriented programs Comprehensive selection of proprietary nursing programs	• User-friendly interface • Exceptional customer service • Many free programs developed by working nurses to assist in the clinical area • Access through personal computer

SAFEGUARDS IN DRUG DEVELOPMENT, MANUFACTURE, AND DISTRIBUTION IN THE UNITED STATES

Most nurses administer drug therapy as part of their daily routine, and advanced practice nurses (such as nurse practitioners) may prescribe and dispense medications as well. Every state has its own Nurse Practice Act that fully describes nursing activities involving drug therapy. Nurses should be familiar with the Nurse Practice Act in their state because these acts define nurses' roles and responsibilities. Similarly, familiarity with governmental safeguards that promote drug safety, reliability, and uniformity helps nurses administer drug therapy safely and appropriately. These regulations help to ensure that commercially available drugs are safe and effective.

New drugs are being developed at an unprecedented rate. Any new drug that comes to market undergoes years of testing to determine the drug's pharmacologic properties and its potential for toxicity.

Standards for Drug Purity and Content

Since 1820, the **United States Pharmacopeia** (USP) has been the source for standards of strength, quality, purity, and preparation of medicinal compounds. In 1888, the American Pharmaceutical Association began publishing another resource, the **National Formulary** (NF), which expanded this effort to set national standards for drug quality. Before that time, there was little need for standard resources because of the scarcity of effective drugs. In 1906, the Pure Food and Drug Act was passed, and the USP and NF compendiums became the official drug standards in the United States. Passage of the Pure Food and Drug Act in 1906 and the Food, Drug, and Cosmetic Act in 1938 protected the public from adulterated or mislabeled drugs and empowered the federal government to enforce these standards. The legislation required drug manufacturers to follow these standards to ensure that drugs were uniform, pure, and reliable. Later, amendments (1941–1945) to the Pure Food and Drug Act required that biologic products used as drugs (such as insulin and some antibiotics) be certified on a batch-by-batch basis by a government agency.

The USP is the current authoritative source for drug standards and is revised every 5 years by a group of experts in chemistry, microbiology, nursing, pharmaceutics, and pharmacology. Drugs are deleted when their clinical use shows unacceptably high toxicity or when newer, more effective agents are developed. Originally, the USP restricted its data to single drugs, and the NF was a reference for mixtures and formulas. Gradually, both reference books were expanded to include both single drugs and multiple-drug mixtures, and the two books have since been combined; the reference is now called the *United States Pharmacopeia–National Formulary*.

Legislation for Drug Safety and Efficacy

Federal legislation protects the public from drugs that are impure, toxic, ineffective, or not tested before marketing. The primary purpose of federal legislation is to ensure safety.

Pure Food and Drug Acts

The history of drug regulation reflects several medical and public health events. The **Pure Food and Drug Act of 1906** became law mostly because of revelations of unsanitary and unethical practices in the meatpacking industry and because of the many potent and dangerous drugs on the market. Although many of these drugs contained opioids (e.g., opium, morphine, or heroin), no law required the manufacturer to list the ingredients on the product label. In addition, the Pure Food and Drug Act designated the USP and NF as the official standards and empowered the federal government to enforce those standards.

The **Federal Food, Drug, and Cosmetics Act of 1938** (FFDCA) was enacted largely in response to a considerable number of deaths (more than 100) caused by the marketing of a drug called elixir of sulfanilamide, which was not adequately tested for safety before marketing. Elixir of sulfanilamide contained the solvent diethylene glycol, which investigations later revealed to be nephrotoxic. The FFDCA established the Food and Drug Administration (FDA) as the agency for monitoring and controlling drug manufacturing and marketing, allowed the FDA to prohibit the marketing of any drug judged to be incompletely tested or dangerous, and stipulated that drugs must be labeled.

According to the FFDCA, the drug label must contain the following:

- No false or misleading statements
- The suggested dose and frequency of use
- The name and business address of the manufacturer/packer or distributor
- The amount of all dependency-producing drugs in a product and the statement, "Warning: May Be Habit Forming"
- The kind, quantity, and percentage of certain specified ingredients that could be harmful (e.g., drugs containing alcohol, atropine, or digitalis)
- Complete, understandable directions for safe use and warnings against unsafe use by children, pregnant women, and people with contraindicating pathologic conditions

Kefauver-Harris Amendment

In the early 1960s, a drug-related tragedy altered drug-testing methods and expanded the scope of legislation regulating drugs. Based on results of animal testing, the sedative drug thalidomide was marketed across Europe as a nontoxic hypnotic. Hundreds of pregnant women who took the drug gave birth to infants with phocomelia, a condition characterized by severely shortened, deformed, or missing limbs. Thalidomide was not a widespread problem in the United States because the drug had been withheld by the FDA. Nonetheless, some babies with thalidomide-associated deformities were born in the United States to women who used the drug after obtaining it outside the country.

The thalidomide tragedy was one of the events that led to substantial changes in how drugs are regulated in the United States: requirements for more extensive testing of new drugs for teratogenic effects, stipulations that manufacturers prove both drug safety and efficacy, and passage of the 1962 Kefauver-Harris Amendment to the 1938 FFDCA. The Kefauver-Harris Amendment tightened controls on drug safety, especially experimental drugs, stating that adverse reactions and contraindications must be cited and included in the literature. Additionally, the amendment ordered evaluation of the testing methods used by manufacturers, specified the process for withdrawal of approved drugs when safety and effectiveness were in doubt, and mandated the establishment of the clinical efficacy of new drugs before marketing. The law applied to both new and existing drugs. Furthermore, all drugs marketed between 1938 and 1962 were required to be tested for effectiveness to remain on the market. The Kefauver-Harris Amendment also authorized the FDA to establish official names for drugs, and in the early 1960s, the United States Adopted Names Council was established to ensure uniform drug nomenclature.

Procedure for Drug Development and Approval

Years of research and millions of dollars go into the development of a new drug. The first step in the development of a new drug is in the discovery or synthesis of a potential new drug molecule. Once a potential new drug molecule is developed, it must be subjected to a battery of preclinical tests and clinical trials before it can be approved for use as a therapeutic agent. **Preclinical trials** are designed to provide basic safety, bioavailability, pharmacokinetic, and initial efficacy data about the drug and are carried out in animal subjects in the laboratory setting. Preclinical testing lasts approximately 3½ years. For every 1,000 compounds that enter laboratory testing, only one makes it to human testing.

Clinical Trials

At the conclusion of preclinical testing, the drug manufacturer submits the safety and effectiveness data from animal studies to the FDA in what is known as an investigational new drug (IND) application. The IND includes the following:

- All known information about the biologic, chemical, pharmacologic, and toxicologic properties of the new agent
- Precise details of how the drug is manufactured and storage requirements to preserve its stability

- The name and qualifications of each investigator who will participate in the clinical trial
- A signed affidavit by each investigator attesting that the study will be adequately supervised and that study volunteers have given informed consent
- Study protocols (guidelines) that clearly define how the drug is to be administered to study subjects (e.g., dose, route, duration) and what specific observations will be made during the clinical trial

If approved, the investigational new drug then undergoes clinical trials in humans. **Clinical trials** occur in four phases (I–IV) and may require from 5 to 9 years for completion (Figure 2.2). Phases I through III take place before a new drug is marketed. Phase IV testing is completed after marketing begins. Recently, the FDA has changed its policy to include women in early clinical trials (phases I and II), to determine whether differences in female physiology (e.g., menstrual cycle, menopause) influence pharmacotherapeutics, pharmacodynamics, and pharmacokinetics.

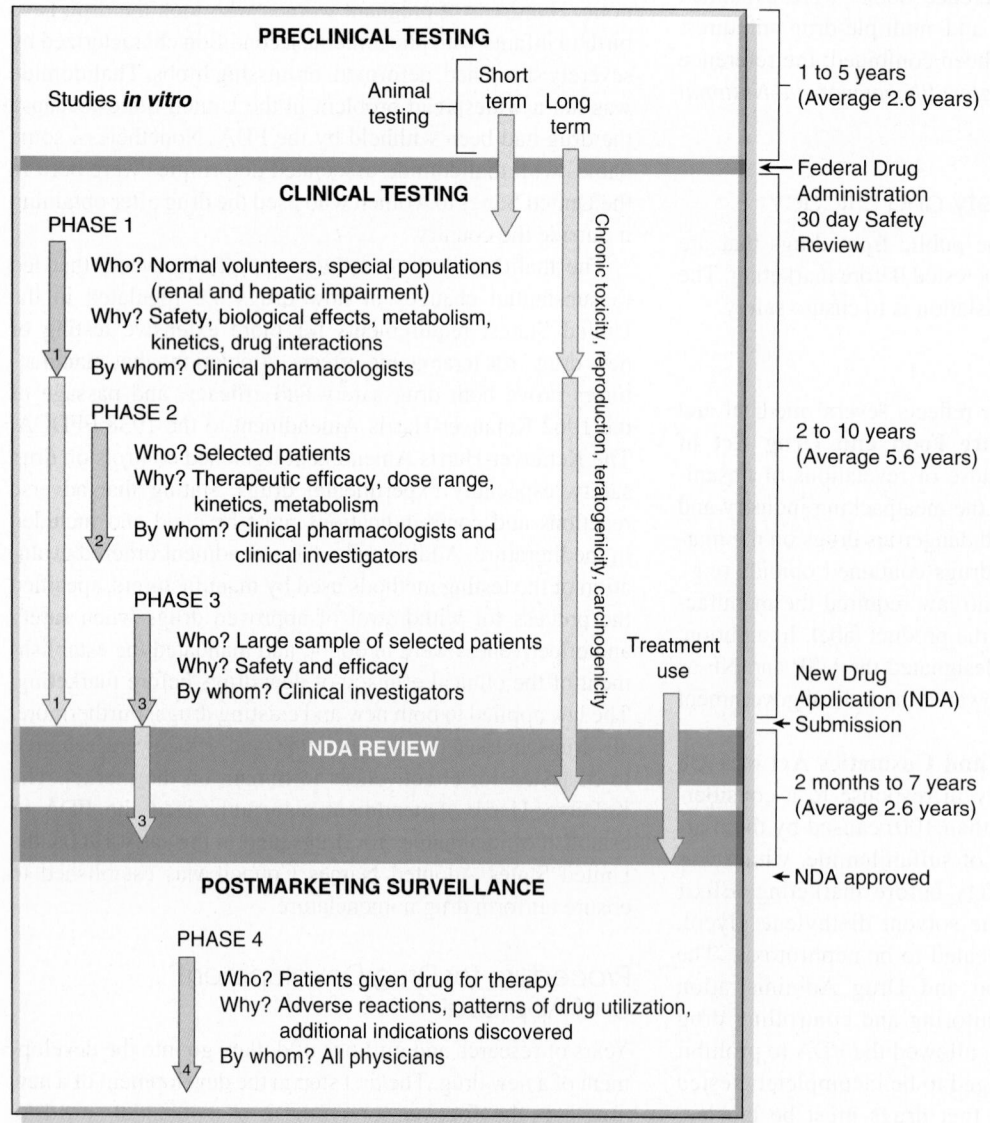

• FIGURE 2.2   Phases of Drug Development in the United States

Phase I

Phase I testing introduces the drug into humans. While most testing is done on healthy volunteers, some patients may also participate in phase I testing. The goal of this testing is to determine the metabolic and pharmacologic actions of the drug in humans as well as the adverse effects that occur with increasing doses, and, if possible, to gain early evidence of the drug's effectiveness. This information is used to design well-controlled, scientifically valid phase II studies. The Center for Drug Evaluation and Research (CDER) can prohibit the study drug from continuing to phase II testing for reasons of safety.

Phase II

Phase 2 studies are well-controlled, closely monitored, and conducted in a small cohort of several hundred people. The goal is to obtain some preliminary data on the effectiveness of the drug for a particular indication or indications in patients with the disease or condition. Results from the long-term animal studies are reviewed and compared with the human results—especially concerning the effects, if any, on fertility and reproduction.

Phase III

Phase III testing includes both controlled and uncontrolled trials. This widespread testing is also intended to uncover some infrequent or even rare adverse effects that sometimes affect only a small portion of the population. In this phase, several hundred to several thousand patient volunteers are enrolled in double-blind studies (studies in which neither the patient nor the researcher knows whether the drug or a placebo was given) and crossover-design studies (studies comparing the study drug with an existing drug). These studies are monitored closely to evaluate the safety and effectiveness of the drug.

Nurses are generally most involved in this phase of clinical trials and may be responsible for administering investigational drugs to patients. Patients must be fully informed about the potential risks and benefits associated with the intended study. One of the nurse's roles is to address how patients feel about the clinical trial, because these feelings may affect the quality and integrity of the investigation. Individual personal responses to an investigational drug may vary considerably. Some patients taking an investigational drug may believe that it is better than existing forms of therapy because it is new. These patients may have unrealistic expectations about the drug's usefulness or actions. Others may be more reluctant to participate in the study because they feel like "guinea pigs." Most patients tend to respond in a positive way to any therapeutic intervention by interested and caring health care personnel. This positive result is called the **placebo response** and may involve objective physiologic and biochemical changes as well as changes in subjective complaints (e.g., stomach upset, insomnia, sedation) associated with the disorder being treated. The placebo response occurs relatively consistently in 20% to 40% of patients in almost all studies.

If the drug proves safe and effective through the first three phases of the clinical trial, the manufacturer may then apply for a new drug application (NDA). All clinical data, as well as the earlier preclinical data, are reviewed by the FDA. Approval of the NDA means that the drug may be marketed. The FDA now requires analysis by gender in almost all NDAs. Research has identified pharmacokinetic differences between men and women that may be harmful to women if dosages are not adjusted accordingly. Because the distribution patterns of fat differ in men and women, many dosing schedules have been found to be excessive, and even harmful, in women.

Phase IV

Once a drug goes on the market, the FDA conducts postmarketing surveillance to monitor the drug for safety and any new developments while it is in widespread distribution. If safety problems appear, the agency limits the drug's approved uses or removes the drug from the market. In addition to postmarketing surveillance, the FDA may direct the drug company to do additional clinical drug trials during phase IV, especially for those drugs approved on the fast track. Another area of considerable interest in this phase is the effect of the drug on elderly patients and children, because these groups are usually excluded from early clinical trials.

During phase IV, the pharmaceutical company that markets the drug keeps careful records on the results of therapy and must advise the FDA of any adverse effects and other effects on therapy. Occasionally, reports of toxicity occur with enough frequency that precautions for use are expanded and emphasized. For example, felbamate (Felbatol), a drug used to treat seizures, was found to cause aplastic anemia. Sometimes a drug is removed from the market because of serious side effects, as was the case with terfenadine (Seldane).

In recent years, the FDA and the USP have begun several programs to ensure adequate postmarketing surveillance of drugs. These programs rely heavily on health care practitioners, including nurses, pharmacists, and physicians, to report problems or suspected problems with drug products to the FDA or USP. Examples of these programs include MedWatch and the Practitioners' Reporting Network.

MEDWATCH

The MedWatch program, sponsored by the FDA, encourages voluntary reporting from health professionals and consumers about adverse effects from drug products or medical devices directly to the FDA by mail, electronic mail (*www.fda.gov/medwatch*), or fax. Suspicion that a medical product may be related to a serious event is sufficient cause for a health professional to submit a MedWatch report. The goals of MedWatch are to increase awareness of serious reactions caused by drugs or medical devices, to facilitate the reporting of adverse reactions, and to provide the health care community with regular feedback about product safety issues.

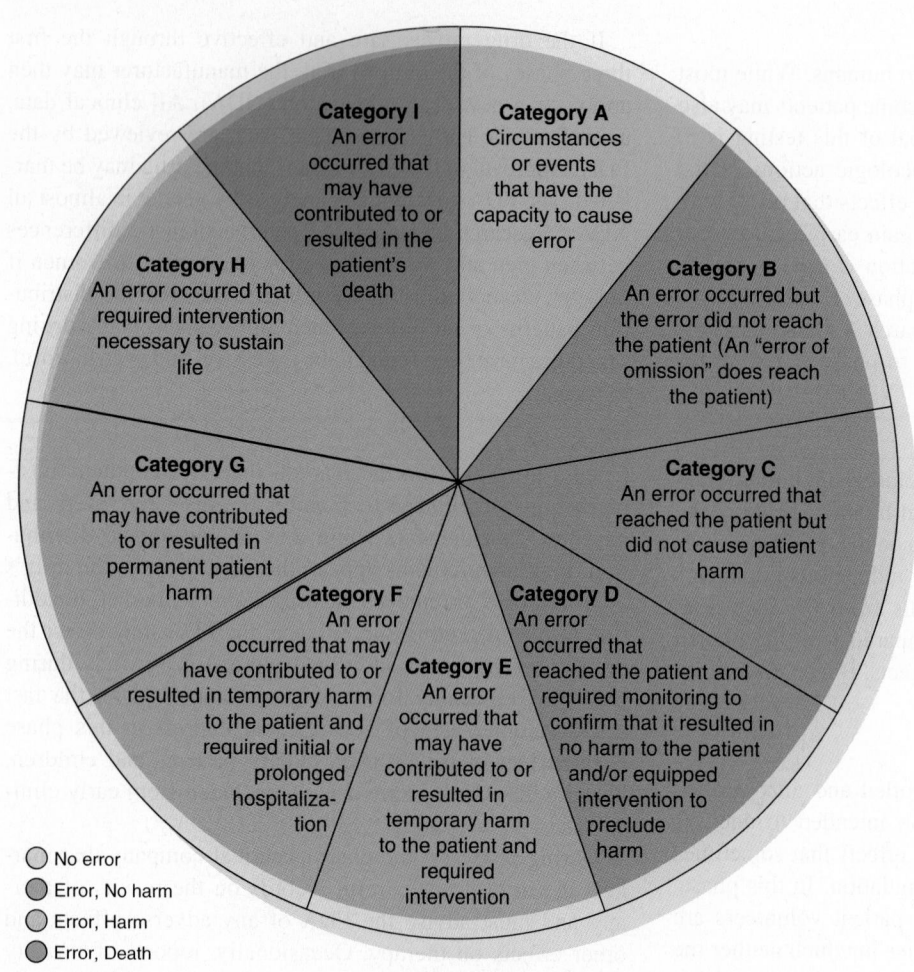

DEFINITIONS

Harm
Impairment of the physical, emotional, or psychological function or structure of the body and/or pain resulting therefrom.

Monitoring
To observe or record relevant physiological or psychological signs.

Intervention
May include change in therapy or active medical/surgical treatment.

Intervention Necessary to Sustain Life
Includes cardiovascular and respiratory support (e.g., CPR, defibrillation, intubation, etc).

• FIGURE 2.3 Medication Error Index (Reproduced with permission from the National Coordinating Council for Medication Error Reporting and Prevention.)

PRACTITIONERS' REPORTING NETWORK

The **Practitioners' Reporting Network** sponsored by the USP involves four coordinated reporting programs:

• The USP Drug Product Problem Reporting Program specifically targets drug packaging and is dedicated to reporting problems with unclear labeling, defective packaging, poor product quality, suspected counterfeiting, or product tampering.
• The USP Drug Product Problem Reporting Program for Radiopharmaceuticals targets problems with adverse effects or quality of radioactive drugs.
• The Medication Errors Reporting Program looks for actual or potential medication errors that may involve labeling, packaging, miscalculations, or misinterpretation, as well as other problems in drug nomenclature, marketing,

advertising, or use of abbreviations. To rank medication errors according to severity, the National Coordinating Council for Medication Error Reporting and Prevention developed the Medication Error Index to assist health care professionals in evaluating the extent of harm caused by an error (Figure 2.3).
• The Medical Device and Laboratory Product Problem Reporting Program looks at quality, performance, and safety of medical devices.

The Approval Process

Only about 10% of new drugs that begin clinical trials prove safe and effective enough to win regulatory approval. Approving a drug for therapeutic use involves a long, complex, and expensive process. On average, it takes 12 years and

Box 2.1 STREAMLINING THE DRUG APPROVAL PROCESS

Because of the high cost of research and development, many new and promising drugs never become available for consumers, primarily because of money: Manufacturers project that not enough revenue will be generated by drug sales to cover the cost of drug development.

Orphan Drugs

The 1982 Orphan Drug Act provides certain tax benefits to companies that invest in drugs useful in the diagnosis, treatment, or prevention of rare diseases, termed **orphan drugs**. Other legislation defined these rare diseases as those affecting fewer than 1 of every 200,000 people in the United States or diseases that may affect more than 1 of every 200,000 people but with no reasonable expectation that the company will recover development costs from sales within the United States.

Treatment Investigational New Drugs (Compassionate Use Protocol)

This process allows an investigational drug to be administered to patients who are desperately ill but are not enrolled in its clinical trial.

Drugs that qualify for a Treatment IND have demonstrated preliminary evidence of the drug's efficacy and the drug is intended to treat a serious or life-threatening illness or disease.

Accelerated Development/Review

This is a highly specialized mechanism for speeding the use of drugs that promise significant benefit over existing therapy for serious or life-threatening illnesses. The manufacturer must continue clinical testing after the drug is approved to provide proof that the drug provides therapeutic benefit to the patient.

Parallel Track

Under this policy, patients with AIDS whose condition prevents them from participating in controlled clinical trials can receive investigational drugs shown in preliminary studies to be promising.

$350 million for a new drug to be approved. The preclinical, clinical, and FDA review processes may be accelerated (fast-tracked) when an urgent need is perceived. In recent years, certain laws and protocols have been initiated to speed the drug approval process (Box 2.1).

Legislation to Promote Truth in Advertising

In 1912, Congress passed the Sherley Amendment to the 1906 Federal Pure Food and Drug Act, which prohibited drug manufacturers from making fraudulent therapeutic claims about their products. The FFDCA of 1938 bolstered this amendment by providing labeling requirements for the first time. Manufacturers were required to use standard drug nomenclature, and the presence and amount of certain potentially toxic drugs (including atropine, alcohol, or opiates) had to be disclosed. Directions for safe use and dosage had to be listed, and the manufacturer's or distributor's name had to be clearly marked. False or misleading statements were prohibited from appearing on the label.

Today, the Federal Trade Commission regulates the advertisement of medications aimed at the general public. The FDA regulates advertising of medications to medical personnel and relies on reports from practitioners and its own investigators to uncover abuses and fraud. Drug companies can be sanctioned for promoting the use of drugs in a manner that is not consistent with the agency-approved package insert.

The stated intent of the FDA is not to regulate medical practice but to guarantee the safety, purity, effectiveness, and reliability of drugs sold in the United States. However, the agency also aims to prevent manufacturers from promoting so-called off-label or unlabeled uses of drugs, in part to encourage the development of proper safety and efficacy data.

Sanctions may also be imposed if a manufacturer advertises exaggerated claims of efficacy or reduced adverse effects in its product.

Legislation Regarding Controlled Substances

The Harrison Narcotic Law of 1914 legally defined the term *narcotic* and provided the first effective regulation regarding the manufacture and distribution of certain drugs known for their abuse potential, including cocaine, marijuana, and opium. The 1970 Comprehensive Drug Abuse Prevention and Control Act (also called the Controlled Substances Act, or CSA) established the Drug Enforcement Agency (DEA), formerly known as the Bureau of Narcotics and Dangerous Drugs (BNDD) of the United States Department of Justice, as the regulatory body responsible for the safe distribution and control of potentially addictive drugs. This act, which was designed to remedy the escalating problem of drug abuse, categorized and controlled drugs according to their abuse potential and medical usefulness on a scale of I to V, hence the term **controlled substance.** This act also defined the terms

CRITICAL THINKING SCENARIO

CANDIDATE FOR A NEW DRUG

Steve Smith has had AIDS for the past 10 years. He is being considered for treatment with a new drug during phase III clinical trials. Steve expresses concern about taking a new drug, especially in view of his declining health status and what he has heard about a shortened clinical evaluation process for AIDS drugs; he asks you, "What does the term 'new drug' mean?" What is your response?

| TABLE 2.2 | Schedule of Controlled Substances | | | |

Category	Abuse Potential	Dependance Liability	Examples	Rules Governing Prescription
C-I	High	Severe	Heroin, hashish, LSD, GHB	• No accepted medical use in the U.S. • There is a lack of accepted safety for use of the drug or other substance under medical supervision.
C-II	High	Severe	Amphetamines, some opioid narcotics (e.g., morphine, meperidine), dronabinol, short-acting barbiturates (e.g., pentobarbital, secobarbital)	• Requires tamper-proof prescription. • Telephone orders not accepted • Refills not allowed. Additional medication requires new prescription.
C-III	Moderate	Moderate	Some opioid narcotics (e.g., codeine, hydrocodone), some CNS stimulants, anabolic steroids	• A written or telephone order is acceptable. • May be refilled 5 times within 6 months from the date of issue • Prescription must be rewritten after 6 months or 5 refills.
C-IV	Low	Limited	Benzodiazepine anxiolytics, anticonvulsants, muscle relaxants, and sedatives; nonbenzodiazepine hypnotics and intermediate-acting barbiturates. Opioid narcotics such as propoxyphene or pentazocine	• Same as C-III drugs
C-V	Limited	Lowest	Antidiarrheal preparations with diphenoxylate and loperamide; small amounts of narcotics such as codeine used as antitussives	• Many of these drugs may be obtained without a prescription.

drug dependency and *drug addiction* and established education and treatment programs for drug abuse.

Under the CSA, five categories, known as schedules, were established, and controls were placed on prescribing, dispensing, and storing drugs in health care facilities according to the scheduled category (Table 2.2).

Drugs may be moved from one schedule category to another. For example, propoxyphene, which was originally assigned a C-V rank, was reassigned to the more restrictive C-IV category because of its popularity for misuse, abuse, and overdose. Tetrahydrocannabinol (THC, the active ingredient in marijuana)—ranked in the C-I category for many years—was moved to C-II because of its legitimate clinical use as a powerful antiemetic to relieve the adverse effects of cancer chemotherapy.

Nursing Management of Controlled Substances

The prescribing, dispensing, and storing of controlled substances is subject to considerably greater governmental control than the use of conventional prescription drugs. Procedures are precisely defined by law for virtually every step from manufacture to administration to wasting or discarding. Many hospitals use an automated system to electronically track the use of stock drugs, including controlled substances. In some health care environments, these automated systems are not used, and the nurse must document the administration of a narcotic on a narcotic log sheet. When using a narcotic log sheet, the nurse must document the following:

• Date and time of administration
• Drug name and dose
• Patient's name
• Prescriber's name
• Administering nurse's name

In a health care facility that does not use an automated system, stock supplies of narcotics must be kept in double-locked storage cabinets. Keys to the cabinet are restricted to licensed nurses, who are also responsible for the accurate accounting of all narcotics. The nurse finishing a shift and the nurse beginning a shift generally perform the narcotic count together to ensure an accurate account of all controlled substances.

The handling of controlled substances is a nursing responsibility that should never be taken lightly. Transfer of a C-II, C-III, or C-IV drug to anyone other than the person for whom it is prescribed is a crime. Violation of the CSA can result in a fine, imprisonment, or both. Any nurse who violates the CSA is also subject to loss of the nursing license and the right to practice nursing.

Legislation Regarding Drug Distribution

The Durham-Humphrey amendments (1952) to the 1938 FFDCA separated drugs for the first time into two major classifications: nonprescription drugs and prescription drugs.

Prescription drugs, also known as **legend drugs**, must be identified by the legend (inscription) on the container: "Caution: Federal law prohibits dispensing without a prescription." Containers of controlled substances must also display an additional warning label: "Caution: Federal law prohibits the transfer of this drug to any person other than the patient for whom it was prescribed." The Durham-Humphrey amendments further specify procedures for the distribution of prescription drugs. A prescription from a licensed practitioner is required before the drug can be dispensed, and refills are not permitted without authorization of the prescriber.

Labeling

Labeling, according to the USP, is the written, printed, or graphic matter affixed to an immediate container, package, or wrapper in which the medication is enclosed. Informational sheets that are not attached (such as patient information/ instruction sheets) are not considered part of the label. The prescription label remains a primary source of information to patients about the proper use of their medications. Cautions regarding use and storage are usually on auxiliary labels, and some medications require their use. The following are examples of auxiliary labels:

- Avoid prolonged or excessive exposure to sunlight or sunlamp while taking this medication.
- Avoid the use of grapefruit juice with this product.
- Avoid the use of laxatives with this product.
- Do not take this drug if you are pregnant or suspect that you may be pregnant.
- Do not take with dairy products or antacids, or ingest these products within 1 hour before or 2 hours after taking this medication.
- Do not use past the expiration date.
- May cause drowsiness. Alcohol may intensify this effect. Use care when operating a car or dangerous machinery.
- Must be refrigerated/do not freeze.
- Take all of this medication/complete the full course of therapy.
- Take on empty stomach, at least 1 hour before or 2 hours after meals.
- Take with full glass of water.

Online Pharmacies

Consumers are increasingly going online to meet their prescription drug needs. While online pharmacies are convenient, they are not always safe. A recent analysis of 118 online pharmacies found that only 51 (43.2%) of them stated their precise location and that ninety-six (81.4%) did not require a medical prescription from the customer's physician (Orizio, 2009). Selling prescription drugs without a valid physician–patient relationship is a consumer health risk. For example, Ryan Haight, 18, died on February 12, 2001, after overdosing on Vicodin, which he had purchased from an Internet pharmacy without a prescription. H.R. 6353, The Ryan Haight Internet Pharmacy Consumer Protection Act of 2008 amends the Controlled Substances Act with respect to the sale of controlled substance drugs through the Internet. The overall effect of this law is to restrict the delivery, distribution, or dispensing of controlled substances by means of the Internet without a valid prescription obtained through a provider in a one-to-one in-person medical evaluation.

Nongovernmental Institutional Controls

Health care institutions, such as hospitals and skilled nursing facilities, may adopt additional regulations to ensure safe drug therapy and drug distribution. The Joint Commission for accreditation of hospitals and healthcare organizations is a watchdog group that provides the impetus for additional regulation. The Joint Commission sets the standards for quality of patient care and accreditation of health care institutions.

Generally, regulations to meet these standards of care for drug therapy vary greatly among institutions, but most guarantee that the therapy prescribed for any patient is continually reviewed for appropriateness, safety, and efficacy. Examples of these regulations include automatic discontinuation of antibiotic orders after 7 to 10 days of treatment or automatic discontinuation of narcotic or controlled substance orders after 48 to 72 hours. Institutional regulations exist to prevent prolonged, costly, and sometimes inappropriate administration of drugs. Development and implementation of such policies usually requires a collaborative effort among the nursing, pharmacy, and medical staffs.

EFFECT OF LEGAL AND INSTITUTIONAL CONTROLS ON NURSING MANAGEMENT OF DRUG THERAPY

Nurses need to be familiar not only with institutional protocols for safe and effective drug administration but also with official and professional regulations and laws. Drug laws and nurse practice acts vary from state to state, and these regulations define nursing responsibilities related to drug safety and effectiveness in patient care. Nurses must be familiar with the current regulations in their states and in their practice settings. Nurses can stay up to date by regularly consulting with representatives of regulatory bodies, arranging in-service training and information sessions, and understanding the policies of their own agencies.

In professional practice, nurses must adhere to and obey established drug control laws and protocols. They must avoid advising patients on the use of drugs, and they cannot provide drug therapy without proper authorization. Within the institution, nurses are responsible not only for drug security (to prevent unauthorized use or accidental loss) but also for the safe administration of drugs. Infraction of the laws and protocols that protect and promote patient safety may result in the loss of one's nursing license.

PATIENT EDUCATION AS A SAFEGUARD IN DRUG THERAPY

Educating patients is a key safeguard in drug therapy. Educating patients about drug therapy improves adherence to drug therapy and promotes therapeutic outcomes. In other words, patients who understand the prescribed drug regimen have the best chance of achieving the maximum benefit from it.

Patient education requires a nurse to have skills in gathering data, individualizing instructions, prompting and supporting the patient, and assessing and evaluating the pharmacotherapeutic response for determining patient outcomes. An effective patient teaching program parallels the nursing process—the nurse assesses the patient's learning needs, formulates a diagnosis, identifies a desired outcome, develops and implements a teaching plan, and evaluates the teaching and learning that have occurred. Strategies for enhancing patient education are given in Box 2.2.

Patient Learning Needs

Learning needs for drug education vary among patients, as does each patient's adherence to the prescribed treatment regimen. Some variations result from clinical factors, such as the nurse–patient relationship. Others are related to the scope or complexity of drug therapy in relation to pharmacotherapeutic, pharmacokinetic, and pharmacodynamic parameters; contraindications, precautions, and adverse effects of therapy; and the potential for drug interactions with undesired effects. Variations may also relate to core patient variables: health status (Box 2.3); life span and gender; lifestyle, diet, and habits; environment; and culture and inherited traits.

Teaching Focus and Content

Because each patient processes information differently, the nurse attempts to individualize and communicate information so that the patient or the caregiver can understand it and act on it appropriately. If possible, the nurse prepares written or audiovisual materials for the patient to consult as needed (see Chapter 1, Box 1.4).

Box 2.2 STRATEGIES FOR ENHANCING PATIENT EDUCATION

- Avoid jargon; communicate in short words and sentences.
- Include written information using diagrams and illustrations.
- Promote understanding with repetition and reinforcement.
- Relate new information to the patient's existing knowledge and previous experiences.
- Highlight and recap important information. Ask the patient to repeat the instructions or demonstrate new techniques.

Box 2.3 ASSESSMENT: ANOTHER SAFEGUARD

To ensure the patient's safe adherence to drug therapy and to formulate an effective, relevant drug teaching plan, the nurse needs not only to assess the patient's learning needs, but also the patient's health history, asking about the following:

- Allergies or idiosyncratic reactions to drugs or foods
- Chronic conditions
- Drugs and other medications currently used (including vitamins, other supplements, and over-the-counter drugs)
- Pregnancy status now and future plans (for women of childbearing age)
- Use of alcohol, caffeine, nicotine, or illicit substances

Evaluating and Documenting Educational Outcomes

Evaluation and documentation of patient education include time of teaching, content of teaching, the patient's response to the teaching session, an evaluation of the patient's grasp of the subject matter, and an assessment of unmet or future learning needs. Like documentation of drug therapy and other nursing care, documentation of patient education activities becomes part of the clinical and legal record, serving as a reference for other health care professionals and helping guide future educational efforts.

Consumer Drug Information on the Internet

Patient education about drug therapy is particularly important in light of the explosive growth of the Internet, which has created countless opportunities for patients to access health-related information, products, and services. The Internet has forever changed the way many consumers obtain prescription drugs and health information. Opting for the convenience and privacy of the information-rich Internet, consumers have increasingly gone online for information on diseases and medications.

The quality of information provided on some Internet sites has become a concern for health care providers. Consumers may have difficulty recognizing the difference between accurate drug information and personal web pages that have biased opinions from nonmedical personnel. Because sites with the most accurate drug information frequently charge for their services, consumers may not be as likely to access these sites. Because information obtained from an Internet site may conflict with information provided by the health care provider, patients are counseled to discuss contradictory information they obtain from a website with the health care provider before changing a medication regimen.

IMPORTANCE OF NURSING MANAGEMENT OF DRUG THERAPY

The importance of pharmacotherapy in nursing practice continues to grow. Nurses are legally responsible for the drugs they administer and for safe drug administration. When caring for patients with acute health problems, the nurse is the health care provider who usually administers drugs. This function becomes substantially more demanding as more new drugs enter the marketplace, multiple-drug therapies grow more complex, and drug delivery systems become more sophisticated. Safe drug administration requires a thorough understanding of therapeutic drug actions and adverse drug reactions.

In some clinical settings, nurses are allowed to modify drug regimens according to specifically designed protocols, and almost all states now allow advanced practice nurses to prescribe drugs. Future nursing practice will likely involve the prescribing of selected drugs.

Application of the nursing process to the pharmacologic aspects of patient care is especially important because long-term use of drug therapy is frequently necessary to control chronic disease processes. Nursing management in drug therapy may be considered an applied science because it relies on knowledge and principles from many different disciplines, such as anatomy and physiology, anthropology, biochemistry, mathematics, microbiology, organic chemistry, psychology, and sociology.

CHAPTER SUMMARY

- Sources of drugs include plants, animals, minerals, and chemical substances.
- Each drug is identified by at least three names, including the chemical name; the generic (nonproprietary) name, which is a contraction or shortening of the chemical name; and the trade or brand (proprietary) name. In the United States, official names are assigned by the government and are usually the same as the generic name.
- Drugs that share similar characteristics are classified in several ways: by clinical indications, effects on body systems, or chemical composition.
- Drug classifications (also known as families) emphasize common characteristics of each grouping, usually identify a prototype drug, and facilitate the association of new drugs within an established family as new drugs become available.
- Sources of drug information include pharmacopeias, which are official sources; compendiums, which are unofficial sources; product-insert literature from pharmaceutical firms; published reports; and findings in journals and electronic databases.
- The development and delivery of drugs are guided by federal legislation that is continually being updated.
- The approval process for a new drug is lengthy and expensive. It involves four phases of clinical trials.
- The FDA program MedWatch takes reports from health professionals and consumers about adverse reactions and disseminates information about those reactions as well as information about labeling changes and other safety issues.

- Educating patients is a key safeguard in drug therapy. The nurse implements strategies that optimize patient learning.

QUESTIONS FOR STUDY AND REVIEW

1. What is the purpose of the USP and the NF?
2. What is the purpose of the "omics" technologies?
3. How are drugs classified? What is the purpose of placing drugs in classifications?
4. Discuss the purpose and intent of government regulations, such as the Food, Drug, and Cosmetics Act, and the Durham-Humphrey amendments,. What safeguards do these laws provide?
5. Explain the purpose and extent of clinical trials. Identify some advantages and disadvantages to clinical trials.
6. What are controlled substances? What are some nursing implications related to administering a controlled substance? What special precautions are required for handling controlled substances?
7. Identify some points about safe drug use that should be taught to all patients.
8. What kinds of information about drugs should be included in the patient teaching plan?

NEED MORE HELP?

Chapter 2 of the Study Guide to Accompany *Drug Therapy in Nursing*, 4th Edition, contains NCLEX-style questions and other learning activities to reinforce your understanding of the concepts presented in this chapter. For additional information or to purchase the study guide, visit thePoint.

REFERENCES

Bhathena, A., & Spear B. B. (2008). Pharmacogenetics: improving drug and dose selection. *Current Opinion in Pharmacology*, 8(5):639–646.

Food and Drug Administration. (2006). New drug approval process. Retrieved from *http://www.fda.gov/cder/handbook/develop.htm*

Food and Drug Administration. (2000). Drug prescription labels. Retrieved from *http://www.fda.gov/cber/rules/labelreg.pdf.*

Food and Drug Administration (1982). Orphan Drug Act. Retrieved from *http://www.fda.gov/orphan/index.htm*

Food and Drug Administration (1982). Title II of the comprehensive drug abuse prevention and control act of 1970 *http://www.ask.com/bar?q=controlled+substances+act&page=1&qsrc=178&ab=2&u=http%3A%2F%2Fwww.fda.gov%2Fopacom%2Flaws%2Fcntrlsub%2Fctlsbtoc.htm*

GovTrack.us. H. R. 6353–110th Congress (2008). Ryan Haight Online Pharmacy Consumer Protection Act of 2008, *GovTrack.us (database of federal legislation)* <http://www.govtrack.us/congress/bill.xpd?bill=h110-6353> (accessed Mar 17, 2009)

Gomez A. & Ingelman-Sundberg M. (2009). Pharmacoepigenetics: its role in interindividual differences in drug response. *Clinical Pharmacology and Therapeutics*,

Gurwitz D. & Lunshof J. E. (2008). Personalized pharmacotherapy: genotypes, biomarkers, and beyond. *Clilnical Pharmacology and Therapeutics*, 85(2):142.

Leake C. D. (1975). *A historical account of pharmacology to the twentieth century.* Springfield, IL: Charles C Thomas Press.

Montoya I. D. (2008). The root cause of patient safety concerns in an Internet pharmacy. *Expert Opinion on Drug Safety,* 7(4):337–341.

Orizio G., Schulz P., Domenighini S., et al, (2009), Cyberdrugs: a cross-sectional study of online pharmacies characteristics. *Europen Journal of Public Health,* 16 pp.

Streetman D. S. (2007). Emergence and evolution of pharmacogenetics and pharmacogenomics in clinical pharmacy over the past 40 years. *The Annals of Pharmacotherapy,* 41(12):2038–2041.

Wasinger, V. C., Cordwell, S. J., Wilkins, M. R., et al. (1995). Progress with gene-product mapping of the Mollicutes: Mycoplasma genitalium. *Electrophoresis,* 16(7):1090–1094.

Drug Administration

Learning Objectives

At the completion of this chapter the student will:

1. Describe the three routes for administering drugs.
2. Differentiate systemic and local effects related to the various routes of drug administration.
3. Describe the variety of oral forms of enteral drugs.
4. Differentiate the three main methods of parenteral drug administration.
5. Describe the methods of topical administration.
6. Describe how the route of administration interacts with core drug knowledge.
7. Describe how the route of administration interacts with the core patient variables.
8. Describe nursing interventions to maximize therapeutic and minimize adverse effects based on drug administration route.

Key Terms

buccal	intramuscular	suspension
capsules	intrathecal	sustained release
elixir	intravenous	syrup
emulsion	intravenous piggyback	systemic effect
enteral route	intravenous push	tablet
enteric coating	local effect	topical route
intra-arterial	parenteral route	troches
intra-articular	subcutaneous	
intradermal	sublingual	

Drug therapy can be administered by several different routes or methods. These routes of administration require different preparations or forms of a drug. Most drugs are available from the drug manufacturer in multiple forms. The selection of the route and form is based on the interaction between core drug knowledge and core patient variables. In managing drug therapy, nurses use this information to assess patient needs, plan care, administer drugs, and evaluate the effectiveness of therapy. This chapter describes the different routes of drug administration, explains the different forms of drug preparations, and shows how the route and drug form interact with the core drug knowledge and the core patient variables.

DRUG ADMINISTRATION ROUTES: GENERAL CONSIDERATIONS

The three basic routes of drug administration are enteral, parenteral, and topical. (Some authorities place topical in the parenteral category.)

- The **enteral route** uses the gastrointestinal (GI) tract for the ingestion and absorption of drugs. The most common method of administering drugs through the enteral route is orally. The enteral route also includes drugs that are administered through a nasogastric (NG) or a gastrostomy (G) tube.
- The **parenteral route** avoids or circumvents the GI tract and is associated with all forms of injections: intramuscular (IM), subcutaneous (SC or SQ), and intravenous (IV). Less commonly used parenteral routes than IM, SC, and IV are intradermal (into the dermis), intrathecal (into the cerebrospinal fluid), intra-articular (into a joint), and intra-arterial (into an artery).
- The **topical route** is technically another parenteral route because it also bypasses the GI tract. Drugs administered topically are applied to the skin or mucous membranes, including those of the eyes, ears, nose, vagina, rectum, and lungs.

Drugs are administered for their local or systemic effects. For example, most drugs applied topically to the skin or mucous membranes exert their effect at that site, which is called a **local effect.** An example is corticosteroid cream applied to relieve the itch from a rash. However, certain drugs given topically are absorbed by the skin and distributed throughout the body systems to produce a **systemic effect.** Drugs given for a systemic effect by any route must be capable of being transported into the blood and distributed through the body to a location distant from the administration site. An example is fentanyl, the narcotic used for pain relief, which is imbedded in a transdermal patch and applied to the skin.

Drugs administered by a route other than the enteral route have the advantage of avoiding the first-pass metabolism in the liver. Drugs administered enterally are absorbed from the stomach and small intestine. However, they first pass through the liver, the primary organ for drug metabolism, before being distributed throughout the body. Drugs administered parenterally and even some topical drugs are transported directly into the blood, thereby bypassing the liver. (See Chapter 4 for a complete discussion of the first-pass effect and the processes of pharmacokinetics.)

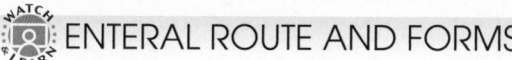

ENTERAL ROUTE AND FORMS

The enteral route involves using the GI tract for the administration and absorption of drugs. Enteral drugs, particularly oral drugs, are manufactured and prepared in a variety of forms, including solid tablets and capsules and liquid elixirs and syrups. Because the oral route of administration is the most common enteral route, oral dosage forms are the most common preparations. They are convenient, economical, and easy to use.

Some oral drugs, such as antacids and laxatives, are given for their local effect in the GI tract, but most are given to achieve a systemic effect. In most cases, patients can reliably self-medicate with oral drug forms.

Oral Drug Forms
Tablets

A **tablet** is a solid dosage form that is prepared by compressing or molding a drug into various sizes and shapes. In many cases, tablets are scored; that is, designed to be easily broken at a point so that one half or one quarter of the dose may be given. Unless a tablet is scored, it should never be broken because doing so could result in inaccurate dosage.

The active ingredients in tablets are commonly mixed with lactose or other sugars, binding agents, or other inert materials to facilitate manufacturing and ensure stability of the preparation. When the patient swallows the tablet, esophageal peristalsis propels it to the stomach, where it dissolves and releases the drug into the gastric contents.

Drugs that are appropriate for use in tablet form have some limitations. First, the drug must be stable in gastric contents. Because gastric juices may be highly acidic, drugs that rapidly degrade in acid environments may not be administered as conventional tablets. An additional consideration is flavor because the tablet will begin to dissolve as soon as it is placed in the mouth. Drugs determined by the pharmaceutical company to be bitter, irritating, or unpleasant tasting are not usually manufactured in conventional tablet form because they would be accepted poorly by patients. These limitations can be overcome by using a special coating on the tablet.

An **enteric coating** is a wax-like layer that is used on some tablets. This layer resists the acid environment of the stomach but dissolves in areas in which the local pH is neutral or slightly alkaline (e.g., the small intestine). Enteric coatings may be used to protect acid-labile drugs, to provide a sustained-release dose, or to guard against local adverse effects from a drug. Other types of commonly used coatings include film or sugar. Both of these coatings are used to protect the patient from bitter or unpleasant-tasting drugs. These coatings do not impart any time-release characteristics.

Sustained-release (also called controlled-, timed-, extended-, or prolonged-release) tablets are formulated to release a drug slowly over an extended period, rather than rapidly like conventional tablets. Sustained release occurs by several methods:

- Layers of enteric coatings may be applied, and the drug is released in response to changes in the surrounding pH of the GI fluid.
- The tablet may be formulated to release the drug in a steady, controlled manner.
- The tablet may be formulated to release the drug in a series of pulsations.

In most cases, the total dose of drug in a sustained-release preparation is higher than that found in a regular tablet. The patient may safely take the higher dose because it is released in a controlled fashion, thereby preventing any adverse effects from overdosage.

Sublingual and Buccal Tablets

Sublingual and buccal preparations are tablet forms that are not used as often as oral tablets. These small, hard, compressed tablets are designed to dissolve rapidly in the vascular mucous membranes of the mouth. **Buccal** tablets are placed in the buccal pouch (between the cheek and gum), and **sublingual** tablets are placed under the tongue. Sublingual and buccal tablets must be relatively nonirritating, flavorless, and highly water soluble.

Because the buccal and sublingual areas are highly vascular, drugs are quickly absorbed into the bloodstream, and a rapid onset of drug effect occurs. At the same time, drugs administered in this way avoid the first-pass phenomenon because they are not ingested into the GI tract. Although these formulations typically are considered oral forms because they are placed in the mouth, most experts think of the sublingual and buccal forms as parenteral preparations because they are not absorbed in the GI tract. Others consider them a variation of the topical route.

Troches

Troches, also called pastilles or lozenges, are commonly used to achieve a local effect in the mouth or pharynx (throat). The drug is embedded in hard candy or another suitably flavored vehicle that the patient holds within the mouth, where it slowly dissolves. Antitussives, anti-infectives, local anesthetics, antihistamines, and analgesics are administered this way.

Capsules

Capsules are solid dosage forms in which the drug is usually encased in a shell of hard or soft gelatin. When the patient swallows the capsule, the drug is carried to the stomach, where the gelatin capsule quickly dissolves and releases the drug into the gastric contents. Because the active ingredients are enclosed in gelatin, foul-tasting drugs can be easily administered in

capsules. Another advantage is that many patients find gelatin capsules easier to swallow than tablets. Unlike tablets, capsules cannot be easily divided or broken into equal pieces, so one disadvantage is that dosage may not be as flexible.

The most common capsules encase a powdered drug. Soft, elastic capsules are somewhat thicker and may be used to encase a drug paste, semiliquid, or liquid (provided the drug itself does not dissolve the capsule). In addition, the contents may be altered in one of several ways to produce a sustained-release dosage form as follows:

- Layers of enteric coatings may be applied to the drug particles, producing what is commonly known as micro-encapsulation. The drug is released in response to changes in the surrounding pH of the GI fluid. The rate of release is controlled by varying the thickness of the layers around the drug particles.
- The capsule may be formulated to release the drug in a steady, controlled manner from a matrix of drug encased in a slowly dissolving substance, such as wax.
- The drug is bound to ion-exchange resins, chemical compounds that form insoluble complexes within the capsule. Changes in the local environment, such as altered electrolyte content or pH, cause the drug to be released slowly from the resin matrix.

Like their tablet counterparts, sustained-release capsules may contain higher doses than those found in regular-release forms, but the patient may safely take the higher dose because the drug is released in a controlled fashion.

Syrups

A concentrated solution of sugar, such as sucrose, in water is known as a **syrup.** Most syrups that contain 65% or more sucrose are also resistant to mold, yeasts, and other microorganisms, and they have a reasonable shelf life with no need for refrigeration. Occasionally, sucrose may crystallize out of solution, clouding the syrup or giving it the appearance of particulate matter.

Elixirs

An **elixir** is a clear hydroalcoholic mixture that is usually sweetened or otherwise pleasantly flavored. Most elixirs contain ethanol and water, but glycerin, sorbitol, propylene glycol, flavoring agents, aspartase, and even syrups may also be found in elixirs. The alcohol content of elixirs varies greatly and can exceed 25%. Elixirs are stored at room temperature, and the alcohol content usually prevents the growth of any mold or other microorganisms. Elixirs should always be clear. Cloudiness indicates contamination.

Emulsions and Suspensions

Many drug preparations use mixtures of two chemically incompatible substances. These preparations may be administered orally. Rarely, they may be used topically.

An **emulsion** is created when two liquids that do not mix well are combined, and one liquid distributes uniformly through the other. Because these mixtures tend to separate rapidly, remember to shake the preparation well immediately before measuring a dose and to administer the dose soon after pouring and measuring. To enhance the stability of the mixture, an emulsifying agent is added. Most emulsions consist of a nonaqueous agent (oil or lipid phase) dispersed with an aqueous (water) agent. In general, nothing should be added to emulsions because additives may adversely affect the stability of the mixture.

A **suspension** is a drug preparation consisting of two agents: a finely divided solid dispersed within a liquid. The stability of the preparation depends on the ability of the dispersing medium to wet the solid particles. Surface-active agents may be used.

Nasogastric or Gastrostomy Tube Forms

Patients who cannot swallow but who have a functioning GI tract may have an NG (nasogastric) or G (gastrostomy) tube in place. An NG tube is a soft, flexible tube that is advanced through a nostril and into the stomach for administering food, fluids, and drugs, usually for a short time. An NG tube presents a risk for aspiration from gastric reflux because the tube prevents the gastroesophageal sphincter from closing. A G tube is surgically inserted into the stomach for administering food, fluids, and drugs to patients who need long-term care. Sometimes a G tube is inserted via a procedure called a percutaneous endoscopic gastrostomy; these tubes are then referred to as PEG tubes. Providing drugs and foods through a G tube is preferred over an NG tube because the G tube method leaves the gastroesophageal sphincter intact. Regurgitation is less likely with a G tube than with an NG tube.

Drugs administered through a tube should be either liquid or crushed and in a liquid vehicle. A liquid drug form is preferred because research has shown that this form causes less clotting of tubes than crushed and dissolved drugs. However, if a liquid form is not available, the tablet may be crushed as long as it is not an enteric-coated or sustained-release preparation. Sustained-release or enteric-coated tablets are never crushed.

Nursing Management in Enteral Drug Administration

Core Drug Knowledge

Although the oral method of drug delivery is most common, not all drugs can be administered orally. Gastric acids and enzymes destroy many drugs; others simply may not be absorbed.

Absorption may begin in the stomach, but most absorption of orally administered drugs occurs in the small intestine. Food may interfere with the dissolution and absorption of certain drugs, especially enteric-coated drugs, because of the considerable variation in individual gastric emptying times and therefore in the length of time a drug spends in the stomach.

Assessment of Relevant Core Patient Variables

Health Status

A primary consideration for administering an oral drug is the patient's condition. Can the patient tolerate an oral drug? Patients who are vomiting, uncooperative, or unconscious or whose condition requires that they receive nothing by mouth (i.e., no oral food or fluid) are not suited for oral drug therapy. Alternate routes should be used. If the patient cannot swallow at all but has a working GI system, the drug may be given through an NG or a G tube. If patients can take oral drugs but have difficulty swallowing tablets, pills, and capsules, the drugs may be crushed and mixed in a few milliliters of water or liquid or in a tablespoon of jelly, applesauce, or pudding. Large volumes of fluid or food are avoided because the patient must consume the full volume to receive the full drug dose. Alternately, a liquid drug form may be substituted. Sublingual drugs may be administered even to unconscious patients because these drug forms are so rapidly absorbed by the vasculature.

Life Span and Gender

The high sugar content of syrups can mask unpleasant drug flavors, making syrups useful vehicles for administering drugs orally to both adults and children. Because they usually contain little or no alcohol, syrups are especially good vehicles for drugs administered to children. Because of the potentially high alcohol content, elixirs are usually not used in children or in adults who should avoid ethanol.

Environment

Oral drug forms are easily self-administered by patients and can be used in home environments and acute or long-term care settings.

Planning and Intervention

Maximizing Therapeutic Effects

Capsules with sustained-release pellets in them can be opened and the pellets sprinkled on food or mixed with a liquid; the patient must eat or drink all the food or fluid.

Because emulsions and suspensions have a tendency to separate, they should be shaken well immediately before measuring a dose and then administered promptly.

Drugs administered through an NG or G tube are instilled slowly without excessive force. Some may be allowed to flow in by gravity. The tube is flushed with 10 to 30 mL of water before and after drug administration to ensure that the patient receives the full dose and to maintain the patency of the tube.

Minimizing Adverse Effects

Drugs that have enteric coatings and drugs in sustained-release form should never be chewed, crushed, or broken. Doing so increases the risk for adverse effects, including toxicity, because a higher dosage of the drug is available all at once.

Repeated doses of sucrose-containing syrups may increase the risk for gingivitis or dental caries. Good oral hygiene should accompany the use of syrups. Also, patients

Box 3.1 — FIVE RIGHTS OF DRUG ADMINISTRATION

In managing drug therapy safely and effectively, the nurse must heed the five rights of drug administration:

right	Patient
right	Drug
right	Time
right	Dose
right	Route

TABLE 3.1 — Abbreviations Related to Medication Administration

Abbreviation	Meaning
a.c.	before meals
p.c.	after meals
qam	every morning
bid	twice a day
tid	three times a day (usually limited to hours awake)
qid	four times a day (usually limited to hours awake)
q4h	every four hours
q6h	every six hours
qh	every hour
prn	as needed
ad lib	as desired
IM	Intramuscularly
IV	Intravenously
SQ or SC	Subcutaneously
PO	by mouth
SL	Sublingually
OD	right eye
OS	left eye
OU	both eyes
STAT	Immediately

with diabetes may need to monitor their glucose levels closely if they are receiving large doses of drugs in syrups.

Before administering drugs through an NG or G tube, the tube is assessed for proper placement. In addition, the head of the patient's bed is elevated to help prevent aspiration from reflux. If the patient is also receiving tube feedings, the nurse reviews information on the specific drug because some drugs are not absorbed well with tube-feeding formulas. When a tube-fed patient needs such a drug, the feeding must be shut off for a time both before and after drug administration.

To help maintain safety during drug administration, the nurse must closely follow the cardinal rules of drug administration (Box 3.1). These rules are known as the Five Rights; recently some authors have added a sixth right: documentation, and others have added a seventh: right reason for administration to improve patient safety. Adding additional "rights," however, provides no guarantee of increased patient safety from drug therapy. The Institute for Safe Medication Practices states that the five rights should only be considered as broadly stated goals or desired outcomes of safe medication practices. The five rights in themselves do not ensure medication safety. Neither do they offer procedural direction on how to achieve these goals. Most importantly they ignore the larger issues of interdisciplinary actions and the system problems which produce most medication errors (Institute for Safe Medication Practices, January 2007). The nurse assumes individual accountability for safe drug administration by engaging in behavior that follows nationally accepted standards of practice and institutionally prescribed behaviors designed to achieve the goals of the five rights. These accepted standards of practice include the following:

To administer a drug to "the right patient" the nurse should use two unique patient identifiers (such as the name and the patient history number, never the room number). To administer the "right drug," at the "right time" using the "right route," the nurse must be able to read and interpret the medication order correctly. Standard abbreviations are frequently used in medication orders (Table 3.1). The nurse must know these abbreviations. Some abbreviations are likely to be misinterpreted and cause medication errors, these should be avoided. (Joint Commission on Accreditation, 2005) (Table 3.2) Additionally, nurses need to confirm that every ordered drug is appropriate for

TABLE 3.2 — The Joint Commission Official "Do Not Use" List 2005

Do Not Use	Potential Problem	Use Instead
U (unit)	Mistaken for "0" (zero), the number "4" (four) or "cc"	Write "unit"
IU (International Unit)	Mistaken for IV (intravenous) or the number 10 (ten)	Write "International Unit"
Q.D., QD, q.d., qd (daily) Q.O.D., QOD, q.o.d, qod (every other day)	Mistaken for each other Period after the Q mistaken for "I" and the "O" mistaken for "I"	Write "daily" Write "every other day"
Trailing zero (X.0 mg)* Lack of leading zero (.X mg)	Decimal point is missed	Write X mg Write 0.X mg
MS MSO₄ and MgSO₄	Can mean morphine sulfate or magnesium sulfate Confused for one another	Write "morphine sulfate" Write "magnesium sulfate"

* Applies to all orders and all medication-related documentation that is handwritten (including free-text computer entry) or on pre-printed forms.

TABLE 3.3	Measurement Equivalents
Metric	**Household**
5 milliliters	1 teaspoon
15 milliliters	1 tablespoon
30 milliliters	2 tablespoons or 1 ounce
500 milliliters	1 pint
1,000 milliliters or 1 liter	1 quart or 2 pints
1 kilogram or 1,000 grams	2.2 pounds

this person. Errors in listing the correct medications for a patient frequently occur as the patient moves between environments, such as from an intensive care unit to a general unit, or from the hospital to an extended care facility. For information on reducing errors related to changing environments, see Chapter 11.

To administer the "right dose," dosage calculation is often necessary. The most accurate method for doing dosage calculations is to use a calculator. Any drug dosage calculation book contains all of the necessary specific information. Many institutions require that all drug calculations be confirmed by two nurses before drug administration to prevent drug errors. Information about calculating pediatric doses is provided in Chapter 6. Occasionally, the nurse may need to convert the unit of measurement for the drug to another unit of measurement (Table 3.3).

PARENTERAL ROUTE

The parenteral route is associated with all forms of drugs administered by a syringe, needle, or catheter. The three most commonly used parenteral routes are intramuscular, subcutaneous, and intravenous.

 Intramuscular Administration

The **intramuscular** (IM) technique involves injecting drugs into certain muscles. This method requires specific knowledge of anatomy and aseptic technique. Because muscles have a good blood supply, drugs that are injected into a muscle move directly into the bloodstream without having to be broken down and absorbed, as oral drugs processed by the GI tract must be. Thus, the onset of action with intramuscular injections is faster than with oral administration. Similarly, because muscles have more blood vessels than subcutaneous tissue, the onset of action after IM injection occurs more rapidly than after subcutaneous injection.

Drugs such as oils or irritating chemicals can be administered intramuscularly in solutions or suspensions. Many injectable drugs are dry powders and must be reconstituted before administration, possibly requiring a specific amount of diluent. Thin and watery solutions given intramuscularly move promptly into the blood vessels. Because suspensions

or drugs with an oil base are thicker or more viscous than water-based solutions, they do not move as quickly into the blood vessels. With these oil-based suspensions, a deposit of the drug is formed within the muscle that is slowly released into the bloodstream.

The sites for IM injection are the ventrogluteal, deltoid, rectus femoris, and vastus lateralis muscles (Figure 3.1). Site selection is based on characteristics of the drug, such as viscosity, and characteristics of the patient, such as age and size. While the dorsogluteal site was used frequently in the past, injection in the dorsogluteal site carries a risk for damaging the sciatic nerve if the injection site is not located properly. Many experts and nursing fundamental texts no longer recommend using this site, and some state that it should be used only as a last resort. For a number of years the ventrogluteal site has been the most recommended in the literature (as it is the safest deep muscle), but it continues to be the least used in practice (Floyd, S. & Meyer, A., 2007; Greenway, K., 2004; Nicoll, L. & Mesby, A., 2002; Roger, M. A. & King, L., 2000; Beyer, S. & Nichol, L., 1996). The ventrogluteal is free of major nerves and blood vessesls, can accommodate large volumes of medication, and all types of medications including highly viscous and irritating medications. So why have nurses been hesitant to utilize this site? Research indicates the reasons are diverse but include: insufficient teaching about site use during nursing education, lack of confidence in identifying the site, students imitating the practices of older nurses instead of practices taught in school, old habits, and lack of belief that it is safer than other sites (Floyd & Meyer, 2007).

The needle length chosen for injection should be long enough to enter the muscle, not the subcutaneous tissue. Patients who are overweight or obese may need longer needles than other patients to correctly place the medication (Zaybak, Gunes, Tamsel et al, 2007). Consult your nursing practice textbooks for more information on the specific techniques used for administering intramuscular injections.

Subcutaneous Administration

Subcutaneous (SC) drugs are administered under the skin into fat and connective tissue. These drugs must be highly soluble, low volume (less than 2 mL in a good-sized adult), and nonirritating (to prevent tissue damage, tissue necrosis, and sterile abscess formation). Distribution of the drug is through the capillaries and is less rapid than by the IM route. Distribution slows if the patient has inadequate peripheral circulation or if the drug is administered into scar tissue, which is avascular; onset will therefore be delayed.

The SC route may be used for vaccines, insulin, heparin, and narcotics. The sites used for this route are the upper, lateral arm; anterior thigh; abdomen; and midback above the scapula (although this last is infrequently utilized) (Figure 3.2). Not all medications given subcutaneously utilize all of these sites for administration. Correct administration into the subcutaneous tissue and not the muscle requires an assessment of the amount of subcutaneous tissue and correct needle

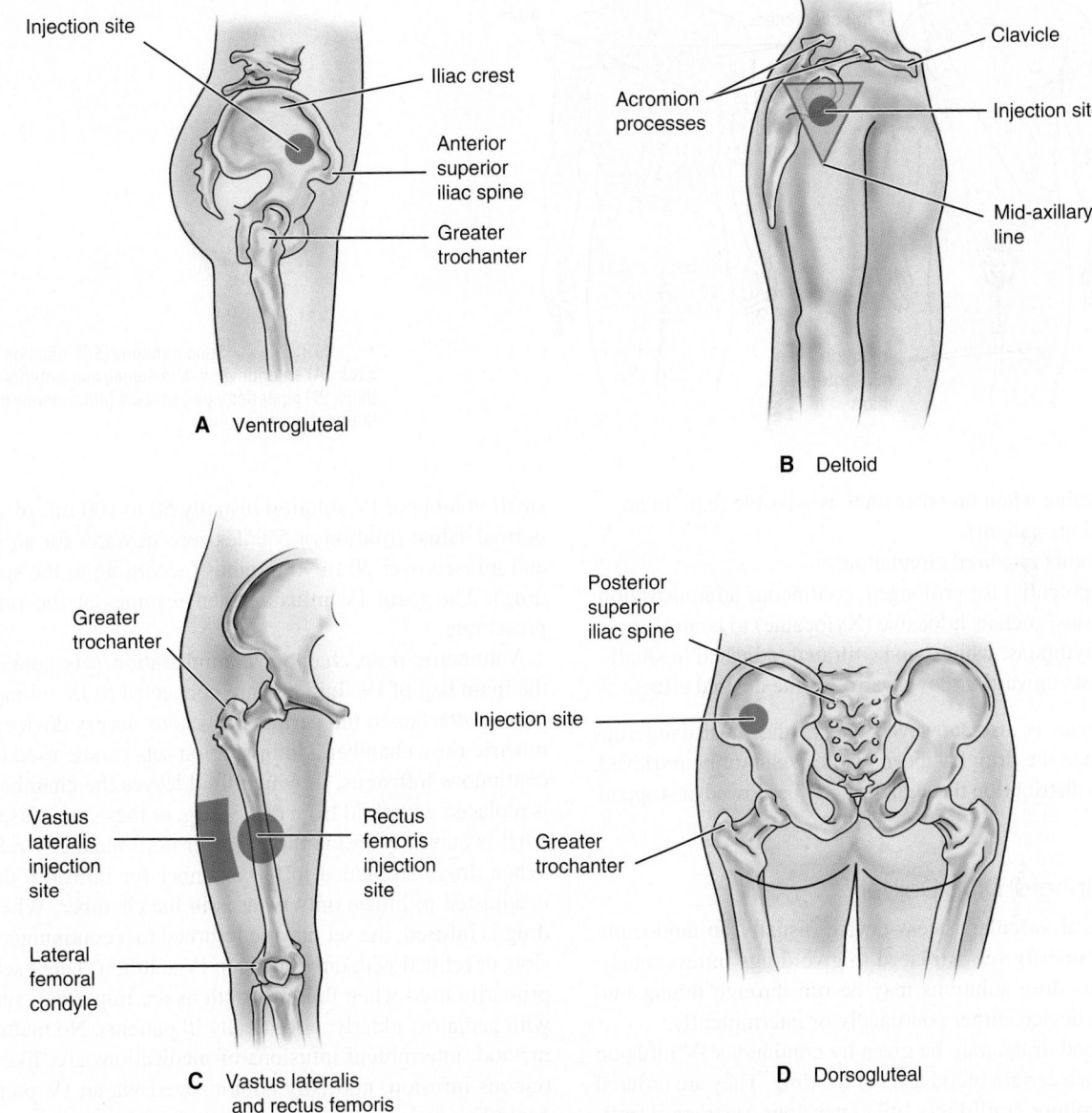

A Ventrogluteal

B Deltoid

C Vastus lateralis and rectus femoris

D Dorsogluteal

- FIGURE 3.1 Anatomic landmarks and intramuscular (IM) injection sites: (**A**) ventrogluteal; (**B**) deltoid; (**C**) vastus lateralis and rectus femoris; (**D**) dorsogluteal (site of last resort; use should be limited).

length selection (Annersten & Willman, 2005). The size of the individual determines the angle of injection. Refer to nursing practice textbooks to review SC injection techniques. Specific information on administration of special drugs, such as insulin and heparin, are included in the chapters on these drugs (Chapters 49 and 32, respectively).

Intravenous Administration

The **intravenous** technique administers a drug directly into the bloodstream, bypassing the need for absorption from the GI tract or transportation from other parts of the body, such as muscle or subcutaneous tissue. IV administration ensures

prompt, sometimes immediate, onset of action and eliminates the uncertainty associated with varied absorption rates from other routes. The IV route is advantageous in that it

- Has immediate effect (e.g., nitroprusside lowers blood pressure in hypertensive crisis).
- Allows administration of a large volume of drug (e.g., with certain antibiotics, such as cefoxitin).
- Avoids tissue irritation or injury resulting from IM or SC administration (e.g., with chemotherapeutic drugs, vasopressors such as norepinephrine [Levophed], or cardiac glycosides such as digoxin [Lanoxin], because the blood buffers the drug).

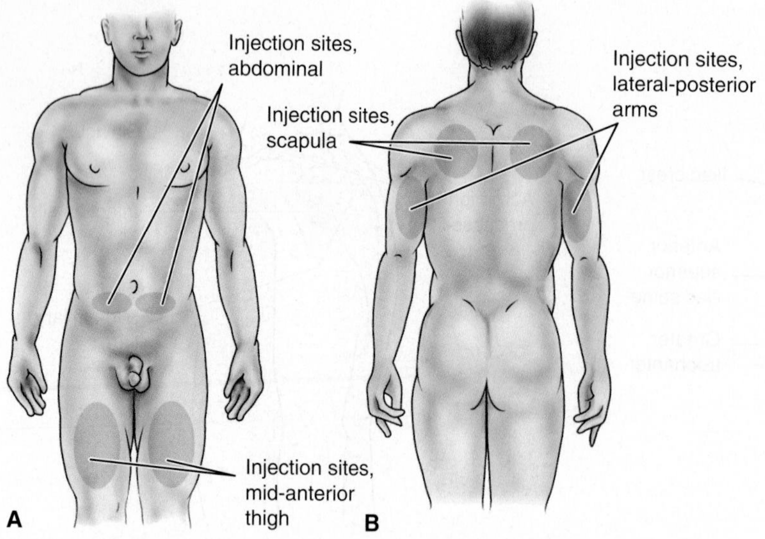

• FIGURE 3.2 Subcutaneous (SC) injection sites: (**A**) anterior view: abdominal, mid-anterior thigh; (**B**) posterior view: scapula (infrequently used), lateral-posterior arms.

• Is acceptable when no other route is possible (e.g., in an unconscious patient).
• Circumvents impaired circulation.
• Has the potential for prolonged, continuous administration of solutions, such as lidocaine (Xylocaine) to control cardiac arrhythmias, which can be titrated (adjusted in small increments upward or downward) for the desired effect.

The IV route is also, however, one of the most dangerous routes. Once the drug has been given, it cannot be retrieved, nor can its distribution through the body be slowed or stopped.

Peripheral Drug Delivery

A peripheral vascular access device, usually an angiocatheter or a butterfly set, is placed to give drugs intravenously. Intravenous drug solutions may be run through tubing into the access device, either continually or intermittently.

Prescribed drugs may be given by continuous IV infusion to maintain a certain blood level of the drug. They are ordered either in volume (milliliters [mL]) per hour or strength (milligrams [mg], micrograms [mcg], or units [U]) per hour. Aminophylline, lidocaine, and heparin are examples of drugs that are given continuously to achieve maximum therapeutic effect. The rate of continuous infusion for drugs should be maintained by use of an IV pump or controller.

IV drugs may also be given intermittently. When the patient receives continuous IV fluids and is also receiving intermittent IV drug therapy, the drug is given through a secondary IV tubing or through a volumetric dose chamber administration set, also called a metered-dose infusion set. When a secondary IV tubing is used to administer an IV drug, the tubing is added to the main line tubing, usually at a Y port. Adding secondary tubing is called "piggybacking" because the tubing with the drug rides on top of the primary fluid tubing. Antibiotics are frequently given intermittently by **intravenous piggyback** (IV piggyback). Such drugs are diluted in a small volume of IV solution (usually 50 to 100 mL of sterile normal saline solution or 5% dextrose in water for an adult) and infused over 30 to 90 minutes (according to the specific drug). The main IV infusion then resumes at the original preset rate.

Volumetric-dose chamber administration sets connect to the main bag of IV fluid and are connected to IV tubing that in turn attaches to the peripheral venous access device. Volumetric-dose chamber administration sets can be used to run continuous infusions, in which fluid leaves the chamber and is replaced with fluid from the IV bag, or they can infuse only what is currently inside the chamber until manually refilled. When drugs are added to the chamber for infusion, the set is adjusted to infuse only what is in the chamber. When the drug is infused, the set may be returned to a continuous infusion, or refilled with only the main IV solution. These sets are primarily used when fluid restrictions are important, such as with pediatric, elderly, or critically ill patients. No matter the method, intermittent infusions of medications are, like continuous infusion, normally administered via an IV pump or controller.

Certain IV drugs, whether given by piggyback or through a metered-dose infusion set, may be incompatible with an existing continuous IV infusion. If this situation arises, the tubing should be flushed with 10 mL of an appropriate solution (usually sterile normal saline) before and after administration of the drug.

If intravenous drugs are prescribed intermittently, and other fluids are not running constantly, the access device is capped to prevent blood from coming out and bacteria from entering the body. This cap may be permanently attached to a small extension tubing set. This tubing is secured to the peripheral device. An access device equipped this way is called "locked," or the patient is said to have a "lock" in place.

Drug infusion locks are used for patients who require intermittent IV drugs but do not need continuous IV fluid administration. As with piggybacks, the drug is usually diluted in 50 to 100 mL of solution. When the drug infusion is complete, the tubing is disconnected from the lock, allowing the patient increased ease of movement. The lock is kept patent (open, without blood clotting occurring), with small volumes of either normal saline (0.9% sodium chloride) solution or heparin pushed through the lock on a routine basis, usually every 8 hours. Depending on the solution that is used for flushing, the lock device is commonly called a saline lock or a heparin lock. Saline locks are flushed with 0.5 to 2 mL of sterile normal saline solution. Heparin locks are flushed with 10 to 100 U heparin. The nurse should be familiar with established institution protocols regarding the exact method for flushing drug infusion locks.

Direct administration into a vein or an established drug infusion lock of a concentrated drug in a very small amount of solution (usually 1 to 2 mL) is called an **intravenous push** (IVP or IV push). The drug is pushed into the vein very slowly over at least 1 minute. The exact amount of time depends on the drug and the dose. Drugs given by IVP may be used for intermittent dosing or for treating emergencies, such as cardiac arrest.

Central Access

Certain patients may require IV access for a prolonged time, or they may not be able to have peripheral vascular access devices inserted. Devices used for these patients include single or multilumen central venous catheters and implantable venous access ports. A central venous catheter is inserted by the health care provider into a vein (jugular or subclavian) near the heart. The catheter may have as many as three lumens to allow the administration of various solutions and drugs. Peripherally inserted central lines (PICs) or peripherally inserted midlines can be inserted by nurses specifically skilled in the technique. These also may be multilumen lines, and drugs may be delivered continuously, intermittently, or by IVP.

An implantable vascular access port (VAP) is surgically implanted under the skin with the distal end inserted into a large central vein. A special needle (a Huber needle) is used to suffuse the drug into the port. These ports are used for intermittent infusions of, for example, antineoplastic drugs. Use of a VAP requires advanced skills and expertise on the part of the nurse.

Other Parenteral Delivery Routes

Other parenteral routes are the intradermal, intra-articular, intra-arterial, and intrathecal routes. These routes of parenteral administration are not as common as the IM, SC, and IV routes.

Intradermal injections are made into the dermis just below the epidermis. This technique is used primarily for local anesthesia and for sensitivity tests, such as allergy and tuberculin tests. A small needle (25- or 27-gauge) and small-volume syringes (less than 1 mL) are used for intradermal injections.

The most common sites for intradermal injections are the medial forearm and the back over the scapula because the skin is thinner there.

An **intra-articular** injection is performed only by a skilled practitioner and involves injecting a drug into a joint. Corticosteroids are typically administered by intra-articular injection to relieve pain in an acutely inflamed joint. The effect is local. Nurses do not commonly administer medications by this route.

Intra-arterial drug administration requires a surgeon to insert a catheter into an artery leading directly to the targeted treatment area. The drug is delivered under positive pressure through the catheter. The positive pressure overcomes the pressure within the arterial system. For example, powerful undiluted chemotherapeutic agents can be delivered directly to a tumor by way of the artery that feeds it. Intra-arterial ports can also be implanted by a surgeon.

In **intrathecal** administration, a drug is delivered into the cerebrospinal fluid. It may be administered directly into the spinal subarachnoid space (a spinal) or outside the subarachnoid space (an epidural). Drugs are introduced into these areas by a catheter placed by specially trained health care providers. The drugs most commonly administered by this route are local anesthetics, antibiotics, and radiographic contrast media. This route is commonly used to deliver an anesthetic during labor and delivery. Pain relief can also be achieved with drugs given via this route by the nurse or by the patient using a patient-controlled analgesia device.

Nursing Management in Parenteral Drug Administration

Parenteral administration may be selected for a variety of reasons. This route allows drugs to be distributed directly to the vascular system without having to be absorbed by the GI tract and sent to the liver before circulating. This route also avoids the erratic absorption associated with the movement of the drug through the GI tract. Drugs that are highly metabolized by the first-pass mechanism can be given in smaller doses when given parenterally rather than orally because the parenteral route presents more drug to the vascular system initially than the enteral route does. Some drugs are almost completely metabolized during the first pass, so the parenteral route is chosen exclusively for these drugs. Moreover, drugs that are rapidly destroyed by GI secretions can be given parenterally to promote their effectiveness. Parenteral routes may also be necessary because of the GI irritant nature of the drug. Drugs administered by the parenteral routes have a faster onset of action than those administered orally or topically.

Assessment of Relevant Core Patient Variables
Health Status

A parenteral route may be chosen because the patient cannot tolerate oral drugs, cannot swallow, or has a condition that warrants resting the GI tract or keeping it empty.

Muscle mass must be sufficient for the volume of a drug given intramuscularly. The gluteal muscle mass can deteriorate if the person does not walk (e.g., because of paralysis), and in such cases it should be avoided as a site for IM injections. The patient's veins must be able to accept a venous access device if drugs are to be given intravenously. When peripheral access devices cannot be inserted, central venous access devices may be used.

Life Span and Gender

Infants have small muscle mass. The largest muscle mass at birth is the vastus lateralis, which is the preferred site for IM injections in infants, although the rectus femoris may also be used. The deltoid is never used for IM injections in infants. The gluteal muscles develop with walking and usually are not used for injections until the child has been walking for 1 year.

Elderly people have decreased muscle mass overall and decreased tissue elasticity, which may result in drugs oozing from injection sites. Muscle mass must be determined before IM injections.

Lifestyle, Diet, and Habits

Parenteral forms of drugs are more expensive than oral forms. Parenteral administration requires specialized skills, equipment, and education. Placing IV access devices into peripheral veins may be difficult in patients who are IV substance abusers.

Environment

Patients, particularly diabetic patients who receive insulin, can be taught to give themselves SC injections at home. The techniques for IM injections can also be taught to patients and their families for home use, although this practice is not as common. IV administration of drugs usually occurs in an acute or a long-term care setting; however, it can also be performed in the home setting with a home health nurse administering the drug therapy.

Planning and Intervention

Maximizing Therapeutic Effects

Selecting the appropriate-sized syringe and needle is key to administering an IM or SC injection. Selection is based on the patient, the type of required injection, the administration site, and characteristics of the drug (how viscous, how irritating, and how much volume).

CRITICAL THINKING SCENARIO

CHOOSING THE RIGHT DRUG ADMINISTRATION SITE

Georgia Govans, 79 years old, is admitted with osteomyelitis of the hip, a severe infection, after a recent repair of a hip fracture. She has a temperature of 101°F (38.3°C) on admission and a history of severe peripheral vascular disease.

1. Which route will most likely be chosen to administer antibiotics to this patient?

2. Select and support a choice of drug delivery method based on the patient's history and her drug requirements.

A continuous IV drug infusion should be monitored to ensure that therapeutic blood levels are achieved and that drug therapy is effective. After administration of an intermittent IV drug, the lock must be flushed to maintain patency. If heparin is used to keep the lock patent, flushing the lock is usually necessary before drug infusion with sterile normal saline solution, and then again after the infusion before flushing with the heparin. Flushing is necessary because many drugs are incompatible with heparin.

Minimizing Adverse Effects

To minimize adverse effects and drug errors, the nurse follows the five rights of drug administration when administering parenteral drug therapy. To prevent infections, the drug, all parts of the syringe that have come into contact with the drug, and the shaft of the needle that enters the patient's body must be sterile. Meticulous administration technique is necessary because most parenteral drugs enter the bloodstream readily, quickly spreading any organisms introduced with the injection.

Site selection is important because incorrect placement of the needle may damage blood vessels or nerves. Knowledge of the muscles, visible or palpable anatomic landmarks, and location of major nerves and blood vessels in the underlying tissue is an absolute necessity for safe administration.

The oils and irritating chemicals found in the solutions or suspensions of some parenteral drugs may be dangerous if given intravenously. Care must be taken by careful site selection and aspiration before injection to prevent inadvertently administering an IM drug into a blood vessel.

To prevent bacterial growth, reconstituted drugs usually require refrigeration if they are not completely used after dilution. The reconstituted drug container must be labeled with the patient's name, dilution date, and volume and type of diluent used.

When administering drugs that are very irritating to the tissues, the nurse may use an injection technique known as the Z-track method to prevent the drug from seeping up from the muscle into the subcutaneous tissue. Subcutaneous tissue is displaced to one side before inserting the needle into the muscle. The drug is then injected, the needle is withdrawn, and the subcutaneous tissue is allowed to go back into place. Consult your nursing practice texts for more detailed information.

Patients receiving drugs with powerful effects on the body such as dopamine (which increases cardiac output), and heparin (an anticoagulant) by continuous IV infusion must be closely monitored. The adverse effects of these drugs can be serious or life threatening. The rate at which such drugs are administered must be regulated carefully by using an IV pump or controller. Newer forms of pumps have "smart" software that help prevent medication errors because they are programmed with the hospital defined dosing limits and other clinical advisories to help nurses remember the "rules" regarding safe administration of high risk drugs. If nurses bypass the safety technology imbedded in the pump then medication errors can still occur (Institute for

Safe Medication Practices, April 2007). Because the drug enters the bloodstream directly, blood levels of the drug can rise above desired therapeutic levels quickly. Blood levels, therefore, should be closely monitored.

TOPICAL ROUTE AND FORMS

The topical route of drug administration involves applying drug preparations to the skin or mucous membranes, including the eyes, ears, nose, rectum, vagina, and lungs. The primary advantage is that topical drugs usually act locally, although some can have systemic effects. A disadvantage of topical drugs is that most are intended for only one specific site. For example, ophthalmic drugs are used only in the eyes, and dermatologic drugs are used only on the skin. Drugs that can be administered in topical forms include antibiotics, antiseptics, antifungals, anti-inflammatory agents, antipyretics, vasodilators, hormones, antismoking agents, analgesics, antiemetics, and débriding agents.

The most common and widely used topical agents are applied to the skin. Dermatologic preparations come in several forms: lotions, creams, liquids, ointments, and emollients. Emollients are applied liberally to dry skin. Most drugs applied to the intact skin have primarily local effects because little drug is absorbed through the outer epidermis. Absorption increases under the following circumstances:

- The skin is abraded or denuded.
- The drug is added to a specific solvent because only lipid-soluble substances are absorbed through the intact skin.
- The medicated skin is covered by an occlusive dressing (e.g., in treatment for psoriasis).

Most dermatologic drugs are applied in a thin layer or in a measured amount (topical nitroglycerin is applied in inches). Single-dose, adhesive-backed drug applications, called transcutaneous or transdermal drug delivery systems, are currently available. Some examples of the transdermal drug delivery route include nitroglycerin (Nitro-Dur) for patients with coronary artery disease, scopolamine (Transderm-Scop) for patients who suffer from motion sickness, and fentanyl (Duragesic) for patients with severe pain. Although this drug form can be expensive, its ability to avoid first-pass effects is an advantage. The transdermal system is convenient and usually requires less frequent application than other forms.

Drugs administered to the eye take the form of drops or ointments that are applied to the rim of the lower lid. Drugs administered in the ear are in the form of drops. Drugs administered through the rectum are either in suppositories (waxy, bullet-shaped systems that dissolve in the body from body heat) or ointments. Drugs administered into the vagina are in the form of suppositories, creams, foams, liquids, or tablets (moistened before insertion to promote dissolving inside the body).

Drugs given into the nose are in liquid sprays, drops, or aerosol preparations. Inhalers, another form of aerosolized therapy, are used for respiratory conditions and have an

effect on the lungs but are inhaled through mouth breathing. Patients should shake the inhaler well, exhale fully, and then inhale while pushing down on the inhaler to activate it. They should breathe in the puff of drug and hold the breath for several seconds before exhaling. The timing of this technique is difficult for many patients. The use of a spacer, which acts as a reservoir for the drug, is helpful for many patients. The patient activates the inhaler, and the drug enters the spacer. The patient then breathes in from the spacer. If multiple puffs of the inhaler are ordered, the patient should wait 1 to 2 minutes between puffs. The inhaler and the patient's mouth should be rinsed after drug administration.

Nursing Management in Topical Drug Administration
Assessment of Relevant Core Patient Variables

For the most part, assessment involves inspecting the skin for integrity. If the skin is not intact, aseptic technique becomes an important factor in infection control.

Planning and Intervention

To maximize therapeutic effects and minimize adverse effects, the nurse should wear gloves or use an applicator when administering dermatologic drugs, to avoid infecting the patient and to protect his or her own skin from the drug. If the skin is broken, the nurse needs to use sterile technique when applying a dermatologic drug to prevent introducing bacteria and other organisms into the body. If an adverse effect occurs with drugs given by a transdermal system, removing the patch usually relieves the symptoms.

To promote safe administration of topical drugs, the nurse must again observe the five rights of drug administration (see Box 3.1).

CHAPTER SUMMARY

- The three routes of drug administration are enteral, parenteral, and topical.
- The drug route may produce systemic effects, local effects, or both.
- Oral drugs may be available in sustained-release or enteric-coated form to delay onset of action of the drug.
- Food, fluids, and other drugs may alter the absorption of enteric drugs.
- The parenteral route avoids the GI tract and the irregularities of absorption, including the first-pass effect. The most common methods of parenteral drug administration are the IM, SC, and IV routes.
- Onset of drug action is more rapid with the parenteral than with the enteral route.
- Patient characteristics (age, weight, muscle mass) and drug characteristics (volume, viscosity, irritability) are considered when selecting a site for IM drug administration.
- Administration of IV drugs may be through continuous drip, intermittent infusion, or IVP methods into peripheral

or central venous access devices. IV drugs are normally administered via a pump or controller to maintain a steady, safe rate of drug delivery.

• Topical drugs include those that are applied to the skin and mucous membranes of the eyes, ears, nose, rectum, and vagina.

QUESTIONS FOR STUDY AND REVIEW

1. Which route of drug administration is most frequently used?
2. What is the advantage of an enteric-coated tablet?
3. Why might a parenteral route of a drug be prescribed instead of an enteral route?
4. Which parenteral technique poses the greatest risk for rapid drug toxicity to a patient?

NEED MORE HELP?

Chapter 3 of the Study Guide to Accompany *Drug Therapy in Nursing*, 4th Edition, contains NCLEX-style questions and other learning activities to reinforce your understanding of the concepts presented in this chapter. For additional information or to purchase the study guide, visit thePoint.

REFERENCES

Annersten, M. & Willman A. (2005). Performing subcutaneous injections: a literature review. *Worldviews on evidence-based nursing / Sigma Theta Tau International, Honor Society of Nursing*, 2(3):122–130.

Beyer, S. & Nichol, L. (1996). Back to basics. Administering IM injections the right way. *American Journal of Nursing*, 96(1): 34–35.

Joint Commission on Accreditation of Healthcare Organizations. (2005). Official "do not use" abbreviation list. Retrieved March 14, 2009, from *http://www.jointcommission.org/PatientSafety/DoNotUseList/facts_dnu.htm*

Floyd, S. & Meyer, A. (2007). Intramuscular Injections: What's Best Practice. *Kai Tiaki Nursing New Zealand*, 13(6):20–22.

Greenway, K. (2004). Using the ventrogluteal site for intramuscular injection. *Nursing Standard*, 18(Z5):39–42.

Institute for Safe Medication Practices. The five rights: A destination without a map. January 25, 2007. http://www.ismp.org/newsletters/acutecare/articles/20070125.asp. Retrieved March 13, 2009.

Institute for Safe Medication Practices (2007). Smart pumps are not smart on their own. Retrieved from http://www.ismp.org/Newsletters/acutecare/articles/20070419.asp?ptr=y: on March 14, 2009.

Nicoll, L. & Mesby, A. (2002). Intramuscular injection: an integrative research review and guideline for evidence based practice. *Applied Nursing Research*, 16(2):149–162.

Roger, M. A. & King, L. (2000). Drawing up and administering intramuscular injections: A review of the literature. *Journal of Advanced Nursing*, 31(3):574–582.

Zaybak, A., Gunes, U. Y., Tamsel, S., et al. (2007). Does obesity prevent the needle from reaching muscle in intramuscular injections? *Journal of Advanced Nursing*, 58(6):552–556.

UNIT 2
Core Drug Knowledge

Pharmacotherapeutics, Pharmacokinetics, and Pharmacodynamics

Learning Objectives

At the completion of this chapter the student will:

1. Define pharmacotherapeutics, pharmacokinetics, and pharmacodynamics.
2. Describe the processes used as drugs move throughout the body.
3. Understand how the chemical makeup of a drug and the internal chemistry of the body affect a drug's ability to cross cell membranes.
4. Identify factors that affect absorption of drug molecules.
5. Describe factors that influence the distribution of drug molecules.
6. Discuss factors that may alter metabolism.
7. Identify how drug molecules are excreted from the body.
8. Identify the main mechanism drugs use to produce their effects on the body.
9. Describe the variables that influence the dose of a drug that is administered.

Key Terms

absorption	excretion	pharmacodynamics
affinity	first-pass effect	pharmacokinetics
agonist	half-life	pharmacotherapeutics
antagonist	intrinsic activity	potency
biotransformation	loading dose	prodrug
blocker	maintenance dose	receptor
blood–brain barrier	metabolism	steady state
clearance	metabolites	therapeutic index
distribution	off label use	therapeutic range
efficacy	P-450 system	

The nurses' role in drug therapy involves more than passing the appropriately ordered drug to the right patient. The nurse must understand how drug therapy creates its effects in the body (both positive and negative) and be able to critically assess the patient's response to drug therapy. In order to do this, the nurse needs to know basic pharmacologic facts. These facts make up the Core Drug Knowledge related to a particular drug. As in all bodies of knowledge, there is a "language" of words that is specific to pharmacology and drug therapy. The nurse needs to understand this language and be able to correctly use the words in order to read and interpret written drug material and scholarly articles as well as to clearly communicate with pharmacists, physicians, and other health professionals about drug therapy. This chapter examines the pharmacotherapeutics, pharmacokinetics, and pharmacodynamics in Core Drug Knowledge; it is the basis, along with Chapter 5, for understanding all of the drug information presented in the rest of the text.

PHARMACOTHERAPEUTICS

Pharmacotherapeutics is the achievement of the desired therapeutic goal from drug therapy. Essentially, it is the clinical purpose—the indication—for giving a drug. The terms *indications* and *therapeutics* are often substituted for the more formal term *pharmacotherapeutics*. For example, when a person has hypertension, we give drugs to lower the blood pressure to a normal level. In this way we treat, or manage, a chronic condition. The desired pharmacotherapeutics can also be used to induce a cure. For example, when a patient has a bacterial infection, we give an antibiotic that kills the infecting organism. The desired therapeutic effect of a drug can also be to prevent a problem. An example of this type of use is when a patient has had total joint replacement surgery. Because this procedure increases the patient's risk for developing a thrombus (blood clot), drug therapy with anticoagulants is used to prevent this undesirable outcome. Whatever the clinical or medical reason is for prescribing a drug, the pharmacotherapeutics is the desired outcome of administering that drug.

Generally, the pharmacotherapeutics of a drug is determined through clinical drug trials. Findings from these studies are submitted to the governmental agency that oversees approval of new drugs. In the United States, this agency is the Food and Drug Administration (FDA). If the clinical studies indicate that the effect a drug has on the desired outcomes of treatment is statistically significantly better than that achieved by a placebo (an inactive substance), the drug is approved for a particular indication or indications. This information is included when labeling the drug and in printed material about the drug. (For more information on clinical trials see Chapter 2)

After a drug is approved, however, it may be legally prescribed for a use that is not indicated on the label (referred to as **off label use**), if the prescriber believes it to be of benefit. Many "off label" uses of drugs are based on the findings of additional research studies that are performed and reported in the professional literature. Case reports published in the literature may also support off-label uses of a drug. Off label uses may become standard pharmacotherapeutic uses of a drug. The official drug label is modified only if the drug company goes back to the FDA with additional information and requests that a new pharmacotherapeutic indication be added. After an official review, the FDA may decide to alter the drug label. Because this process can be lengthy and expensive for the drug company, the company may not seek relabeling, even if the drug is commonly used in practice in this way. Nurses should not be overly concerned about off-label uses as long as the literature supports such use or the prescriber can explain why this drug is being used for a patient who does not have a condition for which the drug is indicated. Nurses do need to question all orders if the intended pharmacotherapeutics of a drug does not correlate with the patient's reason for receiving drug therapy. Such questions are necessary to help prevent medication errors in which the wrong drug has been prescribed. Nurses are also legally responsible for understanding the pharmacotherapeutics of all drugs that they administer.

PHARMACOKINETICS

Pharmacokinetics is the movement of the drug particles inside the body and the processes that occur during this movement. In general, pharmacokinetics is the effect of the body on the drug. Pharmacokinetics is made up of four phases: absorption, distribution, metabolism, and excretion. **Absorption** is the movement of the drug from the site of administration into the bloodstream. **Distribution** is movement of the drug through the bloodstream, into the tissues, and eventually into the cells. **Metabolism** is the conversion of the drug into another substance or substances. **Excretion** is the removal of the drug, or what the drug became after metabolism, from the body. The effects from metabolism and excretion of the drug together are technically referred to as elimination; however, in practice most clinicians use the term elimination in place of excretion.

Drug molecules move during all phases of pharmacokinetics. To move throughout the body, the drug must cross membranes. Cells in most membranes are very close together, without much space between the cells. The membrane of the cell itself is made up mostly of lipid molecules. Drugs cross cell membranes in one of three ways. First, they can pass between the spaces or channels between the molecules in the membrane. Drug molecules can only cross a cell membrane this way if they are very small. Second, drugs can pass through the membrane with the help of a transport system. This method may or may not require the use of energy. Third, drugs can penetrate the membrane directly. To be able to penetrate the membrane, the drug must be lipophilic (soluble in lipids). Direct penetration is the method used by most drugs to cross the cell membrane.

The chemistry of the drug particles will also affect the movement of particles throughout the body. A drug particle is a molecule formed from different elements; the electrons are shared between the atoms in the molecule. In some drug molecules, although the elements are bound together, the positive charges (protons) and the negative charges (electrons) are grouped away from each other. These charged molecules are termed polar molecules. Although the charge in polar molecules is unevenly distributed (a region of the molecule is negatively charged and another region is positively charged), such molecules have an equal number of positive and negative charges, so that they have no net charge. Polar molecules are hydrophilic (soluble in water), not lipophilic. Therefore, polar drug molecules are not able to penetrate cell membranes. Nonpolar molecules are lipophilic; therefore, nonpolar molecules are able to penetrate cell membranes.

Ions are molecules that carry a net charge (either positive or negative). Very small ions move through the channels on the cell membranes (the spaces between molecules). Other ions do not cross the cell membrane. Some molecules that normally do not carry a charge can be induced to carry a charge, depending on their environment. The process of inducing a molecule to carry a charge is called ionization because ions have a net charge. Acids give up a positive charge in a basic (alkaline) environment. Bases accept a positive charge in an acidic environment. Movement of molecules through a membrane occurs as long as the environment does not cause the molecules to ionize (i.e., become charged molecules). For most molecules, once they have become ionized they cannot pass through the cell membrane. If the environment promotes ionization, movement through the membrane stops. When the pH on either side of a membrane differs, drug molecules tend to move to the side where ionization will occur. Once the molecules become ionized they cannot move back through the membrane. This process is termed ion trapping or pH portioning. Altering the pH on one side of a membrane thus alters the movement of the drug molecules.

Absorption

Several variables affect the completeness and rate of drug absorption. The completeness of absorption is the portion of the drug that is absorbed. Drugs given orally may not be completely absorbed because of other drugs or food that the patient is ingesting. The rate of absorption of a drug depends on the route of administration. The rate of absorption is also affected by the speed at which the drug dissolves, known as the rate of dissolution.

- Drugs that are administered orally generally take the longest to be absorbed because they must be broken down into small particles before they can move into the bloodstream. The presence of other drugs or food may also impair the rate of oral drug absorption.
- Drugs given parenterally are already dissolved and in a liquid form and therefore are absorbed more rapidly than drugs given orally.
- Drugs that are administered subcutaneously or intramuscularly are absorbed into the small capillaries fairly rapidly. Intramuscular absorption is somewhat more rapid than subcutaneous absorption.

- Drugs that are administered intravenously are placed directly into the bloodstream and are not technically absorbed, although some sources refer to intravenous drugs as being instantly absorbed.

Large surface areas increase the rate of absorption. Drugs administered orally are thus absorbed primarily in the small intestine, which has a larger surface area than the stomach, although some absorption occurs in the stomach. Blood flow also affects the rate of absorption—the greater the volume of blood flow, the faster the rate of absorption. Absorption speeds up with increased blood flow because increased flow carries more absorbed drug molecules away into the general circulation; in its place is blood without any particles of drug. Thus, the high concentration of drug moves into the blood where there is a low concentration of drug. Patients who have impaired circulatory systems absorb drugs less rapidly than those with normally functioning systems. Lipid solubility also alters absorption. Drugs that are more lipid soluble usually are absorbed more rapidly than others because they can cross the lipid cell membranes easily. Finally, when pH differences between the site of administration and the plasma favor the drug molecules becoming ionized in the plasma, absorption is more rapid than when the molecules do not become ionized.

Finally, the physiologic condition of the patient affects drug absorption. Core patient variables that affect drug absorption are summarized in Box 4.1.

Distribution

The distribution of a drug throughout the body depends on three factors: blood flow to the tissues, the drug's ability to leave the blood, and the drug's ability to enter cells.

Once a drug is absorbed, it is transported to the tissues and cells through the circulatory system. In healthy individuals, all tissues are well perfused; thus, drug molecules can easily be distributed throughout the body. However, pathophysiologic changes in the vascular system (such as narrowed, stiff, or occluded vessels) impair the distribution of drug molecules. This impairment may or may not affect distribution enough to decrease the therapeutic effect of the drug. For example, in a patient with peripheral vascular disease, circulation to the heart is not usually greatly impaired, although circulation to the legs and feet is. In this patient, a drug given for an altered cardiac rhythm may not be distributed well into the tissues in the legs, but plenty of drug molecules reach the heart, so that the drug is capable of achieving the desired pharmacotherapeutic effect. However, a drug given to treat cellulitis of the foot may not have adequate distribution to achieve the desired pharmacotherapeutic effect because of the impaired circulation in the lower extremities.

Some tissues have little or no blood supply. Scar tissue is avascular, and adipose (fat) tissue has a poor blood supply. Two types of pathologic conditions—abscesses (pus-filled pockets surrounded by normal tissue) and solid tumors—have very limited blood supply, especially to their centers. Because drug therapy does not distribute well to these areas,

Box 4.1 **DRUG ABSORPTION AND CORE PATIENT VARIABLES**

Health Status

- Any change in health status related to circulation, condition of the GI tract, or pH of body fluids (e.g., disease, trauma, strenuous physical exercise, or drug therapy) can reduce drug absorption. The condition of the gastric and intestinal surfaces affects oral drug absorption.
- Contact time, surface area of contact, and the condition of the absorptive surface may increase or decrease the amount of drug absorbed. For example:
  - Large surfaces (e.g., pulmonary alveolar epithelium, intestinal mucosa) absorb drugs rapidly.
  - Decreased absorptive surface from damage (e.g., radiation), disease (e.g., inflammatory bowel disease), or surgery (e.g., surgically shortened intestine) lessens drug absorption.
- Absorption from the GI tract depends on factors such as gastric volume, GI pH, gastric emptying time, intestinal transit rate, gastric motility, and GI enzyme levels.
  - Delayed transport from the stomach to the intestine (e.g., food in the stomach) will dilute the drug and increase the contact time by slowing gastric emptying.
  - Decreased GI motility (e.g., constipation) permits increased drug contact time with the GI mucosa, enhances drug dissolution, and allows extra time for absorption, which may lead to increased drug effects and toxicity.
  - Increased intestinal motility (e.g., diarrhea), will move a drug very quickly through the GI tract, reducing the amount of time the drug remains in contact with the GI mucosa and impairing drug absorption.
- The quality of blood flow to the site of absorption affects how much of the drug is absorbed.
  - Increased blood flow (e.g., application of heat or massage) enhances intramuscular and subcutaneous drug absorption because of the resulting increase in circulation.
  - Absorption slows when blood flow decreases (e.g., shock or vasoconstriction).
  - Some muscles normally have greater blood supply; for example, a drug injected into the deltoid muscle will be absorbed faster than one injected into the gluteus muscle because of the greater blood flow to the deltoid muscle.

Life Span and Gender

- Ingested solids versus liquids empty more slowly from women's stomachs.
- Gastric acidity is lower in women.
- Women have lower gastric levels of alcohol dehydrogenase.

Lifestyle, Diet, and Habits

- Diet may stimulate digestive enzymes and alter the gastric and intestinal mucosa.
- Generally, drugs ingested with food are absorbed slower than drugs taken on an empty stomach.
- Some drugs and food form complexes that cannot pass through the mucosal lining of the GI tract (e.g., tetracycline antimicrobials that bind with calcium, magnesium, iron, aluminum), and thus effective blood levels may not be reached.
- Some drugs are destroyed by the high acidity and peptic activity of gastric digestive enzymes.

it is difficult to treat problems that may develop (such as infections in the adipose tissue) or the pathology itself (i.e., the abscess or tumor) by drug therapy alone.

Once the drug has moved through the blood to the tissues, it must leave the bloodstream to enter the tissue itself. This transition is necessary because most drugs do not produce their effect while in the blood. The drug leaves the vascular space in the capillary bed. Because the cells of the capillary walls have fairly wide spaces between them, the drug molecules simply move between the cells to leave the capillaries and enter the tissues.

Protein Binding

Protein binding of drugs affects their distribution and is an important concept to understand. Drug particles form reversible bonds with proteins in the blood, most specifically albumin. Because albumin is a large molecule, it cannot pass through capillary walls. Therefore, when the drug particle is attached to the albumin, the drug is prevented from passing through the capillary walls. Different drugs have different affinities, or attractions, to protein molecules. Some drugs are so attracted to protein that almost all of the drug will bind with protein if the protein is available. These drugs are classified as highly protein bound. Other drugs have so little attraction that hardly any of the drug will bind with the available protein. Only drug molecules that are unattached to protein are capable of moving to their site of action (distribution) and achieving the desired therapeutic effect.

Another way of saying this is that only the free drug is active. Consider two drugs, A and B. Drug A is 95% protein bound; Drug B is 25% protein bound. This means that for every 100 molecules of Drug A, 95 molecules will be bound

Variation in Protein Binding

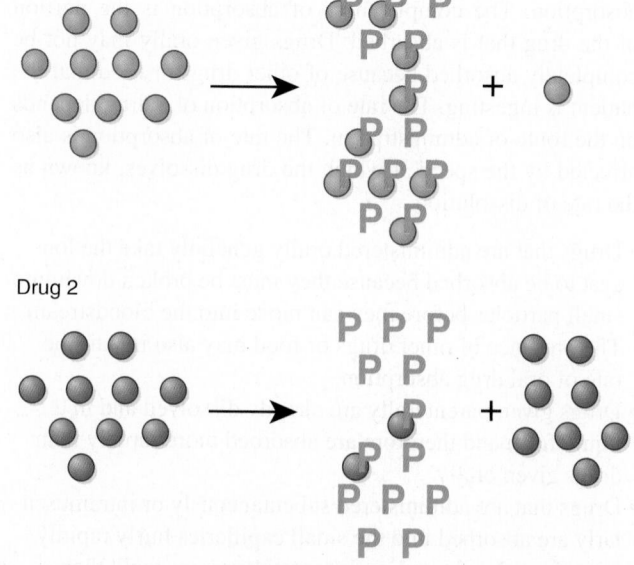

• FIGURE 4.1 Drug 1 (•) is highly protein (P) bound. Little of the drug is free and active. Drug 2 (•) has low protein binding. A great deal of the drug is free and active.

Effect of Protein Levels on Drug Binding

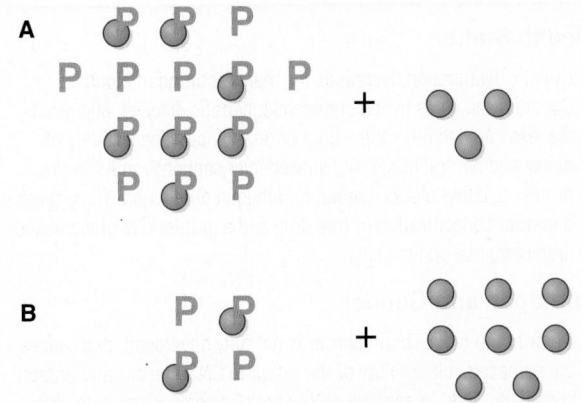

• FIGURE 4.2 **(A)** High protein binding (P) of a drug allows only a few drug molecules to be free and active. **(B)** When serum protein levels are below normal, the drug molecules have nowhere to bind. The number of drug molecules that are free is thus greater than would be normally expected. More therapeutic effects and adverse effects are likely to occur.

with protein, and 5 molecules will be free and active. For every 100 molecules of Drug B, however, 25 will be bound to protein, and 75 will be free and active. Drug A may therefore require a larger dose than Drug B to achieve the same therapeutic effect, because not as many of the molecules from each dose can distribute through the body and be active (Figure 4.1).

Protein binding can be compared with ninth-grade students at a school dance. If most of the students are interested in dancing, only a few of them are free to do as they please and to move about (and potentially cause trouble). If, however, most of the students are not that interested in dancing, then many

are free to do as they please. The odds are increased that what they choose to do may be seen as troublesome to the teachers.

The bonds between the drug and protein molecules are not permanent. The bonds will dissolve in time, and the drug molecules will become free and active. Other drug molecules may then form a bond with the protein molecule. The length of time the drug is bound varies, based on properties of the drug. In keeping with our analogy of a dance, students may dance with each other for quite some time, or for only one song. They then separate and choose new partners, or they may remain free.

Drug dosages are calculated by the drug manufacturer based on the protein-binding characteristics of the drug. When the recommended dose is determined by the manufacturer, it is based on normal protein levels being available in the blood. When the patient has a lower-than-expected protein level (e.g., as a result of malnutrition, liver failure, or severe burns), the distribution of the drug is altered. Even if the drug normally has a high affinity for protein (i.e., it is highly protein bound), if protein is lacking, not as much drug can be bound. Less drug is bound because there is no place for the drug molecule to go. When less drug is bound, more drug is free and can be distributed to its site of action, thereby causing increased therapeutic, and possibly increased adverse, effects (Figure 4.2).

Because different drugs have different affinities for albumin, the administration of more than one drug simultaneously may also alter protein binding and consequently affect distribution of both drugs. For example, a particular drug is being administered. Part of that drug is bound to protein. Now, a second drug is also given, and it has a higher attraction to albumin than the first drug has. The second drug will bump or displace the first drug in order to bind with the protein (Figure 4.3).

• FIGURE 4.3 Consequence of drug displacement from albumin and other plasma proteins. Some drugs (e.g., "Drug 1") are greater than 90% bound to plasma proteins. The "free" (unbound) drug molecules, but not the bound molecules, are available to act at receptors. "Drug 2" displaces only five molecules of Drug 1, which more than triples the serum concentration of free (active) Drug 1. This increase could be fatal if Drug 1 has a narrow margin of safety. Displacement of drugs that are less highly protein bound is less significant. For example, if Drug 1 were 50% bound and 50% free, displacement of 10% of the bound fraction would increase the free fraction from 50% to 55%. This small increment is unlikely to be clinically relevant.

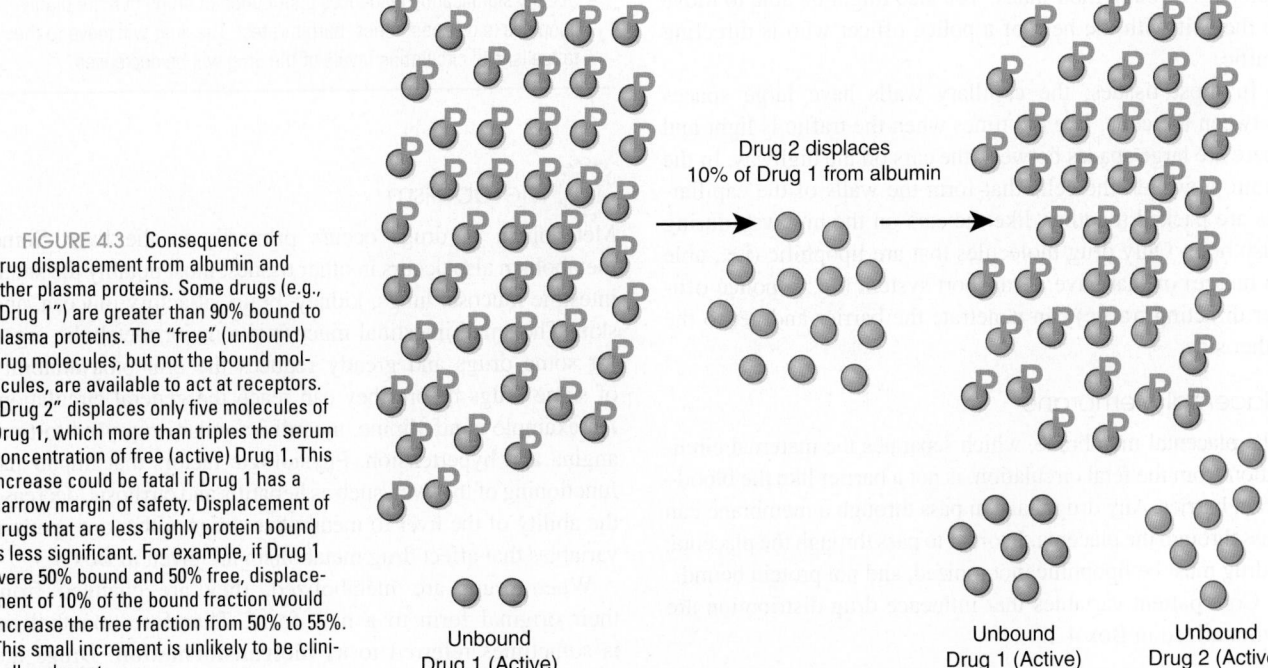

Protein Bound
Drug 1 (Inactive)

Protein Bound
Drugs 1 and 2 (Inactive)

Drug 2 displaces
10% of Drug 1 from albumin

Unbound
Drug 1 (Active)

Unbound
Drug 1 (Active)

Unbound
Drug 2 (Active)

Displacement means that more of the first drug is free and active and will be distributed (compared to the distribution that occurred when the first drug was the only drug being administered). The dosage of the first drug may have to be decreased to prevent excessive therapeutic or adverse effects as long as the second drug is simultaneously prescribed.

In summary, protein binding plays an important role in distribution of active drug molecules. Changes in the expected protein-binding capabilities of a drug, either from pharmaceutical properties of other drugs or from patient-related variables, alter the effectiveness of drug therapy.

Blood–Brain Barrier

The capillary bed that services the brain is different from other capillary beds and affects distribution of a drug to the brain. Instead of wide spaces between the cells in the capillary walls, the cells are packed tightly together. This structure prevents drug molecules, and other foreign substances, from passing through and entering the brain. This system is called the **blood–brain barrier.** The purpose of the blood–brain barrier is to keep toxins and poisons from reaching the brain. This protective mechanism normally promotes health, but occasionally it prevents treatment of problems. For example, many antibiotics cannot cross the blood–brain barrier, making treatment of life-threatening infections of the brain, such as bacterial meningitis, difficult.

The way the blood–brain barrier works can be likened to a driver trying to exit a highway during rush hour. Imagine that you are driving in the far left lane of a three-lane highway. To exit the highway at one of the exit ramps, you must cross two lanes of traffic. If the traffic is light and there are great distances between the cars, exiting the highway can be accomplished easily. However, if the traffic is heavy and bumper to bumper, it is almost impossible to cross the other lanes to exit. In order to exit, you need to convince other drivers to let you pass through their lanes. You also might be able to move to the exit with the help of a police officer who is directing traffic.

In most tissues, the capillary walls have large spaces between the cells, like the times when the traffic is light and there are large spaces between the cars on the highway. In the brain, however, the cells that form the walls of the capillaries are packed together, like the cars on the highway during rush hour. Only drug molecules that are lipophilic (i.e., able to merge) or that have a transport system (i.e., a police officer directing traffic) can penetrate the barrier and get to the other side.

Placental Membrane

The placental membrane, which separates the maternal circulation from the fetal circulation, is not a barrier like the blood–brain barrier. Any drug that can pass through a membrane can pass through the placenta. In order to pass through the placenta, a drug must be lipophilic, not ionized, and not protein bound.

Core patient variables that influence drug distribution are summarized in Box 4.2.

 ## Metabolism

Metabolism of drugs occurs primarily in the liver. Some metabolism also occurs in other tissues, most notably the small intestine mucosa, lungs, kidney, brain, olfactory mucosa, and skin. The small intestinal mucosa is a major metabolic organ for some drugs and greatly reduces the oral bioavailability of some drugs before they can reach the general circulation. An example is nifedipine, a cardiovascular drug used to treat angina and hypertension. Physiologic factors that impair the functioning of the liver, such as hepatitis and cirrhosis, decrease the ability of the liver to metabolize drugs. Other core patient variables that affect drug metabolism are given in Box 4.3.

When drugs are metabolized, they are changed from their original form to a new form. Therefore, metabolism is sometimes referred to as **biotransformation**. Drugs are

Box 4.3 DRUG METABOLISM AND CORE PATIENT VARIABLES

Life Span and Gender

- Drug metabolism in patients whose enzymatic metabolic systems are either immature or functioning less efficiently (e.g., neonates, children, and older adults) is highly variable but is usually diminished. Decreased drug metabolism places the patient at increased risk of adverse effects from the drug.

Lifestyle, Diet, and Habits

- Malnutrition may prolong drug effects as a result of poor hepatic microsomal metabolism.
- In obese people, phase II transformations tend to occur more rapidly, thereby necessitating higher drug dosages.
- Drug effects may be intensified if the specific drug places the person at nutritional risk by producing anorexia, increased appetite, nausea and vomiting, nutritional deficiencies, stomatitis, or toxic reactions, for example.
- Diet may contribute to individual variations in drug metabolism. Charcoal-broiled foods and cruciferous vegetables induce one CYP isoenzyme, whereas grapefruit juice inhibits one.
- Exposure to cigarette smoke and pesticides may cause a more rapid metabolism of some drugs because of enzyme induction.

Environment

- Reduced partial pressure of oxygen at higher altitudes may affect enzymatic reduction systems.
- Environmental pollutants may affect induction or inhibition of hepatic enzymes.
- Light is a key modulator in the regulation of metabolic pathways and in specific settings may affect drug response (e.g., intensive care units that commonly remain constantly lit).

generally metabolized from substances that are lipophilic into substances that are hydrophilic. The ability of a drug to become soluble in water is important because it allows the drug to be excreted through the renal system.

Metabolites

A product of metabolism is called a **metabolite**. *Drugs that are metabolized are generally changed into an inactive form*, having no effect on the body as they travel throughout the body waiting to be excreted. *Occasionally, a drug is metabolized into an active metabolite*. This active substance can achieve an independent effect on the body, which can be either therapeutic or adverse. For example, after metabolism, codeine is changed to morphine, which is a stronger analgesic than codeine. So the active metabolite of codeine provides additional pain relief to the patient. Metabolism can convert a drug that has little or no therapeutic effect in its original form into the active, helpful form. Drugs that are inactive until metabolized into an active form are called **prodrugs.** An example of a prodrug is primidone, used to control seizures. Primidone's primary anticonvulsant effect comes from the drug being metabolized into phenobarbital and PEMA, both strong anticonvulsants. Finally, an active metabolite may cause a different and potentially harmful effect from that of the original drug. An example of a drug with a harmful metabolite is meperidine, an analgesic, whose active metabolite is neurotoxic and without pain-relieving properties.

Rates of Metabolism and the First-Pass Effect

Metabolism occurs at different rates for different drugs. Some drugs are highly metabolized, meaning that every time drug molecules are circulated to the liver (about 25% of the cardiac output is sent to the liver), a large percentage of the drug molecules is metabolized. Other drugs are metabolized at slower rates, and a smaller percentage is metabolized each time the drug molecules circulate through the liver. Keep in mind that the percentage of drug that is metabolized each time the drug circulates, or passes, through the liver is the same, but the total number of drug molecules that are metabolized will be different (Table 4.1). The percentage of the drug that is metabolized with each pass through the liver is

TABLE 4.1 Effect of the Liver on Drug Metabolism

Number of Drug Molecules Throughout the Body (Other Than Liver)	Number of Drug Molecules Sent to the Liver	Number of Passes Through the Liver	Number of Drug Molecules Metabolized in Liver	Percentage of Drug Metabolized	Number of Drug Molecules Leaving Liver After Metabolism	Total Number of Drug Molecules (Molecules Leaving Liver plus Molecules in General Circulation)
—	100	First	25	25%	75	75
56.25	18.75	Second	4.68	25%	14.07	70.32
52.74	17.58	Third	4.40	25%	13.18	65.92
49.44	16.48	Fourth	4.12	25%	12.36	61.80
46.35	15.45	Fifth	3.86	25%	11.59	57.94

For this hypothetical drug given orally, 25% of the drug is metabolized every time the drug circulates to the liver for metabolism. Note that the percentage of drug metabolized stays the same each time but the total number of drug molecules metabolized varies. Why is there less drug returning to the liver than was left after the previous pass and metabolism? This is because only about 25% of any given cardiac output will be sent to the liver; the rest of the drug is sent elsewhere in the body from the heart. Note that the most extensive metabolism occurs with the first pass of the drug through the liver.

an inherent trait of the drug itself. Highly metabolized drugs may lose their therapeutic effectiveness quickly, especially drugs that are administered orally. After an oral drug is broken down and absorbed into the circulatory system, the first place the blood travels is to the liver, through the portal vein. Thus, drugs that are highly metabolized lose much of their effectiveness during this first pass through the liver, before they reach general circulation. This loss of effectiveness is called the **first-pass effect.** Drugs that experience a high first-pass effect may need higher oral doses to achieve a therapeutic level of circulating drug. To avoid the first-pass effect or the need for high oral doses of a drug, drugs that are highly metabolized are often given by another route that bypasses the liver initially. For example, the drug may be given intravenously. None of the drug given intravenously will initially go to the liver; all of it will return to the heart. From the heart, slightly more than 25% of the drug will be sent to the liver, where a percentage of it is metabolized.

P-450 System

Metabolism is predominantly achieved by specific microsomal enzymes called the cytochrome P-450 system, or, more commonly, the **P-450 system.** This system is a combination of several types of cytochromes, called families. Of these, only three families—CYP1, CYP2, and CYP3—are involved in drug metabolism. The other enzymes in the P-450 group metabolize naturally occurring substances, such as fatty acids. Scientists have been able to identify specific members of each cytochrome family. These members are identified by a number representing "family" a letter (representing the subgroup) and another number (representing the specific isoenzyme) (e.g., CYP1A2). Most of the P-450 system is located in the liver and this is the primary site of drug metabolism. Isoenzymes can also be found in other organs, however, such as those in the small intestine mucosa, and are responsible for the metabolism that occurs in these locations.

The total number of isoenzymes present in the body is not divided equally between the three families. The enzyme subgroup CYP3A is the most common in both the liver and in the small intestine and is responsible for the metabolism of most drugs; the next most prevalent subgroup in both sites is CYP2C (Paine et al., 2006) (Figure 4-4).

Some drugs either induce or inhibit the P-450 system, altering metabolism of other drugs (see Appendix G online). Usually, just one P-450 family is affected. Drugs that induce a hepatic enzyme increase the amount of that enzyme present in the liver. Induction is accomplished most frequently by stimulating enzyme synthesis. When a large quantity of one of these enzymes is present, more metabolism can occur through this pathway. Drugs that are metabolized by this pathway (also referred to as substrates of the enzyme) will therefore be metabolized more rapidly than drugs that are not. This increase in metabolism rapidly decreases the amount of circulating, active drug. Some drugs can induce the enzymes necessary for their own metabolism and thus can increase the rate of their own metabolism. Drugs that

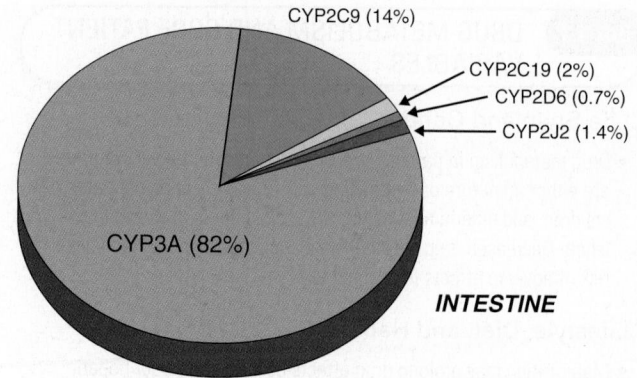

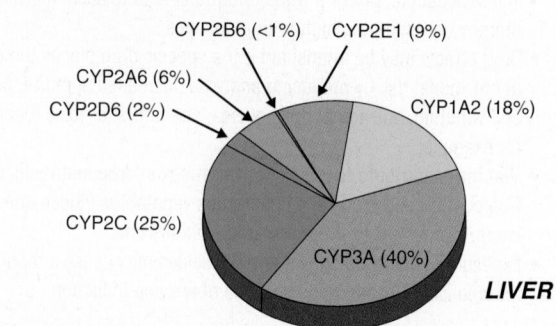

• FIGURE 4.4 Prevalence of P-450 isoenzymes in the small intestine compared to the liver. From Paine, M. et al. (2006). The humanintestinal Cytochrome P450 "pie." *Drug Metabolism and Disposition,* 34(5):880–886. Dr Paine cites that the values for the liver pie were derived from Shimada et al. (1994). Interindividual variations in human liver cytochrome P-450 enzymes involved in the oxidation of drugs, carcinogens and toxic chemicals: studies with liver microsomes of 30 Japanese and 30 Caucasians. *Journal of Pharmacology and Experimental Therapeutics,* 270:414–423.

inhibit a particular hepatic enzyme slow the metabolism that occurs through this pathway, causing an increase in the amount of circulating, active drug. Metabolism returns to normal after the inducing or inhibiting drug is no longer administered, although it may take several days after an inducer is discontinued.

When two or more drugs are metabolized by the same hepatic enzymatic pathway, the drugs compete with each other for action from the enzyme. This competition results in at least one of the drugs having its metabolism impaired. To understand this concept entirely, consider the analogy of using the Internet through a dial-up connection. When there are few customers online, getting connected and using the online services is easy. However, when demand is very high, it may be difficult to get connected at all, and once connected, you may be abruptly disconnected, losing your ability to use the online services. Similarly, when the demand is high for the services of a particular hepatic enzyme, not every drug will receive attention immediately.

Drugs that affect the P-450 system are responsible for many drug interactions, as discussed in more detail in Chapter 5.

A number of patient related variables influence the presence and activity of the P-450 system. Genetic variations of the specific isoenzymes account for differences in rate of metabolism and drug clearance in some individuals receiving drug therapy. Multiple genes regulate the activity of P-450 enzymes. The isoenzyme CYP2D6, while it accounts for only 2% to 5% of all hepatic P-450 isoenzymes, is very important to consider because it metabolizes about one fourth of all clinically used medications (Harvard Mental Health Letter, 2009). Genetic polymorphisms (variations) of this isoenzyme result in people being poor metabolizers, intermediate metabolizers, extensive metabolizers, or ultrarapid metabolizers of drugs. The majority of the population are extensive metabolizers via this isoenzyme, so this is considered the norm. About 5% to 10% of American whites are poor metabolizers via this enzyme; about 1% to 10% are ultrarapid metabolizers (Mulder et al., 2007; Bernard et al., 2006). In comparison, between 2% and 7% of African Americans are poor metabolizers, and about 5% are ultrarapid metabolizers. Asian populations have an extremely low incidence (1% or less) of the genetic variations that create poor metabolizers or ultrarapid metabolizers (Data on Asian Americans is not specifically available.) (Bernard et al., 2006). Patients who are poor metabolizers of a particular drug will have higher circulating levels of that drug than would be normally anticipated. These higher levels can produce additional therapeutic as well as adverse effects. Patients who are ultrarapid metabolizers of a drug will have lower circulating levels of the drug than would be normally anticipated and may not achieve the desired therapeutic response from a dose; larger doses may be warranted.

The presence and activity of different isoenzymes, varies by the sex of the patient. For example there is more CYP 3A4 in the liver of women than in men, but this difference does not seem apparent in the GI system (Paine et al., 2005). Women are known to have more active 3A4, 2A6, and 2B6, less active 1A2,2E1 and no difference in activity with 2C9 and 2D6 (Anderson, 2008), although these differences may or may not be clinically significant. Some research indicates that sex alone does not contribute substantially to the large variation of metabolism via P-450 that is seen between individuals. (He et al., 2006). More research is needed to confirm the exact interaction between sex, P-450 variations, and drug metabolism.

Some foods and herbs may also interact with the P450 system. Grapefruit and its juice is well known to decrease the amount of the P-450 isoform 3A that is available in the intestines, but not in the liver. Consequently it decreases the metabolism of drugs that rely on that enzyme system for metabolism and raises circulating levels of that drug. St John's Wort, an herb used to treat depression, has the opposite effect from grapefruit. See Chapter 5 for more discussion of drug interactions via the P-450 system. While most of the research has been done on the effect of a food or herb on drug effectiveness, it should be remembered that P-450 reactions may go both ways, and that a drug may decrease the therapeutic effects that may occur naturally from some herbs or foods (Yarnell & Abascal, 2007).

It has been postulated that inflammation may alter the presence of some P-450 isoenzymes. One study of children with inflammatory bowel disease (Crohn's disease) found that they had significantly higher levels of CYP 3A4 and CYP3A5 than children without Crohn's disease. These variations may explain why medication given to treat Crohn's doesn't always achieve a therapeutic response (Fakhoury et al., 2006)

Decreased internal temperature of a patient may alter the action of the P-450 during metabolism. A review of the literature by Tortorici et al. (2007) found that

> …mild to moderate hypothermia decreases the systemic clearance of cytochrome P-450 metabolized drugs between 7% and 22% per degree Celsius below 37°C during cooling. The addition of hypothermia decreases the potency and efficacy of certain drugs… [there is] evidence that the therapeutic index of drugs is narrowed during hypothermia.

As hypothermia is sometimes intentionally induced in patients who have cardiac arrest out of the hospital, these patients should be screened carefully for drug adverse effects once they are in the hospital.

 Excretion

Excretion is the process of removing a drug, or its metabolites, from the body. The most common route for drug excretion is through the urine. Other routes include bile in the GI tract, expired air from the lungs, breast milk, sweat from the skin, and saliva. Sweat and saliva are not therapeutically important routes of excretion, however.

Diseases and pathophysiologic changes in the kidney, such as renal failure, decrease the effectiveness of the kidney in drug excretion. Other patient variables that affect drug excretion are discussed in Box 4.4.

Processes Involved in Renal Excretion

Three processes are involved in renal excretion of drugs. The first is glomerular filtration. Drugs come to the kidney

---

 Box 4.4 DRUG EXCRETION AND CORE PATIENT VARIABLES

Health Status

- Renal impairment or renal failure decreases a drug's elimination from the body. If renal excretion is an important route of its elimination and the drug is given on a regular dosing schedule, its slowed removal from the body will produce a greater accumulation of drug in the body with an increased likelihood of additional therapeutic and adverse effects.
- If cardiac output is decreased, the kidney may not be perfused adequately, decreasing the glomerular filtration rate as well as excretion of drugs.
- Hepatic compromise or dysfunction will also decrease the elimination of drugs.
- Drug therapy may produce nephrotoxicity as an adverse effect. Therefore, the renal elimination of all other drugs may be decreased.

Life Span and Gender

- In elderly patients, the rate of drug clearance is reduced.
- Some drugs have different rates of clearance depending on the sex of the patient.

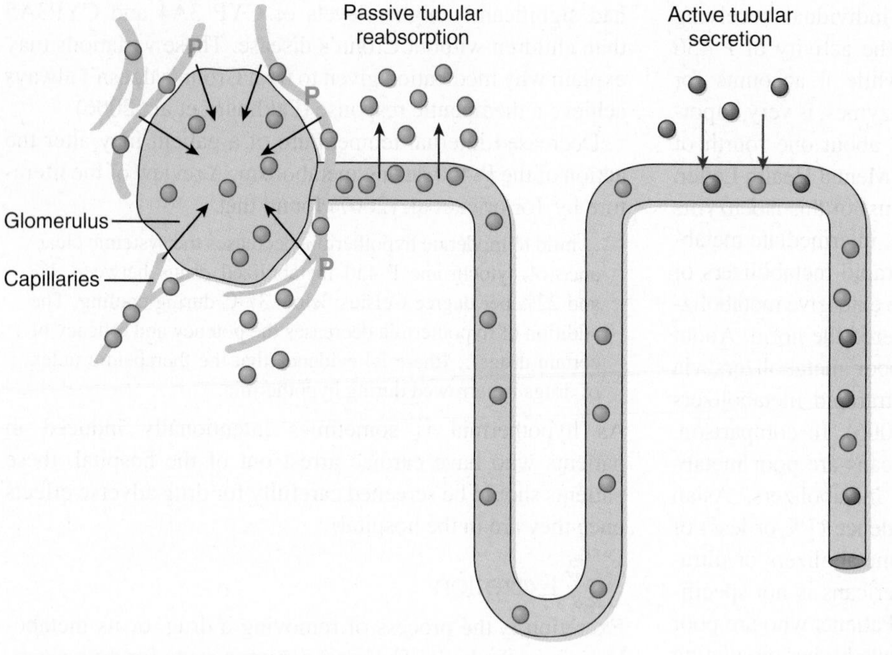

Passive tubular
reabsorption

Active tubular
secretion

Glomerulus

Capillaries

• FIGURE 4.5 Renal excretion of drugs.
Most drugs pass easily through the capillary
walls and enter the tubules of the nephrons.
Large molecules, such as proteins, cannot pass.
Because of concentration gradients, some drug
molecules will passively move back into the
circulatory system (passive tubular reabsorption). Some drugs are actively moved into the
tubule to be excreted.

through the capillaries surrounding Bowman's capsule. This
capillary network is the glomerulus. Most drug particles pass
easily through the spaces of the capillary walls into the urine
in the proximal tubule. Only very large particles, such as
proteins, cannot pass. Drug molecules bound to protein will
therefore also not be filtered.

The second process is passive tubular reabsorption. Because
a concentration gradient now exists, with more drug particles
in the urinary tubule than in the bloodstream, the drug particles will try to move from the area of greater concentration
to that of lesser concentration. Remember that for a drug to
move through a membrane, it must be lipophilic. Therefore,
for a drug to be able to move through the membranes
separating the tubular and vascular structures, it must still be
lipophilic. If it has been changed by metabolism into a form
that is not lipid soluble (meaning that it is now an ion or a
polar compound), passive tubular reabsorption cannot occur.
Instead, the drug remains in the urine and is excreted.

The third process that affects excretion is active tubular secretion. Active transport systems in the renal tubule
work to move some drugs from the blood and into the urine
(Figure 4.5). There is one active transport system for organic
acids and one for organic bases.

Factors That Affect Renal Excretion

Because ions cannot be passively reabsorbed from the tubule,
drug excretion can be increased if the pH of the urine encourages the drug to become an ion. Remember that acids will
ionize in basic environments and bases will ionize in acidic
environments. Therefore, if another drug or some other agent
is introduced that makes the urine more basic, acidic drugs
will be ionized and not reabsorbed. Drug overdosage or
ingestion of a poison is often treated in this way to promote
excretion of the drug before it can harm the patient.

Overuse of the active transport system also affects excretion.
Two drugs that rely on the active transport system for excretion
will compete with each other for places on the transport system. As the transport system becomes overloaded, some of the
drug particles will remain in the blood until they can be moved
by the transport system. This residual portion will increase
the circulating time of active drug in the body and slow the
excretion of both drugs. This process is much like people waiting to ride a shuttle from the parking lot to a building. The
shuttle bus has a limited number of seats and can travel only
so fast between the two points. During the times when crowds
are infrequent, everyone can find a seat on the shuttle without
waiting. However, during rush hour, when crowds are large,
not everyone can find a seat on the shuttle immediately. Some
people will have to wait for their transportation to the building.

Two drugs can be given together to deliberately slow the
rate of excretion of one or both of the drugs. A common
example of this approach is giving probenecid, a drug used
to treat gout, along with a penicillin or cephalosporin, antibiotics that are used to treat infections. In this situation, the
probenecid is used not for its normal pharmacotherapeutic
effect but solely to slow the rate of active transport and excretion of the antibiotic. This means that the antibiotic remains
in the blood and can continue to be active for a longer time
than when given without the probenecid.

Factors That Affect Biliary Excretion

A factor that affects excretion of drugs through bile is enterohepatic recirculation. Some of the bile that leaves the liver
and enters the intestine is reabsorbed back into the portal circulation and returned to the general circulation. Drug molecules that are in the bile are also reabsorbed. This process
lengthens the time the drug is present in the bloodstream and
can produce an effect.

Other Pharmacokinetic Concepts

Half-Life

The combined processes of metabolism and excretion are responsible for elimination of a drug from the body. The amount of time that is required to remove half (50%) of the blood concentration of a drug is called **half-life**. Drugs have various half-lives, based on their pharmacologic properties and rate of metabolism and excretion. Some drugs have half-lives measured in minutes; others have half-lives measured in days. It is important to understand that in one half-life, a set percentage of the drug molecules present in the blood will be eliminated, not an absolute set number of drug molecules. For example, if 1,000 drug molecules are present in the blood, 500 drug molecules will be left after one half-life. If there are 500 molecules, 250 will be left after one half-life. If there are only 10 drug molecules, 5 molecules will be left after one half-life. Each half-life removes 50% of the drug stored in the body; the number of molecules varies depending on the total load of drug in the body. If the rate of metabolism and excretion of a drug is slower than normal in an individual (for example if a patient has liver or renal failure) then the time to achieve a half life may be lengthened.

Steady State

There is a point at which the amount of drug being administered and the amount being eliminated balance off. Essentially, this balance means that what comes in equals what goes out. This balance creates a stable level of the drug in the blood called **steady state.** Technically, a 100% steady state cannot be achieved if a particular drug is given more than one time. However, the balance is almost even between the drug amount administered and that eliminated. At five half-lives, 97% of steady state will be achieved; therefore, steady state has been traditionally defined as five half-lives. However, most of steady state (94%) is achieved in four half-lives. In terms of clinical response from a given drug level, a drug at 94% of steady state will not achieve substantially less therapeutic effect than a drug at 97% of steady state. Because of this similarity in clinical response, it is now frequently stated that it takes four to five half-lives for steady state to be achieved.

When a particular dosage of one drug (i.e., a dose) is given at set repeated intervals (i.e., dosing intervals), it takes between four and five half-lives of the drug for the dose to equal the elimination rate of the drug. Imagine that the half-life of Drug A is 1 day and that 10 mg of Drug A is administered daily. On the second day, after one half-life, 5 mg of the drug is eliminated. An additional 10 mg dose is taken, raising the total amount of the drug in the body to 15 mg (50% × 10 = 5; 5 + 10 = 15). The next day (after two half-lives), 7.5 mg of drug remains in the body. When that day's dose is administered, the total amount of drug in the body becomes 17.5 mg. The following day (after three half-lives), the body has 8.75 mg left. When the daily dose is given, the total amount in the body becomes 18.75 mg. The next day, four half-lives will have taken effect, leaving 9.375 mg of the drug in the body, which is 94% of the daily dose of 10 mg. Another dose is administered, bringing the amount to 19.375 mg. On the fifth day (after five half-lives), 9.6875 mg of the drug remains, which is 97% of the 10-mg daily dose. Thus, somewhere between four and five half-lives, the daily dosage is essentially the same as the amount left in the bloodstream after elimination (in = out) (Figure 4.6).

Although a larger amount (dose) of a given drug elevates the drug level found in the blood after steady state is achieved, increasing the dose has no effect on how *quickly* steady state can be achieved. Achievement of steady state is not based on drug dose. Steady state is achieved based on the amount of *time* required for four to five half-lives to occur,

Answers for Critical Thinking Scenarios are found on the website: http://thepoint.lww.com/Aschenbrenner4e

CRITICAL THINKING SCENARIO

HALF-LIFE AND DRUG DOSING

Gayle Herbert is 80 years old and has a history of renal insufficiency and chronic heart failure. She is receiving digoxin, a drug that strengthens the force of the heart's contraction, for chronic heart failure. Digoxin undergoes almost no metabolism but is primarily eliminated by renal excretion. The dose of the digoxin is to be increased, starting today. The half-life of digoxin is 30 to 40 hours.

1. If the new dose of digoxin were given orally once a day, how long would it take for the drug to reach steady state? Will Ms. Herbert's renal insufficiency affect the time to reach steady state?
2. Ms. Hawkins is also 80 years old and receives digoxin, but she does not have renal insufficiency. Would you expect Ms. Herbert's dose to be the same, less than, or greater than Ms. Hawkins' dose of digoxin? Why?

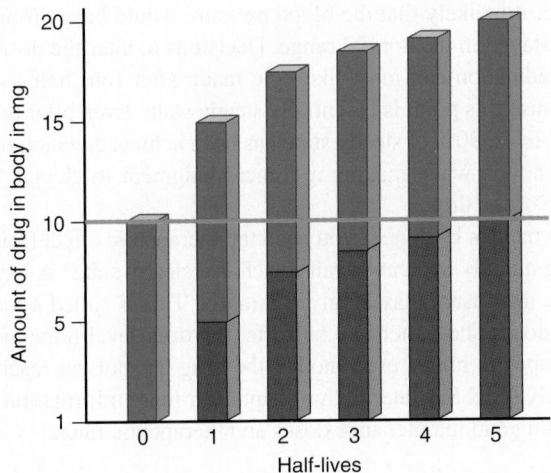

• FIGURE 4.6 With each half-life, 50% of the drug in the body is eliminated. Note that steady state (in = out) is achieved in four to five half-lives.

and half-life is related to the rate of elimination of the drug, which is an inherent property of the drug. Similarly, increasing the frequency of drug administration (i.e., dosing) *does not affect how quickly* the drug achieves steady state. Steady state is still achieved in the same amount of time: four to five half-lives. The full pharmacotherapeutic response of a particular drug dose is measured when the drug has achieved steady state. Every time the dose is adjusted, it takes between four and five half-lives before the drug achieves steady state for that dose and for the full therapeutic effect to be assessed. This fact is important to remember when dose adjustments (up or down) are being considered in order to achieve a desired therapeutic effect. If the dose is modified before steady state is achieved, it is difficult to predict exactly what blood level will be achieved and, in turn, what therapeutic effect will be achieved from a drug dose. The result may be a blood level that is too low to be therapeutic or one that is too high, leading to adverse effects.

Consider, for example, giving captopril to treat a hypertensive episode. The half-life of captopril is about 2 hours. This half-life means that in 10 hours, half of the drug administered will have been eliminated and the full effect of the initial dose of captopril will be evident. Let's say, however, that 4 hours after the drug is administered, the patient's blood pressure remains somewhat elevated. Two half-lives have occurred in this time. The physician orders a larger dose of captopril to be administered now. Twenty-five percent of the first dose remains in the patient's body after two half-lives. This residual drug is added to the new, larger dose. Later, the patient is found to be hypotensive, from too much effect of the medicine. In this particular case, not enough of the first dose had been eliminated before a second, but larger, dose was given. The combination created too high a blood level of the captopril. The drug did what it was intended to do: it lowered the blood pressure. But it lowered it too much. Had the dose been the same during the second administration of the drug, it is likely that the blood pressure would have dropped but stayed in the normal range. Decisions to alter the dose of a medication can most likely be made after four half-lives, because this point is essentially steady state. Even after three half-lives, 90% of steady state has been achieved, which may be enough when making a clinical judgment to change the dose of the drug.

What can be done if you need the therapeutic effect from a drug quickly and can't wait to achieve steady state? A larger dose than usual may be given initially. This is called a loading dose. Then after one half life, the drug level remains in therapeutic range, even though the drug has not yet reached steady state. See later in this chapter for more information on loading and maintenance doses and therapeutic range.

Clearance

Several pharmacokinetic factors work together to affect the rate at which drug molecules disappear from the circulatory system. This rate is called **clearance** or clearance rate of a drug. Renal excretion and hepatic metabolism are the major modes of clearance. Some drugs are primarily cleared by one mechanism rather than the other. For other drugs, the two mechanisms are both actively involved in clearance.

The gender of the patient can also alter the clearance of some drugs. Some drugs are cleared more rapidly in women (e.g., clozapine, erythromycin, and theophylline), whereas others are cleared more rapidly in men (e.g., lorazepam, acetaminophen, and digoxin). Slower clearance means that the drug particles stay in the circulation longer, increasing the half-life and the potential for increased therapeutic and adverse effects from the drug. It is important to recognize that even though a drug's clearance is shown to be statistically altered, this statistical difference does not necessarily create a clinical difference.

PHARMACODYNAMICS

Pharmacodynamics is the biological, chemical, and physiologic actions of a particular drug within the body and the study of how those actions occur. Essentially, it is how the drug affects the body. The pharmacodynamics of a drug are responsible for its therapeutic effects and sometimes its adverse effects. The pharmacodynamics of a drug can be affected by the age of the patient (Box 4.5).

Drugs cannot create new responses in the body; they can only turn on, turn off, promote, or block a response that the body is inherently capable of producing. Understanding the pharmacodynamics of a drug is critical to being able to understand and critically assess a patient's response to drug therapy.

Drug–Receptor Interactions

Most drugs create their effects in the body by attaching to special sites, called **receptors,** on cells. At the receptor site, the drug is able to stimulate the cell to act in a way that the cell is designed to act. Drugs do this by attaching to the body's receptors for intrinsic elements such as hormones, neurotransmitters, or other internal methods of regulating cell function. Although each cell has many different receptor sites, the receptor sites do not all produce the same effects

---

Box 4.5 PHARMACODYNAMICS: EXAMPLES OF AGE-RELATED CHANGES

- Increased myocardial sensitivity to anesthesia
- Increased analgesic effect from opioids
- Increased sedative effect from benzodiazepines (or other CNS depressants)
- Increased anticoagulant effect from anticoagulant therapy
- Exaggerated responses to cardiovascular drugs (normal homeostatic responsiveness is altered)

Note: When administering drug therapy to an older adult, the nurse should be alert to the possibility of moderate reductions in drug clearance and the potential for exaggerated pharmacodynamic responsiveness.

when stimulated. Each type of receptor is responsible for producing a particular effect in the cell. Drug molecules are able to attach only at certain receptors, and the receptors to which they attach determine the effect produced. Other drugs match up with different receptors, thus producing different effects.

When drug molecules attach to a receptor, they can stimulate the cell to act. Drugs that act in this way are described as **agonists,** meaning that they promote a function. Alternately, by attaching to a receptor, drug molecules can prevent something else from attaching and causing an effect. Drugs that act in this way are described as **antagonists** or **blockers.** Consider a busy parking garage at a mall. If other drivers have parked in all of the parking spaces before you get there, you are prevented from parking and going into the mall to shop. As you circle around waiting for a driver to leave a spot, you are in competition with all of the other drivers who are circling, looking for spots. At some point, a driver will vacate a parking space. If you are close by, you will be able to park and go in and shop. If other cars are closer, they will get the spot and again block you from parking. This scenario is similar to how drugs block receptor sites.

A drug may latch onto a site to prevent a hormone or a neurotransmitter from attaching to the cell and turning on a function. If the drug is on the receptor, the other chemical cannot also be on the receptor. This fact is helpful when excessive internal stimulation of the cell causes the patient to experience pathologic changes. For example, in a patient with excessive stomach acid, the receptors in the stomach known as histamine-2 (H_2) receptors are overactivated, and the patient feels GI distress. When drugs called H_2 antagonists are given that attach to H_2 receptors and block the acid from attaching to the receptors, the person has a decrease in symptoms and feels better. The example of the parking garage also brings up an important point about drugs at receptor sites. The bonds that are formed are almost always temporary. When the drug molecule is no longer attached to the receptor, other drug particles may then attach, or the internal substance may then attach, to the receptor. Because there is competition for the receptor sites, the chemical that is present in the largest amount, either the drug or the internal regulator, is the most likely to be near an open receptor and attach to the receptor site. Most drugs that are antagonists are competitive; only a very few are not.

There are two theories about drug–receptor interactions: the single occupancy theory and the modified occupancy theory.

Single Occupancy Theory

The single occupancy theory has two aspects. First, the intensity of the body's response to the drug is directly related to the number of receptors occupied by the drug. The more receptors occupied, the stronger the response that is produced. Second, the maximum response occurs when all of the receptors have drug molecules attached. This theory does not explain, however, how two different drugs, each of which can attach to the same type of receptors, can produce

different degrees of effect from stimulating the receptor. We know from common usage that different drugs need different doses to achieve their therapeutic effects. If you have two drugs that each relieve headaches, but the standard dose of Drug A is 20 mg and the standard dose of Drug B is 100 mg, there are obviously more drug molecules of Drug B than of Drug A. Thus, Drug B is attaching to and stimulating more receptors than Drug A, yet they both work to relieve a headache. Additionally, we know that, with some drugs, a ceiling effect occurs: at some point, no matter how much more drug you give, you cannot get any additional therapeutic response. Yet it would seem that if all of the receptors are occupied, a maximal effect should be seen. The single occupancy theory, which assumes that all drugs have identical abilities to bind with receptors and that all drugs, once bound, have identical abilities to influence the functioning of the receptor, cannot be the only explanation for the way that drugs create an effect at receptor sites.

Modified Occupancy Theory

The modified occupancy theory is based on different assumptions about how drugs work at receptors. It states that different drugs have different strengths of attractions, or **affinity,** for receptor sites. Drugs with high affinity are strongly attracted to a receptor; drugs with low affinity are not very strongly attracted to a receptor. Drugs with strong affinity attach to a receptor even if not many drug particles are available. Drugs with low affinity attach only if large numbers of drug molecules are present. A comparison can be made with going to a movie. If you are very interested in seeing a particular movie, you'll make sure you go, even if you go alone or with only one friend. If you're not too interested in a movie, you'll go, but only if all your other friends are going, too. Thus, low doses of a drug with high affinity for a receptor will bind with that receptor and produce an effect.

Another assumption of the modified occupancy theory is that drugs, once attached to a receptor, have different abilities to stimulate the receptor. A drug's ability to stimulate its receptor is termed its **intrinsic activity.** Drugs with high intrinsic activity cause strong reactions from the receptor; drugs with low intrinsic activity cause low reactions from the receptor. A drug with high affinity and high intrinsic activity is able to produce a strong effect from a small amount of drug.

Changes in Receptor Sensitivity

Receptors are not static; they can change or modify their response to a stimulus. Such change occurs when a receptor is continuously stimulated to act or continually inhibited from action. Receptor response can be modified either by changing the number of receptors on the cell or by changing the sensitivity of the current receptors.

Continual stimulation from an agonist usually makes the receptor desensitized to the drug and thus less active. Continual blockage from an antagonist usually makes the receptor become hypersensitive and much more likely to react.

Nonreceptor Responses

Although most drug effects are related to drug–receptor responses, some drugs exert their effect by reacting physically or chemically with other molecules in the body. For example, antacids create their effect by mixing with stomach contents to raise the pH, making it less acid. Another example is heparin, an anticoagulant. Heparin interferes with the conversion of prothrombin to thrombin (which is needed to form a stable clot) by inactivating factor X.

VARIABLES THAT INFLUENCE THE DOSE OF A DRUG

Potency and Efficacy

From the drug–receptor theories, we see that the dose and characteristics of a drug have some relation to the pharmacotherapeutic effect achieved with drug therapy. A certain level of drug must be present in the body to produce an effect at all. This level is called the minimum effective concentration (MEC). After the MEC is reached, the strength of the response to a drug increases proportionately as more drug is given, until a plateau is reached and no additional therapeutic effect can be achieved, no matter the dose. When this relation between drug dose and response is plotted on a graph, it is referred to as a dose–response curve (Figure 4.7).

The amount of a drug that must be given in order to produce a particular response—its relative pharmacologic activity—is called the **potency** of a drug. A drug that is highly potent requires little of the drug to produce its effect. The affinity of a drug is related to its potency. Drugs with high affinity for a receptor need little drug to bind to the receptor and are thus highly potent drugs. How well a drug produces its desired effect is called **efficacy**. The efficacy of a drug is related to

its intrinsic activity. Drugs with high intrinsic activity have greater efficacy.

Potency is not the same as efficacy. Two drugs may have different potencies but the same efficacy. For example, it might take 25 mg of Drug A to lower elevated blood pressure but 50 mg of Drug B to lower blood pressure by the same amount. Both drugs have equal efficacy, but Drug A is more potent than Drug B because fewer milligrams are needed to achieve the effect. Is the more potent drug the better drug? Not necessarily. Rarely is potency the most important consideration when selecting a drug. If the less potent drug, which is equal in efficacy, can be administered in a similarly sized pill as the more potent drug, patients and prescribers will view the drugs similarly. Other important considerations include the cost of each drug and the adverse effects from each one. If the less potent but equally effective drug is less expensive or is better tolerated by the patient, it will be the preferred drug. If the necessary route of administration is different, this consideration may also make one drug more desirable than the other. For example, if the more potent drug is administered only intravenously, but the less potent drug can be given orally, the less potent drug will usually be preferred when the patient is receiving drug therapy at home.

If drugs have similar potencies, but different efficacies, the drug that has better efficacy is usually preferred because this drug does a better job of achieving the desired therapeutic effect. However, if the largest effect that the drug can achieve (the maximal efficacy) is greater than the patient's clinical status warrants, a drug with a lower maximal efficacy may be chosen. For example, morphine has a higher maximal efficacy for relieving pain than acetaminophen. If the patient has postoperative pain at a surgical incision site, the morphine, with a higher maximal efficacy, is appropriate. If the patient has only a mild headache, the morphine is not appropriate, but the acetaminophen is.

ED_{50}, Maintenance, and Loading Doses

Because people are unique, how individuals respond to a drug dose varies. To determine what dose of a medicine should be given as the "usual dose," the distribution of doses needed to produce a response in a large and varied number of people is statistically calculated. The dose that is required to produce the therapeutic response in 50% of the population is called the effective dose 50% (ED_{50}). This dose is considered the standard or typical dose and is usually chosen as a starting dose. Once a dose is chosen and administered consistently over time (e.g., every day), it is called the **maintenance dose.** Patients who are started on drug therapy using the standard maintenance dose arrive at steady state after four to five half-lives. The full therapeutic effect of any dose is achieved at steady state. For drugs that have long half-lives, achieving steady state may take days or weeks. The patient's medical condition may warrant immediate and full drug effect, however, in order to maintain health or life. When this is the case, a larger dose than usual is given initially. This initial large

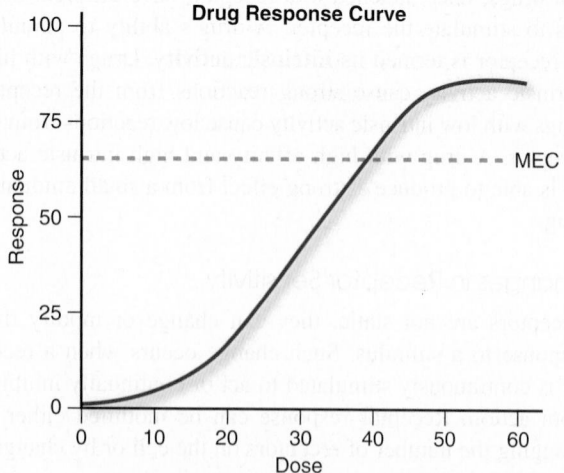

• FIGURE 4.7   As the dose of a drug is increased, more response from the drug is achieved. Once the drug reaches the minimum effective concentration (MEC), a therapeutic effect can be observed. At a certain point, increasing the drug's dose fails to produce any greater response, and the curve flattens out. This point is the maximal efficacy of the drug.

dose is called a **loading dose.** After one half-life, half of the administered dose is still available. The loading dose is computed so that after some of the drug is eliminated, the drug concentration in the body is still in the therapeutic range. The large initial loading dose is often divided into two or three portions, which are given more frequently than maintenance doses are administered. This dosing prevents the initial amount circulating in the patient from being so high that the patient experiences adverse effects.

Therapeutic Index

Just as people vary in the dose of a drug they need to achieve an effective therapeutic response, they vary as to the dose that will produce death. The lethal dose is computed in a laboratory setting and analyzed statistically. The point at which the dose would be fatal in 50% of the population receiving that dose is called lethal dose 50% (LD_{50}). To determine the safety of a drug, the LD_{50} is compared with the ED_{50}. The relation of LD_{50} to ED_{50} is called the **therapeutic index**. Therapeutic index can be explained by this equation, where TI represents the therapeutic index:

$$TI = \frac{ED_{50}}{LD_{50}}$$

If the amount of a drug required to be the ED_{50} is similar to the amount that is the LD_{50}, the mathematical ratio of the two values will equal a number close to one. For example, if the ED_{50} is 99 mg and the LD_{50} is 100 mg, the therapeutic index would be computed this way:

$$TI = \frac{99}{100} \text{ or } TI = 0.99, \text{ which can be rounded to 1}$$

When the ED_{50} and the LD_{50} do not differ by much, the drug is considered to have a narrow therapeutic index. These drugs are not very safe and are therefore difficult to dose because the dose needed to be effective in half of the population will also kill half of the population. Drugs used in practice do not have a therapeutic index as narrow as in this example. However, the closer the two numbers are to each other, or the closer that the TI is to 1.00, the more difficult it is to use the drug to treat patients. For some types of conditions, however, the only appropriate drug is one that has a narrow therapeutic index. When patients receive these drugs, they must be closely monitored for adverse effects because adverse effects will become evident before death occurs. The current blood level of the drug is also monitored closely to make sure that the drug stays in the therapeutic range.

Thankfully, most drugs have a wide therapeutic index. A wide therapeutic index means that the amount required to be effective is very small, compared with the amount required to be lethal; for example:

$$TI = \frac{25}{1000} \text{ or } 0.025$$

In this example, the disparity between the ED_{50} and the LD_{50} is large. The therapeutic index is not close to 1.0. This drug is easy to dose; fatal effects are unlikely to occur because the LD_{50} is 400 times greater than the ED_{50}. Although this patient should be monitored for adverse effects, he or she is not at high risk for experiencing a problem, unlike the patient receiving a drug with a narrow therapeutic index.

Nurses will not need to compute the therapeutic index. Furthermore, the numerical quotient of the comparison of the ED_{50} and the LD_{50} will not be published in the drug literature. Rather, the drug literature will state that the drug has a narrow therapeutic index. If the drug does not have a narrow therapeutic index, usually no mention is made.

DRUG DOSAGE AND BLOOD CONCENTRATION

As previously stated, a minimum effective concentration of a drug (the MEC) is required to achieve the desired pharmacotherapeutic effect. As drug levels within the body increase, the patient is more likely to experience adverse effects from drug therapy. For some drugs, these adverse effects may be very serious and potentially harmful to the patient. The goal of drug dosing is to give a dose that places the drug concentration above the MEC but below the level at which adverse effects occur. This range is called the **therapeutic range**.

To help determine whether a drug's dose is adequate to be in the therapeutic range, but not so high as to cause adverse effects, blood levels of the drug are often measured. Although most drugs do not achieve their therapeutic effect within the blood, blood samples are used because they are fairly easy to obtain. For many types of drugs, it would be too difficult to measure samples at the site of drug action. For example, drugs that alter cardiac function would require samples of tissue from the heart. Blood levels of a drug can be used, however, only if the relationship between the amount of drug circulating in the blood and the effects of the drug in the body are known. This information is not known for all drugs; therefore, blood samples are not drawn for every type of drug therapy. Acceptable target blood levels have been determined for most drugs that produce serious adverse effects.

Nurses need to monitor drug blood levels if samples are drawn and must notify the physician or nurse practitioner if the level indicates that the patient is not in the therapeutic range or is greatly above the therapeutic range. Nurses should also seek orders for a blood level of a drug if a patient appears to be experiencing adverse effects. Because blood levels reflect the changes that have occurred from drug metabolism and excretion, it is important to note the exact time the last dose of the drug was administered on the drug blood level specimen slip. This record enables the laboratory to consider the pharmacokinetics of the drug during analysis.

The therapeutic range can only be considered an average, much like the temperature of 98.6°F is an average normal body temperature. Some patients experience the therapeutic effects from a drug when their blood levels show that the drug is at "subtherapeutic" levels, whereas others experience adverse effects while the blood levels of the drug are in the "normal" range. This is due to genetic variations in individuals that alter the body's pharmacokinetic responses to a drug. The drug blood level is only one piece of data that must be considered when evaluating the patient's response to drug therapy. Changes to a drug's dose should be based on the total picture of the patient's response to therapy. Treat the patient, not the lab value.

CHAPTER SUMMARY

- Pharmacotherapeutics is the clinical purpose or indication for giving a drug.
- Pharmacokinetics is the effect of the body on the drug. It is made up of four phases: absorption, distribution, metabolism, and excretion. Absorption is the movement of the drug from the site of administration into the bloodstream. Distribution is movement of the drug through the bloodstream and eventually into the cells. Metabolism refers to the changing of the drug into another substance or substances (i.e., metabolites). Excretion is the removal of the drug or its metabolites from the body. Metabolism and excretion are considered together as elimination of a drug. Most commonly in practice, however, the clinician uses the term elimination as a synonym excretion.
- The blood–brain barrier is the body's natural defense to keep toxins and poisons from reaching the brain. It also may prevent the distribution of needed drug molecules from reaching their target.
- Drugs have different affinities for protein molecules, especially albumin, in the blood. Drugs that are highly protein bound have a lower proportion of their molecules available to produce the desired therapeutic effect. Only the free drug is active.
- Metabolism of drugs occurs primarily in the liver. Liver metabolism is predominantly achieved by specific liver enzymes, known as the P-450 system. The P-450 system also metabolizes some drug in the small intestine. Some drugs can induce this system, increasing their own or other drugs' metabolism. When multiple drugs are metabolized by the same P-450 family, the metabolism of all the drugs is normally decreased. Anything that impairs liver functioning also decreases drug metabolism. Decreased metabolism leads to increased circulating levels of the drug, more therapeutic effect, and possibly more adverse effects.
- Drugs that are administered orally pass through the liver before going to the general circulation. If the drug is highly metabolized, a high first-pass effect occurs. This effect substantially decreases the amount of drug that is distributed to the body.
- The kidney is the primary organ responsible for drug excretion. There are three processes that affect the excretion of drugs in the urine: glomerular filtration, passive tubular reabsorption, and active tubular secretion. Anything that decreases kidney function decreases drug excretion, leading to increased circulating blood levels of the drug.
- Half-life of a drug is the amount of time needed to eliminate (by metabolism and excretion) half of the drug molecules currently in the body.
- Steady state is when the continuing dose of a drug is in balance with the elimination rate of the drug, that is, when the amount of drug entering the body equals the amount being removed. Steady state is achieved after four to five half-lives. Achievement of steady state is not related to the dosage of the drug or the frequency of drug administration.
- Most drugs create their effects in the body by attaching to special sites, called receptors, on cells. At the receptor site, the drug is able to stimulate the cell to act in a way that the cell is designed to act. Drugs that stimulate the cell to act are known as agonists. Drugs that attach to receptors to prevent other substances from attaching and "turning on" the cell are called antagonists or blockers.
- The single occupancy theory and the modified occupancy theory help to explain how drugs achieve their effects at receptors.
- Potency of a drug refers to how *much* of a drug is needed to create the desired therapeutic effect. Efficacy of a drug refers to how *well* the drug creates the desired therapeutic effect. Drugs may have different potencies but the same efficacy. Efficacy is a more important consideration than potency when selecting a particular drug.
- Loading doses are larger-than-normal doses used when therapy is initiated with drugs that have very long half-lives. The purpose of the loading dose is to achieve quickly a blood level of the drug that is in therapeutic range even though the drug has not reached steady state.
- Maintenance doses are the doses administered regularly throughout therapy.
- The therapeutic index is a measurement of the safety of the drug. Drugs that are described as having a narrow therapeutic index do not have much difference between the effective dose and the toxic or lethal dose. Patients receiving these drugs need to be monitored very closely for adverse effects. They also need to have their drug blood levels monitored closely.
- Drug dosages are adjusted to maintain a therapeutic level of the drug. Drug blood levels are one way of determining whether a dose needs to be either increased or decreased.

QUESTIONS FOR STUDY AND REVIEW

1. What is the difference between pharmacokinetics and pharmacodynamics?
2. What is the advantage of a drug being lipophilic during the distribution phase of pharmacokinetics?
3. Why are drugs metabolized to a hydrophilic form?
4. How do most drugs achieve their effect within the body?
5. Why would a drug that has a high first-pass effect be given by a route other than the oral route?

6. If a patient has renal insufficiency or poor hepatic functioning, how might the dose of a drug be adjusted? Why?

7. Your patient is receiving a drug that is known to be highly protein bound. The laboratory reports for this patient indicate that the albumin level is below normal. How might this affect the patient's risk for adverse effects of the drug therapy? Why?

NEED MORE HELP?

Chapter 4 of the Study Guide to Accompany *Drug Therapy in Nursing,* 4th Edition, contains NCLEX-style questions and other learning activities to reinforce your understanding of the concepts presented in this chapter. For additional information or to purchase the study guide, visit thePoint.

REFERENCES

Anderson, G. D. (2008). Gender differences in pharmacological response. *International Review of Neurobiology*, 83;1–10.

Bernard, S., Neville, K. A., Nguyen, A. T., & Flockhart, D. A. (2006). Interethnic differences in genetic polymorphisms of CYP2D6 in the U.S. population: clinical implications. *The Oncologist*, 11(2):126–135.

Fakhoury, M., Lecordier, J., Medard, Y., Peuchmaur, M., & Jacqz-Agrain E. (2006). Impact of inflammation on the duodenal mRNA expression of CYP3A and P-glycoprotein in children with Crohn's disease. *Inflammatory Bowel Diseases*, 12(8):745–749.

Harvard Mental Health Letter. February 2009. Retrieved from www.health.harvard.edu March 14, 2009.

He, P., Court, M. H., Greenblatt, D. J., & von Moltke, L. L. (2006). Factors influencing midazolam hydroxylation activity in human liver microsomes. *Drug Metabolism and Disposition*, 34(7):1198–1207.

Mulder, H., Heerdink, E., Iersel, E. E., Wilmink, F. W., & Egberts A. C. G. (2007). Prevalence of patients using drugs metabolized by cytochrome P450 in different populations: a cross-sectional study. *The Annals of Pharmacotherapy*, 41:408–413.

Paine, M. F., Ludington, S. S., Chen, M. L., Stewart, P. W., Huang, S. M., & Watkins, P. B. (2005). Do men and women differ in proximal small intestinal CYP3A or P-glycoprotein expression? *Drug Metabolism Disposition*, 33(3):426–433.

Paine, M. F., Hart, H. L., Ludington, S. S., Haining, R. L., Rettie, A. E., & Zeldin, D. C. (2006). The human intestinal Cytochrome P450 "pie." *Drug Metabolism and Disposition*, 34(5):880–886.

Shimada, T., Yamazaki, H., Mimura, M., Inui, Y., & Guengerich, F. P. (1994). Interindividual variations in human liver cytochrome P-450 enzymes involved in the oxidation of drugs, carcinogens and toxic chemicals: studies with liver microsomes of 30 Japanese and 30 Caucasians. *J Pharmacol Exp Ther*, 270:414–423.

Tortorici, M. A., Kochanek, P. M., & Poloyac, S. M. (2007). Effects of hypothermia on drug disposition, metabolism, and response: A focus on hypothermia-mediated alterations on the cytochrome P450 enzyme system. *Critical Care Medicine*, 35(9):2196–2204.

Yarnell, E. & Abascal, K. (2007). Interaction of Herbal Constituents with Cytochrome P450 enzymes. *Alternative & Complementary Therapies*, 13(5):239–247.

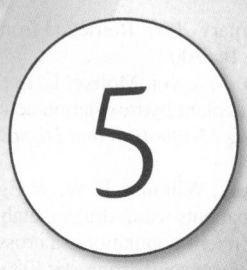

Adverse Effects and Drug Interactions

Learning Objectives

At the completion of this chapter the student will:

1. Identify the core drug knowledge of adverse effects and drug interactions.
2. Identify how adverse effects and drug interactions may alter the pharmacokinetics and pharmacodynamics of drug therapy.
3. Define the major toxicities that may occur as adverse effects.
4. Identify core patient variables related to adverse effects and drug interactions.
5. Relate the core drug knowledge of adverse effects and drug interactions to core patient variables.
6. Generate a nursing plan of care based on the interactions between core drug knowledge and core patient variables for adverse effects and drug interactions.
7. Describe nursing interventions to maximize therapeutic effects and minimize adverse effects and drug interactions in drug therapy.
8. Determine key points for patient and family education about adverse effects and drug interactions.

Key Terms

additive effect	cardiotoxicity	nephrotoxicity
adverse effect	drug interaction	neurotoxicity
allergic response	hepatotoxicity	ototoxicity
anaphylaxis	idiosyncratic response	potentiation
antagonistic drug interaction	immunotoxicity	synergistic effect

n a perfect world, a perfect drug would produce only its desired therapeutic effect. Its effective dose would be easy to determine, it would be totally safe, and it would be so well tolerated that everyone who took it would adhere to and comply with the prescribed therapy. Alas, this is not a perfect world, and there is no perfect drug. All drugs can produce undesirable effects, some of them mild and annoying, others life threatening. Drugs also can produce altered effects because of interactions with other drugs, foods, or substances such as herbs and botanicals. These unexpected and nontherapeutic effects from drug therapy cause many patients to stop taking their prescribed drug therapy.

An **adverse effect** of drug therapy is a usually undesirable effect other than the intended therapeutic effect. It may occur even with normal drug dosing. An adverse effect may result from too much of a therapeutic effect (e.g., hypotension that may result from antihypertensive drug therapy) or from other pharmacodynamic effects of the drug (e.g., beta blockers are given for their effect on the heart, but they also have an effect on the bronchial tree). These effects are usually dose dependent and predictable. Adverse effects may also occur independently of the dose and be unpredictable. The term *adverse effect* encompasses all nontherapeutic responses to drug therapy and is used throughout this text.

A **drug interaction** occurs when two drugs or a drug and another element (such as food) have an effect on each other. This interaction may increase or decrease the therapeutic effect of one or both of the drugs, create a new effect, or increase the incidence of an adverse effect.

To maximize therapeutic effect, minimize adverse effects and drug interactions, and plan for appropriate patient and family education, nurses need to understand adverse effects and drug interactions and use this knowledge in their management of drug therapy. This chapter deals with these aspects of core drug knowledge.

ADVERSE EFFECTS

Every drug can produce adverse effects. Many adverse effects, such as nausea, are mild and bothersome perhaps only to the patient. Others, including liver failure, are serious or even life threatening. Serious adverse effects lead to the withdrawal of a small number of drugs from the market every year. A drug is withdrawn not because it was approved without testing—clinical studies are done on all drugs under development, and all adverse effects in the study participants are identified. Sometimes, however, complete knowledge of adverse effects cannot be obtained until the drug has been used for a longer time than the length of the trial or by more people than were included in a trial. Sometimes, adverse effects can be identified only when used extensively by patient populations that may not have been adequately represented in the study population, such as older adults, or patients with certain disease processes (e.g., renal disease).

It is important for nurses and other health care professionals to be alert for adverse effects from drug therapy. Sometimes, determining whether an adverse effect has occurred as a result of drug therapy is difficult. Adverse effects may be mistaken for changes associated with aging or disease pathology. For example, slight memory loss may be attributed to changes with aging, or hyperglycemia may be attributed to uncontrolled diabetes rather than to an adverse effect.

Serious adverse reactions (e.g., death or potential fatality, significant disability, requires or prolongs hospitalization, congenital anomaly, or requires intervention to prevent permanent damage) from a drug, especially a newly approved drug, should be reported to a national database, such as the MedWatch reporting system sponsored by the FDA through its website (FDA website)Reporting of serious adverse effects is necessary for corrective action to take place; examples of actions that may be taken to protect the public include revising the drug label, adding Black Box warnings for health care providers to highlight the most serious warnings (Box 5.1), creating patient Medication Guides that are dispensed with each filled prescription of a drug, or, if needed, withdrawing the drug from the market. Medication Guides are provided for drugs with potential serious adverse effects (Box 5.2). Alternative therapy without these potential serious adverse effects may not exist for many drugs. The underlying assumption is that these drugs may be safely used if patients know what symptoms warrant immediate consultation with the prescriber.

Box 5.1 BLACK BOX WARNINGS

What Exactly is a Black Box Warning?

- A method of flagging a serious warning so that prescribers do not miss seeing it
- The warning is placed at the top of the drug label information with a black border printed around it.
- Printed materials and online databases that provide information about drugs all must show the Black Box warning.

Does a Black Box Warning Mean That the Drug is Too Dangerous to Use?

- No, it means that special and careful monitoring for onset of a problem is required for its appropriate use. All drugs carry risks of adverse effects, and many of these may be small but serious or life threatening, such as blood dyscrasias or liver failure.
- Sometimes the warning is used to emphasize that the use of the drug should be limited to patients only with certain conditions or who meet certain guidelines.
- Examples of drugs that have Black Box warnings:
  - SSRIs and other antidepressants
  - Most chemotherapeutic drugs
  - Some antibiotics (e.g., the aminoglycosides such as gentamicin, chloramphenicol, and the lincosamides such as clindamycin)
  - Some antiarrhythmic drugs (e.g., procainamide, tocainide, and amiodarone)
  - The antidiabetic drug metformin

Allergic Responses

Adverse effects that are not predictable or dose related are caused by allergic or idiosyncratic responses. An **allergic response** is an immune system response. If the body interprets the drug as a foreign substance (antigen) and forms antibodies against the drug, the immune system initiates the antigen–antibody response when the drug is taken again. This response involves the release of histamine, which is responsible for many symptoms of allergy: redness, itching, swelling, rash, and hives. The allergic response may change over time, and symptoms may become more severe each time the drug is introduced into the body. The most serious allergic response is called **anaphylaxis.** During anaphylaxis, changes occur throughout the body, including constriction of bronchial smooth muscles (bronchospasms), vasodilation, and increased vascular permeability. The symptoms of anaphylaxis include acute respiratory distress, marked hypotension, edema (most importantly laryngeal edema), rash, tachycardia, cyanosis, and pale, cool skin. Convulsions may occur. If anaphylaxis is untreated, death is likely. Treatment includes the administration of vasopressor agents to increase the blood pressure; bronchodilators to open the airway (most often epinephrine, which is both a vasopressor and a bronchodilator); antihistamines to block the effects of the released histamine (such as diphenhydramine); corticosteroids, which have anti-inflammatory effects and reduce swelling; oxygen therapy to treat cyanosis; and intravenous fluids to help support blood pressure. Endotracheal intubation and mechanical ventilation are often needed to support an open airway and respiration.

Idiosyncratic Responses

Idiosyncratic responses to a drug are another form of adverse effect. These responses are unusual and in fact may be the opposite of what is anticipated. They are sometimes called *paradoxical effects*. Idiosyncratic responses are related to an individual's unique response to a drug, rather than to the dose of a drug. They are considered to be genetically predetermined. The genetically inherited trait of responding to general anesthetics by developing malignant hyperthermia is an example of an idiosyncratic response to drug therapy.

Historically, different terms have been used to differentiate mild from serious nontherapeutic drug effects. The term *side effect* typically referred to a minor effect (such as nausea), whereas the term *toxic effect* referred to a more serious, potentially life-threatening effect (such as impaired renal function). In reality, the distinction between the terms is often blurry, and classification in one or the other category is somewhat arbitrary. For that reason, the newer, current term in pharmacologic literature is *adverse effect,* which is used to describe all undesired effects. Some practitioners still use the term *side effect* as a synonym for *adverse effect.*

Toxicities

Specific patterns or groups of symptoms related to drug therapy that carry risk for permanent damage to an organ or system and that may result in death are called *toxicities*. The organ or system that is affected is used to name the toxicity (as in neurotoxicity, nephrotoxicity, cardiotoxicity). Drug toxicities are now listed *as a type of adverse effect* from a drug (e.g., nephrotoxicity is an adverse effect of aminoglycoside antibiotics). When two or more drugs taken by a patient can produce the same toxicity, the risk that the patient will develop the drug toxicity increases. The most commonly referenced drug toxicities are: neurotoxicity, hepatotoxicity, nephrotoxicity, ototoxicity, cardiotoxicity, and immunotoxicity A description of these drug toxicities follows.

Neurotoxicity, sometimes referred to as central nervous system (CNS) toxicity, is a drug's ability to harm or poison a nerve cell or nerve tissue. Signs and symptoms of neurotoxicity include drowsiness, auditory and visual disturbances, restlessness, nystagmus (involuntary cyclic movement of the eyeballs), and tonic-clonic (grand mal) seizures. Neurotoxicity can occur after exposure to drugs and other chemicals and gases (e.g., alcohol, solvents, insecticides, industrial vapors, and pollutants). Injury to the CNS is largely irreversible because the highly differentiated neurons of the brain cannot divide and regenerate. Immature nervous systems (e.g., fetal and neonatal nervous systems) can easily be damaged by drugs that produce neurotoxicity.

Hepatotoxicity is damage to the liver. Manifestations of hepatotoxicity include hepatitis, jaundice, elevated liver enzyme levels, and fatty infiltration of the liver. Hepatic anatomy and hepatic function both contribute greatly to the high susceptibility of the liver to toxicants. Blood draining from the stomach and small intestines is delivered directly to the liver by the hepatic portal vein. As a result, the liver is exposed to relatively large concentrations of ingested drugs or other potentially toxic substances. If the drug that was absorbed and is now present in the blood is hepatotoxic, liver damage will likely occur because of the large number of drug molecules presented to the liver. The liver is also responsible for metabolizing most drugs. If liver damage occurs, the drug will not be metabolized as efficiently, leaving more circulating drug to cause further liver damage.

Damage to the kidneys is called **nephrotoxicity.** Decreased urinary output, elevated blood urea nitrogen, increased serum creatinine, altered acid-base balance, and electrolyte imbalances can all occur with kidney damage. The renal system is similar to the hepatic system in that it is susceptible to poisoning because of its anatomy and function. The cells within the proximal tubule are frequently damaged by nephrotoxic drugs. These cells are responsible for filtering, concentrating, and eliminating toxic as well as nontoxic materials; as water is reabsorbed instead of eliminated, the concentration of drug molecules in the tubule rises, thereby increasing the potential for damage.

Ototoxicity is damage to the eighth cranial nerve. Structures of the inner ear that may be affected include the cochlea (responsible for hearing) and the vestibular and semicircular canals (responsible for balance). Ototoxicity may or may not be reversible. Signs and symptoms of ototoxicity include tinnitus, which is a buzzing or ringing sound in the ear, and sensorineural hearing loss. Also called nerve deafness, sensorineural hearing loss usually begins with the loss of high-frequency sound and may worsen until low-frequency sound is also difficult to hear. Other signs and symptoms, particularly of vestibular toxicity, include light-headedness, vertigo, a spinning sensation from a seated position, and nausea and vomiting.

Irregularities in cardiac rhythms and conduction, heart failure, and even damage to the myocardium may result from an adverse effect known as **cardiotoxicity.** Exactly how some drugs produce cardiotoxicity is unknown. Older adults, who have less effective hearts than younger adults, and children younger than 2 years, whose hearts are still growing, are most susceptible to cardiotoxicity from drugs.

When the immune system is significantly affected by drug therapy, the condition is called **immunotoxicity.** A wide variety of drugs can affect the immune system. Some may cause immunosuppression, whereas others may directly destroy immune system components. The effect of both kinds of immunotoxicity may be an increased incidence of bacterial, viral, and parasitic infections.

DRUG INTERACTIONS

Drug interactions occur when one drug (Drug A) is affected in some way by another drug (Drug B), a food, or some other substance that is taken concurrently. The effect may be to increase the therapeutic or adverse effects from Drug A or to decrease the therapeutic or adverse effects from Drug A. Rarely, a new and different effect may be induced.

Drug interactions may be beneficial (e.g., when the interaction increases the therapeutic effect of a drug or decreases its adverse effects). Sometimes, drugs are ordered specifically to bring about the desired drug interaction. For example, probenecid, a drug used to treat gout, is given to patients without gout to prevent the renal excretion of penicillin, thus allowing the penicillin to circulate longer and produce additional therapeutic effects.

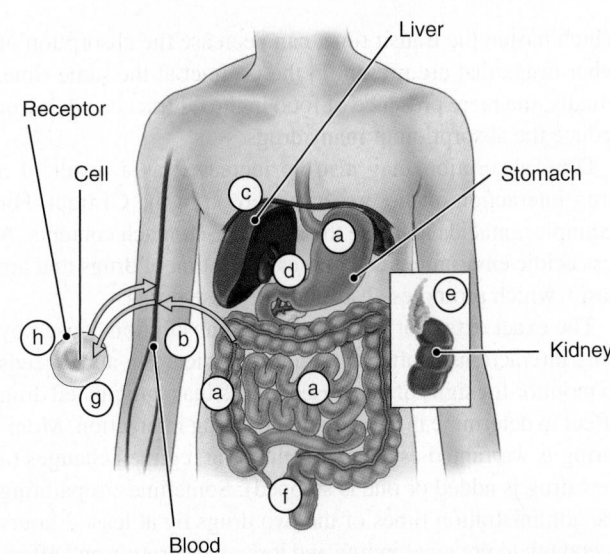

• FIGURE 5.1 Drug interaction sites within the body. Drug interactions can occur in numerous body sites. Absorption can be enhanced or reduced in the gut (**a**); protein binding can be affected within the vasculature (**b**); metabolism can be affected in the liver (**c**); excretion can be affected through bile (**d**), through the kidney (**e**), or in feces (**f**); tissue binding of one drug can be affected by another (**g**); and finally, drugs may have an effect through action on specific receptors (**h**).

Negative effects from drug interactions are those that decrease the therapeutic effect or increase the adverse effects of a drug. For example, consuming foods high in tyramine (such as smoked meats) while taking a monoamine oxidase inhibitor (MAOI) antidepressant can lead to pronounced elevation of blood pressure and may induce a hypertensive crisis. Drug interactions that alter the circulating level of one of the drugs are especially worrisome if the drug has a narrow therapeutic index (see Chapter 4). In this case, a slight elevation of the blood level of the drug may produce serious adverse effects, whereas a slight decrease in the blood level may cause the drug to become nontherapeutic.

Drug interactions may take place in any phase of pharmacokinetics—absorption, distribution, metabolism, or excretion. Drug interactions can also change the pharmacodynamics of a drug or the adverse effects of the drugs. When two drugs can both independently cause the same adverse effect, there is an increased risk for that adverse effect when both drugs are taken. Drug interaction sites in the body are shown in Figure 5.1 and are discussed throughout the sections that follow.

Drug Interactions Affecting Pharmacokinetics
Drug Interactions Affecting Absorption

Drug absorption is often decreased because of drug interactions. If a drug binds with another substance in the gastrointestinal (GI) tract, less of the drug is available to be absorbed. For example, milk and antacids bind with the antibiotic tetracycline and prevent its absorption. This binding of a drug is termed *chelation*. Because drug absorption is related to how long the drug is present in the GI tract, changes in GI transit time alter drug absorption. Therefore, drugs such as laxatives, which hasten the transit time, can decrease the absorption of other drugs that are present in the GI tract at the same time. Finally, the mere presence of food in the GI tract can delay or reduce the absorption of many drugs.

Drug absorption may also be increased as a result of a drug interaction or the presence of food in the GI tract. For example, antacids increase the pH of the stomach contents. A less acidic environment decreases ionization of drugs that are basic, which promotes absorption of these drugs.

The exact extent of changes in drug absorption caused by drug interactions is often difficult to predict. The nurse needs to monitor for signs of decreased or less than anticipated drug effect to determine if there might be a drug interaction. Monitoring is warranted especially if the drug regimen changes (a new drug is added or one is stopped). Sometimes, separating the administration times of the two drugs by at least 2 hours is enough to prevent binding and loss of absorption and effectiveness. Other times, an increased dose of the affected drug may be indicated.

Drug Interactions Affecting Distribution

Distribution is affected by two types of drug interactions. The first is competitive protein binding. When two drugs compete for the same protein receptors, the drug that has a higher affinity for the site will displace the other drug. Thus, one of the drugs will have more free and active molecules to be distributed through the body than would normally be anticipated. (Protein binding is discussed in more detail in Chapter 4.)

The second way that drug distribution can be affected by drug interactions is when a drug alters the extracellular pH. A drug that increases the pH of the extracellular fluid (i.e., makes the extracellular fluid more basic) increases the ability of acidic drugs to ionize in the extracellular space. Remember that drugs will cross a membrane in order to be ionized, but once ionized the drug cannot move back through the membrane. In the example above, acidic drugs move from the low-pH (acidic) environment found within the cells into the higher-pH (basic) environment in the extracellular space in order to be ionized. Once ionized, the drugs are trapped on that side of the membrane. Thus, drug distribution is altered.

Drug Interactions Affecting Metabolism

Probably the most important and common drug interaction is one that alters the metabolism of a drug. Most metabolism occurs in the liver, some also occurs in the small intestine. As you recall from Chapter 4, metabolism of drugs is related to the cytochrome P-450 system. Some drugs either induce or inhibit the P-450 system (see Appendix G online), thus altering the metabolism of other drugs (Figure 5.2). Usually, just one P-450 family is affected.

Drugs that induce a hepatic enzyme increase the amount of that enzyme in the liver. Induction of the P-450 system is accomplished most frequently by stimulating synthesis of the enzyme. When one of the hepatic enzymes is present in greater quantities than the others, more metabolism by this pathway can occur. Drugs that are metabolized by this pathway (also referred to as drugs that are substrates of the enzyme) are therefore metabolized more rapidly, which in turn rapidly decreases the amount of circulating, active drug. Some drugs can induce the enzymes necessary for their own metabolism and thus can increase the rate of their own metabolism. Drugs that inhibit a particular hepatic enzyme slow the metabolism that occurs through this pathway, causing an increase in the amount of circulating, active drug. Metabolism will return to normal after the inducing or inhibiting drug is no longer administered, although the return to normal may not occur until several days after an inducer is discontinued.

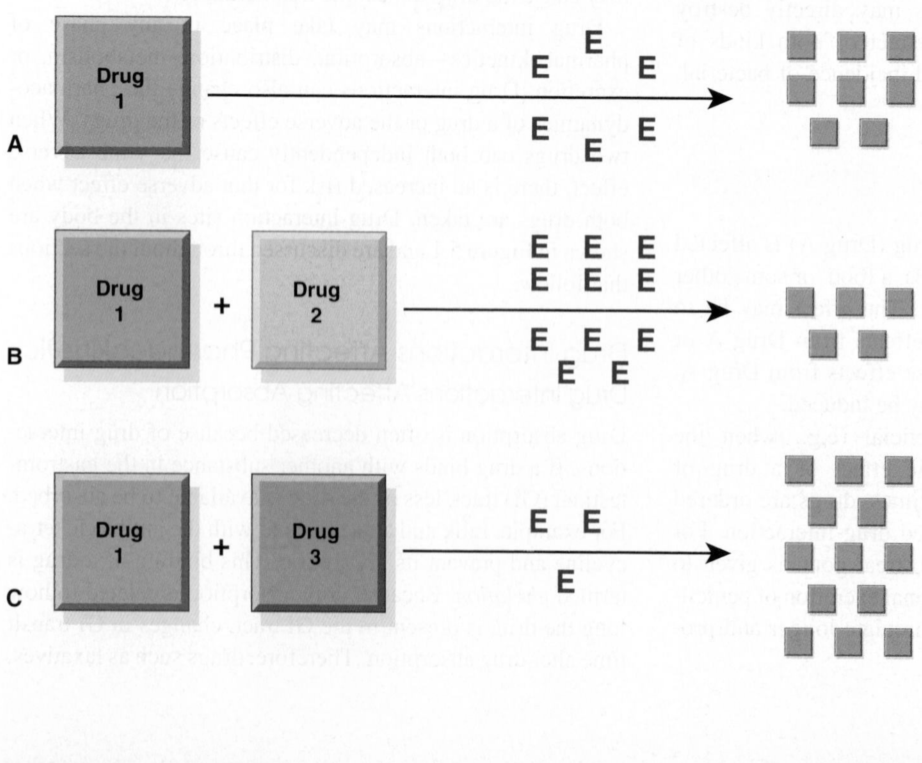

• FIGURE 5.2 Drug interactions affecting P-450 metabolism. (A) Normal drug metabolism through the P-450 iso-enzymes for Drug 1. (B) Drug 2 induces the P-450 system, increasing metabolism of Drug 1. Less Drug 1 than normal is left to circulate after this drug interaction. (C) Drug 3 inhibits the P-450 system; thus, metabolism is decreased for Drug 1. More Drug 1 than normal is left to circulate after this drug interaction.

If two drugs that affect the cytochrome P-450 system must both be administered to a patient, the dose of one of the drugs may have to be adjusted. When two or more drugs are metabolized by the same hepatic enzyme pathway, they compete with each other for the action of the enzyme. This competition results in impaired metabolism of one or more of the drugs. Consider the analogy of using the Internet through a dial-up connection. When few customers are online, it is easy to be connected and to use the online services. However, when there is very high demand, getting connected may be difficult, and once connected, you may be abruptly disconnected, losing the ability to use the online services. Similarly, when the demand is high for the services of a particular hepatic enzyme, not every drug will receive attention immediately.

In addition to drugs altering the metabolism of other drugs, grapefruit juice is known to inhibit CYP3A4. Remember that the P-450 isoenzymes responsible for drug metabolism are found not only in the liver but also in the intestinal wall. Grapefruit juice has an effect on CYP3A4 found in the intestinal wall, but not in the liver, and acts by blocking its function. The inhibition of CYP3A4 decreases the GI metabolism of many drugs, which allows more of the drug to be absorbed, resulting in substantially higher blood levels than if grapefruit juice were not consumed. Metabolism of many varied drugs such as calcium channel blockers (used to treat hypertension), statins (used to lower blood lipid levels), and antihistamines (used to prevent allergic reactions) is effected by grapefruit juice. Because the amount of CYP3A4 in the intestine varies among individuals based on genetic variations, the degree to which grapefruit juice alters drug metabolism also varies. In some people, the effect is great; in others, the effect is minimal. The more CYP3A4 that is present in the GI tract, the more drug metabolism can be increased. The effect also appears to be dose dependent (i.e., the more grapefruit juice a person drinks, the more inhibition of CYP3A4 that occurs). If the patient regularly drinks grapefruit juice before drug therapy is started, the drug dosage can be adjusted to obtain a therapeutic level or therapeutic effect. In this case, the patient can safely continue to drink grapefruit juice. Problems arise, however, when a patient intermittently drinks grapefruit juice or starts to drink it after drug therapy has been started. In these situations, the grapefruit juice may alter drug levels unpredictably, and the potential exists for substantial elevations that may cause adverse effects. Patients who did not consume grapefruit juice before the initiation of drug therapy should avoid drinking it once drug therapy has begun. See Appendix F online for a list of drugs that interact with grapefruit juice.

Some herbs and botanicals may also affect the CYP3A4 enzyme. St. John's Wort, for example, is a potent inducer of CYP3A4 and enhances the metabolism of drugs that are substrates of this enzymatic pathway. Drugs that are substrates of the CYP3A4 enzymatic pathway include protease inhibitors (used to treat AIDS), oral contraceptives, tricyclic antidepressants, and the immunosuppressant cyclosporine. Table 10.2 lists other possible drug interactions with herbs.

Alcohol and nicotine also alter the metabolism of some drugs. Nicotine is known to induce some isoenzymes in the P-450 system. A high blood alcohol level impairs the liver's ability to metabolize other drugs. Chronic use of alcohol may also induce some hepatic isoenzymes. Chronic alcoholism damages the liver permanently, decreasing drug metabolism.

Age also appears to decrease either the effectiveness of the P-450 enzymes or the number of enzymes available. The half-life of drugs processed by hepatic P-450 enzymes is typically 50% to 75% longer in adults older than 65 years than in younger adults (Ginsberg et al., 2005). This longer half-life is likely related to decreasing liver function that occurs with aging.

Inherited genetic variations of P-450 isoenzymes (termed genetic polymorphism) also effect how quickly or slowly a drug may be metabolized as well as its potential to cause drug interactions. These variations can often be attributed to the ethnicity of the patient (Bernard et al., 2006). Genetic profiling to determine whether a person has a CYP isoenzyme variation that produces poor metabolism of a drug (leading to higher than normal circulating levels, increased therapeutic effects, and increased adverse effects) or ultrarapid metabolism of a drug (leading to lower than normal circulating levels and failure to achieve the therapeutic response) could be used to determine the best drug dose for an individual. The dose would thus be tailored to decrease the risk of adverse effects and drug interactions and to promote optimal desired effects.

Genotyping for specific isoenzymes will not, however, indicate whether a particular drug will or will not work in a given patient (Pestka et al., 2007). Genetic profiling is currently expensive and still in its infancy. For genotyping to be relevant for patient care, specific patient populations (those most likely to have P450 interactions from drug therapy) should be screened, rather than all patients. For example, CYP 2D6 is known to be responsible for the metabolism of many drugs, and there are many normal variations to its presence. Psychiatric, psychogeriatric, and geriatric populations are commonly treated with at least one drug that is metabolized by CYP 2D6, so this group may be more likely to benefit from genotyping before drug therapy is started (Mulder et al., 2007; Pestka et al., 2007). CYP 2C9 variation is responsible for much of the adverse effects from the anticoagulant warfarin. See Box 5.3 to learn how research on this genetic variation is shaping dosing patterns for warfarin.

Drug Interactions Affecting Excretion

Drugs can alter renal filtration, renal reabsorption, or renal secretion. In doing so, they may alter the excretion of other drugs. Glomerular filtration is dependent on blood flow to the kidney. Drugs that decrease cardiac output decrease the amount of circulating blood that is sent to the kidneys. Renal reabsorption of a drug is dependent on whether a drug is ionized. Drug-induced changes in urinary pH affect whether other drugs are ionized and excreted or remain nonionized and are reabsorbed. Renal secretion uses a transport system to move the drug molecules into the urine for excretion.

If two drugs are dependent on the same transport system, the excretion rate of both is slowed.

Drug Interactions Affecting Pharmacodynamics

Drug interactions may affect the pharmacodynamics of one or both drugs administered. The overall effect may be positive or negative. Drug interactions can occur when both drugs act at the same receptor or at different receptors. Drugs that act at the same receptor compete to be attached to the receptor. The drug that has the weaker affinity for the receptor will not be able to exert its therapeutic effect, as discussed in Chapter 4. Drugs that act in different ways, or at different receptors, can interact in several ways. They may create an additive effect, a synergistic effect, a potentiated effect, or an antagonistic effect.

Additive Effect

An **additive effect** occurs when two or more "like" drugs (in terms of therapeutic effect) are combined, and the result is the sum of the drugs' effects. If written as an equation, this concept would be expressed as: 1 (Drug A) + 1 (Drug B) = 2. An additive effect may be intentional or may unintentionally cause harm. Consider the following two examples:

• Codeine and acetaminophen work differently to reduce pain. When these two analgesic drugs are combined, the additive effect is better control of pain (compared with that resulting from the use of either drug alone).
• Alcohol and salicylates, such as aspirin, can both cause GI bleeding. When a salicylate and alcohol are consumed together, the risk for GI bleeding is greatly increased because each agent independently can cause GI bleeding.

Synergistic Effect

A **synergistic effect** occurs when two or more "unlike" drugs (in terms of therapeutic effect or mechanism of action) are used together to produce a combined effect, and the outcome is a drug effect greater than either drug's activity alone. As an equation, this concept would be expressed as: 1 (Drug A) + 1 (Drug B) = 3. Just like an additive interaction, a synergistic interaction may be intentional or may unintentionally cause harm. Consider the following examples:

• A beneficial synergistic effect occurs when two different types of antibiotics that work in very different ways are combined, such as penicillin G and an aminoglycoside antibiotic. This approach is commonly used in the treatment of subacute bacterial endocarditis.
• When three different types of antihypertensive drugs—an alpha-adrenergic blocker (a vasodilator), a beta-adrenergic blocker (a sympatholytic), and a diuretic—are combined, the antihypertensive effect is better than with any drug alone.
• A harmful synergistic effect is represented by the interaction between drugs that depress the CNS, such as morphine and alcohol; this interaction causes additional CNS depression that may be fatal.

Potentiated Effect

Potentiation best describes an interaction in which the effect of only one of the two drugs is increased. In other words, a drug that has a mild effect enhances the effect of a second drug. As an equation, this concept would be represented as ½ (Drug A) + 1 (Drug B) = 2. For example, when the antiemetic drug hydroxyzine, which has some CNS depressant effects and produces mild analgesic effects, is combined with a narcotic analgesic such as morphine, the pain-relieving ability of the morphine is increased without increasing the dose of the morphine.

Antagonistic Effect

An **antagonistic drug interaction** is the opposite of a synergistic effect. It results in a therapeutic effect that is less than the effect of either drug alone because the second drug either diminishes or cancels the effects of the first drug. As an equation, this concept would be expressed as: 1 (Drug A) + 1 (Drug B) = 0. For example, when the heparin antagonist protamine sulfate (a strong basic anticoagulant) is given as an antidote for heparin (a strong acidic anticoagulant) to halt heparin-induced bleeding, a stable salt forms, resulting in a loss of anticoagulant activity for both drugs. Antagonistic interactions can also occur at receptor sites when one drug is an agonist and the other drug is an antagonist for the same receptor, such as with morphine, a narcotic agonist, and naloxone, a narcotic antagonist used to correct narcotic overdosage.

DRUG INCOMPATIBILITIES

Drug incompatibilities are similar to drug–drug interactions in that a chemical inactivation or physical reaction occurs. This reaction may involve two or more drugs, inside the body or outside, before they are administered. While administering drugs parenterally (intravenously, intramuscularly, or subcutaneously), the nurse is especially alert to the possibility of drug incompatibilities and drug interactions. The most common kinds of incompatibilities are chemical and physical.

Chemical Incompatibilities

Chemical incompatibilities between drugs change both the drug's structure and its pharmacologic properties. The alteration may be beneficial. For example, heparin and protamine sulfate (a heparin antagonist) form an ionic bond that lacks any anticoagulant activity. Conversely, the chemical incompatibility may also be harmful; for example, combining multivitamins and antibiotics in the same intravenous (IV) solution changes the solution's pH and inactivates the antibiotic.

Physical Incompatibilities

Physical incompatibilities occur when two drugs are mixed together. The mixture results in the formation of a precipitate. Phenytoin and a diluent containing dextrose, for example, produce a cloudy, white precipitate. This kind of reaction usually interferes with the pharmacologic activity of one or both drugs.

This is one of the reasons that manufacturers provide specific instructions for preparation, dilution, and addition of drugs to other solutions. These instructions should be followed carefully.

IMPLICATIONS FOR NURSING MANAGEMENT

When administering drug therapy, the nurse's main focus is on ensuring a beneficial outcome by maximizing therapeutic effects, minimizing adverse effects and drug interactions, and providing appropriate drug education for the patient and family. Beneficial outcomes are achieved by relating core drug knowledge to core patient variables throughout the nursing process. Understanding how core drug knowledge and core patient variables interact to affect outcome is important because these interactions may predispose the patient to adverse effects from drug therapy.

Nursing Management of the Patient Receiving Drug Therapy
Assessment of Core Patient Variables
Health Status
Concurrent medical conditions may increase the risk for adverse effects from drug therapy. For example, if a patient has diminished renal function and then takes a drug that may cause nephrotoxicity, the patient is more likely to develop adverse effects, even with a therapeutic dose. A patient's chronic health condition may also necessitate drug therapy that may interact with other drug therapy or promote adverse effects. For example, a patient with AIDS may be taking drug therapy that carries the risk for hepatotoxicity. If this patient develops tuberculosis, he or she will need to take additional drug therapy, which also may cause hepatotoxicity.

Life Span and Gender
A patient's age can greatly increase the risk for adverse effects from drug therapy. The liver and kidneys of both young children and older adults do not function as well as those of young adults. As a result, those populations are at increased risk for adverse effects and drug interactions. In addition, older adults are more likely to be receiving polypharmacy for multiple chronic illnesses and thus are more likely to experience drug interactions.

In some drug therapy women are known to have more significant adverse effects than men. This may be related to a sex difference in pharmacokinetics (including P-450 differences), pharmacodynamics, or even the dose concentration within the body. This is because the dose of most drugs are not based on weight; when men and women receive the same dose of a drug the circulating concentration of a drug will be less in men because men generally weigh more than women (Anderson, 2008). The P-450 system is altered with pregnancy; CYP1A2 activity is decreased and CYP2D6 and CYP3A activities are increased during pregnancy. The nurse should assess how any drug therapy received by a pregnant woman is metabolized. Drugs that are metabolized via these pathways may need dosage adjustments by the physician (Tracy et al. 2005). Adverse effects from drug therapy taken by a pregnant woman may affect the unborn child. Many drugs can also be passed in breast milk, causing adverse effects in the infant. Life span issues are discussed in more detail in Chapters 6, 7, and 8.

Lifestyle, Diet, and Habits
What and when a patient eats and drinks and the patient's various habits and choices (e.g., the use of tobacco, alcohol, caffeine, street drugs, or over-the-counter herbs and botanicals) may influence the effects of drug therapy, either positively or negatively. For this reason, remember to ask patients about diet and other habits when performing a drug history or when providing patient education on prescribed drug therapy. Then inform patients about possible interactions and describe how to maximize therapeutic effects or prevent or minimize adverse effects and drug interactions. (For more information on how lifestyle, diet, and habits influence drug therapy, see Chapters 9 and 10.)

Environment
The patient's environment may increase the likelihood that a certain adverse effect will occur. For instance, some antibiotics can cause the adverse effect of photosensitivity. Even brief exposure to sunlight or strong ultraviolet light can cause severe sunburn, hives, or a rash. Other drugs (e.g., anticholinergics, belladonna alkaloids) reduce the body's tolerance to heat or inhibit the body's ability to reduce temperature by perspiration. These types of drugs may make the patient vulnerable to heat stroke in hot weather or during exercise.

The environment in which drug therapy is administered can also play a role in the early detection of adverse effects. For example, a critically ill patient receives drug therapy under close supervision, which could lead to early detection of any adverse effects. However, a person who is receiving drug therapy in a community setting may be more at risk for adverse effects because the early signs of the adverse effect may not be identified as easily as they would be in a clinical setting. The relationship of environment to drug therapy is discussed in more detail in Chapter 11.

Culture and Inherited Traits
Researchers are beginning to study responses to drug therapy that are genetically determined in various ethnic and racial populations. These responses may place the patient at greater risk for adverse effects or drug interactions than the rest of the global population. Box 5.3 describes one study that focused on the metabolic activity of the P-450 system in Caucasian, African American, and Hispanic men and women. Culture and inherited traits and the ways that they influence drug therapy are discussed in more detail in Chapter 12.

Nursing Diagnoses and Outcomes
Nursing diagnoses are related to specific adverse effects of the ordered drug therapy and to drug interactions. Outcomes

BOX 5.2 FOCUS ON RESEARCH

Moving Research Findings Into Clinical Practice

Sanderson S, Emery J, Higgins J. (2005). CYP2C9 gene variants, drug dose, and bleeding risk in warfarin-treated patients: A HuGEnet™ systemic review and meta-analysis. *Genetics in Medicine: Official Journal of the American College of Medical Genetics,*7:97–104.
FDA News. August 16, 2007 FDA Approves Updated Warfarin (Coumadin) Prescribing Information *New Genetic Information May Help Providers Improve Initial Dosing Estimates of the Anticoagulant for Individual Patients*
http://www.fda.gov/bbs/topics/NEWS/2007/NEW01684.html

The Study

It has been known for years that getting the correct dose of the anticoagulant drug warfarin can be difficult in many people and many people suffer with significant bleeding from warfarin therapy. These problems are related to changes in the metabolism of warfarin via CYP 2C9. One-third of patients receiving warfarin metabolize it quite differently than expected. Research has shown that some of the unexpected response to warfarin depends on a patient's variants of the genes CYP2C9. A systematic review of clinical trials examining two variant allelels of CYP 2C9 and the consequent effect on warfarin metabolism was conducted. Nine studies (2,775 patients) were included in the meta- analysis. Twenty percent of the patients carried a genetic variation on CYP2C9. These patients required a mean reduction of 27% in the dose of warfarin from "standard doses" to achieve therapeutic effects without adverse effects (such as serious bleeding). Patients with genetic variations of CYP2C9 had a higher relative risk for bleeding than patients without the genetic variation.

Nursing Implications

In 2007 the US Food and Drug Administration modified the label of warfarin to highlight these findings, and other research findings relative to genetic variation increasing the risk of adverse effects from warfarin in patients. This relabeling was unique in emphasizing how genetic variation of a P450 isoenzyme alters patient response to therapy and should be considered when starting warfarin therapy. Currently, FDA sponsored research is still underway to determine which patients would most benefit from genetic testing, and if a dosing algorithm can be devised to decrease unintentional bleeding while still achieving therapeutic effectiveness. In the near future it is likely that nurses will play a role in genetic testing of patients and may need to confirm that genetic testing has been accomplished prior to starting a patient on warfarin therapy.

---

are directed at preventing or minimizing either occurrence without harm to the patient. Some examples include the following:

- Risk for Infection related to drug-induced myelosuppression
  Desired outcome: The patient will not develop infection while on drug therapy.
- Imbalanced Nutrition: Less Than Body Requirements, related to drug-induced nausea, vomiting, anorexia, stomatitis
  Desired outcome: Despite adverse effects, the patient will receive enough nourishment to meet physiologic needs.
- Risk for Poisoning (Toxicity) related to use of drug with a narrow therapeutic index
  Desired outcome: The patient will receive drug therapy without harmful or poisonous effects.

Planning and Intervention

Maximizing Therapeutic Effects

When drug interactions are intentional and desirable, it is important to give the drugs at the prescribed time intervals. They should be administered at the same time if necessary to achieve the interaction. When drug interactions are not desired but both drugs are needed for therapy, the doses must be administered at different times to promote the therapeutic effect of each drug.

Minimizing Adverse Effects

To help protect the patient from serious adverse effects and drug interactions, obtain a drug history from the patient, beginning with a list of all drugs that the patient has taken. Drug references or databases may then be consulted for complete descriptions of known or suspected drug interactions.

If a patient is taking a drug that may interact in the GI tract (including P-450 interaction from grapefruit juice) with another drug in the current regimen, the drugs should not be coadministered but their administration times should be staggered. If that is not sufficient to minimize an interaction contact the prescriber about changing one of the ordered drugs. If the drug interaction occurs systemically (such as in the P-450 system in the liver) staggering the doses will not be sufficient. Contact the prescriber about possibly changing one of the ordered drugs: sometimes a different drug in the same drug class does not pose the interaction. If both drugs are required, additional monitoring of the patient or dose adjustment of one of the drugs may be warranted. If the interaction is potentially serious, the prescriber should be consulted before you or the patient begins administering the new drug. When a patient is receiving two or more drugs and either unexpected effects or no therapeutic effects occur, you should suspect that a drug interaction may have occurred and investigate fully.

If administering two or more medications parenterally, check the label information for drug compatibility to determine if the same IV tubing or syringe can be used for both medications. Do not check for drug interactions on the label as this is referring to systemic interactions (e.g, via the P-450 system).

Throughout therapy, monitor the patient for signs and symptoms of interactions and adverse effects and for alterations in health status that increase the risk for adverse effects. If a drug interaction is known to increase or decrease the circulating level of one of the drugs, serum drug levels are monitored to determine whether therapeutic levels are being maintained.

Providing Patient and Family Education

Before and throughout drug therapy, inform the patient and family about adverse effects and drug interactions. Initial instruction includes teaching the patient how to minimize the occurrence of these effects and how to cope with them. In addition, teach the patient which effects to expect, which to report to the prescriber, and which require immediate medical attention.

SUSPECTED ADVERSE EFFECTS

You are a nurse working in an emergency room of a community hospital. A patient with diabetes is brought in with complaints of nausea and abdominal pain. On physical assessment, she is found to have an enlarged, tender liver. Her liver enzymes are substantially elevated. She is to be hospitalized. During your assessment, you learn that the patient was started on a newly approved drug for her diabetes 3 months ago.

1. How would you determine whether her symptoms were known adverse effects from the drug therapy?

2. You determine that her symptoms are not listed as known adverse effects, but you still feel concerned that they may be related to her drug therapy. What action would be appropriate based on your suspicion?

Ongoing Assessment and Evaluation

During drug therapy, continue to monitor for adverse effects and drug interactions, including allergic responses. Also consider the possibility of a drug interaction each time a new drug is added to the treatment plan. If none of these effects occurs and the therapeutic effect has been achieved, drug therapy is evaluated as successful.

CHAPTER SUMMARY

- Adverse effects are all unintended effects of drug therapy. All drugs have adverse effects. Adverse effects may be very mild and merely bothersome or serious and life threatening.

- Adverse effects are usually predictable or dose related. Adverse effects that are not predictable or dose related are attributable to allergic responses or idiosyncratic responses. The most serious allergic response is called anaphylaxis, which can be fatal if not treated.

- Adverse effects that carry the risk for permanent damage or death and form specific patterns or groups of symptoms related to drug therapy are called toxicities. The major drug toxicities are hepatotoxicity, nephrotoxicity, neurotoxicity, cardiotoxicity, ototoxicity, and immunotoxicity.

- Drug interactions occur between two drugs or a drug and food or another substance, such as alcohol. Some drug interactions are beneficial, whereas others are harmful.

- Drug interactions may affect any aspect of pharmacokinetics: absorption, distribution, metabolism, or excretion.

- An important and common drug interaction is one that alters the metabolism of a drug by either inducing or inhibiting the P-450 system. Drug–drug interactions usually alter the P-450 system in the liver, whereas interactions between drugs and grapefruit juice primarily alter the P-450 enzymes in the GI tract.

- Drug interactions may also alter the pharmacodynamics of drug therapy. Two or more drugs may compete for the same receptor site, or they may work in different ways in the body with conflicting or cumulative results. Drugs that act in different ways, or at different receptors, may create an additive effect, a synergistic effect, a potentiated effect, or an antagonistic effect.

- Nurses must understand the core drug knowledge of adverse effects and drug interactions because these phenomena interact with the core patient variables during drug therapy. Recognizing the potential for these interactions allows the nurse to plan care in a way that will maximize the therapeutic effects, minimize the adverse effects, and provide effective patient and family education.

QUESTIONS FOR STUDY AND REVIEW

1. You are assessing a patient's drug history. The patient tells you that she is allergic to a particular drug. List the symptoms that would indicate that the response was a true allergic response and not an adverse effect of drug therapy.

2. Your patient is 75 years old and is receiving a drug that may cause ototoxicity. Describe why it may be difficult to determine whether adverse effects are occurring.

3. Your patient is receiving two drugs. Drug A is metabolized by the CYP3A4 hepatic system. Drug B induces the CYP3A4 hepatic system. What effect will Drug B have on the circulating blood level of Drug A?

4. Two patients each receive the same dose of the same drug that is metabolized in the GI tract by the CYP3A4 system. Each patient drinks a glass of grapefruit juice. Will the effect of the grapefruit juice on circulating drug levels be identical in both patients? Why or why not?

5. Describe why hepatotoxic drugs may produce more liver damage when given orally than when given parenterally.

6. Your patient receives three different drugs that all produce CNS depression. Explain what effect this combination will have on the pharmacodynamics of these drugs.

7. Your patient has been on Drug A to lower his blood pressure and has been obtaining a therapeutic effect from the drug. The patient's blood pressure has been in a normal range for several days. Then, the patient develops an infection and is started on Drug B. Within 24 hours, the patient is hypertensive again. What assessment would you make?

NEED MORE HELP?

Chapter 5 of the Study Guide to Accompany *Drug Therapy in Nursing*, 4th Edition, contains NCLEX-style questions and other learning activities to reinforce your understanding of the concepts presented in this chapter. For additional information or to purchase the study guide, visit thePoint.

REFERENCES

Anderson, G. D. (2008). Gender differences in pharmacological response. *International Review of Neurobiology*, 83:1–10.

Bernard, S., Neville, K. A., Nguyen, A. T., & Flockhart, D. A. (2006). Interethnic differences in genetic polymorphisms of CYP2D6 in the U.S. population: clinical implications. *The Oncologist*, 11(2):126–135.

Ginsberg, G., Hattis, D., Russ, A., & Sonawane, B. (2005). Pharmacokinetic and pharmacodynamic factors that can affect sensitivity to neurotoxic sequelae in elderly individuals. *Environmental Health Perspectives*, 113(9):1243–1249.

Pestka, E. L., Hale, A. M., Johnson, B. L., Lee, J. L., & Poppe, K. A. (2007). Cytochrome P450 testing for better psychiatric care. *Journal of Psychosocial Nursing*, 45(10):15–18.

Mulder, H., Heerdink, E., Iersel, E. E., Wilmink, F. W., & Egberts, A. C. G. (2007). Prevalence of patients using drugs metabolized by cytochrome P450 in different populations: a cross-sectional study. *The Annals of Pharmacotherapy*, 41:408–413.

Tracy, T. S., Venkataramanan, R., Glover, D. G., & Caritis, S. N. (2005). Temporal changes in drug metabolism (CYP1A2, CYP2D6 and CYP 3A activity) during pregnancy. *American Journal of Obstetrics and Gynecology*, 192:633–639.

U.S. Food and Drug Administration. MedWatch website. Retrieved from *www.fda.gov/medwatch*. *http://www.fda.gov/medwaTCH/report/DESK/advevnt.htm* on March 18, 2009.

UNIT 3
Core Patient Variables

Life Span: Children

Learning Objectives

At the completion of this chapter the student will:

1. Identify key areas of core drug knowledge for children that differ from those for adults.

2. Explain why calculating drug dosages for children is different from calculating dosages for adults.

3. Describe methods for calculating dosages for children of different ages.

4. Identify key core patient variables for children and explain how they differ from those for adults when considering drug therapy.

5. Discuss key developmental variables for each of the pediatric age groups (infant, toddler, preschooler, school-aged, and adolescent) that affect how the nurse administers drug therapy.

6. Propose some common nursing diagnoses related to drug therapy in children.

7. Describe key nursing interventions to promote maximal therapeutic effects and minimal adverse effects during pediatric drug therapy.

8. Identify key points to include in educating patients and families about pediatric drug therapy.

Key Terms   body surface area   nomogram   play therapy
                kernicterus   pediatric patient

When implementing pediatric drug therapy, the nurse must remember that children are different from adults in many ways. Although some drugs and administration routes are similar in adults and children, the nursing management of drug therapy varies greatly. For example, physiologic differences in children and the child's immature body systems, greater fluid composition, and smaller size all affect the core drug knowledge. These differences can exaggerate or diminish the pediatric patient's response to drug therapy, making some drug actions and outcomes less predictable in the child than in the adult.

Additionally, in children, core patient variables differ from those in adult patients and from child to child because of the differences across the developmental stages of childhood. The **pediatric patient** is usually defined as younger than 16 years and weighing less than 50 kilograms.

This chapter focuses on core drug knowledge that is relevant and unique to pediatric patients and on core patient variables that emphasize children's needs according to developmental changes. Special issues in managing pediatric drug therapy are explored, including maximizing therapeutic effects, minimizing adverse effects, and educating patients and families.

Nursing Management of the Pediatric Patient
Core Drug Knowledge Related to Children
Pharmacotherapeutics
Therapeutic indications and effects for many drugs are similar for children and adults. Not all drugs that are labeled as safe

for adults, however, have been labeled as safe for children; of all approved drugs, only about 20% are approved for pediatric use (Luo et al., 2007). One reason for this is that few drugs have been adequately tested in clinical trials on pediatric patients. Historically, it was considered unethical to enroll children in randomized, controlled drug studies. Because drugs in development were not tested on children, they were not labeled as approved for use in children. As a result, pediatricians must often prescribe medications for off-label uses in children (Aschenbrenner, 2006). An off-label use is when a drug is used for a purpose not clearly stated on its label but the prescriber has reason to believe the drug will produce the desired therapeutic effect (see Chapter 4 for a complete discussion of off-label use of drugs). A recent study of hospitalized children found that at least one drug was used off label in almost 79% of these patients (Shah et al., 2007).

Compounding this problem of off-label uses was a lack of financial incentives for drug manufacturers to retest drugs already on the market to obtain approval for use in children. In recent years, however, the thinking has changed so that it is now considered unethical to *exclude* children from drug studies and not to include child-specific prescribing information on labels for drugs used in children. To meet this need, the United States Congress passed the Best Pharmaceuticals for Children Act in 2001; this Act was reauthorized in 2007 (Aschenbrenner, 2006). This act provides several avenues for drugs already on the market to

---

Box 6.1 CALCULATING PEDIATRIC DRUG DOSAGES

Body Surface Area Method

Step 1. Determine the body surface area (BSA) of the child. It is measured in meters squared. A standard formula is used. Computations should be made with a calculator.

$$BSA = \sqrt{\frac{Weight\ in\ kg \times Height\ in\ cm}{3,600}}$$

Example: Child weighs 10 kg and is 45 cm tall

1. Multiply weight in kilograms by height in centimeters.

$$BSA = \frac{10 \times 45}{3,600}$$

2. Divide product by 3,600.

$$= \frac{450}{3,600}$$

3. Enter square root sign on calculator.

$$= \sqrt{0.125}$$

4. Round the BSA to the nearest hundredth.

$$= 0.35\ m^2$$

Step 2. Determine dose using the computed BSA and this formula:

$$\frac{Child's\ BSA}{1.7\ m^2\ (average\ adult\ BSA)} \times Usual\ adult\ dose = Child's\ dose$$

Example: Child's BSA = 0.35 m², and usual adult dose is 100 mg.

$$= \frac{0.35\ m^2}{1.7\ m^2} \times 100$$

$$= 20.588\ (20.59)\ mg\ is\ child's\ dose.$$

Body Weight Method

Usual dose (in mg): 1 kg :: needed dose (in mg): weight of child in kg, solve for the needed dose

Example:

Usual dose is 10 mg/1 kg and child weighs 18 kg

$10\ mg : 1\ kg :: \chi\ mg : 18\ kg \quad \chi = 180\ mg$

be tested in clinical drug trials in children. Labeling changes are occurring based on findings from these new studies. At the end of December 2008, 159 drugs had been tested for use in children and been relabeled. The list of the drugs that have been studied for use in children and the summaries of medical and clinical pharmacology reviews is available on the FDA website (http://www.fda.gov/cder/pediatric/label-change.htm). Until all drugs have been tested and labeled for use in children, nurses need to be aware that off-label use will occur. When a drug is prescribed off-label, the full therapeutic and adverse effects, as well as appropriate dosing, may be unknown.

Even when a drug has the same labeled therapeutic uses in adult and children, a major difference is the appropriate drug dosage for different age groups. Committing drug dosages to memory is difficult and unnecessary because child weights vary considerably. Unlike most adult drug dosages, almost all pediatric drug dosages are based on the weight of the child in kilograms. Dosage is usually specified in milligrams of drug per kilogram of body weight (mg/kg).

When a child dose is not specified, it can be determined from the adult dose based on the body surface area of the child. The **body surface area** is the external surface of the body expressed in square meters. The ratio of body surface area to weight is inversely proportional to length; therefore, the infant or young child who is shorter and weighs less than the adult has relatively greater surface area than would be expected from the weight. Body surface area is calculated using a standard formula, found in Box 6.1.

Body surface area can also be determined by using a nomogram (Figure 6.1). A **nomogram** is a chart or a graph that shows relationships between numerical variables. A representative nomogram used to estimate body surface area in children may have several columns of calibrated measures representing height, surface area, and weight. Body surface area is calculated by drawing a line across the columns to connect the patient's height with the patient's weight. The point at which the line intersects the central surface area column is the patient's *estimated* body surface area. Using a nomogram is less accurate than using the formula to determine body surface area.

Once body surface area is determined, the dosage can be computed using the formula in Box 6.1. A child's drug dosage may also be determined by comparing the child's weight to the recommended dose per kilograms of weight. Administering the correct drug dosage is crucial in pediatric drug therapy. The child's small and immature body systems make overdosages potentially lethal. Drugs with high potential for toxicity, such as anticancer drugs, are more likely to have their dosage determined by body surface area than by only the weight of the child.

Pharmacodynamics

A drug's mechanism of action is the same in all individuals at all ages. However, what distinguishes individual responses is the ability of the organ systems to function

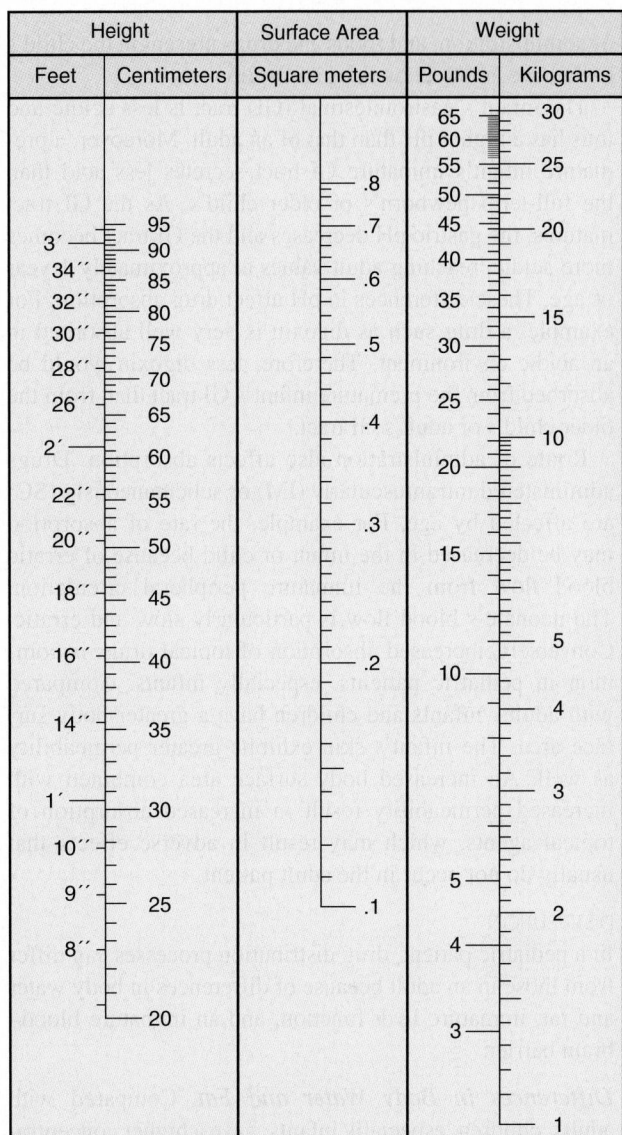

Height		Surface Area	Weight	
Feet	Centimeters	Square meters	Pounds	Kilograms

• FIGURE 6.1 A pediatric nomogram is a device for estimating body surface area in children. To use it, draw a line from the child's height to the child's weight. The point at which this line intersects the surface area in the middle is the child's estimated body surface area.

fully and appropriately. In very young children, immature organ systems have less than optimal functioning, which may necessitate increasing or decreasing drug doses to prevent toxicity and to achieve a therapeutic drug level.

Pharmacokinetics

A child's age, growth, and maturation can affect how the body absorbs, distributes, metabolizes, and excretes a drug. By understanding how drugs affect pediatric patients differently from adult patients, the nurse can help maximize the therapeutic effects of a drug and minimize adverse effects. Dosages must often be lowered to account for immature or impaired body systems in neonates and infants.

ABSORPTION

Absorption of a drug depends on various factors. In the pediatric patient, age, disease process, dosage form, route of administration, and foods and drugs present in the child's body have an effect on drug absorption.

The infant's gastrointestinal (GI) tract is less acidic and thus has a higher pH than that of an adult. Moreover, a premature infant's immature GI tract secretes less acid than the full-term newborn's or older child's. As the GI tract matures, the gastric pH decreases and the GI tract becomes more acidic, reaching adult values at approximately 1 year of age. These differences in pH affect drug absorption. For example, a drug such as digoxin is very well absorbed in an acidic environment. Therefore, less digoxin would be absorbed from the premature infant's GI tract than from the older child's or adult's GI tract.

Route of administration also affects absorption. Drugs administered intramuscularly (IM) or subcutaneously (SC) are affected by age. For example, the rate of absorption may be decreased in the infant or child because of erratic blood flow from the immature peripheral circulation. The neonate's blood flow is particularly slow and erratic. Conversely, increased absorption of topical drugs is common in pediatric patients, especially infants. Compared with adults, infants and children have a greater body surface area. The infant's skin exhibits greater permeability as well. An increased body surface area combined with increased permeability result in increased absorption of topical agents, which may result in adverse effects that usually do not occur in the adult patient.

DISTRIBUTION

In a pediatric patient, drug distribution processes can differ from those in an adult because of differences in body water and fat, immature liver function, and an immature blood–brain barrier.

Differences in Body Water and Fat. Compared with adults, children, especially infants, have a higher concentration of water in their bodies and a lower concentration of fat. Newborns have the greatest proportional water content, followed by infants, children, and then adults (Table 6.1). Because infants and children have a greater proportion of body water, water-soluble drugs are diluted to a greater degree, and for this reason, it is important to assess the amount of water in the body of an infant or child before administering water-soluble drugs. The drug moves to areas of water throughout the body, not just in the blood, resulting

in lower concentrations of the drug in the blood. With drugs such as gentamicin, proportionately increased dosages may be required to achieve or maintain therapeutic levels.

To a lesser degree, fat-soluble drugs are affected by the proportionately lower fat in the infant and child. Fat distribution increases with age; thus, fat-soluble drugs are distributed to a greater degree in the adult. Because fat-soluble drugs are not widely distributed in the infant's or child's body, greater blood concentrations may result, leading to toxicity.

Immature Liver Function. In the infant and especially in the neonate, immature liver function affects drug distribution. The neonate's immature liver produces fewer plasma proteins, especially albumin; acidic drugs bind strongly to albumin. Pharmacologic effects of drugs result from unbound (i.e., free) drug. In the neonate and infant, more free drug is available because less drug is bound to plasma proteins. The result is increased blood levels of drugs, which in turn can cause greater adverse effects and toxicity in infants. Drug binding to serum proteins reaches adult levels by 6 months of age.

Multiple drugs administered to an infant may compete for the same binding sites, resulting in higher blood concentrations of both drugs or of the drug with less affinity for the binding site. Other naturally occurring substances in the body can also compete for fewer binding sites in the pediatric patient. For example, bilirubin, which may increase during the neonatal period, binds with plasma proteins. When a sulfonamide is administered to the neonate who has an increased bilirubin level, it competes with bilirubin for binding sites, leaving more bilirubin free in the blood. Rarely, the bilirubin level can increase to a dangerous level, resulting in bilirubin accumulation in the central nervous system (CNS), a life-threatening condition called **kernicterus.**

Immature Blood–Brain Barrier. The blood–brain barrier prevents drugs in the general circulation from passing to the circulation of the brain, thereby protecting the brain from toxic substances. At birth, the blood–brain barrier is not fully developed. Therefore, newborns are particularly vulnerable to CNS toxicity. In the newborn, the effect of drugs that act on the CNS (e.g., phenobarbital and morphine) is intensified. In addition, infants experience exaggerated CNS responses to other drugs targeted for other body systems.

METABOLISM

The liver metabolizes most drugs. However, the immaturity of the neonatal and infant liver results in decreased or incomplete metabolism of many drugs, which may necessitate lower drug dosages or an increased interval between doses to achieve appropriate blood levels. In children with liver disease, drug metabolism is further complicated by the liver's inability to detoxify drugs. A child with an immature liver or compromised liver function is at risk for drug toxicity.

Drugs requiring oxidation for metabolism are frequently more rapidly metabolized in children than in adults because

TABLE 6.1	Proportional Water Content Across the Life Span
Age	**Percentage of Body Water**
Newborn	75%–85%
Infant	Approximately 85%
One year old	65%
Two years old	60%
Adult	50%–60%

children have a faster resting respiratory rate. These drugs include phenobarbital, phenytoin, and the methylxanthines (e.g., theophylline and caffeine). With these types of drugs, children may require higher dosages or more frequent administration schedules than adults do to maintain therapeutic blood levels.

EXCRETION

Most drugs are eliminated from the body through the urine. Drug elimination requires a functioning renal system, and its effectiveness depends on glomerular filtration rate, tubular reabsorption, and maturity of the renal system. In children with impaired renal function, drug dosages should be altered to achieve and maintain therapeutic drug levels.

The neonate, especially the preterm infant, has immature kidneys, and renal excretion of drugs is slow. Drug dosages and therapeutic drug levels must therefore be monitored closely to prevent toxicity. In addition, the reduced glomerular filtration rate and decreased tubular secretion and reabsorption during the first 6 months of life extend the half-life of many drugs (e.g., penicillins, sulfonamides, and cephalosporins). Drugs with a narrow margin between effective and toxic doses must be administered at longer dosage intervals to prevent toxicity. At about 3 months of age, the infant's kidneys can concentrate urine at the adult level, but urinary excretion remains low until the child is about 30 months old, when the kidneys become functionally mature.

A few drugs are excreted through the biliary tree into the intestinal tract. Biliary blood flow is decreased during the first few days of life, during which careful monitoring of drug levels and signs and symptoms of toxicity is imperative.

Contraindications and Precautions

As stated above, most drugs prescribed to children are prescribed off-label and have never been clinically tested for efficacy, unique pharmacokinetics, or adverse effects in children. Off-label usage therefore requires cautious administration and careful, frequent assessments of the child. Some drugs are known to be dangerous in children and are labeled as such; these drugs are contraindicated. The core drug knowledge must be determined for each drug before the drug can be administered to a child.

Adverse Effects and Drug Interactions

Adverse effects of some drugs are more severe and more likely to occur in children because of the immature body systems of children. Newborns and young children may experience serious adverse effects either from direct administration of a drug or through their mother's use of a medication. In a review of adverse effects in infants and children younger than 2 years that were reported to the United States Food and Drug Administration (FDA) between 1997 and 2000, approximately 3.5% of the adverse effects accounted for half of the reported deaths in children. About one fourth of the total adverse effects reported were related to exposure from the mother during pregnancy, delivery, or lactation (Moore et al., 2002).

Other adverse effects on body systems occur only at specific phases of development. For example, tetracycline administered to a child between the ages of 4 months and 8 years will stain the permanent teeth. Glucocorticoids given to a child of any age will suppress growth if the child has not matured to full adult size. Drug receptor sensitivity varies with age; it may be increased or decreased for certain drugs. This variability may promote adverse effects and may necessitate lower or higher drug dosages than would normally be expected (see Chapter 5).

Drug interactions in children are similar to those occurring in adults.

Assessment of Core Patient Variables Related to Children

Health Status

A child's disease process can affect absorption of drugs from the GI tract. Diarrhea, for example, decreases intestinal transit time and therefore decreases the time available for drug absorption. Children with hepatic or renal disease cannot metabolize or excrete drugs as easily as other children and are more prone to adverse effects from drugs. As with adults, any chronic disease or condition may alter the effects of certain drugs and must be seriously considered in drug therapy.

Life Span

Always consider the developmental stage of the pediatric patient. In planning appropriate drug administration methods, explain the treatment and enlist the child's cooperation. If doing so is not possible, seek appropriate assistance to administer the drug therapy safely. Developmental considerations are especially important when communicating with the child. To elicit cooperation and obtain necessary information, communication must be at an appropriate level of understanding for the child. The following are age-appropriate considerations in administering drugs to infants and children. Box 6.2 provides more information regarding pediatric drug routes.

INFANTS (BIRTH TO 12 MONTHS)

Some infants with a well-developed sucking reflex may willingly swallow a pleasant-tasting liquid drug through a bottle nipple. Other babies may spit out oral medicine, making it difficult to administer a full dose. Administer infant drops by gently squeezing the child's cheeks to open the mouth, and then placing the drops in the buccal pouch to ensure they will be swallowed. Drugs may be given to infants in rectal

CRITICAL THINKING SCENARIO

CALLING ON CORE DRUG KNOWLEDGE FOR CHILDREN

You are caring for a premature newborn in the nursery. The newborn is receiving intravenous antibiotic therapy to treat an infection. Which specific aspects of core drug knowledge do you think will most help you anticipate any adverse effects of drug therapy?

Box 6.2 SPECIAL PRECAUTIONS FOR PEDIATRIC DRUG ROUTES

One way to promote a good outcome when administering drug therapy is to call on your knowledge of normal growth and development in children and your knowledge of safe administration techniques for specific routes.

Oral Route

- Drug volume should not exceed that which can be swallowed by a very small mouth. The drug dose should be mixed in a small amount of liquid so all of the dose is taken.
- Avoid adding a drug dose to formula. The infant may refuse future feedings because of the foul taste.
- Balance dosage schedules with feeding schedules. Consider whether the drug should be given with meals or on an empty stomach. Check for the possibility of a food-drug interaction.

Intramuscular Route

- Assess whether a less painful route is possible.
- If the IM route is unavoidable, apply a topical, local anesthetic, such as a lidocaine and prilocaine combination (EMLA cream), to numb the injection site.
- Locate anatomic landmarks and boundaries of injection sites.
- Evaluate muscle mass, skin condition, and potential complications related to the child's diagnosis.

- Rotate injection sites as needed, and use appropriate equipment and techniques.
- Seek help to hold the child still while administering the IM injection.

Intravenous Route

- Minimize initial pain on starting the IV by applying a topical anesthetic.
- Check the IV insertion site hourly for infiltration in infants and children.
- Monitor fluid status for signs of overload (risk is greatest in neonates and young infants because of their immature kidney function).
- Double check dosage calculations with another nurse.
- Control the IV infusion rate by using either a volumetric pumps with a microdrip calibrated chamber or a syringe pump. If the infusion pump is one of the new "smart" pumps (i.e., containing computer software that includes specific drug information and policies and procedures related to administering that particular drug) do not "work around" or turn off the safety features.
- Supply no more than 1 hour's worth of fluid when administering a continuous IV drip with an infusion pump (in case the pump malfunctions).
- Engage the lock feature on a volumetric pump to prevent unauthorized changes in the drop rate.

---

suppository form if necessary. However, to avoid expulsion of the suppository before the drug is absorbed, you may need to hold the child's buttocks together for a short time.

If the IM route must be used, choose the smallest gauge of needle appropriate for the drug. The preferred injection site for infants and children up to age 3 years is the vastus lateralis. This muscle is on the side of the thigh in the upper outer quadrant of the area between the greater trochanter and the knee. The vastus lateralis has few nerves and blood vessels and forms the largest muscle mass in this age group.

Normally, a ⅜-inch needle is used for the vastus lateralis in infants; if one is not available, a needle no larger than ⅝ inch should be used. With the longer needle, modify the angle of injection from the usual 90 degrees to 45 degrees toward the frontal plane of the knee. The 45-degree angle ensures that the needle does not traverse the blood vessel.

The rectus femoris is another possible injection site. This muscle is located near the vastus lateralis but is anterior mid-thigh; inject the needle at a 90-degree angle at this site.

In infants, neither the deltoid nor the dorsogluteal muscle site is used because the muscle masses are too small and undeveloped. The ventrogluteal muscle site, which is large at birth, is not recommended for use in infants because problems encountered in positioning the child make it difficult to locate the muscle site accurately.

Drugs may be administered intravenously to the infant through a peripheral site. These intravenous (IV) sites differ from those used for adults. Ideally, select a site that is easy to access and that poses the least risk to the patient. In the neonate and infant, the scalp's many superficial veins offer easy access. The superficial temporal vein just

in front of the pinna of the ear and the metopic vein in the middle of the forehead are relatively easy to find and are less risky for patients (Figure 6.2). Other suitable IV sites for infants and older children include the vessels in the nondominant hand, forearm, upper arm, feet, and antecubital fossa. Distal IV sites are used first and are moved proximally as necessary. The feet also provide good IV sites and are used in infants.

TODDLERS (13 MONTHS TO 3 YEARS)

Toddlers can swallow liquid forms of drugs, and older toddlers can chew oral drugs. Because toddlers experience

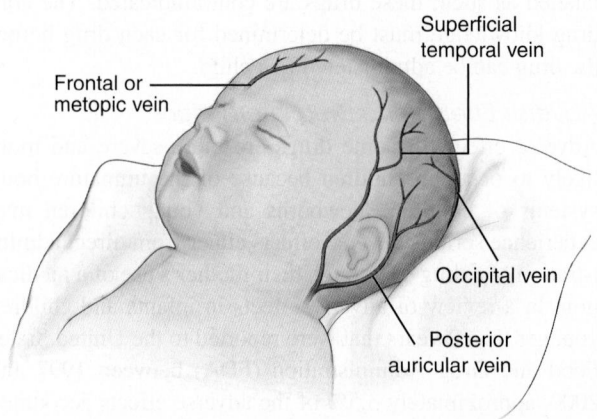

• FIGURE 6.2 The scalp is an excellent site for intravenous (IV) therapy in the neonate and infant. The superficial temporal vein and the metopic vein in the central forehead are the preferred sites because they are easy to find and reasonably safe.

anxiety when separated from their parents, having a parent nearby usually helps the child's cooperation during drug therapy. Attempt to elicit cooperation from the toddler but be prepared for the toddler to resist. A toddler's resistance may be associated with a past experience, such as unpleasantly flavored drugs or a painful injection.

Toddlers are also likely to be anxious or uncooperative during administration of rectal suppositories because of their experiences with toilet training and sphincter control. Toddlers have vivid imaginations but limited understanding of how the body works. A common fear is that important body contents will leak out from an injection site. As with infants, the vastus lateralis and rectus femoris remain the IM injection sites of choice for toddlers.

When IV drug therapy is necessary for toddlers, the scalp veins are still appropriate and can be used up to age 18 months. By this time, hair follicles mature and skin layers thicken, making IV access more difficult. Although the scalp provides excellent IV access, it is not the first choice because of the anxiety it causes parents. Parents feel uneasy because of the scalp's close proximity to the brain and because the area must be shaved at the IV site. If a scalp vein must be used and the site shaved, ask the parents whether they would like to save the hair, and collect it for them if desired. Saving their child's hair makes the procedure less distressing to some parents. For toddlers, as for infants, other peripheral IV sites are also used. If possible, try to avoid using the foot so as not to impede the toddler's mobility or cause undue frustration. The foot veins are used, however, in children who need to be immobile.

PRESCHOOLERS (3 TO 5 YEARS)

Preschoolers are often uncooperative during drug administration. Strategies for enlisting cooperation include offering choices (e.g., between liquid medicines or chewable tablets) when feasible. Heightened awareness and the fear of punishment or body mutilation in this age group may influence the child's perception of and cooperation with drug therapy. Nurses (and parents) should always reassure preschoolers that the drug is to help them feel better and keep them healthy.

When an IM injection must be given, the use of topical anesthetic creams (e.g., EMLA) to numb the site reduces pain in preschoolers during the injection. Several sites may be used for IM injections in preschoolers, most commonly the vastus lateralis, rectus femoris, and ventrogluteal sites. The ventrogluteal site is free of major nerves and blood vessels and is characterized by deep muscle mass. It is located above the greater trochanter between the anterior superior iliac spine and the posterior iliac crest. The drug is injected into the gluteus medius muscle, which is in the ventrogluteal site. Injection in the gluteus medius is less painful than injection in the vastus lateralis. *The dorsogluteal site is generally not recommended because of potential damage to the sciatic nerve if the site is not chosen with precision.* When IV drug therapy is necessary, peripheral sites are selected for the preschooler. Scalp veins are no longer used.

SCHOOL-AGED CHILDREN (6 TO 12 YEARS)

The school-aged child is often very cooperative. As with the preschooler, offer choices to help the school-aged patient exercise control. The school-aged child's greatest fears of drug therapy are usually related to negative past experiences. School-aged children can tolerate warning of drug therapy without becoming fearful and anxious. The school-aged child takes pride in accomplishments such as receiving an injection without incident.

Oral drugs may still be provided in liquid form or chewable tablets. Many school-aged children can also swallow pills. Generally, if rectal drug forms must be used, the school-aged child will feel embarrassment. School-aged and older children, like adults, must be ensured privacy at all times throughout the procedure.

The ventrogluteal site is recommended for an IM injection in the school-aged child, but the vastus lateralis and rectus femoris sites may also be used in this age group. The dorsogluteal site is again not generally recommended. Although it is not the preferred administration site, the deltoid muscle may also be used for small volumes of drugs (0.5 mL) or vaccines. This site is often considered less painful than the ventrogluteal site.

ADOLESCENTS (13 TO 16 YEARS)

An adolescent's ability to cooperate is highly developed and much like an adult's. Offer adolescents control whenever possible and let them make choices. Also offer support and encouragement without treating adolescents like children. Adolescents are more likely to cooperate and participate in drug therapy when they have a complete understanding of the treatment regimen. Adolescents are particularly sensitive about their bodies and their independence. Therefore, privacy and control are important issues to consider when administering drug therapy to this age group.

Routes of administration are similar to those for adults. Oral forms of drug therapy include tablets or pills. Suppositories can be used, but the adolescent is likely to be embarrassed. IM injection sites are usually the same as for adults unless the adolescent is particularly small. Careful examination is necessary to ensure that adequate muscle mass is available for IM injection. Any of the muscles may be used depending on patient size and drug characteristics. The dorsogluteal site should be used *only as a last resort*. Site selection for IV therapy in adolescents is the same as for adults.

Lifestyle, Diet, and Habits

The infant's primary food intake is milk and formula. These substances decrease acidity and thus increase gastric pH. Drug absorption is usually affected by pH levels; therefore, food and drug interactions are a primary concern when administering oral drug therapy to infants.

In school-aged children and adolescents, assess for the use and abuse of substances such as caffeine, alcohol, tobacco, and street drugs. During drug therapy, these substances cause the same complications in children as in adults. Adolescence is a time of experimentation, which may include experimentation with legal and illegal substances. Preadolescents may also experiment with these substances. Try to elicit this information from all school-aged or adolescent patients throughout drug therapy because potential adverse effects or interactions of these substances may cause serious complications. Regardless of the patient's age and appearance, never assume that the child does or does not use or abuse certain substances. Pose questions regarding substance use in the health assessment interview in a nonjudgmental, matter-of-fact manner.

Question the parent regarding the use of herbal therapy. Use of alternative therapies has become common, and their use is frequently not reported to the primary care provider. Studies of pediatric patients in various settings indicate that 8% to 45% of the patients had received herbal preparations from their families (Soo et al., 2005; Martel et al., 2005; Lanski et al., 2003) Patients and their families often do not consider these therapies "medications" or may not realize how they can interact with prescribed drug therapy. One study in a pediatric emergency department found that most of the parents did not know if the herbal products had any adverse effects or if they could interact with prescribed medication. Less than half of the parents had discussed the use of herbs with their child's primary care provider (Lanski et al., 2003).

Also consider the economic circumstances of the patient and family. Are the parents concerned about paying for the child's drug therapy? Are insurance and other resources available?

Environment

Children may receive drug therapy in any setting, although some types of drugs may be administered primarily in one setting or another, just as in the adult population. Children receiving drug therapy at home need to have a parent or guardian responsible for ensuring that the child receives the prescribed therapy. General considerations about the home need to be assessed just as they are assessed for adults. Does the home have electricity, a refrigerator, and indoor plumbing?

An important additional question to ask of the parent or caretaker is whether the home has a safe place to store prescription and nonprescription drugs away from children. Childhood ingestion of drugs is a serious concern because many drugs have serious adverse effects or may cause poisoning in children. Unintentional ingestion of over-the-counter drugs is a serious problem. McFee and Caraccio (2006) found that a grandparent was often the source of unintentional exposures to medications in children under six years of age. They found that the most important factor was the accessibility of the drug to the child; the sites with easiest access were tables or countertops (46%), low shelves (29%), and pocketbooks left on the floor or furniture (17%). Whether or not the drug was in a childproof container did not significantly affect whether accidental ingestion occurred.

Culture and Inherited Traits

The family's beliefs greatly affect a child's attitude and adherence to the therapeutic regimen. Questions and assessment concerns to consider include the following:

- Does the child's cultural background suggest suspicions about or taboos against drug therapy?
- Do health practices in the child's family rely on other forms of healing, such as using herbal or natural medicines, acupuncture, prayer, or mysticism?
- Do family religious beliefs directly conflict with the use of drug therapy?

The child's cultural background and heritage must be considered quite seriously when planning drug therapy (see Chapter 12). Additionally, some children may have inherited genetic differences in their P-450 systems which may alter drug therapy.

Nursing Diagnoses and Outcomes

Nursing diagnoses and outcomes related to specific drug therapy for children are much the same as they are for adults. However, many drug therapies are burdensome for families to maintain, present special concerns, or pose risks to a child's normal growth and development. Common nursing diagnoses and outcomes may include the following:

- Delayed Growth and Development
  Desired outcome: The patient will achieve normal growth and development during drug therapy.
- Ineffective Family Therapeutic Regimen Management
  Desired outcome: Family members will master effective management strategies of the patient's drug regimen.
- Caregiver Role Strain
  Desired outcome: The patient and family will develop effective coping skills to avoid, reduce, or relieve stress on family caregivers.

Planning and Intervention
Maximizing Therapeutic Effects

Administering drugs safely and effectively to children requires an understanding of pediatric anatomy and physiology, the patient's developmental and cognitive levels, and the child's diagnosis and prognosis. Use this knowledge to select appropriate drug administration sites, equipment, and administration techniques. When offering a child choices for the sake of gaining his or her cooperation during drug administration, present only those choices that truly exist. For example, do not ask a preschooler if he or she would like to take medicine now if the child does not really have the choice to refuse. Instead, ask which drug the child wants to take first or how many bandages the child would like to apply after an injection.

ORAL DRUG THERAPY

Although usually not painful, administration of oral medications can be traumatic, especially when the drug flavor is foul and the child protests. Many pediatric drugs come in liquid form and are drawn up into a syringe (without a needle) for accurate measurement. The drug can then be transferred to a medicine cup for older, cooperative children who prefer this way of receiving the drug.

If the patient cannot swallow pills, some pills can be crushed and dissolved in a liquid or soft food (such as applesauce, gelatin, or ice cream) that masks the flavor of the drug. Dilute the drug in the smallest amount of liquid or food possible to ensure that the child receives the full dose and does not leave any in the residue. Another method of masking bad-tasting drugs for children is to offer a flavored ice pop or ice chips to help numb the taste buds and promote cooperation.

Work carefully with the child to ensure that all of the drug is taken. If the child drools or spits out some of the drug, calculate the amount of drug lost. If the total is considerable, report the estimated amount lost to the prescriber and obtain an order for a replacement dose. For drugs that pose a high risk for toxicity, another dose is unlikely to be ordered. For example, when digoxin (which slows the heart) is given to children with congestive heart failure, an overdose can be lethal.

PARENTERAL DRUG THERAPY

To ensure accurate parenteral drug delivery, choose age-appropriate equipment. For example, the length and gauge of a needle must be suited to the child's age and growth level. A needle that is too long for the child's size delivers a drug into the muscle rather than into the subcutaneous tissue, thereby speeding the rate of absorption. An institution's adoption of standard drug concentrations for infusions and purchasing the new "smart" infusion pumps (which contains computer software that includes specific drug information and policies and procedures related to administering that particular drug) have also been found to be valuable in reducing IV medications errors.

RECTAL DRUG THERAPY

Always give the patient and family a full explanation of the need to administer a drug rectally and ask the child to attempt to retain the drug for as long as possible. As always, take into consideration the developmental level of the child with the rectal administration of drugs. To allow time for the drug to be absorbed, dissuade young children from going to the bathroom and encourage them to participate in a quiet activity. Older children and adolescents need to have their privacy maintained during the administration of rectal suppositories.

Minimizing Adverse Effects

PREVENTING MEDICATION ERRORS

Medication errors are the most common type of error in the medical care of children. Most of these errors can be prevented through appropriate actions by the individual healthcare providers (physician, pharmacist, and nurse) and by health care systems, such as hospitals. Medication errors in children are more likely to be life threatening than medication errors in adults, even though their rate of occurrence is similar. Children are more at risk because they have not

physiologically matured. Immature liver or renal function, for example, can increase the circulating level of a drug beyond what would be expected in adults. The younger the child, the less likely the body organs function maximally, so infants and premature infants are at the highest risk of serious adverse effects from drug therapy and medication errors. Hughes and Edgerton's (2005) research review identifies the children most likely to be involved in a medication error. These include children:

- Younger than two years old
- In intensive care units, especially neonatal intensive care units
- In Emergency Departments between the hours of 4 and 8 AM or on weekends, with the highest risk for those children who are seriously ill
- Who are receiving chemotherapy
- Who are receiving IV medication
- Whose weight was not documented

Pediatric medication errors are most likely to occur in the prescribing phase and the administration phase of drug therapy. One study of rural, northern California emergency rooms found that in the most acutely ill children more than half of medications prescribed were associated with some sort of medication error (Marcin et al., 2007). As mentioned previously, many drugs are not specifically labeled for use in children. Therefore, the efficacy, correct dose, and possible adverse effects may not be known for the drug when used in pediatric patient populations, and medication errors may result. Incorrect dosage is the most common error. When determining a drug dosage, remember that muscle mass, body water, fat content, gastric pH levels, and liver function vary greatly from the child to the adult. These variations affect the pharmacokinetics of the drug and must be considered when determining the correct dosage. Overdosage of many drugs can cause serious or even fatal effects in children. Also remember that the pediatric drug dosage is not merely a reduced adult dosage; rather, it is calculated by specific equations adjusted to the child's weight and body surface area (see Box 6.1). It is important to be proficient at using these mathematical formulas in computing the correct dose.

Of all the problems that may contribute to an incorrect dose, the most common involve errors in math during dosage calculation. Dosage calculation can involve several steps, and a mathematical error can occur at each step. Because a pediatric dose is calculated as a percentage of an adult dose, the computed pediatric dose often includes a decimal point. Misplacement of the decimal point results in a tenfold error: either too much drug (ten times as much), or too little drug (one tenth of what it should be). *Ten-fold errors are the most common dosing error in children.* Because infants and young children require extremely small doses due to their size and immature body systems, a dose that is ten times too large may be lethal. Because mathematical computation of a drug dose is common in pediatric dosing but rare with adults, children are most likely to incur a ten-fold medication error. In addition to misplaced decimal points, errors in computing can also lead to serious medication errors. Most of the problems in dosage calculation are related to the following:

- Inability to identify the correct mathematical calculation or sequence of calculations to perform to obtain the correct answer
- Poor math skills related to using fractions, percentages, decimals, and ratios
- Infrequent use of calculation formulas
- Inexperience in applying dosage calculation formulas to actual clinical practice (Hughes & Edgerton, 2005)

Even when the pediatric drug dose is calculated correctly, it may be incorrect for a particular child based on the child's illness or current physiologic state. For example, drug calculations for premature newborns (those born at less than 30 weeks' gestation) must consider not only their current weight, but also physiologic characteristics found in this age group: lower gastrointestinal motility, higher levels of extracellular body water, lower total body fat, and decreased plasma protein binding. Because of these factors, premature newborns require much smaller doses than if only weight or body surface area were considered. Children who weigh between 40 and 50 kg (the cutoff size for a pediatric patient) may in some cases be eligible for adult doses; the standardized pediatric dose conversion formulas may be less useful for these patients (Hughes & Edgerton, 2005).

Strategies to reduce the incidence of medication errors in children require efforts from both the individual health care provider and the health care system. These strategies include:

- *Always weigh the child before administering any medication.* Since most pediatric dosage is based on the weight of the child, it is not safe to give any medication without knowing the child's accurate weight. Documenting the patient's weight in kilograms, not pounds, should be standard procedure throughout the institution. Reweigh the child as indicated by disease or physical condition if the weight is likely to change (e.g., a child with cancer may lose weight due to his disease process or from an adverse effect of drug therapy) (Hughes and Edgerton, 2005; US, Pharmacopeia, 2009; American Academy of Pediatrics Guideline, 2003, reaffirmed 2007).
- *Standardize as much as possible throughout a health care system.* Standardized medication order sheets should include entry spaces for weight, age, and allergies. Standardized concentrations of high-risk drugs administered by IV infusion, such as opioids, heparin, insulin, potassium, and chemotherapy, should be used whenever possible as these prevent computation errors. Avoid use of nonapproved abbreviations and the apothecary system of measurement, as these are likely to be misinterpreted and cause errors. Standardization of equipment, such as scales and infusion pumps, will prevent errors between units or services. See Box 6.3 for research on this topic

BOX 6.3 FOCUS ON RESEARCH

Standardization and Technology Decrease Medication Errors

Taylor, J. A., Loan, L. A., Kamara, J., Blackburn, S., & Whitney, D. (2008). Medication administration variances before and after implementation of computerized physician order entry in a neonatal intensive care unit. *Pediatrics*, 121(1):123–128.

The Study

The frequency of medication administration variances before and after the implementation of computerized physician order entry (CPOE) was studied via a prospective before/after observational study in one neonatal intensive care unit (NICU). A medication administration variance was defined as a discrepancy between the physician order and the medication given. Medication administration variances included: drug ordered but not given, drug given but not ordered, drug given at the wrong time (i.e., more than 1 hour before or after ordered time), wrong dose given (i.e., more than 10% greater than prescribed dose), or given via the wrong route. The reasons for variances in medication administration were attributed to: intentional violation (generally when a nurse delayed an oral medication to coincide with infant's feeding schedule), pharmacy problem (delay in drug delivery, delivery of wrong drug), prescribing problem (incomplete or confusing order), administration mistake, intravenous access issues, and nurse busy with acutely ill child. Nurses were observed administering medications in the NICU before and after the introduction of CPOE in the unit. Variances related to administration via the wrong route were completely eliminated after implementation of CPOE and variances due to the wrong time were significantly lower after the implementation of CPOE. Administration of

medications at the wrong time accounted for more than half of all observed variances and almost half of these were from pharmacy problems or prescribing problems. Although the initial period after roll out of the CPOE had higher incidences of variance than pre CPOE, when this initial period was not considered, there was more than a two fold reduction in the rate of administration variances after CPOE compared to before CPOE start up. Even with these decreases, a variance occurred approximately 10% of the time after CPOE use.

Nursing Implications

While CPOE have built in warnings and blocks to help prevent many common errors of prescribing such as ordering the wrong dose, the final step where an error can be made or prevented is in the actual administration of the drug by the nurse. This research shows that healthcare technology such as the CPOE can help to decrease much of the errors that occur in this phase of drug therapy. Most of the errors that still occur are due to a dose being given late. Understanding that this problem can be related to pharmacy or prescribing problems helps to identify system wide concerns that impair drug administration accuracy. When a dose is given late intentionally, it can be argued that this "error" is not dangerous, but rather a reflection of the nurse's professional judgment. This indicates that standardized times for drug administration may need to be modified at times to be in the patient's best interest. Nurses should be involved in CPOE software development to help differentiate these reasons for late drug administration. The fact that variance still occurs after CPOE use indicates the complexity of drug administration. More research in this area in warranted.

(Hughes & Edgerton, 2005; US Pharmacopeia, 2009; American Academy of Pediatrics (AAP) Guideline, 2003, reaffirmed 2007; Kozer, Scolnik et al., 2005; Coco, King & Slattery, 2005; White, Veltri, & Fackler, 2005; and Larsen & Parker et al., 2005).

• *Use computerized drug order entry systems where possible.* These systems help prevent medication errors made by misinterpreting illegible handwriting. These systems also can compute the correct dose based on built-in algorithms as well as built-in safety checks to confirm appropriateness of ordered drug dosages (US Pharmacopeia, 2009 and AAP Guideline, 2003, reaffirmed 2007).

• *Use reliable drug information sources to determine the recommended dose.* If the drug label does not include a recommended pediatric dose, a computerized pharmacology database or current printed drug information references may be used. Although many nursing drug references give dosage ranges for children as well as adults, they usually do not include dosages specific to preterm and full-term neonates. When administering drugs to these patients, use a pediatric drug guide that gives ranges of pediatric dosages in mg/kg of body weight or by dose for all children.

• *Double-check each calculated dose for accuracy.* It is recommended that the pharmacist check the dose, even if it was ordered via a computer order entry system. As the nurse is the last person involved in drug delivery, the nurse is the last person to find a potential drug calculation error as well as the last person who might make an error. The nurse is responsible for ensuring the accuracy of a prescribed drug dose before it is administered. For safety, even when drug doses were previously computed by the physician, pharmacist, or both, *always double-check dosage calculations before administering any dose to a child.* Certain hospital protocols may require two nurses to independently double-check a dose prior to administration of medications that pose a high risk of injury to the child, such as chemotherapy, anticoagulants, insulin, or opioids. Inservice programs can be provided to ensure that all health care professionals are capable of accurately performing pediatric dosage calculation (Hughes & Edgerton, 2005; US Pharmacopeia, 2009; AAP Guideline, 2003, reaffirmed 2007).

• *Measure and deliver oral medications via oral syringes only, never via syringes used to administer parenteral injections.* This precaution prevents oral medications from accidentally being given by the wrong route (US Pharmacopeia, 2009).

• *Involve the family in drug administration.* Families of children need to be aware of the drug therapy that is prescribed for the child. By being knowledgeable about the indication, dose, and frequency of medication administration, families become active partners with the rest of the health care team in preventing medication errors (Hughes & Edgerton, 2005).

• *Communicate the drug therapy plan clearly when different nurses will be caring for the patient.* Medication errors are most likely to occur at points of transition such as at shift change or in patient transitions between units or from the hospital to another institution or to home (Hughes & Edgerton, 2005). (See Chapter 11 for more information.)

Nurses are viewed by all members of the health care team as having primary responsibility for ensuring patient safety. Thus, you are essential in decreasing the incidence of pediatric medication errors. Nurses have a responsibility to do two things. The first is to incorporate the above recommendations into daily practice. The second is to participate in hospital-wide safety committees to help institute system-wide recommendations.

While many of the serious adverse effects and medication errors in pediatric patients occur in acute care settings, many also occur in the home setting. See the discussion under Patient and Family Education for more information on preventing these types of errors.

REDUCING PSYCHOLOGICAL STRESS AND ANXIETY
Some adverse effects in pediatric drug therapy involve psychological distress of the child or parent. Consider age-related emotional needs when selecting appropriate communication techniques to help allay anxiety and negative, stress-provoking feelings regarding drug therapy. For school-aged children and adolescents, address feelings and discuss and answer questions as simply and honestly as possible.

Although infants do not converse, they do communicate nonverbally. Parents are helpful in providing a history of the infant's experiences, behaviors, and schedule, and they can also provide an interpretation of the infant's nonverbal cues. Infants are very much in tune with their parents and can sense their feelings. If the parents are anxious, the infant is likely to be anxious as well. Therefore, offer parents reassurance and full explanations regarding procedures and rationales. During therapy, the parents may comfort the infant by maintaining eye contact, gently stroking the head, or talking in soothing tones. Parents are not asked to restrain the infant but should be at hand to comfort the child. After drug therapy is administered, they should cuddle and comfort the child.

Because toddlers need to view drug therapy as positively as possible, they should be comforted and praised after receiving a drug regardless of whether they were cooperative or uncooperative. Whatever their behavior, they should never be referred to as a "bad boy" or "bad girl." Toddlers take pride in their accomplishments, and positive feedback and praise enhance their sense of self-esteem.

Play therapy is useful for reducing a child's anxiety and promoting understanding of drug therapy. To familiarize the child with an administration procedure, encourage role-playing with dolls and appropriate medical equipment.

During role-playing, further encourage the child to express any feelings of anxiety or anger.

For preschoolers and school-aged children, take care to explore the child's experiences with the health care system. These experiences strongly influence the behavior of these children, which, like the behavior of toddlers, are accepted without value judgments. Similarly, take advantage of opportunities to provide positive feedback and avoid negativity.

Providing Patient and Family Education

A crucial step in administering pediatric drug therapy is educating the child, the parents, and other family members or caregivers. Providing honest and detailed explanations and rationales helps reassure those caring for the child. Patient and family education is especially important if drug therapy continues when the child returns home. Many pediatric medication errors occur unintentionally in the home setting because the parent does not adequately understand the drug, its effects, and the best manner to dose the drug. Parents need to be taught specific drug information, including the name of the drug, what it is for, how it works, its adverse effects, and the exact dose for the child. This information should be provided in writing. Parents should be taught exactly how to measure and administer the medication to their infant. Teach the parent to use a measured-oral-dosing syringe, and have the parent demonstrate dosing with the equipment. Include the child in drug education and provide age-appropriate explanations. Children have a right to appropriate information regarding any medicine they take. Including children in drug education, starting at an early age, helps them to grow into the role of informed consumers. The position paper *Ten Guiding Principles for Teaching Children and Adolescents About Medicines* issued by the United States Pharmacopeia encourages educating children about drug therapy. Additional resources for teaching children about medications, including guidelines for creating age-appropriate teaching materials, are also available from the United States Pharmacopeia website.

Education for infant patients is directed solely toward the parent. Medication errors can result in serious adverse effects in infants. Overdosing can result from a miscalculation of the dose, an incorrectly measured dose, double-dosing (from multiple caregivers each providing a dose), administration of doses too closely together, or administration of the drug by the wrong route. For toddlers, fully explain the rationale for drug therapy and type of administration in private, away from the toddler. Give toddlers a very brief, straightforward, honest explanation immediately before they receive drug therapy and especially before an invasive procedure. The information is supplied just before a procedure so that little time is left for their fears and anxiety to escalate.

Preschoolers require simple explanations. They often understand more than they can articulate. The information on the drug therapy should be accurate but brief. Giving preschoolers a simple description of the medication administration procedure and calmly informing them—for example, telling them that they might feel a momentary "pinch" or "stick"—is generally sufficient to prepare them. For preschoolers, just as for toddlers, supply the information immediately before a procedure so that there is little time for their fears and anxiety to escalate. Parents or primary caregivers are usually permitted to be with the child during the procedure.

The school-aged child can understand somewhat more in-depth explanations and will ask many specific questions regarding drug therapy. Answers and explanations are honest and as detailed as necessary for the patient and parents. Information is provided on what the child wants to know, not just what the health care provider believes the child should know.

Adolescents are treated like adults with regard to full explanations and rationale for drug therapy. Invite adolescents to be involved in these discussions and encourage them to ask questions and express their feelings. Stress the importance of therapeutic adherence because adolescents are at the age when they assume more responsibility for their own health and well-being. Many adolescents take responsibility for scheduling and administering their own drug therapy.

At a minimum, include the following in initial education for school-aged children, adolescents, and parents:

- Generic and trade names of drugs
- Rationale for drug therapy
- Description of the intended therapeutic drug effect
- Route by which drug will be administered
- Schedule and duration of administration
- Potential adverse effects
- Special drug-related precautions or restrictions (e.g., relating to exercise or diet)

In addition, educate as many family members or other caregivers as possible. Doing so promotes accurate and safe drug administration to the child at home and ensures that sources of information about the child's drug history are easily found, especially in an emergency.

School-aged children and adolescents typically require instruction in proper techniques for self-administering drug therapy. For example, children with diabetes need to learn how to select injection sites and administer injections. Children with asthma need instruction in using respiratory inhalers. Other patients may need instruction in how to mix, shake, or otherwise prepare drugs before measuring the dose.

Give parents and pediatric patients as much opportunity to practice drug administration techniques as possible while you observe and offer feedback. For example, techniques are re-evaluated frequently during admissions to the hospital or at scheduled medical visits, because problems related to poor

COMMUNITY BASED CONCERNS

Minimizing accidental ingestion and overdosing in children:

- Measure drug with medication spoon or cup not with a household spoon.
- Keep all drugs (including OTC drugs) out of the reach of children (more than 3 feet off of the ground). Be sure all family members and caregivers are aware of this need.
- Do not throw used transdermal patches of medication where a child can reach it because young children will likely put it into their mouths.
- Do not tell children that medicine is candy.

technique frequently arise. Providing parents with a dosing spoon or syringe with a line marked at the correct dose and asking them to again demonstrate how they measure the dose is an effective technique for teaching how to measure a dose properly. Spoken instructions on administering the drug are much less effective.

Emphasize to parents and children the importance of administering a drug at the appropriate times and continuing therapy for the full course of treatment. Sometimes, parents stop administering a drug once the child no longer exhibits signs or symptoms of an illness, which is especially true if the child protests or has difficulty taking the drug. Stress to the parents that interrupting drug therapy before treatment is completed may cause problems such as recurrence of an infection or development of a drug-resistant infection.

As accidental drug ingestion and poisoning in young children frequently is from a grandparent's medication, nurses should assess ALL patients as to whether they have exposure to young children. All parents and grandparents should be taught to keep medications out of the reach of children (i.e., higher than 3 feet). (See Box 6.4 Community Based Concerns)

The best way to prevent adverse effects from drug therapy is to minimize the need for it. The importance of general health education to parents (such as the importance of vaccination, use of safety seats, and hand washing to prevent infections) cannot be overemphasized.

Ongoing Assessment and Evaluation

Nursing management of drug therapy in a child is considered effective when the developmental needs of the patient have been met, the care has involved the family, and the drug has achieved its therapeutic effect without adverse effect to the child. Children who are receiving drug therapy for chronic conditions need to be reassessed frequently and evaluated during regular yearly pediatric checkups to ensure that they are safely adhering to prescribed drug therapy, self-administering drug therapy as indicated, and growing and developing normally while undergoing drug therapy.

CHAPTER SUMMARY

- Children are different from adults both physically and emotionally, and these differences seriously affect the planning of safe and effective drug therapy.
- Most drugs have not been tested for efficacy or safety in children and thus are prescribed off-label to children. Additional monitoring for adverse effects from drug therapy is necessary when drugs are used off-label.
- A child's age, growth, and development are crucial considerations in relating core drug knowledge with core patient variables in drug therapy.
- A child's age, weight, body surface area, water content, and fat content must be considered when determining the proper dose of a drug. Drug dosage is calculated for each child, using mathematical formulas. Most drug dosages are calculated based on the child's weight. No medication should be administered unless the current weight is documented on the chart.
- Pediatric dosages must be accurate because even small errors can cause adverse effects, toxicity, or death. A misplaced decimal point results in a ten-fold dosing error. This is the most common dosage calculation error occurring in children. The nurse independently verifies all dosage calculations made by other health care providers prior to administering each dose.
- To maximize the therapeutic effect of any drug, the nurse must ensure that all of the appropriate dose is administered by the desired route.
- Many of the adverse effects of drug therapy can be avoided or minimized by ensuring that the child receives the appropriate drug dosage calculated specifically for him or her. Nurses should have access to a pediatric drug reference, guide, or electronic data base that gives the pediatric ranges for drug doses, including those for preterm and full-term neonates.
- In addition to determining the correct dose for a child, pediatric medication errors can be prevented by standardizing as much as possible within a hospital setting, using computerized order entry whenever possible, using the appropriate administration equipment, involving the family in medication administration, and carefully communicating the drug therapy plan at points of transition in care.
- One of the adverse effects in pediatric drug administration is psychological distress in the child or parent. The nurse who uses knowledge of age-related emotional needs and communication techniques can greatly help relieve this emotional distress and enhance compliance with drug therapy.
- Patient and family education regarding drug therapy should include information needed to help the child take the drug safely and effectively. Teaching involves giving honest and straightforward explanations about drug therapy, answering questions, allaying patient and family anxiety, and emphasizing the importance of drug compliance. Parents should be taught how to measure a correct dose at home and how to use the appropriate measuring/dosing tool.

QUESTIONS FOR STUDY AND REVIEW

1. How does the neonate's and infant's liver function affect drug distribution?

2. What is body surface area? How is body surface area utilized in pediatric drug therapy?

3. What dose adjustment might be expected when a water-soluble drug is given to an infant?

4. Are all drugs that are safe for adults also safe for children?

5. A three-year-old child is hospitalized and is to receive amoxicillin, an antibiotic. The recommended dose is 25 mg/kg/day in divided doses every 12 hours. The child weighs 20 kg. What is the correct dose that should be administered every 12 hours? What should you do to prevent the most common pediatric medication error when administering the amoxicillin?

6. What is the appropriate site of an IM injection for an infant?

7. Why is it important to assess the preschooler's or school-aged child's past experience with health care providers and drug therapy? Why is patient and family education important with pediatric patients?

NEED MORE HELP?

Chapter 6 of the Study Guide to Accompany *Drug Therapy in Nursing,* 4th Edition, contains NCLEX-style questions and other learning activities to reinforce your understanding of the concepts presented in this chapter. For additional information or to purchase the study guide, visit the**Point**.

REFERENCES

American Academy of Pediatrics. Policy statement: prevention of medication errors in the pediatric inpatient setting (2003). *Pediatrics,* 112(2):431–436.

Reaffirmed May 1, 2007. *Pediatrics,* 119(5):1031.

Aschenbrenner, D. S. (2006). Drug watch: Pediatric drug information. *American Journal of Nursing,* 106(4):34.

Hughes, R. G. & Edgerton, E. A. (2005). Reducing pediatric medication errors: Children are especially at risk for medication errors. *American Journal of Nursing,* 105(5): 79–84.

Lanski, S. L., Greenwald, M., Perkins, A., et al. (2003). Herbal therapy use in a pediatric emergency department population: Expect the unexpected. *Pediatrics,* 111(5 Pt 1):981–985.

Luo, X., Doherty, J., Cappelleri, J. C., Frush, K. (2007). Role of pharmacoepidemiology in evaluating prescription drug safety in pediatrics. *Current Medical Research and Opinion,* 23(11): 2607–2615.

Marcin, J. P., Dharmar, M., Cho, M., Seifert, L. L., Cook, J. L., Cole, S. L., Nasrollahzadeh, F., & Romano, P. S. (2007). Medication errors among acutely ill and injured children treated in rural emergency departments. *Annals of Emergency Medicine,* 50(4):361–367.

Martel, D., Bussieres, J. F., Theoret, Y., Lebel, D., Kish, S., Moghrabi, A., & Laurier, C. (2005). Use of alternative and complementary therapies in children with cancer. *Pediatric Blood & Cance*r, 44(7):660–668.

Shah, S. S., Hall, M., Goodman, D. M., Feuer, P., Sharma, V., Fargason, C. Jr., Hyman, D., Jenkins, K., White, M. L., Levy, F. H., Levin, J. E., Bertoch, D., & Slonim, A. D. (2007). Off-label drug use in hospitalized children. *Archives of Pediatric and Adolescent Medicine,* 161(3):282–290.

Soo, I., Mah, J. K., Barlow, K., Hamiwka, L., & Wirrell, E. (2005). Use of complementary and alternative medical therapies in a pediatric neurology clinic. *The Canadian Journal of Neurological Sciences,* 32(4):524–528.

United States Food and Drug Administration. (2009). Pediatric Exclusivity Labeling Changes. http://www.fda.gov/cder/pediatric/labelchange.htm. Accessed March 19, 2009.

United States Pharmacopeia. Position statement. Ten guiding principles for teaching children and adolescents about medicines. Retrieved March 20, 2009, from *http://www.usp.org/audiences/consumers/children/principles.html*

United States Pharmacopeia. Error-avoidance recommendations for medications used in pediatric populations. Retrieved March 20, 2009, from *http://www.usp.org/hqi/patientSafety/resources/pedRecommnds2003-01-22.html?USP_Print*

Life Span: Pregnant or Breast-Feeding Women

Learning Objectives

At the completion of this chapter the student will:

1. Identify how core drug knowledge of drug therapy in pregnant or breast-feeding patients may vary from core drug knowledge in other life-span groups.

2. Identify how normal physiologic changes with pregnancy alter the pharmacokinetics of drug therapy.

3. Define teratogenic effect and its relevance in managing drug therapy in the pregnant patient.

4. Differentiate the classifications of drugs for use in pregnancy.

5. Describe why adverse effects of drug therapy may be overlooked in pregnant patients.

6. Identify how the pregnant or breast-feeding patient's core patient variables in drug therapy may vary from the core patient variables of other life-span groups.

7. Relate the core drug knowledge to core patient variables when providing drug therapy in pregnant or breast-feeding patients.

8. Generate a nursing plan of care from the interactions between core drug knowledge and core patient variables for drug therapy in pregnant or breast-feeding patients.

9. Describe nursing interventions to maximize therapeutic effects and minimize adverse effects in drug therapy in pregnant or breast-feeding patients.

10. Determine key points for patient and family education in drug therapy for pregnant or breast-feeding patients.

Key Terms

eclampsia	gestational diabetes	organogenesis
fetal alcohol syndrome	hyperemesis	preeclampsia
fetal hydantoin	gravidarum	teratogenic
syndrome	lactation	

Although the prevalence varies, drug therapy during pregnancy is common. Nursing management of drug therapy for pregnant women is challenging for several reasons. The main issue is that nursing care is needed for both the patient and the fetus because most drugs pass through the placental membrane to the fetus (usually by diffusion) or through breast milk to the infant.

Drug therapy in pregnant women is used primarily for two reasons: to treat a preexisting medical condition or to treat complications that arise during pregnancy. Although drug therapy may be indicated during pregnancy or during **lactation** (the secretion of breast milk), nursing management must focus on both the therapeutic effects on the patient and the potential adverse effects on the developing fetus or infant being breast-fed.

The nurse must know about the physiologic changes that occur during pregnancy and how they may alter the patient's response to a drug. The nurse must also understand the adverse effects of certain drugs on the developing fetus. Although adverse effects of drug therapy to the breast-fed infant are generally less severe than those to the fetus during pregnancy, the nurse must also be familiar with the potential adverse effects from drug therapy during lactation.

This chapter presents core drug knowledge and core patient variables that pertain to pregnancy and lactation. In addition, some general guidelines are presented for maximizing therapeutic effects, minimizing adverse effects, and providing patient and family education for any drug therapy.

Nursing Management of the Pregnant or Breast-Feeding Patient
Core Drug Knowledge
Pharmacotherapeutics
Pharmacotherapeutics are no different in a pregnant woman than in a woman who is not pregnant. The important consideration in drug therapy for pregnant women is the potential adverse effects on the developing fetus. A clear clinical indication for drug therapy must exist before a drug is prescribed or self-administered. Although the range for most drug dosages remains the same for the pregnant patient, the nurse must always consider the risk for fetal effects. The lowest therapeutic dose of a drug should be administered to the pregnant woman to help minimize fetal effects.

Some health problems occur secondarily to pregnancy and require drug therapy. These problems include **preeclampsia** (a serious hypertensive condition that can develop during pregnancy) or **eclampsia** (a life-threatening condition resulting from uncontrolled preeclampsia, involving cerebral edema and convulsions). **Gestational diabetes,** a form of diabetes that develops during pregnancy, may also occur. Occasionally, if the fetus has a health problem, drugs are administered to the pregnant woman with the intent of treating the fetus as the drug passes through the placenta. For example, digoxin (a drug that slows the heart rate and strengthens the force of contraction) is administered to the

mother to treat fetal tachycardia and congestive heart failure in the fetus.

Pharmacokinetics
Several physiologic and anatomic changes occur during pregnancy. They can alter the pharmacokinetics of drugs and involve the endocrine, gastrointestinal (GI), cardiovascular, circulatory, and renal systems.

ABSORPTION
Changes in the GI system are influenced by pregnancy hormones and mechanical pressure from the growing uterus. Progesterone decreases gastric tone and motility and prolongs stomach emptying time, which may alter the pharmacokinetics of orally administered drugs. Progesterone also promotes functional respiratory system changes during pregnancy. Tidal volume increases 30% to 40%, with a 50% increase in minute volume by term. These increases, along with the pulmonary vasodilation that occurs during pregnancy, enhance the absorption of drugs that are inhaled.

DISTRIBUTION AND METABOLISM
Hemodynamic changes in the cardiovascular system alter heart rate, cardiac output, venous and arterial blood pressures, blood volume, circulation, and coagulation. The heart rate increases about 10 to 15 bpm above baseline as a result of a 40% increase in blood volume. A 50% increase in plasma volume causes a hemodilution of plasma albumin, which potentiates changes in drug distribution. Plasma lipid levels increase throughout pregnancy as a result of the more complete absorption and decreased elimination of fats during pregnancy. These changes in lipid levels may alter drug transport mechanisms and drug distribution. Drugs are distributed by the circulatory system to the fetus by passing through the placenta, usually by diffusion. Drugs may compete with the hormones of pregnancy for albumin-binding sites, which may result in a larger amount of unbound (or free) drug in circulation, leaving the drug available to cross the placental membrane and enter the fetal circulation. Drugs that are lipophilic (fat soluble) and not bound to protein pass easily through the placenta's lipid membrane.

Drugs are also distributed into breast milk. Drugs that are widely distributed throughout the mother's body are usually minimally passed into breast milk, producing low drug concentrations in breast milk. Other drugs, such as those with increased lipid solubility and low protein binding (e.g., central nervous system [CNS] agents), pass more easily and may produce high drug concentrations in breast milk. Lipophilic drugs pass easily because breast milk contains a high percentage of fat. Drugs that are not highly protein bound have more active, free drug molecules in the bloodstream, which can then diffuse into breast milk. Other drugs that are more likely to diffuse into breast milk include drugs with lower molecular weights and those with organic bases; these drugs may become "trapped" in breast milk because of its low pH, producing high drug concentrations.

Not all drugs present in breast milk are well absorbed by the neonate. Drug levels in breast milk are not equivalent to drug levels in the mother's blood, and so drugs with poor bioavailability usually do not achieve high concentrations in the neonate's circulation. A breast-feeding infant usually ingests less than 2% of the mother's total dose.

Drug metabolism is not altered by pregnancy or breast-feeding.

EXCRETION

Changes in renal function during pregnancy result from changes in renal plasma flow, glomerular filtration rates, and renal tubular reabsorption. By the third trimester, the renal blood flow has increased 40% to 50% from the pre-pregnancy level. Increases in renal plasma flow cause greater capillary pressures, requiring an increase in filtration through the glomerulus. The glomerular filtration rate increases by approximately 50% and contributes to increased excretion rates. Therefore, drug excretion rates may be increased during pregnancy.

Pharmacodynamics

Two dramatic physical changes occur in the mother during pregnancy: by 32 weeks' gestation, cardiac output is increased by 50%; and from the second trimester on, arterial blood pressure is decreased. These conditions necessitate careful evaluation of a drug's pharmacodynamics.

Contraindications and Precautions

Some drugs and vaccines are contraindicated during pregnancy, and others should be given with caution if they pose a threat to the developing fetus by passing through the placenta (Box 7.1). Some drugs and vaccines can cause **teratogenic** effects (physical defects) in the developing fetus. See Table 7.1 for a list of known teratogenic drugs. For example, antiepileptic, phenytoin (Dilantin), a hydantoin, is known to cause **fetal hydantoin syndrome.** This syndrome is characterized by craniofacial abnormalities, limb defects, growth deficiency, and mental deficiency (Hansen & Smith, 1975). These abnormalities are believed to occur because phenytoin competes for folic acid–binding sites.

The precise effects of drug therapy on the fetus are mostly undetermined. A review of all drugs approved in the United States between 1980 and 2000 found that the teratogenic risk in human pregnancy was still undetermined for more than 90% of those drugs. The longer the drug had been on the market, the more likely it was that the exact teratogenic risk was unknown (Lo & Friedman, 2002).

A drug is traditionally identified as a teratogen based on the findings of animal teratology studies. This method is problematic because animal models are frequently poor predictors of whether a drug is a human teratogen. Nonhuman primates are good predictors of human teratogenicity because they are the most genetically similar to humans; however, nonhuman primates are rarely used in experiments because of the expense involved. Rodents are used

---

BOX 7.1   COMMUNITY BASED CONCERNS

Smallpox Vaccine

In collaboration with the Food and Drug Administration (FDA) and the Department of Defense in the United States, the Centers for Disease Control and Prevention (CDC) established the National Smallpox Vaccine in Pregnancy Registry. In 2003 after the military began vaccinating military personnel against smallpox. The registry includes women found to be pregnant when vaccinated, those who became pregnant within 28 days of vaccination, and those who, while pregnant, were in close contact with a person who had received the smallpox vaccine within the past 28 days. Women reported to this registry will are monitored throughout the pregnancy and at the conclusion of the pregnancy to document pregnancy outcomes. Fetal vaccinia, a rare but serious infection manifested by skin lesions and internal organ involvement, can result in fetal or neonatal death or premature birth. Historically, there have been 50 reported cases world wide of fetal vaccinia. Evaluation of pregnancy registry data from 376 exposed women from 2003 to 2006 did not find an increased incidence of: pregnancy loss, preterm birth, or birth defects. And no cases of fetal vaccinia were identified (Ryan & Seward, 2008).

While the analysis of the pregnancy registry data is reassuring, it is a very small sample size and should not be construed to mean there are no risks if a pregnant woman receives the vaccine. The CDC and the FDA continue to recommend that women should be screened for pregnancy before vaccination. Women who are pregnant or might become pregnant within 4 weeks after vaccination should not be vaccinated against smallpox unless there is active circulating disease because of the risk for fetal vaccinia, which is a rare but serious infection of the fetus. Fetal vaccinia is manifested by skin lesions and internal organ involvement and can result in fetal or neonatal death or premature birth. Smallpox vaccine has not been clearly shown to cause other teratogenic effects or other adverse effects in the fetus or newborn. People who have close personal contact with a pregnant woman should also not be vaccinated.

The CDC has recommended that screening for pregnancy before vaccination is paramount to preventing exposures in pregnant women. The screenings that have occurred as part of the current immunization campaign against smallpox appear to have been effective in minimizing exposure of pregnant women to the vaccine.

Sources: Centers for Disease Control. (2003). *Women with smallpox vaccine exposure during pregnancy reported to the national smallpox vaccine in pregnancy registry—United States, 2003* [Electronic version]. *MMWR,* 52(17):386–388. Available: *http://www.cdc.gov/mmwr/preview/mmwrhtml/mm5217a3.htm Accessed March 22, 2009.*
Ryan, M. A. & Seward, J. F.; Smallpox Vaccine in Pregnancy Registry Team (2008). Pregnancy, birth, and infant health outcomes form the National Smallpox Vaccine in Pregnancy Registry, 2003-2006. *Clinical Infectious Diseases,* 46 (Suppl 3):S221–S216.

most frequently in teratology studies, but unfortunately they are very dissimilar to humans in terms of their physiology, metabolism, and ontogenetic development. Although animal studies do not provide all of the information in determining teratogenicity of a drug, they currently are the most-used tool to screen drugs for their potential to cause human birth defects. Clinical studies in pregnant women have not been done because of ethical concerns about experimentation on the fetus.

The ultimate assessment of drug safety during pregnancy, unfortunately, comes from the use of the drugs in humans. To address the need for more information about how

TABLE 7.1 Examples of Drugs or Drug Classes Known or Highly Suspected to Be Teratogenic

Teratogenic Drug or Drug Class	Indication
Alkylating agents (cyclophosphamide)	Cancer
Androgenic hormones(danazol)	Hormone replacement
Antiepileptics (valproic acid, carbamazepine, phenytoin)	Seizure control in epilepsy
Antimetabolities (methotrexate)	Cancer; Crohn's disease; rheumatoid arthritis; ectopic pregnancy; termination of early pregnancy (combined with misoprostol)
Anti–thyroid (propylthioracil, methimazole)	Hyperthyroidism
Anxiolytic (diazepam)	Anxiety, seizure control, pre-procedure relaxation
Coumarin (warfarin)	Anticoagulant
Estrogens (diethylstilbestrol)	Hormone replacement
Fluconazole	Anti-fungal
Lithium	Mood stabilizer in bipolar disease
Misoprostol	Intestinal ulcer from NSAID use; off label use for cervical ripening and induction of labor; medical termination of early pregnancy (when combined with mifepristone)
Oral contraceptives	Birth control
penicillamine	Cystinuria and rheumatoid arthritis
Retinoids (isotretinoin)	Recalcitrant cystic acne
Radioactive iodine (sodium iodide-128)	Hyperthyroidism
SSRI antidepressants (paroxetine, fluoxetine, sertraline)	Depression
Thalidomide	Cancer; leprosy

Data from Buhimschi, C. S. & Weiner, C. P. Medications in pregnancy and lactation. In Queenan, J. T., Spong, C. Y., Lockwood, C. J. (eds). *Management of high-risk pregnancy: an evidence-based approach.* 5th ed. Malden, MA: Blackwell Publishing Ltd., 2007:38–58.

drugs affect a pregnancy, the United States Food and Drug Administration (FDA) has established Pregnancy Registries. There are also pregnancy registries in other countries, and there are some that are global, with enrollees from around the world. Women who take medication during pregnancy for a chronic or acute condition may elect to join one of these registries. A complete list is found on the FDA web site. The information gleaned regarding pregnancy outcomes is added to a national database, whose purpose is to provide more definitive information about the teratogenic affects of various drug therapies and the margins of safety with drug exposure during pregnancy. There are several limitations of these registries. These include: small sampling size that doesn't represent the desired population; voluntary enrollment which may skew the results; enrollment in more than one registry could lead to over or under estimation of risk; medical records are not always examined to validate data; small sample sizes may not be able to detect small or moderate risks; and the inability to detect that the underlying maternal condition and not the drug is the cause of the fetal injury because women with the condition but not receiving drug therapy are excluded from the registry (Wyszynski, 2009). Compiling data from multiple registries can be problematic because the statistical analysis performed on reported data are not identical, and some registries may provide poorer quality information due to protocols that are not epidemiologically sound (Kennedy, Uhl, & Kweder, 2004)

PREGNANCY CATEGORIES

Drug manufacturers are required by law to include information in a drug's label about possible risks if the drug is administered to a pregnant or breastfeeding woman. In 1980, the FDA developed a categorical ranking based on research findings to help classify drugs by the risks posed to the fetus, weighed against the potential benefits to the pregnant woman. The categories are A, B, C, D, and X (Box 7.2).

Box 7.2 FDA PREGNANCY CATEGORIES

Category A: Controlled human studies in pregnant women fail to demonstrate a risk to the fetus.

Category B: Animal studies fail to demonstrate fetal risk, but there are no controlled human studies in pregnant women; or animal studies demonstrate fetal risk that was not confirmed in controlled human studies in pregnant women.

Category C: Animal studies demonstrate fetal risk, and there are no controlled human studies in pregnant women to rule out fetal risk, or there are no animal or human studies. Drugs are given if the benefit justifies risk.

Category D: Controlled human studies demonstrate positive evidence of fetal risk. In life-threatening situations, the benefit may be acceptable despite the risk.

Category X: Controlled human studies demonstrate fetal risk. The fetal risk outweighs any possible benefit. Use in pregnant or potentially pregnant women is contraindicated.

Categories A and B (and to some extent, C) are generally based on increasing risk. Categories D and X (and to some extent, C) are based on risk versus potential benefit. These categories have been found to be confusing to health care providers for a number of reasons including:

- The categories do not supply enough information for providers and consumers to make informed decisions about drug therapy.
- The FDA, in trying to keep the categories simple, has grouped together drugs that do not have identical risks.
- The alphabetical progression leads people to believe that the seriousness of the risk increases with each letter, which is not correct.

To provide clearer and more relevant information for a prescriber to use in decision making, the FDA announced in 2008 that elimination of the five categorical rankings (A, B, C, D, and X) would begin in 2009. In its place the FDA will include on drug labels a narrative summary of effects for both pregnancy and lactation. Under both the revised pregnancy and lactation subsections of the label there will be a fetal/newborn risk summary, clinical considerations (such as points for patient education or management while on drug therapy), and a data section (where clinical trial data is described in detail). Information from pregnancy exposure registries will be included, if available. The new labels are appearing first for newly approved drugs. Drugs that were approved for use prior to 2009 will have their labels updated over several years. This means that nurses will see two different forms of pregnancy and lactation information on drug labels for awhile, and thus must be familiar with both (Aschenbrenner, 2008).

So why does every nurse need to understand this? While its importance might seem most obvious for those who work clinically with pregnant women, women of child bearing age are in every specialty and environment, be it a medical-surgical unit, oncology unit, operating room, home health, or outpatient center… [The] nurse is the last person to check the medication's appropriateness before the patient receives the drug. And because it is has been estimated that nearly half of all pregnancies are unplanned (FDA. Briefing document, 2003) nurses must know the ramification of giving any drug to a pregnant woman. If a drug has serious teratogenic risks then the patient must be screened for pregnancy prior to starting drug therapy. One final contributing reason as to why this is important information is that nurses are asked about drug safety in pregnancy and lactation from everyone- from patients, family members, friends, and neighbors. If nurses are going to be able to explain these changes to patients, they have to understand them (Aschenbrenner, 2008).

LACTATION CATEGORIES

In 2005, the American Academy of Pediatrics Committee on Drugs published its updated recommendations on drugs and breast-feeding (American Academy of Pediatrics, 2005). The report identifies several categories of drugs (and other agents) and their potential to cause problems with breast-feeding, which are as follows:

- Cytotoxic drugs that may interfere with cellular metabolism of the nursing infant (including cyclophosphamide, cyclosporine, doxorubicin, and methotrexate)
- Drugs of abuse for which adverse effects on the infant during breast-feeding have been reported (including amphetamines, cocaine, heroin, marijuana, and phencyclidine)
- Radioactive compounds that require temporary cessation of breast-feeding
- Drugs for which the effect on nursing infants is unknown but may be of concern (Table 7.2)
- Drugs that have been associated with significant effects on some nursing infants and should be given to nursing mothers with caution (Table 7.3)
- Maternal medication usually compatible with breast-feeding
- Food and environmental agents that may also have effects on breast-feeding

All contraindicated drugs have been reported to cause signs and symptoms in the infant or produce an adverse effect with lactation. The American Academy of Pediatrics states that this list is not complete and recommends that all drugs of abuse should be avoided by lactating women, even though reports of neonatal adverse effects are not found in the literature for all substances. If a breast-feeding woman is receiving any radioactive compounds, such as those used for treating malignant tumors or an overactive thyroid gland, the patient should pump her breasts during the time that breast milk is radioactive and discard that milk in a biohazard container designed for radioactive materials. Breast-feeding can resume when the drug is stopped and the breast milk contains no radioactivity.

Drugs with unknown effects on the neonate that may be of concern include psychotropic drugs (antianxiety drugs, antidepressants, and antipsychotic drugs). These drugs appear in low concentrations in breast milk after maternal ingestion. However, these drugs have long half-lives, and because of immature hepatic and renal function in newborns, the drugs or some of their metabolites may reach measurable amounts in nursing babies' plasma and tissues and in organs such as the brain. The longer the nursing mother receives psychotropic drugs, the greater is the risk of harmful effects in the infant. Nursing mothers should be informed that if they take one of these drugs, the infant will be exposed to it. These drugs affect neurotransmitter function in the developing CNS, and the long-term neurodevelopmental effects that can occur from newborn exposure are unknown. It is possible that psychotropic drugs may impair the short-term or long-term function of the CNS. See Table 7.2 for a full list of drugs for which the effect on nursing infants is unknown but may be of concern.

Drugs that are associated with significant neonatal effects after breast-feeding and that should be used with caution include the over the counter drugs aspirin and

TABLE 7.2 **Drugs for Which the Effect on Nursing Infants is Unknown but May Be of Concern**

Drug Class and Drug	Reported Possible Effect
Antianxiety	
alprazolam	Unknown
diazepam	Unknown
lorazepam	Unknown
midazolam	Unknown
prazepam	Unknown
quazepam	Unknown
temazepam	Unknown
Antidepressant	
amitriptyline	Unknown
amoxapine	Unknown
bupropion	Unknown
clomipramine	Unknown
desipramine	Unknown
dothiepin	Unknown
doxepin	Unknown
fluoxetine	Colic, irritability, feeding and sleep disorders, slow weight gain
fluvoxamine	Unknown
imipramine	Unknown
nortriptyline	Unknown
paroxetine	Unknown
sertraline	Unknown
trazodone	Unknown
Antipsychotic	
chlorpromazine	Galactorrhea in mother; drowsiness and lethargy in infant; decline in developmental scores
chlorprothixene	Unknown
clozapine	Unknown
haloperidol	Decline in developmental scores
mesoridazine	Unknown
trifluoperazine	Unknown
Antiarrhythmic	
amiodarone	Possible hypothyroidism
Anti-infective	
chloramphenicol	Possible idiosyncratic bone marrow suppression
clofazimine	Potential for transfer of high percentage of maternal dose; possible increase in skin pigmentation
Metronidazole tinidazole	In vitro mutagen; may discontinue breastfeeding for 12–24 hours to allow excretion of dose when single-dose therapy given to mother
Antiepileptic	
lamotrigine	Potential therapeutic serum concentrations in infant
GI Stimulant	
metoclopramide	As dopaminergic blocking agent may potentially block these neuroreceptor sites in infant

Based on the American Academy of Pediatrics policy statement on the transfer of drugs and other chemicals into human milk, 2001, remains current policy as of March 21, 2009.

TABLE 7.3	Drugs That Have Been Associated with Significant Effects in Some Nursing Infants and Should Be Given to Nursing Mothers with Caution
Drug Class and Drug	**Reported Effect**
Beta Blocker	
***As a class, breast fed infants remain normotensive**	
acebutolol	bradycardia, tachypnea
atenolol	Cyanosis; bradycardia
5-Aminosalicylic Acids	
mesalamine	Diarrhea
olsalazine	
balsalazide	
sulfasalazine	Bloody diarrhea
Anti-inflammatory	
aspirin	Metabolic acidosis (from large chronic doses, such as with arthritis)
Antihistamine	
clemastine	Drowsiness, irritability, refusal to feed, high-pitched cry, neck stiffness
Antimigraine	
ergotamine	Vomiting, diarrhea, convulsions
Mood Stabilizer	
lithium	One-third to one-half therapeutic blood concentration in infant
Antiepileptic	
phenobarbital	Sedation; infantile spasms after weaning from milk containing phenobarbital; methemoglobinemia
primidone	Sedation; feeding problems

Based on the American Academy of Pediatrics policy statement on the transfer of drugs and other chemicals into human milk, September 2001, current as of March 21, 2009. And data from Buhimschi, C. S., & Weiner, C. P. (2009b). Medications in pregnancy and lactation Part 2. Drugs with minimal or unknown human teratogenic effect. *Obstetrics & Gynecology,* 113(2 Pt 1):417–432.

clemastine (Tavist). The blood concentration of these drugs may become high enough to be of clinical importance in the breast-fed infant. The reported effects for these drugs include CNS changes, cardiovascular changes, and GI problems. See Table 7.3 for a full list of drugs associated with significant neonatal effects.

Infant exposure via breast milk may be of concern for a larger numbers of infants than previously believed, although there is limited research on this. A recent survey at one US hospital found that breastfeeding women were much more likely to use medications than pregnant women (p<0.0001) and a third of these women took medications rated as possible or probably unsafe or whose safety was unknown (Stultz et al., 2007).

Often, drugs identified as being compatible with breast-feeding are not part of large research studies. Rather, information is obtained from single case reports or a small series of reports. However, *most drugs that are taken by the mother for treatment are believed to pose no harm to the breast-fed newborn.* Breast-feeding confers many advantages to the baby and is encouraged by health professionals and public health officials.

Adverse Effects

The two major considerations when evaluating adverse effects of drug therapy in pregnant women are common side effects of pregnancy and the adverse effect that maternal drug therapy can have on the fetus. Symptoms such as nausea and vomiting, light-headedness or hypotension, constipation, heartburn, urinary frequency, heart palpitations, and fatigue may mask the adverse effects of drug therapy in pregnant patients, making adverse effects more difficult to assess. When considering the effects of drugs on the fetus, several factors are important, including dose and duration of drug therapy, the type of adverse effect that may appear, and when during pregnancy the drug is taken. The timing of drug exposure is critical because. Teratogens act during critical periods of embryonic or fetal development.

BOX 7.3 FOCUS ON RESEARCH

Pregnancy and Prescribed Teratogenics

Andrade, S. E., Raebel, M. A., Morse, A. N., Davis, R. L., Chan, K. A., Finkelstein, J., et al. (2006). Use of prescription medications with a potential for fetal harm among pregnant women. *Pharmacoepidemiology and Drug Safety*, 15(8):546–554.

The Study

This study was designed to estimate the prevalence of pregnant American women taking a prescription drug that has a potential for fetal harm. This was a retrospective study using the automated databases of eight health maintenance organizations in the United States. Women who delivered a baby between January 1996 and December 2000 were included in the study. Women who had received ovulation stimulants or who had a preterm delivery were excluded from the analysis. Of the 114,165 women whose records were examined, 1.1% of them received a teratogenic drug within the 270 days before delivery. A larger percentage (5.8%) received an FDA category D or X drug; these drugs were mostly prescribed and used in early pregnancy.

Nursing Implications

Using a teratogenic drug during pregnancy has potential risks for the infant. Many women are prescribed these drugs in early phases of pregnancy when the developing fetus may be most at risk of congenital defects. Nurses should look up the pregnancy information related to all drugs they administer. Nurses need to confirm the pregnancy status of any patient of childbearing age prior to dispensing any drug that has known teratogenic effects. Nurses also need to educate women desiring to become pregnant about the risks of teratogenic drug effects to help prevent exposure to a teratogen prior to the woman knowing she is pregnant.

Teratogens that create injury to large number of cells in the early embryo in the preimplantation phase most likely will result in loss of the pregnancy (Buhimschi & Weiner, 2008).

The critical period of **organogenesis,** during which the major fetal organs form, is from implantation up to approximately day 58 to 60 after conception. If drugs that cause teratogenic effects are administered during this period, major malformations of fetal organ systems may result (see Table 7.1). If possible, drug therapy should be delayed until after this time. Unfortunately, most women do not realize they are pregnant or do not seek prenatal care until after this early period; thus, accidental exposure to teratogens may occur (Box 7.3).

After 60 days, the embryonic phase is complete, and the fetal phase begins. This phase continues through the remainder of the pregnancy, during which fetal exposure to drugs continues to have the potential for harm. The fetal effects that may occur are of four primary types:

• Damage to structures or organs that were formed normally during organogenesis
• Damage to systems undergoing tissue development
• Growth retardation
• Fetal death or stillbirth

Combinations of these effects may also occur. Damage to the fetus may be caused by teratogens but may also be caused by agents that have no apparent potential to produce abnormal development. An example is coumarin derivatives used as anticoagulants, which may produce eye and brain defects from hemorrhagic accidents in the fetus. Growth retardation is the most common fetal effect. However, it is difficult to determine whether this effect is caused by the drug therapy or the primary condition for which the drug therapy is prescribed. For example, there are case reports of fetal growth retardation when the mother received the antihypertensive drug propranolol, but untreated hypertension is also associated with this condition.

Additionally, some drugs create adverse neonatal effects (Table 7.4). These agents do not normally cause teratogenic effects but instead create a situation that makes it difficult for the neonate to adapt to life outside the uterus. Examples

TABLE 7.4	Selected Nonteratogenic or Minimally Teratogenic Drugs with Adverse Fetal Effects or Breast Feeding Effects	
Nonteratogenic Drug or Class	**Adverse Fetal Effects**	**Breast Feeding Effects**
acetaminophen	Possible link between drug, gastroschisis, and small bowel atresia if mother is genetically predisposed and fetal exposure occurs during early pregnancy	Compatible with breast feeding
corticosteroids	Cleft lip (evidence is weak); increased risk of neonatal sepsis (suggested but not confirmed); suppression of fetal breathing, movement, impaired myelination, intrauterine grown restricitohn, and microcephaly	No adequate reports or well controlled studies in breast feeding
diphenhydramine	No evidence of fetal risk; May cause neonatal depression if given during labor	Infant may demonstrate irritability
labetalol	Large doses given IV can cause bradycardia, hypoglycemia, hypotension, pericardial effusion, myocardial hypertrophy, and fetal death due to acute hypotenison	Breast fed infants are normotensive
tetracycline	cause yellow-gray-brown discoloration of the permanent adult teeth	Considered compatible with breast feeding

Data from Buhimschi, C. S., & Weiner, C. P. (2009b). Medications in pregnancy and lactation Part 2. Drugs with minimal or unknown human teratogenic effect. *Obstetrics & Gynecology*, 113(2 Pt 1):417–432.

are floppy infant syndrome from the use of benzodiazepines (antianxiety agents) near the time of delivery and premature closing of the ductus arteriosus from the use of nonsteroidal anti-inflammatory drugs (NSAIDs) such as indomethacin (Indocin).

The risk for adverse effects of drug therapy on the breast-feeding infant are not as great as those relating to drug therapy during pregnancy because the breast-feeding infant usually ingests less than 2% of the total dose of the drug given to the mother. The dose the infant receives depends on the amount of drug excreted into breast milk, the daily volume of milk ingested, and the average plasma concentration of the mother. Unfortunately there has been limited research on drug concentrations in breast milk. How the infant metabolizes and excretes the drug also contributes to the circulating volume of the drug in the infant (Buhimschi & Weiner, 2009a). At this time there are limited numbers of drugs that are contraindicated with breast feeding (see lactation categories above). More research is needed to know whether the administration of a particular drug poses a risk to the breast-feeding infant.

Drug Interactions

Drug interactions are unchanged during pregnancy and breast-feeding.

Assessment of Core Patient Variables Relevant to Pregnancy and Breast-Feeding

Health Status

Several considerations must be taken into account when assessing health status during pregnancy. First, if the patient has a preexisting condition that requires drug therapy, the health care providers must consider whether the prescribed drug therapy will have adverse effects on the fetus. Second, any adverse effects the pregnancy may have on the mother's health must be identified because they may require changes in drug therapy. Third, if the pregnancy does induce changes in health status that require new drug therapy, any adverse effects of this drug therapy on the fetus will have to be determined.

Pregnant women, especially those being treated with drug therapy, must be assessed for preexisting conditions. Give special attention to any cardiovascular problems because the cardiovascular system undergoes many changes and stresses during pregnancy. The pregnancy may necessitate changes in drug selection or dosage. Also assess the woman's use of over-the-counter drugs, which may pose risks to the fetus.

Seizure disorder is important to consider during pregnancy. A woman with a seizure disorder who is planning a pregnancy must first seriously consider how antiepileptic drug therapy might affect the fetus. Many traditional, established antiepileptics are commonly believed to have teratogenic potential because of their mechanism of action. These teratogenic effects include congenital abnormalities such as neural tube defects, specific facial and other deformities, and mental impairment. However, stopping all drug therapy for the pregnant woman with epilepsy is not necessarily advisable because seizures and status epilepticus, which can occur when drug therapy is stopped, are responsible for most excess maternal deaths in women with epilepsy (i.e., deaths in women with epilepsy beyond what would be expected to occur statistically). Controversy exists regarding what harm maternal seizures can cause the fetus. Some clinical experts have hypothesized that seizures in a pregnant woman may cause fetal hypoxia, leading to CNS damage. This "between a rock and a hard place" reality demonstrates the difficulty of making drug therapy decisions that are in the best interest of both the mother and the baby.

If antiepileptics must be continued during pregnancy, drug selection is important. However, the literature offers limited clear guidance as to drug selection based on risk to the infant. Typical or classic antiepileptic drugs such as phenytoin have generally been considered to be teratogenic since the 1970s (Hansen & Smith, 1975) and the drugs carry warnings on their labels related to risks of teratogenicity. Newer research seems to indicate that phenytoin use during pregnancy increases the risk of congenital malformation at about the same rate as not treating epilepsy during pregnancy.(Harden, 2008; Vajda, 2008; Battino & Tomson, 2007).

Most of the newer classes of anti epileptic drugs do not have a high risk for teratogenetic effects, with one exception. There seems to be agreement that valproic acid (Depakote) should be avoided, as it has been linked to higher incidences of congenital abnormalities, especially neural tube defects, than other antiepileptic drugs. Teratogenic risk increases with the daily dose of valproic acid with higher risk from daily dosage over 1,000 mg/d. The risk from valproic acid is compounded with low serum folate levels (Buhimschi & Weiner, 2009a). Exposure to multiple antiepileptic drugs (polytherapy) increases the risk of adverse effects in the fetus; combining valproic acid with any other drug increases the risk the most (Harden, 2008; Pennell, 2008; Battino & Tomson, 2007). The literature also supports that valproic acid, as well as phenytoin and phenobarbitol diminish cognitive ability of the child exposed in utero; polytherapy also increases this risk (Harden, 2008). *The safest choice appears to be for women to maintain therapy to control their seizures with the smallest dose and monotherapy when at all possible* (Harden, 2008; Vajda, 2008; Battino & Tomson, 2007). Antiepileptics may be discontinued for select patients upon medical consultation.

Another health condition that may warrant assessment is depression. Pregnancy and postpartum periods are considered times of high risk for depression due to hormonal changes, especially if the woman has a previous history of depression. Untreated depression can impair the mother–infant bond and create emotional problems in the child. Research indicates that only 18% of women with depression disorder seek treatment during pregnancy and postpartum (Marcus, 2008). Untreated depression can have negative effects during pregnancy such as: inadequate weight gain, under utilization of prenatal care, increased substance use, and premature birth. Infants of depressed mothers may have lower birth weight, a decreased Apgar score, smaller head circumference, and be small for their gestational age (Marcus, 2008; McClanahan, 2009). Antidepressants treat depression, but with the increased use of antidepressants, concerns have arisen about the effects these drugs might have during pregnancy and breast-feeding. There is little definitive information on this subject to date. A literature review found such inconsistent findings regarding whether or not selective serotonin reuptake inhibitors (SSRI), a class of antidepressants, increase teratogenic risks that the only conclusion was that the teratogenic potential of these drugs was unproven (Gentile & Bellantuono, 2009).

Diabetes, whether preexisting or developed during pregnancy, is another important condition to consider. Women may have type 1 or type 2 diabetes before pregnancy or they may develop diabetes temporarily during pregnancy, this is called gestational diabetes. In gestational diabetes, the secretion of placental hormones (human placental lactogen, cortisol, progesterone, and catecholamines) causes the pregnant woman to develop insulin resistance as the pregnancy progresses. Whatever the type of diabetes, hyperglycemia may result, which requires either an increase in insulin therapy for those women already receiving it (i.e., type 1) or initiation of insulin therapy for those with type 2 or gestational diabetes. Because hyperglycemia is believed to increase the incidence of congenital anomalies (particularly during the first trimester), the primary goal for the pregnant patient is to maintain normal blood glucose levels. Historically, insulin is the drug of choice for controlling blood glucose levels because it does not cross the placenta and does not pose concerns for adverse effects. Recently research supports the use of the oral anti-hyperglycemic drug glyburide to treat gestational diabetes. Glyburide, unlike other drugs in its class, has been found to have a very low incidence of moving through the placenta into the fetal circulation; the exact mechanism of this is unknown currently (Kimber-Trojnar et al., 2008). Glyburide may have altered pharmacokinetics in pregnant women, as one study showed 50% less plasma concentrations in this possible (Herbert et al., 2009). This may account for why glyburide has a reported success rate in gestational diabetes of 80% to 85% (Kimber-Trojnar et al., 2008). Evidence in the literature supports the use of glyburide for gestational diabetes and does not show a higher incidence of maternal or fetal complications from using it instead of insulin (Coustan, 2007; Nicholson et al., 2008; Moretti et al., 2008; and Nicholson et al., 2009) Some experts disagree about the safety of glyburide (Kimber-Trojnar et al., 2008). The use of another oral antihyperglycemic, metformin, has not been studied as much as glyburide, and the limited findings are inconclusive as to whether it is an appropriate treatment for gestational diabetes (Coustan, 2007; Nicholson et al., 2009). After the neonate is delivered, maternal glucose levels should return to baseline levels, and insulin or glyburide therapy is usually no longer necessary for women who did not need them before becoming pregnant.

Another change in health status that may occur during pregnancy is **hyperemesis gravidarum,** commonly called pernicious vomiting of pregnancy. While nausea and vomiting are common in up to 80% of normal pregnancy, hyperemesis gravidarum is potentially life threatening and affects up to 1.5% of pregnant women (Bottomley & Bourne, 2009). Dehydration, ketonuria, and vitamin deficiency can be complications. When hyperemesis gravidarum is severe, antiemetic drug therapy is needed to control the vomiting. Although there is insufficient research evidence to demonstrate the most effective therapy, safety data supports the use of antihistamines (such as diphenhydramine (Benadryl), Meclizine, Dramamine, which also has antiemetic effects), phenothiazines (a drug class with antiemetic and antipsychotic properties that block dopamine receptors), and metoclopramide (a drug that promotes gastric emptying and promotes peristalsis; it is used as an antiemetic because it blocks peripheral dopamine receptors which cause nausea) (Bottomley & Bourne, 2009). The literature also supports the use of steroids such as prednisolone (Sheehan, 2007). Some sources have shown that the selective serotonin antagonist antiemetics such as ondansetron may be helpful and do not appear to cause teratogenic effects, but the research is very limited with these drugs (Einarson et al., 2004; Sheehan, 2007).

Preeclampsia is another serious condition that can develop and require drug therapy during pregnancy. This hypertensive condition of pregnancy typically develops after the 24th gestational week. Preeclampsia is characterized by a triad of symptoms—hypertension, edema, and proteinuria. Uncontrolled preeclampsia may lead to eclampsia, a condition characterized by cerebral edema and convulsions. The primary goal of preeclampsia treatment is to prevent eclampsia and stabilize the patient until the fetus reaches maturity. Treatment for preeclampsia is aimed at decreasing CNS irritability and reducing maternal blood pressure to enhance placental and maternal circulation to the organs. Drug therapy for preeclampsia includes magnesium sulfate, which is the drug of choice for preventing convulsions, and hydralazine, a drug used to treat hypertension. Other drugs used in treating hypertension in preeclampsia include diazoxide, nifedipine, and labetalol.

Another condition secondary to pregnancy that may occur is thrombus formation. The decreased venous return and increased levels of clotting factors and fibrinogen that are characteristic in pregnancy produce a state of hypercoagulation, which increases the risk for clot formation. Pregnant women who develop thrombosis are treated with the anticoagulant heparin.

Life Span and Gender

Teenage pregnancy continues to be a problem in the United States. Adolescents are prone to experimentation with various substances, both legal and non-legal. Teenagers may also not realize they are pregnant or may not admit to pregnancy till late in the pregnancy, therefore not receiving adequate prenatal care. These issues combined may create problems for the mother and infant. Nurses assess for these behaviors.

Lifestyle, Diet, and Habits

The lifestyle, diet, and habits of pregnant or breast-feeding women can have a serious impact on the course of the pregnancy and the development of the fetus or infant. For example, alcohol is a known human teratogen. **Fetal alcohol syndrome** is a serious pattern of teratogenic effects seen in infants born to women who may have consumed alcohol chronically during pregnancy. Fetal alcohol syndrome is marked by specific physical malformations at birth and severe growth retardation, mental retardation, and microcephaly. Cocaine abuse is also known to cause adverse fetal effects and is suspected to be a human teratogen. Opiate abuse does not appear to significantly increase the risk for congenital anomalies, but other adverse outcomes are associated with the use of opiates, including abruptio placentae, neonatal withdrawal, preterm birth, and fetal growth retardation. Smoking tobacco also has adverse fetal effects, most notably fetal growth retardation.

Environment

Although some changes in health status that occur in pregnancy require drug therapy administered in the hospital setting, such as magnesium sulfate for preeclampsia, most drug therapy given during pregnancy or breast-feeding is administered in the patient's home.

Culture and Inherited Traits

Cultural beliefs may affect whether a woman accepts certain drug therapies while she is pregnant or breast-feeding. Assess for these beliefs when managing drug therapy in the pregnant or breast-feeding woman. For more about the effects of culture on pharmacotherapeutics (see Chapter 12).

Nursing Diagnoses and Outcomes

Nursing diagnoses formulated for the pregnant or breast-feeding patient receiving drug therapy are similar to diagnoses made for patients with other concerns relating to life span. The main difference is that for the pregnant or breast-feeding woman, the nursing diagnosis must address the needs of both the patient and her child. Relevant nursing diagnoses may include the following:

- Risk for Injury to the fetus related to adverse effects of maternal drug therapy
  Desired outcome: The patient will demonstrate therapeutic drug effects with minimal adverse effect to the fetus or infant by avoiding unnecessary drugs throughout pregnancy and lactation and by using nonpharmacologic measures to relieve common discomforts of pregnancy.
- Anxiety related to perceived danger of drug therapy to fetus or infant
  Desired outcome: The patient's anxiety will be minimal during drug therapy.
- Risk for Injury to the patient related to failure to receive needed drug therapy because of its potential adverse effects on the fetus or infant
  Desired outcome: The patient will not sustain an injury from choices made about receiving drug therapy.

Planning and Intervention

The nurse and other health care providers have a responsibility to the pregnant patient to consider the risk-to-benefit ratio of drug therapy, to educate the childbearing patient regarding possible teratogenic effects, and to support the patient's decision to accept or refuse drug therapy.

Maximizing Therapeutic Effects

If a prescribed drug therapy does not have adverse effects for the developing fetus or the child of the breast-feeding woman, emphasize this absence of known risk when teaching patients. Women may be reluctant to take needed drug therapy if they believe it may be harmful to the fetus.

Minimizing Adverse Effects

Limiting drug use in pregnancy decreases maternal and fetal adverse effects. No drug can be considered absolutely safe when administered during pregnancy, although general guidelines can assist the health care provider with decisions relating to drug therapy. Women of childbearing age should always be assessed for pregnancy before any drug therapy is initiated. During pregnancy, nonpharmacologic alternatives to drug therapy should be used if possible, especially for common discomforts of pregnancy, such as nausea and vomiting, light-headedness or hypotension, constipation, heartburn, urinary frequency, heart palpitations, and fatigue. If drug therapy is required, first check the drug's FDA pregnancy category or drug label information to determine safety. An evaluation of the risks versus the benefits shows whether administering a drug is justified. When a drug is to be administered, consult with the prescriber so that the minimum therapeutic dose is used for as short a time as possible. If possible, drug therapy is delayed until after the first trimester of pregnancy, during which all major fetal organ systems are forming, especially if the drug has the potential for causing teratogenic effects.

Monitor the pregnant woman and the fetus for both therapeutic and adverse effects of drug therapy. If prolonged drug use is necessary and poses risk to the woman or fetus, monitor serum levels of the drug to detect elevations that may lead to adverse effects. Dosage adjustments or discontinuation of the drug may be needed to reverse adverse effects or prevent toxicity. To reduce the risk for adverse effects, only drugs that are absolutely necessary are administered when complications of pregnancy occur. To help relieve typical discomforts of pregnancy, teach the patient

---

CRITICAL THINKING SCENARIO

ENSURING DRUG SAFETY DURING LACTATION

Your patient, a breast-feeding mother, tells you that she frequently gets stress headaches and takes aspirin for them. She would like the aspirin to have as little effect on the baby as possible. What questions might you ask her? What advice can you offer her?

how to use nonpharmacologic strategies, such as eating dry crackers first thing in the morning to prevent nausea.

When evaluating a patient, be careful to distinguish discomforts of pregnancy (e.g., nausea, vomiting, heartburn, light-headedness, urinary frequency, heart palpitations) from possible adverse drug effects. In addition, the pediatrician should be informed about maternal drug therapy. Knowledge of fetal exposure to drugs assists the pediatrician in making appropriate health care decisions regarding the neonate.

When questions and concerns arise regarding drug therapy and breast-feeding, similar strategies are used to prevent adverse effects. The various approaches include using nonpharmacologic remedies, determining the safest drug possible based on the amount of the drug that is transferred to breast milk and the possible neonatal effects, and assessing blood concentrations of the drug in the breast-feeding infant. Each drug administered to the lactating patient is evaluated for its potential adverse effects on the neonate, and the nurse also assesses the infant for adverse effects of the drug. Other methods used to reduce neonatal drug exposure include scheduling drug therapy just after breast-feeding or before the infant is going to sleep for a long time. Some drugs, such as antineoplastic drugs and drugs of abuse, are contraindicated during lactation, and breast-feeding is discontinued if the patient is taking any of these drugs. Agents such as general anesthetics, sedatives, and radioactive compounds required for a short-term diagnostic test should be cleared from the patient's circulation before she resumes breast-feeding. The nurse must know the drug's half-life and duration of action to be able to determine when breast-feeding can begin again. The risks to the neonate must be balanced against the advantages of the drug to the woman.

Providing Patient and Family Education

The nurse's role in counseling about pregnancy and fetal drug effects ideally begins before pregnancy. This counseling helps women make informed choices about drug therapy and helps minimize the risk for accidental exposure to teratogens in the early stages of pregnancy (from conception to day 60). Informing women of childbearing age about fetal drug effects can help them make decisions about planning pregnancy and about what to do when they become pregnant. The Organization of Teratology Information Specialists produces patient education sheets about many medications. These sheets are available online, and many are in Spanish and French in addition to English.

Patient and family education during pregnancy and breast-feeding is primarily focused on adverse effects to the fetus and infant. If the woman has used a drug before learning that she is pregnant, she will need information regarding to what degree of risk the fetus has been exposed, if any. Each pregnant patient should be given information on a drug's effects, both therapeutic and adverse, and should be permitted to make an informed decision about whether to receive the drug therapy.

The pregnant patient should also be taught how to anticipate adverse effects of drug therapy and distinguish them from normal pregnancy-related problems. Instruct the patient to notify the health care provider if adverse drug effects occur. The woman who is lactating also is informed of possible adverse effects of drug therapy on the infant and is instructed to report those findings immediately to the health care provider.

Ongoing Assessment and Evaluation

Nursing management of drug therapy during pregnancy and lactation is considered effective when maternal therapeutic needs have been met without harm to the fetus or the breast-feeding infant. Other measures of effective drug therapy include successful patient- and family-oriented drug education and assessment findings indicating that the mother and child are not experiencing adverse drug effects.

CHAPTER SUMMARY

- Drug therapy may be indicated for pregnant or lactating women to manage preexisting or newly developed conditions. Although therapeutic effects may be achieved in the woman, drug therapy may adversely affect the fetus or infant.
- The physiologic changes that occur during pregnancy may alter drug absorption, distribution, and elimination.
- Some drugs are contraindicated in pregnancy, and caution is advised for using others because drugs may pass through the placenta to the fetus and cause teratogenic effects. The potential fetal risks must be compared with maternal benefits when drug therapy is required.
- The effects of most approved drugs on a developing human fetus are not known. Voluntary enrollment by pregnant women in Pregnancy Registries for different drug therapies is one new mechanism for gaining knowledge about drugs and their effects on the developing fetus.
- Drugs may be excreted into breast milk, although the total received by the infant is a small percentage of the maternal dose. The nurse should be familiar with the prescribed drugs and the substances of abuse that are contraindicated during breast-feeding.
- Symptoms of pregnancy may mask adverse effects of drug therapy in the mother. Discomforts commonly associated with pregnancy, such as nausea and vomiting, light-headedness or hypotension, constipation, heartburn, urinary frequency, heart palpitations, and fatigue, are also frequent adverse drug effects.
- Limiting drug use during pregnancy and lactation decreases maternal and fetal adverse effects. Nonpharmacologic alternatives to drug therapy should be used if possible, particularly when treating the common discomforts of pregnancy.
- Substances of abuse are contraindicated during pregnancy and lactation because they can cause serious teratogenic effects, such as fetal alcohol syndrome, or harm the breast-feeding infant.
- The minimum therapeutic dose should be used for as short a time as possible during pregnancy. If possible, drug therapy should be delayed until after the first

trimester of pregnancy, during which the fetal organ systems are forming.

• Both the pregnant patient and the fetus should be monitored for therapeutic and adverse effects of drug therapy, and that practice should continue for the lactating patient and breast-feeding infant.

QUESTIONS FOR STUDY AND REVIEW

1. Which FDA pregnancy category rating includes the criterion "The fetal risk outweighs any possible benefit," and what does that mean?
2. Explain what types of drugs are most easily transferred across the placenta to the fetus.
3. Explain why gestational weeks 3 through 8 are considered critical when drug administration is considered during pregnancy.
4. Describe the physiologic changes in the renal system that increase drug excretion rates.
5. Why are lipophilic drugs more likely to enter breast milk than nonlipophilic drugs?

NEED MORE HELP?

Chapter 7 of the Study Guide to Accompany *Drug Therapy in Nursing*, 4th Edition, contains NCLEX-style questions and other learning activities to reinforce your understanding of the concepts presented in this chapter. For additional information or to purchase the study guide, visit thePoint.

REFERENCES

American Academy of Pediatrics. (2001). (current as of 2009) Policy statement. The transfer of drugs and other chemicals into human milk. Retrieved from *http://aappolicy.aappublications.org/cgi/content/full/pediatrics;108/3/776* Accessed March 21, 2009.

American Academy of Pediatrics. (Revised 2005). Policy Statement. Breastfeeding and the use of human milk. Pediatrics, *115*(2);496–506. Retrieved March 21, 2009 from *http://aappolicy.aappublications.org/cgi/content/abstract/pediatrics;115/2/496.*

Aschenbrenner, D. S. (2008). Drug Watch. FDA revises pregnancy information. *American Journal of Nursing*.nov 1008

Bottomley, C. & Bourne, T. (2009). Management strategies for hyperemesis. *Best Practice & Research. Clinical Obstetrics & Gynaecology*, March 2, 2009.

Buhimschi, C. S. & Weiner, C. P. (2009a). Medications in pregnancy and lactation Part 1. Teratology. *Obstetrics & Gynecology*; 113(1):166–188

Buhimschi, C. S. & Weiner, C. P. (2009b). Medications in pregnancy and lactation. Part 2. Drugs with minimal or unknown human teratogenic effect. *Obstetrics & Gynecology,* 113(2 Pt 1):417–432.

Coustan, D. R. (2007). Pharmacological management of gestational diabetes: an overview. *Diabetes Care*, (Suppl 2):S206–S208.

Einarson, A., Maltepe, C., Navioz, Y., Kennedy, D., Tan, M. P., & Koren, G. (2004). The safety of Ondansetron for nausea and vomiting of pregnancy: a prospective comparative study. *BJOG: An International Journal of Obstetrics and Gynaecology*, 111(9):940–943.

Gentile, S. & Bellantuono, C. (2009). Selective serotonin reuptake inhibitor exposure during early pregnancy and the risk of fetal major malformations: focus on paroxetine. *Journal of Clinical Psychiatry,* pii:ej08r04468 (Epub ahead of print).

Hansen, J. W. & Smith, D. W. (1975). The fetal hydantoin syndrome. *Journal of Pediatrics,* 87(2):285–290.

Herbert, M., Ma, X., Naraharisetti, S., Krudys, K, et al. (2009). Are we optimizing gestational diabetes treatment with glyburide? The pharmacologic basis for better clinical practice. *Clinical Pharmacology and Therapeutics,* March 18.

Kennedy, D. L., Uhl, K., & Kweder, S. L. (2004). Pregnancy exposure registries. *Drug Safety: an International Journal of Medical Toxicology and Drug Experience,* 27(4):215–228.

Kimber-Trojnar, Z., Marciniak, B., Leszczynsk-Gorzelak, B., Trojnar, M., & Oleszczuk, J. (2008). Glyburide for the treatment of gestational diabetes mellitus. *Pharmacological Reports,* 60(3):308–318.

Lo, W. Y. & Friedman, J. M. (2002). Teratogenicity of recently introduced medications in human pregnancy. *Obstetrics and Gynecology,* 100(3):465–473.

Marcus, S. M. (2008). Depression during pregnancy: rates, risks and consequences–Motherisk Update 2008. *Canadian Journal of Clinical Pharmacology*, 16(1):e15–e22.

McClanahan, K. K. (2009). Depression in pregnant adolescents: considerations for treatment. *Journal of Pediatric and Adolescent Gynecology,* 22(1):59–64.

Moretti, M. E., Rezvani, M., & Koren, G. (2008). Safety of glyburide for gestational diabetes: a meta-analysis of pregnancy outcomes. *The Annals of Pharmacotherapy,* 42(4):483–490.

Nicholson, W., Bolen, S., Witkop, C. T., Neale, D., Wilson, L., & Bass, E. (2009). Benefits and risks of oral diabetes agents compared with insulin in women with gestational diabetes: a systemic review. *Obstetrics and Gynecology,* 113(1):193–205.

Nicholson, W., Wilson, L. M., Witkop, C. T., et al. (2008). Therapeutic management, delivery, and postpartum risk assessment and screening in gestational diabetes. *Evidence Report Technology Assessment (full report),* 162:1–96.

Organization of Teratology Information Specialists. Fact sheets. Retrieved from *http://www.otispregnancy.org/hm/inside.php?id=41#1. Accessed March 21, 2009.*

Sheehan, P. (2007) Hyperemesis gravidarum–assessment and management. *Australian Family Physician,* 36(9):698–701.

Stultz, E. E., Stokes, J. L., Shaffer, M. L., Paul, I. M., & Berlin, C. M. (2007). Extent of medication use in breastfeeding women. *Breastfeeding Medicine: The Official Journal of the Academy of Breastfeeding Medicine,* 2(3):145–151.

U.S. Food and Drug Administration, Office of Women's Health. List of pregnancy registries. Retrieved March 21, 2009, from http://www.fda.gov/womens/registries/default.htm.

U.S. Food and Drug Administration. FDA News. May 28, 2008. FDA Proposes New Rule to Provide Updated Information on the Use of Prescription Drugs and Biological Products during Pregnancy and Breast-feeding. Retrieved March 21, 2009, from *http://www.fda.gov/bbs/topics/NEWS/2008/NEW01841.html.*

U.S. Food and Drug Administration. (December16, 2003). Briefing document. Nonprescription Drugs and Reproductive Health Drugs Advisory Committee meeting; page 9. Retrieved March 21, 2009, from http://www.fda.gov/ohrms/dockets/ac/03/briefing/4015B1_01_WCC-Briefing%20Document.pdf.

Wyszynski, D. F. (2009). Pregnancy Exposure Registries: Academic Opportunities and Industry Responsibility. *Birth Defects Research (Part A): Clinical and Molecular Teratology,* 85:93–101.

8

Life Span: Older Adults

Learning Objectives

At the completion of this chapter the student will:

1. Identify how core drug knowledge of drug therapy in older adults may vary from core drug knowledge for younger adults.
2. Identify how normal physiologic changes with aging alter pharmacokinetics of drug therapy.
3. Define polypharmacy and its relevance in managing drug therapy in the older adult.
4. Describe why adverse effects of drug therapy may be overlooked in older adults.
5. Identify how the older adult's core patient variables in drug therapy may vary from the younger adult's core patient variables.
6. Relate the interaction of core drug knowledge to core patient variables when providing drug therapy in older adults.
7. Generate a nursing plan of care based on the interactions between core drug knowledge and core patient variables for drug therapy in older adults.
8. Describe nursing interventions to maximize therapeutic and minimize adverse effects in drug therapy in older adults.
9. Determine key points for patient and family education in drug therapy for older adults.

Key Terms

benefit: risk ratio
frail elderly
geriatric patient

medication reconciliation
nonadherence
older adult

paradoxical excitement
polypharmacy

he **older adult** (or **geriatric patient**) is defined as a person who is 65 years of age or older. This population is divided into three subgroups: the young-old (65 to 74 years), the middle-old (75 to 84 years), and the old-old (85 years and older). Of these, the old-old group is the fastest growing and most medically needy and will generate the greatest consumption of societal resources for the next half century. Older adults comprise about 15% of the U.S. population, and this percentage is rising, but they receive more than one-third of all the drugs that are prescribed (Fulton, 2005; Ballentine, 2008).

Many older adults are independent and in generally good health. They may receive drug therapy for chronic conditions (many of them related to normal aging changes), but their physiologic conditions are well controlled, and they do not consider themselves "sick." However, some older adults are not independent and are in poor or compromised health. These are the **frail elderly,** a term that describes all people older than 65 years who have one or more debilitating conditions. Being frail and elderly places a person at higher risk for developing serious adverse drug effects.

Many physiologic changes occur with normal aging, which is accompanied by a decline in general organ and system function. In general, aging organs and body systems are less responsive than young ones to a drug's effect. Age-related changes affect the patient's response to drug therapy because both the therapeutic and the adverse effects are altered. This state creates specific risks and needs for the older adult receiving drug therapy. To manage drug therapy safely and effectively in the older adult, the nurse must be aware of these changes. The nurse also needs to be aware that many older adults take multiple prescribed and over-the-counter (OTC) drugs. Taking several drugs simultaneously is called **polypharmacy**. Polypharmacy is also considered taking more medications than are clinically indicated. It is not uncommon for older adults to receive 5 or more prescription drugs as well as over-the-counter drugs. Polypharmacy is increasing even though it is known to increase the risk for morbidity and mortality in older adults (Hajjar et al., 2007)

This chapter presents the ways that core drug knowledge and core patient variables may be altered because of age. This chapter also presents general guidelines for maximizing therapeutic effects, minimizing adverse effects, and providing patient and family education for the older adult.

Nursing Management of Older Adults
Core Drug Knowledge
Pharmacotherapeutics

The pharmacotherapeutics of drug therapy for older adults is similar to that for younger adults. Some drug therapies are more frequently used than others in older adults because their therapeutic effects offset the decreased functioning of body organs and systems that occurs with normal aging. Older adults are prone to certain disease processes or pathologic conditions, such as chronic heart failure, chronic renal disease, and hypertension; certain drug therapies used to treat these conditions are used frequently in older adult patients.

Box 8.1 PHARMACOKINETIC CHANGES IN OLDER ADULTS

Physiologic Changes Related to Normal Aging
Absorption

Increased gastric pH
Decreased absorptive surface
Decreased blood flow
Decreased gastrointestinal motility

Distribution

Decreased cardiac output
Decreased total body water
Decreased lean body mass
Decreased serum albumin
Increased alpha-1-acid glycoprotein
Increased body fat

Metabolism

Decreased hepatic mass
Decreased hepatic blood flow

Excretion

Decreased renal blood flow
Decreased glomerular function
Decreased tubular secretion

Pharmacokinetics

The processes of drug absorption, distribution, metabolism, and excretion may be affected or impaired by the normal physiologic changes of aging. Changes in the gastrointestinal (GI), cardiovascular, and circulatory systems; reduced body mass; and disturbances in liver and kidney function can alter the pharmacokinetics of drug therapy. Box 8.1 identifies these age-related physiologic changes in the older patient. Such changes ultimately affect the extent and duration of systemic availability of a drug and the possibility and probability of adverse drug effects.

ABSORPTION

Although absorption seems to be the least affected pharmacokinetic process during aging, several physiologic changes related to absorption affect drug therapy. In the older adult, increased gastric pH levels, decreased rate of blood flow, decreased GI motility, and reduced body surface area may influence the rate of absorption. However, the degree to which these factors affect absorption is unclear. Disease processes are more likely than age-related changes to alter an older adult's absorption patterns.

With age, the GI tract undergoes several changes that can alter oral drug absorption or affect bioavailability. For example, the stomach's response to food decreases, typified by reduced gastric acidity. Drugs that require an acidic environment to dissolve may take longer to disintegrate and be absorbed by the body; this delay may ultimately decrease systemic availability of a drug.

Circulation problems (e.g., reduced blood flow to organs) and reduced surface area of the GI tract are common in older adults. Drug absorption from the GI tract is highly dependent on both blood flow to the GI tract and the surface area of the GI tract; consequently, the extent or rate of drug absorption may be decreased in older adults. Additionally, decreased blood flow to tissues and muscles can alter the absorption of drugs administered subcutaneously or intramuscularly in older adults. Altered absorption can be further complicated by disease processes, such as peripheral vascular disease. Therefore, an intramuscular (IM) drug injection in the older adult may produce erratic blood concentrations because of changes in tissue perfusion and reduced muscle mass (another common age-related change).

Because GI motility decreases in older adults, substances take longer to move through the GI tract. Because of the extended GI transit time, a drug is in contact with the GI membranes for a longer time; therefore, the extent of drug absorption increases. For many drugs, the effects of increased contact time with the GI membranes are balanced by the effect from the decreased surface area.

The overall effects of aging on the GI tract result in a slowed drug absorption rate yet allow for the extent of drug absorption to be almost as complete as that in younger adults. However, this slowing in the rate of absorption not only results in slower onset of action but also alters the intensity of peak response because peak serum drug concentrations are blunted by the slowed absorption. Such an effect on the rate and extent of drug absorption may or may not have immediate clinical consequences, but the patient may require an increase in drug dosage if therapeutic effects decrease substantially below desired levels.

DISTRIBUTION

Several physiologic factors affect the distribution of a drug in older adults, including decreased body mass, reduced levels of plasma albumin, and a less effective blood–brain barrier. Other age-related factors that may affect drug distribution include declining cardiac output, extreme changes in body weight, poor nutrition, dehydration, inactivity, and extended bed rest.

The body mass of a person decreases with age. In the older adult, the proportion of body fat increases as the percentage of lean muscle mass decreases. Consequently, body water decreases in proportion to the total body weight. The higher proportion of body fat to lean muscle mass and decreased body water can substantially alter the distribution patterns of most drugs, depending on whether they are fat-soluble or water-soluble. In older adults, a highly fat-soluble drug (e.g., diazepam [Valium], an antianxiety drug) exhibits an increased volume of distribution; this increase results in a prolonged distribution phase, a prolonged half-life, and an increased duration of action. The increased volume of distribution for a given drug dose means that concentrations are lower in the blood but higher in the tissues. Therefore, when diazepam is given to older patients, one can anticipate

a greater response to the drug and a greater likelihood of adverse effects than in a young adult.

In contrast to fat-soluble drugs, highly water-soluble drugs (e.g., gentamicin, an antibiotic) exhibit a decreased volume of distribution because of the decrease in total body water in the older patient. Even at standard doses, more of these drugs circulate in the blood, making toxic blood levels a potential hazard.

Plasma levels of the protein albumin, which is produced by the liver, also are reduced in the elderly, often by as much as 13%. The reduced plasma albumin level reflects declining metabolic activity in the liver. Plasma albumin is responsible for binding, transporting, and distributing many drugs throughout the body, particularly acid-based drugs. In contrast, amounts of plasma alpha-1-acid glycoproteins, which principally bind and transport alkaline-based drugs, are not depressed in older adults. Hence, the acid or alkaline base of drugs can cause significant alterations in the older patient's response to drugs. In addition, when plasma albumin levels decline in the older adult, fewer binding sites are available for drugs. This scarcity of binding sites results in higher concentrations of unbound forms of a drug, which increases target organ exposure, pharmacologic activity, and the risk of adverse effects. Although higher concentrations of free drug also increase the amount of the drug available for metabolism and renal excretion, normal age-related decreases in liver and kidney function offset any increase in these pharmacokinetic processes. Overall, low plasma protein levels place older adults at increased risk of adverse effects from drug therapy. This risk is especially high when the drug is normally highly protein bound. An example is the anticonvulsant phenytoin (Dilantin), a highly protein-bound drug. Polypharmacy further complicates the effects of decreased albumin levels in older adults. Recall that highly protein-bound drugs compete for protein-binding sites even in younger patients. When fewer sites are available to start with, and several drugs must compete for fewer sites, the drugs may be unable to locate a protein-binding site. Ultimately, the effects of drug therapy increase because more free or unbound drug is available to be active.

Age-related changes in the central nervous system (CNS) can alter drug distribution. Normally, the blood–brain barrier prevents drugs from affecting the brain, but with advancing age, the efficiency of the blood–brain barrier declines. This decline permits higher levels of drug than normal to penetrate the brain.

METABOLISM

The liver's efficiency at metabolizing substances gradually declines throughout the aging process. In the older adult, three major physiologic changes greatly affect the efficiency of the liver. First, the size of the liver changes, and the number of metabolically active hepatocytes may decrease as much as 50%. Most change occurs when adults are in their 60s or 70s. Second, because cardiac output declines with age, blood flow to the liver declines as well. With less blood-borne oxygen available, the liver's capacity to remove many metabolic by-products is reduced. Third, the overall ability of the liver to metabolize drugs and other chemicals is reduced.

Normal hepatic metabolism of substances occurs in two major phases. Phase I metabolic reactions include oxidation, reduction, and hydrolysis of drug molecules. During phase I, the liver creates metabolites that may retain some degree of pharmacologic activity. Phase II reactions combine the drug or other metabolites produced in phase I with highly water-soluble forms of acetate, glucuronic acid, sulfate, or an amino acid. These reactions produce an inactive metabolized form of the drug that is excreted in the urine or feces. Ultimately, most phases I and II reactions make drugs more water-soluble, which restricts their access to the tissues, promotes removal from the body, and thereby terminates pharmacologic activity.

Aging affects the efficiency of both phases of metabolic activity but tends to alter phase I more than it alters phase II reactions. Because drug metabolism is slowed by reduced oxidation in phase I, drug blood levels are higher and drug half-lives are extended in older adults. This effect usually alters the appropriate dose and dosing interval and the duration of adverse effects. For example, when elderly adults receive a benzodiazepine (e.g., to relieve anxiety or promote sleep), they may experience associated cognitive impairments, such as sedation, confusion, and decreased mental alertness, for a longer time than normal after drug therapy ceases. Often, standard half-life parameters are inaccurate for the elderly patient. Nurses obtain age-related drug half-life information to evaluate drug responses accurately in older patients. Nurses who are unfamiliar with age-related differences may mistakenly interpret an older patient's altered cognitive function as a normal sign of aging rather than as a residual drug effect.

EXCRETION

Efficient renal function is a crucial factor in ensuring drug clearance from the blood and excretion from the body, and in terminating drug action. Aging can substantially decrease renal efficiency by altering the two main processes by which the kidneys remove drugs from the blood: glomerular filtration and renal tubular secretion. Both of these processes decline in efficiency with age and ultimately result in slower drug excretion and altered drug half-life.

One of the standard markers for renal function is the serum creatinine concentration, which reflects creatinine clearance from the blood by way of glomerular filtration. Despite the decline in the efficiency of glomerular filtration in the older patient, serum creatinine levels often remain in the normal range (Table 8.1). The normal range is maintained because creatinine production declines in the older patient as muscle mass decreases; therefore, less creatinine overall exists in the older adult to be filtered. These so-called normal creatinine levels can be misleading and should not be interpreted as an indication of normal renal function in elderly patients.

TABLE 8.1	Age-Related Differences in Creatinine in Men	
Age (Yr)	Creatinine Clearance Levels*	Serum Creatinine
17–24	140	0.808
25–34	140	0.808
35–44	133	0.813
45–54	127	0.829
55–64	119	0.837
65–74	109	0.825
75–84	96	0.843

*$Ccl_{cr} = (140 - age)(weight)/(72)(serum\ creatinine)$

NOTE: Women also demonstrate a similar decline in Ccl_{cr} with age. Ccl_{cr} for women is about 85% of values in men.

Pharmacodynamics

Decreased organ efficiency in the older adult alters pharmacodynamic responses. Because absorption is prolonged in the older adult, response to single doses of drugs is commonly delayed substantially. For example, the older adult taking aspirin for intermittent joint pain usually experiences a longer onset of action than normal. This delayed onset is not experienced for drugs that the older adult takes on a regular basis because doses taken at regular intervals maintain steady blood levels.

Most drug responses are based on the drug–receptor interaction. A patient's response to a particular drug depends on how efficiently that drug's receptor system operates or on the number of available receptors for that drug. An example of this interrelationship is the elderly patient and the beta-adrenergic receptor system. As a result of aging, the beta-adrenergic receptor system seems to operate less efficiently and possibly with fewer receptors. This decline in efficiency explains why the older adult is typically less responsive to beta-adrenergic agonists (stimulants), such as isoproterenol (Isuprel), a bronchodilator. Age-related changes affect the parasympathetic muscarinic-receptor system as well. Generally, the older adult has an increased response to anticholinergic drugs, such as atropine, and to the anticholinergic effects of drugs such as tricyclic antidepressants.

Decreases in the number of receptors are also associated with decreases in the respective neurotransmitters themselves. Older patients, for example, have decreased amounts of the neurotransmitters dopamine and acetylcholine.

Contraindications and Precautions

Although drug contraindications are generally similar for older adults and younger adults, some drugs carry label warnings specific to older adults. Some diseases or conditions that may contraindicate certain drug therapies are more likely to occur in older adults. Moreover, because of the older adult's decreased renal function and possibly metabolic function, many drugs should be used with caution. Some drugs or drug classes cause substantially more adverse effects in older adults than in other age populations. These drugs are generally considered inappropriate for older adults; however, with proper clinical management, monitoring, and dose limitations, these drugs may be used if necessary.

The Beers Criteria are an evidenced based, standard tool for the identification of potentially inappropriate medications in older adults. Originally formulated in 1997, this reference was updated in 2003. Based on a thorough review of the literature, questionnaires sent to practitioners, and review of an expert panel, it lists 48 medications or classes of medications that should generally be avoided in older adults. These drugs either are ineffective or pose unnecessary higher risks for older adults, and safer alternatives are available. See Table 8.2 for the updated Beers Criteria. The criteria also name 20 diseases or conditions in which specific medications should be avoided (Fick et al., 2003).

Use of inappropriate drugs may be a substantial problem in the current health care system. Small studies have found that between 32% and more than 50% of community-dwelling adults received at least one inappropriate prescribed drug (Gallagher et al., 2008; Rossi et al., 2007), and a large retrospective study of nearly 18,000 people found that 40% of the community-dwelling older adults had filled prescriptions for at least one inappropriate drug and 13% had filled two or more inappropriate prescriptions. Furthermore, those who received an inappropriate drug were significantly more likely to experience an adverse effect than those who received only appropriate drugs (14% versus 4.7%, p<0.001) (Fick et al., 2008). Polypharmacy (5 or more drugs) increased the risk for receiving an inappropriate drug Research has found that between 30% and 50% of patients receiving an inappropriate drug came to the emergency room and/or became hospitalized (Nixdorff et al., 2008). And a recent study of hospital prescribing showed that almost half of older adults were prescribed at least one potentially inappropriate drug; 6% received three or more potentially inappropriate drugs. These drugs are more likely to be prescribed to patients with myocardial infarction or heart failure, and to men rather than women. Cardiologists were much more likely than geriatricians or hospitalists to prescribe a potentially inappropriate drug that could produce severe adverse effects (Rothberg et al., 2008). Some small research studies argue that while the Beers' criteria of potentially inappropriate drugs is one important factor contributing to adverse effects, emergency room visits, and hospitalization for older adults in the community, it may not be the best single predictor of adverse drug effects that occur in a hospital setting; rather, polypharmacy upon admission is the best predictor (Page & Ruscin, 2006; O'Mahony & Gallagher, 2008). Larger clinical research studies are needed to clarify the best practice for minimizing adverse drug effects for hospitalized older adults.

The nurse needs to work closely with physicians, nurse practitioners, and pharmacists to minimize the use of drugs that are generally contraindicated in older adults, by seeking safer alternative drug therapy as well as minimizing unnecessary polypharmacy.

At the same time, the nurse must realize that there will be occasions when an "inappropriate" drug will be used because it is the best therapy to treat the older adult. During these occasions, the nurse will need to work closely with the rest of the health care team, the patient, and the family in providing clinical care to minimize potential adverse outcomes to the patient.

Adverse Effects

Although the same adverse effects from any given drug therapy will occur in older adults as in other age groups, physiologic changes in older adults place them at greater risk for certain adverse effects. Adverse drug effects are an important cause of hospital admissions in older adults. Adverse drug effects are also a serious concern for older adults who receive medication in ambulatory care settings.

Because of the less effective blood–brain barrier, older adults may be more vulnerable to CNS adverse effects, such as increased depressant or sedative activity of drugs. Research also indicates that CNS drugs decrease cognitive functioning of older adults (Box 8.2). In addition, decreased dopamine concentrations in the brain of older adults render them more susceptible to parkinsonian effects of dopamine antagonists, such as the phenothiazine antipsychotics and metoclopramide. Older adults are also more responsive to anticholinergic drugs and drugs with anticholinergic adverse effects (see Chapter 14).

Depending on the severity of these adverse responses, drug dosages may be limited or contraindicated for a particular patient.

Drug-induced behavioral changes often affect the older adult. Sometimes, they occur unexpectedly. For example, when beginning drug therapy with a sedative or a benzodiazepine to treat anxiety, the older patient may experience an effect that is the opposite of the intended effect. This effect is known as **paradoxical excitement,** whereby the patient is wide awake and hyperactive rather than calm and relaxed.

Determining whether an older patient is experiencing an adverse effect or a normal age-related health problem is difficult. Age-related health problems often mimic the adverse effects of drug therapy. For example, hearing loss can be a sign of aging, or it can be a serious adverse effect of some antimicrobial drugs (e.g., gentamicin). Loss of balance and unsteadiness while walking are often experienced by older patients and may be confused with the adverse effects of some drugs that cause dizziness or light-headedness. Clearly, the nurse needs to distinguish between these two conditions.

Drug Interactions

Drug interactions are the same for older adults as for other populations, but because older adults tend to take more drugs, they are at higher risk for interactions. It is

TABLE 8.2 **Revised Beers Criteria for Potentially Inappropriate Medication Use in Older Adults: Independent of Diagnoses or Conditions**

Drug Class and Specific Agent	Concern	Severity Rating (High or Low)
Analgesics and Anti-inflammatories		
propoxyphene (Darvon) and combination products (Darvon with ASA, Darvon-N, and Darvocet-N)	Drug that offers few analgesic advantages over acetaminophen, yet has the adverse effects of other narcotics.	Low
indomethacin (Indocin and Indocin SR)	Of all available NSAIDs, this drug produces the most CNS adverse effects.	High
pentazocine (Talwin)	Narcotic analgesic that causes more CNS adverse effects, including confusion and hallucinations, more commonly than other narcotic drugs. Additionally, it is a mixed agonist and antagonist.	High
meperidine (Demerol)	This drug is not an effective oral analgesic in doses commonly used. It may cause confusion and has many disadvantages compared to other narcotic drugs.	High
ketorolac (Toradol)	Immediate and long-term use should be avoided in older people, because a significant number have asymptomatic GI pathologic conditions.	High
Long-term use of full-dosage, longer half-life, non-COX- selective NSAIDs: naproxen (Naprosyn, Avaprox, and Aleve), oxaprozin (Daypro), and piroxicam (Feldene)	These have the potential to produce GI bleeding, renal failure, high blood pressure, and heart failure.	High
Antiemetics		
trimethobenzamide (Tigan)	One of the least effective antiemetic drugs, yet it can cause extrapyramidal adverse effects.	High
Muscle Relaxants and Antispasmodics		
methocarbamol (Robaxin), carisoprodol (Soma), chlorzoxazone (Paraflex), metaxalone (Skelaxin), cyclobenzaprine (Flexeril), and oxybutynin (Ditropan) (Do not consider the extended-release Ditropan XL.)	Most muscle relaxants and antispasmodic drugs are poorly tolerated by elderly patients, because they cause anticholinergic adverse effects, sedation, and weakness. Additionally, their effectiveness at doses tolerated by elderly patients is questionable.	High
orphenadrine (Norflex)	This drug causes more sedation and anticholinergic adverse effects than safer alternatives.	High
Benzodiazepines (used for sleep, anxiety, seizures)		
flurazepam (Dalmane) [sleep]	This hypnotic has an extremely long half-life in elderly patients (often days), producing prolonged sedation and increasing the incidence of falls and fractures. Medium- or short-acting benzodiazepines are preferable.	High
Doses of short-acting benzodiazepines: doses greater than lorazepam (Ativan), 3 mg; oxazepam (Serax), 60 mg; alprazolam (Xanax), 2 mg; temazepam (Restoril), 15 mg; and triazolam (Halcion), 0.25 mg	Because of increased sensitivity to benzodiazepines in elderly patients, smaller doses may be effective as well as safer. Total daily doses should rarely exceed the suggested maximums.	High
Long-acting benzodiazepines: chlordiazepoxide (Librium), chlordiazepoxide-amitriptyline (Limbitrol), chlordiazepoxide-clidinium (Librax), diazepam (Valium), quazepam (Doral), halazepam (Paxipam), and clorazepate (Tranxene)	These drugs have a long half-life in elderly patients (often several days), producing prolonged sedation and increasing the risk of falls and fractures. Short- and intermediate-acting benzodiazepines are preferred if a benzodiazepine is required.	High
Antidepressants		
amitriptyline (Elavil), chlordiazepoxide-amitriptyline (Limbitrol), and amitriptyline-perphenazine (Triavil)	Because of its strong anticholinergic and sedation properties, amitriptyline is rarely the antidepressant of choice for elderly patients.	High
doxepin (Sinequan)	Because of its strong anticholinergic and sedating properties, doxepin is rarely the antidepressant of choice for elderly patients.	High
Daily fluoxetine (Prozac)	This drug has a long half-life, which increases the risk of excessive CNS stimulation, sleep disturbances, and increasing agitation. Safer alternatives exist.	High

(Continued)

TABLE 8.2 — **Revised Beers Criteria for Potentially Inappropriate Medication Use in Older Adults: Independent of Diagnoses or Conditions** *(continued)*

Drug Class and Specific Agent	Concern	Severity Rating (High or Low)
Antianxiety (other than benzodiazepines)		
meprobamate (Miltown and Equanil)	This is a highly addictive and sedating anxiolytic. People using meprobamate for prolonged periods may become addicted and may need to be withdrawn slowly.	High
Antipsychotics		
thioridazine (Mellaril)	This drug has a greater potential for CNS and extrapyramidal adverse effects.	High
mesoridazine (Serentil)	This drug has CNS and extrapyramidal adverse effects.	High
Sedatives (non-benzodiazepine)		
All barbiturates (except phenobarbital) except when used to control seizures	When used in this way, these drugs are highly addictive and cause more adverse effects than most sedative or hypnotic drugs in elderly patients.	High
Other Psychotropic Drugs		
ergot mesyloids (Hydergine)	These agents have not been shown to be effective in the doses studied.	Low
Antiarrhythmics		
disopyramide (Norpace and Norpace CR)	Of all antiarrhythmic drugs, this is the most potent negative inotrope and therefore may induce heart failure in elderly patients. It is also strongly anticholinergic. Other antiarrhythmic drugs should be used.	High
digoxin (Lanoxin) (should not exceed 0.125 mg/d except when treating atrial arrhythmias)	Decreased renal clearance may lead to increased risk of toxic effects.	Low
amiodarone (Cordarone)	This drug is associated with QT interval problems and a risk of provoking torsades de pointes. It has a lack of efficacy in older adults.	High
Other Cardiovascular Drugs		
cyclandelate (Cyclospasmol)	This drug has not been shown to be effective in the doses studied.	Low
isoxsupine (Vasodilan)	This drug is ineffective.	Low
Anticoagulants/Antiplatelets		
Short-acting dipyridamole (Persantine). Do not consider the long-acting form (which has better properties than the short-acting form in older adults), except for patients with artificial heart valves.	This drug may cause orthostatic hypotension.	Low
ticlopidine (Ticlid)	This drug has been shown to be no better than aspirin in preventing clotting and may be considerably more toxic. Safer, more effective alternatives exist.	High
Antihypertensives		
methyldopa (Aldomet) and methyldopa-hydrochlorothiazide (Aldoril)	These drugs can cause bradycardia and can exacerbate depression in elderly patients.	High
reserpine at doses >0.25 mg	This drug can induce depression, impotence, sedation, and orthostatic hypotension.	Low
guanethidine (Ismelin)	This drug causes orthostatic hypotension. Safer alternatives exist.	High
guanadrel (Hylorel)	This drug causes orthostatic hypotension.	High
doxazosin (Cardura)	This drug may cause hypotension, dry mouth, and urinary problems.	Low
Short-acting nifedipine (Procardia and Adalat)	This drug may cause hypotension and constipation.	High
clonidine (Catapres)	This drug may cause orthostatic hypotension and CNS adverse effects.	Low
Antidiabetic		
chlorpropamide (Diabinese)	It has a prolonged half-life in elderly patients and could cause prolonged hypoglycemia. Additionally, it is the only oral hypoglycemic agent that causes syndrome of inappropriate antidiuretic hormone (SIADH) secretion.	High

TABLE 8.2 **Revised Beers Criteria for Potentially Inappropriate Medication Use in Older Adults: Independent of Diagnoses or Conditions** *(continued)*

Drug Class and Specific Agent	Concern	Severity Rating (High or Low)
Gastrointestinal Drugs		
GI antispasmodic drugs: dicyclomine (Bentyl), hyoscyamine (Levsin and Levsinex), propantheline (Pro-Banthine), belladonna alkaloids (Donnatal and others), and clidinium-chlordiazepoxide (Librax)	GI antispasmodic drugs are highly anticholinergic and have uncertain effectiveness. These drugs should be avoided (especially for long-term use).	High
Long-term use of stimulant laxatives: bisacodyl (Dulcolax), cascara sagrada, and Neoloid except in the presence of opiate analgesic use	These drugs may exacerbate bowel dysfunction.	High
Mineral oil	This agent has the potential for aspiration and adverse effects. Safer alternatives are available.	High
cimetidine (Tagamet)	This drug has CNS adverse effects, including confusion.	Low
Anticholinergics and Antihistamines		
chlorpheniramine (Chlor-Trimeton), diphenhydramine (Benadryl), hydroxyzine (Vistaril and Atarax), cyproheptadine (Periactin), promethazine (Phenergan), tripelennamine, dexchlorpheniramine (Polaramine)	All nonprescription and many prescription antihistamines may have potent anticholinergic properties. Non-anticholinergic antihistamines are preferred in elderly patients when treating allergic reactions.	High
Diphenhydramine (Benadryl)	This drug may cause confusion and sedation. It should not be used as a hypnotic, and when used to treat emergency allergic reactions, it should be used in the smallest possible dose.	High
Amphetamines and Anorexics		
	These drugs have potential for causing dependence, hypertension, angina, and myocardial infarction.	High
Anti-infectives		
nitrofurantoin (Macrodantin)	This drug has the potential to cause renal impairment. Safer alternatives are available.	High
Vitamins, Minerals, Electrolytes		
ferrous sulfate (>325 mg/d)	Doses >325 mg/d do not dramatically increase the amount absorbed but greatly increase the incidence of constipation.	Low
Hormones		
methyltestosterone (Android, Virilon, and Testred)	This drug is associated with the potential for prostatic hypertrophy and cardiac problems.	High
desiccated thyroid	There are concerns about cardiac effects from this hormone preparation. Safer alternatives are available.	High
estrogens only (oral)	There is evidence of the carcinogenic (breast and endometrial cancer) potential of these agents and lack of cardioprotective effect in older women.	Low
Diuretics		
ethacrynic acid (Edecrin)	This agent may cause hypertension and fluid imbalances. Safer alternatives are available.	Low

Adapted from *Archives of Internal Medicine 163*, 2719 (2003). ©2003 American Medical Association. Retrieved from http://www.archinternmed.com.

BOX 8.2 FOCUS ON RESEARCH

Inappropriate Drugs in Older Adults and Cognitive Decline

Wright, R. M., Roumani, Y. F., Boudreau, R., et al. (2009). Effect of central nervous system medication use on decline in cognition in dommunity-dwelling older adults: findings form the Heatlh, Aging, And Body Composition Study. *Journal of the American Geriatric Society, 57*(2): 243–250.

The Study

The Health, Aging and Body Composition Study, begun in 1996, examined how age-related changes in weight and body composition (e.g., amount of muscle present in the body) influenced health. Two thousand seven hundred thirty-seven healthy older adults were enrolled in the study sponsored by the National Institutes of Health. The study was a longitudinal cohort study set in Pittsburgh, Pennsylvania and Memphis, Tennessee. This aspect of the study evaluated whether combined use of multiple central nervous system (CNS) medications over time was associated with cognitive changes. The subjects had normal cognitive level at the start of the study as measured by the Modified Mini-Mental State Examination (referred to as 3MS); their scores were 80 or better out of a possible 100. Use of a CNS medication (benzodiazepine, opioid, antipsychotics, or antidepressants), the duration of use, and the dose were determined at baseline, (year one) and years three and five. The 3MS was administered at each of those times. By year five, more than one-fourth of them demonstrated cognitive decline and CNS use increased from 13.9% at baseline to 15.3% and 17.1% at years three and five. Combination use of more than one CNS drug and a higher dose of the drug were associated with more cognitive decline in the older adults studied.

Nursing Implications

This research highlights the risks to older adults when potentially inappropriate drugs are given to them. CNS drugs such as the ones monitored are included in the potentially inappropriate medication list in the Beer's Criteria. However, the Beer's Criteria does not list cognitive decline from these drugs, so these findings add to the potential concerns related to using these drugs in older adults. Adverse effects from drug therapy cause substantial morbidity and mortality in older adults. Although many adverse effects cannot be prevented, nurses should be vigilant to help protect patients from those that *are* preventable. Nurses should question any medication order in which an inappropriate drug appears to have been ordered for the patient. If patients require a drug that is on the Beer's list, especially a CNS drug, the dose should be kept as low as possible and the duration of use should be as short as possible to minimize adverse effects. Patients who demonstrate a cognitive decline should have their drug therapy carefully evaluated. It should not be assumed that changes in cognitive function are related to aging, as it may be a drug-related effect.

not uncommon for older adults to be taking between 8 and 12 prescribed and OTC drugs to treat a variety of diseases. Often, the combination of so many different drugs causes serious drug interactions. For example, a patient who is taking a total of 10 different prescriptions and OTC drugs risks 45 different two-drug combinations that could interact to produce an adverse effect. Drug interactions can decrease the effectiveness of one or both of the drugs or increase the risk of adverse effects. Drug interactions are common in older adults.

Assessment of Relevant Core Patient Variables Related to Older Adults

Health Status

Aging is associated with a decline in normal bodily maintenance and function. The major organ systems (cardiovascular, respiratory, GI, genitourinary, endocrine, and others) all become much less efficient with advancing age and cause a multitude of health problems that often require drug therapy. When assessing the older patient's health status, assess for polypharmacy, which has the potential for causing serious drug interactions and adverse effects. The compromised health status of the older adult can further alter the pharmacokinetics of certain drugs and is of equal concern. In such cases, assess the functional ability of the older adult's body systems and determine whether the patient has any diseases that may affect prescribed drug therapy. Pay particular attention to cardiovascular, hepatic, and renal problems, because these problems can greatly alter the patient's responses to drug therapy.

When assessing the older patient's renal function status, remember that normal laboratory value ranges may be deceptive. As discussed, the older patient with compromised renal function may have serum creatinine levels or blood urea nitrogen (BUN) levels in the normal range. Hence, normal serum creatinine or BUN levels are not a true indicator of the older patient's renal status.

Assessment should always include a thorough inventory of all the drugs the patient is currently taking, dosage, and dosing schedule. This inventory helps alert the nurse to any possible drug interactions. The nurse also should confirm that the medications the patient is taking matches the prescribed therapy listed in the health care record. This assessment should occur at every visit, in all health care settings, and every time the patient transitions from one setting to another (e.g., from intensive care to a general unit, from hospitalization to discharge home, or to a long-term care facility). This type of assessment is termed **medication reconciliation**. It may be done via a list of drugs or via direct observation by having the patient present all of their medications to the nurse. Determine if the patient can identify

CRITICAL THINKING SCENARIO

THINKING ABOUT AGE-RELATED CORE PATIENT VARIABLES

Antonio Mendez, a 70-year-old man with type 1 diabetes mellitus, has been admitted to your unit for the second time in a month with diabetic ketoacidosis. His blood glucose level on admission is elevated, at 600 mg/dL. The prescriber writes an order for 15 U of NPH insulin mixed with 5 U of regular insulin every morning. As the patient's nurse, you are assessing why this patient continues to have elevated blood glucose levels. What relevant core patient variables should you investigate with this patient?

each drug and its purpose. Older adults frequently identify their pills by appearance rather than name. Use of generic drugs may confuse older adults as these drugs do not have the distinctive shape and colors found in trade name drugs (Ballentine, 2008). Gaps in the knowledge of older adult patients indicate that teaching about drug therapy is needed.

In addition, assess whether the older adult patient is taking the medication as prescribed. When taking a drug at home, older adults may take the medication more often than indicated or less often than indicated. This is termed **nonadherence**. Nonadherence with therapy is not usually related to a patient's refusal to take the drug therapy as prescribed, but usually is associated with a variety of other reasons. Medication adherence rates can be as low as 50% for chronic conditions (Bazian Report, 2005; Roehl et al., 2006). This is because there are a high number of daily prescribed medications required, making the regimen confusing as well as expensive. Adherence is therefore difficult in patients who have difficulty remembering to take all of their different drugs, or who may have difficulty remembering which drug to take for which health problem at what time. Another reason for nonadherence or poor adherence when there is polypharmacy is if patients do not feel they can afford a medication. Other reasons for nonadherence include physical deficits that prevent accurate self administration (e.g., poor eyesight, or decreased fine motor ability to open pill bottles), anticipation of or actually experiencing adverse effects, and a general lack of understanding of the rationale for drug therapy. If a generic drug is prescribed by one prescriber and the identical trade name drug by another prescriber, the older adult may take both if they are unaware that they are the same drug. If a patient does not have the physical ability to travel to a pharmacy, he or she may not be able to obtain a filled prescription. All of these reasons can contribute to nonadherence. Information from the assessment indicates what information the nurse needs to emphasize in patient education.

Ask the older adult patient about all OTC drugs, because many patients do not consider these medicines "drugs" and may not mention them unless specifically asked. For example, many older adults take laxatives to relieve constipation, a common problem associated with age-related slowing of GI motility. Most older patients are unaware that laxatives can interact with and complicate prescribed drug therapy by decreasing absorption of some drugs. Unless specifically asked about laxative use, the patient may not volunteer the information.

Lifestyle, Diet, and Habits

Because lifestyle, diet, and habits of the older adult affect the pharmacokinetics and pharmacodynamics of drug therapy, assess several basic areas of daily living, such as how active the patient is and what his or her daily routine includes. Moderate, regular exercise promotes circulation, absorption of drugs given intramuscularly or subcutaneously, and distribution of drugs through the GI tract.

Dietary patterns and habits are also important. If older adults have difficulty swallowing solid food and eat only soft or chopped foods, they may need to have oral drugs (such as pills or tablets) crushed and mixed with a diluent for swallowing or have the drugs prescribed in a liquid form.

The use of alternative medications, such as herbs and botanicals, has increased with older adults as it has with the general population. Almost 13% of older adults use herbal products such as glucosamine, echinacea, or garlic, yet half do not report this use (Roehl et al., 2006; Bruno & Ellis, 2005). Because older adults tend to take more prescribed medications than other age groups, they are at higher risk for drug interactions if they take alternative medications. Ask the older patient if he or she takes any alternative medications and then document the findings. Documentation is important to help all health care providers identify any potential drug–herb interactions.

Another important assessment is how drug therapy and the related adverse effects have altered the older adult's lifestyle or impaired the quality of life. How have the activities of daily living been impaired? How have adverse effects interfered with the patient's involvement in community or family events? Some drugs place the older adult at risk for injury and therefore can greatly limit the quality of life. For example, drugs that cause dizziness or light-headedness when standing put the older patient at great risk for falls and broken bones. Drugs that cause postural hypotension, such as many antihypertensives, have been associated with falls and hip fractures.

The mental status of older patients is extremely important to their quality of life. Many older patients are depressed because they are lonely or have limited ability to function and participate in life's enjoyments. Sometimes, drug therapy can further decrease the older patient's quality of life because of adverse drug effects. Depression, delirium, dementia, and low self-esteem are commonly cited adverse effects of drug therapy.

Habits regarding drug therapy should be considered when planning drug administration in the hospital. Assess whether the older adult patient has a preferred schedule for taking drug therapy at home, because it may be more therapeutic to maintain the patient's established routine and dosage schedule than to readjust them to fit hospital routines. Maintaining the same drug schedule not only promotes similar drug actions and reactions but also helps reduce stress and anxiety in older patients who may have difficulty adjusting to changes in routine.

Because older adults typically have fixed incomes, question patients to determine whether their health insurance includes payment or partial payment for drug therapy. Coverage may influence whether the older patient can afford the prescribed drug therapy. As mentioned, many older patients take several drugs for various health problems, and drug therapy may be extremely costly; therefore, patients may not be taking the drugs as prescribed because they do not feel they can afford them. Confirm that patients are able to afford needed medications. If the patient does not have adequate financial resources or does not have health insurance with a prescription benefit, help the patient gain access to reduced-price medications. Pharmaceutical companies have programs that provide assistance to those with very low incomes, and government assistance programs are also available. It may be necessary to work with social workers to meet this patient need.

Environment
Assessing the older patient's environment is another important element when considering drug therapy. Determine whether the patient lives alone or with other family members or caregivers who can help obtain and administer drug therapy if needed. Other considerations are as follows:

• Is the pharmacy accessible to the older adult?
• Can the patient drive or take a bus to the pharmacy, or is someone available to go for him or her?
• Does the pharmacy make deliveries?

If ready access is not available, it may be necessary to make referrals to other sources for drug therapy, such as mail-order pharmacies.

Culture and Inherited Traits
Whenever assessing older adults, be sensitive to beliefs and cultural values that may have an effect on drug therapy. Some ethnic or cultural groups still practice folk medicine, preferring home remedies or herbal treatments to traditional drug therapy. These patients may be skeptical or afraid of new or unfamiliar methods of drug therapy. Moreover, they may not understand the drug regimen. Among cultural groups that may practice folk medicine are Eastern Europeans, Hispanic Americans, Native Americans, Asians, some African Americans, and some patients from remote or rural areas of the United States, such as Appalachia, the Ozark Mountains, or Alaska. Additionally, the number of some of the cytochrome P-450 isoenzymes, needed for drug metabolism, may vary based on genetic inherited traits that are not transmitted along race or ethnic lines. This may place some older adults at increased risk for adverse effects from some medications.

Nursing Diagnoses and Outcomes
Nursing diagnoses specific to drug therapy in older adults are similar to those for patients in other age groups. However, because of age-related health problems of older patients, decreased organ functioning, and polypharmacy, some diagnoses more commonly apply. They include the following:

• Risk for Injury related to adverse effects of drug therapy stemming from polypharmacy, inappropriate prescribing, or drug interactions secondary to increased therapeutic effect, delayed elimination, and prolonged drug half-life from altered pharmacokinetics.

Desired outcome: *The older adult patient will not sustain an injury while on drug therapy.*
• Ineffective Therapeutic Regimen Management because of impaired memory, lack of financial resources, impaired physical abilities, complex drug regimen, inability to physically obtain prescribed drugs, or lack of understanding of drug regimen.
Desired outcome: *The patient will effectively manage the therapeutic regimen with the help of appropriate resources.*

Planning and Intervention
Maximizing Therapeutic Effects
For any drug therapy to be therapeutic, the appropriate dose must be taken at the appropriate times. The more complicated the overall therapeutic regimen, the greater the likelihood of poor adherence to the drug therapy. Remember, nonadherence does not always mean that the patient directly refuses to follow the recommended drug therapy schedule. It may indicate that the patient cannot adhere to the prescribed drug course for various reasons. It is necessary to determine the true cause of nonadherence in order to make an appropriate plan of care.

Nurses and prescribers can improve adherence by making drug regimens as easy to follow and as uncomplicated as possible. For example, some drugs are available in sustained-release forms that can be taken once or twice a day, rather than four or more times a day. Some combination drug forms are available that incorporate two drugs, allowing the patient to take only one preparation instead of two. Consult the health care provider for appropriate orders if such options are available for the patient's specific drug therapy.

When new drug therapy begins, plan a new drug schedule to coincide with other prescribed schedules whenever possible. If the patient already takes a drug three times a day with meals, and the new drug must be taken once a day, the patient should take the new drug with breakfast when other drugs are taken. In this way, the patient need not remember another time to take a drug. This kind of planning promotes therapeutic adherence.

After simplifying drug therapy as much as possible, verify that the patient can remember to take the drug. If an older adult patient is having trouble remembering which drug should be taken at which time, assist the patient by creating memory aids. Pill boxes are available with compartments labeled by the hours of the day or by meal times (B, L, D), as are pill boxes labeled with days of the week. The patient places each drug in its appropriate slot at the beginning of the day and can then easily check whether each dose was taken on schedule. An inexpensive adaptation of the commercial pill box is an egg carton with hand-labeled hours of the day on each egg compartment.

When recommending types of drug preparations for each patient, consider which form can be self-administered easily. A chewable tablet or a liquid may be easier to take if the patient has difficulty swallowing pills. If a choice of dosage forms is possible, consult the prescriber about selecting the form that is most easily used. To improve the ability to self-administer drug therapy correctly, advise the patient of options that can be requested from the dispensing pharmacy. For example, containers with easy-to-remove, non-childproof caps and large-print labels promote therapeutic adherence for patients with arthritis or vision impairments. Also, verify that the patient can obtain prescriptions and refills from the pharmacy independently or has the necessary assistance.

Older adults must be monitored diligently for initial and continuing therapeutic drug effects. To detect improvements or deterioration in the patient's condition, perform periodic comparative assessments of current and previous status and identify changes in therapeutic effectiveness that may necessitate a dosage adjustment.

Patients cannot benefit from drug therapy if they do not receive the proper prescribed drug therapy. As medication regimens become more complex, it is likely that the patient's medical record may not accurately reflect the current drug therapy that the patient is receiving. Medications that have been newly added may be missing, or medications that were discontinued may still appear. Inaccurate drug names, doses, routes, or frequency of administration may also be present. Every time patients change the environment where they receive drug therapy, an error can occur. This is true whether a patient is transferring from one hospital inpatient unit to another, is being admitted to or discharged from the hospital to home or an extended-care facility, or is being seen at an outpatient clinic or office where drug therapy is prescribed and then will return home. The nurse at each point of care should be responsible for medication reconciliation. Although electronic records are generally considered to be more reliable than paper records, research has found that electronic records are not 100% accurate either (Kaboli et al., 2004), so medication reconciliation is still indicated. (For more information on medication reconciliation, see Chapter 11.)

Minimizing Adverse Effects

Some older adults are more at risk of medication-related problems. Those most at risk include: those over age 85, those who take 1 or more medications or more than 12 doses of a medication per day, or those who have at least 6 active chronic medical diagnoses, especially renal impairment (Roehl et al., 2006), as chronic conditions change the pharmacokinetics of drug therapy and chronic conditions frequently require 3 or more drugs for treatment. Whenever possible, alternatives to drug therapy should be considered as the initial treatment for problems. For example, if the older adult complains of difficulty sleeping, encouraging some mild exercise during the day (e.g., walking) or suggesting minor dietary changes (e.g., avoiding large meals near bedtime) may be enough to promote sleep. Sedatives and other drug therapy should be used only if absolutely necessary, and then in low doses (see Table 8.2). Reducing the number of prescribed medications decreases the risk of adverse drug effects and drug interactions.

Drugs should be used with great caution in older adults because these patients exhibit a narrower **benefit: risk ratio** than younger adults. A benefit: risk ratio is the margin between desired therapeutic effects and adverse consequences of drug therapy. Obviously, the beneficial therapeutic outcomes must be considered in relation to the associated physical risk factors.

Because the renal and metabolic systems of most older adults do not function as efficiently as those of younger patients in metabolizing and eliminating drugs from the body, older adults are at increased risk for drug overdose or toxicity. Because of diminished renal function in older patients, closely monitor for signs and symptoms of possible drug toxicity when the patient is taking drugs (e.g., digoxin, a drug that slows the heart rate) that do not undergo significant metabolism. When potentially nephrotoxic drugs (e.g., gentamicin, certain cephalosporin antibiotics, and nonsteroidal anti-inflammatory drugs) are used, be particularly careful because the older adult is especially prone to rapid onset of action and severe nephrotoxicity. Monitor serum blood levels to detect whether toxic drug levels are developing.

Additionally, distinguish carefully between the normal signs and symptoms of aging and the onset of adverse effects from drug therapy. Some adverse effects—impaired cognition or memory, or alterations in mood—mimic signs of aging. For example, the patient who falls repeatedly may be experiencing drug-induced light-headedness or drowsiness from benzodiazepines, used to treat anxiety or as sleep aids. Those with difficulty communicating may be experiencing aphasia as a result of antipsychotic drug therapy. Refer to a computerized drug data base or consult with the pharmacist for assistance in determining whether behaviors or symptoms exhibited by the older adult stem from adverse drug reactions or drug interactions.

Many older patients demonstrate atypical adverse effects that mimic signs of aging and paradoxical effects. If drug-induced symptoms are misinterpreted by the nurse, proper interventions may be neglected, and the older adult may unnecessarily suffer long-term effects. Unless the nurse knows the patient's history, health status, and potential adverse effects of the drugs the patient is taking, he or she will not be able to distinguish between drug-induced symptoms or excessive therapeutic effect and age-related problems.

Obtain a current drug profile and an accurate history of the patient's usual abilities and changes in abilities or health status. By establishing this baseline information, it is possible for the nurse to be alert to any new signs and symptoms in the patient that could be drug related. Ask older adults if they believe they are having adverse effects from drug therapy because they are frequently correct in recognizing such effects. If the older adult patient has any communication impairments, talk with family members or others who know the older adult patient well to determine the patient's baseline behaviors.

BOX 8.3 COMMUNITY BASED CONCERNS

Identification and Management of Polypharmacy Problems

- Question the patient about any and all drug therapy that he or she is taking or has taken in the past. Remember to ask about any non-prescribed, over-the-counter (OTC) preparations.
- Ask to see the drug bottles to verify the physician's or nurse practitioner's orders and evaluate the patient's knowledge about the drugs. Frequently, patients will pull out plastic bags or boxes full of drugs.
- Read the labels carefully. Attempt to identify drugs unknown to the patient or unclear prescriptions. If the prescriptions have changed frequently, or the patient has a long history of chronic health problems, the drug labels may be worn, faded, or difficult to read.
- Determine which drug prescriptions and OTC preparations are for current use. Some patients keep drugs for problems they no longer have. Due to expense, patients may not want to dispose of these; if you cannot get rid of them, then at least separate them from drugs currently in use.
- Determine if there are any duplications of a prescription. Many times patients see more than one physician or nurse practitioner, who may each prescribe the same medication. The patient may not realize this, especially if one of the prescriptions is listed with a generic name and another with a trade name.
- Determine whether therapy can be simplified. Consult with the physician or nurse practitioner as indicated.
- Look up all drugs to determine if any drug interactions are possible between the drugs currently being used. Consult with the physician or nurse practitioner as indicated.
- Assess the patient and family carefully for changes that have occurred since drug therapy began. The onset of new problems may actually be adverse effects from a medication.
- Assist the patient in creating a time schedule to take all prescribed drugs appropriately but in accordance with the patient's lifestyle. Use memory aids as needed.

In addition, become familiar with the core drug knowledge regarding possible adverse effects and drug interactions of the patient's specific drug therapy. Monitor the older patient carefully for development of adverse effects caused by physiologic changes or polypharmacy. If the older adult shows any signs of adverse effects, seek appropriate changes in the drug therapy. Box 8.3 discusses the identification and management of polypharmacy problems.

Help devise a drug schedule that minimizes the risks of adverse effects. For example, if the patient is to take a drug that causes sedation, the dose may be given at bedtime, if possible, to avoid daytime drowsiness and to lessen the risk of falling. In general, the prescriber may start the older adult's therapy with a low dose and increase the dose gradually as needed to reach a therapeutic level. Once the desired therapeutic effects occur, the dosage can be stabilized at that level. Using the minimal therapeutic dosage minimizes the risk for adverse effects.

Providing Patient and Family Education

Educate patients about drug therapy in various ways. Written instructions regarding drug use and times of administration may be developed and emphasized to help prevent confusion. This education is especially important when patients are receiving several drugs.

Also, teach patients and families about expected or possible adverse effects and how to differentiate between them and normal signs of aging. Help patients understand which adverse effects should be reported immediately to the health care provider or nurse practitioner. In addition, teach patients and families methods to assist with accurate dosage and administration of drugs. Because the post-hospital regimen of drug therapy may be complex for the older adult, efforts should be made to determine as early as possible which drugs will be prescribed for home use to allow adequate time for thorough patient and family education about the drug therapy.

Ongoing Assessment and Evaluation

Because the physiologic changes associated with aging often greatly alter the pharmacologic properties of drug therapy, assess the older patient continually for therapeutic and adverse effects of drug therapy. In many situations, also assess the home environment and family support to determine the older patient's ability to adhere to drug therapy. Consistent and regular monitoring of the older patient is extremely important because of polypharmacy, which is common in older patients and puts them at high risk for drug interactions, decreased therapeutic effects, and nonadherence. Drug therapy is effective in the older adult when therapeutic effects are achieved without serious adverse effects that diminish quality of life.

CHAPTER SUMMARY

- Older adults share common age-related changes and risk factors that alter drug administration, dosage, and expected response to drug therapy.
- Aging alters all of the pharmacokinetic processes, placing older adults at increased risk for adverse drug effects.
- Serum creatinine levels often remain in the normal range despite impaired kidney function.
- Pharmacodynamics of drug therapy may be decreased in older adults because of changes in the receptor systems. Older adults also have decreased amounts of the neurotransmitters dopamine and acetylcholine.
- Some drugs or drug classes produce more adverse effects in the older adult, partly related to decreased organ functioning. Dose modifications and close clinical monitoring are necessary if these drugs must be used in older adults.
- Many signs and symptoms of health problems in older adults result from the normal aging-related decline in organ or system function. These symptoms often mimic the adverse effects of drug therapy. The nurse must be careful to distinguish between the normal signs and symptoms of aging and the onset of adverse effects from drug therapy.

- Three main concerns with drug therapy in older adults are polypharmacy, inappropriate drug prescription, and nonadherence with therapy.
- Polypharmacy is an important concern in older adults because it greatly increases the risk of drug interactions and adverse effects
- Inappropriate drugs are all too frequently included in the older adult's drug regimen. These drugs are described in the Beer's criteria; they increase adverse effects, emergency room visits, and hospitalizations for older adults. They are more likely to be prescribed if the patient is receiving polypharmacy.
- Nonadherence with drug therapy is when a patient does not take a drug as prescribed but takes too much or too little of a prescribed drug. Multiple factors contribute to nonadherence such as forgetfulness, complexity of the drug regimen, cost of drug therapy, physical inability to open medication packaging, and inability to travel to the pharmacy.
- Nurses can promote older patients' adherence to prescribed drug therapy by minimizing the use of drug therapy when possible, simplifying the therapeutic regimen as much as possible, titrating doses upward gradually as prescribed to minimize adverse effects, helping with drug administration scheduling, assisting with memory aids if needed, and providing teaching and instructions in writing.
- Medication reconciliation will help to rectify inappropriate drug prescription, prevent drug interactions, and correct accidental overuse of a prescribed drug.
- Nurses need to assess patients' circumstances and cultural preferences or barriers to determine whether patients have the means and ability to obtain and comply with prescribed treatments, dietary recommendations, daily routine, and activity levels that can affect drug therapy.

QUESTIONS FOR STUDY AND REVIEW

1. Describe the effects of aging on the liver and its functioning.
2. How do normal changes in the renal system place the older adult at risk for adverse effects from drug therapy?
3. What is polypharmacy? Why is it an important issue for the nurse to consider in older adult patients?
4. Why are adverse drug effects often overlooked in older adults?
5. Why is it important to consider the core patient variables of lifestyle, diet, and habits with older adults receiving drug therapy?

NEED MORE HELP?

Chapter 8 of the Study Guide to Accompany *Drug Therapy in Nursing,* 4th Edition, contains NCLEX-style questions and other learning activities to reinforce your understanding of the concepts presented in this chapter. For additional information or to purchase the study guide, visit the**Point**.

REFERENCES

Ballentine, N. H. (2008). Polypharmacy in the elderly: maximizing benefit, minimizing harm. *Critical Care Nursing*, 31(1):40–45.

Bazian Report. (2005). The effects of education on patient adherence to medication. *Evidence-Based Health & Public Health*, 9(6):398–404.

Bruno, J. J. & Ellis, J. J. (2005). Herbal use among US elderly: 2002 National Health Interview Survey. *The Annals of Pharmacotherapy*, 39(4):643–648.

Fick, D. M., Cooper, J. W., Wade, W. E., Waller, J. L., Maclean, J. R., & Beers, M. H. (2003). Updating the Beers criteria for potentially inappropriate medication use in older adults. *Archives of Internal Medicine*, 163:2716–2724.

Fick, D. M., Mion, L. C., Beers, M. H., & Waller, J. L. (2008). Health outcomes associated with potentially inappropriate medication use in older adults. *Research in Nursing & Health*, 31:42–51.

Fulton, M. & Allen, E. (2005) Polypharmacy in the elderly: a literature review. *Journal of the American Academy of Nurse Practitioners*, 17(4):123–132.

Gallagher, P. F., Barry, P. J., Ryan, C., Hartigan, I. & O'Mahony, D. (2008). Inappropriate prescribing in an acutely ill population of elderly patients as determined by Beers Criteria. *Age and Ageing*, 37(1):96–101.

Hajjar, E. R., Cafiero, A. C., & Hanlon, J. T. (2007). Polypharmacy in elderly patients. *The American Journal of Geriatric Pharmacotherapy*, 5(4):345–351.

Kaboli, P. J., McClimon, B. J., Hoth, A. B., & Barnett, M. J. (2004). Assessing the accuracy of computerized medication histories. *American Journal of Managed Care*, 10(11 Pt 2): 872–877.

Nixdorff, N., Hustey, F. M., Brady, A. K., Varji, K., Leonard, M., & Messinger-Rapport, B. J. (2008). Potentially inappropriate medications and adverse drug effects in elders in the ED. *American Journal of Emergency Medicine*, 26(6):697–700.

O'Mahony, D. & Gallagher, P. F. (2008). Inappropriate prescribing in the older population: need for new criteria. *Age and Ageing*, 37(2):138–141.

Page, R. L. & Ruscin, J. M. (2006). The risk of adverse drug events and hospital-related morbidity and mortality among older adults with potentially inappropriate medication use. *The American Journal of Geriatric Pharmacotherapy*, 4(4):297–305.

Roehl, B., Talati, A., & Parks, S. (2006). Medication Prescribing for Older Adults. *Annals of Long Term Care, 14*(6). Retrieved from http://www.annalsoflongtermcare.com/article/5779

Rossi, M. I., Young, A., Maher, R., et al. (2007). Polypharmacy and health beliefs in older outpatients. *The American Journal of Geriatric Pharmacotherapy*, 5(4):317–323.

Rothberg, M. B., Pekow, P. S., Liu, F., et al. (2008). Potentially inappropriate medication use in hospitalized elders. *Journal of Hospital Medicine*, 3(2):91–102.

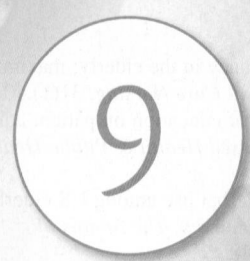

9

Lifestyle: Substance Abuse

Learning Objectives

At the completion of this chapter the student will:

1. Describe the scope of substance abuse in the United States.

2. Identify etiologic factors associated with substance abuse.

3. Identify frequently abused drugs and list common medical problems associated with abuse of these drugs.

4. Describe the pharmacologic basis for physical and psychological drug dependence, tolerance, and addiction.

5. Explain the adverse effects associated with chronic abuse of alcohol, cocaine, marijuana, and opioids.

6. Discuss the nursing management of patients who abuse substances, including alcohol, cocaine, marijuana, hallucinogenics, and opioids.

Key Terms

abstinence syndrome	habituation	psychological dependence
addiction	physical dependence	substance abuse
cross-dependence	psychedelic	tolerance
cross-tolerance	psychoactive	withdrawal syndrome

lifestyle, diet, and habits are core patient variables that exert some of the most important effects on a patient's response to drug therapy. The use of substances such as alcohol, tobacco products, and illicit or "street" drugs can seriously complicate drug therapy as well as the patient's general condition. Box 9.1 summarizes highlights from a national survey concerning the use of alcohol, tobacco, and illicit drugs in the United States.

Substance abuse is the inappropriate and usually excessive self-administration of a drug substance for nonmedical purposes. Drugs with a high abuse potential have the ability to stimulate compulsive drug-seeking behavior. Contemporary substance abuse has pervasive economic, legal, medical, moral, psychological, religious, and social implications. Substance abuse occurs throughout the life span and cuts across all racial, socioeconomic, ethnic, and cultural groups. Furthermore, factors in the patient's environment, family, or community can influence susceptibility to substance abuse and lead to drug addiction.

Drug **addiction** is a complex process involving interactions among the drug (availability, cost, pharmacology, toxicology); the user (personal resources, psychiatric profile, temperament); and society (family and peer influences, positive and negative advertising, and social attitudes). Broadly speaking, drug addiction alters the patient's life in a harmful way; for example, drug-related activity may result in a jail sentence.

Substance use and abuse interact with drug therapy in several ways:

- Drug therapy may become drug abuse.
- Chronic abuse may create health problems that require treatment with additional drug therapy.
- Treating or preventing symptoms of withdrawal from a substance may require drug therapy.
- Concurrent use of a substance may interact with drug therapy prescribed for a physiologic problem.

This chapter discusses various factors involved in substance abuse, several commonly abused drug categories and how they affect the body, and nursing management of substance-abusing patients.

CAUSES OF SUBSTANCE ABUSE

Dopamine Hypothesis

Scientists have demonstrated that a link exists between the neurotransmitter dopamine (especially DA-D3) and drugs of abuse and that dopamine plays a key role in a wide range

BOX 9.1 COMMUNITY BASED CONCERNS

How Many Substance Abusers?

Substance Abuse and Mental Health Services Administration (SAMHSA) National Survey on Drug Use & Health is the primary source of information on the prevalence, patterns, and consequences of alcohol, tobacco, and illegal drug use and abuse in the general U.S. civilian noninstitutionalized population, aged 12 years and older. The following information is highlighted in the 2009 report:

- In 2009, an estimated 21.8 million Americans, or 8.7% of the population aged 12 years or older, were current illicit drug users. Current drug use means use of an illicit drug during the month preceding the survey interview.

Drug	Number of Users
Marijuana	16.7 million
Psychotherapeutics (pain relievers, stimulants, tranquilizers, sedatives)	7 million
Cocaine	1.6 million
Hallucinogens	1.3 million
Inhalants	0.6 million
Heroin	0.2 million

- Gender
  - Males (10.8%) more than females (6.6 %).
- Age
  - The highest rate was among persons aged 18 to 20 (22.2 %).
  - Ages 12–17: 10 %
  - Ages 18–25: 21.2%
  - Ages 26–29: 14.4%
  - Ages 65 or older: 0.9 %.
- Race/ethnicity
  - American Indian or Alaska Native: 18.3%
  - Two or more races: 14.3%
  - Black or African American: 9.6%
  - White: 8.8%
  - Hispanic or Latino: 7.9%
  - Asian: 3.7%
- Educational status
  - college graduates: 6.1%
  - attended college but no degree: 9.8%
  - high school graduates: 8.8 percent
  - Non-high school graduates: 10.2%
- Employment status
  - unemployed: 17%
  - part time employment: 11.5%
  - full time employment: 8%
- Geographical Area
  - West: 10.3%
  - Northeast: 9.2%
  - Midwest: 7.9%
  - South: 7.8%
- In 2009, an estimated 69.7 million Americans aged 12 or older were current users of a tobacco product. This represents 27.7 percent of the population in that age range.
- In 2009, slightly more than half of Americans aged 12 or older reported being current drinkers of alcohol (51.9%). Approximately 6.8% of these drinkers defined themselves as a "heavy drinker" defined as 5 or more drinks on the same occasion on each of 5 or more days per week.

Source: U.S. Department of Health and Human Services Substance Abuse and Mental Health Services Administration Office of Applied Studies Results from the 2009 National Survey on Drug Use and Health. Retrieved from http://oas.samhsa.gov/NSDUH/2k9NSDUH/2k9Results.htm#1.1 on April 14, 2011.

of addictions. Dopamine is associated with feelings of pleasure and elation. Dopamine levels can be elevated by a hug or kiss, a word of praise, a winning poker hand, or the effects of a drug. Cocaine use stimulates a surge of dopamine in an addict's brain, which essentially triggers the cocaine high. Research studies have demonstrated that in dopamine-rich areas of the brain, nicotine behaves in a manner remarkably similar to that of cocaine. Brain imaging technology can track increases in dopamine and link them to feelings of euphoria. This dopamine hypothesis gives rise to the recognition that there may be a clear biologic basis for drug dependence.

Current research focuses on the persistence of addiction, despite pharmacological and psychosocial treatment. The current hypothesis is that chronic addiction changes molecular and cellular mechanisms within a number of forebrain circuits, resulting in the deterioration of neural processes that normally serve affective and cognitive functioning.

The major drugs of abuse mimic the structures of neurotransmitters. Neurotransmitters serve as a basis for every thought and emotion, for memory, and for learning; they carry the signals between all the neurons in the brain. At a purely chemical level, every enjoyable experience amounts to an explosion of dopamine in the brain.

Several other factors, including physiologic, genetic, developmental, and environmental factors, play a role in determining why some people abuse substances. Box 9.2 explores factors that may place people at risk for substance abuse.

Physiology

The physiologic effects of drugs with a high potential for abuse involve the body's adaptation to the toxic effects of the drugs at the biochemical and cellular level. Several physiologic changes characterize this process: tolerance, physical dependence, and psychological dependence. It is important to note that tolerance or physical dependence alone does not imply addiction.

Box 9.2 WHO'S AT RISK FOR SUBSTANCE ABUSE?

- Family factors that influence early childhood:
  - Chaotic home environment
  - Ineffective parenting
  - Lack of nurturing and parental attachment
  - Child abuse or sexual assault
- Factors outside of the family:
  - Poor social coping skills
  - Poor school performance
  - Association with a deviant peer group
- Individuals with chronic pain (e.g., back, joint, musculoskeletal disorders) who may occasionally misuse or abuse their prescribed drugs
- Individuals with a family history of substance abuse
- Teenagers—especially if they are dealing with self-esteem issues
- The socioeconomically disadvantaged—they may be desperate to "escape their world," selling and using drugs to survive
- Health care professionals (e.g., physicians, nurses, pharmacists) who have easy access to drugs and may begin using drugs or substances to promote sleep or arousal, decrease physical discomfort, and manage stress and anxiety

Tolerance

With drug use over time, tolerance develops. **Tolerance** occurs when the body develops a natural resistance to the drug's physical or euphoric effects, making it necessary to take increasing doses more frequently to achieve the desired effect. When a patient becomes tolerant to a class of drugs, **cross-tolerance** may also occur, meaning that tolerance to a drug in a particular class may also occur to other drugs in the same class. For example, tolerance to clonazepam (Klonopin) may result in tolerance to diazepam (Valium). Cross-tolerance does not extend to drugs in another class. For example, tolerance to clonazepam, a benzodiazepine, would not induce tolerance to meperidine (Demerol), an opiate drug.

Physical Dependence

Physical dependence occurs when changes in body cells, secondary to tolerance, cause the body to "need" the drug for homeostasis. Abstinence results in a withdrawal syndrome. Physical dependence is related to the amount and duration of drug abuse. The higher the dose and the longer the duration, the more physically dependent the patient becomes. Drugs associated with a high degree of physical dependence include heroin, morphine, alcohol, benzodiazepines, barbiturates, nicotine, and caffeine.

Physical dependence alone does not define addiction. A patient may be physically dependent on a drug without showing behavior patterns associated with addiction. For instance, a patient with chronic pain syndrome may be dependent on opioid drugs. However, this dependence on opioid drugs does not constitute an addiction. In reality, taking these drugs enhances the patient's quality of life.

Patients may also experience **cross-dependence.** When patients are dependent on a specific drug in one drug class, they may also be dependent on a similar drug in the same class. For example, if a patient who is dependent on clonazepam does not have access to that drug but is able to obtain diazepam, the patient will not experience a withdrawal syndrome.

Abstinence syndrome, or **withdrawal syndrome,** develops when dependent drug use is stopped abruptly. This interruption results in physical signs and symptoms of withdrawal as the body tries to return to "normal." Signs and symptoms of withdrawal syndrome are specific to the class of drug abused and are generally the opposite effects of the drug action. The severity of withdrawal syndrome is directly correlated with the degree of physiologic dependence and duration of use.

Psychological Dependence

Psychological dependence, thought by some experts to be the most important factor in addiction, involves the compulsive use of, and craving for, a drug. It results from the direct influence of drugs on brain chemistry. The drug causes an altered state of consciousness and distorted perceptions that are pleasurable and satisfying to the user. The recollection of these pleasurable feelings, along with the physiologic changes caused by tolerance and the fear of withdrawal symptoms, reinforces continued use of the drug. Thus, patients with a psychological addiction are motivated by the feelings the drug provides, rather than the body's need for the drug.

Genetics

Genetic factors also play an important role in drug dependence, and this genetic vulnerability varies. For example, certain genes may predispose a person to, or protect the person from, alcoholism.

Several studies emphasize the effects of heredity and maintain that the disease of addiction—a chronic, progressive, recurrent, incurable, and potentially fatal condition—is a consequence of genetic deficiencies in brain tissues or neurotransmitters. For example, a vast body of evidence from studies of alcoholism suggests that genetic factors are more influential than environmental factors and that alcoholism is a multifactorial disorder in which biologic and genetic factors interact. These conclusions are supported by animal research (breeding of "alcoholic" rats), studies of twins (alcohol metabolism, alcohol drinking patterns, each twin's response to alcohol), and studies of adoptees whose biologic parents suffered from alcoholism.

Development and Environment

Developmental and environmental influences can trigger changes in brain hormones. For example, chronic stress can decrease brain levels of neurotransmitters, such as metenkephalin, dopamine, norepinephrine, and serotonin. Many sociologic studies suggest that physical or emotional stress caused by abuse, anger, peer pressure, and other environmental stressors can cause people to seek and sustain use of mind-altering drugs, leading to drug dependence. Several kinds of developmental and environmental factors may influence a person's substance abuse, including personality traits, mood disorders, availability of drugs, cultural attitudes, and socioeconomic circumstances.

Personality Traits

No absolute addictive personality has been identified, and the ability to respond to stress and peer pressure varies among people. However, substance abusers are frequently described as having a low tolerance for frustration, being impulsive and manipulative, and experiencing fears of failure. Feelings of inadequacy, resentment, hostility, and anger are other common characteristics thought to predispose a person to substance abuse. People with one or several of these personality traits may use substances to escape from reality or to relieve emotional discomfort.

Mood Disorders

The literature and clinical findings provide evidence that mood disorders have a major effect on health status, quality of life, and likelihood of substance abuse. Patients with mood disorders (e.g., depression and anxiety, dependent personality, antisocial personality) are more likely to become substance dependent or substance abusers at some time in their lives.

Patients who have depression or anxiety and who cannot cope with life's daily pressures and problems may try to escape from a mental or physical environment perceived as anxiety ridden, bleak, and joyless. People with a dependency disorder are unable to face everyday experiences independently. Instead, they use drugs to help them feel powerful and secure. Often, this behavior pattern becomes a vicious cycle. Larger or stronger amounts of drug may be needed to resolve the discomfort. People who have an antisocial personality may initially use substances to help them relate socially and to relieve their loneliness. The effects of alcohol and drugs may provide the courage to be social and have fun.

Availability of Drugs and Drug Diversion

Availability of a drug is an important factor in developing and maintaining abuse. Drugs are readily available in hospitals and clinics, which helps explain, in part, the potential for drug abuse among health care providers, nurses, and pharmacists. Although diversion of prescription drugs is a relatively small aspect of the overall drug abuse problem, drug diversion is estimated to cost employers and insurance companies $25 billion annually.

The most commonly diverted prescription medications are scheduled controlled substances, including stimulants (e.g., methylphenidate), narcotic analgesics (e.g., oxycodone), and central nervous system (CNS) depressants, especially benzodiazepines. The most abused, nonscheduled drug in the United States is carisoprodol (Soma), a centrally acting muscle relaxant. Carisoprodol is metabolized to meprobamate—a C-IV antianxiety agent. Illicit uses of carisoprodol include taking it with diphenhydramine, hydrocodone, or methadone; the combination of these drugs produces a heroin-type high.

Socioeconomic Circumstances

Economic circumstances have made drug abuse a major problem in many cities and towns across the United States. Some people may use or traffic drugs to escape harsh surroundings of poverty and illiteracy and change their perceptions of reality. In contrast, those who are not economically disadvantaged may use psychoactive drugs as a form of recreation, rather than an escape from their environment. Common reasons for using drugs include altering mood, exploring feelings, promoting social interaction, escaping boredom, stimulating creativity, improving physical performance, or enhancing the senses.

SUBSTANCE ABUSE AND THE CENTRAL NERVOUS SYSTEM

Virtually all abused drugs have some effect on the CNS and, with continued use, result in a physiologic or a psychological dependence, otherwise known as **habituation**. However, used with medical supervision, many drugs that affect the CNS have a therapeutic influence. These drugs are invaluable therapeutically because of the very specific physiologic and behavioral changes that result. Drugs that selectively affect

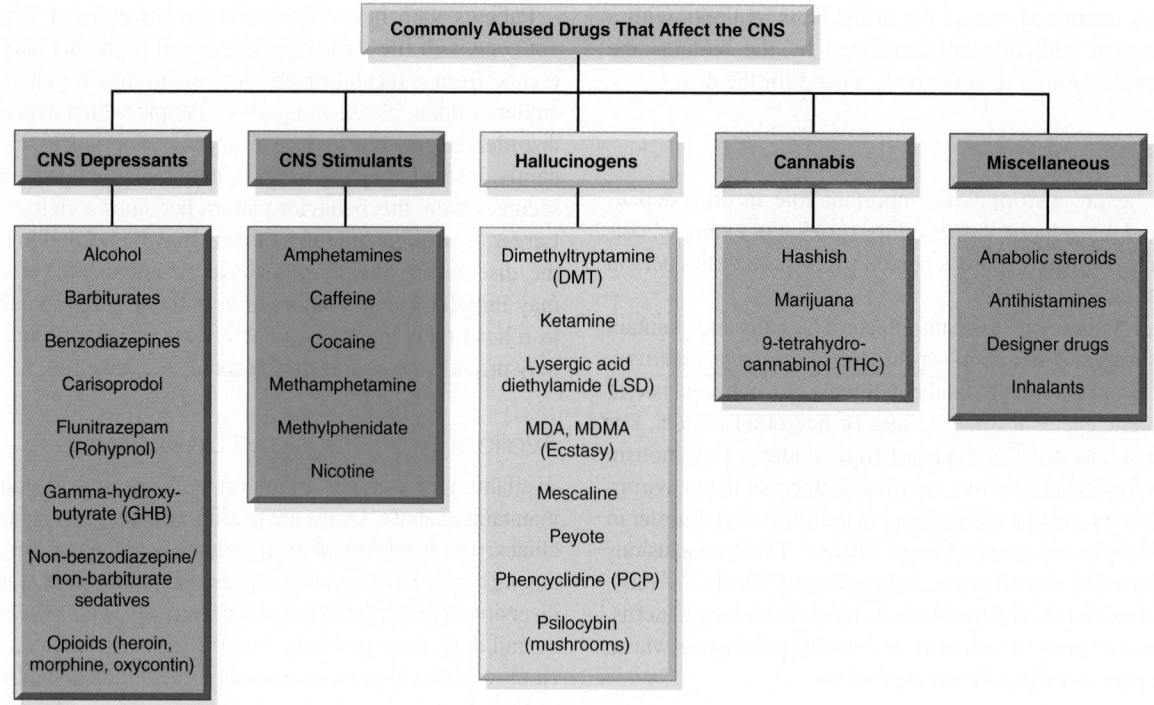

Commonly Abused Drugs That Affect the CNS

CNS Depressants	CNS Stimulants	Hallucinogens	Cannabis	Miscellaneous
Alcohol	Amphetamines	Dimethyltryptamine (DMT)	Hashish	Anabolic steroids
Barbiturates	Caffeine	Ketamine	Marijuana	Antihistamines
Benzodiazepines	Cocaine	Lysergic acid diethylamide (LSD)	9-tetrahydro-cannabinol (THC)	Designer drugs
Carisoprodol	Methamphetamine	MDA, MDMA (Ecstasy)		Inhalants
Flunitrazepam (Rohypnol)	Methylphenidate	Mescaline		
Gamma-hydroxy-butyrate (GHB)	Nicotine	Peyote		
Non-benzodiazepine/non-barbiturate sedatives		Phencyclidine (PCP)		
Opioids (heroin, morphine, oxycontin)		Psilocybin (mushrooms)		

• FIGURE 9.1   Selected drugs of abuse.

the CNS may be used for analgesic, antiepileptic, antipyretic, antiemetic, or anorectic purposes or to suppress movement disorders. These drugs can also be used without altering consciousness to treat mood and thought disorders.

However, the excessive use of these drugs can have adverse effects when their use leads to dependence. In combination with alcohol, additive pharmacologic effects may occur after administration of all antihistamines, anxiolytics, CNS depressants, and opioids. Commonly abused drugs that affect the CNS are classified into five main categories:

1. CNS depressants
2. CNS stimulants (**psychoactive** drugs)
3. Hallucinogens (**psychedelic** drugs)
4. Cannabis
5. Miscellaneous drugs

A miscellaneous category of abused substances includes inhalants such as airplane or model glue, gasoline, or nitrous oxide; designer drugs such as analogues of fentanyl;

CONSIDERING SUBSTANCE ABUSE AMONG PROFESSIONALS

As a nursing student, you may become aware of health care professionals who jeopardize their careers and their patients' safety by using drugs inappropriately.

1. Give some reasons why you think that a colleague might misuse drugs.

2. What is your responsibility when you know a colleague is misusing drugs?

antipsychotic drugs such as lithium; anabolic or androgenic steroids such as testosterone analogues; and over-the-counter (OTC) drugs, such as diet pills and antihistamines, that contain caffeine and phenylpropanolamine. Figure 9.1 depicts selected drugs of abuse.

Central Nervous System Stimulants

The most commonly abused CNS stimulants include cocaine and methamphetamine. These CNS stimulants initially increase heart rate and blood pressure. The more potent stimulants energize muscles, decrease appetite, cause some degree of mental and physical alertness, produce feelings of self-confidence, and induce some degree of euphoria. Psychoactive drugs, particularly cocaine and methamphetamine, affect nerve impulses by disrupting the normal functioning of stimulatory neurotransmitters—dopamine, norepinephrine, and serotonin. The body responds to more frequent and higher doses of the drug by releasing smaller quantities of these neurotransmitters. Excess amounts can cause insomnia, hypertension, and cardiovascular problems—especially if a person has a sensitivity to the drug. Intoxication with amphetamines, cocaine, hallucinogens, and marijuana may cause panic attacks. Prolonged use may lead to anxiety, confusion, dependency, depression, exhaustion, anhedonia (inability to experience normal pleasure), irritability, paranoia, and violence as the body's own neurotransmitters are depleted. Synthesis of the depleted neurotransmitters may take months to occur after chronic, heavy use.

The CNS stimulants have a wide range of effects that increase their potential for abuse. Caffeine, nicotine, amphetamines, and cocaine increase alertness and energy, lessen drowsiness and fatigue, increase concentration and thinking, alleviate moodiness, and impart a "high" or happy feeling. All stimulant drugs pose a risk of both physical and psychological dependence.

Caffeine is categorized as a mild CNS stimulant. It is found in coffee, tea, cocoa, colas and other soft drinks, and chocolate. It is also found in many OTC products, such as analgesics and weight-control products.

Nicotine is a highly addictive drug found in tobacco products such as cigarettes, cigars, pipe tobacco, and snuff. Tobacco use is the principal cause of preventable morbidity, disability, and premature death in the United States. Studies indicate that lung and oral/pharyngeal cancer and cardiovascular disease mortality from tobacco use is lower in states that have adopted a comprehensive tobacco control program; California and New Jersey are two examples. Because nicotine is highly addictive, many people require nicotine replacement in order to successfully stop smoking. Nicotine is available in a variety of formulations including a nasal spray, buccal lozenge, buccal chewing gum, and transdermal patch. Some of these formulations require a prescription, but many are available OTC.

Amphetamines are anorexiants used medically in short-term use for treating obesity, narcolepsy (a chronic disorder characterized by recurrent attacks of drowsiness and sleep during daytime), and attention deficit hyperactivity disorder (ADHD). Drug abusers typically take large oral doses or inject amphetamine—known as "speed"—for an intense "rush" that lasts only a short time. Studies have demonstrated that abnormal brain chemistry associated with methamphetamine abuse is evident months after the drug abuse has stopped. Brain scans have demonstrated reduced N-acetyl-aspartate compounds in the basal ganglia. Although no direct correlation is known, these reduced N-acetyl-aspartate levels are associated with a variety of diseases, including dementias, epilepsy, multiple sclerosis, brain tumors, and cerebral infarction.

Cocaine, another popular drug of abuse, produces a powerful but short-acting effect. Cocaine is not only psychologically addicting but also physically addicting because of its effect on neurotransmitters. The life-controlling effect of cocaine can lead an addict to exclude everything from his or her life except the pursuit of cocaine. A cocaine habit can cost an addict thousands of dollars a week to maintain.

Methamphetamine (meth), a psychostimulant drug, has become a national problem. It is the most frequently abused stimulant. Meth is easily produced using household chemicals and basic chemistry laboratory instruments. The "recipe" is found readily on the Internet. Meth targets the central nervous system by stimulating the release of dopamine. It also stimulates the release and blocks the reuptake of both norepinephrine and serotonin, but to a lesser degree than dopamine. It is more powerful than cocaine and has a longer half-life, which prolongs its intoxicant effects.

As a general rule, intoxication with stimulant drugs is more dangerous than withdrawal. Acute intoxication may cause severe and prolonged seizure activity, whereas withdrawal symptoms include nausea, sleep disorders, cravings, depression, irritability, agitation, and fatigue. Withdrawal symptoms occur within 24 hours and can last as long as 1 week or more.

Central Nervous System Depressants

Small doses of CNS depressants decrease heart rate, respiration, and reaction time, although initially they induce some euphoria. They relax the muscles, suppress physical and mental pain, diminish inhibitions, and promote sedation. CNS depressants, such as the opioids, can also decrease muscular coordination and energy and cause constipation, depression, nausea, vomiting, physical dependence, and withdrawal symptoms if used to excess.

Commonly abused CNS depressants include alcohol, barbiturates, and benzodiazepines. Sedative-hypnotic drugs can cause physical and psychological dependence. Regular use of these drugs over a long period leads to drug tolerance and a need for larger and larger doses to achieve the desired effect.

Alcoholism is the number one drug problem in America. Alcohol abuse and dependence are associated with 100,000 deaths annually in the United States, cause 30% of all traffic fatalities, and affect approximately 10% of Americans at some point in their lives (Up to Date, 2008). Because of its complex nature, alcoholism is difficult to define. Generally, people are considered alcoholics if their lifestyle is dominated by acquiring and consuming alcoholic beverages and if this behavior interferes with personal, professional, social, or family responsibilities and relationships. The Diagnostic and Statistical Manual of Mental Disorders (DSM IV) defines alcoholism as a maladaptive pattern of use associated with 3 or more of the following:

- Tolerance
- Withdrawal
- Substance taken in larger quantity than intended
- Persistent desire to cut down or control use
- Time is spent obtaining, using, or recovering from substance
- Social, occupational, or recreational tasks are sacrificed
- Use continues despite physical and psychological problems

Barbiturates, once the mainstay of sedative-hypnotic drugs, are also used as anesthetics and antiepileptics. Many barbiturates are short-acting drugs, which helps explain the problem with abuse; that is, the person needs to use more drug to sustain the desired effect. Examples of barbiturates habitually used include pentobarbital, secobarbital, and amobarbital. Methaqualone has been withdrawn from the market and is no longer legally manufactured.

Benzodiazepines, which were initially developed as an alternative to the highly dependency-producing barbiturates, are longer-acting drugs. However, they still cause physical and psychological dependence if taken regularly over a prolonged period. Benzodiazepines, which are used primarily to relieve anxiety and to provide a hypnotic, or sedative, effect, are widely prescribed and therefore readily available. Some common benzodiazepines habitually used are diazepam, alprazolam, clorazepate, clonazepam, and lorazepam.

TABLE 9.1	Clinical Findings in Alcohol Withdrawal

Symptoms	Onset After Last Drink
Tremulousness, anxiety, headache, nausea/vomiting, diarrhea, palpitations, anorexia, diaphoresis	6–36 hours
Tonic-clonic seizures	6–48 hours
Hallucinosis (visual, auditory or tactile)	12–48 hours
Delirium tremens (delirium, agitation, tachycardia, hypertension, fever, and diaphoresis	48–96 hours

Abrupt withdrawal from long-term use of sedative-hypnotic drugs should never be attempted because withdrawal symptoms are serious and potentially fatal. Withdrawal symptoms include agitation, dysphoria, insomnia, vomiting, diarrhea, ataxia, hallucinations, acute psychosis, muscle and abdominal cramps, anorexia, and seizures. These symptoms may occur 12 to 72 hours after the last use of the drug and may last up to 14 days.

Like the sedative-hypnotic drugs, abrupt withdrawal from long-term alcohol abuse may trigger a withdrawal syndrome that ranges from simple tremors to seizure activity and delirium. Symptoms may occur in as little as 6 hours or as long as 96 hours (see Table 9.1).

Opioids

Opioids (also known as narcotic analgesics) are commonly prescribed to relieve pain, suppress coughing, enhance anesthetic effect for surgery, and relieve severe diarrhea. These narcotic drugs have a high potential for abuse and are extremely addicting both physically and psychologically. Frequently used and abused opioids include heroin, opium (paregoric), morphine, meperidine (Demerol), hydromorphone (Dilaudid), codeine, pentazocine (Talwin), and propoxyphene (Darvon). Administered orally, heroin and morphine undergo first-pass metabolism and have only one third to one sixth the effect of heroin or morphine administered parenterally. Therefore, abusers of these drugs usually administer them by injection or inhalation.

All opioids affect the CNS and cause cerebral changes, mood changes, confusion, euphoria, and analgesia. Regular use of narcotics over several weeks usually results in tolerance to the drug's effects. Withdrawal effects from narcotics induce muscle pain, nausea and vomiting, abdominal cramps, and diarrhea. Although these symptoms can be severe, they are not generally lethal. However, death may occur if the patient becomes severely dehydrated and experiences profound electrolyte imbalances. Withdrawal symptoms occur within 8 to 12 hours and can persist for up to 10 days.

Tranquilizers

Certain tranquilizing drugs, known as "date rape" drugs, have made headlines. They are Rohypnol and gamma-hydroxybutyrate (GHB). Rohypnol is the trade name for flunitrazepam—a sedative-hypnotic benzodiazepine that produces muscle relaxation and amnesia. Although this drug is classified as a depressant, it can induce aggression, excitability, and even death. Outside the United States, Rohypnol is legally manufactured and is prescribed for the short-term treatment of severe sleep disorders. It is widely available in Europe, Mexico, and Colombia but is neither manufactured nor approved for sale in the United States. Rohypnol is 10 times more potent than diazepam (Valium). Rohypnol is a tasteless and odorless drug that dissolves clear in liquids, making it difficult to detect. Because of its illicit use, the manufacturers of Rohypnol reformulated the drug so that it turns blue in liquids. Unfortunately, many mixed drinks and punches are themselves dark in color, making these drinks ideal vehicles for administering the drug to unsuspecting victims. Rohypnol induces slowing of psychomotor performance, muscle relaxation, decreased blood pressure, sleepiness, and amnesia. Some of the adverse effects associated with use are drowsiness, headaches, memory impairment, dizziness, nightmares, confusion, and tremors.

GHB is a powerful, rapidly acting CNS depressant initially developed as an anesthetic agent in the 1960s. Produced naturally by the body in small amounts, the physiologic function of GHB is unclear. GHB, which became an FDA Schedule I Controlled Substance in March 2000, is abused for its ability to produce euphoric and hallucinogenic states and for its alleged function as a growth hormone, which releases agents to stimulate muscle growth. The popularity of GHB stems from its ease of manufacture—home chemistry kits and instructions can be found on the Internet. Like Rohypnol, GHB is a colorless, tasteless, and odorless drug that dissolves in liquids. Effects occur in 15 to 30 minutes and last for 3 to 6 hours. Adverse effects associated with GHB include nausea, vomiting, delusions, depression, vertigo, hallucinations, seizures, respiratory distress, loss of consciousness, slowed heart rate, lowered blood pressure, amnesia, and coma. The margin between GHB's anesthetic dose and its lethal dose is very narrow. Since 1995 there have been 73 documented deaths related to GHB. Between 1998 and 2000, there were 4,969 GHB emergency room admissions reported.

Because of concern about Rohypnol, GHB, and other similarly abused sedative-hypnotics, Congress passed the Drug-Induced Rape Prevention and Punishment Act of 1996 in October of that year. This legislation increased federal penalties for using any controlled substance to aid in sexual assault.

Hallucinogens

Hallucinogenic drugs have pronounced mental and emotional effects because they distort the way the brain interprets sensory information. They can also mimic certain mental illnesses such as schizophrenia. Included in this category are the naturally occurring substances (marijuana, mescaline, and psilocybin) and the synthetic substances (lysergic acid diethylamide [LSD], dimethyltryptamine [DMT], and phencyclidine hydrochloride [PCP]). Psychedelic drugs are, with the exception of marijuana, not used medically. Psychedelics do not cause physical dependence, and only marijuana has been shown to produce psychological dependence.

Relatively new amphetamine-derivative drugs with special stimulatory effects on the brain are termed hallucinogenic amphetamines (e.g., 3,4-methylenedioxymethamphetamine [MDMA], "Ecstasy"). These drugs can be inhaled, injected, or swallowed. They cause a long-lasting reduction in the brain's supply of serotonin and produce powerful psychic changes.

Another drug, ketamine, an anesthetic used in animals, is used frequently for conscious sedation in humans. It produces some emergent hallucinogenic effects (hallucinations and sensory distortion) that immobilize the user and detach him or her from reality. Ketamine does not depress the circulatory or respiratory systems. Its effects are equivalent to those of being severely inebriated.

Inhalants

The term "inhalants" refers to products that can be abused by inhaling them through the nose or mouth to achieve an intoxicating effect (Box 9.3). Because they are easily accessible, inexpensive, and easy to conceal, inhalants are some of the first substances abused. These substances can be inhaled in various ways. Common methods include inhaling directly from containers (products such as rubber cement or correction fluid), sniffing fumes from plastic bags held over the mouth and nose, or sniffing a cloth saturated with the substance.

Effects of inhalant use resemble alcohol inebriation. As the user inhales, the body becomes starved of oxygen. As a compensatory effect, the heart rate increases in an attempt to increase blood flow to the brain. The user initially experiences stimulation, a loss of inhibition, and a distorted perception of reality and spatial relations. After a few minutes, the senses become depressed, and a sense of lethargy arises as the body attempts to stabilize blood flow to the brain, usually referred to as a "head rush." Users can become intoxicated several times over a few hours because of these chemicals' short-acting, rapid-onset effect. Many users also experience headaches, nausea, vomiting, slurred speech, loss of coordination, and wheezing.

Box 9.3 COMMONLY ABUSED COMMERCIAL PRODUCTS

Adhesives: Model airplane glue, rubber cement, household glue
Aerosols: Spray paint, hair spray, air freshener, deodorant, fabric protector
Anesthetics: Nitrous oxide, ether, chloroform
Cleaning agents: Dry cleaning fluid, spot remover, degreaser
Food products: Vegetable cooking spray, whipped cream, and other products in aerosol containers (nitrous oxide "whippets")
Gases: Butane, propane, helium
Solvents: Nail polish remover, paint thinner, typing correction fluid and thinner, toxic markers, pure toluene, toluol, cigarette lighter fluid, gasoline

---

The nurse should suspect inhalant abuse when observing paint or stains on the body or clothing, spots or sores around the mouth, red or runny eyes and nose, chemical odor on the breath, a drunken or dazed appearance, loss of appetite, excitability, and irritability.

Tolerance and physical dependence may occur with heavy or long-term use. Withdrawal symptoms may include sweating, rapid pulse, hand tremors, insomnia, nausea, vomiting, physical agitation, anxiety, hallucinations, and grand mal seizures.

Designer Drugs

These drugs are similar in chemical structure to existing drugs and are developed with relative ease in illegal laboratories. They are extremely potent, and when used recreationally, they have addictive capabilities greater than those of existing drugs. For example, alpha-3-methyl fentanyl (the street version of fentanyl), which may be represented as "China white" (heroin), is 35 times more potent than heroin. Fentanyl, a narcotic analgesic legitimately used during and after surgery, is an example of an existing drug "designed" into another form. These analogues of existing substances, which offer similar psychoactive properties, are primarily designed to bypass federal regulation and control by means of their chemical formulations, which differ from those of existing drugs and are thus not covered by existing laws. Two meperidine analogues that have appeared on the street include MPPP (1-methyl-4-phenyl-4-propionoxypiperidine) and PEPAP (1-[2-phenylethyl]-4-acetyloxypiperidine). They are often marketed as "new heroin." MPPP is popular among drug abusers because when it is injected, it produces a euphoria similar to that produced by heroin. An impurity formed during the illicit manufacture of MPPP, called MPTP (1-methyl-4-phenyl-1,2,3,6-tetrahydropyridine), destroys brain cells and much of voluntary muscular movement. MPTP produces a crippling condition that closely resembles Parkinson disease.

Anabolic Androgenic Steroids

Anabolic androgenic steroids are synthetic formulations of the male hormone testosterone. The abuse of these drugs in men and women to increase strength and enhance athletic performance is widespread. Anabolic androgenic steroids also have a dramatic effect on emotions and make the user feel more confident and aggressive. Continued use of anabolic androgenic steroids may lead to emotional instability, rage, depression, or psychosis. Serious health problems are associated with both short- and long-term use of anabolic androgenic steroids. These problems include sex hormone imbalances (including amenorrhea or erectile dysfunction), changes in secondary sexual characteristics (e.g., gynecomastia, hypomastia, testicular atrophy, and ovarian atrophy), permanent sterility, hepatic cancer, and myocardial infarction. In light of the risks associated with these substances, many athletic organizations have banned their use.

Nursing Management In Commonly Abused Drugs

The nurse's role in substance abuse involves having core knowledge related to specific drugs and to abuse prevention, assessing potential or actual abuse, and formulating nursing diagnoses related to the assessment findings. Once the nurse has gathered the data and developed nursing diagnoses, outcome criteria can be identified, and interventions can be implemented. Finally, the nurse evaluates whether the outcome criteria have been met and what further patient care is needed. It is important for the nurse to have open, unbiased observation for the potential abuse of drugs by all patients, regardless of gender, age, ethnicity, education, or socioeconomic status.

Core Drug Knowledge in Alcohol Abuse

Pharmacokinetics

Alcohol, known clinically as ethanol (ETOH), does not require digestion before absorption. It is completely absorbed by the stomach and small intestine within 2 hours of ingestion. However, food in the stomach decreases the effects of alcohol, delays gastric emptying time, and retards absorption from the small intestine. Once in the systemic circulation, alcohol is immediately distributed to the rest of the body at a rate proportional to blood flow and water content. Consequently, high concentrations in the brain, liver, lung, and kidney develop rapidly. Once absorption is complete, brain and blood alcohol levels are very similar.

The liver metabolizes alcohol by two different pathways—using the enzyme alcohol dehydrogenase and the microsomal ethanol-oxidizing system (MEOS). In the average adult, 90% to 98% of an ingested dose of alcohol is converted to acetaldehyde by alcohol dehydrogenase. The acetaldehyde is then oxidized to acetate by aldehyde dehydrogenase. The acetate is finally oxidized in the liver to carbon dioxide and water. These actions primarily take place in the cytoplasm and mitochondria of the hepatocyte. The remaining 2% to 10% is excreted unchanged in the urine and expired air. The average rate of metabolism of alcohol by non-tolerant people is 100 mg/kg of body weight per hour (or 7 g/h in a person who weighs 70 kg).

People with chronic alcoholism metabolize alcohol by way of the MEOS, which occurs primarily in the endoplasmic reticulum. Metabolism of ethanol by this pathway produces an end product of acetaldehyde and free radicals, both of which damage liver cells. Metabolism by this pathway is also dangerous because cytochrome P-450, an enzyme that is integral to the pathway, is required by the liver to transform toxins, drugs, and excess fat-soluble vitamins. If P-450 is being used to metabolize alcohol, it cannot perform its other tasks. The result is susceptibility to organ damage from other toxins, drugs, and vitamins. Alcohol is excreted in urine by the kidneys, in the breath by the respiratory system, and in sweat by the skin.

Box 9.4 HEALTH PROBLEMS RELATED TO ALCOHOL ABUSE

Cardiac arrhythmias and cardiomyopathy
Cancers of the upper GI tract, liver
Cirrhosis of the liver
Gastritis and GI bleeding
Hepatic dysfunction and hepatitis
Hypertension
Impotence
Malnutrition and vitamin deficiencies
Increased incidence of peptic ulcer disease
Pancreatitis
Peripheral neuritis
Pregnancy complications and neonatal drug dependency
Seizures
Wernicke-Korsakoff syndrome

Pharmacodynamics

Alcohol adversely affects many body systems (Box 9.4). Alcohol is thought to interfere with the transmission of nerve impulses at synaptic junctions, although this exact mechanism is unclear. It is similar in action to that of general anesthetics and probably exerts its action on the brain by dissolving in neuronal plasma membranes rather than by acting on a specific receptor.

Like the general anesthetics, alcohol sequentially depresses the CNS (i.e., the cerebrum, cerebellum, spinal cord, medulla). However, the excitatory stage of alcohol is longer, and the anesthetic stage is equivalent to toxicity. The margin between alcohol's anesthetic dose and its lethal dose is very narrow.

Adverse Effects

Alcohol depresses the CNS. However, the depressant effects may appear to be stimulatory because alcohol depresses the higher centers of the brain, causing people to shed behavioral and social inhibitions. The degree of depression produced is directly proportional to the quantity of alcohol consumed. Table 9.2 presents blood alcohol levels and stages of intoxication.

Awareness of these two effects may depend on the excitability of the CNS at the time of drug administration, which is influenced by the environmental setting in which the drug is used and the personality of the user. For example, in a quiet, nonsocial environment, the excitatory influence may be impaired, and the drug's CNS depressant effects of sedation and drowsiness may dominate. In a social setting, where sensory input is increased, the effects of low doses of alcohol may be perceived as stimulation because the drinker may demonstrate talkativeness, increased self-confidence, and a release of usual inhibitions.

Alcohol impairs muscular coordination. It increases the heart rate and dilates the blood vessels, causing body heat loss and, in low doses, lowers the blood pressure, which is thought to reduce the risk for myocardial infarction in patients with high levels of high-density lipoproteins. However, with large

TABLE 9.2	Blood Alcohol Levels and Stages of Intoxication
Blood Alcohol Level (mg/dL)	Physical and Behavioral Effects
<50	Body sway, euphoria, excitement, impaired judgment, incoordination, increased sociability, loss of inhibitions
50–100	Disturbed gait, impaired ability to operate machinery (e.g., motor vehicles), increased reaction time, increasingly impaired judgment, distractibility, slurred speech
100–140	Ataxia, increasingly impaired mental and motor skills, impaired short-term memory
140–200	Inability to operate a motor vehicle, staggering gait
200–300	Blackouts; in combination with other CNS depressants, death secondary to additive effects
>300	Severe respiratory and cardiovascular depression, coma, death

doses of alcohol, dangerous levels of cardiovascular depression can occur. Prolonged alcohol use causes hypertension and cardiovascular damage such as alcoholic cardiomyopathy.

Alcohol irritates the gastrointestinal (GI) tract by causing an increase in digestive enzymes. Ulceration of the gastric mucosa is a serious complication of excessive alcohol consumption. Alcohol also causes altered bowel function, inducing either constipation or diarrhea. The risk of developing alcoholic liver disease is related to the quantity and duration of alcohol consumption. Excessive alcohol consumption creates fatty deposits in the liver. These deposits can damage and scar the liver and lead to complications, such as cirrhosis, ascites, esophageal varices, and portal hypertension. Excess alcohol consumption inhibits antidiuretic hormone and therefore increases urine production. Finally, alcohol disrupts endocrine functions, causing alterations and fluctuations in blood glucose, catecholamine, and aldosterone levels. Alcoholics are frequently immunologically compromised, with an increased risk of mortality resulting from cancers of the upper GI tract and liver. Additionally, patients with alcohol abuse behaviors are frequently malnourished, resulting in hypoalbuminemia. Patients with hypoalbuminemia have altered protein-binding ability. Thus, the potential for adverse effects and drug toxicity during any type of drug therapy is increased.

Drug Interactions
Alcohol has no nutritional value, and it interferes with the absorption of vitamins and minerals. Alcohol can affect iron absorption, folate activities, and platelets. These harmful effects can result in a variety of anemias. Table 9.3 gives more information about drug interactions with alcohol.

Core Drug Knowledge in Cocaine Abuse
Cocaine is derived from the leaves of *Erythroxylon coca*. It is available in two forms: crystalline cocaine hydrochloride and highly purified cocaine alkaloid. Cocaine hydrochloride is usually administered orally, intravenously, or by nasal insufflation because it is water soluble and unstable when exposed to heat. The alkaloid form of cocaine—called "crack" because of the popping sound it makes when the crystals are heated—is stable on exposure to heat but is water insoluble; therefore, it is usually administered by inhalation. On the street, pure cocaine is diluted or "cut" with other substances to increase its quantity and thereby increase profits to the sellers.

Freebasing consists of converting the cocaine alkaloid to a freebase rock form using a solvent such as diethyl ether. This rock is then heated, and the fumes are inhaled. This practice is potentially dangerous because the fumes are potent and diethyl ether is flammable; in addition to the risk of burns, many users report being addicted after only one use. Treatment for cocaine addiction is difficult because of the extreme physical and psychological dependence associated with its use.

Pharmacokinetics
Cocaine is rapidly absorbed into the bloodstream, regardless of whether it is snorted, inhaled, or injected. Cocaine has a 1- to 2-minute onset of action and a 30-minute duration of action after smoking or intravenous (IV) injection; peak effects after inhaling cocaine occur in 30 to 60 minutes, with a duration of action of several hours. Cocaine is only 30% to 40% bioavailable after oral administration, and GI absorption may continue for several hours. Orally administered cocaine has a slower onset of action, approximately 1 hour.

Cocaine is extensively metabolized in the liver and the blood. Metabolites may be detected in the urine for 2 or more days. Because cocaine is so rapidly metabolized in the liver, the user must inhale, inject, or smoke the drug approximately every 30 minutes to maintain the high. Cocaine is characterized by tachyphylaxis (a rapidly decreasing response to a physiologically active substance following administration of a few doses). Therefore, its psychoactive effects diminish rapidly, despite its continued presence in the plasma.

The elimination half-life for cocaine is similar for all forms of administration—about 50 minutes for the oral route, 80 minutes for the intranasal route, and 60 minutes for the IV route.

Cocaine enters breast milk and may have negative effects on nursing infants. Potential adverse effects include irritability, vomiting, diarrhea, tremors, and seizure activity.

Pharmacodynamics
Cocaine has pronounced effects on the central and peripheral nervous systems. It impairs the uptake of norepinephrine and epinephrine by presynaptic nerve endings, thus activating the adrenergic systems and causing hypertension, tachycardia, and vasoconstriction. Cocaine interferes with serotonin uptake, causing dramatic alterations in the sleep–wake cycle

TABLE 9.3   Agents That Interact with Alcohol

Interactants	Effect and Significance	Nursing Management
Analgesics (e.g., aspirin)	Combination may cause severe stomach irritation	Monitor for upper or lower GI bleeding.
Anesthetics*	Potentiation of the anesthetic effect	Observe during patient's recovery from anesthetic effects. Recovery may be prolonged.
Anticoagulants	Potentiation of the anticoagulant effect, leading to possible hemorrhage	Observe for signs of bleeding: bruising, black tarry stools.
Antiepileptics	Accelerated antiepileptic drug metabolism	Monitor for poor seizure control. Also monitor for seizures and provide for patient safety.
Antidiabetics, hypoglycemics	Unpredictable; rise or fall of blood glucose level	Monitor blood glucose levels regularly.
Antihistamines	Additive sedative effects; increased incidence of accidents due to drowsiness and increased response time	Ensure patient safety.
Antihypertensives	Additive hypotensive effects	Monitor blood pressure. Explain strategies for coping with orthostatic hypotension.
Antipsychotics* (e.g., phenothiazines)	Significant respiratory depression	Monitor breathing. Provide respiratory assistance if needed.
Barbiturates	Significant synergistic effects with alcohol	Monitor for severe respiratory depression.
Diuretics	Significant increased hypotensive effects due to antidiuretic hormone and diuresis	Monitor fluid and electrolyte levels. Caution patient about orthostatic hypotension.
Narcotics*	Synergistic, intensified CNS depressant effects	Provide respiratory support if significant respiratory depression occurs.
Sedative-hypnotics*	Additive effects; adverse effects on alertness and performance	Ensure patient safety.
Vitamins	Continuous alcohol use interferes with vitamin absorption and synthesis	Monitor for nutritional deficiencies (thiamine, folate, B_{12}) and paresthesias.

*These are potentially hazardous when ingested by a heavy drinker, patient with long-term alcoholism, or patient recovering from alcoholism.

and evoking feelings of intense energy. It also impairs dopamine reuptake, thus activating the dopaminergic system and causing euphoria, thereby strongly reinforcing use. With long-term use, dopamine becomes progressively depleted from nerve endings, causing the dysphoria that is so prominent during withdrawal. Dopamine depletion and dysphoria frequently lead to drug craving, causing a very high rate of relapse. Cocaine also interferes with sodium ion activity in peripheral nerves, causing local anesthetic actions.

Adverse Effects

Adverse reactions to cocaine include:

- CNS stimulation, including severe agitation, anxiety, excitement, paranoid psychosis, and seizures
- Cardiovascular effects, including atrioventricular arrhythmias, severe hypertension, cardiomyopathy, coronary and peripheral vasoconstriction, myocardial infarction, and intestinal or renal ischemia
- Pulmonary complications, including pneumothorax, pulmonary edema, and respiratory arrest

- Metabolic complications, including disseminated intravascular coagulation, hepatotoxicity, hyperthermia, renal failure, and rhabdomyolysis
- Complications of nasal inhalation, including anosmia, nasal mucosal atrophy, nasal septal necrosis, and rhinorrhea

High doses of pure cocaine in freebase form (crack) can overtax the cardiovascular system and cause sudden death from acute myocardial infarction or rupture of the aorta. Cocaine sensitizes cardiac cells and causes an increase in contractility. Corresponding high levels of epinephrine secondary to excitement from cocaine cause the person to be particularly susceptible to cardiac arrest.

Core Drug Knowledge in Opioid Abuse

Heroin, the most abused opioid in the United States, is a synthetically manufactured drug that possesses morphine-like pharmacologic activity. It has a poor oral availability; therefore, abusers often begin by smoking the drug. As the abuser becomes tolerant to the drug, he or she begins to use the drug by IV injection. When abusers can no longer find a site for IV injection, they will start subcutaneous administration, also known as "skin-popping." Pure heroin is very expensive and dangerously powerful. For these reasons, street heroin is usually mixed with fillers, such as sugars, starches, or quinine, resulting in a mixed substance that contains only 1% to 10% heroin.

Pharmacokinetics

The rate of heroin's absorption by the bloodstream depends on the method of administration. Absorption rate increases from oral use to IV injection. Typically, effects are felt within about 30 minutes after oral administration and within a range of 5 to 15 minutes after smoking or injecting. Depending on the dose, the effects of injected heroin persist for approximately 4 to 6 hours. Most heroin is converted to morphine and excreted by the kidneys. Insignificant quantities of unconverted heroin may be found in urine and feces. Heroin also enters breast milk. The nursing infant may experience tremors, restlessness, vomiting, and poor feeding.

Pharmacodynamics

Heroin acts on the body in a manner similar to that of other opioids. An intense rush follows IV administration of heroin. This rush subsides in a few minutes, and the effects resemble those following oral dosing. The abuser feels relaxed, carefree, and somewhat dreamy but is able to carry on with many normal activities. Taking daily doses of heroin (at least 24 mg) usually results in a clinically significant dependence in a few weeks.

Adverse Effects

The pathophysiologic effects of heroin are also similar to those of the other opioids (see Chapter 23); however, the degree of some effects is greater. An overdose of heroin may result in severe respiratory depression, pulmonary edema, coma, and possibly death. Some pathophysiologic effects specific to IV heroin use include infection with human immunodeficiency virus (HIV) or hepatitis from contaminated needles, toxic reactions to contaminants injected along with the heroin, vasculitis, and thromboembolic complications.

Core Drug Knowledge in Marijuana Abuse

The most commonly abused psychedelic drug is marijuana, which is derived from the hemp species, *Cannabis sativa*. Marijuana refers to the entire plant chopped and dried; the more potent hashish is the dried resinous exudate of the flowering tops.

The major ingredient of marijuana is 9-tetrahydro-cannabinol (THC). The THC concentration in the average marijuana cigarette has increased substantially during the past 3 decades. A typical marijuana cigarette delivers a dose of THC ranging from 2.5 to 5 mg.

Pharmacotherapeutics

An oral form of marijuana, dronabinol (Marinol), is now used in the United States to treat anorexia in patients with acquired immunodeficiency syndrome (AIDS) and for reducing nausea and vomiting in patients with cancer who are undergoing chemotherapy. Studies are ongoing related to its effectiveness in reducing intraocular pressure associated with glaucoma.

Pharmacokinetics

The systemic availability of THC after smoking is about 25%, with a peak plasma concentration occurring after 10 to 30 minutes. The duration of the entire effect is about 2 to 3 hours. The effectiveness of THC after oral ingestion is less than after smoking it: systemic availability is less (6% to 20%), onset of CNS effects is 30 to 60 minutes, peak plasma concentrations are reached within 2 to 3 hours, and the duration of action is about 4 to 6 hours for psychoactive effects and more than 24 hours for appetite stimulant effects.

THC is converted quite rapidly to a pharmacologically active metabolite, 11-hydroxy-9-THC. Further metabolism yields an inactive metabolite (11-nor-9-carboxy-9-THC), which is excreted in the urine. The plasma half-life of THC is approximately 13 days, and the urinary elimination half-life of 11-nor-9-carboxy-9-THC is approximately 10 days. However, the concentrations of these metabolites do not correlate well with THC's clinical effects and are poor predictors of behavioral impairment or intoxication. The slow urinary elimination provides an ideal marker for detecting marijuana use in drug testing.

Pharmacodynamics

The mechanism of action of THC is unknown; however, antiemetic and other pharmacologic effects occur within minutes of use. THC produces minor cognitive effects, such as an altered sense of time, a period of euphoria followed by sedation, less discriminate hearing, and enhanced visual stimuli.

Adverse Effects

Some of the adverse effects of THC include decreased myocardial oxygen supply, a dose-related increase in heart rate (20 to 50 bpm after one or two marijuana cigarettes), and impaired fertility. Cannabinoid receptors are concentrated most heavily in the cerebellum, the part of the brain that controls motor coordination, and in the hippocampus, which governs learning and memory. Large numbers are also found in the cerebral cortex, the seat of higher thinking, and lesser numbers are scattered in the immune system. They are largely absent from the brainstem regions that govern heartbeat and respiration. At high levels of intake, a cannabis psychosis may occur, and regular heavy cannabis users may suffer repeated psychotic episodes and personality changes. Chronic use of THC appears to cause permanent brain damage, as evidenced by loss of short-term memory, decreased motivation, impaired performance of simple and complex motor tasks, development of acute anxiety that may reach panic proportions, and severe psychological dependence.

Although smoking marijuana is often thought to be relatively safe compared with smoking tobacco, the smoke is virtually identical in both cases. Smoking marijuana involves inhaling larger volumes of smoke and holding the breath as much as four times longer than with tobacco, which ultimately makes smoking three to four marijuana joints a day equivalent to smoking one pack of tobacco cigarettes a day.

Tolerance to the effects of marijuana develops quite slowly. Evidence that marijuana is addictive has been obscured partly because THC is readily stored in body fat, and marijuana users who quit are often "weaned" off the drug slowly as small amounts continue to filter into the bloodstream. However, several studies have shown that a "flu-like" syndrome occurs during withdrawal from marijuana. The National Institute of Drug Abuse (which funds most of the marijuana research in the United States) estimates that 100,000 people seek treatment every year for marijuana dependency.

Core Drug Knowledge in Hallucinogen Abuse

Although often associated with the 1960s, LSD and PCP are still used. LSD is taken orally, and PCP can be taken orally, smoked, or injected. Tolerance develops with continued use of these drugs. However, psychological dependence is rare, and physical dependence does not occur. In addition, no specific withdrawal syndrome is associated with these drugs. LSD and PCP have no accepted medical use and are classified as FDA Schedule I drugs.

Pharmacokinetics

The effects of LSD and PCP usually occur 30 to 90 minutes after ingestion or inhalation and can last between 8 and 12 hours. The effects depend on the amount taken, the user's personality, the user's mood and expectations, and the setting in which the drug is used.

PCP is rapidly metabolized in the liver to inactive metabolites. Large doses of PCP may result in accumulation of large amounts of non-metabolized PCP in the urine. PCP has a half-life of 30 minutes to 1 hour in small amounts and of 1 to 4 days in large doses.

Pharmacodynamics

The mechanism of action is unclear, although some experts think serotonin-antagonistic activity within the brain is responsible for its hallucinogenic properties. Alterations in sensory perception, distortions of size, body image distortions, and surreal feelings of separation of body parts are prominent features of LSD intoxication. Sensory input is also enhanced, which creates vivid visual illusions, hallucinations, and intensely colored visual images.

Adverse Effects

Subjective effects and mood changes are quite variable with LSD. A dream-like state with feelings of good humor, euphoria, relaxation, and a sense of wonderment may predominate. Conversely, "bad trips" may occur. These consist of dysphoria, nervousness, anxiety, disorientation, hallucinations, panic attacks, and severe psychotic attacks. LSD produces adrenergic effects, most notably hypertension, hyperpnea, tachycardia, hyperthermia, pupillary dilation, and hyperreflexia. Diaphoresis, salivation, lacrimation, nausea, and vomiting may also occur.

Dopaminergic and anticholinergic effects on the body occur with PCP use. In addition, this drug shares some of the dysphoric properties of the opioids. After low doses, the user has a sense of thinking and acting swiftly. Moods may range from euphoria and a sense of "bouncing" to depression. Larger doses cause changes in mood, which are quite unpredictable and labile. A sense of unreality predominates. Under the influence of PCP, a person may experience a "bad trip" and become irrational, extremely combative, and violent. The lack of pain secondary to its anesthetic effect seems to exaggerate the person's perception of his or her own strength. In some cases, PCP can cause severe psychoses, seizures, respiratory depression, intracerebral hemorrhage, hyperpyrexia, and death.

Flashbacks—hallucinatory episodes that occur days to years after taking the drug—occur with LSD and PCP use. Prolonged psychotic episodes (lasting several days to several months) with visual hallucinations have been precipitated by LSD and PCP.

Core Drug Knowledge in Inhalant Abuse

Inhalants, another type of psychedelic drug, are volatile chemicals and gases that produce behavioral effects and are subject to abuse. Commonly abused inhalants include model glue, spray paint and hair spray propellants, cleaning solvents, gasoline, and kerosene (see Box 9.3). Nonmedical nitrous oxide is another popular inhalant.

These substances are generally sniffed from rags, paper or plastic bags, gauze, or ampules. Long-term inhalant abuse can cause permanent CNS, hepatic, renal, and bone marrow damage and greatly reduced mental and physical abilities.

Pharmacokinetics

Inhalants are rapid-acting substances. Their effects are almost immediate. The duration of the effect depends on the substance used. For example, the effects of glue, paint, or gasoline usually last several or more hours, whereas the effects of nitrous oxide typically last less than 5 minutes. The effects of amyl nitrate (or butyl nitrate) last from a few seconds to several minutes.

Pharmacodynamics

Inhaling volatile chemicals and gases produces a short-lived, mild intoxication that typifies the early stages of anesthesia. These agents produce a sense of exhilaration and light-headedness. Judgment, vision, memory, and perception of reality are impaired. These substances are slightly hallucinogenic and cause CNS depression because of the hypoxia they induce. Abusive, violent behavior has also been known to occur in people who abuse inhalants.

Adverse Effects

Psychological dependence can develop, but physical dependence is rare. Tolerance to the substance can develop over time, and more of the substance is needed over time to produce the same effect.

Toxicities depend on the properties of the individual solvents. The consequences of inhaling these substances can be severe. Abuse of inhalants has been implicated in severe brain damage, cancer, neuropathies, kidney failure, liver damage, respiratory failure, and cardiac arrest.

Assessment of Core Patient Variables in Substance Abuse

Health Status

When the nurse suspects that a patient may be abusing substances, a physical, psychological, and functional health assessment is performed. Focus on the physical, psychological, emotional, and functional status of the patient (Table 9.4).

Substance abuse screening may be easily incorporated into a health habits survey, with questions moving from legal and less stigmatized substances, such as caffeine, nicotine, and alcohol, to inquiries about street drugs. Ask questions about drug use or abuse, which should cover lifetime experience, because recovering users remain at risk for relapse. In addition, take a complete health and drug history. During this time, try to obtain as much information about legal and illegal drug use as possible. When providing this information, the patient may use street names to refer to particular drugs or drug classes. Therefore, it is necessary to be familiar with commonly used street names for legal and illicit drugs (Table 9.5). At this time, also ask the patient about any family history of substance abuse. During the physical assessment, convey a nonjudgmental attitude, which may encourage the patient to communicate. A person is more likely to open up to someone who appears open and nonjudgmental. Do not assume someone is or is not a drug user. There is no stereotypical drug user. People who abuse drugs are from all socioeconomic and cultural backgrounds.

Life Span and Gender

Substance abuse throughout the life span poses serious problems for patients, families, and the community.

EFFECTS IN PREGNANCY

An estimated 10% of infants are exposed to illicit drugs during the gestational period. When alcohol, caffeine, and nicotine are considered, some researchers report as many as 33% of all pregnant women have used a psychoactive drug during pregnancy.

Alcohol use during pregnancy increases the risks of spontaneous abortions, fetal demise, problematic pregnancies, lower birth rate, and neonates who are slower to grow postnatally. Specific toxic effects of alcohol on the developing fetus are known as fetal alcohol syndrome (FAS). The incidence of FAS in some parts of the United States is estimated to be as high as 1 in 300 births. It is a common cause of preventable birth defects. FAS causes growth deficiency, CNS dysfunction, craniofacial abnormalities, microcephaly, and other major organ defects. Neither has any amount of alcohol been established as safe during pregnancy or lactation, nor has any time during pregnancy been determined as safe for drinking it. Alcohol is teratogenic, but unlike other teratogens, alcohol does not uniformly affect all fetuses exposed to it.

Fetal physiology differs from neonatal and adult physiology. These differences suggest that maternal ingestion of psychoactive substances may produce a more dramatic effect in the fetus.

Fetal nourishment occurs through the placenta. To reach the fetus, drugs in the maternal environment must cross over the continuous lipid membrane of the placenta. Substances with a molecular weight of less than 600 (such as alcohol and cocaine) cross over easily. Drug effects may persist for a greater length of time in the fetal environment because fetal blood is moderately acidotic and contains fewer protein-binding sites, and undeveloped hepatic function decreases the fetus' ability to metabolize and excrete the substance. Although excretion occurs through the placenta, the drug may be recirculated throughout the amniotic fluid before it is excreted.

The effects of opioid abuse during pregnancy include preterm birth, intrauterine growth retardation, and low birth weight. Cocaine use during pregnancy has disastrous effects on the fetus; it causes potent vasoconstriction that reduces placental blood flow by about 50%. This reduction results in fetal hypoxia and alters the maternal–fetal nutrient exchange. Fetal effects of maternal cocaine and methamphetamine use include abruptio placentae, preterm labor and delivery, intrauterine growth retardation, microcephaly, low birth weight, and cerebral infarction. Fetal exposure can be recognized in a neonate who exhibits a withdrawal syndrome characterized by tremor, poor feeding, increased muscle tone, abnormal sleep patterns, and high-pitched crying.

Women who use alcohol, opioids, cocaine, and methamphetamine should be counseled to avoid breast-feeding because these drugs are concentrated in breast milk.

EFFECTS IN INFANCY

Opioid-exposed infants experience several common complications: hypoglycemia, septicemia, and hyperbilirubinemia. In addition to metabolic problems, term infants are at risk for pneumonia and meconium aspiration. Preterm and full-term infants alike experience withdrawal symptoms. Narcotic abstinence syndrome, which contributes substantially to neonatal morbidity, is characterized by CNS hyperirritability, GI dysfunction, increased muscle tone, respiratory distress, tremor, and vague autonomic symptoms such as fever, skin mottling, sneezing, and yawning. Initially, some infants may require drug therapy and treatment in the neonatal intensive care unit. Some symptoms may persist for 3 or 4 months or more.

TABLE 9.4	Characteristics of Selected Drugs of Abuse			

Drug	Method of Use	Intoxication Effects	Symptoms of Overdose	Health Consequences
Alcohol	Oral	Bloodshot and watery eyes, alcohol breath, motor incoordination, slurred speech, elevated blood pressure, nystagmus, mood swings and irritability, sedation	Severe vomiting or vomiting while "sleeping" or passed out and not waking up after vomiting; not responding to verbal or tactile stimulation; ataxic gait; slow, labored breathing; cold, clammy skin; rapid pulse; respiratory depression or arrest	Hypertension, GI bleeding, liver dysfunction, pancreatitis, gastric cancer
Benzodiazepines	Oral IV	Same as barbiturates	Same as barbiturates	Confusion, dizziness, impaired coordination/memory/judgment, fatigue, addiction
Cannabis	Smoked Oral	Euphoria, slowed thinking/reaction time, confusion, impaired balance/coordination	Fatigue, paranoia, acute psychosis	Impaired memory/learning, anxiety, panic attacks, cough, frequent respiratory infection, increased heart rate, addiction
Cocaine	Snorted Smoked Injected	Increased heart rate/blood pressure/temperature, mental alertness, feelings of exhilaration, energy, pupil dilation, motor agitation	Agitation, paranoia, acute psychosis, seizures, respiratory failure, stroke, death	Reduced appetite, nausea, headaches, rapid/irregular heartbeat, chest pain, heart attack, stroke, convulsions
Flunitrazepam (Rohypnol)	Oral	Reduced pain/anxiety, feelings of well-being, lowered inhibitions, slowed pulse/breathing, decreased blood pressure, poor concentration	Respiratory depression and arrest, death	Confusion, fatigue, memory loss for time under the drug's effects, impaired coordination/memory/judgment, visual/gastrointestinal disturbances, urinary retention
Methamphetamine	Oral Injected Snorted Smoked	Euphoria, hallucinations, hyperthermia, hyperreflexia, increased alertness, increased physical activity, insomnia, paranoia, tachycardia, restlessness	Restlessness, tremor, muscle twitches, rapid breathing, confusion, hallucinations, panic, aggressiveness, unexplained muscle pain or tenderness, muscle weakness, fever or flu symptoms, irregular heartbeat, seizure activity, and dark-colored urine.	Long-term neuron damage, heart attack, stroke, seizure disorder, fetal harm during pregnancy, xerostomia, progressive periodontitis, requires long-term psychological therapy to overcome intense cravings.
Methylphenidate	Oral Injected Snorted Smoked	Increased or decreased blood pressure/heart rate, mental alertness, energy, feelings of exhilaration	Vomiting, agitation, tremors, hyperreflexia, muscle twitching, convulsions (may be followed by coma), euphoria, confusion, hallucinations, delirium, sweating, flushing, headache, hyperpyrexia, tachycardia, palpitations, cardiac arrhythmias, hypertension, mydriasis, dryness of mucous membranes	Reduced appetite, digestive problems, rapid/irregular heartbeat, heart failure
Nicotine	Smoked Chewed	Increased heart rate/blood pressure, mental alertness, energy, feelings of exhilaration	Agitation, anxiety, seizures	Reduced appetite, rapid/irregular heartbeat, adverse pregnancy outcomes, chronic lung disease, cardiovascular disease, stroke, cancer, addiction
Opioids	Oral Injected Smoked Snorted	Apathy, euphoria, pinpoint pupils, sedation	Unconsciousness, respiratory depression and arrest, death	Collapsed veins, infection of the heart lining and valves, abscesses, cellulitis, liver disease and pulmonary complications such as pneumonia.
PCP and analogues	Oral Injected Smoked Snorted	Increased or decreased heart rate and blood pressure, impaired motor function, numbness	Violent behavior, paranoia, seizures, acute psychosis, heart failure, death	Memory loss, nausea or vomiting, loss of appetite, depression, panic, aggression, violence
Hallucinogens	Oral Snorted Smoked	Altered perception and feelings, tremor, numbness, insomnia, loss of appetite, weakness	Acute psychosis, death (frequently from trauma)	Chronic mental disorders, flashbacks

TABLE 9.5	Selected Drug Street Names
Drug	**Selected Street Names**
CNS depressants	
Barbiturates	Downers, reds, red devils, RDs, yellows, blues, rainbows, Christmas trees
Benzodiazepines (general)	Coral, idiot pills, M&Ms, tranq, Uncle Milty, ups & downs
Chlordiazepoxide (Librium)	Green and whites, libs, roaches
Diazepam (Valium)	V, vals
Flunitrazepam (Rohypnol)	Circles, forget me drug, getting roached, La Rocha, lunch money drug, Mexican Valium, pingus, R-2, reynolds, rib roach-2, roapies, robutal, roofies, rope, rophies, row-shay, ruffles, wolfies
Nonbenzodiazepines (general)	Ludes, Qs, 714s, vitamin Q
Gamma Hydroxybutyric Acid (GHB)	Liquid X, fantasy, organic quaalude, Georgia home boy, grievous bodily harm, liquid E, liquid ecstasy
Opioids	
Fentanyl	China white, king ivory, dance fever, jackpot
Heroin	Smack, Horse, Black Tar, *Chiva, Negra,* Mexican brown, train, white boy, downtown
Hydromorphone	Drug stores
Methadone	Dolls, dollies
Morphine	Miss Emma, Mort, M
CNS stimulants	
Amphetamines	Uppers, whites, minibennies, hearts, dexies, black beauties
Cocaine	Snow, flake, blow, crack, Coke, Coca, Blanca, Nieve, Soda, uptown
Methamphetamine	Crank, cristal, glass, go-fast, ice, meth, methlies, quick, Mexican crack, speed, stove-top, West Coast
Inhalants	
General	Air blast, bagging, discorama, glading, gluey, kick, Medusa, moon gas, Oz, poor man's pot, snorting
Amyl nitrite	Rush, locker room, pearls, poppers
Isobutyl nitrite	Aroma of men, bolt, climax, quicksilver, rush, snappers, thrust, whiteout
Nitrous oxide	Buzz bomb, laughing gas, shoot the breeze, whippets
Cannabis	Pot, grass, weed, joint, roach, honey, reefer, Grifa, Mota, Blunts, Yerba
Other	Adhesives, spray paint, hair spray, dry cleaning fluid, spot remover, lighter fluid
Hallucinogens	
Ketamine	Special K, super K, super acid, vitamin K, cat Valium, jet, K
LSD	Acid, L, microdots, sunshine, windowpane, boomers
MDA (Ecstasy)	Speed for lovers, X Adam, B-bombs, cristal, disco biscuit, Eve, iboga, pollutants, sweeties, Bens, love drug, scooby snacks, wheels, clarity, dex, essence, hug drug, morning shot, speed for decadence, E, go
Peyote	Button, mesc, mescal, cactus
Psilocybin	Shrooms, magic mushrooms
PCP	Angel dust, Hog, love boat

EFFECTS IN CHILDHOOD

Children of people with alcoholism face a broad range of problems that vary in severity and are associated with all phases of the life span. They are at risk for a range of cognitive deficits, especially those related to verbal ability, ADHD, antisocial personality disorder, anxiety, and depression. The prevalence of alcoholism is higher than normal in all first-degree relatives of patients with alcoholism, and on average, children of people with alcoholism are three to five times more likely to develop alcoholism than children of people who do not have alcoholism. Many children of alcoholics develop intensely resilient personalities.

EFFECTS IN ADOLESCENCE

The greatest physical and emotional changes occur during adolescence. The struggle toward independence is a time of great conflict, and rebellion is common during this period. Common forms of rebellion include style of dress and appearance, although rebellion can take destructive forms, such as illicit drug use and excessive alcohol drinking.

Several risk factors have been identified for adolescent substance abuse:

• Family constitution and stressful family events
• Poor parent–child relationships
• Low self-esteem
• Psychological disturbances, such as depression
• Low academic motivation
• Other problem behaviors
• Absence of religion
• High level of thrill-seeking behavior
• High family and peer substance use
• Early tobacco use

EFFECTS IN OLDER ADULTS

In the United States, adults who are 65 years and older are the fastest-growing segment of the population. Retirement often brings changes in the older person's societal role as well as a decrease in social and financial status. Declining health, financial problems, and illness and death of family and friends are common losses of aging. Depressive symptoms related to these losses are common in older people. For some, alcohol or drug use becomes a way of coping with age-related changes, which normally cause physiologic changes. These changes have an important effect on how the body metabolizes drugs. Reductions in blood flow with age may result in an inability of the liver and kidneys to process drugs as efficiently as in youth; benzodiazepines, for example, are metabolized at about half the rate seen in a younger person, making these drugs more difficult to use in the older population.

Alcohol- and drug-related medical problems may not be recognized because multiple medical problems are common in the elderly, and they may be mistaken for age-related problems. Confusion, depression, falls and other accidents, idiosyncratic reaction to prescribed drugs, inattention to self-care, incontinence, labile moods, and malnutrition are all conditions that can be related either to normal age-related changes or to the use of alcohol or drugs.

Environment

As with other chronic drug use, heavy and chronic use of cocaine and methamphetamine is especially accompanied by dysphoria and anhedonia. Former substance abusers are at risk for relapse because the perceived cure for the dysphoria is more drug use. Recurrence of symptoms and intense drug craving may occur even after long abstinence. Environmental triggers may produce intense desire for the drug even after years of recovery.

Culture and Inherited Traits

Some populations, most notably East Asians and American Indians, exhibit an unusual response of facial flushing, vasodilation, and tachycardia after consuming ethanol. These people have a genetic deficiency in the enzyme aldehyde dehydrogenase, which leads to an accumulation of acetaldehyde even after consuming relatively small amounts of ethanol.

Nursing Diagnoses and Outcomes

A comprehensive nursing assessment yields subjective and objective data helpful in formulating nursing diagnoses and desired outcomes relevant to short- or long-term drug history and actual or potential health problems related to substance abuse. Nursing diagnoses may vary according to which substances are used and what symptoms appear. In addition to Deficient Knowledge, Disturbed Sensory Perception (Visual and Auditory), and Risk for Poisoning, additional typical nursing diagnoses and outcomes may include the following:

• Ineffective Denial related to impaired ability to accept consequences of behavior
Desired outcome: The patient will acknowledge an alcohol or substance abuse problem; explain the psychological and physiologic effects of alcohol or drug use; abstain from alcohol and drug use; state recognition of the need for continued treatment; express a sense of hope; use alternative coping mechanisms to cope with stress; and have a plan for high-risk situations for relapse.
• Risk for Other-Directed Violence related to drug or alcohol abuse
Desired outcome: The patient will demonstrate control of behavior with assistance from others; have a decreased number of violent responses; and describe causation and possible preventive measures.
• Ineffective Health Maintenance related to substance abuse
Desired outcome: The patient will identify barriers to health maintenance and will engage in (or verbalize an intent to engage in) health maintenance behaviors, including abstinence and sobriety.
• Self-concept Disturbance related to self-destructive behavior (substance abuse)
Desired outcome: The patient will appraise self-situations in a realistic manner without distortions; verbalize and demonstrate increased positive feelings; and demonstrate healthy adaptation and coping skills.

Planning and Intervention

In general, nursing interventions involve maximizing the therapeutic effects of the treatment plan, minimizing factors that may contribute to resumption of substance abuse, and providing patient education to help the patient cope with denial and recognize the importance of his or her substance abuse problem.

Maximizing Recovery

Initial nursing interventions in acutely intoxicated patients are generally directed toward preventing life-threatening or debilitating effects from the substance itself or its withdrawal. These nursing interventions evolve from the specific physiologic and psychological effects of the particular substance. For example, if the patient is experiencing hallucinogenic and CNS-stimulant intoxication or withdrawal, monitor vital signs and mental status and provide a quiet, dim, nonstimulating, nonthreatening environment. Additional monitoring focuses on emotional status and possible seizure activity.

Because physical or psychological withdrawal symptoms may follow abrupt cessation of a substance, the first intervention is medical detoxification if the person entering treatment is currently under the influence of drugs. Physiologic symptoms associated with drug withdrawal may be treated with various pharmacotherapies. For example, diazepam or lorazepam is used to modify the symptoms of alcohol withdrawal and prevent the seizures it can precipitate. Clonidine (Catapres) is frequently used to manage the symptoms of opioid and cocaine withdrawal.

Minimizing Relapse

For alcohol, cocaine, or narcotic abusers, treatment is life-long, and relapses do occur. However, several therapies may promote motivation to remain substance free and increase the patient's chances for success. They include psychotherapy, support groups, and administration of withdrawal and anticraving drugs. Nursing management strategies in alcoholism are summarized in Box 9.5.

Some patients who have withdrawn from alcohol and who desire to achieve continued sobriety may elect to take the drug disulfiram (Antabuse). Its effects rely on a drug interaction (between ethanol and disulfiram) to produce unpleasant and undesirable symptoms as a deterrent to alcohol ingestion. The very unpleasant symptoms of a disulfiram–ethanol reaction include facial flushing, throbbing headache, hyperventilation, tachycardia, palpitations, nausea and copious vomiting (within 60 minutes after alcohol ingestion), hypotension, shortness of breath, vertigo, syncope, confusion, and profuse diaphoresis. In very severe reactions, myocardial infarction, cardiovascular collapse, unconsciousness, convulsions, and even death may occur.

Another drug used to assist with continued sobriety is naltrexone (ReVia). Naltrexone is available as an oral tablet that is given three times per week or an injectable drug that is administered monthly. This drug is also used to manage opiate addiction. Although the mechanism of action is not fully understood, it is theorized that blocking the opioid receptors by naltrexone may result in the blockade of the neurotransmitters in the brain that are believed to be involved with alcohol dependence. The most common adverse effects associated with naltrexone are dizziness, headache, anorexia, and nausea.

Box 9.5 NURSING MANAGEMENT STRATEGIES IN ALCOHOLISM

Nursing interventions are modified according to the problems and complications encountered in patients with alcoholism. Some general interventions follow.

Acute Alcohol Intoxication

- Maintain an open and adequate airway.
- Support respiration and blood pressure.
- Alleviate hypoglycemia, ketoacidosis, dehydration, and neurologic deficit by administering glucose and IV fluids containing potassium, magnesium, phosphate, and vitamins (thiamine, pyridoxine, and folic acid).

Alcohol Withdrawal Syndrome

- Administer drug therapy as prescribed (e.g., primarily benzodiazepines—chlordiazepoxide or lorazepam) to suppress the withdrawal syndrome.

Chronic Alcoholism

- Inform the patient of the necessity for complete abstinence from alcohol use, including alcohol in "benign" products such as cough syrups and food flavoring (vanilla extract).
- Refer the patient and family to social and environmental support groups, such as Alcoholics Anonymous, Alateen, Al-Anon.
- Teach about preventive medical and pharmacologic treatments, such as aversion therapy with disulfiram (Antabuse), hypnotherapy, psychotherapy, and treatment programs in private or public clinics outside of a hospital setting.

The newest drug approved by the FDA for the treatment of alcoholism is acamprosate (Campral). Acamprosate works by stabilizing the balance between CNS glutamate and GABA. Common adverse effects include GI distress and CNS effects such as anxiety, insomnia, and depression.

Patients withdrawing from cocaine addiction may be treated with amantadine (Symmetrel), bromocriptine (Parlodel), buprenorphine (Buprenex), carbamazepine (Tegretol), desipramine (Norpramin), and lithium. These drugs have been used clinically with varying degrees of success.

Treatment for heroin addicts is possible. However, the process is slow, and some methods used are somewhat controversial. Box 9.6 discusses the treatment of heroin addiction.

Treatment for marijuana abuse consists mainly of nonpharmacologic interventions combined with an exercise program to help deal with withdrawal symptoms and cravings for the drug.

Because no addiction results from LSD or PCP use, no withdrawal syndrome results, and no treatment is required. Treatment for LSD and PCP abuse is necessary only when the user experiences a bad trip. Box 9.7 provides guidelines for intervening on a "bad trip."

Treatment for acute inhalant intoxication is similar to that for CNS depressant overdose. Patients need oxygen and other respiratory assistance. They should not receive any

Box 9.6 TREATING HEROIN ADDICTION

For many substance abusers, overcoming heroin or other opioid addiction is a long and difficult process. Over the years, many treatment interventions have been proposed and used with varying degrees of success, failure, and controversy.

Methadone (Dolophine, Methadose)

Oral methadone is substituted for heroin at a dose sufficient to suppress opioid withdrawal and then, theoretically, reduced by 50% every other day. This treatment effectively suppresses withdrawal symptoms and has a long duration of action (24 hours). About 1 mg of methadone is equivalent to 1.5 mg heroin.

Methadone treatment is controversial for several reasons: some practitioners argue that methadone therapy simply substitutes one addicting substance for another. Although the goal is to be drug free, many patients continue to take methadone rather than be tapered from the drug. Additionally, illicit methadone markets have developed because of the widespread use of methadone programs and the fact that patients are allowed to take larger quantities home and make fewer clinic visits.

Clonidine (Catapres)

Clonidine, an adrenergic agonist and antihypertensive drug, is useful in treating mild heroin dependence and withdrawal. It suppresses the sensory nervous system and the hyperactivity that accompanies withdrawal. Clonidine facilitates withdrawal in two ways: it may be substituted for methadone (after methadone facilitates withdrawal) and then withdrawn, or it may be used with the long-acting opioid antagonist naltrexone (ReVia) as a substitute for methadone. Ultimately, the clonidine is withdrawn, leaving the patient solely on naltrexone.

Naltrexone (ReVia)

A recent treatment option for heroin addiction is long-term naltrexone. Naltrexone is a long-acting narcotic antagonist. An oral dose of 50 mg effectively blocks the receptors for 24 hours so that heroin has no effect and the patient experiences no real pleasure from taking the drug. The decision to "do drugs" must be made a day in advance.

Buprenorphine (Buprenex, Suboxone, Subutex)

Buprenorphine, a semisynthetic mixed opiate agonist-antagonist, is the first therapy approved for in-office prescribing for opioid dependence under the federal Drug Addiction Treatment Act of 2000. In supervised drug rehabilitation programs, it is administered as a sublingual tablet. In unsupervised programs, buprenorphine is given as an oral drug combined with naloxone (an opioid antagonist). If the buprenorphine tablet is dissolved in water and injected, the full antagonistic effect of naloxone occurs. This effect does not occur when the drug is taken orally. In contrast to methadone, buprenorphine is given three times per week.

Psychiatric Treatment and Support Programs

Traditional psychiatric treatment has been relatively ineffective for heroin and other opioid addicts. Therapeutic communities led by health care professionals and ex-addicts appear to be somewhat more effective in treating recently detoxified users. These organizations help restructure the addict's lifestyle and orientation through leadership, group help, and self-help.

Box 9.7 INTERVENING ON A "BAD TRIP"

Nursing interventions for managing the terrifying perceptions and hallucinations or "bad trips" resulting from LSD or PCP use rely on decreasing sensory stimuli and providing comfort and support. Some guidelines follow:

LSD

- Place the patient in a quiet room to decrease sensory stimuli.
- Remain with the patient, and help the patient to calm down by talking to him or her while panic and agitation are at a peak. This approach will help to alleviate fear and anxiety.
- Administer tranquilizers, barbiturates or benzodiazepines, or nicotinic acid as prescribed to counteract the chemical effects of LSD. Do not administer phenothiazines. They may induce hypotension, confusion, and an increased panic reaction because of their influence on the anticholinergic-like effects of LSD.

Ketamine (or PCP)

- Put the patient in a dark, quiet room, and closely observe him or her.
- Avoid verbal communication because any sensory stimuli may cause further reaction and agitation.
- If pharmacologic therapy is prescribed (e.g., benzodiazepines), administer as directed. As with bad LSD trips, phenothiazines should be avoided because of their addictive anticholinergic effects.

vasopressor therapy, such as injected epinephrine, because the interaction between a vasopressor and an inhalant may trigger serious arrhythmias.

Providing Patient and Family Education

After identifying a substance abuse problem, intervene by assisting the patient and family to develop ways to prevent substance abuse, such as communicating and reinforcing healthy coping strategies and stress-reduction behaviors; recognizing the patient's values, beliefs, and support systems; and identifying and encouraging contact with self-help groups, community resources, rehabilitative organizations, and support groups.

Help family members identify their feelings and responses to the substance abuse problem and cope with these feelings. Refer them to counseling services and emotional support groups. Entry into substance abuse treatment programs is frequently through an evaluation and referral center.

This is also an opportune time to teach the family more about the hazards of substance abuse. Explain that relapses may occur and that support groups (e.g., Alcoholics Anonymous, Alateen, Narcotics Anonymous) exist for helping the patient and family members to deal with relapses and to work through new problems related to recovery and altered relationships. The goal of treatment—longer and longer periods of abstinence and sobriety—is emphasized. Relapse prevention includes teaching patients to identify and manage feelings, recognize high-risk situations, and develop effective coping strategies.

Ongoing Assessment and Evaluation

Health consequences of substance abuse are usually manifested by changes in physiologic and behavioral functioning; therefore, evaluative guidelines related to detoxification, withdrawal, and rehabilitation correspond to signs that the patient has returned to normal physiologic and psychological functioning.

Nurses and other health care professionals have a community responsibility to provide information about substance abuse. Meeting this responsibility may involve providing information and counseling or referring patients, friends, and neighbors to treatment resources. Be familiar with the community resources, and keep up-to-date on common drug abuse problems and their treatment.

Recovery is lifelong and requires total abstinence from the abused substance. The recovering person can never return to controlled use without rekindling the addiction.

CHAPTER SUMMARY

- Substance abuse is a substantial problem nationwide and worldwide.
- Strong evidence supports a dopamine hypothesis of drug abuse and addiction and a biologically inherited tendency toward alcoholism.
- Drug abuse is a complex biopsychosocial problem that does not lend itself to simple solutions.
- Characteristics of drug abuse include tolerance, physical dependence, and psychological dependence.
- Drugs of abuse are categorized as CNS stimulants, CNS depressants, hallucinogens, cannabis, and miscellaneous drugs.
- The most commonly abused drugs are alcohol, cocaine, heroin, marijuana, caffeine, and nicotine.
- The nurse's role in substance abuse involves understanding core drug knowledge related to specific drugs, preventing abuse, assessing potential or actual abuse, and formulating nursing diagnoses related to the assessment findings.
- The nurse is pivotal in maximizing recovery, minimizing relapse, and providing patient and family education.

QUESTIONS FOR STUDY AND REVIEW

1. What adverse effects can occur if alcohol is taken concurrently with barbiturates, benzodiazepines, or other CNS depressants?
2. Define the following: drug abuse, drug misuse, addiction, physical dependence, and psychological dependence.
3. What factors place a person at high risk for substance abuse?
4. Methadone maintenance for opioid addiction is controversial. Why is this so?
5. Describe nursing interventions for a person experiencing a hallucinogenic "bad trip."
6. Name several drugs that are frequently associated with abuse, and propose some reasons that they are abused.

NEED MORE HELP?

Chapter 9 of the Study Guide to Accompany *Drug Therapy in Nursing*, 4th Edition, contains NCLEX-style questions and other learning activities to reinforce your understanding of the concepts presented in this chapter. For additional information or to purchase the study guide, visit thePoint.

REFERENCES

Anonymous Author (2009). Top 10 misused drugs in the world. Retrieved from http://www.streetdrugs.org/html%20files/Top%2010.html

Ago, Y., Nakamura, S., Baba, A., Matsuda, T. (2008). Neuropsychotoxicity of abused drugs: effects of serotonin receptor ligands on methamphetamine- and cocaine-induced behavioral sensitization in mice, *Journal of Pharmacological Science*, 106(1):15–21.

Agrawal, A. & Lynskey, M. T. (2008). Are there genetic influences on addiction: evidence from family, adoption and twin studies, *Addiction*, 103(7):1069–1081.

American Psychiatric Association. (2000). *The Diagnostic and Statistical Manual of Mental Disorders*, Text Revision (4th Ed), Washington DC, American Psychiatric Association.

Ball, D. (2008). Addiction science and its genetics, *Addiction*, 103(3):360–367.

Bevilacqua, L., & Goldman, D. (2009). Genes and addictions. *Clinical Pharmacology and Therapeutics*, 85(4):359–361.

Brown University Health Education. Retrieved from http://www.brown.edu/Student_Services/Health_Services/Health_Education

Clark, J. (2008). The danger next door: methamphetamine. *RN*, 71(5):22–28.

Ducci, F. & Goldman, D. (2008). Genetic approaches to addiction: genes and alcohol. *Addiction*, 103(9):1414–1428.

Heidbreder, C. (2008). Selective antagonism at dopamine D3 receptors as a target for drug addiction pharmacotherapy: a review of preclinical evidence. *CNS and Neurological Disorders Drug Targets*, 7(5):410–421.

Hoffman, R. S. & Weinhouse, G. L. (2010). Management of moderate and severe alcohol withdrawal syndromes. Retrieved from http://www.uptodate.com/online/content/topic.do?topicKey=neonatol/27541&selectedTitle=15~52&source=search_result-ttp://www.uptodate.com/online/content/topic.do?topicKey=ad_tox/4456&selectedTitle=1~52&source=search_result

Kelsch, N. (2009). Why meth? Not in my town: never forget identifying signs of methamphetamine abuse. *RDH*, 29(1):62.

Li, M.D. & Burmeister, M. (2009). New insights into the genetics of addiction, Nature Reviews. *Genetics*, 10(4), 225–231.

O'Brien, C. (2008). A 50-year-old woman addicted to heroin: review of treatment of heroin addiction. *Journal of the American Medical Association*, 300(3):314–321.

Pascual, M., Boix, J., Felipo, V., et al. (2009). Repeated alcohol administration during adolescence causes changes in the mesolimbic dopaminergic and glutamatergic systems and promotes alcohol intake in the adult rat. *Journal of Neurochemistry*, 108(4):920–931.

Pinto, S. & Schub, T. (2008). Substance Abuse: Inhalants. Retrieved from CINAHL Plus with Full Text database.

Polednak, A. P. (2009). Trends in incidence rates of tobacco-related cancer, selected areas, SEER Program, United States, 1992-2004. *Preventing Chronic Disease*, 6(1):A16.

Rahman, S. (2008). Drug addiction and brain targets: from preclinical research to pharmacotherapy. *CNS and Neurological Disorders Drug Targets*, 7(5):391–392.

Rush, B., Koegl, C. J. (2008). Prevalence and profile of people with co-occurring mental and substance use disorders within a comprehensive mental health system. *Canadian Journal of Psychiatry,* 53(12):810–821.

Spiga, S., Lintas, A., & Diana. M. (2008). Addiction and cognitive functions. *Annals of the New York Academy of Sciences*, Oct, 1139:299–306.

Schuckit, M. A. (2009). An overview of genetic influences in alcoholism. *Journal of Substance Abuse Treatment,* 36(1): S5-14.

Sielski, L. (2010). Infants of mothers with substance abuse. Retrieved from http://www.uptodate.com/contents/infants-of-mothers-with-substance-abuse?source=search_result&selectedTitle=1~150

Xian, H., Scherrer, J. F., Grant, J. D., et al. (2008). Genetic and environmental contributions to nicotine, alcohol and cannabis dependence in male twins. *Addiction*, 103(8):1391–1398.

Yu, Y., Kranzler, H. R., Panhuysen, C., et al. (2008). Substance dependence low-density whole genome association study in two distinct American populations. *Human Genetics*, 123(5):495–506.

Yücel, M., Lubman, D. I., Solowij, N., & Brewer, W. J. (2007). Understanding drug addiction: a neuropsychological perspective. *Australian & New Zealand Journal of Psychiatry*, 41(12):957–968.

Lifestyle, Diet, and Habits: Nutrition and Complementary Medications

Learning Objectives

At the completion of this chapter the student will:

1. Discuss the role of nutrition in health maintenance.
2. Identify common nutritional factors affecting drug efficacy.
3. Identify common ways that drug therapy may alter nutritional status.
4. Differentiate prescribed uses of vitamins and herbal and botanical preparations from nonprescribed uses.
5. Identify core patient variables that increase the risk of the occurrence of drug–nutrient interactions.
6. Identify key aspects of nursing management to maximize therapeutic effect and minimize adverse effects from drug interactions with diet, diet supplements, and herbal and botanical preparations.

Key Terms

alternative therapy
botanical preparations
complementary therapy
glycemic index

glycemic load
herbal preparations
mineral cations
phytomedicinals

trace elements
vitamins

The core patient variable of lifestyle, diet, and habits represents the way a person lives his or her life and the choices he or she makes to accept or reject behaviors that influence health. In drug therapy, this variable is assessed according to how these factors interact with the prescribed drug therapy. This chapter focuses on normal dietary habits, including the use of herbal, botanical, and nutritional supplements.

The core patient variable of diet interacts with the patient's health in several ways. First, a well-balanced diet may prevent chronic illness and therefore indirectly decrease the need for drug therapy. Additionally, a well-balanced diet influences the pharmacokinetics of many drugs. Second, the nutritional status of a patient can be altered by a chronic disease or as an adverse effect of drug therapy. Nutritional supplements and herbal or botanical preparations may also be taken to increase wellness or to meet normal nutritional needs. Lastly, certain foods, beverages, dietary supplements, and herbal or botanical preparations can affect the absorption and effectiveness of some drugs or produce an adverse effect. These points are discussed in this chapter.

DIETARY FACTORS AFFECTING DRUG EFFICACY

Health status in general has a nutritional base. A proper, well-balanced diet provides a healthy person with an adequate supply of nutrients. Predicted drug response in the body is based on the ideal of a body that has the normal balance of elements, including dietary factors. When dietary factors are altered, drug therapy may produce different effects in the body than would normally occur.

Several factors related to malnutrition are believed to alter drug disposition. Box 10.1 describes various pharmacokinetic and nutrient interactions. Protein levels are one important factor. Diminished protein status results in lower amounts of plasma proteins and can substantially increase the concentration of free drug available. Because only free drug is active, this increase in free drug increases the drug's pharmacologic effect and the risk of adverse effects. Adequate protein levels are especially important for drugs that are normally highly protein bound. As explained in Chapter 4, albumin is the most important protein, in terms of drug action, because most protein binding by drugs occurs with albumin molecules. Drug binding to albumin is also affected by high-fat meals and fasting. Both of these situations lead to high serum levels of free fatty acids that compete with the drug for albumin-binding sites. Additionally, a diet poor in proteins may inhibit the biotransformation of drugs because protein deficiency may make drug-metabolizing systems less effective.

Malnourished people exhibit decreased oxidative metabolism and reduced glomerular filtration rate, potentially increasing blood concentrations of the drug or an active metabolite. This nutritional state increases the effect of the drug and the potential for adverse effects.

Box 10.1 PHARMACOKINETIC AND NUTRIENT INTERACTIONS

Absorption

- Changing the acidity of the digestive tract (e.g., rapid-acting carbohydrates, such as candy, cause sustained- or timed-release medication to dissolve too quickly)
- Stimulating secretion of digestive enzymes (e.g., griseofulvin is absorbed better when taken with foods—especially fat—that stimulate the release of digestive enzymes)
- Altering the rate of absorption (e.g., acidic foods and beverages interfere with nicotine absorption from nicotine gum used for smoking cessation; aspirin is more slowly absorbed when taken with food)
- Binding to drugs (e.g., calcium binds to tetracycline, limiting drug absorption)
- Competing for absorption sites in the intestines (e.g., dietary amino acids interfere with levodopa absorption)

Distribution

- Changing binding of drug allows more free drug in bloodstream (low protein)

Metabolism

- Acting as structural analogues (e.g., anticoagulants and vitamin K)
- Competition for metabolic enzyme systems (e.g., phenobarbital and folate)
- Altering enzyme activity and contributing pharmacologically active substances (e.g., monoamine-oxidase inhibitors and tyramine)

Excretion

- Changing the acidity of the urine (e.g., vitamin C can alter urinary pH and limit the excretion of aspirin)

Dietary factors that promote obesity have an indirect effect on drug therapy. Body composition is an important consideration in determining drug response. For example, distribution of fat-soluble drugs is increased in obese and the elderly because of the increased proportion of adipose tissue to lean body mass.

Excessive intake of vitamins may also adversely affect the action of some drugs. For example, increased

---

CRITICAL THINKING SCENARIO

MALNUTRITION AND DRUG ACTION

Larry Willis, a 35-year-old homeless man, is brought to the emergency department by the police, who found him collapsed and having a seizure on the street. He is malnourished. He is admitted to the hospital and started on a standard dose of phenytoin, a drug used to prevent seizures, which is a highly protein-bound drug. He is showing signs of adverse effects from the phenytoin.

Use your knowledge of the effect of diet on drug actions to determine why this man is having adverse effects.

pyridoxine intake may adversely affect the therapeutic effect of levodopa by increasing its metabolism. Increased or decreased intake of some elements may alter the absorption or reabsorption of a drug. For example, changes in the dietary intake of sodium alter the reabsorption of lithium in the renal tubule. Significant decreases in dietary sodium result in extra lithium being reabsorbed, higher circulating levels of lithium, and potential drug toxicity from elevated lithium levels.

Food and nutrient intake can affect drug excretion by changing the urinary pH. For example, acidic drugs are more rapidly excreted in alkaline urine. A diet rich in meat or in vegetables may also influence the urine pH— either acidic or basic—and in this way the renal excretion of drugs may be changed considerably because drugs are generally either weak organic acid or bases. Conversely, drugs may also interfere with the availability and use of certain nutrients (e.g., vitamins, electrolytes, or trace elements); this interaction may occur with the long-term administration of certain drugs (e.g., antibiotics, oral contraceptives, anticonvulsants, laxatives) or the chronic consumption of alcohol. Deficiency of certain nutritional factors or even diseases may be the consequence of such interactions.

A particular food, or the manner in which food is prepared, can also affect drug disposition. For example, grapefruit juice is a potent inhibitor of the intestinal cytochrome P-450 3A4 system (specifically, CYP3A4-mediated drug metabolism), which is responsible for the first-pass metabolism of many medications. This interaction can lead to increases in bioavailability and corresponding increases in serum drug levels. Appendix G describes drugs that interact with grapefruit or its juices. Cruciferous vegetables (broccoli, brussels sprouts, cabbage, cauliflower, rutabaga, turnips, kohlrabi, and kale, as well as greens such as mustard and collards) markedly induce chemical oxidations when added to the diet and increase drug metabolism. The polycyclic hydrocarbons—similar to those found in cigarette smoke—generated from charcoal broiling of foods may increase drug metabolism. As you remember, inducing drug metabolism results in a lower serum concentration (or a subtherapeutic level) of the drug.

Finally, the time that food and beverages are consumed in relation to the time drugs are taken may alter the effectiveness of the drug therapy. Some drugs must be taken on an empty stomach to promote absorption; some drugs bind with certain types of foods, which prevents drug absorption; and some drugs must be taken with food for best results.

DRUG THERAPY AND NUTRITIONAL STATUS

Drugs potentially affect the status of almost every nutrient. Particularly important to consider are vitamin A and the B vitamins folate and pyridoxine because intake of these vitamins is often marginal and many commonly used drugs affect them. Some drugs affect nutrient metabolism and excretion by an "antivitamin" process. They inhibit the synthesis of specific enzymes by competing for the vitamins or vitamin metabolites necessary to their structure. For example, the antineoplastic drug methotrexate is a folic acid antagonist. Without folic acid, synthesis of deoxyribonucleic acid (DNA) is inhibited, cell replication ceases, and cell death results. A drug may also form a complex with a nutrient, thereby making it unavailable for use by the body. For example, the antituberculosis drug isoniazid forms a complex with pyridoxine, interfering with its metabolism and resulting in vitamin B_6 deficiency.

Other "antivitamin" drugs include hydralazine and L-dopa (which affect levels of vitamin B_6) and the coumarin anticoagulants (which block the action of vitamin K to prolong bleeding time).

Some commonly used drugs have nutrition-related actions. For example, chronic phenytoin therapy is associated with folate deficiency and megaloblastic anemia. Folic acid and phenytoin are structurally similar and are thought to compete with each other for the same surface receptors. Diuretic drugs increase the excretion of nutrients by interfering with reabsorption in the renal tubules. Chronic use may result in depletion of potassium, magnesium, and zinc because renal excretion of these minerals is increased.

COMPLEMENTARY NUTRITIONAL THERAPIES

The use of nutritional supplements and herbal and botanical preparations is often considered an **alternative therapy** for health. Although these choices have been traditional in some non-Western cultures, they are now being used more frequently in Western cultures, where they have come to be viewed less as alternative practices to Western medicine and more as augmentations or supplements to health care. The term **complementary therapy** is now often used for these choices. Complementary nutritional therapies include supplements of basic food elements, vitamins, and minerals, as well as the use of herbs and botanicals.

Nutritional Supplements

If patients do not have enough of a nutrient, oral supplements of that nutrient may be prescribed as adjuncts to drug therapy.

Protein

Protein, which provides 4 kcal/g, is one of the most important and abundant substrates in the body. Generally, a patient requires 0.8 grams of protein per kilogram of body weight. The body may draw on dietary or tissue protein to obtain needed energy when the supply from carbohydrates and fats is inadequate. Proteins are polymers of essential amino acids, nonessential amino acids, or both. Although animal proteins generally contain sufficient essential amino acids, many plant proteins do not, and vegetarians may not eat a wide enough variety of plants to ensure an adequate supply. Quality protein should provide approximately 10% to 15% of a healthy person's well-balanced diet.

People wishing to build muscle mass may take amino acid supplements and eat excess protein in the belief that increased protein intake facilitates the deposition of protein into muscles. However, ingested amounts exceeding those needed to replace body losses are simply converted into fat and stored. Some amino acids (e.g., L-carnitine) have gained popularity as preventive or therapeutic agents and are taken as dietary supplements. Their use may be hazardous in that there may be competition for transport with other amino acids into cells or the central nervous system (CNS). The research supporting their use is nonexistent or considered marginal by many nutritional experts. Supplements containing the essential amino acids lysine and arginine, promoted as regulators of body composition and muscle growth because these amino acids stimulate growth hormone secretion, have been proved clinically to lack these effects. Tryptophan has been used to enhance brain serotonin concentrations as a sleep inducer and in conjunction with weight-loss regimens.

Carbohydrates

Carbohydrates—especially sugars and starches—are the most common dietary component; they provide 4 kcal/g and constitute the body's primary source of fuel for heat and energy. A well-balanced diet for a healthy person supplies approximately 50% to 55% of the total kilocalories from carbohydrates. Carbohydrates are subdivided into simple or complex, depending on the size of the molecule. Simple sugars (e.g., fructose, sucrose) and refined sugars used primarily in soft drinks and baked goods are absorbed rapidly and quickly increase blood glucose. Conversely, starches are complex carbohydrates that must be digested; thus, absorption of glucose is slower, and serum levels of glucose, insulin, and triglycerides remain more stable.

The **glycemic index** represents how quickly the carbohydrate increases the blood glucose level. Simple carbohydrates have a high glycemic index while complex carbohydrates have a low glycemic index.

Some foods with a low glycemic index may actually be less healthy than some foods with a high glycemic index. For instance, potato chips have a lower glycemic index than brown rice. While the glycemic index is important, the glycemic load of a food is more important. The **glycemic load** includes both the glycemic index and the amount of carbohydrates in a particular food. For example, carrots have a high glycemic index but a limited amount of carbohydrates, thus it has a low glycemic load.

Fat

Dietary fats from animal and plant sources provide the body's alternate or storage form of heat and energy. Fat—a more concentrated fuel—supplies 9 kcal/g. Fat should supply no more than 30% of the total intake of a well-balanced diet in a healthy person (or fewer than 90 g/d). Triglycerides are the predominant dietary lipids. Other important natural and dietary lipids include cholesterol and its esters and phospholipids. Cholesterol is an important component of cell membranes and a precursor of steroid hormones. Phospholipids, like cholesterol, are important components of cellular membranes and intracellular organelles. Although the body is able to synthesize adequate amounts of phospholipids, phospholipid compounds are marketed as over-the-counter (OTC) health aids (e.g., lecithin) for treating or preventing aging, cancer, heart disease, obesity, and other conditions. Data to support these claims are limited or nonexistent.

Essential fatty acids—linolenic acids (omega-3; derived from corn, peanuts, soybeans) and linoleic acids (omega-6; derived from halibut, salmon)—must be supplied in the diet. Patients who are receiving all of their nutrition parenterally need to have fats administered to meet all their nutritional needs.

Dietary Fiber

Dietary fiber—a group of plant substances resistant to human digestion—is categorized by the food industry as soluble (dissolves in neutral or acid detergent) or insoluble (does not dissolve). Important characteristics of fiber are its water-retention ability, cation exchange properties, and antioxidant actions. Fiber added to the diet may be recommended to treat or prevent constipation, which can be an adverse effect of some drug therapies. If the patient cannot consume sufficient oral dietary fiber, drug therapies of bulk-producing laxatives, such as psyllium, may be prescribed.

Recommended Intake of Vitamin and Minerals

The Institute of Medicine (IOM) of the National Academy of Sciences is responsible for determining the recommended amount of vitamin and minerals required to keep a person healthy. Dietary Reference Intake (DRI) is the general term for a set of reference values used for planning and assessing nutrient intakes of healthy people. DRI is determined by evaluation of three important types of reference values: Recommended Dietary Allowances (RDA), Adequate Intakes (AI), and Tolerable Upper Intake Levels (UL). The RDA recommends the average daily intake that is sufficient to meet the nutrient requirements of nearly all (97% to 98%) healthy individuals in each age and gender group. An AI is set when there is insufficient scientific data available to establish a RDA. AIs meet or exceed the amount needed to maintain a nutritional state of adequacy in nearly all members of a specific age and gender group. The UL is the maximum daily intake that is unlikely to result in adverse effects.

Vitamins

Vitamins are a chemically diverse group of organic compounds needed by the body to maintain health by regulating metabolism and assisting in the biochemistry of food digestion as cofactors for enzymes. Small quantities of each necessary vitamin must be obtained exogenously, either because the vitamin cannot be synthesized in humans or because its rate of synthesis is too slow to produce sufficient quantities. The Food and Drug Administration considers nearly all vitamin products to be dietary supplements, and they are controlled by the Dietary Health and Supplement Education Act. Vitamins are generally classified as water soluble or lipid soluble. There are 13 vitamins—A, D, E, K (lipid soluble), vitamin C, and 8 B-complex vitamins (water soluble). Water-soluble vitamins are stored in the body only to a limited extent, and frequent consumption of these compounds is needed to maintain adequate body levels. Conversely, lipid-soluble vitamins are maintained in the body much longer, do not require such frequent ingestion, and have a greater potential for toxicity if taken in excess.

Vitamins may be prescribed when general nutritional status is poor, oral intake is insufficient, or the body has additional demands for a vitamin, such as vitamin C to promote wound healing. Vitamin supplements may also be prescribed to correct for general malnutrition to achieve optimal health or to maximize the therapeutic effects and minimize the adverse effects from drug therapy. When vitamins and minerals are taken in excess, potential adverse effects may occur. At the same time, many drugs can contribute to the deficiency of many vitamins.

Minerals

Major Mineral Cations

Major **mineral cations** include calcium, magnesium, potassium, and sodium. Their movement across cell membranes is highly regulated; they function in energy metabolism, membrane transport, and maintenance of membrane potential.

Potassium is the principal intracellular cation in body tissues. It has an important role in many physiologic processes, including transmission of nerve impulses; contraction of cardiac, skeletal, and smooth muscle; acid-base balance; and maintenance of normal renal function. Sodium functions to maintain the body's balance of calcium and potassium. It has an important effect in cardiac function, regulating osmotic pressure in the cells and fluids, acting as an ion balance in the tissues, producing a buffering action in the blood, and guarding against excessive loss of water from the tissues. No DRI for potassium and sodium has been established. Calcium is a critical component of the skeleton and is vital to neuromuscular transmission, cellular signaling, and blood clotting. The adult DRI is 1300 mg. Magnesium is involved in a great number of enzymatic reactions. Deficiency produces osteomalacia, neuromuscular disorders, seizures, and cardiac dysrhythmias. The adult DRI is 420 mg daily. Excess magnesium may cause CNS changes, hypotension, and cardiac toxicity including cardiac arrest.

If a patient is severely deficient in one or more of these electrolytes, intravenous (IV) replacement is used to prevent serious complications, and oral replacements may be ordered to treat less severe deficits. Electrolyte imbalances may increase the risk for adverse effects from some drug therapies. They may also occur as an adverse effect resulting from some drug therapies. Supplements are often used as adjuncts to drug therapy for these reasons.

Trace Elements

There are a number of essential **trace elements,** also known as microminerals. The most important of these include chromium, copper, iron, selenium, and zinc. Trace elements are present in minute amounts in body tissues and are essential to optimal growth, health, and development. Seafood is usually rich in nearly all micronutrients except manganese, which is readily available from plant sources.

Chromium improves insulin action, and a deficiency may cause elevated levels of blood sugar, cholesterol, and triglycerides. Copper is used in making blood cells and is active in the metabolism of iron. Copper-containing enzymes are involved in immune functions. Severe illness, high-dose zinc supplementation, and antacids can reduce absorption of copper. Supplementation may be necessary with zidovudine treatment (because zidovudine reduces copper levels) and with total parenteral nutrition.

Iron is an essential nutrient. It is needed to make red blood cells; deficiency results in anemia. Iron participates in oxidation and reduction reactions. It must be tightly bound to serum proteins to prevent potentially destructive oxidant effects. Bound to serum proteins, it is first stored and then distributed throughout the body.

Selenium is an especially important antioxidant. Its levels correlate with immune function—specifically, albumin levels, lean body mass, and total lymphocyte count. Deficiency occurs in infection and increased metabolic rates. Deficiency is also associated with heart disease and anemia.

Zinc is absorbed in the small intestine; high-fiber diets limit its absorption. Zinc promotes wound healing and functions in antibody production. Deficiency impairs protein metabolism and the immune response.

The trace minerals may be administered if dietary intake is low or the patient is malnourished. They are usually included in a multivitamin formula. Correction of generalized malnourishment is often an adjunct to drug therapy to achieve maximum therapeutic effect from the drug or to prevent adverse effects from drug therapy.

Herbal and Botanical Preparations

Herbal preparations and **botanical preparations** are those substances derived from a plant source and used as a dietary supplement or as a medication. Although herbal and botanical preparations have been traditional in some non-Western cultures, they are now being used more frequently in Western cultures as augmentations or supplements to health care. To illustrate this point, United States sales of herbal supplements increased to over 4 billion dollars in 2007. This revival of interest in herbal, botanical, and dietary supplements in the United States during the past two decades can be attributed to an aging population with a large number of chronic diseases. Many of these diseases have no satisfactory conventional medical treatments, or the conventional treatment for them involves severely limiting adverse effects. Interest can also be attributed to a pervasive "back to nature" movement in a society increasingly attracted to good nutrition, exercise, and preventive health care as a means of remaining young and active.

Plants have historically been used for medicinal purposes. Many drugs used today are derived from plants. Therapeutic agents derived from plants or the preparations made from them are called **phytomedicinals**. Aspirin, for example, comes from the bark of the willow tree, and digoxin is derived from digitalis or purple foxglove. Today, many herbs and other plant substances are being sold as OTC preparations. Many of the most popular herbal, botanical, and dietary preparations are marketed as a means of preventing aging-associated disorders, providing energy enhancement and a feeling of well-being, and assisting with weight loss; they are also sold for more traditional therapeutic uses. Regulation of these products may be limited because they are considered food sources rather than drug therapies. The bioavailability, or activity, of a preparation may vary widely between manufacturers. Consumers tend to think of these substances as harmless because they are sold over the counter. In actuality, like prescription drugs, herbal preparations can cause substantial adverse effects (Table 10.1). Furthermore, herbs may interact with prescribed drugs in ways that affect their therapeutic response. Table 10.2 presents selected herbs and possible drug interactions.

Because of the increased OTC use of herbs and botanicals, Western medicine has recently examined many of these substances in clinical studies. Some findings support using these substances to treat or manage disease or altered physiology. For example, a health care provider may prescribe an herb such as St. John's wort for depression or saw palmetto for benign prostatic hypertrophy.

Nursing Management of the Patient With Dietary Considerations

Assessment of Relevant Core Patient Variables

Abnormal dietary intake and the use of herbs and nutritional supplements may have a bearing on drug therapy; therefore, question the patient during an initial drug assessment to uncover relevant information. If the assessment reveals an abnormal dietary intake, such as low protein

TABLE 10.1	Herbal and Botanical Preparations and Potential Adverse Effects
Borage	Possible hepatotoxicity from toxic alkaloids
Calamus	Nephrotoxicity and seizures
Chaparral	Acute hepatitis, hepatic failure, and renal failure
Coltsfoot	Hepatotoxicity, photosensitivity, and possible carcinogenicity
Comfrey	Hepatotoxicity, possible carcinogenicity
Ephedra/ephedrine (ma huang)	Arrhythmias, cerebrovascular accident, heart failure, hypertension, myocardial infarction, nephrolithiasis, psychosis, and seizures
Germander	Hepatitis and hepatic cell necrosis
Hemlock	Seizures and respiratory failure
Kava	Oculogyric crisis and exacerbation of Parkinson disease
Life root	Veno-occlusive disease
Lily of the valley	Digitalis-like toxicity
Pennyroyal	Abortifacient and hepatic failure
Sassafras	Hallucinations, hepatotoxicity, and possible carcinogenic activity
Senna	Syncope, loss of bowel function, and death from cardiac dysrhythmias
Willowbark	Reye syndrome

or malnutrition, the deficiency must be corrected in some way. Determine why the patient is malnourished. Does the patient make poor choices as to what to eat, or is there a lack of money to buy food? Is there insufficient knowledge about what types of food should be in a balanced diet? Is the patient unable to feed himself because of muscle weakness? Is impaired cognition causing the patient to forget to eat? Does the patient have nausea or loss of appetite either from a disease process or as an adverse effect of drug therapy?

To assess the use of herbs and nutritional supplements, focus data collection on what substances the patient takes (e.g., drugs, nutritional supplements, herbs, and other preparations); why the patient takes them; which brands are used; and who recommended their use. This information is important and will help determine whether the desired effect of self-administered drug therapy is based on fact, fad, or tradition.

Also, document the patient's age and life span status, because many of these therapies are not recommended for use with children, during pregnancy, or during lactation. Carefully assess older adults, patients who are chronically ill, those with a history of marginal or inadequate nutritional intake, and anyone receiving multidrug therapy over an extended period, because such patients are likely to have drug-induced nutritional deficiencies. Because the effects of drug therapy can be altered by specific foods, the

TABLE 10.2 Selected Herbs and Possible Drug Interactions

Herb	Possible Drug Interactions
Bromelain	Increases the risk for bleeding with anticoagulants Increases the effects of antibiotics
Chamomile	Increases the risk for bleeding with anticoagulants
Cranberry	Decreases the elimination of many renally excreted drugs
Echinacea	May interfere with or counteract immunosuppressant therapy
Ephedrine (ma huang)	May increase CNS stimulation and adverse effects from caffeine, decongestants, sympathomimetics, bronchodilators, and CNS stimulants
Evening primrose	May interact with antipsychotic agents Increases the risk for temporal lobe epilepsy
Garlic	May interfere with hypoglycemic therapy May potentiate the antithrombotic effects of anti-inflammatory drugs May increase bleeding times with antiplatelet or anticoagulant therapy
Ginger root	High doses may interfere with cardiac, antidiabetic, or anticoagulant therapy
Ginseng	May increase the effect of monoamine oxidase inhibitors, antihypertensives, and hypoglycemics May interfere with the action of steroids Red ginseng may increase the CNS stimulant effects of coffee or tea
Hawthorn	Can potentiate the cardiac glycoside actions of digitalis
Kava	May intensify the effect of barbiturates and alcohol
Saw palmetto	May change the effects of hormones in oral contraceptives, patches, or hormone replacement therapy
St. John's wort (hypericum)	Serotonin syndrome may occur when used with other serotonergic drugs such as SSRIs, trazodone, tricyclic antidepressants, or amphetamines May produce increased drug effects when given with other antidepressants
Valerian	May potentiate CNS depression from sedatives

SSRI, selective serotonin reuptake inhibitor.

time that a patient normally consumes food and beverages before self-administering drug therapy at home should be determined.

Nursing Diagnoses and Outcomes

Nursing diagnoses and outcomes related to nutritional considerations vary depending on the dietary factor and the drug therapy that the patient is receiving. Some potential general diagnoses include:

• Risk for Injury related to low protein levels and malnutrition
  Desired outcome: Protein levels and malnutrition will be corrected to prevent adverse effects from drug therapy.
• Risk for Injury related to adverse effects from excessive use of vitamins or herbs
  Desired outcome: The patient will not develop any adverse effects while using nutritional supplements.
• Risk for Injury related to drug interactions of vitamins, herbs, or food intake with prescribed drug therapy
  Desired outcome: Drug interactions will be prevented while the patient is on drug therapy.
• Deficient Knowledge related to interactions of vitamins or herbs with drug therapy

  Desired outcome: The patient will obtain sufficient knowledge to make knowledgeable choices about the use of vitamins and herbs while on drug therapy.
• Health-Seeking Behaviors related to the use of nutritional supplements
  Desired outcome: The patient will effectively use nutritional supplements to complement drug therapy to increase health.

Planning and Intervention

Maximizing Therapeutic Effects and Minimizing Adverse Effects

If the patient has been determined to have low protein levels, consult with the physician or nurse practitioner about protein replacement. Oral protein supplements or a high-protein diet may be ordered. If levels are substantially below normal, IV infusions of albumin may be indicated. If the patient is generally malnourished but eating, encourage him or her to eat a well-balanced diet. Verify that the patient is capable of feeding himself or herself and offer appropriate assistance if needed. Work with the physician or nurse practitioner to alleviate nausea, vomiting, or loss of appetite related to disease process or drug therapy that prevents sufficient oral intake.

If the patient cannot take in enough food orally, vitamins or other nutritional supplements may be ordered. In some cases, enteral nutrition (i.e., tube feedings) or total parenteral nutrition may be necessary to correct the imbalances.

If the assessment reveals that the patient is at risk for an interaction among a prescribed drug and foods, nutrients, herbs or nutritional supplements, discuss with the patient the many ways that these interactions affect nutritional status and drug therapy effectiveness. It may also be necessary to discuss these findings with the prescriber of drug therapy.

Many of the nurse's actions to maximize the therapeutic effect or minimize the adverse effects of drug therapy, in relation to dietary factors, are centered around patient education.

Providing Patient and Family Education

- Teach patients about the potential interactions of food, nutrients, and complementary nutritional therapies with prescribed drug therapy.
- Emphasize to patients and families the importance of being well nourished while receiving prescribed drug therapy.
- Teach patients when to take the prescribed drug in relation to meals if timing is relevant for the particular drug (e.g., should the drug be taken on an empty stomach to promote absorption?).
- Encourage patients to inform all their health care providers about all dietary supplements used.
- Teach patients that botanical supplements should be used as treatment for serious health conditions only with the advice and supervision of a qualified health practitioner.
- Instruct the parents of children and pregnant women or breast-feeding mothers not to use botanical products unless advised to do so by a qualified health practitioner, particularly if using these products is associated with toxicity or drug and food interactions.
- Counsel patients about the variable quality of nutritional products.
- Advise patients to watch for any unusual reactions to any medication and to report them to the health care provider.

Ongoing Assessment and Evaluation

Assess for potential drug interactions when a patient is taking any dietary supplement or herbal preparation in addition to prescribed drug therapy. These interactions may reduce the therapeutic effect of the prescribed drug, or cause adverse effects from either the prescribed drug or the supplemental therapy. Drug therapy can be evaluated as effective if dietary factors have not impaired drug action or produced adverse effects. Dietary treatments may be evaluated as effective if they return the patient to a normal physiologic status, or if they work efficiently as adjuncts to drug therapy.

CHAPTER SUMMARY

- Numerous medications and nutrients interact, which can lead to imbalances or interfere with drug effectiveness.
- Supplementary use of vitamins, herbals, and botanicals may be prescribed by a health care provider to meet normal nutritional needs or to treat diseases or pathologies. The use of these nutritional supplements may also be self-prescribed by the patient.
- Foods and nutrients can alter the absorption, distribution, metabolism, and excretion of medications.
- Adverse drug–nutrient interactions are most likely to occur with medications taken for chronic conditions, if several medications are taken, or if nutrition status is poor or deteriorating.
- When assessing for the extent of drug–nutrient interactions, it is important that the nurse consider the patient's age, drug dose, and duration of therapy with medications known to have an adverse effect on nutrients.
- The glycemic index and the glycemic load offer important information to guide the patient to a well-balanced, healthy diet.
- Dietary Reference Intake (DRI) is the general term for a set of reference values used for planning and assessing nutrient intakes of healthy people. DRI includes the Recommended Dietary Allowances (RDA), Adequate Intakes (AI), and Tolerable Upper Intake Levels (UL).
- Patients may not recognize the importance of mentioning their use of dietary supplements or their normal dietary patterns during a drug history. Nurses need to be aware of this lack of awareness and routinely ask patients about this information.

QUESTIONS FOR STUDY AND REVIEW

1. What factors in a patient's drug history suggest a likelihood of drug–nutrient interactions?
2. Describe how drugs and nutrients can interact and alter metabolism.
3. Describe how foods can alter drug absorption.
4. Why is it important for the nurse to routinely assess patients for their use of dietary supplements or herbal preparations?

NEED MORE HELP?

Chapter 10 of the Study Guide to Accompany *Drug Therapy in Nursing*, 4th Edition, contains NCLEX-style questions and other learning activities to reinforce your understanding of the concepts presented in this chapter. For additional information or to purchase the study guide, visit thePoint.

REFERENCES

American Botanical Council. (2009). Herb Supplement Sales Show Growth in Multiple Market Channels. Retrieved from http://newhope360.com/herbs-medicinals/herb-supplement-sales-show-growth-multiple-market-channels

Bush, T. M., Rayburn, K. S., & Holloway, S. W., et al. (2007). Adverse interactions between herbal and dietary substances and prescription medications: a clinical survey, *Alternative Therapies in Health and Medicine*, 13(2):30–35.

Cannon, J. P. (2006). *Nutritional supplements: what works and why—a review from A to Z.* West Conshohocken, PA: Infinity Publishing.

Council for Responsible Nutrition. (2009). Vitamin and Mineral Recommendations. Retrieved from http://www.crnusa.org/about_recs2.html

Merck Manuals Online Medical Library. (2008). Carbohydrates, Proteins, and Fats. Retrieved from http://www.merck.com/mmhe/sec12/ch152/ch152b.html

Tovar, R. T. (2009). Clinical approach to clinical herbal toxicity, *Seminars in Diagnostic Pathology*, 26(1):28–37.

Willett, W. C. & Skerrett, P. J. (2005). *Eat, drink, and be healthy: The Harvard Medical School guide to healthy eating.* New York, NY: Simon and Schuster.

Environment: Influences on Drug Therapy

Learning Objectives

At the completion of this chapter the student will:

1. Identify environmental settings appropriate for pharmacotherapy.
2. Identify limitations for drug therapy for each specific environmental setting.
3. Discuss the importance of medication reconciliation in relationship to patient safety.
4. Discuss environmental influences on drug stability and effectiveness.
5. Discuss environmental influences on adverse effects of drug therapy.
6. Identify the relationship between environment and occupation.
7. Identify the role of the nurse regarding environmental influences on drug therapy.

Key Terms

environment
hepatic drug-metabolizing enzymes

industrial chemicals
medication reconciliation

pollutants

The core patient variable of **environment** also is relevant to drug therapy. There are three aspects of environment related to drug administration. The first aspect of environment is the physical setting in which the drug is administered. The second aspect of environment is environmental influences that may affect the stability or efficacy of certain drugs or drug classes. The third aspect of environment is the factors that may increase the risk of adverse effects, injury, or toxicity from drug therapy (Figure 11.1).

These aspects of environment as well as the nurse's role regarding environment and pharmacotherapy are discussed in this chapter.

PHYSICAL SETTINGS FOR DRUG THERAPY

Drug therapy may be administered in a variety of settings. These settings include acute care hospitals, acute rehabilitative units, transitional care units, outpatient units, long-term care facilities, and the home or community environment. Many factors influence whether a particular drug or class of drugs may be administered safely in a specific physical setting.

Acute Care Hospitals

Although most types of drugs are administered in acute care hospitals, certain drugs or drug classes are given in specific areas of these hospitals. For instance, the patient receiving

intravenous (IV) digoxin (Lanoxin) requires continuous heart monitoring. This requirement necessitates that the drug be administered in a critical care unit, step-down unit, or other specialized area that has both a specially trained nurse and the appropriate equipment, such as cardiac monitors, to assess the patient continuously.

Surgical patients receive inhaled anesthetics such as tubocurarine (Tubarine) only in the surgical suite, where the anesthesiologist or nurse anesthetist monitors the patient. Patients in active labor or immediately after delivery receive drugs such as oxytocin (Pitocin) in the delivery suite or postpartum unit. Alternatively, in an emergency, oxytocin may also be administered in the emergency department. Although these drugs are used for different medical problems, the common theme is that they require specialized nurses to administer them in a specialized unit of the acute care hospital.

Although most oncology drugs, such as 5-fluorouracil (5-FU), may be given on any medical unit, the administration of these agents is restricted to specially trained nurses. These nurses must understand specifics about handling chemotherapeutic drugs, recognizing and administering rapid treatment of severe adverse effects, and properly disposing of oncologic drugs (see Chapters 55 and 56).

Acute Rehabilitative Units

Acute rehabilitative units (ARUs) may be located in a portion of the acute care facility or another site off the main campus of the hospital. Although drugs given by most routes,

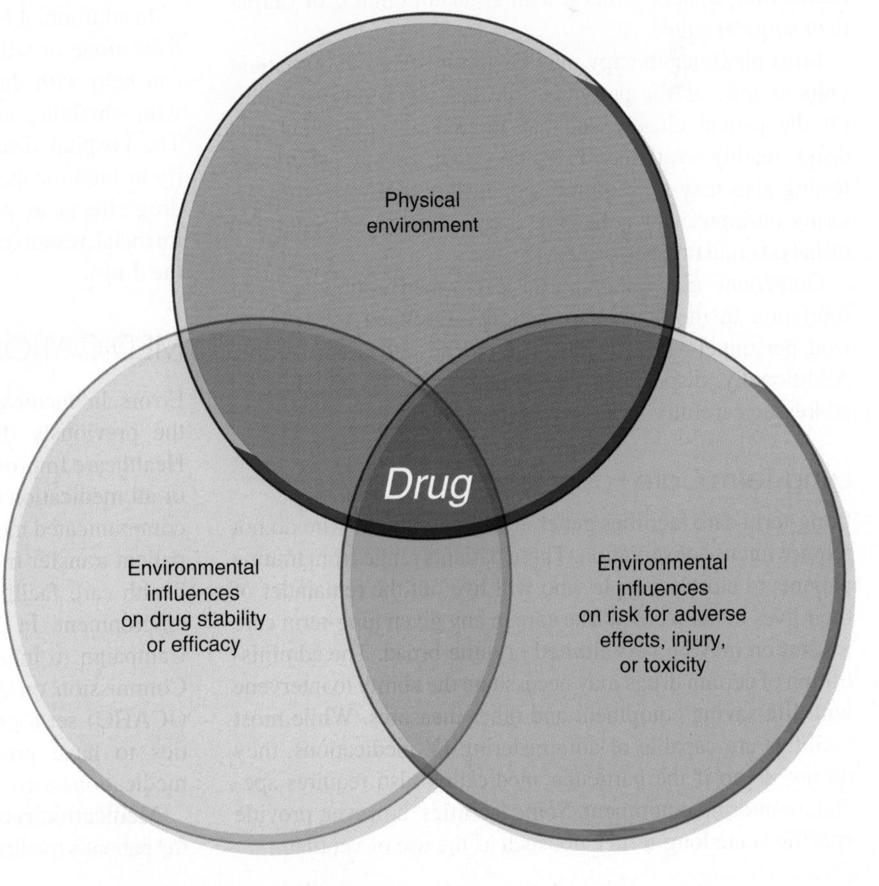

• FIGURE 11.1 The physical environment, environmental influences on drug stability or efficacy, and environmental influences that increase the patient's risk of adverse effects, injury, or toxicity intersect to affect the action of a drug.

including IV drugs, can be administered on these units, ARUs are developed to focus on the physical rehabilitation of the patient. Therefore, if the patient needs medication that requires close monitoring, or equipment such as cardiac monitors, the patient is moved back into the acute care hospital.

Transitional Care Units

Transitional care units (TCUs) have been developed to continue care of patients who are well enough to be discharged from the acute care facility but may not be eligible for a long-term facility because they need IV drug therapy or intense physical therapy. Like an ARU, these units may be in a portion of the acute care facility or in a different location. Because the patient-to-nurse ratio is higher in the TCU, drug therapy that requires close monitoring or equipment such as cardiac monitors limits the type of pharmacotherapy administered in this type of unit.

Outpatient Units

In the acute care facility, the term *outpatient* refers to the patient who arrives in the morning for a procedure with the expectation of returning home after the procedure is completed. Occasionally, the patient has a complication that requires that she or he be admitted to the acute care facility after the procedure.

In the community, *outpatient* refers to a patient who receives health care in an environment other than the acute care setting. These environments may include urgent care centers, physicians' offices, mental health clinics, or outpatient surgical suites.

Most pharmacotherapy may be administered in outpatient units as long as the particular site has the ability to monitor the patient closely and has life-saving equipment and drugs readily available. In some cases, on-site laboratory testing also may be required. For instance, before administering intramuscular gold salts, a complete blood count and urinalysis must be performed.

Outpatient chemotherapy is performed routinely. The limitation in the acute care setting—the need for specialized personnel—is also pertinent in the outpatient setting. Additionally, disposal of chemotherapeutic agents must be addressed carefully in this environment.

Long-Term Care Facilities

Long-term care facilities generally admit patients who do not require intense observation. These patients range from trauma patients to elderly people who will live out the remainder of their lives in the facility. The care in any given long-term care institution may be very limited or quite broad. The administration of certain drugs may necessitate the ability to intervene with life-saving equipment and other measures. While most facilities are capable of administering IV medications, they do not do so if the particular medication also requires special monitoring equipment. Some facilities, however, provide specific acute long-term care, such as the use of ventilators.

CRITICAL THINKING SCENARIO

Your patient has been involved in a major automobile accident and sustained a fracture of his femur. While talking with the patient, he remarks, "I feel like I am going to jump out of my skin. I haven't had my Ativan in 2 days." How would you respond?

Home Environment

Most drug routes are safe for administering medication in the home environment. Limiting factors include the need to monitor the patient closely and the need for special monitoring equipment. Although some patients receive pharmacotherapy from a home health nurse, many other patients are taught to self-administer medications, or family members and friends are taught to deliver the drugs safely.

The decision to teach the patient or family to administer drugs is made after a careful evaluation of the home environment by the home health nurse. Assessing the patient's environment may give important clues to its potential influence on therapeutic effectiveness, the patient's adherence to the drug regimen, and the potential risks from drug therapy itself. For example, if a patient is receiving a drug that causes dizziness as an adverse effect, stairs in the home may pose a risk for falls or injury. General factors to consider in the home include cleanliness; lighting; adequate heat, water, and refrigeration; and walkways in and around the house that are unobstructed and in good repair.

In addition, it is necessary to determine whether the patient lives alone or with other family members or caregivers who can help with the responsibilities of health care and assist with obtaining and administering drug therapy if needed. The hospital discharge planner assesses the patient's ability to monitor therapeutic effects and recognize any adverse drug effects, as well as whether the patient has the required financial resources, transportation, and knowledge to obtain the drugs.

MEDICATION RECONCILIATION

Errors in medication administration may occur in any of the previously described environments. The Institute for Healthcare Improvement (IHI) estimates that as many as 50% of all medication errors in hospitals occur because of poorly communicated medical information, which may occur during patient transfer from one location to another within the same health care facility or during transfer to a new health care environment. In 2001, the IHI launched its 100,000 Lives Campaign to improve patient outcomes. In 2006, the Joint Commission on Accreditation of Healthcare Organizations (JCAHO) set a goal requiring all JCAHO-accredited facilities to have protocols for documenting and reconciling medications across the environmental continuum.

Medication reconciliation is a systematic process in which the patient's medication history is compared to the current list of prescribed medications. In most facilities, this process is done by the nurse, however, in some hospitals the process may be done by the pharmacist as well. Medication reconciliation also may be done in an outpatient setting, such as a provider's office. The goal of medication reconciliation is to improve patient outcomes by potentially preventing serious adverse effects.

The nurse is responsible for collecting the patient's medication history, including over-the-counter medications, vitamins, and herbs or other supplements, from the patient or patient's family. After that information is obtained, the nurse compares the medications ordered by the health care provider with the list of medications obtained from the patient or family. The nurse communicates any discrepancies between these lists to the health care provider, including any differences in the appropriate dose of medications. This process continues each time the patient is transferred from one setting to another, even within the same facility. When the patient is discharged, the nurse compares the medications administered in the hospital with the discharge medication orders and again discusses any discrepancies with the health care provider. Finally, the nurse teaches the patient, the patient's family, or the patient's caregiver the name, dose, and frequency of the medication to be taken at home, potential adverse effects, and what adverse effects necessitate contact with the health care provider.

ENVIRONMENTAL INFLUENCES ON DRUG STABILITY AND EFFECTS

Many drugs are sensitive to the physical environment. Excess heat, light, or moisture or sudden temperature changes can affect the stability of a drug, and many drugs lose their potency when exposed to these elements. For example, nitroglycerin, a drug used for acute anginal pain, is affected by air, light, and moisture. Because of these environmental interactions, the nurse is responsible for the safe storage of the drug away from elements that can decrease its effectiveness. In addition, patient education must include the importance of keeping the drug in its original container and the need to replace the patient's supply frequently.

The environment can also modify drug effects. For example, temperature affects drug activity. Heat relaxes peripheral vessels, accelerates the circulation, and thus intensifies the actions of some drugs such as vasodilators; cold has the opposite effect—it retards drug action by constricting the blood vessels and slowing circulation. High altitude puts the body under stress, and relative oxygen deprivation at high altitudes may make some drugs ineffective, whereas it increases the sensitivity to others, such as alcohol and central nervous system depressants.

Environmental influences can affect pharmacotherapy in any environmental setting, not just the home environment. For instance, some IV drugs that are administered in the acute hospital setting, such as nitroprusside and amphotericin B, must be covered in aluminum foil or with a brown bag during administration to avoid light sensitivity.

ENVIRONMENTAL INFLUENCES ON ADVERSE EFFECTS AND INJURY

Environmental chemicals are increasingly being recognized as agents that cause substantial drug interactions in some people. For example, polychlorinated biphenyls (found in industrial solvents or used as flame retardant), polycyclic aromatic hydrocarbons (caused by incomplete combustion of organic materials and found in cigarette smoke), chlorinated hydrocarbons (found in pesticides), and consumption of ethanol are active inducers of **hepatic drug-metabolizing enzymes.** People chronically exposed to these chemicals metabolize some drugs (e.g., cimetidine, theophylline) more rapidly than normal.

A patient's environment may also influence the relationship between physiologic function, drug effects, and adverse effects or injury. Alcohol, tobacco, or pesticides may alter the pharmacokinetics of certain drugs and increase the patient's risk for adverse drug effects. For example, benzodiazepines such as lorazepam (Ativan), in combination with alcohol, may increase the adverse effect of respiratory depression to such an extent that death may occur. Another example is heat and antihypertensive drugs. Almost all of the antihypertensive drugs may cause the adverse effect of orthostatic hypotension. The combination of pharmacotherapy for hypertension with soaking in a spa or hot tub may lead to syncope. Photosensitivity is another potentially adverse effect that is associated with many different types of drugs. When a patient is taking a drug that causes photosensitivity, the nurse assesses the patient's life style for potential exposure to sunlight and emphasizes ways to minimize this potential adverse effect. Appendix G lists common drugs that may induce photosensitivity.

The role of the home health nurse is to assess the physical environment of the patient to determine the limitations for home pharmacotherapy. That assessment should also extend to finding ways to decrease the potential for injury related to pharmacotherapy. For example, many patients receive narcotic analgesics to control pain when they return home. Some of the most frequent adverse effects to narcotic analgesics are sedation and dizziness. The home health nurse identifies potential hazards in the home environment, such as stairs and loose rugs, to teach the patient to avoid these potential hazards when feeling sedated or dizzy.

Simple daily activities also may be affected by environmental influences of pharmacotherapy. For instance, the patient who is a stay-at-home mother may not recognize that the heat of her home can increase the adverse effects of sedation and weakness when taking certain drugs. When she attempts to make dinner, a simple task such as cutting up vegetables may become hazardous.

In the broad context of environmental influences, the patient's occupation also must be considered. Certain types of adverse effects, such as sedation and dizziness, are enhanced by environmental influences and can lead to serious or deadly harm to patients with certain occupations. For instance, sedation or dizziness in a patient who works as a taxicab driver may lead to accident and injury to the patient as well as others in his or her cab. Drugs that cause photosensitivity may actually cause partial-thickness burns in a patient who works as a lifeguard. Before the patient is discharged from the hospital, the nurse evaluates the patient's risk for adverse events based on his or her life style.

Patients who work in an environment that exposes them to **industrial chemicals** and pesticides have the highest risk for adverse effects and drug toxicity because these environmental **pollutants** affect drug biotransformation. These factors are thought to be responsible for decreased efficacy, prolonged pharmacologic effects, and increased toxicity.

A large number of drugs and chemicals, environmental pollutants, and endogenous substances are extensively metabolized in the liver before being excreted from the body. The environment can influence the metabolism of these substances. A variety of factors in the environment can influence the metabolism of chemicals by CYP450-dependent enzymes. These include concurrent drug treatment, cigarette smoking, and exposure to occupational and environmental pollutants.

THE NURSE'S ROLE

The nurse's role is extending more frequently beyond inpatient hospital settings to homes, schools, and industry. The nurse's role now includes the expanded range of health care concerns of health education, home health care, hospice, and public health because people are now being discharged from health care institutions at increasingly early stages in their treatment. Nurses monitor drug response and provide patient education about medication in a variety of patient care environments.

Nursing Management of the Patient with Environmental Considerations

Assessment

Drug action is not exclusively a biologic phenomenon. Environment is an important determinant of drug response. A number of components of the institutional environment are under the control of nursing. In the hospital, assess factors that influence drug outcome, such as a new or strange environment; unfamiliar people, noises, and equipment or procedures; and lack of physical activity. All of these factors may increase the need for some medications, such as analgesics, laxatives, and sedative-hypnotics. For example, providing a quiet, cool environment and reducing external stimuli to decrease tension and stimulation enhances the anxiolytic effects of sedative drugs.

Controlling the environment after discharge is a much more difficult task for the nurse. It is necessary to determine the environment in which the drug will be administered because drug therapies may occur in multiple environments. For example, patients may start chemotherapy or antidiabetic therapy in one environment, such as the acute care hospital, and continue therapy in the home environment.

People may not realize that environmental factors may affect their prescribed drug therapy. With that possibility in mind and to safeguard patients, conduct a complete drug assessment focusing on environmental and occupational influences.

Nursing Diagnoses and Outcomes

• Risk for Injury related to environmental hazards such as falls from stairs or loose rugs
Desired outcome: The patient will remain without a fall.
• Risk for Injury related to decreased drug stability stemming from environmental factors
Desired outcome: The patient will store drugs as directed.
• Impaired Skin Integrity related to environmental exposure to sunlight
Desired outcome: The patient will take measures to control the amount of direct sunlight to exposed skin and use sunscreen at all times.

Planning and Intervention

The planning and intervention phases of the nursing process contain short- and long-term goals. Often, these goals are modified as therapy proceeds. When working with patients to blend the element of environment into a regimen that promotes health maintenance and disease prevention, the nurse's role may be broad and include elements of advocacy, education, referral, consultation, clinical care, management, organization, research, and evaluation. However, at this stage of the nursing process, the nurse's primary role usually focuses on patient education.

The rapport established early in the nurse–patient relationship provides the basis for the trust that is needed as the nurse continues to collaborate with the patient. To maximize the benefits of drug therapy as it is affected or changed by environment, teach the patient about safe therapy and promote collaboration among health care providers and the patient. It may be necessary to teach patients how to evaluate their personal and occupational environments for hazardous chemicals and, if appropriate, suggest wearing or using protective equipment. Another aspect of patient education is teaching the patient about the proper way to discard medications. Therapeutic drugs can contaminate the environment through metabolic excretion, improper disposal, or industrial waste.

The extent of teaching varies, depending on the environment in which the patient will receive the drug (e.g., home, clinic, group home, hospice). Although some education is required whatever the setting, more information is necessary if the patient will be taking the drug at home than if the patient receives the drug in a rehabilitation center or other facility. The patient must be knowledgeable about all aspects of the drug regimen so that it can be self-administered safely and effectively. If another person—a family member or someone else—will be responsible for the patient's drug therapy at home, that person needs to be included in the educational process.

Ongoing Assessment and Evaluation

Evaluate the patient for increased or decreased drug effectiveness related to environmental stimuli. Assess the patient for signs of adverse effects that may have been induced by environmental factors. Review measures to control environmental factors with the patient at each clinic visit.

CHAPTER SUMMARY

• Environmental settings include acute care hospitals, acute rehabilitative units, transitional care units, outpatient units, home, and community.
• Limitations of pharmacotherapy for any setting include need for close monitoring of the patient, need for specialized equipment, need for life-saving equipment and drugs, and need for specialized personnel.
• Medication reconciliation must occur whenever a patient is admitted, transferred to a new environment, or discharged.
• The environment can affect the stability of a drug.
• The environment can affect the effectiveness of a drug.
• Environmental influences can increase the risk of adverse effects, toxicity, and patient injury.
• Environmental influences can increase the risk of injury in specific occupations.
• The nurse's role is to identify possible environmental influences on pharmacotherapy and institute appropriate patient education.

QUESTIONS FOR STUDY AND REVIEW

1. Identify elements of the environment essential for the nurse to assess regarding drug therapy.
2. How can smoking, alcohol, or environmental chemical exposures influence a patient's drug response?
3. What is the nurse's role in managing the patient with environmental considerations?
4. Explain the process of medication reconciliation.

NEED MORE HELP?

Chapter 11 of the Study Guide to Accompany *Drug Therapy in Nursing,* 4th Edition, contains NCLEX-style questions and other learning activities to reinforce your understanding of the concepts presented in this chapter. For additional information or to purchase the study guide, visit thePoint

REFERENCES

Boddice, S. D., & Kogan, P. (2009). Research on patient safety: falls and medications. *Home Health Nurse,* 27(9):555–560.
Clay, B. J., Halasyamani, L., Stucky, E. R., et al. (2008). Results of a medication reconciliation survey from the 2006 Society of Hospital Medicine national meeting, *Journal of Hospital Medicine,* 3(6):465–472.
Facts and Comparisons. (2010). *Drug facts and comparisons.* Philadelphia, PA: Lippincott Williams & Wilkins.
Gardner, B., & Graner, K. (2009). National patient safety goals. Pharmacists' medication reconciliation-related clinical interventions in a children's hospital. *Joint Commission Journal on Quality & Patient Safety,* 35(5):278–282.
The Joint Commission. (2011). National patient safety goals. Retrieved from *http://www.jointcommission.org/standards_information/npsgs.aspx*
Karch, A. M. (2010). *Nursing Drug Guide,* Philadelphia, PA: Lippincott, Williams & Wilkins.
Koda-Kimbal, M. A, Young, L.Y., Kradian, W. A., et al. (2008). *Applied therapeutics: the clinical use of drugs,* Philadelphia, PA: Lippincott Williams & Wilkins.
Tatro, D. S. (2009). *Drug interaction facts.* Philadelphia, PA: Lippincott Williams & Wilkins.

12

Culture: Considerations in Drug Therapy

Learning Objectives

At the completion of this chapter the student will:

1. Identify the influences that culture and ethnicity have on health and illness.

2. Recognize similarities and differences among the five major ethnic groups in the United States.

3. Describe why it is important to assess a patient's culture and inherited traits when managing his or her drug therapy.

4. Describe techniques that can be used in nursing management in drug therapy when working with patients and families of different cultures and ethnicities.

5. Describe how a person's genetic makeup can alter the pharmacokinetics of a drug.

Key Terms
biocultural ecology
cultural blindness
cultural competence

culture
ethnicity
ethnocentrism

pharmacogenetics
pharmacogenomics
stereotyping

North America has been called a "melting pot." A better expression might be "cultural mosaic," because this term signifies that people who emigrate to North America blend into society while retaining their individuality in terms of their culture. **Culture** is the shared customs and traditions, norms and values, institutions, arts, history, and folklore of a group. Similarly, **ethnicity** refers to a group that shares a common cultural heritage and that is linked by race, nationality, or language. An ethnic group is part of a larger social group.

The United States is becoming an increasingly multicultural society. In terms of nursing management and drug therapy, this diversity means that a patient's basic beliefs about health and disease may vary based on his or her cultural heritage. American society is primarily composed of five major ethnic population subgroups: white Americans, black Americans, Asian–Pacific Islander Americans, Hispanic Americans, and Native Americans. Each native and immigrant group has specific cultural attitudes about health, illness, and health care practices. Within each group, cultural attitudes, customs, and values may also vary widely (i.e., not all members of a culture have identical beliefs and practices). Members of minority cultures also tend to assume some or all of the practices and beliefs of the majority. Some aspects of minority cultures also become assimilated into the practices of the majority, producing a blend of cultural beliefs and attitudes.

Nurses today are being challenged to learn more about how cultural differences affect health, influence health-seeking behaviors, influence a patient's adherence or nonadherence to treatment regimens, and alter their responses to drug therapy. Nurses already realize that language and economics continue to be the main barriers to appropriate health care for many culturally diverse populations.

As patient populations become more culturally diverse, cultural competence becomes another feature of skillful nursing. **Cultural competence** requires maintaining awareness of one's own values and beliefs without letting them have undue influence on those of other backgrounds, demonstrating knowledge and understanding of another's culture, accepting and respecting cultural differences, and considering a patient's culture carefully.

Nurses must be aware that patients with various cultural and ethnic backgrounds may have beliefs and practices that differ from their own. These beliefs and practices are not wrong or inferior, merely different. Regardless of the patient's ethnicity or cultural background, nurses must be mindful of patients' beliefs and practices and consider them respectfully when managing drug therapy.

Ethnic groups share similarities in biologic and cultural characteristics. The term **biocultural ecology** (Purnell & Paulanka, 2003) refers to specific inherited physical, biologic, and psychological variations in ethnic and racial groups. These variations include skin color; physical body differences; genetic, endemic, and topographic diseases; individual psychological makeup; and biologic differences that affect the ways drugs are metabolized.

Recent pharmaceutical research has revealed that drug metabolism, dosing requirements, therapeutic response, and adverse effects differ among racial and ethnic groups. Additionally, research has found genetic variations within apparently homogeneous populations. For the purposes of this text, the core patient variable of culture and inherited traits is to be interpreted extremely broadly. In this text, the term *culture* refers to religious practices and beliefs, the use of medical or other health practices, and ethnicity—all of which may influence a patient's behavior in health and in illness. *Inherited traits,* or genetic variations, are also part of this core patient variable.

WORLD VIEW

Culture represents a way of perceiving, behaving in, and evaluating the world. A person's cultural identity influences his or her perception of the environment. Beliefs about the causes and effects of illness, health practices, and health-seeking behaviors are all influenced by a person's or group's perception of the environment—their world view. Three kinds of world-view health beliefs have been identified. These perspectives are known as biomedical health beliefs, magicoreligious health beliefs, and holistic health beliefs.

Biomedical Health Beliefs

In general, North Americans describe health from the scientific point of view. Scientific thinking underlies the biomedical view of health, in which life and life processes are controlled by physical and biochemical processes that can be manipulated by humans. For example, specific causes (bacteria, viruses) for an illness can be identified, and a specific treatment (drug therapy, surgery) can be developed to effect a cure.

Magicoreligious Health Beliefs

Predominant themes of magicoreligious health beliefs among some cultural groups focus on the concept of supernatural forces controlling health and illness and on the idea that illnesses are the result of "being bad" or "opposing God's will." Those who subscribe to these views perceive health as a gift from God and illness as an opportunity to realign with God. Prayer to God is used to cope with disease and to seek intervention for healing. Some cultures (e.g., West Indian) believe that magic, voodoo, or a hex or spell by a sorcerer or witch can cause illness. Some Mexican American and other Latin American groups believe that illness results from selection by the evil eye, or *mal ojo*. In these cases, the person seeks treatment from a traditional or folk healer, perhaps in addition to scientific therapies. The person's subscription to magicoreligious health beliefs influences his or her approach to health care.

Holistic Health Beliefs

A harmonious balance of the forces of nature is the basis of holistic health beliefs. According to this view, everything in the universe has a place and a function to perform according to natural laws that maintain order. Disturbing these laws creates imbalance, chaos, and disease. Four facets of the person's nature—physical, mental, emotional, and spiritual—must be in balance and harmony for the person to be healthy.

Traditional Native American and Chinese American cultures have a holistic belief system. Disease occurs when an imbalance exists in the person's nature. An example of holistic health beliefs among Chinese American groups is the yin and yang theory of health and illness; among Mexican American and other Hispanic groups, it is the hot and cold theory of illness. Therapies that may be used to restore a state of balance may include exercise, herbal remedies, meditation, and nutritional or dietary changes.

For example, within the biomedical world view of health, tuberculosis is clearly defined as an infection caused by mycobacteria. However, according to a holistic world view, in which disease results from multiple environmental "hot" interactions, tuberculosis is caused by the interrelationships of poverty, malnutrition, overcrowding, and mycobacteria.

EFFECT OF CULTURAL DIVERSITY ON HEALTH CARE

Purnell's Model for Cultural Competence

To understand any culture thoroughly, examining it with the use of a conceptual framework is helpful. Purnell's model for cultural competence (Purnell, 2009) is an example of a conceptual framework that is geared specifically to health care providers. This model identifies 12 aspects (or domains) of every culture that health care providers should consider. The domains are:

1. Overview (heritage and residence)
2. Communication
3. Family roles and organization
4. Workforce issues
5. Biocultural ecology
6. High-risk health behaviors
7. Nutrition
8. Pregnancy and childbearing practices
9. Death rituals
10. Spirituality
11. Health care practices
12. Health care practitioners

This text does not present comprehensive descriptions of every culture in the United States, nor does it provide instructions for performing a comprehensive cultural assessment. The intention of this text is to provide general knowledge of cultural concerns relevant to nursing management in drug therapy, using a brief description of those factors in the five most common cultures in the United States. Although Purnell's model may continue to evolve, certain domains are easily applicable to nursing management in drug therapy. These aspects are overview (heritage and residence), communication, family roles and organization, spirituality, health care practices, and biocultural ecology.

According to Purnell's model, heritage describes where the people come from, and residence describes where they currently live. Heritage and residence are important factors to consider because they provide clues about potential illnesses or conditions that may be present in the patient and require drug therapy. For example, new immigrants to the United States who have lived in areas where malaria is prevalent (e.g., Egypt, Italy, Turkey, Vietnam) may need to be screened for malaria, and if they test positive, to receive drug treatment. Another example is patients who currently live in crowded, poor urban areas who may need to be screened for tuberculosis.

Communication is an important part of culture for the nurse to assess. Communication includes verbal language (including dominant language; dialects; contextual use of words; and paralanguage variations, such as voice volume, tone, and inflection) and nonverbal language (e.g., eye contact, facial expression, use of touch, and temporality of world view). Temporal relationships are defined according to whether a culture is oriented to the past, present, or future (Purnell, 2009). Past-oriented cultures (e.g., German) may value the importance of providing historical background before presenting new information. Present-oriented cultures (e.g., Chinese) place more importance on the "here and now" than on the past or future. Future- oriented cultures (e.g., white American, European) believe it is important to prepare for what lies ahead. Punctuality is also part of temporal relationships; some cultures see promptness as important for all aspects of life, whereas others may be more relaxed about time, especially in social situations. The nurse needs to be mindful of all of these issues when working with patients. The ability to communicate effectively with a patient has a major effect on assessment, teaching, and the entire nurse–patient relationship.

The domain of family roles and organization defines the relationships among those inside and outside the family. Family roles and organization include head of household and gender roles; family goals and priorities; developmental tasks of children and adolescents; roles of the aged and extended family; social status; and acceptance or non-acceptance of nontraditional lifestyles (e.g., divorce, single parenting, same-sex relationships). This information is important for the nurse to consider when providing teaching to the patient and family. For example, some Middle Eastern men may feel that the health care provider does not respect them as the head of the family if patient education is directed toward a female family member (even if the woman is the patient).

Spirituality includes all formal religious beliefs and the use of prayer. It also includes all behaviors that provide meaning to life and strength to the person. Spirituality may influence nutrition, health care practices, and the other cultural domains. Identifying sources of strength and comfort for patients is important because these resources assist in promoting health and high-level wellness. The nurse considers spirituality to treat the patient holistically.

Health care practices include the focus of typical care (acute or preventive); the basis for health care (traditional, magicoreligious, or biomedical); beliefs about individual responsibility for health; self-medicating practices; views about mental illness, chronic illness, rehabilitation, organ donation, and transplantation; and responses to pain and the sick role. These practices influence not only how a patient responds to health and illness but also his or her acceptance of drug therapy. Drug interactions may occur from self-medication or the use of alternative therapies (e.g., herbs). The knowledge of health care practices not only assists the nurse in assessing the patient but also provides a basis for appropriate patient education.

Biocultural ecology identifies specific physical, biologic, and physiologic variations that stem from ethnic and racial background. Some diseases have a genetic predisposition, placing certain ethnic groups at increased risk. These diseases may require drug therapy. For example, African Americans are more likely to develop hypertension than are white European Americans (Centers for Disease Control, 2009). Most important for nurses managing drug therapy, some racial and ethnic variations alter drug metabolism. Active pharmacokinetic processes (e.g., protein binding and metabolism) are more likely to be affected by ethnic differences than passive pharmacokinetic processes (e.g., absorption).

Although data in this field are limited, more studies are being done to examine drug therapy for interracial variations.

Pharmacogenetics, Pharmacogenomics, and Drug Therapy

That different people respond to a particular drug in different ways (e.g., some have little or no response to therapy, and others endure adverse effects) has long been a well-known, if puzzling, fact. As the study of genes and DNA has progressed,

pharmacogenes, which are genes involved in the response to a drug, have been identified. There are 30,000 genes but an unknown number of pharmacogenes. Pharmacogenetics to Pharmacogenomics—the study of drug response in the context of the entire genome.

Pharmacogenetics is the study of inherited differences of a specific gene in response to clinical drug therapy (Pharmacogenetics and Pharmacogenomics Knowledge Base, 2011). People with some variations of genetically carried traits can have alterations in the following processes: drug metabolism, drug transportation, ion channels, or drug receptors. These alterations may increase or decrease drug levels that can be achieved from a dose, or increase or decrease the effectiveness of a drug's dose from that which normally occurs, placing these patients at risk for developing adverse effects or for clinical failure of drug therapy (even if they are taking a "standard" dose). These genetic factors therefore alter the dose necessary to be therapeutic but to avoid toxicity. This link between genetic makeup and drug response may be related to race or ethnicity; however, research increasingly shows individual variation within population groups that is not related to race or ethnicity. Understanding how different people respond to a particular drug and adjusting the drug dose to meet each person's unique needs is essentially the concept of "one drug for many people." The difficult challenges in analyzing and using pharmacogenetic data involve linking information about the variation in human genes to the variation in drug response, and determining if the cost of genetic testing is offset by savings from preventing serious drug adverse effects. Figure 12.1 is a visualization of the relationship between genes and drug therapy. Already there are over 50 drugs with pharmacogenetic discoveries listed

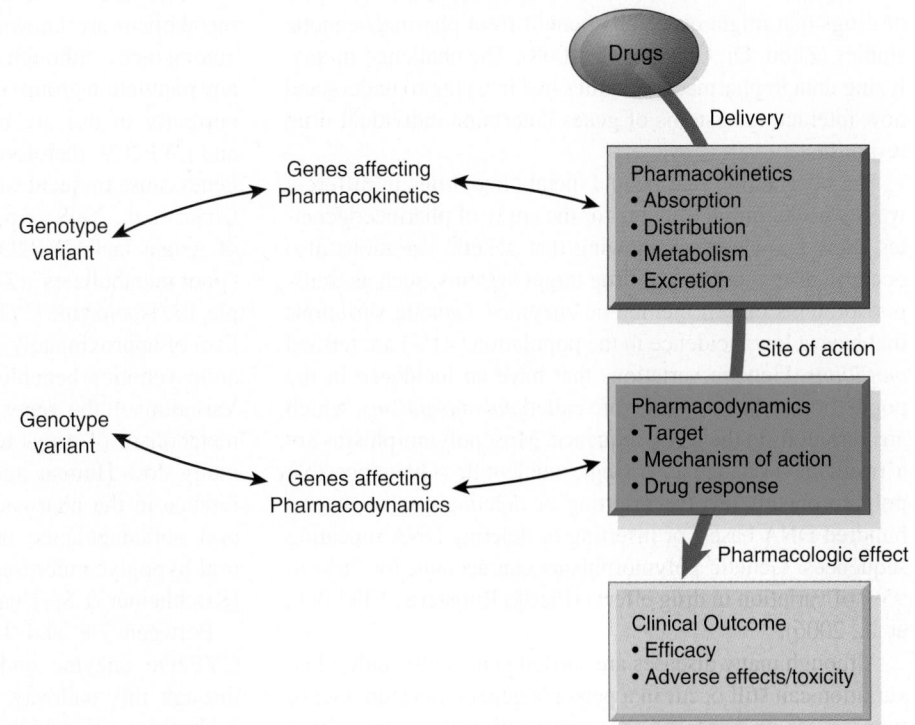

• FIGURE 12.1 Genotype and phenotype variations can alter a drug's effect from what is expected. Phenotype variations alter pharmacokinetics, pharmacodynamics and drug responses, clinical outcomes, and molecular and cellular functional assays. (©PharmGKB, 2006. Used with permission.)

in their drug label information (Shin, Kayser, & Langaee, 2009). The FDA lists pharmacogenetic information (which is termed "genomic biomarkers") that will help to: identify those patients likely to have a positive therapeutic response to a drug versus those likely to have a poor response; identify those patients likely to experience adverse effects (especially serious adverse effects); and determine the best dose to optimize the safe and effective treatment of a disease (FDA Table of Valid Genomic Biomarkers in the Context of Approved Drug Labels).

Pharmacogenomics is the study of drug response in the context of the entire genome. The genome of an organism contains all of its genetic information. In other words, it is the study of all genes in a group of individuals simultaneously to determine the basis for drug response variations (Pharmacogenetics and Pharmacogenomics Knowledge Base).

Pharmacogenomics entails the use of databases to identify disease-relevant drug targets in the human genome at the molecular level and to target drugs to clinical populations that share unique genetic profiles. This approach is essentially the concept of "many drugs for many people." With pharmacogenomics, researchers are able to look at variations in all the genes in a group of individuals simultaneously to determine the basis for variations in drug response. Ideally, those who prescribe drug therapy will use knowledge from pharmacogenomics as well as non-genetic factors (such as environment) to know how the patient is likely to react to a particular drug. They will therefore choose a drug that will achieve the maximum therapeutic effect but not produce adverse effects.

Pharmacogenomics, although still in its infancy, may become an important tool in developing new drugs in the future. Drugs with narrow therapeutic indexes (and therefore with high potential for serious adverse effects) are examples of drugs that might especially benefit from pharmacogenetic studies (Zhou, Di, Chan, et al., 2008). The challenge in analyzing data in pharmacogenomics lies in trying to understand how interacting systems of genes determine individual drug responses.

The observation that people metabolize drugs in different ways was the initial impetus for the study of pharmacogenetics. New knowledge is showing that genetic variations also occur in drug receptors or drug target systems, such as transport proteins or cell membrane enzymes. Genetic variations that have a low incidence in the population (<1%) are termed *mutations*. Genetic variations that have an incidence in the population of 1% or greater are called *polymorphisms,* which are variations in the DNA sequence. Most polymorphisms are a result of a change in a single nucleotide. Other possible polymorphisms involve inserting or deleting one or several hundred DNA bases, or inserting or deleting DNA repeating sequences. Genetic polymorphisms can account for 20% to 95% of variation in drug effects (Pierik, Rutgeerts, Vlietinck, et al., 2006).

Although many diseases are carried genetically, individual variation can still occur in a person's genetic makeup. Genotype is a person's specific gene composition; this composition

reflects any variations unique to that person. Phenotype is the observable or measurable expression of a genotype. All people with a similar phenotype will experience a particular disease or disorder, but they will not necessarily have the identical genotype. These variations in genotype account for different responses to drug therapy. For example, a chromosomal variation known as the Philadelphia chromosome is present in most, but not all, patients with chronic myeloid leukemia. Chronic myeloid leukemia is a type of cancer in which large numbers of mature myeloid cells are found in the peripheral blood and in the bone marrow. The variation in genotype expressed as the Philadelphia chromosome produces a certain abnormal protein. Cells with this abnormal protein do not respond to drug therapy but continue to reproduce. Research that explained how this particular protein malfunctioned enabled creation of a specific drug, imatinib (Gleevec), with a mode of action aimed specifically at the dysfunctional protein. This drug is much more successful than others in treating chronic myeloid leukemia, but only if the genotype variation of the Philadelphia chromosome is present.

When there is variation in genotyping of a particular disease, the disease is sometimes referred to as a heterogenic disease. One example is inflammatory bowel disease. This variation in genotyping of a disease makes it difficult to predict how people with the same disease will react to drug therapy. Treatment responses in people with a heterogenic disease are influenced by many confounding factors, such as disease severity or duration, as well as polymorphisms (Pierik, Rutgeerts, Vlietinck, et al., 2006).

Because drug metabolism through the P-450 hepatic enzymes has been studied the longest, some conclusions about genetic variations in the enzymes responsible for drug metabolism are known. Some of these data show variation among races, although great individual variation exists within any population group (i.e., specific race). Nearly 80% of drugs currently in use are metabolized by CYP2D6, CYP2C19, and CYP2C9, therefore variations (polymorphisms) in these genes cause frequent variations in drug metabolism (Zhou, Di, Chan, et al., 2008). Approximately 5% of Europeans and 1% of Asians lack CYP2D6 activity and are therefore known as "poor metabolizers" (Zhou, Di, Chan, et al., 2008). For example, the isoenzyme CYP2D6 is known to be active in metabolism of approximately 20% drugs, including antidepressants, antipsychotics, beta blockers, and some chemotherapy drugs. Variations in the genes controlling this isoenzyme can cause metabolism of drugs to be either abnormally fast or abnormally slow. Human studies have revealed up to a 10-fold difference in the pharmacokinetics of various antidepressants, oral anticoagulants, nonsteroidal anti-inflammatories, and oral hypoglycemic drugs due to polymorphism of CYP2C9 (Kirchheiner & Seeringer, 2007).

Between 7% and 10% of white people lack an active CYP2D6 enzyme and therefore metabolize drugs poorly through this pathway. A small percentage of whites have a phenotype in which the CYP2D6 gene is duplicated, so that they have two active genes, making them ultra-rapid metabolizers. Interethnic variability has been shown with Asian and black African/African American populations, who have reduced CYP2D6 activity compared with whites. Other unique ethnic groups are known to have variations of CYP2D6 that make them ultra-rapid metabolizers. One study of the isoenzyme CYP2C19 shows that 3% to 4% of whites and African Americans are poor metabolizers via this pathway, compared with 14% to 21% of Asians (Shilbayeh & Tutunji, 2006). A small recent study of Vietnamese found that they had similar variation in CYP2D6, CYP3A4, and CYP2C19 as other Asian populations (Veiga et al., 2009). One study examined the prevalence of the variation in CYP2C19 in Jordanian Arabs. It found that the majority of Jordanian Arabs are extensive metabolizers, although a subset are poor metabolizers (Shilbayeh & Tutunji, 2006).

Patients who respond to drugs differently based on their ethnic and genetic heritage may be at risk for a higher incidence of morbidity and mortality from a disease, because the prescribed therapy may not be as effective for them in controlling their disease. When one considers ethnic variation in drug activity, it is important to consider the route by which the drug is administered. Pharmacokinetic responses to drug therapy may be altered by different routes—for example, a drug that has a high first-pass effect when given orally does not exhibit this concern when given parenterally. Thus, if a patient had a racial genetic variation that altered their ability to metabolize (and have a first-pass effect), then giving the same drug by a different route may negate the ethnic genetic differences in drug metabolism (Chen, 2006). Given the multitude of factors that can influence a drug's dose will require long-term use of both knowledge of genetic factors as well as non-genetic factors that impact pharmacokinetics and pharmacodynamics (Shin, Kayser, & Langaee, 2009).

Although some genetic variation can be explained by race or ethnicity, these data cannot be solely relied on in cultures where genetic mixing of ethnic populations occurs. Interethnic mixing is becoming increasingly more common globally, which means that it is risky to apply knowledge that has been gleaned from pure ethnic groups to mixed populations. Ethnic subgroups of a larger ethnic group may also have unique genetic differences because they may have been geographically isolated in the past. For example, although Chinese, Malaysian, and Indian subgroups can all be considered Asians, one study found that genetic variations among them accounted for the fact that the Chinese and Malaysians required less warfarin (an oral anticoagulant) than Indians to achieve a therapeutic response without adverse effects. The authors believed that these differences reflected the ethnogeographic distinctions among the three groups (Lee et al., 2006).

Some data support individual genetic variation in CYP3A4 and CYP2C9 and the effects these variations have on drug interactions, drug metabolism, and drug dosing. Data are also being gathered on other isoenzymes in the P-450 family. (See also Chapters 4 and 5 for more information.) Identification of the genotype and/or the phenotype for these isoenzymes

promises much therapeutic value, especially if the drug that is to be administered has a narrow therapeutic index (Zhou et al., 2008).

Genetic testing for some CYP alterations is available and is used increasingly at many clinical sites. Genetic variations which alter drug metabolism or drug effectiveness may exist, for which there is no created test yet. Thus patients may be at risk even if their genetic testing indicates that they are "normal" metabolizers. Other limitations on the tests include the cost of testing and the need for physician education related to ordering genetic testing as well as interpreting and utilizing the results. As more drugs become labeled with statements relevant to potential adverse effects or loss of effectiveness related to polymorphisms, with a recommendation to perform genetic testing prior to prescribing the drug, the testing for these genetic markers will become more common.

In addition to the P-450 family of isoenzymes, two other mechanisms of drug metabolism involve enzymes: N-acetyltransferases (NATs) and thiopurine methyltransferase (TPMT). NATs speed up the rate of the chemical reaction in which an acetyl group is transferred to a particular drug, increasing its water solubility and promoting renal excretion. Mutations or polymorphisms of NAT genes are responsible for slowing the metabolism of drugs such as isoniazid (an antitubercular agent) and some cardiovascular drugs, among others. Patients with genetic variations that affect these enzymes are at risk for higher circulating levels of drug and adverse effects. Tests to predict these variations are not currently part of routine clinical practice.

TPMT is necessary for the metabolism of certain types of drugs, known as thiopurine drugs. This chemical class of drugs is used for a variety of purposes, such as treating rheumatoid arthritis, preventing rejection of transplanted organs, treating pediatric acute lymphoblastic leukemia, and treating steroid-resistant inflammatory bowel disease. These drugs are highly toxic and have a narrow therapeutic index; thus, finding the proper dose for a patient is crucial to prevent adverse effects and injury. In some clinical areas, laboratory analysis for TPMT—rather than the conventional method of using the patient's weight—is considered the current standard for determining the proper dose of a thiopurine drug. Patients with an alteration in TPMT gene begin therapy at a much lower dose than the usual standard dose.

Another way that genetic variation can alter drug response is to alter the sensitivity of a target receptor to a specific drug molecule; if the receptor site is more or less sensitive to the drug then the therapeutic effectiveness may go down or the risk for adverse effects may go up. For example, the beta 2 receptor is one receptor target where genetic modification is clinically significant (Zhou et al., 2008).

Currently, pharmacogenetics is still a relatively new area of study; pharmacogenomics is even more in its infancy. Although these disciplines are actually two different fields of study, they can be considered interdependent and to have some outcomes in common. Indeed, the literature may use the terms almost interchangeably, causing potential problems

BOX 12.1 FOCUS ON RESEARCH

Cost Effectiveness of Warfarin Genotyping

Eckman, M.H., Rosand, J., Greenberg, S.M., & Gage, B.F. (2009). Cost-effectiveness of using pharmacogenetic information in warfarin dosing for patients with nonvalvular atrial fibrillation. *Annals of Internal Medicine*, 150(2), 73–83.

The Study

In order to determine the cost effectiveness of using pharmacogenetic testing before starting the anticoagulant warfarin in patients, a Markov state transition decision model was used by the researchers. They created an ideal "base case" of a 69-year-old man with newly diagnosed nonvalvular atrial fibrillation (these patients require long-term anticoagulation therapy) who has no contraindications to warfarin therapy. The effectiveness was measured in quality adjusted life years and costs were in 2007 U.S. dollars. They found that the patient had better outcomes if the genotype was assessed and dosing was based on the genotype. However, this increase in patient outcomes was expensive ($170,000 per quality adjusted life year). The researchers concluded that for 90% of patients with nonvalvular atrial fibrillation, it was not cost effective to perform genotyping to determine the dose of the warfarin. However, for patients with high risk of hemorrhage from the anticoagulant, which could lead to cerebral hemorrhage or other severe events, genotyping may be cost effective to determine the best dose of warfarin.

Nursing Implications

It has been long known that finding the correct therapeutic dose of the anticoagulant warfarin is difficult in some patients. They either have subtherapeutic levels of the drug or they have higher than normal levels and therefore bleed very easily. In 2007, the FDA revised the label for warfarin and suggested that genetic testing be considered before starting therapy to identify those patients who would be likely to have serious adverse effects from a "standard" dose of warfarin. This research brings up an important but not always considered point related to pharmacogenomics: the economic costs of testing may be too great to consider using the technology for everyone. In a time of economic difficulty and the need to constrain health care costs, the health care system cannot afford to increase the costs of drug therapy. Just because genetic testing of an individual (to find the best drug or the best dose before starting therapy) may be possible, does not necessarily mean it must be done. Nurses should be aware of the pros and cons related to pharmacogenetic testing. When patients would truly benefit (such as those at high risk for serious, life-threatening adverse events), nurses should consult with the prescriber about obtaining this testing before starting drug therapy.

when applying some of the pharmacogenetic/pharmacogenomic study findings. First, the findings may only relate to patients with one specific disease who have received a particular drug, and the data may not be applicable when the same drug is prescribed to patients with different diseases than the one originally studied. Second, therapeutic responses to a drug may vary among individuals because of variability of the disease (e.g., how long the patient has had the disease or the severity of the disease), or variability of drug response due to polymorphisms, or both. Third, many pharmacogenetic/ pharmacogenomic studies lack explicit statements concerning how to translate the study's findings into clinical practice (Pierik, Rutgeerts, Vlietinck, et al., 2006). As more information becomes available and technology develops to identify genetic variations easily and accurately, it is anticipated that drug therapy will be individualized to meet each patient's needs optimally while minimizing risks for adverse effects (Box 12.1).

Cultural Differences Among Major Ethnic Groups

The following sections describe some of the differences in the five predominant ethnic groups in the United States, using the parameters described in Purnell's model. Every culture includes variations; therefore, these are general characteristics. Any statement that describes a general characteristic of a culture risks being considered stereotypical. Therefore, these descriptions must not be considered applicable to every person in any given culture. Indeed, many aspects of the dominant culture are usually also present in the nondominant cultures of our society. Every patient needs to be assessed individually for beliefs and practices.

White Americans

The most prevalent culture in the United States is that of whites. The people in this cultural group trace their ancestors to various European countries. Although they exhibit differences, white Americans have many common cultural traits.

White Americans speak English; a few may also speak a second language. White Americans tend to be future oriented and encourage work and sacrifice today as an investment for the future. People in this cultural group expect to delay the purchase of nonessential items to provide for drug therapy, medical treatment, and other health care needs, in the belief that doing so will help ensure a healthier future. White Americans have a linear sense of time (e.g., this action or event happens at this time followed by another action or event at a particular time). Time is highly valued, and people in this cultural group tend to be punctual for meetings, appointments, and social gatherings (Purnell, 2009).

Married white Americans generally live in traditional nuclear families of a man and woman and their children. However, nontraditional, nonnuclear families are becoming more common. Although historically men worked and women stayed at home to care for children, this division of labor now occurs less frequently, and more households have two working spouses.

The predominant religious belief is Christianity, with multiple denominations represented (e.g., Protestant, Roman Catholic). However, some white Americans are Jewish. Some religious beliefs may affect a patient's acceptance of certain drug therapies. For example, Roman Catholicism does not support the use of birth control. This doctrine could alter a woman's acceptance of oral contraceptives, even when given for medical management of irregular menstrual periods.

Most white Americans share a bioscientific view of disease and health management, although nontraditional health care practices are becoming more accepted and common. Some white Americans hold strong religious views and rely on prayer to regain health. Many white Americans hold a combined belief in the abilities of science and prayer or faith to restore health. Health care practices are based primarily on traditional Western medicine, although alternative therapies are also used to some extent.

White Americans have been found to have more acid glycoproteins than other ethnic groups. Therefore, when they take drugs that bind to these proteins, they have lower amounts of free (or active) drug than when the same dose is given to someone of another ethnic group (Johnson, 2000). Most clinical drug studies have been performed on white men; therefore, the pharmacokinetic information from the study may or may not be applicable to white women or to other ethnic groups. More studies are now being done that include white women.

Black Americans

The largest group of black Americans is African American. This group will be discussed as illustrative of black Americans, although some differences exist among African-American and non–African-American blacks. African Americans trace their ancestors to Africans who were brought to North America as slaves. African Americans speak English and may also speak a black dialect of English. Generally, African Americans tend to be more present oriented than past or future oriented. Having a circular view of time, rather than a linear view, they are more relaxed about time than whites. It may be more important for some African Americans to have made an appointment than to be punctual. However, many African Americans share the dominant culture's belief in linear time (Purnell & Paulanka, 2003).

African Americans may have extended families, with the grandmother having an important role. Historically, the families tend to be matriarchal, although patriarchal families are not uncommon now.

Some African Americans tend to be very spiritual and actively practice their religions. Most African Americans are practicing Christians, with Baptist and Methodist being the most common denominations. However, several other Christian denominations are represented in African American culture, as are the Nation of Islam and other Islamic sects. Islamic lifestyle is strictly regulated, and important parts of this lifestyle include cleanliness pertaining to specific religious beliefs. During times of crisis (e.g., critical illness, imminent death), these patients and their families turn to religion. Because they believe that life is precious, they perceive almost any medical treatment (e.g., transfusion) needed to support survival as acceptable, unless it is contradicted by their religious beliefs.

Historically, access to traditional health care for African Americans was uncertain. As a result, folk medicine became a necessity for treating illness. Even today, some African Americans may turn to folk medicines and practices much as their ancestors did, viewing health as a state of harmony of body, mind, and spirit and illness as a state of disharmony resulting from natural causes, evil spirits, or divine punishment. Health-related folk practices are intended to restore harmony. The art of healing stems from a fundamental belief that healing power is a gift from God; prayer, rituals, or the laying on of hands often accompanies the use of home remedies. Certain people within the community may be identified as having this power to cure. The traditional healers of the African American community are usually women, who are proficient in using home remedies. Some African Americans may also seek advice from a voodoo practitioner. Additionally, African Americans use bioscientific medicine to treat disease and illness. Traditional or folk medicines may be used before, or concurrently, with Western medicine.

In general, African Americans respond to some drugs differently than whites. For example, they are less responsive to beta blockers (e.g., propranolol) and more responsive to monotherapy for hypertension than whites. The pathology of hypertension, a substantial health problem in this group, is caused by volume expansion, decreased levels of renin, and increased intracellular concentration of sodium and calcium. Because African Americans usually have dark eyes, their eyes dilate less than the eyes of people with light eyes in response to mydriatic drugs used during ophthalmologic procedures. Other biomedical differences include a higher incidence of extrapyramidal effects from tricyclic antidepressants and the antipsychotic haloperidol and greater susceptibility to tricyclic antidepressant delirium and other adverse effects of psychotropic drugs. These differences are based on pharmacogenetic differences in drug metabolism.

Asian and Pacific Islander Americans

Asian and Pacific Islander Americans have their ancestral origins in China, Japan, Korea, Vietnam, Cambodia, and other Asian countries and in the various Pacific Islands. Cultural differences among Asian–Pacific Islander Americans are many because of their diverse backgrounds. However, because the Chinese American population is the largest, it is discussed here.

Generally, Chinese Americans speak English. Older Chinese Americans may speak a Chinese dialect as their first language and may or may not speak English. Younger Chinese Americans speak predominantly English and may or may not also speak some Chinese.

The Chinese concept of time is related to the natural cycles of birth, life, and death. Therefore, time is to be integrated into life, rather than mastered (as whites attempt to do). Some Chinese Americans see little value in punctuality, whereas others, who view tardiness as a sign of disrespect and therefore as unharmonious, are prompt and expect the same promptness from others.

Traditional Chinese Americans place great significance on family and family roles. They emphasize the male relatives: fathers, sons, and uncles. Usually, the established head of the household—a man—has great authority and assumes all major responsibilities for the family.

Many Chinese Americans consider formal religion to be superstition, whereas others practice Buddhism, Roman Catholicism, Protestantism, Taoism, or Islam. Religion is considered a personal expression, prayer is a source of comfort, and formal group services are minimal.

Chinese Americans believe that harmony with nature is essential for physical and spiritual well-being and that harmony comes from a balance among the cycles and elements of nature (fire, water, wood, earth, and metal) and the cycles of life. Traditional Chinese Americans view the body and spirit as a gift given to them by their parents and ancestors. Therefore, the body and spirit must be cared for and well maintained. Care and maintenance are accomplished through the powers that govern the universe: yin and yang. Although these forces are in opposition to one another, they function in unison. A person whose yin is flourishing and whose yang is steadily active or energized is considered to be healthy.

Yang represents the positive male energy that produces light, warmth, and fullness or satisfaction. Matters that are ascending, brilliant, dynamic, and external belong to yang. Yin, in contrast, represents the negative female energy of darkness, cold, and emptiness. Things that are descending, dull, internal, regressive, and static belong to yin. For example, the surface of the body and the back are yang; the inside of the body and the front are yin.

Yin also represents the five viscera of the five solid organs (heart, kidney, liver, lungs, and spleen; referred to as *ts'ang*), which collect and store secretions. Diseases of winter and spring are thought to be yin. Yang represents five hollow organs (bladder, gallbladder, large intestine, small intestine, and stomach), referred to as *fu,* and the diseases associated with the warmer seasons of summer and fall.

The pulses are controlled by both yin and yang. For example, if yin is too strong, the person is nervous, apprehensive, and catches colds easily. Disease is caused by an upset in the balance of yin and yang, and weather has an effect on the body's balance (e.g., heat is injurious to the heart; cold is injurious to the lungs). According to this culture, improper balance of yin and yang will shorten a person's life span.

Chinese American health care practices vary. Younger Chinese Americans usually seek Western medical care first and traditional Chinese treatment as a follow-up. Older Chinese Americans may seek health care in the reverse order. Traditional Chinese health care is based on the concept of harmonious yin and yang.

Herbal medicines and Western foods and drugs may affect some Chinese Americans in important ways. Chinese Americans are also more likely than most other Americans to have certain inherited conditions. For example, alpha thalassemia, an inherited disorder of hemoglobin metabolism, affects Chinese Americans with greater frequency than it affects other cultural groups (except those of Mediterranean origin), placing them at greater risk for anemia. In addition, a sex-linked genetic

disease—a deficiency of glucose-6-phosphate dehydrogenase (G6PD)—is common in the Chinese American. This disease is characterized by a lack of the G6PD enzyme and results in anemia. Chinese American populations also have a relatively high incidence of lactose intolerance, which leads to gastric symptoms, such as diarrhea, when milk or other dairy products are consumed. Certain drugs are metabolized differently and have different effects in Chinese Americans. Among these drugs are mephenytoin (Mesantoin); diazepam (Valium; poorly metabolized in 15% to 20% of Chinese Americans); beta blockers, atropine (Sal-Tropine), and alcohol (increased sensitivity); antidepressants and neuroleptics (increased responses at lower doses); and analgesics (decreased sensitivity, but increased gastrointestinal [GI] adverse effects). Specific variations of drug metabolism among Chinese Americans are difficult to determine because most clinical drug studies have not differentiated them from other Asians.

Some variation of drug response among Chinese Americans is unrelated to differences in drug metabolism. Lithium carbonate (Eskalith), used in managing bipolar disorder, is a drug that is not metabolized, but it has a different effect in Chinese Americans than in Europeans and whites. Chinese Americans require lower levels of lithium to achieve a therapeutic response. Part of the explanation for the differences in drug responses lies in the number and type of drug receptors present. Just as different drugs can be metabolized only by specific liver enzymes, receptors are custom designed to accept only certain drug configurations. As with enzymes, the number and type of receptors are influenced by genetics. Chinese Americans, and other Chinese people, appear to have a greater number of lithium-activated receptors than other groups.

Hispanic Americans

Hispanic Americans are a large minority in the United States because of birth rates and immigration. Members of the Hispanic American community have their origins primarily in Puerto Rico, and in Mexico, Cuba, and other Latin American countries. The culture of Mexican Americans is described here.

Mexican Americans may speak either Spanish or English as their primary language. They may also be bilingual. Historically, Mexican Americans have been more present oriented than future oriented. Because time is viewed as relative, punctuality is relaxed, especially in social situations, although in modern society, the trend is toward greater punctuality. Mexican American families tend to be patriarchal, with the male head of the household as the primary decision maker. These roles too are changing, with greater responsibility being shared with female family members.

Although some Mexican Americans tend to view life as chance, believing that health is purely the result of good luck (if one's luck changes, so does one's health), others have a dominant fatalism and hold the opinion that God is responsible for delivering health or illness, and that good health should not be taken for granted. Still others are deeply involved in formal religions, primarily Catholicism, but some worship with the Church of Jesus Christ of Latter Day Saints (LDS), Jehovah's Witnesses, Seventh Day Adventists, Presbyterians, and Baptists. In this context, appropriate ways of preventing ill health involve using herbs and spices, praying and wearing religious artifacts, and maintaining a balanced diet and physical activity. Socioeconomic and educational backgrounds influence the beliefs held by the individual Mexican American.

People are expected to maintain equilibrium by eating and working properly. Good health exists when the biologic, psychosocial, and spiritual natures are holistically balanced in relation to the environment. The more serious physical and mental-emotional illnesses are brought to the male *curandero* or female *curandera,* who is a holistic healer in the community. The use of herbs (commonly in the form of teas and poultices) is a popular treatment offered by folk healers. Western medicine is also used.

As with other cultural groups, Mexican Americans believe that disease occurs when there is an imbalance between opposing life forces. For Mexican Americans, these forces are perceived as hot, cold, wet, and dry. The body is composed of four kinds of fluids (also known as humors), which may vary in temperature and moisture content. They are blood (hot and wet), yellow bile (hot and dry), phlegm (cold and wet), and black bile (cold and dry). Imbalances may exist among these fluids, and these imbalances are manifested as illness. Maintaining a balance between these fluids is important to promote wellness. When the four humors are balanced, the body is healthy.

These concepts provide a way of determining the remedy for a particular illness. Illness is thought to be caused by prolonged exposure to hot or cold; to cure the illness, the opposite quality of the etiologic agent is applied to absorb the hot or cold. For example, a cold substance is used to treat a hot illness. Hot conditions include constipation, diarrhea, fever, infections, kidney problems, liver problems, rashes, skin ailments, sore throat, and ulcers. Cold foods include barley water, chicken, fish, dairy products, fresh vegetables, goat meat, honey, raisins, and tropical fruits. Cold herbs and medicines include linden, milk of magnesia, orange-flower water, sage, and sodium bicarbonate.

Conversely, hot substances are used to treat cold conditions. Cold conditions include cancer, colds, dysmenorrhea, earache, headache, joint pains, malaria, paralysis, pneumonia, rheumatism, stomach cramps, teething pain, and tuberculosis. Hot foods include aromatic beverages, beef, cheese, chili peppers, chocolate, eggs, pork, liquor, goat milk, onions, peas, temperate-zone fruits, and whole grains (except barley). Hot herbs and medicines include anise, aspirin, cinnamon, castor oil, cod-liver oil, iron preparations, garlic, ginger, penicillin, tobacco, and vitamin preparations.

Hot and cold do not refer to temperature but are descriptive of the nature of a particular substance. Food, beverages, animals, and people possess the characteristics of hot and cold in varying degrees. Other Hispanic groups also consider items as hot or cold, but different substances are classified into these categories.

Few clinical drug studies have separated Mexican Americans from other Hispanic groups, so that information about variations in drug metabolism must be generalized from findings in Hispanic groups. Some studies have shown that Hispanics may metabolize some drugs differently from other cultural groups. For example, studies indicate that Hispanics need lower doses of antidepressants than do other groups and experience greater adverse effects from these drugs. Further complicating the issue is the fact that many Mexican Americans have mixed heritage. Therefore, generalizations may not be accurate for all Mexican Americans.

Native Americans and Alaska Natives

The Native American and Alaska Native population in the United States consists of more than 500 tribes that are recognized by the federal government and many others that are not. Native Americans (or American Indians) and Alaska Natives are the original inhabitants of North America, and each tribal community is unique in its cultural beliefs. The Navajo Indians are the largest tribe. A person must have at least one quarter Navajo blood to be considered part of the tribe. The Navajo Indians are presented as the example of Native Americans and Alaska Natives.

The Navajo tribe lives in a large reservation that consists of portions of Arizona, Utah, and New Mexico. In New Mexico, the Navajo tribe is scattered and lives with Zuñi Indians and settlers from the LDS church. A nomadic people, the Navajo tribe travels great distances searching for adequate grazing grounds for their sheep. Navajo Indians speak Navajo, which until the 1970s was only a spoken language. A few older Navajo people speak some English or Spanish; younger Navajo people are usually bilingual and speak Navajo and English. The Navajo and Apache have similar languages, but their dialects are different. Minor variations in the pronunciation of Navajo words may change the meaning of the word or phrase spoken. Navajo Indians believe that silence is an appropriate way to communicate nonverbally, and feel comfortable even during long silences. Navajos, especially older people, take their time to respond carefully and thoughtfully to what is said to them.

In contrast to whites, who view time in a present–future–past sequence, Navajo Indians view time in a present–past–future sequence. This outlook means that Native Americans attach little value to planning for the future, often considering it foolish. Time has little meaning or importance. Activities begin when people or members of a group gather.

The Navajo, like most other Native Americans, are matrilineal. Men are important, but grandmothers and mothers are the center of society. No decisions are made unless the appropriate older woman is present.

Native American religion predominates among the Navajo, although some have been converted to Christian religions, such as the LDS church, Jehovah's Witnesses, and some evangelical groups. The Navajo view spirituality as being in a state of harmony with one's surroundings. Prayer is important. Spirituality cannot be separated from healing and is

DIVERSITY, DRUG THERAPY, AND IMPLICATIONS FOR TEACHING

Forty-nine-year-old Maria Alvarez is a bilingual Mexican American for whom English is a second language. She is newly diagnosed with type 2 diabetes with prescribed "diabetic teaching" related to diet, exercise, and oral drug therapy. The nurse reviews cultural phenomena affecting health and health care among Mexican Americans and adult teaching-learning principles before working with Mrs. Alvarez.

1. What are some of the most significant considerations for the nurse to explore prior to teaching Mrs. Alvarez?

2. During one of the teaching sessions, the nurse plans to use pamphlets to teach Mrs. Alvarez about her disease and the prescribed drug therapy. What may be a limitation of printed material?

---

important in healing ceremonies. Illnesses result from not being in harmony with nature; from the spirits of an evil person, such as a witch; or from violating tribal taboos. Healing ceremonies restore mental, physical, and spiritual balance. The Navajo may use Western medicine in addition to healing from tribal ceremonies.

Type 2 diabetes is very common among Navajo people, as it is among all Native Americans and Alaska Natives. Other health problems common to the Navajo people are severe combined immunodeficiency syndrome (failure of antibody response and cell-mediated immunity, not related to acquired immunodeficiency syndrome [AIDS]), Navajo neuropathy (an inherited condition in which myelinated fibers are completely absent, and death occurs before the age of 24 years), albinism, and genetic blindness. Although little research has been conducted on variation in drug metabolism in Navajos, or other Native Americans and Alaska Natives, it is known that Navajo people can have increased adverse effects to some medications. For example, adverse reactions to lidocaine (Xylocaine), an anesthetic and antiarrhythmic, occur in 29% of Navajos but in only 11% to 15% of whites.

Nursing Management of Culturally Diverse Groups

In administering drug therapy to culturally diverse patient populations, it is necessary to respect each patient's cultural heritage, beliefs, and practices. A health care provider not fully aware of a patient's background may be unable to understand many of the patient's health beliefs and practices. Lack of knowledge or misunderstanding may unintentionally turn what should be a therapeutic experience into a degrading and humiliating experience for patients of other cultures. If possible, every effort should be made to accommodate the patient's traditional practices with standard drug therapy while providing nursing care to maximize therapeutic effects, minimize adverse effects, and promote health and safety for the patient and the family.

When caring for patients, be conscious of ethnocentrism, stereotyping, and cultural blindness. Because culture influences people so strongly in the way they feel, think, act, and judge the world, people often subconsciously restrict their view of the world to the point of being unable to accept other cultures. This inability is called **ethnocentrism.** Ethnocentrism inhibits acceptance of others and may lead to a clash of values and poor communication. Health care providers exhibit ethnocentricity when they act from the mistaken belief that only their own cultural and ethnic beliefs are normal, superior, or right. **Stereotyping** refers to the assumption that all patients of a particular culture or ethnic group will have the same response. Health care providers may exhibit **cultural blindness** if they proceed as if differences do not exist. Because the American health care system is based on the dominant pattern of Western scientific health beliefs and practices, it is not uncommon for health care providers to dismiss any deviations from the established pattern. The implication of all this is clear—throughout care, remember to be nonjudgmental and to convey respect.

Nursing Diagnoses and Outcomes

When developing nursing diagnoses, be aware of cultural beliefs, values, and behaviors that may influence the patient's situation. Although all nursing diagnoses may have related cultural factors, some can be specifically identified as having strong cultural implications. Patients with identified genetic polymorphisms are at risk for alterations in the effectiveness of the drug (either more than normal or less than anticipated) and increased risk of adverse effects from drug therapy. Box 12.2 presents nursing diagnoses and outcomes related to drug therapy, cultural diversity, and inherited traits.

Planning and Intervention

After the beliefs of the patient and family about health and disease, drugs and drug therapy, personal health habits, and chronic illness are assessed, planning and implementation may proceed.

Maximizing Therapeutic Effects

When drug therapy is recommended, make an effort to determine whether prescribed therapies are consistent with the patients' physical needs, cultural backgrounds, religious preferences, dietary preferences, and self-care practices. Then incorporate these aspects into nursing practice whenever possible and when not contraindicated for health reasons.

Minimizing Adverse Effects

Nurses and patients need to be aware that certain cultural practices (e.g., using herbal preparations in addition to conventional drug therapy) may create drug toxicity or herb–drug interactions. Conventional prescribed drugs may have actions similar or antagonistic to an herb or herbal product. For example, overmedication may result when ginseng (a tonic stimulant and an antihypertensive) is taken in combination with antihypertensive drugs. Some foods may also

Box 12.2 **NURSING DIAGNOSES AND OUTCOMES RELATED TO DRUG THERAPY, CULTURAL DIVERSITY, AND INHERITED TRAITS**

Impaired Verbal Communication

Desired outcome: Effective communication about drug therapy will be established among the patient, patient's family, and health care providers, despite possible language differences.

Anxiety related to new drug treatment

Desired outcome: Patient will recognize and express feelings of anxiety and will identify potential and actual sources of anxiety when health care practices during drug therapy interfere with cultural habits and health practices.

Fear of Health-Seeking Behaviors related to barriers to

health care (e.g., caregiver's judgments of nonadherence or deviant behaviors) or fear of being criticized for traditional practices and inability to communicate these needs effectively in the English language

Desired outcome: Patient will recognize and express feelings of spiritual distress when health care practices, such as drug therapy, interfere with spiritual beliefs.

Ineffective Health Maintenance

Desired outcome: Patient (and family) will verbalize an understanding of beneficial, neutral, and harmful cultural health practices as they relate to drug therapy.

Ineffective Coping or Disabled Family Coping

Desired outcome: Individual (or family) will more effectively deal with stress after talking with a health care provider who explains the reason for, or expected outcome of, planned drug therapy as it relates to cultural beliefs and practices.

Spiritual Distress

Desired outcome: Patient will recognize feelings of spiritual distress when health care practices, such as drug therapy, interfere with traditional beliefs and habits.

Risk for Injury related to inherited altered response to drug therapy

Desired Outcome: Genetic variations that are known to be related to increased incidence of adverse effects of drug therapy or related to loss of effectiveness of drug therapy will be identified in the patient prior to the onset of such therapy to allow for its safe and effective use.

Box 12.3 **COMMUNICATING WITH PATIENTS WHO SPEAK ANOTHER LANGUAGE**

Use an interpreter (preferably) or a translator. Use dialect-specific interpreters (if possible) trained in health care. If possible, use an interpreter of the same age and same gender as the patient.

- Look at the patient when you speak, not at the interpreter.
- Speak slowly.
- Do not raise your voice or exaggerate your mouth movements.
- Provide time for interpretation or translation.
- Allow time for the patient to think before he or she responds.
- Avoid using relatives and children as interpreters; they may not be objective and the patient or relative may be embarrassed by the content of the discussion.
- Listen attentively.

If an interpreter or translator is not available:

- Remember that patients often understand more language than they can speak.
- Limit the number of words you use, and include as many words of the patient's language as possible.
- Speak slowly, but not loudly.
- Use nonverbal language.

---

interact with some drug therapies; normal dietary patterns must be assessed to help prevent food–drug interactions (see Chapter 10).

Providing Patient and Family Education

The communication style of the patient should be considered when preparing to provide patient education. The reasons for a treatment plan must be shared with patients and families and explained in language and at levels they can understand. When planning educational materials for patients whose primary language is not English, make every effort to obtain interpreters or translations of written materials. Interpreters are preferred to translators because

an interpreter makes sure that the meaning behind the message is the same; translators merely change the words from one language to another. Box 12.3 provides guidelines for communicating with patients who speak another language. Pictures that reinforce the content of the verbal and written instructions are also helpful. Many computer systems are available that can automatically translate instructions into other languages (e.g., Spanish). Computer programs can also alter the level of language to make it appropriate for the patient's educational background. Compile and maintain a list of community resources that are available to assist patients of different cultures.

If the patient is present oriented, his or her understanding of acute and chronic illness may be affected by the perception of time. In such cases, teaching a patient about drugs for a chronic disease (e.g., hypertension) may be more successful if emphasis is placed on short-term problems (e.g., what may happen if the drug is not taken on time) than long-term problems, such as stroke and myocardial infarction.

In addition, consider gender roles and the importance of various family relationships to the patient when teaching about drug therapy. Ascertain that the appropriate person is present before beginning. For example, this person might be the grandmother of a Navajo Indian patient or the husband of a Mexican American woman.

Ongoing Assessment and Evaluation

To evaluate the effectiveness of nursing care for a patient of another culture, determine the extent to which the goals have been met by comparing the patient's current status with the identified outcome criteria.

CHAPTER SUMMARY

- Pharmacogenetics accounts for individual variation in the response to drug therapy. This variation is related to genetic alterations known as polymorphisms. Understanding the unique genetic makeup of an individual patient can ideally allow custom tailoring of the dose of a drug to promote therapeutic effect and prevent adverse effects.

  Pharmacogenetics is a new field, and knowledge about genetic variations affecting drug therapy is still somewhat limited, although it is rapidly growing. Some pharmacogenetic differences are inherited along ethnic or racial lines; other differences are unique to people and not inherited by ethnicity or race.

- Pharmacogenomics examines how all genes can affect drug therapy. The hope is that by understanding human genome variations, drugs can be developed that are more effective in different patient populations and predictions can be made concerning whether or not patients will have altered pharmacologic responses to a drug.

- Genetic variations of specific P-450 isoenzymes are known to influence drug metabolism. The variations include ultra-rapid metabolizers, extensive metabolizers, intermediate metabolizers, and poor metabolizers. Ultra-rapid metabolizers biotransform drugs using a particular isoenzyme more rapidly and thus may be at risk for subtherapeutic system levels of a prescribed drug. Poor metabolizers do not biotransform drugs using that isoenzyme, which means that systemic drug levels will rise higher than anticipated, producing more adverse effects.

- Genotype testing is now available for some of the P-450 isoenzymes and is used in clinical practice for some drugs.

- Many cultural groups in North America embrace both their original culture and the dominant North American culture.

- Although generalizations may be made about the beliefs of different cultural groups, these statements cannot be applied to all people sharing a cultural background. Every person must be assessed to determine his or her unique beliefs.

- Individual health-seeking behaviors and health practices exist and differ, sometimes markedly, among the major cultural groups in the United States.

- Medicinal plants and symbolic rituals play important roles in the health practices of many cultural groups.

- Patients should be advised of the potential for chemical interactions between folk medicine or herbal remedies and traditional (Western) drug therapy.

- Factors related to communication, time, and environmental control influence the relationship between the nurse and the patient whose backgrounds are culturally different.

- Individual variation in response to the effects of drugs and pharmacokinetic drug differences may occur because of biologic and genetic differences among people. For example, some patients may metabolize certain drugs more slowly because of a genetically induced enzyme deficiency.

- Nursing management emphasizes a thorough assessment of a patient's health beliefs, traditional practices, and cultural influences, so that the nurse and other health care providers may implement interventions that complement the patient's values. Therapeutic regimens that accommodate a patient's cultural values (and traditional rituals) are more likely to foster adherence to drug therapy and discourage alienation from the health care system.

- Cultural, ethnic, and environmental influences add complex issues to pharmacotherapy.

QUESTIONS FOR STUDY AND REVIEW

1. How does culture differ from ethnic group?
2. How is an awareness of cultural differences helpful when providing nursing management in drug therapy?
3. Describe strategies that can be used when your patient does not speak the same language as you.
4. Explain how an individual's concept of time will influence patient teaching about drug therapy.
5. Why are clinical drug studies that describe a drug's altered pharmacokinetic process in Hispanics not always applicable to Mexican Americans?
6. A patient is receiving a drug with a narrow therapeutic index that is highly metabolized by CYP2D6. Genetic testing has indicated that this patient is a poor metabolizer via CYP2D6. Is this patient more at risk for reduced therapeutic effects or increased adverse effects? What nursing actions would you use to either maximize the therapeutic effect or minimize adverse effects?

NEED MORE HELP?

Chapter 12 of the Study Guide to Accompany *Drug Therapy in Nursing*, 4th Edition, contains NCLEX-style questions and other learning activities to reinforce your understanding of the concepts presented in this chapter. For additional information or to purchase the study guide, visit thePoint.

REFERENCES

Centers for Disease Control and Prevention. (2009). High blood pressure: facts and statistics. Retrieved from http://www.cdc.gov/bloodpressure/facts.htm

Chen, M. L. (2006). Ethnic or racial differences revisted: impact of dosage regimen and dosage form on pharmacokinetics and pharmacodynamics. *Clinical Pharmacokinetics*, 45(10): 957–964.

Food and Drug Administration. (2011). Table of Valid Genomic Biomarkers in the Context of Approved Drug Labels. Retrieved from http://www.fda.gov/Drugs/ScienceResearch/ResearchAreas/Pharmacogenetics/ucm083378.htm

Kirchheiner, J. & Seeringer, A. (2007). Clinical implications of pharmacogenetics of Cytochrome P450 drug metabolizing enzymes. *Biochimica et Biophysica Acta*, 1770(3):489–494.

Lee, S. C., Ng, S. S., Oldenburg, J., et al. (2006). Interethnic variability of warfarin maintenance requirement is explained by VKORC1 genotype in an Asian population. *Clinical Pharmacology and Therapeutics*, 79(3):197–205.

Pierik, M., Rutgeerts, P., Vlietinck, R., et al. (2006). Pharmaco-genetics in inflammatory bowel disease. *World Journal of Gastroenterology*, 12(23):3657–3667.

Purnell, L. D. (2009). *Guide to culturally competent health care* (2nd ed.). Philadelphia, PA: F. A. Davis.

Shilbayeh, S. & Tutunji, M. F. (2006). Possible interethnic differences in omeprazole pharmacokinetics: Comparison of Jordanian Arabs with other populations. *Clinical Pharmacokinetics*, 45(6):593–610.

Shin, J., Kayser, S. R., & Langaee, T. Y. (2009). Pharmaco-genetics: from discovery to patient care. *American Journal of Health System Pharmacy*, 66(7):625–637.

The Pharmacogenetics and Pharmacogenomics Knowledge Base. (2011). Retrieved, from http://www.pharmgkb.org.

Veiga, M. I., Asimus, S., Ferreira, P. E., et al. (2009). Pharmacogenomics of CYP2A6, CYP 2B6, CYP2C19, CYP2D6, CYP3A4, CYP3A5 and MDR1 in Vietnam. *European Journal of Clinical Pharmacology*, 65(4):355–363.

Zhou, S. F., Di, Y. M., Chan, E., et al. (2008). Clinical pharmacogenetics and potential application in personalized medicine. *Current Drug Metabolism*, 9(8):738–784.

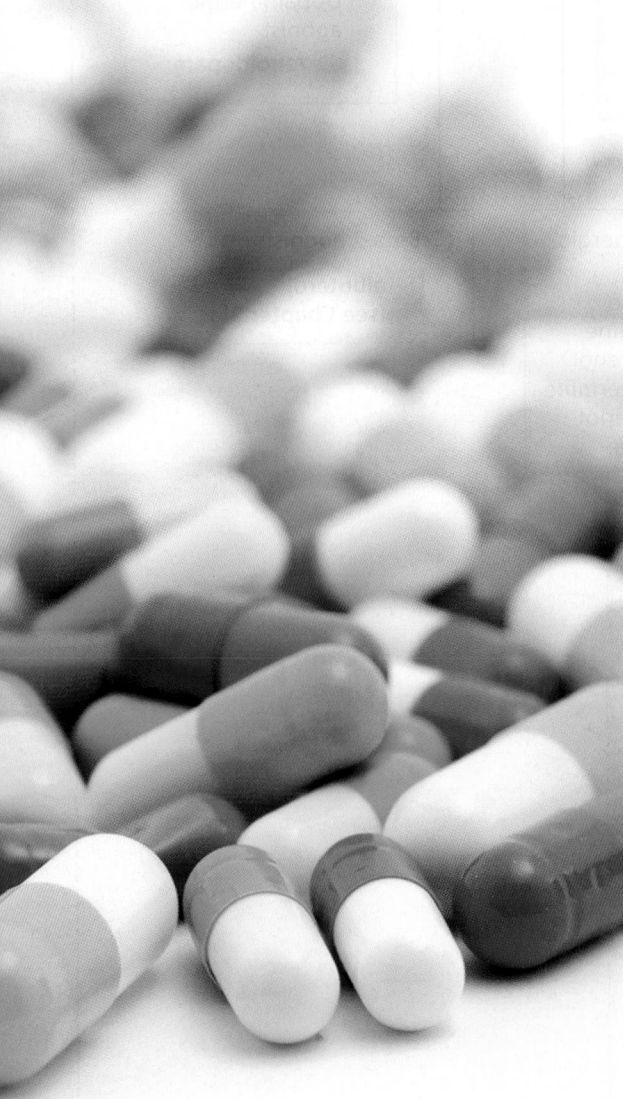

Drugs Affecting Adrenergic Function

Learning Objectives

At the completion of this chapter the student will:

1. State the neurotransmitters that stimulate the sympathetic nervous system
2. Understand how adrenergic drugs create their therapeutic effects in the sympathetic nervous system.
3. Differentiate adrenergic agonist from adrenergic antagonist drugs.
4. Identify core drug knowledge about drugs that act as adrenergic agonists or antagonists.
5. Identify core patient variables relevant to drugs that act as adrenergic agonists or antagonists.
6. Relate the interaction of core drug knowledge to core patient variables for drugs that act as adrenergic agonists or antagonists.
7. Generate a nursing plan of care from the interactions between core drug knowledge and core patient variables for drugs that act as adrenergic agonists or antagonists.
8. Describe nursing interventions to maximize therapeutic effects and minimize adverse affects for drugs that act as adrenergic agonists or antagonists.
9. Determine key points for patient and family education for drugs that act as adrenergic agonists or antagonists.

Key Terms

adrenergic nervous system
agonists
antagonists
autonomic nervous system
central nervous system

neurotransmitters
nonselective-acting drugs
parasympathetic nervous system
peripheral nervous system
selective-acting drugs

shock
sympathetic nervous system
synaptic transmission

Drugs Affecting Adrenergic Function

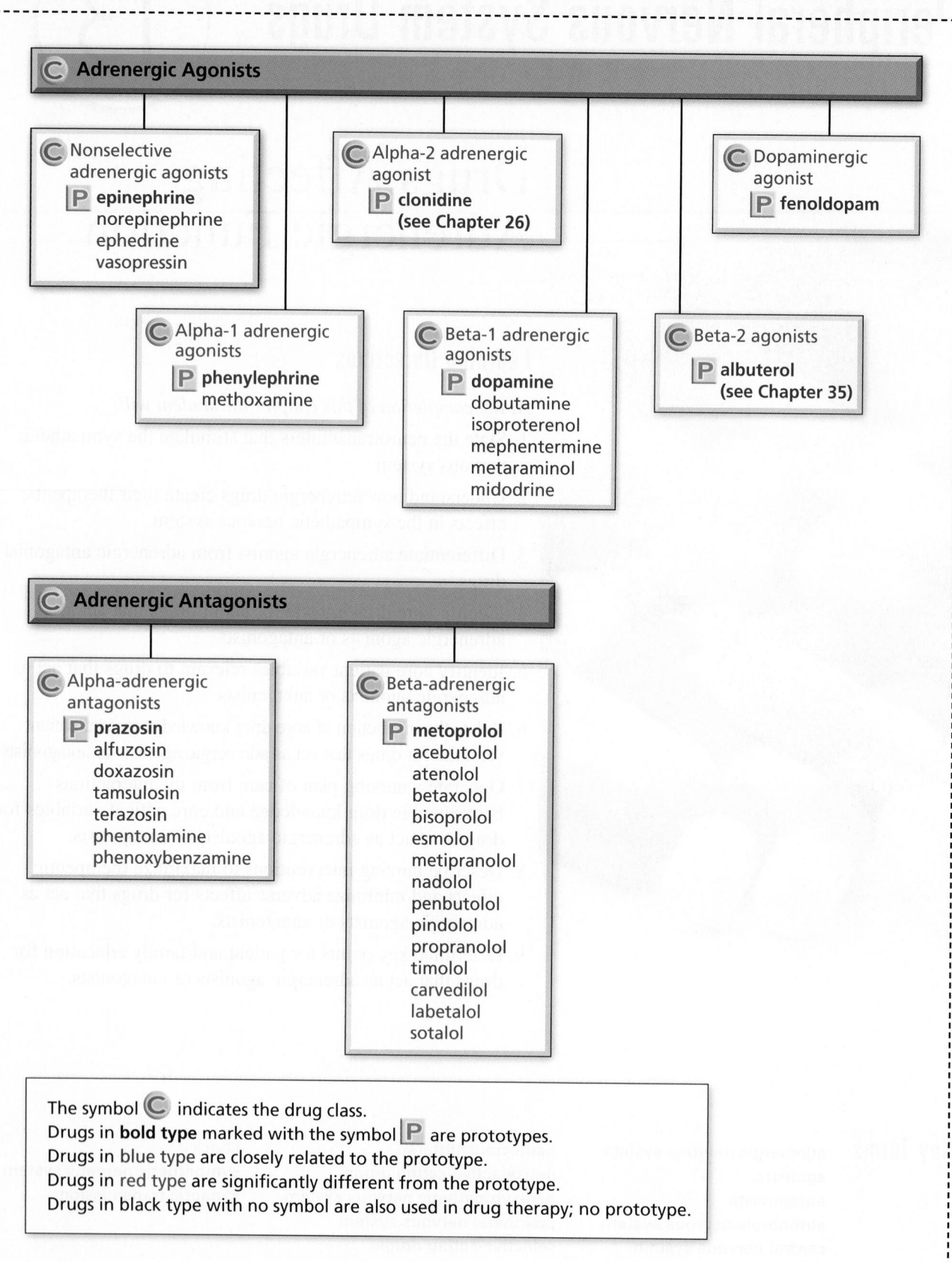

Adrenergic Agonists

Nonselective adrenergic agonists
P epinephrine
norepinephrine
ephedrine
vasopressin

Alpha-2 adrenergic agonist
P clonidine
(see Chapter 26)

Dopaminergic agonist
P fenoldopam

Alpha-1 adrenergic agonists
P phenylephrine
methoxamine

Beta-1 adrenergic agonists
P dopamine
dobutamine
isoproterenol
mephentermine
metaraminol
midodrine

Beta-2 agonists
P albuterol
(see Chapter 35)

Adrenergic Antagonists

Alpha-adrenergic antagonists
P prazosin
alfuzosin
doxazosin
tamsulosin
terazosin
phentolamine
phenoxybenzamine

Beta-adrenergic antagonists
P metoprolol
acebutolol
atenolol
betaxolol
bisoprolol
esmolol
metipranolol
nadolol
penbutolol
pindolol
propranolol
timolol
carvedilol
labetalol
sotalol

The symbol **C** indicates the drug class.
Drugs in **bold type** marked with the symbol **P** are prototypes.
Drugs in blue type are closely related to the prototype.
Drugs in red type are significantly different from the prototype.
Drugs in black type with no symbol are also used in drug therapy; no prototype.

The nervous system is a complex and amazing interconnected web that stimulates a physiological response and then curtails the same physiological response in the body to create just the right balance to support life. The normal function of the nervous system depends on the actions of neurotransmitters. Neurotransmitters are released from storage, stimulate particular receptors to cause an effect and then their effect is terminated as they are degraded or recycled and stored for future use.

The nervous system is responsible for maintaining our vital functions, such as breathing and keeping our hearts beating, while also allowing us to move voluntarily and to respond to environmental stimuli. It is easy to understand how important a properly functioning nervous system is to each individual. When the fine balance of stimulation and cessation of stimulation in the nervous system is disrupted, the individual can experience a wide variety of problems or pathologies. Many drug therapies work in the nervous system to either mimic the action of these neurotransmitters (when there is not enough intrinsic stimulation), or to block the receptor where the neurotransmitter attaches, thus preventing the effect from the neurotransmitter (when there is excessive stimulation from the neurotransmitter). Remember that drug therapy cannot produce any new effects in the body, it can only turn on or prevent effects for which the body is already capable.

This chapter focuses on drugs that affect the sympathetic nervous system. These drugs either stimulate sympathetic receptors or they block these sympathetic receptors. Those that stimulate the receptors are referred to as adrenergic **agonists** (stimulators) and those that block are referred to as adrenergic **antagonists** (blockers). Prototypes have been selected that stimulate or block specific sympathtetic receptors. Some drugs are relatively specific for the receptor on which they act, while others affect more than one receptor. The prototype nonselective adrenergic agonist is epinephrine. The prototype alpha-1 adrenergic agonist is phenylephrine, and the prototype alpha-2 adrenergic agonist is clonidine. The prototype beta-adrenergic agonist is dopamine. The prototype beta-1 agonist is albuterol; it is discussed in Chapter 35. The prototype dopaminergic agonist is fenoldopam.

The adrenergic antagonists are categorized similarly. Prazosin is the prototype alpha antagonist, whereas the prototype beta-blocker is metoprolol.

PHYSIOLOGY

Function of the Autonomic Nervous System

The nervous system is divided into two main branches: the **central nervous system** (CNS) and the **peripheral nervous system** (PNS) (Figure 13.1). The CNS is composed of the brain and spinal cord. The PNS consists of all neurons that are found outside the brain and spinal cord and is further subdivided into two major divisions: efferent and afferent. The efferent division has neurons that carry signals away from the brain and spinal cord to the periphery, whereas the afferent division contains neurons that carry impulses from

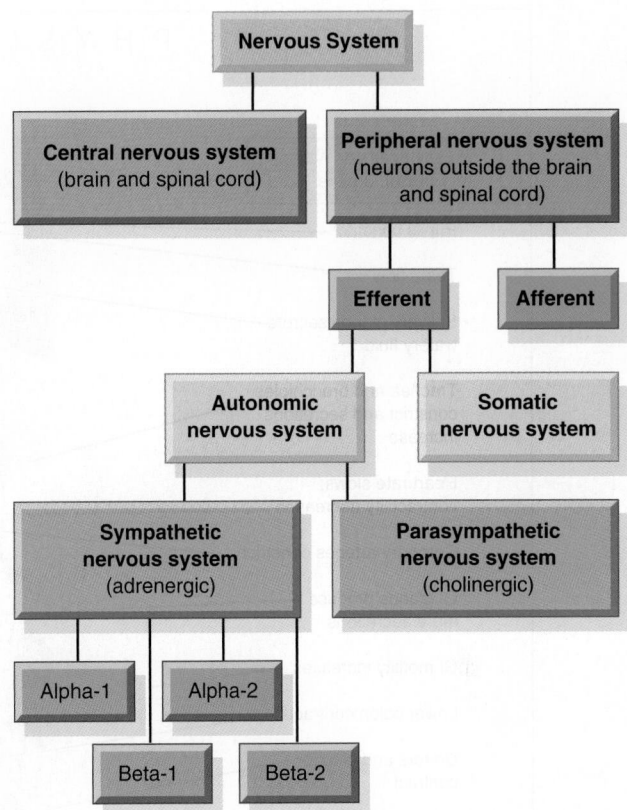

● FIGURE 13.1 The human nervous system.

the periphery to the CNS. The efferent division may be further subdivided into the somatic nervous system (which works on the skeletal muscles and is responsible for voluntary movement) and the **autonomic nervous system** (ANS) which is responsible for nonvoluntary nervous system control. The ANS is in turn subdivided into the **sympathetic nervous system** (SNS), also known as the **adrenergic nervous system**, and the **parasympathetic nervous system** (PSNS), also known as the cholinergic nervous system. See Figure 13.1 to help you visualize the branches of the nervous system.

The ANS has been identified as an involuntary system responsible for the control of smooth muscle (e.g., in bronchi, blood vessels, and the gastrointestinal [GI] tract), cardiac muscle, and exocrine glands (e.g., gastric, sweat, and salivary glands). These regulatory functions of the body are monitored by both the sympathetic and parasympathetic branches of the ANS. Some organs and tissues are regulated by both systems. When both the SNS and PSNS stimulate a particular organ or tissue, the action may be oppositional or complementary. Figure 13.2 presents the major effects of the SNS and PSNS on the body. The cholinergic system and drugs which affect it are discussed in Chapter 14. The sympathetic system is responsible for the "fight or flight" response. In other words, it allows our bodies to be ready to act quickly to situations perceived as potential threats. Sympathetic stimulation will increase our heart rate, dilate our pupils, mobilize our energy, and redirect our blood flow from non-essential organs to our skeletal muscles.

PHYSIOLOGY

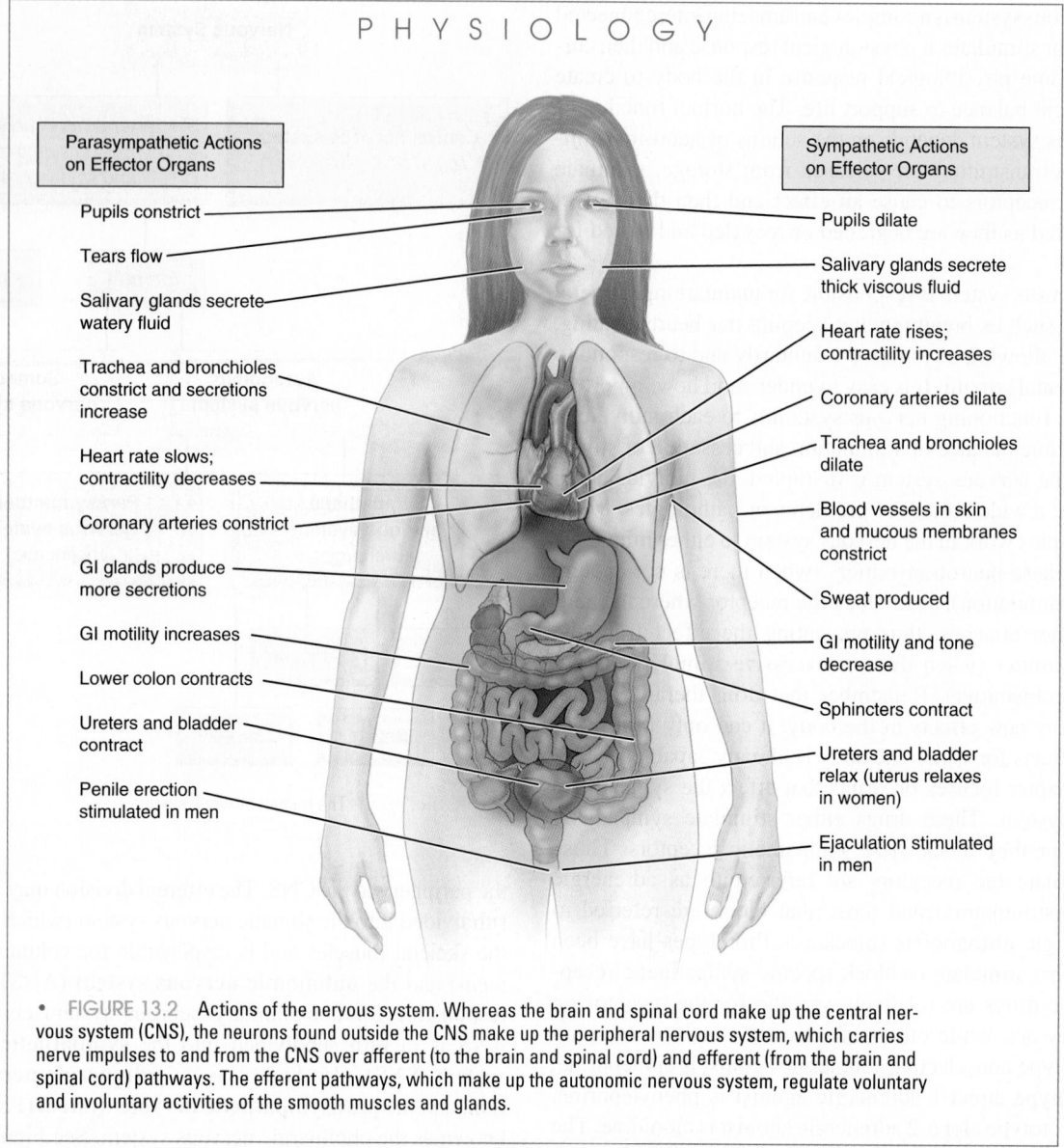

Parasympathetic Actions on Effector Organs

- Pupils constrict
- Tears flow
- Salivary glands secrete watery fluid
- Trachea and bronchioles constrict and secretions increase
- Heart rate slows; contractility decreases
- Coronary arteries constrict
- GI glands produce more secretions
- GI motility increases
- Lower colon contracts
- Ureters and bladder contract
- Penile erection stimulated in men

Sympathetic Actions on Effector Organs

- Pupils dilate
- Salivary glands secrete thick viscous fluid
- Heart rate rises; contractility increases
- Coronary arteries dilate
- Trachea and bronchioles dilate
- Blood vessels in skin and mucous membranes constrict
- Sweat produced
- GI motility and tone decrease
- Sphincters contract
- Ureters and bladder relax (uterus relaxes in women)
- Ejaculation stimulated in men

• FIGURE 13.2 Actions of the nervous system. Whereas the brain and spinal cord make up the central nervous system (CNS), the neurons found outside the CNS make up the peripheral nervous system, which carries nerve impulses to and from the CNS over afferent (to the brain and spinal cord) and efferent (from the brain and spinal cord) pathways. The efferent pathways, which make up the autonomic nervous system, regulate voluntary and involuntary activities of the smooth muscles and glands.

How does the body actually achieve stimulation of either the sympathetic or parasympathetic system? The actual connection between neurons and effector organs or tissues relies on **neurotransmitters** and **synaptic transmission**. The neurotransmitters in the ANS include acetylcholine (ACh), norepinephrine (NE), and epinephrine (Epi). Dopamine (DA) is the precursor to NE and is sometimes also considered in this group. Synaptic transmission initially involves the synthesis of neurotransmitters in the nerve terminal, with subsequent storage of the neurotransmitter awaiting an action potential that allows the neurotransmitter to be released. After release, the neurotransmitter diffuses across the synaptic gap and reversibly (i.e., not permanently) binds to a receptor on the postsynaptic cell. After binding and exerting an effect, the neurotransmitter is dissociated from its binding site by a variety of mechanisms that allow the neurotransmitter to be degraded or to undergo reuptake for reuse (Figure 13.3). To

effect an action, the neurotransmitter needs to bind with an appropriate receptor site on the effector organ or tissue.

In the SNS, preganglionic transmission is mediated by ACh, whereas postganglionic transmission is mediated by NE. ACh also stimulates the adrenal medulla to release Epi. Once the postganglionic neurons are stimulated by neurotransmitters and transmit their impulse to the effector organs or tissues, several events may occur. For example, beta-1 stimulation by NE increases the heart rate, while at the same time beta-2 stimulation induces bronchodilation.

Neurotransmitters
Acetylcholine

Acetylcholine is the preganglionic neurotransmitter in the SNS and both the preganglionic and postganglionic

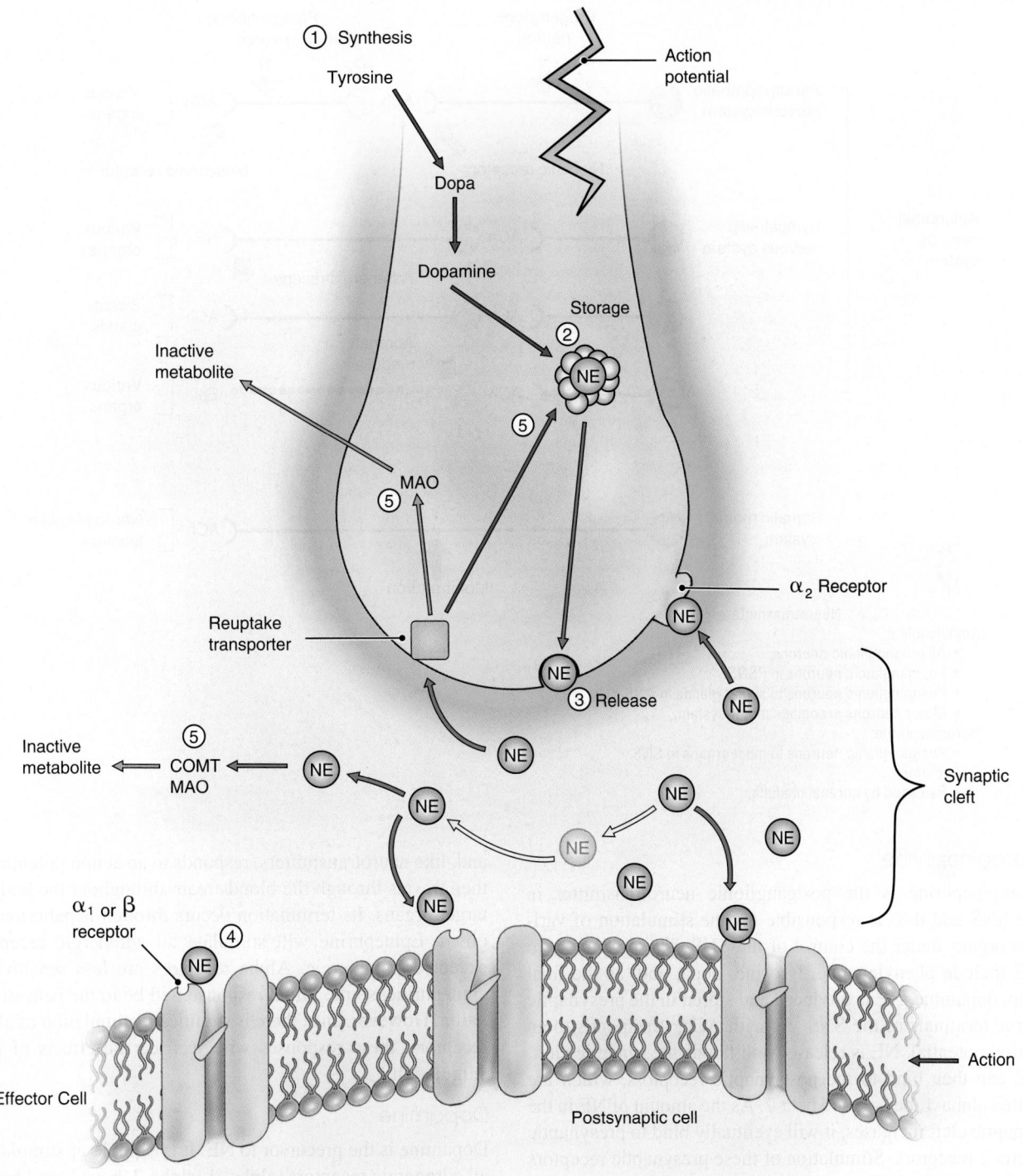

- FIGURE 13.3   Norepinephrine (NE) release and degradation. (1) NE is stored; (2) NE is released from the nerve terminal in response to an action potential and diffuses across the synaptic cleft; (3) NE binds to receptor site to stimulate an action; (4) NE is inactivated by COMT or (5) undergoes reuptake back to the nerve terminal for reuse or inactivation by MAO.

neurotransmitter in the PSNS (Figure 13.4). The precursors to ACh are choline and acetyl coenzyme A. After formation and storage, ACh is released in response to an action potential, and then binds to cholinergic receptors on the target organs or tissues. After dissociation, ACh is degraded by acetylcholinesterase (AchE) into two inactive products, acetate and choline, or it undergoes reuptake back to the nerve terminal, where it is re-stored for further use.

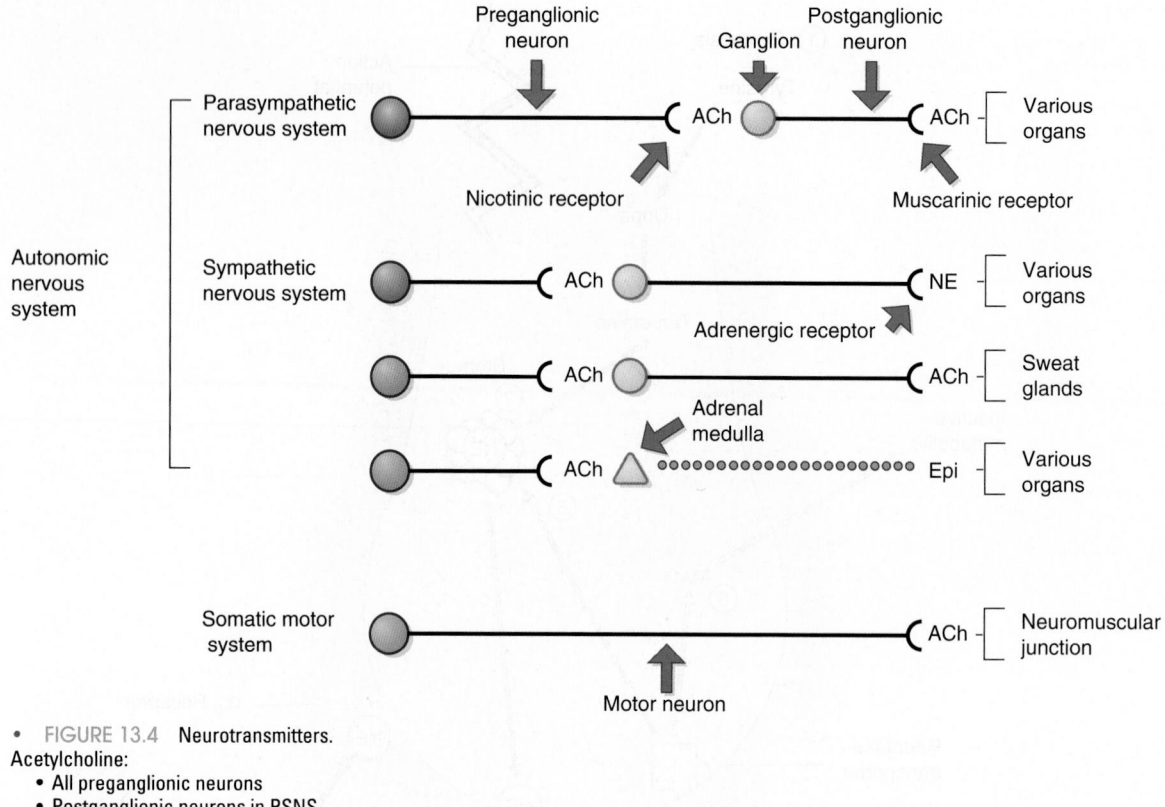

• FIGURE 13.4 Neurotransmitters.
Acetylcholine:
- All preganglionic neurons
- Postganglionic neurons in PSNS
- Postganglionic neurons to sweat glands in ANS
- Motor neurons in somatic motor system.
Norepinephrine:
- Postganglionic neurons to most organs in SNS.
Epinephrine:
- Released by adrenal medulla.

Norepinephrine

Norepinephrine is the postganglionic neurotransmitter in the SNS and thus is responsible for the stimulation of various organs under the control of the SNS. The precursors to NE include phenylalanine, tyrosine, dopa, and, as the final step, dopamine. NE is produced and stored in the presynaptic nerve terminals of the SNS. As with ACh, it responds to an action potential. NE is released and floods the synaptic cleft. NE can then bind to the postsynaptic receptors, which are called alpha-1, beta-1, and beta-2. As the amount of NE in the synaptic cleft increases, it will eventually bind to presynaptic alpha-2 receptors. Stimulation of these presynaptic receptors acts as a negative feedback loop to shut off the flow of NE into the synapse. The NE in the synaptic space either is transmitted back into the nerve terminal (called reuptake) where it can be restored for further use, or the NE can be degraded by one of two enzymes, either monoamine oxidase (MAO) in the nerve ending or catechol-O-methyltransferase (COMT) within the synaptic cleft (see Figure 13.3).

Epinephrine

Epinephrine is actually a hormone that is converted enzymatically from NE in the adrenal medulla. Epinephrine is also referred to as adrenalin. It is stored in the adrenal medulla

and, like neurotransmitters, responds to an action potential. It then travels through the bloodstream throughout the body to target organs. Its termination occurs through hepatic metabolism. Epinephrine will stimulate all adrenergic receptors except dopaminergic. Alpha receptors are less sensitive to epinephrine, so the initial response will be to the beta stimulation. However, once there is significant stimulation of alpha receptors, these responses will override the effects of beta stimulation.

Dopamine

Dopamine is the precursor to NE. It is capable of stimulating all adrenergic receptors (alpha -1, alpha-2, beta-1, and beta-2 as well as specific dopamine receptors.

Adrenergic Receptors

Receptors are that are stimulated by NE are called adrenergic receptors; those that are stimulated by acetylcholine are called cholinergic. In the SNS, there are several types of adrenergic receptors, including alpha-adrenergic and beta-adrenergic receptors.

There are also subtypes of alpha- and beta-adrenergic receptors. The current pharmacologically significant adrenergic subtypes are alpha-1, alpha-2, beta-1, and beta-2 receptors (there is also a beta-3 receptor). Alpha-1 and alpha-2 receptors also can be further divided into additional subtypes. Alpha-1 receptors are located in the eyes, blood vessels, bladder, male sex organs, and prostatic capsule. Alpha-2 receptors are located in presynaptic nerve terminals. Alpha-1 receptors are primarily responsible for vasoconstriction of coronary arteries and veins and decrease smooth muscle motility in the GI tract (to slow down digestion during flight or fight). Alpha-2 receptors are responsible for shutting off the release of NE. Beta-1 receptors are found primarily in the heart but also in the kidney. Beta-1 receptors are primarily responsible for increasing cardiac output by increasing the speed of conduction, increasing the force of contraction, and increasing the pulse rate. They also play a role in renin release from the kidney. Beta-2 receptors are located in the arterioles of the heart, lung, and skeletal muscles as well as in the bronchi, uterus, liver, and skeletal muscle. Beta-2 receptors are responsible for many effects: bronchial dilation (to promote breathing); creating energy from the breakdown of fats stored in fat tissue (lipolysis) or from providing glucose to the cells through new creation of glucose (gluconeogenesis) or the breaking down of glycogen into glucose (glycogenolysis) and promoting the release of insulin so that the new glucose can enter into cells to be used as energy; dilation of smaller coronary arteries, the hepatic artery, and arteries to skeletal muscle (to provide additional perfusion of the organs; contraction of skeletal muscle, relaxation of the uterus, relaxing the detrusor muscle of the bladder to allow urine storage in the bladder; to slow GI motility (to delay digestion) and contraction of GI tract sphincters to prevent defecation; increase renin release from the kidney; to thicken secretions of salivary glands; and inhibit the release of histamine from mast cells. Beta-3 receptors have also been identified. Beta-3 receptors help to break down fats in fat tissue for energy metabolism and for heat production; thus beta-3 has an active role in regulation of weight. It is hoped that this function could be tapped to create drugs for weight loss. Unfortunately, beta-3 receptors also cause tremors, and thus are not pharmacologically useful at this time.

The various adrenergic receptors respond to stimulation by one or more neurotransmitters. Alpha-1 and beta-1 receptors respond to all three sympathetic neurotransmitters (Epi, NE, and dopamine). Alpha-2 and beta-2 receptors respond to epinephrine and NE. The relative selectivity of various adrenergic agonists can be used to therapeutic benefit in determining which effector organs or tissues should be targeted (Table 13.1).

In addition to alpha-1 and beta-1 receptors, dopamine also affects dopaminergic receptors. As stated above, the dopaminergic receptor is related to adrenergic receptors in that dopamine is the precursor to NE. As such, it can activate both alpha- and beta-adrenergic receptors.

Stimulation of dopamine receptors in the brain controls both voluntary movement as well as neurocognitive functions. Although the number of dopamine receptors in the brain is limited, they are extremely important to normal brain function. Many dopamine receptors are located within the kidney In low amounts, dopamine binds with vascular and renal receptors, dilating blood vessels, increasing blood flow to renal, mesenteric, and coronary arteries, and increasing overall renal perfusion. As the presence of dopamine increases, beta-1 receptors are stimulated, increasing heart rate and strength of contraction. Dopamine in even higher concentrations acts on alpha-1 receptors, leading to vasoconstriction and elevated blood pressure. Dopaminergic receptors are known to exist as subtypes, and at least five have been identified. Dopaminergic receptors in the periphery are located primarily in the kidney.

PATHOPHYSIOLOGY

Diverse tissues and organs are innervated by the ANS, and few discrete disorders are directly related to compromise of the SNS. There are disorders or conditions that can benefit from additional stimulation of the adrenergic receptors (either in total or relatively selectively for one subtype of receptor) or the blockade of those receptors. Thus, the therapeutic uses of sympathetic drugs are related to providing extra-adrenergic stimulation or blockade of normal ANS functioning. Because adrenergic receptors are distributed throughout the body and because adrenergically innervated organs and tissues show a predominance of one type of receptor over another, it is important to examine the major effects mediated by the different types of receptors to understand the implications of drug treatment in differing pathologic states (see Table 13.1).

One of the most frequent indications for adrenergic agonist drugs is **shock.** Shock is the result of inadequate tissue perfusion, leaving the cells without the oxygen and nutrients they need to function normally and survive. When cell dysfunction is widespread, the patient can die. Shock has multiple causes. *Hypovolemic* shock results from a decrease in circulating blood volume from bleeding or hemorrhage. It occurs when intravascular volume decreases more than 15% and as much as 25%. *Cardiogenic* shock is the result of the heart's inability to pump enough blood to adequately perfuse the vital organs. This type of shock may be caused by myocardial infarction, ventricular arrhythmias, severe cardiomyopathy, or chronic heart failure. *Septic* shock occurs when a severe infection brings about circulatory insufficiency. *Obstructive* shock is caused by a massive blockage in blood flow that results in inadequate tissue perfusion. Obstructive shock can originate with a large pulmonary embolus, cardiac tamponade, restrictive pericarditis, or severe cardiac valve dysfunction. *Neurogenic* shock is uncommon. It occurs because of a blockade of neurohormonal outflow that may be induced by drugs (e.g., spinal anesthesia) or trauma to the spinal cord.

Shock has two phases—early (compensated) and late (noncompensated). In early shock, the body tries to compensate for the decreased perfusion. The heart and respiratory rates increase, and blood pressure is generally maintained, or it may be low-normal. The body begins to shunt some blood

TABLE 13.1	Adrenergic Receptor Subtypes' Location and Action	
Location	Response to Stimulation (Agonist Effect)	Response to Blockade (Antagonist Effect)
Alpha-1		
Arteries and veins	Constriction	Dilation
Bladder neck	Contraction	Relaxation
Eyes	Mydriasis (dilation) of the pupil	Miosis (constriction) of the pupil
Male sex organs	Ejaculation	Inhibits ejaculation
Prostatic capsule	Contraction	Relaxation
Alpha-2		
Central nervous system	Inhibits release of norepinephrine	Extends activity of norepinephrine
Beta-1		
Heart	Increased rate	Decreased rate
	Positive inotropic action (increased force of contraction)	Negative inotropic action (decreased force of contraction)
	Increased atrioventricular speed of conduction	Reduced atrioventricular speed of conduction
Kidney	Release of renin	Inhibits release of renin
Beta-2		
Arterioles	Dilation	Constriction
Bronchi	Dilation	Constriction
Liver	Glycogenolysis (breakdown of glycogen)	Inhibits breakdown of glycogen
Skeletal muscle	Contraction, glycogenolysis	Relaxation, inhibits breakdown of glycogen
Uterus	Relaxation	Stimulates contractions
Dopamine-1 (DA-1)		
Vessels	Peripheral vasodilation	Peripheral vasoconstriction
Proximal tubule	Maintain or increase GFR	Decreases GFR
Renal tubules	Natriuresis (more sodium excreted in urine)	Sodium retention
	Diuresis	Reduced urine production
Dopamine-2 (DA-2)		
Vessels	Peripheral vasodilation	Peripheral vasoconstriction
Glomerulus	Deceased renal blood flow	Increased renal blood flow
Renal nerves	Decreased glomerular filtration rate (GFR)	Increased GFR
Adrenal cortex	Decreased Na and H2O excretion	Natriuresis and diuresis
	Decreased aldosterone	Increased aldosterone

flow away from the skin, although the skin is still perfused. Urine output decreases slightly as renal blood flow is reduced. Emotionally, the patient may be anxious or confused. When the body is no longer able to make up for changes brought on by shock, the patient develops late, or uncompensated, shock. Tachycardia persists, but the blood pressure falls dramatically, and the rate of respiration falls. Venous constriction occurs, and with the circulation shut off, the skin becomes cold and clammy. Urine output declines dramatically and may cease when the kidneys are no longer perfused. The patient becomes nonresponsive and unconscious.

Pharmacological Effects on the SNS

Understanding how the complex nervous system works can be overwhelming. Still, in consideration of pharmacology there is really only one question that students and nurses need to answer. And that is: How does drug therapy create a specific effect in the nervous system? And here, the answer is fairly direct. Drugs create their effect on the nervous system by either stimulating a neuroreceptor, or by blocking it to prevent the intrinsic neurotransmitter from attaching and creating an effect. So to understand drugs that affect the nervous system, we only need to concern ourselves with the receptors

TABLE 13.2	Sympathetic Nervous System Terminology Synonyms
Stimulation of Adrenergic Receptors These words mean the same thing:	**Blocking of Adrenergic Receptors** These words mean the same thing:
Adrenergic agonist = Sympathetic agonist = Sympathomimetic	Adrenergic antagonist = Sympathetic antagonist = Sympatholytic = Antiadrenergic
Alpha-adrenergic agonist = alpha agonist = alpha stimulant	Alpha-adrenergic antagonist = alpha antagonist = Alpha blocker
Beta-adrenergic agonist = beta agonist = beta stimulant	Beta-adrenergic antagonist = beta antagonist = Beta blocker
epihephrine = adrenalin	

on the postganglionic side. The physiology on the preganglionic side, while important, is not where drugs create their therapeutic effect. In this light, nurses need to know what happens when you stimulate or block alpha-1, alpha-2, beta-1, beta-2, and dopaminergic receptors to understand the pharmacodynamics of adrenergic drugs. Many drugs attach to these receptors, and they have many diverse uses in pharmacology. Because of the diversity of uses, students can find studying this content daunting. The facts appear random and include almost everything. It is recommended that students first memorize what occurs with receptor stimulation and blockade, then consider the given prototypes to be examples of stimulating and blocking those receptors. Throughout the rest of the text, there will be discussion of drugs that affect the nervous system. Thus it is important to gain a basis of what happens with stimulation and blockade of neuroreceptors to be a foundation of your knowledge for much of drug therapy. An additional point students should understand concerning drugs that act on the nervous system is that while you will learn what happens with each unique receptor when it is stimulated or blocked, drugs do not just affect one receptor. They may affect multiple receptors equally or they may be relatively selective in what they stimulate or block. This may account for a wide variety of actions and adverse effects from a particular drug. A final factor that makes studying nervous system drugs difficult is that multiple names seem to be used to mean the same thing. Students need to recognize these synonyms when they are used interchangeably. See Table 13.2 for this information.

Ⓒ ADRENERGIC AGONISTS

Adrenergic agonists are drugs that mimic the action of the SNS; thus, they are also known as sympathomimetic agents. They exert their effects by direct or indirect stimulation of adrenergic receptors. Indirect mechanisms include increasing the transmission of NE, inhibiting NE reuptake, and inhibiting MAO or COMT. Inhibiting the reuptake of NE or

inhibiting MAO or COMT is related to the dissociation and termination of NE binding to adrenergic receptors, which results in the continuation of the effects of NE.

These drugs are generally divided into two groups: catecholamines and noncatecholamines. Catecholamines are so named because of a chemical structure they have in common. Because of this chemical similarity, they also possess three similar characteristics. First, they have a short duration of action, resulting in their need to be administered in a continuous fashion (i.e., by intravenous [IV] infusion). Second, they cannot be given orally. As oral agents, they cannot be given continuously, and certain substances in the body (MAO and COMT) would degrade them before they reached systemic circulation. Third, because of their chemical structure, they do not cross the blood–brain barrier. Noncatecholamines have directly opposite characteristics. They have a longer duration of action, may be given orally, and do cross the blood–brain barrier.

Adrenergic agonists are also classified according to their selectivity. Drugs that stimulate multiple adrenergic subtype receptors are called **nonselective-acting drugs**. Nonselective adrenergic agonists stimulate both alpha and beta receptors. Drugs that target a specific subtype receptor are called **selective-acting drugs**. To maximize therapeutic effects and minimize adverse effects, selective-acting drugs are used more frequently than nonselective drugs. It is important to remember that selectivity is not absolute. Although a selective-acting drug is preferential to a given subtype receptor, when given in higher doses it may also stimulate other subtype receptors.

• Ⓒ NONSELECTIVE ADRENERGIC AGONISTS

Nonselective adrenergic agonists stimulate most receptors; therefore, they have a multitude of uses. It is important to remember that these drugs stimulate all of the subtypes, regardless of which subtype would be most helpful for a specific pathology.

The prototype for nonselective adrenergic agonists is epinephrine. This drug stimulates alpha-1, alpha-2, beta-1, and beta-2 receptors. The only adrenergic receptor subtype it does not stimulate is the dopamine receptor.

Nursing Management of the Patient Receiving Ⓟ Epinephrine
Core Drug Knowledge
Pharmacotherapeutics
Epinephrine has a wide variety of indications; some of the most common include: anaphylactic shock, hypersensitivity reaction; asthma, cardiopulmonary resuscitation, and ventricular fibrillation. Self-injectable epinephrine is prescribed in community settings for anaphylactic shock associated with allergies to foods, especially nuts, seafood, milk and eggs, as well as insect bites, bee stings, venom, and asthma.

Additionally, epinephrine can be used in the treatment of congestion of mucosa; blood coagulation disorder; excessive uterine contractions; syncope due to heart block or carotid sinus hypersensitivity; simple glaucoma; cataracts; chloroquine poisoning; cluster headaches; croup; GI hemorrhage; herpes simplex infection; hyperkalemia; hypothermia; mastocytosis; obstetric analgesia; priapism; septic shock; and wheezing in infants. It is also used in open heart surgery and as an adjunct in topical anesthesia (Table 13.3).

Pharmacokinetics

Epinephrine may be administered parenterally, topically, or by inhalation. Depending on the administration method, epinephrine exerts its effects very quickly and is metabolized rapidly. It is well absorbed after intramuscular (IM) or subcutaneous (SC) injection, and its duration of action ranges between 1 and 4 hours. It is metabolized in the liver and excreted through the kidneys.

Pharmacodynamics

Epinephrine is a potent sympathomimetic drug with profound effects on a variety of organ systems. It stimulates all adrenergic receptors and causes the greatest adverse effects in the cardiovascular system and CNS. It acts directly on the postsynaptic adrenergic receptors.

After activation of the receptor, epinephrine is terminated by reuptake into adrenergic nerves or inactivated by the enzymes COMT and MAO. Depending on the location and distribution of receptors, epinephrine exerts a variety of responses in different effector organs and tissues. In the cardiovascular system, epinephrine exerts positive (or increased) inotropic (force or energy of contraction) and chronotropic (heart rate) effects on the myocardium by stimulating beta-1 adrenergic receptors. Although it might seem that stimulation of beta-2 receptors (which cause vasodilation) and stimulation of alpha-1 receptors (which cause vasoconstriction) would cancel each other out and create no effect, this is not true. Initially the beta-2 receptor stimulation is prevalent in the body effects and there will be vasodilation in skeletal muscles as well as other organs. As the dose increases, then the alpha-1 effects are evident, and these override the beta-2. In the skin and viscera, epinephrine stimulates alpha-adrenergic receptors, causing vasoconstriction. The overall effect is to increase systolic pressure and slightly decrease diastolic pressure. In the respiratory system, epinephrine causes bronchodilation by stimulation of beta-2 adrenergic receptors and is used in this way to treat patients with asthma or to manage anaphylactic shock.

Contraindications and Precautions

Absolute contraindications to epinephrine include hypersensitivity, sulfite sensitivity, closed-angle glaucoma, and its use during labor. It is also absolutely contraindicated in patients with severe organic cardiac disease, and in patients receiving cyclopropane, chloroform, or trichloroethylene general anesthesia and in shock states other than

anaphylactic shock. In septic shock, epinephrine should be reserved for only extreme cases of cardiac collapse if other catecholamines have failed, as it also impairs gastric blood flow and increases lactate (Coons & Seidl, 2007). The action of epinephrine can exacerbate the symptoms of closed-angle glaucoma. As a beta-2 agonist, epinephrine administered during labor can delay progression to the second stage. The cardiovascular effects of epinephrine, such as increased myocardial oxygen demand, increased heart rate, vasoactivity, and potential to induce arrhythmias, may be detrimental to patients with severe cardiac disorders. These same cardiovascular effects may worsen shock states, although epinephrine is used to manage anaphylactic shock and ventricular fibrillation. There are no absolute contraindications for patients requiring emergency therapy for anaphylactic reaction. In patients receiving general anesthetic agents, epinephrine may induce myocardial sensitization to catecholamines, resulting in cardiac irritability.

Relative contraindications include cerebrovascular disease, such as cerebral arteriosclerosis or organic brain syndrome. The alpha effects of epinephrine have the potential to induce cerebrovascular hemorrhage with these disease states, especially when epinephrine is administered intravenously. Another relative contraindication is hypertension because the vascular effects of epinephrine can worsen this condition. Patients with hyperthyroidism may become more sensitive to catecholamines, resulting in cardiotoxic symptoms. Epinephrine also increases glycogenolysis in the liver. Patients with diabetes mellitus are monitored for hyperglycemia. Use with caution in patients having longstanding asthma co-occurring with emphysema and degenerative heart disease, psychiatric conditions, preexisting seizures, difficulty urinating, and concurrent use of MAOI and tricyclic antidepressants or sympathomimetic drugs.

Adverse Effects

Adverse effects are frequent because of epinephrine's ability to stimulate the four major adrenergic subtypes. Potential severe adverse effects include hypertensive crisis, angina, cerebral hemorrhage, and cardiac arrhythmias. If extravasation occurs during parenteral administration, necrosis may result because of epinephrine's potent vasoconstrictive properties.

Patients with hyperthyroidism or hypertension are more susceptible to headaches, anxiety, fear, and palpitations after taking epinephrine. In others, the main adverse effects are tremor, weakness, dizziness, anxiety, pallor, palpitations, apprehensiveness, sweating, nausea, and vomiting. Because of the breakdown of glycogen that is stimulated in response to epinephrine's effect on beta-2 receptors in the liver and in skeletal muscle, epinephrine may increase blood glucose levels in patients with diabetes.

Drug Interactions

Epinephrine interacts with a variety of classes of compounds, including tricyclic antidepressants, oxytocics, halogenated anesthetics, and beta blockers (Table 13.4). In

TABLE 13.3 Summary of Selected Ⓒ Adrenergic Agonists

Drug (Trade) Name	Selected Indications	Route and Dosage Range	Pharmacokinetics
Ⓒ Nonselective Adrenergic Agonists			
Ⓟ epinephrine (Adrenalin, Epinephrine)	Asthma/COPD Anaphylactic reaction	*Adult:* SC, IM, 0.1–0.5 mg (not to exceed 1 mg per dose). May repeat every 15–20 min. Auto-injector: 0.3 mg IM or SC. *Adult IV:* 0.1–0.25 mg (not to exceed 1 mg per dose) every 5–15 min, followed by a 1–4 mcg continuous infusion *Adult and child inhalation:* Nebulizer: 8–15 drops in reservoir; Administer 1–3 inhalations 4–6×/d MDI: 1 inhalation with onset of symptoms; May repeat after 1–5 min *Child:* SC, 0.01 mg/kg or 0.3 mg (not to exceed 0.5 mg per dose). May repeat every 15 min × 2 doses, then every 4 h *Child IV:* 0.1 mg; may be followed by 0.1 mcg/kg/min continuous infusion	*Onset:* IV, instant; SC > 1 h *Duration:* 20–30 min; SC, 4 h $t_{1/2}$: NA
	Cardiac arrest (ACLS, PALS)	*Adult:* 1 mg IV every 3–5 min *Child:* 0.01 mg/kg IV every 3–5 min *Endotracheally:* 2.0–2.5 mg diluted in 10 mL NS	
	Ophthalmic agent (0.1%, 0.5%, 1%, and 2%)	1–2 drops in eyes 1–2× d	
ephedrine	Asthma, enuresis, nasal congestion, rhinorrhea, sinusitis Hypotension	*Adult:* PO, 25–50 mg every 6 h (max 150 mg daily) *Adult:* IM, SC, 25–50 mg every 4–6 h; IV, 5–25 mg IV slow push	*Onset:* PO, 15–60 min; IM, 10–20 min; IV, instant *Duration:* PO, 3–5 h; IM/IV, 1 h $t_{1/2}$: 3–6 h
norepinephrine (Levophed)	Hypotension/shock Ventricular fibrillation/cardiac arrest	*Adult:* IV, 8–12 mg/min *Child:* 0.05–0.3 mcg/kg/min 0.5–1.0 mcg/min titrated to effect	*Onset:* 1–2 min *Duration:* 1–2 min $t_{1/2}$: 7–18 h
Ⓒ Alpha-1 Adrenergic Agonists			
Ⓟ phenylephrine (Dristan, Dimetapp, Neo-Synephrine, others;)	Nasal congestion, common cold, glaucoma, shock, hypotensive crisis, anesthetic adjunct, PSVT	*Adult:* Topical, 1–2 sprays of 0.25%–1% solution q3–4h; IM, SC, 2–5 mg; IV, 0.2–0.5 mg (IM/IV titrated to patient response) PO 10-20 mg q4h; 1 drop of 2.5% ophthalmic solution; Child IV: 0.1–0.5 mcg/kg/min titrated to patient response	*Onset:* IM, 10–15 min; IV, immediate *Duration:* IM 30–120 min; IV, 15–20 min $t_{1/2}$: 2–3 h
methoxamine (Vasoxyl)	Hypotension, blood pressure maintenance during anesthesia, shock, SVT	*Adult:* IM, 10–15 mg; IV, 3–10 mg by slow push depending on condition	*Onset:* 30–120 s *Duration:* 60 min $t_{1/2}$: NA
Ⓒ Alpha-2 Adrenergic Agonists			
Ⓟ clonidine (Catapres)	Cancer pain (epidural), anti-hypertensive, alcohol withdrawal, diabetic diarrhea, menopausal flushing, opiate detoxification, herpetic neuralgia, ulcerative colitis	*Adult:* PO, 100–300 mcg bid; IM/IV, 150 mcg; epidural, 75–150 mcg	*Onset:* 30–60 min *Duration:* 24 h $t_{1/2}$: 12–16 h

(Continued)

TABLE 13.3 Summary of Selected © Adrenergic Agonists *(continued)*

Drug (Trade) Name	Selected Indications	Route and Dosage Range	Pharmacokinetics
© Beta-Adrenergic Agonists			
P dopamine (Intropin)	Hemodynamic imbalances	*Adult:* IV, 0.5–1 mcg/kg/min Seriously Ill Adult: IV, initial, 2 to 5 mcg/kg/min; increase in 5 to 10 mcg/kg/min increments; max 50 mcg/kg/min Child: initial, 2 to 5 mcg/kg/min; increase in 5–10 mcg/kg/min increments; max 30 mcg/kg/min.	*Onset:* IV, 1–2 min *Duration:* IV, length of infusion $t_{1/2}$: 2 min
dobutamine (Dobutrex)	Cardiac decompensation due to decreased contractility	*Adult:* IV infusion, 2.5–20 mcg/kg/min	*Onset:* 1–2 min *Duration:* Unknown $t_{1/2}$: 2 min
isoproterenol (Isuprel)	Cardiac arrhythmias Shock Bronchodilation	*Adult:* IV, 20–60 mcg IV push followed by continuous IV infusion; 2–20 mcg titrated to patient response *Child IV:* 0.1–1 mcg/kg/min titrated to patient response *Adult IV:* 0.05–0.2 mcg/kg/min titrated to patient response *Adult and Child Inhalation:* 0.5% solution 5–15 inhalations; may repeat in 5–10 min up to a maximum of 5× d *Adult Inhalation:* 1% solution 3–7 inhalations; may repeat in 5–10 min up to a maximum of 5× d *Adult and Child MDI:* 1–2 inhalations 1–5 min apart up to 6× day (5× d for child) *Adult SL:* 10–20 mg every 3–4 h up to 3× d; 60 mg/d max *Child SL:* 5–10 mg every 3–4 h up to 3× d; 30 mg/d max *Adult:* IM, 0.2 mg followed by 0.02–1.0 mg contingent on response; *Adult:* SC, 0.2 mg followed by 0.15 to 0.2 mg contingent on response. *Child:* IV, 0.1 mcg/kg/min titrated to patient response	*Onset:* Rapid *Duration:* 2 h $t_{1/2}$: Unknown
mephentermine (Wyamine)	Prophylaxis to prevent hypotension secondary to spinal anesthesia Hypotension following spinal anesthesia Shock	*Adult:* IM, 30–45 mg 10–20 min prior to procedure *Adult:* IV, 30–45 mg as a single injection *Adult:* IV, 0.5 mg/kg	*Onset:* IM, 10–15 min; IV, immediate *Duration:* IM, 1–2 h $t_{1/2}$: 15–20 min
metaraminol (Aramine)	Prevention and/or treatment of acute hypotensive state	*Adult:* Prevention, IM or SC 2–10 mg; treatment, IV infusion, 15–100 mg	*Onset:* IM, 10 min; SC 5–20 min; IV, 1–2 min *Duration:* IM, SC; 20–60 min $t_{1/2}$: Unknown
© Dopamine Agonists			
P fenoldopam (Corlopam)	Severe hypertension, renal vasodilation	*Adult:* PO, 100 mg 4×/d; IV, 0.03 mcg/kg/min initially, increased by 0.05–0.1 mcg/kg/min every 15 min, up to 1.6 mcg/kg/min for up to 48 h. *Children:* IV, 0.2 mcg/kg/min initially, increased by 0.3–0.5 mcg/kg/min every 20–30 min, up to 0.8 mcg/kg/min for up to 4 h.	*Onset:* 15 min *10 min* *Duration:* 1 h 1 h $t_{1/2}$: 5 min $t_{1/2}$: 5 min

TABLE 13.4   Agents That Interact with P Epinephrine

Interactants	Effect and Significance	Nursing Management
beta blockers	Alpha-adrenergic activity of epinephrine predominates when beta-blockade is present allowing for hypertension followed by reflex bradycardia	Monitor blood pressure; avoid concurrent use if possible.
halogenated anesthetics	Arrhythmias resulting from sensitization of the myocardium to catecholamines	Monitor patient's cardiovascular status and ECG carefully during and after anesthesia.
lithium	May decrease the peripheral vasoconstrictive effects of epinephrine	Monitor BP and assess for hypotension.
methyldopa	Potentiation of epinephrine's vasopressor effect	Monitor BP and assess for arrhythmias. Consult prescriber about adjusting epinephrine dosage.
oxytocic drugs used in labor and delivery	Synergistic vasoconstriction, resulting in hypertension	Monitor patient's blood pressure and vital signs carefully.
phenothiazines	May decrease the peripheral vasoconstrictive effects of epinephrine	Monitor BP and assess for hypotension.
tricyclic antidepressants	Potentiation of epinephrine's vasopressor effect	Monitor BP and assess for arrhythmias. Consult prescriber about adjusting epinephrine dosage.

addition, because epinephrine increases blood glucose levels and promotes hepatic glycogenolysis, it may interfere with blood glucose determinations.

Assessment of Relevant Core Patient Variables

Health Status

Document preadministration vital signs. If epinephrine is being given for respiratory distress, auscultate and document the patient's lung sounds. In patients with diabetes, obtain a baseline glucose level.

Before administering epinephrine in a nonemergency situation, evaluate for diseases, disorders, or medications that contraindicate the safe use of epinephrine or require special monitoring. If possible, assess the patient for a history of sulfite sensitivity because some epinephrine formulations contain sulfites that may induce a reaction (Box 13.1). It is also important to evaluate the use of over-the-counter (OTC) or herbal medications because these agents may contain sympathomimetic ingredients. However, when epinephrine is administered during an emergency, the potential benefits always outweigh the risks associated with it. If allergic anaphylaxis is suspected, assess to verify the triggers by obtaining a comprehensive history, investigating the circumstances of the episode, and perform allergen skin tests and measurement of allergen-specific IgE in serum (Simmons, 2006).

Life Span and Gender

Document the age and gender of the patient and assess women of childbearing age for pregnancy and lactation. Epinephrine is in the U.S. Food and Drug Administration

(FDA) pregnancy risk category C, and its use should be avoided in pregnant or lactating women. It must be administered carefully to infants, small children, and very old patients because adverse drug effects may be more pronounced in these age groups. In children with asthma, epinephrine may produce hypotension and syncope.

Lifestyle, Diet, and Habits

Document the patient's occupation and daily activities. Patients treated for glaucoma with epinephrine may develop corneal pigmentation, which may impair their vision. This condition may have a significant impact on people working in transportation (e.g., airline flight crew, truck drivers) and those working at night in low-light conditions.

Patients with diabetes who receive epinephrine for chronic conditions (e.g., asthma) should monitor blood glucose closely. Insulin dosages may need to be adjusted.

Environment

Be aware of the environment in which the drug will be administered, and assess the home or other relevant setting if appropriate. When epinephrine is administered intravenously, it is given in a hospital setting or possibly by trained emergency personnel in the community. In community settings where no health care providers are available, individuals with allergies, asthma, or other conditions that put them at risk for anaphylactic shock must carry self-injectable epinephrine and know how to use it (Simmons, 2007). Patients with severe allergies also may carry self-injectable epinephrine for treatment prior to the arrival of emergency medical personnel. It may be administered by other routes in any setting.

BOX 13.1 COMMUNITY BASED CONCERNS

Teaching for Patients Prescribed Self-Injectable Epinephrine

Epinephrine is commonly prescribed in the community setting as an auto-injector for self-treatment of insect bites, stings, venom, and food allergies. All patients who have experienced anaphylaxis in the community should have access to epinephrine. Health care providers must teach patients how and when to use epinephrine and encourage its appropriate use by reassuring concerns about adverse effects. In most patients, adverse effects are minor and transient. They include tremor, dizziness, palpitations, anxiety, restlessness, and headache. Accidental self-injection, most frequently in the hand, typically does not have serious implications and resolves within 2 to 24 hours. Self-injectable epinephrine is marketed as EpiPen, EpiPen Jr and Twinject with premeasured doses for children and adults. Very large or obese individuals should have at least two doses. The number of auto-injectors dispensed should allow for a dose for every 10 to 20 minutes travel time to a medical facility.

Ensure that patients prescribed self-injectable epinephrine understand the following:

- Anaphylaxis is unpredictable. Subsequent exposures to an allergen can result in an increased reaction.
- Self-injectable epinephrine is the best treatment and will enable immediate relief.
- Carry the injector at all times. Risk for anaphylaxis occurs even outside of normal routines. Store in multiple settings or carry everywhere.
- Use the auto-injector without delay when exposed to an allergen at the first signs of trouble breathing, tightness in the throat or lightheadedness. Teach to distinguish exposures that are not likely to cause anaphylaxis, such as skin contact with a food allergen that is not ingested.
- Inject into the muscle of the outer thigh for more rapid systemic absorption.
- Antihistamines and inhalers are not sufficient treatment for anaphylaxis.
- Store at room temperature, do not refrigerate, and replace injectors yearly.

Nursing Diagnoses and Outcomes

- Imbalanced Nutrition: Less Than Body Requirements, related to drug-induced anorexia or nausea
  Desired outcome: The patient will maintain adequate nutrition by learning how to cope with adverse effects or use an antiemetic agent if recommended.
- Disturbed Sleep Pattern, Insomnia, related to CNS excitation secondary to adrenergic drug therapy
  Desired outcome: The patient will learn about and practice sleep hygiene or take bedtime sedatives as prescribed so that normal sleep patterns will be maintained.
- Disturbed Sensory Perception related to impaired vision
  Desired outcome: The patient will notify the provider if vision changes occur.
- Ineffective Tissue Perfusion (Cardiopulmonary) related to cardiovascular effects of epinephrine
  Desired outcome: The patient will notify the provider if tachycardia, chest pain, or palpitations occur.

Planning and Intervention

Maximizing Therapeutic Effects

In addition to therapeutic monitoring, administering adrenergic agonists requires close monitoring of vital signs and careful monitoring for adverse effects. Physical measures to treat a stopped heart, such as chest compressions, are used before epinephrine. The IV route is preferred for treatment of cardiac arrest, although intramyocardial injection or insertion through an endotracheal tube may be done by trained personnel if IV access cannot be established. For treatment of respiratory problems, the SC or IV routes may be used. Encourage patients who receive epinephrine for other (nonemergency) uses to take the epinephrine exactly as prescribed and at the required dosage frequency to enhance therapeutic potential.

Minimizing Adverse Effects

When epinephrine is given to treat anaphylactic shock or cardiac arrest, monitor the patient's blood pressure carefully for hypertension. Monitor the patient's pulse and electrocardiogram (ECG) for changes in rhythm. If given intravenously, check the site frequently for patency to prevent extravasation. Should extravasation occur, infiltrate the region with phentolamine to minimize injury.

Patients receiving epinephrine for its cardiovascular effects are placed on continuous cardiac monitoring. Be prepared to intervene if adverse effects to epinephrine occur during therapy. For symptoms such as angina, tachycardia, or cardiac arrhythmias, be prepared to administer beta-adrenergic blocking agents. For hypertension, be prepared to administer alpha-adrenergic blocking agents.

Nursing strategies to minimize adverse effects include providing the patient with light, comfortable bedding, soothing baths, and optimal skin care. Patients receiving epinephrine for bronchodilation may experience restlessness and sweating. If the patient tires easily, you may need to help with self-care activities to minimize fatigue. In addition, promotion of sleep hygiene is important so that the patient can overcome the CNS stimulation that may occur with epinephrine.

Assisting the patient with menu planning may help to promote appetite and counteract the anorectic effect of epinephrine. Monitor the patient for signs of sulfite sensitivity. Finally, key interventions for patients with cardiovascular problems include monitoring for anginal pain and arrhythmias, whereas interventions for asthma patients include regular auscultation of lung sounds and assessment of respiratory functioning.

Epinephrine may be used for its vasoconstrictive properties in conjunction with local anesthetic agents to decrease bleeding during laceration repair. Read the label carefully to avoid administering epinephrine to an area of the body where vasoconstriction may cause damage, such as the fingers, toes, nose, ears, or male genitalia.

Providing Patient and Family Education

- Many patients who take epinephrine are acutely ill; therefore, it is inappropriate to provide complex instructions. Teaching should be brief, simple, and supportive. Once the acute illness resolves, the patient and family members may realize a greater benefit from instruction, particularly if the patient will be discharged on epinephrine or a similar adrenergic drug.
- For patients taking epinephrine for bronchodilation, explain the proper use and care of a nebulizer or a metered-dose inhaler and advise patients and families about common adverse effects. Emphasize the timing of doses to prevent disrupting sleep.
- For patients at risk for anaphylactic shock in the community setting, teach the proper use of self-injectable epinephrine and emphasize the importance of wearing a Medic Alert bracelet.
- For patients taking epinephrine in ophthalmic form, teach how to instill topical eye drugs properly.
- Advise patients to avoid OTC drugs containing sympathomimetic ingredients, which may potentiate the effects of epinephrine.
- Remind patients with diabetes to monitor their blood glucose levels carefully.

Ongoing Assessment and Evaluation

Assess the patient for resolution of the presenting problem. For example, when epinephrine is administered for the management of bronchoconstriction, the effect of treatment is a decrease in wheezing. Regardless of the presenting problem, the patient is constantly monitored for adverse effects related to the action of epinephrine. It is important to remember that epinephrine is a nonselective adrenergic agonist. Therefore, all receptor subtypes (alpha-1, alpha-2, beta-1, and beta-2) are stimulated, and the potential for adverse reactions is high.

Drugs Closely Related to [P] Epinephrine

Norepinephrine (Levophed) is very similar to epinephrine. Like epinephrine, NE is a catecholamine and may not be administered orally. The major difference is that NE does not stimulate beta-2 receptors. Adverse effects and drug interactions are identical to those of epinephrine, with the exception that NE does not promote hyperglycemia. Clinically, NE is used in the management of hypotension and cardiac arrest.

Drugs Significantly Different From [P] Epinephrine

Ephedrine

Like epinephrine, ephedrine stimulates alpha-1, alpha-2, beta-1, and beta-2 receptors. Unlike epinephrine, it is not a catecholamine. Ephedrine, also known as *ma huang,* is

derived from plants of the genus *Ephedra* and has been used in Chinese medicine for more than 5,000 years. Ephedrine is metabolized to norephedrine, which is responsible for the stimulating effects of the drug on the CNS.

In Western medicine, ephedrine is primarily used intravenously to prevent or treat hypotension associated with spinal anesthesia and topically for the treatment of sinus congestion. Ephedrine is used extensively in OTC medications because of its ability to stimulate multiple adrenergic receptors. It is a frequent ingredient in OTC bronchodilators as well as in many drugs used for colds and flu. Oral ephedrine and pseudoephedrine have been misused as an agent for weight loss and is often included in herbal products and dietary supplements that supposedly increase strength, decrease weight, and produce an "herbal high." One of its more recent uses is as a substrate for the illegal synthesis of amphetamine and methamphetamine. The U.S. Department of Justice, Drug Enforcement Agency has added both ephedrine and pseudoephedrine to the list of substances subject to the Controlled Substances Act (Drug Enforcement Agency, 2008). Consequently, as of 2008 commonly used OTC medications containing ephedrine or pseudoephedrine must be obtained behind the counter and quantities are limited for each transaction. When used inappropriately, potential severe adverse effects of ephedrine include heart attack, stroke, paranoid psychosis, vomiting, fever, palpitations, convulsions, and coma.

Vasopressin

Vasopressin, also known as antidiuretic hormone, is classified as an endocrine-metabolic or gastrointestinal agent as large doses will stimulate peristalsis. It is also used in the management of shock states due to ventricular fibrillation, hypovolemia, sepsis, and cardiopulmonary bypass. During these shock states, exogenous vasopressin increases blood flow to the heart and brain and reduces blood flow to the skin, skeletal muscle, small bowel, and fat. According to the American Heart Association Advanced Cardiac Life Support Guidelines (AHA, 2005) a single dose of vasopressin (40 U IV) may be used to replace the first or second dose of epinephrine in the management of pulseless ventricular tachycardia (VT) or ventricular fibrillation (VF). However, recent studies have found that in the case of out-of-hospital cardiac arrest, vasopressin administered with epinephrine showed no improvement in outcomes over epinephrine alone (Gueugniaud et al., 2008). During in-hospital postresuscitation in refractory cardiac arrest, adding the glucocorticoids methylprednisolone and hydrocortisone to the combinations of vasopressin and epinephrine can improve survival (Mentzelopoulos et al., 2009).

• Ⓒ ALPHA-1 ADRENERGIC AGONISTS

The alpha-1 adrenergic agonists are drugs that stimulate the alpha-1 receptor directly. Phenylephrine (Allerest) is an ideal prototype for the alpha-1 adrenergic agonists.

Nursing Management of the Patient Receiving ℗ Phenylephrine

Core Drug Knowledge

Pharmacotherapeutics

Phenylephrine may be used parenterally for treatment of vascular failure in shock, shock-like states, or drug-induced hypotension. Other parenteral uses include overcoming paroxysmal supraventricular tachycardia, prolonging spinal anesthesia, maintaining blood pressure during spinal and inhalation anesthesia, and vasoconstriction in regional anesthesia. Although approved for these uses, phenylephrine is generally not the drug of choice for management of these conditions. More commonly, phenylephrine is used topically for relief of nasal and nasopharyngeal mucosal congestion and to produce mydriasis (dilation of the pupil) for ophthalmologic procedures. Phenylephrine for nasal congestion is marketed as an OTC alternative to the now-regulated ephedrine and pseudoephedrine products, although its effectiveness at nonprescription doses has not been proven (Hatton et al., 2007).

Pharmacokinetics

Phenylephrine is poorly absorbed orally and is usually given parenterally or topically. Following IM administration, a vasopressor effect is apparent within 15 to 20 minutes and lasts for 1 to 2 hours (see Table 13.3). The drug is metabolized in the liver and excreted mainly in urine. It has an elimination half-life of 2 to 3 hours. Even if phenylephrine got into breast milk, it would probably be destroyed in the infant's intestines before absorption.

Pharmacodynamics

Phenylephrine is structurally similar to epinephrine and is a powerful alpha-1 adrenergic agonist with very little activity at beta-adrenergic receptors. The predominant actions of phenylephrine are in the vascular system, where it acts as a vasopressor by stimulating alpha-1 vascular receptors and thus causes vasoconstriction. As a result, renal perfusion and cardiac output are decreased, and blood pressure is increased by the heightened peripheral resistance. When used in nasal sprays or cold preparations, the vasoconstriction decreases nasal congestion temporarily.

Contraindications and Precautions

The main contraindications to phenylephrine are drug hypersensitivity, sulfite sensitivity, severe hypertension, ventricular tachycardia, and closed-angle glaucoma. Precautions need to be observed for hyperthyroid states and pregnancy and in patients who are elderly or have diabetes, myocardial disease, arteriosclerosis, uncorrected hypovolemia, or asthma.

Adverse Effects

The main adverse effects of phenylephrine are headache, restlessness, excitability, and reflex bradycardia following an increase in blood pressure. Restlessness and excitability are experienced by many people who take OTC nasal decongestants containing sympathomimetics, with effects similar to those of phenylephrine. Rebound nasal congestion is a common adverse effect.

Drug Interactions

Phenylephrine interacts with monoamine oxidase inhibitors (MAOIs), tricyclic antidepressants, and oxytocics used in labor and delivery (Table 13.5).

Assessment of Relevant Core Patient Variables

Health Status

Assess for medical disorders such as diabetes, hyperthyroidism, heart disease, cerebral arteriosclerosis, bronchial asthma, idiopathic orthostatic hypotension, chronic bronchitis, and chronic obstructive pulmonary disease. Phenylephrine may increase airway resistance and bronchial smooth muscle tone and therefore should be given only if absolutely necessary. Also assess for a history of sulfite sensitivity because some formulations of phenylephrine contain sulfites that may induce a reaction. Finally, assess for recent use of prescription drugs (e.g., tricyclic antidepressants and MAOIs). Communicate positive findings to the health care provider in nonemergency situations before phenylephrine is administered.

Obtain pretreatment vital signs to establish a baseline for therapeutic monitoring and detection of potential adverse effects. During therapy, monitor therapeutic effects to evaluate the decrease in frequency or severity of target symptoms or the resumption of functions that were previously changed.

Life Span and Gender

Document the age and gender of the patient and assess women of childbearing age for pregnancy and lactation. Phenylephine is a pregnancy category C drug. During pregnancy, phenylephrine is used only if absolutely necessary because it is not known whether phenylephrine causes fetal

TABLE 13.5	Agents That Interact with P Phenylephrine	
Interactants	**Effect and Significance**	**Nursing Management**
methyldopa	Methyldopa may increase the pressor response of phenylephrine	Monitor patient's blood pressure and vital signs carefully.
monoamine oxidase inhibitors	Increased amount of norepinephrine available for release, resulting in headache, hypertension, hyperpyrexia, and possibly in hypertensive crisis	Avoid concurrent use if possible.
oxytocics	Synergistic vasoconstriction, resulting in hypertension (when epinephrine is administered to correct hypotension)	Monitor patient's blood pressure and vital signs carefully.
tricyclic antidepressants	Inhibition of reuptake of norepinephrine in the neuron and diminished pressor effect of phenylephrine	Anticipate dosage adjustment of phenylephrine. Monitor patient carefully for hypertension and cardiac arrhythmias.

abnormalities. If the patient is breast-feeding, the infant is monitored for adrenergic stimulation. If such stimulation occurs, the drug may have to be discontinued.

Elderly patients may be at increased risk for blurring of vision from mydriasis. The topical 10% ophthalmic phenylephrine solution is avoided in infants and used cautiously with the elderly because there is an increased risk for systemic absorption.

Lifestyle, Diet, and Habits
Document the patient's occupation and activities of daily living. It is important to advise the patient to exercise caution when driving or operating machinery at night or under very bright light because mydriasis may cause temporary blindness. Additionally, ask the patient about his or her use of OTC cough, cold, or herbal remedies containing sympathomimetic ingredients, which intensify the effects of phenylephrine.

Environment
In the acute care hospital, phenylephrine is administered in a closely monitored area, such as the intensive care unit, for treatment of hypotension or shock. For other uses, it may be self-administered by the patient in any environment.

Nursing Diagnoses and Outcomes
- Impaired Gas Exchange related to bronchoconstriction or bronchospasm
  Desired outcome: Gas exchange will remain unimpaired by coughing or drug-induced bronchoconstriction.
- Imbalanced Nutrition: Less Than Body Requirements, related to anorexia or nausea secondary to use of an adrenergic drug
  Desired outcome: The patient will take sufficient nourishment, manage diet adequately, and use antiemetics if necessary.
- Disturbed Sleep Pattern, Insomnia, related to CNS excitation secondary to phenylephrine use
  Desired outcome: The patient will maintain normal sleep patterns by practicing sleep hygiene measures and using a sedative at bedtime if necessary.

Planning and Intervention
Maximizing Therapeutic Effects
Blood loss or volume deficits are corrected before IV phenylephrine is used to treat hypotension. Phenylephrine may be used concurrently with replacement therapy if necessary to prevent cerebral or coronary artery ischemia. For topical use, the following factors are considered:
- To produce optimal mydriasis, be careful to instill the ophthalmic form of phenylephrine into the conjunctival cul-de-sac.
- If the phenylephrine is in the form of a nasal spray, demonstrate the proper way to administer the spray. The patient can then perform a repeat demonstration.
- Encourage the patient to use phenylephrine exactly as prescribed and at the required dosage frequency to enhance therapeutic effects.

Minimizing Adverse Effects
When given to treat hypotension, IV phenylephrine is administered through a large vein, preferably in the antecubital space. This method will help prevent extravasation, which may cause necrosis as a result of vasoconstriction. Check the IV site frequently for patency. If extravasation does occur, the antidote is the potent alpha blocker phentolamine (Regitine), which is injected subcutaneously into the affected tissue with a fine-gauge needle. Also monitor for signs of sulfite sensitivity.

Teach the patient the following strategies to minimize adverse effects during topical drug therapy:
- Avoid driving at night because blurred vision can be hazardous. Wearing sunglasses, however, may relieve the glare of bright lights and reduce photophobia.
- Time doses to prevent disrupting sleep, and use effective sleep hygiene measures (dimmed lights, reduced noise, soothing music).
- Avoid OTC drugs that contain sympathomimetic ingredients that potentiate the effect of phenylephrine.

Providing Patient and Family Education

- Stress the hazards associated with driving and operating heavy or dangerous machinery until the effects of the drug on the individual are known.
- Teach the patient about drug interactions and advise not to use phenylephrine if he or she is taking MAOIs, tricyclic antidepressants, or drugs that treat glaucoma.
- Teach the patient to recognize and report signs and symptoms of adverse effects requiring medical attention, such as a fast, pounding, or irregular heartbeat; chest pain that lasts longer than 5 minutes; trouble breathing; or tingling in the hands or feet.
- Teach patients that prolonged use for nasal congestion for more than 3 to 5 days can cause rebound congestion.

Ongoing Assessment and Evaluation

Determining whether therapy is successful for patients taking phenylephrine and other adrenergic drugs is relatively straightforward. Because the contraindications and precautions for phenylephrine are many, it is important to assess lifestyle and occupation and be able to recognize and manage adverse effects. Completing a detailed and thorough history and physical examination on any patient anticipating long-term adrenergic drug therapy is essential.

Drug Closely Related to P Phenylephrine

Methoxamine (Vasoxyl) is a parenteral vasopressor agent used for blood pressure support during surgery and for terminating some supraventricular tachycardias. It increases blood pressure by increasing peripheral resistance through the alpha receptors.

Methoxamine is contraindicated for use in patients with sulfite sensitivity, severe hypertension, hyperthyroidism, bradycardia, partial atrioventricular block, myocardial disease, severe arteriosclerosis, or sulfite hypersensitivity.

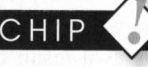

MEMORY CHIP

P Phenylephrine

- Alpha-adrenergic agonist and vasopressor (constricts blood vessels, raises blood pressure)
- Treats hypotension, shock related to vascular failure, nasal congestion; also used during anesthesia
- Major contraindications: hypersensitivity, severe hypertension, ventricular tachycardia, and closed-angle glaucoma
- Most common adverse effects: hypertension, headache, sleep disturbances
- Most serious adverse effect: reflex bradycardia
- Important drug–drug interaction: possible life-threatening interaction with monoamine oxidase inhibitors
- Maximizing therapeutic effects: Instill eye drops in conjunctival cul-de-sac.
- Minimizing adverse effects: Avoid situations that increase blurred vision.
- Most important patient education: Stress safety related to blurred vision.

Like phenylephrine, methoxamine may interact with MAOIs, tricyclic antidepressants, and oxytocics. In addition, methoxamine may interact with bretylium, which results in arrhythmias. It may partially or fully reverse the antihypertensive effects of guanethidine. Lastly, use of methoxamine with halogenated hydrocarbon anesthetics can sensitize the myocardium to the effects of catecholamines.

Potential adverse effects include hypertension, ventricular ectopic beats, nausea and vomiting, headache, anxiety, sweating, pilomotor response, uterine hypertonus, fetal bradycardia, and urinary urgency.

C ALPHA-2 ADRENERGIC AGONISTS

As you recall from previous discussion, the alpha-2 receptors are located on the presynaptic side of the synapse. A significant release of NE is needed to flood the synapse and allow for stimulation on the presynaptic side. Stimulation of alpha-2 receptors act as a negative feedback loop for the release of the SNS neurotransmitter NE. In other words, stimulation of alpha-2 receptors in the SNS decreases sympathetic outflow by inhibiting the release of norepinephrine. The prototype alpha-2 adrenergic agonist is clonidine (Catapres), which has a narrow range of specific clinical indications and has fallen out of favor in many practice arenas. For this reason, although it can be considered a prototype, only a condensed discussion of it will appear in this text.

Clonidine

Clonidine's approved pharmacotherapeutic use is for the treatment of hypertension. Clonidine's alpha-2 stimulation results in decreased heart rate, decreased blood pressure, decreased vasoconstriction, and decreased renal vascular resistance. However, renal blood flow and glomerular filtration rate remain unchanged essentially. Clonidine is considered a secondary or supplemental antihypertensive; its antihypertensive uses are actually quite limited and are discussed in Chapter 26. Off-label uses are varied but mostly relate to its sympathetic inhibition effects from alpha-2 stimulation. They include preventing symptoms of alcohol, methadone, or opiate withdrawal during detoxification (perhaps the most common current use for the drug); reduction of allergen-induced inflammatory reactions in patients with extrinsic asthma; smoking cessation; and ulcerative colitis. Clonidine also can be administered via an epidural line to control pain; it appears to prevent pain transmission from the spinal cord to the brain.

Clonidine may be administered orally, parenterally, or, most frequently, transdermally. When administered transdermally, the drug is released at a constant rate for 7 days. Patients need to be taught how to apply the patch and how to safely dispose of it.

Some adverse effects of clonidine, such as dry mouth, drowsiness, dizziness, sedation, and constipation, are fairly common. Dry mouth and drowsiness also occur frequently when clonidine is administered transdermally. Rebound hypertension may occur if the drug is discontinued abruptly. Erythema is a common adverse effect.

Because clonidine can be used to prevent the symptoms of narcotic withdrawal, a black market exists for clonidine in some communities and the patient may be tempted to sell the prescription. Nurses and other health care providers should be alert to patients returning for a duplicate prescription of clonidine, claiming to have lost the original shortly after it was prescribed. This may indicate the patient has sold or stored the prescription. In such cases, the prescriber may be notified and consulted about a change in the prescription, particularly if it appears that the patient is not taking the clonidine.

● Ⓒ BETA-ADRENERGIC AGONISTS

Beta-adrenergic agonists also mimic the action of the SNS; therefore, they are also known as sympathomimetic agents. They exert their effects by stimulation of one or both beta-adrenergic receptors. Like the alpha-adrenergic drugs, they are classified as either a catecholamine or noncatecholamine.

Beta-adrenergic agonists are also labeled according to their selectivity. Drugs that stimulate both beta-1 and beta-2 receptors are nonselective. Those that target either beta-1 or beta-2 are selective. To maximize therapeutic effects and minimize adverse effects, selective drugs are used most frequently. Again, as with alpha-adrenergic drugs, selectivity is preferential but not exclusive.

Beta-1 Agonists

The prototypical beta-1 agonist is dopamine (Intropin). Dopamine also can stimulate dopaminergic receptors, but it is chosen as the beta-1 agonist prototype as it clearly effects beta-1 receptors and is a drug widely used for cardiovascular problems.

Nursing Management of the Patient Receiving Ⓟ Dopamine

Core Drug Knowledge

Pharmacotherapeutics

Dopamine is used to correct the hemodynamic imbalances present in shock due to myocardial infarction, trauma, endotoxic septicemia, open heart surgery, renal failure, and chronic cardiac decompensation (i.e., chronic heart failure) (see Table 13.3). For the treatment to be most effective, the patient should not be experiencing severe disruptions in urine production, myocardial function, and blood pressure. In other words, the earlier the signs of shock are recognized and treatment is started with fluids and dopamine, the more successful the therapy will be. There is debate that dopamine provides only transient improvements in renal perfusion in patients with renal failure, and low doses for nephroprotective purposes are discouraged (Drieghe et al., 2008). Dopamine is used off-label for cardiac catheterization, acute hypotension, and organ transplant.

Pharmacokinetics

The onset of dopamine's action is within 5 minutes. Duration of action is less than 10 minutes. The drug is distributed widely in the body but does not cross the blood–brain barrier. Dopamine is metabolized in the liver, kidneys, and plasma by MAO and COMT to inactive compounds. About one fourth of it is taken up into adrenergic nerve terminals that are specialized neurosecretory vesicles. There, through hydroxylation, it becomes norepinephrine. Dopamine is excreted mainly by the kidneys.

Pharmacodynamics

Dopamine is a naturally occurring catecholamine and a precursor to norepinephrine. It stimulates alpha-1 and beta-1 receptors through direct methods and indirectly through the release of stored epinephrine. It also has dopaminergic effects. Beta-1 stimulation produces increased cardiac output by increasing the force of contraction and heart rate. Although dopamine causes the oxygen needs of the myocardium to increase, this effect is less pronounced than when isoproterenol is administered. Tachyarrhythmias usually do not occur. Systolic blood pressure increases, whereas if any increases in diastolic pressure occur, they are usually minimal. Total peripheral resistance (from alpha effects) is not changed substantially if dopamine is given at low or intermediate levels. Although blood flow to the peripheral beds may decrease, blood flow to the mesenteric beds increases. Dopamine dilates renal and mesenteric vasculature as well as the cerebral and cardiac beds. This dilation, which is believed to arise from stimulation of dopaminergic receptors, produces an increase in renal blood flow, glomerular filtration rate, and urinary output. The dopaminergic zero effect in the peripheral resistance is lost as the dose becomes high because the alpha stimulation takes precedence. The alpha stimulation produces increased peripheral resistance, raising blood pressure as the dose of dopamine increases. The drug's dosage is titrated upward until adequate perfusion of vital organs is achieved.

Contraindications and Precautions

Dopamine is contraindicated in pheochromocytoma, uncorrected tachyarrhythmias, and ventricular fibrillation. Any underlying hypovolemia is corrected before therapy begins. Acidosis decreases the effectiveness of dopamine and other vasopressors. It is important to correct acidosis before starting therapy or as soon as it occurs. Dopamine must be administered in an environment where blood pressure, cardiac output, urinary flow, and pulmonary wedge pressure can be monitored closely.

Adverse Effects

The most frequent adverse effects from dopamine are ectopic beats, nausea and vomiting, tachycardia, angina, palpitations, dyspnea, headache, hypotension, and vasoconstriction. Infrequent effects are abnormal conduction, bradycardia, widened QRS complex, and piloerection. High

TABLE 13.6 Agents That Interact with P Dopamine

Interactants	Effect and Significance	Nursing Management
guanethidine	Partial or total reversal of the antihypertensive effects of guanethidine. This may be desirable if hypotension from shock is present.	Monitor blood pressure.
halogenated hydrocarbon anesthetics	May sensitize the myocardium to the effects from a catecholamine. This may cause a serious arrhythmia	Use a cardiac monitor and assess cardiac function carefully. Use extreme caution.
methyldopa	Coadministration may result in an increased pressor response resulting in hypertension	
monoamine oxidase inhibitors; furazolidone	Increase the pressor effect of dopamine 6- to 20-fold as dopamine metabolism is inhibited	Avoid this combination. If given by mistake, administer phentolamine.
oxytocic drugs	Severe persistent hypertension	Avoid combination if possible. Monitor BP closely if must be given.
phenytoin	Simultaneous infusion has led to seizures, severe hypotension, bradycardia, and possible cardiac arrest	Monitor BP closely if coadministration is necessary. Discontinue phenytoin and provide supportive measures if hypotension occurs.
tricyclic antidepressants	The pressor response of dopamine may be decreased, causing it to be less effective	Increase dosage of dopamine if necessary

doses may cause ventricular arrhythmias and dilated pupils. High doses given over a long time have caused gangrene. Gangrene has also occurred in patients receiving low doses who had occlusive vascular disease.

Overdosage is evidenced by excessive hypertension. If overdosage occurs, reduce the rate or stop the infusion until the patient is stabilized.

Drug Interactions

A few drugs are known to interact with dopamine (Table 13.6).

Assessment of Relevant Core Patient Variables

Health Status

The absence of pheochromocytoma, uncorrected tachyarrhythmias, and ventricular fibrillation must be confirmed because these conditions are contraindications to the use of dopamine. Verify that existing volume deficits have been corrected. Also assess for drug use known to cause interaction, especially MAOIs. It is important to determine whether the patient has a history of occlusive vascular disease (such as arteriosclerosis, arterial embolism, Raynaud disease, or frostbite), because such a patient may be more likely to develop necrosis from vasoconstriction with dopamine. If possible, assess for a history of sulfite sensitivity, because some dopamine formulations contain sulfites.

Life Span and Gender

Assess for pregnancy because dopamine is a risk category C drug. Whether dopamine is excreted into breast milk is unknown. Also note the patient's age before administering dopamine. Dopamine's effect and safety in children has

not been established, although it has been used in a limited number of pediatric cases.

Environment

Because dopamine is an IV drug, it is administered only in acute care settings, where continuous monitoring of the patient's cardiovascular status can occur.

Nursing Diagnoses and Outcomes

- Risk for Ineffective Tissue Perfusion to Vital Organs related to drug effect
  Desired outcome: The patient will maintain sufficient perfusion of vital organs to prevent serious damage.
- Risk for Injury related to adverse effects of drug therapy
  Desired outcome: Adverse effects of drug therapy will not occur or will be minimized to prevent injury.

Planning and Intervention

Maximizing Therapeutic Effects

Administer IV dopamine using an infusion pump to regulate flow. It is important to start at low doses and titrate up until the desired renal or hemodynamic response is attained. Oxidizing agents, iron salts, or alkaline solutions such as 5% sodium bicarbonate are not added because these substances deactivate dopamine.

Minimizing Adverse Effects

If the drug is not prediluted, follow the manufacturer's instructions for dilution, because dopamine is a potent drug that may cause extravasation. It is imperative to use an infusion pump. Before treatment, correct hypovolemia with whole blood or plasma as indicated. Monitor the blood pressure, urinary flow, cardiac output, and pulmonary wedge pressure closely throughout therapy.

Assess for a disproportionate rise in diastolic blood pressure, which may indicate predominant vasoconstriction. Patients with a history of occlusive vascular disease are monitored closely for changes in temperature or color of skin or extremities. If these changes occur, consult with the physician to determine the benefits of dopamine compared with the risk for developing necrosis.

Monitor the insertion site for patency, free flow, and signs of extravasation. Using a large vein such as the antecubital fossa decreases the potential for extravasation. Should extravasation occur, inject the affected area with phentolamine in the subcutaneous space to minimize the potential for necrosis or sloughing of tissues.

When discontinuing dopamine, gradually decrease the dose and then monitor the resulting effects. Sudden discontinuation of dopamine may induce hypotension.

Providing Patient and Family Education

- Dopamine is administered during an acute medical crisis. Patient education is therefore limited at that time.
- If the patient is awake and alert, inform the patient that his or her blood pressure is low and that the medication will raise blood pressure to a normal level.
- Instruct patient to report signs of chest pain, palpitations, rapid heart rate, and extravasation.
- Advise patient that this drug may cause headache, anxiety, nausea, vomiting, oliguria, and difficulty breathing.
- Reassure the patient and family that the patient will be monitored closely during administration of the drug.

MEMORY CHIP ❗

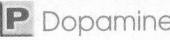 Dopamine

- Used to treat the hypotension resulting from shock because it stimulates alpha and beta receptors to increase cardiac output, blood pressure, and renal perfusion
- Correct hypovolemia before administering.
- Major contraindications: pheochromocytoma, uncorrected tachyarrhythmias, and ventricular fibrillation
- Most common adverse effects: ectopic beats, nausea and vomiting, tachycardia, angina, palpitations, dyspnea, headache, hypotension, and vasoconstriction
- Most serious adverse effect: ventricular arrhythmias
- Important drug–drug interaction: monoamine oxidase inhibitors
- Maximizing therapeutic effects: Use infusion pump, titrate drug until desired effect is obtained.
- Minimizing adverse effects: Monitor blood pressure, urinary output, cardiac output, and pulmonary wedge pressure throughout therapy.
- Most important patient education: Reassure patient that close monitoring will be maintained.

Ongoing Assessment and Evaluation

Dopamine therapy is effective if blood pressure stabilizes, urinary output returns to normal, cardiac output returns to normal, and the patient does not have serious adverse effects from the drug.

Drugs Closely Related to P Dopamine

Dobutamine

Dobutamine (Dobutrex) is chemically similar to dopamine. Like dopamine, its primary influence is on beta-1 receptors, with similar effects on the force of contraction. Dobutamine is somewhat less effective than dopamine at increasing the rate at the sinoatrial (SA) node. Also like dopamine, dobutamine's beta-2 effects on vasodilation are minimal. Unlike dopamine, dobutamine has almost no effect on alpha receptors to cause vasoconstriction. Although cardiac output and blood pressure are similarly increased with both drugs, dobutamine does not produce the increased renal output that dopamine does. Furthermore, dobutamine always increases peripheral resistance, whereas dopamine may increase or decrease peripheral resistance. Dobutamine does not cause the release of endogenous norepinephrine that dopamine causes.

The pharmacotherapeutic uses of dobutamine differ from those of dopamine. Dobutamine is indicated in the short-term treatment and support of patients experiencing cardiac decompression because of depressed contractility. The decreased contractility may be secondary to either organic heart disease or cardiac surgery. Patients with atrial fibrillation and a rapid ventricular rate are treated with digoxin before dobutamine treatment to protect the ventricles.

Dobutamine is metabolized by two methods: methylation of the catechol and conjugation. By-products are excreted in the urine. Onset of action is 1 to 2 minutes, but up to 10 minutes may be needed for the peak effect to occur. A contraindication unique to dobutamine is the presence of idiopathic hypertrophic subaortic stenosis. Although elevated pulse usually does not occur when using dobutamine, tachycardia can occur. Accompanying the tachycardia is a rapid and substantial increase in blood pressure, with the systolic pressure rising 50% or more. These adverse effects are usually dose related, and reducing the dose promptly corrects the problem. Interestingly, dobutamine also can cause significant hypotension if given in excessive amounts; again, decreasing the dose usually corrects the problem. Dobutamine may cause or exacerbate ventricular ectopic beats, although ventricular tachycardia is rare. Other rare adverse effects include nausea, headache, anginal pain, nonspecific chest pain, palpitations, and shortness of breath. Phlebitis and local inflammation at the IV site may occur; a large vein is chosen to minimize the patient's risk for developing these complications. Coons and Seidl (2007) identify a decreased responsiveness to dobutamine in elderly patients, and recommend that hemodynamic endpoints be targeted instead of using a specific dose. Doses of 2.5 to 10 mcg/kg per minute can increase cardiac output without significantly increasing heart rate, but doses over 20 mcg/kg per minute increase the risk of tachycardia and hypotension in all patients.

As with dopamine, patients receiving dobutamine require continuous cardiac monitoring while receiving the drug. Blood pressure is checked frequently. Pulmonary wedge pressure and cardiac output (assessed on a cardiac monitor that reads the information from inside the heart via a catheter inserted into the pulmonary artery) are checked whenever possible.

Isoproterenol

Like dopamine, isoproterenol (Isuprel) has a strong effect on beta-1 receptors and produces similar increases in contractility. However, isoproterenol's effects on heart rate and vasodilation are much greater than those of dopamine. Isoproterenol does not stimulate the alpha receptors for vasoconstriction. Like dopamine, isoproterenol increases cardiac output. Renal perfusion is also affected, although unlike dopamine, isoproterenol can either increase or decrease it. Peripheral resistance always is decreased, but blood pressure may go up or down from isoproterenol. Although isoproterenol may be used to treat shock, the practice is uncommon because of the tachycardia that may occur. Isoproterenol is an ingredient in respiratory drugs used to manage asthma, bronchitis, and emphysema.

Mephentermine

Mephentermine (Wyamine) has a weaker effect than dopamine on the beta-1 receptors, causing less increase in contractility and heart rate. However, it has a stronger effect on the beta-2 receptors, producing moderate vasodilation. It has only a weak effect on alpha-1 receptors, causing a small increase in vasoconstriction. The pharmacodynamics of mephentermine, when compared with those of dopamine, are in some ways similar. It increases cardiac output and blood pressure. It may have no effect on peripheral resistance or it may increase it, and renal perfusion may increase or decrease. Mephentermine is used to treat hypotension from ganglionic blockade or spinal anesthesia. It can be used on an emergency basis to maintain blood pressure during hypovolemic shock, but only until blood or blood substitutes become available.

Metaraminol

Metaraminol (Aramine) is similar to mephentermine in that it has only minor effects on beta-1 receptors, creating mild increases in contractility and heart rate. It has more effect on vasoconstriction from alpha-1 stimulation than mephentermine, but less than dopamine has. It has no effect on vasodilation from beta-2 stimulation. It primarily increases blood pressure by increasing peripheral resistance. Unlike dopamine, it lowers cardiac output and renal perfusion. Although it stimulates the sinoatrial node somewhat (which theoretically should increase the heart rate), the net effect on the heart is bradycardia, resulting from a strong reflexive response to the significant vasoconstriction. Metaraminol is

used in the prevention and treatment of acute hypotensive states occurring with spinal anesthesia. It is an adjunct treatment for hypotension due to hypovolemia, reactions to drug therapy, surgical complications, and shock associated with brain damage due to trauma or tumor. Unlike dopamine, it can be given by IM or SC injection, in addition to being given as an IV infusion.

Drugs Significantly Different From P Dopamine

Midodrine

Midodrine (ProAmatine) raises blood pressure, but it is not used as a vasopressor in shock. Instead, it is used in the symptomatic treatment of orthostatic hypotension in patients whose lives are impaired significantly despite standard clinical treatment. An unlabeled use is in the treatment of urinary incontinence. It is administered orally. Midodrine is a prodrug that becomes active when it changes into the metabolite desglymidodrine. The metabolite is an alpha-1 agonist that increases the tone of the arteriolar and venous vasculature, increasing peripheral resistance. It results in increased standing, sitting, and lying blood pressures in orthostatic hypotension. Because it increases supine blood pressure, midodrine is not given less than 4 hours before bedtime. Suggested dosing times are shortly before or just after rising in the morning, midday, and late afternoon. This dosing schedule helps the patient maintain his or her normal daytime activities and prevent supine hypertension during the night. If supine hypertension does occur, it may be controlled by preventing the patient from lying completely flat (e.g., by lying with the head of the bed elevated).

Beta-2 Agonists

Drugs that are selective for beta-2 stimulation are used in the management of chronic airway limitation (CAL) diseases such as asthma. They may be given orally, parenterally, by nebulizer, or by metered-dose inhalers. While historically nonselective beta-2 agonist drugs were used in these conditions, they produced significant cardiac adverse effects. To minimize adverse effects, use of beta-2 selective drugs has become the community standard. Beta-2 respiratory agonists differ from each other in the way they are delivered as well as in their onset and duration of action. The prototype respiratory beta-2 agonist is albuterol. Albuterol as well as other respiratory beta-2 agonist drugs are discussed in Chapter 35.

• C DOPAMINERGIC AGONISTS

Although there are five types of dopamine receptors, only dopamine-1 (DA1) and dopamine-2 (DA2) receptors mediate responses in the adrenergic nervous system. Stimulation of DA1 and DA2 receptors results in peripheral vasodilation; however, stimulating both receptors may have either complementary or opposing effects. Fenoldopam (Corlopam) is a DA1 agonist and the prototype for dopaminergic agonist drugs. It was chosen as the prototype over dopamine as it only stimulates dopaminergic receptors.

Nursing Management of the Patient Receiving [P] Fenoldopam

Core Drug Knowledge

Pharmacotherapeutics

Fenoldopam is used for in-hospital, short-term (up to 48 hours) management of severe hypertension when rapid and selective but quickly reversible emergency reduction of blood pressure combined with renal vasodilation is necessary.

Pharmacokinetics

Fenoldopam is administered as a constant infusion. Steady-state concentrations are achieved within 20 minutes. There is a predictable relationship between the dose and the plasma concentration of fenoldopam. Metabolism of fenoldopam is by conjugation in the liver without involvement of the cytochrome P-450 enzymes. Ninety percent of infused fenoldopam is eliminated in urine and 10% in feces.

Pharmacodynamics

Fenoldopam is a selective peripheral DA1 agonist. Unlike dopamine, it does not bind with DA2, alpha, or beta receptors. It provides rapid vasodilation to the coronary, renal, mesenteric, and peripheral arteries. The pharmacokinetics of fenoldopam is not influenced by age, gender, or race in hypertensive emergency patients (see Table 13.3).

Contraindications and Precautions

Fenoldopam is contraindicated in patients with known hypersensitivity to sulfites because it is in a solution containing sodium metabisulfate (Varon, 2008). Patients with a history of glaucoma or intraocular hypertension are monitored closely because fenoldopam may increase intraocular pressure during infusion. Increases in intraocular pressure are dose-dependent (Varon, 2008). Patients with hypokalemia also require close monitoring because fenoldopam may reduce serum potassium when administered for more than 6 hours. Fenoldopam is given cautiously to patients with acute cerebral infarction or hemorrhage because it may cause hypotension.

Adverse Effects

Fenoldopam may induce symptomatic hypotension; therefore, close monitoring of blood pressure is essential. Fenoldopam may also cause dose-related tachycardia, especially with infusion rates greater than 0.1 mcg/kg/min. Tachycardia diminishes over time but remains elevated with higher doses. Patients may also experience flushing of the face, neck, or upper chest; headache; nausea; and vomiting. Less common adverse effects include abdominal or back pain, GI effects, sweating, and CNS effects such as insomnia, dizziness, nervousness, or anxiety.

Drug Interactions

No formal drug–drug interaction studies have been done with fenoldopam. Fenoldopam should be avoided with beta blockers and diuretics (Table 13.7). Theoretically, the potential exists for drug–drug interactions with the concomitant administration of antihypertensive agents such as alpha blockers, calcium-channel blockers, or angiotensin-converting enzyme (ACE) inhibitors.

Assessment of Relevant Core Patient Variables

Health Status

Assess for a history of sulfite sensitivity, because fenoldopam contains sulfites that may induce a reaction. Also assess for a history of glaucoma or intraocular hypertension and determine whether antihypertensive medications were used recently. Document preinfusion baseline vital signs, especially the blood pressure and heart rate. In a nonemergent situation, obtain a baseline serum potassium level.

Life Span and Gender

Fenoldopam is a pregnancy risk category B drug; however, because animal reproduction studies are not always predictive of human response, fenoldopam is used during pregnancy only if clearly needed. Whether fenoldopam is excreted in breast milk is unclear. Its safety and efficacy in pediatric use have not been established.

Environment

Fenoldopam is administered only in the acute care hospital setting. When used for antihypertensive emergent therapy, the drug is administered in a critical care environment.

Nursing Diagnoses and Outcomes

- Risk for Ineffective Tissue Perfusion related to hypotension, tachycardia, or increased intraocular pressure
  Desired Outcome: *The patient will maintain adequate tissue perfusion throughout therapy.*

TABLE 13.7	Agents That Interact with [P] Fenoldopam	
Interactants	**Effect and Significance**	**Nursing Management**
Beta-adrenergic blocking agents	Potential inhibition of reflex tachycardia resulting in decreased cardiac output	Advise provider if patient has been on recent beta-blocker therapy. Avoid concomitant use.
Diuretics	The natriuretic and diuretic properties of fenoldopam could lead to worsening volume depletion.	Advise provider if patient has been on recent diuretic therapy. Avoid concomitant use.

- Risk for Injury related to hypokalemia
  Desired Outcome: *The patient will maintain a serum potassium level within normal limits throughout therapy.*

Planning and Intervention

Maximizing Therapeutic Effects

Dilute the fenoldopam ampule concentrate with 0.9% sodium chloride or 5% dextrose. The drug is administered with an infusion pump to regulate flow. Fenoldopam is never administered as an IV push. The initial dose is titrated upward or downward, no more frequently than every 15 minutes and less frequently as goal blood pressure is approached. The recommended increments for titration are 0.05 to 0.1 mcg/kg/min to a maximum of 1.6 mcg/kg/min.

Minimizing Adverse Effects

Visually inspect the drug ampule. If particulate matter or cloudiness is observed, discard the medication. Start at low doses and titrate up to avoid reflex tachycardia. Monitor the heart rate and blood pressure continuously throughout the infusion. Fenoldopam may be abruptly discontinued in the presence of hypotension. In patients receiving fenoldopam for more than 6 hours, obtain baseline and periodic electrolyte levels, especially for potassium. Monitor intraocular pressure in patients with intraocular hypertension or glaucoma. Discard diluted solution that is not used within 24 hours of preparation.

Providing Patient and Family Education

- Explain to the patient and family the rationale for the use of fenoldopam.
- Emphasize the importance of reporting adverse effects, especially those associated with hypotension, during the infusion.
- Explain the necessity of frequent heart rate and blood pressure measurement.
- Reassure the patient that close monitoring will be maintained throughout drug therapy.

Ongoing Assessment and Evaluation

It is important to monitor vital signs throughout fenoldopam infusion. In the hypertensive patient, evaluate the efficacy of fenoldopam by monitoring the reduction in blood pressure.

Drugs Significantly Different from P Fenoldopam

Carbidopa-levodopa

Carbidopa-levodopa is also a dopaminergic drug but it works on the dopamine receptors in the brain, D_1, D_2, D_3. These dopamine receptors help to maintain a balance of stimulation versus non-stimulation of the basal ganglia in the brain. This balanced stimulation (with counter-balance from ACh stimulation) is required for normal, smooth, coordinated motor function. When there is a lack of this dopamine stimulation, the patient experiences Parkinson disease.

MEMORY CHIP

P Fenoldopam

- Used to treat severe hypertension by stimulating dopamine-1 receptors, resulting in peripheral vasodilation
- Major contraindications: sulfite hypersensitivity
- Most common adverse effects: hypotension, tachycardia, facial flushing, headache, nausea
- Most serious adverse effect: hypotension angina, cardiac dysrhythmia, heart failure
- Important drug–drug interaction: beta-blocking agents and diuretics
- Maximizing therapeutic effects: Titrate the drug slowly.
- Minimizing adverse effects: Continuously monitor heart rate and blood pressure; administer by continuous IV infusion (do not use bolus).
- Most important patient education: Reassure the patient that close monitoring will be maintained.

Carbidopa-levodopa is discussed as a prototype for treating Parkinson disease in Chapter 21.

C ADRENERGIC ANTAGONISTS

• C Alpha-Adrenergic Antagonists

Alpha-adrenergic antagonists block the stimulation of alpha receptors. Alpha-1 receptors have three distinct subtypes: alpha-1a, alpha-1b, and alpha-1d. Alpha-1a receptors mediate human prostatic smooth muscle contraction, whereas alpha-1b and alpha-1d receptors are involved in vascular smooth muscle contraction. Clinically relevant drugs in current use block alpha-1 receptors in the vasculature and the prostate. The prototype alpha-adrenergic antagonist is prazosin (Minipress).

Nursing Management of the Patient Receiving P Prazosin

Core Drug Knowledge

Pharmacotherapeutics

Prazosin is primarily used to treat hypertension as a second-line drug when combined with other drugs. It also may be used in the treatment of refractory chronic heart failure, Raynaud syndrome, post-traumatic stress disorder (PTSD), and benign prostatic hyperplasia (BPH).

Pharmacokinetics

Prazosin is given orally. It is metabolized in the liver without involvement of the P-450 enzymes and is excreted in the bile, feces, and urine. Prazosin is highly protein bound. It crosses the placenta and may enter breast milk. A single oral dose has a 10-hour duration of action and a half-life of 2 to 4 hours (Table 13.8).

Pharmacodynamics

Prazosin selectively and competitively blocks postsynaptic alpha-1 adrenergic receptors, decreasing sympathetic tone

TABLE 13.8 Summary of Selected C Adrenergic Antagonists

Drug (Trade) Name	Selected Indications	Route and Dosage Range	Pharmacokinetics
C Alpha-Adrenergic Antagonists			
P prazosin (Minipress)	Hypertension	*Adult:* PO, for HTN 3–15 mg daily in divided doses 2-4 times/day; max daily dose 20 mg; dosing varies for other uses	*Onset:* 2–4 h *Duration:* 10–24 h $t_{1/2}$: 2–4 h
doxazosin (Cardura)	BPH / HTN	*Adult:* PO, 1–8 mg daily according to individual response / *Adult:* PO, 1–4 mg daily	*Onset:* 2 h *Duration:* 24 h $t_{1/2}$: 22 h
dutasteride (Avodart)	BPH	*Adult:* PO, 0.5 mg daily	*Onset:* Unknown *Duration:* 2–3 h $t_{1/2}$: 5 wk
alfuzosin (Uroxatral)	BPH	*Adult:* PO, 10 mg daily (extended release); 7.5–10 mg/d in 3–4 divided doses (immediate release)	*Onset:* 1.5 h (immediate release); 8 h (extended release) *Duration:* 4 d $t_{1/2}$: 5 h
tamsulosin (Flomax)	BPH	*Adult:* PO, 0.4 mg 30 min following a meal	*Onset:* 4–8 h *Duration:* Unknown $t_{1/2}$: 9–15 h
terazosin (Hytrin)	HTN / BPH	*Adult:* PO, 1–10 mg/d / PO, 10–20 mg/d	*Onset:* 1–2 h *Duration:* 24 h $t_{1/2}$: 12 h
phentolamine (Vasomax)	Drug infiltration	Infiltrate area with small amount of solution made by diluting 5–10 mg in 10 mL 0.9% sodium chloride	*Onset:* 15–20 min; IV, immediate *Duration:* IM, 30–45 min; 15–30 min $t_{1/2}$: 19 min
	Pheochromocytoma-induced HTN and sweating, micturitional disorders, Raynaud vasospasm / Erectile dysfunction	*Adult:* IV, 2.5–5 mg *Child:* IV, 0.05–0.1 mg/kg / *Adult:* PO, 40–80 mg	
phenoxybenzamine (Dibenzyline)	Pheochromocytoma-induced HTN and sweating, micturitional disorders, Raynaud vasospasm, impotence	*Adult:* PO, 10–30 mg bid; can be given IV, but not IM or SC, because drug is an irritant	*Onset:* 2 h *Duration:* 1 wk $t_{1/2}$: 24 h
C Beta-Adrenergic Antagonists			
Nonselective			
P metoprolol (Lopressor, Toprol XL)	Angina, HTN, post-MI, heart failure	*Adult:* PO, 100–450 mg/d depending on patient's condition and response; IV, 2–20 mg titrated to response *Child:* PO, 1–2 mg/kg/d in 2 divided doses	*Onset:* PO, 15 min; IV, immediate *Duration:* 15–19 h $t_{1/2}$: 3–4 h
propranolol (Inderal)	Cardiac arrhythmias, MI, hypertrophic subaortic stenosis, HTN, pheochromocytoma, prophylaxis of migraine, angina, essential tremor	*Adult:* PO, 80–320 mg/d in divided doses; IV, 1–3 mg at 1 mg/min with monitoring	*Onset:* PO, 20–30 min; IV, immediate *Duration:* PO, 6–12 h; IV, 4–6 h $t_{1/2}$: 3–5 h
metipranolol (OptiPranolol)	Glaucoma / Ocular HTN	*Adult:* topical, 1 drop 0.3% solution in affected eye(s) bid / *Adult:* PO, 10–40 mg bid	*Onset:* 0.5–3 h *Duration:* <24 h $t_{1/2}$: 3 h
nadolol (Corgard)	Angina, HTN, cardiovascular disorders	*Adult:* PO, 40–320 mg daily; IV, 0.01–0.05 mg/kg at 1 mg/min to 10 mg maximum	*Onset:* Varies *Duration:* 17–24 h $t_{1/2}$: 20–24 h
penbutolol (Levatol)	HTN	*Adult:* PO, 10–40 mg/d	*Onset:* Varies *Duration:* 20 h $t_{1/2}$: 5 h

(Continued)

TABLE 13.8   Summary of Selected © Adrenergic Antagonists *(continued)*

Drug (Trade) Name	Selected Indications	Route and Dosage Range	Pharmacokinetics
pindolol (Visken)	HTN, hyperthyroidism Angina	*Adult:* PO, 15–40 mg daily *Adult:* PO, 2.5–5.0 mg/d up to 40 mg/d	*Onset:* Varies *Duration:* 24 h $t_{1/2}$: 3–4 h
sotalol (Betapace)	Ventricular arrhythmias, angina, HTN	*Adult:* PO, 80–320 mg daily in divided doses; IV, 0.2–1.5 mg/kg over 5 min with monitoring	*Onset:* 2–3 h *Duration:* 24 h $t_{1/2}$: 7–18 h
timolol (Timoptic, Blocadren)	HTN, angina, arrhythmias, post-MI, prophylaxis of migraine	*Adult:* PO, 10–60 mg daily or bid in divided doses; IV, 0.5 2×/d followed by oral dosing	*Onset:* 0.5–3 h *Duration:* 3–4 h $t_{1/2}$: NA
	Glaucoma	*Adult:* topical, 1 drop of 0.25% solution in affected eyes bid	*Onset:* 15–20 min *Duration:* 24 h $t_{1/2}$: 3–4 h
Cardioselective atenolol (Tenormin)	Angina, HTN, post-MI, arrhythmias, CHF, anxiety, irritable bowel syndrome, alcohol withdrawal	*Adult:* PO, 50–100 mg daily IV: 5 mg over 5 min; second 5-mg dose 10 min later *Child:* PO, 0.3 to 1.4 mg/kg/d	*Onset:* PO, 3 h *Duration:* 24 h $t_{1/2}$: 6–7 h
acebutolol (Sectral)	Ventricular arrhythmias HTN Angina	*Adult:* PO, 200 mg bid (maximum 2,600 mg/d in 2–3 divided doses) *Adult:* PO, 400–800 mg/d *Adult:* PO, 600–1,600 mg/d in 2–3 divided doses	*Onset:* 1.5–3 h *Duration:* 6–8 h $t_{1/2}$: 3–4 h
betaxolol (Betopic, Kerlone)	HTN, cardiovascular disorders	*Adult:* PO, 10–40 mg/d	*Onset:* 30–60 min *Duration:* 12–15 h $t_{1/2}$: 14–22 h
	Glaucoma	*Adult:* topical, 1 drop 0.5% solution in affected eye(s) bid	*Onset:* Unknown *Duration:* Unknown $t_{1/2}$: 14–22 h
bisoprolol (Zebeta)	Angina CHF HTN	*Adult:* PO, 5–20 mg daily *Adult:* PO, 1.25–10 mg daily *Adult:* PO, 2.5–20 mg daily (40 mg maximum)	*Onset:* 30–60 min *Duration:* 12–15 h $t_{1/2}$: 9–12 h
esmolol (Brevibloc)	Acute MI, Post-op HTN, supraventricular arrhythmia Rapid-sequence intubation	*Adult:* IV, 500 mcg/kg over 1 min followed by maintenance of 50–300 mcg/kg/min *Child:* IN, 300–1,000 mg/min *Adult:* IV, 2 mg/kg 1.5–3 min prior to intubation	*Onset:* immediate *Duration:* 10–30 min after discontinuation $t_{1/2}$: 9 minutes
metoprolol (Lopressor, Toprol XL)	Angina, HTN, post-MI	*Adult:* PO, 100–450 mg/d depending on patient's condition and response; IV, 2–20 mg titrated to response *Child:* PO, 1–2 mg/kg/d in 2 divided doses	*Onset:* PO, 15 min; IV, immediate *Duration:* 15–19 h $t_{1/2}$: 3–4 h

© Alpha/Beta-Adrenergic Antagonists

Drug (Trade) Name	Selected Indications	Route and Dosage Range	Pharmacokinetics
labetalol (Normodyne, Trandate)	HTN	*Adult:* 100–400 mg 2–3×/d; IV: 1 to 2 mg/kg *Child:* PO, 1–3 mg/kg/d in two divided doses; IV: 0.25 to 1.5 mg/kg/h	*Onset:* PO, 20 min; IV, 2–5 min *Duration:* PO, 8–24 h; IV, 2–4 h $t_{1/2}$: 2.5–8 h
carvedilol (Coreg)	HTN	*Adult:* 6.25 mg PO bid 7–10 d, then increase to 12.5 mg PO bid, maximum 25 mg PO bid *Child:* Not approved	*Onset:* 1–2 h *Duration:* 24 h $t_{1/2}$: 7–10 h
	Heart failure	*Adult:* 3.125 mg PO bid × 2 wk; then 6.25 mg PO bid; maximum 25 mg PO bid *Child:* Not approved.	
	Static angina Post-MI	*Adult:* 25–50 mg PO bid *Adult:* 6.125–12.5 mg PO, increase to maximum of 25 mg/d	

of the vasculature, dilating arterioles and veins, resulting in decreased peripheral resistance and decreased supine and standing blood pressure.

Contraindications and Precautions
The main contraindication to prazosin use is hypersensitivity. Prazosin is used cautiously in patients with angina pectoris because severe hypotension may cause or worsen angina. Prazosin is also used cautiously in patients who are pregnant or who have chronic heart failure or renal failure.

Adverse Effects
The most common adverse effects of prazosin are lightheadedness, dizziness, headache, drowsiness, weakness, lethargy, nausea, and palpitations. These effects may spontaneously resolve or be alleviated with a decreased dosage. Other common adverse effects include reflex tachycardia, orthostatic hypotension, nasal congestion, and inhibition of ejaculation.

Prazosin is well known for causing "first-dose syncope." This adverse effect is more likely with higher doses and with patients who are volume-depleted (Sica, 2005) and may be avoided by administering a lower first dose with food. Prazosin-induced syncope is unpredictable and does not correlate with serum prazosin levels. Syncope may be preceded by tachycardia (120 to 160 bpm) and occurs more frequently with dosage increases alone or when increases are combined with the adjunctive use of other antihypertensive agents.

Prazosin may cause adverse effects in practically any body system. Adverse effects include edema, dyspnea, and angina. Prazosin therapy may also induce rash, pruritus, priapism, urinary frequency, incontinence, blurred vision, dry mouth, pancreatitis, liver function test abnormalities, diaphoresis, fever, arthralgia, and mental depression.

Drug Interactions
Prazosin has many potential drug interactions. Prazosin may interact with other antihypertensive medications, especially other alpha- or beta-blocking agents. It may also interact with drugs for erectile dysfunction, resulting in profound hypotension. Certain herbal supplements such as dong quai, ephedra, yohimbe, ginseng, saw palmetto, and garlic may also interact with prazosin. Alcohol should be avoided as well, as it may increase vasodilation.

Assessment of Relevant Core Patient Variables
Health Status
Assess the patient's history for diseases or disorders that may contraindicate the use of prazosin. Communicate positive findings to the provider before the drug is given. Before and throughout therapy, closely monitor the patient's heart rate and blood pressure and assist the patient with position changes and ambulation.

Life Span and Gender
Document the age and gender of the patient and assess women of childbearing age for pregnancy and lactation.

If the patient is pregnant, prazosin must be used cautiously if at all because it is in FDA pregnancy risk category C. Safety and efficacy have not been established in pediatric patients. Elderly patients are more likely than other adults to be affected by postural hypotension and syncope.

Lifestyle, Diet, and Habits
Document the patient's occupation and daily activities. Patients should be cautious when operating machinery, exercising, driving, changing positions, or climbing stairs. Assess the patient for use of herbal supplements, which may interact with prazosin and for alcohol use, which may increase vasodilation.

Environment
Be aware of the environment in which the drug will be administered and assess the home or living environment, if appropriate. Prazosin may be administered in any setting, by health care providers, nurses, or the patients themselves.

Nursing Diagnoses and Outcomes
- Ineffective Tissue Perfusion related to prazosin-induced hypotension
  Desired outcome: *The patient will maintain adequate tissue perfusion.*
- Imbalanced Nutrition: Less Than Body Requirements, related to nausea secondary to prazosin use
  Desired outcome: *The patient will receive adequate nourishment by practicing appropriate dietary management.*
- Risk for Injury related to orthostatic hypotension
  Desired outcome: *The patient will remain free of injury.*

Planning and Intervention
Maximizing Therapeutic Effects
Emphasize the importance of taking the prescribed dose on a daily basis exactly as instructed. Explain the importance of refraining from OTC drug use because many OTC drugs contain ingredients that may decrease or dangerously enhance the effectiveness of prazosin.

Minimizing Adverse Effects
Nursing strategies to minimize adverse effects include having the patient take the first dose just before bedtime, having the patient lie down if syncope occurs, monitoring the patient's weight, and checking for edema. Explain the importance of changing position slowly to avoid orthostatic hypotension.

Providing Patient and Family Education
- Advise patients to take the drug as prescribed and to avoid operating machinery or driving for about 4 hours after the first dose.
- Teach the patient about additional adverse effects, such as dizziness and weakness (after changing position rapidly, in hot weather, after exercising, and after drinking

MEMORY CHIP

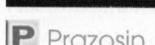 Prazosin

- Vasodilator
- Treats, hypertension, Raynaud syndrome, prostatic obstruction, PTSD
- Major contraindication: hypersensitivity
- Most common adverse effects: lightheadedness, dizziness, headache, drowsiness, weakness, lethargy, nausea, and palpitations
- Most serious adverse effect: "first dose syncope"
- Maximizing therapeutic effects: Refrain from administering any OTC drug in combination with prazosin.
- Minimizing adverse effects: Stress safety issues regarding CNS effects; check drug interactions.
- Most important patient education: safe ways to cope with postural hypotension; use caution driving or using heavy machinery.

---

alcohol). To avoid injury from these effects, the patient may need to avoid driving or engaging in tasks that require alertness until the body adjusts to the drug, to change positions slowly, to use caution when climbing stairs, to cool down when exercising, and to avoid consuming alcoholic beverages.

- Highlight the symptoms that should be reported to the provider if they occur. These symptoms include blurred vision, difficulty breathing, fainting spells, light-headedness, irregular heartbeat, palpitations or chest pain, mental depression, swelling of the legs and ankles, protracted vomiting, and prolonged, painful erections.

Ongoing Assessment and Evaluation

Monitoring of blood pressure, heart and lung sounds, and edema is important. To identify significant potential drug interactions, also determine whether any other drugs are being taken concurrently with prazosin.

Drugs Closely Related to P Prazosin

Alfuzosin (Uroxatral), doxazosin (Cardura), tamsulosin (Flomax), and terazosin (Hytrin) are also alpha-adrenergic antagonists. They differ from each other in pharmacokinetics and their specificity to alpha-1a subtype receptors. All of these drugs are used to manage benign prostatic hyperplasia (BPH). With the exception of alfuzosin, they all require dose titration when beginning therapy.

Alfuzosin is used primarily to treat symptoms of BPH. It is given cautiously to patients with hepatic dysfunction and is metabolized mainly by the P-450 system. It is also given cautiously to patients with pre-existing cardiac disorders because it may prolong the QT interval. Alfuzosin is the least likely of the alpha blockers to cause ejaculatory problems. It should be given with food. Doxazosin is also used in the management of hypertension as well as the treatment of BPH symptoms and CHF. Doxazosin, like prazosin, may also induce first-dose syncope. It is used cautiously in patients with hepatic dysfunction.

Tamsulosin is a once-a-day capsule that should be taken with a meal. The nurse teaches the patient not to open, crush, or chew the capsule, to maintain its prolonged action. Tamsulosin causes less hypotension than other alpha blockers and may be given concurrently with antihypertensive agents. Additionally, tamsulosin is the alpha blocker most likely to cause ejaculatory problems.

Terazosin is another alpha blocker that may cause first-dose syncope. It also alters lipid metabolism, decreasing the levels of total cholesterol, low-density lipoprotein (LDL) cholesterol, and very-low-density lipoprotein (VLDL) cholesterol. Terazosin is also used in the management of hypertension.

Drugs Significantly Different From P Prazosin

Phentolamine

Unlike prazosin, phentolamine (Regitine, Oraverse) blocks both alpha-1 and alpha-2 receptors. It is used in the management of tissue necrosis caused by extravasation of parenterally administered alpha-adrenergic (e.g., epinephrine) drugs and in the management of symptoms from a pheochromocytoma, an adrenaline-secreting tumor of the adrenal gland that causes severe hypertension. Phentolamine may induce adverse effects similar to those of prazosin, but it is more likely to cause reflex tachycardia because of its ability to block alpha-2.

Phentolamine is contraindicated in patients with a known hypersensitivity or renal impairment. It is also contraindicated for use in patients with a history of acute myocardial infarction or any evidence of coronary artery disease because of its cardiac-stimulating effects and resultant increase in myocardial oxygen demand. Also, reflex tachycardia can exacerbate angina. Phentolamine is used with caution in patients with gastric and duodenal ulcers because the drug has a histamine-like effect. Phentolamine can stimulate secretion of gastric acid and pepsin in the stomach, which can aggravate peptic ulcer disease.

Phentolamine should not be used in conjunction with epinephrine. Phentolamine can antagonize epinephrine's alpha receptor–mediated actions and exaggerate its beta-adrenergic responses, resulting in hypotension, vasodilation, and tachycardia. Potential adverse reactions are similar to those of prazosin.

Phenoxybenzamine

Like phentolamine, phenoxybenzamine (Dibenzyline) blocks both alpha-1 and alpha-2 receptors. Its approved use is for the treatment of sweating and hypertension associated with pheochromocytoma. It has additional off-label uses for treatment of urinary symptoms associated with BPH, neurogenic bladder, and functional outlet obstruction and hypertensive crises brought on by sympathomimetic amines. The effects of phenoxybenzamine are similar to those of phentolamine. Phenoxybenzamine has a slower onset of action and a longer duration of action than phentolamine—its effects begin several hours after administration, and the effects of a single dose may last 3 to 4 days.

• C BETA-ADRENERGIC ANTAGONISTS

Beta-adrenergic antagonists are frequently and more commonly called beta blockers. They comprise a significant group of drugs that can be grouped according to their specificity of action at the beta-1 and beta-2 receptors. If the predominant actions of stimulation of each of the two groups of beta-adrenergic receptors are considered, it follows that sometimes a therapeutic effect will require stimulation of beta-1 only (tachycardia, increased lipolysis, inotropy) or sometimes of both beta-1 and beta-2 receptors (vasodilation, decreased peripheral resistance, bronchodilation). Metoprolol (Lopressor, Toprol XL) is the prototype nonselective beta blocker.

Nursing Management of the Patient Receiving P Metoprolol

Core Drug Knowledge
Pharmacotherapeutics
Metoprolol is approved for the treatment of hypertension, angina, and controlled congestive heart failure. (For a complete discussion of beta-blocker therapy in heart failure, see Chapter 29). It is also used to treat irregular cardiac rhythms. It is used after myocardial infarction. It has been used to treat essential tremor when first-line medications are not effective (Lyons & Pahwa, 2008). Metoprolol also is used for the prevention of migraines (Schellenberg, Lichtenthal, Wohling, Graf, & Brixius, 2008),

Pharmacokinetics
Metoprolol is well absorbed following oral administration, and peak serum levels are observed within 1.5 to 4 hours of ingestion; however, hypotensive stability may not occur for 2 to 3 weeks. Beta blockade may occur within 1 to 2 hours. Parenteral dosing speeds the onset and lowers the duration. Much of an ingested dose is subjected to first-pass metabolism in the liver. Metabolites are excreted through urine. Metoprolol crosses the placenta and is excreted into breast milk. It has a half-life of 3 to 8 hours.

Pharmacodynamics
Metoprolol is a relatively selective beta-blocking drug that is selectively active on beta-1 (cardiac) receptors. It may also block beta-2 (bronchial, vascular smooth muscle) receptors at higher doses (greater than 100 mg). Some patients are more sensitive to these effects than other patients. Beta-1 blockade decreases heart rate and myocardial contractility during periods of high sympathetic activity (such as during physical exercise), which results in decreased cardiac output. As cardiac output decreases, so does blood pressure. In cardiac conduction tissue, beta blockade results in slowing of atrioventricular conduction and suppression

of automaticity. These actions result in decreased oxygen demand, thus suggesting its use as an antianginal agent. As metoprolol decreases cardiac output, it may seem contradictory for it to be used in heart failure, where typically the left ventricle does not have the normal ejection fraction. However, the slower heart rate means that the heart does not have to work as hard, and this has benefits for an overstressed heart in heart failure.

Contraindications and Precautions
Metoprolol carries a black box warning that abrupt cessation of therapy will cause an exacerbation of angina and in some patients a myocardial infarction has occurred. This black box warning is similar to other beta blockers.

The main contraindications for metoprolol are related to pre-exisiting cardiac problems. These include severe bradycardia, complete heart block, cardiogenic shock, uncompensated cardiac failure, sick sinus syndrome (unless using a pacemaker), severe peripheral arterial disease, hypersensitivity, and pheochromocytoma. The action of metoprolol depresses conduction through the atrioventricular node and decreases contractility. These actions can exacerbate cardiac disorders. In Raynaud disease, symptoms can be exacerbated secondary to a reduced cardiac output and a relatively increased alpha stimulation. Beta blockers like metoprolol have been associated with major depression, although the mechanism is unclear. Abrupt discontinuation of metoprolol in patients with hyperthyroidism may induce a thyroid storm.

Metoprolol must be used cautiously if the patient has a history of narrowed airway or bronchospastic disease such as asthma as the beta-2 blockade (although limited) may exacerbate this problem. Caution is used in patients with pheochromocytoma and vasospastic angina because unopposed alpha stimulation may result in paradoxical hypertension. Metoprolol is used cautiously in patients with diabetes because beta blockade can mask the signs of hypoglycemia, especially palpitations, tachycardia, and tremors. Patients receiving metoprolol during surgery are monitored closely because of the cardiodepressant effects prevents the heart from responding to adrenergic stimulation from situations that require an increase in heart rate such as blood loss. Patients also require cautious use of metoprolol if they receive calcium channel blocking drugs. Patients with renal and hepatic diseases also require close monitoring to ensure clearance of the drug from the body.

Adverse Effects
If metoprolol or a similar beta blocker is withdrawn abruptly, severe hypertension, angina, myocardial ischemia, infarction, or ventricular arrhythmias may occur. Other common adverse effects are hypotension, bradycardia, heart block, pruritus, rash, diarrhea, dizziness, fatigue, headache, depression, and dyspnea. Major adverse effects include bronchospasm and cardiac complications. Respiratory complications are not as common with metoprolol as with nonspecific beta

blockers but are still possible. In the CNS, metoprolol may cause cognitive dysfunction or depression. Hallucinations and psychosis have been reported with high doses of the drug. These CNS effects are seen more frequently in elderly patients and resolve after discontinuation. The drug predisposes patients with type 1 diabetes to hypoglycemia and may trigger hyperthyroidism in susceptible individuals. In the GI system, diarrhea is common and may be severe enough to require discontinuation of the drug. Sexual dysfunction is possible but not as common in metoprolol as it is in non-selective beta blockers such as propranolol.

Drug Interactions
Beta antagonists have many interactions with other drugs. Some of the more significant interactions include those with clonidine, epinephrine, verapamil, aminophylline, barbiturates, phenothiazines, cimetidine, ergot derivatives, hydralazine, NSAIDs, insulin, lidocaine, prazosin, quinidine, and rifampin (Table 13.9).

Assessment of Relevant Core Patient Variables
Health Status
Assess for conditions for which the drug is contraindicated or for which special precautions might be necessary (e.g., uncontrolled asthma or chronic obstructive lung disease, severe sinus bradycardia, right ventricular hypertrophy or failure secondary to pulmonary hypertension, second- or third-degree atrioventricular block, cardiac failure, or cardiogenic shock). It is also important to determine whether any other drugs are being taken concurrently to identify significant potential drug interactions.

Because metoprolol is used mainly to treat angina, hypertension, CHF, cardiac arrhythmias, and migraine headaches, the physical assessment includes blood pressure, cardiovascular status, genitourinary function, and mental and neurologic status. Heart and lung sounds are auscultated as well.

Life Span and Gender
Document the age and gender of the patient and assess women of childbearing age for pregnancy and lactation. If the patient is pregnant, metoprolol is administered only if necessary. This drug is classified as FDA pregnancy risk category C, and the possibility of inducing fetal abnormalities is not established. Although metoprolol is excreted in breast milk, there have been no reports of adverse effects on infants; metoprolol is considered compatible with breast feeding. Elderly patients may be at risk for injury resulting from blurred vision related to metoprolol use.

Lifestyle, Diet, and Habits
Document the patient's occupation and daily activities. Advise patients, particularly those in hazardous occupations, to exercise caution when driving or operating machinery until the effects of the drug are known, as the drug

may cause dizziness or drowsiness. Blurred vision also is possible.

Environment
Be aware of the environment in which the drug will be administered and assess the home or living environment, if appropriate. Metoprolol may be administered in any setting by health care providers, nurses, or patients themselves.

Nursing Diagnoses and Outcomes
• Risk for Ineffective Tissue Perfusion related to hypotension, bradycardia, or decreased cardiac output
Desired Outcome: The patient will maintain adequate tissue perfusion throughout therapy.
• Risk for Injury related to dizziness secondary to beta blockade
Desired outcome: The patient will not sustain injury and will learn safe methods for dealing with dizziness and postural hypotension.
• Disturbed Sleep Pattern, Insomnia and Drowsiness, secondary to beta blockade
Desired outcome: The patient will sleep normally and awaken rested.
• Activity Intolerance related to lethargy and weakness secondary to beta blockade
Desired outcome: The patient will maintain a satisfactory activity level.
• Risk for Fluid Volume excess related to decreased cardiac output
Desired outcome: The patient with chronic heart failure will not develop worsening of symptoms while on metoprolol.

Planning and Intervention
Maximizing Therapeutic Effects
Instruct the patient to take metoprolol exactly as prescribed and at the required dosage frequency to enhance the therapeutic potential. Advise patients taking metoprolol in sustained-release form to swallow the whole drug and not to chew, crush, or break it. Patients may also take the drug with food to increase the drug's bioavailability and to avoid possible GI upset (e.g., diarrhea).

Inform patients about what to do if they miss a dose. If the next dose is more than 4 hours away (8 hours for sustained-release forms), the patient is advised to take the missed dose as soon as possible. If the next dose is scheduled to occur within the next 4 hours (8 hours for sustained-release forms), the patient should skip the missed dose and return to the regular schedule.

Minimizing Adverse Effects
• Metoprolol should not be used during acute exacerbation of CHF. Until the patient's heart failure is stabilized the drug should be withheld; contact the physician or nurse practitioner if a patient is admitted to the hospital with

TABLE 13.9	Agents That Interact with P Metoprolol	
Interactants	**Effect and Significance**	**Nursing Management**
alcohol	Decreased absorption and increased elimination of metoprolol, resulting in tachycardia and possible increase in hypertension	Advise patient to avoid ethanol. Monitor blood pressure and heart rhythm.
aminophylline	Reduced elimination of theophylline	Monitor for signs and symptoms of theophylline toxicity.
barbiturates	Decreased metoprolol levels resulting from barbiturate induction	Monitor for increased blood pressure. Monitor respiration.
cimetidine	May increase metoprolol level twofold	Monitor cardiac function carefully (i.e., blood pressure, heart rate), and lower dosage of metoprolol as prescribed.
clonidine	Life-threatening increases in blood pressure after discontinuation of clonidine therapy	When clonidine is to be withdrawn from concomitant therapy with a beta blocker, discontinue the beta blocker first, and monitor blood pressure carefully.
epinephrine	Initial hypertension followed by bradycardia	Consult with prescriber: Labetalol (alpha/beta blocker) or alpha blockers (e.g., prazosin, doxazosin) may prevent rebound hypertension.
ergot derivatives	Peripheral ischemia and cold extremities	If used together, monitor for peripheral ischemic effects (i.e., cold extremities), and substitute a selective beta blocker (e.g., atenolol) if ischemia occurs.
hydralazine	Increased levels of both drugs	If concurrent therapy is required, administer with food or switch to a sustained-release beta blocker. Monitor blood pressure carefully.
insulin	Prolonged hypoglycemia with masking of symptoms	Monitor blood glucose level regularly. Anticipate adjustment in drug dosages. Consult prescriber about lowering metoprolol dosage, and monitor impact on blood glucose level.
lidocaine	Increased, potentially toxic lidocaine level	Consult prescriber about lower lidocaine dosage. Monitor for enhanced inotropic effect of metoprolol.
nonsteroidal anti-inflammatory drugs	Decreased metoprolol level	Monitor blood pressure.
phenothiazines	Increased levels of both drugs; phenothiazines inhibit first-pass metabolism of metoprolol	Administer concomitant therapy with caution. Monitor phenothiazine level, and decrease dosage if prescribed.
prazosin	Increased postural hypotension from prazosin	Monitor blood pressure. Caution patient to rise slowly from seated position and use hand railings, particularly on stairs.
quinidine	Moderate increase in drug levels	Use caution with concomitant administration. Monitor for hypotension, bradycardia, arrhythmias, and heart failure.
rifampin	Rifampin-induced enzymes that decrease beta blocker levels by increasing metabolism and clearance	If concurrent therapy is required, monitor blood pressure carefully. A higher dose of metoprolol may be required in patients receiving rifampin for longer than 1 to 2 wk. Or the prescriber may substitute atenolol or nadolol for metoprolol.
verapamil	Increased hypotensive effects of both drugs	Monitor blood pressure carefully for serious hypotension.

acute uncompensated CHF and the metoprolol is not temporarily stopped.

- Check the apical and peripheral pulses before giving metoprolol. If the pulse is irregular or if there is bradycardia, withhold the drug and notify the prescriber because signs may be early indications of adverse or cardiotoxic effects.
- Monitor for peripheral edema or weight gain as these may indicate worsening of heart failure from the metoprolol.
- Monitor blood pressure, pulmonary wedge pressure, and cardiac rhythm and conduction (by ECG), particularly when adrenergic antagonists such as metoprolol are administered intravenously, because altered cardiac output may result from adrenergic blockade.
- In patients with impaired renal or hepatic function, monitor for signs of drug accumulation and potential toxicity.

Providing Patient and Family Education

- Sympatholytic drugs interfere with compensatory and homeostatic mechanisms regulated by the normal functioning of the SNS, particularly in response to stress. Therefore, it is crucial to identify and monitor environmental stressors for patients receiving adrenergic antagonists, such as metoprolol.
- Careful teaching about adverse effects is important. This includes teaching patients how to take their own pulses and detect irregular rhythms or bradycardias, to monitor for worsening of CHF, and to monitor for depression.
- Promote therapeutic adherence by reminding patients and their family members that drug therapy is meant to control certain life-threatening or debilitating conditions and should be continued even when the patient is feeling well and has no symptoms.
- If drug therapy is being discontinued, stress tapering or gradual withdrawal to prevent rebound symptoms and to adjust the activity levels to suit the reduced blockade.
- As another safety factor, teach the patient to change position slowly to reduce dizziness and light-headedness and to avoid operating machinery or driving until full adaptation to side effects has occurred. Factors known to enhance postural hypotension (e.g., heat, exercise, and alcohol consumption) should be avoided.

Ongoing Assessment and Evaluation

The same assessment focus is used for adrenergic antagonists as for the adrenergic agonists. All patients with cardiovascular disorders are considered worthy of extra attention when taking an adrenergic antagonist such as metoprolol. When evaluating the success of nursing management in metoprolol therapy, anticipate the absence of signs and symptoms for the condition being treated, as well as minimal adverse effects.

If metoprolol is being given for angina or hypertension, blood pressure should be within normal limits, the frequency of anginal attacks should be reduced, and there should be tolerance to reasonable activity. Moreover, the patient should be free from injury resulting from postural hypotension or dizziness. If metoprolol is used in chronic heart failure then the patient should have a decrease in symptoms. For antiarrhythmic indications, no arrhythmias should be evident on ECG findings. The patient may report sexual adjustment. Ideally, the patient and family can understand, recognize, and cope with adverse effects.

Drugs Closely Related to Metoprolol

Beta-1 selective drugs include acebutolol (Sectral), atenolol (Tenormin), betaxolol (Betoptic), bisoprolol (Zebeta), and esmolol (Brevibloc). These drugs are used to manage angina, hypertension, and chronic heart failure. Acebutolol and esmolol are also used in the management of cardiac arrhythmias. Esmolol is used post-acute MI and prior to rapid sequence intubation.

Nonselective beta-1 antagonists include propranolol (Inderal), metipranolol (OptiPranolol), nadolol (Corgard), penbutolol (Levator), pindolol (Visken), and timolol (Blocadren). These drugs have the same core drug knowledge and core patient variables as metoprolol. Pindolol is used in the management of hyperthyroidism. Nadolol is also used for GI hemorrhage, hyperthyroidism, migraine headaches, and cardiac arrhythmias. Metipranolol and timolol

---

MEMORY CHIP

P Metoprolol

- Selective Beta-2 blocker
- Treats hypertension, angina, chronic heart failure, cardiac arrhythmias, post-MI
- Decreases heart rate and contractility, slows conduction, suppresses automaticity
- Major contraindications: cardiovascular abnormalities (e.g., bradycardia, complete heart block, cardiogenic shock, uncompensated cardiac failure).
- Most common adverse effects: cardiac (hypotension, bradycardia, heart block, worsening of heart failure), depression
- Most serious adverse effect: heart block, bronchoconstriction/bronchospasm
- Maximizing therapeutic effects: Take the medication exactly as prescribed, never double a dose.
- Minimizing adverse effects: Assess pulse and blood pressure before giving a dose; assess for weight increases and fluid retention
- Most important patient education: to never abruptly stop taking the medication; how to check their own pulse and blood pressure; to monitor for weight gain or swelling in extremities, or worsening of CHF symptoms (if have CHF)
- **Black box warning: Suddenly stopping metaprolol can exacerbate angina and may lead to myocardial infarction.**

CRITICAL THINKING SCENARIO

THINKING CRITICALLY ABOUT BETA-BLOCKER THERAPY

Mr. DiGiovanni is a 65-year-old man with hypertension and angina. He was recently ill with a GI virus and had vomiting and diarrhea for 3 days. During this time he did not eat much and did not take his prescribed metoprolol as he could keep nothing down. He develops chest pain and is taken to the emergency room, where his vital signs are 98-118-22, 150/90.

1. What do you think has caused him to have chest pain, tachycardia, and hypertension?

2. Mr DiGiovanni is admitted, treated, and stabilized. What discharge teaching will he need related to his metoprolol therapy?

are used to manage ocular hypertension and glaucoma. Timolol is also used for post–myocardial infarction (MI) syndrome and supraventricular arrhythmias. Propranolol's uses are similar to metoprolol. These drugs also stimulate beta-2 receptors so there are respiratory effects which may be problematic for those with respiratory conditions such as asthma or COPD.

Drugs Significantly Different From
P Metoprolol
Carvedilol

Carvedilol (Coreg) is a combined alpha selective and nonselective beta blocker. Although it has some pharmacologic similarities to labetalol, the ratio of beta-1 to alpha-1 effects is much greater for carvedilol than for labetalol. Carvedilol also possesses antioxidant properties (an effect not shared by other beta blockers). Carvedilol has multiple actions that make it a useful cardiovascular drug. Similarly to labetalol, carvedilol antagonizes both alpha-1 and beta receptors. However, the ratio of beta blockade to alpha-1 blockade for carvedilol is in the range of 10:1 to 100:1. The ratio for labetalol is 1.5:1. Carvedilol is indicated for the management of hypertension, heart failure, and stable angina and as post–myocardial infarction prophylaxis. It is frequently administered with other antihypertensive agents to gain additive therapeutic effects.

When carvedilol therapy is initiated, the patient should have a standing blood pressure measurement 1 hour after dosing. An initial dose of 6.25 mg should be maintained for 7 to 14 days; then, the patient should be evaluated for the effectiveness of the dose. If further control of diastolic blood pressure is needed, the dosage may be increased to 12.5 mg orally twice daily for an additional 7 to 14 days. If needed, the dosage may be further increased to the maximum recommended dosage of 25 mg orally twice daily if tolerated. If the pulse rate drops below 55 bpm, the dosage of carvedilol should be reduced. Doses should be taken with food to slow the rate of absorption and reduce the risk for orthostatic hypotension.

Labetalol

Labetalol (Normodyne) is a competitive nonselective beta-adrenergic and selective postsynaptic alpha-1 adrenergic receptor blocker that can be given orally and parenterally. Labetalol blocks beta-1 receptors in the heart, beta-2 receptors in bronchial and vascular smooth muscle, and alpha-1 receptors in vascular smooth muscle. The beta-blocking activity is three to seven times as potent as the alpha-blocking ability. The result of labetalol's actions at alpha and beta receptors leads to vasodilation and decreased total peripheral resistance, which results in decreased blood pressure without a substantial decrease in resting heart rate, cardiac output, or stroke volume.

Sotalol

Sotalol (Betapace) is an oral, nonselective beta-adrenergic blocking agent. Unlike other beta blockers, sotalol has no sympathomimetic activity or membrane-stabilizing effects but does possess class III antiarrhythmic properties similar to those of amiodarone. As a result, sotalol is used as an antiarrhythmic. It is primarily used in the management of atrial fibrillation or flutter, ventricular arrhythmias, and angina.

CHAPTER SUMMARY

- Regulation of physiologic processes in the autonomic nervous system (ANS) is managed by oppositional or complementary stimulation by the sympathetic (adrenergic) and parasympathetic (cholinergic) nervous systems.
- To effect an action, a neurotransmitter needs to bind with an appropriate receptor site on the effector organ or tissue.
- The primary neurotransmitter of the SNS is norepenephrine (NE). Additionally, epinephrine and dopamine stimulate adrenergic receptors.
- The sympathetic nervous system (SNS), commonly referred to as the fight-or-flight system, increases cardiovascular and respiratory function, increases metabolism, diverts blood to muscles, and decreases GI activity.
- SNS receptors with pharmacological relevance are subdivided into alpha-1, alpha-2, beta-1, and beta-2 subtypes. Alpha-1, beta-1, and beta-2 receptors are located on the post-synaptic side of the synapse, while alpha-2 receptors are located on the pre-synaptic side of the synapse. Stimulation of alpha-2 receptors acts as a negative feedback and shuts off the flow of NE, stopping sympathetic stimulation.
- Adrenergic agonists stimulate the adrenergic receptors, whereas adrenergic antagonists block adrenergic receptors within the SNS, preventing endogenous neurotransmitters from attaching to the receptor. There are multiple terms for these categories of drugs.
- Alpha-1 agonists, such as phenylephrine, stimulate alpha-1 receptors directly. They are most commonly used as nasal

decongestants and in ophthalmology to achieve mydriasis. They may also be used as vasopressors to treat vascular failure and related shock.

- Alpha-2 agonists such as clonidine shut off the sympathetic release of NE and sympathetic stimulation. They are used in the treatment of substance abuse to prevent withdrawal symptoms and have a minor use in the treatment of hypertension.
- Nonselective adrenergic agonists, such as epinephrine, are used to treat anaphylactic shock, asthma, hemorrhage, and ventricular fibrillation. The nonselective activity stimulates all four adrenergic subtypes.
- Dopamine, a vasopressor, is used to correct the hemodynamic imbalances present in shock. Dopamine is a naturally occurring catecholamine and a precursor to norepinephrine. It stimulates alpha and beta receptors directly and indirectly (by releasing the stored epinephrine). It also has dopaminergic effects, including increased renal perfusion, increased cardiac output, increased or decreased peripheral resistance (depending on the dose), and increased blood pressure.
- Drugs that are relatively selective for beta-2 stimulation are used to treat asthma.
- Fenoldopam, a dopamine-1 agonist, is used in the management of acute hypertension for rapid reduction of blood pressure.
- Alpha-1 antagonists, such as prazosin, cause vasodilation and are used to treat hypertension and benign prostatic hyperplasia (BPH).
- Beta-blockers, such as metoprolol, are relatively selective for beta-1 receptors in the heart; in larger doses they also have effects on beta-2 receptors. They are used to treat hypertension, angina, controlled chronic heart failure, cardiac arrhythmias, hyperthyroidism, and migraine headache.

QUESTIONS FOR STUDY AND REVIEW

1. How do drugs that stimulate the SNS create their effect?
2. What happens when beta-1 receptors are blocked?
3. How is it possible that epinephrine creates both vasodilation and vasoconstriction?
4. Why is dopamine dosage determined by urinary output and cardiovascular response?
5. How does prazosin decrease blood pressure?
6. How does phenylephrine create its desired effects?

NEED MORE HELP?

Chapter 13 of the Study Guide to Accompany *Drug Therapy in Nursing*, 4th Edition, contains NCLEX-style questions and other learning activities to reinforce your understanding of the concepts presented in this chapter. For additional information or to purchase the study guide, visit the Point.

REFERENCES

American Heart Association. (2005). Guidelines for cardiopulmonary resuscitation and emergency cardiovascular care. Dallas, TX: Author.

Coons, J. C., & Seidl, E. (2007). Cardiovascular pharmacotherapy update for the intensive care unit. *Critical Care Nurse Quarterly,* 30(1):44–57.

Drieghe, B., Manoharan, G., Heyndrickx, G. R., Madaric, J., Bartunek, J., Sarno, G., et al. (2008). Dopamine-induced changes in renal blood flow in normals and in patients with renal dysfunction. *Catheter cardiovascular interventions,* 72(5):725–730.

Drug Enforcement Administration (DEA), Department of Justice. (2008). Elimination of exemptions for chemical mixtures containing the list I chemicals ephedrine and/or pseudoephedrine. Final rule. *Federal Register,* 73(133):39611–39614.

Gueugniaud, P. Y., David, J. S., Chanzy, E., et al. (2008). Vasopressin and epinephrine vs. epinephrine alone in cardiopulmonary resuscitation. *New England Journal of Medicine,* 359(1):21–30.

Hatton, R. C., Winterstein, A. G., McKelvey, R. P., et al. (2007). Efficacy and safety of oral phenylephrine: systematic review and meta-analysis. *Annals of Pharmacotherapy,* 41(3):381–389.

Lyons, K. E., & Pahwa, R. (2008). Pharmacotherapy of essential tremor: an overview of existing and upcoming agents. *CNS Drugs,* 22(12):1037–1045.

Mentzelopoulos, S. D., Zakynthinos, S. G., Tzoufi, M., et al. (2009). Vasopressin, epinephrine, and corticosteroids for in-hospital cardiac arrest. *Archives of Internal Medicine,* 169(1):15–24.

Schellenberg, R., Lichtenthal, A., Wöhling, H., et al. (2008). Nebivolol and metoprolol for treating migraine: an advance on beta-blocker treatment? *Headache,* 48(1):118–125.

Sica, D. A. (2005). Alpha1-adrenergic blockers: current usage considerations. *The Journal of Clinical Hypertension,* 7(12):757–762.

Simmons, F. (2006). Anaphylaxis, killer allergy: long-term management in the community. *Journal of Allergy and Clinical Immunology,* 117(2):367–377.

Simmons, F. (2007). Anaphylaxis: evidence-based long-term risk reduction in the community. *Immunology & Allergy Clinics of North America,* 27(2):231.

Tatro, D. S. (2006). *Drug interaction facts.* Philadelphia, PA: Lippincott Williams & Wilkins.

Varon, J., & Marik, P. (2008). Perioperative hypertension management. *Vascular Health and Risk Management,* 4(3):615–627.

Weber, M. A. (2006). Hypertension treatment and implications of recent cardiovascular outcome trials. *Journal of Hypertension,* 24(Suppl 2):S37–S44.

Drugs Affecting Cholinergic Function

Learning Objectives

At the completion of this chapter the student will:

1. State the neurotransmitter that stimulates the parasympathetic nervous system.
2. Understand how cholinergic drugs create their therapeutic effects in the parasympathetic nervous system.
3. Differentiate cholinergic agonist from anticholinergic drugs.
4. Identify core drug knowledge about drugs that act as cholinergic agonists or anticholinergics.
5. Identify core patient variables relevant to drugs that act as agonists or anticholinergics.
6. Relate the interaction of core drug knowledge to core patient variables for drugs that act as cholinergic agonists or anticholinergics.
7. Generate a nursing plan of care from the interactions between core drug knowledge and core patient variables for drugs that act as cholinergic agonists or anticholinergics.
8. Describe nursing interventions to maximize therapeutic and minimize adverse affects for drugs that act as cholinergic agonists or anticholinergics.
9. Determine key points for patient and family education for drugs that act as cholinergic agonists or anticholinergics.

Key Terms

anticholinergic
autonomic nervous system
cholinergic agonists

cholinergic antagonists
cholinergic crisis
miosis

muscarinic receptor
nicotinic receptor
parasympathetic nervous system

Drugs Affecting Cholinergic Function

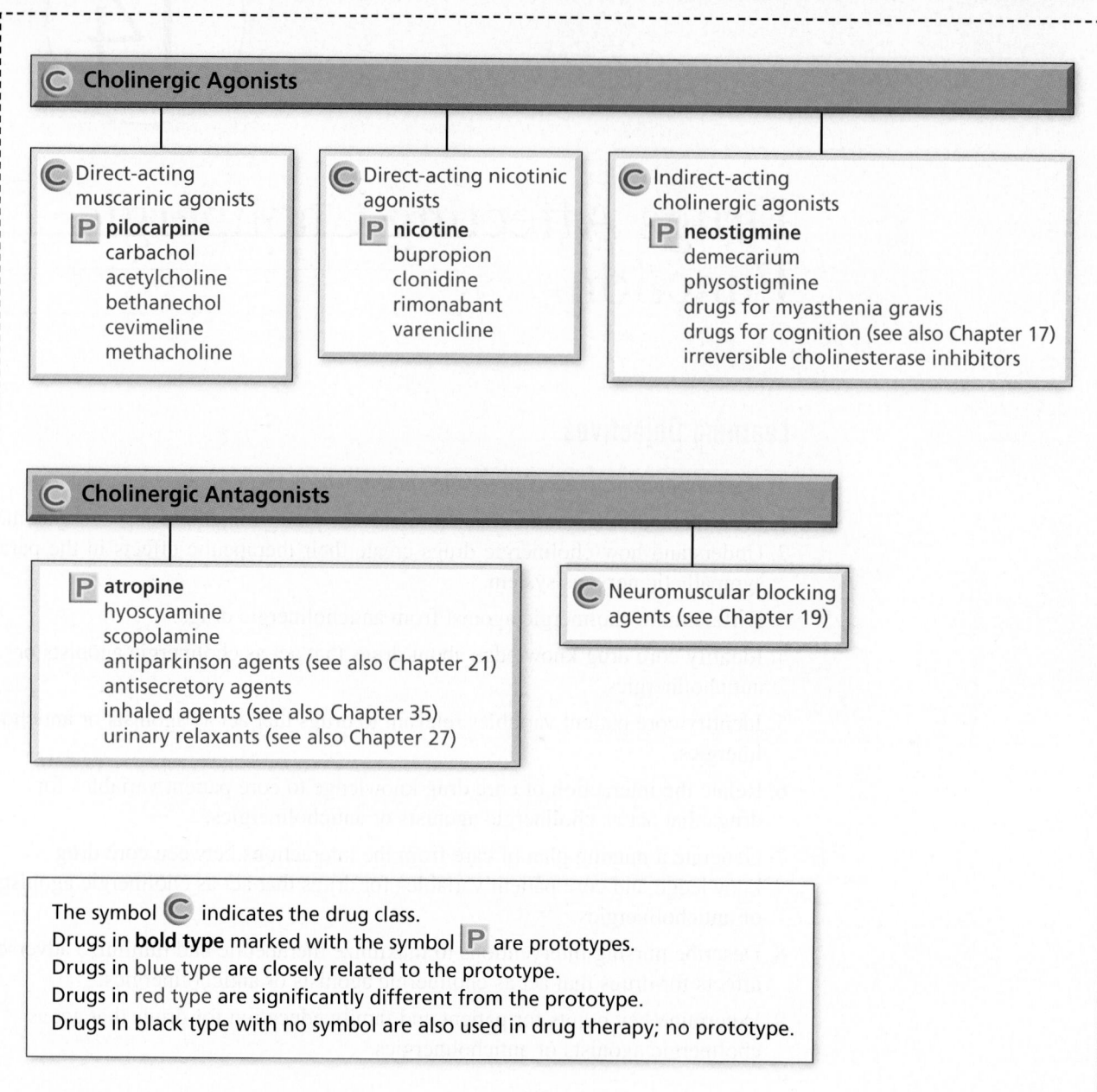

C Cholinergic Agonists

C Direct-acting muscarinic agonists
- **P** **pilocarpine**
  - carbachol
  - acetylcholine
  - bethanechol
  - cevimeline
  - methacholine

C Direct-acting nicotinic agonists
- **P** **nicotine**
  - bupropion
  - clonidine
  - rimonabant
  - varenicline

C Indirect-acting cholinergic agonists
- **P** **neostigmine**
  - demecarium
  - physostigmine
  - drugs for myasthenia gravis
  - drugs for cognition (see also Chapter 17)
  - irreversible cholinesterase inhibitors

C Cholinergic Antagonists

P **atropine**
- hyoscyamine
- scopolamine
- antiparkinson agents (see also Chapter 21)
- antisecretory agents
- inhaled agents (see also Chapter 35)
- urinary relaxants (see also Chapter 27)

C Neuromuscular blocking agents (see Chapter 19)

The symbol **C** indicates the drug class.
Drugs in **bold type** marked with the symbol **P** are prototypes.
Drugs in blue type are closely related to the prototype.
Drugs in red type are significantly different from the prototype.
Drugs in black type with no symbol are also used in drug therapy; no prototype.

As described in Chapter 13, the **autonomic nervous system** (ANS) is divided into the sympathetic (adrenergic) and parasympathetic (cholinergic) nervous systems. These systems work in combination or in opposition to maintain homeostasis within the body. As in the SNS, the PSNS effects occur in response to a neurotransmitter stimulating a receptor. Acetylcholine (ACh) is the neurotransmitter that produces parasympathetic effects. Because the receptor is stimulated by Ach, it is referred to as a cholinergic receptor. This chapter identifies drugs used to treat the major disorders that are affected by deficiencies or excesses in cholinergic neurotransmission. It also discusses the wide range of therapeutic uses of cholinergic drugs. This chapter presents the cholinergic drugs that are categorized into **cholinergic agonists** (i.e., they stimulate cholinergic receptors) and **cholinergic antagonists**, also known as anticholinergics (i.e., they block the cholinergic receptor and prevent ACh from attaching to the receptor).

The cholinergic drugs are also categorized by the type of cholinergic receptor they affect. For example, pilocarpine (Akarpine) is the prototype direct-acting muscarinic agonist, whereas nicotine (Nicotrol, ProStep) is the prototype direct-acting nicotinic agonist. Neostigmine (Prostigmin) is the prototype indirect-acting cholinergic agonist, also known as an anticholinesterase or cholinesterase inhibitor. The prototype representing the anticholinergics, is atropine (Atropine Sulfate).

PHYSIOLOGY

Function of the Autonomic Nervous System

As mentioned in Chapter 13, the autonomic nervous system is an involuntary system responsible for the control of smooth muscle, cardiac muscle, and exocrine glands. These regulatory functions of the body are monitored by both the **sympathetic nervous system** and the **parasympathetic nervous system.** The sympathetic and parasympathetic nervous systems work either as complementary or oppositional systems to maintain the involuntary functions of the body. Chapter 13 includes a discussion of synaptic transmission and regulation of physiologic processes; review that if necessary. The parasympathetic nervous system is sometimes referred to as the "rest and digest" system; it is responsible for normal physiological processes that are present when the SNS is not active. For example, stimulation of the PSNS receptors by ACh is responsible for increased salivation, increased GI tone and motility, and increased gastric secretions; all of these assist in the digestion of food. An acronym of SLUDD can be used help remember the functions of the PSNS (**S**alivation, **L**acrimation, **U**rination, **D**igestion, and **D**efecation). The PSNS regulates the body's visceral organs via the innervation of three kinds of tissues: smooth muscle, cardiac muscle, and glands. Although the stimulation of some of the muscarinic cholinergic receptors causes vasoconstriction, acetylcholine causes endothelial cells to produce nitric oxide, which diffuses to smooth muscle and results in vasodilation and perfusion of the organs.

Cholinergic Neurotransmitters

Cholinergic drugs act on the parasympathetic nervous system, one of the subdivisions of the ANS. Acetylcholine (ACh) is the presynaptic and postsynaptic neurotransmitter in the parasympathetic nervous system (see Figure 13.4). The precursors to ACh are choline and acetyl-coenzyme A. After formation and storage, ACh is released in response to an action potential, diffuses across the synaptic cleft, and binds to cholinergic receptors on the target organs or tissues. After dissociation, ACh is degraded into two inactive products, acetate and choline, by acetylcholinesterase (AChE) (Figure 14.1).

Cholinergic Receptors

There are three types of cholinergic receptors: nicotinic$_N$ (neuronal-type), nicotinic$_M$ (muscle-type), and muscarinic (Table 14.1).

Nicotinic Receptors

The **nicotinic receptors** (nicotinic$_N$ and nicotinic$_M$) are called *nicotinic* because they are stimulated primarily by nicotine, a plant alkaloid, but they will also respond to acetylcholine. They have a very low affinity for muscarine.

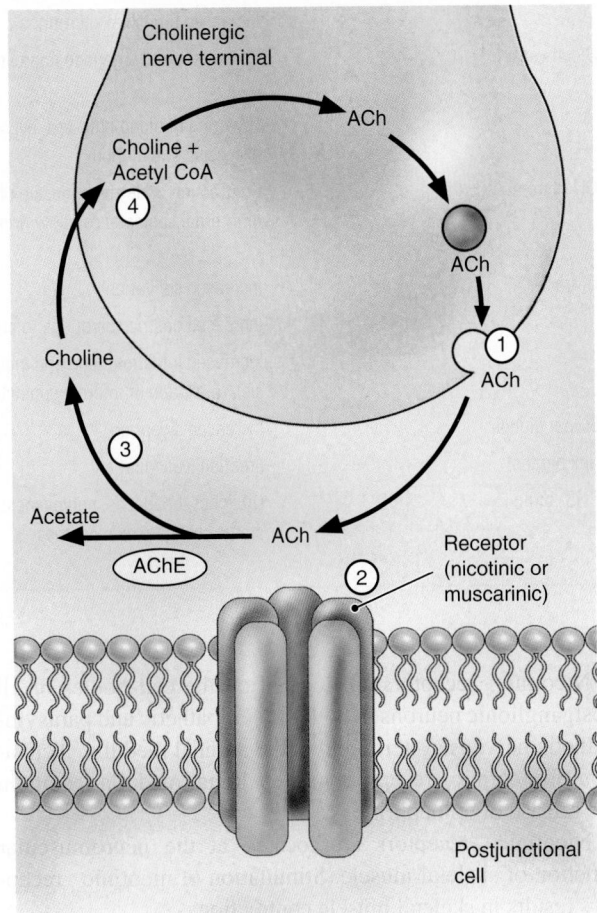

• FIGURE 14.1 Acetylcholine release and degradation. (1) Stored acetylcholine (ACh); (2) acetylcholine is released from the nerve terminal in response to an action potential and diffuses across the synaptic cleft; (3) binds to muscarinic or nicotinic receptor site to stimulate an action; and (4) is degraded by acetylcholinesterase into acetate and choline.

TABLE 14.1 Cholinergic Receptor Subtypes' Location and Action

Location	Response to Stimulation	Response to Blockade (all actions return the PSNS to baseline, they are NOT SNS effects)
Nicotinic$_N$		
All autonomic nervous system ganglia	Stimulation of sympathetic and parasympathetic *postganglionic* transmission	Prevents stimulation of sympathetic and parasympathetic *postganglionic* transmission
Adrenal medulla	Release of epinephrine	Prevents release of epinephrine
Nicotinic$_M$		
Neuromuscular junction	Contraction of skeletal muscle	Relaxation of skeletal muscle
Muscarinic		
Eye	Miosis (pupillary constriction)-poor night vision	Mydriasis (pupil dilation)-good night vision but decreased vision in daylight (photophobic)
	Improved accommodation	Decreased accommodation
Heart	Decreased rate	Increased rate
	Decreased force of contraction	Increased force of contraction
	Decreased speed of conduction	Increased speed of conduction
	All of these actions decrease cardiac output, contributing to a decrease in blood pressure	All of these lead to an increase in cardiac output and increase in blood pressure
Lung	Bronchoconstriction- difficulty breathing	Bronchodilation-improved ease of breathing
	Increased bronchial secretions	Decreased bronchial secretions
Blood vessels	Vasodilation to organs to improve perfusion and function	Vasodilation to peripheries and skin-causing flushed, red, warm skin
	Lowering of blood pressure, hypotension possible with excessive stimulation	Increase in blood pressure to baseline; hypertension possible with excessive blockade
GU system	Contraction of detrusor muscle of bladder and relaxation of internal sphincter to allow urination	Relaxation of detrusor muscle of bladder and Contraction of internal sphincter to prevent emptying the bladder Urinary retention
GI tract	Increased salivation	Dry mouth
	Increased gastric secretions to promote digestion	Decreased gastric secretions to prevent digestion
	Increased intestinal tone and motility (increased peristalsis), relaxation of internal sphincter to allow defecation	Decreased intestinal tone and motility leading to constipation
Sweat glands	Increased sweating	Decreased sweating
Sex organs	Erection (vasodilation)	Lack of erection, prevent sexual intercourse
CNS- brain	Dizziness, headache, nervousness, confusion, mental status changes, memory loss	Disorientation, agitation, anxiety, hallucination, delusions, delirium, psychosis, seizures, prolonged sedation, coma

Nicotinic$_N$ receptors are located on the cell bodies of all postganglionic neurons in both the sympathetic and parasympathetic nervous systems and in the adrenal medulla. Activation of nicotinic$_N$ receptors in the adrenal medulla results in the release of epinephrine.

Nicotinic$_M$ receptors are located at the neuromuscular junction of skeletal muscle. Stimulation of nicotinic$_M$ receptors results in skeletal muscle contraction.

Muscarinic Receptors

Muscarinic receptors respond to acetylcholine and also bind muscarine, an alkaloid substance isolated from mushrooms.

There are five subtypes of muscarinic receptors (M$_1$–M$_5$). They are located on postsynaptic cells regulated by the PSNS and on sweat glands. Of interest is the presence of muscarinic receptors on blood vessels; however, these receptors are not associated with the nervous system. Although their physiologic activation is unclear, their pharmacologic response is vasodilation, resulting in decreased blood pressure.

PATHOPHYSIOLOGY

The tissues and organs that are innervated by the ANS are diverse, and few discrete disorders are directly related to

TABLE 14.2	Parasympathetic Nervous System Terminology Synonyms	
Drugs That Stimulate Parasympathetic Receptors	**Drugs That Block Parasympathetic Receptors**	
Parasympathetic agonist = Parasympathomimetic = Cholinergic agonist = Cholinergic stimulant = Cholinomimetic	Parasympathetic antagonist = Parasympatholytic = Cholinergic antagonist = Cholinergic blocker = Anticholinergic	
Direct acting nicotinic agonists = ganglionic stimulating agents	Acetylcholinesterase = cholinesterase. indirect-acting cholinergic agonists = cholinesterase inhibitors = anticholinesterase agents	

compromise of the parasympathetic nervous system. Instead, the therapeutic uses of parasympathetic drugs are related to providing extra cholinergic stimulation or blockade of normal ANS functioning. Disorders of the bronchi, cardiovascular system, gastrointestinal or genitourinary tract, skeletal muscle, eyes, and various glands may respond to cholinergic stimulation through their muscarinic and nicotinic receptors.

Pharmacological Effects on the PSNS

How do drugs create their therapeutic effect in the PSNS? Similar to their action in the SNS, drugs create their therapeutic effects in the PSNS by stimulating cholinergic receptors or by blocking the receptor so that acetylcholine cannot attach to the receptor. So in order to understand how these drugs work, it is again necessary to first learn what happens when these receptors are stimulated or blocked. See Table 14.2 for help in learning these different effects. Students should then consider the prototype drugs listed in this chapter as examples of what happens with cholinergic stimulation or blockade. Cholinergic and anticholinergic drugs will be presented throughout the text, so understanding what happens at the receptor is crucial to building a knowledge of pharmacology. Students also should be aware that although the cholinergic receptors are technically divided into two subtypes, all of them will respond to ACh. Therefore, in practice these receptors often are just referred to as "cholinergic" and the drugs that effect them as "cholinergic" or "anticholinergic." As in the SNS, several words are used as synonyms related to the PSNS. For assistance in learning these terms, see Table 14.1. *Students must be careful not to think of drugs that produce PSNS blockade as being the same as drugs that cause SNS stimulation. Although there are similarities, this is not correct.* Instead, think of anticholinergic effects of drugs as returning the patient to the baseline so that the PSNS can be stimulated again.

Because the anticholinergic effects may be more familiar to students due to their presence in over-the-counter products, some students may wish to read this chapter "backwards," starting with the anticholinergics and then finishing with the cholinergics. However, conceptually for most students it is best to think of what happens with stimulation and then to consider blockade, so the drug prototypes are arranged in this manner.

C CHOLINERGIC AGONISTS

Cholinergic agonists include direct-acting muscarinic agonists, direct-acting nicotinic agonists, and indirect-acting cholinergic agonists (Table 14.3).

• C DIRECT-ACTING MUSCARINIC AGONISTS

Direct-acting muscarinic agonists are drugs that bind to the muscarinic receptors located in various tissues and organs throughout the body. Their activation elicits a response that resembles the action of the parasympathetic nervous system; therefore, they are also called parasympathomimetic agents. Although pilocarpine (Akarpine) has limited therapeutic scope, it is the ideal prototype for the direct-acting muscarinic agonists.

Nursing Management of the Patient Receiving P Pilocarpine
Core Drug Knowledge
Pharmacotherapeutics
Pilocarpine is a direct-acting cholinergic agonist with ophthalmic uses. The major indications for pilocarpine are open-angle glaucoma, acute treatment of angle-closure glaucoma, induction of **miosis** (pupillary constriction) to counteract mydriatic effects of sympathomimetics used in surgery, and miosis induction following ophthalmoscopy to counteract the effects of cycloplegics and mydriatics. Oral pilocarpine is used to treat xerostomia (dry mouth) caused by hypofunction of the salivary gland arising from radiotherapy for cancer of the head or neck.

Pharmacokinetics
Pilocarpine may be applied topically by solution or in an ocular system that allows sustained release over 7 days. With topical administration, miosis occurs within 10 to 30 minutes, and a maximal decrease in intraocular pressure occurs within 2 to 4 hours. When pilocarpine is given as an oral agent, peak effects are achieved in about 1 hour. Peak effects may take longer if the drug is taken with food. The mechanism for inactivation of pilocarpine is not clear but is thought to occur at the neuronal synapses and in plasma. Pilocarpine and its degradation products are excreted in the urine.

Pharmacodynamics
Pilocarpine directly stimulates cholinergic receptors. It produces miosis by contracting the iris sphincter. In open-angle glaucoma, pilocarpine contracts the ciliary muscle, increasing the outflow of aqueous humor, which reduces intraocular pressure. In closed-angle glaucoma, pilocarpine-induced miosis opens the angle of the anterior chamber of the eye, allowing the aqueous humor to exit. Pilocarpine also counteracts the mydriatic effects of sympathomimetic agents used in ophthalmologic examinations. When administered

TABLE 14.3 Summary of Selected C Cholinergic Agonists

Drug (Trade) Name	Selected Indications	Route and Dosage Range	Pharmacokinetics
C Direct-Acting Muscarinic Agonists			
P pilocarpine (Isopto Carpine, Pilopine HS, Salagen)	Dry mouth from chemotherapy Open-angle glaucoma, changes in intraocular pressure, reversal of mydriasis	*Adult:* PO, 5 mg tid for chemotherapy-induced dry mouth (xerostomia) *Adult:* intraocular, 1 drop of 1%–2% solution q6–8 h or 20–40 mg/h by intraocular delivery device (Ocusert)	*Onset:* 10–30 min *Duration:* 4–8 h $t_{1/2}$: 3/4–1–1/2 h
acetylcholine (Miochol-E)	Cataract extraction, iridectomy, iris incarceration, keratoplasties, ophthalmic surgery, peripheral iridectomy, parotitis, renal failure, respiratory distress syndrome	*Adult:* intraocular, 5–20 mg as 0.5–2.0 mL solution	*Onset:* 10–30 min *Duration:* 10 min $t_{1/2}$: Minutes
bethanechol (Urecholine)	Decompensated bladder, lower motor neuron lesions, neurogenic bladder, postpartum urinary retention, urinary retention, postoperative urinary retention, atonies, sexual dysfunction, bladder dysfunction, parotitis, motion sickness	*Adult:* PO, 10–50 mg tid or qid	*Onset:* 30–90 min *Duration:* 1–6 h $t_{1/2}$: Variable
carbachol (Isopto Carbachol, Miostat)	Glaucoma	*Adult:* topical, 2 drops of 0.75%–3.0% solution tid for glaucoma	*Onset:* 10–20 min *Duration:* 8 h $t_{1/2}$: Minutes
cevimeline (Evoxac)	Xerostomia associated with Sjögren's syndrome	*Adult:* PO, 30 mg	*Onset:* 60–90 min *Duration:* Unknown $t_{1/2}$: 5 h
methacholine (Provocholine)	Diagnosis of bronchial airway hyperactivity	Individualized	*Onset:* Rapid *Duration:* 15–75 m $t_{1/2}$: Unknown
C Direct-Acting Nicotinic Agonists			
P nicotine (Nicotrol, Commit, NicoDerm, Nicorette, Nicotrol)	Smoking cessation	*Adult:* PO, 2 mg chewing gum prn; transdermal, 5–22 mg daily depending on number of weeks without cigarettes	*Onset:* Transdermal 1–2 h *Duration:* 2–24 h $t_{1/2}$: 3–4 h
C Indirect-Acting Cholinergic Antagonists			
P neostigmine (Prostigmin)	Myasthenia gravis (MG) Neuromuscular blockade reversal Paralytic ileus and urinary retention	*Adult:* PO, 150 mg/d *Adult:* SC/IM, 0.5 mg *Adult:* 0.5 mg, then 0.5 mg q3h up to five times	*Onset:* PO, 2–4; SC/IM, 20–30 min; IV, 60 s *Duration:* PO, 2.5–4 h; IV 1–2 h $t_{1/2}$: 50–90 min
ambenonium (Mytelase)	MG, parotitis	*Adult:* PO, 5–25 mg tid or qid	*Onset:* 20–30 min *Duration:* 3–8 h $t_{1/2}$: Unknown
demecarium (Humorsol;)	Glaucoma	*Adult:* 1–2 gtt 1–2 × d *Child:* 1 gtt daily	*Onset:* less than or equal to 1 h *Duration:* 1 min $t_{1/2}$: Unknown
donepezil (Aricept)	Alzheimer Dementia	*Adult:* PO, 5–10 mg/d at bedtime	*Onset:* varies *Duration:* 2 wk $t_{1/2}$: 70 h
edrophonium (Tensilon, Enlon, Reversol)	Diagnosis of MG, differentiation between cholinergic and myasthenic crises, antagonism of neuromuscular blockade, parotitis, supraventricular tachycardia, Eaton-Lambert syndrome	*Adult:* IV, 1–10 mg depending on the indication; IM, 10 mg	*Onset:* IV, 30–60 s *Duration:* IV 5–10 min $t_{1/2}$: 5–10 min

TABLE 14.3	Summary of Selected © Cholinergic Agonists *(continued)*		
Drug (Trade) Name	**Selected Indications**	**Route and Dosage Range**	**Pharmacokinetics**
galantamine (Razadyne)	Alzheimer Dementia	*Adult:* PO, 16–24 mg/d	*Onset:* Varies *Duration:* 8 h $t_{1/2}$: 60–80 h
memantine (Namenda)	Alzheimer Dementia	*Adult:* PO, 5–20 mg/d in 2 divided doses	*Onset:* Varies *Duration:* Unknown $t_{1/2}$: 7 h
pralidoxime (Protopam)	Anticholinesterase or organophosphate poisoning	*Adult:* IV initially, 1–2 g/100 mL in normal saline solution over 30 min, then PO, 1–3 g repeated in 5 h	*Onset:* IV, rapid *Duration:* Not applicable $t_{1/2}$: 0.8–2.7 h
physostigmine (Antilirium, Isopto Eserine)	Alzheimer disease Antidote for anticholinergic overdose Glaucoma, parotitis, acute myelogenous leukemia, chronic pain	*Adult:* PO, 6–18 mg in four to nine divided doses daily *Adult:* IV, 2 mg slow push over 2 min or more *Adult:* 0.25% or 0.5%, 1 drop up to four times daily or 1 cm 0.25% ointment one to three times daily	*Onset:* IV, 3–5 min *Duration:* 30–60 min $t_{1/2}$: 15–40 min
pyridostigmine (Mestinon, Regonol)	Motion sickness MG Reversal of nondepolarizing neuromuscular blockade	*Adult:* PO, 30 mg tid *Adult:* PO, 600 mg paced throughout the day *Adult:* IV, 0.1–0.25 mg/kg	*Onset:* PO, 35–45 min; IV, 5 min *Duration:* 3–6 h $t_{1/2}$: 1.9–3.7 h
tacrine (Cognex)	Alzheimer disease, anticholinergic overdose	*Adult:* PO, 10 mg qid increasing by 40 mg/d every 6 wk; IV slow push, 0.25–0.5 mg/kg	*Onset:* Varies *Duration:* Unknown $t_{1/2}$: 2–4 h

orally, pilocarpine stimulates secretions of the exocrine glands. All secretory glands may be affected, with results including an increase in salivary flow.

Contraindications and Precautions

Some contraindications may not be applicable to ophthalmic use, and others are not applicable to oral use. Hypersensitivity is a contraindication regardless of the formulation utilized.

Ophthalmic pilocarpine is contraindicated for use in patients with a history of retinal detachment. Miotics can precipitate detachment of the retina, resulting in a sudden drop in intraocular pressure. Ophthalmic pilocarpine is also contraindicated for use in patients with acute iritis or other conditions that would be exacerbated by pupillary constriction.

Oral pilocarpine has more contraindications and precautions because of its systemic effects, specifically its ability to mimic the effects of the parasympathetic nervous system. For example, patients with asthma, chronic bronchitis, or chronic airway limitation may have exacerbations of these conditions because pilocarpine stimulates the mucous cells of the respiratory tract and increases bronchial smooth muscle tone and airway resistance. Pilocarpine causes contractions of the gallbladder or biliary smooth muscle, possibly resulting in biliary obstruction, cholangitis, or cholecystitis. Patients with cardiac disease may not be able to compensate for the transient changes in heart rhythm or hemodynamics caused by oral pilocarpine. Pilocarpine increases ureteral smooth muscle tone and may precipitate renal colic,

especially in patients with nephrolithiasis. Oral pilocarpine may induce dose-related central nervous system (CNS) effects that could exacerbate conditions of psychiatric disturbances or cognitive disturbances.

Pilocarpine is classified as a pregnancy category C drug. The oral dosage form should only be used in pregnant women if the benefits outweigh the risks to the fetus.

Finally, patients using ophthalmic or oral preparations of pilocarpine should be cautioned about nighttime driving, particularly the elderly and those with opaque lenses. Loss of visual acuity and accommodation is greater in poor light.

Adverse Effects

The ophthalmic adverse effects of pilocarpine include transient stinging and burning, tearing, and ciliary spasm. The ocular system (Ocusert) may cause conjunctival irritation. Systemic adverse effects include hypertension, tachycardia, bronchiolar spasm, pulmonary edema, salivation and sweating, and nausea and vomiting. CNS effects include dizziness, headache, nervousness, memory loss, and exacerbation of a current psychosis. When systemic effects occur with other cholinergic agonists, a **cholinergic crisis** may arise. Cholinergic crisis must be recognized quickly and managed effectively. It is caused by cholinergic toxicity and results in medullary paralysis (central respiratory paralysis), peripheral respiratory paralysis, excessive tracheobronchial and salivary secretions, bronchospasm, and laryngospasm. These effects may cause respiratory failure,

	TABLE 14.4 Agents That Interact with P Pilocarpine		
Interactant	Effect and Significance	Nursing Management
Cholinergic drugs	Enhanced cholinergic effect	Monitor increased and prolonged cholinergic stimulation.
Anticholinergic drugs	Decreased cholinergic effect	Keep in mind that a dosage adjustment may be needed.

which can be reversed with the maintenance of a patent airway. Muscle twitching, fasciculations, and paralysis may also occur. All symptoms of cholinergic crisis may be reversed with atropine, an anticholinergic drug.

Drug Interactions

There are no known important interactions between pilocarpine and other drugs, although other cholinergic agonists or blockers may enhance or antagonize its effects (Table 14.4).

Assessment of Relevant Core Patient Variables

Health Status

Cholinergic agonists such as pilocarpine do not have a wide range of therapeutic uses, but when they are used, they may cause systemic side effects and interact with preexisting disorders in life-threatening ways. A careful history and physical assessment will identify contraindications and precautions necessary for the person taking pilocarpine.

Determine whether the patient has uncontrolled asthma or acute iritis, which are contraindications to pilocarpine therapy. Assess patients for significant cardiovascular disease because they may be unable to compensate for transient changes in hemodynamics or rhythm induced by pilocarpine. Pilocarpine should be used cautiously in patients with chronic bronchitis or chronic airway limitation because it may increase airway resistance, bronchial smooth muscle tone, and bronchial secretions. Patients with a history of biliary disease or nephrolithiasis are also closely monitored.

Life Span and Gender

Document the age and gender of the patient and assess women of childbearing age for pregnancy and lactation. If the patient is pregnant, this drug should be used only if necessary because it is not known whether pilocarpine causes fetal abnormalities. If the patient is breast-feeding, the infant is monitored for cholinergic stimulation; if such stimulation occurs, the drug may need to be discontinued. Elderly patients may be at higher risk for injury because of blurred vision.

Lifestyle, Diet, and Habits

Document the patient's occupation and daily activities. Advise patients to exercise caution when driving or operating machinery at night or in low light because miosis compromises dark adaptation.

Environment

Be aware of the environment in which the drug will be administered and assess the home or living environment if appropriate. Pilocarpine may be administered in any setting by a health care provider, nurse, or the patient.

Nursing Diagnoses and Outcomes

- Risk for Injury related to blurred vision
  Desired outcome: The patient will remain free of injury.
- Disturbed Sensory Perception (Visual) secondary to instillation of topical miotic.
  Desired outcome: The patient will adapt to blurring and adapt activity accordingly.
- Acute Pain related to local corneal irritation by miotic instillate
  Desired outcome: The patient will remain free from irritation.

Planning and Intervention

Maximizing Therapeutic Effects

Because pilocarpine is usually instilled, demonstrate how to instill drops into the conjunctival sac. To obtain the optimal intraocular hypotensive effect using the Ocusert system, also demonstrate the placement and insertion of the system into the inferior conjunctival sac.

If both the solution and gel are used, the solution is applied first, and the gel is applied 5 minutes later. Following administration of the solution, finger pressure is applied on the lacrimal sac for 1 to 2 minutes.

Oral pilocarpine is administered at regular intervals throughout the day.

Minimizing Adverse Effects

As with all cholinergic agonists, the use of pilocarpine requires the availability of an antidote in case of systemic overdose or cholinergic crisis. Atropine is the usual agent for this purpose. For patients with known allergies or suspected hypersensitivity, life support measures must be available in case of bronchial spasm or allergic reactions. Systemic side effects include stimulation of sphincters, so that patients may need access to a bedpan or urinal.

Contact lenses should be removed before ophthalmic treatment. If pilocarpine drops are applied to the eyes when soft contact lenses are in place, the lenses can deteriorate or absorb the drug. It also is possible that hard contact lenses can cause corneal abrasion or roughening of the corneal surface. Corneal abrasion can increase systemic absorption, possibly causing toxicity.

Providing Patient and Family Education
• Caution patients about blurred vision and its hazards.
• Teach patients to recognize systemic adverse effects and how to manage them.
• Instruct patients using the Ocusert system on inserting and removing the ocular device safely and antiseptically.

Ongoing Assessment and Evaluation

During therapy, monitoring of therapeutic effects should reveal the decrease in frequency or severity of target symptoms or the resumption of the problem for which pilocarpine was prescribed. Nurses familiar with ophthalmic surgery and conditions are adept at continuous assessment and evaluation of changes in intraocular pressure. Moreover, they can use a tonometer to gauge substantial changes in intraocular pressure. Other evaluations include whether adverse side effects are effectively minimized.

Drug Closely Related to P Pilocarpine

Carbachol (Isopto Carbachol) is another topical miotic agent used in the management of glaucoma. It is administered as an ophthalmologic solution up to three times daily. Like pilocarpine, it works by direct stimulation of the muscarinic cholinergic receptors in the eye. Contraindications and adverse effects are similar to pilocarpine.

Drugs Significantly Different From P Pilocarpine

Acetylcholine

Acetylcholine (Miochol-E) is a topical miotic agent. As a drug, acetylcholine is limited to use in the management of

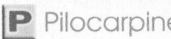 **MEMORY CHIP**

 Pilocarpine

• A direct-acting muscarinic agonist used for simple and acute glaucoma, preoperative and postoperative intraocular tension, mydriasis, and xerostomia
• Major contraindications (ophthalmic): hypersensitivity, history of retinal detachment, and acute iritis
• Major contraindications (oral): hypersensitivity, severe respiratory diseases
• Most common adverse effects: blurred vision, myopia
• Most serious adverse effects: cholinergic crisis, bronchospasm
• Maximizing therapeutic effects: Administer ophthalmic solution into the conjunctival cul-de-sac.
• 6Minimizing adverse effects: availability of antidote, aseptic technique for ophthalmic administration
• Most important patient education: symptoms of cholinergic crisis and need for immediate medical attention

ophthalmologic surgery. It produces complete miosis in cataract surgery, keratoplasty, iridectomy, and other anterior segment surgery in which rapid miosis is required. Because it is given topically, systemic adverse effects rarely occur. However, it may cause problems for patients with acute cardiac failure, bronchial asthma, peptic ulcer, hyperthyroidism, gastrointestinal spasms (cramps), urinary tract obstruction, or Parkinson disease. It is contraindicated for use in patients with acute iritis and acute inflammatory disease of the anterior chamber of the eye.

Bethanechol

Bethanechol (Urecholine) is an oral synthetic muscarinic stimulant with primary effects on the urinary and gastrointestinal tracts. Its effect on the bladder results from stimulation of muscarinic receptors in the detrusor muscle. As the detrusor contracts, the bladder capacity decreases, resulting in micturition. Bethanechol also stimulates ureteral peristalsis and relaxes the trigone and external sphincter. Because bethanechol is a direct-acting agonist, spinal cord injury does not compromise its actions. Stimulation of muscarinic receptors in the gastrointestinal tract restores peristalsis, increases motility, and increases the resting lower esophageal sphincter pressure. Bethanechol also stimulates the lower gastrointestinal tract, resulting in defecation. It is the preferred drug in the treatment of postpartum and postoperative nonobstructive urinary retention. It is also used in the management of urinary retention related to phenothiazine or tricyclic antidepressant therapy. Bethanechol may induce systemic adverse effects similar to those of pilocarpine. As with pilocarpine, drug interactions include other cholinergic or anticholinergic drugs. In addition, bethanechol in conjunction with ganglionic blocking agents may result in a critical decrease in blood pressure.

Cevimeline

Cevimeline (Evoxac) is a cholinergic agonist that is indicated for the treatment of symptoms of dry mouth in patients with Sjögren syndrome (Kruszka & O'Brian, 2009). It binds with muscarinic receptors and increases secretion of exocrine glands such as salivary and sweat glands. Cevimeline is contraindicated in patients with known hypersensitivity, uncontrolled asthma, acute iritis, or narrow-angle (angle-closure) glaucoma. It is used with caution in patients with cardiovascular or pulmonary diseases. Cevimeline can alter cardiac conduction or heart rate; therefore, patients with significant cardiovascular disease may be unable to compensate for transient changes in hemodynamics or rhythm. Also, cevimeline can increase airway resistance, bronchial smooth muscle tone, and bronchial secretions; hence, patients with asthma, chronic bronchitis, or chronic obstructive pulmonary disease should be closely monitored.

Methacholine

Methacholine (Provocholine) is a parasympathomimetic inhalation agent used to help diagnose bronchial airway hyperreactivity in patients who do not have clinically apparent asthma. Methacholine induces bronchoconstriction in asthmatic patients more readily than in nonasthmatic patients.

Contraindications and precautions include hypersensitivity to parasympathomimetic agents, concurrent beta-antagonist therapy, epilepsy, cardiovascular disease characterized by bradycardia, peptic ulcer disease, thyroid disease, urinary tract obstruction, and clinically apparent asthma, wheezing, or very low baseline pulmonary function test results.

Prior to administering methacholine to women of childbearing age, determine the patient's pregnancy status. Methacholine testing should be done within 10 days of the first day of menses or within 2 weeks following a negative pregnancy test result. Methacholine should not be administered to women who breast-feed because it is unknown whether the drug is excreted in breast milk. When given to patients receiving beta blockers, the effects of methacholine can be exaggerated or prolonged. Common adverse effects include headache, throat irritation, light-headedness, and pruritus. Because acute respiratory distress may occur, emergency equipment and medications should be at the bedside during this diagnostic test.

• Ⓒ DIRECT-ACTING NICOTINIC AGONISTS

The direct-acting nicotinic agonists are also called ganglionic stimulating agents. These drugs create their effect by attaching to the nicotinic receptor. The two significant classes of nicotinic stimulants are the ganglionic stimulants (e.g., nicotine) and the neuromuscular nicotinic stimulants that are discussed in Chapter 19.

Nicotine is the obvious selection as the direct-acting nicotinic receptor agonist prototype. Its pharmacological use is limited to products designed to help in the cessation of smoking tobacco. Non-pharmacologically it is used and abused in smoking and chewing tobacco.

Nursing Management of the Patient Receiving Ⓟ Nicotine

Core Drug Knowledge

Pharmacotherapeutics

Nicotine replacement is used as an adjunct to smoking cessation programs. Various formulations are available, such as gum, transdermal patches, and nasal spray. The nicotine gum and transdermal patches are available over the counter (OTC) in the United States. The patches are preferred for maintenance therapy during smoking cessation programs, unless the patient is allergic to the patches. Gum, nasal spray, or lozenges may be useful for episodic or bolus effects of nicotine and in institutional settings in which smoking is not allowed (Frishman, 2007).

Pharmacokinetics

When delivered as a chewing gum, nicotine is readily absorbed through the buccal mucosa when the gum is chewed. However, the amount of nicotine absorbed depends on how long the saliva remains in the mouth and by the pH. "A low pH suppresses the buccal absorption of nicotine" (Frishman, 2007). Very little nicotine is absorbed from the gastrointestinal tract because of extensive first-pass metabolism through the liver. Regular use of the gum provides steady-state blood levels of nicotine similar to those achieved by smokers. However, peak plasma levels occur much more slowly than when tobacco smoke is inhaled. Nicotine levels reach the brain within 7 seconds of a single puff on a cigarette, but peak concentrations of the gum can take 14 to 20 minutes; the transdermal patch can require as long as 4 hours to reach peak concentrations.

Nicotine is widely distributed in the body tissues, particularly the CNS. It crosses the placenta and is secreted in milk. The concentrations of nicotine in amniotic fluid and fetal serum exceed those in maternal serum. Detectable amounts also appear in the serum and urine of infants of nursing mothers who smoke.

Nicotine is metabolized in the liver by oxidation and excreted by the kidneys as unchanged nicotine and metabolites.

Pharmacodynamics

Nicotine is a potent ganglionic and CNS stimulant, with actions that are mediated through specific nicotine receptors. In small doses, it stimulates all autonomic ganglia; in larger doses, initial stimulation is followed by blockade. The dependency potential of nicotine is based mostly on its CNS stimulant effects (Fant, 2009).

Contraindications and Precautions

Nicotine in any dosage form should not be used in patients immediately after myocardial infarction, or in those with life-threatening arrhythmias or severe or worsening angina pectoris. It should not be used in patients who have allergies to any of the components of the delivery system, including gum, nasal spray, and transdermal patches. Smoking should be avoided during nicotine therapy because of the potential for overdose and toxicity (with manifestations including dizziness, nausea, and headache).

Adverse Effects

The adverse effects of nicotine in the cardiovascular system include peripheral vasoconstriction and tachycardia. In the CNS, the effects may include headache, paresthesias, fatigue, insomnia, nervousness, nausea, hot flashes, and nightmares. Diarrhea, dry mouth, nausea, and dyspepsia are adverse effects on the gastrointestinal system. Use of Nicotrol spray may cause nasal irritation, lacrimation, throat irritation, sneezing, and coughing. The transdermal patches may cause erythema, pruritus, edema, or rash at the site of administration.

The nicotine transdermal system and nasal spray are classified as FDA pregnancy category D, although the benefits of nicotine replacement therapy during pregnancy appear to outweigh the risks of continued smoking during pregnancy.

TABLE 14.5	Agents That Interact with Ⓟ Nicotine	
Interactants	**Effect and Significance**	**Nursing Management**
adenosine	Enhanced cardiovascular effects of adenosine	Advise patients undergoing stress tests to avoid chewing nicotine gum or reduce adenosine dosage to avoid angina.
lithium	Potentiates effects of nicotine	Monitor for increased effect.

Drug Interactions

Adenosine and lithium carbonate interact with nicotine (Table 14.5).

Assessment of Relevant Core Patient Variables

Health Status

A careful history and physical examination will identify contraindications and precautions pertaining to the person beginning nicotine replacement therapy. The patient's desire to cease smoking or the requirement not to smoke usually prompts nicotine replacement therapy. Before therapy begins, ensure that the patient has had neither a recent myocardial infarction nor symptoms of significant cardiovascular disease (e.g., arrhythmias and angina pectoris) because these conditions are contraindications to therapy. Before application of transdermal nicotine patches, skin test results should be reviewed to determine sensitivity to the drug.

Life Span and Gender

Document the age and gender of the patient and assess women of childbearing age for pregnancy and lactation. If the patient is pregnant, nicotine therapy should be used only if necessary—for example, in cases in which the benefits of smoking cessation are important. If the patient is breast-feeding, the infant should be monitored for respiratory or CNS stimulation. If such stimulation occurs, the timing of breast-feeding or the administration of the nicotine may need to be staggered to minimize adverse effects. Older adults undergoing nicotine therapy may be at increased risk for dizziness and sleep disturbances resulting from CNS stimulation.

Lifestyle, Diet, and Habits

Document the patient's occupation and daily activities. Advise patients not to smoke during nicotine therapy to avoid overdosage and adverse effects. Patients whose jobs require shift work should be aware that sleep disturbances may disrupt their rest. In addition, inspect the patient's oral cavity for dentures and other significant dental work. Nicotine gum is heavier and stickier than regular gum and may affect artificial teeth or other dental work.

Environment

Be aware of the environment in which the drug will be administered. Nicotine in any of its dosage forms may be administered in any setting by health care providers, nurses, or patients themselves.

Culture and Inherited Traits

Explore the patient's underlying cultural beliefs and values regarding smoking. In many cultural groups, such as Japanese American, Austrian, Polish immigrant, and highly acculturated Latino, smoking tobacco is popular and widely accepted. It is important to recognize that some patients may have more difficulty giving up smoking than others because of cultural influences.

Nursing Diagnoses and Outcomes

- Risk for Injury to mouth, teeth, or dental work related to gum viscosity, and sore throat or mouth related to use of the intranasal spray
  Desired outcome: *The patient will remain free of injury or problems related to adverse effects of therapy.*
- Disturbed Sleep Pattern related to drug-induced insomnia
  Desired outcome: *The patient will experience undisturbed sleep.*

Planning and Intervention

Maximizing Therapeutic Effects

The following nursing interventions may help to maximize the beneficial effects of nicotine therapy:

- Encourage the patient to adhere to the recommended dosage schedule because it is the one most likely to reduce craving.
- Encourage patients to avoid carbonated drinks, coffee, beer, wine, and other acidic drinks 15 minutes prior and during use of Nicorette gum or lozenge, as these may inhibit absorption (Frishman, 2007).
- Because nicotine replacement therapy is an adjunctive measure in smoking cessation programs, all other program measures are promoted and encouraged.
- Because craving is substantially increased when patients are exposed to others who smoke (promoting effects from secondary smoke inhalation, reinforcing old habits, and prompting recollection of pleasurable sociocultural influences), encourage the patient to minimize exposure to these influences initially.

Minimizing Adverse Effects

Overstimulation of the CNS may be counteracted by promoting good sleep hygiene and adjusting the dosage and timing of the last nicotine dose of the day. Other adverse effects may require the episodic use of analgesics for headaches.

Avoiding gastrointestinal effects requires good mouth care (particularly for the patient using nicotine gum) and possibly the use of antiemetics (for nausea) or antidiarrheals, as needed. For patients using the transdermal nicotine patches, good skin care and rotation of patch sites will help to minimize skin reactions. Upper respiratory tract effects may be counteracted with a room humidifier. Adverse effects that cannot be managed and that may be specific to the delivery system warrant a change to a different system on a trial basis.

Clinical research trials are exploring whether a vaccine could decrease cardiovascular risks from smoking. See Focus on Research, Box 14.1.

Providing Patient and Family Education

- Caution patients receiving nicotine replacement therapy about adverse effects and the possibility of overdosing with concomitant use of tobacco smoking during therapy.
- Watch the patient demonstrate the correct use of sprays or transdermal patches to ensure safe, optimal self-dosing.
- Instruct the patient on how to manage adverse effects and encourage the patient to contact the health care provider if self-management is ineffective or if serious or persistent adverse effects continue.
- If toxicity or overdosing is suspected, the therapy must be discontinued until the effects abate and then a decreased dosage or frequency of dosing can be reintroduced.
- Encourage the patient to avoid other stimulants during nicotine therapy, including caffeine-containing beverages, because they may lead to exaggerated CNS stimulation experienced as irritability and nervousness.
- Encourage patients to avoid carbonated drinks, coffee, beer, wine, and other acidic drinks 15 minutes prior and during use of Nicorette gum or lozenge, as these may inhibit absorption.
- Caution the patient and family to keep nicotine out of the reach of children.
- Incorporate all other smoking cessation program measures in the educational effort because replacement therapy is only a short-term adjunct measure.

BOX 14.1 FOCUS ON RESEARCH

Wagena, E.J., Vos, A., Horwith, G., et al. (2008). Immunogenicity and safety of a nicotine vaccine in smokers and nonsmokers: results of a randomized, placebo-controlled phase 1 / 2 trial I. *Nicotine & tobacco research: official journal of the Society for Research on Nicotine and Tobacco*, 10 (1):213–218.

Background
The Study

Can you prevent the adverse effects from smoking by administering a vaccine? As smoking is responsible for much morbidity and mortality in this county, researchers are trying to find a new way to help patients who smoke and have been examining the possibility of a vaccine that could be used. The idea was that after receiving a nicotine vaccine, the nicotine would be targeted as an antigen by the immune system of the patient. After vaccination, any subsequent exposures to nicotine should result in an immunologic response where by the patient's antibodies will bind with the nicotine molecule. Binding the nicotine in this way will prevent its passage through the blood–brain barrier and any physiologic response (both pleasurable and harmful) to the nicotine from taking place.

This purpose of this early-phase clinical trial was to determine if the vaccine would indeed alter the immune system. Thirty subjects were chosen, 21 of whom smoked at least 15 cigarettes per day and admitted to having no desire to quit smoking during the study. Smoking status of these 21 was confirmed as nicotine was found in their urine upon initial screening. The other 9 subjects chosen were ex-or nonsmokers. The 30 study participants were randomly assigned to either the placebo or the active group. Smokers and nonsmokers were randomized separately. This study did not include women of childbearing potential.

A single dose of 100 mcg of active vaccine (NicVAX) or an identical placebo was injected by the study nurses into the deltoid muscle of the participants. All participants received four immunizations of either the active vaccine or the placebo on day 0, 14, 28, and 182. The participants were required to return after each injection for assessment of their antibody assay and smoking status. Smoking status was assessed by performing an alveolar carbon monoxide test and a urinary nicotine test.

All participants in the active group showed significant levels of nicotine-specific antibodies after receiving the fourth injection, most showed significant levels of antibodies after three rounds of injections. No nicotine-specific antibody was found to be present in the placebo group after all four injections. Results also showed that the immunogenicity of the vaccine was not affected by the presence of nicotine at the time of the injections. The adverse effects most frequently reported by both the active and placebo groups were bad taste, dry mouth, and tenderness at the injection site. Weight gain was also a frequent adverse effect, but only in the active group. In conclusion, the study found that the vaccine was safe and effective in generating an immune response to nicotine molecules in the blood in both smokers as well as nonsmokers.

Nursing Implications

While these early clinical trials are promising, there is a great deal of research that still needs to be done to develop a nicotine vaccine, As many people complain of weight gain when they stop smoking, the weight gain by the vaccinated group appears to support the hypothesis that by developing antibodies to nicotine the patient does not have their nicotinic receptors simulated, much as if they were stopping smoking. Nurses should stay abreast of these research trials and the development of a vaccine. If a vaccine could be developed, it would be very helpful in preventing the adverse effects of smoking even if patients did smoke. As pleasurable sensations from smoking should also be prohibited, people should be able to stop smoking easier if they received a vaccine. Until the development of a vaccine, patients should be encouraged to participate in smoking cessation counseling programs. Nurses should continue to educate their patients on the risk of nicotine during pregnancy. If a vaccine is developed, nurses should encourage their patients to maintain a healthy diet and exercise program in order to prevent weight gain after receiving the vaccine.

COMMUNITY BASED CONCERNS

How to Help Your Patient to QUIT SMOKING

Tobacco dependence is the most preventable cause of death (Fant, 2009). Research shows that nurses are an underutilized resource in helping to reduce smoking rates worldwide. One reason more nurses don't participate in this important patient education is a lack of nursing education about nicotine replacement therapy (NRT) and other smoking cessation techniques (Sarna, 2009). So, how should you plan and implement patient education for smoking cessation? Here are some tips:

ASSESSMENT

Assess patient's level of addiction by asking two important questions.

1. *How many cigarettes do you smoke a day?*
2. *How long after awakening do you have your first cigarette of the day?*

For patients that only smoke one to two cigarettes per day or who wait until the afternoon for their first cigarette, smoking should still be strongly discouraged, although NRT may not need to be used. Patients who smoke early in the day and who smoke several cigarettes throughout the day may need more than one kind of NRT (Tonstad, 2009).

Additional assessment questions include;

3. How do you feel about your smoking?
4. What do you like about it?
5. What are your concerns?"

These questions will help you determine how to tailor any smoking cessation program to the individual patient.

SET MUTUAL GOALS

1. Help the patient see their concerns about smoking as strengths. For example, if a patient says, "I don't want to be a bad example or my kids (or grandkids)." Then recognize, "It sounds like you want the best for your family. I can tell you about your options for reducing and eventually stopping your smoking."

INTERVENTIONS

1. Describe benefits of smoking cessation that are specific to that patient (Tonstad, 2009). For example:
   - If the patient has elevated lipid levels tell them these benefits of stopping smoking: HDL levels increase, even more than they would with moderate exercise and LDL levels decrease, decreasing the risk for sudden cardiac death
   - If the patient has a cardiovascular history tell them these benefits: Pulse decreases by an average of 7–8 beats/min when you stop smoking and pulse rate is inversely correlated with age of death; Even one cigarette a day can cause platelet aggregation, increasing risk for pulmonary embolism or other cardio-vascular events
   - If the patient is concerned about cancer tell them: Risks for cancer dramatically decrease with smoking cessation as damaged respiratory cells are able to recover
2. Provide information on therapies to stop smoking. The options are as follows:
   - Patch–21 mg/24 hours for 4 weeks, then 14 mg/24 hours for 2 weeks, then 7 mg/24 hours for 2 weeks, then 15 mg/24 hours for 8 weeks (Frishman, 2007).

- Gum–9 to 12 pieces daily for 8 to 12 weeks or more. The gum should be chewed slowly and with periods of rest, to provide a steady absorption rate of the nicotine through the buccal mucosa (Tonstad, 2009).
- Lozenge–Use up to 24 pieces per day for 6 weeks and then down-titrate. Use if gum is not tolerated because of taste or headache (Frishman, 2007).
- Inhaler–Inhale deeply and frequently in order to achieve 30% blood level of nicotine as smoking. 80 puffs = 4 mg nicotine (Frishman, 2007).
- Bupropion–150 mg two times a week, started one week before cessation and titrated up to desired dose. Schedule for 12 weeks or more (Tonstad, 2009).
- Nortryptiline–a tricyclic anti-depressant that has beneficial impact on withdrawal symptoms. Not FDA approved for nicotine withdrawal, so should only be used as second-line treatment (Frishman, 2007).
- Varenicline–Start 1 week before smoking cessation 0.5 mg/d for day 1 to 3, 0.5 mg two times per day for days 4 to 7, then up to 1 mg two times per day for 12 weeks. If the patient is successful after 12 weeks, continue for 12 more weeks to prevent risk of relapse (Frishman, 2007).
- Clonidine–100 mcg twice a day, started a week before cessation and titrated up to 400 mcg twice a day according to tolerance. 3 to 4 weeks of therapy. Controls withdrawal symptoms (Frishman, 2007).
- SSRIs (specific serotonin reuptake inhibitors)– for example, fleuxotrine, 60 mg/day may be helpful, although not as effective in smokers who are already depressed (Frishman, 2007).
- MAOIs (monoamine oxidase inhibitors)—for example, moclobemide 400 mg/d for 2 months and then 200 mg/d for the third month of cessation (Frishman, 2007).

3. Encourage the patient to be seen by a certified counselor if possible. Combining a form of talk therapy with pharmacotherapy increases quit rates. If a counselor is not available, help the patient establish a support network that will encourage him/her to engage in some behavioral changes, such as avoiding second-hand smoke and drinking more than two alcoholic drinks at a time.

Evaluation

In order to establish further structure for a patient's cessation program, establish a quit date and *follow up*, especially if therapy is not an option for the patient (Tonstad, 2009).

References

Fant, R. V., Buchhalter, A. R., Buchman, A. C., & Henningfield, J.E. (2009). Pharmacotherapy for tobacco dependence. *Handbook of Experimental Pharmacology*, 192:487–510.

Sarna, L., Bialous, S. A., Rice, V. H., & Wewers, M.E. (2009). Promoting tobacco dependence treatment in nursing education. *Drug and Alcohol Review*, 28(5), 507–516.

Tonstad, S. (2009). Smoking cessation: How to advise the patient. *Heart (British Cardiac Society)*, 95(19):1635–1640.

Frishman, W. H. (2007). Smoking cessation pharmacotherapy–nicotine and non-nicotine preparations. *Preventive Cardiology*, 10(2 Suppl 1):10–22.

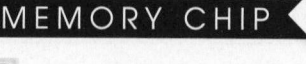

P Nicotine

- A direct-acting nicotinic agonist used as an adjunct to smoking cessation programs
- Major contraindications: immediately post MI, life-threatening dysrhythmias, severe angina
- Most common adverse effects: erythema, pruritus, burning, headache, insomnia
- Most serious adverse effect: vasculitis
- Maximizing therapeutic effects: adherence to the recommended dosing
- Minimizing adverse effects: Limit timing of last dose to promote rest and sleep.
- Most important patient education: correct use of multiple administration routes, avoidance of other stimulants

Ongoing Assessment and Evaluation

During therapy, symptoms of tobacco craving should gradually subside. Throughout therapy, remain alert for signs and symptoms of overdosing, which indicate that the patient is "cheating" and smoking tobacco while taking the nicotine replacement. Dizziness, nausea, and headaches may result and promote nonadherence to the therapeutic use of nicotine. Other evaluative measures include assessing the quantitative decrease of adverse effects and promoting therapeutic adherence.

Drugs Significantly Different From **P** Nicotine

Bupropion

Bupropion (Zyban) is a lower dose of the antidepressant Wellbutrin. It is considered a first-line drug for smoking cessation. Bupropion is discussed in Chapter 16.

Clonidine

Clonidine (Catapres) is an alpha-2 agonist generally used for hypertension. It is considered a second line drug for smoking cessation. Clonidine is covered in depth in Chapter 28.

Rimonabant

Rimonabant (Zimulti, Acomplia) is a selective cannabinoid-1 receptor blockers used in the management of weight loss. During clinical trials for weight loss, it was found to be also helpful in smoking cessation as well as post-cessation weight loss (Fagerstrom, 2006). Rimonabant is also discussed in Chapter 22.

Varenicline

Varenicline (Chantix) is a partial agonist with high affinity and selectivity for alpha-4-beta-2 nicotinic acetylcholine receptor subtypes. Its binding produces agonist activity at a subtype of the nicotinic receptor, but at a significantly lower level than nicotine. Varenicline also prevents nicotine binding to alpha-4-beta-2 receptors, decreasing stimulation of the central nervous mesolimbic dopamine system, which is thought to be responsible for the reinforcement and reward experience associated with smoking. Varenicline is used in a 12-week pharmacologic intervention that may be extended an additional 12 weeks if the patient continues to abstain from smoking. Adverse effects include rash, gastrointestinal (GI) disturbances, headache, insomnia, dream disturbances, and lethargy. Varenicline is classified as a pregnancy category C drug and should not be taken when breast-feeding.

C INDIRECT-ACTING CHOLINERGIC AGONISTS

Synaptic transmission of neurotransmitters was discussed in Chapter 13. To review, the final step of synaptic transmission is termination. After the neurotransmitter crosses the synaptic gap and binds to a receptor, the neurotransmitter is cleared from the synaptic gap by enzymatic degradation, reuptake, or diffusion. Acetylcholine, the neurotransmitter of the cholinergic nervous system, is cleared from the synaptic gap by acetylcholinesterase, also known as cholinesterase. Any drug that inhibits acetylcholinesterase (i.e., inhibits the breakdown of acetylcholine) will prolong the activity of acetylcholine at the synapse. Thus these drugs will indirectly increase the stimulation at the cholinergic receptor. For this reason, some indirect-acting cholinergic agonists are also known as *cholinesterase inhibitors* or *anticholinesterase agents*. It is important to remember that acetylcholine stimulates both nicotinic and muscarinic receptor sites; therefore, cholinesterase inhibitors prolong the action of acetylcholine throughout the body.

The two major groups of indirect-acting cholinergic receptor stimulants are the reversible and "irreversible" cholinesterase inhibitors. Neostigmine (Prostigmin) is the prototype for reversible cholinesterase inhibitors. As the "irreversible" cholinesterase inhibitors have minimal pharmacological properties, they are discussed under the section Drugs Significantly Different From Neostigmine below.

Nursing Management of the Patient Receiving **P** Neostigmine

Core Drug Knowledge

Pharmacotherapeutics

The most significant indication for neostigmine therapy is myasthenia gravis. In this disease, the neuromuscular junction is affected by an autoimmune process that diminishes the number of functional nicotinic receptors at the junction. The result is the characteristic weakness and fatigue that accompany exercise in people with this disease. The use of neostigmine effectively increases the amount of acetylcholine available at the myoneural junction, resulting in enhanced strength of muscle contraction.

Other clinical indications include urinary retention and paralytic ileus. Neostigmine is also used as an antidote for nondepolarizing neuromuscular blocking agents (Table 14.6).

TABLE 14.6	Agents That Interact with P Neostigmine	
Interactants	**Effect and Significance**	**Nursing Management**
Aminoglycoside antibiotics (neomycin, streptomycin, kanamycin)	Mild nondepolarizing blocking action	Monitor for increased neuromuscular blockade.
Corticosteroids	Decreases effect of anticholinesterase therapy in myasthenia gravis	Ensure respiratory support if needed.
Depolarizing muscle relaxants (succinylcholine) and mivacurium	Increased, prolonged neuromuscular blockade	Avoid use if possible. If not, administer these drugs only as directed and only if indicated. Provide emergency respiratory support.
Magnesium	Antagonizes and counteracts beneficial effects of neostigmine	Avoid magnesium-containing drugs and foods.
Anticholinesterase drugs	Excessive GI stimulation and symptoms of cholinergic crisis or underdosage in patients with myasthenia gravis	Have antidote (atropine or belladonna) available to treat overdosage.

Pharmacokinetics

Neostigmine is administered both orally and parenterally. It is poorly absorbed when given orally. Onset of action occurs within 2 to 4 hours when taken orally, and within 10 to 30 minutes when given parenterally. The drug is metabolized by microsomal liver enzymes and hydrolyzed by cholinesterases. Duration of effect varies considerably among patients. Approximately 80% of neostigmine is excreted in the urine within 24 hours as unaltered drug and metabolites.

Pharmacodynamics

Neostigmine is a reversible inhibitor of postsynaptic cholinesterase and therefore acts as a cholinergic agent by increasing the synaptic presence of acetylcholine.

Contraindications and Precautions

Neostigmine is absolutely contraindicated in patients with gastrointestinal obstruction or ileus and urinary tract obstruction because it increases contractions of smooth muscle. It should not be used in patients with peritonitis because it increases gastrointestinal motility, which would exacerbate the disorder. Neostigmine should be used with caution in patients with peptic ulcer disease because it stimulates gastric acid secretion, again inducing an exacerbation of the disorder. The CNS stimulation induced by neostigmine may exacerbate hyperthyroidism or seizure disorders.

Neostigmine should be used cautiously in patients with hypotension and bradycardia because it can further decrease blood pressure and heart rate by increasing vagal tone. Neostigmine also has direct stimulatory effects on the myocardium, which can increase oxygen demand. This state can be dangerous for patients with cardiac disease, particularly coronary artery disease alone or in association with cardiac arrhythmias. In the respiratory system, neostigmine may induce bronchoconstriction; therefore, it should be used cautiously in patients with asthma, chronic bronchitis, or chronic airway limitation.

Adverse Effects

The most serious adverse effects result from overactity of the cholinergic system, which may be life threatening. This excessive cholinergic stimulation is termed cholinergic poisoning or cholinergic crisis. Think of this as "too much of a good thing," or more of the cholinergic effects than is normally desired from stimulation. Usually the cause is dose related; the dose of neostigmine is too high, leading to too much degradation of acetylcholinesterase, so excessive receptor stimulation results. Symptoms include nausea and vomiting, diarrhea, salivation, sweating, peripheral vasodilation, bronchial constriction, and respiratory arrest.

The most common unwanted effects of neostigmine's cholinergic stimulation of end organs are nausea and vomiting, diarrhea, abdominal pain, miosis, salivation, diaphoresis, sinus bradycardia, bronchospasm, and increased bronchial secretions.

Drug Interactions

Neostigmine and the anticholinesterase drugs in general interact with steroids, aminoglycoside antibiotics, depolarizing muscle relaxants, local anesthetics and some general anesthetics, and magnesium, all of which have an influence on the neuromuscular junction (Table 14.6). Steroids may decrease the anticholinesterase effects of neostigmine, with a resulting worsening of the myasthenic condition. This exacerbation may require an increased dose of neostigmine or alternate dosing of each class of agent. Some of the aminoglycosides cause a mild neuromuscular blockade, which may antagonize the effects of neostigmine. For the depolarizing muscle relaxants, such as succinylcholine, neostigmine may increase the time of neuromuscular blockade; thus, concurrent usage in people with myasthenia is contraindicated.

Assessment of Relevant Core Patient Variables

Health Status

Before administering the drug, perform a baseline physical assessment to document the current status of the patient, especially respiratory status and muscle strength. Myasthenia affects the muscles of respiration and other muscle groups; therefore, respiratory function may be further compromised in the presence of upper respiratory tract infections or allergies. Undertreatment or overtreatment is of particular concern because it can lead to life-threatening crises.

Also assess for a history of diseases or disorders that contraindicate the use of neostigmine. Communicate positive findings to the health care provider before neostigmine is administered.

Life Span and Gender
Document the age and gender of the patient. Because they have lower body mass than other adults and decreased renal functioning, elderly patients may be more prone to the psychotogenic effects of cholinergic overdose, including restlessness, anxiety, and agitation. Also determine whether the patient is pregnant or breast-feeding because these patients should avoid neostigmine.

Lifestyle, Diet, and Habits
Document the patient's occupation, daily activities, and rest and exercise patterns. Patients taking neostigmine for myasthenia gravis may need to pace their daily activities to allow the peak and duration effects of neostigmine dosing to support their muscular and respiratory work.

Environment
Be aware of the environment in which the drug will be administered and assess the home or living environment, if appropriate. Neostigmine in its oral form may be administered in any setting by health care providers, nurses, the patient, or family members.

Nursing Diagnoses and Outcomes
- Impaired Gas Exchange related to drug-induced bronchospasm, increased secretions, or respiratory paralysis
  Desired outcome: The patient will maintain effective gas exchange.
- Ineffective Airway Clearance
  Desired outcome: The patient will maintain effective airway clearance.
- Ineffective Breathing Pattern related to drug dosage
  Desired outcome: The patient will maintain effective breathing patterns.
- Self-Care Deficit (Feeding, Bathing/Hygiene, Dressing/Grooming, Toileting) related to the impact of neuromuscular weakness secondary to overdose
  Desired outcome: The patient will seek assistance in carrying out self-care as needed.

Planning and Intervention
Maximizing Therapeutic Effects
Neostigmine is administered at regular intervals throughout the day to ensure effective blood levels. If the patient has difficulty swallowing or breathing, the parenteral form of neostigmine should be administered until oral therapy can be tolerated.

Minimizing Adverse Effects
As with other cholinergic stimulants, the use of neostigmine requires the availability of an antidote in case of systemic overdose or cholinergic crisis. Atropine, as an anticholinergic, is the usual antidote. In patients with myasthenia gravis, it is sometimes necessary to distinguish between a cholinergic crisis and a myasthenic crisis. In the case of a cholinergic crisis, it is likely that too much anticholinesterase has been given, whereas a myasthenic crisis may be the result of inadequate dosages failing to control myasthenic symptoms. A challenge IV dose of edrophonium (Tensilon), another anticholinesterase drug, will differentiate the two states. Edrophonium is used because it has a very quick onset (30 to 60 seconds) and the duration of action is only 10 minutes. If the symptoms of a patient with myasthenia gravis improve after the dose, it means they needed more cholinergic stimulation and their standing treatment for myasthenia gravis is inadequate; they can be considered to have been experiencing a myasthenic crisis. If there is no relief of symptoms or if an increase in muscle weakness follows (i.e., the patient gets worse), then the patient is receiving too much anticholinesterase and is experiencing a cholinergic crisis. In this case the antidote is necessary.

For patients with known allergies or suspected hypersensitivity, life-support measures must be available in case of bronchial spasm or hypersensitivity reactions. Because adverse systemic effects include stimulation of sphincters, patients may need access to a bedpan or urinal in case of rapid responses.

If the patient has a history of allergies or asthma or chronic obstructive lung disease, careful monitoring of the first few doses of neostigmine is required to ensure that respiratory difficulties do not occur.

Providing Patient and Family Education
The key considerations for patient and family education include managing serious adverse effects and recognizing crisis states that may require prompt and expert intervention:

- Explore aspects of long-term therapy that sometimes escape the attention or resources of acute care staff, such as decreased libido.

CRITICAL THINKING SCENARIO

NEOSTIGMINE THERAPY

Amy Rose, a 27-year-old legal assistant, has been admitted to your unit with a diagnosis of myasthenia gravis. She has been started on neostigmine therapy, and you are wondering how to differentiate between a myasthenic crisis and a cholinergic crisis.

1. Explain the key differences between the two situations, and propose a nursing management strategy that you could use for either situation.

2. Discuss the implications of a health care provider-ordered edrophonium test. Why do you think this test would be ordered?

MEMORY CHIP

P Neostigmine

- An indirect-acting cholinoceptor stimulant used in the management of myasthenia gravis
- Major contraindications: GI obstruction or ileus, urinary tract obstruction, peritonitis
- Most common adverse effects: nausea or vomiting, diarrhea, abdominal pain, miosis, salivation, diaphoresis, sinus bradycardia
- Most serious adverse effects: cholinergic crisis, cardiac arrest
- Maximizing therapeutic effects: Administer at regular intervals throughout the day to ensure adequate blood levels
- Minimizing adverse effects: availability of atropine, the antidote for cholinergic crisis
- Most significant nursing responsibility: Differentiate between cholinergic crisis and myasthenic crisis
- Most important patient education: symptoms of cholinergic crisis and need for immediate medical attention

- Assist patients and their families in understanding how to recognize myasthenic crisis (undermedication) and distinguish it from cholinergic crisis (overmedication), and in knowing how to respond to either situation. In myasthenic crisis caused by undermedication, muscle weakness becomes pronounced and may cause quadriparesis, quadriplegia, shortness of breath, respiratory insufficiency, and difficulty swallowing. Conversely, in a cholinergic crisis caused by overmedication, there is an increase in gastrointestinal motility with diarrhea and cramping, bradycardia, muscle fasciculation, pupillary constriction, and increased salivation and sweating. Advise the patient and family to seek immediate care if any of these symptoms occur.

Ongoing Assessment and Evaluation

Be familiar with procedures for detecting and managing myasthenic or cholinergic crises. Monitor changes in neuromuscular functioning, vital signs, respiratory rate and capacity, mobility, self-care levels, and self-esteem.

An important component of the ongoing assessment is the patient's neuromuscular status. The focus is on vital capacity (respiratory status), presence of ptosis, presence of diplopia, ability to chew and swallow, strength of hand grip bilaterally, and quality of gait if the patient is ambulatory. Acute care settings often provide a detailed assessment sheet designed specifically for the person with myasthenia gravis. Other data should include baseline and ongoing measurements of blood pressure and pulse and respiratory rates.

Drugs Significantly Different From P Neostigmine

Demecarium

Demecarium (Humorsol) is a long-acting cholinesterase inhibitor and potent miotic used in the management of glaucoma. It increases the amount of fluid that drains from the eye, resulting in reduced pressure in the eye. It also causes the pupil to become smaller and reduces its response to light or dark conditions.

Demecarium is a category X drug because it may cause fetal deformities. It is given cautiously to patients with cardiovascular disorders, asthma, seizure disorders, and hyperthyroidism.

Demecarium may cause local or systemic adverse effects. Local effects include burning, redness, stinging, or other irritation of the eyes. More serious local effects include eye pain and retinal detachment. Systemic effects are infrequent when demecarium is instilled carefully. Compression of the lacrimal duct for several seconds immediately following instillation minimizes drainage into the nasal chamber, where extensive absorption may occur.

Physostigmine

Physostigmine (Antilirium) is a parenteral and ophthalmic cholinesterase inhibitor. Physostigmine is most commonly used as an ophthalmic agent in the treatment of open-angle glaucoma. It is also used to counteract toxic anticholinergic effects (both central and peripheral) of other drugs, particularly in overdose situations. In the past it was used to treat tricyclic antidepressant overdose, but this use has lost favor because of physostigmine's own potentially harmful effects.

Drugs for Myasthenia Gravis

Ambenonium chloride (Mytelase), edrophonium (Tensilon), and pyridostigmine (Mestinon) are used to improve muscle strength in patients with myasthenia gravis and so also are indirect-acting cholinergic drugs. Ambenonium has a longer duration of action than neostigmine and is more potent. However, it is not used as frequently. Pyridostigmine is an analogue of neostigmine and is marketed in both regular and sustained-release tablets and is the most commonly used agent of the group for oral treatment of myasthenia gravis. It is also available in a form for intravenous administration. Other therapeutic uses are as prophylaxis in organophosphate poisoning and reversal of neuromuscular blockade. It is less potent than neostigmine. Edrophonium is the drug of choice for diagnosing myasthenia gravis because of its rapid onset (30 to 60 seconds) of action and short duration of action (about 10 minutes). It must be given IV. Because of the short duration of action and the need for IV therapy, it is not appropriate for long-term treatment of myasthenia gravis. It works by binding with acetylcholinesterase to prevent it from attaching to the cholinergic receptor. It is also used to differentiate cholinergic crisis from myasthenic crisis and to reverse the effects of nondepolarizing neuromuscular blockers after surgery. Contraindications, adverse effects, and drug interactions are similar to those of neostigmine.

Drugs for Cognition

Several indirect-acting cholinergic agonists are approved for improving cognitive symptoms, such as problems with memory, attention, reason, language, and ability to perform simple tasks, associated with Alzheimer disease. Elevated levels of acetylcholine in the cerebral cortex are believed to be responsible for improvement in cognition; however, intact cholinergic neurons must be present. Currently, rivastigmine (Exelon), tacrine (Cognex), galantamine (Razadyne), donepezil (Aricept), and memantine (Namenda) are approved for the management of Alzheimer disease. These drugs work by enhancing cholinergic neurotransmission in relevant parts of the brain by the use of cholinesterase inhibitors to delay the breakdown of acetylcholine released into synaptic clefts (Birks et al., 2009). A full discussion of drugs used to treat Alzheimer disease is in Chapter 17. Neostigmine is not indicated for use in disorders of cognition, although the drugs used for cognition fall under the same class of drugs (Birks, 2006).

Irreversible Cholinesterase Inhibitors

Most of the irreversible cholinesterase inhibitors are in the organophosphate category. Because of the phosphate element of these drugs, they are highly lipid soluble and are easily absorbed from any administration site. Their ease of absorption, coupled with their potential toxicity, is the basis for their use as insecticides and chemical warfare agents.

There are a few therapeutically useful irreversible inhibitors, such as echothiophate and isoflurophate (Floropryl), which are used for glaucoma that is refractory to the usual miotics.

Overdose or accidental overexposure to irreversible anticholinesterase drugs is characterized by cholinergic crisis. The antidote of choice is pralidoxime (Protopam, PAM). Pralidoxime is not effective in reversing overdose of reversible anticholinesterase drugs. It works best when given immediately after the exposure. It does not cross the blood–brain barrier and, therefore, is ineffective in reversing anticholinesterase in the CNS.

Ⓒ CHOLINERGIC ANTAGONISTS

The cholinergic antagonists are drugs that antagonize, or block, muscarinic or nicotinic receptors directly. They are generally referred to as anticholinergics. They may be clustered into three categories: antimuscarinic drugs (the largest group), antinicotinic drugs (with two subcategories: ganglionic blockers and neuromuscular blockers), and cholinesterase regenerators.

Antinicotinic Ganglionic Blockers

The ganglionic blockers include mecamylamine (Inversine) and trimethaphan (Arfonad). Mecamylamine inhibits acetylcholine at the autonomic ganglia, causing a decrease in blood pressure. Mecamylamine is no longer recommended for treatment of hypertension as newer and more effective drugs have been created which have been found to decrease mortality from hypertension. Mecamylamine also blocks central nicotinic cholinergic receptors, which inhibits the effects of nicotine and may suppress the desire to smoke.

Trimethaphan blocks the ganglionic receptors so that acetylcholine cannot attach. It is used in treating hypertensive crisis and has been used in the emergency control of

hypertension in patients with acute dissecting aortic aneurysm. It is discussed further in Chapter 26.

Neuromuscular Blockers

The neuromuscular blockers, which are covered in Chapter 19, include the prototype nondepolarizing agent tubocurarine, as well as cisatracurium, doxacurium, pancuronium, and vecuronium, as well as the prototype depolarizing agent succinylcholine. These drugs compete with acetylcholine for cholinergic receptors. They are used as adjuncts to anesthesia and assist in entubation.

Antimuscarinic/Anticholinergic Drugs

Atropine is an anticholinergic drug that specifically targets the muscarinic cholinergic receptors. Atropine is the ideal prototype for the antimuscarinic group of cholinergic antagonists.

Nursing Management of the Patient Receiving Ⓟ Atropine

Core Drug Knowledge

Pharmacotherapeutics

Atropine has a multitude of therapeutic uses and a variety of preparations. It is used in emergency situations, such as symptomatic bradycardia, pulseless electrical activity, ventricular asystole, or cardiopulmonary resuscitation. Preoperatively, it is used to decrease respiratory secretions, and during surgery, it is used to block cardiovagal reflexes and succinylcholine-induced arrhythmias. Other uses include reversal of organophosphate insecticide toxicity or neuromuscular blockade, as well as the antidote to overdosage with a cholinergic drug or from eating poisonous mushrooms (which attach to muscarinic receptors). Ophthalmic solutions are used to change pupil size or activity of the ciliary muscle, and in the treatment of iritis or uveitis. Atropine-containing solutions are used to manage traveler's diarrhea or gastric spasms. Oral forms can also be used as treatment for ureteric colic. Off-label atropine might be used as an adjunct for treating asthma. Atropine is available as oral tablets and in oral solutions, as parenteral solutions for SC, IM, or IV administration, as an ophthalmic drop, and as a liquid for nebulization.

Pharmacokinetics

Following intramuscular administration, onset of effect is usually rapid, peaking at 30 minutes and lasting up to 5 hours (Table 14.7). Topical administration to the eyes may take 30 to 40 minutes to produce cycloplegia (paralysis of ciliary muscles), whereas intravenous (IV) administration produces rapid effects. Atropine is partially metabolized in the liver, with about 60% of a dose eliminated unchanged through the kidneys.

Pharmacodynamics

Atropine is a competitive inhibitor at autonomic postganglionic cholinergic receptors. Atropine attaches and blocks all cholinergic receptors throughout the entire body.

TABLE 14.7	Summary of Selected Ⓒ Cholinergic Antagonists		
Drug (Trade) Name	**Selected Indications**	**Route and Dosage Range**	**Pharmacokinetics**
Ⓟ atropine (Atropine Sulfate)	Anesthesia induction, premedication for surgery Bradycardia Biliary spasm, GI radiography, irritable bowel syndrome, peptic ulcers, urinary incontinence, asthma, bronchitis, reversal of bronchospasm, hiccups, organophosphate poisoning, arrhythmias (e.g., angiography induced, postmyocardial infarction, succinylcholine induced), myelodysplasia, neuromuscular blockade reversal, hyperhidrosis, hypothermia, rhinorrhea, tetanus asystole, dental procedures	*Adult:* SC, IM, or IV, 0.3–0.6 mg 60 min before inducing anesthesia *Adult:* IV, 0.5–2.0 mg *Adult:* 0.3–1.2 mg q4–6h any route for GI or anticholinergic uses	*Onset:* SC, varies; IM, 10–15 min; IV, immediate *Duration:* 4 h $t_{1/2}$: 2.5 h
benztropine (Benztropine Mesylate, Cogentin)	Drug-induced extrapyramidal symptoms, akathisia, dystonic reactions, haloperidol-induced acute dystonic reaction, parkinsonism, drooling, myoclonus, priapism	*Adult:* PO, IM, IV, 1–4 mg daily or bid	*Onset:* PO, 1 h; IM, IV, 15 min *Duration:* PO, IM, IV 6–10 h $t_{1/2}$: 4–8 h
darifenacin (Enablex)	Overactive bladder	*Adult:* PO, 7.5–15 mg daily	*Onset:* Slow *Duration:* Unknown $t_{1/2}$: 13–19 h
dicyclomine (Bentyl, Antispas;)	Irritable bowel syndrome	*Adult:* PO, 80–160 mg/d in equally divided doses	*Onset:* 1–2 h *Duration:* 4 h $t_{1/2}$: 9–10 h
flavoxate hydrochloride (Urispas)	Overactive bladder	*Adult and Child >12 y:* PO, 100–200 mg 3–4×/d	*Onset:* 1 h *Duration:* 24 h $t_{1/2}$: Unknown
glycopyrrolate (Robinul)	Inhibit salivation and excessive respiratory tract secretions	*Adult:* IM, 4 mcg/kg 30–60 min prior to procedure	*Onset:* 15–30 min *Duration:* 2–7 h $t_{1/2}$: 2.5 h
hyoscyamine (Cystospaz)	Abdominal cramps, anticholinesterase poisoning, biliary disorders, colic, diverticulitis, dysentery, enterocolitis, GI disorders, irritable bowel syndrome, neurogenic bowel disturbances, Parkinson disease, peptic ulcer, pylorospasm, spastic colon, splenic flexure syndrome, pancreatitis, rhinitis	*Adult:* PO, 0.125–0.25 mg q4h; PO (sustained-release product), 375–0.75 mg q12h; SC, IM, IV push, 0.25–0.5 mg	*Onset:* PO, 5–20 min; IV, 2 min *Duration:* 4–12 h $t_{1/2}$: Not applicable
ipratropium (Atrovent;)	Asthma, chronic bronchitis, chronic obstructive lung disease, rhinorrhea	*Adult:* Inhaler, 36 mcg qid	*Onset:* 15 min *Duration:* 3–4 h $t_{1/2}$: 1.6 h
oxybutynin (Ditropan, Ditropan XL, Oxytrol)	Overactive bladder	*Adult:* PO, 5 mg 3–4× d; XL 5–30 mg daily; syrup, 1 tsp bid–tid; transdermal patch 3.9 mg/d placed 2× wk *Children under 5 y:* PO, 5 mg bid syrup, 1 tsp bid	*Onset:* 30–60 min *Duration:* 6–10 h $t_{1/2}$: Unknown
propantheline (Pro-Banthine, Propantheline Bromide;)	Duodenal ulcer, GI spasmolytic, hyperhidrosis, sialorrhea, urinary incontinence	*Adult:* PO, 15–30 mg 30 min before meals and 30 mg at bedtime or 15–30 mg q4–6h	*Onset:* 30–60 min *Duration:* 6 h $t_{1/2}$: 3–4 h
scopolamine (Scopolamine Hydrobromide, Hyoscine Hydrobromide)	Motion sickness Preanesthetic premedication, obstetric amnesia, antidelirium Glaucoma, ophthalmology, uveitis	*Adult:* PO or transdermal patch, 0.6–1.0 mg *Adult:* PO, 1 mg 1–4 h before anesthesia; IM, 0.4–0.6 mg 45–60 min before anesthesia *Adult:* topical, 1–2 drops of 0.25% solution in eye 1 h before refraction; 1–2 drops up to four times daily for uveitis	*Onset:* PO/IM, 30 min *Duration:* 4–6 h $t_{1/2}$: 8 h

(Continued)

TABLE 14.7	Summary of Selected Ⓒ Cholinergic Antagonists	*(continued)*	
Drug (Trade) Name	**Selected Indications**	**Route and Dosage Range**	**Pharmacokinetics**
solifenacin (Vesicare)	Overactive bladder	*Adult:* PO, 5–10 mg every day	*Onset:* Unknown *Duration:* Unknown $t_{1/2}$: 2–3 d
tiotropium (Spiriva)	Bronchospasm	*Adult:* Inhaler, 18 mcg daily	*Onset:* 30 min *Duration:* 24–48 h $t_{1/2}$: 5–6 d
tolterodine (Detrol, Detrol LA)	Overactive bladder	*Adult:* PO, 1–2 mg 2×/d LA: 2–4 mg daily	*Onset:* 1–2 h *Duration:* 6–8 h $t_{1/2}$: 1.9–3.7 h
trihexyphenidyl (Artane)	Alzheimer dementia Drug-induced EPS	*Adult:* PO, 5–15 mg/d in 3–4 divided doses	*Onset:* 1 h *Duration:* 6–12 h $t_{1/2}$: 5.6–10.2 h
trospium (Sanctura)	Overactive bladder	*Adult:* PO, 20 mg 2×/d	*Onset:* 3 h *Duration:* Unknown $t_{1/2}$: 20 h

These receptors are found in gastrointestinal and pulmonary smooth muscle, exocrine glands, the heart, and the eye. The principal actions of atropine are: increase in heart rate; a reduction in salivary, bronchial, and sweat gland secretions; mydriasis (enlarged pupils); paralysis of the ciliary muscle; contraction of the bladder detrusor muscle and of the gastrointestinal smooth muscle; decreased gastric secretion; and decreased gastrointestinal motility.

The action of atropine on the heart rate is dose dependent. In doses of 0.4 to 0.6 mg, atropine causes a slight sinus bradycardia through vagal stimulation. In larger doses (1 to 2 mg), it causes sinus tachycardia secondary to inhibition of vagal control of the sinoatrial node in the heart. Atropine is mostly given for its ability to increase the heart rate.

Contraindications and Precautions

Contraindications to atropine use include hypersensitivity to anticholinergics or sulfites. Atropine is contraindicated in myasthenia gravis because the drug competes with the small amount of acetylcholine that has potential to act in the body. Atropine is relatively contraindicated in acute myocardial infarction because the drug can potentiate arrhythmias. In addition, the increase in heart rate caused by atropine increases the oxygen demand on the heart and can exacerbate myocardial ischemia. Precautions should be observed with patients who drive or perform hazardous tasks for a living (because of the adverse effects of drowsiness and blurred vision). Precautions are also needed for the elderly as well as those with glaucoma, severe forms of hepatic disease, ulcerative colitis, renal disease, prostatic hypertrophy, coronary artery disease, chronic heart failure, arrhythmias, tachycardia, hypertension, asthma, and allergies. Finally, precautions are needed for anyone with increased sensitivity (e.g., infants and small children) and for patients with

brain damage, hyperthyroidism, and hyperthermia. All of these circumstances may be exacerbated with atropine and other anticholinergics.

Adverse Effects

The most common adverse effects of atropine are blurred vision, dry mouth, constipation, and urinary retention. The most serious potential adverse effect is an anticholinergic overdose. This overdose is characterized by the phrase "mad as a hatter (CNS psychotic effect), dry as a bone (salivary), red as a beet (peripheral vasodilation), and blind as a bat (mydriasis)."

In the CNS, the predominant effect is drowsiness, but more serious CNS effects are possible, especially in the elderly. These include: confusion, disorientation, delusions, hallucinations, and psychosis. Other potential adverse effects include elevation of intraocular pressure, decreased ability to sweat, and tachycardia. Although anticholinergic drugs are used in the management of asthma, the drying of respiratory secretions may result in mucus plugs that may actually induce bronchospasm and asthma attacks.

Atropine is a FDA pregnancy category C drug and should be avoided by pregnant and lactating women.

Drug Interactions

Atropine interacts with phenothiazine antipsychotics and with haloperidol (Table 14.8). Cardiac status, as measured by electrocardiography (ECG), may be affected by atropine. Atropine may interfere with ECG measurements through its cardiovascular effects and result in spurious cardiac findings. The ECG interpretation should note the atropine therapy.

Assessment of Relevant Core Patient Variables

Health Status

Because atropine has many actions on the body, carefully assess the patient for contraindications or precautions to its

TABLE 14.8	Agents That Interact with P Atropine	
Interactants	Effect and Significance	Nursing Management
phenothiazines	Decreased antipsychotic efficacy of phenothiazines	Adjust phenothiazine dosage.
haloperidol	Decreased serum haloperidol levels, worsening of symptoms, onset of tardive dyskinesia	Avoid concurrent atropine or lower haloperidol dosage; monitor carefully.

use before administering the drug. It is important to determine whether the patient has acute angle-closure glaucoma, obstructive disease of the gastrointestinal tract, paralytic ileus, obstructive uropathy, intestinal atony (particularly in elderly or debilitated patients), megacolon complicating ulcerative colitis, unstable cardiovascular status in acute hemorrhage, tachycardia secondary to cardiac insufficiency of thyrotoxicosis, myasthenia gravis, toxemia of pregnancy, or previous exposure to high temperatures.

Communicate positive findings to the health care provider. Also determine whether the patient has chronic obstructive lung disease, severe heart disease, hypertension, ulcerative colitis, ileus, chronic lung disease, hyperthyroidism, autonomic neuropathy, hepatic or renal disease, prostatic hypertrophy, esophageal reflux, or hiatal hernia. Because these conditions may be exacerbated with atropine therapy, monitor these patients closely. Also assesses the patient's use of OTC or herbal medications. These drugs frequently contain atropine-like ingredients that may induce severe adverse effects.

Life Span and Gender
Document the age of the patient. Atropine must be used carefully with infants, young children, and anyone older than 40 years because the adverse effects may be more pronounced in these age groups.

Environment
Document the patient's occupation and daily activities. People treated with atropine may experience mydriasis and hence difficulties adjusting to changing light intensities. These effects may have considerable impact on people working in transportation (airline flight crew, drivers) and those working at night (because of photophobia and temporary blindness in response to bright lights).

Nursing Diagnoses and Outcomes
- Urinary Retention related to adverse effects of drug
  Desired outcome: The patient will eliminate without difficulty.
- Constipation related to adverse effects of drug
  Desired outcome: The patient will continue baseline elimination pattern.
- Risk for Injury related to drug-induced drowsiness and blurred vision
  Desired outcome: The patient will understand adverse effects and develop a repertoire of strategies for their management.

- Ineffective Sexuality Patterns or Sexual Dysfunction related to anticholinergic impact on erection and ejaculation in men and on vaginal secretions in women
  Desired outcome: The patient and partner will adjust sexual functioning and develop a repertoire of strategies to maintain satisfaction.

Planning and Intervention
Maximizing Therapeutic Effects
Two factors should be considered for the person receiving atropine, because they arise directly from the interactions between core drug knowledge and core patient variables. First, patients taking atropine for peptic ulcer disease should adhere to dietary restrictions established to prevent exacerbations of the disease, thereby allowing the therapeutic potential of the atropine to be achieved. Suggest administering the larger dose at bedtime to decrease sleep-disturbing pain. Second, patients need to be encouraged to take their atropine exactly as prescribed and at the required dosage frequency to enhance therapeutic potential.

Minimizing Adverse Effects
Because a prominent anticholinergic effect is dry mouth, good oral hygiene is important. Dryness may be relieved with hard candies, chewing gum, or lip balm. Blurred vision and mydriasis can be hazardous for drivers, particularly at night; therefore, driving is best avoided. Bright lights and photophobia may be counteracted with sunglasses. For patients with a complaint of dry eyes, artificial tears should be administered.

Atropine alters the body's ability to regulate temperature; therefore, minimize extremes of heat and strenuous exercise, and adequately and deliberately hydrate the patient. Constipation is a troubling adverse effect that may be managed by adding fiber to the diet, promoting hydration, and exercising moderately.

In longer-term therapy, stress the importance of mouth care and monitor the need for urinary catheterization or measures to relieve constipation and abdominal distention. A distressing adverse effect for many patients relates to their preferred modes of sexual expression, which may be dramatically changed with anticholinergic drugs. If appropriate, supportive counseling or directive teaching about alternatives to intercourse may be useful, although many of these issues are better managed by a sex therapist.

Providing Patient and Family Education
Important aspects of patient and family teaching include recognizing and managing adverse effects:

MEMORY CHIP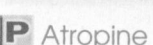

P Atropine

- An anticholinergic drug given in emergency situations such as severe bradycardia or during CPR. Used routinely as a preoperative medication to reduce intraoperative pulmonary secretions
- Major contraindications: hypersensitivity to sulfites, myasthenia gravis, acute myocardial infarction
- Most common adverse effects: blurred vision, constipation, dry mouth, urinary retention
- Most serious adverse effect: cardiac arrhythmias
- Maximizing therapeutic effects: Take the medication exactly as prescribed and at the required dosage
- Minimizing adverse effects: good oral hygiene, fluid replacement
- Most important patient education: safety issues for blurred vision; avoid OTC and herbal medications without the direct approval of the health care provider.

- Inform older men of the need to report any changes in urinary stream because it may be a prodromal symptom of prostatic hypertrophy.
- Suggest aids to elimination, including adequate exercise, added dietary fiber, and increased fluid intake.
- Stress the hazards associated with driving, especially at night, because night vision may be altered significantly by atropine.
- Remind the patient to avoid all OTC and herbal medications without the direct approval of the health care provider. As previously mentioned, these medications frequently contain atropine-like ingredients.

Ongoing Assessment and Evaluation

Assessment of goal attainment is relatively straightforward for patients receiving anticholinergic therapy with atropine. Ongoing assessment includes data about elimination patterns, sexual functioning and adjustment, and recognition and management of side effects. The ongoing assessments may be tailored to the clinical indications for which atropine or other anticholinergics are prescribed, but they should include any concurrent drug therapy to rule out the possibility of drug interactions. Vital signs measured at onset of therapy are compared with vital signs throughout therapy and are used to monitor and detect adverse effects.

Assess bowel and bladder function on an ongoing basis because of the profound impact that drug therapy may have on elimination. Because of the potential for confusion, anyone at risk for adverse CNS effects should have a mental status assessment.

Drugs Significantly Different From P Atropine
Hyoscyamine

Hyoscyamine (Cystospaz) relaxes smooth muscle spasm resulting from parasympathetic stimulation. It inhibits gastrointestinal propulsive motility and decreases gastric acid secretion. It also controls excessive pharyngeal, tracheal, and bronchial secretions. It requires only half the dose of atropine; therefore, it has a lower potential to induce adverse effects.

Scopolamine

Scopolamine (Isopto Hyoscine) is a naturally occurring anticholinergic agent found in belladonna leaf. Compared with atropine, scopolamine is more potent in its anticholinergic effects on the iris, ciliary body, and the salivary, bronchial, and sweat glands. It is less potent than atropine on the heart and on bronchial and gastrointestinal smooth muscle. In contrast to atropine, scopolamine at therapeutic doses produces CNS depression characterized by drowsiness, euphoria, amnesia, fatigue, and dreamless sleep resulting from decreased periods of rapid eye movement. Paradoxical CNS excitation manifested as restlessness, hallucinations, or delirium can occur, especially when the patient is experiencing severe pain. Scopolamine is very effective for the prevention of motion sickness, and this indication represents the most common clinical use. Other uses for scopolamine include treatment of iritis, uveitis, and Parkinson disease.

Antiparkinson Agents

Trihexyphenidyl (Artane) and benztropine (Cogentin) are centrally acting anticholinergics used adjunctively to treat all types of parkinsonian syndromes, including antipsychotic-induced extrapyramidal symptoms. In general, anticholinergic agents can help control tremors but are less effective for treating bradykinesia or rigidity.

Trihexyphenidyl (Artane) is effective in 50% to 75% of patients. Additionally, it can block dopamine reuptake, thereby prolonging dopamine's effects.

Benztropine (Cogentin) can be given both orally and parenterally. It produces less CNS stimulation than does trihexyphenidyl. Benztropine may be helpful in geriatric patients who cannot tolerate cerebral-stimulating agents. Antiparkinson drugs are discussed more in Chapter 21.

Antisecretory Anticholinergics

Glycopyrrolate (Robinul) and propantheline (Pro-Banthine) are oral agents used to decrease the secretion of gastric acid. Since the advent of histamine-2 blockers and proton pump inhibitors, these antisecretory anticholinergics have fallen out of favor because they induce myriad adverse effects. However, for patients unresponsive to histamine-2 blockers or proton pump inhibitors, these drugs may be effective.

Inhaled Agents

Ipratropium bromide (Atrovent) and tiotropium (Spiriva) are inhaled anticholinergic drugs that are structurally very similar to atropine. These drugs have greater antimuscarinic activity on the bronchial smooth muscle, and systemic effects are minimal. Compared with atropine, they are roughly twice as potent as a bronchodilator. Both drugs are used in the management of chronic obstructive pulmonary disorders such as chronic bronchitis, emphysema, and asthma.

Intranasal administration of ipratropium produces a localized parasympatholytic effect. This action reduces watery hypersecretion from mucosal glands of the nose, thereby relieving rhinorrhea associated with the common cold or allergic or nonallergic perennial rhinitis. These drugs are discussed more fully in Chapter 35.

Urinary Relaxants

In overactive bladder (OAB), the bladder or detrusor muscle contracts prior to the bladder being full, causing the patient to feel a sense of urgency to void. OAB can occur with or without urinary incontinence. Cholinergic antagonists such as darifenacin (Enablex), flavoxate hydrochloride (Urispas), oxybutynin, (Ditropan, Ditropan XL, or Oxytrol), solifenacin (Vesicare), tolterodine (Detrol, Detrol LA), and trospium (Sanctura) are used for OAB (Lam, 2007). These drugs are preferential to M_2 and M_3, but they may also stimulate the other muscarinic receptors, resulting in adverse effects. The most common adverse effect is dry mouth.

Oxybutynin is the only drug available in a generic formulation and as a transdermal patch. Its long-acting formulation causes dry mouth in approximately 60% of patients. For patients who cannot tolerate adverse effects of oxybutynin, trospium chloride is preferred (Biastre & Burnaski, 2009). The anticholinergics used in treating OAB are discussed further in Chapter 27.

CHAPTER SUMMARY

- The parasympathetic (cholinergic) nervous system stimulates the GI system and decreases metabolism and cardiovascular and respiratory function to preserve energy. It is considered the "rest and digest" system.
- In the parasympathetic system, the transmitter is acetylcholine, and the receptors are considered cholinergic. Cholinergic may be further divided into muscarinic or nicotinic.
- Parasympathetic or cholinergic drugs can be stimulating or blocking in their action. The cholinergic stimulating drugs are known as cholinergic agonists, and the cholinergic blocking agents are known as cholinergic anticholinergics. There are additional terms for these drugs (see Table 14.1).
- Acetylcholine is inactivated by acetylcholinesterase, which is sometimes referred to as cholinesterase.
- Drugs that interfere with acetylcholinesterase's breakdown of acetylcholine (i.e., they inhibit the action of acetylcholinesterase) are known as anticholinesterase agents.
- Therapeutic uses of cholinergic drugs are varied and related to providing extra cholinergic stimulation or blockage to normal autonomic nervous system functioning.
- Excessive stimulation of cholinergic receptors is known as cholinergic poisoning or cholinergic crisis. The symptoms of this overstimulation can be remembered by the saying: Red as a beet, dry as a bone, blind as a bat, and mad as a hatter. Overdosage with a cholinergic drug can produce this condition.
- A prototype of a direct-acting muscarinic agonist is pilocarpine, which is used for simple and acute glaucoma, preoperative and postoperative intraocular tension, and mydriasis.

- A prototype direct-acting nicotinic agonist is nicotine, which is used as an adjunct to smoking cessation programs.
- A prototype indirect-acting cholinergic receptor stimulant is neostigmine, which is used to control the symptoms of myasthenia gravis. It inhibits the action of acetylcholinesterase. As with any of the cholinergic drugs, adverse effects involve many of the major organ systems.
- Atropine is the prototype of the antimuscarinic anticholinergic drugs. It is most commonly used to raise heart rate in cardiac emergencies and preoperatively to dry oral secretions.

The most common adverse effects of anticholinergic drugs are blurred vision, dry mouth, constipation, and urinary retention.

QUESTIONS FOR STUDY AND REVIEW

1. What happens when you stimulate cholinergic receptors in the eye after administering pilocarpine eye drops?
2. What happens when you stimulate cholinergic receptors in the GI and GU tract?
3. If you administered a cholinergic drug, what adverse effects might occur in the cardiovascular system?
4. How does neostigmine create its therapeutic effect?
5. What signs and symptoms indicate a cholinergic crisis? What is the antidote?
6. You may have encountered a way of remembering excessive anticholinergic effects through the terms "mad as a hatter, blind as a bat, red as a beet, and dry as a bone." How does "dry as a bone" relate to adverse anticholinergic effects?
7. How does atropine cause both bradycardia and tachycardia? Which effect is the most common desired effect from the drug: raising the pulse rate or slowing it?

NEED MORE HELP?

Chapter 14 of the Study Guide to Accompany *Drug Therapy in Nursing*, 4th Edition, contains NCLEX-style questions and other learning activities to reinforce your understanding of the concepts presented in this chapter. For additional information or to purchase the study guide, visit thePoint.

REFERENCES

Biastre, K., & Burnaski, T. (2009). Trospium chloride treatment of overactive bladder. *The Annals of Pharmacotherapy*, 43(2): 283–295.
Birks, J. (2006). Cholinesterase inhibitors for Alzheimer's disease. *Cochrane Database of Systematic Review*. Retrieved from *http://www.mrw.interscience.wiley.com/cochrane/clsysrev/articles/CD005593/ frame.html*.
Birks J., Grimley Evans J., Iakovidou, V. et al. (2009). Rivastigmine for Alzheimer's disease. *Cochrane Database Syst Rev*.(2):CD001191.
Evans, J. G., Wilcock, & G., Birks, J. (2004). Evidence-based pharmacotherapy of Alzheimer's disease. *International Journal of Neuropsychopharmacology*, 7(3):351–369.
Fagerstrom, K., & Balfour, D. J. (2006). Neuropharmacology and potential efficacy of new treatments for tobacco dependence. *Expert Opinion on Investigational Drugs*, 15(2):107–116.

Fant, R. V., Buchhalter, A. R., Buchman, A. C., et al. (2009). Pharmacotherapy for tobacco dependence. *Handbook of Experimental Pharmacology,* 192:487–510.

Foulds, J., Steinberg, M. B., Williams, J. M., et al. (2006). Developments in pharmacotherapy for tobacco dependence. *Expert Opinion on Investigational Drugs,* 15(2):107–116.

Frishman, W. H. (2007). Smoking cessation pharmacotherapy—nicotine and non-nicotine preparations. *Preventive Cardiology,* 10(2 Suppl 1):10–22.

Jonsson, R., & Lockhart, P. B., et al. (2007). Salivary dysfunction associated with systemic diseases: Systematic review and clinical management recommendations. *Oral Surgery, Oral Medicine, Oral Pathology, Oral Radiology, and Endodontics,* 103(Suppl S57.e1–15):13, 41.

Kruzska, P., & O'Brian, R. J. (2009). Diagnosis and management of Sjogren syndrome. *American Family Physician,* 79(6): 465–470.

Lam, S., & Hilas, O. (2007). Pharmacologic management of overactive bladder. *Clinical Interventions in Aging,* 2(3): 337–345.

Update on drugs for overactive bladder syndrome. (2007). *Drug and Therapeutics Bulletin,* 45(6):44–48.

Von Bultzingslowen, I., Sollecito, T. P., Fox, P. C., et al. (2007). Salivary dysfunction associated with systemic diseases: Systematic review and clinical management recommendations. *Oral Surgery, Oral Medicine, Oral Pathology, Oral Radiology, and Endodontics,* 103(Suppl):S57.e1–S57.e15.

UNIT 5

Central Nervous System Drugs

15

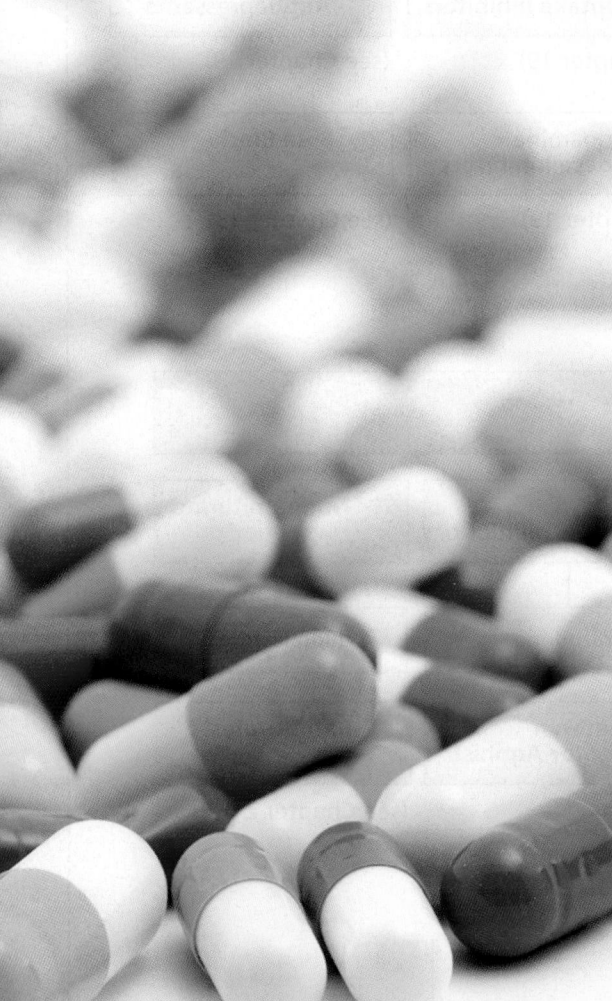

Drugs Relieving Anxiety and Promoting Sleep

Learning Objectives

At the completion of this chapter the student will:

1. Describe the varied therapeutic uses of benzodiazepines.
2. Identify core drug knowledge about drugs that relieve anxiety and promote sleep.
3. Identify core patient variables related to drugs that relieve anxiety and promote sleep.
4. Relate the interaction of core drug knowledge to core patient variables for drugs that relieve anxiety and promote sleep.
5. Generate a nursing plan of care from the interactions between core drug knowledge and core patient variables for drugs that relieve anxiety and promote sleep.
6. Describe nursing interventions to maximize therapeutic and minimize adverse effects for drugs that relieve anxiety and promote sleep.
7. Determine key points for patient and family education for drugs that relieve anxiety and promote sleep.

Key Terms

anxiety	insomnia	REM
anxiolytics	neuroplasticity	
GABA	NREM	

Drugs Relieving Anxiety and Promoting Sleep

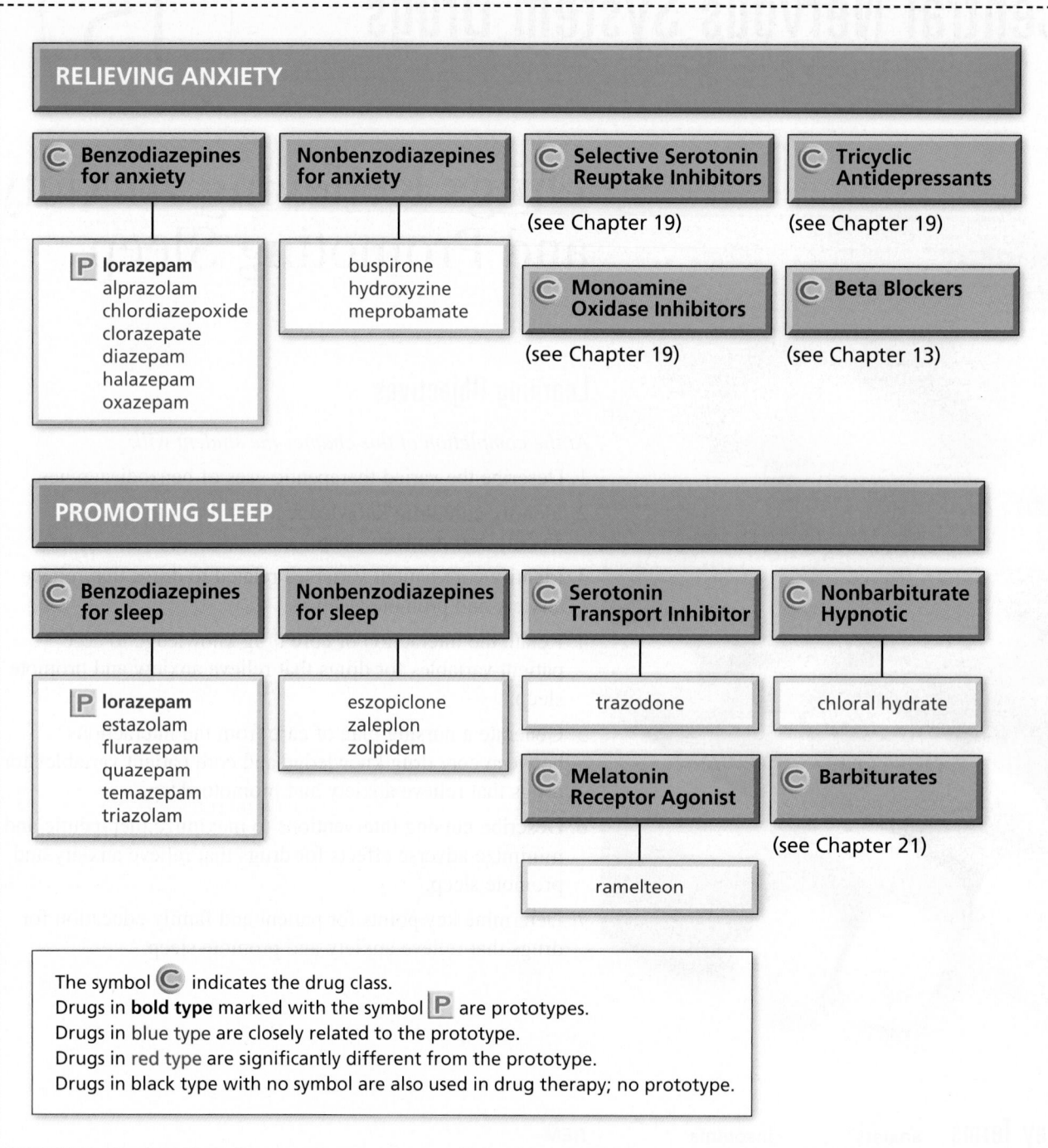

RELIEVING ANXIETY

C Benzodiazepines for anxiety

P lorazepam
alprazolam
chlordiazepoxide
clorazepate
diazepam
halazepam
oxazepam

Nonbenzodiazepines for anxiety

buspirone
hydroxyzine
meprobamate

C Selective Serotonin Reuptake Inhibitors

(see Chapter 19)

C Monoamine Oxidase Inhibitors

(see Chapter 19)

C Tricyclic Antidepressants

(see Chapter 19)

C Beta Blockers

(see Chapter 13)

PROMOTING SLEEP

C Benzodiazepines for sleep

P lorazepam
estazolam
flurazepam
quazepam
temazepam
triazolam

Nonbenzodiazepines for sleep

eszopiclone
zaleplon
zolpidem

C Serotonin Transport Inhibitor

trazodone

C Melatonin Receptor Agonist

ramelteon

C Nonbarbiturate Hypnotic

chloral hydrate

C Barbiturates

(see Chapter 21)

The symbol **C** indicates the drug class.
Drugs in **bold type** marked with the symbol **P** are prototypes.
Drugs in blue type are closely related to the prototype.
Drugs in red type are significantly different from the prototype.
Drugs in black type with no symbol are also used in drug therapy; no prototype.

Drugs that depress the central nervous system (CNS) cause a continuum of effects ranging from producing relaxation and relieving anxiety to producing anesthesia and loss of consciousness. Some drugs that depress the CNS, such as the benzodiazepines, can produce multiple effects depending on the dose and the route of administration. Two of those effects, relieving anxiety and promoting sleep, are discussed in this chapter. The prototype benzodiazepine for this chapter is lorazepam (Ativan). Lorazepam is primarily used to treat anxiety, although it may also be used to promote sleep and rest. This chapter also discusses drugs outside the benzodiazepine class that are used to relieve anxiety or induce sleep. Benzodiazepines used as muscle relaxants are mentioned in Chapter 20, and those used in seizure disorders are presented in Chapter 18.

PHYSIOLOGY

Emotions and Neurotransmitters

The brain governs all physiological and psychological functions of the body including cognition, thoughts, memory, motivation, and emotion. Human emotions, although universal, are not well understood. The limbic system in the brain is known to be primarily responsible for emotions, but why a particular situation might create a severe psychological response in one person but not in another is dependent on environmental and internals factors that are unique to the individual. Much of the neurophysiologic research that has been done on the emotions of fear and anxiety has centered on the amygdala, an almond-shaped structure, and on the hippocampus, both located within the brain. The amygdala receives incoming sensory signals and then communicates with the frontal lobes of the brain where information is interpreted. It is believed that the central part of the amygdala is the storage site for emotional memories. The amygdala can signal the brain that a threat is present and set off a fear response or anxiety. When a stimulus is interpreted as highly threatening, the amygdala floods the brain with danger messages, demanding immediate action and not allowing time for the rest of the brain to process the information with rational and systematic thought.

The systems of the brain do not operate in isolation and its structures undergo frequent refinement in response to the internal and external environment. This process is known as neuroplasticity. To illustrate the point of how functions of the brain adapt during its constant interaction with the environment, imagine what would happen if you were in the pathway of a falling tree. The cerebral cortex of your brain would interpret the sight, compare it to known past experiences, determine that the tree will hit you if you do not move out of the way, and send messages to various body systems to respond. In this case, the heart will beat faster to provide more blood supply to the muscles, and the muscles will contract to run. However, the amygdala determines that the tree is extremely dangerous to the body's well-being and demands that the body respond and *run now,* think later.

Another part of the brain, the hippocampus, is responsible for processing threatening or traumatic stimuli. The hippocampus helps encode information into memories.

To continue with the above example, the next time you encounter a stimulus similar to the falling tree (such as the cracking noise the tree made before it began to fall), the hippocampus will remember this traumatic stimulus and send the message to the amygdala, which will then sense immediate danger and flood the brain with messages to flee for safety.

The brain sends its messages by a complex process in the nervous system that involves a release of neurotransmitters that assist in the movement of impulses along nerve pathways._. Neurotransmitters either inhibit or excite the receptor cell. One of those inhibitory neurotransmitters is gamma-aminobutyric acid, better known as **GABA.** The inhibitory action of GABA works in opposition to the excitatory neurotransmitter glutamate. GABA is released into the synapse, crosses the synapse, and then attaches to a postsynaptic receptor site. Once it is attached, an influx of negatively charged chloride ions enters the postsynaptic neuron. Hyperpolarization of the cell occurs, which in turn leads to an increase in the firing threshold. This produces an inhibitory effect on the nerve cell. A drug such as lorazepam acts by enhancing the actions of GABA (Mayers & Baldwin, 2006). Figure 15.1 depicts the action of GABA on the cell's receptors.

Sleep

Although sleep was once thought of as a time of inactivity, it is now known that the process of sleep involves active physiologic changes in which all major organs and regulatory systems continue to function. The activities that occur in the brain during sleep are essential for the maintenance of mental and physical health.. Circadian processes driven by the brain's biological clock cause sleep and wakefulness to occur at predictable times and are influenced by the physical environment such as light and darkness as well as social or work schedules. The sleep–wake cycle generally consists of eight hours of nocturnal sleep and sixteen hours of wakefulness in response to the release of the hormones melatonin and cortisol (National Sleep Foundation, 2006). While the eyes are closed during sleep, periodic rapid eye movements can be observed. Sleep, therefore, has two phases; the first has no rapid eye movements (**NREM**), and the second has rapid eye movements (**REM**). NREM sleep is further sub-divided into four stages:

- Stage 1—light sleep; muscles relax; brain waves are irregular and rapid.
- Stage 2—brain waves are larger than in stage 1, with bursts of electrical activity.
- Stages 3 and 4—deep sleep, with even larger, slower brain waves called delta waves; this stage is often referred to as slow-wave sleep.

After stage 4 sleep, the body begins REM sleep. During REM sleep, brain waves are almost the same as they are during waking hours, and dreaming occurs. The body becomes essentially paralyzed during REM sleep, so that it cannot act out the dreams. After a period of REM sleep, the person cycles through the NREM stages before again returning to REM sleep. A complete sleep cycle consists of NREM and REM

PHYSIOLOGY

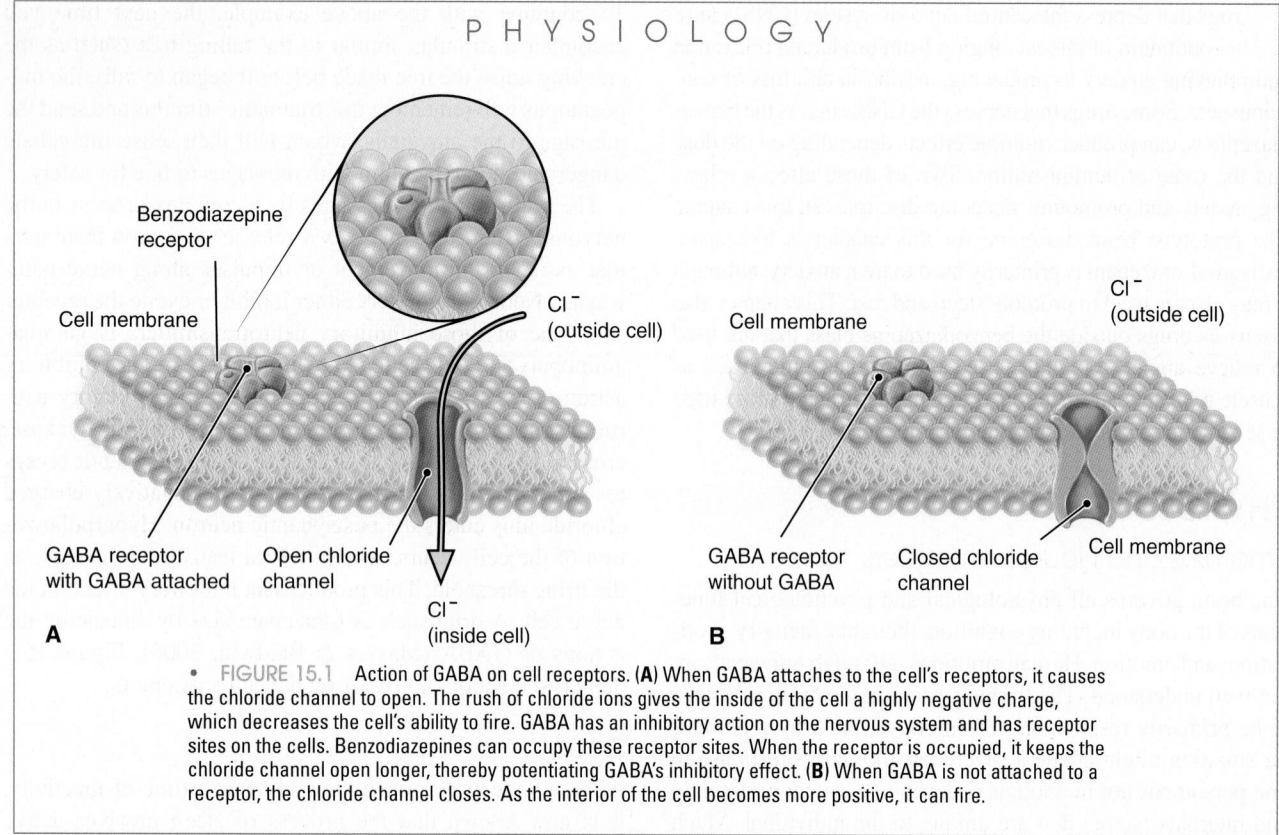

Benzodiazepine
receptor

Cell membrane

Cl⁻
(outside cell)

Cell membrane

Cl⁻
(outside cell)

GABA receptor
with GABA attached

Open chloride
channel

GABA receptor
without GABA

Closed chloride
channel

Cell membrane

A

Cl⁻
(inside cell)

B

- FIGURE 15.1   Action of GABA on cell receptors. (**A**) When GABA attaches to the cell's receptors, it causes the chloride channel to open. The rush of chloride ions gives the inside of the cell a highly negative charge, which decreases the cell's ability to fire. GABA has an inhibitory action on the nervous system and has receptor sites on the cells. Benzodiazepines can occupy these receptor sites. When the receptor is occupied, it keeps the chloride channel open longer, thereby potentiating GABA's inhibitory effect. (**B**) When GABA is not attached to a receptor, the chloride channel closes. As the interior of the cell becomes more positive, it can fire.

cycles that alternate every 90 to 110 minutes and is repeated four to six times per night (National Sleep Foundation, 2006). Arousal from sleep is fairly easy when in REM but can be difficult from NREM. A person awakened from NREM sleep may be confused and disoriented until completely awake, a process that can take up to 5 minutes. Approximately 75% of sleep time is non-REM sleep, and 25% is REM sleep. REM periods generally become longer and more frequent during the later part of the sleep cycle.

A number of physiologic changes occur within the different stages of sleep. The low point of the 24-hour cycle for temperature occurs at night during sleep, although sleep does not cause the decrease. Urine secretion falls during sleep. The heart rate and respirations are slower and more regular during NREM sleep and then more rapid and less regular during REM sleep. Blood flow to the brain is increased during REM sleep. Autonomic nervous functions tend to be active during REM, with irregular breathing, variable pulse rate and blood pressure levels, and an increased metabolic rate. Hormones affecting growth, energy level, and metabolic function are secreted during sleep. Secretion of growth hormone increases during the first 2 hours, and surges of adrenocorticotropic hormone and cortisone secretion occur in the second half of the sleep period. Penile erections can occur during sleep and are more frequent during REM sleep. Luteinizing hormone secretion is increased for both boys and girls during puberty, and prolactin is secreted at an increased rate in both men and women, especially immediately after the onset of sleep.

The amount of sleep needed by a person varies throughout the life span, with infants requiring the most sleep and adults requiring the least. The time in each phase of the sleep cycle also varies throughout the life span. Although sleep requirements among people vary greatly, just as important as the quantity of sleep is getting the right mix of REM and NREM sleep (National Sleep Foundation, 2006).

PATHOPHYSIOLOGY

Anxiety

Anxiety is a universal experience among humans characterized by a feeling of unease that something bad or undesirable may happen. Anxiety functions as a protective mechanism that has evolved to help people recognize danger and take action for self-preservation. It has both physiological and emotional characteristics triggered by events that could be threatening, disruptive, or dangerous. Anxiety is considered to be pathologic however, if it develops when no actual threat exists, when it occurs chronically, and it interferes with the ability to function in daily life.

Anxiety disorders are differentiated by their own distinctive features, but they all share characteristics of excessive and irrational fear and dread. Anxiety is a serious illness that affects approximately 40 million American adults each year (National Institute of Mental Health, 2007), making it one of the most common mental conditions that often goes untreated.

Development of anxiety disorders is related to the combination of stressful life experiences, psychological characteristics, and/or genetic inherited traits (U.S. Public Health Service, 2009).

Anxiety disorders can occur with other physical and emotional problems and the symptoms of either can be difficult to differentiate. Depressive disorders, substance abuse disorders, and eating disorders are only of a few of the mental illnesses in which symptoms can be masked or exacerbated by anxiety disorders. People with anxiety disorders are two to three times more likely to have an alcohol or other substance abuse disorder at some point in their lives than the general population. Treatment may include psychosocial modalities such as cognitive behavioral therapies, exposure therapy, relaxation therapy, or psychotherapy, as well as drug therapy (Anxiety Disorders Association of America, 2009).

The following are some types of anxiety disorders:

• Panic disorder—sudden feelings of terror that come on suddenly and repeatedly without warning. Panic attacks are usually accompanied by physical changes such as heart pounding, sweating, weakness, faintness, or dizziness. A fear of impending doom, fear of losing control, and a loss of touch with reality are common in panic attacks. Because patients cannot understand or explain the physical changes that are occurring, they can have great concern about these symptoms, believing they are dying or losing their minds. Occurring at any time, even during sleep, the symptoms of a panic attack usually peak in 10 minutes but may continue for a while longer.

Panic attacks often begin in adolescence or early adulthood, and panic disorder affects about 6 million American adults yearly. It is twice as common in women as in men. There appears to be a genetic predisposition to developing the condition, and comorbid disorders often include depression, drug abuse, or alcoholism, which need to be treated separately. People with panic disorder may develop phobias and avoid places or situations where a previous attack has occurred; some people may be so affected that they do not leave the house.

Phobic disorders are persistent, unrealistic fears of situations or objects that do not realistically pose a significant threat or danger. Phobias may be severe and incapacitating. Some specific phobias are further discussed in this chapter.

• Social phobia (also called social anxiety disorder)—overwhelming anxiety and excessive self-consciousness in everyday social situations. It is characterized by persistent, intense, and chronic fears of being watched and judged by others and by being embarrassed by one's own actions. Physical symptoms that often accompany social phobia include blushing, profuse sweating, trembling, nausea, and difficulty talking. Social phobia affects about 15 million adult American women and men. Onset usually occurs during childhood or early adolescence. Like other anxiety disorders, there is some evidence that genetic makeup may make a person more at risk of having social phobia. Comorbid conditions often include other anxiety disorders or depression. People with social phobia may resort to substance abuse in an effort to self-medicate their anxiety yet can respond successfully to psychotherapy and or medication.

• Specific phobia—an intense, irrational fear of a particular thing or situation that poses little or no actual danger. Common examples are fear of heights, elevators or enclosed spaces, or flying. The anxiety is not generalized to other situations. For example, a person who becomes extremely anxious if they are in a tall building may be able to climb a mountain without any anxiety.

Specific phobias affect an estimated 19.2 million adult Americans and are twice as common in women as men. Onset of specific phobias is usually in childhood or adolescence, and the phobias persist into adulthood. The causes of specific phobias are not well understood, but there is some evidence that the tendency to develop them may run in families. If help is sought, specific phobias respond very well to carefully targeted psychotherapy.

• Obsessive-compulsive disorder (OCD)—recurrent, unwelcome thoughts with rituals attempting to control the anxiety resulting from these thoughts. For example, a patient may be filled with doubts and repeatedly check situations of concern (e.g., whether doors are locked). The recurring thoughts are obsessions; the behaviors that deal with those thoughts are compulsions. The compulsive behavior ends up taking over the person's life, providing little help in dealing with the anxiety from the obsessive thinking, and is distressing to the patient.

OCD affects about 2.2 million American adults; men and women are equally affected. The disorder usually first appears in childhood, adolescence, or early adulthood. Comorbid conditions include eating disorders, other anxiety disorders, or depression. Research suggests that OCD may be inherited.

OCD usually responds to pharmacologic treatment and/or psychotherapy that involve controlled exposure to the situation that produces fear or anxiety.

• Post-traumatic stress disorder (PTSD)—a debilitating condition that can develop following a terrifying event that involved physical harm or threat of physical harm to either oneself or to another. Events that can trigger PTSD include war experience, kidnapping, robbery, man-made disasters (e.g., bombings, fires), or natural disasters (e.g., hurricanes). A person experiences persistent frightening thoughts and memories of the ordeal, termed flashbacks. People with PTSD may feel emotionally numb and have difficulty relating to people they were once close to. They may startle easily, lose interest in things they used to enjoy, have trouble feeling affectionate, be irritable, become more aggressive, or even become violent. They avoid situations that remind them of the original incident, and anniversaries of the incident are often very difficult. PTSD symptoms seem to be worse if the event that triggered them was deliberately initiated by another person, such as in a mugging or a kidnapping.

PTSD affects about 7.7 million American adults, but it can occur at any age, including childhood. Women are more likely to develop PTSD than men, and there is some evidence that susceptibility to the disorder may run in families. Comorbidities that often accompany PTSD are depression, substance abuse, and one or more of the other anxiety disorders.

Psychotherapy and medication are usually effective in treating PTSD.

- Generalized anxiety disorder (GAD)—chronic anxiety that lasts more than 6 months and causes the person to have exaggerated worry and tension every day. In this disorder, the person always anticipates disaster and worries excessively over issues such as health, money, work, and family. Symptoms include inability to relax, startling easily, difficulty concentrating, and trouble falling asleep or staying asleep. Severe GAD can make it difficult to partake in ordinary daily activities.

GAD affects about 6.8 million adult Americans. Women have a higher prevalence of GAD than men, and although it can begin anytime during life, it most frequently begins between childhood and middle age. Again, there is evidence that genes play a modest role in GAD. Comorbid conditions normally include other anxiety disorders, depression, and substance abuse.

GAD is commonly treated with medication or cognitive-behavioral therapy, but comorbidities must also be treated appropriately.

The development of anxiety disorders may occur from a complex set of risk factors including genetics, brain chemistry, and life events. Neuroemotional memories stored in the amygdala are believed to play a role in disorders involving very distinct fears, such as phobias. Other parts of the brain may be involved with other types of anxiety. The hippocampus, for example, shrinks in people who have experienced severe stress because of child abuse or military combat, which may explain why people with PTSD have flashbacks, deficits in explicit memory, and fragmented memory of details of the traumatic event. Other research indicates that the basal ganglia and striatum in the brain are involved in obsessive-compulsive disorder (National Institute of Mental Health, 2006).

Neurotransmitters are known to play a role in anxiety, although exactly how they do so is not known. GABA has long been known to have a role in diminishing anxiety, and antianxiety drugs (**anxiolytics**) enhance the action of GABA. Serotonin and norepinephrine have also recently been discovered to function in anxiety, and other neurotransmitter systems, such as corticotropin-releasing factors and substance P, appear to be abnormally regulated in patients who have anxiety. More research is needed to determine whether drugs that are antagonists to these systems might be helpful in treating anxiety. Also, because GABA works to counteract glutamate, decreasing glutamate or diminishing its activity might decrease anxiety.

Sleep Disorders

It is estimated that between 50 and 70 million Americans are affected by chronic sleep disorders and intermittent sleep problems. Sleep deprivation has a profound impact on mental and physical health. Relationships have been shown between sleep disturbances and cardiovascular disease, obesity, diabetes, and a decreased immune response (National Sleep Foundation, 2006). Disordered sleep is not only a common symptom of many psychiatric illnesses, it can increase one's perception of stress, ability to manage stressors, and can dramatically influence one's quality of life (Leblanc, 2007). Sleep disorders are many and may include the following problems:

- Narcolepsy—sudden irresistible sleep attacks of unknown origin lasting from seconds to minutes, two to six times a day
- Sleep apnea—a group of disorders characterized by cessation of breathing during sleep, lasting 10 seconds or longer and occurring 30 or more times during a night's sleep
- Sleepwalking—getting up and walking about while still asleep, although the eyes are open; usually occurs in children
- Night terrors—occur only in children, with periods of fright, crying, moaning, or screaming after a brief time asleep; episodes usually do not last long and are not generally remembered in the morning
- Excessive daytime sedation
- Insomnia—problems with initiating and/or maintaining sleep

Across the lifespan, sleeplessness or lack of restful sleep has an effect on a person's ability to physically, cognitively, and emotionally function in the daytime. Sleep loss results in an accumulation of sleep debt that must eventually be repaid by either napping or sleeping longer in later cycles (National Sleep Foundation, 2006). In a large survey of adult Americans which focused on the sleep habits of working adults, 65% reported having at least one symptom of a sleep problem a few nights a week or more within the past month (National Sleep Foundation, 2008). The most common problems reported were frequent waking during the night and waking up feeling unrefreshed, followed by difficulty falling asleep and waking up early and being unable to return to sleep Within this survey, 44% reported one or more of these problems occurring almost every night, 26% reported high levels of daytime sleepiness, and 39% had driven while drowsy within the past year (National Sleep Foundation, 2008). Sleep problems also affect adolescents and children. Nearly half (45%) of adolescents surveyed reported a sleep problem at least one night a week (National Sleep Foundation, 2006). Parents surveyed about their infant to school-aged children reported that 69% had sleeping problems, including difficulty falling asleep and frequent awakening during the night (National Sleep Foundation, 2004). Sleeping difficulties are a common occurrence in the elderly. Aging is associated with a more fragmented sleep; waking more frequently during the night, going to sleep earlier in the evening, and awakening earlier in the morning (Wolkove, 2007).

Of these disorders, **insomnia** occurs most frequently. Insomnia is the perception or complaint of inadequate or poor-quality sleep. It has many presentations, which include:

• Difficulty falling asleep or staying asleep
• Waking up too early in the morning without being able to return to sleep
• Waking up frequently during the night with difficulty returning to sleep
• Not sleeping long enough
• Feeling that sleep was not restful
• Sleeping poorly

Because people vary greatly in their need for sleep and their satisfaction with sleep, insomnia cannot be defined merely by the number of hours a person sleeps or by how long it takes to fall asleep. Insomnia is instead classified by frequency of occurrence: acute (often due to a temporary situation such as jet lag or stress and lasting up to one month), or chronic (occurring for a month or longer).

Insomnia has many causes. Acute insomnia is often related to stress, environmental noise, extreme temperatures, change in the surrounding environment, sleep–wake schedule problems such as jet lag, or adverse effects of drug therapy. Chronic insomnia is more complex and often results from more than one cause, including underlying physical or mental disorders, as well as adverse effects of drug therapy. Not only is chronic insomnia a common cause of depression and a symptom of many mental illnesses, it is now thought that sleep problems increase the risk of developing depression (Mayers, Baldwin, 2006). Other underlying causes of insomnia include arthritis, kidney disease, heart failure, asthma, sleep apnea, narcolepsy, restless legs syndrome, Parkinson disease, hyperthyroidism, and hormonal changes during menopause. Insomnia tends to occur more often in women than men, especially after the women reach menopause.

In addition, chronic insomnia may be "primary," which means that it is not caused by other medical, psychiatric, sleep, or medication factors. Factors such as increased body temperature, metabolic rate, or brain metabolism may cause primary insomnia. Poor sleep habits may also contribute to primary and other forms of insomnia.

Chronic insomnia may also be related to the core patient variable of life span, diet, and habits. The following behaviors are associated with chronic insomnia: overuse of caffeine, misuse of alcohol or other substances, disrupted sleep–wake cycles such as from shift work, and chronic stress. Some people also have insomnia related to smoking cigarettes just before bedtime, excessive napping in the afternoon or evening, and expecting or worrying about sleep difficulties.

Although lifestyle changes can prevent insomnia in most people with acute insomnia, some patients need short-term drug therapy to help them sleep. Chronic insomnia can be treated by diagnosing and treating any underlying medical or psychological problems. Stopping behaviors that contribute to insomnia is also helpful. Patients may also need to apply behavioral techniques such as relaxation therapy, sleep restriction therapy, and reconditioning to overcome chronic insomnia. Relaxation techniques such as progressive relaxation and rhythmic breathing allow the muscles to relax and the mind to stop "racing," thereby allowing natural sleep to occur. Sleep restriction may be used when people spend too much time in bed trying to fall asleep. These patients are allowed only a few hours in bed at night for a while, and then the time in bed is gradually increased until a more normal night's sleep occurs. Reconditioning helps people reconnect being in bed and bedtime with sleeping. They need to avoid using their beds for any activity besides sleeping or sex. If they are unable to sleep, they are instructed to get out of bed and return to bed only once they are sleepy, so that eventually the body will associate the bed with sleeping. They are also coached to avoid naps and to continue going to bed and getting up in the morning at the same time every day. The use of drug therapy to treat chronic insomnia is very controversial. Generally, it is considered best to use drug therapy for the shortest duration possible.

DRUGS TO RELIEVE ANXIETY

Various drug therapies can be used in treating anxiety disorders. Treatment with drug therapy does not cure the anxiety but keeps it under control. The person with anxiety usually receives psychotherapy in addition to drug therapy. Many drugs that were originally designed to treat other conditions have been found to be helpful in treating some of the anxiety disorders, because they have an effect on the neurotransmitters involved in anxiety.

• SELECTIVE SEROTONIN REUPTAKE INHIBITORS

Selective serotonin reuptake inhibitors (SSRIs) are a class of antidepressant drugs, some of which are now considered first-line therapy for anxiety disorders such as panic disorder, OCD, PTSD, GAD, and social phobia. Low serotonin levels are known to be present in severe stress and in many mood and anxiety-related disorders, and SSRIs indirectly increase the amount of the neurotransmitter serotonin available in the synapses. SSRIs that are prescribed for anxiety include citalopram (Celexa), fluvoxamine (Luvox), paroxetine (Paxil), fluoxetine (Prozac), and sertraline (Zoloft). (Venlafaxine, a drug closely related to the SSRIs, is also used in treating GAD.) The prototype SSRI is sertraline (Zoloft), and it is discussed in Chapter 16.

SSRIs are generally well tolerated with few adverse effects. Unlike the benzodiazepines, they do not cause diminished alertness or ataxia. Although SSRIs can produce some nausea or jitteriness when first started, these adverse effects usually go away with continued use. However, SSRIs can also cause sexual dysfunction. Unlike the benzodiazepines, which can reduce anxiety from one dose, the SSRIs must be taken for several weeks for their full anxiety-relieving effect to be evident.

TRICYCLIC ANTIDEPRESSANTS

The tricyclic antidepressants (TCAs), another class of antidepressants, are not used as frequently as the SSRIs. Except for OCD, TCAs are as effective as the SSRIs in treating most anxiety disorders, most likely because they act similarly. TCAs work by affecting the regulation of serotonin or norepinephrine in the brain. The TCAs used to treat anxiety, panic disorder, and PTSD are doxepin (Adapin), nortriptyline (Aventyl), amitriptyline (Elavil), imipramine (Tofranil), maprotiline (Ludiomil), desipramine (Norpramin), trimipramine (Surmontil), and protriptyline (Vivactil). Clomipramine (Anafranil) is used to treat OCD. The tricyclics are discussed in Chapter 16. The prototype TCA is nortriptyline (Pamelor).

TCAs have a higher adverse effect profile than SSRIs, which limits their use as antidepressants. Adverse effects include dizziness, drowsiness, dry mouth, and weight gain. Overdosage with a TCA is much more likely to result in death than overdosage with an SSRI. As with the SSRIs, several weeks of therapy on TCAs are necessary before anxiety begins to diminish.

MONOAMINE OXIDASE INHIBITORS

Monoamine oxidase inhibitors (MAOIs) are the oldest class of antidepressants. The MAOIs used to treat anxiety disorders are phenelzine (Nardil), tranylcypromine (Parnate), and isocarboxazid (Marplan). These drugs are occasionally prescribed for panic disorder and social phobia. Monoamine oxidase is the enzyme that degrades serotonin in the synapse. By inhibiting the enzyme, higher levels of serotonin can remain in the synapse and be active. The prototype MAOI is phenelzine (Nardil). Further information about MAOIs also appears in Chapter 16.

The MAOIs are associated with a significant risk of a serious drug–food interaction. If the patient taking an MAOI consumes food or drink that is high in tyramines, such as aged, cured meats, blue cheese, and Chianti wine, a hypertensive crisis (a potentially life-threatening condition) can develop. The newest MAOI is a transdermal patch (selegiline [Emsam]); the lowest available dose does not have the same risk of food–drug interactions, although higher doses may still have some risk.

BETA BLOCKERS

Beta blockers are adrenergic drugs most frequently used for a wide variety of cardiac conditions, such as angina, hypertension, and arrhythmias. Among other actions, they slow the heart rate. This helps patients with some types of anxiety who may be uncomfortable and highly aware of the tachycardia and palpitations that can occur in anxiety. Beta blockers are sometimes prescribed to control this symptom in social phobia. The prototype beta blocker propranolol is discussed in Chapter 13.

C BENZODIAZEPINES

Benzodiazepines are used for a number of therapeutic effects, including anxiety relief, sleep promotion, antiepileptic effects, muscle relaxation, treatment of acute alcohol withdrawal, induction of general anesthesia, preoperative sedation, and conscious sedation. Some of these drugs have other specific uses, many of them off label. As a class, benzodiazepines appear to potentiate the effects of GABA. Because GABA is an inhibitory neurotransmitter, this benzodiazepine-mediated intensification of the effects of GABA leads to more CNS depression than would normally be found.

Benzodiazepines bind to specific receptor sites to produce their effects. At least two types of these receptors are believed to exist: BZ_1 and BZ_2. Sleep mechanisms are thought to be related to BZ_1, and memory, motor, sensory, and cognitive functions related to BZ_2. Activity of the benzodiazepines may involve the following sites: spinal cord (muscle relaxation), brainstem (antiepileptic activity), cerebellum (ataxia effects), and the limbic and cortical areas (emotional behavior). The antianxiety effects of benzodiazepines are separate from those that nonspecifically depress the CNS (leading to sedation and motor impairment). Much larger doses of benzodiazepines are required to produce the effects of ataxia and sedation than to produce antianxiety effects.

As a drug class, benzodiazepines have a high margin of safety (i.e., a wide therapeutic index) and are therefore often the drug class of first choice to treat some types of anxiety, most commonly GAD. All of the benzodiazepines have similar efficacy; they differ by pharmacokinetics and cost. Lorazepam is the prototype benzodiazepine used to treat anxiety. Other drugs in this class represented by the prototype are alprazolam (Xanax), chlordiazepoxide (Librium), clorazepate (Tranxene), diazepam (Valium), halazepam (Paxipam), and oxazepam (Serax).

Nursing Management of the Patient Receiving P Lorazepam

Core Drug Knowledge

Pharmacotherapeutics

Lorazepam (Ativan) is used in treating anxiety disorders, most frequently in GAD, for short-term relief of anxiety that occurs with depression and for insomnia. Day-to-day stress and anxiety should not be treated with antianxiety drugs. Lorazepam, when given intramuscularly or intravenously preoperatively and before anesthesia, produces sedation, relieves anxiety, and decreases the patient's ability to recall events surrounding surgery. Off-label uses of lorazepam include treating status epilepticus, chemotherapy-induced nausea and vomiting, the symptoms of acute alcohol withdrawal, and psychogenic catatonia. Although there is no consensus for a benzodiazepine of choice for treatment of alcohol withdrawal, lorazepam can effectively be used to reduce the risk of seizures and decrease alcohol withdrawal symptoms (Vincent, et al., 2007). The use

CRITICAL THINKING SCENARIO

LORAZEPAM AND ANXIETY

Lena Hawthorne, 18 years old, was started on lorazepam for anxiety 3 days ago. She calls the clinic and tells you that the dosage must not be large enough because her symptoms of anxiety have increased. She complains of feeling so anxious that she feels she "might jump out of her skin." She also complains of having insomnia since she started taking lorazepam.

1. What is your assessment of her problem?
2. What interventions would you carry out or suggest at this time?

---

of benzodiazepines to treat seizures is further discussed in Chapter 18.

Pharmacokinetics

Lorazepam, like other benzodiazepines, is readily absorbed from the gastrointestinal (GI) tract. Unlike some of the other benzodiazepines, lorazepam is readily absorbed when it is given intramuscularly. Because of its high lipid solubility, lorazepam is widely distributed in the body tissues, and it is also highly protein-bound (85%). Compared to other benzodiazepines, lorazepam has an intermediate speed of onset when taken orally. Lorazepam is hepatically metabolized to an inactive substance, making it—along with oxazepam (Serax)—unusual among the drugs in the class, which are otherwise metabolized to active compounds. This easy inactivation is an advantage for patients with liver disease and for older adults. Lorazepam is eliminated through the urine.

Intravenous lorazepam is distributed quickly to the brain, which makes it effective in treating status epilepticus (discussed further in Chapter 18). Unlike diazepam, another benzodiazepine given for status epilepticus, lorazepam redistributes out of the brain slowly, providing prolonged protection against further seizures. Although the half-life of lorazepam in the blood is rather short, its effectiveness in controlling seizures is related to how long it is at the site of action—the brain, not the bloodstream. Lorazepam has been proven to be more effective than diazepam in controlling status epilepticus (Prasad, al-Roomi, Krishnan, et al., 2005). Table 15.1 provides a summary of selected benzodiazepines and a comparison of their pharmacokinetic properties.

Pharmacodynamics

Like all benzodiazepines, lorazepam increases the effects of GABA, which has an inhibitory effect on the CNS. However, none of the benzodiazepines act like GABA or increase the amount of GABA present. The intrinsic amount of GABA is limited; hence, the effects from benzodiazepines are also limited. Tolerance to lorazepam and the other benzodiazepines can occur if they are used long-term, requiring larger doses to achieve a therapeutic effect. Thus, it is recommended that they be limited to short-term use.

Contraindications and Precautions

Contraindications to administration of lorazepam, which apply to all the benzodiazepines, are hypersensitivity, psychoses, acute narrow-angle glaucoma, intra-arterial use, and use in children younger than 6 months. Prolonged administration of lorazepam or any other benzodiazepine produces physical dependence, and withdrawal symptoms occur if the drug is stopped suddenly. Like most other benzodiazepines, lorazepam is a pregnancy category D drug. Benzodiazepines, have been found in maternal and cord blood, indicating transfer to the fetus; therefore, they should not be used for obstetric uses during labor and delivery.

Paradoxical reactions have been reported with lorazepam and other benzodiazepines, evidenced by excitement, stimulation, and acute rage. These effects have been noted mostly in patients with psychiatric disorders and in hyperactive, aggressive children. But older adults are also at risk of paradoxical effects. Other symptoms that may occur are acute hyperexcited states, anxiety, hallucinations, increased muscle spasticity, insomnia, and sleep disturbances. These effects usually occur within the first 2 weeks of therapy.

Adverse Effects

Lorazepam, like other benzodiazepines, is generally well tolerated, with few adverse effects. Mild drowsiness is common but transient, occurring in the first few days of therapy and then dissipating. Ataxia and confusion may also occur, especially in older adults and in debilitated patients. Dose adjustments should be made if these effects persist. Respiratory disturbances and partial airway obstruction may occur if excessive lorazepam is given intravenously before a procedure. A number of other adverse effects are possible, although they are rare. Many relate to the CNS depression that occurs with the drug therapy. These adverse effects are as follows:

- *Cardiovascular:* bradycardia, tachycardia, cardiovascular collapse, hypertension, hypotension, decreased systolic blood pressure, palpitations, edema, and phlebitis and thrombosis at intravenous (IV) sites
- *CNS:* problems with arousal and energy (sedation, sleepiness, depression, lethargy, apathy, fatigue, hypoactivity, restlessness, stupor, coma); balance and movement (light-headedness, syncope, rigidity, tremor, dystonia, vertigo, dizziness, unsteadiness, ataxia, impaired coordination, weakness, akathisia, hemiparesis, hypotonia, psychomotor retardation, seizures); mood and emotions (crying, sobbing, euphoria, nervousness, irritability, agitation); cognitive (memory impairment, disorientation, delirium, anterograde amnesia, confusion, difficulty in concentration, inability to perform complex mental functions); speech (slurred speech, aphonia, dysarthria); other (vivid dreams, "glassy eyed" appearance, headache, extrapyramidal symptoms, paradoxical reactions)
- *Dermatologic:* urticaria, pruritus, rash, dermatitis, hair loss, hirsutism, ankle and facial edema

TABLE 15.1 Summary of Selected Ⓒ Benzodiazepines

Drug (Trade) Name	Selected Indications	Route and Dosage Range	Pharmacokinetics
Ⓟ lorazepam (Ativan)	Anxiety, anesthetic premedication, status epilepticus, alcohol withdrawal, chronic insomnia	*Adult:* PO, 2–6 mg/d; IM, 0.05 mg/kg; IV, 2 mg *Child:* Not recommended; IV/IM, oral dose not established	*Onset:* PO, 1–3 h; IM, 15–30 min; IV, 1–5 min *Duration:* 12–24 h $t_{1/2}$: 10–20 h
alprazolam (Xanax)	Anxiety, panic disorder, agoraphobia	*Adult:* PO, 0.25–1.0 mg tid *Child:* Not established	*Onset:* 30 min *Duration:* 4–6 h $t_{1/2}$: 6.3–26.9 h
chlordiazepoxide (Librium)	Anxiety, alcohol withdrawal, anesthetic premedication	*Adult:* PO, 5–10 mg tid–qid (50–100 mg for alcohol withdrawal); IM/IV, 50–100 mg *Child* >6 y: PO, 5 mg bid–qid; IM/IV, 25–50 mg; not recommended under 6 y	*Onset:* PO, varies; IM, 10–15 min *Duration:* 48–72 h $t_{1/2}$: 5–30 h
diazepam (Valium);	Anxiety, status epilepticus, skeletal muscle relaxant	*Adult:* PO, IM, 2–10 mg/bid–qid; rectal, 0.2 mg/kg daily–bid; IV, 5–10 mg prn *Reduced dosage in geriatric or debilitated patients* *Child* >2 y: PO, 1–2.5 mg tid–qid; IM and IV, up to 0.25 mg/kg; Rectal, 0.5 mg/kg	*Onset:* PO, 30–60 min; IM, 15–30 min; rectal, rapid; IV, 1–5 min *Duration:* 3 h (1 h IV) $t_{1/2}$: 20–50 h
flurazepam (Dalmane);	Insomnia	*Adult:* 15–30 mg at bedtime *Child:* Not for use <15 y	*Onset:* 15–30 min *Duration:* 7–8 h $t_{1/2}$: 2–3 h; 47–100 h (active metabolite)
	Preoperative sedation, anxiolysis, amnesia Sedation Anesthesia	*Adult:* IM, IV: 1–5 mg *Child:* 0.025–0.15 mg/kg *Dose individualized/reduced in patients >60 y of age, debilitated, or chronically ill.*	*Onset:* IM, *Adult:* 15 min; *Child:* 5 min; IV, 1–3 min *Duration:* 6 h $t_{1/2}$: 1.8–6.4 h
Ⓒ Benzodiazepine Antagonist			
flumazenil (Romazicon);	Benzodiazepine antagonist	*Adult:* IV, 0.2 mg q 60 s up to 1 mg (reversal of conscious sedation); 0.2 mg, then 0.3 mg q 30 sec up to 3 mg (management of benzodiazepine overdose).	*Onset:* 20–30 s *Duration:* 72 h $t_{1/2}$: 7–15 min; 41–79 min (repeated doses)

- *GI:* constipation, diarrhea, dry mouth, coated tongue, sore gums, nausea, anorexia, change in appetite, vomiting, difficulty swallowing, increased salivation, gastritis
- *GU:* incontinence, changes in libido, urinary retention, menstrual irregularities
- *Ophthalmic:* visual disturbances, diplopia, nystagmus
- *Psychiatric:* behavioral problems, hysteria, psychosis, suicidal tendencies
- *Hematologic:* elevated liver enzymes, leukopenia, blood dyscrasias, anemia, thrombocytopenia, eosinophilia
- *Miscellaneous:* decreased hearing, nasal congestion, auditory disturbances, hiccups, fever, diaphoresis, gynecomastia, changes in weight, dehydration, lymphedema, joint pain, and burning or pain at the intramuscular injection site

Drug Interactions

Several drug interactions are possible with lorazepam, the most important of which occur when lorazepam is coadministered with other drugs or substances that also depress the CNS. When lorazepam or other benzodiazepines are administered with alcohol, narcotics, barbiturates, or other CNS depressants, the effect on the CNS is additive. These combinations may depress respiratory drive, create severe hypotension or bradycardia, and substantially alter level of consciousness. Although lorazepam and other benzodiazepines are very safe when taken by themselves, even in large doses, the effects can be deadly when they are combined with other CNS depressants, especially in large quantities. Table 15.2 presents agents that interact with lorazepam.

TABLE 15.2	Agents That Interact with ℗ Lorazepam	
Interactants	**Effect and Significance**	**Nursing Management**
alcohol, CNS depressants (opioid narcotics, barbiturates)	Increased CNS effects of lorazepam	Evaluate patient for additive CNS-depressant effects. Monitor serum levels (if appropriate) for therapeutic levels. Avoid concomitant administration if possible.
antacids	Altered rate of absorption of lorazepam, but generally not the extent of absorption	Administer antacid 1 h before or 2 h after lorazepam.
digoxin	Increased serum concentration of digoxin and possible toxicity	Assess serum digoxin levels closely. Monitor the patient's cardiac status frequently for changes.
levodopa	Decreased control of parkinsonian symptoms	Administer lorazepam cautiously to patients receiving levodopa for Parkinson disease. Assess patient for increasing muscle rigidity, tremors, and drooling.
oral contraceptives	Increased clearance of lorazepam may affect symptom management	Change in lorazepam dosage may be needed.
phenytoin	Increased serum concentration of phenytoin leading to possible toxicity	Monitor serum phenytoin levels closely.
probenecid	Interference with hepatic conjugation leading to more rapid onset or prolonged effect of lorazepam	Assess patient for continued sedative effects. Assess for dosage change as indicated.
rifampin	Increased hepatic microsomal enzyme metabolism of lorazepam leading to decreased effectiveness of lorazepam	Assess for dosage change of lorazepam as indicated. Assess patient for changes in seizure control or decrease in sedative effect.
scopolamine	Increased sedation when administered with parenteral form of lorazepam	Institute safety measures. Assess patient for signs of increased drowsiness, dizziness, and ataxia.
theophylline	Possible antagonism of sedative effects of lorazepam	Assess for lorazepam dosage adjustment.

Assessment of Relevant Core Patient Variables

Health Status

Assess the patient for any contraindications to using lorazepam before initiating therapy. Assess for renal and hepatic impairment, which may alter the circulating levels of the drug. In patients who have depression along with anxiety, assess for risk for suicide. Obtaining a baseline level of hepatic enzymes and a complete blood count provides a reference for comparison when these levels are checked throughout long-term therapy.

Life Span and Gender

Assess the patient's age. IV lorazepam is not recommended in children younger than 18 years of age because data regarding its effects are minimal. Similarly, the efficacy and safety of oral lorazepam have not been established for children younger than 12 years of age. When it is used in children, the initial dose should be small, and it should be increased in very small increments. Lorazepam is contraindicated in children younger than 6 months of age. Lorazepam and other benzodiazepines should be used with extreme caution

in the elderly. Compared with younger adults, older adults taking lorazepam or other benzodiazepines are more likely to exhibit adverse effects than younger adults, therefore they are usually started at half the dose recommended for younger adults, titrated slowly, and used for only short periods (Wolkove, Elkholy, Baltzan, Palayew, 2007). According to the Beers Criteria for potentially inappropriate drugs in older adults, lorazepam and other benzodiazepines pose a high risk of severe adverse effects. Therefore, the dose of lorazepam should be limited to no more than 3 mg per day (Fick, Cooper, Wade, et al., 2003).

Specifically, lorazepam, like other benzodiazepines, may cause excessive ataxia or lethargy in older adults. In a systematic review medications as risk factors for fall, it was found that one of the main group of drugs associated with this risk were benzodiazepines (Hartikainen, Lonnroos, Louhivuori, 2007). Older adults taking benzodiazepines have been found to be at higher risk of developing impaired mobility or losing their ability to be independent in performing their activities of daily living than older adults who do not receive benzodiazepines (Gray, LaCroix, Hanlon, et al., 2006). Risk factors must be carefully assessed when using benzodiazepines in older adults.

It is not clear from the literature whether benzodiazepines affect women differently than men. Some sources state that women metabolize all benzodiazepines differently, have a higher risk of developing physical dependency from benzodiazepines, and experience the desired and adverse effects of the drug differently. But other sources have not found any difference between men and women related to benzodiazepine use. Benzodiazepines, such as lorazepam, may be prescribed more for women than for men.

When lorazepam is prescribed to a woman, assess whether she is pregnant, because lorazepam is a pregnancy category D drug and should generally be avoided during pregnancy. It is not known whether lorazepam enters breast milk, although other benzodiazepines do. The post-partum period is a time of heightened risk for developing or relapse of mental illness (Menon, 2008), therefore more studies are indicated with use to determine the true of effect on the nursing infant.

Lifestyle, Diet, and Habits

Assess the patient for the use of alcohol, narcotics, and other CNS depressants, which have an additive effect with lorazepam. The patient who has a history of alcohol or substance abuse may be a poor candidate for lorazepam because of the likelihood of developing dependency on the drug. Studies have shown a higher rate of death from overdose when benzodiazepines are used with opiate abuse (Kenna et al., 2007). Determine whether the patient regularly drives, operates heavy machinery, or participates in other activities that require mental alertness. These activities may be dangerous during the initial period of drug use, because of drowsiness caused by the drug.

Environment

Oral lorazepam may be administered in any environment. IV infusions of lorazepam require that the patient be in a monitored environment. Equipment to maintain a patent airway should be at the bedside.

Culture and Inherited Traits

Studies have shown that some benzodiazepines have a longer half-life in Asians than in Caucasians due to differences in hepatic enzymes (Bray, et al., 2008). These results suggest that Asians should receive lower doses of the drug than whites, although no specific studies with lorazepam in Asians have been performed.

Nursing Diagnoses and Outcomes

- Risk for Injury related to drowsiness and other adverse effects
  Desired outcome: *The patient will not sustain an injury while on lorazepam.*
- Anxiety related to disease process
  Desired outcome: *The patient will achieve symptom control.*

MEMORY CHIP

P Lorazepam

- Used to treat anxiety disorders
- Works by increasing the inhibitory effects of GABA
- Major contraindications: psychoses and acute narrow-angle glaucoma
- Most common adverse effects: mild drowsiness, ataxia, confusion
- Most serious adverse effects: paradoxical reactions
- **Life span alert: contraindicated in children under 6 months; pregnancy category D; older adults more likely to develop ataxia and confusion, so give smaller doses**
- Maximizing therapeutic effects: Daily dose should be split into two or three doses to give sustained daily therapeutic effect; counseling ("talk therapy") should be given while on drug therapy.
- Minimizing adverse effects: Assess for suicidal tendencies; discontinue long-term treatment by tapering dose slowly.
- Most important patient education: Avoid taking alcohol and other CNS depressants while on lorazepam to prevent additive CNS depression.

- Deficient Knowledge related to newly prescribed drug therapy
  Desired outcome: *The patient will learn the actions and adverse effects of lorazepam and how to safely self-administer the drug.*

Planning and Intervention

Maximizing Therapeutic Effects

Lorazepam has a fairly short duration of action; therefore, divide the daily dosage for treating anxiety into two or three doses and administer the drug throughout the day to achieve continued therapeutic effect. If one of the symptoms of anxiety experienced is difficulty sleeping, give the largest dose of the day at bedtime to promote sleep. If the drug is given solely as a sleep aid, give the entire dose at bedtime. Protect IV solutions of lorazepam from light and store them in the refrigerator to prevent loss of potency.

To help the patient learn coping skills and further decrease anxiety on a more permanent basis, talk therapy or counseling should accompany drug therapy with lorazepam.

Minimizing Adverse Effects

If GI distress occurs, administer lorazepam with food. Monitor for paradoxical reactions such as increased agitation or hallucinations and stop the drug if they occur. Hepatic function and blood cell counts should be assessed periodically during therapy to determine whether any adverse effects have occurred. To prevent undue adverse effects, older adults and children should be started on small doses of lorazepam, and the dose should then be increased slowly as necessary. Coadministration of lorazepam with other CNS depressants should be avoided if possible. If it is necessary to coadminister these agents, assess the patient carefully for signs of significant CNS depression.

BOX 15.1 FOCUS ON RESEARCH

Cost-Effectiveness of Benzodiazepine
Tapering Methods

Oude Voshaar, R. C., Krabbe, P. F., Gorgels, W. J., et al. (2006). Tapering off benzodiazepines in
long-term users: An economic evaluation. *Pharmacoeconomics*, 24(7):683–694.

The Study

The focus of this randomized, controlled study was to compare the relative costs and outcomes of tapering off long-term benzodiazepine use versus tapering off combined with cognitive behavioral therapy. Factors included in the cost analysis included the intervention treatment, prescribed drugs, health care services, productivity loss, and patient expenses. Patients (180) were divided between the two treatment groups and a control, in which benzodiazepine use continued. The findings showed a reduction in benzodiazepine costs in both treatment groups. Tapering off alone was slightly more cost-effective, but the difference was small. Addition of cognitive behavioral therapy to tapering did not appear to offer any clinical or economic advantages.

Nursing Implications

Long-term benzodiazepine use creates additional costs to the patient and to the health care system. Additionally, it places the patient at risk of adverse effects. Tapering off the dose of a benzodiazepine not only reduces the risk of withdrawal symptoms but also is a financial benefit to the patient. Commonly, cognitive behavior therapy accompanies this tapering. Although the study found that tapering off alone and tapering off with cognitive therapy were similarly effective clinically (stopping drug therapy led to no significant withdrawal complications), some patients may benefit from the support a group therapy session can offer. Therefore, nurses should assess patients' individual needs relative to using group therapy for benzodiazepine withdrawal.

Dilute injectable lorazepam with an equal volume of compatible solution, such as sterile water for injection, sodium chloride for injection, or 5% dextrose solution, and inject at a rate not to exceed 2 mg/min. Give IV lorazepam only in a monitored environment with equipment at the bedside to maintain a patent airway. Monitor patient closely during administration.

Carefully assess patients with depression and anxiety for suicidal tendencies. The number of pills dispensed to the patient should be the least amount feasible.

To prevent withdrawal symptoms when lorazepam is to be discontinued, the drug should be slowly tapered off if the patient has been on the drug for a long time or if a high dose of the drug was being taken. Withdrawal effects include insomnia, anxiety, loss of appetite, tremor, perspiration, tinnitus, and perceptual disturbances (Anwar, 2008). Craving for benzodiazepines will occur during the tapering-off period; however, the severity will decrease over time to negligible proportions (Mol, et al., 2006). See Focus on Research Box 15.1.

Providing Patient and Family Education

- To prevent additive CNS depression, teach patients to avoid taking alcohol and other CNS depressants while on lorazepam.
- Warn patients that drowsiness, sedation, and ataxia may occur when the drug is first started, but that these effects should disappear once they accommodate to the drug. Until the effects of the drug on a particular patient are known, the patient should avoid driving, operating machinery, or any other tasks that require mental alertness and concentration.
- If patients experience GI distress from lorazepam, instruct them to take the drug with food.
- Warn women of childbearing age to avoid becoming pregnant while on lorazepam because it is a pregnancy category D drug. Women should not breast-feed while on lorazepam because it is not known whether the drug distributes into breast milk, although other benzodiazepines do.
- Inform patients of the importance of returning for follow-up blood work if lorazepam therapy is to continue for an extended period.
- Teach patients and family what the paradoxical effects of lorazepam are and explain that if they occur, patients should stop taking the drug and immediately contact the prescriber.

Box 15.2 provides teaching guidelines for the patient who is prescribed benzodiazepines to be taken at home.

Ongoing Assessment and Evaluation

Lorazepam therapy is effective if the patient reports a reduction in feelings of anxiety and begins to develop other, more positive coping mechanisms for life problems. For lorazepam therapy to be effective, adverse effects either should not occur or should be tolerable and manageable so that the patient does not need to stop therapy. Throughout therapy, assess for therapeutic response and onset of adverse effects.

BOX 15.2 COMMUNITY BASED CONCERNS

Teaching for Patients Prescribed Home Benzodiazepine Therapy

Patients are often prescribed benzodiazepines, such as lorazepam, to be taken at home. In addition to the initial drowsiness that the drug can cause, CNS depression may also impair cognition and processing of information and may slow response time, all of which place these patients at considerable risk for having an accident while driving. This risk increases with the additive CNS depression that can occur if benzodiazepines are taken with alcohol and other CNS depressants, including prescription medications. Patients may forget about additive effects from alcohol use once they adapt to lorazepam therapy or if they do not experience drowsiness in the first place. Ensure that patients who are to start on lorazepam understand the following precautions:

- They should avoid driving until the effects of the drug on them are known.
- They should avoid drinking alcohol.
- If they ingest alcohol, they should have someone else (who has not been drinking) drive.
- If it is necessary to start another CNS depressant medication, they should again use extra caution driving until the combined effects of the drugs are known.

• NONBENZODIAZEPINES

Buspirone

Buspirone (BuSpar) is an azaspirodecanedione that is not chemically or pharmacologically related to the benzodiazepines or any other sedative or anxiolytic drug. It is used to treat symptoms of anxiety, although exactly how it works is unknown. In laboratory studies, it shows a high affinity for serotonin receptors, but it has no effect on GABA receptors. Buspirone also has moderate affinity for one type of brain dopamine receptor; it may act as a presynaptic dopamine agonist. It also increases norepinephrine metabolism in the locus ceruleus.

Optimum relief of anxiety usually occurs after 3 to 4 weeks of treatment, although some improvement is often seen within 7 to 10 days of starting therapy. Although buspirone is intended for short-term therapy, patients who have been treated with buspirone for up to 1 year have not required a dosage increase to maintain therapeutic effect, and withdrawal symptoms did not occur if the drug was stopped suddenly. This is an advantage over benzodiazepines, including the prototype, lorazepam. Buspirone produces much less sedation than lorazepam and does not produce substantial functional impairment. However, it can cause dizziness, nausea, headache, nervousness, light-headedness, or excitement as adverse effects. Because it is difficult to predict what effects any particular patient will experience, patients should be cautioned to avoid driving or operating machinery until the effects of the drug on them are known.

Hydroxyzine

Hydroxyzine (Vistaril) is a miscellaneous antianxiety drug that exerts CNS depressant activity in subcortical areas. It rapidly produces a feeling of calm and relieves anxiety without impairing mental alertness. Hydroxyzine also has bronchodilatory, antihistamine, analgesic, antispasmodic, and antiemetic effects. It can be administered intramuscularly or orally. It may be coadministered with a narcotic to control pain while minimizing the nausea that may be an adverse effect from the narcotic. Adverse effects of hydroxyzine include dry mouth, drowsiness (usually transient in continuous therapy), and involuntary motor activity (which usually occurs at higher-than-recommended doses).

Meprobamate

Meprobamate (Equanil) is also used for short-term management of anxiety symptoms. Meprobamate has selective effects at multiple sites within the CNS, including the thalamus and the limbic system. It may also inhibit multineuronal spinal reflexes. It has mild tranquilizing properties and some antiepileptic and muscle-relaxant properties.

Meprobamate can produce several CNS adverse effects, such as drowsiness, ataxia, dizziness, slurred speech, headache, vertigo, weakness, impaired visual accommodation, euphoria, overstimulation, paradoxical excitement, and fast electroencephalographic activity. Cardiovascular adverse effects include tachycardia, arrhythmias and palpitations, transient electrocardiographic changes, syncope, and hypotensive crisis. Nausea, vomiting, and diarrhea are possible, as are potentially severe allergic responses.

Meprobamate is a pregnancy category D drug that is associated with congenital malformations if taken in the first trimester. It is also excreted into breast milk at levels two to four times that found in the maternal plasma. It should therefore be avoided in pregnant women, women who might become pregnant, and breast-feeding women.

DRUGS TO PROMOTE SLEEP

Drugs to promote sleep come from several different classes. They include the benzodiazepines, nonbenzodiazepines that interact with the GABA-benzodiazepine receptor complex; melatonin receptor agonists; trazodone, an atypical antipsychotic; chloral hydrate, a nonbarbiturate hypnotic; and barbiturates. Although not discussed in this chapter, many over-the-counter sleep aids contain antihistamines such as diphenhydramine and doxylamine.

Benzodiazepines

In addition to their use in treating anxiety, benzodiazepines are used to treat insomnia or in situations in which a restful sleep is desired, such as the night before surgery. The benzodiazepine receptor subtype BZ_1 is thought to be associated with sleep mechanisms; BZ_1 receptors are specific GABA receptors located in the limbic, neocortical, and mesencephalic reticular systems in the brain. All of the benzodiazepines decrease the number of times the person awakens during the night. Stage 2 sleep is lengthened by all benzodiazepines. Most benzodiazepines shorten stages 3 and 4 (slow-wave sleep). Almost all benzodiazepines decrease the amount of time spent in REM sleep.

Five of the benzodiazepines have been approved for use as sleep aids (hypnotics). These are estazolam (ProSom), flurazepam (Dalmane), quazepam (Doral), temazepam (Restoril), and triazolam (Halcion). The major difference among these drugs is their half-life. Triazolam has the shortest half-life, at 1.5 to 5.5 hours, whereas quazepam has the longest half-life, at 41 hours. Table 15.3 presents the indications and half-lives for selected benzodiazepines. The drugs with shorter half-lives cause fewer problems with daytime sedation, although they may produce more early-morning insomnia.

The use of benzodiazepines as sleep aids should be short term. If benzodiazepines are used for as long as 3 or 4 weeks and then discontinued, REM rebound may occur (i.e., the REM sleep will occur more than usual in the sleep cycle). Abruptly discontinuing triazolam may produce rebound sleep disorder, in which the insomnia is worse than it was before treatment. The rebound effect is less likely to occur with estazolam, flurazepam, or quazepam, which have longer half-lives.

TABLE 15.3	Labeled Therapeutic Indications and Half-Lives of Benzodiazepines						
Name	$t_{1/2}$ (h)	Anxiety	Insomnia	Seizures	Muscle Spasms	Alcohol Withdrawal	Anesthesia Induction
alprazolam	6.3–26.9	✓					
chlordiazepoxide	5–30	✓				✓	
clonazepam	18–50			✓			
Clorazepate	40–50	✓		✓		✓	
diazepam	20–80	✓		✓	✓	✓	✓
estazolam	8–28		✓				
flurazepam	2–3 (47–100 metabolites)		✓				
Halazepam	14	✓					
lorazepam	10–20	✓		✓		✓	✓
midazolam	1.8–6.4						✓
oxazepam	5–20	✓				✓	
quazepam	41 (47–100 metabolites)		✓				
temazepam	3.5–18.4 (9–15 metabolites)		✓				
triazolam	1.5–5.5		✓				

Anterograde amnesia (inability to remember events that occur after the drug is taken) is more likely to occur with high doses of triazolam, but it may also occur with lower doses of triazolam or with the other benzodiazepines. When patients with depression or other underlying psychiatric disorders take benzodiazepines for sleep, their conditions may worsen. Triazolam is especially likely to cause problems. Unusual or bizarre behavior has been noted in some patients who take benzodiazepines such as triazolam. These behaviors include loss of inhibition, aggressiveness, agitation, hallucinations, and depersonalization. Some European countries removed triazolam from the market in the early 1990s because of these adverse effects. Reducing the dose tends to limit the occurrence of these adverse effects.

Unlike lorazepam, benzodiazepines used to promote sleep are classified as pregnancy category X. These drugs are teratogenic when used during the first trimester, and if they are given to the mother during the last weeks of pregnancy, their distribution through the placenta results in neonatal CNS depression. Other adverse effects and characteristics of benzodiazepines are similar to those for lorazepam.

The use of benzodiazepines in older adults to treat insomnia, like their use in treating anxiety, places the older adult at increased risk for falls and other accidents. They have been associated with mobility problems and decreased ability to perform ADLs. Short-acting benzodiazepines do not appear to be any safer for older adults than longer-acting benzodiazepines (Gray, et al., 2006). Older patients taking benzodiazepines should be carefully monitored for daytime sedation and impaired motor coordination.

Nonbenzodiazepines

Eszopiclone

Eszopiclone (Lunesta) is a nonbenzodiazepine hypnotic. The drug induces sleep quickly, prevents waking during the night, and creates feelings of refreshment after a night's sleep; thus it is useful for a variety of insomnia problems. Eszopiclone is believed to achieve its therapeutic effect from interaction with GABA receptor–benzodiazepine receptor complexes. It is the only drug for insomnia that is approved for long-term use (up to 6 months of use). Unlike the benzodiazepines, eszopiclone does not seem to produce tolerance, even with long-term use. Withdrawal symptoms are possible after discontinuation, but they are mild. Caution should be used with individuals who have problems with drug addiction. Addicts report that ingesting zopiclone with alcohol heightens euphoria and in the United Kingdom, the street name for the drug is zim-zims (Cimolai, 2007).

Eszopiclone has a rapid onset (within 1 hour) and is metabolized in the liver and excreted in the urine. If taken with a high-fat or heavy meal the onset of action may be delayed. Because of its rapid onset, eszopiclone should be taken immediately before bedtime. Older adults are more sensitive to the effects of eszopiclone, as they are to other sedative/hypnotics; therefore, they should receive a lower dose than younger adults.

The most common adverse effects of eszopiclone after 6 weeks of use were headache, prolonged drowsiness, and an unpleasant taste. Eszopiclone is a pregnancy category C drug. It should not be used in labor and delivery, and whether it is known to cross into breast milk (Menon, 2008). Clinical trials have not been conducted in children under 18 years of age; effects in this age group have not been identified.

Zaleplon

Zaleplon (Sonata) is a sedative for short-term use (up to 28 days). Although a nonbenzodiazepine and not chemically related to the benzodiazepines, it does interact with the GABA-benzodiazepine complex. Zaleplon is prescribed to people who have trouble falling asleep. Because it has a fairly high first-pass effect, approximately 30% of an oral dose is metabolized prior to the drug's reaching the systemic circulation. Therefore, the half-life of zaleplon is short. Sedatives with short half-lives may be more likely to cause early morning waking, and zaleplon may do this, although there are not sufficient data to confirm this. However, if the patient has had problems with early morning waking or frequent waking prior to starting drug therapy, zaleplon will not decrease their occurrence; it should not be used if frequent waking is the presenting sleep problem. Additionally, zaleplon does not increase the total sleep time but only decreases the amount of time needed to fall asleep.

The most common adverse effects of zaleplon are drowsiness, dizziness, light-headedness, and difficulty with coordination. Zaleplon is a pregnancy category C drug.

As with other sleeping aids, zaleplon carries the warning that worsening of insomnia and emergence of new thinking or behavior abnormalities (starting as aggressiveness, agitation, hallucinations, and depersonalization) after starting treatment are possible and may be related to an unrecognized psychiatric or physical disorder. This adverse effect seems to be dose dependent, so the smallest effective dose possible should be used, especially in older adults and debilitated patients who may be more sensitive to these adverse effects. Additionally, next-day amnesia may occur. The risk of this adverse effect can be minimized if patients take the drug only when they know they will be able to sleep for at least 4 hours.

The effects of zaleplon may be reduced if it is taken with or immediately after a high-fat or heavy meal. Therefore the patient should be instructed to avoid taking this medication with meals. The circulating levels of the drug are increased with severe hepatic impairment. Affected patients should not receive zaleplon, and patients with minor hepatic impairment should receive a lower dose.

Like benzodiazepines, zaleplon may lead to dependency, and rebound insomnia is possible the first one or two nights after stopping the drug. Unlike the benzodiazepines, zaleplon is not known to cause withdrawal symptoms, although they are possible. Zaleplon has an abuse potential similar to benzodiazepines. Tolerance does not seem to develop when the drug is used for as long as 4 weeks, which is different from long-term use of benzodiazepines. Like other sleep-inducing drugs, zaleplon may have additive CNS depressant effects when coadministered with other CNS depressants. A smaller dose of zaleplon may be necessary when given with other CNS depressants. Alcohol should be avoided. Zaleplon contains FD&C Yellow No. 5 (tartrazine), which can cause allergic-type reactions (including bronchial asthma) in those susceptible; this sensitivity often occurs in those who also have aspirin hypersensitivity. Because a drug interaction occurs through the P-450 system, the dose of zaleplon should be reduced if the patient is receiving cimetidine (OTC Zantac). Cimetidine greatly increases the level of circulating zaleplon. It also is found to cross into breast milk (Menon, 2008).

Zolpidem

Zolpidem (Ambien) is used for short-term treatment of insomnia—generally not for more than 7 to 10 days. It induces sleep rapidly and should be taken immediately before going to bed and should not be given with meals. Although zolpidem is not chemically related to the benzodiazepines, it does interact selectively with the GABA-BZ receptor complex and shares some pharmacologic properties with the benzodiazepines. Zolpidem generally preserves all of the sleep stages and has only minor effects on REM sleep. Zolpidem is rapidly absorbed from the GI tract and has a short half-life. Hepatic dysfunction prolongs its half-life, but renal failure does not seem to increase the circulating level of zolpidem. The drug is available in both quick-onset and continuous-release oral forms. Two new forms of zolpidem have been recently made available, Edluar which is a sublingual form and Zolpimist which is an oral spray. Zolpidem does not seem to produce residual effects the next morning or cause a prolonged rebound effect when the drug is discontinued, although rebound insomnia is possible the first night after drug discontinuation. However, withdrawal symptoms can be seen if the drug is stopped abruptly, although this appears to be rare. Tolerance is possible.

The most common adverse effects from zolpidem are headache, prolonged drowsiness, and dizziness. Caution the patient that the drug may produce drowsiness and that he or she should take precautions until the effects of the drug are known. Zolpidem causes CNS depression, and as with all other CNS depressants, an additive effect is seen if zolpidem is combined with alcohol or other CNS-depressant drugs.

Zolpidem is a pregnancy category C drug. It is not recommended for use during labor and delivery or lactation. Clinical information is not available to determine the exact effect on children under 18 years of age. Older adults may be more susceptible to adverse effects, and their dose should be half of that given to younger adults (6.25 mg versus 12.5 mg). In addition, zolpidem, like other sedative/hypnotics, can produce visual or auditory hallucinations and behavior changes (including agitation or bizarre behavior) in certain patients. Patients who are known to have an underlying psychiatric illness as well as insomnia should take this drug cautiously, with the dosage kept as low as possible until the individual effects are known.

Melatonin Receptor Agonist

Melatonin is a hormone that is secreted by the pineal gland in a circadian cycle. Melatonin is released in response to darkness and is believed to be involved in the maintenance of circadian rhythm underlying the normal sleep-wake cycle. During the daylight hours, secretion is low. Release of the hormone begins around 9 PM and peaks during the night hours (2 to 4 AM). Over-the-counter melatonin is not regulated by the Food and Drug Administration and may vary in its strength and purity. Over-the-counter melatonin is used to promote sleep and to re-establish normal sleep cycles when traveling (i.e., to prevent jet lag).

Ramelteon

Melatonin receptor agonists stimulate the same receptor sites as endogenous melatonin. The only prescription drug currently in this class is ramelteon. Ramelteon (Rozerem) is used in the treatment of insomnia when the patient has difficulty falling asleep. Unlike the benzodiazepines and other sleep aids, ramelteon has high affinity at two specific melatonin receptors, MT_1 and MT_2. Ramelteon's action at these receptors is therefore believed to be responsible for its ability to induce sleep. It does not have any significant affinity for GABA receptor complex or receptors that bind neuropeptides, cytokines, serotonin, dopamine, noradrenaline, acetylcholine, or opiates. Ramelteon has not been found to cause rebound insomnia or withdrawal symptoms, unlike benzodiazepines; neither does it seem to pose a risk for abuse or tolerance. Thus, unlike other hypnotics, ramelteon is not a controlled substance.

Ramelteon has a high first-pass effect and is absorbed rapidly, with a peak effect occurring usually in less than 1 hour. Because of its rapid onset, teach patients to take the drug no more than 30 minutes prior to going to bed. Ramelteon has a short half-life (2 to 5 hours). The isoenzyme CYP1A2 is most involved with its metabolism (the CYP2C and CYP3A4 subfamilies are also involved but only to a minor degree); drug molecules not metabolized are eliminated via the kidneys. Mild to moderate liver impairment increases the circulating level almost four-fold, and caution must be used if giving the drug to these patients.

Common adverse effects of ramelteon include headache, daytime sleepiness, dizziness, tiredness, nausea, worsening insomnia, and colds. Ramelteon may affect reproductive hormones by increasing prolactin, possibly decreasing testosterone levels. These changes may cause missed monthly periods, nipple drainage, decreased sex drive, or problems getting pregnant. If patients experience these problems, they should have blood tests to check their hormone levels. A high-fat meal significantly decreases the effectiveness of ramelteon; thus, it should not be taken either with or immediately after a high-fat meal. Ramelteon is a pregnancy category C drug.

Ramelteon may interact with other drugs. Fluvoxamine, which is a strong inhibitor of CYP1A2, increases the circulating levels of ramelteon so much that the two drugs should not be taken together. Other strong inhibitors of CYP1A2 should also be avoided, because they increase the risk of adverse effects; the effects of mild or moderate inhibitors have not been studied and are not known at this time. Other drug interactions via the P-450 system are possible.

Drugs From Other Classes

Trazodone

Trazodone (Desyrel) is an atypical antidepressant. This drug causes significant sedation as an adverse effect; thus, it is sometimes used as a sleep aid, unlike other atypical antidepressants. Trazodone is most commonly used to promote sleep if the patient is receiving an antidepressant that causes insomnia. See Chapter 16 for more discussion of trazodone.

Chloral Hydrate

Chloral hydrate is a nonbarbiturate hypnotic used to induce sleep and to cause preoperative sedation in order to lessen anxiety. It can be used as an adjunct to opiates and analgesics in pain control; it can also suppress or prevent alcohol withdrawal symptoms when given by rectal suppository. It is for short-term use only because it loses much of its effectiveness in producing and maintaining sleep after 2 weeks of use. Its exact mechanism of action is not known, although it is known to produce mild cerebral depression and quiet, deep sleep.

In therapeutic doses, chloral hydrate has little effect on respirations, blood pressure, or reflexes. It does produce numerous adverse effects in the CNS, including disorientation, incoherence, paranoid behavior, excitement, delirium, nightmares, and confusion, among others. Prolonged use may result in psychological and physical dependency and tolerance. Sudden withdrawal may cause CNS excitation with tremor, anxiety, hallucinations, or even delirium, and may be fatal. Chloral hydrate has largely been replaced by other drugs that promote sleep in a safer and more effective manner.

Barbiturates

Barbiturates such as phenobarbital (Bellatal), secobarbital (Seconal), and pentobarbital (Nembutal) were used to treat insomnia before the availability of the benzodiazepines. Although they are effective for short-term treatment of insomnia, they are also highly habit forming. Patients can develop tolerance and physical and psychological dependence on the drugs. Withdrawal symptoms can be severe and can lead to death. Patients who develop tolerance to a barbiturate are likely to overdose in an attempt to self-medicate and obtain therapeutic response. Overdosage results in severe respiratory depression as well as general CNS depression, likely followed by death. Because of these problems, barbiturates are not generally used to treat insomnia.

Phenobarbital is sometimes used as an adjunct for seizure disorders (see Chapter 18). Phenobarbital, as well as other barbiturates such as pentobarbital and secobarbital, is used parenterally as an adjunct to anesthesia.

CHAPTER SUMMARY

- Benzodiazepines, such as lorazepam, are used frequently to treat anxiety and sleep disorders. They work by intensifying the effects of GABA at specific receptors. They have fewer adverse effects and are generally better tolerated than older drug classes used for these conditions. They are generally very safe to use because they have a large therapeutic index.

- Benzodiazepines can also be used in treating seizures and muscle spasms, as adjuncts to anesthesia, and in managing acute alcohol withdrawal. They are currently the drug class of first choice in treating status epilepticus and treating or preventing seizures from alcohol withdrawal. Specific benzodiazepines are approved for different uses.

- Benzodiazepines differ mainly by their onset of action and half-life. They are generally recommended for short-term use in anxiety and insomnia, although their use in practice may vary. Only five benzodiazepines are specifically labeled to be used to treat insomnia: estazolam, flurazepam, quazepam, temazepam, and triazolam.

- Older adults are more sensitive to the adverse effects of benzodiazepines and should receive a smaller dose than younger adults. When benzodiazepines are used in older adults, drugs with shorter half-lives should be selected.

- Other drug classes used to treat anxiety are the selective serotonin reuptake inhibitors (SSRIs) and the tricyclics, both classes of antidepressants. Their effectiveness in anxiety treatment, irrespective of whether the patient has depression, is believed to be attributable to their effect on serotonin levels. For some anxiety disorders, SSRIs and tricyclics are now considered the first choice for treatment.

- Buspirone is another drug used to treat anxiety. It is not chemically related to the benzodiazepines. Tolerance and withdrawal do not occur with buspirone as they do with the benzodiazepines.

- Zolpidem and eszopiclone are newer agents used to treat insomnia. Zolpidem is for short-term use; tolerance may develop. Eszopiclone is unique in that it is labeled for long-term use up to 6 months, and tolerance does not develop even after long-term use. Both zolpidem and eszopiclone achieve their therapeutic effects by interacting selectively with some of the GABA-BZ receptor complexes and share some pharmacologic properties with the benzodiazepines, although they are not chemically related.

- Ramelteon is a hypnotic that works uniquely by stimulating melatonin receptors. It does not cause tolerance, dependency, or withdrawal and is not a controlled substance, unlike other hypnotics. It is approved for short-term use.

- The use of barbiturates and chloral hydrate for insomnia is now limited because other drugs depress the CNS more safely and effectively. Barbiturates are sometimes used for treating seizure disorders.

QUESTIONS FOR STUDY AND REVIEW

1. How does lorazepam, a benzodiazepine, decrease anxiety?

2. If a patient has been taking lorazepam regularly for several weeks, would the same dose continue to be effective? If the same patient suddenly stopped taking lorazepam, what physiologic effects might occur?

3. Why might lorazepam be the benzodiazepine of choice for a patient with anxiety and decreased liver function?

4. Why might an older adult be more at risk for falls than a younger adult when taking lorazepam at home?

5. Explain why triazolam, used to treat patients who have difficulty falling asleep, may also cause the adverse effect of early-morning insomnia.

6. Explain the advantages of eszopiclone over benzodiazepines used to promote sleep.

NEED MORE HELP?

Chapter 15 of the Study Guide to Accompany *Drug Therapy in Nursing*, 4th Edition, contains NCLEX-style questions and other learning activities to reinforce your understanding of the concepts presented in this chapter. For additional information or to purchase the study guide, visit thePoint.

REFERENCES

Anwar, A. (2008). Benzodiazepines: uses, mode of action and prescribing issues. *Nurse Prescribing*, 6(12):544–548.

Anxiety Disorders Association of America. *Facts and statistics*. Retrieved May 14, 2011, from http://www.adaa.org/about-adaa/press-room/facts-statistics

Bray, J., Clarke, C., Brennan, G., Muncey, T. (2008). *Journal of Psychiatric and Mental Health Nursing*, 15:357–364.

Cimolai, N., (2007). Zopiclone: Is it a Pharmacologic Agent for Abuse? *Canadian Family Physician*, 53(12):2124–2129.

Fick, D. M., Cooper, J. W., Wade, W. E., et al. (2003). Updating the Beers criteria for potentially inappropriate medication use in older adults. *Archives of Internal Medicine*, 163:2716–2724.

Glass, J., Lanctot, K., Hermann, N., Sproule, B., Busto, U. (2005). Sedative hypnotics in older people with insomnia: meta-analysis of risks and benefits. *British Medical Journal*, 331(7526):1169.

Gray, S. L., LaCroix, A. Z., Hanlon, J. T., et al. (2006). Benzodiazepine use and physical disability in community-dwelling older adults. *Journal of the American Geriatrics Society*, 54(2):224–230.

Hartikainen, S., Lonnroos, E., Louhivuori, K. (2008). *The journals of Gerontology Series A: Biological Sciences and Medical Sciences*, 62:1172–1181.

Kenna, G., Nielsen, D., Mello P., Schiesl, A., Swift, R. (2007). Pharmacotherapy of Dual Substance Abuse and Dependence. *CNS Drugs*, 21(3):213–237.

Leblanc, M., Beaulieu-Bonneau, S., Merette, C., Savard, J., Ivers, H., Morin, C. (2007). Psychological and Health related quality of life factors associated with insomnia in a population based sample. *Journal of Psychosomatic Research*, 63(2):157–166.

Mayers, A. G., Baldwin, D. S., (2006). The relationship between sleep disturbance and depression. *International Journal of Psychiatry in Clinical Practice*, 10(1):2–16.

Menon. S. (2008). Psychotropic medication during pregnancy and lactation. *Archives of Genecological Obstetrics*, 277:1–13.

Mohr, W. (2009). *Psychiatric-Mental Health Nursing Evidence-Based Concepts, Skills, and Practice (7th ed)*. Philadelphia: Lippincott Williams & Wilkins.

Mol, A. J., Oude Voshaar, R. C., Gorgels, W. J., et al. (2006). The absence of benzodiazepine craving in a general practice benzodiazepine discontinuation trial. *Addictive Behaviors,* 31(2):211–222.

National Institute of Mental Health. (2009). *Anxiety disorders*. Retrieved from http://www.nimh.nih.gov/health/publications/anxiety-disorders/introduction.shtml.

National Sleep Foundation. (2004). *Sleep poll in America*. Retrieved from http://www.sleepfoundation.org/sites/default/files/2004SleepPollFinalReport.pdf.

National Sleep Foundation. (2005). *Sleep poll in America*. Retrieved from http://www.sleepfoundation.org/sites/default/files/2005_summary_of_findings.pdf.

National Sleep Foundation. (2006). *Sleep poll in America*. Retrieved from http://www.sleepfoundation.org/sites/default/files/2006_summary_of_findings.pdf

National Sleep Foundation. (2006). *Sleep-wake cycle: Its physiology and impact on health. Retrieved from http://www.sleepfoundation.org/sites/default/files/SleepWakeCycle.pdf.*

National Sleep Foundation. (2008). *Sleep in America Poll*. Retrieved from http://www.sleepfoundation.org/sites/default/files/2008%20POLL%20SOF.PDF.

Prasad, K., Al-Roomi, K., Krishnan, P. R., et al. (2005). Anticonvulsant therapy for status epilepticus. *Cochrane Database Systematic Review* (4):CD003723.

Ramakrishnan, K., Scheid, D. (2007). Treatment Options for Insomnia. *American Family Physician,* 76(4):517–526.

Simpson, K., et al. (2006). Medications and Sleep in Nursing Home Residents with Dementia. *Journal of the American Psychiatric Nurses Association,* 12(5):279–285.

The brain from top to bottom. Retrieved September 2009, from http://thebrain.mcgill.ca/flash/a/a_04/a_04_cr/a_04_cr_peu/a_04_cr_peu.html

U.S. Food and Drug Administration. (2008). Retrieved from http://www.accessdata.fda.gov/drugsatfda_docs/label/2008/022196lbl.pdf.

U.S. Food and Drug Administration. (2009). Retrieved from http://www.accessdata.fda.gov/drugsatfda_docs/label/2009/021997lbl.pdf.

U.S. Public Health Service. *Mental health: A report of the surgeon general. Etiology of anxiety*. Retrieved from http://www.surgeongeneral.gov/library/mentalhealth/chapter4/sec2.html.

Vincent, W. K., Smith, K., Winstead, S., Lewis, D. (2007). Review of alcohol withdrawal in the hospitalized patient: management. *Orthopedics,* 30(6):446–449.

Wolkove, N., Elkholy, O., Baltzan, M., Palayew, M. (2007). Sleep and aging: 1. Sleep disorders commonly found in older people. *Canadian Medical Association Journal,* 176(9):1299–1304.

Wolkove, N., Elkholy, O., Baltzan, M., Palayew, M. (2007). Sleep and aging: 2. Management of sleep disorders in older people. *Canadian Medical Association Journal,* 176(10):1449–1454.

16

Drugs Treating Mood Disorders

Learning Objectives

At the completion of this chapter the student will:

1. Identify risk factors for the development of depression.
2. Identify the symptoms of major depression.
3. Identify the symptoms of dysthymic disorder
4. Identify the symptoms of bipolar disorder.
5. Identify the core drug knowledge of drugs used to treat mood disorders.
6. Relate the interaction of core drug knowledge to core patient variables for drugs used to treat mood disorders.
7. Generate a nursing plan of care from the interactions between core drug knowledge and the core patient variables for drugs used to treat mood disorders.
8. Describe nursing interventions to maximize therapeutic and minimize adverse effects for drugs that affect mood.
9. Determine key points for patient and family education for drugs that affect mood disorders.

Key Terms

antidepressants
bipolar disorder
depression
dysregulation
mania

mood
mood stabilizers
neurogenesis
neurotransmitters
psychotropic

serotonin reuptake
inhibitor withdrawal
syndrome
serotonin syndrome

Drugs Treating Mood Disorders

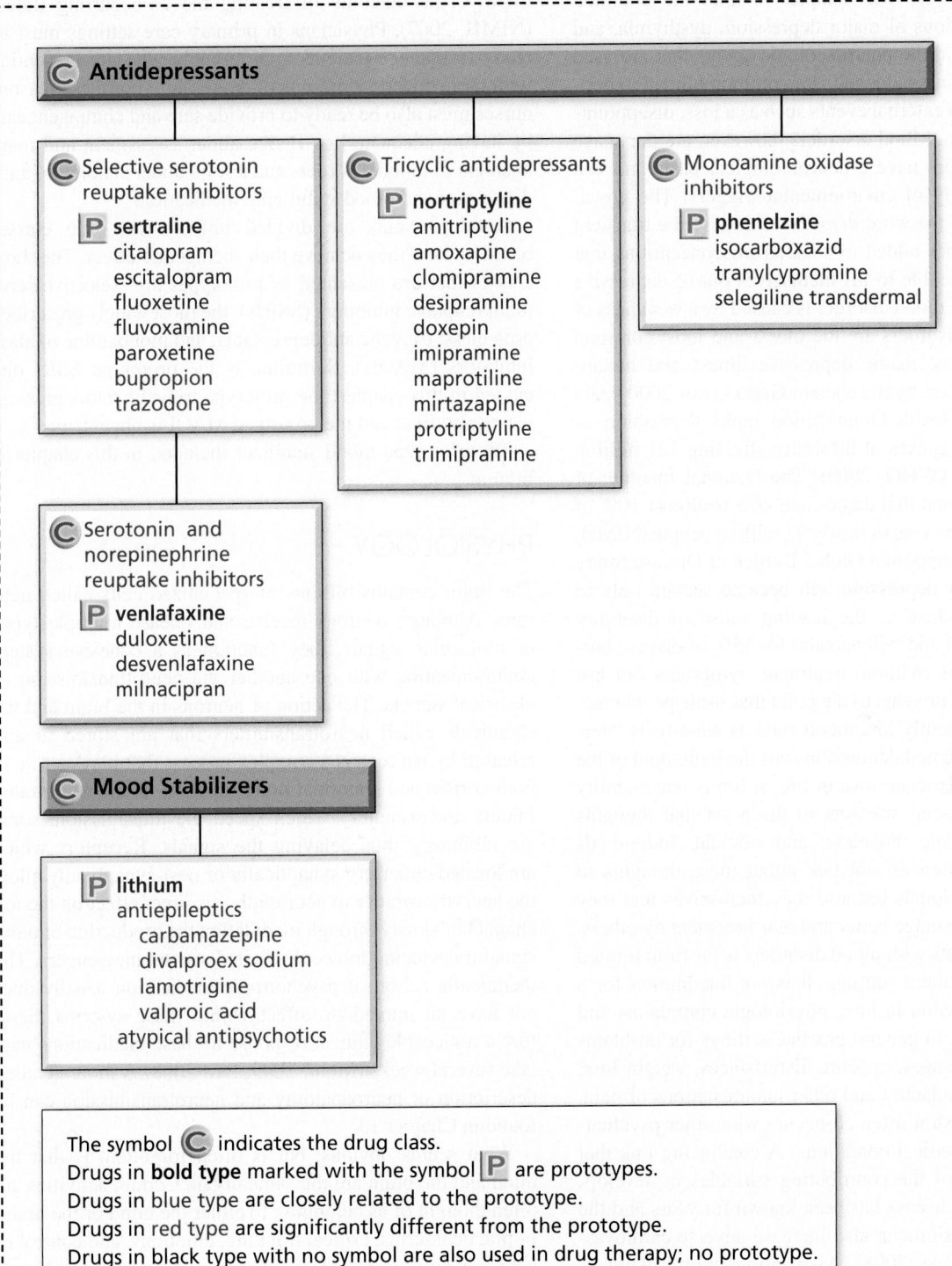

C **Antidepressants**

C Selective serotonin reuptake inhibitors
- **P** **sertraline**
- citalopram
- escitalopram
- fluoxetine
- fluvoxamine
- paroxetine
- bupropion
- trazodone

C Tricyclic antidepressants
- **P** **nortriptyline**
- amitriptyline
- amoxapine
- clomipramine
- desipramine
- doxepin
- imipramine
- maprotiline
- mirtazapine
- protriptyline
- trimipramine

C Monoamine oxidase inhibitors
- **P** **phenelzine**
- isocarboxazid
- tranylcypromine
- selegiline transdermal

C Serotonin and norepinephrine reuptake inhibitors
- **P** **venlafaxine**
- duloxetine
- desvenlafaxine
- milnacipran

C **Mood Stabilizers**

- **P** **lithium**
- antiepileptics
  - carbamazepine
  - divalproex sodium
  - lamotrigine
  - valproic acid
- atypical antipsychotics

The symbol **C** indicates the drug class.
Drugs in **bold type** marked with the symbol **P** are prototypes.
Drugs in blue type are closely related to the prototype.
Drugs in red type are significantly different from the prototype.
Drugs in black type with no symbol are also used in drug therapy; no prototype.

Mood disorders are complex and serious biological illnesses that affect patterns of thinking, memory, energy levels, impulse control, sleep and appetite, and many other physiologic processes. This chapter reviews the common clinical manifestations of major depression, dysthymia, and bipolar disorder and the pharmacologic agents that are used to treat them. Feeling saddened is a common human experience in response to external events such as a loss, disappointment, or frustration. Mood disorders, however, are pervasive emotional states that have a neurobiological basis and can occur independently of environmental triggers. The prevalence of the use of the word *depression* to describe transient states of sadness has added to societal misconceptions that a person should be able to lift themselves out of depressive symptoms or that a mood disorder is caused by a weakness of character. Mood disorders are the oldest and most common psychiatric illnesses, manic depressive illness and melancholia were described by the ancient Greeks over 2000 years ago. The World Health Organization ranks depression as one of the leading causes of disability affecting 121 million people worldwide (WHO, 2009). The National Institute of Mental Health reports that depression affects almost 10% of Americans in a given year or nearly 21 million people (NIMH, 2009). The WHO supported Global Burden of Disease Study predicts that major depression will become second only to ischemic heart disease as the leading cause of disability worldwide by 2020 and will account for 15% of disease burden (WHO, 2009a). Without treatment, symptoms can last for weeks, months, or years to the point that some people recognize their persistently low mood state as what feels "normal" to them. Untreated depression robs the individual of the ability to fully experience joys in life, it limits one's ability to handle psychosocial stressors to the point that thoughts can become fatalistic, hopeless, and suicidal. Individuals with depression often do not talk about these thoughts to health care professionals because they themselves feel they should be able to manage better and fear judgment by others. Treatment of patients with mood disorders is far from limited to psychiatric treatment settings. It is not uncommon for a person with depression to have physiologic complaints and first seek treatment in general practice settings for problems such as GI disturbances, appetite disturbances, weight loss, sleep problems, headaches and other manifestations of pain. In addition, depression often co-occurs with other psychiatric illnesses and medical conditions. A convincing link that depression is one of the contributing variables in developing cardiovascular disease has been known for years and the presence of depression can also increase adverse cardiovascular events (Sansone, 2008). Associations with inflammatory illnesses such as rheumatoid arthritis have been made (Pav, 2008). In patients with diabetes the risk of depression appears to be higher (up to twice as much) than in those without diabetes (Williams, et. al, 2007). Studies have shown that people who have depression in addition to another serious medical illness tend to have more severe symptoms of both depression and the medical illness, more difficulty adapting

to their medical condition, and more medical costs than those who do not have coexisting depression. Research has yielded increasing evidence that treating the depression can also help improve the outcome of treating the co-occurring illness (NIMH, 2007). Physicians in primary care settings must be ready to manage patients appropriately who are presenting with more covert symptoms of depression. For these reasons nurses must also be ready to provide safe and competent care by having adequate knowledge about assessment and management of mood disorders and a solid understanding of antidepressant and mood stabilizing medication.

Antidepressants are divided into several drug classes based on how they achieve their therapeutic effect. The three classes that are presented as prototypes are: selective serotonin reuptake inhibitors (SSRIs), the most widely prescribed drug class; tricyclic antidepressants; and monoamine oxidase inhibitors (MAOIs). Sertraline is the prototype SSRI discussed in this chapter; the prototype tricyclic antidepressant is nortriptyline; and the prototype MAOI is phenelzine.

The prototype mood stabilizer included in this chapter is lithium.

PHYSIOLOGY

The brain contains billions of specialized cells called neurons. Although neurons receive and release multiple types of molecular signals, they function as a cohesive system communicating with one another via neurotransmission of electrical signals. The action of neurons in the brain and the chemicals called neurotransmitters that are stored in and released by neurons is a complex process that plays a role in both normal and abnormal brain function. Some neurotransmitters are excitatory which speed the transmission, some are inhibitory thus delaying the signals. Receptors which are located either pre-synaptically or post-synaptically allow the neurotransmitter to act rapidly by direct effect on the ion channel or slowly through modulating the production of other signal transducing molecules called second messengers. The therapeutic action of psychotropic medication usually does not have an immediate effect within these systems therefore a noticeable clinical response to these medications may take several weeks.(Mohr, 2009; Pav, 2008) A more detailed description of neuroanatomy and neurotransmission can be found in Chapter 13.

What seems obvious, but is often forgotten, is that the mind and the brain are the same organ. Certain activities are often thought of as belonging to either the mind or the brain. In practical terms, critical thinking, emotions, and control of behavior are thought of as occurring in the mind, whereas activities such as controlling muscles of the body and regulating breathing, digestion, and body temperature are thought of as occurring in the brain. Conceptualizing the information in this way makes it easier to understand how illnesses in the brain can affect not only the emotions that a person experiences but also bodily functions such as movement and digestion.

PATHOPHYSIOLOGY

The National Institutes of Health declared the 1990s as the decade of the brain. During this time, unprecedented research about the brain and how it works improved the lives of people suffering with mood disorders. Research has been focused on creating medication that specifically targeted the neurotransmitters that are believed to affect mood. Illnesses resulting in mood disorders are associated with an imbalance or **dysregulation** of neurotransmitters, specifically, serotonin and norepinephrine. Improved techniques of brain imaging brought about greater understanding of the neurochemical processes at work as well as the structural changes that occur in the brain when a person experiences depression or stress. Research is also shedding light to the similar effects depression and stress share on immune and stress responses. Changes in the brain that are linked to these conditions include atrophy and structural remodeling in the limbic system, changes in the length and number of neuronal processes and a decline in neurogenesis (production of new neurons). Brain imaging studies show reductions of hippocampal volume with people who have been depressed most of their lives. This effect becomes more prominent when the depressive person was exposed to trauma during childhood (Pav, 2008). Antidepressant medications have been shown to target these abnormalities (Pav, 2008; Duman, 2002). The development of genetic studies has identified a specific gene that predisposes some people to develop depression when exposed to emotional stressor and it has been shown that all forms of mood disorders have genetic susceptibility and a hereditary component. There have been encouraging developments in resolving the problems in diagnosing and treating mood disorders but much remains to be discovered about the illness's exact etiology, its' prevention and treatment.

Major Depressive Disorder

Symptoms that characterize major depression are outlined by the American Psychiatric Association in the *Diagnostic and Statistical Manual for Mental Disorders,* fourth edition, text revision (DSM-IV-TR), which helps health care providers differentiate psychiatric illnesses.

Diagnosing major depression is partly a process of elimination. A patient's symptoms cannot be the result of a general medical condition such as cancer or hypothyroidism, nor can they be the result of drug abuse or an adverse effect of medication, although some drug classes are associated with depression. Box 16.1 lists these drug classes.

Box 16.1 DRUG CLASSES ASSOCIATED WITH DEPRESSION

- Alcohol
- Antiepileptics
- Antihypertensive agents
- Antiparkinsonian agents
- Antituberculosis agents
- H2 antagonists
- Narcotic analgesics
- Oral contraceptives
- Psychotropic agents
- Steroids

A pattern of other signs and symptoms must be present to complete an accurate diagnosis of major depression. Within a 2-week period, a person must manifest a depressed, even tearful mood or report or demonstrate to others a diminished interest or lack of pleasure in all activities most of the day. The symptoms must cause impairment at work or other social functions. Additionally, four other symptoms must be present from the following: changes in appetite, weight, sleep, or energy; a decrease in concentration; recurring death wishes; or thoughts of suicide. Thus, in addition to mood, major depression affects a person's body and ability to think. In cases of severe major depression, psychotic symptoms such as delusions may also occur.

Major depressive disorder affects approximately 14.8 million American adults, or about 6.7% of the U.S. population age 18 and older, in a given year (NIMH, 2008). Median age of onset of major depression is age 32 and the disorder is more prevalent in women than in men.

Risk factors for depression include:

- Having previously been depressed
- Having a first-degree relative diagnosed with depression
- Being a woman, an adolescent, or a young adult

Research indicates that alterations in neurotransmitters such as serotonin are associated not only with depression but also with the risk of suicide. Diminished levels of this brain chemical have been found in patients with depression, impulse control disorders, or a history of violent suicide attempts, and also in postmortem brains of suicide victims (NIMH, 2009a). In 2006, suicide was the 11th leading cause of death in the United States across all age groups. Depression accounts for about 60% of suicides of both youths and adults. Untreated depression is often associated with suicide. Less than 20% of depressed adults, and only about 2% of youths, are taking antidepressants at the time they commit suicide (Mann, Emslie, Baldessarini, et al., 2006). More than four times as many men as women die by suicide (CDC, 2009), although women report *attempting* suicide during their lifetime about three times as often as men (NIMH, 2008). Suicide attempts are an additional significant problem in depressed patients. In the population at large, it has been estimated that 12 to 25 attempted suicides may occur for every successful suicide (NIMH, 2008). It is also estimated that more than 90% of people who kill themselves have a diagnosable mental disorder, most commonly, a depressive or substance abuse disorder (NIMH, 2008).

Depression and suicide are problems across the lifespan. Depression affects about 3% to 5% of American youth annually. Suicide is the third leading cause of death among 15- to 24-year-olds, (CDC, 2009) about 0.01% of all youths will commit suicide per year. In 2005, one fifth of all high school students reported seriously thinking about committing suicide in the past 12 months, half of these attempted suicide. Although adolescent females were more likely to attempt suicide, the rate of completed suicides was higher in males (CDC, 2007). Suicide was also determined to be the second leading cause of death among 25 to 34 year olds (CDC, 2009).

Although depression frequently occurs in older adults, it should not be considered a normal part of aging. It is often a comorbidity with stroke, diabetes, cancer, and Parkinson disease, and older adults are more likely to experience these illnesses. Of the nearly 35 million Americans 65 years of age and older, an estimated 2 million have a depressive illness (including major depressive disorder, dysthymic disorder [mild, chronic depression], or bipolar disorder).

Older Americans are disproportionately likely to die from suicide. Comprising only 12% of the U.S. population, individuals 65 years of age and older accounted for 14% of all suicide deaths in 2006 (NIMH, 2009a). The highest suicide rates in the United States are found in white men older than 85 years of age followed by males aged 75 to 84 (CDC, 2009). Many studies have pointed to depression as the leading cause of suicide in the elderly (Garand, 2006). Frequently, polypharmacy confounds the diagnosis and treatment of mental disorders in the elderly (Crumpacker, 2008).

Dysthymic Disorder

Dysthymia and major depression have many common symptoms, including depressed mood, sleep disturbance, low energy, and poor concentration. Whereas in major depression the symptoms can be quite severe, the defining feature of dysthymia is the chronicity of symptoms. Depressive symptoms must persist for 2 years in adults and a minimum of 1 year in children and adolescents. From 3% to 6% of the U.S. population has suffered with this disorder at some time in their life, and the rate was found to be higher in primary care treatment settings (Sansone, 2009). Dysthymia is a serious disorder, it can be very disabling and often occurs with other psychiatric disorders such as major depression, anxiety, and substance abuse disorders (Sansone, 2009). Other symptoms that characterize dysthymia include low self-esteem, inability to make decisions, and feelings of hopelessness. The Greek word *dysthymia* means " bad state of mind." People with this disorder often see themselves as incapable, and their thoughts are filled with self-criticism and excessive guilt. Like *EEyore*, a character from "Winnie the Pooh," a person with dysthymia has a black rain cloud over them most of their days and aspects of their family and occupational life are profoundly affected. The long duration of these thoughts and feelings can result in the lack of clinical recognition of this type of depression; high rates of people with dysthymia go on to having a major depressive episode (Sansone, 2009).

Bipolar Disorder

Bipolar disorder is a brain disorder that not only causes unusual shifts between low and elevated mood but affects energy, activity levels, sleep, thought process, and judgment in extreme ways. Symptoms can occur on a spectrum from severe mania to hypomania to periods of being symptom free to mild to moderate depression and more severe depression (NIMH, 2009b). People with this disorder need to manage symptoms throughout their lives and if left untreated, bipolar

disorder usually worsens in frequency and intensity of mood shifts and psychosocial consequences. There is a 90% recurrence rate with this disorder.

Mania, a characteristic symptom of bipolar disorder, is diagnosed when a person has an elevated or irritable mood lasting at least 1 week (or less if hospitalization is necessary) and at the same time has three or more of the following symptoms:

- Grandiosity
- Distractibility
- Decreased sleep
- More goal-directed activities or psychomotor agitation
- Rapid speech patterns
- Subjective expression of racing thoughts with changing topics or interjecting unrelated topics
- Excessive involvement in pleasurable activities that have a high potential for painful consequences (American Psychiatric Association, 2000)

In people diagnosed with bipolar disorder, depressive symptoms occur three times more frequently than manic symptoms (Noonan, 2007). This links the illness with a higher risk of suicide: 25% to 50% of people with this disorder attempt suicide at least once in their life time, and the majority of these suicide victims die by their first attempt (Foutoulakis, 2008). When a patient presents with symptoms of depression it is important to obtain a history back to school age to determine if there were previous episodes of mania. Persons often suffer for 10 to 12 years before a correct diagnosis and treatment for bipolar disorder begins (Noonan, 2007). The frequency of cycling between periods of mania and depression, along with the severity levels of each phase, differentiate between the subtypes of bipolar disorder.

This mood disorder affects approximately 5.7 million American adults in a given year, or about 2.6% of the U.S. population aged 18 and older (NIMH, 2008). Bipolar disorder runs in families and is inheritable. Close relatives of people suffering from this condition are 10 to 20 times more likely to develop either depression or manic-depressive illness than those in the general population. Because of this strong familial link, bipolar disorder is believed to have a genetic component; however, the exact gene or genes have not yet been identified.

Unlike major depression, with which women are diagnosed more frequently than men, bipolar disorder affects men and women equally. Most diagnoses are made in early adulthood. The median age of onset is 25 years.

It is not uncommon for bipolar disorder to occur with other psychiatric illnesses such as anxiety disorders, attention deficit disorder, and substance abuse disorders. Studies have also linked bipolar disorder with physical disorders such as diabetes, heart disease, migraines, and asthma (Schwartz, 2009). Throughout his or her lifetime, each person will establish a particular pattern of illness. Treatment usually takes a multifaceted approach with pharmacotherapy, symptoms management, and family therapy and education; with treatment, 70% to 80% of people are able to live meaningful, productive lives.

© ANTIDEPRESSANTS

Imagine going to a physician and explaining that you are experiencing a particular pain. The physician responds that he or she knows exactly what you are experiencing, can prescribe something to treat it, but will tell you it will be several weeks before the pain is gone. For patients experiencing emotional pain, such as depression, this is their very experience.

Most antidepressant drugs have a lag period of 10 days to 4 weeks before a therapeutic response is noted. Increasing the dose will not shorten this period but rather increases the incidence of adverse reactions Although antidepressants can bring about an immediate change at neuroreceptor sites, it is unclear why a corresponding immediate relief of depressive symptoms does not occur. A current hypothesis about antidepressant medication is that a correction of dysregulation of neurotransmitters occurs. Post-synaptic receptors, which participate in neurotransmission, may have as important a role as do the pre-synaptic receptors where regulation of neurotransmitter release and reuptake occur. Long-term antidepressant therapy produces changes in both pre- and post-synaptic neuroreceptors, which results in a higher level of available neurotransmitters. The decrease in sensitivity to the neurotransmitter at the pre-synaptic receptor sites is a process that takes days to achieve with antidepressant therapy. The effect of the antidepressant medication when administered for longer periods is a down-regulation, or decrease, in number of post-synaptic receptor sites, thus potentially explaining why the medication exerts a delayed response (Mohr, 2009; Pav, et al., 2008; Duman, 2002).

Research has demonstrated that the action of antidepressants may not wholly involve neurotransmitters. Antidepressants may also function to realign the connections between the cortical and limbic areas of the brain. One small study showed that depressed patients did not have normal connections between these two areas of the brain. Treatment with an antidepressant (specifically, sertraline) increases these connections and possibly increases the regulatory influence of the cortical mood-regulating regions over the limbic regions of the brain (Anand, Li, Wang, et al., 2005). This suggests the possible connection between depression and chronic stress responses. Antidepressant medication could be reversing the structural alterations in these regions of the brain affected by depression and stress. Recent studies have demonstrated an increase in neurogenesis in the hippocampal regions of the brain and the ability to refine genetic expression (Duman, 2002).

For the patient with an acute depressive disorder, this delay in the remission of depressive symptoms is difficult to accept. By the time a person seeks treatment for these illnesses, he or she wants immediate relief from pain. It is important to educate the patient to continue taking their medication despite the delay in symptom reduction or feeling completely

recovered. Ongoing assessment of the patient should occur regularly while treated pharmacologically for depression as patients may only be achieving a reduction in their depressive symptoms. Only 30% of patients achieve a full remission of symptoms with an initial trial of antidepressant medication taken at adequate doses for a sufficient duration of time. This means a decision to either switch medications or to augment the treatment with another medication must be made by the treatment provider (Sussman, 2007; Rush, 2006).

Although the full therapeutic effect of mood lifting does not occur for up to 4 weeks, antidepressants begin to have some effect earlier in the course of treatment. Energy levels are likely to return to predepressive levels prior to a complete lifting of the depression. Suicidal patients are at great risk at this point because it is theorized that the medication gives the patient the energy to act on their suicidal thoughts and there are select patients who seem to be more vulnerable to this potential. Therefore it is essential for the patient to be reassessed at regular intervals for presence of suicidal thinking, intent, and plan, especially within the early stages of treatment (Crumpacker, 2008).

As discussed earlier, there are three main classes of antidepressants: SSRIs, tricyclics, and MAOIs. There are several other miscellaneous classes of antidepressant medication, such as the SNRIs (serotonin norepinephrine reuptake inhibitors). Each type of antidepressant works a little differently, but they all change the brain chemistry to improve neurotransmission. Table 16.1 presents a summary of selected drugs used to treat depression and other mood disorders.

All types of antidepressants are similarly effective in treating depression. However, if a patient does not demonstrate a therapeutic response to a particular drug, he or she may respond positively to another antidepressant, including another drug in the same pharmacologic class. Research has found that about one in four patients has remission of depressive symptoms after switching from one SSRI to another antidepressant (Rush, Trivedi, Wisniewski, et al., 2006). Alternately, similar positive response to drug therapy can be achieved by augmenting the original drug with a drug from a different class (Rush et al., 2006; Sussman, 2007).

Although antidepressants all act similarly, each type has unique adverse effects. The goal in antidepressant therapy is to bring about the greatest relief of symptoms while minimizing any unpleasant adverse effects as much as possible. Table 16.2 compares the adverse effects of selected antidepressant drugs, and Table 16.3 describes methods of managing these adverse effects.

• © SELECTIVE SEROTONIN REUPTAKE INHIBITORS

Currently, the selective serotonin reuptake inhibitors (SSRIs) are the first choice for treating depression. They are preferred over the tricyclics and the MAOIs because they can be less damaging to the heart and have minimal anticholinergic and hypotensive effects. Selection of one SSRI over another is based on individual patient response to a drug and prescriber

TABLE 16.1   Summary of Selected C Drugs for Treating Mood Disorders

Drug (Trade) Name	Selected Indications	Route and Dosage Range	Pharmacokinetics
C Selective Serotonin Reuptake Inhibitors (SSRIs)			
P sertraline (Zoloft)	Major depression, obsessive-compulsive disorder, PTSD	*Adult:* PO, 50–200 mg/d *Child:* OCD use, 25–200 mg/d	*Onset:* 4.5–8.4 h *Duration:* 12–20 h $t_{1/2}$: 26 h (104 h for active metabolite)
citalopram (Celexa)	Major depression	*Adult:* 20–40 mg/d *Child:* Safety and efficacy have not been established for <18 y	*Onset:* Slow *Duration:* Unknown $t_{1/2}$: 35 h
escitalopram (Lexapro)	Major depression, generalized anxiety disorder	*Adult:* 10–20 mg/d *Adolescent:* 10–20 mg/d (MDD only) *Child:* Safety is and afficacy have not been established for <12 y of age	*Onset:* slow 5 h *Duration:* unknown $t_{1/2}$: 27–32 h
fluoxetine (Proza)	Major depression, obsessive-compulsive disorder, panic disorder, post-traumatic stress disorder, bulimia nervosa	*Adult:* PO, 20–60 mg/d not to exceed 80 mg/d *Child:* PO, 10–20 mg/d	*Onset:* Slow *Duration:* 10–12 h $t_{1/2}$: 1–3 d (7–9 d for S-norfluoxetine, active metabolite)
fluvoxamine (Luvox)	Obsessive-compulsive disorder, social anxiety disorder	*Adult:* PO, 50–300 mg/d *Child:* Safety and efficacy have not been established for <18 y	*Onset:* Rapid *Duration:* 4–16 h $t_{1/2}$: 13.5–15.6 h
paroxetine (Paxil)	Major depression, obsessive-compulsive disorder, panic disorder	*Adult:* PO, 20–50 mg/d *Child:* Safety and efficacy have not been established for <18 y	*Onset:* 5.2 h *Duration:* 12–16 h $t_{1/2}$: 21 h
C Serotonin and Nonepinephrine Reuptake Inhibitors (SNRIs)			
P venlafaxine (Effexor)	Major depression, generalized anxiety disorder, social anxiety disorder (extended release only)	*Adult:* PO, 75 mg/d in 2–3 divided doses—max 225 mg/d Extended release: 37.5–75 mg/d up to 225 mg/d (MDD only) *Child:* Safety is and afficacy have not been established for <12 y of age	*Onset:* varies *Duration:* varies $t_{1/2}$: 5–7 h
desvenlafaxine (Pritiq)	Major	*Adult:* PO, 50 mg/d—max 400 mg/d Extended release: 37.5–75 mg/d up to 225 mg/d (MDD only) *Child:* Safety and afficacy have not been established for <12 y of age	*Onset:* 7.5 h *Duration:* varies $t_{1/2}$: 11 h

duloxetine (Cymbalta)	Major depression, diabetic neuropathic pain, generalized anxiety disorder	*Adult:* MD—20–30 mg/d BID
		  Neuropathic pain: up to 60 mg/d
		  Generalized anxiety: 60 mg/d
		Extended release: 37.5–75 mg/d up to 225 mg/d (MDD only)
		Child: Safety and afficacy have not been established for <12 y of age
			Onset: 6 h
			Duration: varies
			$t_{1/2}$: 8–17 h

C Tricyclic Antidepressants			
P nortriptyline (Pamelor)	Major depression	*Adult:* PO, 75–150 mg/d *Child:* Use not recommended	*Onset:* Varies *Duration:* 2–4 wk $t_{1/2}$: 18–44 h
amitriptyline (Elavi)	Major depression	*Adult:* 75–150 mg/d; IM, 20–30 mg qid *Child:* Not recommended for <12 y	*Onset:* Varies *Duration:* >20 h $t_{1/2}$: 31–46 h

TABLE 16.1 **Summary of Selected Ⓒ Drugs for Treating Mood Disorders** *(continued)*

Drug (Trade) Name	Selected Indications	Route and Dosage Range	Pharmacokinetics
amoxapine (Asendin)	Major depression	*Adult:* PO, 200–300 mg/d *Child:* Not recommended for <16 y	*Onset:* Varies *Duration:* 2–4 wk $t_{1/2}$: 8–30 h
clomipramine (Anafranil)	Obsessive-compulsive disorder	*Adult:* PO, 25–100 mg/d *Child:* PO, 25 mg/d with gradual increases to a maximum of 3 mg/kg/d or 100 mg/d	*Onset:* Slow *Duration:* 1–6 wk $t_{1/2}$: 19–37 h
desipramine (Norpramin)	Major depression	*Adult:* PO, 100–200 mg/d *Child:* Not recommended for <12 y	*Onset:* Varies *Duration:* 3–4 d $t_{1/2}$: 12–24 h
doxepin (Sinequan)	Major depression Depression, associated anxiety	*Adult:* PO, 75–150 mg/d *Child:* not recommended for <12 y	*Onset:* Varies *Duration:* Unknown $t_{1/2}$: 8–24 h
imipramine (Tofranil)	Major depression	*Adult:* PO, 75–150 mg/d; IM, 100 mg/d *Child:* PO, 1.5 mg/kg/d	*Onset:* Varies *Duration:* Unknown $t_{1/2}$: 11–25 h
protriptyline (Vivactil)	Major depression	*Adult:* PO, 15–40 mg/d divided into 3 or 4 doses *Child:* Use not recommended	*Onset:* Slow *Duration:* Unknown $t_{1/2}$: 67–89 h
maprotiline (Ludiomil)	Major depression, bipolar disorder	*Adult:* PO, 75–225 mg/d *Child:* Use not recommended; safety and efficacy have not been established	*Onset:* Slow *Duration:* 2–3 wk $t_{1/2}$: 61 h
mirtazapine (Remeron)	Major depression	*Adult:* PO, 15–45 mg/d single dose at bedtime *Child:* Safety and efficacy have not been established	*Onset:* Slow *Duration:* 2–4 wk $t_{1/2}$: 20–40 h
trimipramine (Surmontil)	Major depression	*Adult:* PO, 75–150 mg/d *Child:* Use not recommended	*Onset:* Varies *Duration:* Unknown $t_{1/2}$: 7–30 h

Ⓒ Monoamine Oxidase Inhibitors (MAOIs)

Drug (Trade) Name	Selected Indications	Route and Dosage Range	Pharmacokinetics
Ⓟ phenelzine (Nardil)	Major depression	*Adult:* PO, 15 mg tid, increasing to 60 mg/d; maximum 90 mg/d	*Onset:* Approximately 4 wk *Duration:* 48–96 h $t_{1/2}$: Unknown
trancyclopromine (Parnate)	Major depression	*Adult:* PO, 30 mg/d; maximum dose 60 mg/d in divided doses	*Onset:* 7–10 d *Duration:* Unknown $t_{1/2}$: 2.5 h
seligiline (Emsam)	Major depression	*Adult:* transdermal patch—daily 6 mg, 9 mg, or 12 mg patches each 24 h period	*Onset:* varies *Duration:* 25–30% of transdermal med delivered over 24 h $t_{1/2}$: unavailable

Ⓒ Mood Stabilizers

Drug (Trade) Name	Selected Indications	Route and Dosage Range	Pharmacokinetics
Ⓟ lithium (Eskalith)	Mania of bipolar disorder	*Adult:* 1,800 mg/d (slow release) for acute mania; 900–1,200 g/d for maintenance *Child:* Safety and efficacy have not been established for <12 y	*Onset:* 5–7 d *Duration:* Unknown $t_{1/2}$: 10–50 h

Ⓒ Other Antidepressants

Drug (Trade) Name	Selected Indications	Route and Dosage Range	Pharmacokinetics
trazodone (Desyrel)	Major depression	*Adult:* PO, 150–600 mg/d *Child:* Safety and efficacy have not been established	*Onset:* Varies *Duration:* Varies $t_{1/2}$: 4–9 h

TABLE 16.2 Adverse Effects of Selected Antidepressant Drugs

	Anticholinergic*	Agitation, Insomnia	Drowsiness	Cardiac Arrhythmia	Orthostatic Hypotension	Gastrointestinal Distress	Weight Gain
SSRIs							
sertraline	0	2	0	0	0	3	0
citalopram	1	3	0	0	0	3	0
fluoxetine	0	2	0	0	0	3	0
fluvoxamine	0	2	0	0	0	3	0
paroxetine	0	2	0	0	0	3	2
Tricyclics							
nortriptyline	1	0	1	2	2	0	1
amitriptyline	4	0	4	3	4	0	4
clomipramine	4	1	4	3	1	1	3
doxepin	3	0	4	2	2	0	3
imipramine	3	1	3	3	4	1	3
trimipramine	1	0	4	2	2	0	3
amoxapine	2	2	2	3	2	0	1
desipramine	1	1	1	2	2	0	1
protriptyline	2	1	1	2	2	0	0
maprotiline	2	0	4	1	0	0	2
mirtazapine	1	1	4	0	2	1	2
Other							
nefazodone	1	1	3	0	2	3	0
bupropion	0	2	0	1	0	1	0
trazodone	0	2	0	1	0	1	0
venlafaxine	0	0	4	1	1	1	1
MAOIs							
phenelzine	1	2	1	0	2	1	1
trancyclopromine	1	2	1	0	2	1	1

*Dry mouth, blurred vision, urinary hesitancy, and constipation.
0, absent or rare, to 4, common.

preference. It is important to note that if a medication from one class of antidepressants such as an SSRI is discontinued and switched to a different class of medication such as an MAOI, a washout period (waiting period) must occur. This period can vary between 7 and 14 days and will depend on the type of antidepressant being discontinued.

In 1987, fluoxetine (Prozac) became the first SSRI approved by the Food and Drug Administration (FDA) for use as an antidepressant in the United States. It immediately became popular because of its ease in dosing and few adverse effects. Its effectiveness, combined with the increasing social acceptance of antidepressant use, led many patients to ask their physicians for Prozac. Its great marketing success is thought to have stimulated widespread research and subsequent introduction of other, newer antidepressants. Fluoxetine has been around long enough that its patent has now expired, resulting in generic availability of this drug. But in the United States, the cultural impact is such that most people still think of Prozac when they think of antidepressants.

Currently, sertraline (Zoloft) is one of the most widely prescribed SSRIs in the United States. Because of its widespread use, sertraline has been chosen as the prototype SSRI.

Nursing Management of the Patient Receiving P Sertraline

Core Drug Knowledge

Pharmacotherapeutics

Sertraline was approved by the U.S. FDA in 1991 for treating depression in adults. Treating acute depressive disorder with sertraline requires several months or longer of drug therapy, just as it does with other antidepressants.

TABLE 16.3 — Management of Adverse Effects of Antidepressants

Symptoms	Strategies for Management
Gastrointestinal	
Nausea, anorexia	Administer with food (or antacids) if drug absorption is unaffected.
Diarrhea	Use antidiarrheal medication (if not contraindicated).
Constipation	Diet change (increase fiber and fluids), exercise, stool softener (avoid laxatives); wait for tolerance to drug effects.
Sexual dysfunction	Discuss methods available for satisfactory sexual expression.
Anorgasmia	Encourage talk with health care provider regarding dosage reduction or drug holiday.
Erectile dysfunction	
Impaired ejaculation	
Orthostatic hypotension	Use calf exercises, wear support hose, increase fluid intake.
Anticholinergic effects (dry eyes and mouth)	Use artificial tears, frequent dental hygiene, sugar-free chewing gum; wait to develop tolerance to drug effects.
Tremor/"jitteriness"	Slow, gradual titration of increasing dosages; encourage discussion with health care provider regarding dosage reduction or drug holiday.
Insomnia	Take medication in the morning (exception is trazodone).
Sedation	Caffeine (if not contraindicated), take medication at bedtime (exception is bupropion in afternoon).
Headache	Evaluate diet, stress, other drugs used; suggest dosage reduction to health care provider.
Weight gain	Decrease carbohydrate intake; consume low-fat diet; exercise.

Additional approved uses for sertraline include obsessive-compulsive disorder (adults and children), panic disorder, and post-traumatic stress disorder.

Although sertraline is not approved by the FDA for treating depression in children at this time, the SSRI is widely used on an unlabeled basis to treat pediatric depression. Several studies have demonstrated that sertraline is safe and effective for treating major depressive disorder in children (Rynn, Wagner, Donnelly, et al., 2006; March, Klee, & Kremer, 2006).

Pharmacokinetics
Sertraline is well absorbed following oral administration, with peak plasma levels occurring within 4.5 to 8.4 hours. It has a 26- to 104-hour elimination half-life (with metabolites) and reaches a steady state within 7 days. SSRIs such as sertraline are extensively metabolized by the liver and should be used with caution in patients with severe liver impairment. Food may increase the onset of the peak effect from sertraline, but this result is not clinically significant, and no recommendations are made to take the drug with food.

Pharmacodynamics
Sertraline is a potent and selective inhibitor of neuronal serotonin (5-HT) reuptake and has a weak effect on norepinephrine (NE) and dopamine (DA) neuronal reuptake. Because the SSRIs do not have a high affinity for muscarinic (Ach), histaminergic (H₁), and alpha-adrenergic receptors, their capacity for causing anticholinergic, sedative, cardiac, and orthostatic hypotensive effects is considerably less than that of the tricyclics. Achieving antidepressant effects from sertraline, as with other antidepressants, can take anywhere from 10 days to 4 weeks. Some symptoms of depression,

such as loss of energy, may be corrected before the mood is fully elevated.

Contraindications and Precautions
Sertraline should be administered with caution in patients with compromised liver function. Adjustments such as a lower or less-frequent dosing schedule may be made for these patients. Although no studies have been conducted specifically in patients with seizure disorders, the incidence of seizures in patients taking sertraline is 0.2%, which is similar to other antidepressant and placebo studies. A history of seizures therefore requires cautious use of sertraline

As previously mentioned, some concern exists that SSRI antidepressants such as sertraline, or other antidepressant drugs, may increase the risk of suicidal thinking or attempts at suicide in some children and adults. At this time, it is debatable whether sertraline or any other antidepressant actually induces suicidal ideation, or whether the drugs' ability to restore energy levels before elevating mood provides depressed patients with the ability to act on their depressed mood. The FDA has revised the warning labels of all antidepressant drugs with a standardized class warning to indicate that when taking sertraline as well as any other SSRI, both children adolescents and young adults ages (18 to 25) should be closely monitored for worsening of depression and the emergence of suicidal thoughts and tendencies. This warning is prominently displayed in a Black Box warning on the drug label (for more information on Black Box warnings, see Box 5.1 in Chapter 5). For many years, the SSRIs have carried on their label a precaution that close monitoring of patients was necessary in the early stages of treatment. Only the significance of the warning has changed.

The issue of whether SSRIs and other antidepressants increase the risk of suicidality is still debated as some studies have shown that antidepressant medication may have a protective factor against suicide in adults—including young adults ages 18 to 25. The need for carefully designed research studies is imperative because it has been postulated that as a result of having the more significant FDA warning label, there has been a decrease in *treated* depression in some age groups. See Box 16.2 for a discussion of these current studies on the relationship between SSRI antidepressants and the risk of suicidal behavior. For the most recent labeling information on specific antidepressant medication, visit the FDA website: *http://www.fda.gov*.

Adverse Effects

Compared with the tricyclics, sertraline and other SSRIs have fewer adverse anticholinergic and cardiovascular effects and usually do not cause weight gain. Adverse effects, which are mild and brief, include gastrointestinal distress (anorexia, nausea, vomiting, and diarrhea), headache, fatigue, insomnia, and sexual dysfunction (delayed ejaculation, inability to achieve orgasm). Some of these adverse effects are transient, subsiding within the first 1 to 2 weeks of therapy. Other adverse effects may include hematologic problems, such as blood dyscrasias, leukopenia, and altered platelet function. Since serotonin is released by platelets to promote aggregation, use of SSRIs leads to depletion of serotonin in platelets which may result in decreased coagulation.

Syndrome of Inappropriate Anti-Diuretic Hormone Secretion or SIADH is another potential adverse side effect of sertraline or any SSRIs. The condition results in hyponatremia and it usually happens in the first week of SSRI treatment. A study of SSRI use in an elderly population found as many as 12% to 25% having hyponatremia and 12% having the syndrome. Symptoms of hyponatremia are nonspecific initially and could include malaise, nausea, headache, lethargy and myalgia, but could progress to loss of consciousness and convulsions. Age and female gender are possible risk factors for developing this complication (Looper, 2007).

For some patients, the most limiting adverse effects of SSRIs are the disturbances in sexual function. This effect may not be a concern to the depressed patient beginning therapy, but it may become a greater concern as the patient regains interest in sexual activity. The presence of this adverse effect is a frequent reason that patients consider stopping drug therapy. In clinical trials, only 10% to 15% of patients required discontinuation of treatment because of an adverse event. As noted earlier, sertraline and other SSRIs may increase the risk of suicide, although the incidence of suicide is extremely small. Suicidal thoughts or attempts that occur early in the course of therapy may be related to the drug's beginning to work; remember that the energy level of the patient increases before the depression is fully relieved.

Drug Interactions

Sertraline is highly bound (98%) to plasma protein. If it is administered with another drug that is highly protein bound, increased free concentrations of either drug may result. The activity of isoenzyme cytochrome P-450 2D6 may be substantially inhibited by sertraline. Any drug that is metabolized by this isoenzyme should therefore be administered with caution, because expected plasma levels will be altered. Consuming caffeinated beverages can increase the stimulant sensation experienced by the patient taking sertraline and other SSRIs. Nicotine intake from cigarette smoking may cause an increase in the metabolism of sertraline and other SSRIs. The FDA has issues a safety alter regarding the combined intake of sertraline and other drugs that enhances serotonergic neurotransmission and tryptans, medications used to treat migranes (FDA, 2009g). Even when prescribed on its own, a rare, life-threatening event called **serotonin syndrome** can occur as a result of overactivation of the central serotonin receptors. Symptoms to watch for are sweating, fever, increased blood pressure, tachycardia, abdominal pain, diarrhea, muscle spasm, increased motor activity, irritability, hostility, and altered mental state. In its most severe presentation, cardiovascular shock or even death may result This rare but serious side effect can occur with initiation or increase of dosage of any SSRI or SNRI (Looper, 2007). Table 16.4 summarizes potential drug interactions with sertraline.

Assessment of Relevant Core Patient Variables

Health Status

Review the patient's drug history for current drugs used, health history for any illnesses that may complicate therapy, and mental status. Assess for a history of seizures because SSRIs such as sertraline are used with caution in patients with such a history. The drug should be discontinued if seizures occur. Additionally, because anxiety, nervousness, and insomnia occur in 2% to 22% of patients treated with SSRIs, careful consideration should be given to the use of these antidepressants in patients who already exhibit one or more of these symptoms. SSRIs, such as sertraline, may not be the antidepressant drug class of choice for the extremely underweight depressed patient, because approximately 3% to 9% of patients treated with SSRIs experience substantial weight loss. However, only rarely has weight loss required patients to discontinue therapy.

Also, assess for the presence of suicidal ideation before starting therapy, and closely monitor the patient for evidence of worsening depression or onset of suicidal ideation while receiving sertraline or other SSRIs. The most critical time to closely monitor the patient for behavioral changes is during the first few weeks of drug therapy.

As previously mentioned, depression is commonly seen in patients with other medical conditions. The efficacy of antidepressant treatment with co-occurring disorders has yielded some interesting research which suggests that treatment of depression also can result in improvement of existing medical conditions. A finding from a study of diabetic

TABLE 16.4	Agents that Interact with P Sertraline	
Interactants	Effect and Significance	Nursing Management
alcohol	Additive CNS depression may occur.	Monitor for adverse effects.
benzodiazepines	Decreased metabolism of benzodiazepines through hepatic oxidation route. Significance not known.	Monitor for adverse effects of benzodiazepines.
cimetidine	Increases half-life, AUC, and C_{max} of sertraline, but clinical significance is unknown.	Adjust sertraline doses as necessary.
clozapine	May elevate clozapine levels.	Monitor for adverse effects of clozapine.
cyproheptadine	May decrease or reverse pharmacologic effects of SSRIs.	Monitor for reduced efficacy of sertraline.
drugs metabolized by P-450 2D6	Sertraline or other SSRIs may substantially inhibit the activity of P-450 2D6 (especially during the beginning of therapy); metabolism of these other drugs may be reduced, potentially resulting in adverse effects.	Monitor for adverse effects. Lower doses of sertraline may be needed.
drugs that are highly protein bound	Because sertraline and other SSRIs are highly protein bound, sertraline may displace the other drug from the protein, causing increased circulating levels of the other drug and possibly adverse effects. If other drugs are started while the patient is on sertraline, the sertraline may be displaced from the protein, resulting in higher circulating levels of sertraline, and possibly adverse effects.	Monitor for adverse effects.
hydantoin	Sertraline may increase hydantoin levels.	Monitor for increased hydantoin levels.
MAOIs, St. John's wort	Serotonin syndrome, with serious, sometimes fatal, reactions such as hyperthermia, rigidity, vital sign changes, mental status changes, and autonomic nervous system instability.	Avoid sertraline and other SSRIs when MAOIs are used and within 14 days of stopping an MAOI. Teach patients not to self-medicate with St. John's wort if taking sertraline.
phenytoin	May increase phenytoin levels.	Monitor for adverse effects of phenytoin. Check blood phenytoin levels when starting therapy or changing dose of sertraline.
sumatriptan	Concurrent use increases serotonin levels, potentially leading to serotonin syndrome.	Avoid concurrent use.
sympathomimetic drugs	Increases sensitivity to the effects of sympathomimetics. Serotonin syndrome is more likely to occur.	Monitor for adverse effects.
tolbutamide	Coadministration has been shown to decrease the clearance of tolbutamide. Clinical significance unknown.	Monitor tolbutamide levels.
TCAs	May increase serum TCA levels.	Monitor for adverse effects. Monitor TCA blood levels. TCA dose may have to be reduced.
tryptophan	Concurrent use increases serotonin levels, potentially leading to serotonin syndrome.	Avoid concurrent use.
warfarin	Increases prothrombin time and may cause bleeding.	Monitor prothrombin time.

AUC, area under the curve; C_{max}, maximum concentration.

patients using sertraline for depression supported use of the medication following a remittance of depressive symptoms as it was found to delay the onset of another episode of depression and improve the interval of time before another episode of depression occurred. Recovery from depression also was associated with improved long-term glucose control, as measured by glycosylated hemoglobin levels (Lustman, Clouse, Nix, et al., 2006). Exactly how or why this occurs is not known at this time. Another study compared the use of sertraline in younger (below age 55) and older (above age 55) diabetic patients and found that the younger group had a more positive response to sertraline in the prevention of recurrence of depression. The authors speculated that there were variables they did not account for in the older group; nonetheless, this study also correlated improved glycosylated hemoglobin levels during the depression-free intervals (Williams, et al., 2007). In addition, depression is associated with acute coronary syndrome (ACS). Sertraline has been the most studied medications used for the treatment of depressed patients with cardiac disease. The benefits demonstrated are that it is an antidepressant that is well tolerated in this group of patients and appears to improve the quality of life (Sansone, 2008). One study found that an episode of major depression associated with ACS is as likely to occur before the ACS as after it. Predictors of success in treating depressed patients with diabetes using sertraline were as follows: current episode of depression began before development of ACS; history of a previous depressive episode; or depression rated as severe. The likelihood of successful antidepressant effects from sertraline was increased if the patient had more than one of these three predictors (Glassman, Bigger, Gaffney, et al., 2006). More research is necessary in this area.

Life Span and Gender

Consider the patient's age. As previously discussed, although some research indicates that sertraline has been proved safe and effective for use in children, this drug is not approved for use in children to treat depression. When it is used in children, the pediatric dose is usually half that for adults because of children's smaller body size. Concern exists that sertraline, like all other antidepressants, may increase depression and risk of suicidal thinking or behaviors in children. Treatment with sertraline for depression appears to increase the risk of suicidality more in children than in adolescents (March, Klee, & Kremer, 2006). Clinical trials have not shown that the use of sertraline increases suicidality at all in children or adolescents treated for obsessive-compulsive disorder (March, Klee, & Kramer, 2006). See Box 16.2 for further discussion of the suicide risk with SSRI antidepressant medication.

The adverse effect profile in the elderly patient is similar to that in younger healthy adults. However, because of decreased clearance of the drug in the older patient, smaller doses and slower increases should be made when prescribing sertraline or other SSRIs. A pilot study of 37 mildly depressed elderly patients compared the use of sertraline with regular (facility-based, three times weekly for 60 minutes) exercise demonstrated that both were almost equally effective in decreasing symptoms of mild depression for this group of patients. The exercise group developed an improvement in physical strength and endurance not achieved by the group using only medication. Although this study used a small group of subjects, previous studies have suggested that combining exercise with antidepressant

medication yields improved benefits in elderly patients (Brenes, 2007).

Ask female patients of childbearing age whether they are pregnant, intend to become pregnant, or are breast-feeding. The FDA classifies sertraline in pregnancy risk category C. Sertraline, however, is recommended as first-line treatment for breastfeeding woman in the United States because it exhibits undetectable levels in the breast fed infant (Menon, 2008; Field, 2008). Sertraline and two other SSRIs (Fluoxetine and Paroxetine) have been studied to determine if they can provide symptomatic relief in treating PMS and Premenstrual Dysphoric Disorder, the results show that these medications are most effective for ameliorating symptoms when the medication is used continuously rather than intermittently over the course of a woman's menstrual cycle (Shah, 2008).

Lifestyle, Diet, and Habits

The SSRIs can affect sexual functioning. Men may report delayed ejaculation or ejaculatory failure, whereas women may report the inability to achieve orgasm. However, sexual functioning can also be adversely affected by the very depression that the SSRI is prescribed to treat. Therefore, a baseline assessment of sexual functioning should be performed before starting treatment with sertraline.

Also, assess the normal use of caffeine in patients who will be starting sertraline, because caffeine interacts with sertraline. In addition, assess for alcohol use and determine whether the patient smokes cigarettes, because these agents also interact with sertraline. Alcohol abuse is a frequent co-occurring disorder with depression. Patients who stopped using alcohol and then began taking sertraline not only were less likely to be depressed but were less likely to relapse into drinking. Research indicated that if their depression was not controlled, they were much more likely to begin drinking again (Oslin, 2005).

Culture and Inherited Traits

Consider the patient's cultural background. Some people with a polymorphism in the P-450 isoenzyme 2D6 may lack this enzyme and therefore would be poor drug metabolizers, would have higher circulating drug doses, and could possibly experience adverse effects from the SSRIs, even at low doses. A range of 2D6 levels has been identified globally among various ethnic groups. Their findings suggest that poor metabolizing is least common in East Asians, followed by African Americans and then Hispanics, with whites exhibiting this condition most frequently. For this reason, an East Asian patient may respond more than an African American patient, a Hispanic patient, or even a white patient, even if they all receive the same dose of an SSRI. A small pharmacokinetic/pharmacodynamic study appears to support this finding. The researchers compared the dosage needed to achieve therapeutic effect in depressed Chinese and Caucasians treated with sertraline and the steady-state plasma concentrations of the two groups. The Caucasian patients required a higher dose of sertraline to achieve relief of depression and had a higher plasma level of sertraline than the Chinese patients (Hong,

BOX 16.2 COMMUNITY BASED CONCERNS

SUICIDALITY AND ANTIDEPRESSANT MEDICATION

Over the past years the possible relationship between the use of antidepressants and the increased risk of suicidality (defined as the combination of new suicide attempts, new onset of suicidal ideation, and worsening of pre-existing suicidal ideation) has been the topic of much debate. In 2003 and 2004 U.S. and European regulators issued public health warnings about this possible association. In the early 1990s, similar reports emerged of suicidal behavior in adults who received Prozac, the first SSRI, for depression. The belief was that Prozac had an early activating effect on depressed people and gave them enough energy to follow through on suicidal impulses before there was a mood elevating effect. In 1991, the US Food and Drug Administration had a psychopharmacologic drug advisory meeting and concluded there was no clear evidence of this risk. In 2003, anecdotal case reports of suicidality and suicide in adolescents receiving SSRIs (paroxetine) prompted the FDA to review 25 randomized controlled clinical trials involving SSRIs. The FDA's review reexamined the adverse effects reported from all pediatric clinical trials in which any SSRI was used. It is important to note that no pediatric suicides occurred in any of these trials and the definition of suicidality was not identical in all of the studies. The outcome of this review resulted in the addition of Black Box warnings to the labels of SSRIs (and other classes of antidepressants). This is the FDA's most serious drug label warning. Subsequent studies found the same risk with young adults population, ages 18 to 25 years. The current warning states: antidepressant medicine may increase suicidal thoughts or action in some children, teenagers and young adults within the first few months of treatment (Prescriber's Letter, 2008). There are many reports in the news that peak the public's concern and leads to fear of the use of antidepressant medication.

The scientific community is often split when interpreting findings of clinical research. Large scale reviews of data ensued to establish if these findings would be repeated in adult clinical trials. A review of 372 controlled trials of adults (nearly 100,000 subjects) using SSRI and non SSRI antidepressant medication concluded that antidepressant medication had a protective effect rather than causing an increase in suicidal ideation and behavior. There were eight suicides during the course of the reviewed trials involving almost 100,000 people. Data from this study did suggest there was a higher rate of suicide was found in adults under the age of 25 once antidepressant therapy had begun (Stone, 2009). Thus the FDA has since expanded the labeling of all antidepressants to include young adults under the age of 25 as well as adolescents and children in this Black Box warning.

Another analysis within the Veterans Health Administration looked at a cohort of about 226,866 veterans and compared suicide rates within the subjects before and after SSRI treatment. The results concluded that antidepressants may decrease the risk of suicide; they found no greater risk of suicide with use of SSRIs when compared to other antidepressants and there was no significant difference between adult age groups (Gibbons, 2007). Another study looking specifically at older patients and found that initiation of SSRI therapy is the most closely associated time period that

could increase the risk of suicidal behavior when compared with other antidepressants (Juurlink, et al., 2006).

A recent large scale meta-analysis of 200,000 patients of all ages from eight observational studies had been analyzed to specifically look at the correlation between exposure to SSRI antidepressants and the increased rate in suicide completion or attempt. The findings of this study found that not only do SSRIs have a protective effect against suicide in patients age 65 and older, this is true in adults and even in young adults ages 18 to 25 years. This study did find a higher rate of suicide attempts and completions with the adolescent groups when SSRIs were used and supports the FDA's warning of use of antidepressant medications within this age group (Barbui, 2009).

A concern is that as a result of the FDA's antidepressant label warnings, depression is being undertreated in the pediatric community. There is another concern that this trend will be repeated in the young adult group as well. Rates of SSRI prescriptions and suicides were examined in the United States and in the Netherlands after the warnings were issued in 2003 and 2004. In the Netherlands, suicide rates increased by 49% between the years 2003 and 2005. In the United States, this rate increased by 14%. There was an inverse association between suicide rates with SSRI prescriptions. The conclusion that cannot be disputed is that suicide is more common in children with untreated major depression (Gibbons, 2007).

Any nurse involved with treating depressed patients in the community should reach one clear conclusion from these studies: **Safe and successful treatment of a depressed patient depends on much more than merely giving the correct dosage of an antidepressant.** It is not disputed that SSRIs can be physically activating in the initial stages of therapy, but the patient must be kept safe regardless of when the medication was initiated. To achieve this outcome in the community, it is essential to make critical interventions: the first is rooted in the development of a trusting therapeutic relationship with the patient with the goal of facilitating honest communication. This bond encourages the patient to take active responsibility for his or her own safety. Another is to conduct regular neuropsychiatric assessments of patients treated for depression. Can you imagine treating a patient for diabetes and not monitoring blood glucose levels, or giving electrolyte replacement therapy without looking at associated serum levels? Educating the patient and involving the family will play an integral role in providing a safe environment for the patient. Reports in the media may be misinterpreted and there may be a reluctance to seek treatment or take antidepressant medication if prescribed. Depressed patients are at risk of suicide and there seems to be select groups of patients that are more vulnerable to suicidal behavior at the initiation of antidepressant treatment. All precautions must be taken to maintain patient safety. There is much more to treating depressed patients than suggesting that they just take a pill a day and be on their way. Nurses working with patients who take antidepressant medication in the community or in any practice setting should assume that the assessment of the clinical response to antidepressant medication as well as the presence of suicidal thoughts or behavior is *their* responsibility.

Norman, Naing, et al., 2006). However, additional and larger research studies are still necessary to confirm these findings. Also, Native Americans must be included in further reports, because very few data exist for this group.

Other researchers have found that a polymorphism in a gene is linked with therapeutic response to SSRI treatment. Patients with a polymorphism that has the L (or

long) allele have better response to an SSRI than patients who have the polymorphism of the S (or short) allele (Yu, Tsai, Chen, et al., 2002; Lotrich, Pollock, & Ferrell, 2003). The L allele is more highly prevalent in African Americans (77% to 87%) than in European Americans (56% to 60%) (Lotrich et al., 2003). Patients who have been identified as having the L allele should receive an SSRI, such as sertraline, as a drug of first choice for treatment of depression, because they are likely to obtain therapeutic effects from this therapy. Some studies have shown that the outcome of antidepressant treatment runs in families but individual variation to treatment with antidepressant medication has been largely unpredictable. A search for a genetic predictor of response to treatment was reviewed in a prospective study of the 1,953 patients with major depessive disorder treated with the antidepressant citalopram in the Sequenced Treatment Alternatives for Depression Study (STAR D* study). A significant association was found between treatment outcomes with use of citalopram and the presence of the genetic markers which encode HTR2A (Serotonin 2A receptor). Serotonin 2A receptors downregulate with the SSRI medication citalopram and this study suggested this is a genetic variation that could help predict the effectiveness of an antidepressant medication (McMahon, 2006).

Nursing Diagnoses and Outcomes

- Risk for Suicide related to increased energy from sertraline without relief of suicidal ideations or low mood
  Desired outcome: The patient will identify alternative coping mechanisms.
- Restlessness related to psychomotor agitation secondary to sertraline use
  Desired outcome: The patient will identify appropriate interventions to promote relaxation.
- Sleep Pattern Disturbance: Less than Body Requirements, related to psychomotor agitation secondary to sertraline use
  Desired outcome: The patient will identify appropriate interventions to promote sleep.
- Nausea, Abdominal Pain, or both related to abnormal peristalsis secondary to sertraline use
  Desired outcome: The patient will report a decrease of nausea.
- Diarrhea and Loose Stools related to adverse effects of medication secondary to sertraline use
  Desired outcome: The patient will re-establish and maintain normal pattern of bowel functioning.
- Sexual Dysfunction related to disrupted sexual response pattern, such as impotence or anorgasmia, secondary to sertraline use
  Desired outcome: The patient will identify satisfying and acceptable sexual practices and some alternative ways of dealing with sexual expression.

Planning and Intervention

Maximizing Therapeutic Effects

By the time patients begin drug therapy, they may be at their most hopeless state. This state sometimes can even be compounded by their initial response to the medication. Equally important to remember is that the patient does not experience the maximum therapeutic effect for several weeks. Routine, consistent measurement of symptoms and adverse effects needs to occur at each treatment visit. The patient should be assessed using a standardized tool such as the Hamilton Rating Scale for Depression or the Quick Inventory of Depressive Symptomatology–Self Report (Rush et al., 2006). To maximize the therapeutic effect of antidepressant therapy, establish a therapeutic, trusting relationship with the patient by offering the hopeless patient hope for the future by being candid about the therapeutic effects and adverse effects of the medication. Properly administering the medication at regular times, without missing doses, is important as well.

Minimizing Adverse Effects

Remember that any possible adverse effects of sertraline often occur immediately or early in the treatment course. Restlessness or even insomnia may be reported by patients at the beginning of therapy. To minimize these effects, give the medication early in the day, when the patient is most active and least likely to be bothered by such effects. The adverse effects of nausea and diarrhea can be minimized as well by giving the medication with food or even by dividing the daily dose into more frequent, smaller doses. Carefully assess the patient on drug therapy for worsening of depression or signs of suicidal ideation. *Close monitoring of all patients, but especially children, teens and young adult, s is imperative to minimize the risk of suicide.* Closest monitoring needs to be done during the beginning of therapy and at each dose change. To further guard against suicide, sertraline and other SSRIs should be administered only in addition to counseling and therapy, not in its place.

To help the patient minimize any sexually related adverse effects, demonstrate a willingness to discuss these matters with the patient in an open and honest manner. Inquire about any changes in sexual functioning, because changes associated with medication use may lead to nonadherence to drug therapy. Patients should always be discouraged from consuming alcohol while undergoing sertraline therapy because increased central nervous system (CNS) depression may result. It is also important to protect the patient from ultraviolet light until his or her individual photos Sertraline can be associated with developing Serotonin Discontinuation Syndrome; you must consider the length of time the patient has been taking any SSRI, the dosage, and the half-life of the drug before stopping an SSRI. This can occur in 20% to 25% of patients stopping SSRIs abruptly and may last 1 to 2 weeks (Looper, 2007).

The symptoms of this syndrome can be remembered by using the mnemonic FLUSH:

Flu-like (e.g., fatigue, myalgia, loose stools, nausea)
Light-headedness, dizziness, or both
Uneasiness, restlessness, or both
Sleep and sensory disturbances
Headache

Symptoms of sertraline toxicity or overdose are dilated pupils, tachycardia, electrocardiographic (ECG) changes, anxiousness with decreased level of consciousness, and vomiting. No deaths have been reported by overdose involving sertraline alone. However, a few fatalities have occurred when sertraline was mixed with alcohol or other drugs in a deliberate overdose. Management of overdose should include treating presenting symptoms. There are no specific antidotes. Activated charcoal may be as effective as emesis or lavage.

Providing Patient and Family Education

- Educate patients and families about realistic expectations for antidepressant therapy. Include information about the delay in relief of symptoms and the necessity of continuing with the medication even after relief of symptoms is achieved.
- Educate patients and families about potential suicidal ideation. Families need special help to learn how to recognize behavioral changes that may indicate suicidal ideation, because patients may not recognize it in themselves.
- Teach the patient and family to read the Medication Guide that accompanies the filled prescription. They should read it each time they receive a refilled prescription because new information may be included (see Chapter 5, Box 5.2, What is an FDA Medication Guide?).
- Emphasize the risk for SSRI withdrawal syndrome if patients abruptly stop taking their medication.
- Inform patients about possible adverse effects (e.g., nausea, restlessness, insomnia, sexual dysfunction) and advise them on how to minimize disruption to their lifestyle. Emphasize that adverse effects may occur before therapeutic effects and that many of them are transient.
- Discuss the increased stimulant effect that results when sertraline and caffeine are combined and advise patients to modify their diet accordingly.
- Teach patients to avoid alcohol and other CNS depressant drugs to avoid any cumulative depressant effect.
- Caution patients about using heavy machinery or driving until individual response to the drug is known.

Ongoing Assessment and Evaluation

Continue to assess the patient's mood and observe any increase in anxiety, nervousness, restlessness, or insomnia. If the patient becomes physically energized yet experiences little improvement in mood, assess the patient especially closely for suicidal thoughts because he or she is at greater risk of acting on these thoughts under these conditions. Periodically monitor laboratory tests that assess liver function and measure total blood cholesterol and triglycerides to assess the patient for any possible changes. As sertraline therapy continues, expect patients to report an increased interest in their surroundings and more energy to participate in daily activities. Sertraline therapy is considered effective when depression is fully relieved and no serious adverse effects occur.

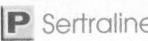

MEMORY CHIP

P Sertraline

- Selective serotonin reuptake inhibitor used to treat depression, obsessive-compulsive disorder, panic disorder, and post-traumatic stress disorder
- Major contraindications: Cautious use in patients with decreased liver function
- Most common adverse effects: gastrointestinal distress, headache, sleep disturbance, and abnormal ejaculation
- Most serious adverse effect: may possibly increase the risk for suicide, especially in pediatric populations
- **Life span alert: pregnancy category C, see black box warning**
- Maximizing therapeutic effects: Encourage patient to continue medicine, even though immediate response does not occur, and continue medication well after an improvement is experienced.
- Minimizing adverse effects: Give with food; avoid ultraviolet light.
- Most important patient education: Teach that a lag time occurs between beginning therapy and relief of symptoms; avoid alcohol and drugs.
- **Black box warning: may increase the risk of suicidal thoughts or behaviors in children, adolescents, and young adults**

Drugs Closely Related to P Sertraline

Other SSRIs closely related to sertraline include citalopram (Celexa), escitalopram (Lexapro), fluoxetine (Prozac), fluvoxamine (Luvox), and paroxetine (Paxil). Fluoxetine and escitalopram are the only SSRIs that are labeled for use in children, although they carry the same label warning about the potential for increasing suicidal ideation as the other SSRIs. (US FDA, 2009c) Fluoxetine has some unique pharmacokinetic properties. It has a much longer half-life than the other SSRIs. Unlike the others, which are excreted unchanged via the urine and feces, like sertraline, fluoxetine is metabolized in the liver.

Drugs Significantly Different From P Sertraline
Bupropion

Bupropion (Wellbutrin) is a weak blocker of neuronal uptake of norepinephrine and serotonin. It also inhibits, to some extent, neuronal reuptake of dopamine. Bupropion has the benefit of being somewhat energizing for patients with major depression. It also may be coadministered with other SSRIs to decrease the effect of the primary medication when sexual functioning is adversely affected. Research has found that bupropion is successful as a second-line drug when treatment with an SSRI alone has not been totally effective. Patients receive equal benefit from switching to bupropion or having the drug added to their regimen of an SSRI.

Bupropion should be administered with caution to any patient who has an increased seizure risk. Missed doses should never be doubled; seizure may result. Although the usual dose is 300 mg/d, the risk of seizure may be four times greater when bupropion is given at doses between 300 and 450 mg/d.

This risk further increases almost 10 times at doses of between 450 and 600 mg/d. A new salt form of buproprion called Aplenzin (buproprion hydrobromide) has recently been approved and is used in once-a-day dosing. Caution should be taken in patients with renal or hepatic impairment, and like other forms of bupropion, it is contraindicated for patients with any type of seizure disorder (FDA, 2009a).

A form of bupropion called Zyban has been available and is widely used for smoking cessation. Although not indicated for management of depression, it carries the same risks in taking bupropion as an antidepressant and prescribers should monitor patients for neuropsychiatric changes when taking this medication. Taking Zyban for smoking cessation with other forms of bupropion is contraindicated (US FDA, 2009b).

Trazodone

Trazodone (Desyrel) is a weak serotonin transport inhibitor as well as a serotonin receptor (5-HT$_2$) blocker. This combined action diminishes some of the troubling adverse effects associated with 5-HT transporter inhibitors, such as insomnia, jitteriness, and sexual dysfunction. Trazodone is also an adrenergic receptor blocker that affects both alpha-1 and alpha-2 receptors, so it can cause dizziness and orthostatic changes. It is not recommended for use by patients during the initial recovery phase of a heart attack. Patients with pre-existing cardiac disease should also be monitored closely, particularly for cardiac arrhythmias.

Trazodone may cause priapism, a prolonged and often painful penile erection rarely associated with sexual arousal. Trazodone also causes sedation. For this reason it is often prescribed as a supplemental therapy to other antidepressants that cause insomnia as an adverse effect. Trazodone should be taken at bedtime to help promote sleep

Therapeutic response to trazodone usually occurs within 2 weeks. Administered orally, the drug is well absorbed; food enhances its absorption. Metabolism in the liver is extensive; none of its metabolites is believed to be pharmacologically active.

Serotonin and Norepinephrine Reuptake Inhibitors (SNRIs)

This is a class of medication that blocks the reuptake of both serotonin and norepinephrine with differing selectivity. It comprises several drugs: velafaxine (Effexor), duloxetine (Cymbalta), mirtazepine (Remeron), milnacipran (Savella), and desvenlafaxine (Pristiq). They have many similarities to the SSRIs therefore they carry the same risks, such the possibility of serotonin syndrome. These risk factors are described in detail under SSRIs and sertraline. Use of an SNRI or SSRI with an MAOI is strictly contraindicated and a washout period must occur between using these drugs.

Venlafaxine

Venlaflaxine (Effexor) is a mixed norepinephrine and serotonin reuptake inhibitor. It has no significant affinity for adrenergic receptor blockade (alpha-1 or alpha-2), H$_1$, or Ach receptors.

Its pharmacologic effects are dose related, and it exhibits triphasic pharmacologic effects within its dosage range. At the lowest effective dose, venlafaxine primarily affects 5-HT reuptake. Its effects on NE and DA occur at higher concentrations (dosages of more than 300 mg/d). It may cause constipation, diaphoresis, dizziness, hypertension, nausea, nervousness, somnolence, and disturbance in sexual function.

When increasing the dosage, gradual titration is important to maximize venlafaxine's therapeutic effect. Minimizing adverse effects may be accomplished by giving an extended-release formulation of venlafaxine (Effexor XR), which provides more stable plasma and CNS drug levels than the rapidly absorbed and rapidly eliminated immediate-release drug formulation.

Venlafaxine is the most studied of all the SNRIs; many studies suggest that it is superior to SSRIs in treating the severely depressed because is exerts "dual action" inhibiting reuptake of serotonin and norepiphrine. However, when compared with other serotonin and norepinephrine reuptake inhibitors (SNRIs), such as duloxetine and milnacipran, venlafaxine seems to be the least well tolerated, causing serotonergic side effects of nausea, sexual dysfunction, withdrawal problems, and dose-dependent hypertension. It is also more cardiotoxic when compared with duloxetine and milnacipran (Stahl, 2005). Overdosage with venlafaxine has occurred, most commonly when it is used in combination with alcohol or other drugs. It can produce tachycardia, potentially life-threatening ECG changes, hypotension, changes in level of consciousness, mydriasis, seizures, rhabdomyolysis, liver necrosis, serotonin syndrome, vertigo, vomiting, and even death. Death from venlafaxine overdosage is more likely than from SSRIs but not as likely as from tricyclics. Patients should receive a small quantity of capsules when they are first started on drug therapy and are still depressed, in order to minimize the risk of intentional overdosage.

Duloxetine

This SNRI has been approved for treatment of major depression, generalized anxiety disorder, diabetic peripheral neuropathic pain and it has recently been approved for treatment of fibromyalgia. Typical dosing is 40–60 mg/d, in divided doses. It is not recommended for patients with severe hepatic or renal impairment. Common side effects include nausea, dry mouth, constipation, somnolence and decreased appetite (US FDA 2009d).

Desvenlafaxine

Desvenlafaxine (Pristiq) is an SNRI approved for treatment of major depression; it is available in 50 mg and 100 mg tablets. Common side effects are nausea, headache, dizziness, dry mouth, constipation, and decreased libido. Caution should be used in patients with hypertension or history of seizure (FDA, 2009e).

Milnacipran

Milnacipran (Savella) is an SNRI that has been approved for the management of fibromyalgia. All SNRIs show usefulness in relieving chronic pain, a condition that frequently co-occurs with depression (US FDA, 2009f).

Treatment Challenges

Symptoms of depression may not improve with initial treatment. When patients don't respond, there is a risk of stopping an antidepressant too soon or using a subclinical dose, thus preventing a sufficient trial of this medication. The results of a study called Sequenced Treatment Alternatives to Relieve Depression (STAR D*) helped develop treatment guidelines to manage patients with depressive symptoms that do not remit after initial therapy with an SSRI. It was found that two-thirds of the participants of this study did not achieve remission with initial treatment with an SSRI. The study examined the usefulness of switching to other antidepressants, using psychotherapy, or augmenting the original SSRI with medications from different classes: buspirone, bupropion, lithium, or triiodothyroxine were used. For patients who did not attain a full clinical response following these steps in treatment, a change to different antidepressant medication was tried: venlafaxine and mirtazepine (SNRIs), tricyclic antidepressants, or an MAO inhibitor.

To *not* experience improvement of symptoms is a very frustrating experience for patients. The lessons learned from the study help providers to use empirically based strategies to find pharmacologic solutions for patients with major depression that do not initially respond to an SSRI (Sussman, 2007). The addition of second generation antipsychotic medication to an SSRI can be used when psychotic features manifest during a major depressive episode. In cases of severe, chronic depression that does not respond well to medication, a biologic therapy, such as electroconvulsive therapy, is considered.

• C TRICYCLIC ANTIDEPRESSANTS

The tricyclics were named for their molecular structure, which features a three-ring nucleus. They are generally categorized as secondary or tertiary amines. Most secondary amines (e.g., amoxapine, desipramine, maprotiline, mirtazapine, nortriptyline, and protriptyline) are better tolerated than tertiary amines (e.g., amitriptyline, clomipramine, doxepin, imipramine, and trimipramine). Although the tricyclics are similar in treating depression, they differ in potency and selectivity. Patients taking tertiary amines generally experience an increased incidence of anticholinergic effects, cardiovascular adverse effects, and impaired memory and cognition. The tertiary amines have a very narrow therapeutic index; even a moderate overdose, such as a dose greater than 1 g, is toxic and can be fatal. These are a few of the reasons secondary amine tricyclics are preferred over the tertiary amine tricyclics.

All tricyclics enhance the activity of norepinephrine and serotonin by blocking neuronal reuptake of these neurotransmitters. Their lack of specificity affects other receptor systems and is associated with anticholinergic, neurologic, and cardiovascular adverse effects.

The prototype tricyclic is nortriptyline (Pamelor), a secondary amine. Although secondary amines do not have as many of the adverse effects as the tertiary amines, they do share the same potential for cardiovascular toxicity. It is

because of this risk that the tricyclics are not considered a first-choice treatment for depression.

Nursing Management of the Patient Receiving P Nortriptyline
Core Drug Knowledge
Pharmacotherapeutics

Nortriptyline is used to relieve the symptoms of depression. It is also used off-label at dosages of 75 to 300 mg/day as adjunctive analgesia for phantom limb pain and chronic pain (such as in migraine, chronic tension headache, diabetic neuropathy, trigeminal neuralgia, cancer pain, painful peripheral neuropathy, postherpetic neuralgia, and arthritic pain) and for cocaine withdrawal, panic disorder, bulimia nervosa, and premenstrual syndrome.

Pharmacokinetics

Nortriptyline is well absorbed from the gastrointestinal tract, achieving peak plasma concentrations in 2 to 4 hours. It undergoes a substantial first-pass effect and is highly bound (more than 90%) to plasma proteins, lipid soluble, and widely distributed in tissues, including the CNS. Wide individual variation occurs in steady-state plasma levels at a given dosage, primarily because of differences in the rate of metabolism or first-pass effect. Effective dosage levels vary greatly and must be individualized. Metabolism of nortriptyline and the other tricyclics occurs in the liver, through the P-450 enzyme system.

Pharmacodynamics

Nortriptyline specifically blocks reuptake of NE into nerve terminals, thereby allowing increased concentration at postsynaptic receptor sites. The chemical structure and pharmacologic activity of nortriptyline resemble those of the phenothiazine antipsychotics (see Chapter 17). Three major pharmacologic actions of nortriptyline are blocking of the amine pump, sedation, and peripheral and central anticholinergic action. Other pharmacologic and clinical effects include inhibition of histamine, sedation, and mild peripheral vasodilator effects.

Contraindications and Precautions

Nortriptyline should be used with extreme caution in patients with cardiovascular disorders because of the possibility of conduction defects, arrhythmias, chronic heart failure, sinus tachycardia, myocardial infarction, stroke, and tachycardia. These patients require cardiac surveillance at all dosage levels of the drug. In high doses, nortriptyline may produce arrhythmias, sinus tachycardia conduction defects, and prolonged conduction time. Elderly patients and patients with a history of cardiac disease are at special risk for developing cardiac abnormalities. Patients with hyperthyroidism or those receiving thyroid medications require close supervision because of the possibility of cardiovascular toxicity, including arrhythmias.

Nortriptyline can slow cardiac conduction and cause arrhythmias. It is possible that a patient will be sensitive to any of the tricyclics once he or she has developed sensitivity to one of them.

Because nortriptyline, like other tricyclics, lowers the seizure threshold, it should be used with caution in patients with a history of seizures or other predisposing factors (e.g., brain damage of varying etiology, alcoholism, concomitant drugs known to lower the seizure threshold). However, seizures have also occurred following administration of tricyclics to patients with no history of seizure disorders. Because of its anticholinergic effects, nortriptyline should be used with caution in patients with a history of urinary retention, glaucoma, or increased intraocular pressure because even an average dose may precipitate a recurrence. Human fetal risk has been demonstrated during clinical trials and postmarketing surveillance, which puts nortriptyline in FDA pregnancy category D. With other tricyclics such as amitriptyline and imipramine, there have been clinical reports of congenital malformations and limb-reduction anomalies.

Adverse Effects

Adverse effects are related to nortriptyline's effects on neurotransmitters. In comparison to drugs in this class that are tertiary amines, nortriptyline and other secondary-amine tricyclics have less effect on the histamine, cholinergic, and alpha-1 adrenergic receptor sites. At usual therapeutic concentrations, they block NE reuptake. Patients report sedation and anticholinergic effects most frequently, although they usually develop tolerance to these effects. Other adverse effects include disturbed concentration and confusion (especially in older adults), headache, tremors, nausea, vomiting, bone marrow depression, urinary retention, sexual function disturbances, skin rash, nasal congestion, and weight gain, which may be significant. In agitated patients, increased anxiety or agitation may occur. Schizophrenic or paranoid patients may exhibit a worsening of their psychoses. Because photosensitivity may occur, patients receiving nortriptyline should avoid sun exposure or use protective measures to prevent skin reactions.

Nortriptyline can cause skin rashes or "drug fever" in susceptible people. These allergic reactions are rarely severe. They are most likely during the first few days of treatment but may also occur later. If a patient develops rash or fever, the drug should be discontinued.

At the upper limit of the therapeutic range, serious and potentially life-threatening cardiac and CNS effects may begin to develop. Overdosage produces symptoms that are primarily an extension of the common adverse reactions. Cardiac irregularities, especially tachycardia and conduction disturbances, are common and create the most serious hazards. Fatal arrhythmias may occur as long as 56 hours after overdose. Other problems include metabolic acidosis, respiratory depression, seizures, and extremely high fever. Box 16.3 describes emergency measures for tricyclic overdose.

DRUG INTERACTIONS

Nortriptyline is associated with multiple drug interactions because it, like other tricyclics, is metabolized through

---

> **Box 16.3 EMERGENCY MEASURES FOR TCA OVERDOSE**
>
> - Provide symptomatic and supportive care.
> - Monitor cardiac changes continually.
> - Administer phenytoin, lidocaine, or propranolol as prescribed for life-threatening cardiac arrhythmias.
> - Avoid giving drugs such as quinidine, procainamide, and disopyramide. These agents depress myocardial conductivity and contractility.
> - Reserve administration of the cholinergic agonist physostigmine for life-threatening, refractory anticholinergic symptoms.

the P-450 liver enzyme system. Drugs with potential for interaction with nortriptyline include sedative-hypnotics, alcohol, antihypertensives, antiarrhythmics, and anticholinergics. Nortriptyline and other highly protein-bound substances, such as aspirin, phenytoin, and phenothiazines, may compete for binding sites. Other drugs, such as methylphenidate, oral contraceptives, and antipsychotics, may interfere with the metabolism of nortriptyline. Nortriptyline may prevent the antihypertensive action of some drugs by their primary and secondary effects at the NE synapses. Administering nortriptyline with an MAOI may result in severe CNS toxicity. Nortriptyline potentiates the sedative effects of alcohol. Table 16.5 summarizes interactions that can occur with nortriptyline.

Assessment of Relevant Core Patient Variables

Health Status

Assess patients for pre-existing cardiovascular disease because these patients are especially sensitive to the potential cardiotoxicity of nortriptyline. Assess patients carefully for a history of seizure activity or organic brain disease because nortriptyline lowers the seizure threshold.

Life Span and Gender

Consider age-related factors associated with nortriptyline therapy. Lower dosages are recommended for adolescents and older adults. The dosage should be increased slowly depending on the clinical response and any evidence of intolerance.

Children are especially susceptible to the cardiotoxic and seizure-inducing effects of high doses of nortriptyline. Because of these safety issues and the uncertain benefit to children and adolescents, other types of antidepressants should be considered before nortriptyline or other tricyclics. Elderly patients may be especially sensitive to the anticholinergic adverse effects of nortriptyline, and this sensitivity can result in confusion, disorientation, delusions, and hallucinations. The combination of these symptoms can continue to worsen to the extent that the patient even becomes delirious. Older adults may be at an increased risk for falls during drug therapy with nortriptyline.

TABLE 16.5	Agents that Interact with ℗ Nortriptyline	
Interactants	**Effect and Significance**	**Nursing Management**
alcohol	Increased sedative effects	Avoid coadministration
anticholinergic agents	Increased anticholinergic effects	Assess patient for increasing tachycardia, dry mouth, blurred vision, constipation, and urinary retention. Coadminister with caution.
barbiturates	Decreased serum concentration of nortriptyline Potential additive CNS depression	Anticipate need for increase in nortriptyline dosage. Institute safety measures. Monitor neurologic status closely.
cimetidine, haloperidol, SSRIs	Increased plasma concentration of nortriptyline	Monitor serum levels as appropriate. Assess for signs of nortriptyline toxicity.
clonidine	Increased risk for hypertension and hypertensive crisis Increased anticoagulant effects	Monitor blood pressure closely. Avoid coadministration.
dicumarol		Assess for signs and symptoms of bleeding. Anticipate need for decreased dosage of dicumarol. Avoid coadministration.
guanethidine	Antagonism of guanethidine action	Monitor blood pressure closely.
disulfiram	Increased risk for organic brain syndrome Increased effect of nortriptyline	Avoid coadministration.
levodopa	Delayed levodopa absorption and decreased bioavailability	Assess for therapeutic effects of both drugs.
MAOIs	Hyperpyrexia, sweating, confusion, seizures, tachycardia, tachypnea, hypotension, coma, DIC, and death	Avoid coadministration. Discontinue MAOIs 7–10 days before starting nortriptyline.
oral contraceptives, phenothiazines	Inhibition of hepatic enzyme system metabolism of nortriptyline leading to increased plasma levels	Monitor for signs and symptoms of nortriptyline toxicity.

Assess women of childbearing age for pregnancy or intention to become pregnant, Neonatal toxicity in the forms of anticholinergic effects: urinary retention and bowel obstruction can develop with use of tricyclic antidepressants. Of all the tricyclic antidepressants, Desipramine is the preferred medication because of it relatively lower anticholingergic effects. Therefore, the drug should be used only when potential benefits to the mother outweigh potential hazards to the fetus. Also, ask if female patients are breast-feeding. Tricyclic antidepressants, with the exception of Doxepin, do not accumulate in breast-fed babies. Amitriptyline and imipramine appear to be the most appropriate drugs when needed during breast feeding (Menon, 2008).

Lifestyle, Diet, and Habits

Adverse effects of nortriptyline can be very similar to the symptoms of depression. For this reason, it is important to evaluate the patient's symptoms within the context of his or her lifestyle before starting nortriptyline therapy.

Ask the patient whether he or she performs activities that require mental alertness, manual dexterity, or motor coordination. Nortriptyline may impair concentration and coordination; hence, the patient receiving nortriptyline should perform such activities with caution until actual drug effects on the individual patient are known.

Photosensitivity may also develop as a result of nortriptyline therapy. Patients whose lifestyles expose them to the outdoors need to protect themselves from overexposure to sunlight.

Culture and Inherited Traits

Keep in mind inherited traits relevant to therapy with nortriptyline. Very little published information exists concerning differences in antidepressant pharmacology among African Americans, Hispanic Americans, and white Americans of European descent (Wood & Zhou, 1991); however, some studies have suggested that ethnicity influences the pharmacokinetics, pharmacotherapeutics, and pharmacodynamics of **psychotropic** drugs (agents that affect the mind, emotions, or behavior). For example, results of one study showed that plasma nortriptyline levels were 50% higher in African American patients than in white Americans. Another reported that Hispanic American patients have greater sensitivity than others to the anticholinergic effects of tricyclics and therefore require a lower dosage. Collected survey data from multiple Asian countries indicated that imipramine and amitriptyline dosages were much lower than those customary in the United States, suggesting that Asians achieve significantly higher plasma concentrations of tricyclics and have lower clearance rates than whites. Although these studies have been criticized for improper control of independent variables, such as dosage for body weight or smoking and even diet or alcohol consumption, it is prudent to consider a patient's ethnic background, at least in part, until more conclusive studies prove otherwise.

As nortriptyline is metabolized by the P-450 system, it is helpful to identify inherited differences in these isoenzymes which can alter drug metabolism. Genotypes for two P-450 isoenzyme genes, P-450 2D6 and P-450 2C19, can be identified using the AmpliChip CYP450 laboratory test (de Leon, Susce, & Murray-Carmichael, 2006). This test classifies patients into two phenotypes for P-450 2C19 (extensive metabolizers and poor metabolizers). Three to four percent of Caucasians and African American are poor metabolizers of P-450 2C19, in comparison with 14% to 21% of Asians. Using the AmpliChip test, it is possible to identify four phenotypes of P-450 2D6: ultrarapid metabolizers, extensive metabolizers, intermediate metabolizers, and poor metabolizers. Ultrametabolizers have unusually high activity, extensive metabolizers are considered "normal," intermediate metabolizers have low activity of P-450 2D6, and poor metabolizers have no activity. For the isoenzyme P-450 2D6, 7% of Caucasians and 1% to 3% of other ethnic group are poor metabolizers. Downward adjustment in the dose of nortriptyline or other tricyclics is most likely needed by those who are poor metabolizers for each of these isoenzymes.

Nursing Diagnoses and Outcomes

Several nursing diagnoses may apply to the depressed patient receiving nortriptyline therapy. Examples include:

• Constipation or Diarrhea related to medication use
Desired outcome: The patient will establish normal bowel habits.
Disturbed Sleep Pattern related to medication-induced somnolence or insomnia
Desired outcome: The patient will report a satisfactory balance of rest and activity.

In addition to these, selected nursing diagnoses for treatment with nortriptyline include the following:

• Risk for Poisoning related to TCA toxicity
Desired outcome: The patient will identify factors that increase the risk for and verbalize practices to prevent poisoning.

• Risk for Injury related to adverse effects (e.g., blurred vision, drowsiness, and hypotension) secondary to nortriptyline use
Desired outcome: The patient will identify factors that increase the risk for and relate intent to practice safety measures to prevent injury.
• Imbalanced Nutrition: More than Body Requirements, related to adverse effects of nortriptyline
Desired outcome: The patient will verbalize reasons for a risk for weight gain, identify normal nutritional needs, and discuss methods to control weight.
• Disturbed Sensory Perception related to chemical alterations secondary to nortriptyline therapy
Desired outcome: The patient will experience normal sensory perception.

Planning and Intervention
Maximizing Therapeutic Effects
Use therapeutic drug monitoring to monitor effective plasma drug levels to achieve the greatest likelihood of antidepressant response and the smallest risk of adverse effects. Optimal serum concentrations for nortriptyline are 50 to 150 ng/mL. For maintenance therapy, a single daily dose of nortriptyline may be used. A single daily dose at bedtime, if convenient, minimizes the daytime adverse effect of sedation. The sedative effect at bedtime may be beneficial in patients with concomitant sleep disorders.

Following remission, the patient may require maintenance medication for a longer time at the lowest dose that maintains remission. Maintenance therapy should continue for at least 3 months to decrease the possibility of relapse.

Minimizing Adverse Effects
Although the half-life of nortriptyline is long enough to permit single daily dosing, adverse reactions may require divided dosing schedules. Because older adults have an increased risk of adverse effects, they should receive initial doses equivalent to one half to one third of the dose administered to younger adults. Ultimately, elderly patients may benefit by receiving nortriptyline in split doses, because they may be unable to tolerate single daily doses. Regular ECG monitoring of cardiac rhythm is essential for any person taking nortriptyline. Therapy may also induce neutropenia; watch for clinical indicators such as fever or sore throat, which may signal serious neutrophil depression; therapy should be discontinued if such evidence of pathologic neutropenia occurs. In addition to serum levels of the drug, periodically monitor blood studies, including a complete blood count with differential, serum glucose level, and renal and hepatic function. Monitoring helps detect adverse effects so that intervention can occur before interrupted drug therapy or nonadherence compromises the therapeutic effect. Closely monitor patients with glaucoma during drug therapy, because nortriptyline may precipitate an acute episode of angle-closure glaucoma.

As with all antidepressant therapy, continue assessing the patient for low mood and suicidal thoughts. When a patient is most depressed, he or she may have thoughts of suicide but at the same time may not have enough energy or concentration to plan and follow through on these thoughts. However, the risk of suicide increases if the suicidal thoughts remain while the patient's concentration and energy improve to the point at which he or she can act on the suicidal thoughts. This fact is particularly important with the patient taking tricyclics because the very drug taken to treat the depression can also be taken in a lethal dose to commit suicide. Ensure patient safety by closely monitoring the number of pills that are accessible to him or her.

Providing Patient and Family Education

- Teach patients and families that the therapeutic response will not be immediate. Several weeks may pass before any measurable clinical effect is noted. The symptoms of depression may come and go during the earliest stages of treatment. If this possibility is not discussed, patients may become even more hopeless, thinking that they will never be symptom-free. Also, discuss the ongoing risk of suicide with patients and families.
- It is also important to teach patients about the need to continue with nortriptyline therapy even after initial relief of depressive symptoms. Inform them that stopping the medication at this time will most likely result in a relapse of the depressive symptoms.
- Stress the importance of taking the drug exactly as prescribed and of not stopping the drug abruptly or without consulting with the health care provider. Abrupt discontinuation may cause nausea, headache, and malaise.
- Help patients stay motivated to continue treatment. To promote adherence to the therapeutic regimen, educate patients and families about the medication effects—both therapeutic and adverse. Advise patients about adverse effects that, if unexplained, may contribute to nonadherence. These effects include sweating, weight gain, and sexual dysfunction.
- Warn patients of the possibility of photosensitivity reactions. Advise them to avoid prolonged exposure to sunlight or bright artificial light, to apply sunscreen before exposure, and to wear protective clothing.
- Emphasize the importance of keeping the drug safely stored and away from curious children. Children are very susceptible to nortriptyline-induced cardiotoxicity.
- Caution patients to avoid operating machinery, driving a vehicle, or engaging in activities that require focus and concentration until they are aware of their own individual response to the medication. Most antidepressants cause some degree of sedation and may impair mental alertness and physical coordination. Because certain drug combinations produce an additive CNS depressant effect, patients should not use antidepressants concurrently with alcohol or sleep-inducing drugs such as sedative-hypnotics.
- Advise patients to wear or carry medical identification, such as a Medic Alert tag, regarding antidepressant therapy because nortriptyline can interact with many other drugs.

Ongoing Assessment and Evaluation

Continually assess depressed patients for suicidal thoughts during nortriptyline therapy. As with all antidepressant therapy, the depressed patient with suicidal thoughts is at greatest risk for self-harm once he or she has become sufficiently energized to act on the thoughts. Because of the potential for drug-related toxicity to the heart, all patients, particularly those receiving higher than usual dosages of nortriptyline or other tricyclics, should have periodic ECG examinations regardless of normal cardiac functioning before treatment. Patients with pre-existing cardiovascular disease should be closely monitored, with ECG tracings performed routinely.

Patients taking multidrug therapies should be monitored for other effects as well because other drugs, such as antihypertensives, alcohol, and therapeutic hormones, may cause depression.

Obtain baseline and periodic laboratory blood tests to monitor leukocyte counts, differential blood cell counts, and liver function studies. Also, monitor drug serum levels to ensure that therapeutic levels are maintained. Nortriptyline therapy is considered effective when depression is relieved and adverse effects either do not occur or are minimal.

MEMORY CHIP

P Nortriptyline

- Tricyclic secondary amine antidepressant used to treat symptoms of depression
- Major contraindication: cautious use in patients with pre-existing cardiovascular disease
- Most common adverse effects: drowsiness, dry mouth, constipation, hypotension
- Most serious adverse effect: arrhythmias caused by changes in atrioventricular conduction
- **Life span alert: not recommended for children; decrease or divide the dosage for elderly patients, see black box warning**
- Maximizing therapeutic effects: Maintain a therapeutic serum plasma level; continue therapy at least 3 months to prevent relapse.
- Minimizing adverse effects: Give entire dose at bedtime to decrease drowsiness.
- Most important patient education: Symptom relief is not immediate and may take several weeks; when symptoms are relieved, medication must be continued.
- **Black box warning: may increase the risk of suicidal thoughts or behaviors in children, adolescents, and young adults**

BOX 16.4 FOCUS ON RESEARCH

Recovery from Major Depression in the Older Adult.

Dew, M., Whyte, E., Lenze, E., Houck, P., Mulsant, B., Polluck B., Stack, J., Bensasi S., Reynolds, C., (2007). Recovery from major depression in older adults receiving augmentation of antidepressant pharmacotherapy. *American Psychiatric Association.* 164(6):892–899.

This study used recommendations from the STAR D study (Rush, 2006) to examine if older adults could attain the same benefit of augmenting SSRI type antidepressant medication with an addition of another type of antidepressant if there was a poor initial clinical response. With this study, 195 older adults were treated for major depression disorder using paroxetine and psychotherapy. Subjects in the study were regularly evaluated, out of the 195 participants 105 were deemed to have an inadequate response to paroxetine and psychotherapy or had experienced a relapse after an initial promising response to these therapies. These 105 participants were offered a next step at treatment, some declined and fell out of the study and some could not continue with the study because of co-morbid illnesses. This left 69 participants to receive augmentation with either sustained released bupropion, notriptyline or lithium carbonate added to the participant's regime of paroxetine or psychotherapy.

The findings of this study were as follows:

- About 50% of these 69 participants experienced improvement in symptoms using the augmentation protocol outlined in the study.
- Poor sleep patterns at the beginning of the study was found to be the most significant variable associated with the participants who required augmentation.
- The recovery of the participants who did not respond to initial treatment with paroxetine and psychotherapy was much slower than the individuals who initially showed clinical remission of symptoms but then experienced a relapse.
- The recovery of participants with more medical complications and anxiety was also slower than other participants.

- The participants who required augmentation had a higher frequency of side effects with the addition of another antidepressant medication.

The authors of the study concluded that older adults can benefit from augmentation. They did concede however, that switching to a different antidepressant medication if the first one did not work (given at appropriate dosages and duration), may be just as effective a strategy for elderly patients; it is a simpler medication regime, it has less possibility of drug-drug interactions and would have lower economic costs.

Nursing implications

Although enormous gains have been made in understanding and treating major depressive disorder, this mental illness is typically very resistant to treatment. Confounding the diagnosis and treatment of major depression in the older adult are the physiologic complications of aging and co-morbid medical illnesses. Untreated depression results in poor quality of life, a higher incidence of co-morbid medical problems and ultimately higher rates of mortality. The conclusions of this study supported the practice of using an evidenced based protocol outlined by the STAR D* Study with elderly patients who do not respond to initial antidepressant and psychotherapy. The practice of adding additional medication however, is not without inherent risks to the elderly patient. Since poor sleep was a significant variable that correlated with the participant's lack of response to initial therapy, this should be a symptom that nurses listen to in all patients rather than dismissing it's significance. Additionally, a little prevention could go a very long way: patients with chronic medical illnesses are at risk for developing major depression, these patients should have regular screening before significant symptoms of major depression develop because of the high rates of resistance to treatment. Given our numbers in practice and exposure to the elderly in many practice settings, registered nurses are well poised at identifying patients who are at risk for depression and should have a watchful eye for potential complications in treatment.

C MONOAMINE OXIDASE INHIBITORS

The monoamine oxidase (MAO) enzyme system is widely distributed throughout the body. This system is responsible for metabolizing amines such as dopamine, epinephrine, norepinephrine, and serotonin. Drugs described as MAOIs inhibit MAO enzymes, thereby increasing the concentration of those amines.

There are two subtypes of MAO. MAO A, found primarily in the gastrointestinal tract, liver, and peripheral adrenergic nerves, predominantly metabolizes norepinephrine, serotonin, and tyramine. MAO B, found in the brain, primarily metabolizes dopamine. Although the precise antidepressant mechanism of MAOIs is unclear, it is thought that the increases in norepinephrine and serotonin or changes in other amine concentrations in the CNS are responsible. MAOIs were initially used to manage tuberculosis. It was observed that patients taking these drugs often experienced an elevation in their mood and hypotension. Although they are effective as antidepressants and antihypertensives, their use is limited by their potential to cause intense adverse effects and potentially fatal interactions, such as hypertensive crisis. Potentially fatal pharmacodynamic drug–drug interactions can occur with MAOIs when they are combined with a variety of drugs that are norepinephrine or serotonin agonists or with foods rich in tyramine, such as air-dried, aged, and fermented meats, sausages, and salamis, aged cheeses, tap beers, and soy sauce. Because MAOIs are irreversible inhibitors of monoamine oxidase, up to 2 weeks may be required for normal amine metabolism to be restored once the drug is discontinued.

In general, nonselective MAOIs are indicated for patients who are unresponsive to other antidepressant pharmacotherapy. They are rarely first-choice drugs. The prototype MAOI is phenelzine (Nardil).

Nursing Management of the Patient Receiving P Phenelzine

Core Drug Knowledge

Pharmacotherapeutics

Phenelzine is used mainly to treat depression that is unresponsive to other drug therapy or treatments. Patients may have mixed anxiety and depression with phobic or hypochondriacal features. In some cases, phenelzine is used to treat bulimia, cocaine addiction, and panic disorder associated with agoraphobia.

Pharmacokinetics

Phenelzine appears to be well absorbed following oral administration, and peak levels of phenelzine are reached in 2 to 4 hours. However, maximum inhibition of phenelzine does not occur for 5 to 10 days. Antidepressant action can take from 7 days to 8 weeks. Phenelzine is excreted in the urine, mostly as metabolites.

Half-life is fairly short and unrelated to the length of enzyme inhibition, which is prolonged: The clinical effects of phenelzine may continue for up to 2 weeks after therapy is discontinued.

Pharmacodynamics

Phenelzine increases the concentrations of DA, NE, and serotonin within the neuronal synapse because it inhibits the enzyme monoamine oxidase. Phenelzine, a hydrazine derivative, irreversibly inhibits both MAO A and MAO B.

Contraindications and Precautions

Poor liver function is a contraindication for using phenelzine because hydrazine compounds damage the functional tissues of the liver. Phenelzine is also contraindicated in patients with chronic heart failure. Cautious use is advised in patients with ischemic heart disease or a history of stroke or myocardial infarction because phenelzine may produce cardiovascular depressing effects, such as orthostatic hypotension, bradycardia, and decreased contractility of the heart muscle.

Adverse Effects

Toxic drug levels, which may damage the liver, can occur and appear to be unrelated to phenelzine dosage or treatment duration. Other adverse effects are anticholinergic, including blurred vision, constipation, and dry mouth. These effects are more pronounced at dosages above 45 mg/d. CNS-related adverse effects include akathisia, ataxia, dizziness, drowsiness, headache, insomnia, and nystagmus. Adverse effects related to other systems include agranulocytosis, anemia, leukopenia, thrombocytopenia, sexual function disturbances, and urinary retention.

The most serious adverse reactions involve changes in blood pressure and hypertensive crisis. Use of these drugs in elderly or debilitated patients or in patients with hypertension, cardiovascular problems, or cerebrovascular disease is inadvisable.

Drug Interactions

Pseudoephedrine and phenylpropanolamine, which are examples of mixed-acting sympathomimetics, are common ingredients in over-the-counter (OTC) decongestants, appetite suppressants, and weight-loss products. They release NE from adrenergic nerve endings. The indirect-acting sympathomimetics also trigger NE release. Acute, severe, and potentially fatal hypertensive crises are possible when combining phenelzine with drugs from either of these classes, tyramine, or tryptophan. Table 16.6 lists drugs that can interact with phenelzine.

These drug–drug or drug–food interactions occur because phenelzine and the other agents act in peripheral adrenergic nerve endings to increase the buildup of NE, although they prevent the release of NE in response to normal nerve activity. However, when phenelzine is combined with the mixed-acting and indirect-acting sympathomimetics, NE release is not inhibited. The result is an intense adrenergic response because of the extra supply of NE. Ingesting a tyramine-containing food or a sympathomimetic drug may precipitate a hypertensive crisis. Normally, MAO enzymes in the liver metabolize these substances rapidly. However, when MAO enzymes are inhibited, tyramine metabolism decreases and triggers the release of accumulated NE, triggering a hypertensive episode. The earliest symptom may be a severe headache. The necessity of avoiding these substances to prevent a life-threatening hypertensive crisis is the major limitation of MAOIs. Table 16.7 lists the tyramine-rich foods that should be avoided by patients taking MAOIs.

Assessment of Relevant Core Patient Variables

Health Status

Perform a baseline cardiovascular assessment and complete blood count and liver function tests for the patient taking phenelzine. Assess the patient's orientation, mood, and affect because phenelzine may cause memory and emotional changes, irritability, and nervousness.

Life Span and Gender

Consider the patient's age and its relation to phenelzine therapy. Phenelzine is not recommended for patients younger than 16 years. Because patients older than 60 years may be more prone to adverse drug effects, dosages (less than 60 mg/d) should be increased gradually and adjusted accordingly.

Ask women of childbearing age if they are pregnant, intend to become pregnant, or are breast-feeding. Phenelzine is in FDA pregnancy category C. It crosses the placenta and enters breast milk.

Lifestyle, Diet, and Habits

Assess the patient's lifestyle to determine whether he or she performs activities requiring alertness, physical coordination, or manual dexterity. Because of possible associated adverse effects such as ataxia, drowsiness, and blurred vision, patients need to exercise caution when driving or operating machinery. Also, evaluate the patient's nutritional status. Pyridoxine deficiency, frequently observed as numbness and swelling, is associated with phenelzine use. For this reason, the patient may need a pyridoxine (vitamin B_6) supplement. Ask the patient about his or her participation in outdoor activity, because phenelzine may cause photosensitivity. The patient should wear sunscreen and protective clothing in prolonged outdoor exposure, such as recreational or occupational pursuits.

TABLE 16.6   Agents That Interact with P Phenelzine

Interactants	Effect and Significance	Nursing Management
anesthetics	Adverse cardiovascular effects from sympathetic stimulation	Monitor heart rate, rhythm, and blood pressure for adverse effect from sympathetic stimulation.
antihypertensives (e.g., guanethidine, methyldopa)	Loss of antihypertensive effects	Monitor blood pressure for degree of control.
beta-adrenergic blockers	Bradycardia possible during concurrent use of MAOIs and beta-adrenergic blockers	Monitor heart rate, rhythm, and cardiac output for adverse effect from bradycardia.
dextromethorphan	Hyperpyrexia, hypotension, and death associated with this combination*	Caution patients taking MAOIs to avoid OTC cold and cough preparations.
levodopa	Hypertensive reactions with combinations of levodopa and MAOIs	Avoid concurrent administration. Monitor cardiovascular status for adverse effect.
L-tryptophan	Coadministration resulting in hyperreflexia, confusion, disorientation, amnesia, ataxia, and Babinski signs	Caution the patient taking MAOIs to avoid food supplements, herbal/homeopathic, or home remedies without approval from the health care provider.
meperidine	Coadministration may result in agitation, seizures, fever, apnea, and death with possible adverse reactions weeks after MAOI withdrawal	Avoid concomitant administration of MAOIs and meperidine. For analgesia, administer other narcotic analgesics with caution.
SSRI, TCA, or venlafaxine antidepressants	Potential serious (occasionally fatal) reactions, including hyperthermia, rigidity, autonomic instability with labile blood pressure, myoclonus, and extreme agitation	Monitor neurologic and cardiovascular status for adverse effect.
sulfonamide compounds	Coadministration may cause either sulfonamide or MAOI toxicity	Avoid concurrent administration.
sulfonylurea anti-diabetic agents	Possible potentiation of hypoglycemic response and delayed recovery from hypoglycemia	Monitor patients with diabetes for level of control and incidence of hypoglycemic episodes.
sumatriptan	Coadministration may cause sumatriptan toxicity	Avoid concurrent administration.
sympathomimetics (mixed acting or indirect acting, including anorexiants)	MAOI potentiation of sympathomimetic substances may cause severe headache, hypertension, hyperpyrexia possibly resulting in hypertensive crisis	Avoid concurrent administration.†
thiazide diuretics	Exaggerated hypotensive effects may result from concurrent use	Avoid concurrent administration. Monitor cardiovascular status and blood pressure for degree of control.

*Interaction inconclusive due to lack of adequate patient data.
†Direct-acting agents appear to interact minimally (if at all).

Assess the patient for willingness to adhere to the dietary restrictions required with phenelzine therapy. Assess for use of herbal preparations such as St. John's wort, L-tryptophan, and ginseng because they can interact with phenelzine.

Environment

Consider the environment in which phenelzine will be administered. The drug should be kept in a tightly closed container away from light and heat.

Culture and Inherited Traits

Consider the patient's ethnic background when beginning drug therapy with phenelzine. Acetylation inactivates phenelzine and its metabolites. About one half of Americans and Europeans (and more in Asia) are slow acetylators of hydrazine-type drugs, including phenelzine. This fact may contribute to the exaggerated effects observed in some patients who receive standard doses of phenelzine.

TABLE 16.7	Tyramine Dietary Modifications and MAOIs	
Type of Food or Drink	Tyramine-rich Foods and Drinks to Avoid	Acceptable Foods and Drinks Containing No or Little Tyramine
Meat, Poultry, Fish	Air-dried, aged and fermented meats, sausages, and salamis Pickled herring Any spoiled or improperly stored meat, poultry, and fish (i.e., foods that have a change in color or odor or have become moldy)	Fresh meat, poultry, and fish. Fresh processed meats (lunch meats, hot dogs, breakfast sausage, and cooked sliced ham)
Vegetables	Broad bean pods (fava beans)	All other vegetables
Dairy Products	Aged cheeses (e.g., cheddar, Swiss, blue, camembert, and cheese spreads)	Other cheeses, including processed cheeses, mozzarella, ricotta, and cottage Yogurt
Alcoholic Beverages	All tap beers Other beers that have not been pasteurized	Bottled and canned beer All wines (All alcohol should be in moderation)
Other	Concentrated yeast extract (e.g., Marmite) Sauerkraut Most soybean products (including soy sauce and tofu) Over-the-counter supplements containing tyramine	Brewer's yeast, baker's yeast Soy milk Pizzas from commercial chain restaurants prepared with cheeses low in tyramine

Based on the Food and Drug Administration drug label for selegiline transdermal (Emsam). http://www.fda.gov/cder/foi/label/2006/ 021708s000_021336s000lbl.pdf

Nursing Diagnoses and Outcomes

- Risk for Injury related to drug–nutrient, drug–drug, or drug–environment interactions or hypertensive crisis secondary to phenelzine antidepressant therapy
  Desired outcome: The patient will remain safe and injury-free during drug therapy.
- Ineffective Therapeutic Regimen Management related to MAOI-required dietary restrictions
  Desired outcome: The patient will acknowledge an understanding of the need to follow a low-tyramine diet and demonstrate appropriate dietary choices.
- Imbalanced Nutrition: More than Body Requirements, related to adverse effect of phenelzine
  Desired outcome: The patient will understand and acknowledge the risk for weight gain, identify normal nutritional needs, and discuss methods to control weight.

Planning and Intervention

Maximizing Therapeutic Effects

Before phenelzine therapy is initiated, platelet MAO enzyme activity (mostly B subtype) is usually measured. After therapy is under way, an inhibition of more than 85% is associated with therapeutic response. However, platelet enzyme inhibition exceeding 95% increases the risk of serious drug and food interactions.

Minimizing Adverse Effects

The primary difficulties with phenelzine are the numerous dietary and medication restrictions that the patient must obey to avoid drug–food and drug–drug interactions. Taking phenelzine with foods high in tyramine or with certain drugs (e.g., ephedrine, dextromethorphan, cocaine, decongestants, appetite suppressants) increases the potential for a hypertensive crisis. The symptoms of hypertensive crisis include severe occipital headache, stiff neck, nausea, vomiting, diaphoresis, and extremely elevated systolic and diastolic blood pressure.

Advise the patient to avoid herbal preparations such as St. John's wort, L-tryptophan, and ginseng because they can interact with MAOIs. Encourage the patient to consult with the prescriber of the medication before using any OTC products. Alcohol (especially beer, ale, sherry, and Chianti wine), stimulants, and illicit drugs should never be used because they increase the likelihood of adverse effects or hypertensive crisis. Dosages exceeding 30 mg/d may result in postural hypotension, leading to syncope. If dosage increases are necessary, they should be made gradually. Other measures to minimize adverse effects include maintaining a tyramine-restricted diet during and for at least 2 weeks after phenelzine therapy and giving the drug with food or milk if gastrointestinal discomfort is problematic. If the patient has been on fluoxetine therapy, at least 6 weeks should elapse before phenelzine therapy begins.

Providing Patient and Family Education

- Warn all patients taking phenelzine against eating foods with high tyramine content or consuming alcohol during and for 2 weeks following phenelzine treatment. Ensure that the patient taking phenelzine understands and follows the special required dietary guidelines (see Table 16.7 for a list of foods to avoid). Any aged food has the potential to produce a hypertensive crisis in patients taking phenelzine.

- Caution patients against self-medication with certain proprietary agents such as cold, hay fever, or weight-reduction preparations containing sympathomimetic amines while undergoing phenelzine therapy.
- Stress the importance of not discontinuing the phenelzine, adjusting the dosage, or ingesting any other medication, even OTC preparations, except on the advice of the prescriber. Alert patients that the medication may cause drowsiness or blurred vision and warn them to exercise caution when driving or performing other tasks that require alertness, coordination, or physical dexterity until effects of the drug are known.
- Alert patients to the possibility of dizziness, weakness, or fainting when arising from a sitting position.
- Emphasize to patients and families that antidepressant effects may be delayed a few weeks. Caution them to notify the health care provider if the patient develops severe headache, palpitations, tachycardia, a sense of constriction in the throat or chest, sweating, dizziness, neck stiffness, nausea, vomiting, or other unusual symptoms.

Ongoing Assessment and Evaluation

Observation of the patient is necessary to identify the therapeutic effects of phenelzine. These effects may occur within 7 days after therapy begins, although in some patients, a therapeutic response may not occur for up to 6 to 8 weeks. Effectiveness of phenelzine is demonstrated by improved mood and increased

MEMORY CHIP

 Phenelzine

- Monoamine oxidase inhibitor used to treat depression unresponsive to other treatments or drug therapy
- Major contraindications: chronic heart failure, impaired liver or kidney function
- Most common adverse effects: restlessness, orthostatic hypotension, blurred vision
- Most serious adverse effect: hypertensive crisis
- **Life span alert: Avoid giving to children 16 and younger; reduce dosage for older adults, see black box warning**
- Maximizing therapeutic effects: Platelet monoamine oxidase inhibition activity should be monitored to achieve a goal between 85% and 95%.
- Minimizing adverse effects: Avoid tyramine-rich foods and over-the-counter cold remedies with dextromethorphan.
- Most important patient education: Adhere strictly to a tyramine-free diet (MAOI diet) during and 2 weeks after medication is stopped; antidepressant effect may take several weeks; take only as prescribed and do not stop abruptly.
- **Black box warning: may increase the risk of suicidal thoughts or behaviors in children, adolescents, and young adults**

social activity in depressed patients. The patient's appetite, energy, and sleep pattern will improve as well.

During therapy, blood pressure should be monitored frequently to detect any abnormal response. Periodic liver function tests, such as aspartate transaminase, alanine transaminase, and bilirubin, should be performed. Phenelzine should be discontinued at the first sign of liver failure. Therapy should be discontinued immediately if the patient reports palpitations or frequent headaches, because these signs may signal a hypertensive crisis. Drug therapy with phenelzine is considered effective if depression is alleviated and serious adverse effects are avoided.

Drugs Closely Related to P Phenelzine
Isocarboxazid and Tranylcypromine

Isocarboxazid (Marplan) and tranylcypromine (Parnate) are also MAOIs and are very similar to phenelzine. The differences of these drugs from the prototype are in two areas; neither is indicated for treating bulimia nervosa; and they have three serious, although rare, adverse effects not found with phenelzine: agranulocytosis, anemia, and thrombocytopenia.

Selegiline Transdermal

Selegiline transdermal (Emsam) is a new treatment for depression. It is effective in treating major depression as well as preventing relapses of depression. Like phenelzine, it is an irreversible MAO inhibitor, inhibiting both MAO A and MAO B, primarily MAO B. MAO A enzymes are distributed into the brain, gut, liver, placenta, and skin. MAO B enzymes are distributed in the brain, platelets, and lymphocytes. Oral selegiline is not approved as an antidepressant but is used in the treatment of Parkinson disease (see Chapter 17). Transdermal dosing of selegiline prevents the first-pass effect and thus produces higher systemic levels of the drug and fewer metabolites than the oral formulation. Selegiline transdermal systems are available in three sizes: 20 mg/20 cm^2, 30 mg/30 cm^2, and 40 mg/40 cm^2, which deliver 6, 9, or 12 mg, respectively, of selegiline over 24 hours.

Although selegiline remains active after 24 hours of wearing the transdermal patch, the absorption rate may become variable, so the patch should be changed daily. Increased drug absorption via the skin is possible based on individual factors; some patients may absorb up to one third more drug than is listed on the label. Absorption may potentially be increased with vasodilation, so patients should be instructed to avoid exposing the patch site to external sources of direct heat (such as a heating pad, electric blanket, heat lamp, saunas, hot tubs, heated water beds, or prolonged direct sunlight).

Like the prototype phenelzine, selegiline transdermal may cause serious drug interactions when used with other drugs that affect monoamine activity. Induction of serotonin syndrome may occur if the following drugs are used concomitantly with selegiline transdermal: SSRIs, dual serotonin and norepinephrine reuptake inhibitors, tricyclics, oral selegiline, other MAOIs, mirtazapine, bupropion, some analgesics (meperidine, tramadol, methadone, propoxyphene, pentazocine), the antitussive dextromethorphan, cyclobenzaprine, buspirone, or the herbal supplement St. John's wort. Concomitant use with any of the following agents may cause hypertensive crisis: sympathomimetic amines (cold products, weight-loss preparations containing vasoconstrictors such as pseudoephedrine, phenylephrine, phenylpropanolamine, and ephedrine), general anesthetics, cocaine, and local anesthetics containing vasoconstrictors, or any herbal or dietary product containing tyramines. If a patient has been taking any of these drugs before they are to start therapy with selegiline transdermal, a wash-out period equal to 4 to 5 half-lives, approximately 1 week, should be allowed before starting treatment with selegiline transdermal. Fluoxetine, an SSRI with a longer half-life, should be stopped at least 5 weeks before starting selegiline transdermal therapy. If selegiline transdermal therapy is to be stopped, at least 2 weeks should be allowed before beginning treatment with any of the above-mentioned contraindicated drugs, because it creates a nonreversible effect on MAO enzymes; two weeks allows the body to produce new MAO so that there will not be a drug interaction.

A major advantage of selegiline transdermal over phenelzine is that this form of selegiline does not pose the risk of a drug–food interaction from dietary tyramine *when the 6 mg/24-hour dose is administered.* Because the MAO B enzymes do not appear in the gut, blocking them does not cause the typical drug–food interactions that can cause hypertensive crisis. Remember that selegiline transdermal blocks both MAO A and MAO B, but primarily B. There is a theoretical possibility that patients taking higher daily doses of selegiline transdermal can still experience hypertensive crisis if they consume dietary tyramines, so patients receiving these doses should still be advised to avoid dietary sources of tyramine. In clinical trials, no patients developed hypertensive crisis.

Adverse effects from selegiline transdermal include the risk of postural hypotension and skin reactions at the site of patch application. To minimize these effects, instruct patients to change positions gradually after lying down and to apply the patch to clean, dry, intact skin. Older adults are more at risk of orthostatic hypotension. Patches should be applied daily at approximately the same time but using a different location; upper chest or back (below the neck but above the waist), upper thigh, or outer upper arm are all appropriate sites. Only one patch at a time should be worn, and the patches should never be cut. Because active drug remains in the discarded patch, teach patients to fold the patch in half after removal and to dispose of it in a manner in which it is not accessible to children or pets.

C MOOD STABILIZERS

When a person has been diagnosed with bipolar disorder and is experiencing a manic episode, he or she is treated with drugs that are categorized as mood stabilizers. Treatment with these drugs decreases the extreme range of mood experienced by the patient. In addition to mood, a manic episode also increases energy and disorganizes cognition.

Lithium carbonate (Eskalith), usually simply called lithium, is the prototype mood stabilizing or antimanic drug. Other drugs used to treat bipolar disorder and to stabilize mood include carbamazepine, gabapentin, and valproic acid. These drugs may be combined with lithium for a greater therapeutic effect.

Nursing Management of the Patient Receiving P Lithium

Core Drug Knowledge

Pharmacotherapeutics

Lithium is called a mood stabilizer because its primary action is to prevent extreme mood swings. Lithium is also thought to help control symptoms of mania and depression during periods of remission. Some studies have shown that lithium is efficacious in preventing suicide (Noonan, 2007). The therapeutic range for the drug is 0.6 to 1.2 mEq/L. The drug also has several unlabeled uses. It increases the neutrophil count in patients with cancer chemotherapy–induced neutropenia and in patients with acquired immunodeficiency syndrome (AIDS) who receive zidovudine therapy. It also is useful in preventing cluster headache and in treating bulimia, alcoholism, and postpartum-affective and corticosteroid-induced psychoses. Lithium has also been used as an adjunctive medication when there is limited response to antidepressant medication.

Pharmacokinetics

The intestinal tract provides nearly complete absorption of lithium within 6 hours. Food does not substantially slow absorption. Peak plasma levels occur in 0.5 to 3 hours, and plasma half-life is about 20 hours. Onset of action is slow (5 to 7 days, with full therapeutic effects established in 10 to 21 days). Lithium is not protein bound or biotransformed into metabolites. Excretion occurs almost entirely in the urine (95%) and varies with pregnancy, age, and renal status. Lithium and sodium compete for resorption in the proximal renal tubule, where 80% of lithium is reabsorbed. Many factors, such as sodium imbalance, dehydration, or diuretic use, can affect lithium clearance because of the competition between lithium and sodium for resorption. Dose-related adverse effects are not usually serious if serum levels are maintained below 1.5 mEq/L.

Distribution approximates total body water and is complete within 6 to 10 hours. Higher concentrations occur in the bones, thyroid gland, and portions of the brain than in the serum. Although distribution across the blood–brain barrier is slow, the cerebrospinal fluid level is 40% of the plasma concentration. Elimination half-life is 24 hours, with a range between 10 and 50 hours. A steady state is reached after 5 to 7 days without dose changes.

Pharmacodynamics

Lithium competes with calcium, magnesium, potassium, and sodium in body tissues and at binding sites. It alters sodium transport in nerve and muscle cells. It also affects the synthesis, storage, release, and reuptake of central monoamine neurotransmitters, including acetylcholine, DA, gamma-aminobutyric acid, NE, and 5-HT. Although the contributions of these effects are uncertain, its antimanic effects are thought to result from increases in NE reuptake and increased serotonin receptor sensitivity. Lithium has a very narrow therapeutic index

Contraindications and Precautions

Lithium is contraindicated in patients with severe cardiovascular or renal disease and in patients who are pregnant (category D) or breast-feeding.

Adverse Effects

The adverse effects of lithium can be classified as acute, chronic, and toxic. Acute effects include increased thirst, nausea, increased urination, and a fine hand tremor. Chronic adverse effects include increased urination, weight gain, hair loss, acne, and cognitive impairment. Low thyroid function and lack of kidney response to antidiuretic hormones may also occur in patients receiving long-term lithium therapy. However, discontinuing lithium treatment reverses these effects. Long-term lithium therapy (exceeding 10 years) commonly impairs the ability of the kidneys to concentrate urine, although this effect is not associated with a reduced glomerular filtration rate or with renal insufficiency. Lithium toxicity is dose related; the higher the circulating blood level of lithium, the more likely the patient will experience adverse effects and toxicity.

The most serious adverse effects associated with lithium occur when serum concentrations exceed 2 mEq/L, although some patients may experience toxicity even if their serum drug measurements are considered to be in the normal range (remember that the therapeutic range for the drug is 0.6 to 1.2 mEq/L).

Early symptoms include a coarse hand tremor, severe gastrointestinal upset (vomiting and diarrhea), blurred vision, drowsiness, mental dullness, slurred speech, confusion, muscle twitching, and a dizzy or spinning sensation. Serious, later symptoms include seizures, coma, arrhythmias, and permanent neurologic impairment. A serious lithium overdose can be life threatening.

Drug Interactions

Lithium interacts substantially with other drugs that deplete sodium. Examples of such drugs include thiazide diuretics and angiotensin-converting enzyme inhibitors. This interaction may lead to toxicity secondary to decreased renal elimination of lithium. Table 16.8 lists agents that can interact with lithium.

Assessment of Relevant Core Patient Variables

Health Status

Take a complete health history that includes a complete physical assessment and a complete drug history. Lithium's interaction with many other drugs makes this thoroughness essential. Health conditions that increase sodium resorption, such as chronic heart failure or cirrhosis of the liver, may also increase lithium resorption and lead to lithium toxicity. It is essential that patients who are taking lithium inform all health care providers, including dentists, that they are using this drug. Assess the patient's work history, because bipolar disorder can disrupt a person's ability to function at work or cause absenteeism

Life Span and Gender

Consider the patient's age, keeping in mind that lithium clearance in the kidneys decreases as a person ages. Elderly patients should use lithium cautiously because older adults experience more profound or toxic CNS effects. Older adults also are more likely to develop clinical hypothyroidism, lithium-induced goiter, and nephrogenic diabetes insipidus. Ask women of childbearing age whether they are pregnant, intend to become pregnant, or are breast-feeding. Lithium is classified in FDA pregnancy risk category D. It crosses the placenta, and serum concentration is equal in the mother and fetus. Lithium may cause fetal harm when given to a pregnant woman. Data from lithium birth registries suggest an increase in cardiac and other anomalies. Breast-feeding should be avoided by women taking lithium; valproic acid is better tolerated by breast-feeding infants (Menon, 2008).

Lifestyle, Diet, and Habits

Review the patient's diet because sudden changes in sodium intake may alter lithium resorption, changing the amount of drug that is available in the bloodstream. Assess the patient's use of alcohol and other drugs, including caffeine. Concurrent drug or alcohol abuse reduces responsiveness to drug therapy. Alcohol and caffeine-containing foods and beverages, such as coffee, tea, and some sodas, increase lithium excretion. Consider the patient's daily activities. Lithium therapy causes drowsiness and may impair activities that require alertness or physical coordination.

Environment

Be aware of the environments in which lithium may be administered. Lithium can be administered safely in acute care, chronic care, and home care settings.

Culture and Inherited Traits

Consider the patient's ethnic heritage. For example, in Japan, lower lithium doses result in the same serum blood lithium levels. This fact would support lower dosing of patients with Japanese heritage here as well.

Nursing Diagnoses and Outcomes

- Ineffective Therapeutic Regimen Management related to questions about the benefits of the regime (a patient

TABLE 16.8	Agents That Interact with P Lithium Carbonate	
Interactants	**Effect and Significance**	**Nursing Management**
alkalinizing agents: potassium acetate, potassium citrate, sodium bicarbonate, sodium citrate, sodium lactate, tromethamine	Increased renal clearance of lithium	Anticipate possible dosage adjustment.
caffeine	Reduced serum lithium concentrations	Counsel patients about possibly decreased effectiveness of therapy, and identify sources of caffeine (coffee, tea, chocolate, carbonated colas, and other beverages).
verapamil	Possible lithium toxicity	Avoid concurrent use.
diuretics	Increased or decreased lithium levels depending on diuretic: enhanced lithium reabsorption with diuretics that act in distal tubule (thiazides, spironolactone, triamterene) or enhanced renal clearance with diuretics that act at the proximal tubule (osmotic diuretics, carbonic anhydrase inhibitors)	Monitor lithium levels carefully; anticipate dosage adjustments accordingly.
methyldopa	Possible lithium toxicity	Coadminister cautiously.
NSAIDs	Elevated lithium serum concentration from reduced excretion	Monitor lithium levels carefully; observe for signs of toxicity.
phenothiazines, haloperidol, carbamazepine	Neurotoxicity (delirium, seizures, encephalopathy, hyperpyrexia, EPS)	Monitor lithium levels carefully; observe for signs of toxicity.
acetazolamide, theophylline	Increased excretion of lithium	Monitor lithium levels closely. Anticipate dosage adjustment.
TCAs	Increased pharmacologic effect of TCAs	Monitor patient carefully for signs and symptoms of TCA toxicity. Anticipate dosage adjustment for TCAs.
neuromuscular blocking agents	Increased neuromuscular blocking effect with severe respiratory depression	Assess respiratory and neurologic status closely. Anticipate dosage reduction of neuromuscular blocking agent. Coadminister with caution.
fluoxetine	Increased lithium levels	Monitor lithium levels closely. Assess for signs and symptoms of lithium toxicity.

experiencing a manic episode may not want to take medicine that will interfere with his or her feelings of grandiosity or boundless energy)

Desired outcome: The patient will adhere to taking lithium as prescribed to maintain a therapeutic serum lithium level.

- Excess Fluid Volume related to water retention secondary to lithium therapy

  Desired outcome: The patient will adopt strategies to restore and maintain proper fluid balance.

- Risk for Poisoning related to effects of lithium toxicity

  Desired outcome: The patient will comply with regular monitoring of blood lithium levels to maintain a therapeutic serum level.

Planning and Intervention

Maximizing Therapeutic Effects

Continue to play an important role in helping patients with bipolar disorder remain in remission. Instruct the patient about early warning signs of a relapse, ways to manage psychosocial problems, and the importance of health-conscious behaviors. Patients may miss the highs of mania, considering life very flat while on lithium therapy. Offer emotional support to patients who feel this way and encourage them to continue with lithium therapy. If the patient cannot abstain from alcohol, advise moderate intake. Help the patient to arrange a work schedule that provides regular eating and sleeping schedules to minimize stress.

Minimizing Adverse Effects

Monitor the patient's blood level of lithium carefully when first starting therapy or whenever the dose is increased, to prevent toxicity from occurring. Patients' serum lithium levels should be monitored once or twice weekly during initiation of therapy and monthly thereafter to ensure dosage is within therapeutic ranges. Obtain a drug blood level at the first symptom of lithium toxicity. Blood specimens should be taken 8 to 12 hours after drug administration.

The risk of lithium toxicity is increased when the patient becomes hyponatremic (e.g., after diarrhea, with diuretic use, or with dehydration), so monitor these patients carefully. To maintain a therapeutic lithium level, patients should be encouraged not to make any major changes in their consumption of water or salt. Consuming lithium with food or dividing the dose minimizes gastrointestinal distress. Lithium is best taken with, or shortly after, meals. Administration should be accompanied by 10 to 12 glasses of water (8 oz) each day to prevent possible dehydration. Hemodialysis is effective in removing lithium from the body and may be indicated in cases of severe overdose or toxicity.

Providing Patient and Family Education

• Teach the symptoms of lithium toxicity and emphasize that patients must report any such symptoms to the prescriber at once.
• Stress the importance of adhering to a schedule of follow-up laboratory and medical appointments.
• Caution patients to avoid OTC products containing nonsteroidal anti-inflammatory drugs (NSAIDs), except for aspirin, because these products decrease renal clearance. Patients should not use NSAIDs without first consulting the health care provider.
• Caution patients against changing sodium intake, starting new drug therapy, or even using OTC drugs without first consulting the prescriber. Changes such as these may result in toxic lithium levels. In addition, explain the relationship between lithium activity and dietary sodium and teach patients how to maintain a constant level of sodium and fluid intake to avoid fluctuations in lithium level.
• Teach strategies to prevent dehydration during lithium therapy.

Ongoing Assessment and Evaluation

Monitor serum lithium levels throughout therapy as described above. Observe the patient's neurologic and psychiatric functioning and assess neuromuscular, gastrointestinal, cardiovascular, kidney, and thyroid function routinely. To evaluate emotional stability, contrast pretreatment behaviors and patient's report of mood state with current observations and patient report. It is equally important to observe the patient's adherence to the therapeutic regimen. Lithium therapy is considered effective when the bipolar disorder is controlled and the patient does not experience serious adverse effects.

P Lithium Carbonate

• Mood stabilizer for treating bipolar affective disorder, particularly manic episodes
• Changes in sodium or fluid intake will alter blood levels of lithium.
• Major contraindications: severe cardiovascular or kidney disease, pregnancy or lactation, sodium imbalance
• Most common adverse effects: increased thirst or urge to drink, frequent urination, nausea, fine hand tremor
• Most serious adverse effects: lithium toxicity (slurred speech, unsteady gait, weakness, drowsiness, diarrhea, vomiting, confusion, and irregular heartbeat, possibly even seizure)
• **Life span alert: Older adults are at greater risk for hypothyroidism, drug-induced goiter, and nephrogenic diabetes insipidus.**
• Maximizing therapeutic effects: Promote a healthy lifestyle (balanced diet and activity level); encourage adherence.
• Minimizing adverse effects: Monitor serum levels regularly.
• Most important patient education: Have serum lithium levels monitored, avoid major changes in sodium and fluid intake, consult with the prescriber before using any other drugs, even over-the-counter products (especially nonsteroidal anti-inflammatory drugs).

Drugs Significantly Different From **P** Lithium

Antiepileptics

Selective antiepileptic agents, such as carbamazepine, valproic acid, and lamotrigine, demonstrate antimanic effectiveness in patients who do not respond or are intolerant of lithium. The antiepileptics are discussed in more depth in Chapter 18.

Carbamazepine

Carbamazepine (Tegretol) is an alternative to lithium for managing acute mania and for maintenance therapy. The sustained-release form is used for these indications. It is thought to reduce the sensitization of the brain to repeated episodes of mood swing. Mood-stabilizing use of carbamazepine does not appear to cause the blood dyscrasias that

CRITICAL THINKING SCENARIO

BUG OR DRUG?

Your patient is a 55-year-old man with a diagnosis of bipolar disorder whose manic symptoms have recently been stabilized using lithium, 600 mg PO once in the morning and once in the evening. He comes to you asking for medicine to treat his diarrhea, stating that he has been experiencing this symptom for 2 days now, and it must be something going around or something he ate.

1. As his nurse, what are your concerns?

2. What further assessments and interventions should you take?

complicate its use as an antiepileptic. However, blood studies should be monitored to confirm that the patient is tolerating the medication without adverse effects.

Valproates

Valproic acid and divalproex sodium (Depakote) appear as effective as lithium in treating mania but are less effective in managing the depressive component of the disorder. Both these drugs are labeled for use in the treatment of acute manic episode or mixed manic-depressive episodes, with or without psychotic features. Long-term therapy appears to reduce the frequency and severity of bipolar episodes.

Valproic acid has been reported to cause serious or fatal hepatotoxicity within the first 6 months of therapy in some patients. Patients should be monitored very carefully for signs of liver damage, which may be rather nonspecific, such as malaise, weakness, lethargy, facial edema, anorexia, and vomiting. Liver function tests should be performed before starting therapy and then regularly throughout therapy, although serum levels will not always be altered even if hepatotoxicity is developing. The drug should be discontinued if there is significant hepatic dysfunction. Thrombocytopenia is also possible from valproic acid; this appears to be more probable if the dose is high. Because valproic acid can produce teratogenic effects (especially neural tube defects), it is an FDA pregnancy category D drug and should generally be avoided during pregnancy.

Lamotrigine

Lamotrigine (Lamictal) is used to prevent the reoccurrence of a mood disorder episode (depression, mania, hypomania, or mixed episode). It is considered maintenance therapy after acute episodes have been treated with other drugs. Lamotrigine has the potential to cause the life-threatening rash of Stevens-Johnson syndrome, although this is rare. Coadministration of lamotrigine with valproic acid may increase the risk of Stevens-Johnson syndrome. Administering too high an initial dose of lamotrigine or titrating the dose upward too quickly may also increase the risk.

Antipsychotics

Several atypical antipsychotics are also labeled for use in bipolar disorder. These drugs are discussed in Chapter 17. Olanzapine/fluoxetine (Symbyax) is used for depressive episodes. The drugs risperidone (Risperdal), quetiapine (Seroquel), aripiprazole (Abilify), and ziprasidone (Geodon) are used for acute mania.

CHAPTER SUMMARY

- Illnesses resulting in mood disorder are associated with an imbalance or dysregulation of neurotransmitters.
- Antidepressant therapy is used to treat depressive disorders. The three major classes of antidepressants are selective serotonin reuptake inhibitors (SSRIs), tricyclic antidepressants, and monoamine oxidase inhibitors

(MAOIs). Several miscellaneous agents are also used as antidepressants.

- Antidepressants appear to relieve depression by creating changes in both presynaptic and postsynaptic neuroreceptors, correcting the neurotransmitter imbalance. The neuroreceptors affected by antidepressant therapy are the serotonin, norepinephrine, dopamine, acetylcholine, histamine, and alpha-1 adrenergic receptors. Antidepressants stimulate these receptors differently, depending on the drug class. The effects at serotonin, norepinephrine, and dopamine receptors are generally responsible for the therapeutic effects, whereas effects at the other receptor sites are generally responsible for adverse effects.
- All antidepressant therapy requires sustained use of the drug to achieve a therapeutic effect, sometime between 10 days and 4 weeks of therapy. Energy levels may return before the depressed mood is elevated, placing patients at great risk for suicide during this time, because they still have the mindset for suicide, but now they have the physical ability to act on their mood.
- No ideal antidepressant exists, because all produce adverse effects. Some adverse effects are mild and transient, whereas others may be serious. The nurse fulfills important functions, including teaching the patient and family safe and effective use of these agents, offering strategies to minimize adverse effects, and offering hope to patients that drug therapy will help lift their mood.
- Sertraline is the prototype SSRI; it is the most frequently prescribed antidepressant and is generally well tolerated by patients. Nortriptyline is the prototype TCA. Its adverse effect profile includes difficulty concentrating, cardiac irregularities, and seizures. Older adults are particularly prone to these adverse effects. Phenelzine is the prototype MAOI. It is the least used of the antidepressants because of its adverse effects. Hypertensive crisis is the most serious toxic effect of phenelzine and other oral MAOIs. It may occur after ingesting certain foods containing high amounts of tyramine or with concomitant use with several other drugs. The transdermal MAOI selegiline, in the lowest dose available, does not appear to carry the risk of tyramine interaction.
- Bipolar disorder is characterized by mood shifts that include mania and depression. The mood stabilizer lithium is considered the drug of choice for bipolar disorder.
- Lithium ions are managed in the body the same way that sodium ions are managed. Changes in either sodium or fluid intake therefore can affect how much lithium the kidney reabsorbs and changes the circulating level of lithium in the bloodstream.
- Lithium has a narrow therapeutic index. Serum drug levels of lithium must be monitored closely throughout therapy to prevent lithium toxicity.
- Some antiepileptic drugs have been approved for use as mood stabilizers. They are frequently better tolerated than lithium in some patients.

QUESTIONS FOR STUDY AND REVIEW

1. Identify the three main classifications of antidepressant drugs.
2. What is an additional assessment that you must make, in addition to medication efficacy, once the depressed patient has begun antidepressant therapy?
3. Identify an important point that you must teach the patient and his or her family to enhance adherence to antidepressant therapy.
4. What teaching can you give to a patient who complains of gastrointestinal distress associated with sertraline therapy?
5. What are common adverse effects produced by nortriptyline?
6. What are some dietary restrictions during phenelzine treatment?
7. What are the symptoms of an MAOI hypertensive crisis?
8. Identify the pharmacologic agents used to treat bipolar disorder.
9. What is the therapeutic range or level for lithium therapy?
10. What are the symptoms of lithium toxicity?

NEED MORE HELP?

Chapter 16 of the Study Guide to Accompany *Drug Therapy in Nursing*, 4th Edition, contains NCLEX-style questions and other learning activities to reinforce your understanding of the concepts presented in this chapter. For additional information or to purchase the study guide, visit thePoint.

REFERENCES

American Psychiatric Association. (2000). *Diagnostic and statistical manual of mental disorders* (4th ed., text revision). Washington, DC: Author.

Anand, A., Li, Y., Wang, Y., et al. (2005). Antidepressant effect on connectivity of the mood-regulating circuit: An FMRI study. *Neuropsychopharmacology, 30*(7):1334–1344.

Brennes, G., Williamson, J., Messier, S., Rejeski, W., Pahor, M., Ip, E., Penninx, B. (2007). Treatment of minor depression in older adults: a pilot study comparing sertraline and exercise, *Aging and Mental Health*, 11(1):61–68.

Crumpacker, D. (2008). Suicidality and Antidepressants in the Elderly. *Baylor University Medical Center Proceedings*, 21(4):373–377.

CDC, US Department of Health and Human Services. (2007). Adolescent Health in the United States. Retrieved from http://www.cdc.gov/nchsdata/misc/adolescent2007.pdf.

CDC Surveillance Summaries, (2009). Surveillance for Reporting Violent Deaths, Nathional Violent Death Reporting System, 16 States, 2006. *Morbidity and Mortality Weekly Report, 58(SS01) 1–44.* Retrieved from http://www.cdc.gov/mmwr/preview/mmwrhtml/ss5801a1.htm.

de Leon, J., Susce, M. T., & Murray-Carmichael, E. (2006). The AmpliChip CYP450 genotyping test: Integrating a new clinical tool. *Molecular Diagnostic Therapy,* 10(3):135–151.

Dew, M., Whyte, E., Lenze, E., houck, P., Mulsant, B., Polluck, B., Stack, J., Bensasi, S., Reynolds, C. (2007). Recovery from major depression in older adults receiving augmentation

of antidepressant pharmacotherapy. *American Psychiatric Association*, 164(6):892–899.

Duman, S. (2002) Structural alternations in depresson: cellular mechanisms underlying pathology and treatment of mood disorders. *CNS Spectrums,* 7(2):140–147.

Field, T. (2008). Breastfeeding and antidepressants. *Infant Behavioral Development*, 31(3):481–487.

Fountoulakis, K. (2008). The contemporary face of bipolar illness: complex diagnostic and therapeutic challenges. *CNS Spectrum*, 13(9):763–774.

Garand, L., Mitchell, A., Dietrick, A., Hijjawi, S., Pan, D. (2006). Suicide in the older adults: Nursing assessment of suicide risk. *Issues in Mental Health Nursing*, 27:355–370.

Gaynes, B., Rush, J., Trivedi, M., Wisniewski, S., Balasubramani. G., McGrath, P., Thase, M., Klinkman, M., Nierenberg, A., Yates, W., Fava, M. (2008). Primary versus specialty care outcomes for depressed outpatients mkanaged with measurement-based care: Results from STAR*D. *Journal of General Internal Medicine,* 23(5):551–560.

Gibbons, R., Brown, H., Hur, K., Marcus, S., Bhaumik, D., Mann, J. (2007). Relationship between antidepressants and suicide attempts: An analysis of the Veterans Health Administration data sets. *American Journal of Psychiatry,* 164(7):1044–1049.

Gibbons, R., Brown, H., Hur, K., Marcus, S., Bhaumik, D., Erkens, J., Herings, R., Mann, J. (2007). Early evidence on the effects of regulator's suicidality warnings on SSRI prescriptions and suicide in children and adolescents. *American Journal of Psychiatry*, 164(9):1356–1363.

Glassman, A. H., Bigger, J. T., Gaffney, M., et al. (2006). Onset of major depression associated with acute coronary syndromes: Relationship of onset, major depressive disorder history, and episode severity to sertraline benefit. *Archives of General Psychiatry*, 63(3):263–268.

Hong, N. C., Norman, T. R., Naing, K. O., et al. (2006). A comparative study of sertraline dosages, plasma concentrations, efficacy and adverse reactions in Chinese versus Caucasian patients. *International Clinical Psychopharmacology*, 21(2):87–92.

Juurlink, D., Mamdani, M., Kopp, A., Redelmeier, D. (2006). The risk of suicide with selective serotonin reuptake inhibitors in the Elderly. *American Journal of Psychiatry*, 163(5):813–823.

Looper, K. (2007). Potential medical and surgical complications of serotonergic antidepressant medications. *Psychosomatics.* 48(1–2):1–9.

Lotrich, F. E., Pollock, B. G., Ferrell, R. E. (2003). Serotonin transporter promoter polymorphism in African Americans: Allele frequencies and implications for treatment. *American Journal of Pharmacogenomics,* 3(2):145–147.

Lustman, P. J., Clouse, R. E., Nix, B. D., et al. (2006). Sertraline for prevention of depression recurrence in diabetes mellitus: A randomized, double-blind, placebo-controlled trial. *Archives of General Psychiatry*, 63(5):521–529.

Mann, J. J., Emslie, G., Baldessarini, R. J., et al. (2006). American College of Neuropsychopharmacology Task Force report on SSRIs and suicidal behavior in youth. *Neuropsychopharmacology,* 31(3):473–492.

March, J. S., Klee, B. J., Kremer, C. M. (2006). Treatment benefit and the risk of suicidality in multicenter, randomized, controlled trials of sertraline in children and adolescents. *Journal of Child and Adolescent Psychopharmacology, 16*(1–2):91–102.

McMahon, F., Buervenich, S., Charney, D., Lipsky, R., Rush, J., Wilson, A., Sorant, A., Papanicolaou, G., Laje, G., Fava, M., Trivedi, M., Wisniewski, S., Manji, H. (2006). Variations in the gene encoding the serotonin 2A receptor is associated with outcome of antidepressant treatment. *American Journal of Human Genetics,* 78(5):804–814.

Menon. S. (2008). Psychotropic medication during pregnancy and lactation. *Archives of Genecological Obstetrics,* 277: 1–13.

Mohr, W. (2009). *Psychiatric-Mental Health Nursing: Evidence-based concepts, skills and practices, 7th Edition.* Philadelphia, PA: Lippincott Williams & Wilkins.

National Institute of Mental Health. (2007). *Depression Publication.* Retrieved from http://www.nimh.nih.gov/health/publications/depression/index.shtml.

National Institute of Mental Health. (2008). *The numbers count: Mental disorders in America.* Retrieved from http://www.nimh.nih.gov/health/publications/the-numbers-count-mental-disorders-in-america/index.shtml#MajorDepressive.

National Institute of Mental Health. (2009a). *Suicide in the U.S. Statistics and Prevention.* Retrieved from http://www.nimh.nih.gov/health/publications/suicide-in-the-us-statistics-and-prevention/index.shtml.

National Institute of Mental Health. (2009b). *Publication Bipolar Disorder.* Retrieved from http://www.nimh.nih.gov/health/publications/bipolar-disorder/complete-index.shtml.

Noonan, P., Jones Warren, B., White, D. (2007). Diagnosis and pharmacologic treatment of bipolar disorder. *Psychiatric Nurse Counseling Points.* 1(4):1–9.

Oslin, D. W. (2005). Treatment of late-life depression complicated by alcohol dependence. *American Journal of Geriatric Psychiatry,* 13(6):491–500.

Pav, M., Kovaru, H., Fiserova, A., Havrdova, E., Lisa, V. (2008). Neurobiological aspects of depressive disorder and antidepressant treatment: Role of glia. *Physiological Research,* 57: 151–164.

Prescriber's Letter. (2008). Medication Guide: Sertraline antidepressant medicine, depression and other serious mental illnesses, and suicidal thoughts or actions. *Prescriber's Letter,* PV7090 am*p.*

Rush, A. J., Trivedi, M. H., Wisniewski, S. R., et al., for the STAR*D Study Team. (2006). Bupropion-SR, sertraline, or venlafaxine-XR after failure of SSRIs for depression. *New England Journal of Medicine,* 354(120):1231–1242.

Rynn, M., Wagner, K. D., Donnelly, C., et al. (2006). Long-term sertraline treatment of children and adolescents with major depressive disorder. *Journal of Child and Adolescent Psychopharmacology,* 16(1–2):103–116.

Sansone, R., Sansone, L. (2009). Dysthymic disorder: Forlorne and overlooked. *Psychiatry,* 6(5):47–50.

Sansone, R., Sansone, L. (2008). Depression and cardiovascular disease: Just and urban legend? *Psychiatry,* 11:45–48.

Shah, N., Jone, J., Aperi, J., Shemtov, R., Karne, A., Borenstein, J. (2008). Selective Serotonin Reuptake Inhibitors for premenstrual syndrome and premenstrual dysphoric disorder: A meta-analysis. *Obstetrical Gynecology,* 111(5):1175–1182.

Stahl, S., Felker, A. (2008). Monoamine Oxidase Inhibitors: A modern guide to an unrequited class of antidepressants. *CNS Spectrums,* 13(10):855–870.

Stahl, S., Grady, M., Moret, C., Briley, M. (2005). SNRIs: Their pharmacology, clinical efficacy, and tolerability in comparison with other classes of antidepressants. *CNS Spectrums,* 10(9):732–747.

Stone, M., Laughren, T., Levenson, M., Holland, C., Hughes, A., Hammand, T., Temple R., Rochester, G. (2009). Risk of suicidality in clinical trials of antidepressants in adults: analysis of proprietary data submitted to US Food and Drug Administration. *British Medical Journal,* August 11, 2009, 339–288.

Sussman, N. (2007). Translating science into service: lessons learned from the sequenced treatment alternatives to relieve depression (STAR*D) study. *Primary Care Companion, Journal of Clinical Psychiatry,* 9(5):331–337.

U.S. Food and Drug Administration. (2009a). Aplenzin prescribing information. Retrieved from http://www.accessdata.fda.gov/scripts/cder/drugsatfda/index.cfm?fuseaction=Search. DrugDetails.

U.S. Food and Drug Administration. (2009b). Safety Release: Zyban Sustained Released Capsules. Retrieved from http://www.fda.gov/Safety/MedWatch/SafetyInformation/ucm176815.htm.

U.S. Food and Drug Administration. (2009c). Lexapro Prescribing Information. Retrieved from http://www.accessdata.fda.gov/drugsatfda_docs/label/2009/021323s030s031,021365s021s022lbl.pdf.

U.S. Food and Drug Administration. (2009d). Cymbalta Prescribing Information. Retrieved from http://www.accessdata.fda.gov/drugsatfda_docs/label/2009/021427s021s027s028lbl.pdf.

U.S. Food and Drug Administration. (2009e). Pristiq Prescribing Information. Retrieved from http://www.accessdata.fda.gov/drugsatfda_docs/label/2009/021992s001s006s007lbl.pdf.

U.S. Food and Drug Administration. (2009f). Savella Prescribing Information. Retrieved from http://www.accessdata.fda.gov/drugsatfda_docs/label/2009/022256s001lbl.pdf.

U.S. Food and Drug Administration. (2009g). Safety Alert: SSRI. SNRI and Tryptans. Retrieved from http://www.fda.gov/Drugs/DrugSafety/PublicHealthAdvisories/ucm053351.htm.

Williams, M., Clouse, R., Nix, B., Rubin, E., Sayuk, G., McGill, J., Gelenberg, A., Ciechanowski, P., Hirsch, I., Lustman, P. (2007). Efficacy of sertraline in prevention of depression recurrence in older versus younger adults with diabetes. *Diabetes Care,* 40(4):801–806.

World Health Organization. (2009a). Depression. Retrieved from http://www.who.int/mental_health/management/depression/definition/en/.

World Health Organization. (2009b). Gender Disparities. Retrieved from http://www.who.int/mental_health/prevention/genderwomen/en/print.html.

Yu, Y. W., Tsai, S. J., Chen, T. J., et al. (2002). Association study of the serotonin transporter promoter polymorphism and symptomatology and antidepressant response in major depressive disorders. *Molecular Psychiatry,* 7(10):1115–1119.

Drugs Treating Psychotic Disorders and Dementia

Learning Objectives

At the completion of this chapter the student will:

1. Identify diseases and disease processes in which psychotic disorders or dementia are present.

2. Identify the symptoms of psychotic disorders or dementia.

3. Identify the "positive and negative symptoms" of schizophrenia.

4. Identify core drug knowledge of drugs used to treat psychotic disorders or dementia.

5. Name the types of drugs that are used to treat psychotic disorders or dementia.

6. Identify core patient variables relevant to drugs that affect psychotic disorders or dementia.

7. Relate the interaction of core drug knowledge to core patient variables for drugs to treat psychotic disorders or dementia.

8. Generate a nursing plan of care from the interaction between core drug knowledge and the core patient variables for drugs to treat psychotic disorders or dementia.

9. Describe nursing interventions to maximize therapeutic and minimize adverse effects for drugs that affect psychotic disorders or dementia.

10. Identify the signs and symptoms of neuroleptic malignant syndrome.

11. Determine key points for patient and family education for drugs that affect psychotic disorders or dementia.

Key Terms   Alzheimer disease   extrapyramidal symptoms   schizophrenia
             delirium   neuroleptic malignant syndrome   tardive dyskinesia
             dementia   psychosis   vascular dementia

Drugs Treating Psychotic Disorders and Dementia

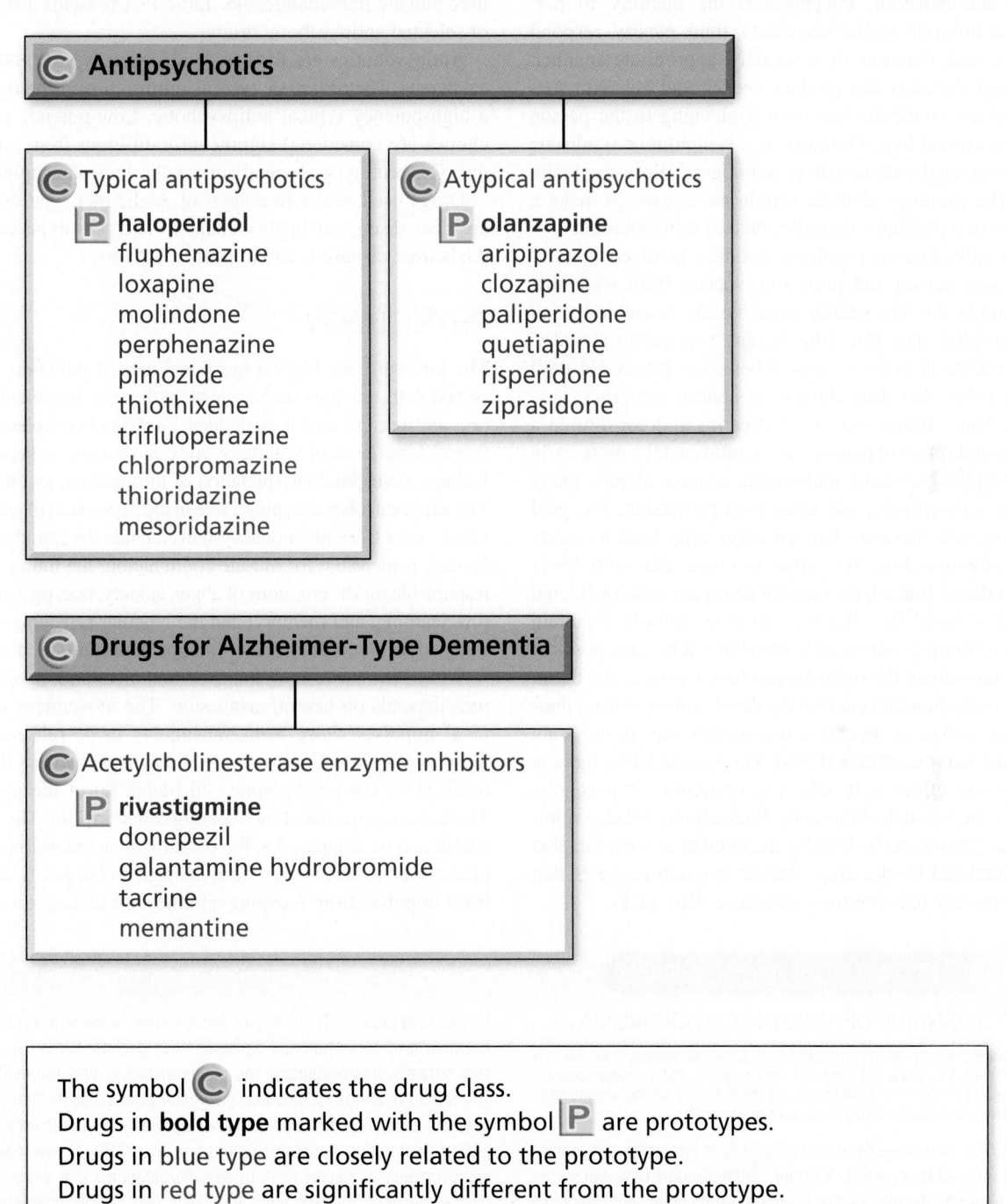

C Antipsychotics

C Typical antipsychotics

P haloperidol
fluphenazine
loxapine
molindone
perphenazine
pimozide
thiothixene
trifluoperazine
chlorpromazine
thioridazine
mesoridazine

C Atypical antipsychotics

P olanzapine
aripiprazole
clozapine
paliperidone
quetiapine
risperidone
ziprasidone

C Drugs for Alzheimer-Type Dementia

C Acetylcholinesterase enzyme inhibitors

P rivastigmine
donepezil
galantamine hydrobromide
tacrine
memantine

The symbol **C** indicates the drug class.
Drugs in **bold type** marked with the symbol **P** are prototypes.
Drugs in blue type are closely related to the prototype.
Drugs in red type are significantly different from the prototype.
Drugs in black type with no symbol are also used in drug therapy; no prototype.

Although it is impossible to read a person's mind, much less to know precisely whether his or her thoughts are ordered or disordered, a person's thoughts influence his or her perception of reality, interpretation of the environment, speech, and behavior. **Psychosis** is the inability to perceive and interpret reality accurately, think clearly, respond correctly, and function in a socially appropriate manner. Disordered thoughts can produce speech and behavior patterns that are confusing and even frightening to the person and those around him. Psychosis is a symptom or syndrome that is associated with certain psychological illnesses (Stahl, 2008). The presence of these symptoms is used to make a diagnosis of a psychotic disorder, such as schizophrenia.

Historically, treating psychotic disorders involved containing the sick person and protecting society from what that person might do. The setting more closely resembled a jail than a hospital. The first drug therapy was aimed at sedating the patient in order to control behavior. It was not until the mid-1950s that drug therapy to control symptoms was devised. These drugs were very effective and constituted a major breakthrough in patient care. Unfortunately, these early drug therapies had many undesirable adverse effects, many of which were chronic, and some even permanent. The goal in creating new therapies has not necessarily been to create a more effective drug, but rather to create one with fewer adverse effects. Indeed, the original drugs are still considered the gold standard for effective symptom control. As brain imaging techniques advanced in the 1990s, it became possible to learn more about the sophisticated functioning of the brain; this new understanding enabled the development of drug therapies that worked at specific neuroreceptor sites in the brain and central nervous system (CNS). This targeted drug therapy not only was effective in relieving symptoms of psychotic disorders, such as delusions and hallucinations, but also minimized adverse effects by limiting the number of receptors that were stimulated by the drug. Recent research suggests that targeted therapy may improve adherence (Box 17.1).

Drugs that relieve symptoms of psychotic disorders are generally referred to as antipsychotics. They are also called neuroleptics, to reflect the fact that the drugs work in the nervous system at neuroreceptor sites. Both terms are currently used and are interchangeable. Table 17.1 presents a summary of selected antipsychotic drugs.

Antipsychotics are further divided into typical and atypical agents. The prototype typical antipsychotic is haloperidol, a high-potency typical antipsychotic. Low-potency antipsychotics are considered significantly different from haloperidol. The prototype atypical antipsychotic is olanzapine.

Drugs used in the treatment of Alzheimer type dementia are also discussed in this chapter. The prototype drug for Alzheimer disease is rivastigmine (Exelon).

PHYSIOLOGY

The cerebrum, the highest functional area of the brain, is concerned with activities such as creative thought, judgment, memory, and reason, and it is divided into two hemispheres. The frontal lobes control voluntary body movement, expression of feelings, perceptual interpretation of information, and thinking. The temporal lobes also play a role in the expression of emotions. Other major CNS functional systems include the extrapyramidal system, responsible for muscle coordination; the limbic system responsible for the emotions of anger, anxiety, fear, pleasure, sorrow, learning, and memory; and the reticular activating system, responsible for consciousness, filtering, and stimulus alert.

Within the nervous system, communication between neurons depends on neurotransmission. The movements of electrical impulses cause neurotransmitters to be released from the presynaptic cell (axon) into the synapse, where they are received by the postsynaptic cell (dendrite) of the next cell. The axons are insulated by a coating called myelin. The myelin sheath can be compared to the coating on an extension cord. It protects the internal wires from damage and prevents the electrical impulses from escaping into the surrounding area.

BOX 17.1 FOCUS ON RESEARCH

NEUROCOGNITIVE DEFICITS IN SCHIZOPHRENIA

Stahl, S. M. (2008) *Stahl's Essential Psychopharmacology*. Cambridge University Press. New York
Ventura, J., Thames, A. D., Wood, R. C., Guzik, L. H., Hellemann, G. S. (2010). Disorganization and reality distortion in schizophrenia: A meta-analysis of the relationship between positive symptoms and neurocognitive deficits. *Schizophrenia Research*. 121: 1–14.

There is a clear neurodegeneration that occurs in late stage schizophrenia, often referred to as stage IV (Stahl, 2008). Studies have been conducted to ascertain the relationship between certain prominent symptoms in schizophrenia and this decline in cognition. One hypothesis is that neurocognitive declines occur due to excitotoxicity and excessive action of the neurotransmitter glutamate (Stahl, 2008). This neurocognitive decline indeed has effects on the ability of schizophrenic individuals to live independently. Ventura et al (2010) conducted a meta-analysis looking at the relationship between positive symptoms and neurocognitive deficits. Specifically, the researchers analyzed the connection between reality distortion (delusions, hallucinations, suspiciousness) and disorganization (conceptual disorganization and bizarre behaviors) as they relate

to cognitive decline. Their results demonstrated a moderate relationship between disorganization and neurocognitive decline, while the relationship between neurocognition and reality distortion was relatively weak. The strong relationship between disorganization suggests that improvements in community function could be improved with treatments that target disorganization symptoms (Ventura et al., 2010). As we look ahead, improvements in neurocognition as schizophrenics age could possibly reduce the need for premature long term care in this population, thus improving independence and quality of life.

Nursing implications
It is important for ongoing evaluation of symptomatology in schizophrenia, closer attention to target symptoms may indeed help aim treatments, both pharmacologic and non-pharmacologic. In patients with schizophrenia, it is appropriate to be aware of potential neurocognitive deficits for promoting independence. Often, as with dementias, early intervention may help promote executive functioning and independence.

TABLE 17.1 Summary of Selected Ⓒ Antipsychotics

Drug (Trade) Name	Selected Indications	Route and Dosage Range	Pharmacokinetics
Ⓒ Typical Antipsychotics			
High Potency			
🅿 haloperidol (Haldol)	Psychotic disorders, hyperexcitability in children	*Adult:* PO, 0.5–2 mg bid to tid; IM, 5–30 mg/d; IM deconate, 50-100 mg IM/mo *Child:* PO, 0.05–0.15 mg/d	*Onset:* PO, varies, IM, 15–30 min *Duration:* PO, 24–72 h; IM, 4–8 h $t_{1/2}$: 21–14 h
acetophenazine (Tindal)	Psychotic disorders	*Adult:* PO, 20–80 mg/d in divided doses *Child:* Not recommended	*Onset:* 2–3 h *Duration:* 36–48 h $t_{1/2}$: 10–20 h
fluphenazine enanthate (Prolixin)	Psychotic disorders	*Adult:* IM/SC, 12.5–25 mg *Child:* Not recommended	*Onset:* 24–72 h *Duration:* 1–3 wk $t_{1/2}$: 3.7 d
perphenazine (Trilafon)	Psychotic disorders	*Adult:* PO, 4–8 mg tid to qid; IM, 5–15 mg/d	*Onset:* Varies *Duration:* 6–12 h $t_{1/2}$: Unknown
thiothixene (Navane)	Psychotic disorders	*Adult:* PO, 2–30 mg/d; IM, 4–30 mg/d	*Onset:* 1–6 h *Duration:* 12–24 h $t_{1/2}$: 34 h
Low Potency			
chlorpromazine (Thorazine)	Psychotic disorders, such as schizophrenia	*Adult:* PO, 10–25 mg, bid, tid, or qid to maximum of 2,000 mg/d; IM, 25–50 mg, repeated in 4 h if needed *Child:* 5–12 y, 23–46 kg, 75 mg/d; 6 mo–5 y (up to 23 kg), 40 mg/d; IM, 0.55 mg/kg q6–8 h	*Onset:* PO, 30–60 min; IM, 10–15 min *Duration:* 4–6 h $t_{1/2}$: 23–37 h
loxapine (Loxitane)	Psychotic disorders	*Adult:* PO, 10–100 mg/d; IM, 12.5–50 mg/d	*Onset:* PO, 30 min; IM, rapid *Duration:* 12 h $t_{1/2}$: 19 h
mesoridazine (Serentil)	Schizophrenia, alcohol withdrawal, acute/chronic alcoholism	*Adult:* PO, 50–400 mg/d (lower dosage for alcohol withdrawal)	*Onset:* Varies *Duration:* 4–8 h $t_{1/2}$: 24–48 h
molindone (Moban)	Psychotic disorders	*Adult:* PO, 50–225 mg/d in divided doses	*Onset:* Varies *Duration:* 24–36 h $t_{1/2}$: 1.5 h
pimozide (Orap)	Tourette syndrome	*Adult:* PO, 1–10 mg/d in divided doses	*Onset:* Varies *Duration:* Unknown $t_{1/2}$: 55–154 h
thioridazine (Mellaril)	Psychotic disorders; agitation, depression, sleep disturbance, and fear in geriatric patients; hyperactivity and related symptoms in children	*Adult:* PO, 50–800 mg/d *Child 2–12 y:* PO, 0.5–3.0 mg/kg/d	*Onset:* Varies *Duration:* 8–12 h $t_{1/2}$: 10–12 h
Ⓒ Atypical Antipsychotics			
🅿 olanzapine (Zyprexa)	Pyschotic disorders Bipolar disorder Agitation in schizophrenia or bipolar I	*Adult:* PO, 5–15 mg/d *Adult:* PO, 5–20 mg/d *Adult:* IM, 10 mg, may repeat if doses are 2–4 h apart, for a total of three doses in 24 h	*Onset:* Unknown *Duration:* Unknown $t_{1/2}$: 21–54 h; average, 30 h
clozapine (Clozaril)	Schizophrenia unresponsive to other antipsychotic drugs	*Adult:* PO, 25–450 mg/d	*Onset:* Varies *Duration:* 4–12 h $t_{1/2}$: 8–12 h
aripiprazole (Abilify)	Schizophrenia, bipolar disorder/mania, major depressive disorder	*Adult:* PO 2–15 mg/d	

(Continued)

TABLE 17.1	Summary of Selected Ⓒ Antipsychotics *(continued)*		
Drug (Trade) Name	**Selected Indications**	**Route and Dosage Range**	**Pharmacokinetics**
ziprasidone (Geodon)	Schizophrenia, bipolar disorder/mania	*Adult:* PO 20–160 mg /d	
quetiapine (Seroquel)	Schizophrenia, bipolar disorder	*Adult:* PO 25–800 mg/d	
Benzisoxazoles			
risperidone (Risperdal)	Psychotic disorders	*Adult:* PO, 1 mg bid to 16 mg/d; IM deconate 25–50 mg/mo	*Onset:* Varies *Duration:* Unknown $t_{1/2}$: 20 h

Thought, like mood, is controlled by neurotransmitters that stimulate neuroreceptors in the brain. The brain has unique receptors, unlike receptors elsewhere in the body. These receptors activate thought processes, and other unique receptors in the brain activate mood response. A combination of neurotransmitters is thought to play a role in the workings of the brain. The primary neurotransmitter related to thought processing is believed to be dopamine. Dopamine is secreted by neurons originating in the midbrain that function in coordination, emotion, and voluntary decision making.

Many areas of the brain secrete acetylcholine; reductions in the amount of this neurotransmitter cause cognitive changes. Acetylcholine has a number of functions, including arousal, coordination of movement, memory acquisition, and memory retention. Research is also being conducted on the extent to which norepinephrine and serotonin might be involved in thought processes. For a complete discussion of acetylcholine and norepinephrine, see Chapters 13 and 14.

PSYCHOTIC DISORDERS

In psychiatry, psychotic disorders are described by different diagnoses. Each diagnosis has its own etiology, symptoms, and treatments, although a given drug may be useful in more than one diagnosis.

Schizophrenia

Schizophrenia is a particular kind of psychosis that is characterized mainly by a clear sensorium but a marked disturbance in thinking. It is a complex illness with uncertain etiology. Schizophrenia interferes with a person's ability to think clearly, manage emotions, make decisions, and relate to others. According to the National Institute of Mental Health (2010), schizophrenia has a 1 year prevalence rate of 1.3 %. Schizophrenia is more likely to occur in men than women, and men tend to have an earlier onset of illness (Messias et al., 2007). The disease typically has an onset between the age of 15 to 24 years. The strongest risk factors appear to be lower social class and family history (Messias et al., 2007).

Schizophrenia is considered to have multiple causes. Current studies imply that one of the causes of schizophrenia is a strong genetic component. Recent research has discovered how two genes, considered schizophrenia risk genes, work

at the molecular level to increase the risk of schizophrenia. The two genes are identified as disrupted-in-schizophrenia-1 (DISC1) and neuregulin 1:

- DISC1, which is involved in the development of the limbic system, has its peak effect in infancy; this suggests that the gene plays an important role in brain development. Three molecules that work in conjunction with DISC1 are reduced in people with schizophrenia. If DISC1 cannot bind to these molecules, this appears to trigger a series of events leading to schizophrenia (Lipska, Peters, Hyde, et al., 2006).
- Neuregulin 1 controls the construction and wiring of the brain during brain development; it also is responsible for communication between nerve cells and a person's ability to adapt to new situations. Genetic variations of neuregulin 1 appear likely to impair the gene from achieving its function and lead to the development of schizophrenia (Law, Lipska, Weickert, et al., 2006).

With a genetic predisposition, the various stressors that may occur in a person's life can trigger the disorder's symptoms. This effect could be compared to what can happen to a bridge made of wooden planks. The structure is strong enough to accommodate light loads safely, but if a heavy truck drove over the bridge, it would be likely to collapse. Other theories for the etiology of schizophrenia include the proposal that the illness is caused by neurodevelopmental changes during brain development. It is suggested that the disease is acquired from the fetal brain's environment. This theory is contradictory to the genetic theory, suggesting that it is not a genetic disease, but acquired (Stahl, 2008). (See Box 17.1 Focus on Research)

Other hypotheses exist for the pathogenesis of schizophrenia, especially with regard to changes in brain chemistry, because schizophrenia is associated with an unusual imbalance of neurotransmitters. The dopamine hypothesis is the most fully developed of these hypotheses. It is based on the unexpected discovery that agents that diminish dopaminergic activity have beneficial effects in reducing the acute symptoms and signs of psychosis, specifically, agitation, anxiety, and hallucinations. However, these agents reduce delusions and social withdrawal less dramatically. Imaging studies have lent credence to the belief that excessive dopamine activity is involved in schizophrenia, particularly on the left side, where the most recognizable "positive" symptoms (e.g., delusions or hallucinations) occur. This imbalance appears to arise not from overproduction of dopamine, but rather from an increase in specific chemical receptors that attract dopamine. Moreover, there appears to be low activity of a subset of dopamine (D_1) receptors in the prefrontal cortex of the brain, where so-called negative symptoms originate. (Positive and negative symptoms are explained later in this chapter.)

The term *schizophrenia* is derived from the Greek words that indicate a broken or shattered personality, separating the cognitive and emotional aspects of the personality. Many people mistakenly believe that schizophrenia involves multiple personalities. People with schizophrenia do not have multiple personalities. Another common misconception is that affected people are prone to violence. Although patients with schizophrenia may sometimes become violent, they are far more likely to withdraw from society. In fact, these people are more often the victims rather than the perpetrators of violence. However, fears and misperceptions persist, and integrating patients with psychotic symptoms into society remains challenging (Box 17.2).

Schizophrenia is characterized by symptoms described as positive, negative, and disorganized. The positive symptoms are so named because they add a layer of something new to the person; they are an excess or a distortion of normal brain function. The positive symptoms of schizophrenia, and the most recognizable symptoms, include delusions (e.g., paranoia or distorted perceptions of other people's intentions) and hallucinations. For example, people with schizophrenia may have beliefs or thoughts that are fixed and false; these beliefs or thoughts are a type of delusion. Hallucinations, on the other hand, can affect any one of the five senses. Auditory hallucinations are the most common type of hallucination; a person with auditory hallucinations might hear voices talking to or about him or her. A person experiencing a visual hallucination may see persons or objects that are not there.

The negative symptoms of schizophrenia include flat or blunted emotions, lack of pleasure or interest in things (anhedonia), and limited speech. These symptoms take away from the person's personality and are thus considered "negative." They also represent a loss or diminishing of normal brain function. For example, people with schizophrenia may have difficulty understanding their feelings or expressing their emotions clearly. Furthermore, they view the world and society as uninteresting and not worth participating in, and they often may not say much or speak unless spoken to. Consequently, an affected person may have trouble relating to others, which in turn can lead to periods of intense withdrawal and profound isolation.

For people with schizophrenia, symptoms of disorganized thinking and speech may cause the following problems:

- Trouble thinking clearly and understanding what other people say
- Using words in a way that makes no sense to anyone else
- Inability to plan ahead
- Inability to solve relatively small problems

The disorganized behavior may make a person do things that do not make sense, such as repeated, rhythmic gestures or ritualistic movements.

Some symptoms of schizophrenia differ between men and women. For example, the negative symptoms are more often present in men; mood symptoms, especially depression, are more commonly seen in women. Additionally, delusions in women appear less bizarre, with more somatic and romantic preoccupation. Men are more concerned with political conspiracy and undercover activities and have more grandiose delusions of power, royalty, and divinity. Many people with schizophrenia have a combination of these symptoms.

Other Psychotic Disorders

Compared with schizophrenia, which is a permanent illness, other psychotic disorders may be short lived. As defined earlier, a psychotic episode is one in which a person loses touch with reality. In addition to being present in schizophrenia, psychosis can also be present in states of depression or mania. The causes of psychosis are varied and can include electrolyte imbalances, metabolic imbalances (e.g., diabetic ketoacidosis), drug abuse (either from drug intoxication or withdrawal), adverse effects from prescribed drug therapy, or hormonal shifts, such as those that occur during the postpartum period.

COGNITIVE DISORDERS

Dementia

Dementia is a clinical syndrome of progressive, degenerative loss of memory and of one or more of these abilities:

- Language skills
- Higher-level skills such as judgment, comprehension, and problem solving
- Ability to recognize or identify objects despite intact sensory function
- Ability to perform motor skills (American Psychiatric Association, 2007)

BOX 17.2 COMMUNITY BASED CONCERNS

Easing Fears About Mental Illness

It is an unfortunate reality that what little attention mental illness receives in the media mostly focuses on episodes of sensational violence, committed by people who are clearly psychotic. However, the overall number of people suffering from mental illnesses, particularly illnesses involving psychosis, is far greater than the number of those who behave violently. Psychotic people most often are the victims, rather than the perpetrators, of injury. Despite this reality, sensational stories of mental illness persist, and prisons fill with untreated mentally ill patients.

All nurses have a responsibility to continue to educate patients, their families, and all members of the community about the symptoms of various mental illnesses and about any resources available for treatment. Rallying the support of the community is crucial to increase the resources that will help patients receive appropriate treatment. More drugs for treating specific symptoms of mental illness are available today than ever before. These advances also mean that there is less need to fear the psychotic patient and more reason than ever before for the patient to be integrated as a functioning member of the community.

Mood and behavior may also be affected in dementia. Agitation or withdrawal, hallucinations, delusions, insomnia, emotional apathy, and loss of inhibitions are also common.

There are many types of dementia, including Alzheimer-type dementia, vascular dementia, and other dementia caused by diseases such as acquired immunodeficiency syndrome (AIDS). Dementia can also be a result of brain damage from substance abuse, such as alcoholism or inhalant use, or from exposure to environmental chemicals. In all of these circumstances, symptoms of dementia develop gradually, and although the deterioration is not necessarily diffuse or "global," it often affects some areas of intellectual functioning while sparing others. Early in the disease, the patient may be aware of changes in intellectual ability and become depressed or anxious and attempt to compensate by writing down information, attempting to structure routines, and simplifying responsibilities. These coping mechanisms may give patients the appearance of intact cognitive abilities for a while, even though they are actually in decline.

Alzheimer Disease

Alzheimer disease is one form of progressive dementia. Alzheimer disease, the most common cause of dementia among people 65 years of age and older, with nearly one in eight older adults affected by Alzheimer Disease. It is the fifth leading cause of death in older adults. An estimated 5.4 million American have Alzheimer Disease, of which 5.2 million are over 65 years of age. (Alzheimer Organization, 2011). The duration of illness, from onset of symptoms to death, averages 8 to 10 years.

At this time, there is no cure or way to prevent Alzheimer disease. As more and more Americans live longer, the number affected by Alzheimer disease will continue to grow, unless a cure or effective prevention is discovered. Alzheimer disease causes a gross, diffuse atrophy of the cerebral cortex. It is associated with extracellular plaques with beta-amyloid protein deposits and neurofibrillary tangles in the cortical neurons, with eventual loss of neurons. The earliest loss of neurons occurs in the nucleus basalis and the entorhinal cortex, where cholinergic neurons are preferentially affected. As the illness progresses, up to 90% of cholinergic neurons in the nucleus basalis baseline may be lost. Cholinergic deficiency in Alzheimer disease is most prominent at the more advanced stages.

Typically, Alzheimer disease begins insidiously with short-term memory loss, whereas long-term memory is initially spared. Eventually, long-term memory is also lost as the disease progresses. In addition to memory loss, other cognitive deficits also impair activities of daily living. People with Alzheimer disease frequently repeat questions, forget phone messages and appointments, do not pay bills, and get lost driving. They may lose weight because they no longer shop for food, cook, or eat. Furthermore, the cognitive deficits are relentlessly progressive; affective, behavioral, and motor signs become more common as the disease advances.

In addition to the cognitive deficits, behavioral and psychiatric symptoms (e.g., abnormal sleep, delusions, depression, hallucinations, mania, violent outbursts, and wandering) tend to occur at some point in most patients with Alzheimer-type dementia.

Vascular Dementia

Vascular dementia results from damage to brain tissue, caused by cerebrovascular events such as transient ischemic attacks or strokes. The areas that experience infarcts are associated with specific neurologic functions, so that an infarct in the cerebellum, for example, can produce problems with motor coordination or balance. Although vascular dementia and Alzheimer dementia differ in cause, many of the symptoms are similar.

Other Dementias

Dementia can also be caused by a variety of medical conditions. The primary mechanism of this diagnosis is the presence of or a noted history of a disease, such as AIDS, Parkinson disease, Huntington chorea, hypothyroidism, normal pressure hydrocephalus, brain tumor, or vitamin B_{12} deficiency. The symptoms caused by these conditions are also similar to those described earlier for Alzheimer disease. Box 17.3 presents risks for and causes of dementia, both irreversible and potentially reversible. Plassman et al. (2007) estimates that 30% of all dementias are caused by syndromes other than Alzheimer's disease.

Delirium

Delirium is a sudden disruption in cognitive functioning, most often caused by a physical change in the body, rather than by changes within the brain. This physical change prevents the

---

Box 17.3 RISK FACTORS AND POSSIBLE CAUSES OF DEMENTIA

Irreversible Risk Factors/Causes

- Age over 65 years
- Cerebral infarction or ischemia
- Diseases such as cardiovascular disorders, type 1 diabetes, degenerative (e.g., Parkinson disease), neoplasms
- Male gender
- Genetic factors such as apolipoprotein E gene on chromosome 19 and chromosome 10

Potentially Reversible Risk Factors/Causes

- Depression
- Diseases such as type 2 diabetes, hyperlipidemia, hypertension, infections
- Drugs with iatrogenic/idiosyncratic effect or polypharmacy
- Lifestyle habits such as excessive alcohol consumption, smoking, illicit drug use, among others
- Metabolic disorders
- Nutritional disorders
- Toxins
- Trauma

brain from receiving some critical element (e.g., blood or oxygen) that it needs to function effectively. This event can be conceptualized as "brain failure," just as any other organ fails as a result of physical impairment. A hallmark symptom of "brain failure" is a disturbance in the level of consciousness that comes and goes throughout the day or days when delirium is present. This disturbance can be either increases in activity (e.g., agitation, aggression, psychosis) or decreases in activity (e.g., somnolence, lethargy, apathy). This pattern is called waxing and waning. Another symptom of delirium, as with dementia, is that psychotic-like symptoms can occur in which the person loses touch with reality. Thus, the patient may experience hallucinations and delusions. Some causes of delirium include substance withdrawal, infection (e.g., septicemia and urinary tract infections), sensory deprivation, metabolic disturbances (arising from renal failure, diabetic ketoacidosis, hypoxia, and fluid or electrolyte imbalance), and adverse effects from some medications. One major difference between delirium and dementia is its onset. Unlike that of dementia, which is slow and gradual, the onset of delirium is rapid.

To treat delirium effectively, the underlying cause must first be identified. *Untreated delirium can be fatal because the underlying condition is not diagnosed and treated.* Although use of an antipsychotic or sedative calms the patient, it does not resolve the cause of the delirium.

Ⓒ ANTIPSYCHOTICS

• Ⓒ TYPICAL ANTIPSYCHOTICS

The typical antipsychotics were the first antipsychotic drugs created. They are sometimes referred to as the conventional antipsychotics. The use of the original drug in this class, chlorpromazine (Thorazine), has become limited because of its substantial adverse effects. Haloperidol (Haldol) is a commonly used typical antipsychotic and is the prototype for the class. No one drug or drug class is preferable for all patients with schizophrenia. The choice of the appropriate antipsychotic therapy, if the typicals and atypicals are equally effective and seem to have similar benefits, is related to the potential adverse effects that might occur. Some patients are willing to risk certain adverse effects but not others. So for some patients, especially those who would be at high risk of long-term cardiovascular impairment from metabolic syndrome, a typical antipsychotic may be the better drug, assuming prophylactic therapy is provided to minimize the risk of EPS. Other patients, who may be more sensitive to the EPS from a typical antipsychotic, may be better candidates for an atypical antipsychotic (Stahl, 2008).

Erik Johnsen and Hugo A. Jørgensen (2008) provide a review of sixteen randomized trials regarding the effectiveness of second generation antipsychotics. They found that olanzapine may have better drug adherence than other second generation antipsychotics, however olanzapine may also have an increase in metabolic side effects.

Nursing Management of the Patient Receiving Ⓟ Haloperidol

Core Drug Knowledge

Pharmacotherapeutics

Haloperidol is used to treat psychotic disorders such as schizophrenia. It is also used to treat Tourette disorder, and it is indicated for pediatric patients with hyperactivity or severe behavioral problems. Off-label, it is used to treat nausea, vomiting, intractable hiccups, psychosis, delirium, and in phencyclidine (PCP)–induced psychosis. Haloperidol can be administered orally, intramuscularly, and intravenously.

Pharmacokinetics

Haloperidol is fairly well absorbed. Its bioavailability from oral doses is 60% to 65%. It is highly protein bound, at 92%. Its exact mechanism of metabolism is unknown, although almost all of it is eliminated by metabolism; about 1% is eliminated in the urine and stool. Research has found that ethnic background influences the pharmacokinetics of haloperidol. Asians achieved a 50% higher plasma concentration of haloperidol than whites who received the same dose. It is hypothesized that this difference is attributable to inherent differences in metabolism, but the precise reason is not known.

Pharmacodynamics

Haloperidol can take several days to reach its full therapeutic effect. The exact cause of this delay is unknown. The delay is frequently more frustrating to the nursing staff than to the patient. Haloperidol produces its effects by blocking dopamine (specifically, D_2), alpha, and serotonin receptors. It has minimal blocking effects at cholinergic and histamine receptors.

Blockade of dopaminergic receptors produces a decrease in movement disorders, relief of hallucinations and delusions, relief of psychosis, worsening of negative symptoms, and release of prolactin. Dopamine blockade also quiets the chemoreceptive trigger zone in the brain that produces nausea and vomiting, thereby relieving these symptoms. Blockade of dopamine receptors may actually create the net effect of too much cholinergic stimulation because the delicate balance between these two systems is altered. Many of the adverse effects from haloperidol are related to this relative imbalance between dopamine and cholinergic neurotransmitters.

Anticholinergic effects from haloperidol are modest but explain adverse effects such as dry mouth. How can haloperidol cause a relative excess of acetylcholine, but also anticholinergic effects? Remember that many drugs are only *relatively selective* for which receptors they stimulate or block. Here, the predominant effect is blockade of dopamine receptors, so the most common adverse effect will be not enough dopamine effects and too much acetylcholine effects. At the same time, *some* cholinergic receptors are also blocked by haloperidol, so there can be some symptoms related to cholinergic blockade (anticholinergic effects).

Other receptors affected by the nonselective actions of haloperidol are the alpha, serotonin, and histamine receptors. Blockade of alpha receptors produces many of the cardiac adverse effects of haloperidol treatment. Other adverse effects, related to alterations in mood, are caused by the blockade of serotonin receptors. Blockade of histamine receptors produces adverse effects such as sedation.

Haloperidol may also decrease the seizure threshold in patients with seizure disorder. Haloperidol controls the positive symptoms of schizophrenia but has no effect on the negative symptoms. Occasionally, the negative symptoms may worsen with haloperidol therapy.

Contraindications and Precautions

Haloperidol is contraindicated if the patient has hypersensitivity to any of the drug's components. It is also contraindicated in Parkinson disease because cholinergic stimulation in that disorder is already excessive.

Haloperidol and other typical antipsychotics carry a black box warning that administration to elderly patients with dementia-related psychosis increases the risk of death in these patients. Deaths are mostly related to cardiovascular events (such as heart failure or sudden death) or infections (such as pneumonia). Haloperidol is not approved for use in patients with dementia related psychosis. This black box warning does not mean that these drugs cannot be used, just that the potential risks and benefits must be weighed. Under certain circumstances prescribers may use the antipsychotics in dementia related psychosis, especially when the psychosis produces aggressive or violent outbursts and other medications have failed (Meeks & Jeste, 2008).

Haloperidol should be administered with caution to patients who:

- Have been exposed to extreme heat or phosphorous insecticides
- Use atropine or other anticholinergic drugs
- Are currently withdrawing from alcohol
- Have any disorder of the skin (dermatosis) or other allergic reactions to phenothiazine derivatives (because of the risk for cross-sensitivity)
- Have experienced an idiosyncratic response to other centrally acting drugs
- Are pregnant, because it is a pregnancy category C drug

Adverse Effects

Adverse effects, which can be perceived as a substantial nuisance or a source of embarrassment to the patient, are the primary reason that patients stop taking haloperidol. Although many adverse effects can be managed or minimized pharmacologically, some patients need to accept that they will experience some adverse effects in order to have their psychotic symptoms controlled.

Adverse effects from haloperidol come from the blockade of various neurotransmitter receptors. The major risk to the patient receiving haloperidol comes from a group of symptoms called **extrapyramidal symptoms** (EPS). The cause of these symptoms is the relative lack of dopamine stimulation (i.e., excess dopamine blockade) and relative excess of cholinergic stimulation. EPS are the most common adverse

effects of haloperidol. The risk of EPS increases if drug therapy is repeatedly and abruptly stopped and then restarted.

There are four major presentations of EPS. The first is Parkinson-like effects (also known as pseudoparkinsonism). With this adverse effect, the patient demonstrates symptoms that are typically seen in Parkinson disease, such as cog-wheeling muscle rigidity, fine tremor, slow motor responses, and a flat affect (a mask-like facial expression). It is important to distinguish this flat affect from the primary symptom of schizophrenia, which is flat affect without the mask-like features, combined with social withdrawal.

The second presentation of EPS is akathisia, a constant feeling of restlessness that the patient cannot control or explain. This presentation must be distinguished from signs of anxiety related to an identifiable source of worry.

The third presentation of EPS is acute dystonia, which involves prolonged muscular contractions and spasms. The spasms may present as arching and twisting of the neck, arching of the back, rolling of the eyes up toward the back of the head, or spasms of the laryngeal-pharyngeal muscles (which may occlude the airway, if the spasms are severe, and can be life-threatening). These symptoms cannot be controlled, occur suddenly, and may be frightening and painful.

The fourth presentation of EPS is called **tardive dyskinesia.** Tardive dyskinesia generally occurs late in haloperidol therapy and usually is irreversible. It is most commonly related to high doses and long-term use. Approximately 1 in 25 patients treated for a period of 1 year develops tardive dyskinesia. After treatment for 7 years, the incidence increases to one in four patients. Symptoms of tardive dyskinesia include involuntary lip smacking, chewing, mouth movements, tongue protrusion, blinking, grimacing, and involuntary muscle twitching of the limbs. Risk factors for developing tardive dyskinesia are listed in Box 17.4.

Other fairly common adverse effects of haloperidol include drowsiness, sedation, somnolence, lethargy, and dysphoria (a decline in mood). It has been hypothesized that the complaints of drowsiness and sedation may actually be signs of drug-induced depression that have been misinterpreted by the patient and the clinician. More research is needed to help devise antipsychotic drugs that do

---

Box 17.4 RISK FACTORS FOR TARDIVE DYSKINESIA (TD)

If the patient is receiving treatment with "typical" antipsychotics, additional factors that place the patient at risk for TD include:

- 6 months of antipsychotic therapy
- Increased length of antipsychotic therapy
- Antipsychotic dosage change—either increased or decreased
- Diagnosis of organic mental disorder or mood disorder
- Increased age
- Diabetes
- Genetic predisposition
- Race (African Americans may be twice as likely to develop TD than whites)

not produce these adverse effects, so that the quality of life can be improved for patients requiring long-term therapy.

Haloperidol used in higher than recommended doses and administration via the intravenous route (a non-approved route) has been associated with serious cardiovascular problems such as QT-prolongation, Torsades de Pointes (a form of ventricular tachycardia), and sudden death.

Use of typical antipsychotics such as haloperidol puts the patient at risk for developing a relatively rare, although potentially fatal, adverse effect called **neuroleptic malignant syndrome.** This syndrome is characterized by fever, sweating, tachycardia, muscle rigidity, tremor, incontinence, stupor, leukocytosis, elevated creatinine phosphokinase levels, and renal failure. Patients are more likely to develop neuroleptic malignant syndrome if they are dehydrated or taking large doses of haloperidol. Neuroleptic malignant syndrome can occur with use of any of the typical antipsychotics. In addition to having an underlying psychotic illness, the patient now also becomes delirious.

Leukopenia and neutropenia have been reported related to antipsychotic use, including haloperidol. This is usually a temporary effect. Another potentially fatal, although extremely rare, adverse effect of haloperidol is agranulocytosis. Although this adverse effect is possible, it is more common with the atypical antipsychotics.

A variety of other uncommon adverse effects can occur as a result of the use of haloperidol. They are categorized as:

• Cardiovascular (tachycardia, hypotension, hypertension)
• CNS (agitation, anxiety, catatonia-like state, confusion, convulsions, depression, euphoria, hallucinations, headache, insomnia, sedation, libido increases, transient dyskinetic signs, vertigo) (mostly from serotonin blockade and histamine blockade)
• Dermatologic (acne, alopecia, maculopapular skin reactions, photosensitivity)
• Gastrointestinal (anorexia, constipation, diarrhea, dry mouth, dyspepsia, nausea, salivation, vomiting) (from cholinergic blockade)
• Genitourinary (breast engorgement, galactorrhea, gynecomastia, impotence, breast pain, menstrual irregularities, priapism [prolonged erection], urinary retention)

• Hematologic and lymphatic (anemia, hyperglycemia, hypoglycemia, hyponatremia, leukocytosis, leukopenia, elevated blood ammonia levels, lymphomonocytosis)
• Hepatic (jaundice, impaired liver function)
• Musculoskeletal (severe spasms causing arching of the body from head to toe)
• Respiratory (bronchospasms, laryngospasm, increased depth of respiration)
• Special senses (cataracts, blurred vision, visual disturbances, retinopathy)
• Miscellaneous (sudden death, withdrawal syndrome, heat stroke, local tissue reactions from injection)

Drug Interactions
A few drug interactions are known to occur with haloperidol. Cigarette smoking has been linked with lower serum levels of haloperidol. Table 17.2 lists agents that interact with haloperidol.

Assessment of Relevant Core Patient Variables
Health Status
Assess the patient to determine whether he or she has an illness that is treated suitably with antipsychotics. Ensure that the patient does not have Parkinson disease, which is a contraindication for use of haloperidol. Also, assess for other conditions that require precautions for haloperidol use. Assess for a history of seizure disorder because haloperidol decreases the seizure threshold. Dehydration places patients at greater risk for developing neuroleptic malignant syndrome.

Life Span and Gender
Assess the patient's age. Determine whether the patient is pregnant or could become pregnant because haloperidol is a pregnancy category C drug. Safety and efficacy in children has not been assessed. Infants should not be breast-fed if the mother is receiving haloperidol. Oral haloperidol should not be used in children younger than 3 years. Young adult males, especially young black males, have the highest risk for the various dystonias. Older adult women have the highest risk of tardive dyskinesia. Older adults with dementia related psychosis are at higher risk of death from haloperidol and other typical antipsychotics.

TABLE 17.2	Agents That Interact with P Haloperido	
Interactants	**Effect and Significance**	**Nursing Management**
anticholinergic agents	Decreased haloperidol serum concentrations	Coadminister with caution
azole antifungal agents	May elevate haloperidol serum concentrations	Adjust dose as needed
carbamazepine	Therapeutic effects of haloperidol may be decreased	Adjust dose as needed
charcoal	Charcoal can decrease absorption	Do not give together
lithium	Alterations in consciousness, encephalopathy, EPS, fever	Discontinue either drug if interaction is suspected
Maalox	Impairs absorption of typical (and possibly atypical) antipsychotics	Do not take within 1 h of taking haloperidol
rifamycins	May decrease haloperidol serum concentrations	Adjust dose as needed

CRITICAL THINKING SCENARIO

WHAT'S WRONG WITH THIS PATIENT?

Your patient, Mr. Jones, has schizophrenia and has been receiving haloperidol, 10 mg twice a day, and benztropine, 2 mg twice a day. His psychotic symptoms are usually well controlled. Today when he comes to the clinic for a checkup he tells you that "the voices" have been speaking to him again, warning him of a plot by terrorists to kill him. You ask to see all of the medications that he has brought with him. In addition to the haloperidol and the benztropine, you find a half-used package of over-the-counter diphenhydramine (Benadryl). He states he is having trouble with seasonal allergies.

1. As this patient's nurse, what do you think is happening to Mr. Jones?
2. As this patient's nurse, what actions should you take?

Lifestyle, Diet, and Habits

Assess the patient's typical daily fluid intake to determine whether the patient is sufficiently hydrated. Determine whether the patient smokes cigarettes, because smoking may decrease the effectiveness of haloperidol. Alcohol may have additive CNS effects with haloperidol, leading to profound CNS depression.

Environment

Assess the environment where the drug will be given. Intravenous (IV) administration is restricted to an inpatient setting and increases the risk of serious cardiovascular adverse effects. Intramuscular (IM) doses may be administered in an outpatient setting. Some formulations act as drug depots and slowly release the drug over several weeks. Other times, IM doses may be administered as an emergency treatment until the person can be admitted to an inpatient setting, or the acute symptoms are controlled. Oral haloperidol can be administered in any environmental setting. Because photosensitivity is a possible adverse effect, assess whether the person is outside frequently.

Culture and Inherited Traits

Assess the patient's ethnicity, because Asians have a 50% higher serum level of haloperidol than whites. This difference may affect the dose required to be effective.

Nursing Diagnoses and Outcome

- Risk for Injury related to EPS from haloperidol
  Desired outcome: The patient will remain injury-free from haloperidol as EPS are prevented or minimized.
- Altered Thought Processes related to hallucinations and delusion
  Desired outcome: The patient's hallucinations and delusions will be controlled by haloperidol therapy.
- Risk for Ineffective Management of Therapeutic Regimen, Individual, related to adverse effects of drug therapy or poor understanding of the need for drug therapy
  Desired outcome: The patient will take haloperidol therapy as directed.

Planning and Intervention

Maximizing Therapeutic Effects

Encourage the patient to take the drug routinely. Ensure that the patient has swallowed the medication when it is administered and that the patient has not kept the medication in his or her cheek (a practice referred to as "cheeking") in order to spit it out and avoid taking the medication. Depot or long-acting injections may be used to ensure medication adherence (Ascher-Svanum et al., 2009)

Minimizing Adverse Effects

Adverse effects are common and dose related. The goal of therapy is to find a dose that effectively controls the psychotic symptoms but produces minimal adverse effects.

Some of the adverse effects (e.g., sedation and drowsiness) are transient, but they can be distressing enough to cause the patient to stop therapy. Encourage patience and continued use of the drug until it can be determined whether the adverse effects dissipate with continued use of the drug. If adverse effects are distressing to the patient, modify the treatment plan to make the therapy more acceptable. For example, instead of giving two equal-sized doses daily to a patient, the larger dose or the entire daily dose could be given at bedtime if daytime sedation is a major problem. Additionally, encourage the patient to be as active as possible during the daytime hours to help ward off sedation.

Many of the adverse effects that are not transient can be minimized to some extent. For example, encourage the patient with akathisia to walk when he or she feels restless. Because many of the adverse effects are related to a relative excess of cholinergic stimulation, anticholinergic drugs—most commonly diphenhydramine, benztropine, *amantidine,* or trihexyphenidyl—may be administered to treat or minimize these effects. The choice of drug and the route of drug administration are dependent on the severity of the EPS present and the degree of patient distress. If the patient is experiencing acute dystonic symptoms, diphenhydramine (Benadryl) or benztropine may be used either intramuscularly or intravenously. Diphenhydramine works rapidly to alleviate acute dystonia, especially those forms that could be life threatening. Once a patient experiences acute EPS, the likelihood increases that acute EPS will recur. To prevent recurrence, benztropine or trihexyphenidyl is added to existing drug therapy on a continuing basis. Sometimes, these drugs are started prophylactically to prevent EPS. However, remember that these drugs have their own adverse effects (see Chapter 21 for more information). EPS are more likely to occur if the patient repeatedly stops and restarts therapy; thus, the patient should be encouraged to stay on drug therapy once started. Akathisia is sometimes difficult to differentiate from anxiety. If this difficulty arises, the prescriber may treat for one or the other, assess the effectiveness of therapy, and change the drugs if the patient does not respond positively to drug therapy.

If the patient develops neuromalignant syndrome, stop the antipsychotic immediately, as this is a potentially life-threatening event. Notify the prescriber that the medication has been stopped for this reason, and obtain orders to treat the syndrome symptomatically. Infuse large volumes of normal saline as quickly as the patient can tolerate, which not only rehydrates the patient but also flushes the drug from the person's body. Antipyretics are also usually administered. Because of the delirium that can occur with neuromalignant syndrome, safety precautions may be required. If necessary, stay with the patient continuously, decrease environmental stimuli, or apply physical restraints (although restraints are usually used only as a last resort).

Providing Patient and Family Education

- Teach patients and families about realistic expectations of antipsychotic therapy. Include information about the delay before relief of symptoms and the necessity of continuing with the medication even after symptom relief is achieved.
- Inform patients and families about possible adverse effects. They need to understand that some adverse effects will have to be managed because it may not be possible to eliminate them completely.
- Encourage patients to report adverse effects so that these effects can be managed appropriately.
- Teach patients to avoid using alcohol and other CNS depressant drugs in order to avoid any additive effects that will produce CNS depression.
- Encourage patients to wear protective covering and sunscreen if they are outside a great deal. Advise them to balance the need to wear clothing to protect from photosensitivity with the need to choose clothing that is cool enough to prevent overheating and heat stroke. Remind patients to drink extra fluids when they are out in the heat in order to prevent dehydration that could lead to neuromalignant syndrome.
- Caution patients about use of heavy machinery or driving until individual response to the drug is known.

Ongoing Assessment and Evaluation

Treatment with haloperidol is considered effective if the psychotic symptoms are controlled or reduced and the patient does not develop serious adverse effects.

Drugs Closely Related to 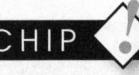 Haloperidol

The other typical antipsychotics are closely related to haloperidol. Molindone (Moban), perphenazine, loxapine (Loxitane), trifluoperazine, fluphenazine (Prolixin), thiothixene (Navane), and pimozide are very similar to the prototype haloperidol in terms of therapeutic uses, pharmacokinetics, pharmacodynamics, and adverse effects. A few exceptions should be noted. The use of pimozide is restricted to treatment of Tourette syndrome. Thiothixene and pimozide have significantly longer half-lives than haloperidol. Unlike haloperidol, some of the typical antipsychotics are metabolized by the P-450 system: pimozide by CYP3A and CYP1A2 and perphenazine by CYP2D6. Molindone and perphenazine create more sedation than haloperidol.

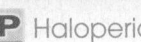

MEMORY CHIP

P Haloperidol

- Typical antipsychotic used to treat schizophrenia and other psychotic illnesses
- Creates its effects by blocking dopamine (specifically D_2), alpha, serotonin, and histamine receptors; minimal blocking effects at cholinergic receptors
- Major contraindication: Parkinson disease
- Most common adverse effect: extrapyramidal symptoms (EPS) such as pseudoparkinsonism, akathisia, acute dystonia, and tardive dyskinesia
- EPS adverse effects are caused by relative lack of dopamine stimulation.
- Most serious adverse effect: neuromalignant syndrome
- **Life span alert: Young adult males, especially young black males, have the highest risk for dystonias. Older adult women have the highest risk for tardive dyskinesia.**
- Maximizing therapeutic effects: Encourage patient to take therapy; check that patient has swallowed drug.
- Minimizing adverse effects: Keep dose as low as possible; avoid going on and off the drug therapy because this behavior increases risk for EPS; administer anticholinergic drugs to treat or prevent EPS adverse effects.
- Most important patient education: importance of continued therapy; how to cope with transient adverse effects and minimize impact of chronic adverse effects
- **Black box warning: related to use in dementia related psychosis due to increased risk for mortality in elderly dementia patients.**

Drugs Significantly Different From **P** Haloperidol

Chlorpromazine (Thorazine), thioridazine (Mellaril), and mesoridazine (Serentil) are all considered low-potency antipsychotics compared with haloperidol, which is a high-potency antipsychotic. This distinction means that a higher dosage of the low-potency drug is necessary to achieve the same antipsychotic effect that is achieved with haloperidol. There is no difference in efficacy between the high-potency and low-potency antipsychotics in treating psychotic symptoms. Recall that the definition of potency is how many milligrams of drug are needed to achieve an effect, and that efficacy refers to how effective the drug is in achieving the therapeutic goal. See Chapter 4 for a complete discussion of these terms. These antipsychotic drugs differ distinctly, however, in their adverse effect profiles. High-potency antipsychotics such as haloperidol cause little sedation or anticholinergic adverse effects such as blurry vision, constipation, dry mouth, urinary hesitation, and delirium, whereas they have a very high likelihood of causing EPS such as dystonias, akathisia, and Parkinson-like effects. Low-potency antipsychotics such as chlorpromazine, on the other hand, tend to produce sedation and frequent anticholinergic adverse effects with a low probability of EPS. Table 17.3 presents a comparison of the risks of various adverse effects with high- and low-potency antipsychotic agents.

Because the high-potency and low-potency antipsychotics alleviate psychotic symptoms to a similar degree, most

TABLE 17.3	Risk for Adverse Effects with High- and Low-Potency Typical Antipsychotics		
	Risk of Adverse Effects		
Drug Name	Anticholinergic	Extrapyramidal	Sedating
High Potency			
fluphenazine			
haloperidol			
loxapine			
molindone			
perphenazine	Low	High	Low
pimozide			
thiothixene			
trifluoperazine			
triflupromazine			
Low Potency			
chlorpromazine			
mesoridazine	High	Low	High
thioridazine			

prescribers consider which type has the least desirable adverse effect profile for each patient. A patient may also express a particular preference for one drug over another. The prescriber chooses the antipsychotic agent accordingly. For example, because an older adult is more sensitive to anticholinergic effects, a drug that produces little anticholinergic effect, such as haloperidol, may be used. Another example is a patient who has previously experienced an EPS such as akathisia from taking haloperidol, who may agree to try thioridazine, which, although more sedating, has much less likelihood of causing EPS.

● C ATYPICAL ANTIPSYCHOTICS

Atypical antipsychotics differ from the typical antipsychotics in that they target only specific dopamine receptors, whereas the typical antipsychotics target all dopamine receptors. This specificity creates a much lower adverse effect profile. Another major advantage of the atypical antipsychotics is that they treat both the negative and positive symptoms of schizophrenia. The first atypical antipsychotic was clozapine. Because this drug causes a serious adverse effect, agranulocytosis, it is not often used in the United States. When it is used, strict guidelines must be followed (Box 17.5). Olanzapine (Zyprexa), which does not carry a risk for agranulocytosis, is the prototype atypical antipsychotic.

Conventional knowledge about typical antipsychotics and atypical antipsychotics is that the atypical agents are more effective, have fewer adverse effects, and are preferable to patients. These beliefs are based on short-term efficacy trials performed when the manufacturers were first developing atypical antipsychotics and seeking FDA approval. Because atypical antipsychotics generally cost more than typical antipsychotics, several recent studies have attempted to determine if the

Box 17.5	CLOZARIL TREATMENT/PATIENT MANAGEMENT SYSTEM

Results of early clinical studies with clozapine (Clorazil) indicated that it was associated with a 1% to 2% incidence of potentially lethal agranulocytosis. To minimize this risk, clozapine is available only through treatment systems that ensure a weekly or biweekly WBC testing prior to delivery of the next supply of medication. During the 5 years of WBC monitoring with the Clozaril National Registry, the risk for agranulocytosis was reduced to approximately 0.38%. Guidelines for the Clozaril treatment/patient management system include:

- Treatment systems may include facilities with on-site pharmacies, facilities without on-site pharmacies, and individual treating physicians.
- Patients taking clozapine are enrolled in the Clozaril National Registry.
- Clozaril is only available through weekly or biweekly distribution systems.
- WBC evaluation is required prior to initiation of therapy, weekly or biweekly during therapy, and for 4 weeks after discontinuation.
- All WBC evaluations (normal and abnormal results) must be promptly reported to the Clozaril National Registry within 7 days of collection.
- The Clozaril National Registry must be promptly notified of all patients who discontinue treatment.

atypical agents are truly better and thus worth the additional cost. These research findings challenge the original assumption and indeed have set off great discussion among the psychiatric scientific community. In general, research has not found atypical antipsychotics to be more effective in managing symptoms than typical antipsychotics yet they are significantly more expensive. While atypical antipsychotics produce less tardive dyskinesia, and less akathisia, they increase the risk of hyperglycemia, hyperlipidemia, and weight gain. (Rosenheck, Perlick, Bingham, et al., 2003; Liebermann, Stroup, McEvoy, et al., 2005; Luft & Taylor, 2006). The impact on quality of life from atypical antipsychotics has not been clearly established as research is somewhat contradictory. Jones, Barnes, Davies, et al. (2006) found that patients who were randomly assigned to receive a typical antipsychotic actually had greater improvement in their quality of life and reduction in their symptoms after one year of treatment than those assigned to receive an atypical agent (other than clozapine). However, Lewis, Davies, Jones, et al. (2006) found atypical and typical antipsychotics to be similar in their effects on quality of life and symptoms in patients who had been previously unresponsive to drug therapy.

The decision to prescribe either a typical or an atypical antipsychotic will need to be based on individual basis for each patient as each can be considered to have benefits and risks.

Nursing Management of the Patient Receiving P Olanzapine

Core Drug Knowledge

Pharmacotherapeutics

Olanzapine is used to treat psychotic symptoms in schizophrenia and for short-term treatment of acute bipolar disorder with either acute mixed or manic episodes. IM forms are used to treat the associated psychomotor agitation, such as threatening, urgently distressing, or self-exhausting behaviors. Olanzapine is also used in combination therapy with lithium or valproate for the treatment of acute manic episodes in bipolar disorder. In addition, it is useful as a maintenance drug for patients with bipolar disease who have responded to acute therapy.

Other off-label uses include Alzheimer-type dementia, other dementias, and obsessive-compulsive disorder that does not respond to selective serotonin reuptake inhibitors. Some research indicates that although olanzapine does have some efficacy in the treatment of Alzheimer disease, the adverse effects offset any therapeutic advantages so its use is not recommended (Schneider, Tariot, Dagerman, et al., 2006).

Pharmacokinetics

Olanzapine is moderately absorbed and achieves a bioavailability of 60%. The drug is highly protein bound, at 93%. It is metabolized by glucuronidation and oxidation through the cytochrome P-450 system, particularly CYP1A2 and CYP2D6. Elimination is through the urine and the feces, with about twice as much being eliminated in the urine. Half-life is between 21 and 54 hours. This long half-life allows the drug to be dosed once a day.

Pharmacodynamics

Olanzapine works by blocking several neuroreceptor sites, including serotonin, dopamine, muscarinic, histamine-1 (H_1), and alpha-1. Olanzapine has high affinity for these sites but lower affinity for gamma-aminobutyric acid (GABA), benzodiazepine, and beta receptor sites, although blockade at these receptor sites also occurs. Olanzapine, like other atypical antipsychotics, affects the negative symptoms as well as the positive symptoms of schizophrenia. (This is in contrast to typical antipsychotics, such as haloperidol, which affect only the positive symptoms.) Olanzapine, as well as other atypical antipsychotics, may elevate blood glucose levels, sometimes to extremely high levels, through an unknown mechanism. Recent research indicates one possibility. A particular brain enzyme from the hypothalamus, known as AMP-kinase, is known to stimulate appetite. What has recently been discovered is that the amount of this enzyme will increase in mice given an atypical antipsychotic. AMP-kinase levels have also been found to increase if histamine receptors (specifically, H_1 receptors) are stimulated. Therefore, blocking the H_1 receptor may prevent weight gain from atypical antipsychotics (Kim, Huang, Snowman, et al., 2007).

Contraindications and Precautions

The only labeled contraindication for olanzapine is known hypersensitivity. Like haloperidol and the typical antipsychotics, olanzapine and the other atypical antipsychotics also carries a black box warning that its use in older adults with dementia related psychosis increases the risk of death from cardiovascular events and infections. Olanzapine should be avoided in older adults with dementia-related psychosis, because of this

increased risk (Salzman et al., 2008). If olanzapine or other atypical antipsychotics are used in treating dementia related psychosis, these drugs should be used for the shortest duration possible. Gradual dose reductions are recommended periodically to ensure that the lowest dosages are used. In the nursing home setting, guidelines require that these drugs are evaluated and gradual dose reductions are considered on an ongoing basis (Meeks & Jeste, 2008).

Olanzapine carries warnings for several other serious effects. Olanzapine, and all other atypical antipsychotics, may create hyperglycemia which may be severe enough to induce ketoacidosis or hyperosmolar coma, or death. Precautions should be taken if the patient has diabetes. Patients who are not diagnosed with diabetes at the start of therapy still remain at risk for developing significant hyperglycemia while taking olanzapine or other atypical antipsychotics. The risk appears to be highest in patients with multiple risk factors for diabetes. All patients should be monitored regularly for evidence of hyperglycemia. Antidiabetic therapy is frequently necessary.

Olanzapine and all other atypical antipsychotics may also induce significant hyperlipidemia and weight gain. The combination of elevated glucose levels, elevated lipid levels, and weight gain is described as metabolic syndrome and is considered a risk factor for serious cardiovascular effects, such as MI.

There is also a warning that olanzapine may induce seizures in patients with a history of seizures or with conditions that potentially lower the seizure threshold. Olanzapine should be used cautiously in patients with a history of seizure disorder because it is known to reduce the seizure threshold.

Olanzapine also carries several other precautions. Olanzapine is a pregnancy category C drug. It may cause hyperprolactinemai (elevated prolactin levels) (Lin, Poland, Lau, et al., 1988). Olanzapine may impair judgment, thinking, and motor skills, and ability to operate machinery.

Olanzapine can also induce orthostatic hypotension; additional precautions should be used if the patient receives other drugs that may cause orthostatic hypotension concurrently with olanzapine. Again, older adults are at increased risk. Caution should be used when treating patients who have hepatic impairment, in patients with pre-existing conditions that are associated with limited hepatic functional reserve, and in patients who are receiving other drugs that may cause hepatotoxicity, because clinically significant elevations of liver enzymes can occur. All antipsychotic drugs have been associated with esophageal dysmotility and aspiration; thus, olanzapine and other antipsychotics should be used cautiously in patients at risk for aspiration pneumonia.

Adverse Effects

In general, atypical antipsychotics are well tolerated and produce few adverse effects. In patients who do experience adverse effects, the most common are CNS related: drowsiness and sedation, insomnia, agitation, nervousness, hostility, and dizziness. The most serious adverse effects with olanzapine are tardive dyskinesia and neuroleptic malignant syndrome, although these effects occur very rarely.

Hyperglycemia can be common in patients with diabetes and may be pronounced enough to require insulin adjustments; diabetic ketoacidosis is possible. Patients without a history of diabetes risk developing diabetes from therapy; the more diabetic risk factors present, the more likely hyperglycemia may develop. In addition to elevated glucose levels, patients may gain weight (a significant number of patients gain more than 7% of their baseline weight), have decreased insulin sensitivity, have lipid elevations, and develop metabolic syndrome (increased visceral fat, as measured by waist circumference, hyperglycemia, hypertension, and dyslipidemia), placing the patient at increased risk for cardiovascular problems. Olanzapine has a higher risk for inducing metabolic disorders than some of the other atypical antipsychotics.

A wide variety of other adverse effects can potentially occur, including:

- Cardiovascular (hypotension, tachycardia, hypertension, bradycardia, cardiac arrest, cerebrovascular accident, chronic heart failure, palpitation, vasodilation, pulmonary embolus, and premature atrial fibrillation)
- CNS (asthenia, abnormal gate, akathisia, akinesia, tremor, amnesia, ataxia, delirium, dysarthria, hypesthesia, hypokinesia, incoordination, increased libido, vertigo, intense or abnormal dreams, euphoria, paresthesia, suicidal thoughts, neuroleptic malignant syndrome, and pseudoparkinsonism)
- Dermatologic (rash)
- Gastrointestinal (constipation, abdominal pain, weight gain, increased appetite, and dry mouth)
- Genitourinary (premenstrual syndrome)
- Musculoskeletal (arthralgia, neck rigidity, twitching, hypertonia, and tremor)
- Ocular (dimmed vision)
- Respiratory (rhinitis, cough, and pharyngitis)
- Metabolic (weight gain, increased glucose levels, increased lipid levels)

Drug Interactions

The risks of using olanzapine in combination with other drugs have not been extensively evaluated. Caution should be used when olanzapine is taken in combination with other centrally acting drugs or alcohol. Coadministering either ethanol or diazepam with olanzapine potentiates the orthostatic hypotension observed with olanzapine. Because of its potential for inducing hypotension, olanzapine may enhance the effects of certain antihypertensive agents. Olanzapine also may antagonize the effects of levodopa and dopamine agonists.

Agents that induce CYP1A2 or glucuronyl transferase enzymes, such as omeprazole and rifampin, may increase olanzapine clearance. Inhibitors of CYP1A2 could potentially inhibit olanzapine clearance. Although olanzapine is metabolized by multiple enzyme systems, induction or inhibition of a single enzyme may appreciably alter olanzapine clearance. Therefore, a dosage increase (for induction) or a dosage decrease (for inhibition) may have to be considered with specific drugs.

Carbamazepine therapy (200 mg twice daily) increases the clearance of olanzapine by approximately 50%, likely because carbamazepine is a potent inducer of CYP1A2 activity. Higher daily doses of carbamazepine may cause an even greater increase in olanzapine clearance. Fluoxetine, a CYP1A2 inhibitor, decreases the clearance of olanzapine, resulting in a mean increase in olanzapine maximum concentration (C_{max}) following fluoxetine of 54% in female nonsmokers and 77% in male smokers. Mean increases in olanzapine area under the curve (AUC) are 52% and 108%, respectively. Lower doses of olanzapine should be considered in patients receiving concomitant treatment with fluoxetine. The combination of olanzapine and the antidepressant fluoxetine increases the risk of suicide due to the increased availability of olanzapine. Table 17.4 lists potential drug interactions with olanzapine.

Assessment of Relevant Core Patient Variables

Health Status

Obtain the patient's baseline vital signs and other measurements, such as weight, serum glucose, triglyceride levels, and complete blood count, before olanzapine therapy begins. It is critical that a patient's serum glucose levels be monitored before and throughout any atypical antipsychotic therapy. Lipids levels should be monitored throughout therapy as well. Also, assess for various individual factors that

TABLE 17.4 Agents That Interact with P Olanzapine

Interactants	Effect and Significance	Nursing Management
carbamazepine	Therapeutic effects of olanzapine may be decreased	Adjust dose as needed
charcoal	Charcoal can decrease absorption	Do not give together
CYP1A2 inducers (e.g., carbamazepine, omeprazole, rifampin)	May decrease olanzapine serum concentrations	May need to increase olanzapine dose
CYP1A2 inhibitors (e.g., fluoxetine)	May increase olanzapine serum concentrations	May need to decrease dose
fluoxetine	Coadministration resulted in a small (16%) decrease in olanzapine clearance	May need to decrease olanzapine dose

can alter drug response, such as liver function and gastric absorption.

Life Span and Gender

Document the age and gender of the patient. Explore the sexual patterns and reproductive goals of the patient, because reproductive effects such as changes in libido, amenorrhea, irregular menses, impotence, and ejaculatory failure may occur. Consider whether the patient is pregnant or could become pregnant, because olanzapine is a pregnancy category C drug. The elderly patient receiving atypical antipsychotics should be considered at higher risk for adverse effects. Older adults with dementia related psychosis are at increased risk of death from infections and cardiovascular events if they receive olanzapine and other atypical antidepressants. This is an off label use of the drug.

Lifestyle, Diet, and Habits

Evaluate the patient's diet. Assess for high fat intake, high carbohydrate and sugar intake, and high overall calorie intake. Assess the baseline exercise level and throughout therapy.

Evaluate the patient's caffeine intake and diet because the efficacy of olanzapine may be affected by fluctuations in caffeine intake. Also assess for use of dong quai and St. John's wort (because these herbal medicines may cause photosensitization) and for the use of kava kava, gotu kola, valerian, St. John's wort, and ethanol (because these agents may increase CNS effects).

Assess the patient's occupational and recreational activities because orthostatic hypotension, drug-related dizziness, and blurred vision may impair coordination and dexterity, and hypotension may occur with hot tubs, hot showers, or tub baths.

Environment

Assess the climate in which the drug will be administered because drug-related heatstroke may occur in hot weather.

Nursing Diagnoses and Outcomes

Several nursing diagnoses may apply to the patient receiving atypical antipsychotics. Examples include:

- Imbalanced Nutrition: More than Body Requirements, related to increased appetite and secondary to olanzapine use
  Desired outcome: The patient will state that there is a risk for weight gain and will identify the effects of a low-fat diet and exercise on weight control.
- Risk for Injury related to drug-induced dizziness, blurred vision, and orthostatic hypotension
  Desired outcome: The patient will identify factors that increase the risk for injury and will relate intent to use safety measures and practices to prevent injury.
- Risk for Fluid and Electrolyte Imbalance and Hyperglycemia related to adverse effects of medication
  Desired outcome: The patient will maintain appropriate fluid and electrolyte balance while receiving medication.

- Risk for Sedation related to adverse effects of the medication
  Desired outcome: The patient will maintain appropriate level of wakefulness while receiving medication.

Planning and Intervention

Maximizing Therapeutic Effects

Maintaining adherence to any medication regimen once a patient experiences relief of symptoms is an ongoing challenge for all health care providers. With patients experiencing disturbances of their thoughts and perceptions, focus from the very start on developing a trusting therapeutic relationship. This trust frequently will be what enables the patient to develop the insight necessary to continue taking medication. This same trust can also form the basis on which you and the patient candidly discuss the many benefits of continuing with the medication, even if adverse effects occur. By focusing on the patient's own hopes and aspirations for the quality of life he or she wishes to have, you help contribute to adherence to the medication regimen.

Minimizing Adverse Effects

Assess fasting blood sugar before drug therapy is initiated. Fasting blood sugar must be monitored throughout therapy, especially if the patient has diabetes. Monitor all patients for signs of hyperglycemia throughout therapy. Diabetic therapy may be indicated. Lipid levels are also monitored during therapy due to the risk of metabolic syndrome related to the use of antipsychotics (Meyer et al., 2008). If older adults with dementia-related psychosis receive the drug off label, assess closely for cardiovascular complications by monitoring their EKG readings and use strict medical asepsis to minimize risk of infection and assess for indications of infection. Early assessment and treatment of these problems may minimize risk of deaths from these adverse effects. To minimize daytime drowsiness, you can give the entire daily dose at night. To prevent orthostatic hypotension, keep patients well hydrated and have them arise slowly from bed.

Providing Patient and Family Education

- Teach the signs of hyperglycemia; patients with diabetes may need to be taught to monitor blood sugar more frequently than before olanzapine therapy.
- Teach patients and families that the therapeutic response will not be immediate.
- Stress the importance of continuing drug therapy even in the absence of psychotic symptoms.
- Help patients stay motivated to continue treatment. To promote adherence to the therapeutic regimen, educate patients and families about the effects of medication—both therapeutic and adverse. Advise patients about adverse effects that, if unidentified, may contribute to nonadherence. An example of this kind of effect is sedation.
- Provide education on a low fat diet and calorie restricted diet (if indicated).
- Ensure that patients understand the importance of keeping the drug safely stored and away from curious children.

MEMORY CHIP

P Olanzapine

- Atypical antipsychotic used to treat schizophrenia and bipolar mania
- Olanzapine works by blocking serotonin, dopamine, muscarinic, H_1, and alpha-1 receptor sites
- Normally well tolerated
- Most common adverse effects: hyperglycemia (especially in diabetic patients), sedation, and drowsiness
- Most serious adverse effects: tardive dyskinesia and neuroleptic malignant syndrome (both rare)
- **Life span alert: Older adults are more at risk for adverse effects.**
- Maximizing therapeutic effects: Encourage patient to take medication regularly.
- Minimizing adverse effects: Monitor glucose levels throughout therapy for all patients; give daily dose at bedtime to decrease daytime sedation.
- Most important patient education: Full therapeutic effect will take time to achieve; patient may need to tolerate some adverse effects until they pass.
- **Black box warning: related to use in dementia related psychosis due to increased risk for mortality in elderly dementia patients.**

Ongoing Assessment and Evaluation

Treatment with an atypical antipsychotic such as olanzapine requires ongoing assessment and evaluation because of the ongoing, chronic nature of most illnesses in which they are used. For this reason, continue to assess the patient for the originally presenting symptoms for which the drug therapy was initiated. Also, evaluate the patient's ability to meet the therapeutic goals identified by the entire treatment team. Throughout this process, persist in monitoring for any adverse effects that the patient may develop, especially hyperglycemia and hyperlipidemia.

Drugs Closely Related to P Olanzapine

Drugs related to olanzapine include risperidone (Risperdal), ziprasidone (Geodon), aripiprazole (Abilify), paliperidone (Invega), clozapine (Clozaril), and quetiapine (Seroquel). Like olanzapine, these drugs are also approved for used in treating bipolar disorder and differ slightly from olanzapine in their adverse effects and half-lives. Risperidone, ziprasidone, and aripiprazole produce fewer anticholinergic effects. Quetiapine produces more sedation than olanzapine. Aripiprazole (Abilify) is a newer atypical antipsychotic and carries an indication for major depressive disorder as an adjunct treatment.

Compared with olanzapine, clozapine causes stronger anticholinergic effects and is more likely to produce sedation and orthostatic hypotension. Clozapine, too, produces significant weight gain; the other drugs closely related to olanzapine produce less weight gain. Clozapine has the unique adverse effect of increasing the risk for agranulocytosis, which can be fatal. Patients receiving clozapine require close watch of their white blood cell count. They are at most risk during the first 6 months of therapy. (See Box 17.5 for more information.)

Compared with olanzapine, aripiprazole has a longer half-life, and the other drugs have shorter half-lives.

DRUGS FOR ALZHEIMER-TYPE DEMENTIA

C ACETYLCHOLINESTERASE ENZYME INHIBITORS

Acetylcholine is a neurotransmitter for several CNS circuits that are located in the basal forebrain, the hippocampus, and parts of the cerebral cortex. Agents that augment this system have been under investigation to treat Alzheimer disease for more than 20 years, and numerous types of drugs that augment levels of acetylcholine to compensate for losses of cholinergic function in the brain have been used in these patients. These drugs have included acetylcholine precursors, muscarinic agonists, nicotinic agonists, and acetylcholinesterase inhibitors. The only Food and Drug Administration–approved drugs to treat the symptoms of Alzheimer disease are the acetylcholinesterase inhibitors. Acetylcholinesterase (AChE) is the enzyme that breaks down acetylcholine. By inhibiting the action of AChE, acetylcholinesterase inhibitors (AChEIs) prolong the activity of acetylcholine on cortical cholinergic receptors and in the synapse. The mechanism of action of the three AChEIs—tacrine, donepezil, and rivastigmine—is essentially the same. These agents increase concentrations of the memory-regulating and cognition-regulating neurotransmitter acetylcholine by reversibly inhibiting the enzyme cholinesterase. Although these drugs have not been shown to alter the course of the dementing process, it is anticipated that disease effects will lessen as the disease process advances and fewer cholinergic neurons remain intact.

The prototype drug used to treat Alzheimer-type dementia is rivastigmine (Exelon). Table 17.5 summarizes selected Alzheimer drugs.

Nursing Management of the Patient Receiving P Rivastigmine

Core Drug Knowledge

Pharmacotherapeutics

Rivastigmine is indicated for treating mild to moderate dementia of the Alzheimer type. In clinical studies, it has been shown to enhance cognition (memory, language, orientation) and improve the ability to perform activities of daily living among patients with mild to moderate Alzheimer disease. Rivastigmine may also be effective in treating vascular dementia. More research is required to confirm this possibility.

Pharmacokinetics

Rivastigmine is rapidly and completely absorbed, with peak plasma concentrations reached in 1 hour. Administering

TABLE 17.5	Summary of Selected Drugs for Alzheimer Disease		
Drug (Trade) Name	Selected Indications	Route and Dosage Range	Pharmacokinetics
[P] rivastigmine (Exelon)	Mild to moderate Alzheimer-type dementia, Mild to moderate Parkinson disease dementia	*Adult:* PO, 3–6 mg bid to a maximum of 12 mg/d, transdermal 4.6–9.5 mg/24 h *Child:* Not currently indicated	*Onset:* Intermediate *Duration:* 10 h $t_{1/2}$: 1.5 h
donepezil (Aricept)	Mild to severe Alzheimer-type dementia	*Adult:* 5–10 mg/d *Child:* Safety and efficacy not established	*Onset:* Unknown *Duration:* Unknown $t_{1/2}$: 70 h
galantamine (Razadyne)	Mild to moderate Alzheimer-type dementia	*Adult:* 4–12 mg/d	
memantine (Namenda)	Moderate to severe Alzheimer-type dementia	*Adult:* 10 mg bid (after titration) *Child:* Safety and efficacy not established	*Onset:* Unknown *Duration:* Unknown $t_{1/2}$: 60–80 h

rivastigmine with food delays drug absorption (by about 1.5 hours) but does not impair it. Rivastigmine may be taken with food if gastrointestinal adverse effects are problematic. Rivastigmine also is formulated for topical use, administered in a daily patch; this formulation decreases the gastrointestinal adverse effects.

Rivastigmine is widely distributed throughout the body. It penetrates the blood–brain barrier, reaching peak concentrations in cerebrospinal fluid in 1.4 to 2.6 hours. Rivastigmine is 40% bound to plasma proteins.

Rivastigmine is rapidly and extensively metabolized by AChE; minimal metabolism occurs by the major CYP450 isozymes. Thus, no CYP450 drug interactions have been observed. It is about equally metabolized through the hepatic cytochrome P-450 enzyme system and excreted as unchanged drug in the urine. The elimination half-life is 1.5 hours, with most elimination as metabolites excreted from the kidneys. The oral solution and capsules may be interchanged at equal doses.

Pharmacodynamics

Rivastigmine is a carbamate derivative that is believed to exert its therapeutic effect by enhancing cholinergic function. This enhancement occurs by increasing the concentration of acetylcholine through reversible inhibition of acetylcholinesterase. Rivastigmine does not alter the course of the underlying dementing process.

Contraindications and Precautions

Rivastigmine is contraindicated in patients with hypersensitivity to carbamate derivatives. No adequate or well-controlled studies have been performed in children or in pregnant or lactating women; therefore, rivastigmine should be used cautiously in these patients. Rivastigmine is in pregnancy category B. It is not known whether rivastigmine is excreted in breast milk. Like other drugs that increase cholinergic activity, rivastigmine should be used with care in patients with a history of asthma or obstructive pulmonary disease.

Adverse Effects

Rivastigmine is associated with substantial gastrointestinal adverse reactions, including nausea and vomiting, anorexia, and weight loss. Other adverse effects include dizziness, headache, chest pain, peripheral edema, vertigo, joint pain, agitation, nervousness, delusion, paranoid reaction, coughing, generalized rash, and urinary incontinence. Rivastigmine may have vagotonic effects on heart rates (resulting in bradycardia) because the drug increases cholinergic activity. These vagotonic effects may be particularly important in patients with "sick sinus syndrome" or other supraventricular cardiac conduction conditions. Because it increases cholinergic activity, rivastigmine may cause urinary obstruction and may have some potential for causing seizures, although seizure activity also may be a manifestation of Alzheimer disease.

Drug Interactions

Pharmacokinetic drug interactions are not believed to occur with rivastigmine because only minimal metabolism of the drug occurs through the major CYP450 isozymes.

Synergistic effects can be expected when AChEIs are given with succinylcholine, similar neuromuscular blocking agents, or cholinergic agonists, such as bethanechol. Because of their mechanism of action, AChEIs have the potential to interfere with the activity of anticholinergic medications.

Assessment of Relevant Core Patient Variables

Health Status

Assess body systems thoroughly. The patient's cardiac status may be adversely affected by AChEIs because these drugs increase cholinergic activity and may cause bradycardia from vagal effects on heart rate. The cholinergic activity of the AChEIs may cause urinary retention or obstruction; men with benign prostatic hypertrophy may be especially at risk.

Evaluate the patient's renal and hepatic function. Dosage adjustments may be necessary in patients with renal or hepatic function impairment. Review the patient's respiratory function because respiratory depression may occur. Carefully assess the patient's gastrointestinal status because AChEIs such as rivastigmine may increase gastric acid secretion, cause gastritis, and exacerbate peptic ulcer disease. Assess and closely monitor individuals with a history of ulcer disease or those receiving nonsteroidal anti-inflammatory drugs for symptoms of active or occult gastrointestinal bleeding.

Life Span and Gender

Assess the age of the patient. The mean oral clearance of rivastigmine is 30% lower in elderly people who take rivastigmine. Rivastigmine therapy is seldom indicated in women of childbearing years. If the drug is needed in a woman of childbearing age, assess for pregnancy and lactation. If appropriate, explore potential benefits of rivastigmine therapy compared with potential risks to the fetus or child.

Lifestyle, Diet, and Habits

Assess the patient for tobacco use because nicotine use moderately increases the oral clearance of rivastigmine (by 23%).

Environment

Be aware of the environment in which the drug will be administered. If appropriate, assess the patient's home or living environment. Secure all medication to avoid accidental inappropriate ingestion by the patient.

Nursing Diagnoses and Outcomes

- Imbalanced Nutrition: Less than Body Requirements, related to decreased desire to eat secondary to nausea and vomiting from drug therapy
  Desired outcome: The patient will ingest daily nutritional requirements in relation to activity level and metabolic needs.
- Risk for Injury related to adverse effect of sedation
  Desired outcome: The patient will establish appropriate sleep and rest patterns, participate in activities, and establish priorities for daily and weekly activities.

Planning and Intervention

Maximizing Therapeutic Effects

It is important to detect and correct any treatable factors that can cause or contribute to cognitive impairment. Be aware that any cognitive impairment may be exacerbated by hearing or visual deficits, depression, delirium arising from a urinary tract infection, heart failure, electrolyte imbalance, or anemia. When the patch form is used, rotation of the site may be necessary to ensure adequate absorption. In patients with moderate dementia, it may be necessary to place the patch on the back where it cannot be removed by them.

Minimizing Adverse Effects

Offer small frequent meals or give the drug with food to offset gastrointestinal effects of nausea and vomiting. Monitor weight throughout therapy. If weight loss occurs, encourage intake of nutrient- and calorie-rich foods that are acceptable to the patient, such as Ensure or Boost beverages, milkshakes, or puddings. When the patch form is used, assess for dermatitis or rash at the site of the patch.

Providing Patient and Family Education

The irreversible nature of Alzheimer disease and its progressive, deteriorating course have devastating effects on affected individuals, their caregivers, and their families. Although drug therapy is directed toward enhancing cognitive and functional abilities, or at least slowing the cognitive decline, teaching considerations reflect more issues regarding the disease process and its progressive nature as well as the burdens facing the caregiver.

- Advise patients and families that nausea and vomiting are likely with rivastigmine use and that anorexia and weight loss may result. Encourage them to monitor for these adverse events and to inform the prescriber if they occur. Inform them that there is a patch form and this may decrease the gastrointestinal adverse effects, thus improving compliance.
- To increase the likelihood that patients will accept the medication from caregivers willingly, teach helpful communication techniques, such as using concrete language, maintaining social greetings and rituals, using a soft tone of voice, and simplifying and repeating instructions frequently.

Ongoing Assessment and Evaluation

Rivastigmine, as with other AChEIs, produces only modest improvement in some measures of cognitive functioning and in other areas of functioning in the patient with mild to moderate Alzheimer disease, apparently slowing the progression of the disease. However, advise patients and their families to maintain realistic expectations regarding what the drug can do.

MEMORY CHIP

P Rivastigmine

- Used in Alzheimer-type dementia
- Works by inhibiting acetylcholinesterase (the enzyme that breaks down acetylcholine), thus increasing the amount of active acetylcholine
- Most common adverse effects: gastrointestinal
- Most serious adverse effect: bradycardia
- Maximizing therapeutic effect: Assess for and correct any treatable factors that may impair cognition.
- Minimizing adverse effects: Offer small, frequent meals; monitor weight; offer nutritional supplements.
- Minimizing adverse effects: consider transdermal option to reduce the gastrointestinal adverse effects.
- Most important patient and family education: that drug therapy will not cure Alzheimer disease but will minimize symptoms; importance of monitoring weight; and techniques to gain patient acceptance of medication

Drugs Closely Related to P Rivastigmine

Donepezil (Aricept), galantamine hydrobromide (Razadyne), and tacrine (Cognex) all have similar pharmacotherapeutics and pharmacokinetics. Donepezil and galantamine are believed to be as effective as rivastigmine in the treatment of Alzheimer disease, although the therapeutic effect is very small. Tacrine may not be as effective as the other drugs. Like rivastigmine, these three drugs may also be effective in treating vascular dementia; more research is necessary to confirm this possibility. In contrast to rivastigmine, which is metabolized by cholinesterase, donepezil, galantamine, and tacrine are metabolized via the P-450 enzyme system. Donepezil seems to cause fewer gastrointestinal adverse effects than either rivastigmine or galantamine. Gradually slowing the titration of rivastigmine and galantamine over at least 3 months may minimize the gastrointestinal effects, making the GI adverse effects from the three drugs similar. The rivastigmine patch may be used to encourage compliance as it is dosed once daily and often reduces gastrointestinal side effects. Donepezil is dosed daily.

Drug Significantly Different From P Rivastigmine

Memantine (Namenda) is a drug for Alzheimer disease that works in a different way than the prototype rivastigmine. *N*-methyl-D-aspartate (NMDA) receptors are believed to be involved in learning and memory, and excessive stimulation of NMDA receptors by the neurotransmitter glutamate is believed to be involved in Alzheimer disease. Normally magnesium ions move away from the receptors, and glutamate then stimulates the receptors. Depolarization occurs at the time glutamate attaches, so calcium is allowed to flow into the calcium channels. Glutamate usually experiences reuptake in the synapse by the glia cell.

However, glutamate reuptake is prevented in Alzheimer disease, and thus glutamate remains in the synapse for a much longer time. Therefore, glutamate continues to stimulate the NMDA receptors, allowing excess calcium to flow into the cell. As the cell normally responds to changes in levels of calcium, this signal is muted with continuous infusion and function declines. Overactivation of glutamate receptors and continuous calcium influx ultimately cause damage to neurons and further decline of cognitive functions. This mechanism may be responsible for both cognitive deficits and neuronal loss in neurodegenerative dementia. Memantine blocks these NMDA receptor sites to prevent the glutamate from overstimulating the receptor. The synaptic level of glutamine does not decrease, but it is prevented from attaching to the NMDA receptor.

The benefits of memantine therapy are modest, and patients can experience a slowing of disease deterioration. Other patients may experience slight improvement in their symptoms. As the drug works in a different way than other drugs for Alzheimer disease, it can be used as combination therapy in disease management. Unlike the prototype rivastigmine, which is for mild to moderate Alzheimer disease, memantine is for moderate to severe disease.

Memantine is generally very well tolerated; in clinical trials the type and rate of adverse effects were similar to those associated with a placebo. Possible adverse effects include dizziness, constipation, headache, and confusion. In clinical trials during drug development, some patients with Alzheimer disease experienced a temporary period of confusion when starting drug therapy or when increasing the dose during the titration period. Memantine is administered orally twice a day.

CHAPTER SUMMARY

- Thought, like mood, is controlled by combinations of neurotransmitters that stimulate neuroreceptors in the brain. The primary neurotransmitter related to thought processing is believed to be dopamine.
- Another important neurotransmitter is acetylcholine. Many areas of the brain secrete acetylcholine; reduction in the amount of this neurotransmitter causes cognitive changes. Acetylcholine has a number of functions including arousal, coordination of movement, memory acquisition, and memory retention. Norepinephrine and serotonin are other neurotransmitters that are believed to be important to normal thought, but their exact mechanisms are not known yet.
- Schizophrenia, a psychotic disorder, has components termed positive and negative symptoms. The term "positive symptom" does not mean that the changes are beneficial to the patient. The positive symptoms of hallucinations and delusions add a layer of something new to the person. They are in excess of or are a distortion of normal brain function. The "negative symptoms" take away from the person's personality and represent a loss or a diminishing of normal brain function. Negative symptoms include flat or blunted emotions, lack of pleasure or interest in things (anhedonia), and limited speech.
- Haloperidol (Haldol) is the prototype typical antipsychotic. It is used to treat psychotic disorders, such as schizophrenia, and relieves primarily positive symptoms. The full therapeutic effect from haloperidol can require several days to develop. Haloperidol creates its effects by blocking dopamine (specifically, D_2), alpha, serotonin, and histamine receptors. It has minimal blocking effects on cholinergic receptors.
- Haloperidol's blockade of dopaminergic receptors produces decreased symptoms of movement disorders, relief of hallucinations and delusions, relief of psychosis, worsened negative symptoms, a release of prolactin, and a quieting of the chemoreceptive trigger zone in the brain. Its blockade of alpha, serotonin, histamine, and cholinergic receptors produces many of its adverse effects.
- The most common reason patients stop taking antipsychotic medications like haloperidol is the occurrence of adverse effects. The higher the dose of haloperidol, the more likely the patient will experience adverse effects. Stopping and starting therapy also increases the likelihood of developing extrapyramidal symptoms (EPS). Encourage the patient to stay with therapy, because some of the adverse effects are transient and can be managed.
- Chlorpromazine (Thorazine), thioridazine (Mellaril), and mesoridazine (Serentil) are all considered low-potency typical antipsychotics, compared with haloperidol, which is a high-potency antipsychotic. A higher dosage of these drugs is necessary to achieve the same antipsychotic affect as those achieved with haloperidol. Both types of typical antipsychotics have the same effectiveness, although they have different adverse effects. High-potency typical antipsychotics, such as haloperidol, have a very high likelihood of causing EPS (e.g., dystonias, akathisia, and Parkinson-like adverse effects). Low-potency typical antipsychotics are more likely to produce sedation and anticholinergic adverse effects but are unlikely to produce EPS.

- Atypical antipsychotics differ from the typical antipsychotics in that they target specific dopamine receptors instead of all of them and that they treat both the negative and positive symptoms of psychotic disorders.
- In general, atypical antipsychotics such as olanzapine are well tolerated and produce few adverse effects, although some patients experience sedation and dizziness. Elevated blood glucose levels can also be problematic, especially for patients with diabetes.
- Drugs that augment levels of acetylcholine, by preventing its breakdown by acetylcholinesterase, compensate for losses of cholinergic function in the brain and are used to treat Alzheimer-type dementia. Rivastigmine (Exelon) is the prototype acetylcholinesterase inhibitor (AChEI).
- Rivastigmine produces modest improvement in some measures of cognitive functioning and in other areas of functioning in the patient with mild to moderate Alzheimer disease, apparently slowing the progression of the disease. The most common adverse effects are gastrointestinal.
- Memantine is also used to treat patients with Alzheimer disease. It works in a unique way to prevent glutamine from overstimulating NMDA receptors. Its effect is also modest.

QUESTIONS FOR STUDY AND REVIEW

1. What are the major differences between high-potency and low-potency typical antipsychotic drugs?
2. Define EPS.
3. What are the differences between typical antipsychotics such as haloperidol and atypical antipsychotics such as olanzapine?
4. Why can acute dystonias be a medical emergency?
5. Describe some of the suggestions that you could offer to a patient to help him or her cope with sedation and drowsiness when haloperidol therapy is first initiated.
6. Describe how rivastigmine produces therapeutic effects in Alzheimer-type dementia.

NEED MORE HELP?

Chapter 17 of the Study Guide to Accompany *Drug Therapy in Nursing*, 4th Edition, contains NCLEX-style questions and other learning activities to reinforce your understanding of the concepts presented in this chapter. For additional information or to purchase the study guide, visit thePoint.

REFERENCES

Alzheimer Organization (2011). Alzheimer's Disease Facts and Figures. Accessed March 25, 2011 online at: http://www.alz.org/downloads/Facts_Figures_2011.pdf

Ascher-Svanum, H., Xiaomei, P., Faires, D., Montgomery, W. & Haddad, P. M. (2009). Treatment patterns and clinical characteristics prior to initiating depot typical antipsychotics for non-adherent schizophrenia patients. *BMC Psychiatry*, 9:46.

American Psychiatric Association (October 2007). APA Practice Guideline: Treatment of Patients With Alzheimer's Disease and Other Dementias, 2nd ed. Accessed online March 25, 2011 at: www.psych.org

Johansen, E. & Jorgensen, H. A. (2008). Effectiveness of second generation antipsychotics: A systematic review of randomized trials. *BMC Psychiatry*. 8:31.

Jones, P. B., Barnes, T. R., Davies, L., et al. (2006). Randomized controlled trial of the effect on quality of life or second- vs first-generation antipsychotic drugs in schizophrenia: Cost

Utility of the Latest Antipsychotic Drugs in Schizophrenia Study (CUtLASS 1). *Archives of General Psychiatry*, 63(10):1079–1087.

Kim, S. F., Huang, A. S., Snowman, A. M., et al. (2007). Antipsychotic drug–induced weight gain mediated by histamine H1 receptor-linked activation of hypothalamic AMP-kinase. *Proceedings of the National Academy of Sciences of the United States of America*, 104(9):3456–3459.

Law, A. J., Lipska, B. K., Weickert, C. S., et al. (2006). Neuregulin 1 (NRG1) transcripts are differentially expressed in schizophrenia and regulated by 5^1 SNPs associated with the disease. *Proceedings of the National Academy of Sciences of the United States of America*, 103(17):6747–6752.

Lewis, S. W., Davies, L., Jones, P. B., et al. (2006). Randomised controlled trials of conventional antipsychotic versus new atypical drugs, and new atypical drugs versus clozapine, in people with schizophrenia responding poorly to, or intolerant of, current drug treatment. *Health Technology Assessment*, 10(17): iii–iv, ix–xi, 1–165.

Liebermann, J. A., Stroup, T. S., McEvoy, J. P., et al. (2005). Effectiveness of antipsychotic drugs in patients with chronic schizophrenia. *New England Journal of Medicine*, 353(12): 1209–1223.

Lin, K. M., Poland, R. E., Lau, J. K., et al. (1988). Haloperidol and prolactin concentrations in Asians and Caucasians. *Journal of Clinical Psychopharmacology*, 8(3):195–201.

Lipska, B. K., Peters, T., Hyde, T. M., et al. (2006). Expression of DISC1 binding partners is reduced in schizophrenia and associated with DISC1 SNPs. *Human Molecular Genetics*, 25(8):1245–1258.

Luft, B. & Taylor, D. (2006). A review of atypical antipsychotic drugs versus conventional medication in schizophrenia. *Expert Opinions in Pharmacotherapy*, 13:1739–1748.

Meeks, T. W. & Jeste, D. V. (2008). Beyond the Black Box: What is the role for Antipsychotics in Dementia? *Current Psychiatry*. 7(6):50–65.

Messias, E., Chen, C. Y., & Eaton, W. W. (2007). Epidemiology of Schizophrenia: Review of Findings and Myths. *Psychiatr Clin North Am*. 30(3):323–338.

Meyer, J. M., Davis, V. G., Goff, D. C., et al. (2008). Change in metabolic syndrome parameters with antipsychotic treatment in the CATIE Schizophrenia Trial; prospective data from phase 1, *Schizophrenia Research*, 101:273–286.

National Institute of Mental Health (n.d.). Epidemiology of Mental Illness Chapter 2. Retrieved August 1, 2010, from http://www.surgeongeneral.gov/library/mentalhealth/chapter2/sec2_1.html

Plassman, B. L., Langa, K. M., Fisher, G. G., et al. (2007). Prevalence of dementia in the United States: the aging, demographics, and memory study. *Neuroepidemiology*. 29(1–2):125–132.

Rosenheck, R., Perlick, D., Bingham, S., et al. (2003). Effectiveness and cost of olanzapine and haloperidol in the treatment of schizophrenia: a randomized controlled trial. *Journal of the American Medical Association*, 290(20):2693–2702.

Salzman, C., Jeste, D. V., Meyer, R. E., et al. (2008). Elderly patients with dementia-related symptoms of severe agitation and aggression: consensus statement on treatment options, clinical trials methodology, and policy. *Journal of Clinical Psychiatry*, 69:889–898.

Stahl, S. M. (2008). *Stahl's Essential physchopharmacology*. New York, NY: Cambridge University Press.

Schneider, L. S., Tariot, P. N., Dagerman, K. S., et al. (2006). Effectiveness of atypical antipsychotic drugs in patients with Alzheimer's disease. *New England Journal of Medicine*, 355(15):1525–1538.

Drugs Treating Seizure Disorders

Learning Objectives

At the completion of this chapter the student will:

1. Identify the three basic mechanisms of action of the antiepileptic drugs.

2. Identify common core drug knowledge about prototype drugs belonging to the major antiepileptic drug classifications.

3. Identify core patient variables of concern related to the major antiepileptic drugs.

4. Generate a nursing plan of care based on the interactions between core drug knowledge and core patient variables for the major antiepileptic drugs.

5. Describe nursing interventions to maximize therapeutic effects and minimize adverse effects for the major antiepileptic drugs.

6. Relate key points for patient and family education for the major antiepileptic drugs.

Key Terms

absence seizure	generalized seizure	seizure
convulsions	glutamate	status epilepticus
epilepsy	partial seizure	tonic-clonic seizure
GABA	postictal	

Drugs Treating Seizure Disorders

Ⓒ Antiepileptics

Antiepileptic drugs that decrease sodium influx

Ⓟ **phenytoin**
ethotoin
fosphenytoin
carbamazepine
felbamate
lamotrigine
levetiracetam
oxcarbazepine
topiramate
valproic acid

Antiepileptic drugs that decrease calcium influx

Ⓟ **ethosuximide**
methsuximide
phensuximide
zonisamide

Antiepileptic drugs that increase the effects of GABA

Ⓒ **benzodiazepines**

Ⓟ **lorazepam (see also Chapter 15)**
clonazepam
clorazepate
diazepam
midazolam
gabapentin
phenobarbital
pregabalin
primidone
tiagabine
vigabatrin

Antiepileptic drugs used in seizures related to pre-eclampsia and eclampsia

Magnesium sulfate (see also Chapter 53)

The symbol Ⓒ indicates the drug class.
Drugs in **bold type** marked with the symbol Ⓟ are prototypes.
Drugs in blue type are closely related to the prototype.
Drugs in red type are significantly different from the prototype.
Drugs in black type with no symbol are also used in drug therapy; no prototype.

pilepsy, a brain disorder, is not a single entity, but rather a group of neurologic disorders in which CNS neurons display hyperexcitability. This excessive neurologic activity produces a wide variety of effects, from loss of consciousness with generalized muscle twitching to mild alterations in consciousness such as confusion or a blank stare with repetitive blinking. All of these effects from altered neurologic activity are termed **seizures.** More than 2 million people in the United States have experienced an unprovoked seizure or have been diagnosed with epilepsy (National Institutes of Neurological Disorders and Stroke, website). Patients with patterns of seizures who are diagnosed with epilepsy are treated with antiepileptic drugs. Many of the antiepileptic drugs, especially the newer drugs, are not chemically related to each other and do not fit into a drug class with other drugs. The three main ways that antiepileptic drugs work are by decreasing the rate at which sodium flows into the cell, inhibiting calcium flow rate into the cell through specific channels, and increasing the effect of the neuroinhibitor gamma-aminobutyric acid (GABA). Some drugs work in more than one way. Three main classes of drugs used to treat seizures are discussed in this chapter: drugs that decrease sodium influx, represented by the prototype phenytoin; drugs that decrease calcium influx, represented by the prototype ethosuximide; and drugs that increase the effectiveness of GABA, represented by the benzodiazepines. The prototype benzodiazepine, lorazepam, is discussed at length in Chapter 15. Magnesium sulfate is a drug used specifically to treat seizures associated with preeclampsia and eclampsia that is significantly different from all of the prototypes. It is discussed at length in Chapter 53.

PHYSIOLOGY

Action potentials within neurons are initiated by an influx of sodium into the cell through special sodium channels in the cell membrane. For sodium to enter through the cell membrane, the channels have to be open and in an active state (also referred to as depolarization). An action potential follows, and neurons fire. As soon as sodium enters, the channels close and return to an inactive state (also known as a refractory period). When the voltage-dependent channel is inactive, sodium cannot enter through the cell membrane. Thus, the sodium channels cannot be further activated by depolarization, and no additional action potential or neuron firing can occur (UpToDate, 2010a).

Influx of calcium through specialized voltage-dependent channels also plays a role in creating an action potential. Usually, this has a limited effect, except in the neurons of the hypothalamus. There are three types of calcium channels in neurons, which differ by their rate of reactivation and their voltage dependency. The movement of these two ions, sodium and calcium, into the cell is controlled by special mechanisms to maintain homeostasis and prevent excessive formation of action potentials. Neurons normally fire at about 80 times a second.

When the cell fires and the action potential spreads across the presynaptic terminal, release of neurotransmitters into the synaptic cleft occurs. Some of these neurotransmitters, such as **glutamate,** produce excitation, and others, such as GABA, inhibit the nervous system. **GABA** normally acts as a counterbalance to glutamate, preventing hyperexcitation, and works at specialized postsynaptic receptors; it is present throughout the brain. When GABA is attached at the receptor, it permits more chloride ions to flow across the cell membrane, inhibiting depolarization. After GABA is released into the synapse, it is taken back up by the nerve cell to be either degraded or re-released. Some GABA is taken up by glial cells, which are nonnerve cells in the supporting tissue around the brain and spinal column. GABA in glial cells is metabolized into the amino acid glutamine, which is used by nerve cells to create more GABA or glutamate (Figure 18.1).

PATHOPHYSIOLOGY

When a group of neurons exhibits coordinated, high-frequency discharge, it is termed a focus. The causes of a focus include head trauma, tumor growth, hypoxia, and inherited birth defects. When the activity from a focus spreads to other areas of the brain, causing other neurons to join in the hyperactivity, seizures result. Seizure may result from either high levels of glutamate or low levels of GABA, which allow the focus to take over in the brain. In epilepsy, the neurons may fire as many as 500 times a second, in great excess of the normal range. A genetic variation of the ion channels for sodium and calcium may allow excess ions to flow through these pathways, inducing seizures (National Institute of Neurologic Disorders and Stroke, website). The classifications of seizures are based on how widespread the neural hyperactivity is within the brain. The two basic types of seizures are partial (also known as focal) and generalized. Figure 18.2 presents the classifications of seizures. Table 18.1 shows which antiepileptic drugs are used for which seizure type. **Partial seizures** occur when focus activity is limited to an area of the brain, within one hemisphere. The hyperactive neurons are in the cerebral cortex, and the effect on the adjacent cortical areas is limited. When the focus activity is within both hemispheres, **generalized seizure** symptoms occur. The spread of focus activity can be compared to teenagers at a party. Although a few partygoers might get hyperactive and a little out of control, the parents in the house inhibit the spread of such behavior, and the party should stay on track. If no parents are present, no direct inhibition on the partygoers' actions occurs, and the hyperactive and wild behavior spreads to more and more people at the party, possibly resulting in a melee.

Partial seizures can be further divided into two main subgroups, simple and complex. The defining difference between them is the degree to which the level of consciousness is altered. Simple partial seizures may manifest as twitching in a particular muscle grouping, for example, in the right leg; no loss of consciousness occurs. Complex partial seizures likely involve some involuntary muscle twitching or movement also, but the patient seems confused or exhibits odd behavior, both of which are evidence of an impaired level of consciousness.

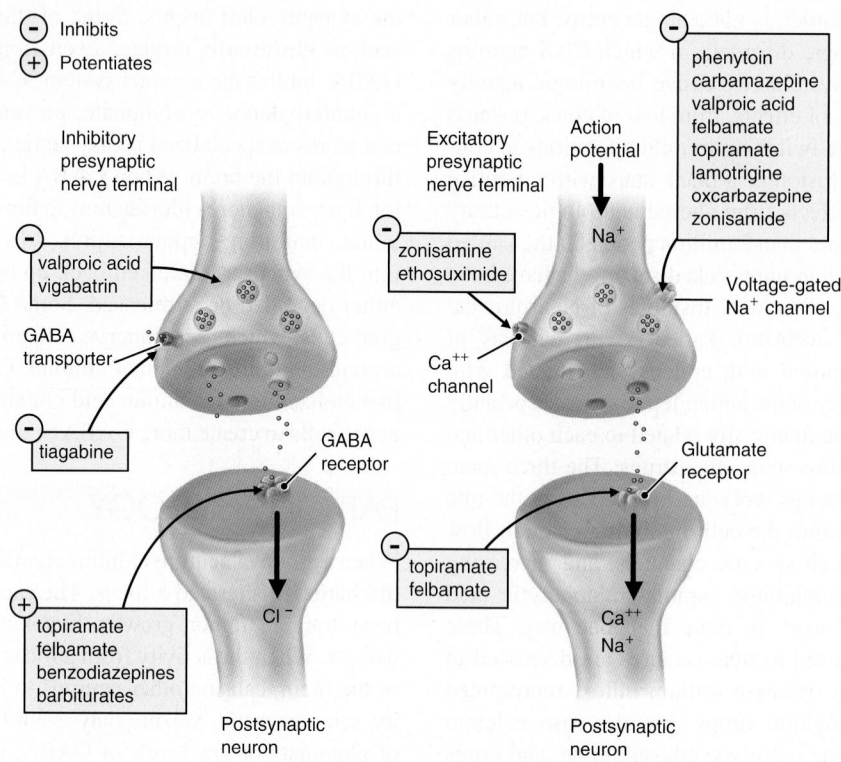

- **FIGURE 18.1** Mechanisms of antiepileptic drugs.

Generalized seizures are divided into several subtypes: tonic-clonic (also referred to as grand mal), absence (also referred to as petit mal), atonic, myoclonic, status epilepticus, and febrile. A brief description of these generalized seizures follows:

- **Tonic-clonic seizure** (grand mal)—the entire cerebral cortex is altered by hyperexcited neurons. Initially, the

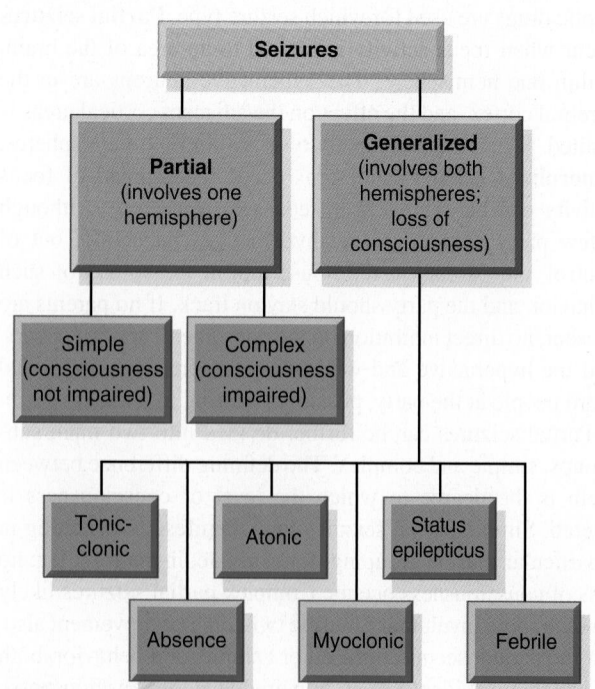

- **FIGURE 18.2** Classification of seizures.

TABLE 18.1	Antiepileptic Drug Therapy Grouped by Therapeutic Use		
Partial Seizures	**Generalized Seizures (Except Status Epilepticus)**	**Status Epilepticus**
Carbamazepine	Carbamazepine	Diazepam
Clonazepam	Clonazepam	Fosphenytoin
Clorazepate	Diazepam	Lorazepam
Diazepam	Ethosuximide	Midazolam
Ethotoin	Ethotoin	Pentobarbital
Felbamate	Felbamate	Phenobarbital
Gabapentin	(Lennox-Gastaut	Phenytoin
Lamotrigine	syndrome)	Propofol
Levetiracetam	Lamotrigine	
Lorazepam	Levetiracetam	
Oxcarbazepine	Lorazepam	
Phenytoin	Methsuximide	
Pregabalin	Oxcarbazepine	
Tiagabine	Phensuximide	
Topiramate	Phenytoin	
valproic acid	Topiramate	
Zonisamide	valproic acid	
	Zonisamide	

Note: Drugs listed alphabetically not in preferred order of use.

person experiences stiffness and rigidity (tonic phase) and falls to the ground. The person loses consciousness, and no movement follows for several seconds. Then, massive muscle spasms (**convulsions**) occur, with the muscles alternating between contracting and relaxing (clonic phase). Urinary or bowel incontinence and biting the tongue can occur during this phase. Premonitions or auras may occur before the onset of tonic-clonic seizures. Following the convulsions, the person gradually regains consciousness. The patient does not remember the events of the seizures and may not fully recover for up to several days. This post-seizure period is referred to as the **postictal** state.

- **Absence seizure** (petit mal)—very brief loss of consciousness, lasting several seconds but less than 1 minute, is characteristic. Some mild symmetric motor activity, such as eye blinking, often occurs. A blank stare and loss of attention may also be observed. Many times, the seizures are so brief that others do not notice them when they happen. These seizures usually occur in children. More than 100 absence seizures may occur in 1 day. The calcium channels that do not require a high voltage and which quickly become inactive are most likely an integral component of the thalamo-cortical circuits associated with absence seizures.

- Atonic seizure—a sudden loss of muscle tone occurs. If the muscles affected are just in the neck, "head drop" is observed. If the loss of tone is more widespread, the patient falls suddenly to the ground in a "drop attack."

- Myoclonic seizure—sudden rapid muscle contractions occur. The contractions can be limited to a body region, such as one limb, or can be generalized throughout the body.

- **Status epilepticus**—one seizure follows another without recovery of consciousness between events or return to baseline clinical state, or lasts longer than 5 minutes. All types of seizures in which consciousness is lost can progress to status epilepticus. The most common causes of status epilepticus are stopping antiepileptic drug therapy and alcohol withdrawal. Other causes include acute brain injury or infection and metabolic disorders. Status epilepticus affects about 195,000 people each year in the United States and results in about 42,000 deaths (National Institute of Neurological Disorders and Stroke, 2006). The longer the period of status epilepticus, the higher the mortality rate. The most life-threatening condition results from generalized tonic-clonic seizures, referred to as generalized convulsive status epilepticus.

Status epilepticus is a medical emergency, and intravenous (IV) drug intervention is needed immediately. Current clinical practice is to begin treatment when a patient has a single seizure lasting at least 5 minutes, or has two or more seizures without recovery. Figure 18.3 presents a treatment pathway for status epilepticus; see Table 18.1 for therapeutic drugs. Treatment failures are usually related to insufficient dosing. A patent open airway may be absent, cardiac function may be altered, and high fever (hyperthermia) can occur. Lactic acidosis and elevated blood levels of carbon dioxide may follow. Patients who remain comatose for more than 30 minutes after generalized clonic status epilepticus is controlled may be experiencing subtle status epilepticus. Generalized

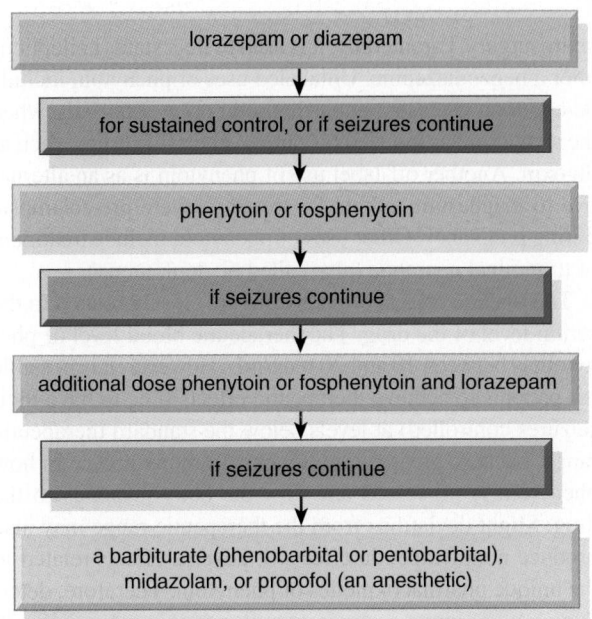

- FIGURE 18.3   Treatment pathway for status epilepticus. The drugs shown in orange are first-line drugs. The drugs shown in yellow are second-line drugs. There is not consensus as to which of the second-line drugs should be used first.

tonic-clonic motor activity is not associated with subtle status epilepticus; diagnosis is based on electroencephalogram (EEG) readings showing persistent ictal discharges.

- Febrile seizures—generalized seizures can also occur as a result of high fevers in infants and young children and are termed febrile generalized seizures. These types of seizures do not increase the risk of developing epilepsy as the child grows.

In addition to epilepsy, seizures may also occur from known and reversible causes—most commonly, metabolic abnormalities (e.g., hypoglycemia and electrolyte imbalance), meningitis, uremia, pre-eclampsia and toxemia of pregnancy, and drug and alcohol abuse.

ANTIEPILEPTIC DRUGS

ANTIEPILEPTIC DRUGS THAT DECREASE SODIUM INFLUX

Phenytoin (Dilantin) is the prototype drug that controls seizures by decreasing sodium influx into the cells. Remember that sodium influx produces an action potential, which then causes the neurons to fire. Phenytoin is representative of a class of drugs called the hydantoins.

Nursing Management of the Patient Receiving [P] Phenytoin

Core Drug Knowledge

Pharmacotherapeutics

Phenytoin is used to control partial and generalized (grand mal) and other psychomotor seizures. It is also used to prevent and treat seizures that occur either during or following neurosurgery. Parenterally, it is used to treat status epilepticus after a benzodiazepine. Unlabeled uses of phenytoin include its common use as an antiarrhythmic drug, especially when the arrhythmia is induced by cardiac glycoside drugs, such as digoxin. Another off-label use of phenytoin is as an alternative to magnesium sulfate for treating severe pre-eclampsia during pregnancy. Other uses of phenytoin include treatment of trigeminal neuralgia (also called tic douloureux).

Therapeutic effects of phenytoin are closely related to the serum level of the drug. The therapeutic blood level of phenytoin is between 10 and 20 mcg/mL. However, it is possible for patients to achieve therapeutic effects (i.e., to have their seizures controlled) at levels below the standard therapeutic range, because great variability exists among people in how phenytoin is processed and how the body responds to the drug. Slight deviations from the therapeutic range may also produce nontherapeutic effects or adverse effects related to the unique pharmacokinetics of phenytoin. Therefore, determining an accurate and effective dose is somewhat difficult. For patients with low albumin levels or for those who are taking highly protein-bound drugs, "free" unbound serum phenytoin levels should be checked and multiplied by 10 to provide an approximation of the target total serum level (UpToDate, 2010b). Adjustments to the initial dose will most likely be needed when therapy is started. Be aware that dosing of phenytoin should be individualized to the patient's needs and that achieving the therapeutic range should be considered a guide but not an absolute rule. Patients who are to start phenytoin therapy orally should receive a loading dose (usually 15 mg/kg divided into three doses) and then a maintenance dose (usually 5 mg/kg/day, which may be given as one dose or divided into two doses) (UpToDate, 2010a).

Pharmacokinetics

Phenytoin is slowly absorbed when given orally. The rate and extent of absorption and bioavailability of phenytoin vary among individuals and also depend on the product formulation. Oral phenytoin reaches peak serum levels in 1.5 hours to 3 hours for prompt-onset preparations and within 12 hours for extended-release products. Intramuscularly administered phenytoin is very slowly and erratically absorbed because the drug precipitates at the injection site within the muscle. Absorption from the site may occur for 5 days or longer. Serum levels reached by intramuscular (IM) injection never equal those reached by oral dosing. Phenytoin is highly protein bound (about 90%). Phenytoin is metabolized in the liver to inactive metabolites, which can be excreted in the urine by tubular excretion. However, the biotransformation of phenytoin to the metabolite has a limit at any given time. In lower doses of phenytoin, complete metabolism occurs fairly easily. However, as the dose increases, not all of the drug can be metabolized at once, and the half-life of phenytoin will increase as the dose increases. At low dosage levels, which are frequently subtherapeutic, the half-life is 6 to 24 hours; as the dose is increased to achieve the therapeutic range, the half-life increases to between 20 and 60 hours.

Because of these pharmacokinetics, small changes in the dose of phenytoin may produce larger than expected changes in the serum concentration of the drug. This variability in the metabolism rate makes phenytoin different from most other drugs. To further complicate the process of metabolism, the rate of metabolism varies greatly among people. This limitation on rate of metabolism is an inherited trait. Table 18.2 summarizes the actions of selected antiepileptic drugs.

Pharmacodynamics

The primary site of action of phenytoin, and of other hydantoins, is believed to be the motor cortex. Phenytoin reversibly binds to sodium channels while they are in the inactive state. This binding delays the return of the channel to an active state. Because sodium can enter the cell to initiate an action potential only when the channels are active, the time between action potentials is greatly lengthened, the neurons cannot fire at an excessive rate, and excessive muscle contractions that occur in grand mal–type seizures are prevented. Phenytoin selectively binds to sites with hyperactive neurons; it does not alter the sodium movement into neurons that fire normally. This ability to selectively work at neurons that are firing abnormally explains why phenytoin is also effective in treating cardiac arrhythmias from ectopic foci.

Contraindications and Precautions

Because of its effects on ventricular automaticity has a black box warning that it must be given slowly intravenously. Phenytoin is contraindicated in patients with sinus bradycardia, sinoatrial block, second- and third-degree atrioventricular (AV) block, or Adams-Stokes syndrome. Phenytoin is also contraindicated if the patient is hypersensitive to hydantoins; phenytoin hypersensitivity reactions are not typical.

Phenytoin and other antiepileptic drugs now carry a warning that their use may increase the risk of suicidal ideation (thinking of suicide) or suicidality (attempting suicide). The Food and Drug Administration's 2008 meta analysis of clinical trials for antiepileptic drugs found that patients taking one or more of these drugs were almost twice as likely to have suicidal ideation or suicidality than those in the trials who received a placebo.

Because phenytoin may cause blood dyscrasias, it should not be administered with other drugs that also have this effect, if at all possible. If such drugs must be used, the patient should be monitored closely for blood dyscrasias. Other precautions include patients with acute intermittent porphyria (rare inherited metabolic disorder characterized by excessive excretion of porphyrins, acute abdominal pain, and neurologic disturbances), because phenytoin may precipitate a crisis. Use caution in diabetic patients because phenytoin may elevate blood glucose levels. Phenytoin use has been associated with osteomalacia, a softening and flexibility of the bones in adults.

Phenytoin should not be abruptly stopped because doing so can precipitate status epilepticus.

Phenytoin is a pregnancy category D drug, and use of the drug during pregnancy is a somewhat complicated and confusing issue. On the one hand, phenytoin, as well as other

TABLE 18.2 Summary of Selected ⓒ Antiepileptic Drugs

Drug (Trade) Name	Selected Indications	Route and Dosage Range	Pharmacokinetics
Drugs That Decrease Sodium Influx			
Ⓟ phenytoin (Dilantin)	Tonic-clonic seizures, psychomotor seizures, status epilepticus	*Adult:* PO, use to serum levels of 5–20 mcg/mL	*Onset:* Slow *Duration:* 6–12 h $t_{1/2}$: 6–24 h
carbamazepine (Tegretol)	Tonic-clonic seizures, mixed seizures, psychomotor seizures	*Adult:* PO, 400–1,000 mg/d *Child 6–12 y:* PO, 200–1,000 mg/d	*Onset:* Slow *Duration:* 4–5 h $t_{1/2}$: 25–65 h initially, 12–17 h with multiple dosing
felbamate (Felbatol)	Adjunctive or monotherapy of partial seizures in adults; adjunctive therapy in children with Lennox-Gastaut syndrome	*Adult (>14 y):* 1,200–3,600 mg/d *Child 2–14 y:* PO, 15 mg/kg/d	*Onset:* Rapid *Duration:* Dose proportional $t_{1/2}$: 20–23 h
fosphenytoin (Cerebyx)	Status epilepticus	*Adult:* IV, dilute in D$_5$W or 0.9% NaCl to a concentration of 1.5–25 mg phenytoin equivalent (PE)*/mL; administer at rate of 150 mg PE/mL	*Onset:* Rapid *Duration:* 1–2 h $t_{1/2}$: 6–24 h
oxcarbazepine (Trileptal)	Adjunctive treatment of partial seizures	*Adult:* PO, 1,200 mg/d as adjunctive therapy; 2,400 mg/d as monotherapy. *Child 4–16 y:* PO, 30–46 mg/kg/d as adjunctive therapy	*Onset:* 1 h *Duration:* 3–13 h $t_{1/2}$: 2*–9**
valproic acid (Depakene)	Sole or adjunctive treatment for simple or complex absence seizures	*Adult:* PO, 10–60 mg/kg/d	*Onset:* Varies depending on dosage form *Duration:* 1–4 h $t_{1/2}$: 5–20 h (average, 10.6 h)
Drugs That Increase Effectiveness of GABA			
Ⓟ lorazepam (Ativan)	Anxiety, anesthetic premedication, status epilepticus, alcohol withdrawal, chronic insomnia	*Adult:* PO, 2–6 mg/d; IM, 0.05 mg/kg; IV, 2 mg *Child:* Not recommended; IV/IM, oral dose not established	*Onset:* PO, 1–3 h; IM, 15–30 min; IV, 1–5 min *Duration:* 12–24 h $t_{1/2}$: 10–20 h
clonazepam (Klonopin)	Myoclonic seizures, absence seizures, akinetic seizures, variant absence seizures (Lennox-Gastaut syndrome)	*Adult:* PO, 1.5–20 mg/d *Child:* PO, 0.01–0.05 mg/kg/d	*Onset:* 20–60 min *Duration:* 6–12 h $t_{1/2}$: 18–60 h
clorazepate (Tranxene)	Partial seizures	*Adult:* PO, 7.5 mg tid *Child:* PO, 7.5 mg bid	*Onset:* 15–45 min *Duration:* 7–8 h $t_{1/2}$: 30–100 h
diazepam (Valium)	Adjunct in convulsant seizures, status epilepticus	*Adult:* PO, 2–10 mg bid or tid *Adult:* IV (initial), 10–15 mg/kg *Child:* IV (initial), 5–10 mg/kg	*Onset:* PO, 30–60 min; IV, 1–5 min *Duration:* PO, 3 h, IV, 15–66 min $t_{1/2}$: 20–80 h, PO
gabapentin (Neurontin)	Partial seizures in adults with and without secondary generalization	*Adult:* PO, 900–1,800 mg/d	*Onset:* Rapid *Duration:* 6–8 h $t_{1/2}$: 5–7 h
phenobarbital	Status epilepticus, cortical local, tonic-clonic seizures	*Adult:* PO, 60–100 mg/d to serum level of 10–40 μg/mL; IM/IV, 200–320 q6h *Child:* PO, 3–6 mg/kg/d; IM/IV, 10–15 mg/kg/d	*Onset:* PO, 30–60 min; IM, 10–30 min; IV, 5 min *Duration:* 8–15 h $t_{1/2}$: 53–140 h
tiagabine (Gabitril)	Adjunctive treatment of partial seizures	Dosage ranges not established	*Onset:* Rapid *Duration:* 6–12 h $t_{1/2}$: Varies (4.5–13.4 h)

(Continued)

TABLE 18.2 Summary of Selected ⊖ Antiepileptic Drugs *(continued)*

Drug (Trade) Name	Selected Indications	Route and Dosage Range	Pharmacokinetics
Drugs That Decrease Calcium Influx			
P ethosuximide (Zarontin)	Absence seizures	*Adult:* PO, 500 mg/d to serum level of 40–100 mcg/mL *Child:* PO, 250 mg/d (3–6 y) or 500 mg/d (6 y or older)	*Onset:* Varies *Duration:* 3–7 h $t_{1/2}$: 40–60 h in adults; 30 h in children 7–9 y
zonisamide (zonegran)	Adjunctive treatment of partial seizures	*Adult:* PO, 100–400 mg/d	*Onset:* 2–6 h *Duration:* More than 105 h $t_{1/2}$: 63 h

antiepeleptic drugs, has been associated with an increased incidence of birth defects in infants whose mothers used the drug. These congenital malformations include cleft lip, cleft palate, and heart malformations. A fetal hydantoin syndrome has been identified that includes prenatal growth deficiency, microcephaly, and mental deficiency. However, these features of intrauterine growth retardation have all been associated with other causes as well as hydantoin use; therefore, phenytoin use may or may not be solely responsible for their onset. Most women taking phenytoin deliver normal, healthy infants. There have also been reports that maternal ingestion of phenytoin can produce bleeding in newborns, usually within 24 hours of birth. The defect is characterized by low levels of vitamin K–dependent clotting factors and by prolonged prothrombin times, partial thromboplastin times, or both. On the other hand, stopping the use of phenytoin and other antiepileptic drugs during pregnancy is likely to induce seizures, including status epilepticus, which places the fetus at risk for being without sufficient oxygen. Even minor seizures may pose a risk to the well-being of the developing fetus, although the exact effects are not known. No easy answer exists to the question of whether to use phenytoin during pregnancy. In general, it is now thought that phenytoin should not be discontinued if the nature, frequency, and severity of the seizures pose a serious threat to either the patient or the fetus. In other words, benefits should outweigh risks. Box 18.1 discusses antiepileptics and pregnancy.

Adverse Effects

The most frequent adverse effects of phenytoin occur in the central nervous system (CNS) and include nystagmus, ataxia, dysarthria, slurred speech, mental confusion, dizziness, insomnia, transient nervousness, numbness, tremor, and headache. Reducing the dose is often effective in eliminating these adverse effects. Other common adverse effects of phenytoin are nausea and gingival hyperplasia (overgrowth of the gums).

Rare but potentially life-threatening adverse effects of phenytoin are dermatologic reactions (Stevens-Johnson syndrome, lupus erythematosus syndrome, and bullous, exfoliative, or purpuric dermatitis), liver damage, and hematopoietic effects (blood dyscrasias). When given intravenously, phenytoin may

CRITICAL THINKING SCENARIO

WHAT HAPPENS WHEN ANTIEPILEPTIC THERAPY STOPS ABRUPTLY?

Rudy Hernandez, a 26-year-old man, is brought to the emergency room by ambulance, accompanied by his wife. He is currently unconscious, is having tonic-clonic convulsions, and has been incontinent of urine. He had two seizures at home without regaining consciousness before the ambulance arrived. His wife states that he was on phenytoin and valproic acid for seizure prevention and that he has been on medication since he was a teenager. She also reports he stopped his medication last week because he didn't like the adverse effects.

1. What type of seizure is Mr. Hernandez exhibiting? What is the likely cause of this seizure?

2. What nursing actions are indicated upon his arrival in the emergency room?

3. What drug therapy or therapies do you expect that he will receive?

Box 18.1 ANTIEPILEPTICS AND PREGNANCY

Teratogenic Effects
- Possible with all antiepileptic drugs
- Risk increases with first-trimester exposure and multidrug therapy
- Little data on new antiepileptic drugs because no studies; do not appear to cause malformation in monotherapy
- Innate ability to metabolize and eliminate antiepileptic drugs increases risk
- Metabolism of hormonal contraceptives is increased by antiepileptic drugs, decreasing their effectiveness, increasing risk for unplanned pregnancy

Competitive Inhibitors of Vitamin K
- Neonatal hemorrhage possible
- Phenytoin, carbamazepine, ethosuximide, phenobarbital, and primidone cause high mortality from hemorrhage
- Transferred in breast milk

Loss of Seizure Control
- Concentration of antiepileptic drugs decreases during pregnancy (even with steady or increasing dose)
- Concentration decreases differently for different antiepileptic drugs
- One fourth to one third of pregnant women will have increased incidence of seizures related to decreased drug concentration

TABLE 18.3 Agents That Interact with P Phenytoin

Interactants	Effect and Significance	Nursing Management
allopurinol, amiodarone, benzodiazepines, cimetidine, clonazepam, disulfiram, ethanol, fluconazole, ibuprofen, isoniazid, metronidazole, miconazole, omeprazole, phenothiazines, salicylates, succinimides, sulfonamides, tricyclic anti-depressants, trimethoprim, valproic acid	Increased pharmacologic effects of phenytoin from inhibition of its metabolism	Monitor patient for changes in seizure control. Monitor serum phenytoin levels. Assess for signs of phenytoin toxicity.
barbiturates, ethanol (chronic ingestion), rifampin, theophylline	Decreased pharmacologic effects of phenytoin due to its increased metabolism	Assess patient for increased seizure frequency and changed seizure control. Monitor serum phenytoin levels at regular intervals.
antacids, charcoal, sucralfate	Decreased phenytoin effects due to decreased absorption	Assess patient for increased seizure frequency and changed seizure control. Monitor serum phenytoin levels at regular intervals.
acetaminophen, carbamazepine, cardiac glycosides, corticosteroids, disopyramide, doxycycline, estrogens (and oral contraceptives), haloperidol, methadone, mexiletine, quinidine, theophylline	Decreased pharmacologic effects of interactants from increased metabolism by phenytoin Analgesic effects of acetaminophen may be reduced by concomitant phenytoin use; the potential hepatotoxicity of acetaminophen may be increased Corticosteroid use may mask systemic manifestations of phenytoin hypersensitivity reactions	Evaluate patient for changed seizure control. Assess patient for evidence of therapeutic effects of interacting drugs. Monitor patient for therapeutic serum levels (if applicable) of interacting drugs.

cause cardiovascular collapse (hypotension, cardiac arrhythmias) if it is administered too rapidly. Phenytoin may increase the risk of suicidal ideation or suicidality.

A number of other adverse effects are possible but not common; these include:

Dermatologic: rash, hirsutism, alopecia
Endocrine: diabetes insipidus, hyperglycemia
Gastrointestinal (GI): vomiting, diarrhea, constipation
Hepatic: hepatitis, jaundice
Respiratory: pneumonia, pharyngitis, sinusitis, hyperventilation, rhinitis, apnea, aspiration pneumonia, asthma, dyspnea, atelectasis, increased cough, epistaxis, hypoxia, pneumothorax, hemoptysis, bronchitis, chest pain, pulmonary fibrosis
Senses: tinnitus, diplopia, taste perversion, amblyopia, deafness, visual-field defect, eye pain, conjunctivitis, photophobia, hyperacusis, mydriasis, parosmia, ear pain, taste loss
Miscellaneous: polyarthropathy, weight gain, chest pain, edema, immunoglobulin A (IgA) depression, fever, photophobia, conjunctivitis, gynecomastia, periarteritis nodosa, pulmonary fibrosis, soft tissue injury at the injection site, lymph node hyperplasia (may represent a hypersensitivity reaction)

Drug Interactions

Numerous drugs interact with phenytoin. Be certain to check for drug interactions when patients are receiving phenytoin and any other drug. These interactions occur because of phenytoin-inducing effects on hepatic microsomal enzyme systems (also referred to as P-450). Pharmacologic induction of these enzymes enhances the metabolism of both endogenous and exogenous substances, including other antiepileptic drugs.

Drug interactions may increase or decrease the effect of phenytoin or the other drug (Table 18.3). Several enteral feeding preparations (tube feedings) may decrease phenytoin levels either by impairing absorption or through some other mechanism. Phenytoin, and other antiepileptic drugs that induce the P-450 system, increase the rate of metabolism of estrogen as well as increase the protein binding of progesterones in oral contraceptives. Both increasing estrogen metabolism and increasing protein binding of progesterone decrease the effectiveness of oral contraceptives, as there is less available estrogen and progesterone. Phenytoin and benzodiazepines precipitate if given via the same IV tubing. In addition, phenytoin may interfere with results of diagnostic endocrine tests that use dexamethasone.

Assessment of Relevant Core Patient Variables

Health Status

Determine whether the patient is hypersensitive to phenytoin or if he or she has any of the cardiac conditions that are contraindications for the use of the drug. Because phenytoin is highly protein bound, assess whether the patient has chronic conditions, such as liver failure, that alter the level of albumin protein. Check ordered blood work to determine whether albumin levels are abnormal.

Before starting therapy, also confirm that the patient has either grand mal or other psychomotor seizures that respond to phenytoin. See Box 18.2 for more information about core patient variables.

BOX 18.2 FOCUS ON RESEARCH

Core Patient Variables and Antiepileptic Drugs

Yeager, K. A., Dilorio, C., Osborne Shafer, P., McCarty, F., Letz, R., Henry, T., & Schomer, D.L. (2005). The complexity of treatments for persons with epilepsy. *Epilepsy & Behavior* 7(4):679–686.

The Study

Medication-management practices of people living with epilepsy were evaluated using data from the 2004 Project EASE (Epilepsy Awareness Support and Education). Data was obtained from self-reports of patients recruited at epilepsy clinics in Atlanta, Georgia, and Boston Massachusetts. Medication complexity was assessed using the Epilepsy Medication and Treatment Complexity Index (EMTCI). The level of complexity for specific medications was based on general medication information, frequency of administration, special instructions (different doses in the same day, changing dose due to menstrual cycle, etc.) and special actions (take with food, crush, must carry at all times, etc.). The medications ranked most complex were forms of carbamazepine and gabapentin. Evaluating the total regimen of all drugs for an individual, higher complexity was positively associated with seizures and hospitalization within the past year.

Nursing Implications

Medication regimens for managing epilepsy are complex and can require extensive memory recall and adjustments to daily routines. These factors certainly contribute to the very high level of medication nonadherence in these patients, which has been reported as high as 70% in some studies. Therefore, it is critical to consider individual patient's abilities and life routines when establishing treatment. Patient education and simplification of regimens is essential as they can influence comprehension of medication and ultimately adherence. Patients need to be involved in setting priorities and establishing a regimen that will work for them.

Life Span and Gender

Before phenytoin therapy begins, assess whether the patient is pregnant. The use of antiepileptic drugs such as phenytoin poses some risk to the developing fetus and, if possible, should not be started during a pregnancy. Women of childbearing age should use birth control to prevent unplanned pregnancy because of those risks, although antiepileptic drugs can reduce the effectiveness of oral hormonal contraceptives (World Health Organization, 2009). However, the effectiveness of oral hormonal contraceptives remains high and superior to intrauterine devices and barrier methods used alone. Exposure to phenytoin during the first trimester of pregnancy increases the risk of malformations in the child; taking multiple antiepileptic drugs increases the risk even more. Teratogenicity may be related to an individual woman's genetic makeup, which influences how well she metabolizes and eliminates antiepileptic drugs. When metabolism and elimination are slower than would normally be predicted, the risk of teratogenic effects increases. Phenytoin, like other antiepileptic drugs, is a competitive inhibitor of vitamin K; this action increases the risk of neonatal hemorrhage in the first 24 hours after birth. Phenytoin is associated with a high mortality rate in neonatal hemorrhage. Suddenly stopping phenytoin carries the risk of inducing seizures, as previously

mentioned. This puts the fetus at risk of hypoxia during the mother's seizure. If possible, the woman should be weaned off phenytoin before becoming pregnant. Phenytoin is passed in breast milk, and so is the competitive inhibition of vitamin K; women taking phenytoin should not breast-feed.

Drug therapy with phenytoin, as with other antiepileptic drugs, need not be lifelong. Box 18.3 presents some guidelines for using and discontinuing antiepileptic drugs.

Older adults are more likely to experience hypotension and cardiac arrhythmias when phenytoin is given intravenously. Nonadherence to antiepileptic drug therapy is particularly high in the elderly, at more than 40% for those over 65 years old (Ettinger et al., 2009).

Lifestyle, Diet, and Habits

Assess for conditions that may make the patient more likely to have decreased blood protein levels. Does the patient have alcoholism? Is the patient malnourished? Is the patient's dietary protein intake severely limited? These conditions put the patient at greater risk for having greater amounts of free, active drug in the blood because less protein albumin is available for binding than would normally be expected. Therefore, the patient is more at risk for having adverse effects from the phenytoin. Chronic ingestion of alcohol also increases the metabolism of phenytoin and therefore alters blood drug levels.

Environment

Oral phenytoin can be administered in any setting. IV phenytoin should be given in a hospital setting, ideally with the patient in a bed with a cardiac monitor.

Nursing Diagnoses and Outcomes

Disturbed Sensory Perception related to adverse effects of drowsiness and sedation

Desired outcome: *The patient will not experience adverse effects to the degree that sensory perception is altered enough to impair quality of life.*

Risk for Injury related to the adverse effects of drowsiness and sedation

Desired outcome: *The patient will not sustain any injury while taking phenytoin.*

Altered Oral Mucous Membrane related to the adverse effect of gingival hyperplasia

Desired outcome: *The patient will demonstrate knowledge of optimal oral hygiene and experience no deterioration in dental health.*

Risk for Injury related to adverse effects of blood dyscrasias

Desired outcome: *The patient will return for follow-up blood work while taking phenytoin and will have no life-threatening blood disorders.*

Planning and Intervention

Maximizing Therapeutic Effects

Therapeutic effect of phenytoin is normally related to achieving a therapeutic blood level of the drug. Monitor blood levels to determine whether they are therapeutic. If the blood level is

BOX 18.3 COMMUNITY BASED CONCERNS

Starting and Stopping Antiepileptic Drug Therapy

Although antiepileptic drug therapy has often been considered lifelong, many patients can be successfully weaned off therapy. Antiepileptic drugs all produce adverse effects; about 1 in 30,000 patients taking an antiepileptic drug experiences a serious adverse effect, and 15% will need to have the drug discontinued because of adverse effects. Some of those adverse effects become more prevalent the longer the drug is taken. Generally, the second-generation antiepileptic drugs (gabapentin, lamotrigine, topiramate, levetiracetam, oxcarbazepine, and zonisamide) have a lower rate of adverse effects. In many patients, the risks of drug therapy may outweigh the risk of occasional seizure activity, and these patients should be considered for drug tapering. After antiepileptic drugs are withdrawn, almost 60% of patients remain seizure-free for 2 years. What follows are some current recommendations regarding the use and discontinuation of antiepileptic drugs.

When to Start Therapy

- After one seizure: usually not necessary, except if there is permanent injury to brain (e.g., cortical stroke, abscess, or tumor); a substantial risk of repeated seizures (abnormal EEG, especially if epileptiform discharges are present); a history of serious brain injury; a brain lesion identified on computed tomography (CT) or magnetic resonance imaging (MRI); focal abnormalities found on neurologic examination; mental retardation; or a first seizure that is a partial seizure.
- After two seizures: almost all patients, because the second seizure proves that patient has substantially increased risk of repeated seizures

When to Stop Therapy

The best time to stop is still somewhat unknown. There is no way to identify which patients will remain seizure-free. Generally, stopping therapy can be considered when the patient:

- Has been seizure-free for at least 2 years (about half of patients who are newly diagnosed with epilepsy become seizure-free after using the first drug prescribed)
- Receives single-drug therapy
- Is able to make individualized decisions
- Has a reasonable understanding of possible risks and benefits of stopping therapy

Withdrawal of drug therapy in some patients is likely to precipitate seizure activity.

Patients Are More Likely To Relapse If They Have:

- Identifiable brain disease
- Mental retardation
- Abnormal neurologic examination
- Seizure onset after age 10
- Multiple seizure types
- Poor initial response to treatment
- Been receiving combination drug therapy
- Some selected epilepsy syndromes, such as juvenile myoclonic epilepsy
- Abnormal EEG
- Family history of epilepsy
- Hippocampal atrophy or abnormal hippocampal signal on MRI

Withdrawal Schedule Recommendations:

- No known optimal tapering regimen
- Slower withdrawal (over 3 to 6 months) less likely to induce seizures; benzodiazepines and barbiturates should be over at least 6 months
- Taper one drug at a time if on combination therapy

---

not therapeutic, and the patient is still having seizures, notify the physician or other prescriber to inquire about increasing the dose. Remember that some patients achieve therapeutic results even when their blood levels of phenytoin are not in the ideal therapeutic range. The drug should be adjusted in very small increments because of the unusual pharmacokinetics of phenytoin. The risk is that a dosage change will move the blood phenytoin level from just marginally therapeutic to toxic. Titrating the dose upward gradually helps minimize this risk. Because of the long half-life, serum levels should be checked within 5 to 7 days after any change in the dose (increase or decrease) in order for the serum level to reflect steady-state levels (UpToDate, 2010a) accurately.

Phenytoin absorption is compromised when administered with enteral tube feedings. Check gastric residuals and refrain from administering the drug for 1 to 2 hours if the residual is greater than 100 mL. Continuous tube feedings should be held for 1 hour before and after administering the phenytoin.

Minimizing Adverse Effects

Adverse effects from phenytoin are frequently related to excessively high blood drug levels. It is important to monitor the patient's blood levels of phenytoin as well as the patient's physical response to drug therapy. Monitor drug levels most closely at the initiation of therapy or after every increase in

the dose. If the patient is demonstrating adverse effects, the drug dosage may need to be decreased. Patients may demonstrate adverse effects even if the serum level of phenytoin is "normal"; it is important to adjust the dose to the clinical response of the patient, not the serum level. Dosage changes downward should also be done in small increments to avoid decreasing the blood level so much that it is below the therapeutic level. Monitor serum levels after any change in phenytoin preparation, because different brands or generic preparations of the drug may have different bioavailabilities that alter serum levels and seizure control. Be especially vigilant during this transitional period (UpToDate, 2010a).

It is important to analyze the patient's mental and neurologic function and behavior regularly for changes from baseline behavior to determine whether CNS adverse effects due to phenytoin are present. If the patient is having difficulty with dizziness, institute safety measures to prevent falls and injury. Assess the patient for depression or changes in mood or behavior which indicate suicidal ideation.

Administer phenytoin with meals if the patient is experiencing nausea and GI distress; avoid antacids because they may impair absorption. Patients with diabetes may experience elevated glucose levels; their glucose levels should be measured more frequently until the effects of phenytoin are determined.

Administer IV push phenytoin no faster than 50 mg/min in adults or 1 to 3 mg/kg/min in neonates; fast administration is associated with cardiovascular collapse. Careful monitoring of the pulse and blood pressure is essential during IV administration. Follow the administration of phenytoin with sterile saline through the same IV catheter to avoid local venous irritation from the alkalinity of the phenytoin. Phenytoin is not given as a continuous IV infusion. IM administration should be avoided because of irregular and delayed absorption. When phenytoin is given after a benzodiazepine to control status epilepticus, a separate IV insertion site and IV tubing must be used for each drug, because the two agents precipitate if they come into contact (UpToDate, 2010c).

Evaluate blood counts, bleeding tendencies, and white blood cell counts regularly to determine whether any hematologic adverse effects have occurred. Notify the prescriber if any abnormalities are detected to prevent serious adverse effects. Vitamin D and calcium supplements are recommended for patients showing symptoms of osteomalacia and also for those at high risk for developing osteomalacia. Report any signs and symptoms of skin rash. Although a rash is usually not serious, phenytoin may need to be discontinued to minimize the risk for severe reactions such as Stevens-Johnson syndrome. Patients of Asian descent should be screened for the HLA-B*1502 allele variant which can increase the risk of Stevens-Johnson syndrome and toxic epidermal necrolysis in those individuals.

Assess the age of a woman and her reproductive status. To offset the increased estrogen metabolism that occurs from phenytoin and other antiepileptic drugs that induce the hepatic enzyme system, women who are concurrently taking hormonal contraceptives may need to have the estrogen dose increased (Zupanc, 2006). To minimize the risk of neonatal hemorrhage, pregnant women taking phenytoin should receive 10 mg/d of vitamin K during the last week of pregnancy.

Providing Patient and Family Education

Much of the patient and family education regarding phenytoin is common to any antiepileptic drug that is prescribed. Box 18.4 contains guidelines for patient and family education common to antiepileptic drugs. Some educational points specific for phenytoin are:

Teach the importance of shaking suspension forms of phenytoin thoroughly before pouring and measuring the dose.
Teach patients and families the importance of good dental hygiene to prevent gingival hyperplasia and gum softening. Encourage patients to brush the teeth at least twice daily with a soft toothbrush and to floss daily.
Suggest that patients take phenytoin with food to minimize GI distress.
Teach patients with diabetes to check capillary blood glucose frequently.
Suggest bleaching or electrolysis if hirsutism is a problem for female patients, because shaving or depilatories often leave stubble.
Teach patients to notify the physician if they experience a change in mood or behaviors that indicate depression or suicidal thoughts or actions. They should also notify the physician if they experience: skin rash, severe nausea or vomiting, swollen glands, bleeding, swollen or tender gums, yellowish discoloration of the skin or eyes, joint pain, unexplained fever, sore throat, unusual bleeding or bruising, persistent headache, malaise, and any indication of an infection or bleeding tendency, which are signs of serious adverse effects. Female patients should also notify the physician if they become pregnant.
Teach women who have delivered an infant about the risks involved in breast-feeding.

Ongoing Assessment and Evaluation

Ongoing assessments include monitoring patients closely for therapeutic responses, seizure control, and adverse effects to drug therapy. Blood levels of the drug should be monitored whenever the dose is changed, or if the patient is having seizures. Because phenytoin interacts with so many drugs through its effect on the enzymes of hepatic metabolism, also determine the likelihood of drug interactions between phenytoin and other newly ordered drugs or newly discontinued drugs. Phenytoin therapy is effective if seizures can be controlled and the patient experiences no serious adverse effects.

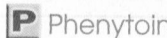 **MEMORY CHIP**

P Phenytoin

- Used to treat generalized tonic-clonic (grand mal) and other psychomotor seizures; status epilepticus
- Binds to receptors on sodium channels, keeping the channels in a closed position longer, preventing influx of sodium ions and excessive firing of the cell
- Major contraindications: sinus bradycardia, sinoatrial block, second- and third-degree AV block, and Adams-Stokes syndrome
- Most common adverse effects: CNS (dizziness, ataxia, blurred vision), nausea, and gingival hyperplasia
- Most serious adverse effects: life-threatening dermatologic reactions, liver damage, and blood dyscrasias; cardiovascular collapse if given too rapidly by IV push
- **Life span alert: can cause fetal hydantoin syndrome, infant death from neonatal hemorrhage, and decreased effectiveness of hormonal contraceptives; circulating level will decrease during pregnancy, increasing risk for seizures**
- Maximizing therapeutic effect: Monitor for therapeutic blood level, avoid coadministration with enteral tube feedings
- Minimizing adverse effects: Change dose upward or downward in small increments; monitor blood levels when dosage is changed or if symptomatic of adverse effects; give IV push very slowly during status epilepticus; vitamin K before date of delivery; monitor mood
- Most important patient education: Be careful driving or operating machinery until effects of drug are known; potential risks to fetus if patient becomes pregnant; may increase suicidal thoughts
- **Black box warning: must be administered ver slowly IV**

Antiepileptic drugs require that much of the same information be shared with patient and family. The nurse providing education for the epileptic patient should include the following information:

- Antiepileptic drug therapy does not cure the seizure disorder; it suppresses seizure activity.
- When seizures recur so frequently that consciousness or normal function cannot be regained in the interval between seizures, the condition is known as status epilepticus; this is a medical emergency.
- Sudden withdrawal of the antiepileptic drug may cause a loss of epileptic control, and the patient may experience seizures or status epilepticus. Prescriptions should not be allowed to run out or expire.
- Failure to take prescribed drug therapy results in recurrent seizures, with increased emergency department and inpatient admissions. Stress the importance of taking drugs on schedule and recommend memory aides, such as written medication schedules and pillboxes, particularly for more complex drug regimens.
- Double dosing of an antiepileptic drug should be avoided. If a dose is missed, instruct the patient to take the dose as soon as it is remembered unless it is close to the time for the next dose.
- All antiepileptic drugs carry a warning that their use may increase thoughts of suicide or suicidal actions. Be alert for changes in behavior or mood that may indicate depression and report this at once to the prescriber. Read the Medication Guide that comes from the FDA with each prescription that is filled for the most up-to-date information on this and other potential adverse effects from drug therapy. Read the Medication Guide each time a prescription is filled as it will have the most up-to-date information contained within it.
- Follow-up appointments with the health care provider and periodic laboratory testing are important because they provide an ongoing record of response (both positive and negative) to antiepileptic drug therapy. Drug levels should be checked at least yearly in patients whose epilepsy is controlled on medication and whose drug dose remains constant. Drug levels need to be monitored more frequently if the patient continues to have seizures or if the dose is adjusted.
- A "seizure record" should be kept. This record can provide information about changes in the type or frequency of seizures over time, the effect of different medications on seizure control, adverse effects of medications, and seizure-provoking factors. This record should include the date and time, as well as the type, of seizure. If a precipitating factor is suspected (e.g., lack of sleep, missed medication, stress, menstrual period, alcohol use), the patient should write it down. For women, it may be helpful to keep track of the relationship between seizures and menstrual cycles. It is also helpful to record the medication, dosage, and blood drug levels (if known). Recommend that the patient and family (or caregiver) show this record to the health care provider during follow-up visits.

- A form of medical identification (e.g., MedicAlert) indicating the medical condition and the drugs prescribed for it, including dosage in case of an emergency, should be carried or worn by the patient.
- Use of OTC preparations, herbal preparations, and dietary supplements may interact with the effectiveness of antiepileptic drugs and should be avoided unless approved by the physician or nurse practitioner. Prescription medications may also interact with the antiepileptic drug, so all providers should be informed of the antiepileptic drug therapy.
- Transient mild drowsiness and dizziness are common in the first few days of therapy, until the patient becomes accustomed to the drug therapy. Observe caution while driving, operating machinery or performing other tasks requiring mental alertness and motor coordination until effects of the drug are known.
- Alcohol consumption should be avoided because it may increase the CNS-depressant effect of the antiepileptic; large amounts of alcohol (three or more drinks per day) are likely to increase the risk of seizures. Small amounts of alcohol (one or two drinks per day) do not usually affect seizure frequency once the patient's condition is well controlled.
- Environmental factors (e.g., flashing lights, alcohol) and physiologic factors (e.g., hypoglycemia, fatigue, stress) may increase the frequency of seizures. If stress aggravates seizure activity, teach the patient to develop effective stress management techniques.
- Antiepileptic drugs can have significant effects on hormonal homeostasis, although epilepsy itself may play a role in causing these problems. Men may experience reduced libido and sexual potency; women may experience sexual arousal disorders. Seizure frequency may increase during menses because of the increase in sex hormones that alter the excitability of cortical neurons.
- Certain P450 enzyme inducing antiepileptic drugs (phenytoin, carbazepine, barbiturates, primidone, topiramate, oxcarbazepine) reduce the effectiveness of oral contraceptives, increasing the risk of unintended pregnancy, and should be used with caution in women of childbearing age (World Health Organization, 2009). Even with changes in the rate of metabolism, oral hormonal contraceptives are still recommended as they offer comparable, if not superior, effectiveness in preventing pregnancy compared to other contraceptive methods, such as intrauterine devices or barrier methods, which are more effective when used in conjunction with oral contraceptives. While oral contraceptives generally do not affect antiepileptic drug activity, studies have shown that serum levels of laotrigine decrease significantly and seizure activity increases with the use of combined oral contraceptives that include estrogen.
- The risk of having a child with a congenital defect may be two to three times greater in epileptic women who received antiepileptic drugs in the early stages of pregnancy. Most antiepileptic drugs are not recommended during pregnancy and lactation. However, the majority of women receiving antiepileptics deliver healthy infants.

Drugs Closely Related to P Phenytoin
Ethotoin

Ethotoin (Peganone) is a hydantoin like phenytoin, with similar pharmacodynamics and pharmacokinetics. It is used in the treatment of tonic-clonic and complex partial seizures. Unlike phenytoin, ethotoin is available only as an oral tablet. Although all hydantoins may cause gingival hyperplasia, the severity of the hyperplasia may be decreased if the patient

is switched to ethotoin. Like phenytoin, ethotoin carries the warning that it may increase suicidal thoughts or actions.

Fosphenytoin

Fosphenytoin (Cerebyx) is actually a prodrug of phenytoin; that is, it is converted to phenytoin. Thus, the actions of the drug are the same as phenytoin. Fosphenytoin creates two unique metabolites when converting into phenytoin: phosphate and formaldehyde. These metabolites are excreted without problems when fosphenytoin is given in recommended amounts. Fosphenytoin is given as doses of phenytoin equivalents. It is administered only as a short-term therapy when other means of IV phenytoin administration are unavailable, inappropriate, or deemed less advantageous. It can also be substituted, short-term, for oral phenytoin. The safety and effectiveness of fosphenytoin sodium when given for more than 5 days are not known. The drug is administered parenterally. Like phenytoin, it carries the warning that it may increase suicidal thoughts or actions.

Drugs Significantly Different From
P Phenytoin

Carbamazepine

Carbamazepine (Tegretol) is used to treat partial seizures with complex symptoms. It can also be used in treating generalized tonic-clonic seizures, mixed seizure patterns, or other partial or generalized seizures. Although effective in all of these types of seizures, carbamazepine seems to produce the most effect in treating partial seizures with complex symptoms. Carbamazepine is also used to treat trigeminal neuralgia. Off-label uses for carbamazepine include its common use in treating several psychiatric disorders (bipolar disorder, depression, schizoaffective illness, schizophrenia resistant to other drug therapies, dyscontrol syndrome associated with limbic system dysfunction, intermittent explosion disorder, post-traumatic stress disorder, and atypical psychosis). Other off-label uses are management of alcohol, cocaine, and benzodiazepine withdrawal; restless legs syndrome; nonneuritic pain syndromes, painful neuromas, or phantom limb pain; neurogenic or central diabetes insipidus; and hereditary or nonhereditary chorea in children. Therapeutic blood level for controlling seizures is 2 to 4 mcg/mL.

Carbamazepine is chemically related to the tricyclic antidepressants. Its mode of action is similar to that of phenytoin; it is believed to suppress the inflow of sodium into the cell, thereby decreasing frequency of action potentials and controlling seizures. It is generally well absorbed. Bioavailability of the drug is essentially the same for conventional tablets, extended-release tablets, and oral suspension. However, peak times differ among these routes, with the quickest peak (about 1.5 hours) from the suspension and the slowest peak (3 to 12 hours) from the extended-release format. Therapeutic blood level for the drug ranges from 4 to 12 mcg/mL for an adult. Carbamazepine is less protein bound than phenytoin, at 76%. Although carbamazepine, like phenytoin, is metabolized by the liver, the characteristics of metabolism are different. The metabolite formed also has antiepileptic activity; its half-life is shorter than that of carbamazepine. The half-life of carbamazepine is initially 25 to 65 hours; with repeated doses of the drug, the half-life decreases to 12 to 17 hours. Excretion of the drug and metabolite are primarily through the urine, but some is also excreted through the feces.

Like phenytoin, carbamazepine is a pregnancy category D drug, and the same concerns exist about its use in pregnancy and sudden discontinuation of the drug during pregnancy.

The most common adverse effects from carbamazepine are similar to those from phenytoin: dizziness, drowsiness, unsteadiness, nausea, vomiting, and diarrhea. A major difference in the adverse effects of these two drugs is the Black Box warning carried by carbamazepine in regard to its potential to cause three fatal blood dyscrasias. These are aplastic anemia (lack of red blood cells caused by disorders of bone marrow), thrombocytopenia (lack of platelets), and agranulocytosis (complete lack of white blood cells). Carbamazepine has been found to increase the risk of developing these fatal disorders; patients taking the drug are between five and eight times more likely to develop these hematologic problems than the general population not taking the drug. Still, even with this increased risk, the likelihood that aplastic anemia, thrombocytopenia, or agranulocytosis will develop is very low. Many patients have transient or persistent decreased red blood cell, platelet, or white blood cell counts and do not develop the more serious conditions. However, patients receiving carbamazepine need to be monitored for these conditions, even more carefully if any changes occur in the blood cell counts. Drug therapy should be discontinued if considerable depression of bone marrow function is apparent. Patients who have hematologic abnormalities should not receive carbamazepine, and those of Asian descent should be screened for the HLA-B*1502 allele variant which can increase the risk of Stevens-Johnson syndrome and toxic epidermal necrolysis in those individuals. Like phenytoin it carries the warning that it may increase suicidal thoughts or actions.

Valproic Acid

Valproic acid (Depakote), also called valproate, is a broad-spectrum antiepileptic drug that is effective against all types of seizures. It is the most widely prescribed antiepileptic drug worldwide. In the United States, the only Food and Drug Administration (FDA)–approved use is for absence seizures, although in practice it is used for tonic-clonic, atonic, myoclonic, and partial seizures. Additionally, valproic acid is approved to treat mania and migraine headaches. Recent randomized experimental trials with valproic acid indicate that it is as effective as phenytoin in treating status epilepticus (Agarwal et al., 2007). The therapeutic blood level for seizure control is 50 to 150 mcg/mL. Valproic acid is available as several formulations, some quick release, some delayed release, and some extended release.

Valproic acid works through a number of different mechanisms. Like phenytoin, it blocks the voltage-gated sodium channels but at different sites than phenytoin or carbamazepine. Unlike phenytoin, it also increases GABA release and concentration. Valproate does not seem to have any direct effect on the GABA receptor. Valproate also inhibits nerve terminal GABA transaminase, which raises presynaptic GABA levels. Valproate may also increase GABA synthesis. Like ethosuximide (to be discussed), valproate acts against special calcium channels to block calcium influx, but has a less favorable adverse event profile (UpToDate, 2010a).

Oral absorption of valproic acid is rapid, and all oral formulations have almost 100% bioavailability. Like phenytoin, valproic acid is highly protein bound, although as the dosage of valproic acid increases, the percentage of drug that is bound decreases. Valproic acid is metabolized through the liver, but, unlike phenytoin, it does not induce hepatic enzymes and does not affect oral hormonal contraceptives. However, it can potentially inhibit the drug metabolism of some drugs. The half-life of valproic acid is between 9 and 18 hours; shorter half-lives of 5 to 12 hours can occur in patients also being medicated with enzyme-inducing agents such as phenytoin, carbamazepine, or barbiturates.

The most common adverse effects of valproic acid are GI problems, tremor, and weight gain. Adverse effects, which are not common but very serious and potentially lethal, are elevated blood ammonia levels (hyperammonemia), possibly with encephalopathy symptoms; platelet disorders; pancreatitis (life threatening); and liver toxicity (including liver failure and death). Liver toxicity, although rare, appears to be more of a risk in children younger than 2 years who are on multiple–antiepileptic drug therapy. Liver function tests should be periodically monitored for patients receiving valproic acid. Other adverse effects that can occur include CNS effects (sedation, ataxia, confusion); dermatologic effects (transient hair loss, skin rash, photosensitivity, Stevens-Johnson syndrome); endocrine effects (irregular menses, breast enlargement); psychiatric effects (depression, psychosis, aggression); and miscellaneous effects (weakness, fever, hearing loss, otitis media).

Valproic acid is a pregnancy category D drug. Case reports in the literature indicate an increased risk of neural tube defects (such as spina bifida) when the drug is used during pregnancy, with about 1% to 2% of births having neural tube defects. This adverse effect is usually associated with the use of higher doses. Compared with phenytoin, carbamazepine, and lamotrigine, valproic acid poses the highest risk of serious fetal adverse effects (Meador et al., 2006).

Valproic acid may cause falsely elevated urine ketone tests when used in patients with diabetes and altered thyroid tests. Like phenytoin, it carries the warning that it may increase suicidal thoughts or actions.

Lamotrigine

Lamotrigine (Lamictal) is approved as an adjunct therapy for treating partial seizures in adults and generalized seizures of Lennox-Gastaut syndrome (the most severe form of childhood epilepsy, characterized by very frequent seizures of several different types; it is usually nonresponsive to other antiepileptic drug therapy) in pediatric and adult patients. This drug has been found effective as adjunct therapy in primary generalized tonic-clonic seizures. In addition, clinical studies have shown that lamotrigine is effective as monotherapy for adolescents and adults with newly diagnosed partial or mixed seizure disorders. It *is* effective in treating children with newly diagnosed absence seizures, the most common pediatric epilepsy syndrome, but less so than ethosuximide and valproic acid (Glauser et al., 2010).

Lamotrigine is not chemically related to other antiepileptic drugs. It appears to act by decreasing the sodium influx into the cells. A standardized serum blood level has not been determined.

Lamotrigine is easily absorbed from the GI tract and has about 98% bioavailability, which is not affected by food. Peak serum levels are reached in 1.4 to 4.8 hours. Lamotrigine is much less protein bound than phenytoin, at about 55%. Lamotrigine does not displace other protein-bound antiepileptic drugs. An unusual feature of lamotrigine is its ability to bind in melanin-containing skin (e.g., in eyes and pigmented skin). Lamotrigine is metabolized by hepatic enzymes and is capable of inducing its own metabolism with repeated administration. When administered with other antiepileptic drugs that induce hepatic enzymes, its elimination is increased. The exception to this effect is when lamotrigine is administered along with valproic acid. Valproic acid more than doubles the half-life of lamotrigine, requiring dose adjustments of lamotrigine.

The most common adverse effects of lamotrigine are CNS effects (dizziness, double vision, ataxia, blurred vision, somnolence, and headache), GI effects (nausea and vomiting, which are dose related), and rash. Although rashes can be common, serious life-threatening rashes, including Stevens-Johnson syndrome, can occur. Life-threatening rashes are more common in children treated with lamotrigine. For this reason, children younger than 16 years should not be treated with lamotrigine unless they have Lennox-Gastaut syndrome that is resistant to other drugs. Administering lamotrigine with valproic acid also appears to increase the incidence of rash. Because it is not possible to distinguish which rashes will become serious, drug therapy should be stopped at the first sign of a rash. Unfortunately, even stopping drug therapy immediately may not prevent a rash from becoming life-threatening or permanently disfiguring. Like phenytoin, it carries the warning that it may increase suicidal thoughts or actions.

Lamotrigine is a pregnancy category C drug. Animal studies have shown maternal and fetal toxicity, but teratogenic effects have not been determined, although lamotrigine is known to decrease the fetal folate concentrations in animals.

Topiramate

Topiramate (Topamax) is used to treat partial-onset seizures and tonic-clonic seizures. There is evidence that topiramate is effective monotherapy in adolescents and adults with newly diagnosed partial or mixed seizure disorders (French et al., 2004). Off-label uses include cluster headaches, infantile spasms, and Lennox-Gastaut syndrome (a severe form of epilepsy). Like phenytoin, topiramate has an effect on the sodium influx into cells, blocking formation of action potentials. Unlike phenytoin, topiramate has two other methods of action. Topiramate enhances the effectiveness of GABA, increasing the inhibitory effects of the neurotransmitter. Topiramate also blocks the receptors for glutamate, a stimulating neurotransmitter. Therapeutic serum levels have not been determined.

Topiramate is easily absorbed when taken orally. Bioavailability of tablets is about 80%; it is not altered by food intake. Peak levels occur in about 2 hours. The half-life of topiramate is 18.7 to 23 hours. Steady state is reached in about 4 days in patients with normal renal function. Unlike phenytoin, topiramate has low protein binding, about 13% to 17%. Also unlike phenytoin, topiramate is mostly excreted unchanged in the urine. Only a small percentage of the drug is metabolized. A drug interaction related to the P-450 system occurs when topiramate is taken with other drugs that induce these enzymes, such as phenytoin. While phenytoin may increase the metabolism of topiramate, topiramate may decrease the metabolism of phenytoin (UpToDate, 2010d. Enzyme induction will also reduce the effectiveness of oral hormonal contraceptives, which may still be the most effective form of contraception and can be augmented with intra-uterine devices or barrier methods.

Topiramate is a weak carbonic anhydrase inhibitor and, like other carbonic anhydrase inhibitors (e.g., acetazolamide and dichlorphenamide), it promotes kidney stone formation by reducing urinary citrate excretion and increasing the urinary pH. The concurrent use of topiramate and other carbonic anhydrase inhibitors increases the risk of kidney stone formation. The renal bicarbonate loss that results from inhibition of carbonic anhydrase can produce metabolic acidosis. Larger doses of topiramate are more likely to result in metabolic acidosis. Baseline and periodic evaluation of serum bicarbonate are recommended for those receiving topiramate (UpToDate, 2010d).

Topiramate carries a warning that oligohidrosis (decreased sweating) and hyperthermia, with potentially serious sequelae, may occur. These adverse effects have infrequently required hospitalization. This warning is based on postmarketing reports that have been received. Most cases have been associated with high environmental temperatures or vigorous exercise. Caution needs to be used if topiramate is prescribed with other drugs that can predispose the patient to heat-related disorders, such as other carbonic anhydrase inhibitors or drugs with anticholinergic effects. Teach all patients, especially parents of children prescribed topiramate, to monitor for decreased sweating and elevated temperature and to seek medical help if these occur. Proper hydration in hot weather, especially before and during exercise or activity, is helpful to decrease the effects from oligohidrosis and hyperthermia.

Topiramate is ranked as a pregnancy category C drug. Animal studies have found that teratogenic effects can occur if given during the time of organ development. No studies have been done with humans.

The most common adverse effects with topiramate are weight loss and the CNS effects (psychomotor slowing; cognitive impairment such as difficulty with concentration, speech or language problems, especially word-finding difficulties; somnolence and fatigue). Other CNS effects are also possible, but not as common. However, generally, the drug is well tolerated.

Topiramate is available in tablets and in sprinkle capsules. Tablets should be swallowed whole because they have a bitter taste if broken. Instruct patients to open the sprinkle capsules and to sprinkle the entire contents onto a teaspoon of soft food, such as applesauce, and swallow (not chew) it immediately. Follow with water to guarantee that all the drug is swallowed.

Oxcarbazepine

Oxcarbazepine (Trileptal) is chemically similar to the metabolite of carbamazepine; it was designed to mimic its efficacy while minimizing adverse effects and risks of drug interactions. Oxcarbazepine is used as either monotherapy or adjunctive therapy in adults with partial seizures and as adjunctive therapy for children 4 to 16 years of age with partial seizures. In addition, there is evidence that oxcarbazepine is effective monotherapy in adolescents and adults with newly diagnosed partial or mixed seizure disorders (French et al., 2004). Although the precise mechanism of action of oxcarbazepine is not known, it is believed to block voltage-sensitive sodium channels, similar to phenytoin. Its effects on increasing potassium conduction and suppressing high-voltage calcium channels may also contribute to the anti-epileptic properties of oxcarbazepine. The drug is rapidly absorbed. It has moderate–low protein binding, at 40%. The drug is rapidly converted to its active metabolite; all of the drug's effects are achieved through the metabolite. The metabolites are excreted through the urine.

There seems to be some cross-hypersensitivity between oxcarbazepine and carbamazepine. Between 25% and 30% of patients who have exhibited hypersensitivity to carbamazepine also have hypersensitivity to oxcarbazepine. Oxcarbazepine is a pregnancy category C drug. Although no human studies exist to confirm the drug's teratogenicity in humans, its similar chemical structure to carbamazepine, a known teratogen, makes it likely that oxcarbazepine also causes human teratogenic effects.

The most common adverse effects of oxcarbazepine are related to the CNS (dizziness, somnolence, diplopia, abnormal vision, fatigue, ataxia, abnormal gait, and tremor) and the GI system (nausea, vomiting, abdominal pain, and dyspepsia). Hyponatremia can also occur with oxcarbazepine use; clinically important hyponatremia generally occurs within the first 3 months of treatment. Routine assessment of sodium levels in patients taking oxcarbazepine is necessary.

Oxcarbazepine is a CYP3A4/5 inducer and can cause substantial drug interactions with some other antiepileptic drugs that are also inducers of this pathway. The circulating levels of oxcarbazepine decrease when it is given with carbamazepine, phenytoin, valproic acid, or phenobarbital. Coadministering these drugs causes only phenytoin and phenobarbital levels to rise. Verapamil, a calcium channel blocker used in several cardiac conditions, causes oxcarbazepine levels to decrease substantially. Oxcarbazepine causes the circulating levels of oral contraceptives to decrease by up to half. Teach women taking oral contraceptives that they need to use an additional form of birth control while taking oxcarbazepine.

Levetiracetam

Levetiracetam (Keppra) is an adjunct antiepileptic drug used to treat partial-onset seizures in adults and children as well as generalized myoclonic seizures in adults and adolescents. Research has shown that levetiracetam monotherapy is as effective as phenytoin, with less undesirable adverse effects and better long-term outcomes, although it is labeled only as an adjuvant therapy (Szaflarski et al., 2010). Levetiracetam is chemically unrelated to other antiepileptic drugs. Unlike phenytoin, its exact mechanism of action is not known, although it does *not* inhibit seizures by any mechanism related to inhibitory or excitatory neurohormones. Levetiracetam may prevent hypersynchronization of epileptiform burst firings and propagation of seizure activity from the hippocampus.

Levetiracetam is rapidly absorbed, and food does not affect the extent of absorption. Two thirds of the drug is renally excreted unchanged. The one third that is metabolized is not metabolized through any of the P-450 isoenzymes, and it does not induce any of the P-450 isoenzymes. An advantage of levetiracetam is that it does not require titration when therapy is started; patients can be started on the maintenance dose. Dosing needs to be decreased if renal impairment develops.

Generally, levetiracetam is well tolerated. The most common adverse effects are usually mild to moderate in intensity, and they are transient, disappearing after initial titration. These effects include fatigue, somnolence, dizziness, upper respiratory infection, and asthenia (weakness). Somnolence can occur in nearly 50% of patients unless the dose is slowly increased upward to the desired dose. Like phenytoin, it carries the warning that it may increase suicidal thoughts or actions.

Unlike phenytoin and other antiepileptic drugs, levetiracetam has no known drug interactions. It is a pregnancy category C drug.

Felbamate

Felbamate (Felbatol) is not a first-line antiepileptic drug. It is approved to treat partial seizures, either with or without generalization in adults, and Lennox-Gastaut syndrome in children, but it is used only if other therapies have not been effective and the epilepsy is considered severe. This restriction is attributable to the fact that felbamate greatly increases the risk of aplastic anemia (lack of red blood cells from bone marrow damage). The incidence of aplastic anemia among patients who are taking felbamate may be more than 100 times the incidence found in the general population. Death occurs in 20% to 70% of the patients who develop aplastic anemia, depending on the severity of the disorder. Aplastic anemia usually occurs as a full-blown syndrome; thus, there are no clinical warning signs or indications, and laboratory work does not indicate early signs of problems. However, monitoring laboratory studies does indicate full-blown aplastic anemia. Felbamate also greatly increases the risk of liver failure. Liver function tests must be monitored during therapy. Because of these serious consequences, felbamate is used only if other therapies have failed and the benefit to the patient outweighs

these considerable risks. Therapeutic blood levels have not been determined.

The exact manner in which felbamate decreases seizure activity is unknown, which is a significant difference from phenytoin.

Felbamate is well absorbed from the GI tract. About half of the drug is metabolized to several metabolites, and the other half is excreted in the urine unchanged. Terminal half-life of felbamate is 20 to 23 hours.

In addition to the serious adverse effects listed previously, felbamate can produce photosensitivity as well as many other adverse effects, all of which are not common. Felbamate is a pregnancy category C drug. Like phenytoin, it carries the warning that it may increase suicidal thoughts or actions.

• ANTIEPILEPTIC DRUGS THAT DECREASE CALCIUM INFLUX

The prototype antiepileptic drug that inhibits influx of calcium is ethosuximide (Zarontin).

Nursing Management of the Patient Receiving [P] Ethosuximide

Core Drug Knowledge

Pharmacotherapeutics

Ethosuximide is used to treat absence (petit mal) seizures. A therapeutic serum level is 40 to 100 mcg/mL. It is available as capsules and as a syrup.

Pharmacokinetics

Readily absorbed from the GI tract, ethosuximide can reach a peak serum level in 3 to 7 hours. Ethosuximide is extensively metabolized to inactive metabolites, and 20% is excreted unchanged by the kidneys. The plasma half-life is 30 hours in children and 60 hours in adults.

Pharmacodynamics

Ethosuximide, one of the succinimides, works by inhibiting the influx of calcium ions when they travel through a special set of channels, known as T-type calcium channels. Although an electric current is generated when the calcium moves through the T-type channels, in most neurons, this current has only a minimal role in creating an action potential. However, in the hypothalamus neurons, this electric current does play an important role in creating an action potential. Because hypothalamic neurons are responsible for absence seizures, control of action potentials in this location reduces the incidence of absence seizures.

Contraindications and Precautions

Hypersensitivity to succinimides is the only contraindication for ethosuximide. Caution should be used if ethosuximide is used as monotherapy in mixed types of epilepsy because it may increase the frequency of tonic-clonic (grand mal) seizures in some patients. Caution should be used if the patient has pre-existing renal or liver disease. Ethosuximide is a pregnancy class C drug. Like phenytoin, ethosuximide carries the warning that it may increase suicidal thoughts or actions.

Adverse Effects

Common adverse effects of ethosuximide are drowsiness, dizziness, and lethargy. The patient usually accommodates to these adverse effects. Nausea and vomiting are also common. Other CNS and GI effects are possible but not common. Serious adverse effects include blood dyscrasias, with and without bone marrow suppression. Some of the cases of blood dyscrasias have been fatal. Another serious adverse effect is the development of systemic lupus erythematosus. Liver or renal function may also be impaired.

Adverse effects, which are uncommon, include:

- *Dermatologic:* pruritus, urticaria, Stevens-Johnson syndrome, pruritic erythematous rashes, skin eruptions, erythema multiforme, alopecia, hirsutism
- *Genitourinary:* urinary frequency, renal damage, vaginal bleeding, microscopic hematuria
- *Psychiatric:* confusion, instability, mental slowness, depression, hypochondriacal behavior, sleep disturbances, night terrors, aggressiveness, inability to concentrate (these are most often in patients who have previously had psychological disorders)
- *Miscellaneous:* periorbital edema, hyperemia, muscle weakness, swollen tongue, gum hypertrophy

Drug Interactions

Ethosuximide is known to interact with some of the other antiepileptic drugs. Table 18.4 describes these interactions, effects and significance, and nursing management.

Assessment of Relevant Core Patient Variables

Health Status

Patients should have absence seizures in order to receive ethosuximide. Confirm that the patient does not have a hypersensitivity to the drug before starting therapy. Determine whether the patient has pre-existing renal

or hepatic disease, both of which indicate caution with ethosuximide use.

Life Span and Gender

Like all antiepileptic drugs, ethosuximide may cause teratogenic effects if given during pregnancy. However, as with other antiepileptic drugs, suddenly discontinuing ethosuximide may cause an increase in seizures. Women of childbearing age should be aware of the risks related to pregnancy. Assess whether a woman is pregnant before starting drug therapy.

Environment

Ethosuximide can be administered in all environmental settings.

Nursing Diagnoses and Outcomes

- Imbalanced Nutrition: Less than Body Requirements, related to adverse GI drug effects of anorexia, abdominal complaints, nausea, and vomiting
  Desired outcome: The patient will not experience major nutritional imbalances while receiving ethosuximide.
- Risk for Injury from falls related to CNS adverse effects of ethosuximide
  Desired outcome: The patient will not sustain an injury while receiving ethosuximide.
- Risk for Injury from blood dyscrasias related to adverse effects of ethosuximide
  Desired outcome: The patient will not experience major changes in his or her complete blood cell counts.

Planning and Intervention

Maximizing Therapeutic Effects

When initiating therapy or changing a dose, monitor the drug serum level to determine whether a therapeutic range has been obtained.

Minimizing Adverse Effects

Assess complete blood counts regularly to determine whether any low blood cell counts are present. If patients develop signs of infection (sore throat, fever), the blood

TABLE 18.4 Agents That Interact with P Ethosuximide

Interactants	Effect and Significance	Nursing Management
valproic acid	Increased pharmacologic effects of ethosuximide Both increases and decreases in ethosuximide levels have occurred	Monitor patient for changes in seizure control. Assess patient for evidence of therapeutic effects of interacting drugs.
phenytoin	Serum hydantoin levels may increase	Evaluate patient for changed seizure control. Assess patient for evidence of therapeutic effects of interacting drugs. Check for therapeutic serum levels of interacting drugs.
primidone	Lower primidone and phenobarbital levels may occur	Evaluate patient for changed seizure control. Assess patient for evidence of therapeutic effects of interacting drugs. Check for therapeutic serum levels of interacting drugs.

cell counts should also be checked at that time. Periodic urinalysis and liver function studies help identify early any complications that might be from ethosuximide therapy. Like all antiepileptic drugs, taper the dose gradually if it is necessary to discontinue the drug to minimize the risk for seizures, including absence status.

Providing Patient and Family Education

Much of the teaching for ethosuximide is similar to that for phenytoin and other antiepileptic drugs. Specific teaching includes the following:

- Teach patients to take the drug with milk or food if GI upset occurs.
- Teach patients to notify the physician if any of the following occurs: changes in mood or behavior that indicate depression or suicidal thinking, skin rash, joint pain, unexplained fever, sore throat, unusual bleeding or bruising, severe drowsiness, severe dizziness, blurred vision, or pregnancy.
- Teach women of childbearing age to use birth control, because drug therapy carries some risks if they become pregnant. Women who wish to become pregnant while taking this drug need to be counseled about the importance of discussing their options with their physicians first.

Ongoing Assessment and Evaluation

Ongoing assessments include monitoring patients closely for therapeutic responses, seizure control, and adverse effects of drug therapy. Blood levels of the drug should be monitored whenever the dose is changed or if the patient is having seizures. Ethosuximide therapy is effective if seizures can be controlled and the patient experiences no serious adverse effects.

Drugs Closely Related to Ethosuximide

Methsuximide (Celontin) has similar actions and adverse effects as ethosuximide. Unlike ethosuximide, it is available

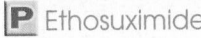 MEMORY CHIP

P Ethosuximide

- Used to treat absence (petit mal) seizures
- Works by inhibiting the influx of calcium ions through T-type calcium channels
- Most common adverse effects: drowsiness, dizziness, lethargy, nausea and vomiting
- Most serious adverse effects: blood dyscrasias, systemic lupus erythematosus
- Maximizing therapeutic effect: Monitor serum levels.
- Minimizing adverse effects: Monitor serum levels and complete blood counts; assess mood
- Most important patient education: Notify the physician of skin rash, joint pain, signs of infection, unusual bleeding or bruising, or pregnancy; may increase suicidal thoughts

only as capsules. Peak concentration levels are reached somewhat more rapidly than for methsuximide—in 1 to 4 hours instead of in 3 to 7 hours.

Phensuximide (Milontin) is very similar to the prototype ethosuximide, with a few exceptions. Like methsuximide, it also peaks in 1 to 4 hours instead of in 3 to 7. Unlike ethosuximide, which is extensively metabolized, phensuximide is excreted in urine and bile, and less than 20% is excreted via the kidneys unchanged. Phensuximide may discolor the urine pink, red, or red-brown. This is not harmful. It may also cause some hematuria. Phensuximide carries an additional warning that when given to patients with acute intermittent porphyria, caution should be used. Like ethosuximide, it carries the warning that it may increase suicidal thoughts or actions.

Drug Significantly Different From P Ethosuximide

Zonisamide (Zonegran) is used as an adjunct drug in treating partial seizures, as well as generalized seizures, in adults. Its therapeutic level has not been determined.

Zonisamide is a sulfonamide drug. Although the exact mechanism of action is not known, it is believed to block calcium flow through T-type calcium channels, like ethosuximide. Additionally, zonisamide appears to alter sodium influx, like phenytoin. Zonisamide also facilitates dopamine and serotonin transmission. It has *not* been shown to increase the effectiveness of GABA.

Absorption of zonisamide is fairly slow with oral administration, and peak levels occur within 2 to 6 hours. If food is present when the drug is administered, the peak does not occur until 4 to 6 hours; however, the bioavailability is not changed with the presence of food. Zonisamide has fairly low protein binding at 40%. Zonisamide binds extensively in erythrocytes as opposed to the plasma. Eight times as much drug is in red blood cells compared with the plasma. The half-life of zonisamide varies; it is 63 hours from the plasma and 105 hours from the red blood cells. A steady state occurs in 14 days. Metabolism occurs in the liver, but most of the drug is eliminated in the urine unchanged. If zonisamide is taken with other drugs that induce hepatic enzymes, its rate of metabolism is increased.

Hypersensitivity to zonisamide or to sulfonamides is a contraindication. Death can occur, although rarely, related to a hypersensitivity reaction to sulfonamides. Zonisamide is a pregnancy category C drug. Like ethosuximide, it carries the warning that it may increase suicidal thoughts or actions.

Common adverse effects of zonisamide include dizziness, somnolence, fatigue, ataxia, decreased mental functioning, nausea, headache, irritability, and renal calculi. Serious adverse effects include Stevens-Johnson syndrome, aplastic anemia, and agranulocytosis. Lack of sweating and elevated temperatures in children were noted during clinical testing. The drug is not approved for use in children.

Zonisamide is known to increase the levels of the following laboratory tests: serum creatinine, blood urea nitrogen, and serum alkaline phosphatase.

● ANTIEPILEPTIC DRUGS THAT INCREASE THE EFFECTS OF GABA

Antiepileptic drugs that affect GABA are designed to increase the supply of GABA by lowering GABA metabolism, reducing reuptake of GABA into the neurons and glia, or increasing the production of GABA. Other antiepileptic drugs imitate the action GABA or improve GABA's inhibition of the nervous system.

Benzodiazepines

Benzodiazepines produce their many effects by potentiating the effects of the neurotransmitter, GABA, which is an inhibitory neurotransmitter. The GABA receptor complex has binding sites for GABA as well as for benzodiazepines and phenobarbital. Certain benzodiazepines are approved for different therapeutic uses, although all of the drugs in the class share many similarities. The prototype benzodiazepine is lorazepam and is discussed in Chapter 15. This chapter highlights diazepam, clonazepam, and clorazepate as antiepileptic drugs. Benzodiazepines are the drugs of first choice in treating status epilepticus. Because benzodiazepines as a class have been associated with the development of tolerance, their usefulness in chronic treatment for epilepsy is limited.

Diazepam

Diazepam is used as an adjunct to other antiepileptic drug therapy in convulsive disorders. It has historically been the drug of first choice to treat status epilepticus, although lorazepam is now often used and has some advantages over diazepam. In fact, research has shown that lorazepam is more effective than diazepam or phenytoin used alone for cessation of seizures and has an effective duration of up to 6 hours compared to 20 minutes for diazepam (Prasad et al., 2007). Both diazepam and lorazepam are an effective adjunctive therapy for myoclonic and atonic seizures, as well as partial and generalized tonic-clonic seizures (UpToDate, 2010a). Diazepam is also used to treat anxiety, as a muscle relaxant, in the treatment of acute alcohol withdrawal, and as a preoperative medication to reduce anxiety, tension, and recall of events. An off-label use is for treatment of panic attacks. The therapeutic blood level of diazepam has not been determined. Diazepam works like all benzodiazepines by increasing the effectiveness of GABA.

Onset of action when taken orally is very rapid for diazepam, and peak plasma levels are reached in 30 minutes to 2 hours. Diazepam is highly lipid soluble, so it rapidly crosses the blood–brain barrier. The drug is very highly protein bound, higher than lorazepam, at 98%. Like lorazepam, diazepam is metabolized through the liver; unlike lorazepam, it is metabolized to an active metabolite. Elimination half-life is 20 to 80 hours; this time is lengthened in obese patients. Like other benzodiazepines, diazepam is excreted in the urine.

Unique pharmacokinetic differences exist between diazepam and lorazepam, which are relevant when the drugs are used to treat status epilepticus. Although both drugs achieve therapeutic effects within a few minutes of IV administration, the onset of action of diazepam is more rapid, with an effect on seizure activity noticeable in as little as 10 to 20 seconds after administration. The onset of action of lorazepam is two minutes or less. The antiepileptic effect of the two drugs differs also; the duration of action of diazepam is short, with seizures often reoccurring 30 to 60 minutes after disruption of status epilepticus, whereas that of lorazepam is long—four to six hours. This phenomenon occurs because diazepam is distributed quickly to the brain, where it creates its effect, but then is rapidly redistributed out of the brain to other body tissues, specifically adipose tissues. On the other hand, lorazepam has a much slower redistribution out of the brain and therefore a longer duration of action in status epilepticus—that is, more than 12 hours (see Chapter 15 for more information).

Diazepam is similar to lorazepam and other benzodiazepines in terms of contraindications, precautions, adverse effects, and drug interactions. Because diazepam is used as an adjunct therapy and coadministered with other antiepileptic drugs, additional CNS depression may occur, and patients need to be cautioned when the drug is added to their therapy. Like the other antiepileptic drugs, diazepam carries the warning that it may increase suicidal thoughts or actions.

Diazepam is administered intravenously during status epilepticus; the small veins in the dorsum of the hand or the wrist should be avoided. It should be injected very slowly, no faster than 5 mg in 1 minute. Diazepam should not be mixed or diluted with other solutions or drugs, either in the syringe or in IV bags of fluid. A separate IV line should be placed to deliver phenytoin after diazepam or other benzodiazepine, because these precipitate if given via the same IV tubing. Diazepam interacts with plastic containers and administration sets, substantially decreasing the availability of drug delivered. If it is not possible to give diazepam directly into the vein, it can be administered through the IV infusion tubing as close to the insertion site into the vein as possible. Although a deep IM route could be used if absolutely necessary, IM injections produce low or erratic plasma levels and may not control status epilepticus easily. For this reason, the IM route is normally avoided.

After status epilepticus is treated with a benzodiazepine such as diazepam or lorazepam, IV phenytoin should be administered.

Clonazepam

Clonazepam is used alone or as adjunctive treatment for Lennox-Gastaut syndrome (absence variety) and atonic and myoclonic seizures. It may be useful in patients with absence seizures who have failed to respond to succinimides, such as ethosuximide. Unlabeled uses include periodic leg movements during sleep, parkinsonian (hypokinetic) dysarthria, acute manic episodes of bipolar disorders, multifocal tic disorders, adjunct treatment for schizophrenia, and neuralgias. Therapeutic serum levels are 20 to 80 mg/mL.

Like other benzodiazepines, clonazepam increases the effectiveness of GABA. Clonazepam suppresses the spike and wave discharge that occurs with absence seizures and decreases the frequency, amplitude, duration, and spread of neuronal discharge in motor seizures. The onset of action of clonazepam is intermediate, with peak plasma level being reached in 1 to 2 hours. Clonazepam is highly protein bound, at 97%. It is metabolized through the liver to five metabolites. The elimination half-life is 18 to 50 hours.

Tolerance to the antiseizure effects of clonazepam can occur within months. Abrupt withdrawal of the drug induces seizures, including status epilepticus.

Clonazepam can produce an increase in salivation as an adverse effect. It should be used with caution in patients for whom increased salivation causes respiratory difficulty. Like diazepam, when given with other antiepileptic drug therapy, clonazepam causes additive CNS depression. Like the other antiepileptics, it carries the warning that it may increase suicidal thoughts or actions.

Other adverse effects, precautions, and drug interactions are similar to the prototype, lorazepam.

Clorazepate

Clorazepate is used as adjunctive treatment for partial and generalized tonic-clonic seizures; it is also used to treat anxiety disorders and for symptom management in acute alcohol withdrawal. The therapeutic blood level for clorazepate has not been determined. It has a fast onset of action, reaches a peak in 1 to 2 hours, and has an elimination half-life of 40 to 50 hours. Clorazepate is highly protein bound at 97% to 98%. It is metabolized in the liver by the same pathway as diazepam. Like all benzodiazepines, it achieves its effects by enhancing the effects of GABA. Additional core drug knowledge about clorazepate is similar to the prototype, lorazepam.

Midazolam

Unlike diazepam, midazolam is primarily used as an anesthetic. Like diazepam, midazolam can stop seizures in status epilepticus quickly (frequently less than one minute); however, because of its short half-life, it needs to be administered as a continuous infusion to maintain an antiseizure effect. It is used in treatment of refractory status epilepticus in which other drug treatment has been unsuccessful, and nasal and buccal administration is useful when IV access is not possible (UpToDate, 2010c).

Drugs Significantly Different From the Benzodiazepines

Gabapentin

Gabapentin (Neurontin) is an adjunct antiepileptic drug used in treating partial seizures, with or without secondary generalization, in patients older than 12 years. Evidence indicates that gabapentin is effective monotherapy in adolescents and adults with newly diagnosed partial or mixed seizure disorders (French et al., 2004). It is also used in treating partial seizures in children 3 to 12 years of age. Off-label uses include multiple sclerosis, amyotrophic lateral sclerosis, neuropathic pain, bipolar disorder, and prophylaxis for migraine

headaches. A therapeutic blood level of gabapentin has not been established.

Gabapentin is structurally related to the neurotransmitter GABA, but it does not interact at GABA receptors. It is believed to promote the release of GABA. It is absorbed through the GI tract, and food does not affect its absorption. It is almost entirely free from protein binding, with only 3% bound. Gabapentin is excreted renally, without undergoing metabolism. Elimination half-life is 5 to 7 hours. Patients with renal failure or renal disease may have additional risks of adverse effects from the drug.

Gabapentin is a pregnancy category C drug. It is secreted into breast milk and should generally be avoided during nursing because the safety and efficacy in children younger than 3 years is not known. The most common adverse effects of gabapentin for patients older than 12 years of age are CNS effects: somnolence, dizziness, ataxia, fatigue, and nystagmus. In children between 3 and 12 years of age, the most common adverse effects of gabapentin are viral infection, fever, nausea and vomiting, somnolence, and hostility. Children younger than 12 years of age could have other neuropsychiatric adverse effects such as behavior problems, aggressive behavior, thought disorders with trouble concentrating or changes in school performance, restlessness, and hyperactivity. Usually, the occurrence of these effects is mild to moderate in intensity.

Because gabapentin does not affect hepatic enzymes responsible for metabolism of other drugs, it is free of drug interactions. This advantage makes it ideal to combine with other antiepileptic drugs for seizure treatment. The only important drug interaction is with antacids, which reduce the bioavailability of gabapentin by 20%; to avoid this interaction, gabapentin should be administered at least 2 hours after antacids are given.

The dose of gabapentin should be increased gradually in older adults, because they may have age-related kidney function deterioration. As with all antiepileptic drugs, gabapentin should be withdrawn slowly and gradually to prevent the onset of seizures. Like other antiepileptic drugs, it carries the warning that it may increase suicidal thoughts or actions.

Pregabalin

Pregabalin (Lyrica) is chemically related to gabapentin. It is used as adjunct therapy to treat partial seizures in adults. It is also used to treat neuropathic pain associated with diabetic peripheral neuropathy and postherpetic neuralgia. Pregabalin modulates the release of several neurotransmitters, including glutamate, noradrenaline, and substance P (which is involved in pain perception). Pregabalin also decreases the influx of calcium into the cell. All of these actions inhibit neuronal excitability.

Pregabalin is taken orally. Steady state is achieved within 24 to 48 hours. Although the plasma half-life is six hours, the effect of pregabalin appears to be much longer. Pregabalin is excreted unchanged; it is not metabolized. The drug has no effect on the P-450 system. Pregabalin does not bind to plasma proteins, so it does not have significant drug interactions with other antiepileptic drugs or other drugs.

The most common adverse effects of pregabalin are CNS effects: dizziness, somnolence, and ataxia. Less common adverse effects include weight gain, peripheral edema, blurred or double vision (which is normally transient), weakness, and impaired concentration. Because pregabalin also may cause euphoria, it is classified as a schedule V controlled substance. Like other antiepileptics, it carries the warning that it may increase suicidal thoughts or actions.

Pregabalin is a pregnancy category C drug.

Phenobarbital

Phenobarbital is used to treat generalized tonic-clonic and cortical focal seizures. Phenobarbital is also used to treat acute convulsive episodes that require emergency intervention (e.g., status epilepticus, eclampsia, cholera, meningitis, tetanus, and toxic reactions to strychnine or local anesthetics), as a preanesthetic, and to induce sleep (see Chapter 15). Phenobarbital is a general CNS depressant that suppresses the sensory cortex; decreases motor activity; alters cerebellar function; and produces drowsiness, sedation, and hypnosis. Phenobarbital's antiepileptic activities are relatively nonselective. Like the benzodiazepines, phenobarbital stimulates GABA receptors, thereby elevating the seizure threshold and limiting the spread of seizure activity by affecting the CNS neuronal pathway neurotransmitters. Tolerance does not occur to the antiepileptic effects of phenobarbital, as it does to the sedative effects. The therapeutic blood level of phenobarbital is 10 to 40 mcg/mL.

Phenobarbital is absorbed through the GI tract; time to reach a peak plasma level varies from 30 minutes to more than 1 hour. It is only moderately protein bound, at 40% to 60%. It is metabolized in the liver and induces the hepatic enzyme system. It can induce its own metabolism. Its half-life is long, 53 to 143 hours. One fourth of phenobarbital is excreted in the urine unchanged.

Phenobarbital is classified as a pregnancy category D drug, and fetal abnormalities are possible if it is used during pregnancy.

Adverse effects are related to CNS depression, and respiratory depression is the most serious. The degree of respiratory depression is dose dependent. The dosage used to control seizures is rarely involved with substantial respiratory depression. Drowsiness occurs commonly with phenobarbital use in the treatment of seizures; however, tolerance to this effect develops with chronic use. Other CNS effects may occur. In some instances, phenobarbital produces CNS effects that are the opposite of what would normally be expected. Therefore, agitation, hyperactivity, insomnia, irritability, and CNS stimulation may occur. Children and older adults are particularly prone to these paradoxical effects. Adverse cognitive effects in children may also include impaired short-term memory and deficits on neuropsychological tests and memory concentration tasks. Fever may occur with chronic use. As with other antiepileptic drugs, status epilepticus may

occur if phenobarbital is stopped suddenly after chronic use. In addition, additive CNS depression occurs if phenobarbital is taken with other CNS depressants. Like other antiepileptic drugs, it carries the warning that it may increase suicidal thoughts or actions.

Because phenobarbital induces the hepatic enzyme system and alters the metabolism of a large number of other drugs, it is characterized by many drug–drug interactions. Enzyme induction will also reduce the effectiveness of oral hormonal contraceptives, which may still be the most effective form of contraception and can be augmented with intrauterine devices or barrier methods.

The drug's many adverse effects, drug interactions, and slow administration mean that its use has greatly decreased since the creation of the newer antiepileptic drugs and it is generally not used a first-line therapy for status epilepticus (UpToDate, 2010c). The reasons phenobarbital is not the best drug for status epilepticus are as follows: When given for emergency use, phenobarbital is administered intravenously and may require at least 15 minutes before peak concentration is reached in the brain to control the seizure. Because of phenobarbital's long half-life, if it is administered continuously until the seizure activity ceases, severe barbiturate-induced CNS depression, including respiratory depression and excessive hypotension, can occur. Because of the length of time needed to reach a therapeutic effect and control status epilepticus, more rapidly acting drugs, such as diazepam or lorazepam, are normally used to treat status epilepticus initially. Phenobarbital is used as a second-line drug after interventions with a benzodiazepine and phenytoin have failed.

Primidone

Primidone (Mysoline) is used to control grand mal, psychomotor, or focal epileptic seizures, either alone or used in combination with other antiepileptic drug therapy. An unlabeled use of primidone is benign familial tremor. Although primidone is actually considered to be an adjuvant antiepileptic drug, one of the active metabolites of primidone is phenobarbital. The other active metabolite is phenylethylmalonamide (PEMA). Although primidone has antiepileptic properties of its own, much of its effect comes from the antiepileptic properties of phenobarbital and PEMA. Animal studies have shown that PEMA also potentiates the effects of phenobarbital. Phenobarbital accounts for between 15% and 25% of the metabolites formed by primidone.

Primidone has a half-life of 5 to 15 hours. PEMA and phenobarbital have longer half-lives (10 to 18 hours and 53 to 140 hours, respectively) and accumulate with chronic use. About 40% of primidone is excreted unchanged in the urine. The remainder of the drug is excreted as unconjugated PEMA and as phenobarbital and its metabolites.

The therapeutic effects and adverse effects of primidone are similar to those of phenobarbital and other antiepileptic drugs. Nursing management of the patient is also similar. It is a potent P450 inducer and will have many drug interactions, including oral hormonal contraceptives.

Tiagabine

Tiagabine (Gabitril) is used as an adjunct therapy in treating partial seizures; thus it is never used as monotherapy. Like the benzodiazepines, it is believed to enhance the effectiveness of GABA. Unlike the benzodiazepines, tiagabine binds to the sites associated with GABA reuptake. By binding to these sites, it inhibits GABA reuptake by presynaptic neurons and glia cells, and the neurotransmitter can further stimulate the receptors on the postsynaptic cells. Tiagabine is sometimes referred to as a GABAergic drug.

Tiagabine is absorbed rapidly and almost completely from the GI tract and peaks in about 45 minutes if taken on an empty stomach; a high-fat meal slows the rate but not the extent of absorption. Tiagabine is highly protein bound, at 96%. Metabolism of tiagabine is in the liver through hepatic enzymatic pathways, mostly CYP3A, although other isoenzymes may also be involved. Although half-life is 7 to 9 hours in healthy adults, it can be decreased considerably (up to 65%) when taken with other antiepileptic drugs that induce hepatic isoenzymes, such as phenytoin, carbamazepine, primidone, or phenobarbital. An unusual feature of the pharmacokinetics of tiagabine is that it exhibits a diurnal effect; steady-state values are 15% lower after the evening dose than after the morning dose. A therapeutic drug level for tiagabine has not been established.

Like all other antiepileptic drugs, tiagabine is not recommended to be used during pregnancy or breast-feeding. It is classified as a pregnancy category C drug because animal studies have indicated teratogenic effects. However, no related controlled studies have been done in women. Tiagabine is excreted in breast milk.

Although tiagabine is usually well tolerated, the most common adverse effects are related to the CNS system. These include dizziness, muscle weakness, somnolence, nervousness, tremor, insomnia, difficulty with concentration or attention, ataxia, and confusion. GI problems of nausea, diarrhea, or vomiting are also common. Although animal studies indicate a risk for visual-field impairment from tiagabine, clinical research has not supported this (see Box 18.4).

Tiagabine is used to prevent seizures, but it now has a warning on its label stating that it may cause seizures if used in patients who do not have epilepsy (FDA, 2005). The FDA lists 59 reports of induced seizures, including seven cases of status epilepticus, which were associated with unlabeled use of tiagabine in patients without epilepsy. Off-label uses include treatment of various psychiatric diseases and chronic pain management. Exactly why tiagabine may induce seizures in such patients is not known, although there are two theories. First, patients who take tiagabine as an antiepileptic are taking it as an adjunct to other antiepileptic drugs, which frequently induce hepatic enzymes that would metabolize tiagabine. Second, it is possible that patients who use tiagabine for an off-label indication are also taking some other medication that may lower the seizure threshold. A drug interaction between these two drugs then results in seizure activity (UpToDate, 2010a). Like the other antiepiletics, it carries the warning that it may increase suicidal thoughts or actions.

Vigabatrin

Vigabatrin (Sabril) is used to treat refractory partial seizures in cases in which other drug therapy has failed to control seizures. The drug has been marketed in Canada and in many European and Asian countries for years, and was approved in 2009 by the U.S. Food and Drug Administration for infantile spasms in children 1 month to 2 years and in combination therapy for refractory complex partial seizures in adults (Food and Drug Administration, 2009). Like tiagabine, vigabatrin is a GABAergic drug. Unlike tiagabine, tiagabine is an irreversible inhibitor of GABA-transaminase (responsible for the metabolism of GABA). Also unlike tiagabine, vigabatrin has been found to significantly increase the risk of visual-field impairment (see Box 18.4). About one third to one half of the patients receiving long-term treatment with vigabatrin develop visual field defects characterized by a bilateral, absolute concentric constriction of the visual field; the severity of the impairment can be mild or severe. Sometimes, the damage to the retina is permanent. Adults seem to be at higher risk for developing the adverse effect (although more research is needed with pediatric populations), and men have about twice the risk of women for developing these problems. Because of these serious adverse effects, patients should receive vigabatrin only if all other combinations of antiepileptic drug therapy have been tried and were unsuccessful. Patients receiving vigabatrin should regularly have their vision tested. As for all other antiepileptic drugs, assess the patient receiving vagabatrin for changes in mood and behavior that may indicate depression or suicidal thoughts.

DRUGS USED IN SEIZURES RELATED TO PRE-ECLAMPSIA AND ECLAMPSIA

Magnesium sulfate is a drug that is completely different from all of the other antiepileptic drugs. Magnesium sulfate is used in treating seizures related to severe pre-eclampsia or eclampsia in pregnant women. It is also used to control preterm labor. Magnesium has a depressive effect on the CNS. It prevents or controls seizures by blocking the neuromuscular transmission of acetylcholine and decreasing the amount of this neurotransmitter liberated at the end plate by motor nerve impulses. This drug is discussed in more detail in Chapter 53.

CHAPTER SUMMARY

- Antiepileptic drugs work by inhibiting influx of sodium ions through sodium channels into the cell, inhibiting calcium ion influx into special calcium channels, or altering the effectiveness of GABA.
- All antiepileptic drugs carry risks for teratogenicity. Stopping drug therapy also carries the risk for inducing seizures, which is risky to the mother and the fetus. Most babies born to epileptic mothers on drug therapy are normal.

- Status epilepticus is a medical emergency and requires IV drug therapy. The first line of treatment is a benzodiazepine, either diazepam or lorazepam. Phenytoin is used next. Phenobarbital is a third-line drug used if neither the benzodiazepine nor the phenytoin is effective.
- Antiepileptic drug therapy can be successfully discontinued in about 70% of people once they are seizure-free for 2 years.
- Nursing management procedures for the antiepileptic drugs are similar in many respects. Patients need to understand the disease process, how the disease and drug therapy may affect their lives, and possible adverse effects of drug therapy.

QUESTIONS FOR STUDY AND REVIEW

1. What is the difference between a seizure and a convulsion?
2. Why is phenytoin useful in treating both seizures and some cardiac arrhythmias?
3. What is the first-line drug of choice in treating status epilepticus?
4. Why should dosage changes of phenytoin be made in small increments?
5. Why would patients with low serum albumin levels be more at risk for adverse effects from phenytoin?
6. How does ethosuximide reduce absence seizures?
7. How do benzodiazepines suppress seizure activity?

NEED MORE HELP?

Chapter 18 of the Study Guide to Accompany *Drug Therapy in Nursing*, 4th Edition, contains NCLEX-style questions and other learning activities to reinforce your understanding of the concepts presented in this chapter. For additional information or to purchase the study guide, visit thePoint.

REFERENCES

Agarwal, P., Kumar, N., Chandra, R., Gupta, G., Antony, A. R., Garg, N. (2007). Randomized study of intravenous valproate and phenytoin in status epilepticus. *Seizure,* 16(6):527–532.

Ettinger, A. B., Manjunath, R., Candrilli, S. D., Davis, K. L. (2009). Prevalence and cost of nonadherence to antiepileptic drugs in elderly patients with epilepsy. *Epilepsy & Behavior,* 14(2):324–329.

Food and Drug Administration. (2000). Complications with the use of anticonvulsants in pregnancy [Slide presentation by M. Yerby]. Retrieved from *http://www.fda.gov/cder/present/clinpharm 2000/Yerby/sld001.htm.*

Food and Drug Administration. (2005). FDA public health advisory: Seizure in patients without epilepsy being treated with Gabitril (tiagabine). Retrieved from *http://www.fda.gov/MEDWATCH/SAFETY/2005/gabitril_DHCP.htm.*

Food and Drug Administration. (2008). FDA public health advisory: Suicidal thoughts and behavior antiepileptic drugs. Retrieved from *http://www.fda.gov/Drugs/DrugSafety/PublicHealthAdvisories/UCM054709*

Food and Drug Administration. (2009). FDA News Release: Sabril Approved by FDA to Treat Spasms in Infants and Epileptic Seizures. Retrieved from *http://www.fda.gov/NewsEvents/Newsroom/PressAnnouncements/ucm179855.htm.*

French, J. A., Kanner, A. M., Bautista, J., et al. (2004). Efficacy and tolerability of the new antiepileptic drugs. 1: treatment of new onset epilepsy: Report of the Therapeutics and Technology Assessment Subcommittee of the American Academy of Neurology; Quality Standards Subcommittee of the American Academy of Neurology; American Epilepsy Society. *Neurology,* 62(8):1252–1260.

Glauser, T. A., Cnaan, A., Shinnar, S., Hirtz, D. G., Dlugos, D., Masur, D., Clark, P. O., Capparelli, E. V., Adamson, P. C. (2010). Ethosuximide, valproic acid, and lamotrigine in childhood absence epilepsy. *New England Journal of Medicine,* 362(9):790–799.

Meador, K. J., Baker, G. A., Finnell, R. H., et al.; NEAD Study Group. (2006). In utero antiepileptic drug exposure: Fetal death and malformations. *Neurology,* 67(3):407–412.

National Institutes of Health, National Institute of Neurological Disorders and Stroke. (2006). *Seizures and epilepsy: Hope through research.* Retrieved from *http://www.ninds.nih.gov/disorders/epilepsy/detail_epilepsy. htm#64163109.*

Prasad, K., Krishnan, P. R., Al-Roomi, K., Sequeira, R. (2007). Anticonvulsant therapy for status epilepticus. *British Journal of Clinical Pharmacology,* 63(60):640–647.

Szaflarski, J. P., Sangha, K. S., Lindsell, C. J., Shutter, L. A. (2010). Prospective, randomized, single-blinded comparative trial of intravenous levetiracetam versus phenytoin for seizure prophylaxis. *Neurocritical Care,* 12(2):165–172.

UpToDate. (2010a). Pharmacology of antiepileptic drugs. Retrieved July 28, 2010 from *www.uptodate.com.*

UpToDate. (2010b). Overview of the management of epilepsy in adults. Retrieved from *www.uptodate.com.*

UpToDate. (2010c). Status epilepticus in adults. Retrieved from *www.uptodate.com.*

UpToDate. (2010d). Topiramate: Drug information. Retrieved from *www.uptodate.com.*

World Health Organization. (2009). Medical eligibility criteria for contraceptive use. 4th edition. Retrieved from http://www.who.int/reproductive-health/publications/mec/cocs.html.

Zupanc, M. L. (2006). Antiepileptic drugs and hormonal contraceptives in adolescent women with epilepsy. *Neurology,* 66(6, Suppl. 3):S37–S45.

Drugs Producing Anesthesia and Neuromuscular Blocking

Learning Objectives

At the completion of this chapter the student will:

1. Describe the physiology of the central nervous system as it relates to anesthesia and neuromuscular blocking.

2. Identify observable changes in stages of anesthesia and neuromuscular blockade.

3. Identify risk and disease factors that may influence a patient's response to anesthetics and neuromuscular blocking agents.

4. Identify core drug knowledge about anesthetic and neuromuscular blocking agents.

5. Identify core patient variables related to anesthetic and neuromuscular blocking agents.

6. Relate the interaction of core drug knowledge and core patient variables for anesthetic and neuromuscular blocking agents.

7. Generate a nursing plan of care based on the interactions between core drug knowledge and core patient variables for anesthetic and neuromuscular blocking agents.

8. Describe nursing interventions to maximize therapeutic effects and minimize adverse effects for anesthetic and neuromuscular blocking agents.

9. Determine key points for patient and family education about anesthetic and neuromuscular blocking agents.

Key Terms

anesthesia
balanced anesthesia
conscious sedation
depolarizing drugs
dissociative anesthesia
motor end plate
general anesthesia
nondepolarizing drugs
paralysis
regional anesthesia
total intravenous anesthesia

Drugs Producing Anesthesia and Neuromuscular Blocking

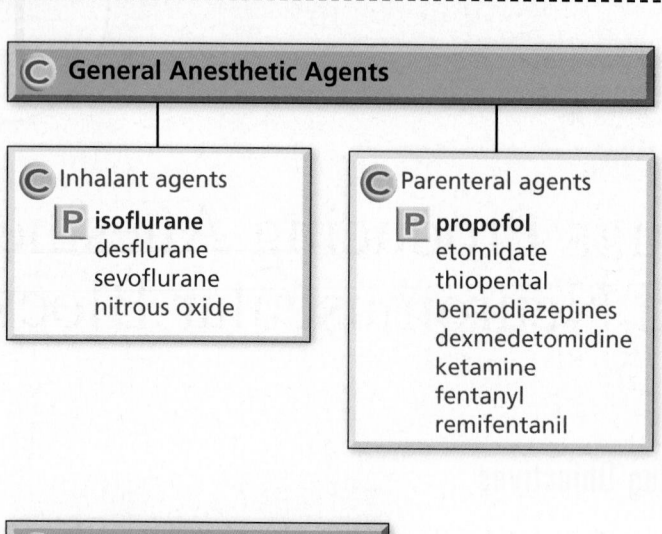

General Anesthetic Agents

Inhalant agents
P isoflurane
desflurane
sevoflurane
nitrous oxide

Parenteral agents
P propofol
etomidate
thiopental
benzodiazepines
dexmedetomidine
ketamine
fentanyl
remifentanil

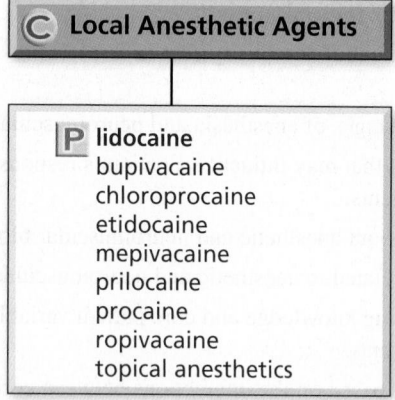

Local Anesthetic Agents

P lidocaine
bupivacaine
chloroprocaine
etidocaine
mepivacaine
prilocaine
procaine
ropivacaine
topical anesthetics

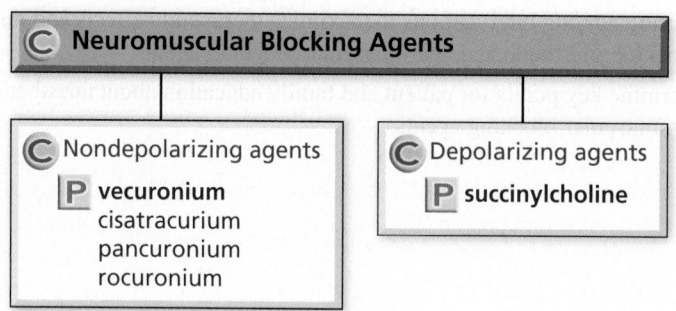

Neuromuscular Blocking Agents

Nondepolarizing agents
P vecuronium
cisatracurium
pancuronium
rocuronium

Depolarizing agents
P succinylcholine

The symbol Ⓒ indicates the drug class.
Drugs in **bold type** marked with the symbol Ⓟ are prototypes.
Drugs in blue type are closely related to the prototype.
Drugs in red type are significantly different from the prototype.
Drugs in black type with no symbol are also used in drug therapy; no prototype.

nesthesia produces a loss of feeling or sensation through administration of a drug or drugs. It is used to avoid sensations (especially pain) and memories associated with surgery and diagnostic procedures. Anesthesia can be classified into two categories: general and regional. **General anesthesia** is characterized by a state of unconsciousness, analgesia, and amnesia. All three states must be present. General anesthetic drugs are subdivided into inhaled agents and intravenous agents. **Regional anesthesia** occurs when sensory transmission from a specific area or region of the body to the central nervous system (CNS) is blocked. This is accomplished through local anesthetic drugs administered in an epidural block, a spinal block, or peripheral nerve blocks. Regional anesthesia is utilized to perform minor surgical procedures for a conscious patient or as an adjunct for general anesthesia. This type of anesthesia is frequently used in ambulatory surgical centers. Local anesthesia is similar to regional anesthesia, but employs its effect on a smaller area of the body. Neuromuscular blocking agents are used to cause **paralysis** (loss of motor function) for surgical procedures or to facilitate mechanical ventilation. These agents are subdivided based on their mechanism of action into **nondepolarizing drugs** (which bind to acetylcholine receptors and function as a competitive antagonist) and **depolarizing drugs** (which closely resemble acetylcholine, binding to the receptor and functioning as an agonist).

This chapter discusses drugs used to induce anesthesia and skeletal muscle paralysis. The focus is not to present the specific anesthetic considerations on how to deliver anesthesia, but rather provide a basic overview of the drugs and their effects on a patient who is recovering from anesthesia in a post-anesthesia care unit (PACU) or on a surgical unit. Inhaled anesthetics are represented by the prototype drug isoflurane (Forane). Intravenous anesthetics are represented by the prototype drug propofol (Diprivan). Local anesthetics, used for regional anesthesia, are represented by the prototype drug lidocaine (Xylocaine). Nondepolarizing neuromuscular junction (NMJ) blockers are represented by the prototype drug vecuronium (Norcuron). Depolarizing NMJ blockers are represented by the prototype drug succinylcholine (Anectine).

PHYSIOLOGY

Central Nervous System Anesthesia

Researchers have yet to identify specifically the mechanism of action of anesthetic drugs. There is simply not one "switch" that anesthetics can turn off and produce amnesia, analgesia, and unconsciousness. However, through different pathways, anesthesia can be accomplished by interrupting the nervous system activity in the CNS. The CNS includes the spinal cord, brain stem, and cerebral cortex—all sites of action in which anesthesia drugs produce their effects. The spinal cord is speculated to be where purposeful responses to painful stimuli are inhibited; the brainstem (specifically the reticular activating system) is probably where consciousness is interrupted; and the cerebral cortex (the site of complex brain functions) is where interference of memory, attention, and awareness probably occur.

At the synaptic level in the CNS, normal arousal mechanisms are affected through presynaptic release of neurotransmitters, such as norepinephrine, serotonin, and dopamine. As described in Chapter 13, these transmitters diffuse across the synaptic cleft to the postsynaptic effector membrane, which is usually another neuron. The postsynaptic membrane contains receptors for the transmitters. The transient combination of the transmitter with the receptor causes membrane changes, leading to propagation of the action potential. An action potential is the brief reversal of electrical polarization of a nerve or muscle cell membrane. In the neuron, the action potential constitutes the nerve impulse. The transmitter can be metabolized by postsynaptic enzymes (such as monoamine oxidase) or removed from further activity through reuptake into the presynaptic storage vesicles. Anesthetics may provoke a decreased release of neurotransmitters or an increased reuptake and inhibition of the postsynaptic enzymes. The result is a diminished postsynaptic response, leading to decreased arousal, decreased sensation (including pain), and loss of consciousness.

Local Anesthetics

Nerve impulses depend on the flow of ion currents through channels in the cell membrane. Nerve cells are negatively polarized at rest, a state that is maintained by active Na^+/K^+ exchange. When a cell is stimulated, it becomes depolarized, and an action potential occurs. Local anesthetics reversibly block all nerve impulses by disrupting membrane permeability to sodium during an action potential. These drugs therefore stop the generation and propagation of the nerve impulse.

Neuromuscular Blockade

Muscle relaxation and paralysis can take place at a variety of sites, including the CNS, somatic nerves, motor nerve terminals, acetylcholine receptor sites, the **motor end plate** (the terminal branch of a motor nerve, which forms part of the NMJ), the muscle membrane, or the internal contractile units of muscle. Normal muscle function involves the arrival of a nerve impulse at the motor nerve terminal, followed by the release of the neurotransmitter acetylcholine into the synaptic cleft. Neuromuscular blockade occurs at acetylcholine receptor sites, where acetylcholine reacts with the muscle cell membrane, causing depolarization and subsequent muscle relaxation.

Nondepolarizing drugs are competitive antagonists preventing the binding of acetylcholine to the receptor; therefore the end plate is unable to depolarize. After administration, muscle fasciculation will not be present, unlike with depolarizing drugs. Depolarizing drugs, structurally similar to acetylcholine, cause continuous muscle depolarization and prevent repolarization. The muscle is unable to repolarize as long as the drug continues to bind to the acetylcholine receptor.

PATHOPHYSIOLOGY

Anesthetics are called functional drugs because they are not used to treat a pathologic disease or disorder. Instead, their effects allow the patient to undergo procedures that either treat or improve a specific disease state. These drugs are utilized in different combinations to achieve the appropriate point along the sedation and anesthesia continuum for a specific procedure. Examples of procedures that anesthetic drugs are used for include general surgery, pediatric dental procedures, electroconvulsive therapy, CT scans, MRI, endoscopy, bronchoscopy, heart catheterization, and complicated dressing changes.

The Joint Commission has identified four levels of sedation and anesthesia on a continuum. These include minimal sedation (anxiolysis), moderate sedation and analgesia (**conscious sedation**), deep sedation and analgesia, and anesthesia. Under conscious sedation, patients respond purposefully to verbal commands alone or with light tactile stimulation and are able to maintain their own airway and breathe spontaneously.

© GENERAL ANESTHETIC AGENTS

The goal of a general anesthetic is to achieve akinesia, analgesia, and amnesia. After administration of a general anesthetic, loss of consciousness and sensation usually follows increasing levels, or stages, of CNS depression. Classic studies with early anesthetics indicate the presence of four stages, which are differentiated through increasing influence on reflex activity, muscle tone, and respiration. Stages I and II constitute anesthetic induction; keeping the patient at stage III is anesthetic maintenance. Reversal of the stages to the conscious state is the process of recovery. The four stages of anesthesia are as follows:

- Stage I, analgesia: From the induction of anesthesia to loss of consciousness. The patient experiences a loss of pain sensation but still remains responsive until the end of the stage.
- Stage II, delirium/excitement: Systolic pressure rises, and the patient may experience excitation, agitation, and restlessness, along with an increased respiratory rate and disconjugate gaze. Potentially dangerous responses can occur during this stage including vomiting, laryngospasm, tachycardia, and uncontrolled movement.
- Stage III, surgical anesthesia: Stage III may have four planes, or levels, characterized by differential responses of the ocular muscles, eye reflexes, and pupils. It begins in plane I with the resumption of regular respiration and the beginning of muscle relaxation. By plane IV, spontaneous respiration ceases. Most surgery occurs when the patient is in planes II or III.
- Stage IV, medullary depression: The respiratory and vasomotor centers are depressed, spontaneous respiration has ceased, and marked hypotension with weak and irregular pulse can occur. Unless rapid intervention and support occur, coma and death follow.

General anesthesia is produced for the most part by a combination of drugs rather than one single agent. This process, called **balanced anesthesia,** is a highly variable technique of general anesthesia using narcotics, analgesics, muscle relaxants, and inhalational agents to produce and maintain the appropriate stage of anesthesia. Constant patient assessment and re-evaluation along with sensitive titration of drugs ensures delivery of an adequate and safe anesthetic.

© INHALED ANESTHETIC AGENTS

The inhalant anesthetics are typified by isoflurane (Forane), a halogenated ether that is the prototype for this group.

Nursing Management of the Patient Receiving P Isoflurane

Core Drug Knowledge

Pharmacotherapeutics

Isoflurane is used to maintain anesthesia and is one of the main components of balanced anesthesia in the operating room for procedures that require amnesia and immobility. It is rarely used for inhalation induction of anesthesia because of its pungency and irritability to the patient.

Pharmacokinetics

The uptake and distribution of isoflurane and all of the volatile anesthetics are influenced by several factors starting with the delivery of the agent from the anesthesia gas machine (Figure 19.1). The gas machine vaporizes the liquid volatile and delivers it at a desired concentration to the patient via the breathing circuit. The agent is absorbed from the alveoli in the lungs into the systemic circulation. The brain (site of action) and other tissues equilibrate with the partial pressure of the volatile delivered to them by the blood.

A tiny fraction of the inhaled dose (<1%) is metabolized and does not result in any end-metabolite toxicities. Alveolar ventilation is responsible for the excretion of isoflurane. Table 19.1 provides a comparison of the pharmacokinetic properties of halogenated general anesthetic agents. However, it is important to recognize that volatile agent pharmacokinetics are more frequently and accurately described by their blood and tissue solubilities than simply by their onset, duration, and half-life times. In addition, other factors, such as the patient's total body fat composition, ventilation, circulation, and the length of anesthesia time, all influence the onset and recovery of the anesthetic.

Pharmacodynamics

The exact mechanism of action of isoflurane—and for the inhaled anesthetics altogether—is unknown. Several theories have been postulated. It is likely that the effects are mediated through physicochemical properties of the gases (lipid solubility, oil-gas, and blood-gas partition coefficients), rather than through specific binding with receptors or through potentiation or inhibition of specific neurotransmitters.

The minimum alveolar concentration (MAC) is a measure of potency. It is the concentration of anesthetic gas required to eliminate movement in 50% of patients challenged by a

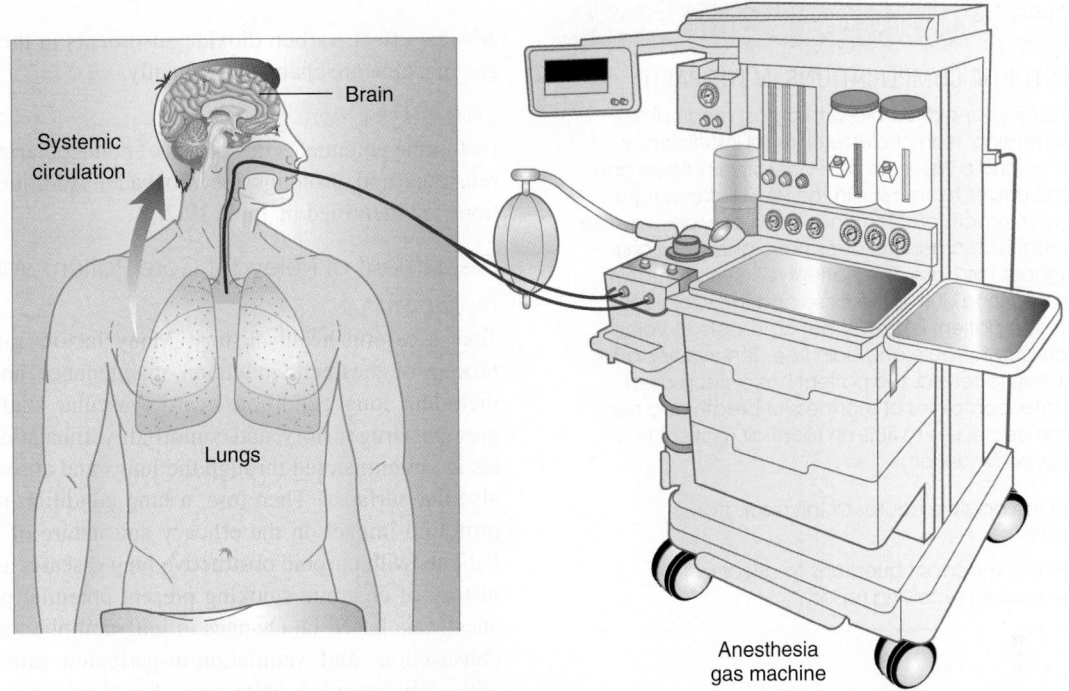

Brain

Systemic
circulation

Lungs

Anesthesia
gas machine

• FIGURE 19.1 Volatile anesthetics are delivered to the patient from the anesthesia gas machine through the breathing circuit. The gas is absorbed by the lungs into the systemic circulation and causes dose-dependent central nervous system depression.

standardized skin incision. The smaller the MAC, the more potent the agent. The concept of MAC can be viewed as a general guide to the overall depth of anesthesia. The MAC of isoflurane is 1.17% for adults when it is administered alone, but it decreases when administered with nitrous oxide.

Contraindications and Precautions

The main contraindications to isoflurane are hypersensitivity to halogenated compounds and predisposition to malignant hyperthermia, which is often determined from the individual or family history (see Chapter 20). Isoflurane and the other volatile agents cause an increase in cerebral blood flow due to their vasodilation effects and therefore increase intracranial pressure (ICP). This is insignificant if the patient has a normal ICP; however, it should be used

with caution in patients with an increased ICP (for example brain mass or hematoma).

Isoflurane is assigned to pregnancy category C and should be used in pregnant women only when the benefits outweigh the risks.

Adverse Effects

Isoflurane along with all of the inhalational agents have adverse effects that are dose dependent and related to their pharmacologic properties. With many anesthetics, blood pressure drops secondary to vasodilation, during induction and returns following surgical stimulation. Like other anesthetics, isoflurane depresses renal function (renal blood flow, glomerular filtration rate, and urine output). However, it is not generally nephrotoxic, and this depressed function can

TABLE 19.1	Summary of Selected ⊖ Inhalant Anesthetic Agents		
Drug (Trade) Name	**Selected Indications**	**Route and Dosage Range**	**Pharmacokinetics**
P isoflurane (Forane)	Anesthesia: induction, maintenance	*Adult:* 1.17% in oxygen or 0.56% with oxygen and 60% nitrous oxide	*Onset:* 7–10 min *Duration:* 7–19 min $t_{1/2}$: minimal biotransformation
desflurane (Suprane)	Anesthesia: induction, maintenance	*Adult:* 6.6% in oxygen or 2.38% in oxygen and 60% nitrous oxide	*Onset:* 2–2.6 min *Duration:* 5–7 min $t_{1/2}$: 2.5 min
sevoflurane (Ultane)	Anesthesia: induction, maintenance	*Adult:* 1.8% in oxygen or 0.66% in oxygen/ 60% nitrous oxide	*Onset:* 1–2 min *Duration:* 4–14 min $t_{1/2}$: 2–3 min

POST-ANESTHETIC COMPLICATIONS IN THE PACU

Mona B., is a 55-year-old female with a past medical history of hypertension, high cholesterol, renal insufficiency, breast cancer, and a history of post-operative nausea and vomiting who arrives to your slot in the PACU after a right mastectomy. In report form the anesthesia provider, you are told this patient had a general anesthetic and was paralyzed throughout the case. The patient received fentanyl and hydromorphone during the case and the vital signs were stable. The patient is drowsy but arousable to voice and appears comfortable and pain free. Ten minutes after report has been received, the patient has a decreased respiratory rate, complains of shortness of breath and her O2 saturation decreases to 88% on room air (patient has taken her oxygen mask off).

1. What are the possible causes of this respiratory depression?

2. What are the important questions to ask or get clarification when receiving report?

---

be avoided with adequate hydration preoperatively. Dose-dependent respiratory depression occurs with all inhaled anesthetics, sometimes resulting in the need for mechanical ventilation throughout surgery. Tremor and shivering may occur in response to a decreased body temperature, but these adverse effects are generally self-limiting. Nausea and vomiting may also occur. If vomiting occurs after surgery in the PACU, the patient is at risk for aspiration pneumonia. Volatile anesthetics produce a dose-dependent decrease in uterine smooth muscle contractility and blood flow.

Isoflurane has been observed to react with carbon dioxide dry adsorbents in anesthetic circle systems to form carbon monoxide and cause carboxyhemoglobinemia. To avoid this

adverse effect, carbon dioxide adsorbents in the anesthesia gas machine are changed frequently.

Drug Interactions

Isoflurane potentiates the effects of nondepolarizing muscle relaxants and prolongs the blockade. Additional interactions are identified in Table 19.2.

Assessment of Relevant Core Patient Variables

Health Status

Take a careful health history. Many factors influence the process of anesthetic induction, maintenance, and recovery, including lung conditions, cardiovascular status, obesity, previous drug history, and comorbidity. Inhalation anesthetics are administered through the lungs and absorbed across alveolar surfaces. Therefore, a lung condition may have a profound impact on the efficacy and nature of anesthesia. Patients with chronic obstructive lung disease, asthma, or a history of cigarette smoking present potential problems in anesthesia based on changes in lung compliance, bronchoconstriction, and ventilation-to-perfusion ratios. Patients with compromised pulmonary function have a substantially increased rate of postoperative complications. Similar issues arise for patients with cardiovascular compromise or disease because absorption, distribution, metabolism, and excretion of inhalant anesthetics are all affected by blood flow through the lungs and the rest of the body.

Life Span and Gender

Document the age of the patient. Challenges with isoflurane administration differ by age group.

In older adults, especially those with failing organ systems, difficulties may occur in detoxification and excretion of administered anesthetic agents, which may lead to increased intensity and duration of drug effects, including toxic effects.

Post-operative Nausea and Vomiting Prevention

White, P., O'Hara, J., Roberson, C., et al. (2008). The Impact of Current Antiemetic Practices on Patient Outcomes : A Prospective Study on High-Risk Patients. *Anesthesia & Analgesia*, 107(2): 452–458.

Background Information

Post-operative nausea and vomiting (PONV) is a common complication to anesthesia that can contribute delays in discharge time from the hospital and a full recovery back to activities of daily living. Studies suggest 25% to 30% of patients will experience PONV during their recovery and in those with risk factors, the incidence increases to 60% to 80%.

Risk factors for PONV are patient-, surgical- and anesthesia-related. These factors include female gender, nonsmoking status, history of PONV or motion sickness, and opioid administration during surgery. Laparoscopic procedures and plastic surgery have a higher incidence of PONV.

The Study

This is a multicenter, prospective, observational study designed to estimate the effectiveness of common antiemetic therapies for prevention and treatment of PONV. There were 376 patients at 11 different sites. Patients had

at least two major risk factors (see above) and underwent either a laparoscopic or plastic surgery. Ninety-two percent of the patients received a prophylactic antiemetic. Thirty-four percent of the patients received a single antiemetic, most often a 5-HT3 receptor antagonist (ondansetron or granisetron), while 35% of the patients received a two-drug antiemetic regimen (5-HT3 and dexamethasone). A 5HT3 receptor antagonist, dexamethasone, and droperidol were administered in combination in 23% of the patients. Emesis rates were lower (18%) when 3 or more antiemetic agents were administered when compared to just one agent (40%). It was demonstrated that the patients who received three or more antiemetics had significantly lower rates of emesis after they were discharged from the PACU.

Nursing Implications

This research study demonstrates the importance of administering an antiemetic for PONV prophylaxis. It also demonstrated that there is a significant difference in the effectiveness of prophylaxis when using more than one antiemetic drug. With this knowledge, nurses can advocate for appropriate PONV prophylaxis and educate patients about the risk of PONV and the medications that can prevent it and improve recovery time and outcomes.

TABLE 19.2	Agents That Interact with Ⓟ Isoflurane		
Interactants	**Effect and Significance**	**Nursing Management**	
nondepolarizing muscle relaxants, such as pancuronium, vecuronium	Potentiates effects of neuromuscular blockers and prolongs blockade	Monitor respiratory function (dosage may need to be reduced). Prepare to provide ventilatory support.	
alfentanil	Prolongs respiratory depression and increases incidence of bradycardia	Monitor respiratory and cardiac function. Provide ventilatory support.	
labetalol	Additive hypotensive effects and decreased cardiac output	Monitor cardiac function. Use extra caution if interaction is anticipated.	
herbal drugs • St. John's wort • *Hypericum perforatum*	Herbal drugs may intensify or prolong the effects of isoflurane.	Advise patient to stop herbal medications 2–3 wk before surgery.	
hepatic inducers • alcohol • barbiturates • carbamazepine • INH • phenytoin • rifampin	Chronic use of agents that induce hepatic enzymes can increase isoflurane metabolism, thus increasing the risk for hepatic injury.	Document the use of these agents in the medical record. Advise the anesthesia provider of the use of these drugs.	

Assess women of childbearing age for pregnancy. Isoflurane has a low pregnancy safety rating (category C). In animal studies, isoflurane showed the potential for fetotoxicity; however, no human studies have been performed. Its use during pregnancy is determined by the balance between potential benefit and harm to both the woman and the fetus.

Lifestyle, Diet, and Habits

Measure the patient's height and weight. The patient with morbid obesity who requires anesthesia may experience problems with isoflurane administration. The obese patient may be particularly prone to longer recovery times and a greater incidence of adverse effects with fat-soluble anesthetics such as isoflurane and methoxyflurane. Other comorbid conditions, such as hypertension, cardiac insufficiency, respiratory difficulties, and diabetes, all of which can generate their own special anesthetic challenges, often occur in obese patients, compounding these difficulties.

One other important category of anesthetic challenge is substance abusers; substance abuse often coexists with disease states that require special attention during anesthesia. For example, alcohol abuse is often associated with an elevated level of hepatic enzymes, which may increase the requirement for anesthetic drugs. In addition, liver dysfunction may lead to changes in the metabolism of such agents. With drug dependency, the postanesthetic period may require more careful monitoring than usual, in case abstinence syndromes develop (see Chapter 9). Take a careful drug history to reveal previous use or abuse of drugs that have the potential to cause severe interactions with isoflurane and other anesthetic agents.

Environment

Isoflurane and other general anesthetics may be administered in special settings by anesthesiologists (a type of specialist physician) and nurse anesthetists (advanced practice nurses trained in anesthesia). Administration usually occurs only in settings that allow for postanesthetic recovery and full life support.

Nursing Diagnoses and Outcomes

• Ineffective Airway Clearance related to suppressed cough reflex and the presence of secretions
  Desired outcome: The patient will maintain effective airway clearance by being suctioned as necessary and by performing deep breathing and coughing exercises.
• Ineffective Breathing Pattern related to respiratory depression secondary to drugs used during anesthesia
  Desired outcome: The patient will maintain effective breathing despite respiratory depression by administration of oxygen as appropriate.
• Risk for Aspiration related to drug-induced nausea and vomiting, gastrointestinal (GI) distention, hypoxia, and stimulation of the vomiting center
  Desired outcome: The patient's nausea and vomiting will be minimized by preanesthetic administration of antiemetics to reduce the risk for aspiration and nausea.
• Ineffective Thermoregulation related to CNS depression secondary to drugs used during anesthesia
  Desired outcome: The patient will be warmed as necessary during the postanesthetic disturbance of thermoregulation.
• Disturbed Sensory Perception, varied, related to CNS depression secondary to drugs used during anesthesia

Desired outcome: *The patient will remain free of sensory or perceptual alterations through careful reorientation, repeated as necessary.*

Planning and Intervention

Maximizing Therapeutic Effects

Preinduction and induction should be carried out in a place where environmental stimuli, particularly noise, are kept to a minimum. Inform the patient about induction procedures and describe measures that are useful for promoting uncomplicated recovery. Also, give preoperative support and reasonable reassurance to concerns voiced by the patient.

Minimizing Adverse Effects

After anesthesia, monitor blood pressure and temperature to detect residual hypotension. Because gaseous or volatile inhalational agents (such as isoflurane) are expired quickly through the lungs, the recovery phase is often short. Manage shivering and tremors, which are common following surgery, with blankets. Until normal respiration resumes, adequate respiratory support must be maintained; take steps such as administering oxygen and asking the patient to cough, to perform deep-breathing exercises, or to change position. After the patient awakens, assess the need for postoperative analgesia.

Recovering patients need to be in a room in which the air supply is continually replaced and exhaled gases are carried out through exhaust vents. Prevent aspiration by helping the patient into a side-lying position and by administering antiemetic drugs. Monitor vital signs frequently to prevent complications such as shock. When the patient returns to the room or unit from the postanesthesia care unit (PACU), continue monitoring vital signs, bowel sounds, and urine output because these signs are directly affected by isoflurane.

Providing Patient and Family Education

Family and patient education falls into preoperative and postoperative categories:

- Provide preoperative teaching to help patients anticipate the surgery and anesthesia without excessive fear and assimilate routines that will aid postoperative recovery.
- Postoperatively, instruct patients to avoid nonprescribed CNS depressants or herbal agents unless approved by the prescriber.
- For outpatient surgery, discharge patients into the care of a responsible adult and instruct patients not to drive or engage in any hazardous activities requiring full alertness or coordination.

Ongoing Assessment and Evaluation

The evaluation of progress in the recovery phase is often carried out in two stages. Initially, the unconscious patient may be transferred to a postanesthesia recovery area. The patient should regain consciousness, orientation, some stability of vital signs, and an ability to cooperate with instructions during this stage. After the immediate postsurgery, and postanesthesia goals have been reached in the PACU, the patient can be transferred back to a room or unit, and a less stringent postoperative protocol may be followed. Other assessments specifically related to the procedure or surgery are distinct from those required for the postanesthesia state. When the patient returns to the room or unit, continue to monitor vital signs, bowel sounds, and urine output, as was done in the PACU.

Drugs Closely Related to 🅿 Isoflurane

Desflurane

Desflurane (Suprane) is similar in molecular structure to isoflurane yet has some distinct advantages to its use. This

---

BOX 19.2   COMMUNITY BASED CONCERNS

Discharge Criteria After Surgery

Whether the patient is being discharged from the post-anesthesia care unit (PACU) to go home or to be admitted to the hospital, discharge criteria must be met. There are two scoring systems (Aldrete and PADSS) that are commonly used in the PACU to assess the patient and determine if the patient is safe for discharge.

The Aldrete Score was developed in 1970 by Dr. Aldrete and is still widely used today. He revised it in 1995 and the modified Aldrete Scoring System is below: (A score ≥9 is required for discharge).

Respiration
  2= Able to take deep breath and cough
  1=Dyspnea/shallow breathing
  0= Apnea

O₂ saturation
  2= Maintain Sp O₂ > 92% on room air
  1= Needs O₂ inhalation to maintain O₂ saturation >90%
  0= O₂ saturation, 90% even with supplemental oxygen

Consciousness
  2= Fully awake
  1= Arousable on calling
  0= Not responding

Circulation (BP= blood pressure)
  2= BP+/– 20 mmHg preop
  1= BP+/– 20-50 mmHg preop
  0= BP+/– 50 mmHg preop

Activity
  2=Able to move four extremities voluntary or on command
  1= Able to move two extremities
  0= Unable to move extremities

It is important for the PACU nurse to be able to appropriately assess for adequate ventilation and oxygenation, vital signs, pain control, nausea and vomiting, and surgical bleeding.

P Isoflurane

- A potent inhalation anesthetic
- Major contraindications: hypersensitivity to halogenated compounds, predisposition to malignant hyperthermia
- Most common adverse effects: hypotension, hypothermia, nausea, or vomiting
- Most serious adverse effect: respiratory depression
- Maximizing therapeutic effects: low-stimulus environment, preoperative teaching regarding anesthetic induction
- Minimizing adverse effects: Monitor need for respiratory support.
- Most important patient education: preoperative teaching regarding anesthesia and surgical procedures

---

volatile has low blood-gas and lipid solubility; therefore, once the gas is discontinued at the end of the case, emergence is rapid because of the decreased saturation in the blood and tissue. Desflurane has a MAC of 6.6%. Desflurane is very pungent and is associated with coughing, increased secretions, and laryngospasm; therefore, it is not used for inhalation induction of anesthesia. At high inspired concentrations, tachycardia and hypertension can occur and for this reason should be avoided in patients that have coronary vascular disease.

Sevoflurane

Sevoflurane (Ultane) offers advantages beyond others in its class. It has a MAC of 1.8%. Induction of and recovery from anesthesia are rapid, and cardiorespiratory depression is minimal, which makes sevoflurane generally safe in patients with coronary artery disease. Additionally, because of its low tissue solubility and nonirritating odor, sevoflurane is an appropriate agent for inhalation induction of anesthesia in the pediatric and adult populations.

Sevoflurane metabolizes to inorganic fluoride and is degraded in soda lime (carbon dioxide absorbents in the anesthesia gas machine) to potentially toxic metabolites, which can be nephrotoxic and hepatotoxic. However, the anesthesia provider can prevent this by delivering the inhaled gas in a specific way.

Drug Significantly Different From P Isoflurane

Nitrous oxide is a colorless, odorless, tasteless, nonflammable, nonirritating, inorganic gas rather than a halogenated ether. It is used commonly as an adjunct in balanced anesthesia to decrease the MAC of halogenated agents. Nitrous oxide is also used for a process called the second gas effect: when two gases (either isoflurane or sevoflurane both slower agents) and nitrous oxide (a faster agent) are administered together, it speeds up the onset time of the slower agent. Nitrous oxide is a powerful analgesic but a relatively weak inhaled anesthetic.

Nitrous oxide is readily absorbed into the blood through the pulmonary capillary system. It has a relatively low solubility in blood and a MAC of 104%. Nitrous oxide is rapidly eliminated in the expired breath, essentially unchanged, with minimal diffusion through the skin. However, nitrous oxide can leave the blood easily and enter an air-filled cavity, causing it to rapidly expand. This chemical property adds limitation to the use of nitrous oxide in specific surgical cases (middle ear, bowel, and intraocular surgeries) or patient disease (pneumothorax). Nitrous oxide can also expand air-filled cuffs of pulmonary artery catheters and endotracheal tubes.

The benefit versus risk ratio should be considered when administering nitrous oxide in pregnant patients undergoing anesthesia, as animal studies show that it can cause fetal death, growth retardation, and skeletal anomalies. Prolonged administration of nitrous oxide can cause inactivation of methionine synthase, a vitamin B_{12}-dependent enzyme, which is necessary for the synthesis of DNA. In the absence of methionine synthase, interference with myelin formation can have significant effects on the rapidly growing fetus.

This effect does not occur within the time frame of clinical surgery, but it poses a potential problem for providers who are chronically exposed to nitrous oxide.

Controversy also exists if nitrous oxide contributes to postoperative nausea and vomiting.

C INTRAVENOUS ANESTHETIC AGENTS

Intravenous (IV) anesthetics are also known as induction agents. Several classes of drugs are used as IV anesthetics in balanced anesthesia and total intravenous anesthesia (TIVA) including barbiturates, benzodiazepines, opioid analgesics, and nonbarbiturate hypnotic agents.

Propofol (Diprivan), a nonbarbiturate hypnotic agent, is the prototype for IV anesthetics (Table 19.3). Often nicknamed "the milk of anesthesia," propofol appears as a milky white solution because it is formulated in a solution with soybean oil, glycerol, and egg phospholipids.

Nursing Management of the Patient Receiving P Propofol

Core Drug Knowledge

Pharmacotherapeutics

Propofol is used for induction and maintenance of general anesthesia and maintenance of sedation in the ICU.

Pharmacokinetics

Propofol is administered intravenously and is rapidly distributed to all tissues in the body. Loss of consciousness usually occurs within 40 seconds and continues for 3 to 5 minutes after a bolus injection. The drug rapidly redistributes throughout the body leading to the advantage of propofol use: the rapid return of consciousness with minimal psychomotor impairment.

Because the metabolic clearance of propofol exceeds hepatic blood flow, it is metabolized through both hepatic and extrahepatic (lung) routes. Continuous infusion of propofol can be administered without a cumulative effect because of its rapid clearance. The kinetics of propofol do not appear to be affected by chronic hepatic or renal disease.

TABLE 19.3 Summary of Selected ⓒ Parenteral Anesthetic Agents

Drug (Trade) Name	Selected Indications	Route and Dosage Range	Pharmacokinetics
Ⓟ propofol (Diprivan)	Anesthesia induction and maintenance, monitored anesthesia care (MAC), sedation for diagnostic and surgical procedures, continuous sedation in intensive care unit	*Adult:* IV, 1.5–2.5 mg/kg for induction, 75–200 mcg/kg/min for maintenance	*Onset:* 30 sec *Duration:* 5–10 min $t_{1/2}$: 2.4 min (distribution); 4–23 h (elimination)
etomidate (Amidate)	Anesthetic induction or adjunct, cardioversion, status epilepticus, head injury	*Adult:* 0.3 mg/kg IV induction	*Onset:* 15–45 sec *Duration:* 4–12 min $t_{1/2}$: 2–4 min (distribution); 2.9–5.3h (elimination)
dexmedetomidine (Precedex)	Preoperative sedation; anxiolysis, sedation in mechanically ventilated patients	Adult: IV, 1 mcg.kg over 10 min; then 0.2–0.6 mcg/kg/h continuous infusion for a max of 24 h. Nonintubated patient: 1 mcg/kg IV over 10 min	*Onset:* 30 min *Duration:* 2.5h $t_{1/2}$: 2–5h
ketamine (Ketalar)	Anesthesia for short surgical or diagnostic procedures not requiring skeletal muscle relaxation	*Adult:* IM, 4–6 mg/kg for induction, 2–4 mg/kg for sedation; IV, 0.5–1.5 mg/kg for induction and 1–3 mg/min for maintenance	*Onset:* IM, 3–4 min; IV, 45–60 sec *Duration:* IM, IV 10–20 min $t_{1/2}$: 11–16 min (distribution); 2–4h (elimination)
midazolam (Versed)	Anesthesia induction, cardiac catheterization, conscious sedation, endoscopy, gastroscopy, premedication	IM, IV 0.2–0.4 mg/kg induction, titrated	*Onset:* IM, 15 min; IV, 30–90 sec *Duration:* 10-30min $t_{1/2}$: 7–15 min (distributive); 1.7–2.6h (elimination)
remifentanil (Ultiva)	Anesthesia induction, analgesia and sedation in mechanically ventilated patients	*Adult:* IV, 0.5–2 mcg/kg/min over 30–60 sec *Child:* IV, 0.05–1.3 mcg/kg/min over 30–60 sec	*Onset:* rapid *Duration:* 20 min $t_{1/2}$: 3–10 min

Pharmacodynamics

The cellular mechanism of action of propofol is unknown, but it is thought to mediate activity of the inhibitory gamma-aminobutyric acid (GABA) receptors. However, the clinical response is clear: anesthesia is immediate and short-lived. Respiratory effects of propofol include dose-dependant respiratory depression (with apnea occurring after induction doses) and a relative bronchodilating effect. Propofol produces cardiac depression and its effects result in hypotension, decreased cardiac output, and systemic vascular resistance. Administration of propofol also produces a decrease in cerebral metabolism, cerebral blood flow, and a decrease in intraocular pressure. Propofol is a weak analgesic agent; therefore, it is generally administered with other analgesics. It also has some anti-emetic properties.

When high-dose propofol is used for long-term (>24 hours) maintenance of sedation as in an ICU, propofol infusion syndrome has been described, yet the incidence is 1% in both pediatric and adult populations. Propofol infusion syndrome is characterized by marked bradycardia (resistant to treatment), combined with fatty liver enlargement, metabolic acidosis, rhabdomyolysis, or myoglobinuria. The syndrome usually leads to fatal cardiac and renal failure.

Contraindications and Precautions

Propofol is contraindicated for patients with a hypersensitivity to propofol or any of the ingredients of its emulsion vehicle. Propofol is relatively contraindicated in patients with a seizure disorder because they are at an increased risk of developing convulsions during the recovery phase.

Propofol should be used with caution in patients with cardiac or peripheral vascular disease because the cardiovascular depressive and hypotensive effects of the anesthetic can aggravate these conditions. In addition, propofol should be used cautiously in patients with cerebrovascular disease, impaired cerebral blood flow, or increased ICP because it can cause a substantial reduction in mean arterial pressure and cerebral perfusion.

Adverse Effects

The most common adverse effect of propofol is pain on injection usually seen when administered in small veins. Preceding the injection it is a common practice to administer lidocaine. The solution in which propofol is prepared can support bacterial growth so it is recommended that aseptic technique is used when administering the drug.

Drug Interactions

Propofol may interact with benzodiazepines and CNS depressants (Table 19.4).

Assessment of Relevant Core Patient Variables

Health Status

Assess the patient for a history of hypersensitivity to propofol, soybean oil, glycerol, or egg phospholipids. Also, assess the

TABLE 19.4	Agents That Interact with P Propofol	
Interactants	**Effect and Significance**	**Nursing Management**
CNS depressants • Alcohol • Anesthetics • Benzodiazepines • Barbiturates • Histamine-1 blockers • Opioids • Phenothiazines • Tricyclic antidepressants	The pharmacologic effects of propofol may be enhanced, resulting in increased sedation and respiratory depression.	Provide continuous patient assessment. Monitor sedation. Monitor respiratory status. Provide supportive therapy as needed.
carbidopa-levodopa	When levodopa is abruptly withdrawn, a symptom complex resembling neuroleptic malignant syndrome may occur.	Administer levodopa as soon as patient is able to resume PO medications. Monitor for muscular rigidity, hyperthermia, mental changes, increased creatine phosphokinase concentration, diaphoresis, and tachycardia.
catecholamines	Propofol and catecholamines may drive each other in a progressively myocardial depressive loop, which could lead to cardiac arrhythmias or cardiac failure.	Monitor cardiovascular status. Follow standing protocols for titrating these drugs.
herbal medications • St. John's wort • *Hypericum perforatum*	Coadministration of propofol with herbal medications may intensify or prolong the effects of propofol.	Advise the patient to discontinue herbal medication 2–3 wk before surgery.

patient for diseases or disorders that contraindicate the use of propofol and for concomitant use of drugs that may interact with propofol. Positive responses should be communicated to the anesthesiologist or nurse anesthetist before surgery.

Life Span and Gender
Document the age of the patient. Elderly, debilitated, and dehydrated patients are typically more sensitive to the effects of propofol than younger patients. In addition, elderly patients typically have reduced total-body clearance of propofol and should be given lower induction doses and slower infusion rates for anesthesia maintenance.

Environment
Propofol must be given in a controlled environment, such as an operating room or ICU. A cardiac monitor, blood pressure monitor, and ventilator generally are required during administration.

Nursing Diagnoses and Outcomes

• Ineffective Breathing Pattern related to respiratory depression secondary to drugs used during anesthesia
  Desired outcome: *The patient will maintain effective breathing despite respiratory depression by administration of oxygen as appropriate.*
• Disturbed Sensory Perception, varied, related to CNS depression secondary to drugs used during anesthesia
  Desired outcome: *The patient will remain free from sensory or perceptual alterations through careful reorientation, repeated as necessary.*

Planning and Intervention

Maximizing Therapeutic Effects
For the surgical patient, preinduction and induction should be done in a low-stimulus environment, as with isoflurane.

It is imperative to educate patients preoperatively to minimize their anxiety, which, in turn, helps maximize the therapeutic effects of propofol.

In the critical care setting, a low-stimulus environment is also important. To avoid overstimulation, interact with the patient only when necessary. Evaluate the depth of analgesia and adjust the infusion of propofol according to the health facility's standing orders.

Minimizing Adverse Effects
Visually inspect the propofol preparation for particulate matter and discoloration before administration. If the emulsion appears to be separated, do not use it. Because the propofol emulsion does not contain preservatives, it is important to limit its duration of administration to avoid bacterial growth. When propofol is used for critical care sedation, it should be discarded after 12 hours if administered directly from the container provided from the pharmacy or within 6 hours if transferred to a syringe or other container.

Providing Patient and Family Education
• Provide preoperative patient education about the induction process to minimize fears of anesthesia.
• In the critical care unit, explain the purpose of the light anesthesia state and reassure patients that they are being constantly monitored.
• For outpatient surgery, discharge patients to the care of a responsible adult and instruct patients not to drive or engage in any activity that requires full alertness or coordination.

Ongoing Assessment and Evaluation
Monitor patients receiving propofol as an induction agent for balanced anesthesia in the postanesthesia recovery room until they are awake and have stable vital signs.

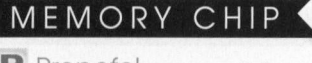

Propofol

- A parenteral anesthetic used in the management of general anesthesia, sedation induction or maintenance, and status epilepticus
- Major contraindications: hypersensitivity to soybean oil, glycerol, or egg phosphatide
- Most common adverse effects: nausea, vomiting, involuntary movements
- Most serious adverse effects: apnea and anaphylaxis
- Maximizing therapeutic effects: low-stimulus environment
- Minimizing adverse effects: Time the administration to avoid potential bacterial growth.
- Most important patient education: Reassure the patient that he or she is being constantly monitored.

When propofol is used to maintain light anesthesia in the critical care unit, continuously monitor blood pressure, cardiac output, and pulmonary capillary wedge pressure. Assess the patient's lung sounds frequently for respiratory depression. Because the patient remains motionless, turn the patient every 2 hours and assess for skin breakdown. Constantly monitor the level of sedation and titrate propofol to maximize sedation. Serum triglycerides should be monitored every 3 to 7 days.

Drugs Closely Related to Propofol
Etomidate

Etomidate (Amidate) is a nonbarbiturate, nonanalgesic anesthetic used primarily for induction, but it can be used for IV anesthesia when supplemented by an opioid analgesic. Induction is rapid, and recovery from a single dose takes only a few minutes (7 to 14 minutes) because of rapid redistribution of drug to other tissues. Etomidate is metabolized by the liver and plasma esterases and has a much shorter elimination time than propofol. There appears to be less respiratory and cardiovascular depression than with barbiturates and propofol. Additionally, etomidate does not release histamine.

The popularity of etomidate has diminished because of its adverse effects, including involuntary movements (myoclonia) during induction, a high incidence of nausea and vomiting during recovery, and adrenocortical suppression. However, it is still utilized in trauma or critically ill patients because of its lack of cumulative response, hemodynamic stability, hypnosis, and lack of histamine release.

Thiopental

Thiopental (Pentothal) is a barbiturate anesthetic agent. Its rapid onset and short duration of action are ideal for an induction agent. Its onset of action after IV administration is less than 1 minute, and the hypnotic action lasts only a few minutes. Metabolism of thiopental takes place in the liver slowly, and the drug accumulates to a toxic level in the tissues after repeated administrations. Thiopental is contraindicated in patients with certain types of porphyria. Thiopental differs from propofol in that it is not used for the duration of anesthesia by continuous infusion, does not provide any analgesia, and can cause an increase in heart rate.

Drugs Significantly Different From Propofol
Benzodiazepines

Benzodiazepines (e.g., diazepam, lorazepam, midazolam) have been used as parenteral agents in balanced anesthesia. Midazolam is water soluble at low pH and has been reported to cause less pain on injection and a lower incidence of venous thrombosis than diazepam. Additionally, midazolam can be administered intramuscularly. Chapter 15 discusses benzodiazepines in depth.

Dexmedetomidine

Dexmedetomidine (Precedex) is an α_2-receptor agonist that produces analgesia, anxiolysis, and sedation without respiratory depression. It is used as an adjuvant in balanced anesthesia, for sedation for procedures other than surgical and for short-term (<24 hours) sedation in the ICU. The use of dexmedetomidine can lead to intraoperative hypotension and bradycardia but it also has been reported to improve hemodynamic stability and post-operative pain control.

Fentanyl

Fentanyl (Sublimaze) is an opioid analgesic used in general anesthesia and conscious sedation (often co-administered with midazolam). Fentanyl produces dose-dependent analgesia, sedation, and respiratory depression with a rapid onset time. The duration of action is short and is eliminated by redistribution when given in a single dose. Chapter 24 discusses opioid agents in depth.

Ketamine

Both chemically and pharmacologically, ketamine (Ketalar) closely resembles phencyclidine, which is a street drug with a pronounced effect on sensory perception. Different from other IV anesthetics, ketamine produces **dissociative anesthesia** characterized by catatonia, amnesia, analgesia yet maintains consciousness and protective reflexes (laryngeal and pharyngeal reflexes). The patient may appear awake and reactive, but under ketamine anesthesia the higher centers of the brain do not perceive auditory, visual, or painful stimuli. Because of the high incidence of postoperative psychological phenomena (sensory and perceptual illusions and vivid dreams) associated with its use, benzodiazepines, barbiturates, or propofol are co-administered with ketamine to decrease these reactions.

Ketamine binds to N-methyl-D-aspartate (NMDA) receptors, in addition to opioid and non-opioid receptors. Also different than propofol, ketamine has analgesic and bronchodilatory properties. It also increases cerebral metabolism, cerebral blood flow, ICP, heart rate, and arterial blood pressure. Because of these unique characteristics of ketamine, it offers an alternative induction agent or as an adjuvant when trying to limit opioid use or when inducing a hemodynamically unstable shock patient or a patient with acute bronchospasm. Ketamine IM can be used for anesthesia induction if obtaining IV access is problematic.

After IV administration, ketamine has an initial half-life of 10 to 15 minutes, which subsequently changes to a longer half-life of 2.5 hours, corresponding with redistribution from the CNS and hepatic biotransformation. The metabolites of ketamine are excreted in the urine. Cardiovascular and respiratory stimulation occurs shortly after injection, peaks after a few minutes, and subsides within 15 minutes.

Ketamine is contraindicated in patients for whom a substantial increase in blood pressure would be hazardous. It is not used for patients with psychiatric disorders, because of the potential for a reaction during emergence from anesthesia, which may include hallucinations and agitation. It also should be avoided in cases of known hypersensitivity. Caution is advised for using ketamine in cases involving mild to moderate hypertension, pregnancy or lactation, alcohol abuse, acute intermittent porphyria, elevated intraocular pressure or ICP, and hyperthyroidism.

Ketamine may enhance the actions of the nondepolarizing neuromuscular blockers (discussed later in this chapter) and prolong respiratory depression. Theophylline should not be coadministered with ketamine because the two interact and may cause unpredictable seizures. Patients on thyroid enhancement therapy may experience hypertension and tachycardia when taking ketamine.

Nursing care of the patient under ketamine anesthesia is largely protective because of the dissociative state that it causes and the likelihood of emergence reactions. Take vital signs and a brief mental status examination as a pretreatment assessment.

The expected outcomes for ketamine anesthesia are effective and safe anesthesia, adequate airway maintenance, and minimal emergence reaction. Emergence reactions may be avoided or diminished if care is taken to reduce external stimuli during the recovery phase and to allow the patient to wake up spontaneously. Frightening emergence symptoms can be stopped with a benzodiazepine such as diazepam. Because emergence reactions may occur up to 24 hours after anesthesia, instruct the patient to avoid hazardous activities, including driving, for at least that long. Ambulatory patients must be discharged into the care of a responsible adult. Instruct the patient to avoid alcohol and other CNS depressants for 24 hours. The nurse in the PACU and the nurse in charge of the patient on his or her return to the unit should evaluate outcomes achieved and compare them with what would be expected under normal conditions.

Remifentanil

Remifentanil (Ultiva) is an ultra-short-acting, selective mu-opioid analgesic, which is used as an adjunctive medication during general anesthesia in both the inpatient and outpatient setting. It has a rapid onset and short half-life even when given as a continuous infusion. It is quickly metabolized by hydrolysis by plasma esterases. Remifentanil is extremely useful during balanced anesthesia because it works rapidly, is titratable, and has a rapid and predictable recovery period.

Ⓒ LOCAL ANESTHETIC AGENTS

Local anesthetic agents are divided into esters and amides based on their chemical structure. Important practical differences exist between these two groups. Esters are rapidly hydrolyzed in the body by plasma cholinesterase and other esterases. One of the main breakdown products is para-aminobenzoic acid, which is associated with allergic phenomena and hypersensitivity reactions. In contrast, amides are slowly degraded in the liver by P-450 enzymes and hypersensitivity reactions are extremely rare.

Local anesthetics produce local or regional anesthesia and analgesia by blocking electrical transmission of pain along nerve fibers (specifically voltage-gated sodium channels) and abolishing sensations in a limited and well-defined area of the body without loss of consciousness (Figure 19.2). The blockade affects all nerve fibers sequentially: autonomic, then sensory, then motor, with effects diminishing in reverse order. Clinically, the loss of nerve function affects temperature first; then pain, touch, and proprioception; and finally, skeletal muscle tone.

Local anesthetics share the same mechanism of action, but they differ in their potency, onset of action, and duration (Table 19.5). Local anesthetic agents include lidocaine, bupivacaine, etidocaine, mepivacaine, ropivicaine, prilocaine, procaine, and chloroprocaine. The prototype discussed in this chapter is lidocaine (Xylocaine), an amide local anesthetic agent.

Nursing Management of the Patient Receiving Ⓟ Lidocaine

Core Drug Knowledge

Pharmacotherapeutics

Lidocaine is used as a local anesthetic in a variety of situations, including regional blocks, peripheral nerve blocks, ophthalmic anesthesia, dental anesthesia, and infiltration anesthesia. It can be applied topically for dental pain, neuropathic pain, and skin disorders that cause inflammation and irritation. When administered intranasally, it is also effective for migraine headaches.

In addition to its uses as a local anesthetic, lidocaine is also used intravenously for ventricular tachycardia and ventricular fibrillation. See Chapter 31 for a discussion of lidocaine as an antiarrhythmic agent.

Pharmacokinetics

Lidocaine may be administered topically, orally, subcutaneously, intradermally, submucosally, and intravenously. Only minimal amounts of lidocaine enter the circulation following subcutaneous injection. The duration of action of subcutaneously administered lidocaine is 1 to 3 hours, depending

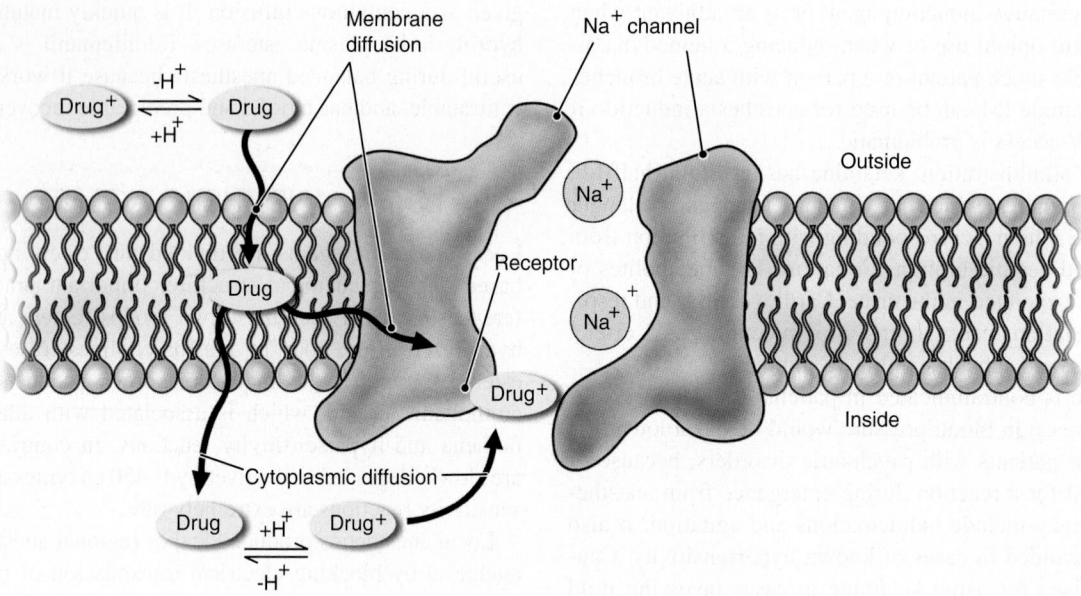

FIGURE 19.2 Local anesthetics' mechanism of action.

on the strength of the lidocaine preparation used. Adding epinephrine to lidocaine in proportions of 1:200,000 to 1:100,000 slows the vascular absorption of lidocaine and prolongs its effects.

Lidocaine is nearly completely absorbed following oral administration but undergoes extensive first-pass metabolism in the liver, resulting in a systemic bioavailability of only 35%. Some systemic absorption is possible when using oral viscous solutions.

Transdermal absorption of lidocaine is related to the duration of application and the surface area over which the patch is applied. When the lidocaine patch is used as directed, very little systemic absorption occurs. After topical administration of viscous solutions or jelly to mucous membranes, the duration of action is 30 to 60 minutes, with peak effects occurring within 2 to 5 minutes.

Pharmacodynamics

Lidocaine produces its analgesic effects through a reversible nerve conduction blockade, which diminishes the nerve membrane's permeability to sodium. This action decreases the rate of membrane depolarization, thereby increasing the threshold for electrical excitability. Direct penetration of the nerve membrane is necessary for effective anesthesia, which is achieved by applying the anesthetic topically or injecting it subcutaneously, intradermally, or submucosally around the nerve trunks or ganglia supplying the area to be anesthetized.

Contraindications and Precautions

Lidocaine is contraindicated in patients with hypersensitivity to amide local anesthetics and in patients with hypersensitivity to sulfites or the preservative methylparaben. To avoid systemic absorption of lidocaine, its administration as a nerve block or as epidural, local, or spinal anesthesia is contraindicated in patients with infection or inflammation at the injection site.

Applying lidocaine preparations to severely traumatized mucosa (large skin abrasions, eczema, burns) can increase its absorption, which in turn increases the risk of systemic toxicity. Application to the oral mucosa can interfere with swallowing and increase the risk of aspiration. Lumbar and caudal epidural anesthesia should be used with extreme caution in patients with existing neurologic disease, spinal deformities, sepsis, and severe hypertension, because the risk of adverse effects increases.

Adverse Effects

Allergic reactions such as urticaria, angioedema, bronchospasm, and anaphylactic shock may occur with lidocaine administration. Some preparations contain sulfites and methylparaben, which can cause severe allergic reactions, including status asthmaticus, in susceptible patients.

Local anesthetic agents are relatively free from adverse effects if they are administered in an appropriate dosage and in the correct anatomic location. However, systemic and localized toxic reactions may occur, usually from accidental intravascular or intrathecal injection, or from an excessive dose of the local anesthetic agent. Systemic reactions to local anesthetics are dose dependent and primarily involve the CNS and the cardiovascular system. Initial symptoms include light headedness, tinnitus, and tongue numbness. Signs of toxicity due to higher doses of absorption progress to patient symptoms of visual disturbances, muscle twitching, seizures, unconsciousness, coma, respiratory arrest, and cardiovascular depression.

Transoral or transdermal application of lidocaine is unlikely to cause systemic adverse reactions because of

TABLE 19.5 Summary of Selected Ⓒ Local Anesthetic Agents

Drug (Trade) Name	Selected Indications	Route and Dosage Range	Pharmacokinetics
Ⓟ lidocaine (Xylocaine)	Infiltration anesthesia Topical anesthesia Peripheral nerve blocks IV regional nerve blocks Epidural and spinal blocks	*Adult and child:* maximum, 3 mg/kg; with epinephrine, maximum: 7 mg/kg	*Onset:* Rapid *Duration:* 1–3 h $t_{1/2}$: 7–30 min
bupivacaine (Marcaine)	Infiltration anesthesia Peripheral nerve blocks Epidural and spinal blocks	*Adult and child:* maximum: 2 mg/kg; with epinephrine maximum: 2 mg/kg	*Onset:* 1–10 min *Duration:* 3–9 h $t_{1/2}$: neonates: 8.1 h $t_{1/2}$: adults: 3.5 h
chloroprocaine (Nesacaine)	Infiltration anesthesia Peripheral nerve block Epidural anesthesia	*Adult:* max safe dose 20 mg/kg *Child:* max safe dose 11 mg/kg	*Onset:* 3–12 min *Duration:* 30–45 min $t_{1/2}$: 1.5–4.7 min
etidocaine (Duranest)	Infiltration anesthesia Peripheral nerve block Extradural blocks	*Adult:* maximum: 4 mg/kg *Child:* maximum dose not established	*Onset:* 2–8 min *Duration:* 4.5–13 h $t_{1/2}$: neonates: 4–8 h $t_{1/2}$: adults: 2.7 h
mepivacaine (Carbocaine, Polocaine)	Infiltration anesthesia Peripheral nerve blocks	*Adult:* 400 mg as a single regional dose not to exceed 1,000 mg/24 h *Child:* 5–6 mg/kg	*Onset:* 5–4 min *Duration:* 1–2 h $t_{1/2}$: neonates: 8.7–9 h $t_{1/2}$: adults: 1.9–3.2 h
prilocaine (Citanest)	Infiltration anesthesia Peripheral nerve blocks IV regional nerve blocks	*Adult and child:* 6 mg/kg; with epinephrine, 9 mg/kg	*Onset:* <2 min *Duration:* 1–2 h $t_{1/2}$: 1.25 h
procaine (Novocain)	Dental anesthesia Infiltration Anesthesia Local anesthesia Peripheral nerve block Regional anesthesia Severe pain Spinal anesthesia Sympathetic nerve block	*Adult:* single dose of 350–600 mg *Child:* 15 mg/kg	*Onset:* 2–5 min *Duration:* 1 h $t_{1/2}$: 7.7 min
ropivacaine (Naropin)	Infiltration anesthesia Peripheral nerve block Epidural anesthesia/analgesia	*Adult:* max safe dose 3 mg/kg *Child:* 2.5 mg/kg	*Onset:* 5–15 min *Duration:* 4–8 h $t_{1/2}$: 1 h

the small amount of lidocaine absorbed. Potential local reactions include erythema, edema, and dysesthesia (abnormal sensations including numbness, tingling, prickling, or burning). These reactions are usually mild and transient, resolving within a few minutes to a few hours.

Drug Interactions

Drug interactions occur most frequently with IV administration of lidocaine. Subcutaneous administration rarely causes drug interactions unless lidocaine is inadvertently administered into an artery or vein.

Local anesthetics can interact with antihypertensive agents, cholinesterase inhibitors, monoamine oxidase inhibitors, and opiate agonists (Table 19.6). These interacting drugs will be discussed in more detail in subsequent chapters.

Assessment of Relevant Core Patient Variables
Health Status

Assess for hypersensitivity to lidocaine or any other drug with "caine" in the name. Communicate positive findings to the provider before administering lidocaine.

Before using topical anesthesia, inspect the area. Do not apply topical anesthesia to abraded or denuded skin. For viscous lidocaine, assess for the patient's ability to swallow before using the drug.

TABLE 19.6   Agents that Interact with P Lidocaine

Interactants	Effect and Significance	Nursing Management
antihypertensive agents	Epidural administration of local anesthetics with antihypertensive agents may result in additive hypotensive effects due to loss of sympathetic tone.	Monitor vital signs.
cholinesterase inhibitors	Local anesthetics can antagonize the effects of cholinesterase inhibitors by inhibiting neuronal transmission in skeletal muscle.	Dosage adjustment of the cholinesterase inhibitor may be necessary to control the symptoms of myasthenia gravis.
monoamine oxidase inhibitors (MAOIs)	Concomitant administration of MAOIs and local anesthetics increases the risk of hypotension.	MAOIs should be discontinued 10 days before surgery requiring a regional block.

opiate agonists
  alfentanil
  fentanyl
  morphine
  sufentanil
	Concomitant use of low-dose local anesthetics with opiate agonists may increase analgesia and decrease opiate dosage requirements.	Monitor for analgesic efficacy.
		Monitor CNS depression.

Life Span and Gender

Lidocaine should be used with caution in patients who are pregnant or breast-feeding. Although lidocaine is a pregnancy category B drug, local anesthetics can cross the placenta rapidly when administered for epidural, paracervical, pudendal, or caudal block anesthesia, resulting in fetal bradycardia. The frequency and extent of toxicity are dependent on the procedure performed. Maternal hypotension can result from regional anesthesia; to alleviate this problem, elevate the feet and position the patient on her left side. When lidocaine is used as epidural anesthesia during labor and delivery, it may prolong the second stage of labor. Monitor for cardiovascular and CNS depression in the fetus or neonate.

Lifestyle, Diet, and Habits

Viscous lidocaine may be provided for patients with stomatitis or chronic ulceration in the mouth. It is important that patients assess their ability to swallow before eating or drinking to avoid biting the interior of the mouth or aspirating foods or fluids.

Environment

Lidocaine is used in a variety of settings, including hospitals, outpatient surgical settings, clinics, private physician's offices, and dental offices. Topical or viscous lidocaine may be administered in the home environment.

Nursing Diagnoses and Outcomes

- Fear related to traumatic injury and concern about pain during the surgical procedure
  Desired outcome: The patient will be assured that pain will not occur during the procedure.
- Risk for Peripheral Neurovascular Dysfunction related to action of drug
  Desired outcome: The patient will refrain from activities that may induce injury while area is numb.
- Impaired Swallowing related to administration of viscous lidocaine

Desired outcome: The patient will refrain from eating or drinking for 1 hour after swallowing viscous lidocaine.

Planning and Intervention

Maximizing Therapeutic Effects

Assist with the administration of lidocaine after the patient is informed about the process. Use a calm, reassuring approach and allow the patient to voice concerns before the procedure begins.

Minimizing Adverse Effects

Read the drug label carefully before helping the provider administer lidocaine. Preparations containing preservatives should not be used for spinal or epidural anesthesia. Preparations with epinephrine should not be administered in areas such as fingers, toes, nose, or penis because prolonged vasoconstriction may damage these areas of the body. Restrict food and fluids for 1 hour after viscous lidocaine is swallowed.

Providing Patient and Family Education

- Tell patients and families how local anesthetics such as lidocaine work. Assure patients that the area will be numb before the procedure begins. Encourage patients to verbalize any discomfort during the procedure.
- Advise patients receiving topical anesthesia at home to place the anesthetic on the dressing first and then to place the dressing on the site. Remind patients receiving viscous lidocaine that it causes numbness of the tongue, cheeks, and throat. Patients should not eat or drink for 1 hour to keep from biting the cheeks or tongue and to avoid aspiration.
- Advise patients of the expected duration of lidocaine's effects. Patients should contact the provider if sensation does not return.

Ongoing Assessment and Evaluation

Evaluate for the lack of sensation before starting a procedure and remind patients to assess for sensation before resuming food or fluid intake.

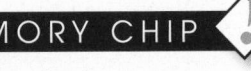
MEMORY CHIP

P Lidocaine

- Used for infiltration anesthesia, regional blocks, nerve blocks, ophthalmic anesthesia, obstetric anesthesia, or dental anesthesia
- Major contraindications: hypersensitivity to amide local anesthetics, sulfites, or methyl paraben; infection or inflammation at the site of administration
- Most common adverse effects: minimal adverse reactions unless accidental intravascular or intrathecal injection occurs
- Most serious adverse effect: allergic reactions
- Maximizing therapeutic effects: calm reassurance by staff
- Minimizing adverse effects: Read labels carefully. Be sure to use the right preparation for the right procedure.
- Most important patient education: safety due to lack of sensation

Drugs Closely Related to P Lidocaine

Bupivacaine, chloroprocaine, etidocaine, mepivacaine, ropivicaine, prilocaine, and procaine have the same mechanism of action but differ in potency, duration and onset of action (see Table 19.5). The potency is based on the lipid solubility of the local anesthetics (the more lipid soluble the more potent the drug). The duration of action is influenced by protein binding and lipid solubility of the drug (increased protein binding and lipid solubility provides a longer blockade time).

Bupivacaine

Bupivacaine (Marcaine) is recommended for local or regional anesthesia. It has the ability to separate sensory and motor blockade because its effect on motor function varies with concentration. With bupivacaine administration, analgesia persists longer than anesthesia, which postpones the need for postoperative narcotics. In combination with narcotics, bupivacaine is also used in epidural patient-controlled analgesia. Bupivicaine is the most cardiotoxic local anesthetic. If systemically absorbed at high doses, it will cause sudden cardiac collapse with ventricular dysrhythmias that are resistant to resuscitation.

Chloroprocaine

Chloroprocaine (Nesacaine) is chemically similar to procaine except for an additional chloride atom which increases the rate of hydrolysis by plasma cholinesterase. Chloroprocaine is a low-potency ester-type local anesthetic that has a rapid onset and a short duration of action.

Etidocaine

Etidocaine (Duranest) is used for epidural, local, and retrobulbar (eye block) anesthesia in surgical and dental procedures. Like lidocaine, etidocaine has a rapid onset of sensory and motor blockade, but the duration of analgesia is 1.5 to 2 times longer. Its profound motor blockade may last up to 9 hours when dosed in an epidural.

Mepivacaine

Mepivacaine (Carbocaine, Polocaine) has an intermediate duration of action. Compared with lidocaine, it produces less vasodilation and has a more rapid onset and longer duration of action. Mepivacaine is indicated for infiltration (administration of a local anesthetic into the area to be numbed) and transtracheal anesthesia and for peripheral, sympathetic, regional, and epidural nerve blocks in surgical and dental procedures.

Ropivicaine

Ropivicaine (Naropin) is a newer local anesthetic that causes less cardiovascular and CNS side effects than bupivacaine. It has an longer duration of action that is used in regional anesthesia. Unlike the other local anesthetics it causes vasoconstriction instead of vasodilation.

Prilocaine

Prilocaine (Citanest) is used primarily for dental anesthesia. It has an intermediate duration of action and is longer acting than lidocaine. Prilocaine causes the least systemic toxicity of the amides but at high doses may cause methemoglobinemia, a condition marked by high levels of a hemoglobin compound that does not carry oxygen.

Procaine

Procaine hydrochloride (Novocain) is a short-acting local anesthetic of the ester type used for local or regional anesthesia and dental applications. It has no topical anesthetic activity. Procaine is more likely to cause a hypersensitivity reaction and vasodilation than amide-type local anesthetics.

Topical Anesthetics

Local anesthetics may be applied to the skin, the eyes, the ears, the nose, and the mouth, as well as to other mucous membranes. In general, cocaine, lidocaine, and prilocaine are the most useful and effective local anesthetics for topical administration, and when used for that purpose, they usually have a rapid onset of action (5 to 10 minutes) and a moderate duration of action (30 to 60 minutes). In addition to its use as a topical anesthetic, cocaine is a potent vasoconstrictor.

Absorption of local anesthetics through intact skin is usually slow and unreliable, and high concentrations are required. EMLA cream is a mixture of local anesthetics (lidocaine and prilocaine in an emulsion) that may be used to provide surface anesthesia of the skin, particularly for children. Cutaneous contact (usually under an occlusive dressing) should be maintained for at least 60 minutes before venipuncture.

C NEUROMUSCULAR BLOCKING AGENTS

Neuromuscular blocking agents interrupt transmission of nerve impulses at the neuromuscular junction causing paralysis. Neuromuscular blocking agents are divided into two categories: non-depolarizing and depolarizing drugs.

Nondepolarizing drugs are competitive antagonists preventing the binding of acetylcholine to the receptor; therefore the

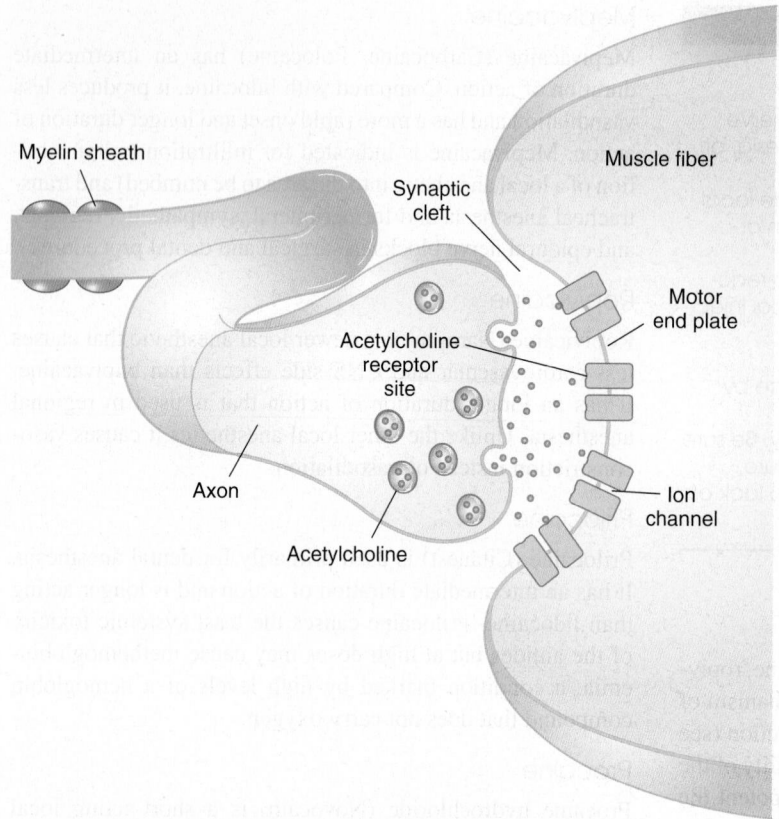

Myelin sheath

Synaptic cleft

Muscle fiber

Motor end plate

Acetylcholine receptor site

Axon

Acetylcholine

Ion channel

• FIGURE 19.3   The neuromuscular junction consists of a prejunctional motor nerve ending (axon), synaptic cleft and the motor end plate. The motor end plates are the terminal branches of motor nerves found on the skeletal muscle. Normally, the neurotransmitter acetylcholine is released from the axon and diffuses toward the receptor site through the synaptic cleft. Muscle contraction occurs when the acetylcholine binds to the receptor. Neuromuscular blockers compete with acetylcholine, not allowing acetylcholine to bind and therefore preventing muscle contraction.

end plate is unable to depolarize. After administration, muscle fasciculation will not be present, unlike depolarizing drugs. Depolarizing drugs, structurally similar to acetylcholine, cause continuous muscle depolarization and prevents repolarization. The muscle is unable to repolarize as long as the drug continues to bind to the acetylcholine receptor. In both categories of drugs, neuromuscular blockade occurs at acetylcholine receptor sites on the motor end plate (Figure 19.3). Doses of neuromuscular blockers need to be carefully titrated for individual patients according to response and may vary with the procedure, the other drugs given, and the state of the patient.

• C NONDEPOLARIZING NEUROMUSCULAR BLOCKING AGENTS

Nondepolarizing neuromuscular blocking agents include vecuronium, rocuronium, pancuronium, and cisatracurium (Table 19.7). The prototype drug is vecuronium (Norcuron).

Nursing Management of the Patient Receiving P Vecuronium

Core Drug Knowledge

Pharmacotherapeutics

Vecuronium, a nondepolarizing muscle relaxant, is an anesthesia adjunct used to provide skeletal muscle relaxation to facilitate intubation and mechanical ventilation and to improve surgical conditions during surgical procedures.

Vecuronium also may be used in the ICU setting to assist with mechanical ventilation.

Pharmacokinetics

Vecuronium, only available for IV use, has an intermediate duration of action (30 to 60 minutes) when compared to other nondepolarizing neuromuscular blocking agents. With an intubating dose of 0.1 mg/kg, onset of muscle paralysis occurs within 2 to 4 minutes. Clinically, the speed of onset and duration of blockage are monitored by using a peripheral nerve stimulator on the facial or ulnar nerve to assess the effect of the neuromuscular blocking agent.

Vecuronium is excreted by the kidney; therefore drug kinetics will be altered with patients who have kidney disease. In addition, a majority of the drug is eliminated in the liver and excreted in the bile. Hypothermia inhibits the means of elimination and alters the pharmacokinetics; keeping the patient normothermic is extremely important.

Pharmacodynamics

As previously discussed, nondepolarizing neuromuscular blocking agents are antagonists of acetylcholine; they compete with the neurotransmitter for the cholinergic receptor sites at the motor end plate. The neuromuscular blocking actions of vecuronium may be reversed with anticholinesterases such as neostigmine, pyridostigmine, and edrophonium. These drugs block the normal breakdown of acetylcholine at the motor end plate, causing the neurotransmitter to accumulate and returning muscle stimulation.

TABLE 19.7	Summary of Selected Ⓒ Neuromuscular Blocking Agents		
Drug (Trade) Name	**Selected Indications**	**Route and Dosage Range**	**Pharmacokinetics**
Nondepolarizing Neuromuscular Junction Blockers			
P vecuronium (Norcuron)	Endotracheal intubation	*Adult and child >10 y:* IV, 80–100 mcg/kg *Child 1–10 y:* IV, Individualized; may need slightly more than adult dose *Infant 7 wk–12 mo:* IV, Individualized *Neonate:* Safe dose not established.	*Onset:* 2–3 min *Duration:* 45–60 min $t_{1/2}$: 70 min
	Neuromuscular blockade as adjunct to general anesthesia with isoflurane	*Adult and child >10 y:* IV, 60–85 mcg/kg; then 10–15 mcg/kg after 25–40 min; then readminister every 12–15 min *Child 1–10 y:* IV, Individualized; may need slightly more than adult dose *Infant 7 wk–12 mo:* 0.08–0.1 mg/kg followed by 0.05–0.1 mg/kg every h as needed *Neonate:* IV, 0.1 mg/kg followed by 0.03–0.15 mg/kg every 1–2 h	
cisatracurium (Nimbex)	Endotracheal intubation, neuromuscular blockade	*Adult:* IV, 0.15–0.20 mg/kg followed by 0.03 mg/kg every 20 min *Child >2 y:* IV, 0.1 mg/kg followed by 1–2 mcg as needed	*Onset:* 5–7 min *Duration:* 35–45 min $t_{1/2}$: 22 min
	Mechanical ventilation	*Adult:* IV, 0.5–10.2 mcg/kg/min	
pancuronium (Pavulon)	Neuromuscular blockade, agitation	*Adult and child:* IV, 0.04–0.1 mg/kg initial dose; may give additional doses of 0.01 mg/kg at 30- to 60-min intervals	*Onset:* 2–3 min *Duration:* 60–90 min $t_{1/2}$: 140 min
rocuronium (Zemuron)	Rapid-sequence intubation Endotracheal intubation	*Adult:* IV, 0.6–1.2 mg/kg *Adult:* IV, 0.6–1.2 mg/kg *Child >3 mo:* IV, 0.6 mg/kg	*Onset:* 1–2 min *Duration:* 30 min $t_{1/2}$: 90 min
	Neuromuscular blockade continuous infusion	*Adult:* IV, 0.01–0.012 mg/kg/min *Child >3 mo:* IV, 0.012 mg/kg/min	
Depolarizing Neuromuscular Junction Blockers			
P succinylcholine (Anectine, Quelicin)	Endotracheal intubation	*Adult:* IV, 2 mg/kg; IM, 3–4 mg/kg *Adolescent and older child:* IV, 1 mg/kg; IM, 3–4 mg/kg *Small child and infant:* IV, 2 mg/kg; IM, 3–4 mg/kg	*Onset IV:* 30–60 sec *Onset IM:* 2–3 min *Duration IV:* 4–6 min *Duration IM:* 10–20 min $t_{1/2}$: <1 min

Vecuronium does not induce histamine release and is considered cardiovascular stable. There have been some reports of bradycardia. Vecuronium does not easily cross the blood–brain barrier or the GI epithelium; hence it does not produce CNS effects, and oral absorption is ineffective. It cannot be stressed enough that neuromuscular blocking agents do not affect consciousness or produce sedation. Patients must be provided adequate anesthesia or sedation before administering muscle skeletal relaxants. Because patients will be paralyzed, they will be unable to spontaneous ventilate and must be mechanically assisted.

Contraindications and Precautions

Vecuronium is contraindicated in patients who have ever shown hypersensitivity to the drug or to any other nondepolarizing blocker. It is classified as a pregnancy category C drug, and is only given if the benefit justifies the risk.

Vecuronium is used with caution in patients with myasthenia gravis or Eaton-Lambert syndrome as small doses have profound effects. Vecuronium should be used with caution in patients with hepatic disease and decreased renal function because the drug is eliminated in the urine and bile. In addition, patients with an electrolyte imbalance may experience altered drug affects.

Adverse Effects

The principal adverse effects of vecuronium result from its blockade of neuromuscular activity at all neuromuscular end plates. Prolonged paralysis can cause immobility that leads to pressure sores (decubitus ulcer formation). Prolonged apnea can result from the paralysis of the respiratory muscles. Therefore, assisted ventilation is needed until the drug's effects resolve or anticholinesterase administration is successful.

Drug Interactions

Drugs that potentiate the action of vecuronium tubocurarine include antibiotics (aminoglycosides, tetracyclines, polymyxin B), inhalation anesthetics, magnesium salts, quinine derivatives, and verapamil. Table 19.8 illustrates these potential drug interactions.

TABLE 19.8 Agents That Interact with P Vecuronium

Interactants	Effect and Significance	Nursing Management

antibiotics
  aminoglycosides
  lincosamide
  polymyxin B
  polypeptides tetracycline
	Potentiate the action of vecuronium, resulting in profound and severe respiratory depression	Avoid combination.
		Provide life support as needed.
		Provide anticholinesterases as indicated.

antiepileptics carbamazepine	In combination, may decrease the duration or efficacy of vecuronium	Monitor for decreased muscle relaxant effectiveness. Titrate drug as necessary.
inhalation anesthetics	Potentiate the actions of vecuronium	Monitor respiratory function. Titrate drug as necessary. Provide life support as needed.
magnesium salts	May enhance the actions of vecuronium, resulting in profound and severe respiratory depression	Monitor respiratory function. Titrate drug as necessary. Provide life support as needed.
quinine derivatives	Have a synergistic action with vecuronium, resulting in profound and severe respiratory depression	Monitor neuromuscular function. Titrate drug as necessary. Provide life support as needed.
verapamil	May enhance the action of vecuronium because of its blockage of calcium channels in skeletal muscle	Avoid combination if possible. Monitor respiratory function. Titrate drug as necessary. Provide life support as needed.

Assessment of Relevant Core Patient Variables

Health Status

Evaluate the patient for a history of hypersensitivity to any NMJ blocker or for any renal or hepatic disease. For patients with a history of any of these disorders, place a note on the chart and the drug administration record (Kardex) identifying the need to monitor them closely.

Before administration, perform a physical assessment. The physical examination should include body weight, temperature, state of hydration (skin turgor, pulses), reflexes and muscle tone, pulse, blood pressure, respiratory rate, and adventitious breath sounds. Assess laboratory tests to establish baseline electrolyte values and renal and hepatic status.

Life Span and Gender

Assess women of childbearing age for pregnancy. Vecuronium is pregnancy category C and should be given only if the potential benefit justifies the risk to the fetus. However, it can be used safely as an adjunct to anesthesia in cesarean deliveries. After birth, closely observe the infant for any signs of respiratory depression, because the drug crosses the placenta.

Environment

Be aware of the environment in which the drug will be administered. As with all neuromuscular blocking agents, vecuronium causes respiratory impairment and reversible paralysis. It should be administered only by a person skilled in airway management.

Necessary equipment for intubation, controlled ventilation, and administration of oxygen must be immediately available.

Nursing Diagnoses and Outcomes

- Impaired Spontaneous Ventilation related to respiratory paralysis
  Desired outcome: The patient will be maintained with artificial ventilation until the ability to sustain spontaneous respirations returns.
- Impaired Skin Integrity related to paralysis
  Desired outcome: The patient will remain free of skin breakdown.
- Fear related to paralysis and helplessness
  Desired outcome: The patient will be reassured and comforted to prevent fear and sympathetic effects of fear during paralysis.

Planning and Intervention

Maximizing Therapeutic Effects

Maximize the therapeutic effects of vecuronium by helping patients understand the reason for the therapy and by helping to decrease their fear and anxiety. Anxiety can be alleviated by reassuring the patient that they will be sedated during the time period in which they are chemically paralyzed with a neuromuscular blocking agent. Monitor patients carefully for pain or distress; responses of the pupils, blood pressure,

MEMORY CHIP

P Vecuronium

- A nondepolarizing neuromuscular junction blocking agent used to facilitate endotracheal intubation and mechanical ventilation
- Major contraindications: hypersensitivity
- Most serious adverse effects: prolonged paralysis, apnea
- Maximizing therapeutic effects: Decrease anxiety and fear.
- Minimizing adverse effects: Have resuscitation equipment and cholinesterase inhibitor antidote at the bedside.
- Most important patient education: Reassure the patient that he or she is being constantly monitored.

and heart rate, although not foolproof, are probably the most reliable guide to their condition. Also, frequently reassure patients that the staff is aware of their feeling of helplessness. The hearing of these patients is not impaired; therefore, explain procedures and interventions.

Minimizing Adverse Effects

Have resuscitation equipment and drugs at the bedside throughout therapy. Evaluate the depth of paralysis by use of a stimulator and use cholinesterase inhibitors to overcome excessive or prolonged neuromuscular blockade.

If paralysis is prolonged, change the patient's position frequently to prevent venous stasis or decubitus ulcer formation and provide frequent skin care to prevent skin breakdown.

Providing Patient and Family Education

- Before administration, explain to patients and families that the drug will paralyze muscles and the patient will be unable to speak, move, or breathe unassisted. It is important to explain that these effects should subside a short time after the drug is discontinued and that the patient will be provided with hypnotic and amnestic drugs as an adjunct.
- Advise patients that adverse effects may occur after administration. These effects include sore muscles, constipation, difficulty voiding, and dizziness on arising. Explain the importance of reporting these symptoms to avoid potential injury.

Ongoing Assessment and Evaluation

Monitor the respiratory and cardiac status of the patient frequently. For patients with prolonged paralysis, monitor skin status frequently. Conscious patients should be monitored for any sign of distress, which is especially important because they are unable to talk or move. However, keep in mind that patients can still hear if inadequately sedated. For patients with prolonged paralysis, turn the patient every 2 hours and monitor for skin breakdown. Provide protection to the corneas by taping eye pads in place and by using artificial tears. Continue use of benzodiazepines and analgesic agents to provide a calm environment for these patients.

Drugs Closely Related to P Vecuronium

Other non-depolarizing intermediate-acting neuromuscular blocking agents include cisatracurium and rocuronium. Pancuronium is structurally similar to vecuronium, however it has a longer duration of action.

Cisatracurium

Cisatracurium besylate (Nimbex) has an intermediate onset and duration of action. It has a unique way of elimination that is different than the other non-depolarizing muscular blocking agents. It undergoes Hoffman elimination, which is pH and temperature dependent. Cisatracurium is very effective and safe for patients who have liver disease and renal failure. Cisatracurium does not cause dose-related increases in histamine release and can be used safely in patients with cardiovascular disease.

Pancuronium

Pancuronium (Pavulon) has a longer duration of action. It is a vagolytic drug and is therefore associated with increases of heart rate, blood pressure and cardiac output. This drug characteristic can be useful in some patients that are bradycardiac and hypotensive as a result of narcotics. Pancuronium produces little histamine release. Pancuronium is contraindicated for use in neonates.

Rocuronium

Rocuronium (Zemuron) has an onset of action is comparable with that of succinylcholine, but its duration of action is considerably longer. Because of its rapid onset, rocuronium may be a useful alternative to succinylcholine for rapid-sequence induction. In addition to its therapeutic actions, rocuronium can cause an increase in heart rate, but this side effect is minimal at normal doses. Rocuronium produces little histamine release and no ganglionic blockade; thus, hypotension and bronchospasm are not associated with its use. Children generally require larger doses per kilogram than adults do to achieve muscle relaxation.

• C DEPOLARIZING NEUROMUSCULAR JUNCTION BLOCKERS

Depolarizing NMJ blockers work by causing the muscle cell membrane to depolarize or become excited, which causes muscle contraction. This action leads to paralysis of the muscle after repeated excitation. This mechanism differs from that of nondepolarizing NMJ blockers, which prevent excitation. Succinylcholine (Anectine) is the prototype depolarizing NMJ blocker (Table 19.8).

Nursing Management of the Patient Receiving P Succinylcholine
Core Drug Knowledge
Pharmacotherapeutics

Succinylcholine is used primarily for rapid endotracheal intubation and other procedures which need a very short-acting paralytic. It is also of value in modifying muscle contractions and preventing fractures during electroconvulsive therapy because it produces a complete neuromuscular blockade within 1 minute that lasts for a few minutes, allowing sufficient time to complete the therapy. The use of succinylcholine as an adjunct to anesthesia or to facilitate prolonged mechanical ventilation has been largely replaced by the use of more effective and less toxic NMJ blockers. However, succinylcholine still plays an important role and is widely used but not without controversy.

Pharmacokinetics

Succinylcholine is administered intravenously and intramuscularly. It has a rapid onset and a short duration of action. Following IV administration, complete muscle relaxation occurs in 30 seconds to 1 minute, lasts for 2 to 3 minutes, and then dissipates within 10 minutes. After intramuscular (IM) injection, muscle relaxation occurs in 2 to 3 minutes and lasts 10 to 30 minutes.

Succinylcholine is distributed in the extracellular fluid but does not readily cross the placental barrier. Succinylcholine has a complex excretion pattern. Approximately 10% of the dose is excreted unchanged in the urine. Succinylcholine is mostly hydrolyzed by plasma pseudocholinesterase to metabolites. One of the metabolites, succinylmonocholine, has nondepolarizing muscle relaxation properties. It is excreted partly in urine, and the remainder is broken down into inactive metabolites. Succinylmonocholine is hydrolyzed slowly.

Pharmacodynamics

Succinylcholine acts as an agonist at the cholinergic nicotinic receptors of the motor end plate. Like the usual neurotransmitter acetylcholine, it depolarizes the postsynaptic membrane, producing repetitive excitation of the motor end plate. Muscular fasciculations (rapid contractions) result, followed by flaccid paralysis. Because of this effect, patients often experience postoperative muscle pain. The ensuing paralysis is short lived because the succinylcholine is hydrolyzed by plasma pseudocholinesterase.

Contraindications and Precautions

Succinylcholine is contraindicated in any patient with a known hypersensitivity to the drug. Because it can induce malignant hyperthermia, it is also contraindicated in any patient with a personal or family history of the disorder. Succinylcholine may interact with acetylcholine to produce

---

Box 19.3 ADVERSE EFFECTS OF SUCCINYLCHOLINE

Hyperkalemia
Elevated intraocular pressure
Elevated intracranial pressure
Elevated intragastric pressure
Dysrhythmias
Myalgia
Myoglobinemia
Malignant hyperthermia
Masseter spasm

---

prolonged apnea; thus, this agent is contraindicated in patients with familial plasma pseudocholinesterase disorders. In addition, succinylcholine is contraindicated in patients with an open eye injury or acute narrow-angle glaucoma because it causes a transient elevation in intraocular pressure immediately after injection (Box 19.3). Succinylcholine may also increase cerebral blood flow and intracranial pressure as fasciculations stimulate muscle fibers and therefore increase cerebral activity. It should be used cautiously in patients with head injuries or pre-existing increased intracranial pressure.

Succinylcholine should be used with caution in patients prone to low pseudocholinesterase levels. Decreased concentrations of serum pseudocholinesterase, the major enzyme that degrades succinylcholine, can lead to very high levels of the drug and prolonged action.

Succinylcholine should also be used with caution in patients who have or are at risk for hyperkalemia. Intense muscle contraction and potassium release from succinylcholine may induce hyperkalemia and provoke complications of hyperkalemia, such as cardiac arrhythmias. Caution is advised especially with children and adults who have compromised cardiac function, degenerative or dystrophic neuromuscular disease, or paraplegia. These patients tend to become severely hyperkalemic when succinylcholine is administered.

Adverse Effects

The principal adverse effects of succinylcholine are associated with muscle paralysis caused by the drug. Prolonged apnea can result from the paralysis of the respiratory muscles, and assisted ventilation is needed until the drug's effects are known. Increased intraocular pressure can aggravate or precipitate glaucoma.

A mild histamine release associated with succinylcholine may result in respiratory difficulty, including wheezing and bronchospasm, cardiac arrhythmias, hypotension, and even cardiac arrest in susceptible patients. Malignant hyperthermia has been reported infrequently. Other metabolic effects include hyperkalemia, with its resultant muscular and cardiac effects, and myoglobinemia and myoglobinuria, which are associated with extreme muscle contraction. Patients may complain of intense muscle pain that may persist for several days after they have received the drug.

Drug Interactions

Succinylcholine interacts with aminoglycosides, anticholinesterases, procaine, and trimethaphan (Table 19.9). It also interacts with drugs that decrease plasma cholinesterase, such as cyclophosphamide, echothiophate, lidocaine infusion, metoclopramide, and quinine derivatives.

Assessment of Relevant Core Patient Variables
Health Status

Assess the patient's personal or family history for low pseudocholinesterase levels. Patients at risk for low

TABLE 19.9 Agents That Interact with [P] Succinylcholine

Interactants	Effect and Significance	Nursing Management
aminoglycosides	Potentiate neuromuscular effects of succinylcholine	Use combination with caution. Delay administration of aminoglycosides as long as possible after recovery of spontaneous respirations. Monitor for respiratory depression. Have mechanical ventilation available.
anticholinesterases	Inhibition of plasma cholinesterase by anticholinesterases may delay hydrolysis of succinylcholine	Use this combination with caution. Monitor patients' spontaneous muscle activity, which must continue for 5 min before longer-acting agents are administered.

plasma cholinesterase inhibitors
  cyclophosphamide
  echothiophate
  lidocaine infusion
  metoclopramide
  quinine derivatives
  oral contraceptives
	Plasma cholinesterase (pseudocholinesterase) necessary to hydrolyze succinylcholine; decreased plasma cholinesterase interferes with the inactivation of succinylcholine, may prolong neuromuscular blockade	Measure serum cholinesterase levels for patients who have been receiving drugs that inhibit plasma cholinesterase.
		Reduce succinylcholine dosage if plasma cholinesterase levels are decreased.
		Monitor for respiratory depression.
		Have mechanical ventilation available.

procaine	Procaine and succinylcholine both hydrolyzed by plasma cholinesterase; competition for the enzyme possibly resulting in prolonged effects of succinylcholine	Monitor for respiratory depression. Have mechanical ventilation available.
trimethaphan	Potent noncompetitive inhibitor of plasma cholinesterase; directly decreases the sensitivity of the respiratory center, increasing risk for respiratory depression	Avoid this combination. Substitute nitroprusside for trimethaphan.

pseudocholinesterase levels include those with severe burns, malnutrition, dehydration, severe hepatic disease, cancer, severe anemia, or myxedema. Also, assess for a history of slow recovery from anesthesia or difficulty during anesthesia.

Before administering succinylcholine, perform a physical assessment. The physical examination should include body weight and temperature, state of hydration (skin turgor, pulses), reflexes and muscle tone, pulse rate, blood pressure, respiratory rate, and adventitious breath sounds.

Life Span and Gender
Document the age and gender of the patient and assesses women of childbearing age for pregnancy. Succinylcholine is used cautiously in children because it can cause severe bradycardia or cardiac arrest. The drug is in pregnancy category C. Although it is uncertain whether it causes fetal harm, it should be used cautiously during pregnancy because the drug places the patient at risk for increased drug effects, such as prolonged apnea. Succinylcholine is commonly used during cesarean section. If repeated dosing is required during delivery, the neonate should be monitored closely for apnea and flaccidity.

Environment
Be aware of the environment in which the drug will be administered. Like vecuronium, succinylcholine causes respiratory impairment and paralysis. It should be administered only by a qualified clinician. Necessary equipment

for intubation, controlled ventilation, and administration of oxygen must be immediately available.

Nursing Diagnoses and Outcomes
- Impaired Spontaneous Ventilation related to respiratory paralysis
  Desired outcome: The patient's breathing will be maintained with artificial ventilation until the ability to sustain spontaneous respiration returns.
- Impaired Physical Mobility related to drug-induced paralysis
  Desired outcome: The patient will remain free from disorders related to immobility, such as skin breakdown.
- Fear related to paralysis and helplessness
  Desired outcome: The patient will be reassured and comforted to prevent fear and sympathetic effects of fear during paralysis.

Planning and Intervention
Maximizing Therapeutic Effects
Maximize the therapeutic effects of succinylcholine by helping the patient understand the rationale for the therapy and by helping decrease fear and anxiety.

Minimizing Adverse Effects
To decrease muscle fasciculations, the patient should receive a small dose of a nondepolarizing NMJ blocker before

MEMORY CHIP

P Succinylcholine

- A depolarizing neuromuscular junction blocking agent used to facilitate endotracheal intubation and short procedures such as endoscopy or electroconvulsive therapy
- Major contraindications: hypersensitivity, history of malignant hyperthermia, familial plasma pseudocholinesterase disorders, and narrow-angle glaucoma
- Most common adverse effects: increased ocular pressure, histamine release, muscle pain
- Most serious adverse effects: prolonged paralysis and apnea
- Maximizing therapeutic effects: Decrease anxiety and fear.
- Minimizing adverse effects: Have resuscitation equipment at the bedside.
- Most important patient education: Reassure the patient that he or she is being constantly monitored.

succinylcholine is given. This step is especially important when succinylcholine is used in children.

Providing Patient and Family Education

- Before administration, explain to patients and families that the drug will paralyze muscles and that patients will be unable to speak, move, or breathe unassisted. It is important to explain that these effects should subside soon after the drug is discontinued.
- Because this drug may be used in an emergency situation, explain the effects of the drug to patients even if they appear to be unconscious.

Ongoing Assessment and Evaluation

Monitor for symptoms of malignant hyperthermia, such as muscle rigidity (especially the jaw), tachycardia, tachypnea, and elevated body temperature. Have dantrolene on standby in case malignant hyperthermia occurs. Also, monitor the cardiac and respiratory status of the patient while succinylcholine is being administered.

CHAPTER SUMMARY

- Anesthesia is a loss of feeling or sensation.
- Balanced anesthesia is a combination of anesthetic agents used to decrease the depth of anesthesia and keep the patient safe.
- Anesthetic agents are divided into inhaled and intravenous agents.
- Isoflurane (Forane) is a halogenated inhaled anesthetic. Nursing management of patients recovering from isoflurane anesthesia includes carefully monitoring residual CNS depression, manifested as respiratory depression.
- Nitrous oxide is an inflammable gas used to increase the effectiveness of halogenated agents without severely depressing the depth of coma.

- Propofol (Diprivan) is the prototype intravenous anesthetic. It has a quick onset and short duration of action.
- Ketamine (Ketalar) causes dissociative anesthesia.
- Local anesthetics such as lidocaine produce local or regional anesthesia by blocking nerve conduction. They are used to facilitate various types of procedures.
- Nondepolarizing NMJ blockers, such as tubocurarine, prevent nerve impulses from exciting muscle; paralysis ensues because the muscle is unable to respond.
- Depolarizing NMJ blockers, such as succinylcholine, cause muscle paralysis by overexcitement (depolarization) and subsequent exhaustion of the muscle.
- The NMJ blockers are primarily used as adjuncts to general anesthesia, to facilitate endotracheal intubation, or to facilitate mechanical ventilation.

QUESTIONS FOR STUDY AND REVIEW

1. What is balanced anesthesia?
2. What environmental safeguards are needed for patients receiving anesthesia?
3. Propofol is administered in a special emulsion vehicle. What problems does this vehicle pose?
4. Describe the potential systemic adverse effects of locally administered lidocaine (Xylocaine).
5. What is the difference in the mechanism of action between non-depolarizing NMJ blockers and depolarizing NMJ blockers?
6. Mrs. Smith has just returned to the intensive care unit after surgery. She is being maintained on pancuronium bromide. The charge nurse comes into the room and starts to discuss Mrs. Smith's prognosis. What should you do?
7. Your patient is scheduled to receive succinylcholine for a surgical procedure. What teaching points would you need to include in a plan for this patient to prepare him or her for the postoperative experience?

NEED MORE HELP?

Chapter 19 of the Study Guide to Accompany *Drug Therapy in Nursing*, 4th Edition, contains NCLEX-style questions and other learning activities to reinforce your understanding of the concepts presented in this chapter. For additional information or to purchase the study guide, visit **thePoint**.

REFERENCES

Aldrete, J. (1995). The post-anesthesia recovery score revisited. *Journal of Clinical Anesthesia*, 7(1):89–91.

Barash, P., Cullen, B., Stoeltling, R., et al. (2009). *Clinical Anesthesia* (6th ed.). New York, NY: Wolters Kluwer Health.

Brush, D., Kress, J. (2009). Sedation and analgesia for the mechanically ventilate patient. *Clinics in Chest Medicine*, 30(1):131–141.

Conway, B. (2009). Prevention and management of postoperative nausea and vomiting in adults. *AORN*, 90(3):391–413.

Facts and Comparisons. (2010). *Drug facts and comparisons*. Philadelphia, PA: Lippincott Williams & Wilkins.

Karch, A. M. (2010). *Nursing Drug Guide*. Philadelphia, PA: Lippincott Williams & Wilkins.

Koda-Kimbal, M. A., Young, L. Y., Kradian, W. A., et al. (2008). *Applied Therapeutics: The Clinical Use of Drugs*. Philadelphia, PA: Lippincott Williams & Wilkins.

Nagelhout, J., and Plaus, K. (2009). *Nurse Anesthesia* (4th ed.). Philadelphia, PA: W. B. Saunders.

Micromedex Healthcare Series. Retrieved August 18, 2010 from *http://www.thomsonhc.com*

Silvay, G., Castillo, J., Chikwe, J., et al. (2008). Cardiac Anesthesia and Surgery in Geriatric Patients. *Seminars in Cardiothoracic and Vascular Anesthesia,* 12(1): 18–28.

Tatro, D. S. (2011). *Drug Interaction Facts 2011: The Authority on Drug Interactions*. Philadelphia, PA: Wolters Kluwer Health/Facts and Comparisons.

Wilhelm, W., Kreuer, S. (2008). The place for short-acting opioids: special emphasis on remifentanil. *Critical Care,* 12(Suppl 3):S5.

Drugs Affecting Muscle Spasm and Spasticity

Learning Objectives

At the completion of this chapter the student will:

1. Correlate the pathophysiology of muscle spasm and spasticity with appropriate pharmacotherapy.

2. Identify core drug knowledge about pharmacologic therapies that affect muscle spasm and spasticity.

3. Identify core patient variables related to drugs that affect muscle spasm and spasticity.

4. Relate the interaction of core drug knowledge with core patient variables for pharmacologic therapies that affect muscle spasm and spasticity.

5. Generate a nursing plan of care from the interactions between core drug knowledge and core patient variables for pharmacologic therapies that affect muscle spasm and spasticity.

6. Describe nursing interventions to maximize therapeutic effects and minimize adverse effects for drugs that affect muscle spasm and spasticity.

7. Determine key points for patient and family education about drugs that affect muscle spasm and spasticity.

Key Terms

centrally acting	spasm	tonic
clonic	spasmolytics	
peripherally acting	spasticity	

Drugs Affecting Muscle Spasm and Spasticity

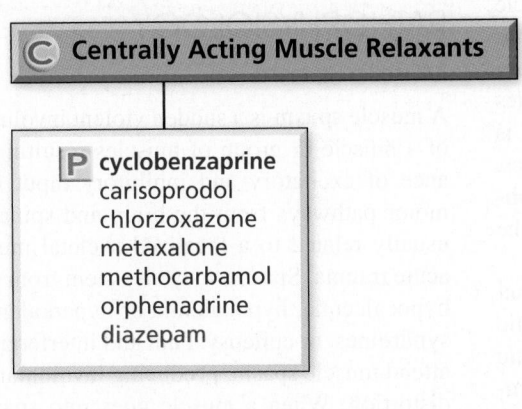

Centrally Acting Muscle Relaxants

P **cyclobenzaprine**
carisoprodol
chlorzoxazone
metaxalone
methocarbamol
orphenadrine
diazepam

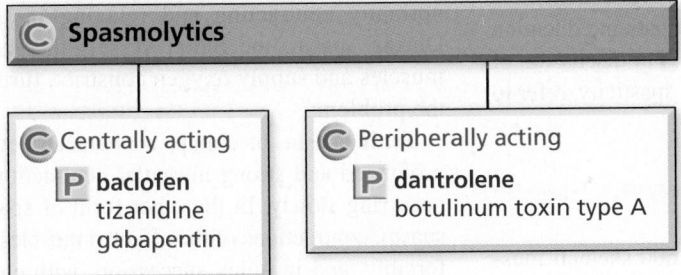

Spasmolytics

Centrally acting

P **baclofen**
tizanidine
gabapentin

Peripherally acting

P **dantrolene**
botulinum toxin type A

The symbol C indicates the drug class.

Drugs in **bold type** marked with the symbol P are prototypes.

Drugs in blue type are closely related to the prototype.

Drugs in red type are significantly different from the prototype.

Drugs in black type with no symbol are also used in drug therapy; no prototype.

rugs used to manage muscle spasm and spasticity can be divided into two major therapeutic groups: skeletal muscle relaxants and **spasmolytics.** Skeletal muscle relaxants are used in combination with physical therapy and anti-inflammatory agents (see Chapter 24) to treat muscle spasms (involuntary contraction of a muscle from a peripheral musculoskeletal condition). Spasticity, an involuntary muscle contraction that is not coordinated with other muscles and is associated with upper motor neuron syndromes, is treated with physical therapy and drugs called spasmolytics. Spasmolytics are categorized as **centrally acting** or **peripherally acting.** As their names imply, these agents act in the brain or in the peripheral muscles.

This chapter discusses the centrally acting muscle relaxant cyclobenzaprine (Flexeril), the centrally acting spasmolytic baclofen (Lioresal), and the peripherally acting spasmolytic dantrolene sodium (Dantrium). Table 20.1 presents a summary of these drugs. In addition, this chapter addresses core drug knowledge, core patient variables, nursing management practices, potential nursing diagnoses, and patient education guidelines related to the use of these drugs. For discussion of physical methods for managing spasm and spasticity, refer to an appropriate medical-surgical textbook.

Ⓒ PHYSIOLOGY

The human body contains approximately 600 skeletal muscles. Skeletal muscle is voluntary, meaning a person can contract it at will. Seen under a microscope, skeletal muscle fibers show a pattern of cross-banding, which gives rise to its other name: striated muscle. The striations are caused by the alignment of bands, the most prominent of which are the A bands, I bands, and Z lines. The unit between two Z lines is called the sarcomere (Figure 20.1).

Striated muscle is composed of two contractile proteins: actin and myosin. The thin filaments are made of actin, which is attached to the Z lines and is found in both A bands and I bands. The thick filaments, found in A bands, are made of myosin. In the process set forth in the sliding filament theory, the sarcomere shortens, and the Z lines move closer together when muscle contracts. The filaments slide together because myosin attaches to, and pulls on, actin. The myosin head attaches to the actin filament, forming a crossbridge. After formation of the crossbridge, the myosin head bends, pulling on the actin filaments and causing them to slide. The result is that the Z lines move closer together, the I band becomes shorter, and the A band stays the same (see Figure 20.1). Muscle contraction is like climbing a rope. The crossbridge cycle is one of grabbing, pulling, and releasing, repeated over and over.

Muscle contraction is triggered by a sudden inflow of calcium ion (Ca^{2+}). In the resting state, the protein tropomyosin winds around actin and covers the myosin-binding sites. The Ca^{2+} binds to a second protein, troponin; this action causes the tropomyosin to be pulled to the side, exposing the myosin-binding sites. With the sites exposed, muscle contracts

in the presence of adenosine triphosphate (ATP). Muscle contraction stops when Ca^{2+} is removed from the immediate environment of the myofilaments.

PATHOPHYSIOLOGY

Muscle Spasm

A muscle **spasm** is a sudden violent involuntary contraction of a muscle or group of muscles resulting from an imbalance of excitatory and inhibitory input from descending motor pathways from the brain and spinal cord. Spasm is usually related to a localized skeletal muscle injury from acute trauma. Spasms may also stem from disorders such as hypocalcemia, hypokalemia or hyperkalemia, chronic pain syndromes, or epilepsy. Pain and interference with function attend muscle spasm, producing involuntary movement and distortion. When a muscle goes into spasm, it freezes in contraction and becomes a hard knotty mass, rather than normally contracting and relaxing in quick succession. During spasm, the blood vessels that normally feed the muscles and supply oxygen constrict, further compounding the problem.

Tonic spasm, or cramp, is characterized by an unusually prolonged and strong muscular contraction, with relaxation occurring slowly. In the other form of spasm, called **clonic** spasm, contractions of the affected muscles occur repeatedly, forcibly, and in quick succession, with equally sudden and frequent relaxations.

Spasticity

Spasticity is a motor disorder that comprises involuntary, velocity-dependent increased muscle tone that is associated with neurologic conditions or trauma to the central nervous system. This contraction causes stiffness or tightness of the muscles and may interfere with gait, movement, or speech. Damage to the portion of the brain or spinal cord that controls voluntary movement usually causes spasticity. Spasticity may be associated with spinal cord injury, multiple sclerosis (MS), cerebral palsy, anoxic brain damage such as a cerebrovascular accident (CVA), brain trauma, severe head injury, and some metabolic diseases, such as adrenoleukodystrophy and phenylketonuria. Symptoms may include hypertonicity (increased muscle tone), clonus (a series of rapid muscle contractions), exaggerated deep tendon reflexes, muscle spasms, scissoring (involuntary crossing of the legs), and fixed joints. The degree of spasticity varies from mild muscle stiffness to severe, painful, and uncontrollable muscle spasms. The condition can interfere with daily activities and with rehabilitation in patients with certain disorders. Goals for treating individuals with spasticity include improving functional activity and mobility, reducing the risk of avoidable complications such as pressure sores and orthopedic deformity, to allow stretching and strengthening of muscles, and alleviating pain.

TABLE 20.1 Summary of Selected Drugs That Affect Muscle Spasm and Spasticity

Drug (Trade) Name	Selected Indications	Route and Dosage Range	Pharmacokinetics
Ⓒ Centrally Acting Muscle Relaxants			
Ⓟ cyclobenzaprine (Flexeril)	Muscle spasms Muscle relaxation	*Adult:* PO, 10 mg tid; maximum 60 mg qid *Child <15 y:* not recommended	*Onset:* 1 h *Duration:* 12–24 h $t_{1/2}$: 8 h
carisoprodol (Soma)	Muscle spasms Muscle relaxation	*Adult:* PO, 350 mg qid *Child:* not recommended	*Onset:* 30 min *Duration:* 4–6 h $t_{1/2}$: 2h
chlorzoxazone (Parafon Forte DSC,)	Muscle spasms Muscle relaxation	*Adult:* PO, 250–500 mg tid/qid *Child:* PO, 20 mg/kg/d in divided doses	*Onset:* 30–60 min *Duration:* 3–4 h $t_{1/2}$: 60 min
metaxalone (Skelaxin)	Muscle spasms Muscle relaxation	*Adult and child >12 y:* PO, 800 mg tid–qid	*Onset:* 1 h *Duration:* 4–6 h $t_{1/2}$: 4–14h
methocarbamol (Robaxin)	Muscle spasms Muscle relaxation Tetanus	*Adult:* 1,500 mg qid; 1,000 mg qid for maintenance *Child:* not recommended *Adult:* IV, 2–4 g up to 3 g/d *Child:* not recommended	*Onset:* 30 min *Duration:* 8 h $t_{1/2}$: 1–2 h *Onset:* rapid *Duration:* unknown $t_{1/2}$: 1–2 h
orphenadrine (Norflex)	Muscle spasms Muscle relaxation	*Adult and child >12 y:* PO, 200–250 mg/d in divided doses; IV, 60 mg q 12 h *Child <12 y:* not recommended	*Onset:* 2–4h *Duration:* 4–6 h $t_{1/2}$: 14–20 h
Ⓒ Centrally Acting Spasmolytics			
Ⓟ baclofen (Lioresal;)	Spasticity	*Adult:* PO, 5–20 mg tid; Intrathecal, 5–25 mcg *Child:* not recommended	*Onset:* 2–3h *Duration:* 24–48 h $t_{1/2}$: 2–4 h
baclofen (Kemstro)		*Adult:* oral disintegrating tablet	
tizanidine (Zanaflex, *Canadian:* Apo-Tizanidine, Gen-Tizanidine)	Spasticity MS Muscle relaxation	*Adult:* 2–4 mg tid; maximum dose 36 mg/d *Child:* not recommended	*Onset:* 1 h *Duration:* 3–6 h $t_{1/2}$: 2.5 h
gabapentin (Neurontin, *Canadian:* Apo-Gabapentin, Gen-Gabapentin, Novo-Gabapentin, Nu-Gabapentin, BCI-Gabapentin)	Spasticity	*Adult:* PO, 600–1,200 mg/d in divided doses *Child:* not recommended	*Onset:* 30 min *Duration:* 8 h $t_{1/2}$: 5–7 h
Ⓒ Peripherally Acting Spasmolytics			
Ⓟ dantrolene (Dantrium)	Athetosis cerebral palsy, MS, hemiplegia, paraplegia, Parkinson disease, spasticity, CVA, spinal cord injury Prevention of malignant hyperthermia Malignant hyperthermia (adult and child) Post-crisis follow-up	*Adult:* PO, 25–100 mg 2–4 times qid *Child <5y:* not approved *Child >5y:* 0.5 mg/kg bid, maximum 100 mg qid IV: 2.5 mg/kg 1 h before surgery PO: 4–8 mg/kg in divided doses 1–2 d before surgery with last dose 3–4 h after surgery IV: 1 mg/kg PO: 4–8 mg/kg in four divided doses for 1–3 d	*Onset:* 4–7 h *Duration:* dose related $t_{1/2}$: 7–9 h
botulinum toxin type A (Botox)	Chronic spasticity	*Adult:* 1 m; extremely individualized	*Onset:* 3 d–2 wk *Duration:* 3 mo $t_{1/2}$: 10 h

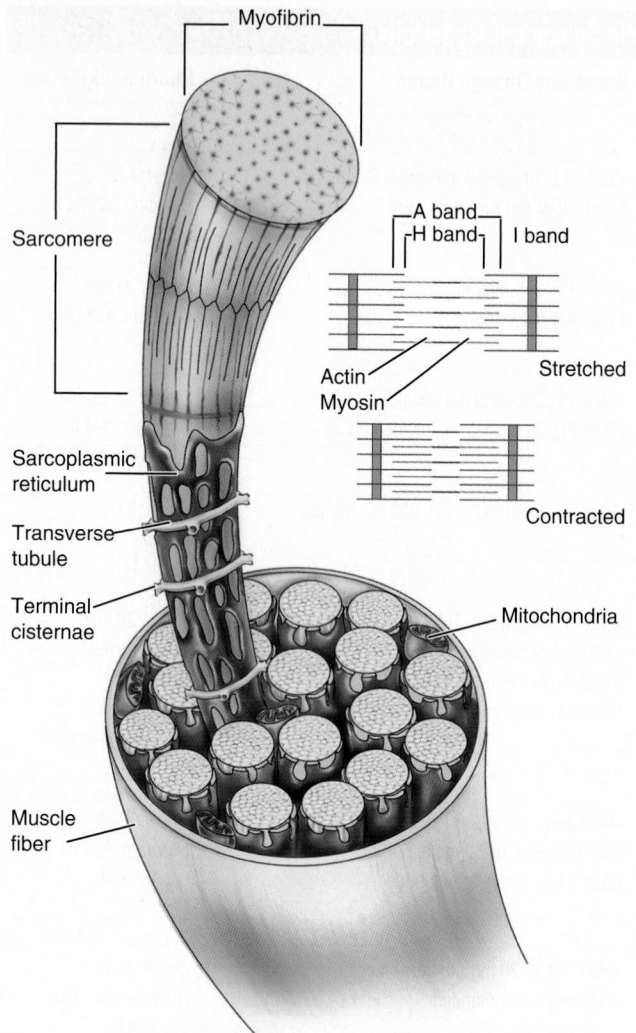

Myofibrin

Sarcomere

A band
H band
I band

Actin
Myosin

Stretched

Sarcoplasmic
reticulum

Transverse
tubule

Terminal
cisternae

Mitochondria

Contracted

Muscle
fiber

• FIGURE 20.1 When stimulation stops, calcium ions are actively transported back into the sarcoplasmic reticulum, resulting in decreased calcium ions in the sarcoplasm. The removal of calcium ions restores the inhibitory action of troponin-tropomyosin; crossbridge action is impossible in this state.

C CENTRALLY ACTING MUSCLE RELAXANTS

The centrally acting muscle relaxants are a group of drugs with similar pharmacologic properties. They act in the central nervous system (CNS). The prototype for centrally acting muscle relaxants is cyclobenzaprine (Flexeril), because evidence indicates that it is the most efficacious (Table 20.1). Diazepam (Valium), a benzodiazepine, is mentioned because it is used in managing both muscle spasms and spasticity. Benzodiazepines are discussed in depth in Chapter 15.

Nursing Management of the Patient Receiving P Cyclobenzaprine

Core Drug Knowledge

Pharmacotherapeutics

Cyclobenzaprine is used to manage muscle spasms associated with acute musculoskeletal disorders, such as low back strain, muscle tenderness, or movement restriction due to

musculoskeletal conditions. It is also used as supportive therapy in patients with tetanus or fibromyalgia.

Pharmacokinetics

Cyclobenzaprine is administered orally. It is well absorbed from the gastrointestinal (GI) tract and probably undergoes first-pass metabolism because plasma levels vary considerably among patients. Onset of skeletal muscle relaxation occurs in about 1 hour, and duration of action ranges from 12 to 24 hours. Optimal effects may take 1 to 2 days to fully develop. Cyclobenzaprine undergoes extensive metabolism and is excreted mainly as conjugated inactive metabolites in the urine and as unchanged drug through bile in the feces. Its half-life ranges from 1 to 3 days.

Pharmacodynamics

Cyclobenzaprine relieves muscle spasms through a central action, possibly at the level of the brain stem, with no direct action on the neuromuscular junction or the muscle involved. It reduces pain and tenderness and improves mobility. Because of its structural similarity to the tricyclic antidepressants (TCAs), cyclobenzaprine may reduce tonic somatic motor activity by influencing both alpha and gamma motor neurons. Cyclobenzaprine is ineffective for treating spasticity associated with cerebral or spinal cord disease or in children with cerebral palsy.

Contraindications and Precautions

Cyclobenzaprine is contraindicated for patients with hyperthyroidism because of a possible increased risk of arrhythmias or an exacerbation of tachycardia. Because of its similarity to the TCAs, cyclobenzaprine is also contraindicated for use within 14 days of administration of monoamine oxidase inhibitors (MAOIs).

In overdoses, TCAs cause conduction disturbances and have been associated with torsades de pointes (an atypical tachycardia) and death. Because it is closely related to the TCA amitriptyline, cyclobenzaprine should be used cautiously in patients with heart failure, cardiac arrhythmias, or atrioventricular block or other conduction disturbances, and in those who are in the acute recovery phase following myocardial infarction (MI).

Cyclobenzaprine possesses anticholinergic activity. Patients with increased intraocular pressure, angle-closure glaucoma, or urinary retention require careful monitoring. In addition, cyclobenzaprine should be used with caution in pregnant or breast-feeding women. Studies for determining safe use during pregnancy have not been performed.

Adverse Effects

The common adverse effects of cyclobenzaprine are related to its CNS depression and anticholinergic activity. The most common adverse effects are drowsiness, dizziness, and dry mouth. Other frequent adverse effects include fatigue, asthenia (loss of strength and energy), nausea and vomiting, constipation, dyspepsia, dysgeusia (unpleasant taste), blurred vision, headache, nervousness, and confusion.

TABLE 20.2	Agents That Interact with P Cyclobenzaprine	
Interactants	**Effect and Significance**	**Nursing Management**
CNS depressants • sedatives • tranquilizers • alcohol • opioids	Cyclobenzaprine, in combination with other CNS depressants, may induce additive effects, resulting in increased CNS depression.	Avoid this combination. Monitor for sedation and dizziness. Provide ambulatory assistance. Ensure patient's safety.
Tramadol	Cyclobenzaprine may react with tramadol, resulting in seizure activity.	Use of tramadol with cyclobenzaprine is not recommended. Monitor for seizure activity.
Guanethidine	Cyclobenzaprine may react with guanethidine, decreasing guanethidine's antihypertensive effect.	Use of guanethidine with cyclobenzaprine is not recommended. Monitor blood pressure. Discuss possible increased dosage of guanethidine with health care provider.
MAOIs	Although the mechanism of action is unknown, it is likely that concurrent administration of cyclobenzaprine and MAOIs enhances adrenergic activity, increasing the likelihood of oretic (hydrochlorothiazide) crisis, severe seizures, and death.	A minimum of 14 days should elapse between the discontinuance of MAOIs and the initiation of cyclobenzaprine therapy. Monitor for elevated temperature, confusion, or seizure activity.
Phytomedicinal herbs • Valerian • *Valeriana officinalis* • Kava kava • St. John's wort • gotu kola	Combination therapy can cause additive effects of sedation and dizziness, which can impair the patient's ability to undertake tasks that require mental alertness.	Monitor for sedation and dizziness. Provide ambulatory assistance. Ensure patient's safety. Dosage adjustments of either or both medications may be necessary.
Tricyclic antidepressants	Cyclobenzaprine is structurally similar to tricyclic antidepressants. When given concurrently, some of the more serious CNS reactions noted with the tricyclic antidepressants may occur.	Monitor for seizure activity. Monitor for arrhythmias.

Serious adverse effects, including arrhythmias, seizures, and MIs, can occur because of cyclobenzaprine's similarity to the TCAs.

Drug Interactions

Interactions between cyclobenzaprine and CNS depressants or antimuscarinic drugs may be extensive. Cyclobenzaprine may also interact with tramadol, guanethidine, MAOIs, histamine-1 blocking agents, and various herbal remedies. These interactions are highlighted in Table 20.2.

CRITICAL THINKING SCENARIO

CYCLOBENZAPRINE IN THE COLLEGE ENVIRONMENT

Katie C., a senior in college is seen at the student health center during finals week, complaining of severe neck spasms. Despite warm compresses and ibuprofen, the spasms have not resolved. She is prescribed cyclobenzaprine.

1. Given the college environment and lifestyle, what information would you include in your patient teaching session about this medication?

2. What in her medical history would be important to identify that could contraindicate being given this prescription?

Assessment of Relevant Core Patient Variables

Health Status

Assess the patient for a history of cyclobenzaprine hypersensitivity or pre-existing diseases such as hyperthyroidism, cardiac dysfunction, recent MI, urinary hesitation/retention, and glaucoma. Caution should be used in patients with mild hepatic impairment. Also, assess for use of medications that may interact with cyclobenzaprine, such as MAOIs. Communicate positive findings to the prescriber before administering the drug. Also, assess for over-the-counter (OTC) drugs used for allergies or hay fever, because these drugs usually have an anticholinergic effect, and additive effects occur when anticholinergic drugs are given concurrently with cyclobenzaprine.

Life Span and Gender

Assess older adult patients for the anticholinergic and CNS depressant effects of cyclobenzaprine, as susceptibility increases with increased age. Safety and efficacy have not been established in patients less than 15 years old.

In addition, it is important to evaluate the female patient's pregnancy and lactation status. Safety during pregnancy has not been documented, although cyclobenzaprine is a pregnancy category B drug. Distribution of the drug into breast milk has not been established, but TCAs are found in breast milk. Because of its structural similarity to the TCAs, cyclobenzaprine may also distribute into breast milk.

Lifestyle, Diet, and Habits

Assess for use of alcohol or any other CNS depressant, which increases the sedating effects of cyclobenzaprine. Advise the patient to assess the depth of sedation related to cyclobenzaprine use before driving a vehicle or attempting activities that require mental alertness or motor coordination. Long-term use of cyclobenzaprine may result in physical dependence. Assess for potential abuse of this drug.

Environment

Cyclobenzaprine may be administered in any environment, but it is most often given on an outpatient basis. Because it can cause sedation, discuss with the patient possible hazards in the home environment.

Nursing Diagnosis and Outcome

• Risk for Injury related to CNS depressant effects and potential cardiovascular effects.
  Desired outcome: *The patient will remain free from injury throughout therapy.*

Planning and Intervention

Maximizing Therapeutic Effects

Have the patient take cyclobenzaprine with a full glass of water at evenly spaced intervals. Coordinate physical modalities such as physical therapy, whirlpool, and cold or hot compresses to the affected area.

Minimizing Adverse Effects

While the patient is hospitalized, ensure the patient's safety by keeping the bed in the lowest position with the side rails up. Accompany the patient during ambulation until the degree of sedation is ascertained. Also, caution the patient about the potential for orthostatic hypotension resulting in dizziness and teach the patient to change positions slowly. Finally, remind the patient of the potential for synergistic effects when cyclobenzaprine is taken with other CNS depressants, especially alcohol. Because cyclobenzaprine can cause physical dependence with long-term use, slowly withdrawing the drug over 1 to 2 weeks is important to prevent abstinence syndrome (see Chapter 9).

Providing Patient and Family Education

• Instruct patients to take cyclobenzaprine exactly as prescribed. If patients miss a dose, they should take it as soon as they remember but should never double the dose.
• Explain that adverse effects such as mild drowsiness, dizziness, or clumsiness may accompany cyclobenzaprine therapy. Although these symptoms will often improve with time, patients must refrain from driving or performing hazardous tasks until their level of sedation is ascertained. Advise patients to contact the prescriber if sedation persists or is bothersome. Also, emphasize the

MEMORY CHIP

P Cyclobenzaprine

• Centrally acting muscle relaxant is used for muscle spasms; ineffective for spasticity
• Most common adverse effect: sedation; safety is a nursing priority
• Most serious adverse effects: occur with abrupt withdrawal and include agitation, auditory or visual hallucinations, seizures, or psychotic symptoms
• **Life span alert: Older adult patients are more prone to sedation and anticholinergic effects.**
• Maximizing therapeutic effects: Take medication exactly as prescribed.
• Minimizing adverse effects: Avoid use of other CNS depressants.
• Most important patient education: Never abruptly stop medication; withdraw medication over a 2-week period.

need to refrain from alcohol, which may exacerbate these adverse effects.
• Advise patients to contact the prescriber immediately if they experience severe headache, confusion, hallucinations, or sudden or increased weakness. Female patients should contact the prescriber immediately if they suspect they may be pregnant.
• Instruct patients to avoid using any OTC or prescription drugs without first consulting the prescriber. Many of these drugs can cause dangerous adverse effects when taken with cyclobenzaprine.
• Finally, instruct patients never to abruptly cease cyclobenzaprine if therapy has been with high doses or over a prolonged period; rather, they should decrease the dosage gradually over 2 weeks.

Ongoing Assessment and Evaluation

Constantly evaluate the patient's safety. Monitor the level of sedation and report to the prescriber if it is severe. In addition to CNS symptoms, monitor for GI symptoms, such as gastric distress or constipation. Provide analgesics for headache, offer small and frequent meals to decrease GI upset, and establish a bowel program if constipation becomes a problem. Successful cyclobenzaprine therapy is marked by decreased muscle spasms and no injury to the patient related to adverse effects.

Drugs Closely Related to P Cyclobenzaprine

Drugs that are similar to cyclobenzaprine include carisoprodol, chlorzoxazone, metaxalone, methocarbamol, and orphenadrine. Like cyclobenzaprine, they all work by affecting the CNS rather than the muscle itself. Thus, patient safety is a priority with all of these drugs.

Carisoprodol

Carisoprodol (Soma) is given orally. Although carisoprodol is itself a nonscheduled drug, it can be very addictive because it is metabolized into meprobamate, a Schedule IV controlled substance. Tolerance and physical dependence may occur with prolonged use; therefore limit use to 2 to 3 weeks. Significant adverse effects include hypomania at higher than recommended doses, withdrawal syndrome, and hypersensitivity. Patients taking carisoprodol may also experience an idiosyncratic reaction inducing weakness, visual or motor disturbances, confusion, or euphoria. Hypersensitivity or idiosyncratic reactions generally occur within administration of the first four doses. Two factors have led to the diminished use of carisoprodol: its ability to produce dependence and the availability of newer agents.

Chlorzoxazone

Chlorzoxazone (Paraflex, Parafon Forte) has been used for many years. It is metabolized in the liver; therefore, it should be used with caution in patients with hepatic disease, because it may cause hepatotoxicity ranging from a mild elevation in hepatic enzymes to hepatic necrosis. In addition, a metabolite of chlorzoxazone is rapidly excreted in the urine, and the drug should be used with caution in patients with renal impairment because it may alter excretion and possibly cause toxicity. Chlorzoxazone requires multiple daily doses and is more expensive than cyclobenzaprine.

Metaxalone

Metaxalone (Skelaxin) is another oral muscle relaxant. It produces less sedation than cyclobenzaprine but requires 4 times a day dosing and is more expensive. Metaxalone is contraindicated in patients with severe renal and hepatic impairment. Before administration, baseline renal and hepatic function should be evaluated, especially if the patient will have long-term therapy. Periodic liver function tests (LFTs) should be performed throughout therapy.

Patients taking metaxalone may experience paradoxical muscle cramps or a mild withdrawal syndrome if the drug is discontinued abruptly.

Methocarbamol

Methocarbamol (Robaxin) may be administered by oral, intramuscular (IM), and intravenous (IV) routes. In addition to its use for muscle spasm, methocarbamol is used in managing tetanus. Methocarbamol may cause brown, brown-black, or green urine. Like chlorzoxazone, it causes less sedation than cyclobenzaprine. Contraindications to methocarbamol include hepatic or renal disorders, age younger than 12 years or older than 60 years, and pregnancy. It is used with caution in patients with seizure disorders because it may exacerbate seizure activity.

When methocarbamol is given intravenously, the rate should not exceed 300 mg/min (3 mL of 10% injection). Because the solution is hypertonic, extravasation may occur, resulting in thrombophlebitis, sloughing, and pain at the injection site.

Orphenadrine

Orphenadrine (Norflex) is another centrally acting muscle relaxant. Administration is oral or parenteral. In addition to having CNS effects similar to those of other centrally acting skeletal muscle relaxants, orphenadrine may induce, although rarely, aplastic anemia or anaphylactic reaction. When given intravenously, it should not be diluted and should be given slowly over 5 minutes.

Orphenadrine should be used with caution in conditions that are affected by its anticholinergic and antihistaminic effects, which include bladder obstruction, prostatic hypertrophy, GI obstruction, peptic ulcer disease, gastroesophageal reflux disease, asthma, glaucoma, and myasthenia gravis. Orphenadrine should also be used with caution in older patients who do not tolerate anticholinergics well. Additionally, caution should be taken when administering to patients with cardiac insufficiency or thyrotoxicosis. The safety of orphenadrine in children or pregnant or breast-feeding women has not been established.

Orphenadrine interacts with haloperidol, worsening schizophrenic symptoms and possibly contributing to the development of tardive dyskinesia. It also interacts with amantadine, with resultant additive anticholinergic effects. Orphenadrine decreases the action of phenothiazines when given concurrently.

Drug Significantly Different From P Cyclobenzaprine

Diazepam (Valium) is a benzodiazepine that can produce any level of CNS depression required, including sedation, hypnosis, skeletal muscle relaxation, antiepileptic activity, or coma. Diazepam and baclofen are the only two centrally acting drugs that are used for spasticity as well as muscle spasm. Although diazepam is an extremely effective muscle relaxant, its use as a maintenance drug for spasms is limited because of its potential for physical and psychological dependence. Additionally, withdrawing diazepam abruptly may induce seizure activity. For further information on benzodiazepines, see Chapter 15.

C CENTRALLY ACTING SPASMOLYTICS

The centrally acting spasmolytics work in the CNS to reduce excessive reflex activity and to allow muscle relaxation. They are used to alleviate musculoskeletal pain and spasms and reduce spasticity in a variety of neurologic disorders. The prototype for the centrally acting spasmolytics is baclofen (Lioresal), which is very effective and inexpensive.

Nursing Management of the Patient Receiving P Baclofen
Core Drug Knowledge
Pharmacotherapeutics
Baclofen relieves some components of spinal spasticity—involuntary flexor and extensor spasms and resistance to passive movements. It is useful in the treatment of spasticity and myoclonus resulting from disorders such as MS,

cerebral palsy, and traumatic injury to the spinal cord. Baclofen is not useful in treating spasms that follow a CVA, or those that occur in Parkinson disease or Huntington chorea. Surgically implanted pumps are used to deliver intrathecal baclofen to patients who have long-term needs or poor control with oral medications. Baclofen has been used in patients with focal dystonic movements, including torticollis (wry neck). It has been used with some success in Meige syndrome (blepharospasm-oromandibular dystonia) and stiff-man syndrome, also known as Moersch-Woltmann syndrome. Stiff-man syndrome occurs primarily in men. It is characterized by muscular rigidity accompanied by paroxysmal painful spasms precipitated by physical or emotional stimuli.

Baclofen has been effective in treating intractable hiccups. It may also be used to manage trigeminal neuralgia and various types of neuropathic pain, including migraine headaches. Neuropathic cancer pain also responds to baclofen therapy.

Pharmacokinetics

Baclofen may be administered orally or intrathecally. It is absolutely contraindicated for intravenous, intramuscular, subcutaneous, or epidural administration. When administered orally, baclofen is rapidly absorbed with peak blood concentrations seen in 2 to 3 hours. It is distributed throughout the body and minimally crosses the blood–brain barrier. Baclofen also crosses the placenta and passes into breast milk. Serum half-life ranges from 2 to 4 hours. The kidneys excrete 70% to 85% of a dose as unchanged drug and active and inactive metabolites. The liver metabolizes the remainder, which is excreted through the feces. Hemodialysis and hemoperfusion have successfully eliminated baclofen from the blood in cases of drug-induced intoxication.

When introduced into the intrathecal space, effective CSF concentrations are reached with plasma concentrations 100 times less than seen following oral administration of baclofen. Though there is considerable interpatient variability, onset of action following intrathecal administration occurs within 1 hour, with peak antispasmodic effect seen at 4 hours. Intrathecal baclofen is cleared by CSF uptake in the CNS.

Pharmacodynamics

Baclofen is a derivative of the inhibitory neurotransmitter gamma-aminobutyric acid (GABA) and acts specifically at the spinal end of the upper motor neurons at $GABA_B$ receptors to inhibit transmission of impulses and cause hyperpolarization. This action reduces excessive reflex activity underlying muscle hypertonia, spasms, and spasticity and allows muscle relaxation. The mechanism of action explains why baclofen is not used for spasticity resulting from CVA or Parkinson disease, because these disorders involve lesional or functional impairment of basal ganglia coordination, in an area of the CNS above the spinal motor neurons.

Contraindications and Precautions

Baclofen is contraindicated in anyone who has demonstrated previous hypersensitivity to it. It is also contraindicated for spasticity of cerebral origin or for reducing the rigidity of parkinsonism or Huntington chorea because it is ineffective in these disorders.

Abrupt discontinuation of baclofen should be avoided, as it may result in severe side effects. Gradual reduction of dosage is recommended. Abrupt withdrawal from oral baclofen may induce confusion, seizures, exacerbation of severe spasticity, hallucinations, and other psychiatric disorders. Abrupt discontinuation of intrathecal baclofen may result in high fevers, hypotension, dysphoria, altered mental status, seizures, rebound spasticity, and muscle rigidity that may advance to rhabdomyolysis, disseminated intravascular coagulation, multi-system organ failure, and death. Withdrawal from intrathecal baclofen may mimic sepsis, autonomic dysreflexia, serotonin syndrome, neuroleptic malignant syndrome, status epilepticus, and toxic or metabolic disorders.

Baclofen is used with caution in patients who have seizure disorders. It has caused deterioration in seizure control and electroencephalographic changes in patients with epilepsy. When given to patients with CNS disorders, such as cerebral hemorrhage or a prior CVA, baclofen may increase the risk for developing CNS, respiratory, or cardiovascular depression and ataxia. Baclofen can increase blood glucose concentrations and should therefore be used cautiously in patients with diabetes mellitus. Patients with pre-existing psychiatric disorders are more likely to develop baclofen-induced psychiatric disturbances. Baclofen should also be used with caution in patients who have renal impairment, because most of the drug is excreted unchanged in the urine.

Baclofen is classified as a pregnancy category C drug and should be used during pregnancy only when the benefits to the pregnant woman outweigh the risks to the fetus. Baclofen appears in small amounts in breast milk; therefore, caution should be used in administering it to breast-feeding women. Baclofen has not been approved for use in children younger than 12 years.

Adverse Effects

The most common adverse effects of baclofen therapy include drowsiness, weakness, dizziness and lightheadedness, headache, nausea and vomiting, hypotension, constipation, lethargy and fatigue, confusion, insomnia, and increased urinary frequency. Other effects in the CNS include euphoria, excitement, depression, and hallucinations. Baclofen may also cause paresthesias, myalgias, or tinnitus. The patient may experience difficulty with coordination, tremors, rigidity, or ataxia. The patient may also experience vision disturbances such as nystagmus, strabismus, miosis, mydriasis, or diplopia. Adverse effects in the GI system include xerostomia, anorexia, dysgeusia, abdominal pain, and diarrhea. Cardiovascular adverse effects, such

TABLE 20.3	Agents That Interact with P Baclofen	
Interactants	**Effect and Significance**	**Nursing Management**
CNS depressants • alcohol • benzodiazepines • barbiturates • opioids	In combination with dantrolene, CNS depressant drugs may have additive effects, increasing CNS depression.	Monitor for increased sedation. Institute safety measures, especially with ambulation.
Nonsteroidal antiinflammatory agents	Baclofen may decrease the clearance of NSAIDs and increase the potential for renal toxicity.	Monitor fluid intake and output.
Phytomedicinals • *Valeriana officinalis* • kava kava • St. John's wort • gotu kola	In combination with dantrolene, phytomedicinals may have additive effects, increasing CNS depression.	Monitor for increased sedation. Institute safety measures, especially with ambulation.
Tricyclic antidepressants	Baclofen and TCAs can potentiate muscle relaxation and enhance anticholinergic effects. This combination may result in severe weakness, memory loss, and loss of muscle tone.	Monitor for adverse effects. Provide ambulatory assistance. Increase fluids or consume sugarless candies for dry mouth. Monitor for urinary retention or constipation.

as palpitations, angina, excessive diaphoresis, and syncope, are possible. Genitourinary (GU) effects may include urinary incontinence or retention, dysuria, erectile dysfunction, ejaculation dysfunction, and nocturia. Integumentary adverse effects may include rash and pruritus.

Drug Interactions

Teach the patient that baclofen may impair his/her ability to perform tasks that require mental alertness or physical coordination. CNS depression may occur when baclofen is administered concurrently with other CNS depressants. Concurrent use with monoamine oxidase inhibitors may increase CNS depression and cause hypotension. Concomitant use of baclofen with other antihypertensive agents may result in hypotension. Baclofen has also been reported to cause false-positive results on tests for occult blood in the stool. Additionally, baclofen may induce elevations in levels of aspartate aminotransferase (AST), alkaline phosphatase, or serum glucose (Table 20.3).

Assessment of Relevant Core Patient Variables

Health Status

Assess for a history of baclofen hypersensitivity or preexisting disorders that contraindicate the use of baclofen. Also assess for muscle spasms and their causes. Baclofen therapy does not affect skeletal muscle spasms resulting from CVA or parkinsonism.

Perform a physical examination that includes baseline assessments of neurologic function, cardiac function, kidney function, and muscle strength and spasticity. Laboratory assessments should include baseline liver and kidney function values and blood glucose level.

Life Span and Gender

Older patients are more susceptible to baclofen-induced sedation and psychiatric disturbances, including hallucinations, excitation, and confusion. Therefore, continually assess older patients taking baclofen for such adverse effects. Evaluate the patient for pregnancy. Baclofen may be used during pregnancy when the benefits to the pregnant woman outweigh the risks to the fetus. Baclofen should not be used in children younger than 12 years.

Lifestyle, Diet, and Habits

Caution the patient about the concurrent use of alcohol and baclofen. Alcohol may increase the risk for CNS depression and other CNS adverse effects. Also, caution patients to assess their level of alertness (which may be affected by CNS depression) before attempting to drive, use machinery, or perform activities that require concentration.

Environment

Oral baclofen can be given in any environment and is generally self-administered in the home. Intrathecal baclofen administration requires a surgical procedure to implant the device. The prescriber refills the reservoir every 4 to 12 weeks, depending on the daily dose.

Nursing Diagnoses and Outcomes

• Acute Pain related to headache, muscle pain, GI disturbances, or rash
  Desired outcome: *The patient will be provided with measures to decrease the discomfort of drug therapy and the possibility of nonadherence.*

- Risk for Disturbed Sensory Perception related to visual changes, vestibular dysfunction, and somatosensory changes
Desired outcome: *The patient will be protected from injury if dizziness, weakness, visual changes, or perceptual changes occur.*

Planning and Intervention

Maximizing Therapeutic Effects

Have the patient take baclofen with a full glass of water at evenly spaced intervals. For the patient with GI distress, coordinate small, frequent meals.

Minimizing Adverse Effects

Ensure the patient's safety by keeping the bed in the lowest position with the side rails up. Assist ambulatory patients with locomotion because sedation and muscle weakness may increase. Advise the patient to change positions slowly to prevent dizziness. Remind the patient to assess his or her sedation level prior to driving or performing tasks that require concentration.

Providing Patient and Family Education

- Education for patients receiving baclofen is similar to that for patients receiving cyclobenzaprine. As with cyclobenzaprine, caution patients to avoid sudden cessation of the drug; instead, patients should taper doses of the drug over 2 weeks.
- Emphasize the importance of safety related to sedation. Be sure patients understand to avoid any activity that requires concentration, especially driving, until their level of sedation is established.
- Remind patients to refrain from alcohol or any other CNS depressant agents.
- Advise patients that it may take up to 1 month to experience the full benefit of baclofen therapy.
- Advise patients of the importance of contacting the prescriber should they experience severe headaches, confusion, hallucinations, or sudden or increased weakness. Advise all female patients to contact the prescriber immediately if they become pregnant.
- Instruct patients with diabetes to use capillary blood glucose monitoring because baclofen may cause blood and urine glucose levels to rise. These patients should notify their prescribers if serum glucose level elevations persist.
- For patients receiving intrathecal baclofen, teach the patient and family aseptic technique and how to assess the integrity of the catheter and infusion system.

Ongoing Assessment and Evaluation

To ensure safety, assess the patient for the CNS effects of baclofen throughout therapy. Monitor for the emergence of hallucinations or psychotic episodes and consult with the prescriber immediately about the possibility of reducing the dose or discontinuing the drug. Also, monitor the patient

MEMORY CHIP

P Baclofen

- Centrally acting spasmolytic is used for muscle spasms or spasticity
- Major contraindication: patients who use spasticity to maintain posture or balance
- Most common adverse effect: sedation; safety is a nursing priority
- Most serious adverse effects: occur with abrupt withdrawal and include agitation, auditory or visual hallucinations, seizures, or psychotic symptoms
- **Life span alert: Older patients are more prone to sedation and other effects on the central nervous system.**
- Maximizing therapeutic effects: Administer at evenly spaced intervals.
- Minimizing adverse effects: Assist in changing positions slowly; withdraw medication over a 2-week period.
- Most important patient education: Never abruptly stop medication.

for integumentary, GI, or GU system complaints. Suggest approaches for dealing with minor symptoms, such as analgesics for headache or small, frequent meals for GI upset. Help establish a bowel program if constipation occurs. For GU effects such as erectile dysfunction, refer the patient to the prescriber and ensure that the patient does not abruptly stop the medication.

Therapeutic monitoring during baclofen therapy will show improvement in symptoms of spasticity and a decrease in resistance to passive movement of limb joints.

Drug Closely Related to **P** Baclofen

Tizanidine (Zanaflex) is an oral agent used to reduce muscle tone and treat spasticity related to cerebral or spinal cord pathology and MS. It is structurally and pharmacologically similar to clonidine and other alpha-2 adrenergic agonists and works at both the spinal and supraspinal levels. Although tizanidine and baclofen are equally effective in treating spasticity, tizanidine is much more expensive. Tizanidine also is effective in reducing the perception of neuropathic, trigeminal, and musculoskeletal pain by regulating central afferent nociceptive signals.

Tizanidine is used cautiously in patients with hypotension, hepatic disease, psychosis, or renal impairment. An important potentiating interaction with tizanidine occurs with oral contraceptives, fluvoxamine, and ciprofloxacin because they are CYP1A2 inhibitors. Tizanidine also has additive effects when given with other antihypertensive agents, alpha-2 agonists, or ethanol. Adverse effects parallel those of other alpha-2 adrenergic agonists, including dry mouth, drowsiness, dizziness, GI disturbances, and liver function abnormalities. Because of its adrenergic action, hypotension and orthostatic hypotension may also occur. Bradycardia may also be seen as well as prolongation of the QT interval on the ECG. Tizanidine produces greater drowsiness and sedation than baclofen but is not associated with the muscle weakness that may occur with baclofen therapy. Slow upward titration of the dose can minimize adverse effects. Patients on long-term therapy should have baseline LFTs performed prior to starting therapy and repeated at 3 and 6 months, and then periodically thereafter.

Drug Significantly Different From P Baclofen

Gabapentin (Neurontin) is a miscellaneous antiepileptic drug that has demonstrated efficacy in the management of neuropathic pain and spasticity. It is useful in managing spasticity associated with MS; this is an off-label indication. It may also be used to treat neuropathic pain associated with postherpetic neuralgia and peripheral diabetic neuropathy. Although its exact mechanism of action is not known, it is thought to interact with voltage-gated calcium channels to decrease pain and spasticity. Gabapentin is orally administered and rapidly absorbed. It is highly lipid soluble, crosses the blood–brain barrier, and is widely distributed in the CNS. Gabapentin is not metabolized and is excreted unchanged in the urine; therefore, monitoring renal function is important. Gabapentin is unusual in that it does not interact with other drugs and does not alter the serum concentrations of other anticonvulsants. Common adverse effects include drowsiness, somnolence, blurred vision, nausea, and fatigue. For additional information regarding gabapentin, see Chapter 18.

C PERIPHERALLY ACTING SPASMOLYTICS

Peripherally acting spasmolytics relax muscles through direct action on the skeletal muscle fibers. They neither interfere with neuromuscular communication nor have CNS effects. Dantrolene (Dantrium) is the most frequently used peripheral agent and the prototype for the peripherally acting spasmolytics

Nursing Management of the Patient Receiving P Dantrolene

Core Drug Knowledge

Pharmacotherapeutics

Dantrolene is an oral and intravenous skeletal muscle relaxant. IV dantrolene is the drug of choice, when accompanied by supportive measures, for acute treatment of malignant hyperthermia, a life-threatening complication of general anesthesia (Box 20.1). Preoperatively, it can be used orally or intravenously to prevent malignant hyperthermia in patients considered at risk.

Dantrolene has several other pharmacotherapeutic uses. It has been used for the treatment of neuroleptic malignant syndrome, though the response to dantrolene in this

COMMUNITY BASED CONCERNS

Dantrolene Therapy and Malignant Hyperthermia

Malignant hyperthermia (MH) is a rare myopathy that is characterized by an acute hypermetabolic state within muscle tissue. It is an autosomal dominant inherited disorder with an incidence of approximately 1:15,000 pediatric patients and 1:40,000 adults. MH is triggered by certain drugs used during general anesthesia and presents with signs including masseter muscle rigidity, tachycardia, hypercarbia due to increased body metabolism, and fever that may exceed 110° F. Severe complications of MH include cardiac arrest, brain damage, internal bleeding, and organ failure. Death can result from these complications.

In order to achieve a successful outcome, an MH crisis must be promptly identified and treated early in the course of the crisis. Treatment strategies aim to terminate the episode and treat complications such as acidosis and hyperkalemia. Intravenous dantrolene is the mainstay of therapy for an MH crisis. Dantrolene directly interferes with muscle contraction by binding the RYR1 receptor calcium channel and inhibiting calcium release from the sarcoplasmic reticulum. The dose of dantrolene administered for an MH crisis is 2.5 mg/kg repeated every 5 minutes until the episode is terminated, up to 10 mg/kg.

Dantrolene may also be given prophylactically to prevent an MH episode in the perioperative period. However, this is not generally recommended as it may worsen muscle weakness in a patient that is already susceptible to muscular disease. Providing a non-triggering anesthetic to patients with a personal or family history of MH is key in prevention of an MH crisis.

The perioperative nurse can assist in preventing an MH episode by obtaining a detailed personal and family history from the patient, inquiring about adverse reactions to anesthesia. Any suspicious findings during the detailed history should be immediately communicated to the rest of the perioperative team including the surgeon and the anesthesia care team. Additionally, the perioperative nurse must be knowledgeable about the protocol for treatment of an acute MH crisis as he or she will frequently be called upon to assist in the treatment of this life-threatening crisis.

---

condition is not always successful. It has been effective in treating upper motor neuron disorders, such as hereditary spastic paraplegia. It has also been used to treat heatstroke and to prevent and treat the rigors associated with amphotericin B. It is useful in managing spasticity resulting from spinal cord and cerebral injuries, MS, cerebral palsy, and possibly CVA. Dantrolene is not effective in treating acute muscle weakness of local origin or muscle weakness resulting from rheumatoid spondylitis, arthritis, or bursitis. Dantrolene use has found favor in the neurologic intensive care unit as an agent to provide neuroprotection by inhibiting serotonin-induced vasoconstriction. This effect is favorable in cerebral vasoconstriction syndromes such as vasospasm after subarachnoid hemorrhage or trauma.

Pharmacokinetics

Approximately 35% of an oral dose of dantrolene is absorbed; peak plasma concentrations are reached in approximately 5 hours. The liver metabolizes dantrolene to weakly active metabolites which are excreted in the urine. The elimination half-life is reported to be about 9 hours in healthy adults and 7.3 hours in children. Therapeutic effects in patients being treated for upper motor neuron disorders may not appear for 1 week or more. Dantrolene crosses the placenta and enters breast milk.

Pharmacodynamics

Dantrolene's mechanism of action differs from that of other oral skeletal muscle relaxants. Dantrolene reduces the force of contraction of skeletal muscle inhibiting the RYR receptor, which in turn reduces the amount of Ca^{2+} released from the sarcoplasmic reticulum, thereby uncoupling (relaxing) muscle contraction from excitation. Interference with the release of Ca^{2+} from the sarcoplasmic reticulum may prevent the increase in intracellular Ca^{2+}, which activates the acute catabolic events of malignant hyperthermia. Dantrolene has little or no effect on contraction of cardiac or intestinal smooth muscle. It may decrease hyperreflexia, muscle stiffness, and spasticity in patients with upper motor neuron disorders.

Contraindications and Precautions

Dantrolene is contraindicated in patients with active liver disease because of its associated liver toxicity. Dantrolene causes weakness because of its generalized reduction of muscle contraction. Thus, it is given very cautiously in patients who rely on spasticity to maintain an upright posture and balance, such as patients with cerebral palsy. Additionally, each vial of IV dantrolene contains 3 g of mannitol. Therefore, IV dantrolene may be inappropriate for patients with mannitol hypersensitivity.

No contraindications apply to IV administration of dantrolene to prevent or acutely treat malignant hyperthermia crisis in the perioperative period. Dantrolene should be used with caution in patients with pre-existing myopathy or neuromuscular disease with respiratory depression. The risk of perioperative complications is increased in patients with these conditions who receive dantrolene for prevention of malignant hyperthermia.

Dantrolene should also be used with caution in patients with cardiac disease and pulmonary dysfunction, particularly chronic obstructive pulmonary disease. For patients with cardiac disease, dantrolene can precipitate pleural effusions or pericarditis. In patients with pulmonary dysfunction, dantrolene can precipitate respiratory depression. Dantrolene is classified as a pregnancy category C drug; therefore, pregnant or lactating women should avoid its use.

Adverse Effects

The most common adverse effect of dantrolene therapy is muscle weakness. Manifestations of such muscle weakness may include drooling, dysphagia, slurred speech, drowsiness, dizziness, malaise, and fatigue. Serious adverse effects seen with dantrolene therapy include potentially fatal hepatitis, seizures, and pleural effusion with pericarditis. There are also rare reports of pulmonary edema following IV dantrolene administrations in which the diluent volume and mannitol needed to deliver the dantrolene may be the contributing factor.

In the GI system, symptoms include diarrhea, constipation, GI bleeding, anorexia, difficulty swallowing, abdominal cramps, and nausea and vomiting. Diarrhea is usually dose-dependent and transient, but in some cases it can be severe, and the drug may have to be withheld. Hematologic adverse reactions with dantrolene therapy include aplastic anemia, leukopenia, and lymphocytic lymphoma.

Rash, acne, abnormal hair growth, and photosensitivity are possible integumentary effects. IV dantrolene may cause edema and thrombophlebitis. Rarely, IV administration may cause erythema and urticaria.

Drug Interactions

Because dantrolene is metabolized by the liver, it is possible that metabolism may be enhanced by drugs that are known to induce hepatic enzymes. Drugs that interact with dantrolene include CNS depressants, clofibrate, estrogens, verapamil, methotrexate, and warfarin. Table 20.4 discusses these potential interactions.

Assessment of Relevant Core Patient Variables
Health Status

Elicit a comprehensive health history, including any history of active hepatitis, estrogen use in women older than 35 years, impaired cardiac or pulmonary function, any liver disease, or spasticity used to sustain upright posture and balance in locomotion or to obtain or maintain increased function. Communicate positive findings for any of these factors to the prescriber.

Perform a physical examination before initiating therapy. Assessment of the musculoskeletal system should include the patient's posture, ability to walk, reflexes, and muscle tone. Document the amount and location of spasticity. Other assessments should include the CNS and GI systems. Laboratory tests should include a complete blood count (CBC) and AST, alanine aminotransferase, alkaline phosphatase, and total bilirubin levels.

Life Span and Gender

Consider the patient's age relative to dantrolene therapy. Hepatotoxicity occurs most commonly in patients older than 30 years of age, especially women older than age 35 who are taking estrogens. It generally occurs 3 to 12 months after starting dantrolene therapy. Children younger than 5 years should not receive dantrolene. Older patients are more vulnerable to the adverse effects of dantrolene. Before giving dantrolene, assess the patient for pregnancy and breast-feeding, because the safety of dantrolene therapy has not been established for pregnant or lactating women.

TABLE 20.4 Agents That Interact with ℗ Dantrolene

Interactants	Effect and Significance	Nursing Management
Calcium channel blockers • diltiazem • verapamil	In combination with dantrolene, calcium channel blockers may increase hyperkalemia and myocardial depression.	Avoid coadministration, if possible. Monitor cardiac function. Monitor potassium levels.
Clindamycin	In combination with dantrolene, clindamycin may increase neuromuscular blockade.	Monitor for increased effects of dantrolene.
Clofibrate	Clofibrate may decrease plasma protein binding of dantrolene, resulting in decreased effects of dantrolene.	Monitor for efficacy of dantrolene therapy.
CNS depressant drugs • alcohol • benzodiazepines • barbiturates • opioids	In combination with dantrolene, CNS depressant drugs may have additive effects, increasing CNS depression.	Monitor for increased sedation. Institute safety measures, especially with ambulation.
Estrogens	Mechanism of interaction is unknown; women older than 35 y are at risk for hepatotoxicity when estrogens and dantrolene are coadministered.	Monitor for signs of hepatotoxicity. Coordinate periodic liver function tests for long-term therapy.
Nondepolarizing Neuromuscular blocking drugs • Rocuronium • Vecuronium • Cisatracurium • Pancuronium	Nondepolarizing neuromuscular blocking drugs are potentiated by dantrolene	Monitor for signs of neuromuscular weakness or incomplete reversal of blockade following general anesthesia. Signs may include respiratory impairment and muscle weakness
Phytomedicinals • *Valeriana officinalis* • kava kava • *Piper methysticum* • gotu kola	In combination with dantrolene, phytomedicinals may have additive effects, increasing CNS depression.	Monitor for increased sedation. Institute safety measures, especially with ambulation.
Psychotropic drugs • MAOIs • phenothiazines	In combination with dantrolene, psychotropic drugs may increase neuromuscular blockade.	Monitor for increased effects of dantrolene.
Methotrexate	The combination of dantrolene and methotrexate may increase methotrexate concentrations. Clearance of methotrexate is impaired by dantrolene or its metabolite 5-hydroxydantrolene	Monitor for increased effects of methotrexate.
warfarin	Warfarin may decrease plasma protein binding of dantrolene, resulting in decreased effects of dantrolene.	Monitor for efficacy of dantrolene therapy.

Lifestyle, Diet, and Habits

Dantrolene capsules contain lactulose. Therefore, assess the patient for lactose intolerance before the drug is given. Assess for alcohol consumption because alcohol increases the sedative properties of dantrolene.

Environment

Caution the patient about the potential for photosensitivity and advise wearing appropriate clothing and sunscreen whenever in direct sunlight. Because dantrolene causes muscle weakness, also discuss with the patient any barriers in the home (such as stairs) that may be affected by dantrolene therapy. In addition, caution the patient to assess the drug's effects before attempting to ambulate without assistance.

Nursing Diagnoses and Outcomes

• Risk for Injury related to muscular weakness
  Desired outcome: *The patient will be injury free despite muscular weakness.*

FOCUS ON RESEARCH

Potential Abuse of Muscle Relaxants

Owens, C., Pagmire, B., Salness, T., et al. (2007). Abuse potential of carisoprodol: a retrospective review of idaho medicaid pharmacy and medical claims data. *Clinical Therapuetics, 29*(10): 2222–2225.

The Study

Carisoprodol is a frequently prescribed muscle relaxant to treat acute painful musculoskeletal conditions. This retrospective review of claims data looks at potential indicators of abuse in long-term users of carisoprodol vs. other skeletal muscle relaxants. Patients in both groups were similar in age, gender, and skeletal muscle relaxant-related indications. Researchers identified that patients taking carisoprodol used concomitant opioids more frequently, more commonly had a previous drug abuse diagnosis, and continued to pay out of pocket when insurance coverage was discontinued as compared to those patients taking other skeletal muscle relaxants. Collectively these factors suggest the abuse potential of carisoprodol.

Nursing Implications

This research study demonstrates the potential for patients to abuse carisoprodol over other skeletal muscle relaxants. It is important for the nurse to recognize this possible drug characteristic and assess for indications of abuse. Likewise, educating patients of the potential to abuse this drug and the risk of becoming physically dependent is important. Addiction has psychosocial, environmental, and behavioral dimensions that the nurse must be able to assess and easily recognize.

- Diarrhea or Constipation related to drug effects
  Desired outcome: *The patient will maintain baseline bowel habits.*
- Risk for Disturbed Sensory Perception: Kinesthetic, related to dizziness, malaise, and fatigue
  Desired outcome: *The patient will remain free of injury from adverse effects.*
- Disturbed Body Image related to drug-related dermatologic effects
  Desired outcome: *Any adverse effects will be resolved by the end of therapy.*

Planning and Intervention

Maximizing Therapeutic Effects

Administer dantrolene with food or milk to avoid gastric distress. For patients with difficulty swallowing, mix the contents of the capsule with fruit juice and administer immediately. If extended-release capsules or tablets are prescribed, do not open or crush them.

Minimizing Adverse Effects

To avoid injury, supervise the transfer or ambulation of patients taking dantrolene. Also, provide frequent skin care and hygiene measures to prevent skin breakdown and request treatment for acne if appropriate. Protecting the patient from exposure to ultraviolet light is important, as is providing sunscreen if exposure is inevitable.

Therapy is initiated at low doses and gradually increased to minimize dose-related side effects. This practice also determines the minimum effective dose and allows a smooth induction of antispastic effects.

Providing Patient and Family Education

- Before the drug is given, explain to patients and family that the drug is being used to relieve spasticity and that muscle weakness may occur. Family members should be instructed to assist patients with ambulation and ensure safety precautions.
- Inform patients that one of the most dangerous adverse effects of dantrolene therapy is hepatitis. Write down a list of symptoms for patients to report to the prescriber immediately, including loss of appetite, nausea, vomiting, yellowed skin or eyes, and changes in color of urine or stool. Also, explain that regular follow-up medical care, including blood tests, is necessary to monitor the effects of the drug on the body.
- Advise patients that other adverse effects may occur, such as drowsiness, dizziness, GI upset, diarrhea or constipation, or rash. Discuss self-care measures to alleviate common symptoms and urge patients to contact the prescriber if the symptoms do not abate. To avoid photosensitivity, advise patients to wear appropriate clothing and use sunscreen when in direct sunlight.

Ongoing Assessment and Evaluation

Monitor for improvement in symptoms of spasticity and decrease in resistance to passive movement of the limb joint. Beneficial effects in spasticity may take 1 week or more to appear. Assist ambulatory patients with locomotion, because muscle weakness may increase.

Monitor for signs of adverse effects, especially hepatitis and hematologic effects. Coordinate periodic laboratory tests to evaluate liver function and the CBC. Withhold dantrolene and contact the prescriber if clinical signs of hepatitis appear.

Drug Closely Related to P Dantrolene

Botulinum toxin type A (Botox) is a neurotoxin used for its muscle-relaxing properties. It is a protein that is produced by the anaerobic bacterium *Clostridium botulinum*. As many as seven serotypes of botulinum neurotoxin exist, but only types A and B are in clinical use at this time. Botulinum toxin type B (Myobloc) is less potent and shorter-acting than botulinum toxin type A.

Botulinum toxin type A is produced under controlled laboratory conditions and is given in extremely small therapeutic doses (0.05 to 0.1 mL per injection site). It blocks neuromuscular conduction by binding to receptor sites

MEMORY CHIP

P Dantrolene

- Peripherally acting spasmolytic is used for muscle spasms or spasticity.
- Drug of choice for preventing or treating malignant hyperthermia
- Major contraindications: patients who use spasticity to maintain posture or balance (such as patients with cerebral palsy) or who have active hepatic disorders
- Most common adverse effect: muscle weakness; safety is a nursing priority
- Most serious adverse effect: fatal hepatitis, especially in women older than 35 years who are taking estrogens
- Maximizing therapeutic effects: Give with food or milk to decrease GI distress.
- Minimizing adverse effects: Assist with ambulation.
- Most important patient education: Advise patients of symptoms of hepatitis and the importance of notifying the prescriber should any occur.

on motor nerve terminals, entering nerve terminals, and inhibiting the release of acetylcholine. Conditions that are treated with botulinum toxin injections include muscle contraction, headaches, chronic muscle spasms in the neck and back, torticollis (severe neck muscle spasms), myofascial pain syndrome, and spasticity from MS or CVA. Botulinum toxin type A is given as an IM injection. Gradual relaxation of muscle spasm develops 1 to 2 weeks after the injection. The reduction of muscle spasm lasts for 3 to 4 months, and pain relief can last even longer. Potential adverse effects from the injection may include temporary increase in pain, weakness in the muscles injected, body aches, dry mouth, hoarseness, and flu-like symptoms. It is contraindicated in the presence of infection at the proposed injection site.

Additionally, botulinum toxin type A reduces contractions associated with blepharospasms and corrects eye alignment in patients with strabismus. It may also treat primary axillary hyperhidrosis (severe underarm sweating), excessive drooling associated with neurologic disorders, and is considered the second-line therapy for neurogenic bladder.

In 2002, the FDA approved botulinum toxin type A (Botox Cosmetic) for cosmetic use. It has been successfully used to treat severe glabellar (frown) lines and is approved for use in adult patients up to 65 years of age. When botulinum toxin type A is injected into the muscles in a particular area of the face, those muscles cannot "scrunch up" for a period of time because they are paralyzed. The effect lasts for 3 to 6 months. Teach your patient the importance of receiving this type of treatment in a medical facility rather than at a "Botox party."

Formation of antibodies to botulinum toxin type A may reduce the effectiveness of the toxin by inactivating its biologic activity. This can be minimized by injecting with the lowest possible dose and allowing for longer intervals between injections.

CHAPTER SUMMARY

- Drugs used to manage muscle spasm and spasticity are divided into muscle relaxants and spasmolytics. Muscle spasm is a sudden, violent, involuntary contraction of a muscle or group of muscles.
- Cyclobenzaprine (Flexeril) is the prototype for centrally acting muscle relaxants.
- Centrally acting muscle relaxants do not act directly on painful muscles; rather, they work by their CNS depressant activity.
- Most centrally acting muscle relaxants are not effective in treating spasticity.
- In addition to their CNS depressant effects, centrally acting muscle relaxants have anticholinergic and antihistaminic effects.
- Safety is a primary concern for patients receiving centrally acting muscle relaxants and spasmolytics.
- Centrally acting muscle relaxants should be given with caution to older adults. They are not indicated for use in children.
- Spasticity is a prolonged increased tone in muscles that may lead to contraction.
- Baclofen (Lioresal) is the prototype centrally acting spasmolytic drug.
- Gabapentin (Neurontin) is a miscellaneous antiepileptic drug that also has spasmolytic properties.
- Dantrolene (Dantrium) is a peripherally acting spasmolytic that affects spasticity within the muscle fibers.
- Botulinum toxin type A (Botox) is used to manage chronic muscle spasms that do not respond to other treatment methods. It may also be used for cosmetic purposes.
- Spasmolytics should be used cautiously in patients who require spasticity to remain upright.

QUESTIONS FOR STUDY AND REVIEW

1. What is the difference between muscle spasm and muscle spasticity?
2. Your patient, who has a history of depression, rammed his car into a light pole, sustaining multiple contusions and abrasions. The patient is taking amitriptyline (Elavil) four times a day and diazepam (Valium) as needed. The patient is placed on cyclobenzaprine for muscle spasms of the neck and back. What precautions would you take with this patient?
3. Which drugs are effective in managing both muscle spasm and muscle spasticity?
4. Why is baclofen ineffective for spasms from CVA or Parkinson disease?
5. What symptoms suggest hepatitis in the patient who is on long-term dantrolene therapy?
6. Your patient was injured in a motor vehicle crash yesterday. The patient has severe musculoskeletal pain in the upper back. Is botulinum toxin a good choice for the management of this patient?

NEED MORE HELP?

Chapter 20 of the Study Guide to Accompany *Drug Therapy in Nursing,* 4th Edition, contains NCLEX-style questions and other learning activities to reinforce your understanding of the concepts presented in this chapter. For additional information or to purchase the study guide, visit thePoint.

REFERENCES

Brashear, A., & Lambeth, K. (2009). Spasticity. *Current Treatment Options in Neurology,* 11(3):153–161.

Dan, B. et al. (2009). Consensus on the appropriate use of intrathecal baclofen (ITB) therapy in paediatric spasticity. *European Journal of Paediatric Neurology.* Retrieved from doi:10/1016/j.ejpn.2009.05.002.

Facts and Comparisons. (2010). *Drug facts and comparisons.* Philadelphia, PA: Lippincott Williams & Wilkins.

Kamen, L. Henney, H. R., & Runyan, J. D. (2008). A practical overview of tizanidine use for spasticity secondary to multiple sclerosis, stroke, and spinal cord injury. *Current Medical Research and Opinions,* 24(2):425–439.

Karch, A. M. (2010). *Nursing Drug Guide.* Philadelphia, PA: Lippincott, Williams, and Wilkins.

Koda-Kimbal, M. A., Young, L.Y., Kradian, W. A., et al. (2008). *Applied Therapeutics: The Clinical Use of Drugs.* Philadelphia, PA: Lippincott Williams & Wilkins.

Malanga, G., Reiter, R. D., & Garay, E. (2008). Update on tizanidine for muscle spasticity and emerging indications. *Expert Opinion on Pharmcotherapy,* 9(12):2209–2215.

Malignant Hyperthermia Association of the United States (MHAUS). (2011). Retrieved from http://www.mhaus.org.

Micromedex Healthcare Series. Retrieved from http://thomsonhc.com.

Muehlschlegel, S. Rordorf, G., Bodock, M., & Sims, J. R. (2009). Dantrolene mediates relaxation in cerebral vasoconstriction: a case series. *Neurocritical Care,* 10(1):116–121.

Muehlschlegel, S. & Sims, J. R. (2009). Dantrolene: Mechanisms of neuroprotection and possible clinical applications in the neurointensive care unit. *Neurocritical Care* 10(1):103–115.

Mullarkey, T. (2009). Considerations in the treatment of spasticity with intrathecal baclofen. *American Journal of Health-System Pharmacy,* 66(Suppl 5):514–522.

Simpson, D. M., et al. (2009). Botulinum neurotoxin versus tizanidine in upper limb spasticity: a placebo-controlled study. *Journal of Neurology, Neurosurgery, and Psychiatry with Practical Neurology,* 80(4):380–385.

Tatro, D. S. (2009). *Drug interaction facts.* Philadelphia, PA: Lippincott Williams & Wilkins.

Tilton, A. (2009). Management of spasticity in children with cerebral palsy. *Seminars in Pediatric Neurology,* 20:82–89.

Yomiya, K., et al. (2008). Baclofen as an adjuvant analgesic for cancer pain. *American Journal of Hospice and Palliative Medicine,* 26(2):112–118.

Drugs Treating Parkinson Disease and Other Movement Disorders

Learning Objectives

At the completion of this chapter the student will:

1. Correlate the pathophysiology of movement disorders with appropriate pharmacotherapy.
2. Identify core drug knowledge about drug therapies that affect movement disorders.
3. Identify core patient variables related to drugs that affect movement disorders.
4. Relate the interaction of core drug knowledge to core patient variables for therapies that affect movement disorders.
5. Generate a nursing plan of care from the interactions between core drug knowledge and core patient variables for therapies that affect movement disorders.
6. Describe nursing interventions to maximize therapeutic and minimize adverse effects for drugs that affect movement disorders.
7. Determine key points for patient and family education for drugs that affect movement disorders.

Key Terms
akinesia
ballismus
bradykinesia
bradykinetic episodes
bruxism

choreiform
dystonic
dyskinetic
dopaminergics

neuroleptic malignant
 syndrome (NMS)
on–off syndrome
parkinsonism

Drugs Treating Parkinson Disease and Other Movement Disorders

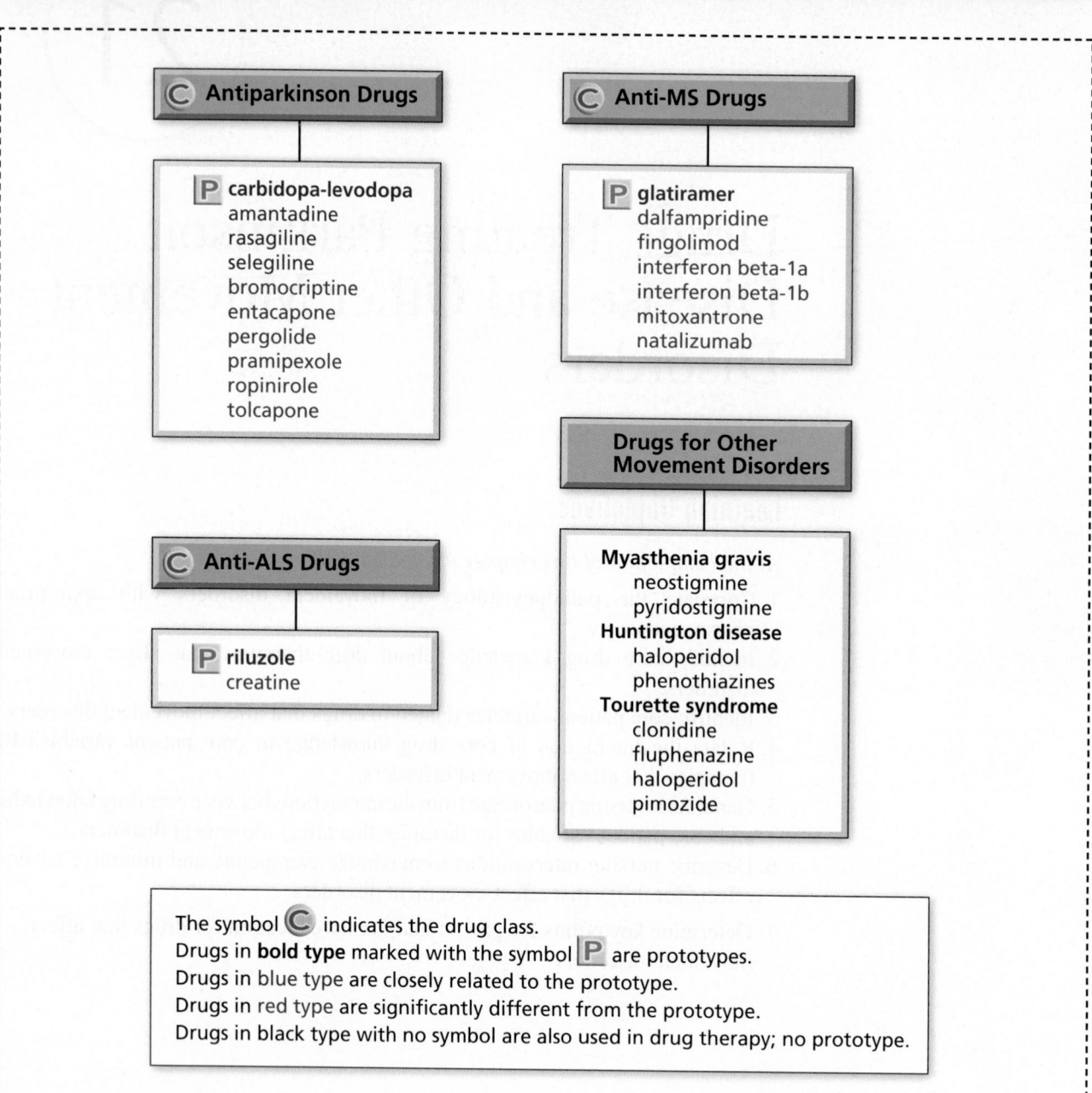

C Antiparkinson Drugs

P carbidopa-levodopa
amantadine
rasagiline
selegiline
bromocriptine
entacapone
pergolide
pramipexole
ropinirole
tolcapone

C Anti-MS Drugs

P glatiramer
dalfampridine
fingolimod
interferon beta-1a
interferon beta-1b
mitoxantrone
natalizumab

Drugs for Other Movement Disorders

Myasthenia gravis
neostigmine
pyridostigmine
Huntington disease
haloperidol
phenothiazines
Tourette syndrome
clonidine
fluphenazine
haloperidol
pimozide

C Anti-ALS Drugs

P riluzole
creatine

The symbol **C** indicates the drug class.
Drugs in **bold type** marked with the symbol **P** are prototypes.
Drugs in blue type are closely related to the prototype.
Drugs in red type are significantly different from the prototype.
Drugs in black type with no symbol are also used in drug therapy; no prototype.

Movement disorders can be chronic, severe, and debilitating. These disorders are incurable, and patients with them have various responses to treatment. As a result of a disorder's progression, patients may become socially isolated and depressed. As patients become increasingly disabled and the drugs become minimally effective, your primary role shifts from one of medical intervention to psychosocial and functional care, with the aim of helping the patient maximize remaining capacities. This chapter limits the discussion to the nurse's pharmacologic role. Information on the nonpharmacologic role of the nurse can be found in a medical-surgical textbook or subject-specific website.

This chapter discusses three major movement disorders—Parkinson disease, amyotrophic lateral sclerosis (ALS), and multiple sclerosis (MS)—focusing on drugs used to inhibit the symptoms associated with these diseases. In addition, it discusses core drug knowledge, core patient variables, nursing management, potential nursing diagnoses, and patient education related to the use of these drugs.

PHYSIOLOGY

The extrapyramidal system is responsible for coarse control of voluntary muscles. This "system" is composed of basal ganglia, cortical areas of the brain that project to the basal ganglia, cerebellar areas of the brain that project to the basal ganglia, and parts of the reticular formation and thalamic nuclei that connect to the basal ganglia. Motor activity requires integration of the actions of the cerebral cortex, basal ganglia, and cerebellum.

The basal ganglia are a group of functionally related nuclei located in paired groups in each cerebral hemisphere. Two primary nuclei are the corpus striatum, located deep within the cerebrum, and the substantia nigra, a group of darkly pigmented cells located in the midbrain. When the basal ganglia are stimulated, muscle tone in the body is inhibited, and voluntary movements are refined.

The regulatory neurotransmitter *dopamine* is produced in the substantia nigra and adrenal glands, and then transmitted to the basal ganglia along a neural pathway for secretion when needed. Recently, five dopamine receptors have been identified in the brain. Three of these receptors (dopamine-1, dopamine-2, and dopamine-3—usually called D_1, D_2, and D_3, respectively) appear to play important roles in properly balancing the stimulation of the basal ganglia involved in normal motor function. Acetylcholine, an excitatory neurotransmitter, is produced by the basal ganglia and in the nerve endings in the periphery of the body. When the body wants to make a movement (e.g., walking or picking up a cup of coffee), the striatum releases dopamine and acetylcholine through the nervous system to the appropriate muscles, which enables initiation, modulation, and completion of smooth, coordinated movement within a fraction of a second.

PATHOPHYSIOLOGY
Parkinson Disease

Parkinson disease occurs with death of the neurons that produce dopamine, a neurotransmitter in the brain. Parkinson disease generally afflicts patients aged 60 years and older, is more apt to affect men than women and progresses slowly to neuromuscular debilitation. Researchers have found that a mutated gene, called a parkin gene, may trigger the disease at an earlier age. Although 13 genes have been linked with Parkinson disease, genetics seems to play only a small role in the development of the disease. Other risk factors associated with Parkinson disease include head trauma, well water consumption and environmental toxins such as herbicides and pesticides. No conclusive evidence exists designating the cause of Parkinson disease; yet scientists believe that the disease occurs due to an interaction of genetics and environment. In Parkinson disease, degeneration of the neurons that supply dopamine to the striatum occurs, resulting in reduced dopamine in the nerve terminals of the nigrostriatal tract. Consequently, an imbalance exists between dopamine inhibition and acetylcholine excitation (Figure 21.1). Additionally, unopposed acetylcholine stimulates the release of gamma-aminobutyric acid (GABA). The combination of excessive acetylcholine and GABA is the basis for most symptoms of Parkinson disease, such as muscle rigidity, tremor at rest, **akinesia** (loss of voluntary movement) or **bradykinesia** (abnormal slowness of movement), and postural instability.

Dopamine is the neurotransmitter that sends information to the parts of the brain that control movement and coordination. As the disease progresses, messages from the brain telling the body how and when to move are delivered more slowly, leaving the patient incapable of initiating or controlling normal movements. Patients may also experience depression, emotional changes, and sleep problems. Memory loss and slow thinking may develop, although the ability to reason usually remains intact.

Parkinsonism is a syndrome with characteristics similar to Parkinson disease that are secondary to other conditions that structurally damage the dopaminergic pathway or interfere with dopamine's action within the basal ganglia. Well-known precipitants of parkinsonism are drugs such as the phenothiazines, metoclopramide, and reserpine. Drug-induced parkinsonism is usually reversible when the drugs are discontinued.

Amyotrophic Lateral Sclerosis

ALS is a progressive neurologic disorder related to degeneration of nerve cells responsible for controlling voluntary movement. It is also known as Lou Gehrig disease, after the famous baseball player who succumbed to the disorder. The etiology of ALS is unknown. It presents in adulthood, usually between ages 40 and 60 years, and affects men two to three times more often than women. ALS affects both the upper

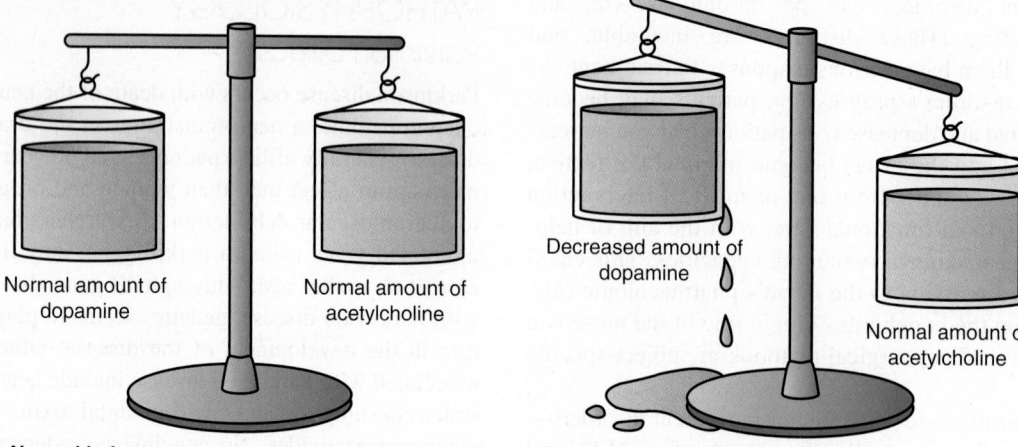

A. Normal balance

Normal amount of dopamine   Normal amount of acetylcholine

B. Imbalance of Parkinson disease

Decreased amount of dopamine   Normal amount of acetylcholine

• FIGURE 21.1 **(A)** Normal balance. This figure depicts the body at rest when the dopamine and acetylcholine systems are balanced. When the body moves, the brain understands the movement the body wants to make and it sends out a balance of dopamine and acetylcholine messages to keep that movement smooth. **(B)** Imbalance in Parkinson disease. This figure represents Parkinson disease, in which the normal levels of acetylcholine and dopamine are imbalanced and abnormal movement affects the body until chemical balance can be restored, to a degree.

motor neurons in the cerebral cortex and the lower motor neurons in the brain stem and spinal cord. Although this disorder is neurologic, one of its classic features is that it spares the entire sensory system and the intellect. Additionally, it spares the cranial nerves that innervate movement of the eye (cranial nerves III, IV, and VI).

The disease begins in the distal neurons and then progresses in a centripetal but asymmetric fashion. The loss of upper motor neurons results in spastic paralysis and hyperreflexia. The loss of lower motor neurons results in decreased muscle tone and reflexes and flaccid paralysis. Ultimately, neuronal cell death leads to muscular weakness, muscle atrophy and fasciculations, spasticity, dysarthria, dysphagia, and respiratory compromise. Although periods of remission may occur, ALS typically progresses rapidly, and death occurs within 5 years for 50% of patients diagnosed with the disease.

Multiple Sclerosis

Multiple sclerosis is an autoimmune disease where the body attacks the myelin sheath resulting in neuromuscular debilitation. MS is a major cause of neurologic disability among young and middle-aged adults. There are four disease courses of MS: relapsing-remitting, primary progressive, secondary progressive, and progressive-relapsing.

At the time of diagnosis, 85% of patients have relapsing-remitting MS, which is characterized by clearly defined relapses (also called exacerbations, flare-ups, or attacks). The relapse is followed by partial or complete recovery periods (remissions). Approximately 10% of MS patients have primary progressive MS. This form of MS is characterized by a slow but nearly continuous worsening of the disease

from the onset of MS, without distinct relapses or remissions. There may be a variation in the rate of progression, an occasional plateau, or a temporary minor improvement. Before the use of disease-modifying drugs, 50% of patients with relapsing-remitting MS developed secondary progressive MS within 10 years of diagnosis. In this subtype, the symptoms of MS change from those of relapsing-remitting MS to a steady progression of the disease with or without intermittent relapse and remission. It is unclear whether the use of disease-modifying drugs will alter the timing of this subtype. Progressive-relapsing MS, which affects only 5% of patients, is rare. This type of MS is characterized by a steady progression of disease, but the patient also has clear acute relapses with or without recovery. This differs from relapsing-remitting MS because of the steady progression of the disease between relapses and remissions.

In MS, more than one area of inflammation and scarring of the myelin in the brain and spinal cord occurs. When myelin is damaged, messages between the brain and other parts of the body are affected. The most common symptoms of MS include fatigue, weakness, spasticity, balance problems, bladder and bowel problems, numbness, vision loss, tremor, and vertigo. The signs and symptoms reflect the location of the lesions; therefore, not every patient experiences every symptom of MS.

C ANTIPARKINSON DRUGS

The relative lack of dopamine, combined with the relative excess of excitatory acetylcholine, causes the symptoms of Parkinson disease. The goal of therapy is to restore the balance between dopamine and acetylcholine, which can

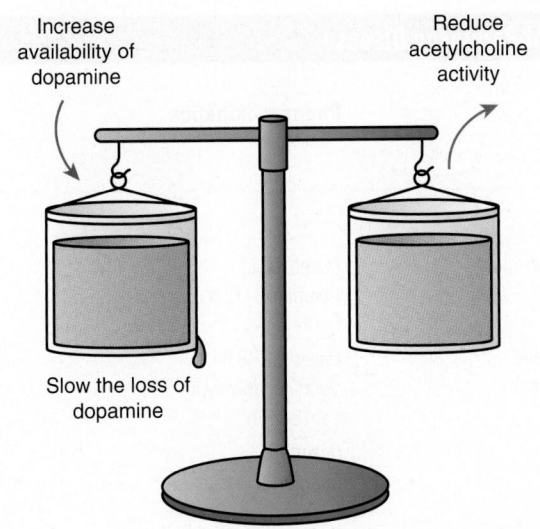

Increase availability of dopamine

Reduce acetylcholine activity

Slow the loss of dopamine

• FIGURE 21.2   The goal of pharmacologic treatment for Parkinson disease is to restore the homeostatic balance between acetylcholine and dopamine, which can be accomplished by increasing the amount or availability of dopamine, slowing the loss of dopamine, or blocking the activity of acetylcholine.

be accomplished by increasing the activity of dopamine or blocking the action of acetylcholine (Figure 21.2).

Drugs used to treat Parkinson disease increase dopamine levels (**dopaminergics**), stimulate dopamine receptors (dopamine agonists), extend the action of dopamine in the brain (dopa decarboxylase [DDC] or catecholamine O-methyl transferase [COMT] inhibitors), or prevent the activation of cholinergic receptors (anticholinergics). Anticholinergics are discussed in depth in Chapter 14; thus they are only briefly summarized in this chapter. Information about antiparkinson agents is given in Table 21.1.

• Ⓒ DOPAMINERGICS

The combination drug carbidopa-levodopa (Sinemet, Parcopa) is the prototype for the dopaminergics.

The logical solution to the imbalance in Parkinson disease is to administer dopamine to the patient; however, dopamine does not cross the blood–brain barrier. Therefore, levodopa, the precursor to dopamine, is the drug of choice, because it does cross the blood-brain barrier and will be converted into dopamine in the brain. Unfortunately, levodopa is largely deactivated in the periphery of the body by two enzymes: dopamine decarboxylase(DDC) and catechol-O-methyl transferase (COMT).

When levodopa is administered as a single drug, approximately 2% actually crosses the blood–brain barrier. To increase the amount of levodopa available to cross the blood–brain barrier, it is combined with the drug carbidopa, a DDC inhibitor. Carbidopa does not cross the blood–brain barrier, but it decreases peripheral destruction of levodopa, allowing 10% of levodopa to reach the brain.

Nursing Management of the Patient Receiving Ⓟ Carbidopa-Levodopa

Core Drug Knowledge

Pharmacotherapeutics

Carbidopa-levodopa (Sinemet, Parcopa) is a combination drug used in treating Parkinson disease. It is also used to treat restless-leg syndrome.

Pharmacokinetics

With oral administration, carbidopa-levodopa may begin to take effect after 1 to 2 months, although some patients require up to 6 months of therapy before noting an effect. The plasma half-life of both carbidopa-levodopa and carbidopa alone is roughly 1 to 2 hours, and the duration of action of a dose is 5 hours. Most carbidopa-levodopa is metabolized into dopamine in the periphery of the body, whereas carbidopa itself is minimally metabolized. Carbidopa-levodopa is eliminated renally as dopamine metabolites and in small amounts as unchanged drug. In addition, carbidopa-levodopa crosses the placenta and is present in breast milk.

Pharmacodynamics

Carbidopa-levodopa diffuses levodopa into the central nervous system (CNS), where it is converted to dopamine. The resulting change in dopamine–acetylcholine balance is believed to improve nerve impulse control and to form the basis of the drug's antiparkinsonian activity. Carbidopa does not cross the blood–brain barrier.

When carbidopa is administered in combination with levodopa, it inhibits the conversion of levodopa to dopamine in the periphery of the body, thereby increasing the amount of levodopa available to diffuse into the CNS. Because the bioavailability of dopamine increases in the CNS, the dosage of levodopa can be reduced. This reduction minimizes the potential for nausea/vomiting adverse reactions from levodopa. The carbidopa-levodopa combination also enables more rapid and even titration of effect.

Contraindications and Precautions

Patients with hypersensitivity to carbidopa-levodopa should not take the drug. Carbidopa-levodopa can activate malignant melanoma; thus, the drug is contraindicated in patients with undiagnosed pigmented lesions or a history of melanoma. Although carbidopa-levodopa may not be used in patients with closed-angle glaucoma, it may be used in patients with open-angle glaucoma if intraocular pressure is closely monitored and controlled. Simultaneous administration of carbidopa-levodopa with monoamine oxidase inhibitors (MAOIs) can result in hypertensive crisis. Therefore, MAOIs should be discontinued 2 to 4 weeks before therapy with carbidopa-levodopa begins.

Precautions to carbidopa-levodopa therapy include cardiac disease (especially arrhythmias or past myocardial infarction [MI]), pulmonary disease, peptic ulcer disease,

TABLE 21.1 Summary of Selected Drugs for the Management of Parkinson Disease

Drug (Trade) Name	Selected Indications	Route and Dosage Range	Pharmacokinetics
Antiparkinson Agents			
Dopaminergics			
carbidopa-levodopa (Sinemet)	Parkinson disease	*Adult:* PO, 25/100 bid–qid to a maximum of 200/2,000 mg/d *Child:* Not recommended	*Onset:* Rapid *Duration:* 6–12 h $t_{1/2}$: 1–2 h
amantadine (Symmetre)	Parkinson disease Antiviral agent	*Adult:* PO, 100–400 mg/d as needed *Adult and child >9 y:* PO, 100 mg bid *Child 1–9 y:* 2–4 mg/lb	*Onset:* 36–48 h *Duration:* Unknown $t_{1/2}$: 15–24 h
rasagiline (Azilect)	Parkinson disease	*Adult:* PO, 1 mg daily *Child:* not recommended	*Onset:* 1 h *Duration:* 6 weeks $t_{1/2}$: 3 hr
selegiline (Eldepryl, Zelapar [oral disintegrating tablet], Emsam [transdermal patch])	Parkinson disease Depression	*Adult:* PO, 5 mg taken at breakfast and lunch *Oral disintegrating tablet:* 1.25–2.5 mg dissolved on the tongue once daily (before breakfast), max of 2.5 mg/d *Child:* Not recommended *Transdermal patch:* 6 mg/24 h patch; max 12 mg/24 h *Child:* Not recommended	*Onset:* 1 h *Duration:* 24–72 h $t_{1/2}$: 9 min; 20.5 h for active metabolites
Dopamine Agonists			
bromocriptine (Parlodel)	Parkinson disease Acromegaly Hyperprolactinemia	*Adult:* PO, 5–50 mg bid *Adult:* PO, 30–30 mg/d *Adult:* PO, 5–7.5 mg/d *Child:* Not recommended	*Onset:* 1 h *Duration:* 14 h $t_{1/2}$: biphasic Initial 6–8 h Terminal 50 h
pergolide (Permax)	Parkinson disease	*Adult:* PO, 1 mg tid *Child:* Not recommended	*Onset:* Varies *Duration:* Unknown $t_{1/2}$: 27 h
pramipexole (Mirapex)	Parkinson disease	*Adult:* PO, 1.5–4.5 mg/d *Child:* Not recommended	*Onset:* Rapid *Duration:* Unknown $t_{1/2}$: 8–12 h
ropinirole (Requip)	Parkinson disease	*Adult:* PO, 1 mg tid *Child:* Not recommended	*Onset:* 30–40 min *Duration:* 16 h $t_{1/2}$: 6 h
COMT Inhibitors			
tolcapone (Tasmar)	Parkinson disease	*Adult:* PO, 100–200 mg tid *Child:* Not recommended	*Onset:* 1 h *Duration:* Unknown $t_{1/2}$: 2–3 h
entacapone (Comtan)	Parkinson disease	*Adult:* PO, 200 g with each dose of carbidopa-levodopa not to exceed 1,600 g daily *Child:* Not recommended	*Onset:* 1 h *Duration:* Unknown $t_{1/2}$: 1–2 h
Combination Drugs			
entacapone, carbidopa-levodopa (Stalevo)	Parkinson disease	*Adult:* PO, individualized to achieve desired therapeutic response; maximum of 8 tablets per day	Same as for individual agents
Anticholinergics			
benztropine (Cogentin)	Parkinson disease	*Adult:* PO/IM/IV, 0.5–6 mg/d *Child:* Not recommended	*Onset:* PO, 1 h; IM/IV, 15 min *Duration:* Unknown $t_{1/2}$: 6–10 h
diphenhydramine (Benadryl)	Parkinson disease	*Adult:* PO, 25–100 mwg/d; IM/IV, 10–50 mg *Child:* PO, >10 kg 12.5–25 g 3–4 times daily, max 300 g qid; IV, 5 mg/kg/d	*Onset:* PO, 15–30 min; IM 20–30 min; IV, rapid *Duration:* 4–8 h $t_{1/2}$: 2.5–7 h
trihexyphenidyl (Artane)	Parkinson disease	*Adult:* PO, 1–15 mg in divided doses *Child:* Safety and efficacy not established	*Onset:* Varies *Duration:* Unknown $t_{1/2}$: 5–10 h

and diabetes mellitus. Carbidopa-levodopa may exacerbate symptoms in patients with these disorders.

Additionally, carbidopa-levodopa may cause mental status changes and should be used with caution in patients with a history of psychiatric disorders. All patients receiving carbidopa-levodopa should be monitored closely for signs of mental disturbances, including depression or suicidal thoughts.

Adverse Effects

Adverse gastrointestinal (GI) effects are common in patients receiving carbidopa-levodopa and include nausea and vomiting, anorexia, and weight loss. Another common adverse effect to carbidopa-levodopa therapy is orthostatic hypotension.

Of the more serious adverse effects of carbidopa-levodopa therapy, abnormal movements are the most common. These abnormal movements result from the increased dopamine in the brain. Abnormal and involuntary movements include the following:

- Continuous rapid jerky involuntary movements resembling a grotesque dance (**chorieform** movements)
- Jerking, twisting movements distinguished by prolonged rhythmic muscle contractions (**dystonic** movements)
- Difficulty executing voluntary movements resulting in tic-like behavior (**dyskinetic** movements)
- Clenching the teeth, associated with forceful lateral or protrusive jaw movements, resulting in rubbing, gritting, or grinding the teeth (**bruxism**)
- Jerking, flinging movements of an extremity (**ballismus**)
- Protrusion of the tongue
- Opening and closing of the mouth
- Bobbing of the head
- Rhythmic movements of the feet or hands
- Quick movements of the shoulder

Abnormal movements are usually dose related and may resolve with a reduction in dose. Unfortunately, with a dose reduction, the symptoms of Parkinson disease may recur.

Psychiatric disturbances may develop with the administration of carbidopa-levodopa. Symptoms include memory loss, anxiety, nervousness, agitation, restlessness, confusion, insomnia, nightmares, daytime somnolence, euphoria, malaise, and fatigue. Patients taking carbidopa-levodopa are also at risk for developing severe mental depression, suicidal tendencies, dementia, hallucinations, paranoid delusion, psychoses, and hypomania.

Cardiac arrhythmias can occur during carbidopa-levodopa therapy because conversion of levodopa to dopamine in the periphery can activate beta-1 receptors. This occurs most frequently in patients with a history of heart disease. Other cardiovascular symptoms include flushing and hypertension.

For patients taking carbidopa-levodopa for a prolonged period, **bradykinetic episodes,** also known as the "**on–off syndrome,**" may occur. Characteristics of this syndrome include akinesia, a sudden return of the effectiveness of the drug, and akinesia paradoxica (an abrupt hypotonic reaction in which the patient usually falls as he or she begins to walk). The akinetic episode can last from minutes to hours. A sudden return of effectiveness may follow, and the cycle can recur many times each day. Recently, the Food and Drug Administration (FDA) approved a new drug to treat these episodes in patients with Parkinson disease (Box 21.1). Loss of response to levodopa may also occur as a more gradual process, usually before the next dose of medication.

Neuroleptic malignant syndrome (NMS, also called parkinsonian crisis) is characterized by an abrupt onset of marked rigidity, akinesia, tremor, and hyperpyrexia. It can follow abrupt discontinuation of carbidopa-levodopa

BOX 21.1 COMMUNITY BASED CONCERNS

Treating Hypomobility in Parkinson Disease

Patients with advanced Parkinson disease who are taking levodopa may experience bradykinetic episodes, also known as "on–off syndrome." These episodes are characterized by a shift from the ability to be mobile (on) to an unpredictable period of immobility (off). The intensity, duration, and frequency of "off" periods vary from patient to patient. Intensity ranges from partial loss of movement to total immobility. On–off syndrome is thought to be related to an increased sensitivity in the brain to small changes in serum levels of dopamine.

Apomorphine hydrochloride (Apokyn) has been approved by the Food and Drug Administration (FDA) as an orphan drug for treating acute, intermittent episodes of hypomobility. Apomorphine hydrochloride helps the patient walk, talk, or move more easily, but it does not prevent hypomobility, nor does it replace the patient's drugs for Parkinson disease. Apomorphine hydrochloride is given as a subcutaneous injection. Symptoms improve within 15 minutes, and the effect lasts for approximately 2 hours. The drug must be given with an antiemetic, because

it can induce nausea and vomiting. It should not be given concurrently with antiemetic agents classified as 5-HT$_3$ antagonists, because this type of antiemetic drug can induce hypotension or loss of consciousness. Examples of these drugs include ondansetron, granisetron, dolasetron, palonosetron, and alosetron. Common adverse effects associated with apomorphine hydrochloride include yawning, dyskinesias, nausea and vomiting, sedation or sleepiness, dizziness, runny nose, hallucinations, edema, chest pain, increased sweating, flushing, and pallor. Apomorphine hydrochloride is an FDA pregnancy category C drug. It is unknown whether it enters breast milk.

When educating patients about apomorphine hydrochloride, you must emphasize the importance of continuing all drugs prescribed for Parkinson disease, despite symptom relief with apomorphine hydrochloride. In addition, emphasize the importance of taking the drug with certain antiemetic drugs. Monitor the first injection to evaluate the patient's or caregiver's ability to administer a subcutaneous injection correctly; emphasize the importance of aspirating before injecting to avoid intravenous (IV) administration.

TABLE 21.2 — Agents That Interact with P Carbidopa-Levodopa

Interactants	Effect and Significance	Nursing Management
Hydantoins	Mechanism of action unknown, but decrease effectiveness of carbidopa-levodopa	Monitor for decreased therapeutic effects. Consider alternative antiepileptic therapy.
iron salts	May form chelates that decreases carbidopa- levodopa absorption	Separate administration of these two drugs as much as possible. Monitor for decreased therapeutic effects.
MAOIs	Inhibit peripheral metabolism of carbidopa- levodopa, resulting in increased levels of dopamine; may result in hypertensive crisis	Do not co-administer these drugs. If accidental administration occurs, phentolamine is the antidote.
phenothiazines	May inhibit dopamine receptors in the CNS	Monitor for decreased therapeutic effects.
tricyclic antidepressants	Delay the absorption of carbidopa-levodopa and may decrease its bioavailability	Monitor for decreased therapeutic effects.

therapy, and it occurs most frequently in patients who are also receiving antipsychotic drugs.

Other adverse effects associated with carbidopa-levodopa include episodic hyperventilation, bizarre breathing patterns, hoarseness, and increased nasal secretions. Urinary retention, polyuria, and urinary incontinence may also occur. Rarely, leukopenia may occur, necessitating discontinuing the drug temporarily.

When levodopa (Dopar) is given alone, it may induce dark-colored sweat or urine.

Drug Interactions

Carbidopa-levodopa can interact substantially with hydantoins, MAOIs, phenothiazines, or tricyclic antidepressants (TCAs). Levodopa alone interacts with pyridoxine. Table 21.2 presents a list of agents that interact with carbidopa-levodopa.

Carbidopa-levodopa administration may cause abnormalities in laboratory tests. Elevations of liver function test values such as alkaline phosphatase, aspartate aminotransferase (AST), alanine aminotransferase (ALT), lactic dehydrogenase (LDH), and bilirubin may occur. Commonly, levels of blood urea nitrogen, creatinine, and uric acid are lower during administration of carbidopa-levodopa. Carbidopa-levodopa may cause a false-positive reaction for urinary ketone bodies when a test tape is used for determination of ketonuria. False-negative tests may result with the use of glucose-oxidase methods of testing for glucosuria.

Assessment of Relevant Core Patient Variables

Health Status

Assess the patient for tartrazine allergy, melanoma, and closed-angle glaucoma. Assess also for a history of psychiatric disorders that necessitate administration of MAOIs. If the patient has any of these disorders, notify the prescriber before administering carbidopa-levodopa.

Assess for previous levodopa or carbidopa-levodopa therapy. After 2 to 5 years of continuous therapy, these drugs lose their overall effectiveness in controlling symptoms of Parkinson disease. Administering a higher dose may affect symptoms but also increases the patient's risk of adverse effects.

Perform a complete physical examination, including mental status. Carbidopa-levodopa can exacerbate diseases or disorders in every body system; therefore, evaluate baseline functioning. Appropriate laboratory or diagnostic tests are determined in part by the patient's pre-existing conditions. Patients with cardiovascular disorders require a baseline electrocardiogram. Patients with pulmonary disorders should have baseline pulmonary function tests. Patients with glaucoma should have intraocular pressure measured at baseline. For patients with diabetes, a glycosylated hemoglobin (HbA_{1C}) level should be obtained. Baseline hepatic function or renal function tests are included for patients with disorders in those body systems.

Throughout the physical examination, document the signs and symptoms of Parkinson disease, such as abnormal posture and gait, muscle rigidity, and tremors. Assess the patient's ability to perform activities of daily living such as dressing, eating, and walking. This baseline information is used to assess the efficacy of carbidopa-levodopa therapy and progression of the disease.

Some patients receiving carbidopa-levodopa have experienced postoperative bleeding episodes; therefore, hematologic studies are recommended for all patients who undergo surgery while receiving the drug (Box 21.2).

Life Span and Gender

Carbidopa-levodopa is a Food and Drug Administration (FDA) pregnancy category C drug and therefore should be used with caution during pregnancy. It should not be given to breast-feeding women because carbidopa-levodopa enters breast milk and may inhibit lactation. Therefore, assess all female patients for pregnancy or breast-feeding. In addition, carbidopa-levodopa should not be administered

BOX 21.2 FOCUS ON RESEARCH

Cohen, J. A., et al. (2010). Oral fingolimod or intramuscular interferon for relapsing multiple sclerosis. *The New England Journal of Medicine*, 362(5), 402–415.

Rationale

Presently, glatiramer acetate and beta interferon are FDA-approved drugs for use in relapse remitting MS and have been shown to reduce relapse rates by approximately 30%; yet both drugs are associated with systemic reactions in up to 60% of patients and need to be given parenterally. Oral fingolimod has been shown to decrease the number of lymphocytes circulating within the body and the lymphocytes ability to initiate an autoimmune reaction on the axons in the myelin sheath. Previous studies on fingolimod have been smaller scale and shorter term investigations.

The Study

A double-blind, double-dummy study comparing fingolimod to interferon beta-1a was conducted on randomly assigned 1,153 relapsing remitting multiple sclerosis patients to determine fingolimod's impact on the relapse rate over one year. This phase 3 clinical trial demonstrated a significantly decreased annualized relapse rate and a decrease in new or enlarged lesions on MRI with 1 year's use of fingolimod versus the use of interferon. No significant findings were obtained related to sustained progressive disability. Adverse effects included hypertension, bradycardia/AV block, increased liver enzymes, macular edema, skin cancer, and two fatal infections from either herpes simplex encephalitis or disseminated primary varicella zoster. Studies transcending longer periods of time are necessary to establish safety and efficacy of this drug in MS patients.

Nursing Implications

The study is a phase 3 clinical trial meaning that the drug is being investigated on large groups of patients using randomized controlled methods at multi-centered sites to compare the 'gold standard' to the experimental drug. The keys for nurses are to become familiar with the process of clinical trials used before the drug is launched on the market, consider the nursing role in clinical trials and to increase nursing knowledge of drugs on the horizon as the drug nears appropriate regulatory agency approval for use by the public.

---

to children younger than 18 years of age, so confirm that the patient is 18 years or older.

Lifestyle, Diet, and Habits

Coordinate a consultation with a nutritionist for patients taking carbidopa-levodopa. Patients should attempt weight control because increased body weight increases the work of the body, especially the muscles. A high-protein diet can slow or prevent absorption of carbidopa-levodopa. Therefore, moderate amounts of protein should be divided equally for consumption throughout the entire day. Pyridoxine (vitamin B$_6$) increases the action of decarboxylases that destroy levodopa in the periphery of the body, resulting in reduced effects of levodopa. Accordingly when taking levodopa alone, patients should avoid foods containing large amounts of pyridoxine, such as avocados, bananas, beef liver, oatmeal, halibut, chicken, pork, mashed potatoes, wheat germ, and sunflower seeds. Because carbidopa inhibits the action of the pyridoxine, patients taking carbidopa-levodopa (Sinemet) may eat foods high in pyridoxine or take pyridoxine supplements. Patients should also increase dietary fiber and fluids to offset the potential for constipation.

Environment

Carbidopa-levodopa is usually administered in the home environment. Assess patients for their ability to understand the prescriber's directions and to physically self-administer drugs. A new formulation of the combination drug (Parcopa), which dissolves rapidly on the tongue, may improve patients' ability to self-medicate. Home care referrals are necessary for patients who cannot self-medicate. Because carbidopa- levodopa does not affect the progression of the disease, coordinate counseling and physical and occupational therapies for the patient to optimize therapeutic outcome.

Culture and Inherited Traits

In decarboxylation, carbidopa-levodopa is metabolized by COMT, which antagonizes the therapeutic effects of carbidopa-levodopa. COMT activity destroys levodopa in the periphery of the body and is found in higher amounts in people of Chinese, Filipino, or Thai descent. Therefore, ask patients about their ethnic heritage as part of the assessment.

Nursing Diagnoses and Outcomes

- Disturbed Thought Processes related to adverse CNS effects
  Desired outcome: The patient will remain oriented and communicate effectively.
- Disturbed Sleep Pattern related to drug therapy
  Desired outcome: The patient will report alterations in sleep patterns affecting activities of daily living.
- Impaired Physical Mobility related to on–off effect
  Desired outcome: The patient will immediately report incidents of the on–off syndrome to the prescriber.
- Risk for Injury related to drug-induced orthostatic hypotension
  Desired outcome: The patient will learn to change position slowly, carefully, and safely to minimize effects of orthostatic hypotension.

Planning and Intervention

Maximizing Therapeutic Effects

Have patients take carbidopa-levodopa on an empty stomach to facilitate absorption of the drug. If the patient has trouble swallowing pills, the rapid-dissolving formulation should be used. Monitor the patient's diet to limit foods high in protein. If the drug causes severe nausea, give the patient a small amount of food 15 to 30 minutes after administering drug therapy.

Minimizing Adverse Effects

Administer carbidopa-levodopa at evenly spaced intervals, and always titrate the dose. Slowly increase the dose to prevent nausea, vomiting, or orthostatic hypotension, and slowly decrease it to prevent NMS (parkinsonian crisis).

Providing Patient and Family Education

- Advise patients that carbidopa-levodopa therapy is palliative and will not cure the disease. Patients must understand that it takes weeks to months to notice benefits from therapy. Caution patients that they should neither change the drug dosage in an attempt to hasten the therapeutic benefits nor discontinue the drug abruptly because they think treatment has failed.
- Advise patients to notify the prescriber about any of the following adverse reactions: uncontrollable movements of the face, eyelids, mouth, tongue, neck, arms, hands, or legs; mood or mental changes; irregular heartbeat or palpitations; difficult urination; severe or persistent nausea or vomiting; appetite loss; difficulty swallowing; or distorted taste.
- Demonstrate how to change positions slowly to avoid dizziness or fainting. Advise patients to assess how the drug affects them before driving, using machinery, or performing tasks that require mental alertness.
- Discuss the potential for "on–off syndrome" described in the section on Adverse Reactions. Ensure that patients understand that they are at risk for injury from falls during the "off" periods. Convey the importance of contacting the prescriber immediately if patients experience an akinetic episode. Advise the patient to report gradual "off" periods before the next dose. Adjustment of medications may decrease this occurrence.
- Include necessary dietary changes in patient education. Patients should avoid high-protein foods when the drug is ingested, and alcohol.
- Caution patients with pre-existing disorders such as arrhythmias, pulmonary diseases, or peptic ulcer disease that carbidopa-levodopa may exacerbate their condition. Patients must contact their prescriber if their symptoms increase in frequency or intensity. Caution patients with diabetes to monitor their glucose by capillary blood testing because carbidopa-levodopa may induce false-positive urinary glucose results. Finally, carbidopa- levodopa sometimes darkens urine and sweat. Assure patients that this effect is no cause for concern.

Ongoing Assessment and Evaluation

Monitor for improvement in the patient's ability to perform daily activities and for decreased muscle rigidity and tremors. During periods of dose adjustment, monitor blood pressure every 4 hours. When dose adjustment is done in the home, teach a family member how to monitor blood pressure.

Monitor for signs of adverse effects from carbidopa-levodopa therapy. Dosage changes may increase adverse effects; thus, notifying the prescriber if these signs occur is important. Monitor for signs of personality, behavioral, or mental changes. Eliciting information regarding these potential changes from the family and patient is important. Patients should also receive a periodic eye examination because carbidopa-levodopa may affect intraocular pressure.

Monitor for signs or symptoms of NMS. If signs or symptoms of NMS develop, assess for adherence to drug therapy to ensure proper dosing. Report any signs of NMS to the prescriber immediately, and instruct the patient and family members that they should report any signs of NMS to the prescriber immediately.

With successful therapy, decreased muscular rigidity, bradykinesias, and tremors, as well as improved mobility, should be observed. The patient should be able to verbalize the importance of contacting the prescriber immediately if any adverse reactions occur and the need for periodic re-evaluation by the prescriber.

Drugs Closely Related to Carbidopa-Levodopa

Amantadine, selegiline, and rasagiline are also dopaminergic agents.

Amantadine

Amantadine (Symmetrel) is an oral antiviral drug that has been found to be effective in treating Parkinson disease. However, this efficacy diminishes within a short time. Amantadine's effects may decrease within as little as 3 to 6 months. Little is known about the precise mechanism of action of this drug in the brain.

Adverse effects of amantadine include insomnia as well as daytime fatigue. Other adverse effects are swollen feet, anxiety, dizziness, urinary retention, depression and hallucinations. The patient may also experience effects similar to those of anticholinergic drugs, such as blurred vision, constipation, urinary retention, and xerostomia (dry mouth). These effects may be enhanced when amantadine is given concurrently with other drugs that have anticholinergic effects. An adverse effect specific to amantadine is "livedo reticularis," a reddish-blue netlike mottling of the skin. Fortunately, this condition is benign and disappears when amantadine therapy is stopped.

Selegiline

Selegiline (Eldepryl) is an MAOI that is selective to monoamine oxidase type–B (MAO-B), a chemical that breaks down dopamine. Selegiline decreases the destruction of dopamine, whether the dopamine is extrinsic, such as the dopamine produced from carbidopa-levodopa, or intrinsic. It is thought to slow the progression of Parkinson disease. Selegiline delays the need for carbidopa-levodopa and effectively prolongs the efficacy of pharmacotherapy. As with amantadine, its action diminishes rapidly; the therapy is viable for only 12 to 24 months.

Selegiline is metabolized in the liver into two metabolites: amphetamine and methamphetamine. These metabolites may be responsible for the most common adverse effect of selegiline, which is insomnia. Concurrent administration of selegiline with carbidopa-levodopa may enhance adverse effects such as orthostatic hypotension, dyskinesias, nausea, and psychological disturbances.

MEMORY CHIP !

P Carbidopa-Levodopa

- Used as dopaminergic agent to treat Parkinson disease
- Most contraindications: known hypersensitivity, allergy to tartrazine, melanoma, closed-angle glaucoma, or breast-feeding
- Most common adverse effects: abnormal movements, orthostatic hypotension, GI effects,
- Most serious adverse effects: neuroleptic malignant syndrome—common with abrupt cessation of drug; precautions with cardiac, pulmonary, and peptic ulcer diseases, diabetes mellitus, psychosis and pregnancy
- Maximizing therapeutic effects: take drug on empty stomach, reduce protein in diet
- Minimizing adverse effects: titrate drug upward to avoid GI effects, titrate drug downward to avoid neuroleptic malignant syndrome
- Most important patient education: caution about hypotension and "on-off syndrome"

Selegiline (Zelapar) is a new orally disintegrating tablet for Parkinson disease for patients with difficulty swallowing. Selegiline (Emsam) is a transdermal system for the treatment of depression (Chapter 19). The transdermal system is ineffective in treating Parkinson disease.

Rasagiline

Rasagiline (Azilect) is the newest FDA-approved drug for symptomatic treatment of Parkinson disease and in non-human subjects has been shown to slow Parkinson disease progression. Like selegiline, it inhibits MAO-B. It is approved for use as an initial single-drug therapy in early Parkinson disease, and as an addition to carbidopa-levodopa in more advanced disease. Rasagiline may interact with tyramine-rich foods or beverages such as cheese and red wine. Drug–drug interactions may also occur with dietary supplements or amines contained in many cough or cold medications. Patients need to avoid these sources of tyramine and amines when taking rasagiline. Like other Parkinson medications, this drug may cause dyskinesias, hallucinations, and hypotension.

Drugs Significantly Different From P Carbidopa-Levodopa

Dopamine Agonists

The various dopamine agonists differ in chemical structure, duration of action, and side effects. The response to a particular dopamine agonist varies considerably between individuals, so that if one dopamine agonist does not offer benefit or causes adverse effects, another agonist may be tried.

Bromocriptine

The pharmacologic action of a dopamine agonist differs from that of carbidopa-levodopa. Bromocriptine (Parlodel), a dopamine agonist, is an oral synthetic agent that has been used to treat Parkinson disease for many years. Its other indications include acromegaly, amenorrhea, galactorrhea,

infertility, and prolactin-secreting pituitary adenomas. It is being investigated for use in treating insulin resistance in patients with type 2 diabetes mellitus.

Bromocriptine works by stimulating D_2 receptors and antagonizing D_1 receptors in the hypothalamus and striatum. For treating Parkinson disease, the effect is to increase the availability of dopamine. Additionally, bromocriptine suppresses prolactin secretion from the anterior pituitary gland, enabling ovulation and ovarian function in amenorrheic patients and suppressing lactation in women with normal ovarian activity.

The adverse effects of bromocriptine therapy limit its use. Symptoms such as psychiatric disturbances, nausea, and orthostatic hypotension are very common. Bromocriptine exacerbates pre-existing conditions such as psychiatric illness, peripheral vascular disease, and peptic ulcer disease. In addition, bromocriptine may cause patients with a history of MI to experience serious cardiac problems.

Bromocriptine should not be administered with drugs that antagonize its actions. Such drugs include those that increase the concentration of prolactin, such as haloperidol (Haldol), loxapine (Loxitane), molindone (Moban), MAOIs, imipramine (Tofranil), amitriptyline (Elavil), methyldopa (Aldomet), phenothiazines, and reserpine (Serpalan). Estrogens or progestins can produce amenorrhea or galactorrhea and should not be given concurrently.

Pergolide

Pergolide (Permax), is another ergot-derived dopamine agonist that is similar to bromocriptine in action, with 10 times the potency of bromocriptine at the D_2 receptors. It has two actions that are different than bromocriptine. It also stimulates D_1 receptors and it affects 5-HT_{2B} receptors on heart valves. Pergolide directly activates dopamine receptors in the striatum and on heart valves, inhibits the secretion of prolactin, and decreases luteinizing hormone. The effects on prolactin secretion persist much longer than the antiparkinsonian action.

Because pergolide is a potent dopamine receptor agonist, it should not be administered with dopamine receptor antagonists (i.e., neuroleptics such as phenothiazines, haloperidol, and thiothixene). Dopamine receptor antagonists can antagonize the effects of pergolide.

Adverse effects of pergolide are nausea, vomiting, confusion, hallucinations, lightheadedness, and fainting. A rare side effect known as fibrosis (thickening or scarring of the membrane lining of body organs) has also been reported. Like cabergoline, it may increase the risk for newly diagnosed cardiac valve regurgitation.

In 2007, pergolide in its brand-name and generic forms was withdrawn from the U.S. market because of studies that implicated the drug in causing serious heart-valve damage. Pergolide may still be available in markets outside of the United States.

Pramipexole

Pramipexole (Mirapex) is the third dopamine agonist used to treat Parkinson disease. Carbidopa-levodopa is converted in the brain into dopamine. In contrast, dopamine agonists such as pramipexole help alleviate the symptoms of Parkinson disease by acting directly on dopamine receptors in the brain. Pramipexole is a selective agonist at D_2 and D_3 receptors in the brain. It is more selective for these receptors than either bromocriptine or pergolide.

Pramipexole has been approved for treating both early and late stages of Parkinson disease. With early-stage monotherapy, pramipexole (like selegiline) delays the need for carbidopa-levodopa, thus extending the pharmacotherapeutic benefits of carbidopa-levodopa when it is used to treat more advanced stages of Parkinson disease. Additionally, in later stages of Parkinson disease, co-administering pramipexole and carbidopa-levodopa can decrease the dosage of carbidopa-levodopa by 25%. This reduction decreases the potential for carbidopa-levodopa's adverse effects.

In the early stages of Parkinson disease, the most frequent adverse effects of pramipexole are nausea, dizziness, drowsiness, insomnia, and postural hypotension. In advanced stages of Parkinson disease, additional adverse effects include dyskinesias, extrapyramidal syndromes (abnormal involuntary movements), and hallucinations. Inform patients that postural hypotension may occur more frequently during initial treatment and that hallucinations can occur at any time during the course of treatment. Pramipexole may cause sleep attacks. Should this occur, the patient should notify the provider and refrain from activities that require mental alertness. Monitor patients with pre-existing renal dysfunction carefully.

Ropinirole

Ropinirole (Requip), the last dopamine agonist, is similar to pramipexole. Like pramipexole, ropinirole may be used in early Parkinson disease or in later stages in conjunction with carbidopa-levodopa. In addition, ropinirole is FDA approved for the treatment of restless legs syndrome. With ropinirole, the dose of carbidopa-levodopa may be reduced, which may in turn help decrease the on–off fluctuations that affect some patients who have been on carbidopa-levodopa for many years.

Administering ropinirole as monotherapy can induce adverse effects in every system of the body. In the autonomic nervous system, the most common adverse effects include diaphoresis, flushing, and dry mouth. In the overall body, the most common adverse effects include weakness, chest pain, dependent edema, fatigue, malaise, pain, and peripheral edema. Cardiovascular adverse reactions include atrial fibrillation, extrasystoles, hypertension, hypotension, orthostatic hypotension, palpitations, sinus tachycardia, and syncope (sometimes with sinus bradycardia). Most cases of syncope occurring with ropinirole therapy are reported more than 4 weeks after initiation and are usually associated with a recent increase in dosage. In the GI system, common adverse effects include abdominal pain, anorexia, dyspepsia, flatulence, and nausea and vomiting. The most common adverse reactions affecting the CNS and peripheral nervous system include dizziness, hyperesthesia, restlessness, and vertigo. The metabolic and nutritional adverse effect is weight loss, whereas respiratory adverse effects include bronchitis, dyspnea, pharyngitis, rhinitis, sinusitis, visual impairment, and xerophthalmia (conjunctival dryness).

Psychiatric adverse reactions include amnesia, impaired concentration, confusion, hallucinations, drowsiness, and yawning. There have been many reports of patients who have fallen asleep while driving or performing other normal daytime activities while taking ropinirole. The episodes have occurred as late as 1 year after initiating treatment. Some patients have reported feeling completely alert before these events. It is not clear whether the medication, the sleep status of the patient, or the Parkinson disease itself contributed to these episodes.

In addition to the above adverse effects, ropinirole in combination with carbidopa-levodopa may induce additional effects, including dyskinesia, falls, headache, hypokinesia, paresis, paresthesias, tremor, constipation, diarrhea, dysphagia, flatulence, hypersalivation, anemia, upper respiratory infections, pyuria, urinary incontinence, and diplopia. Furthermore, anxiety, abnormal dreaming, hallucinations, nervousness, and somnolence (drowsiness) may also occur. The potential advantage of ropinirole over carbidopa-levodopa is a lower incidence of dyskinesia and lower propensity to induce adverse psychiatric effects. Like pramipexole, ropinirole may also cause sleep attacks. Ropinirole is contraindicated during pregnancy because it may cause fetal harm.

Catecholamine O-Methyl Transferase Inhibitors

Tolcapone

Tolcapone (Tasmar) inhibits the enzyme COMT, which degrades dopamine in the periphery of the body. The higher and more sustained plasma concentrations of levodopa that result translate into more constant dopaminergic stimulation in the brain, which in turn leads to greater effects on the signs and symptoms of Parkinson disease. The decreased destruction of levodopa allows a decrease in the daily dosage of carbidopa-levodopa. Tolcapone is indicated for treating Parkinson disease in patients who are experiencing fluctuations in symptoms and are not responding to or are not appropriate candidates for other adjunctive therapies.

COMT also metabolizes medications other than levodopa, including dopamine, dobutamine, epinephrine, norepinephrine, isoproterenol, methyldopa, and bitolterol. The dosage of these agents may have to be reduced in patients who are treated with tolcapone. Because COMT and MAO are the two major enzyme systems involved in the metabolism of catecholamines, the possibility exists that the combined use of tolcapone and a nonselective MAOI such as phenelzine or tranylcypromine would inhibit most pathways involved in normal catecholamine metabolism. Therefore, the concurrent use of these agents should be avoided. However, tolcapone can be used with the selective MAO-B inhibitors selegiline or rasagiline, because these agents have been used together in antiparkinsonian regimens without difficulty.

The most frequent adverse effects of tolcapone are dyskinesia, nausea, increased daytime sleepiness, dystonia, orthostatic hypotension, diarrhea, dizziness, and hallucinations. Tolcapone may elevate liver transaminase concentrations in the blood. Because of reports of fatal liver injury, the manufacturers of tolcapone advise that its use should be reserved for patients who do not respond to or are not appropriate candidates for other available treatments. Extensive liver function testing is required for all patients before and during therapy.

Entacapone

Entacapone (Comtan) is the second COMT inhibitor to be approved and is indicated as an adjunct to carbidopa-levodopa in treating patients with idiopathic Parkinson disease who experience the signs and symptoms of end-of-dose "wearing-off." This agent has no antiparkinsonian effect of its own, and it must be administered with carbidopa-levodopa. Like tolcapone, adding entacapone to a carbidopa-levodopa regimen increases the bioavailability of levodopa. Entacapone is also available as a fixed-dose combination pill with carbidopa-levodopa (Stalevo).

Entacapone has the same adverse effect profile as tolcapone, with the exception that entacapone is not associated with hepatotoxicity or clinically important elevations of liver enzymes. This exception represents an important advantage over tolcapone. Potential drug–drug interactions with entacapone are similar to those for tolcapone.

Centrally Acting Anticholinergic Drugs

The centrally acting anticholinergic drugs work by blocking the access of acetylcholine to cholinergic receptors in the striatum. Centrally acting anticholinergic drugs are less effective than carbidopa-levodopa. They can be used to decrease tremors and rigidity as a monotherapy approach in early Parkinson disease or in combination with dopaminergic drugs in later stages. They are used with caution in older patients because of the potential for severe CNS effects. The anticholinergics used most frequently in treating Parkinson disease are benztropine (Cogentin), diphenhydramine (Benadryl), and trihexyphenidyl (Artane). For additional information concerning anticholinergic drugs, see Chapter 14.

© ANTI-AMYOTROPHIC LATERAL SCLEROSIS DRUGS

Historically, there has not been specific pharmacotherapy for treating ALS. In December 1995, the FDA approved riluzole (Rilutek), the first drug for treatment of ALS (Table 21.3). Riluzole, the prototype anti-ALS drug, does not cure ALS. Rather, it is used to delay the need for tracheostomy or mechanical ventilation in patients who have ALS. Research for additional ALS medications is ongoing.

Nursing Management of the Patient Receiving Ⓟ Riluzole

Core Drug Knowledge

Pharmacotherapeutics

Riluzole is indicated for treating ALS because it slows down the disease's progression by delaying for several months the loss of muscle strength and limb function. The drug is given to extend survival time before tracheostomy is necessary; it is not a cure.

Pharmacokinetics

Riluzole is administered orally in 50-mg doses every 12 hours. Its onset of action is slow, and its duration of action is 3 to 5 days. Well absorbed from the GI tract, riluzole has a half-life of 12 hours. Low protein diets may extend the length of time required to reach stable serum drug levels. Hepatic metabolism of riluzole is extensive, producing six major and several minor metabolites. The cytochrome P-450 enzyme system is involved in hydroxylation and glucuronidation. The main isozyme involved in hydroxylation is CYP1A2. Riluzole crosses the placenta and enters breast milk.

Excretion of riluzole is mainly renal and 5% fecal. Riluzole is largely excreted as metabolites, with about 2% excreted as unchanged drug. Renal clearance of riluzole is individualized, possibly because of the variability of CYP1A2 (see Table 21.3).

Pharmacodynamics

The etiology of ALS is unknown. One of the leading theories of its pathogenesis is that motor neurons are injured by glutamate, a major excitatory brain neurotransmitter.

TABLE 21.3   Summary of Selected Drugs for the Management of Amyotrophic Lateral Sclerosis

Drug (Trade) Name	Selected Indications	Route and Dosage Range	Pharmacokinetics
© Anti-ALS Agents			
Ⓟ riluzole (Rilutek)	ALS	*Adult:* PO, 50 mg q 12 h *Child:* Not recommended	*Onset:* Slow *Duration:* 3–5 d $t_{1/2}$: 12 h
creatine	ALS	*Adult:* PO, 1 packet dissolved 1 fruit juice daily	*Onset:* Rapid *Duration:* Unknown $t_{1/2}$: Unknown

Although the mode of action of riluzole in treating ALS is also unknown, it may work by inhibiting glutamate release and inactivating sodium channels found in damaged neurons which indirectly reduces glutamate receptor stimulation.,

Contraindications and Precautions

The only contraindication to riluzole therapy is a hypersensitivity to any of its components. However, many precautions are issued.

Riluzole has affected fetal development and viability in animal studies; however, adequate studies on human pregnancy have not been completed. It is assigned to FDA pregnancy category C and should be administered only when the benefits to the mother outweigh the risks to the fetus throughout pregnancy. Nursing women need to be advised to avoid breast feeding due to excretion in human breast milk.

Hepatic disease, renal disease, or renal impairment can affect the clearance of riluzole, which is extensively metabolized in the liver and excreted in the urine. Patients with pre-existing hepatic or renal disease should be given riluzole with caution.

Adverse Effects

Evaluating adverse effects caused by riluzole can be difficult because ALS has several manifestations that may be mistaken for adverse effects. In reviewing the adverse effects for patients taking riluzole, consider natural disease progression.

Potential side effects are muscle fatigue, nausea, dizziness, diarrhea, anorexia, vertigo, and somnolence. When these symptoms become troublesome, treatment should be discontinued. Riluzole increases levels of hepatic enzymes in 50% of patients. This increase occurs in patients with no history of hepatic injury. Rarely, jaundice may also occur.

Many potentially adverse reactions have been reported with riluzole therapy, involving every system of the body. However, these adverse reactions have occurred in less than 1% of patients receiving riluzole. One of the most serious potential adverse effects is neutropenia. Although such reactions are rare, a complete blood count (CBC) should be monitored for the patient's safety.

Drug Interactions

As previously mentioned, riluzole may cause hepatic injury. The potential exists for increased risk for hepatic injury when riluzole is used concurrently with potentially hepatotoxic drugs. Additionally, drugs that induce the hepatic enzyme system may also increase the risk for hepatic injury.

The principal isoenzyme involved in the metabolism of riluzole is CYP1A2. Inhibitors or inducers of this enzyme may change plasma concentrations, resulting in toxic or subtherapeutic concentrations of the drug. Table 21.4 presents agents that may interact with riluzole.

Assessment of Relevant Core Patient Variables
Health Status

Elicit a careful history, including any pre-existing hepatic or renal dysfunction. Assess also for a history of cigarette smoking. Communicate any positive findings to the prescriber.

It is important to complete a physical examination of the patient before initiating therapy. Riluzole can induce

TABLE 21.4	Agents That Interact with P Riluzole	
Interactants	Effect and Significance	Nursing Management
CYP1A2 inhibitors • amitriptyline • caffeine • quinolones • theophylline	Administering riluzole with drugs that inhibit CYP1A2 has the potential to increase plasma concentrations of riluzole by decreasing the rate of clearance.	Monitor for toxicity. Monitor serum plasma levels.
CYP1A2 inducers • cigarette smoke • charcoal-broiled foods • omeprazole • rifampin	Administering riluzole with substances that induce CYP1A2 has the potential to increase plasma concentrations of riluzole by increasing the rate of clearance.	Monitor for efficacy of riluzole therapy. Monitor serum plasma levels.
hepatic enzyme inhibitors • barbiturates • carbamazepine	Administering riluzole with hepatic enzyme inducers has the potential to increase the risk for hepatotoxicity.	Monitor liver function tests. Monitor for signs of hepatic dysfunction.
hepatotoxic drugs • allopurinol • aminoglycosides • leflunomide • methyldopa • methotrexate • sulfasalazine	Administering riluzole with other drugs known for their hepatotoxic effects has the potential to increase the risk for hepatotoxicity.	Monitor liver function tests. Monitor for signs of hepatic dysfunction.

adverse effects in every body system. With the exception of hepatic injury, the chance of these adverse reactions is less than 1%. Baseline data are helpful if any of the reactions should occur. Document baseline CBC and renal and hepatic function tests for all patients.

Life Span and Gender

Older patients are more likely to have age-related hepatic and/or renal function changes. Although no specific recommendations for dosage in older adults have been made, older patients need to be more closely monitored for adverse effects.

The metabolism of riluzole depends largely on the activity of a specific isozyme, CYP1A2. This isozyme reportedly is more active in men than women. Higher blood concentrations of riluzole and its metabolites may be present in women, which may increase the risk for adverse effects in women. Continually assess female patients for these effects.

Lifestyle, Diet, and Habits

Evaluate the patient's diet for high fat content, use of caffeine products, and high intake of charcoal-broiled foods, and determine whether the patient is a smoker. The absorption of riluzole may be diminished by up to 20% in patients who consume a high-fat diet. Caffeine products can inhibit CYP1A2, resulting in increased serum concentration of riluzole. Conversely, charcoal-broiled foods and tobacco smoking can induce CYP1A2, which may increase the elimination of riluzole from the body.

Environment

Riluzole is usually administered in the home environment. Assess patients for their ability to understand the prescriber's directions and to physically self-administer drugs. Appropriate home care referrals are necessary for patients unable to self-medicate. Riluzole is extremely expensive. Evaluate patients' financial circumstances and refer patients and families for social services as appropriate.

Culture and Inherited Traits

Determine whether the patient is of Japanese descent. Riluzole clearance in ethnic Japanese patients is 50% less efficient than in whites. It is uncertain whether this effect is related to a difference in metabolic function in ethnic Japanese or to environmental factors such as smoking, alcohol or coffee intake, or diet.

Nursing Diagnoses and Outcomes

- Risk for Injury related to hepatic dysfunction, anemia, and CNS and cardiovascular effects of riluzole therapy
  Desired outcome: *The patient will immediately report any signs of hepatic dysfunction (fatigue, rash, jaundice), anemia (fatigue, sore throat, easy bruising), or CNS or cardiovascular effects to the prescriber.*
- Disturbed Thought Processes related to adverse CNS effects
  Desired outcome: *The patient will remain oriented and able to communicate effectively.*

Planning and Intervention

Maximizing Therapeutic Effects

Administer riluzole with a full glass of water. To increase bioavailability, it is best for riluzole to be taken on an empty stomach, at least 1 hour before or 2 hours after meals. For patients who will be self-medicating, explain the importance of correct administration.

Minimizing Adverse Effects

At the beginning of therapy, riluzole may cause dizziness or sedation. Caution the patient to refrain from driving, using machinery, or performing tasks that require mental alertness until the effects of riluzole have been established.

Providing Patient and Family Education

- It is most important to explain to patients and their families that riluzole will not change the course of the disorder. At best, riluzole will delay the need for tracheostomy and mechanical ventilation. Patients must understand what the eventual sequelae of ALS are and have a legal document in place if they choose to refuse life-sustaining measures.
- Advise patients to take riluzole on an empty stomach at 12-hour intervals. Teach patients to eat a low-protein diet. Also, advise patients to refrain from caffeine, alcohol, and charcoal-broiled foods.
- Advise patients of the potential adverse effects of riluzole. Because progression of the disease may mimic common adverse effects, patients should always contact the prescriber if any symptoms should occur.
- Advise patients about the importance of regular follow-up and the need for periodic blood testing. Present symptoms of hepatic dysfunction and emphasize the importance of contacting the prescriber if any appear.

Ongoing Assessment and Evaluation

Coordinate regular follow-up evaluations of the patient. At each visit, evaluate the patient for the onset of adverse effects and complete a physical examination. CBC and ALT levels should be taken monthly during the first 3 months of treatment, then every 3 months for the remainder of the first year. After the first year, ALT levels should be monitored periodically. Patients with elevated ALT levels require more frequent monitoring. Discontinuation of

CRITICAL THINKING SCENARIO

RILUZOLE AND REALITY

Mrs. Baxter has been diagnosed with ALS. She has moderate weakness in her extremities and uses a walker to ambulate. During your home visit, Mr. Baxter tells you, "I'm so glad they have started my wife on riluzole. I was thinking of having our attorney come over and do all that paperwork about the will because I was so scared. Now I don't have to."

1. How would you respond to Mr. Baxter?

2. What specific topics would you cover with him?

riluzole therapy should be considered when ALT levels become five times the normal range. During each encounter with the patient, reinforce the necessity of dietary and smoking restrictions.

Effective therapy should delay deterioration of the respiratory muscles. The patient should acknowledge the importance of contacting the prescriber immediately if any adverse reactions occur. The patient should also acknowledge the importance of periodic re-evaluation by the prescriber.

Drugs Significantly Different From P Riluzole
Creatine

Creatine monophosphate is a dietary supplement granted FDA orphan drug status for use in patients with ALS. It is similar to the natural compound creatine phosphate, which is an essential component of the energy-converting system in muscle cells. Creatine's primary function is to maintain adenosine triphosphate (ATP) levels within muscle. Muscles use the energy supplied by ATP during anaerobic activity, such as lifting weights. Creatine also promotes an anabolic environment in the muscle, which promotes protein synthesis that is important for muscle growth and repair. Creatine may also be combined with the antibiotic minocycline for managing ALS. Two clinical studies have shown no significant differences in respiratory, motor or functional capacity in ALS populations; although both studies showed an improved survival trend (Shefner, 2004; Rosenfeld, 2009).

Creatine should be used cautiously in people with pre-existing renal disease that produces renal impairment or renal failure. Creatine generates an increased amount of creatinine that must be eliminated by the kidneys. Studies have not been done to show the safety of creatine in children or during pregnancy.

Drugs for Symptom Abatement

Patients with ALS are affected by diverse symptoms, including spasticity, muscle cramping, depression, gastric reflux, excessive salivation, viscous phlegm, pain, constipation, urinary

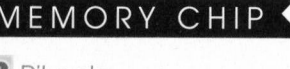
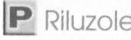

MEMORY CHIP

P Riluzole

- Used to manage ALS delaying need for a ventilator
- Most contraindications: hypersensitivity to riluzole components
- Most comman adverse effects: neutropenia, multiple system impact
- Maximizing therapeutic effects: decrease protein intake; avoid caffeine, charcoal-broiled foods, tobacco, and alcohol
- Minimizing adverse effects: avoid tasks requiring mental alertness until riluzole effects known
- Most important patient education: teach to obtain CBC and ALT levels monthly times 3, then every 3 months

urgency, and in the final stages of the disease, breathing difficulty. Drugs used to decrease spasticity include baclofen, tizanidine, and diazepam (see Chapter 16). For muscle cramps, patients may be prescribed quinine, baclofen, or clonazepam (see Chapters 16 and 18). Gastric reflux is managed with use of histamine-2 blocking agents or proton pump inhibitors (see Chapter 51). For excessive salivation, patients are prescribed anticholinergics or antihistamines (see Chapters 14 and 48). Viscous phlegm can be decreased with guaifenesin (see Chapter 48). Pain is managed initially with acetaminophen or nonsteroidal anti-inflammatory drugs (NSAIDs) such as ibuprofen (see Chapter 24). As the disease progresses, pain management may require narcotic administration (see Chapter 23).

Constipation is a major problem and may be treated with laxatives, prune juice, enemas, or a bowel program (see Chapter 51). Urinary urgency is controlled with tolterodine (see Chapters 14 and 55). Because many of these drugs can be purchased on an over-the-counter basis, educate the patient to consult with the prescriber before using these drugs in an effort to avoid drug–drug interactions.

C ANTI-MULTIPLE SCLEROSIS DRUGS

Although there is no cure for MS, various drugs are available to modify the disease course, treat exacerbations, and manage symptoms (Table 21.5). Pharmacotherapy for MS uses a multilayered approach. Drugs used to affect the progress of the disease are called "ABC therapy." These drugs are interferon beta-1a (Avonex), interferon beta-1b (Betaseron), and glatiramer (Copaxone). The interferons are also used in managing hepatitis C and other disorders and are discussed in Chapter 54. Glatiramer is the prototype drug for managing MS.

Nursing Management of the Patient Receiving P Glatiramer
Core Drug Knowledge
Pharmacotherapeutics

Glatiramer is used to reduce the frequency of attacks in patients with relapsing-remitting MS, It slows the development of new lesions on the myelin sheath and reduces disability. Advantage of glatiramer acetate over interferon beta drugs is the absence of flu-like symptoms.

Pharmacokinetics

The pharmacokinetics of glatiramer in humans has not been studied, and no direct and sensitive analytical method exists for measuring glatiramer in serum. In animal studies, it is readily absorbed after subcutaneous injection, and no evidence exists of any tissue accumulation of glatiramer (see Table 21.5).

Pharmacodynamics

Glatiramer acetate is a synthetic chemical that is similar in structure to myelin basic protein. Its action is unclear; however, the drug is thought to modify immune processes that cause MS by acting as a decoy to locally generated autoantibodies. This effect results in decreased tissue destruction.

TABLE 21.5	Summary of Selected Drugs for the Management of Multiple Sclerosis		
Drug (Trade) Name	Selected Indications	Route and Dosage Range	Pharmacokinetics
C Anti-MS Agents			
P glatiramer (Copaxone)	Relapsing-remitting MS	*Adult:* SC, 20 mg every day	*Onset:* Unknown *Duration:* Unknown $t_{1/2}$: Unknown
interferon beta-1a (Avonex, Rebif)	Relapsing and secondary-progressive MS	*Adult:* Avonex: 30 mcg IM every week Rebif: 44 mcg SC 3× wk	*Onset:* Rapid *Duration:* $t_{1/2}$: Avonex, 8.6–10 h $t_{1/2}$: Rebif, 69 h
interferon beta-1b (Betaseron)	Relapsing MS	*Adult:* SC, 250 mcg every other day	*Onset:* Rapid *Duration:* Rapidly degraded $t_{1/2}$: 8 min–4.3 h
mitoxantrone (Novantrone)	Worsening relapsing-remitting MS and progressive-relapsing or secondary-progressive MS	*Adult:* Four times a year by IV infusion in a medical facility; lifetime limit of 8–12 doses (12 mg/m² every 3 mo)	*Onset:* varies *Duration:* 28 days $t_{1/2}$: 5.8 days (median)
natalizumab (Tysabri)	MS	*Adult:* IV, 3 mg/kg every 4 wk	*Onset:* 1 mo *Duration:* 8 wk $t_{1/2}$: 90–170 h
dalfampridine (Ampyra)	MS	*Adult PO:* 10 mg every 12 h *Child:* Not receeommended	*Onset:* 3–4 h *Duration:* unknown $t_{1/2}$: 5.2–6.5 h
fingolimod (Gilina)	MS, relapsing	*Adult:*	*Onset:* 12–16 h *Duration:* unknown $t_{1/2}$: 5–9 days

Contraindications and Precautions

Absolute contraindications include intravenous (IV) administration and hypersensitivity to mannitol. It should be used with caution in already immunocompromised patients and in patients receiving vaccinations, because the action of glatiramer is to modulate the immune response.

Adverse Effects

Glatiramer may induce chest pain or tightness, breathing difficulties, hives or severe rash, pounding heartbeat, and unusual muscle weakness or tiredness. Patients should be instructed to report these symptoms to the provider immediately.

The most common adverse effects include lumps, pain, and redness at the site of injection. Other common adverse effects include anxiety, bleeding, inflammation, itching, dizziness, flushing, joint aches, muscle stiffness, nausea or vomiting, tremor, and weakness. These symptoms may become quite bothersome, and the patient should contact the provider if they do not subside.

Drug Interactions

Although no known drug–drug interactions occur, glatiramer can alter the results of a Papanicolaou test (Pap smear); therefore, women should tell their obstetrician-gynecologist if they are taking glatiramer.

Assessment of Relevant Core Patient Variables

Health Status

Elicit a patient history, especially questioning hypersensitivity to mannitol or pre-existing immunocompromise. Document patient limitations related to MS to serve as a baseline for evaluating the effectiveness of glatiramer therapy.

Life Span and Gender

Glatiramer is an FDA pregnancy category B drug. It is not known whether glatiramer is excreted into breast milk. Glatiramer has not been studied in patients younger than 18 years.

Lifestyle, Diet, and Habits

Glatiramer has no known interactions with lifestyle, diet, or habits. Much literature has been published on the appropriate diet for a patient with MS, but diet does not affect the use of glatiramer.

Environment

Glatiramer may be used in any environment and is most frequently self-administered at home. It should be kept in the refrigerator before use and should not be exposed to high temperature or intense light. Emphasize the need to place used syringes in a puncture-resistant container and then return the container to the prescriber for proper disposal.

Nursing Diagnoses and Outcomes

- Weakness related to glatiramer injection
  Desired outcome: The patient will recognize weakness and take measures to decrease its impact on activities of daily living.
- Skin Integrity, Impaired, related to injection site reactions
  Desired outcome: The patient will employ strategies to minimize injection site reactions.
- Disturbed Sensory Perception related to anxiety and dizziness
  Desired outcome: The patient will notify the provider if these adverse effects occur.

Planning and Intervention

Maximizing Therapeutic Effects

Explain that glatiramer should be kept in the refrigerator until it is used. Teach the patient and family how to transfer sterile water into the glatiramer using aseptic technique, gently swirl the vial, and then allow the mixture to stand at room temperature until all of the powder is dissolved. Advise the patient and family using glatiramer from prefilled glass syringes to allow the syringe to sit at room temperature approximately 20 minutes before injection.

Minimizing Adverse Effects

Teach the patient and family to administer the subcutaneous injection correctly. It is important to deliver the medication into the subcutaneous tissues and avoid either intradermal or IV administration. Explain the importance of rotating the injection site so that no one spot is used more than once a week.

Providing Patient and Family Education

- Review the potential adverse effects of glatiramer, focusing on how common adverse effects differ from serious effects that should be reported to the provider.
- Review location of subcutaneous injection sites. Subcutaneous sites include the thigh, back of the hip, stomach, and upper arm.
- Review reconstitution procedure of glatiramer powder.
- Review aseptic technique for subcutaneous administration.
- Review appropriate disposal of syringes.

Ongoing Assessment and Evaluation

Elicit a history from the patient at each subsequent visit, focusing on improvement of baseline symptoms or acquisition of new symptoms. Question the patient about adverse effects and document them in the medical record.

Effective therapy should decrease the intensity of baseline symptoms and prolong the intervals between acute exacerbations of MS. The patient should recognize important adverse effects that require contact with the provider.

Drugs Significantly Different From
P Glatiramer

Interferons

Interferon beta is also used in treating MS. Interferon beta is available as interferon beta-1a (Avonex, Rebif) and interferon

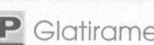

MEMORY CHIP

P Glatiramer

- Used to delay progression of MS
- Most contraindications: IV administration, hypersensitivity
- Most common adverse effects: chest pain/tightness, difficulty breathing, hives/severe rash
- Maximizing therpauetic effects: keep medication refrigerated, reconstitute medication correctly
- Minimizing adverse effects: correct procedure to administer subcutaneous injections
- Most important patient education: avoid accidental IV administration

beta-1b (Betaseron). Interferon beta works by decreasing interferon gamma and other proinflammatory cytokines. Interferon gamma is believed to be one of the major factors responsible for triggering the autoimmune reaction resulting in MS. In MS, T cells migrate across the blood–brain barrier in response to interferon gamma and attack antigens on nervous system tissues. By reducing interferon gamma, T-cell migration is reduced, resulting in less tissue damage. Another action of interferon beta is an increased production of nerve growth factor, which may have a favorable effect of remyelination.

A recombinant process produces both drugs, but in other respects, they differ greatly. In therapy, 1-mg interferon beta-1a represents 200 million units of activity, whereas 1 mg of interferon beta-1b represents 32 million units of activity. Interferon beta-1a shows a reduction in relapse rate and slows disease progression. Interferon beta-1b shows a very substantial clinical benefit in decreasing relapse but has not been shown to slow disease progression. Interferon beta-1a (Avonex) is administered by intramuscular injection, whereas interferon beta-1a (Rebif) and interferon beta-1b (Betaseron) is administered by subcutaneous injection. Interferon beta-1a has not been associated with injection-site necrosis, whereas interferon beta-1b is associated with an injection-site reaction in roughly 85% of patients. Administration of acetaminophen or ibuprofen prior to and 24 hours after interferon beta injections helps to decrease injection-site reactions. Interferon beta should not be administered to patients with hypersensitivity to interferon beta or albumin. It is an FDA pregnancy category C drug and should be avoided during pregnancy because of the risk of spontaneous abortion. It should also be avoided during breast-feeding because serious adverse reactions may occur in the infant. Interferon beta is also used with caution in patients who have a history of cardiac arrhythmias, heart failure, or MI. Suicidal ideation has occurred in patients on interferon beta therapy. It is unclear whether this ideation is related to the drug or to the disease process of MS.

Mitoxantrone

Mitoxantrone (Novantrone) is a chemotherapeutic drug initially developed for certain forms of cancer. An immune system suppressor, it is delivered intravenously in a medical setting. Mitoxantrone is contraindicated for patients with heart disease, liver disease, or certain blood disorders because it may make these problems worse. It is also contraindicated during pregnancy because it may cause birth defects. Mitoxantrone is withheld in patients with hepatic impairment and elevated liver enzymes as no tests exist to predict drug clearance rates to determine dosage adjustments.

Mitoxantrone may cause serious, even fatal, heart damage. To avoid potential heart damage, the drug is typically limited to 12 doses over a period of 2 to 3 years. It may also suppress neutrophils and platelets, increasing the patient's risk of infection or bleeding. Frequent tests are needed to monitor heart function and hematopoietic status while taking mitoxantrone.

Common but less serious side effects of mitoxantrone include nausea, hair loss, increased risk of infections, especially urinary tract infections, menstrual cycle changes, mouth sores, and diarrhea or constipation. Mitoxantrone causes the urine to become blue-green for 24 to 48 hours after each treatment. Although this color change is harmless, the patient should be informed prior to treatment.

The patient taking mitoxantrone should not receive any immunizations without the physician's approval.

Natalizumab

Natalizumab (Tysabri), a monoclonal antibody, is an alpha-4 integrin antagonist in a class known as selective adhesion molecule inhibitors. It is FDA approved to treat patients with relapsing forms of MS to reduce the frequency of symptom flare-ups or exacerbations of the disease. Natalizumab is recommended for patients who have had inadequate response to, or are unable to tolerate, other approved MS therapies.

Natalizumab works by blocking the ability of $\alpha_4\beta_1$ integrin and $\alpha_4\beta_7$ integrin to bind to their receptive vascular-cell adhesion molecules. Binding to adhesion molecules is an important step in white cells crossing arterial blood vessels and entering into the brain to attack myelin in MS. Because of its different mechanism of action, natalizumab is expected to be an important therapeutic option in the management of MS.

Natalizumab was previously taken off the market because some patients developed progressive multifocal leukoencephalopathy (PML). PML, which is caused by a common virus called the JC virus, is characterized by demyelination or destruction of the myelin sheath. Symptoms include speech disturbances, ataxia, vision loss, mental deterioration, paralysis, and, ultimately, coma. Natalizumab is now available under a restricted distribution program called TOUCH, and prescribing physicians and patients must enroll in a mandatory registry program. The drug is given intravenously every 4 weeks at registered infusion centers. The risk of PML rises as the number of natalizumab infusions administered increases. In addition, immune reconstitution inflammatory syndrome (IRIS) has been noted in patients with PML after natalizumab has been discontinued. IRIS is a rare and severe inflammatory problem that results in deteriorating patient status after the immune system has been restored (U.S. Department of Health & Human Services, 2010).

Natalizumab is contraindicated for patients with a compromised immune system and patients taking other drugs that suppress the immune system. Common adverse effects include headache, fatigue, infections, depression, joint pain, and menstrual disorders.

Dalfampridine

Dalfampridine (Ampyra) is one of the newer drugs on the market to treat MS. Indication for the use of dalfampridine is to improve speed of ambulation in patients experiencing any of the four major forms: relapsing-remitting, primary progressive, secondary progressive, and progressive-relapsing. Over 85% of MS patients suffer difficulties with ambulation and perceive this symptom to be one of the most challenging issues of their disease. Dalfampridine may be used as a monotherapy or as an adjunct with above noted MS pharmacotherapeutic therapies.

The demyelinzation of nerves in MS results in potassium channels on nerve surfaces becoming exposed and potassium leaking from the channels resulting in disrupted electrical current. The mechanism of action of dalfampridine is to block the potassium channels on nerve surfaces, which improves nerve impulse conduction leading to improved speed of ambulation.

Common adverse effects of dalfampridine are urinary tract infections, insomnia, headache, and dizziness. The two most serious adverse effects are seizures and hypersensitivity reactions. Due to the risks of seizures, a risk evaluation and mitigation strategy was created to clearly communicate to patients the likelihood of seizures related to the consumption of higher than recommended dosages of the medication.

No drug interactions were identified in clinical trials; yet not all drug interactions have been studied at this time. Complete medication lists need to be obtained from all patients being prescribed this product. Contraindications to the use of dalfampridine include a history of seizures and renal failure. The drug is excreted via the kidneys and renal impairment may lead to toxic levels of the medication within the bloodstream, resulting in an increased risk of seizures. Dalfampridine is a Class C Pregnancy medication, indicating insufficient evidence support for use in humans with potential benefits possibly outweighing the risks. No information is currently available related to the transmission of the drug via breast milk for lactating mothers. Consequently, lactating mothers are advised to discontinue use of dalfampridine when breastfeeding. Safety has not been established in patients less than 18 years of age (Bastings, 2010). An annual expense of greater than $10,000. to the insurer could restrict the use of this medication.

Fingolimod

Fingolimod (Gilena) is a new oral treatment for relapsing remitting MS, which was approved by the US FDA Advisory Council in June 2010 and which it is anticipated will have full FDA approval for use in September 2010. Fingolimod is from a new group of disease-modifying agents from the class of sphingosine 1 phosphate-receptor modulators and is indicated to decrease the number of MS exacerbations and impede the development of physical disabilities. Fingolimod acts on the sphingosine 1 phosphate receptor sites found on thymocytes and lymphocyte surfaces, leading to the impounding of lymphocytes into secondary lymph organs. The reduction of lymphocytes circulating within the body reduces the possibility of autoimmune reactions on the myelin sheath.

Common adverse effects of fingolimod are headache, nasopharyngitis, fatigue, and upper respiratory infections. The more serious adverse effects include bradycardia, AV heart blocks, liver enzyme elevation, and macular edema. As a result of the incidence of the more serious adverse effects, recommendations for use are expected to include first-time dosing in monitored situations, where ECG may be performed to assess for bradycardia and AV heart blocks for six hours after dosing, with atropine/isopreterenol available for treatment as needed. Subsequent monitoring of liver enzymes, ophthalmic assessments, and pulmonary function tests are advised related to the incidence of liver enzyme elevation, macular edema, MS relapse, and risk for decreased pulmonary function. Because of the immunosuppressive effect of fingolimod, more research is needed to more thoroughly determine the risk for malignancies and infections. Further studies are expected to determine the lowest effective dose as current studies have investigated the effects of 0.5 mg and 1.25 mg, with determination that 0.5 mg would be permitted for prescriptive dosing at this time due to the risk for toxicity. Studies have not been conducted on patients with dysrhythmias or diabetes; therefore, the drug should be contraindicated in these populations. Other anticipated contraindicated populations include patients with histories of seizures, malignancies, or cardiac/pulmonary disorders. Pregnancy classification of the drug has yet to be determined. No information is currently available related to use in lactating mothers or children less than 18 years old. Few drug interactions were identified in clinical trials; yet not all drug interactions have been studied at this time. Complete medication lists need to be obtained from all patients being prescribed this product. Drug interactions to be considered include a rise in fingolimod levels with concomitant administration of ketoconazole due to CYP4F2 inhibition. An additional potential drug interaction is the simultaneous administration of beta blockers or calcium channel blockers with fingolimod, which could increase the risk of AV heart blocks and bradycardia.

Drugs for Symptom Abatement

As in ALS, many other classes of drugs are used to manage the symptoms that accompany MS. Pharmacotherapy for symptoms of MS may include glucocorticoids to shorten the duration of an acute attack or delay the progression of optic neuritis. Other drugs useful in managing symptoms include tolterodine for bladder incontinence; carbamazepine or gabapentin for shooting sensory pain; baclofen, carisoprodol, or benzodiazepines for muscle spasticity; and tizanidine for low back pain.

OTHER MOVEMENT DISORDERS AND RELATED DRUG THERAPY

The following disorders and the drugs used to treat them are important to include in any discussion of drugs used to treat movement disorders. The drugs commonly used to treat these disorders are covered in depth in other chapters in this textbook. Therefore, the disorders and drugs commonly used to treat them are discussed briefly in this chapter. For more detailed information about the specific drugs, refer to the appropriate chapter in this textbook.

Myasthenia Gravis

Myasthenia gravis (MG) is an autoimmune disorder that impairs the receptors for acetylcholine at the myoneural junction. It occurs more frequently in young women and men over 50 years of age. In this disease, immunoglobulin G (IgG) antibodies to acetylcholine receptors are formed, then block and ultimately destroy the receptors so that the muscle cannot be stimulated. The patient experiences skeletal muscle weakness and rapid fatigue of the affected muscles. Proximal muscles are affected rather than distal muscles.

The first symptoms of MG are usually weakness of the eye muscles and ptosis. Oropharyngeal muscle weakness and difficulty with chewing, swallowing, or talking may also be the presenting symptoms. The severity of weakness fluctuates throughout the day, generally increasing in the afternoon or as the environmental temperature rises. The course of the disease is usually progressive; however, in some cases, weakness is restricted to the ocular muscles. Spontaneous improvement may occur, but symptoms generally recur as the disease progresses.

Diagnosis of MG is based on the edrophonium (Tensilon) test. In this test, the patient is induced into weakness by being required to maintain a position. Edrophonium, a short-acting acetylcholinesterase inhibitor, is administered intravenously. Intramuscular neostigmine may also be used. With either drug, the patient should have an increase in muscle strength that dissipates after the duration of action of the drug. The most sensitive test for MG is a single-fiber electromyelogram (SFEMG), which measures "jitter" in the involved muscle(s).

As with other movement disorders, MG has no cure. The drugs of choice for MG are cholinesterase inhibitors such as neostigmine (Prostigmin) or pyridostigmine (Mestinon) and are discussed in Chapter 14. Although corticosteroids (Chapter 48), cyclophosphamide (Chapter 57), and immunosuppressants (Chapter 54) such as azathioprine (Imuran) and cyclosporine (Sandimmune) may be used for MG treatment, all of them are used off label except for prednisone.

Huntington Disease

Huntington disease (chorea) is an inherited disorder that remains undiagnosed until midlife, when symptoms first occur. The two main symptoms of the disease are progressive mental status changes leading to dementia and choreiform (rapid, jerky) movements. The inhibitory neurotransmitter GABA is depleted in the basal nuclei and substantia nigra.

Levels of acetylcholine in the brain also appear to be reduced. However, dopamine is unaffected.

Early symptoms of Huntington disease include mood swings; depression; irritability or trouble driving; and difficulty learning new things, remembering facts, or making decisions. As the disease progresses, personality changes, moodiness, and behavior disturbances occur. The dementia, which accompanies progressive disease, may be related to excessive amounts of dopamine. As atrophy of the brain continues, rigidity and akinesia develop.

There is currently no effective treatment to prevent or delay the progression of Huntington disease, and death usually occurs within 10 to 20 years after the appearance of the first clinical symptoms. Treatment of choreiform movements have traditionally included antipsychotic drugs such as haloperidol (Haldol) or phenothiazines, which block dopamine receptors. These drugs are discussed in depth in Chapter 17. In 2008, the FDA approved the first drug in the United States called xenazine (tertrabenazine) for treatment of Huntington Chorea symptoms. Xenazine's mechanism of action is unknown, but believed to reversibly deplete dopamine, serotonin, norepinephrine and histamine from nerve terminals leading to a decrease in chorea or involuntary jerky movements. Adverse effects observed include increasing cognitive impairment, Parkinsonism, rigidity, depression/suicide, sedation and disability. Genotyping for CYP2D6 is necessary for higher dosages to determine the patient's metabolizer status. Poor metabolizers need to have their dose reduced particularly if receiving a strong CYP2D6 inhibitor such as paroxetine (Paxil). Dosing is titrated slowly up with careful assessment for depression, sedation and dysphagia. Xenazine may interfere with their ability to perform complex motor/mental skills leading to difficulty driving a car or operating machinery. Alcohol and CNS depressants may interact with xenazine potentiating sedation. Xenazine is contraindicated in impaired hepatic function, suicidal patients, untreated depression, and patients receiving MOA inhibitors or reserpine and is a category C for pregnancy (Yero & Rey, 2008). Research to find other agents that are useful in treating this disorder is ongoing.

Gilles de la Tourette Disease

Gilles de la Tourette disease (Tourette syndrome, [TS]) is an autosomal dominant inherited tic disorder appearing in childhood and characterized by multiple motor or vocal tics lasting more than 1 year. Patients may also have obsessive-compulsive behavior, attention deficit hyperactivity disorder, or other psychiatric disorders. Coprolalia (involuntary utterances of vulgar or obscene words) and echolalia (involuntary parrot-like repetition of a word or sentence just spoken by another person) can occur but are rare.

Motor and vocal tics from this disease may respond to haloperidol (Haldol) and similar D_2 receptor blockers (see Chapter 17). Up to 80% of patients with TS initially benefit from haloperidol, sometimes dramatically; however, only approximately 20% of patients continue haloperidol for an extended period. Patients often discontinue the drug because of the emergence of side effects such as excessive fatigue, weight gain, dysphoria (affective disorder characterized by anxiety and depression), parkinsonian symptoms, intellectual dulling, memory problems, personality changes, feeling "zombie-like," akathisia (inner restlessness observed with fidgeting and rocking actions), school or social phobias, loss of libido, sexual dysfunction, and, especially after chronic use of high doses, tardive dyskinesia.

Pimozide (Orap) is another drug used for TS. It is chemically distinctive from haloperidol and phenothiazines, with potent dopamine-blocking properties. Its side effects are similar to those of haloperidol but may be less severe and appear in fewer patients. Routine electrocardiographic studies before and periodically during treatment are advised because of potential cardiotoxicity.

Another drug useful in treating TS is clonidine (Catapres), an imidazoline compound with alpha-adrenergic agonist activity. In low doses, clonidine decreases the release of central norepinephrine, resulting in decreased motor tics and improving attention problems. Clonidine has a low incidence of associated side effects, but most important, it does not have the potential to cause tardive dyskinesia. Clonidine is covered in depth in Chapter 28.

CHAPTER SUMMARY

- Movement disorders are chronic, severe, and debilitating.
- Parkinson disease is a naturally occurring disorder characterized by rigidity, rest tremor, bradykinesia or akinesia, and postural instability.
- Parkinsonism is a syndrome of symptoms resembling Parkinson disease but caused by trauma, drugs, or infection.
- Amyotrophic lateral sclerosis (ALS) is a neuromuscular degenerative disease that progresses quickly until the patient experiences respiratory compromise and ultimately death.
- Drugs used to treat movement disorders are not curative.
- Dopaminergic drugs are used to treat Parkinson disease by increasing the action of dopamine in the CNS. The prototype dopaminergic drug is carbidopa-levodopa (Sinemet, Parcopa).
- Dopamine agonists are drugs that stimulate dopamine receptors in the brain. They do not need to be converted into dopamine in order to achieve their effect.
- Drugs that decrease the action of acetylcholine (anticholinergic drugs) are also used to treat Parkinson disease.
- The only FDA-approved anti-ALS drug is the prototype riluzole (Rilutek).
- Riluzole delays the need for tracheostomy and mechanical ventilation.
- Multiple classes of medications are used to manage the symptoms of ALS.
- Multiple sclerosis is generally treated with the "ABC" approach. This term is derived from the names of the drugs interferon beta-1a (Avonex), interferon beta-1b (Betaseron), and glatiramer (Copaxone).

• Other movement disorders and the drugs used to treat them include myasthenia gravis, neostigmine; Huntington disease (chorea), xenazine; haloperidol or phenothiazines; Tourette syndrome, haloperidol, clonidine, and fluphenazine.

QUESTIONS FOR STUDY AND REVIEW

1. How do dopaminergic and anticholinergic drugs work to decrease the symptoms of Parkinson disease?
2. Why is carbidopa-levodopa considered more efficient than levodopa alone?
3. What is neuroleptic malignant syndrome? When is it most likely to occur?
4. What is a bradykinetic episode?
5. What diet restrictions should be discussed when a patient starts carbidopa-levodopa therapy?
6. What assessments should you make throughout carbidopa-levodopa therapy?
7. What is the goal of riluzole therapy?
8. For patients taking riluzole, why is assessing adverse effects difficult?
9. What dietary restrictions should you discuss with the patient starting riluzole therapy?
10. How does glatiramer differ from the interferons in managing multiple sclerosis?
11. What pharmacodynamic similarities of glatiramer and interferon beta may affect patient adherence to therapy?

NEED MORE HELP?

Chapter 21 of the Study Guide to Accompany *Drug Therapy in Nursing*, 4th Edition, contains NCLEX-style questions and other learning activities to reinforce your understanding of the concepts presented in this chapter. For additional information or to purchase the study guide, visit thePoint.

REFERENCES

Bastings, E. (2009). Memorandum to Department of Health & Human Services, Public Health Service, Food and Drug Administration. Subject: NDA 22250 for Fampridine Sustained Release (Amaya). Retrieved from http://www.fda.gov/downloads/Advisory Committees/CommitteesMeetingMaterials/Drugs/PeripheralandCentralNervousSystemDrugsAdvisory Committee/UCM185663.pdf.

Choudry, R. B., Galvez-Jimenez, N., Cudkowicz, M. E. (2010). Pharmacologic treatment of amyotrophic lateral sclerosis. *Up To Date*. Retrieved from http://www.uptodate.com/contents/pharmacologic-treatment-of-amyotrophic-lateral-sclerosis?source=search_result&selectedTitle=6%7E150.

Facts and Comparisons. (2010). *Drug facts and comparisons*. Philadelphia: Lippincott Williams & Wilkins.

Food and Drug Administration. (2010). Center for Drug Evaluation and Research (CDER): Peripheral and Central Nervous System Drugs Advisory Committee Meeting on June 10, 2010. Fingolimod (NDA 22–527) Background Package. Retrieved from http://www.fda.gov/downloads/AdvisoryCommittees/CommitteesMeetingMaterials/Drugs/PeripheralandCentralNervousSystemDrugsAdvisory Committee/UCM214670.pdf.

Koda-Kimbal, M. A., Young, L. Y., Kradian, W. A., et al. (2008). *Applied Therapeutics: The Clinical Use of Drugs (9th Ed)*. Philadelphia, PA: Lippincott Williams & Wilkins.

Olek, M. J. (2010). Treatment of relapsing-remitting multiple sclerosis in adults. *Up To Date*. Retrieved from http://www.uptodate.com/contents/treatment-of-relapsing-remitting-multiple-sclerosis-in-adults?source=search_result&selectedTitle=1%7E15.

Rosenfeld, J., et al. (2008). Creatine monohydrate in ALS: Effects on strength, fatigue, respiratory status and ALSFRS. *Amyotrophic Lateral Sclerosis*, 9(5):266–272. Retrieved from http://www.ncbi.nlm.nih.gov/pmc/articles/PMC2631354/.

Shefner, J. M., et al. (2004). A clinical trial of creatine in ALS. *Neurology*, 63(9):1656–1661. Retrieved from http://www.ncbi.nlm.nih.gov/pubmed/15534251.

Tarsey, D. (2009). Pharmacologic treatment of Parkinson disease. *Up to Date*. Retrieved from http://www.uptodate.com/contents/pharmacologic-treatment-of-parkinson-disease?source=search_result&selectedTitle=4%7E150.

Tatro, D. S. (2011). *Drug interaction facts: the authority on drug interactions*. Philadelphia, PA: Lippincott Williams & Wilkins.

U.S. Department of Health & Human Services: Food and Drug Administration. Tysabri (Natalizumab): Update of Healthcare Information. Retrieved from http://www.fda.gov/SafetyAlertsforHumanMedicalProducts/ucm199965.htm.

Yero, T. & Rey, J. A. (2008). Tetrabenazine (Xenazine), An FDA-approved treatment option for Huntington's disease-related chorea. *Pharmacy and Therapeutics*. 33(12):690–694. Retrieved from http://www.ncbi.nlm.nih.giv/pmc/articles/PMC2730806/.

Drugs Stimulating the Central Nervous System

Learning Objectives

At the completion of this chapter the student will:

1. Describe the physiology of the central nervous system (CNS) as related to arousal and stimulation.

2. Describe the various therapeutic uses of CNS stimulants.

3. Identify core drug knowledge about pharmacotherapies that stimulate the CNS.

4. Identify core patient variables relevant to drugs that stimulate the CNS.

5. Relate the interaction of core drug knowledge to core patient variables for therapies that stimulate the CNS.

6. Generate a nursing plan of care from the interactions between core drug knowledge and core patient variables for therapies that stimulate the CNS.

7. Describe nursing interventions to maximize therapeutic and minimize adverse effects for drugs that stimulate the CNS.

8. Determine key points for patient and family education for drugs that stimulate the CNS.

Key Terms

analeptics
anorectic
attention deficit
   hyperactivity disorder

cataplexy
hypercapnia
hypnagogic hallucinations
narcolepsy

obesity
overweight
sleep paralysis

Drugs Stimulating the Central Nervous System

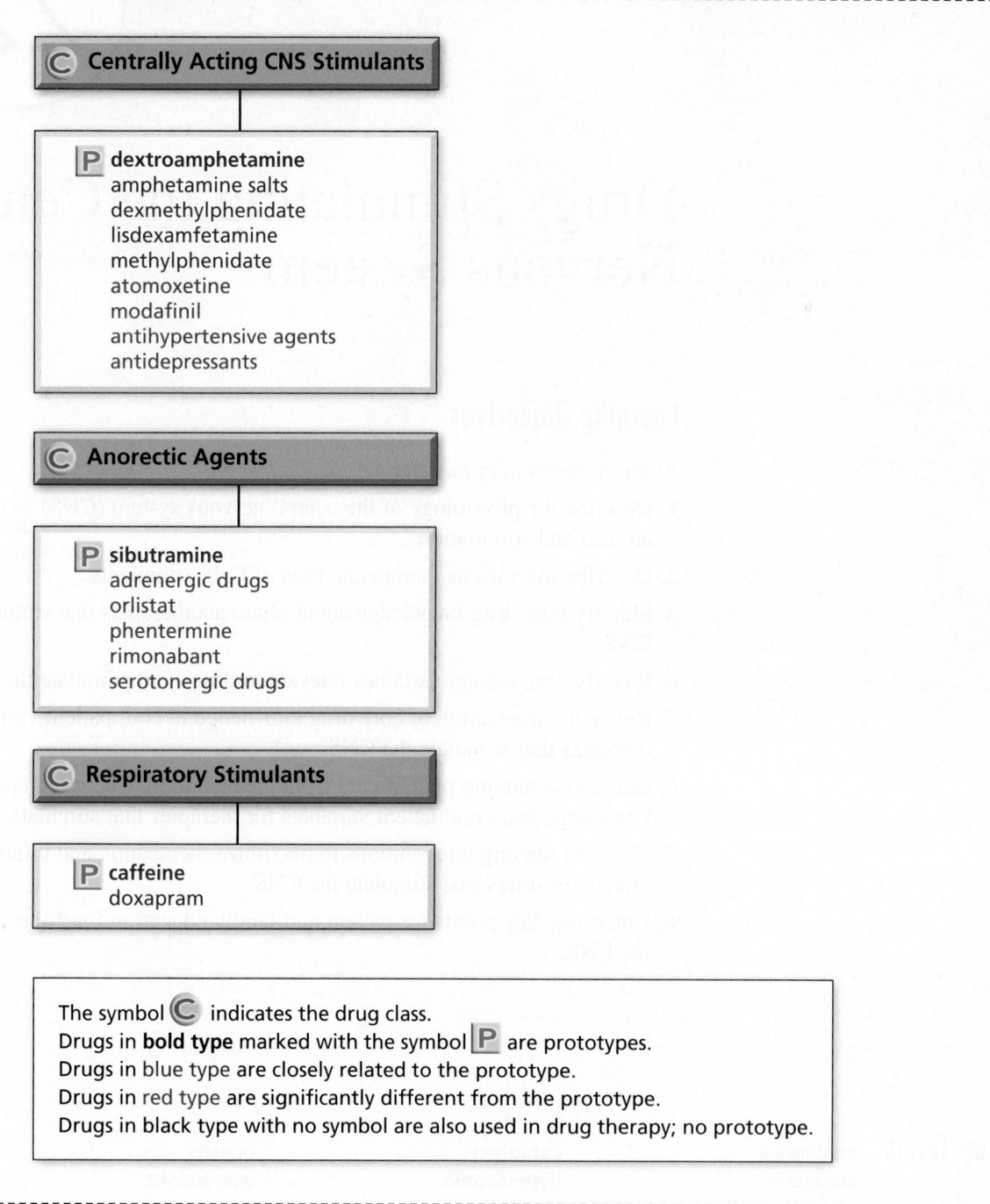

Centrally Acting CNS Stimulants

P **dextroamphetamine**
amphetamine salts
dexmethylphenidate
lisdexamfetamine
methylphenidate
atomoxetine
modafinil
antihypertensive agents
antidepressants

Anorectic Agents

P **sibutramine**
adrenergic drugs
orlistat
phentermine
rimonabant
serotonergic drugs

Respiratory Stimulants

P **caffeine**
doxapram

The symbol C indicates the drug class.
Drugs in **bold type** marked with the symbol P are prototypes.
Drugs in blue type are closely related to the prototype.
Drugs in red type are significantly different from the prototype.
Drugs in black type with no symbol are also used in drug therapy; no prototype.

Many substances are used to stimulate the central nervous system (CNS). These substances, sometimes called **analeptics,** include drugs that are used for therapeutic effects and nontherapeutic effects, both legal and illegal. Substances with therapeutic effects are categorized as central, anorectic, or respiratory stimulants. Central and respiratory stimulants are generally used to stimulate the CNS, whereas **anorectic** agents depress the appetite. The central stimulants are used to treat narcolepsy and as adjuncts in treating attention deficit hyperactivity disorder (ADHD). The anorectic agents suppress appetite or the sensation of hunger, mainly through serotonergic activity or central sympathomimetic effects. They are used as adjuncts to diet and exercise in the short-term management of moderate to severe obesity. The respiratory stimulants are rarely used, but as analeptics, they are representative of drugs that affect the brain stem and respiratory centers.

This chapter presents dextroamphetamine (Dexedrine), the prototype for centrally acting CNS stimulant drugs; phentermine (Adipex-P), the prototype anorectic agent; and caffeine, the prototype respiratory stimulant. In addition, this chapter discusses core drug knowledge, core patient variables, nursing management, potential nursing diagnoses, and patient education related to the use of these drugs.

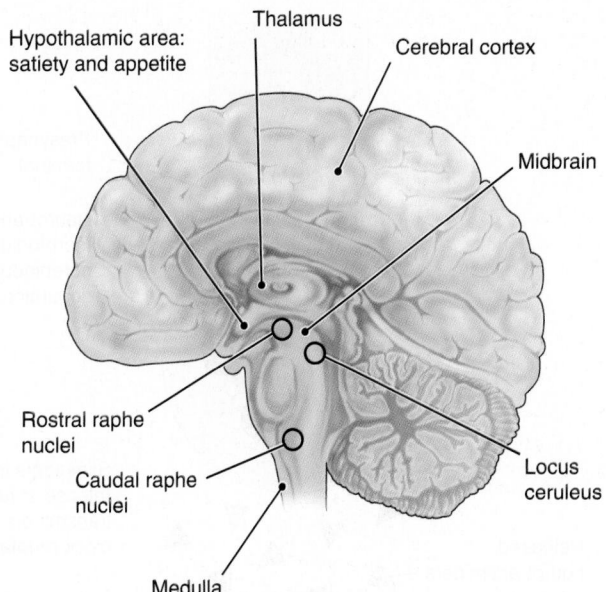

• FIGURE 22.1   Regulatory centers of the brain.

PHYSIOLOGY

The CNS is responsible for providing control systems and surveillance for many vegetative and conscious functions, including appetite, satiety, attention, arousal, activity, and respiration. The hypothalamus mediates appetite and satiety. Various sleep and arousal mechanisms are linked to the raphe nuclei and locus ceruleus in the pons and other parts of the reticular activating system (RAS).

The control of respiration occurs in the pons and medulla. Functional, structural, or lesional disorders may lead to disruptions in the usually smooth regulation of appetite, arousal, and activity. Figure 22.1 is a schema of the brain that shows the location of some regulatory centers involved in appetite, arousal, activity, and respiration.

At a synaptic level in the CNS, normal arousal mechanisms are affected through presynaptic release of neurotransmitters, such as norepinephrine, serotonin, and dopamine (Figure 22.2). These transmitters diffuse across the synaptic cleft to the postsynaptic effector cell, which is usually another neuron. The postsynaptic membrane contains receptors for the transmitters. In normal arousal, the transient combination of the transmitter with the receptor causes membrane changes that lead to propagation of the action potential. The transmitter can be metabolized by postsynaptic enzymes such as monoamine oxidase or removed from further activity through reuptake into the presynaptic storage vesicles. CNS stimulants may provoke an increased release

of neurotransmitters, a decreased reuptake of neurotransmitters, or inhibition of postsynaptic enzymes. The result is a heightened postsynaptic response, leading to increased arousal. Similar mechanisms occur in the sympathetic nervous system, where drugs such as the amphetamines act as indirect adrenergic agonists.

PATHOPHYSIOLOGY

The CNS stimulants are indicated in various disorders and conditions, including narcolepsy, ADHD, obesity, and respiratory stimulation.

Narcolepsy

Narcolepsy, a neurologic condition that affects approximately 1 of every 1,000 people, is characterized by irresistible bouts of rapid-eye-movement (REM) sleep during nonsleep cycles. Associated features include disturbed nocturnal sleep and REM sleep disturbances such as cataplexy, sleep paralysis, hypnagogic hallucinations, and abnormal sleep-onset REM periods. **Cataplexy** is a brief, sudden loss of motor control. In the person with narcolepsy, cataplexy usually manifests itself as a postural collapse to the ground, even though the person maintains full consciousness. **Sleep paralysis** usually precedes the onset of sleep and involves being unable to speak or move, even though awareness of external events remains intact. The elapsed time is usually brief but may seem inordinately long to the person who experiences it.

Hypnagogic hallucinations are auditory, visual, or kinesthetic sensations without stimuli, appearing in the transition period between wakefulness and sleep. For example, the waking person may sense another person in the room but

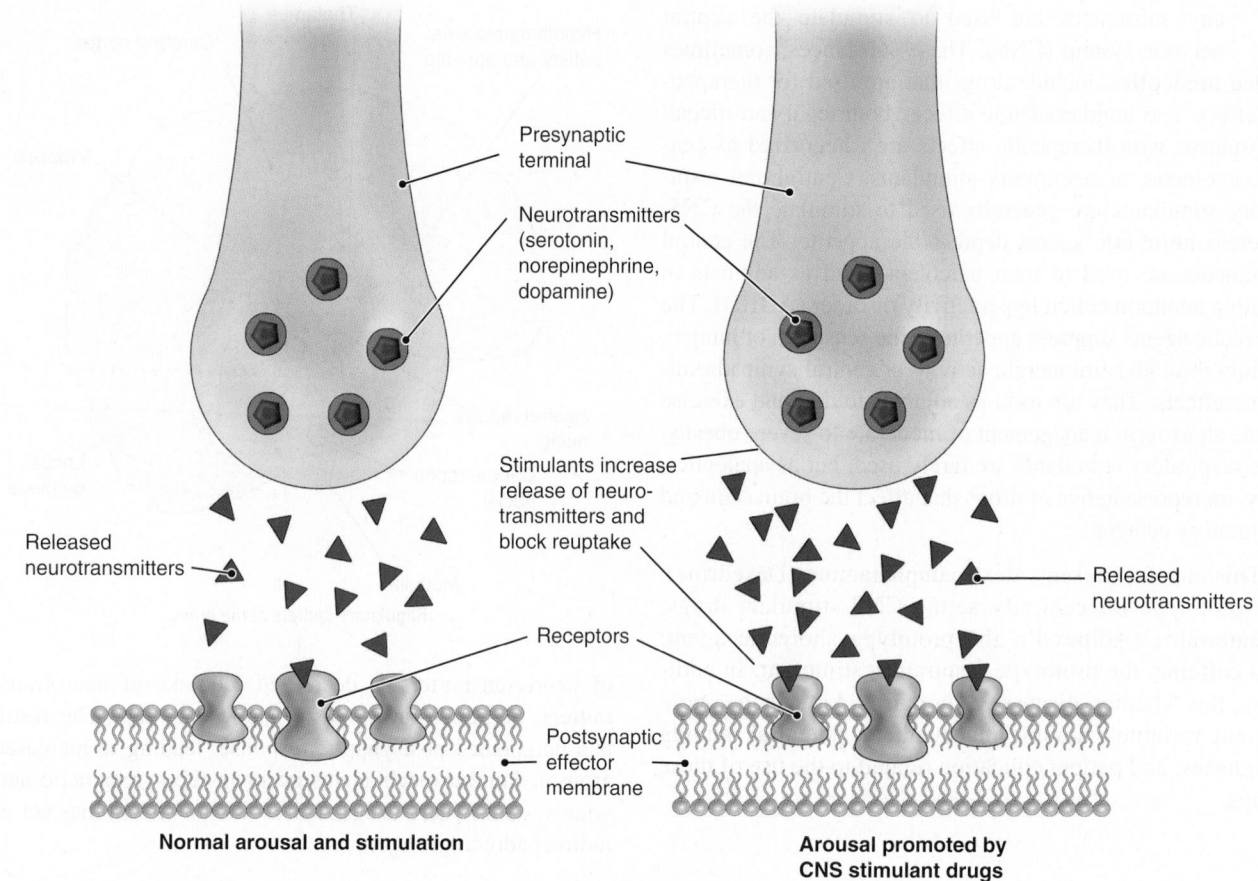

Presynaptic
terminal

Neurotransmitters
(serotonin,
norepinephrine,
dopamine)

Stimulants increase
release of neuro-
transmitters and
block reuptake

Released
neurotransmitters

Released
neurotransmitters

Receptors

Postsynaptic
effector
membrane

Normal arousal and stimulation

**Arousal promoted by
CNS stimulant drugs**

• FIGURE 22.2   CNS arousal.

when fully awake recognizes that he or she is alone. Most people notice such hypnagogic hallucinations occasionally; however, they occur with greater intensity and frequency in patients with narcolepsy. Restoration of more normal physiologic arousal leads to the return of more normal sleep-activity cycles and forms the basis of CNS stimulant pharmacotherapy for narcolepsy.

Attention Deficit Hyperactivity Disorder

Attention deficit hyperactivity disorder (ADHD) is the most prevalent chronic health issue affecting school-aged children. It is characterized by a persistent pattern of inattentiveness, hyperactivity, and impulsivity that is more frequent and severe than typically observed in people of a comparable developmental level (Box 22.1). In the United States, data from the Centers for Disease Control and Prevention indicate that in 2006, about 7.4% of children between 4 and 18 years of age were reported to have a history of ADHD (Bloom, 2007). The prevalence of ADHD in adults is estimated to be 4.4% (Antai-Otong, 2008). Comorbid states that may accompany ADHD include learning disabilities, conduct disorder, oppositional defiant disorder, depression or anxiety, bipolar disorder, and Tourette syndrome.

Current research suggests that ADHD has a biologic basis. Studies involving twins have demonstrated mean

hereditability to be 77% (Spencer, 2007). Genetic studies have shown alterations in several genes that affect the levels or functioning of the neurotransmitters dopamine, norepinephrine, or serotonin at nerve synapses in the brain. Stimulant drugs that are effective against ADHD are thought to work by altering the levels of dopamine and norepinephrine at the synapse. In addition to genetic influences, prenatal factors such as pregnancy or delivery complications, prematurity, and fetal exposure to alcohol or tobacco also increase the risk of ADHD.

The management of ADHD is complex but usually involves pharmacotherapy with one or more of the CNS stimulants, combined with behavior modification.

Overweight and Obesity

Obesity has become one of the major health issues in the United States. The increased number of patients with obesity threatens to overburden our health care system because it is closely associated with comorbid states such as hypertension, coronary artery disease, diabetes mellitus, and osteoporosis. According to the National Health and Nutrition Examination Survey (NHANES), an estimated one-third of adults, or 72 million people, in the United States are obese (NHANES, 2007). The latest reports from NHANES, the show a dramatic increase in obesity in the last 25 years,

Box 22.1 DIAGNOSTIC CRITERIA FOR ADHD

A. Either 1 or 2 applies.
1. Six (or more) of the following symptoms of **inattention** have persisted for at least 6 months to a degree that is maladaptive and inconsistent with developmental level:

Inattention
a) Often fails to give close attention to details or makes careless mistakes in schoolwork, work, or other activities
b) Often has difficulty sustaining attention in tasks or play activities
c) Often does not seem to listen when spoken to directly
d) Often does not follow through on instructions and fails to finish schoolwork, chores, or duties in the workplace (not due to oppositional behavior or failure to understand instructions)
e) Often has difficulty organizing tasks and activities
f) Often avoids, dislikes, or is reluctant to engage in tasks that require sustained mental effort (such as schoolwork or homework)
g) Often loses things necessary for tasks or activities (e.g., toys, school assignments, pencils, books, or tools)
h) Is often easily distracted by extraneous stimuli
i) Is often forgetful in daily activities

2. Six (or more) of the following symptoms of **hyperactivity-impulsivity** have persisted for at least 6 months to a degree that is maladaptive and inconsistent with developmental level:

Hyperactivity
a) Often fidgets with hands or feet or squirms in seat

b) Often leaves seat in classroom or in other situations in which remaining seated is expected
c) Often runs about or climbs excessively in situations in which it is inappropriate (in adolescents or adults, may be limited to subjective feelings of restlessness)
d) Often has difficulty playing or engaging in leisure activities quietly
e) Is often "on the go" or often acts as if "driven by a motor"
f) Often talks excessively

Impulsivity
g) Often blurts out answers before questions have been completed
h) Often has difficulty awaiting turn
i) Often interrupts or intrudes on others (e.g., butts into conversations or games)

B. Some hyperactive-impulsive or inattentive symptoms that caused impairment were present before 7 years of age.
C. Some impairment from the symptoms is present in two or more settings (e.g., at school [or work] or at home).
D. There must be clear evidence of clinically significant impairment in social, academic, or occupational functioning.
E. The symptoms do not occur exclusively during the course of a pervasive developmental disorder, schizophrenia, or other psychotic disorder and are not better accounted for by another mental disorder (e.g., mood disorder, anxiety disorder, dissociative disorder, or personality disorder).

American Psychiatric Association. (2000). Diagnostic and Statistical Manual of Mental Disorders (4th ed.). Text Revision. Washington, DC: Author.

but with little change between 2003–2004 and 2005–2006. Healthy People 2010 target obesity goal is a rate is 15%, which was last reached in 1980 and is far from the 2005 rate of 34.3% (Table 22.1).

Overweight refers to an excess of body weight compared to set standards. The excess weight may come from muscle, bone, fat, or body water. **Obesity** refers specifically to having an abnormally high proportion of body fat. One can be overweight without being obese, as in the example of a bodybuilder or other athlete who has a lot of muscle. However, many people who are overweight are also obese.

To determine obesity, the measurement of choice for researchers and health care providers is body mass index (BMI). BMI is a direct calculation based on height and weight and is not gender specific. To determine BMI, divide a person's weight in kilograms by height in meters squared (weight [kg]/height squared [m^2]). Although BMI does not directly measure percentage of body fat, it provides a more accurate measure of overweight and obesity than weight alone. Box 22.2 lists BMI index categories.

In addition to BMI, health professionals may rely on a person's waist measurement to determine the location of excess body fat and the corresponding health risks. Health risks increase as waist circumference increases. A woman whose waist measures more than 35 inches and a man whose waist measures more than 40 inches may be at particular

TABLE 22.1	Prevalence of Obesity in the United States

More than one third of adults, or over 72 million people, were obese in 2005-2006.

Obesity prevalence, by age and sex, and the Healthy people (HP) 2010 obesity target, adults aged 20 years older: United States, 2005–2006

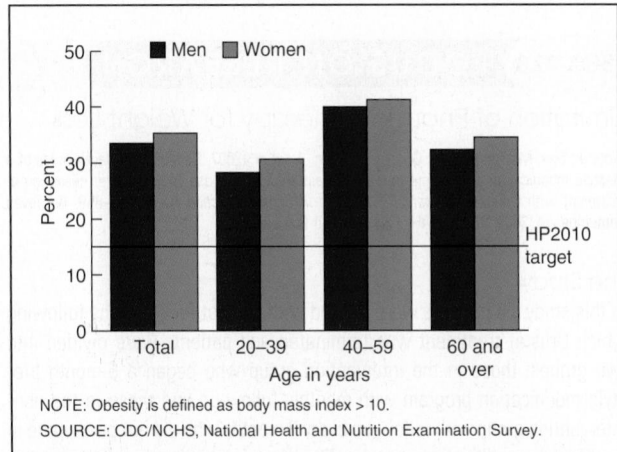

NOTE: Obesity is defined as body mass index > 10.
SOURCE: CDC/NCHS, National Health and Nutrition Examination Survey.

Obesity rates have increased dramatically in the last 25 years and among men, there was an increase in obesity prevalence between 1999 and 2006. There was no siginficant change in obesity prevalence, however, between 2003-2004 and 2005-2006 for men or women.

Box 22.2 **BODY MASS INDEX (BMI) CATEGORIES**

- Underweight: <18.5
- Normal weight: 18.5–24.9
- Overweight: 25–29.9
- Extremely obese: >40
- Children: >95th percentile for age and sex

risk for developing health problems. An increased percentage of abdominal or upper-body fat is related to the risk for developing heart disease, diabetes, high blood pressure, gallbladder disease, stroke, and certain cancers. Body fat concentrated in the lower body (e.g., around the hips) may be less harmful in terms of mortality and morbidity, with the exception of varicose veins and orthopedic problems.

Weight regulation is multifactorial. Key endocrine systems involved in weight regulation include the hypothalamic–pituitary axis, the leptin system, insulin, neuropeptide Y, leptin-regulated hormones, and the autonomic nervous system. Although major endocrine dysfunction may cause obesity, by far the most common causes are overeating and a sedentary lifestyle.

Treating obesity involves a combination of different methods, including modifying eating behavior, implementing and maintaining an exercise program, and using adjunctive pharmacologic therapy to reduce appetite (Box 22.3). Drugs used to manage appetite include serotonin agonists such as phentermine, stimulants such as methylphenidate, lipase inhibitors such as orlistat, and selective serotonin reuptake inhibitors (SSRIs) such as fluoxetine.. In morbidly obese patients, surgical intervention called bariatric surgery has been found to be most effective for long-term weight loss.

Respiratory Stimulation

In patients at risk for postoperative pulmonary complications, respiratory depression may be a complication arising from chronic obstructive lung disease and frequent hypercapnia.

Hypercapnia is a buildup of carbon dioxide levels that may result from pulmonary compromise, frank lung disease, or changes in ventilatory efficacy. The increased levels of carbon dioxide depress the CNS, including the respiratory center, and further compound the problem.

Preterm infants may experience hypercapnia because of their immature respiratory systems. They are prone to postoperative respiratory depression and apnea severe enough to warrant pharmacologic respiratory stimulation. Pharmacologic management of respiratory depression includes administering CNS stimulants such as caffeine and doxapram that act directly on the respiratory center to stimulate effective ventilation and reverse hypercapnia.

Ⓒ CENTRALLY ACTING CNS STIMULANTS

The centrally acting CNS stimulants are drugs that stimulate the CNS directly or indirectly. This group of drugs includes the amphetamines, methylphenidate, pemoline, and cocaine. The ideal and most widely used CNS stimulant is dextroamphetamine (Dexedrine), an amphetamine. This drug is the prototype for the purposes of discussing the central CNS stimulants. Table 22.2 presents a summary of selected CNS stimulants.

Nursing Management of the Patient Receiving Ⓟ Dextroamphetamine
Core Drug Knowledge
Pharmacotherapeutics
The major therapeutic uses of dextroamphetamine include treatment of narcolepsy and ADHD and anorectic adjunct therapy in obesity. Dextroamphetamine is occasionally used to treat refractory depression, which is an unlabeled use. As a stimulant, dextroamphetamine is classified as a Drug Enforcement Administration (DEA) Schedule II drug, which means its use is tightly controlled.

BOX 22.3 FOCUS ON RESEARCH

Limitation of Pharmacotherapy for Weight Loss

Woo, J., Sea, M., Tong, P., Ko, G., Lee, Z., Chan, J., et al. (2007, December). Effectiveness of a lifestyle modification programme in weight maintenance in obese subjects after cessation of treatment with Orlistat. *Journal of Evaluation in Clinical Practice, 13*(6), 853–859. Retrieved September 14, 2009, from CINAHL Plus with Full Text database.

The Study
In this study, 55 patients were treated with Orlistat for 6 months following which Orlistat treatment was terminated and patients were divided into two groups: those in the intervention group who began a 6-month lifestyle modification program with monthly follow-up and those in the non-intervention group with follow-up every 3 months who did not participate in the lifestyle modification program. The lifestyle modification program consisted of monthly group sessions with discussion on dietary management, physical activity, and exercise management, also providing group support.

Patients were given tailored menu plans based on their calculated BMR (basal metabolic rate) at the end of Orlistat treatment and daily food and activity diaries were collected. At the end of the 6-month period, patients from each group were measured. All patients in the non-intervention group had an increase in weight, BMI, waist and hip circumference, and percentage of body fat comparable to the magnitude of reduction obtained during the previous Orlistat treatment, where the intervention group maintained their weight loss.

Nursing Implications
Losing weight and keeping it off is a difficult task. The nurse needs to be a patient advocate. Review the importance of diet and exercise in combination with pharmacotherapy at each visit. Encourage the patient to keep a food and exercise diary and become involved in peer support groups to increase compliance. Be supportive—even if there is only a minimal weight loss.

TABLE 22.2 Summary of Selected Ⓒ CNS Stimulants

Drug (Trade) Name	Selected Indications	Route and Dosage Range	Pharmacokinetics
Stimulants			
Ⓟ dextroamphetamine (Dexedrine Dexedrine Spansules	ADHD, narcolepsy	Dexedrine *Adult:* PO, 5–60 mg/d in divided doses *Child (6–12 y):* PO, 2.5–40 mg/d in divided doses *Child:* Not recommended for children <6 y Dexedrine Spansules *Adult:* PO, 10–60 mg daily	*Onset:* 20–60 min *Duration:* 4–6 h $t_{1/2}$: 12 h
	ADHD, narcolepsy	*Child (6–12 y):* 2.5–5 mg/d to a maximum of 40 mg/day	*Onset:* 60–90 min *Duration:* 6–10 h $t_{1/2}$: 12h
amphetamine salts and dextroamphetamine (Adderall, Adderall XR)	ADHD	Adderall *Adult and adolescent:* PO, 5–60 mg/ 1–2×/d *Child 6–12 y:* 5 mg–40 mg/ 1–2×/d *Child 3–5 y:* PO, 2.5 mg once daily to a maximum of 0.1–0.5 mg/kg/d *Child <3 y:* safety and efficacy not established *Adult and adolescent:* PO, 5–60 mg/d in divided doses	*Onset:* 30–60 min *Duration:* 4–6 h $t_{1/2}$: 10–13 h
	Narcolepsy	*Child 6–12 y:* PO, 5–60 mg/d in divided doses *Child <6 y:* safety and efficacy not established Adderall XR *Adult, adolescent, and child >6 y:* PO, 10–30 mg once daily	
	ADHD	*Child <6 y:* safety and efficacy not established	*Onset:* 30–60 min *Duration:* 10–12 h $t_{1/2}$: 10–13 h
dexmethylphenidate (Focalin, Focalin XR)	ADHD	Focalin *Adult and child ≥6 y:* PO, 2.5–20 mg/d *Child <6 y:* safety and efficacy not established Focalin XR *Adult:* PO, 10–20 mg/d *Child >6 y:* 5–20 mg/d *Child <6 y:* safety and efficacy not established	*Onset:* 1–4 h *Duration:* 5 h $t_{1/2}$: 2.2 h
			Onset: 1–4 h *Duration:* 8–10 h $t_{1/2}$: 2–3 h
lisdexamfetamine (Vyvanse)	ADHD	*Child 6–12 y:* PO, 30–70 mg/d	*Onset:* <1 h *Duration:* 8–10 h $t_{1/2}$: <1 h
methylphenidate (Ritalin, Ritalin SR, Ritalin LA)	ADHD, narcolepsy	Ritalin *Adult:* PO, 5–60 mg/d in 2–3 divided doses, 30–45 min before meals *Child ≥6 y:* PO, 0.3–2 mg/kg/d in 2–3 divided doses, 30–45 min before meals; maximum dosage: 60 mg/d *Child <6 y (weight ≥25 kg):* PO, 2.5–5 mg twice daily before breakfast and lunch; maximum dose: 20 mg tid *Child <6 y (weight <25 kg):* PO, 2.5 mg twice daily before breakfast and lunch; maximum dose: 15 mg tid	*Onset:* 15–30 min *Duration:* 2.5–4 h $t_{1/2}$: 1.5–2.5 h
		Ritalin SR *Adult, adolescent, and child ≥6 y:* PO, 20 mg daily, to a maximum of 60 mg/d *Child <6 y:* safety and efficacy not established	*Onset:* 15–30 min *Duration:* 6–8 h $t_{1/2}$: 4 h
		Ritalin LA *Adult, adolescent, and child ≥6 y:* PO, 20 mg once daily in the morning; maximum of 60 mg/d *Child <6 y:* safety and efficacy not established	*Onset:* 15–30 min *Duration:* 8–10 h $t_{1/2}$: 2–7 h

(Continued)

TABLE 22.2   Summary of Selected ⒸCNS Stimulants *(continued)*

Drug (Trade) Name	Selected Indications	Route and Dosage Range	Pharmacokinetics
methylphenidate (Metadate CD, Metadate ER)	ADHD, narcolepsy	Metadate CD *Adult, adolescent, and child ≥6 y:* PO, 20 mg once daily in the morning; maximum: 60 mg/d *Child <6 y:* safety and efficacy not established	*Onset:* 15–30 min *Duration:* 8–9 h $t_{1/2}$: 6.8 h
		Metadate ER *Adult, adolescent, and child ≥6 y:* PO, 20 mg tid *Child <6 y:* safety and efficacy not established	*Onset:* 15–30 min *Duration:* 6–8 h $t_{1/2}$: 3–4 h
methylphenidate (Concerta)	ADHD	*Adult, adolescent, and child ≥6 y:* PO, initially 18 mg daily; maximum, 54 mg/d *Child <6 y:* safety and efficacy not established	*Onset:* 1 h *Duration:* 12 h $t_{1/2}$: 3.5 h
methylphenidate (Methylin, Methylin Chewable, Methylin ER)	ADHD Narcolepsy	Methylin; Methylin Chewable *Adult:* PO, 20–30 mg in divided doses, preferably before meals; maximum dose: 60 mg/d *Child >6 y:* 5 mg bid before breakfast and lunch; maximum dose: 60 mg/d	*Onset:* Rapid *Duration:* 4–6 h $t_{1/2}$: 3 h
		Methylin ER *Adult:* PO, 20 mg bid; maximum, 60 mg/d	*Onset:* 15–30 min *Duration:* 6–8 h $t_{1/2}$: 3–4 h
methylphenidate transdermal system (Daytrana)	ADHS	*Children 6–12 y:* transdermal patch; apply daily to hip and remove after 9 h	*Onset:* 3 h *Duration:* 12 h $t_{1/2}$: 3–4 h
Nonstimulants			
atomoxetine (Strattera)	ADHD	*Adult and child ≥6 y and weight ≥70 kg:* PO, 40–100 mg/d in 1 or 2 divided doses; maximum: 80 mg/d if administered with other cytochrome P-450 enzyme (CYP) 2D6 inhibitor *Adolescent and child ≥6 y and weight <70 kg:* PO, 0.5–1.2 mg/kg/d in 1 or 2 divided doses *Child <6 y:* safety and efficacy not established	*Onset:* Rapid *Duration:* Unknown $t_{1/2}$: 4–5.2 h
Guanfacine (Intuniv)	ADHD	*Child 6-17 y:* 1–4 mg ER daily	Onset: unknown Duration: 24 h T1/2: 18 h
modafinil (Provigil, Alertec)	Narcolepsy, obstructive sleep apnea, shift work, sleep disorder	*Adult:* 200–400 mg daily	*Onset:* Unknown *Duration:* 15 h $t_{1/2}$: Unknown

Pharmacokinetics

Following oral ingestion, dextroamphetamine has an onset of 20 to 60 minutes and a duration of 5 hours. The sustained-release form of the drug has an onset of 60 to 90 minutes and lasts 6 to 10 hours. The half-life ranges between 10 and 30 hours. Dextroamphetamine is metabolized by the liver and is excreted, partly unchanged and partly in the form of inactive metabolites, in the urine. This process peaks at 12 to 24 hours.

Pharmacodynamics

The exact mechanism of action of dextroamphetamine is unknown, although it is likely that indirect alpha- and beta-adrenergic activity mediates both central and peripheral effects. Dextroamphetamine causes the release of norepinephrine and, in higher doses, dopamine in adrenergic nerve terminals. It also interferes with the reuptake of dopamine. The sites of action in the CNS are the cerebral cortex and the RAS. The drug's anorectic effects are likely secondary to CNS stimulation in the hypothalamic satiety-feeding center.

Contraindications and Precautions

Dextroamphetamine is contraindicated in patients with advanced arteriosclerosis, symptomatic cardiovascular disease, moderate to severe hypertension, hyperthyroidism, known hypersensitivity or idiosyncratic reactions to other sympathomimetic drugs, glaucoma, or a history of drug abuse. Dextroamphetamine use in patients with these disorders places them at risk for hypertension, increased intraocular pressure, or abuse of the drug. Caution is warranted in older adults with even mild hypertension because the adrenergic stimulation of the amphetamines increases blood pressure.

Because of its pressor effects, dextroamphetamine is contraindicated during the first 14 days after discontinuing monoamine oxidase inhibitor (MAOI) therapy, because

MAOI therapy itself may predispose the patient toward elevated blood pressure. Therefore, this 14-day washout period for MAOIs must be observed to prevent hypertensive crisis.

Dextroamphetamine should be given very cautiously to children and adolescents with structural cardiac abnormalities or other serious heart problems. Sudden death and serious cardiac events have occurred in these patients, even with normal doses. Monitoring the growth and development of all children is important because amphetamines have been associated with growth suppression. Stimulant drugs should not be used in children with ADHD and concomitant Tourette syndrome or tics because stimulants exacerbate these motor disorders.

Dextroamphetamine is assigned to pregnancy category C, and women should not use it during the first trimester of pregnancy or during lactation. If its use is required during such periods, the prescriber should monitor treatment carefully to prevent fetal growth abnormalities or irritability in the breast-fed infant.

Some formulations of dextroamphetamine contain yellow dye No. 5 (tartrazine), which may cause allergic-type reactions (including bronchial asthma) in certain susceptible people. This sensitivity is rare, although it is frequently seen in patients who also have aspirin hypersensitivity.

Dextroamphetamine should be used with caution to avoid overdose or drug abuse. The least amount feasible should be prescribed or dispensed at any one time to minimize the possibility of overdosage. Patients should be advised not to discontinue therapy abruptly because rebound symptoms may occur. As tolerance develops, particularly to the anorectic effects of the drug, the recommended dose should not be exceeded in an attempt to increase the effect. Instead, the drug should be discontinued. Patients who have recently ceased smoking cigarettes or using other products that contain nicotine may show hypertensive sensitivity to dextroamphetamine, partly because of the absence of the vasoconstrictive toning effects of nicotine.

Adverse Effects

The most serious potential adverse effects for dextroamphetamine are sudden death, stroke, and MI, which may occur in patients with underlying serious cardiovascular disorders or structural abnormalities. Psychiatric adverse effects such as hearing voices, becoming suspicious for no reason, or becoming manic, even in patients who did not have previous psychiatric problems, have also occurred.

Dextroamphetamine may produce the prototypical effects of all CNS stimulants: decreased appetite, rebound irritability and depression, headache, jittery feeling, gastrointestinal (GI) upset, sleep difficulties, anxiety, and increased blood pressure or heart rate. Blood glucose may also elevate; therefore, patients with diabetes need to monitor their blood glucose closely. Ocular irritation, resulting from decreased lacrimation, and mydriasis are two visual adverse effects that may interfere with activities such as driving. Occasionally, patients with allergic tendencies may experience urticaria when taking dextroamphetamine. Finally, the pronounced sympathomimetic action of dextroamphetamine may lead to an inability to ejaculate and either increased or decreased libido. The FDA has issued a black box warning for dextroamphetamine, as well as other stimulant drugs used for ADHD. There is a high risk for dependency, nontherapeutic use, and the potential to distribute to others.

Drug Interactions

Considerable care must be exercised when administering dextroamphetamine with many other classes of drugs. One noteworthy feature of anorectic drugs is their ability to cause rapid change in nutritional status, which may lead to cachexia and hypoproteinemia and thus possibly alter the pharmacokinetics of other drugs. CNS depressants, if administered with CNS stimulants, counteract each other and leave only residual adverse effects. Table 22.3 lists agents that interact with dextroamphetamine.

Dextroamphetamine may cause elevations in plasma corticosteroid levels beyond normal diurnal variations, which may interfere with serum or urinary steroid determinations.

Maximal absorption of dextroamphetamine occurs in the alkaline environment of the small intestine. Therefore, acidic juices and fruits may impair GI absorption. In addition, foods that acidify urine increase the renal clearance of dextroamphetamine and may lower serum levels. This effect is seen with the anorectic influence of dextroamphetamine, which prompts a form of fasting ketoacidosis and leads to enhanced excretion.

Assessment of Relevant Core Patient Variables

Health Status

Evaluate the patient for pre-existing medical or mental health problems that may exacerbate the symptoms of ADHD. It is important to check the patient's history to rule out any contraindications to the pharmacotherapy, including other drug therapies and drug and alcohol abuse. If the patient is a child or adolescent, ask the parents whether there is a history of cardiac disease or cardiac structural abnormalities. Question the patient regarding the use of nonprescription drugs, particularly those with sympathomimetic effects, because patients often do not report the occasional use of over-the-counter (OTC) drugs unless asked.

Evaluate the patient for advanced arteriosclerosis, symptomatic cardiovascular disease, moderate to severe hypertension, hyperthyroidism, glaucoma, agitated states, a history of drug abuse, a recent history of MAOI use, or known hypersensitivity or idiosyncrasy to the sympathomimetic amines, all of which are contraindications for the use of dextroamphetamine.

Document baseline physical assessment data, including height, weight, and vital signs. In addition, an electrocardiogram (ECG) is important for ruling out any cardiovascular abnormalities that CNS stimulants might exacerbate, especially in children and adolescents.

TABLE 22.3	Agents That Interact with P Dextroamphetamine	
Interactants	Effect and Significance	Nursing Management
Acidifying agents: GI acidifying agents (guanethidine, reserpine, glutamic acid HCl, ascorbic acid, fruit juices) Urinary acidifying agents (ammonium chloride, sodium acid phosphate)	Decreased absorption of dextroamphetamine; lowered blood levels of dextroamphetamine	Instruct patient to avoid acidic foods. Inform patient of possibly reduced effect of medication (especially of the antihypertensive guanethidine).
Alkalinizing agents: Urinary alkalinizing agents (sodium bicarbonate, acetazolamide) GI alkalinizing agents (sodium bicarbonate)	Increase blood levels of dextroamphetamine, potentiating actions	Avoid administering alkaline agents or increase dosing interval.
Antidepressants, tricyclic; SSRIs	Increased sensitivity to the effects of tricyclics and sympathomimetics; increased risk of serotonin syndrome	Avoid combination; monitor for increased CNS effect.
MAO inhibitors	Exacerbation of dextroamphetamine effects, hypertensive crisis, cerebral bleeding	Avoid; allow proper MAOI washout period.
Chlorpromazine	Diminished effects of dextroamphetamine; may increase psychosis	Avoid; may be of therapeutic use in overdose.
Calamus	Reduced amphetamine effects	Inform patient of possibly reduced effect of medication.

Life Span and Gender

Ask whether the patient is pregnant. If the patient is pregnant, dextroamphetamine should be used only if absolutely necessary because it is not known whether dextroamphetamine causes fetal abnormalities (pregnancy category C). If the patient is breast-feeding, monitoring the infant for CNS stimulation is important. In the event of CNS stimulation in the infant, the mother may need to discontinue the drug. Very young and very old patients may be at higher risk for injury because of CNS adverse effects of agitation and restlessness. Monitoring children's growth is important because dextroamphetamine may cause growth suppression.

Lifestyle, Diet, and Habits

Ask the patient about his or her regular consumption of caffeine-containing drinks such as tea, coffee, and cola because they may increase the adverse effects associated with dextroamphetamine.

Support adherence to the drug regimen to enhance the patient's quality of life. People involved in shift work need to adjust the timing of their doses to avoid sleep disturbances and allow for normal appetite. Be mindful of the high abuse potential for dextroamphetamine and assess patients carefully for a history of drug or alcohol abuse.

Environment

Dextroamphetamine may be administered in any setting by physicians, nurses, or patients. Therefore, assess the safety of the patient's environment. When the patient is a child, it is advisable for parents to store and monitor the drugs.

Culture and Inherited Traits

In some immigrant populations, alternative therapies and drug use are a part of religious or cultural practice. Therefore, it is important to determine the nature and type of alternative therapy or ritual drug use to avoid drug–drug interactions and to maximize the therapeutic effects of dextroamphetamine.

Nursing Diagnoses and Outcomes

- Disturbed Sleep Pattern related to drug effects or caffeine use
  Desired outcome: The patient maintains normal sleep patterns through proper use of sleep hygiene measures and bedtime (hour of sleep [HS]) sedation.
- Delayed Growth and Development related to drug effects
  Desired outcome: The patient maintains a normal growth and development profile.
- Disturbed Sensory Perception related to drug response
  Desired outcome: The patient remains free from sensory and perceptual disturbances.
- Imbalanced Nutrition: Less than Body Requirements, related to amphetamine abuse and anorexia
  Desired outcome: The patient maintains adequate nutrition.
- Nonadherence to Therapeutic Regimen related to lack of motivation, poor self-image, or negative effects of prescribed drug
  Desired outcome: The patient adheres to the drug regimen.

Planning and Intervention

Maximizing Therapeutic Effects

It is important to administer dextroamphetamine with food in the morning and no fewer than 6 hours before bedtime, preferably longer for the sustained-release formulations. Inform patients and family members that improvements may not be seen until several weeks after the treatment is initiated. Provide emotional and psychological support during this period: a great deal is necessary, particularly because families often feel guilty about the disorders being treated. It is important to explain to the obese person that anorectic agents are used only to supplement a combined program of calorie reduction, nutritional counseling and adjustment, and systematic exercise of large muscle groups. Enhance support by encouraging the person to attend self-support groups and psychotherapy. Explain that people suffering from narcolepsy, ADHD, or obesity usually benefit from programs designed to foster and enhance self-esteem.

Minimizing Adverse Effects

Monitor for adverse effects of dextroamphetamine and intervene if they occur. In patients experiencing decreased appetite, administer the morning dose of medication before or with breakfast to ensure a good caloric intake at the beginning of the day. Monitor for rebound irritability and depression as the stimulant wears off. Consult with the prescriber to change the time or frequency of dosing if these symptoms are intolerable. Monitor also for headache. Intermittent headaches may be treated with acetaminophen; however, if frequent headaches occur, contact the prescriber to decrease the dose of stimulant or possibly change to a different formulation. To minimize GI distress, administer the medication with meals.

In the event of toxicity or overdose, it is necessary to monitor vital signs and anticipate use of antiepileptics and antipsychotics. Patients who are experiencing drug toxicity or overdose are vulnerable, and they must be placed in a nonstimulating yet supportive environment where they are protected from hurting themselves and kept from injuring others. Reassure the patient with drug toxicity or overdose, particularly because profound depression of systems initially stimulated by the drug may occur.

Providing Patient and Family Education

An important component of health promotion is the encouragement and support of patients taking dextroamphetamine and their families. Ensure that patient and family education includes explaining the importance of adhering to dosing instructions and dosage scheduling, and understanding recommendations regarding possible adverse effects, other drugs to avoid, drug storage, missed doses, abuse potential, and monitoring the effects of therapy.

- It is important to caution all patients treated with dextroamphetamine therapy about adverse effects and the possibility of overdosing. Advise patients and their families about managing adverse effects and about when to consult with their caregivers if self-management is ineffective or if serious and persistent adverse effects continue. If toxicity or overdosing is suspected, it is important to decrease frequency of dosing.
- Provide the patient or the patients' family with a Patient Medication Guide that explains the risk of cardiovascular or psychiatric adverse effects.
- Encourage patients to avoid other stimulants during dextroamphetamine therapy, including caffeinated beverages, because these may lead to exaggerated CNS stimulation, irritability, and nervousness.
- Alert patients and parents or caregivers to keep dextroamphetamine in safe storage, out of children's reach.
- Advise patients to take dextroamphetamine early in the day, unless otherwise instructed, to avoid nighttime insomnia. If the tablets are sustained release or long acting, advise patients not to crush or chew them. Tell patients to notify their prescriber if they experience nervousness, restlessness, insomnia, dizziness, dry mouth, diarrhea, constipation, or an unpleasant taste; a dosage adjustment may be necessary. It is also important to tell patients to avoid all other drugs (including OTC drugs) while taking dextroamphetamine, unless the prescriber recommends them.
- Tell patients and family members what to do if they miss a dose of dextroamphetamine. When patients miss one dose, it is important for them to take that dose as soon as possible to prevent trouble sleeping. However, the dose should be taken no later than 6 hours before bedtime for the short-acting form, and no later than 10 to 14 hours before bedtime for the long-acting form. If patients do not remember the missed dose until the next day, they should skip the missed dose and return to the normal dosing schedule. Patients must never take double doses of the drug.
- Advise patients that dextroamphetamine may impair their ability to engage in potentially hazardous activities, such as operating machinery or driving vehicles, particularly if the effects of drug therapy on the individual patient are not yet known.

Ongoing Assessment and Evaluation

Monitor periodic growth and development data for children throughout therapy. Monitor for adverse effects such as anorexia, irritability, depression, headache, GI distress, anxiety, cardiovascular changes, and sleep deprivation. Review the patient's diet periodically and remind the patient to abstain from caffeine-rich products.

It is important to monitor patients for responses to therapy, including improvements in mental and behavioral symptoms in children, decreased baseline rate of motor activity, weight loss, and decreased frequency of narcoleptic attacks.

The patient should show a reduction in symptoms or symptom severity. Patients receiving dextroamphetamines for ADHD should show improved attention span or decreased impulsivity. Patients receiving dextroamphetamines for obesity should show documented weight loss.

MEMORY CHIP

P Dextroamphetamine

- Releases dopamine and norepinephrine in adrenergic nerve terminals and interferes with the reuptake of dopamine; sites of action in the CNS are the cerebral cortex and the reticular activating system
- Most common adverse effects: restlessness, insomnia, dizziness, overstimulation, palpitations, tachycardia, hypertension, dry mouth, unpleasant taste, and diarrhea
- Maximizing therapeutic effects: Take with food in the morning and not less than 6 hours before bedtime.
- Minimizing adverse effects: Obtain a baseline nursing history and physical assessment to compare with treatment outcomes; important assessment items include sleep disturbances, nervousness, complete diet history (including use of caffeine), height, weight, ECG, and drug or alcohol abuse.
- Most important patient education: importance of adhering to dosing instructions, dosage scheduling, possible adverse effects, other drugs to avoid, drug storage, missed doses, abuse potential, and monitoring the effects of therapy
- **Black box warning: High abuse potential. May lead to dependence, non-therapeutic use, or distribution to others.**

Patients receiving dextroamphetamines for narcolepsy should have fewer or less severe episodes. The patient and family should show an increased understanding of how to recognize and manage adverse effects and be able to explain how to store and administer drug therapy safely.

Drugs Closely Related to P Dextroamphetamine

Amphetamine Salts

Amphetamine salts (Adderall, Adderall XR) are a combination of amphetamine salts and dextroamphetamine. Adderall was formerly marketed as Obetrol, a product used primarily for adjunctive short-term treatment of exogenous obesity. The current formula consists of mixed salts of amphetamine aspartate, amphetamine sulfate, dextroamphetamine saccharate, and dextroamphetamine sulfate. It is approved to treat ADHD or narcolepsy.

CRITICAL THINKING SCENARIO

PHARMACOTHERAPY AND ATTENTION DEFICIT HYPERACTIVITY DISORDER

A family friend has a child who has been diagnosed with ADHD. The friend asks you what you think about treating this disorder with drugs. Instead of giving an opinion, construct a patient teaching plan to help this person understand how to maximize the effects of pharmacotherapy. Present three topics for discussion with the family, and explain how you would prioritize these topics.

Like dextroamphetamine, Adderall has a mechanism of action that is unclear. However, its ability to improve symptoms in ADHD is well documented. These include improved attention span, decreased distractibility, increased ability to follow directions or complete tasks, and decreased impulsivity and aggression. The contraindications and the adverse effect profile of Adderall are similar to those for dextroamphetamine; however, Adderall is also associated with increased cardiovascular adverse effects. It is used with caution for patients with medical conditions that may be compromised by hypertension. The benefit of Adderall is its once-daily dosing and its longer duration of action than that of dextroamphetamine. For patients with difficulty swallowing, the Adderall XR capsule may be opened and the beads sprinkled in applesauce.

Dexmethylphenidate

Dexmethylphenidate (Focalin, Focalin XR) is a CNS stimulant that is chemically similar to the amphetamines and is an isomer of methylphenidate. It is used to manage ADHD. Dexmethylphenidate is thought to block the reuptake of norepinephrine and dopamine into the presynaptic neuron and increase the release of these monoamines into the extraneuronal space. This activity results in improved attention spans, decreased distractibility, increased ability to follow directions or complete tasks, and decreased impulsivity and aggression in patients with ADHD. Although dexmethylphenidate does not produce a physical dependence, it may induce tolerance or psychic dependence. The adverse effects of dexmethylphenidate are similar to those of other stimulant drugs. They occur relatively frequently but are usually mild at normally prescribed dosages. They may be more frequent or severe during the initial days of therapy, but most adverse effects disappear within a few weeks of continued use.

Lisdexamfetamine

Lisdexamfetamine (Vyvanse) is a new drug approved for treatment of ADHD in children 6 to 12 years of age. Lisdexamfetamine is a prodrug of dextroamphetamine, which means that lisdexamfetamine is therapeutically inactive until it is converted to dextroamphetamine in the GI tract. Because it must be metabolized in the GI tract and cannot be given by IV or intranasal routes, this drug may have a lower abuse liability. Studies have also indicated that lisdexamfetamine appears less likely to cause euphoria. Efficacy of lisdexamfetamine is comparable to that of Adderall XR.

Methylphenidate

Methylphenidate (Ritalin, Ritalin SR, Ritalin LA, Methylin, Methylin-ER, Metadate-ER, Metadate-CD, Concerta) is an orally administered CNS stimulant that is chemically and pharmacologically similar to the amphetamines. It is clinically used to treat ADHD and narcolepsy. The CNS actions of methylphenidate are milder than those of the amphetamines and have more noticeable effects on mental activities than on motor activities. Methylphenidate shares the abuse potential of the amphetamines and is a DEA Schedule II controlled substance. Methylphenidate comes in many formulations. Although the active ingredient is the same, these drugs, which are described below, have different pharmacokinetics because of their structure or method of delivery.

Ritalin is the oldest available medication for ADHD and is considered the drug of choice by many prescribers. Its quick onset and short duration make it possible to individualize dosing. Ritalin SR is an extended-release form of methylphenidate with an approximate duration of 8 hours. Ritalin SR tablets must be swallowed whole. Ritalin LA is a long-acting formulation of methylphenidate that provides all-day treatment with one morning dose. This dosing regimen eliminates the social stigma felt by children who have to bring medication to school and decreases the possibility of medication misuse. Advantages include once-daily dosing and the potential for sprinkle administration, if needed.

Methylin is another trade name of methylphenidate. It has three formulations: Methylin and Methylin Chewable tablets, which are comparable to Ritalin; and Methylin-ER, which is comparable to Ritalin SR and Metadate-ER. Methylin Chewable tablets should be taken with 8 ounces of water to minimize the risk of choking.

Metadate-ER is another extended-release form that uses a two-phase process to deliver an initial rapid release of methylphenidate followed by a second, continuous-release phase. Metadate-CD has a controlled delivery system that uses a multiparticulate bead system, with each bead acting as a drug reservoir. The individual beads are coated with different polymers that dissolve and release at different times. Metadate-CD capsules contain immediate-release and extended-release beads in a ratio of 30:70. It has a duration of 12 hours, which is similar to Concerta (see below); however, serum drug levels of Metadate-CD are higher than Concerta for the initial 4 hours of activity. Advantages of Metadate-CD include once-daily dosing, which is especially important for school-aged children, and the ability for sprinkle administration, if necessary. Disadvantages include cost and the fixed ratio of immediate-release to extended-release beads.

Concerta is a once-a-day formulation of methylphenidate that is targeted at patients with moderate ADHD. There is a dose-related size problem with the Concerta capsules. Many patients have difficulty swallowing the larger-dose capsules. The size of the capsule is related to its unique delivery system. The outside of the capsule dissolves and releases the initial methylphenidate within an hour. The inner core has a push layer and a drug layer. Once the capsule is in the GI tract, water enters the osmotic system and dissolves or suspends the drug in the core. The drug is then released by osmotic pressure at a controlled rate through a laser-drilled hole in the membrane. The capsule itself is excreted in the feces. Because of its delivery system, Concerta cannot be crushed, chewed, or opened in any way.

Like Adderall, Concerta is associated with cardiovascular adverse events. Patients with medical conditions that may be compromised by hypertension or tachycardia should not use Concerta. Also, patients with severe ADHD frequently need a larger dose of methylphenidate than can be offered in the Concerta formulation.

In addition to these oral forms of methylphenidate, there is a new delivery system—a transdermal patch (Daytrana). The patch is applied daily but removed after 9 hours to decrease potential adverse effects. If the patient is experiencing severe adverse effects, the patch can be removed early. Warnings and precautions are the same as oral preparations of methylphenidate. Adverse effects are also similar; in addition, the transdermal system may cause skin sensitization. Transdermal patches may fall off with excessive heat or participating in sports activities.

Drugs Significantly Different From P Dextroamphetamine

Atomoxetine

Atomoxetine (Strattera) is a selective norepinephrine reuptake inhibitor initially evaluated for use as an antidepressant. Although it failed to demonstrate efficacy as an antidepressant, further research showed it to be highly effective for ADHD. Atomoxetine is the first ADHD medication that is not a stimulant. Although its true mechanism of action is unknown, it is thought to involve the selective inhibition of the presynaptic norepinephrine transporter. Atomoxetine is metabolized by the cytochrome P-450 2D6 isoenzyme. Concurrent use of drugs that inhibit this pathway, such as SSRIs, increases the serum concentration of atomoxetine and extends its half-life substantially. The only contraindication to the use of atomoxetine is concurrent use of MAOIs. In patients who have been exposed to both drug classes, a 2-week washout period should take place after discontinuing either drug or before starting either drug. Monitor liver enzymes because there is a high incidence of liver damage, elevated liver enzymes, and jaundice requiring discontinuation of the medication for patient recovery. Atomoxetine appears to have a substantial and dose-related effect on growth. Patients may lose weight and gain height while taking atomoxetine. The drug may also increase blood pressure and heart rate and can cause additive cardiovascular effects with albuterol and pressor agents. Atomoxetine should be used cautiously in conditions that predispose patients to hypotension because it has been reported to cause orthostatic hypotension and syncope. The most common adverse effects in adult patients are constipation, dry mouth, nausea, appetite suppression, lethargy, dizziness, insomnia, sexual dysfunction, urinary dysfunction (hesitation or retention), and dysmenorrhea. The most common adverse effects in pediatric patients are lethargy, hypoesthesia, paraesthesia, sensory disturbances, dyspepsia, nausea, vomiting, fatigue, appetite suppression, dizziness, urinary dysfunction (hesitation or retention), and mood swings. The major advantage of atomoxetine is that, because it is not a stimulant, it is not a DEA Schedule II drug—samples can be provided to physicians, prescriptions can be refilled, and the drug does not have be securely stored.

Guanfacine

Guanfacine (Intuniv), a selective alpha-2A adrenergic receptor agonist, is an antihypertensive drugs that has just been approved for the management of ADHD. Because of its selective alpha-2A stimulation, it reduces sympathetic nerve impulses from the vasomotor center to the heart and blood vessels. This results in a decrease in peripheral vascular resistance and a reduction in heart rate, which may also induce its adverse effects. The mechanism by which guanfacine affects ADHD is unclear.

Guanfacine is available as an immediate release or an extended release drug. Only the extended release formulation is approved for ADHD. Common adverse effects associated with its use include syncope, increased weight, depression, and fatigue. Additional adverse effects include hypotension, sedation, headache, and lethargy.

Prior to initiation of therapy, assess heart rate and blood pressure. Continue to monitor during therapy, especially following dose increases. Guanfacine is a pregnancy category B drug.

Modafinil

Modafinil (Provigil) is approved for narcolepsy, obstructive sleep apnea, and shift work sleep disorder. The mechanism of action is unclear. It is theorized that modafinil may alter the balance of gamma-aminobutyric acid and glutamate, resulting in activation of the hypothalamus. Another theory is that is promotes histamine release. Common adverse effects include headache, abdominal pain, anorexia, and insomnia.

Antihypertensive Agents

Antihypertensive agents such as clonidine (Catapres, Kapvay) and guanfacine (Tenex, Intuniv) may be prescribed alone or with a stimulant to manage the symptoms of ADHD, especially in children with tics. These drugs help with impulsivity, sleep problems, frustration tolerance, and activity. They do not have any known effect on inattention. Common adverse effects include drowsiness, dry mouth, and constipation. In-depth information regarding these antihypertensive agents is located in Chapter 28.

Antidepressants

Antidepressants may be used in managing ADHD, especially if comorbid diagnoses are suspected. Tricyclic antidepressants (TCAs), such as desipramine (Norpramin), nortriptyline (Pamelor), and imipramine (Tofranil), improve concentration, mood, and hyperactivity and help regulate emotional ups and downs. It is important to monitor cardiac activity, especially in children, when patients are taking these drugs. SSRIs, such as fluvoxamine (Luvox), paroxetine (Paxil), and fluoxetine (Prozac), are used primarily when mood or anxiety disorders are thought to coexist. SSRIs may increase impulsivity. Venlafaxine (Effexor) is thought to provide the benefits of both TCAs and SSRIs. It is not generally used in children. Common adverse effects with antidepressant drugs include headache, insomnia, weight loss, nervousness, and either constipation or diarrhea. Many of these adverse effects abate after continued use of the drug. For more information regarding antidepressant drugs, see Chapter 16.

© ANORECTIC AGENTS

Obesity is a complex problem that is very difficult to treat. Current views concerning the cause of obesity favor a disturbance in the hypothalamic set-point, which mediates caloric intake and use and energy expenditure. Although drug therapy is helpful, drugs alone cannot manage weight loss. Diet and exercise are equally important. Common agents used as anorectics include phentermine, adrenergic drugs, serotonergic drugs, and orlistat. This section focuses on phentermine (Adipex-P) the prototype anorectic drug. Table 22.4 presents summary of selected anorectic drugs.

TABLE 22.4	Summary of Selected © Anorectic CNS Stimulants		
Drug (Trade) Name	**Selected Indications**	**Route and Dosage Range**	**Pharmacokinetics**
© **Anorectic Stimulants**			
P phentermine (Adipex-P)	Adjunct in obesity	*Adult:* PO, 37.5 mg/d *Child:* safety and efficacy not established in patients 16 years of age and younger	*Onset:* 1–2 wk *Duration:* Multiple dose, 12 wk $t_{1/2}$: 20 h
benzphetamine (Didrex)	Adjunct in obesity	*Adult:* PO, 25–50 mg 1–3 times daily *Child:* Not recommended for children younger than 12 y	*Onset:* NA *Duration:* NA $t_{1/2}$: NA
diethylpropion (Tenuate)	Adjunct in obesity	*Adult:* PO, 25 mg tid 1 h before meals or 75 mg controlled-release at midmorning	*Onset:* Within 1 wk *Duration:* 4–12 h $t_{1/2}$: 8 h
phendimetrazine (Bontril)	Adjunct in obesity	*Adult:* PO, 35 mg tid; sustained release, 105 mg every AM	*Onset:* NA *Duration:* NA $t_{1/2}$: 2–4 h
Orlistat (Xenical, Alli)	Adjunct in obesity	*Adult:* 60–120 mg tid with meals	*Onset:* 24–48 h *Duration:* Unknown $t_{1/2}$: 1–2 h

Nursing Management of the Patient Receiving P Phentermine

Core Drug Knowledge

Pharmacotherapeutics

Phentermine is a DEA Schedule IV drug classified as an indirect sympathomimetic. It is used as an adjuvant to manage obesity by promoting weight loss. It is indicated for patients with an initial BMI greater than or equal to 30 kg/m², or greater than or equal to 27 kg/m² with other risk factors such as diabetes mellitus, dyslipidemia, or hypertension. Tolerance to the anorectic effects of phentermine usually develops within a few weeks of starting therapy; therefore, it is indicated for short-term therapy. When tolerance develops to the anorectic effects, it is generally recommended that phentermine be discontinued rather than increased.

Pharmacokinetics

Phentermine is administered orally as either phentermine hydrochloride or phentermine resin complex. Both formulations are metabolized by the liver and excreted, predominately unchanged, by the kidneys. The resin complex formulation has a slower absorption and longer duration of action.

Pharmacodynamics

Phentermine is structurally and chemically related to the amphetamines, therefore, the pharmacologic effects are also similar. Appetite suppression is believed to occur through direct stimulation of the satiety center in the hypothalamic and limbic regions.

Contraindications and Precautions

Phentermine is contraindicated in patients with advanced arteriosclerosis, agitated states, moderate to severe hypertension, glaucoma, or symptomatic cardiovascular disease, including cardiac arrhythmias. Phentermine is not recommended for use in patients with cardiac disease, including valvular heart disease. Phentermine should not be combined with any other drug class used to decrease weight.

Adverse Effects

Adverse effects can affect several body systems. CNS effects include dizziness, dyskinesia, dysphoria, euphoria, headache, insomnia, overstimulation, restlessness, and tremor. Potential ocular effects include blurred vision, mydriasis, and ocular irritation. Cardiovascular effects include hypertension, palpitations, and sinus tachycardia. GI effects include constipation, diarrhea, dysgeusia, nausea and vomiting, and dry mouth. Other adverse reactions include impotence, libido increase, libido decrease, and urticaria.

Drug Interactions

Drug interactions with phentermine may result in "serotonin syndrome," characterized by CNS irritability, motor weakness, shivering, myoclonus, and altered consciousness. This syndrome may occur when phentermine is used in conjunction with selective serotonin reuptake inhibitors and MAOIs. Table 22.5 presents additional drug interactions.

Assessment of Relevant Core Patient Variables

Health Status

Assess for disorders that contraindicate or require precautions with phentermine therapy. Assess also for current or recent use of medications that may interact with phentermine, especially MAOIs and SSRIs. Communicate positive findings to the prescriber before starting phentermine therapy.

Perform a physical examination that includes calculating the BMI. Phentermine is indicated for use only with morbidly obese patients. Obtain baseline blood pressure and heart rate parameters because phentermine may increase both.

Life Span and Gender

Assess female patients for pregnancy or the intention to become pregnant. Phentermine is classified as pregnancy category C drug because adequate, well-controlled studies with phentermine have not been conducted in pregnant women. Women of childbearing potential should use adequate contraception while taking phentermine. Advise patients to notify their physician if they become or intend to become pregnant during phentermine therapy. Additionally, it is unknown whether phentermine is excreted in breast milk; therefore, phentermine is not recommended for breast-feeding mothers. Accordingly, assess female patients for lactation.

Assess for age-related considerations Dosing in older adults should be done cautiously, because of a greater likelihood of decreased hepatic, renal, or cardiac function.

Lifestyle, Diet, and Habits

Assess the patient's diet and make modifications to optimize therapy. Phentermine is most effective when combined with

TABLE 22.5	Agents That Interact with P Phentermine		
Interactants	**Effect and Significance**		**Nursing Management**
MAOIs	Increased pharmacological effects of phentermine resulting in hypertensive crisis and cerebral hemorrhage.		Avoid combination. Monitor for signs of hypertensive crisis.
SSRIs	Increased sympathomimetic effects and increased risk of serotonin syndrome.		Monitor for increased CNS effects: agitation, anxiety, restlessness.

a low-calorie diet and behavior modification counseling. Assess the use of caffeine and alcohol. Advise the patient to avoid both throughout phentermine therapy.

Environment

Phentermine may be administered in any setting by physicians, nurses, or patients. Assess the patient's environment to ensure safety.

Nursing Diagnoses and Outcomes

- Imbalanced Nutrition: Less than Body Requirements, related to anorexia
  Desired outcome: The patient maintains adequate nutrition.
- Nonadherence to Therapeutic Regimen related to lack of motivation, poor self-image, or negative effects of prescribed drug
  Desired outcome: The patient adheres to drug regimen.

Planning and Intervention

Maximizing Therapeutic Effects

Phentermine should be taken once daily. For the long-acting resin complex, advise the patient to take it at least 10 hours before bedtime; for the immediate-release formulation take at least 4-6 hours before bedtime. It is important to remember that phentermine should be used in conjunction with a low-calorie diet and daily exercise routine for maximum results. Some patients benefit from writing a food journal to assess the amount of food intake and the types of foods consumed.

Minimizing Adverse Effects

Adverse effects are minimized by adhering to the contra-indications and precautions for this medication. Refraining from using drugs that may induce serotonin syndrome or elevate the blood pressure and heart rate is especially important. At least 2 weeks should elapse between discontinuing MAOI therapy and initiating phentermine therapy. Similarly, at least 2 weeks should elapse after stopping phentermine therapy and starting MAOI therapy. It is also important for female patients to take precautions to avoid pregnancy and to contact their prescriber immediately if pregnancy occurs.

Providing Patient and Family Education

- An important component of health promotion is encouragement and support of the patient's commitment to weight loss. Remind patients that phentermine is only one component in the recipe for weight loss. Behavior modification and exercise are equally important for patients to reach their goals.
- Advise the patient to contact the provider if tolerance begins to develop. Taking a larger dose does not increase its effectiveness and increases the risk for severe adverse effects.
- Reinforce avoidance of caffeine and alcohol.

- Educate patients and families about drugs that may interact with phentermine and encourage patients to contact the prescriber before adding any daily medications, even OTC drugs.
- Instruct patients regarding possible adverse effects of phentermine therapy, especially the potential for hypertension. When possible, teach patients and families how to take blood pressure and pulse.
- When working with women, discuss contraception and the importance of notifying the prescriber if the patient becomes pregnant. Discuss also the need to refrain from phentermine therapy if the patient is breast-feeding.

Ongoing Assessment and Evaluation

Calculate BMI at each follow-up visit in addition to obtaining gross weight measurement. Assessing vital signs is equally important, with a focus on blood pressure and heart rate. When possible, review the patient's food journal and assess the progress of the patient's behavior modification. Reinforce the need for daily exercise to complement phentermine therapy. Finally, arrange for serial laboratory tests, including CBC, liver function, and renal function tests.

Evaluating the patient routinely is important for assessing progress. With phentermine therapy, an adequate diet, and regular exercise, the patient should lose between 8 and 10 pounds per month. The patient should not remain on sibutramine therapy if weight loss does not occur. The time frame depends on the person's specific variables.

Drug Significantly Different From
P Phentermine
Adrenergic Drugs

The adrenergic drugs are primarily phenethylamines—drugs similar to amphetamines. These drugs include benzphetamine (Didrex), diethylpropion (Tenuate), and phendimetrazine (Adipost, Bontril). They decrease the appetite by stimulating the CNS. They also have effects similar to those of amphetamines, such as tachycardia, hypertension, nervousness, and anxiety. While they are safer than amphetamines, they still have an abuse potential; thus, they are scheduled drugs. They are not useful for long-term management of obesity because tolerance develops in 6 to 12 weeks.

MEMORY CHIP

P Phentermine

- Used only for patients with a body mass index diagnostic for morbid obesity
- Inhibits dopamine, norepinephrine, and serotonin
- Major contraindications: uncontrolled hypertension
- Most serious adverse effects: "serotonin syndrome" and hypertension
- Most important patient education: Drug must be used in conjunction with a low-calorie diet and exercise plan.

Orlistat

Orlistat (Xenical, Alli) is a GI lipase inhibitor indicated for weight loss and subsequent weight maintenance in morbidly obese patients. As with phentermine, orlistat is used in conjunction with a reduced-calorie diet and physical activity. Orlistat works nonsystemically to block the absorption of dietary fat by approximately 30%. Alli is an over-the-counter formulation of orlistat. A thorough discussion of orlistat appears in Chapter 36.

Off-Label Medications

The antidiabetic drugs pramlintide (Symlin) and exenatide (Byetta) have demonstrated weight loss in diabetic patients. These drugs decrease gastric emptying and increase satiety leading to weight loss. See Chapter 49 for additional information.

Zonisamide (Zonegran) and topiramate (Topamax) are anticonvulsant drugs that are also used off-label for weight loss. Zonisamide acts synergistically by suppressing the NPY/AgRP neuron, which acts in opposition to the POMC (proopiomelanocortin) neuron. The exact mechanism of topiramate is unclear. Several mechanisms have been proposed, including anorexia related to its use, reduction in the activity of salivary enzymes that change taste, reduction in leptin and corticosteroid concentrations, and reduction in serum glucose and insulin concentrations. See Chapter 18 for additional information.

Serotonergic Drugs

Anorectic drugs that affect the serotonergic receptors in the brain include SSRIs, which are generally used as antidepressants. However, they do induce weight loss in the short term. Fluoxetine (Prozac) is the SSRI known best for its ability to induce anorexia. Other serotonergic drugs in this class that cause anorexia are venlafaxine (Effexor) and sertraline (Zoloft). These drugs are discussed in depth in Chapter 16. Bupropion (Wellbutrin), another drug used for depression, is also used for weight control and smoking cessation. Bupropion controls weight by stimulating POMC (proopiomelanocortin) neurons.

© RESPIRATORY STIMULANTS

Respiratory stimulants are used to manage postsurgical respiratory depression and apnea in preterm neonates. Caffeine is the prototype respiratory stimulant (Table 22.6). Because of its CNS stimulation, it is also used to maintain alertness and decrease fatigue. Caffeine is also used nontherapeutically in foods such as cocoa and chocolate and in beverages such as coffee, tea, and colas.

Nursing Management of the Patient Receiving Ⓟ Caffeine
Core Drug Knowledge
Pharmacotherapeutics

Caffeine is used in managing neonatal apnea, asthma, drowsiness, and fatigue. The use of caffeine for apnea of prematurity reduces the rate of bronchopulmonary dysplasia in infants with very low birth weight (Schmidt, 2007).

Caffeine is used in combination with many other drugs such as aspirin, acetaminophen, propoxyphene, and butalbital for treating migraine and other types of headache. Caffeine is also sold without a prescription in products marketed to treat drowsiness or mild water-weight gain.

Caffeine may be administered to patients receiving electroconvulsive therapy (ECT). The desired result from ECT is seizure activity. Seizure augmentation, using proconvulsant agents such as caffeine, is used to overcome resistance to the induction and continuation of seizure activity.

Pharmacokinetics

Caffeine may be administered orally and intravenously. Orally administered caffeine in an adult is well absorbed from the GI tract, reaching peak plasma concentrations within 50 to 75 minutes. In neonates, oral administration results in peak concentrations in 30 to 120 minutes. Formula feedings do not affect the time to maximum concentrations after oral dosing. Caffeine is distributed rapidly to all body tissues and readily crosses the blood–brain and placental barriers. It is distributed into breast milk.

TABLE 22.6	Summary of Selected © Respiratory Stimulants		
Ⓟ caffeine (OTC: Caffedrine, Tirend, NoDoz; prescription: caffeine and sodium benzoate) Caffeine citrate (Cafcit)	Adjunct for analgesia (e.g., headache), stimulant effects Postdural puncture headache Neonatal apnea	*Adult and child >12 y:* PO, 65–200 mg q3–4 h *Adult:* IV/IM, 500–1000 mg caffeine and sodium benzoate (250–500 mg caffeine); not to exceed 2.5 g/d *Child:* IV/PO, 20 mg/kg as loading dose, then 5–10 mg/kg as maintenance dose	*Onset:* PO, 15–45 min *Duration:* NA $t_{1/2}$: 3–5 h
doxapram (Dopram)	Postanesthetic respiratory depression or postanesthetic shivering Drug-induced CNS depression Chronic airway limitation	*Adult:* IV, single injection of 0.18–1 mg/kg, not to exceed 1.5 mg/kg as single dose or 2 mg/kg as multiple doses at 5-min intervals *Adult:* IV, inject priming dose of 1–3 mg/kg/h; to a maximum of 3 g/d *Adult:* IV, 1–3 mg/min; do not use longer than 2 h *Child:* Do not give to children younger than 12 y	*Onset:* 20–40 s *Duration:* 5–12 min $t_{1/2}$: 3.4 h

In adults, caffeine is partially metabolized in the liver. Caffeine metabolism in neonates is limited because of their immature hepatic enzyme systems. Unchanged caffeine and its metabolites are excreted in the urine (see Table 22.6).

Pharmacodynamics

Caffeine is a mild, direct stimulant at all levels of the CNS, which also stimulates the cardiovascular system. Caffeine also stimulates the medullary respiratory center and relaxes bronchial smooth muscle. Caffeine stimulates voluntary muscle and gastric acid secretion, increases renal blood flow, and is a mild diuretic. Caffeine is preferred over theophylline in neonates because of the ease of once-daily administration, reliable oral absorption, and a wide therapeutic window. The cellular mechanism of action is unclear.

Contraindications and Precautions

Caffeine should be used cautiously in patients with anxiety disorders, panic disorder, or both because as a CNS stimulant, it can aggravate these conditions. Caffeine is contraindicated for patients suffering from insomnia because insomnia is one of its most frequent adverse effects. In overdoses, caffeine has been associated with seizures; therefore, it should be prescribed cautiously to any patient with a seizure disorder.

Caffeine may stimulate the force of contraction and increase heart rate and blood pressure. It may also increase left ventricular output and stroke volume. Patients who have cardiac disease, angina, hypertension, or a history of cardiac dysrhythmias should be given caffeine cautiously. Patients should not take caffeine within 14 days of a myocardial infarction.

Patients with chronic disorders such as diabetes mellitus, hyperthyroidism, and peptic ulcer disease should not receive or should minimize their intake of caffeine. In patients with diabetes, caffeine can either increase or decrease blood sugar. In neonates, both hypoglycemia and hyperglycemia have been observed with the use of caffeine. In patients with hyperthyroidism, the stimulatory effects of caffeine can be augmented. Because caffeine can stimulate gastric secretions, it may also aggravate stomach ulcerations.

Caffeine should be used cautiously in patients with hepatic disease or hepatic impairment. Caffeine clearance may be delayed, leading to toxicity. Using caffeine cautiously is especially important in neonates because their hepatic metabolism is underdeveloped. Additionally, renal impairment in premature neonates may delay caffeine clearance because caffeine elimination depends more on renal clearance in neonates than in older infants or adults.

Adverse Effects

Many adverse reactions to caffeine are an extension of caffeine's pharmacologic actions. Caffeine can cause tremor, sinus tachycardia, and heightened attentiveness. Other adverse reactions include diarrhea, excitement, irritability, insomnia, headache, muscle twitches, and palpitations. Because caffeine is a mild diuretic, polyuria is a possibility.

Cardiac arrhythmias, seizures, and delirium are possible after deliberate overdoses. In neonates, intolerance or overdose of caffeine may manifest as tachypnea, hyperglycemia, azotemia, fever, or seizures.

High caffeine intake has been reported to inhibit spermatogenesis in male animals. Adverse effects may also occur when a patient abruptly discontinues use of caffeine. Caffeine withdrawal syndrome is characterized by lethargy, anxiety, dizziness, or headache.

Drug Interactions

Caffeine has many potential drug–drug interactions, including with oral contraceptives, psychostimulants, sympathomimetic agents, fluoroquinolone antibiotics, lithium, and MAOIs. Caffeine may also interact with grapefruit juice. Table 22.7 presents these potential drug interactions.

Assessment of Relevant Core Patient Variables

Health Status

Assess for disorders that contraindicate or require precautions with caffeine therapy. Assess for current or recent use of medications that may interact with caffeine, especially MAOIs and sympathomimetic drugs. Assessing for the use of OTC drugs is important because many of them have sympathomimetic ingredients. Communicate positive findings to the prescriber before starting caffeine therapy.

Obtain baseline vital signs. When caffeine is used for respiratory depression or neonatal apnea, appropriate monitoring equipment should be used.

Life Span and Gender

Ask female patients if they are pregnant or would like to become pregnant. Couples who are pursuing pregnancy should probably limit excessive intake of caffeine. Caffeine drug products are generally classified in pregnancy category B; however, injectable forms are classified in pregnancy risk category C because caffeine easily crosses the placenta. It is generally recommended that pregnant women avoid the intake of caffeine-containing beverages (e.g., coffee, teas, and colas) or limit their use to no more than one or two caffeine-containing beverages per day. Likewise, pregnant women should use caffeine-containing medications only when absolutely necessary.

The American Academy of Pediatrics generally considers the casual use of caffeinated beverages to be compatible with lactation. Lactating women should use caffeine-containing drug products cautiously. When breast-fed infants are prescribed caffeine for apnea, their mothers should avoid the use of caffeine.

In neonates, there is a possible association between the use of methylxanthines like caffeine and the development of necrotizing enterocolitis. All preterm neonates treated with caffeine should be monitored for the development of gastric adverse effects such as abdominal distension, vomiting, bloody stools, and lethargy. In addition, monitoring serum caffeine levels is recommended. Neonates should receive caffeine without sodium benzoate.

TABLE 22.7 Agents That Interact with P Caffeine

Interactants	Effect and Significance	Nursing Management
oral contraceptives	Serum concentrations of caffeine may be increased during concurrent administration with oral contraceptives.	Monitor for nausea or tremors. Limit caffeine intake with oral contraceptives.
fluoroquinolone antibiotics • ciprofloxacin • levofloxacin • norfloxacin • enoxacin	Fluoroquinolone antibiotics decrease the clearance of caffeine, resulting in the potential for caffeine toxicity.	Avoid concomitant use of caffeine with fluoroquinolone antibiotics if possible. Monitor for caffeine toxicity.
lithium	Caffeine reduces serum lithium concentration.	Monitor serum lithium levels. Counsel patients taking lithium regarding caffeine intake.
MAOIs	Dangerous cardiac arrhythmias or severe hypertension may occur because of potentiation of sympathomimetic effects.	Do not administer caffeine within 2 wk of MAOI therapy. Counsel patient taking MAOIs of potential adverse effect with caffeine.
phenylpropanolamine	A combination of caffeine and phenylpropanolamine has resulted in cerebrovascular accident.	Do not combine these agents.
psychostimulants • dextroamphetamine • methylphenidate • modafinil • nicotine • pemoline • pseudoephedrine • sympathomimetic agents	When combined with any of these medications, an additive effect may occur, resulting in nervousness, irritability, insomnia, or cardiac arrhythmias.	Avoid these combinations when possible. Monitor blood pressure and heart rate. Monitor for adverse effects.

The benzoate may displace bilirubin and induce kernicterus. In addition, elevated serum concentrations of benzoate have been associated with neurologic disturbances such as hypotension, gasping respiration, and metabolic acidosis.

Lifestyle, Diet, and Habits
Caffeine is found in many foods and beverages. To avoid toxicity, patients should limit their intake of these foods while taking drugs that contain caffeine. To avoid caffeine withdrawal syndrome, patients should decrease their intake of caffeine daily rather than stop caffeine ingestion abruptly. Patients should never take caffeine tablets with grapefruit juice, which increases the effects of caffeine.

Environment
Oral preparations of caffeine may be administered in any setting by physicians, nurses, or patients. When used for respiratory depression or neonatal apnea, injectable caffeine must be administered in a monitored setting with appropriate life-sustaining equipment available.

Nursing Diagnoses and Outcomes
• Disturbed Sleep Pattern related to insomnia
  Desired outcome: *The patient will maintain adequate sleep and rest cycles.*
• Anxiety related to stimulatory effects of caffeine

  Desired outcome: *The patient will remain calm throughout therapy.*
• Deficient Fluid Volume related to diuretic effect of caffeine and potential diarrhea
  Desired outcome: *The patient will remain well hydrated.*

Planning and Intervention
Maximizing Therapeutic Effects
Ensure that the patient takes the caffeine tablets or caplets as directed. It is very important that the patient does not take more than prescribed. If administering an extended-release form of caffeine, advise the patient to swallow the tablet whole, not to crush or chew it. If administering chewable tablets, advise the patient to chew well and then swallow. Consistent intake of caffeine results in tolerance to its effects. Patients obtain maximum therapeutic effects when they use caffeine intermittently.

Minimizing Adverse Effects
Adverse effects are minimized when patients adhere to the contraindications and precautions for caffeine therapy. Patients taking caffeine for its therapeutic effects should limit their ingestion of caffeine from food and beverage sources. The patient should also refrain from taking OTC products that contain caffeine, especially cold and cough medications that also have a sympathomimetic effect.

Providing Patient and Family Education

- The general public typically does not view caffeine as a drug. Convey to the patient that caffeine is a drug and as such may create serious adverse effects. Review the contraindications and precautions of caffeine therapy with patients and families before initiating therapy. Instruct them about potential drug–drug interactions and explain the importance of refraining from using OTC drugs without the prescriber's knowledge.
- Instruct patients regarding the potential adverse effects of caffeine and ways to minimize their potential. Tell patients to contact the prescriber if symptoms such as anxiety or panic reactions, confusion, dizziness, lightheadedness or fainting spells, fast or irregular breathing or heartbeat (palpitations), muscle twitching, nausea and vomiting, seizures, or trembling occur.
- Alert women of childbearing age to the potential difficulty of becoming pregnant when they ingest large amounts (more than 500 mg/day) of caffeine daily. Inform men of the potential for inhibiting spermatogenesis.
- Review dietary sources of caffeine and explain the importance of limiting caffeine from these sources while taking therapeutic caffeine. Discuss the interaction between caffeine and grapefruit juice to avoid caffeine toxicity.

Ongoing Assessment and Evaluation

Caffeine is indicated for short-term or intermittent therapy. When caffeine is used for respiratory depression or neonatal apnea, monitor the patient's vital signs carefully. When administering caffeine for migraine or other types of headaches, monitor for potential adverse effects, especially CNS and cardiovascular stimulation. Conversely, also monitor for signs of caffeine withdrawal.

Drug Closely Related to Caffeine

Doxapram (Dopram), a parenteral analeptic agent, is used to stimulate postanesthesia respiratory depression or drug-induced CNS depression and to treat chronic pulmonary disease associated with acute hypercapnia. It has an unlabeled use for neonatal apnea. Doxapram works by activating the peripheral carotid chemoreceptors, thereby increasing respiratory rate.

MEMORY CHIP

P Caffeine

- Used therapeutically for neonatal apnea, asthma, drowsiness, and fatigue
- Ingested nontherapeutically in cocoa, chocolate, coffee, tea, and cola
- Stimulates medullary respiratory center, CNS, and cardiovascular systems
- Most common adverse effects: usually an extension of its pharmacologic actions; caffeine withdrawal syndrome occurs with abrupt cessation after long-term or high intake of caffeine

It is not usually the drug of choice because of its narrow margin of safety. Adverse effects include hypertension, sinus tachycardia, arrhythmias, skeletal muscle hyperactivity, dyspnea, headache, dizziness, apprehension, disorientation, pupil dilation, convulsions, cough, tachypnea, laryngospasm, bronchospasm, nausea and vomiting, diarrhea, and urinary retention.

CHAPTER SUMMARY

- The CNS acts as a system of control and surveillance for many unconscious and conscious functions. Normal arousal mechanisms are affected through presynaptic release of neurotransmitters, such as norepinephrine, serotonin, and dopamine.
- The CNS stimulants are used therapeutically to treat several pathologic conditions, including narcolepsy, ADHD, obesity, and respiratory depression. CNS stimulants can be divided into three drug classes according to the specific effects they have on the body: central CNS stimulants, anorectic CNS stimulants, and respiratory CNS stimulants.
- The central CNS stimulants stimulate the CNS directly or indirectly, and drugs in this class include those that are used therapeutically and nontherapeutically. Those that are used therapeutically include dextroamphetamine, amphetamine salts, methylphenidate, pemoline, and cocaine. Those used nontherapeutically include amphetamines, cocaine, nicotine, and caffeine.
- The prototype centrally acting CNS stimulant is dextroamphetamine. It is used to treat ADHD and narcolepsy. Nursing management concerns regarding dextroamphetamine relate to preventing abuse, promoting adherence to the therapeutic regimen, and recognizing and managing adverse effects.
- Another stimulant drug used to treat ADHD is methylphenidate, which has many different trade names. Each proprietary drug has a different vehicle for administration, or pharmacokinetics.
- Other classes of drugs used in the management of ADHD include nonstimulants such as atomoxetine, antihypertensive medications, and antidepressant medications.
- The anorectic CNS stimulants may directly stimulate the satiety center in the hypothalamus. These drugs include phentermine, benzphetamine, diethylpropion, mazindol, phendimetrazine, and phenylpropanolamine. Their mechanisms of action relate to adrenergic or serotonergic inhibition of the hypothalamic satiety center.
- Anorectic drug use is controversial and not effective as monotherapy. These drugs should be used as part of an overall strategy to control obesity.
- All anorectic drugs except phenylpropanolamine are available by prescription only. They all exhibit a wide range of adverse effects.
- Nursing management for anorectic drugs should focus on careful pretreatment assessment, adequate therapeutic monitoring, and proper patient and family education.
- The respiratory CNS stimulants directly affect the brain stem and respiratory centers. Respiratory CNS stimulants include caffeine and doxapram.

QUESTIONS FOR STUDY AND REVIEW

1. Many stimulants are used in the management of ADHD. Develop a learning tool to differentiate between short-acting, intermediate- acting, and long-acting stimulants.

2. You are working in an outpatient setting that specializes in the management of ADHD in children. Develop a series of questions that you would ask parents during follow-up visits. Develop a list of observations that you should document after each visit.

3. You have been telephoned by the daughter of your discharged patient, Mrs. Christo. Mrs. Christo was sent home last week with a diagnosis of narcolepsy and was taking dextroamphetamine, 30 mg/day. Her daughter wants to know how effective this drug is. What questions would you ask her to be able to answer her question properly?

4. You are talking with a colleague who tells you, "I must be allergic to my home. Every weekend I have a terrible headache. I feel tired, dizzy, and lethargic. I never feel this way at work. What could be wrong with me?"

5. Your patient has morbid obesity. She is prescribed phentermine. What are the most important teaching points for this patient?

6. How do phentermine and orlistat differ in their mechanisms of action?

NEED MORE HELP?

Chapter 22 of the Study Guide to Accompany *Drug Therapy in Nursing*, 4th Edition, contains NCLEX-style questions and other learning activities to reinforce your understanding of the concepts presented in this chapter. For additional information or to purchase the study guide, visit thePoint.

REFERENCES

Antai-Otong, D. (2008, July). The art of prescribing. Pharmacological management of adult ADHD: implications for psychiatric care. *Perspectives in Psychiatric Care*, 44(3):196–201. Retrieved from CINAHL Plus with Full Text database.

Attention Deficit Hyperactivity Disorder. Retrieved from *http://www.nimh.nih.gov/health/topics/attention-deficit-hyperactivity-disorder-adhd/index.shtml*

Bloom, B., Cohen, R. A. (2007). Summary health statistics for U.S. children. National health interview survey 2006. *Vital and Health Statistics*. Series 10, Data from the National Health Survey, Sep;(234):1–79.

Bray, G. (2008). Medications for weight reduction. *Endocrinology & Metabolism Clinics of North America*, 37(4):923–942. http://search.ebscohost.com.ezproxy.socccd.edu

DeNoon, D. J. (2009). *Contrave*: New weight loss drug advances. http://www.webmd.com/diet/news/20090608/contrave-new-weight-loss-drug-advances.

Facts and Comparisons. (2010). *Drug facts and comparisons*. Philadelphia, PA: Lippincott Williams & Wilkins.

Karch, A. M. (2010). *Nursing Drug Guide*. Philadelphia, PA: Lippincott Williams & Wilkins.

Koda-Kimbal, M. A., Young, L.Y., Kradian, W. A., et al. (2008). *Applied Therapeutics: The Clinical Use of Drugs*, Philadelphia, PA: Lippincott Williams & Wilkins.

Meijer, W., Faber, A. E., & Tobi, H. (2009). Current issues around the pharmacotherapy of ADHD in children and adults. *Pharmacy World & Science*, 31(5):509–516.

Micromedex Healthcare Series. Retrieved from *http://healthcare.micromedex.com*.

NHANES study. (2007). Retrieved from *http://www.cdc.gov/nchs/nhanes.htm*.

Pineda, D., Palacio, L., Puerta, I., Merchán, V., Arango, C., Galvis, A., et al. (2007). Environmental influences that affect attention deficit/hyperactivity disorder: study of a genetic isolate. *European Child & Adolescent Psychiatry*, 16(5):337–346.

Porth, C. M. (2008). Pathophysiology: *Concepts of Altered Health States (8th Ed)*, Philadelphia, PA: Lippincott Williams & Wilkins.

Prasad, S., Arellano, J., Steer, C., & Libretto, S. (2009). Assessing the value of atomoxetine in treating children and adolescents with ADHD in the UK. *International Journal of Clinical Practice*, 63(7):1031–1040.

Schmidt, B., Roberts, R., Davis, P., et al. (2007). Long-term effects of caffeine therapy for apnea of prematurity. *The New England Journal of Medicine*, 357(19):1893–1902.

Spencer, T., Biederman, J., & Mick, E. (2007). Attention-deficit/hyperactivity disorder: diagnosis, lifespan, comorbidities, and neurobiology. *Ambulatory Pediatrics*, 7(1S):73–81. Retrieved from CINAHL Plus with Full Text database.

Tatro, D. S. (2011). *Drug Interaction Facts: The Authority on Drug Interactions*. Philadelphia, PA: Lippincott Williams & Wilkins.

Visser, S., Lesesne, C., & Perou, R. (2007). National estimates and factors associated with medication treatment for childhood attention-deficit/hyperactivity disorder. *Pediatrics*, 119:s99–s106.

Volkow, N., Wang, G., Kollins, S., et al. (2009). Evaluating dopamine reward pathway in ADHD: clinical implications. *JAMA: Journal of the American Medical Association*, 302(10):1084–1091.

Woo, J., Sea, M., Tong, P., et al. (2007, December). Effectiveness of a lifestyle modification programme in weight maintenance in obese subjects after cessation of treatment with Orlistat. *Journal of Evaluation in Clinical Practice*, 13(6):853–859. Retrieved from CINAHL Plus with Full Text database.

UNIT 6
Analgesic and Anti-Inflammatory Drugs

23

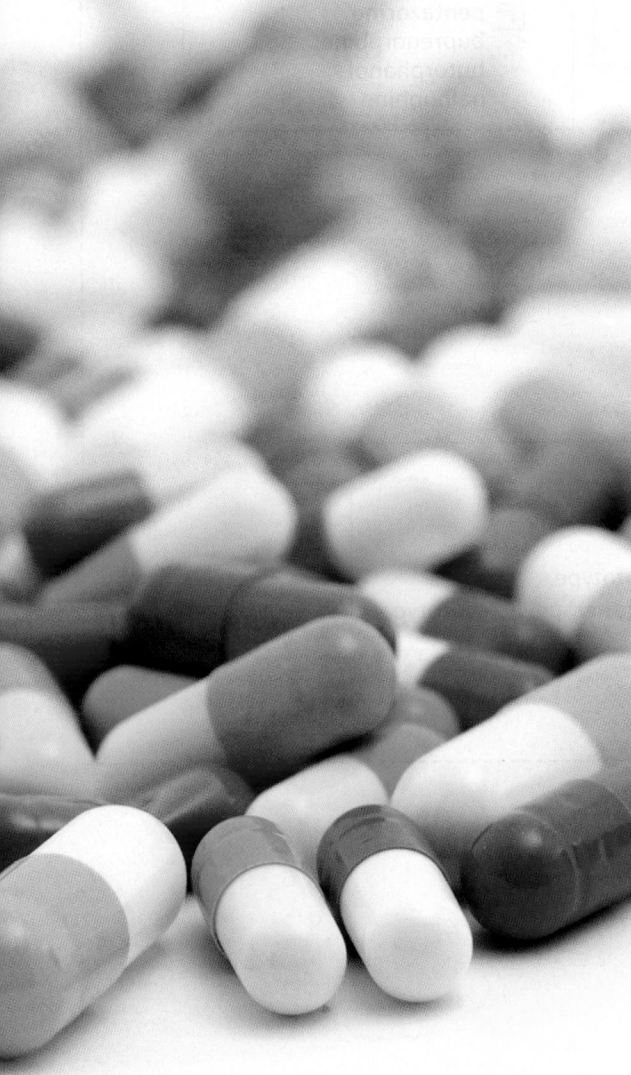

Drugs Treating Severe Pain

Learning Objectives

At the completion of this chapter the student will:

1. Define pain.
2. Describe the physiology of the central nervous system (CNS) as it relates to pain.
3. Differentiate the types of pain.
4. Differentiate the various methods used in pain management.
5. Be able to assess pain.
6. Describe the effects of agonist stimulation and antagonist stimulation at the opiate receptors.
7. Identify core drug knowledge about narcotic drugs.
8. Identify core patient variables related to narcotic drugs.
9. Relate the interaction of core drug knowledge to core patient variables for narcotic drugs that relieve pain.
10. Generate a nursing plan of care from the interactions between core drug knowledge and core patient variables for narcotic drugs used to control pain.
11. Describe nursing interventions that maximize therapeutic effects and minimize adverse effects when narcotics are given for pain management.
12. Describe the key points for patient and family education when narcotics are used in pain management.

Key Terms

acute pain	chronic pain	opioid
addiction	dependence	pain
adjunct analgesics	narcotic	rescue dose
analgesics	neuropathic pain	tolerance
breakthrough pain	nociceptic pain	

Drugs Treating Severe Pain

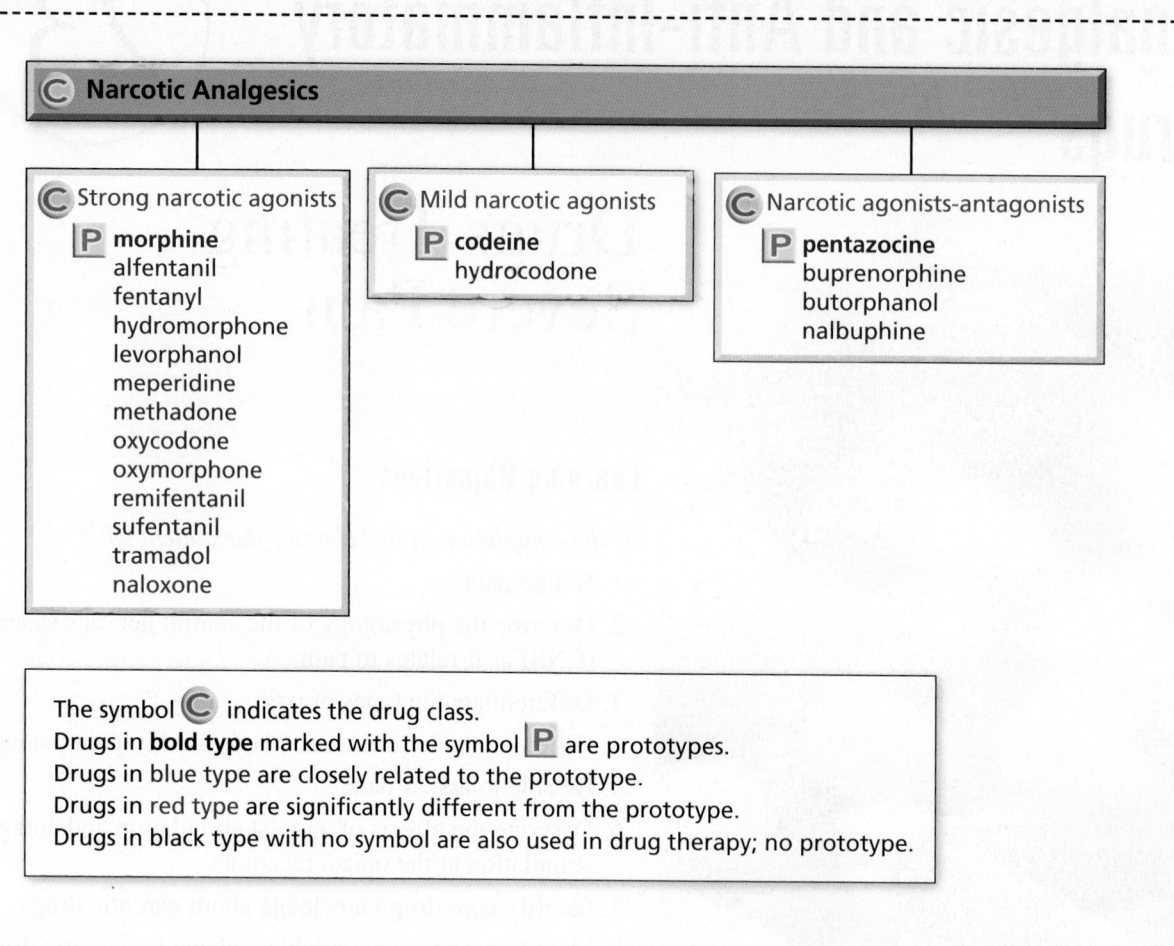

Narcotic Analgesics

Strong narcotic agonists
- **morphine**
  - alfentanil
  - fentanyl
  - hydromorphone
  - levorphanol
  - meperidine
  - methadone
  - oxycodone
  - oxymorphone
  - remifentanil
  - sufentanil
  - tramadol
  - naloxone

Mild narcotic agonists
- **codeine**
  - hydrocodone

Narcotic agonists-antagonists
- **pentazocine**
  - buprenorphine
  - butorphanol
  - nalbuphine

The symbol **C** indicates the drug class.
Drugs in **bold type** marked with the symbol **P** are prototypes.
Drugs in blue type are closely related to the prototype.
Drugs in red type are significantly different from the prototype.
Drugs in black type with no symbol are also used in drug therapy; no prototype.

ain is a multidimensional, subjective experience encompassing the physiologic, sensory, affective, cognitive, behavioral, and sociocultural dimensions of a patient's life. The International Association for the Study of Pain's definition of pain is the most widely used and emphasizes that pain is multidimensional; it defines pain as "an unpleasant sensory and emotional experience associated with actual or potential tissue damage, or described in terms of such damage" (International Association for the Study of Pain). Pain can truly be measured only by subjective data because no objective finding is present in all painful experiences. As early as 1968, the nurse-researcher Margo McCaffery defined pain as "whatever the experiencing person says it is, existing whenever s/he says it does" (McCaffery, 1968). Thus, only the person experiencing pain can accurately state when pain is present and how it is being experienced. Pain may accompany disease or treatment and may change over time. Pain may result from multiple simultaneous causes. If unrelieved, pain can affect the patient's psychological, social, physiologic, and spiritual health and can prevent productive work and enjoyment of personal relationships. Despite the substantial effects that pain has on health status, multiple studies over the years have shown that health care providers undertreat pain, leading patients to suffer needlessly. Approximately one in four Americans age 20 years or older experienced pain lasting a day or longer within the past month (U.S. Department of Health and Human Services, 2006).

Pain may be a major indication for drug therapy, and nurses need knowledge of drug therapy based on core drug knowledge for prescribed drugs. Moreover, pain has an important bearing on multiple core patient variables, which nurses must consider during initial and ongoing assessments and evaluations of drug therapy.

This chapter presents three types of drugs used to treat pain: strong narcotics, mild narcotics, and mixed agonist-antagonists. Morphine is the prototype strong narcotic. Codeine is the prototype mild narcotic. Pentazocine is the prototype mixed agonist-antagonist opioid.

PHYSIOLOGY

The peripheral nervous system and central nervous system (CNS) comprise an integrated system that provides a pathway for pain transmission. The physiologic mechanisms involved in the pain response are complex and are not yet completely understood. Transduction is the term used to describe the phenomena associated with the initiation of a pain signal. Pain receptors are found on the peripheral end plates of afferent neurons. Afferent neurons carry signals into the CNS, whereas efferent neurons carry signals from the CNS to the periphery. The sensation of peripheral pain begins in afferent neurons called nociceptors, which are found in the skin, muscle, connective tissue, circulatory system, and abdominal, pelvic, and thoracic viscera. Nociceptors are preferentially stimulated by a noxious stimulus or to a stimulus that would become noxious if prolonged; these include mechanical, thermal, hormonal (namely prostaglandins), or chemical (namely histamine, bradykinin, and serotonin, which are released during cellular destruction) stimuli. For example, when you stub your toe, pressure in the surrounding tissue causes direct mechanical activation of pain receptors. Potassium, which leaks from the damaged cells into the tissues, then activates the inflammatory response, sending chemical mediators to the site of injury. These mediators are chemically caustic to the nociceptors. Stimulation of the receptors at the end plates then promotes cellular depolarization and generates an action potential.

There are two types of nociceptors: delta fibers and C fibers. Delta fibers are fast traveling, myelinated, and responsive to mechanical stimuli. They sense sharp, stinging, cutting, or pinching pain. C fibers are slow traveling, unmyelinated, and responsive to mechanical, chemical, hormonal, or thermal stimuli. They sense dull, burning, or aching pain. During inflammation, nociceptors become sensitized, discharge spontaneously, and produce ongoing pain. Prolonged firing of the C-fiber nociceptors allows cells to release glutamate, which has a role in the conduction of nerve impulses. Glutamate acts on specialized receptors in the spinal cord, known as N-methyl-D-aspartate (NMDA) receptors. Stimulation of the NMDA receptors causes the spinal cord neurons to become more responsive to all incoming stimuli, leading to a central sensitization to pain impulses.

Once the nociceptor depolarizes, transmission of the pain signal has begun. Transmission is the process whereby the pain information is carried from the receptor end plate along the axon of the afferent neuron. Nociceptors enter the spinal cord and terminate in the dorsal horn, where they synapse in distinct regions. Substance P, a peptide in the unmyelinated fibers entering the dorsal horn, is released in response to painful stimuli. Substance P is a neurotransmitter and neuromodulator that activates special receptor sites. It appears to have a role in interpreting pain and regulating self-produced (endogenous) analgesic responses to nociceptor stimulation (Figure 23.1). The release of excitatory amino acids, such as glutamate and aspartate, also has an important role in carrying the painful stimulus to the brain.

From the dorsal horn, impulses are transferred, through the spinothalamic and spinoreticulothalamic tracts, to various higher brain areas for interpretation. Pain is mediated and modulated through forebrain mechanisms, which act at the spinal, brainstem, cerebral, and limbic levels. Stimulation of these various areas produces an affective response to the painful stimuli based on the individual's previous experience with pain as well as on social, environmental, and cultural influences. Thus, the response to any given painful stimulus is different for different people. The forebrain has the greatest control over nociceptor functioning. Indeed, pathology of the forebrain can cause pain, even if the nociceptors have not been activated peripherally. Pain perception involves multiple cerebral structures. During clinical studies of pain, brain imaging with positron emission tomography (PET) has identified some of the principal structures of this central

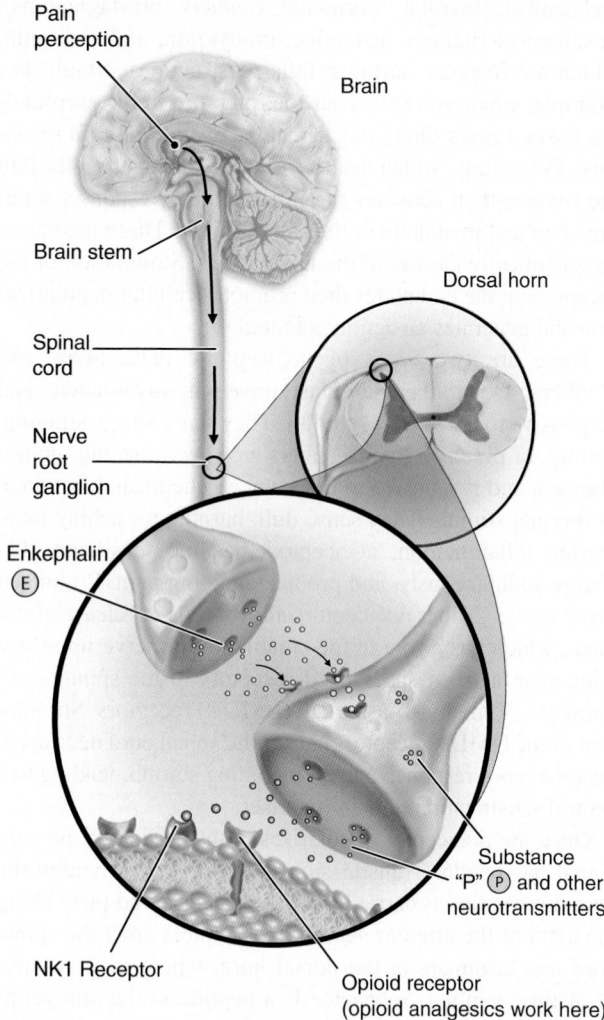

Pain perception

Brain

Brain stem

Dorsal horn

Spinal cord

Nerve root ganglion

Enkephalin
(E)

NK1 Receptor

Substance "P" (P) and other neurotransmitters

Opioid receptor
(opioid analgesics work here)

• FIGURE 23.1 Inhibiting pain perceived over ascending pathways. Once the brain interprets a stimulus as pain, the nervous system responds along descending pathways. From the brain's perception of pain, an impulse is routed through the brainstem and into the spinal cord and travels through the dorsal horn to a dorsal root ganglion. Here, the impulses descending from the raphe nucleus system trigger the release of enkephalin (a peptide or endorphin-like substance). Enkephalin attaches to receptors, causing substance P and other neurotransmitters involved in pain perception to be either released or inhibited from release, depending on the type of receptor to which it attaches. This drawing illustrates that enkephalin is mostly inhibiting the release of substance P and other neurotransmitters. When substance P and other neurotransmitters are released, they attach to neurokinin 1 receptors and the person will sense pain. When substance P and other neurotransmitters are prohibited from release due to extensive enkephalin attachment, the person will not sense pain. The experience of pain can also be diminished by administering opioid analgesics, such as morphine, which attach to the opioid receptors.

network activated by pain. PET imaging has shown synaptically induced increases in regional cerebral blood flow in several regions of the brain when a person is exposed to painful stimuli. The intensity of the blood flow response in the brain correlates parametrically with perceived pain intensity. The areas of the brain involved in interpreting pain include the contralateral insula and anterior cingulate cortex, frontal inferior cortex, posterior cingulate cortex, bilateral thalamus and premotor cortex, and cerebellar vermis. These brain regions

are functionally diverse and are involved with sensation, motor control, affect, and attention.

Components That Influence Pain

Pain has sensory-discriminative (physical) components and affective-motivational (emotional) components. The sensory dimension of pain encompasses pain's location, intensity, and quality. The quality of pain is the way it feels to the patient, for example, burning or gnawing. Affective aspects relate to the way that pain influences a patient's well-being, such as whether it is perceived as annoying, tortuous, or killing pain. Stimulation of the limbic system produces this emotional response to the physical stimulus of pain. Phenomena thought to influence the perception of pain are anxiety, fear, apprehension, attention, motivation, and other cognitive processes. For example, anxiety, fear, or apprehension appears to make the patient more sensitive to pain, allowing the patient to experience stimuli as painful when, under other circumstances, they might not be experienced this way. Conversely, the patient who is aware of his or her condition and wants to control pain may deliberately use techniques (e.g., distraction by talking to others) to cope and decrease the pain experienced. Inhibition of pain and the transmission of painful stimuli occur in various regions of the brain. Inhibitory substances such as endogenous opioids, serotonin, norepinephrine, and gamma-aminobutyric acid (GABA) are released into nerve synapses. These substances bind with receptors on primary afferent and dorsal horn neurons to prevent further transmission of painful stimuli. The ability to release these internal pain modulators varies from person to person; this variation partly explains why, when two people have a similar injury, one may feel a great deal of pain, whereas the other does not.

The peripheral and central nervous systems can become overly sensitized to nociceptive input. When the release of inflammatory mediators or the painful stimulus is intense, repeated, or prolonged, the nociceptors in the periphery generate more nerve impulses than usual and release the impulses more frequently. Central spinal neurons can become overexcited by substantial tissue or nerve injury and by recurrent input from the peripheral nervous system. When overexcitation occurs, the pain response may spread to additional areas in the brain. The patient can then experience an increased pain response to the same stimuli, a pain response to stimuli not previously experienced as painful, or pain from an uninjured area (referred pain). The overstimulation of the central spinal neurons may continue to produce a pain response long after the painful stimulus is gone.

Types of Pain

A number of different terms are used to describe and categorize pain. Pain can be categorized based on its presumed underlying pathophysiology as being either nociceptic or neuropathic. **Nociceptic pain** is caused by the activation of the delta and C nociceptors in response to painful stimuli, such as injury, disease, or inflammation. Pain perception and stimulus intensity are generally closely related to nociceptive pain. Nociceptic pain also indicates real or potential tissue damage. Nociceptic pain is further categorized as either somatic or visceral. Somatic pain results from ongoing activation of peripheral nociceptors found in structural tissues, such as bone, muscle, and soft tissue. It can be further divided as either deep or superficial. It is characterized as well-localized and intermittent, or as constant, aching, gnawing, throbbing, burning, or cramping. The bone and joint pain of arthritis is a common source of somatic pain. Muscle strains after intense physical exertion also result in somatic pain. Both of these are examples of deep somatic pain. Sunburn is an example of superficial somatic pain.

Visceral pain results from stimulation within the deep tissues or organs and surrounding structural tissues. Common visceral pain syndromes include pain associated with cholecystitis, pancreatitis, uterine and ovarian disease, and liver disease. Patients often describe visceral pain as deep, boring, diffuse abdominal pain. Visceral pain is less circumscribed than somatic pain and often has a referred component (e.g., pain from the liver, which can be referred to the right shoulder) or neuropathic processes or causes. Additionally, pain can be described according to its duration (e.g., acute or chronic) or by its underlying pathophysiologic cause (e.g., cancer). Differentiation of pain serves a critical role in diagnostic and therapeutic planning. Adequate pain management is based on accurate pain assessments.

Neuropathic pain is the term used to represent pain in which the underlying pathology is abnormal processing of stimuli in the peripheral or central nervous systems. Thus, neuropathic pain is a result of some injury to the peripheral receptors, afferent fibers, or CNS, or an impairment of the nervous system. Neuropathic pain is unique in character and distribution. It can be described as shooting, burning, or stabbing and generally follows a radicular or radiating pattern. Neuropathic pain is often caused by trauma, inflammation, metabolic disease (e.g., diabetes), infections such as herpes zoster, toxins, and primary neurologic diseases. Several neuropathic pain syndromes may occur in patients with cancer. For example, direct tumor infiltration from adjacent soft tissues or lymph nodes or compression from metastases in the adjacent bony pelvis can damage the lumbosacral plexus. Postmastectomy syndrome is the result of nerve injury, with the development of a traumatic neuroma following surgery. It is characterized by a constricting, burning sensation in the posterior arm, axilla, and anterior chest and is aggravated by movement.

Acute pain, meaning the immediate phase of response to an insult or injury, results from tissue damage. It has cognitive, emotional, and sensory features. Acute pain resolves with the healing of the underlying injury. It is usually nociceptic but can be neuropathic. Acute pain may be related to the treatment of an underlying disease process or to an injury that is expected to resolve. Medical procedures, operations, and trauma are examples of types of treatments resulting in acute pain. Postsurgical pain is the most common treatment-related pain.

Chronic pain is no longer defined purely by how long it is present. In contrast to acute pain, chronic pain may persist well beyond actual tissue injury and healing. The level of identified pathology may be low or insufficient to account for the presence or extent of the pain experienced. Stress and other nonbiologic influences may exacerbate pain intensity, despite a reduction in the physiologic cause of the pain. Chronic pain disrupts sleep and normal living; it does not have an adaptive or useful purpose, as acute pain does. Nearly two thirds of older adults (65 years of age and older) who had pain in the past month stated that their pain has lasted for one year or longer (U.S. Department of Health and Human Services, 2006).

Cancer pain is one type of chronic pain. The pain may be related to the disease itself, or to diagnostic procedures or treatments for the cancer. The pain is usually progressive as the disease advances to end stage and can be severe and debilitating. Additionally, acute episodes may occur, either in response to movement or activity or secondary to therapy or treatment of cancer, such as surgical removal of the tumor or skin irritation from radiation. Cancer pain may also be intermittent. These acute and chronic components make it difficult to classify.

Chronic noncancer pain is another subtype of chronic pain. Chronic noncancer pain usually does not correspond well to identifiable levels of tissue pathology, and it frequently also does not respond well to standard treatments for pain. Chronic noncancer pain may arise from an acute injury that proceeds to chronic pain or from various chronic conditions such as osteoarthritis, migraine headaches, chronic abdominal pain from irritable bowel disease or other conditions, or from neuralgias. Chronic noncancer pain ranges from mild to excruciating.

Whatever the source or classification, pain may delay healing and rehabilitation, prolong other symptoms, and leave the patient immunocompromised. Every effort should be mobilized to manage pain effectively, including stepped pharmacologic intervention (i.e., predetermined, progressive levels of intervention).

DRUG THERAPY TO MANAGE PAIN

When drug therapy is prescribed to treat pain, the pharmacotherapeutics and pharmacokinetics of the drug and relevant core patient variables help govern which drug is selected. Drug therapy may be used to correct the underlying pathophysiologic cause of the pain (e.g., nitroglycerin, a vasodilator, to treat angina pectoris from narrowed coronary vessels), or it may be used to decrease the pain response itself (e.g., morphine to treat postsurgical pain). The degree of pain that the patient is experiencing affects the pharmacodynamics of **analgesics** (drugs used to treat pain). Nowadays, preventing pain is generally accepted to be easier than decreasing pain. It is also easier to treat pain at low levels than at severe levels. Pain that is allowed to escalate requires larger doses of drugs to obtain relief. These interrelationships between pain and core drug variables affect the therapeutic management of pain.

Drug classifications that are normally used for pain management are the **opioid** analgesics and the nonsteroidal anti-inflammatory drugs (NSAIDs). The opioids derive their name from opium because they are natural alkaloids, semisynthetic analogues, or synthetic compounds of opium. Opioids, or **narcotics,** as they are more commonly called, act on the CNS to interfere with the pain experience. Morphine is the standard drug of choice in this category, and all other opioids are compared with it when their efficacy is evaluated. NSAIDs act in the peripheral nervous system, interfering with prostaglandin synthesis and preventing the transmission of pain impulses. Some drugs are combinations of these drug classes, and they act on both the CNS and peripheral nervous system simultaneously. NSAIDs and other nonopiate analgesics, such as acetaminophen (Tylenol), are used to treat mild to moderate pain. Opioids are used in the treatment of moderate to severe pain. For more information on NSAIDs and acetaminophen, see Chapter 24.

The dose and choice of analgesics must be individualized to meet the patient's need for pain relief. However, adverse effects from any given drug may place a ceiling on how large a daily dose can be.

Some other drug classes are used as secondary pain relievers, although their pharmacotherapeutics indicate that their primary uses are for other problems. When drugs are used secondarily for pain relief, they are known as **adjunct analgesics** or co-analgesics. Using multiple types of drugs to treat the exact symptoms of pain experienced is similar to using a combination of drugs (e.g., those that are cell cycle–specific and those that are not cell cycle–specific) to treat cancer. The outcome is more effective than that of any one drug alone. Adjuvant drugs can increase the efficacy of narcotics or provide independent analgesia for specific types of pain. Other CNS depressants that are primarily indicated for other diseases and disorders can be used as adjuncts. Included in this group are drugs that have antiemetic effects (effects against nausea) or mild tranquilizing effects. These CNS depressants are

frequently used in acute pain (e.g., postsurgical pain). Classifications of other adjuvant drugs include antidepressants, corticosteroids, and antiepileptics. Antidepressants are the treatment of choice for neuropathic pain described as burning or numbing. In clinical trials, tricyclic antidepressants are the only antidepressant drugs proved effective in managing neuropathic pain. Antipsychotic drugs, especially atypical antipsychotics, have been used as adjuncts to narcotic treatment for pain, although the literature is somewhat mixed about their effectiveness when used in this manner. Additionally, the adverse effects from antipsychotics may make them unsuitable for use in pain control (Seidel et al., 2010).

Steroids are useful for treating short-term, severe, episodic pain, such as that associated with nerve compression. They are also used in managing cancer pain to relieve chronic pressure-related pain states, such as progressive visceral distention, severe lymphedema, increased intracranial pressure, soft-tissue infiltration unrelieved by NSAIDs and opioids, and continuing nerve compression.

Antiepileptics are important adjuncts for neuropathic pain, particularly that described as stabbing or piercing. The antiepileptics are used for conditions such as trigeminal neuralgia, sciatica, migraine headache, and various neuropathic pain states in patients with cancer. These agents directly affect the peripheral nerve conduction of pain impulses, which is completely separate from their central effect. Research now shows that the antiepileptic gabapentin is helpful in decreasing postoperative pain (Box 23.1).

Finally, in addition to pharmacologic interventions to treat pain, nonpharmacologic methods may be used. These methods are not substitutes for analgesics, especially in moderate to severe pain, but they are valuable adjuncts to therapy. The effective use of nonpharmacologic measures may decrease the dose of narcotic that is required, thereby achieving pain control while minimizing adverse effects. Nonpharmacologic techniques include cognitive strategies for relaxation and

---

BOX 23.1 FOCUS ON RESEARCH

Antiepileptics as Adjuncts for Postoperative Pain Control

Ho, K. Y., Gan, T. J., & Habib, A. S. (2006). Gabapentin and postoperative pain: A systematic review of randomized controlled trials. *Pain, 126*(1–3):91–101.

The Study

This literature review evaluated the efficacy and tolerability of perioperative gabapentin, an antiepileptic drug, for the control of acute postoperative pain when used as an adjunct to opioid therapy. Sixteen randomized controlled clinical trials were identified which compared gabapentin to a placebo control in surgical patients. Meta-analysis of the 16 trials showed that gabapentin decreased reported postoperative pain intensity measured 6 and 24 hours after surgery. Gabapentin also decreased the cumulative opioid dose over 24 hours.

Nursing Implications

Literature reviews of randomized controlled trials provide an overview of the "state of the science" and help nurses and other health care

providers determine if there is any value in a particular intervention. A single research study frequently does not involve enough patients to generalize findings sufficiently, so that they can be applied to all patients in similar circumstances. This review considered the findings from 16 studies together. All these studies were controlled trials with a placebo; this is considered the "gold standard" of a research study, so the findings are most likely to be valid and reliable. Gabapentin has been accepted as an adjunct to chronic pain in the past, but this is new documentation that it may have an important place in the management of acute postoperative pain as well. Nurses might expect to see the use of gabapentin increase in the treatment of postoperative pain. If a particular patient is not a good candidate for receiving opioids (e.g., history of respiratory depression from opioid use, renal or hepatic dysfunction that would impair opioid elimination) or if they have previously had postoperative pain experiences that were difficult to control with an opioid alone, the nurse may consult with the other health care professionals about including gabapentin in the patient's pain management.

TABLE 23.1   Nonpharmacologic Techniques Used in Pain Contro

Technique	Summary Description
Relaxation therapy	Uses progressive muscle relaxation techniques, controlled breathing, and simple hypnosis strategies to help patient achieve physical and emotional relaxation
Guided imagery	Uses visual and auditory imagery selected by the patient and specific to pain-relieving or stress-reducing feelings
Biofeedback	Teaches control of stress through patient's ability to monitor and manipulate some aspects of the autonomic nervous system
Music distraction	Uses music that is selected by the patient for the purpose of distracting the patient from pain and focusing instead on rhythm, tone, harmony, and other aspects of the music
Exercise	Promotes blood flow and tissue oxygenation, prevents muscle atrophy and stiffness, assists in building muscle to stabilize painful joints. An exercise plan defined by a physiatrist is extremely helpful in very debilitated patients. Heat promotes increased blood flow to the affected part, whereas cold reduces swelling associated with the inflammatory response. Take care not to use excessive heat, which can cause burns. Try alternating heat with cold.
Transcutaneous electrical nerve stimulation	Attempts to "confuse" the pain signal by activating other sensory circuits
Massage (various types)	Alleviates muscle stiffness and pain by breaking up fibrous tissue in muscle, increasing circulation, and promoting normal elongation of muscle fibers

physical strategies that interrupt pain transmission. Table 23.1 describes some of the nonpharmacologic techniques used in pain control.

The accepted standard plan for treating pain remains the World Health Organization's model of stepped progression from nonopioid to opioid use, with increasing doses of the opioid until the pain is controlled. Nonopioids, including adjunct medications, may be added to an opioid regimen. Nonpharmacologic methods may also be added. Figure 23.2 illustrates the stepped-progression approach to pain control

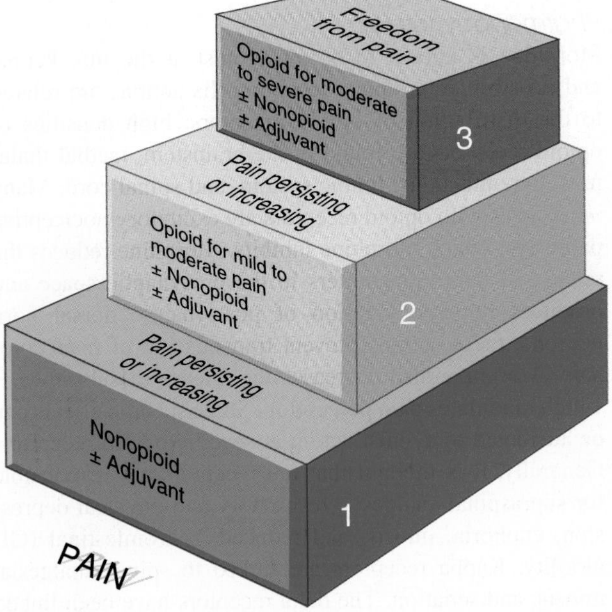

Students need to recognize that the World Health Organization's model is based upon pain starting as mild and then progressing in severity. In an acute care setting, where a patient presents in severe pain for example after surgery) the earliest steps of the model are not employed; instead treatment begins with opioid narcotics. Non-opioids and nonpharmacologic methods can then be added if needed to control pain.

Ⓒ NARCOTIC ANALGESICS

Narcotic analgesics are required for conditions, disorders, or treatments that are accompanied by moderate to severe pain. The narcotic analgesics are the most effective drugs for pain management.

The degree of pain relief that is achieved may be expressed in analgesic equivalents, which is the dose of an analgesic required to produce the same analgesic effect as a 10-mg dose of morphine (the standard measure of pain relief). Some equianalgesic dosages are presented in Table 23.2.

The narcotic analgesics include opiate agonists, mixed agonist-antagonists, and antagonists based on their activity at opioid receptors. Although five types of opiate receptor sites (with the Greek names of mu, kappa, sigma, delta, and epsilon) are known to exist, activity occurs at only three sites (mu, kappa, and delta) with the narcotic analgesics available. From a nursing standpoint, comparing strong with mild to moderate analgesics within the opiate agonist classification may be helpful. This comparison allows examination of two important opiate agonist prototypes: morphine (opiate agonist and strong analgesic) and codeine (opiate agonist and mild to moderate analgesic). Some narcotic analgesics have mixed opioid effects, being agonists at some receptors and antagonists at others. A mixed narcotic agonist-antagonist, pentazocine (Talwin), is also discussed in this chapter.

• FIGURE 23.2   The World Health Organization's three-step analgesic ladder.

TABLE 23.2 Equianalgesic Doses* (mg) of Selected Narcotic Analgesics

Drug	Oral	Parenteral
	Administration Route	
Morphine	30	10
Codeine	200	120–130
Fentanyl	—	0.1–0.2
hydromorphone	7.5	1.3–1.5
meperidine	300**	75
methadone	20 (acute) 2–4 (chronic)	10 (acute) 2–4 (chronic)
oxycodone	30	—
pentazocine	180	60

*In measuring pain relief, the analgesic equivalent compares the degree of pain relief achieved with that obtained by a 10-mg dose of morphine (the standard dose), given parenterally.

** Not a recommended dose.

Narcotics have an important role in pain management and control; however, they are typically underprescribed and underused. Although 26% of American adults reported having pain lasting longer than 24 hours in the past month, only 4.2% of those surveyed reported using a narcotic for pain control (U.S. Department of Health and Human Services, 2006). Research has repeatedly shown that major contributing factors to narcotic underuse are lack of knowledge on the part of health care professionals regarding pain and pain control and misinformation regarding the pharmacokinetics and pharmacodynamics of narcotics. Because patients' pain may be incorrectly assessed and improperly treated, nurses need to be aware of current advances in measuring, classifying, and managing pain.

● Ⓒ STRONG NARCOTIC AGONISTS

Strong narcotic agonists include morphine, hydromorphone, levorphanol, oxycodone, oxymorphone, meperidine, fentanyl, alfentanil, sufentanil, methadone, tramadol, and remifentanil. Table 23.3 presents a summary of selected narcotic analgesics and antagonists. The prototype strong narcotic agonist is morphine. The narcotic antagonist naloxone is significantly different from morphine.

Nursing Management of the Patient Receiving Ⓟ Morphine
Core Drug Knowledge
Pharmacotherapeutics
The most important clinical indication for morphine is moderate to severe acute or chronic pain, including postoperative pain and pain that is nonresponsive to nonnarcotic

analgesics. It can be used to treat chronic pain that is either cancer pain or noncancer chronic pain. Morphine is also used in dyspnea associated with acute left ventricular failure and pulmonary edema; it is the only narcotic agonist used to treat the pain of myocardial infarction (MI). Preoperatively, morphine can be used to sedate a patient, relieve anxiety, facilitate induction of anesthesia, or reduce the amount of anesthetic needed.

Morphine can be administered by multiple routes: oral (PO), subcutaneous (SC), intramuscular (IM), intravenous (IV), epidural, rectal, and topical. Oral forms of morphine are preferred in treating cancer pain, unless the patient is unable to take medication by this route. The sustained-release form (MS Contin, Oramorph, or Kadian) is used only for patients who require an opioid analgesic for more than a few days and need around-the-clock pain control. Of the parenteral routes, the SC and IM routes should be limited to occasions when the drug is to be administered only one time. Repeated injections every 3 to 4 hours should be avoided because they cause additional discomfort, and repeated IM injections risk nerve and muscle injury. To provide continuous, 24-hour administration of morphine through a parenteral route, administer the drug by IV infusion regulated by an infusion-control pump.

Pharmacokinetics
Onset of analgesic effect occurs within 15 to 30 minutes and lasts for about 3 to 7 hours. Morphine is metabolized in the liver and gut wall by conjugation to glucuronide, an active metabolite, which is excreted along with unchanged morphine in urine and breast milk. It is also excreted in the feces through biliary and enterohepatic recycling. It has a half-life of 1.5 to 2 hours.

Pharmacodynamics
Morphine is known to be an agonist at the mu, kappa, and possibly delta opiate receptors. Its actions are related to the distribution of opioid receptors; high densities of opioid receptors are found in the brainstem, medial thalamus, hypothalamus, limbic system, and spinal cord. Many other areas with opioid receptors are excitatory nociceptive pathways, which morphine inhibits. Morphine reduces the release of neurotransmitters in the presynaptic space and produces hyperpolarization of postsynaptic dorsal horn neurons; these actions prevent transmission of nociceptor pain. Morphine also decreases the release of substance P, which modulates pain perception. Some specific effects can be attributed to agonist action at specific opioid receptors. Generally, it is thought that mu receptors are responsible for supraspinal analgesia, respiratory and physical depression, euphoria, miosis, and reduced gastrointestinal (GI) motility. Kappa receptors are linked to spinal analgesia, miosis, and sedation. The delta receptors have been linked with dysphoria and psychotomimetic effects (effects, such

TABLE 23.3 Summary of Selected Ⓒ Narcotic Analgesics and Antagonists in Adults

Drug (Trade) Name	Selected Indications	Route and Dosage Range	Pharmacokinetics
Ⓟ morphine (Roxanol, RMS)	Moderate to severe acute and chronic pain, postoperative sedation, MI, pulmonary edema	Adult: q4h; 10–30 mg PO, IM, SC, 5–20 mg q4–6 h; IV, 2.5–15 mg diluted slow push; rectal, 10–20 mg q4h	Onset: PO, varies; IM, SC, rapid; IV, rapid Duration: 4–7 h $t_{1/2}$: 1.5 h
oxycodone (Roxicodone, Percodan, Percocet)	Moderate to moderately severe pain	Adult: PO, 5 mg q6h	Onset: 15–20 min Duration: 4–6 h $t_{1/2}$: Unknown
fentanyl (Sublimaze)	Analgesia during anesthesia, premedication, induction, maintenance and adjunct in anesthesia	Adult: IM/IV, 50–100 mcg 30–60 min preoperative; adjunct or postoperative, 2–100 mcg/kg; Adult: 12.5–100 mcg/h (system size in cm² = 5–40) Child: 12.5 mcg/h (system size in cm² = 5)	Onset: IM/IV, 7–8 min; transdermal, gradual Duration: IM/IV, 1–2 h; transdermal, 72 h $t_{1/2}$: 11/2–6 h
fentanyl transdermal (Duragesic)	Moderate to severe chronic pain`		
hydrocodone (Hycodan, Lortab)	Cough, analgesia	Adult: PO, 5–10 mg tid or qid for cough; 5–10 mg q4–6h for pain	Onset: 10–20 min Duration: Varies $t_{1/2}$: 3.8 h
hydromorphone (Dilaudid)	Moderate to severe acute pain Moderate to severe chronic pain	Adult: IM/SC, 1–2 mg q4–6 h IV, initial (opiate-naive patients), 0.2–0.6 mg IV (slow) q2–3h as needed ; titrate 1–2 mg IV (slow) q4–6h as needed PO, 2–4 mg q3–4h; IM/SC, 3–4 mg q3–4h	Onset: PO, 30 min; parenteral, 15 min Duration: PO, 3.6 h; parenteral, 4–5 h $t_{1/2}$: 2–3 h
levorphanol (Levo-Dromoran)	Anesthesia adjunct, moderate to severe pain	Adult: IM, slow IV, PO, 1–2 mg; may repeat in 3–8 h	Onset: 30–90 min Duration: 6–8 h $t_{1/2}$: 12–16 h
meperidine (Demerol)	Analgesia, PCA analgesia	Adult: PO, IM, SC, 50–150 mg q3–4h; PCA, 15–35 mg/h	Onset: PO, 15 min; IM, SC, 10–15 min Duration: 2–4 h $t_{1/2}$: 3–8 h
methadone (Dolophine)	Analgesia, narcotic detoxification and withdrawal	Adult: PO, IM, SC, 2.5–10 mg q3–4h for analgesia; PO, 40–120 mg/d as liquid for methadone maintenance	Onset: PO, 30–60 min; IM, SC, 10–20 min Duration: PO, 4–12 h; IM, SC, 4–6 h $t_{1/2}$: 25 h

Moderate Narcotic Analgesics

Ⓟ codeine	Cough, analgesia	Adult: PO, SC, IM, 15–60 mg q4h for pain, 10–20 mg q4h for cough	Onset: 15–20 min Duration: 4–6 h $t_{1/2}$: 3 h

Narcotic Agonist-Antagonist Analgesics

Ⓟ pentazocine (Talwin, Talacen)	Moderate to severe pain, anesthesia adjunct	Adult: PO, 50–100 mg q3–4h; IV, IM, or SC, 30 mg q3–4h	Onset: PO, 15–30 min; IM, SC, 10–20 min; IV, 2–3 min Duration: PO, 3–4 h; IM, SC, 1–3 h; IV, 60 min $t_{1/2}$: 2–3 h

(Continued)

TABLE 23.3   Summary of Selected ⓒ Narcotic Analgesics and Antagonists in Adults *(continued)*

Drug (Trade) Name	Selected Indications	Route and Dosage Range	Pharmacokinetics
buprenorphine (Buprenex)	Pain	*Adult:* IM, IV, 0.3 mg q6h	*Onset:* IM, 15 min; IV, 10 min *Duration:* 6 h $t_{1/2}$: 2–3 h
butorphanol (Stadol)	Pain, anesthesia adjunct	*Adult:* IV, 0.5–2 mg q3–4h for pain; 0.5–4 mg for anesthesia; IM, 2 mg q3–4h for pain	*Onset:* Rapid *Duration:* 3–4 h $t_{1/2}$: 2.1–9.2 h
nalbuphine (Nubain)	Moderate to severe pain, anesthesia adjunct	*Adult:* IM, IV, SC 10 mg q3–6h for pain	*Onset:* IM, SC, <15 min; IV, 2–3 min *Duration:* 3–6 h $t_{1/2}$: 5 h

as hallucinations, that mimic psychosis). The secondary pharmacologic effects of morphine, like those of other narcotic agonists, are related to various effects of receptor stimulation (Box 23.2).

Contraindications and Precautions

Morphine causes respiratory depression. The main contraindications to the use of morphine are hypersensitivity, pre-existing respiratory depression, acute or severe bronchial asthma, and upper airway obstruction. Morphine should also be avoided in premature infants and during labor when delivery of a premature infant is anticipated.

Other contraindications for morphine given by injection or immediate-release oral solutions include heart failure secondary to chronic lung disease, cardiac arrhythmias, increased intracranial or cerebrospinal pressure, head injury, brain tumor, acute alcoholism, or delirium tremens.

Because of its stimulating effects on the spinal cord, morphine should not be used during convulsions.

Caution must be used when administering morphine to patients receiving other CNS depressants because chances for respiratory depression increase. Morphine is generally considered contraindicated in cases of head injury and increased intracranial pressure; if it must be used in such cases, it must be given with extreme caution. Morphine, like all narcotics, may obscure clinical findings; the likelihood of respiratory depression and increased intracranial pressure is greater when morphine is given under these conditions. Caution should also be used when morphine is required for older or debilitated patients or those with renal or hepatic impairment. These patients may have altered pharmacokinetic processes and are more likely than other patients to exhibit adverse effects. Dose reduction may be necessary. Caution should also be used if morphine is

Box 23.2   SECONDARY PHARMACOLOGIC ACTIONS OF MORPHINE AND OTHER NARCOTICS

Provision of analgesia is the primary action of morphine and other narcotics. In addition, these drugs have a wide variety of other effects on the body.

- **Respiration:** Tidal volume is first increased, then decreased because of reduced sensitivity of the respiratory center to carbon dioxide. Depression is dose related. Deaths from overdose usually result from respiratory arrest.
- **Cough reflex:** Cough reflex is reduced because of direct effects on the cough center in the medulla. This may be useful, or it may promote a buildup of secretions, atelectasis, and airway obstruction.
- **Hypotension and orthostatic hypotension:** These result from peripheral vasodilation, reduced peripheral resistance, and inhibition of baroreceptors. Effect is exaggerated in the presence of hypovolemia.
- **Euphoria, dysphoria, alterations in mood, feelings of relaxation, drowsiness, apathy, mental confusion:** These result from stimulation of opioid receptors.
- **Nausea and vomiting:** These develop from direct stimulation of emetic chemoreceptor trigger zone (CTZ) in the medulla.

- **Itching, flushing, red eyes:** These are produced by release of histamine.
- **Miosis (pinpoint pupils):** This results from stimulation of oculomotor nuclei, which increases parasympathetic stimulation of the eye. No tolerance develops to this effect.
- **Abdominal pain, cramps:** These occur from decreased gastric motility; prolonged gastric emptying time; decreased biliary, pancreatic, and intestinal secretions; and delays in food digestion in small intestine. Resting tone of small intestine increases.
- **Constipation:** This happens because of diminished peristalsis, increased tone of large intestine before spasms occur, and inattention to the normal stimuli for defecation reflex.
- **Biliary colic and epigastric distress:** These are due to the constriction of the sphincter of Oddi.
- **Urinary retention, urinary urgency, and difficulty urinating:** These develop from increased tone of smooth muscles in urinary tract and spasms.

given to patients who are sensitive to CNS effects because of concurrent alterations in their health status (e.g., respiratory compromise from chronic obstructive pulmonary disease).

Adverse Effects

The most hazardous adverse effects of morphine relate to excessive CNS depression; they include respiratory depression, hypoventilation, apnea, respiratory arrest, circulatory depression, cardiac arrest, shock, and coma. The most frequent adverse effects of morphine and other agonist narcotics are respiratory depression, apnea, bradycardia, light-headedness, dizziness, sedation, nausea and vomiting, and sweating.

In addition, patients may experience cardiovascular adverse effects (e.g., hypotension, orthostatic hypotension, flushing, peripheral circulatory collapse); CNS effects (e.g., euphoria, dysphoria, delirium, agitation, anxiety, drowsiness, miosis, blurred vision, increased intracranial pressure); GI effects (e.g., abdominal pain, biliary tract spasm, anorexia, constipation); genitourinary (GU) effects (e.g., urinary retention or hesitancy, dysuria, decreased libido, impotence); and decreased cough reflex. Overdoses of morphine may be life threatening and should be treated with naloxone (Narcan), a narcotic antagonist.

Drug Interactions

Generally, providers can anticipate that concurrent therapy of morphine and any other CNS depressant may produce additive CNS adverse effects and substantial clinical effects. Increased respiratory and CNS depression effects are seen when morphine is given with barbiturate anesthetics, monoamine oxidase inhibitors (MAOIs), amitriptyline, cimetidine, clomipramine, and nortriptyline. Because morphine increases biliary tract pressure, levels of serum amylase or lipase may increase. One study showed that the bioavailability of oral morphine increased significantly following a high-fat meal. Parenteral mixtures of morphine with other drugs are often used when treating patients with a terminal disease who have severe pain. Table 23.4 lists drugs that interact with morphine.

Assessment of Relevant Core Patient Variables

Health Status

Assess the patient for respiratory depression. Morphine should not be administered to any patient with respiratory depression because it may precipitate respiratory arrest. It should not be given to anyone with a previous hypersensitivity to morphine.

Assess for current alterations in health status that place the patient at risk for increased sensitivity to CNS depressant effects. These include cardiac, renal, hepatic, or pulmonary disease; hypothyroidism; Addison disease; prostatic hypertrophy; or urethral stricture.

Before therapy, perform a physical examination to establish a baseline in order to monitor the drug's effects. Evaluate orientation, affect, respiratory rate, adventitious sounds, and character of bowel sounds. If prolonged use is anticipated or the patient has a history of hepatic dysfunction, ensure that liver function tests are performed, because morphine is metabolized in the liver.

Assess the patient for the presence and severity of pain. Pain is extremely subjective and unique for each person. The current health status can indicate whether pain might be expected. Physiologic changes that may bring on a pain response and indicate the need for drug therapy with morphine include decreased oxygenation of cardiac cells during an MI, inflamed or infected organs, or inappropriate cell growth from tumors pressing on nerves, vessels, or adjacent organs. Some health states are the source of pain for the patient, whereas others bring pain from their diagnosis or treatment. Postoperative pain is an example of pain caused by treatment.

Life Span and Gender

In using morphine or any other narcotic analgesic, assess for characteristics related to age, pregnancy, labor and delivery, and lactation.

For many years, experts believed that pain perception was absent or diminished in the very young and very old, but this belief is not true. Pain is felt by all humans, regardless of age. However, the inability to express that pain is occurring may impair assessment of pain in both very young and very old patients. Adults older than 65 years of

TABLE 23.4	Agents That Interact With Ⓟ Morphine	
Interactants	**Effect and Significance**	**Nursing Management**
barbiturate anesthetics	Additive respiratory and CNS depression; apnea	Monitor respiratory function.
cimetidine	Additive CNS depression, respiratory depression	Monitor for excessive morphine response and toxicity.
esmolol	Esmolol toxicity—bradycardia, hypotension	Monitor cardiovascular function (may need to decrease esmolol dosage).
other CNS depressants (alcohol, other narcotic analgesics)	Additive CNS depression, respiratory depression	Avoid combinations if possible. Monitor respiratory function.

age are less likely to report pain lasting more than one day than are adults aged 20 to 44 years (U.S. Department of Health and Human Services, 2006). The patient's age also influences the treatment of pain. Age-related factors are important when using morphine because it causes respiratory depression and hypotension.

The very young have impaired organ and system functioning because of immaturity. Therefore, doses of pain-relieving drugs need to be adjusted carefully to the child's body size and weight to prevent overdose and adverse effects.

Older adults are more likely to have age-related deterioration of organs, especially the liver and kidneys. Thus, they are more sensitive to adverse effects and can exhibit signs of overdose unless dose adjustments are made. Older adults should receive a reduced initial dose. Assess their response before additional doses are determined.

Nevertheless, children under 18 years of age and older adults may be undertreated for pain. In U.S. emergency department visits related to pain, children are less likely than adults to receive a narcotic for pain, regardless of the reported pain severity. In the same circumstances, older adults with severe pain are less likely to receive a narcotic than younger adults with severe pain (U.S. Department of Health and Human Services, 2006).

Morphine is assigned to pregnancy category C. Like other narcotics, morphine crosses the placenta rapidly. Abuse of narcotics by pregnant women can cause fetal dependency; infant withdrawal occurs after delivery. If narcotics are given during labor, respiratory depression and psychophysiologic effects may appear in the neonate. Resuscitation equipment and the narcotic antidote, naloxone, should be available. The premature infant is at even greater risk for severe respiratory depression from exposure to morphine. For these reasons, morphine should not be given during labor if the delivery of a preterm infant is expected. Morphine has also been shown to increase the length of labor.

Morphine is secreted in breast milk. Although morphine in breast milk does not usually produce serious problems, withdrawal may be precipitated in breast-fed infants if maternal morphine is discontinued rapidly after prolonged exposure. Waiting 4 to 6 hours after dosing with morphine to breast-feed will decrease the amount transferred to the infant.

The sex of the patient may also have an effect on pain and the need for morphine. Women are more likely than men to report pain (U.S. Department of Health and Human Services, 2006).

Lifestyle, Diet, and Habits

Morphine acts by depressing the CNS. Patients who use morphine to control chronic pain, such as that caused by cancer, or who receive morphine for an extended period eventually need higher doses to control their pain as they become tolerant to the drug's therapeutic effects. **Tolerance**

Box 23.3   DETERMINING OPIOID TOLERANCE

Certain drugs or drug doses are to be used only if the patient is opioid tolerant. To prevent medication errors and adverse effects to opioid-naive patients, nurses should be able to determine if a patient is opioid tolerant or not. Patients can be considered opioid tolerant if they have been receiving for a week or longer any of the following:

- 60 mg or more daily of morphine
- 30 mg or more daily of oxycodone
- 8 mg or more daily of oral hydromorphone
- Equianalgesic dose of any other opioid

---

means that the body has become accustomed to the effects of a substance and that the patient must use more of it to achieve the desired effect. With morphine, chronic usage may result in a degree of tolerance up to 35-fold. Clearly, as patients develop tolerance to morphine, they require larger doses to achieve adequate pain control. In addition to developing tolerance to therapeutic effects, patients also develop tolerance to adverse effects, including lethal effects, of morphine. Patients in whom drug tolerance develops can thus take dosages that would be potentially lethal in patients who are opioid naive. See Box 23.3 for more information about determining opioid tolerance.

Patients who abuse alcohol, prescription drugs that suppress the CNS (e.g., opioid analgesics or benzodiazepines), or street or illicit drugs have special needs when they have pain. When a patient abuses such substances, he or she may develop a cross-tolerance to morphine's pain-relieving effects. Thus, these patients also require higher than normal doses to achieve the desired therapeutic effects of pain relief.

In morphine use that lasts longer than 3 months, physical **dependence** also occurs. Dependence is characterized by a withdrawal or abstinence syndrome when morphine is discontinued; it represents an exaggerated rebound from its acute effects. Dependence may occur during the treatment of cancer pain, and it is important in the clinical management of such pain to allow for proper agonist coverage during changes in drug dosages, schedules, or type of drug therapy. Otherwise, the patient may experience unnecessary pain and the discomfort of abstinence syndrome. Physical dependence is *not* the same as addiction. Unlike tolerance and dependence, addiction is not an intrinsic, predictable drug effect. **Addiction** involves compulsive use of the drug for a secondary gain, not for pain control. The consensus document of the American Academy of Pain Medicine, American Pain Society, and the American Society of Addiction Medicine (2006) defines addiction as a neurobiologic disease characterized by one or more of these behaviors: impaired control over drug use, compulsive use, continued use despite harm, and craving. Genetic, psychosocial, and environmental factors influence the development of addiction. Patients who receive morphine for pain management, even over a long period, do not normally seek morphine once the pain stimulus is gone. However, they do need their morphine doses decreased slowly before the drug is discontinued to prevent withdrawal. Thus, they develop dependence but not addiction. It is very rare for patients who are using morphine, or another narcotic, strictly for relief of pain to develop addiction. Patients who currently abuse or have a history of abusing opioids do have a risk of addiction from drug therapy in pain management. This risk is not a reason to withhold morphine or any other opioid if the patient is experiencing pain. Instead, health care providers, in cooperation with the patient, can accomplish careful drug selection and dosage adjustment. If addiction does occur after therapy concludes, it must be addressed separately. Patients should be helped to wean themselves away from drug use before they are discharged from their providers' care.

Environment

Closely monitor patients receiving morphine as part of monitored anesthesia care (MAC) or postoperatively for signs of serious adverse effects, particularly respiratory depression. Health care providers or patients themselves may administer narcotic analgesics, as in patient-controlled analgesia (PCA). Morphine, like all narcotics, is a controlled substance, and by law every dose must be properly accounted for and documented, including partial doses that may be wasted. Although oral doses may be administered in any setting, doses given by IV infusion, injection, and epidural and intrathecal catheters are normally given only in the hospital, where the patient can be closely monitored. The exception is IV infusions, which may be used in the home during hospice care.

Culture and Inherited Traits

The experience of pain is personal and subjective; however, how people respond to painful stimuli reflects what they have learned about pain from their families, society, and cultures of origin. Learned messages about pain are indirect, and people react to them subconsciously. These messages include reasons that people experience pain and what are considered appropriate responses to it. For example, some religions view pain as a punishment from God for sins. Others view pain as a test from God to develop inner strength and faith. Still others may believe that pain is merely an aspect of life like any other. Some stoic cultures believe that people should tolerate pain without verbal complaints. British, German, and Asian groups are thought of as stoic cultures. Other cultural groups are very expressive about pain, see such expressiveness as acceptable, and may encourage it. Spanish, Italian, and Latin groups are thought to be expressive cultures. Recent studies of Americans show that non-Hispanic white adults reported pain more often than adults of other races and ethnicities (U.S. Department of Health and Human Services, 2006). However, not everyone who shares the same cultural background reacts identically to pain. Consider whether a patient may be reflecting

stoicism or expressionism in their pain reports. Validate the expressive patient's pain, or encourage stoic patients to take needed pain medication. For both types of patient, offer support as well as pain medication.

THINKING CRITICALLY ABOUT DRUG THERAPY IN PAIN MANAGEMENT

Mr. Schneider is 60 years old. He is a second-generation German American. He has worked for 35 years in a local steel mill. He had surgery for a bowel obstruction yesterday. When you assess him, he states he does not have pain, yet he is restless in the bed and moaning. He says he will take something for pain when the pain is very severe. He does not want to get out of bed to ambulate, and he coughs only superficially when asked to demonstrate coughing and deep breathing.

1. Discuss factors that may be contributing to the inconsistencies between the patient's verbal report and nonverbal behavior.

2. Why is appropriate pain management important for this patient?

3. Propose a teaching plan that you think would help this patient with effective pain management.

Nursing Diagnoses and Outcomes

- Ineffective Breathing Pattern, Hypoventilation, related to respiratory depression caused by the drug
  Desired outcome: The patient maintains effective breathing despite respiratory depression.
- Ineffective Airway Clearance secondary to cough suppression by the drug
  Desired outcome: The patient's airway remains patent and clear.
- Constipation secondary to activity of the drug
  Desired outcome: The patient remains free of constipation.
- Urinary Retention related to indirect anticholinergic effects of the drug on the urinary sphincters
  Desired outcome: The patient maintains normal urinary output.
- Risk for Injury related to orthostatic hypotension or sedation secondary to drug effects
  Desired outcome: The patient remains free of injury.
- Acute Pain related to trauma or disease process and insufficient analgesia
  Desired outcome: The patient remains free of pain.
- Deficient Knowledge related to morphine therapy
  Desired outcome: The patient has adequate knowledge of the drug and its adverse effects and their management.

Planning and Intervention

The key issue in morphine therapy is adequate control of pain balanced against the considerable adverse effects of respiratory depression and excessive sedation. Goals of treatment include adequate pulmonary ventilation, a respiratory rate within 12 to 20 breaths per minute, minimal effects of constipation and urinary retention, freedom from injury, and adequate family and patient education for managing drug therapy. It is also important to teach the patient possible adverse effects of morphine and how to manage them. Other goals relate to maintaining safety during potential episodes of orthostatic hypotension.

Maximizing Therapeutic Effects

ASSESSING PAIN

The first step in maximizing the therapeutic effects of drug therapy with morphine or any other narcotic is to complete a full pain assessment. Pain has been greatly underassessed and undertreated. Many professional organizations, clinical guidelines, and accreditation bodies now recommend that pain be routinely assessed for all patients; this recommendation has been likened to making pain a fifth vital sign, which requires assessment whenever the other vital signs are assessed during patient care. Remember that pain is a subjective experience. It is whatever the patient says it is, occurring whenever the patient says it does. Objective data, such as elevated blood pressure or pulse rate, moaning, or grimacing, may accompany pain, but the absence of objective data does not indicate that pain does not exist. Many people actually cope with pain by using distraction techniques, such as smiling, talking, quiet rhythmic breathing,

or watching television. Patients who experience chronic pain are especially likely to use distraction techniques. Every patient has a different level of tolerance for what he or she feels is an acceptable level of pain. Careful assessment enables you to assist the patient in identifying and achieving this level of control. Pain assessment tools allow the individual's pain to be tracked using the same scale or criteria. Although pain can be assessed by asking questions, this approach is not considered a true tool because a tool must be tangible. Verbal assessment may be necessary in a particular situation, but a true tool that has been shown to be valid and reliable is preferable.

To begin the pain assessment, first determine the location of the pain. Location gives possible clues to the source of the pain and can help identify whether the pain is acute or of a more chronic nature. Many pain assessment tools incorporate a representation of the human body from a frontal and posterior view. The tools ask patients to shade or circle on the diagram to show the location of the pain. Such identification helps the patient define what he or she is experiencing and provides a starting point for further assessment. Each pain location should be recorded in the patient's chart along with its associated intensity and quality.

The next step is to determine the pain intensity. Many assessment tools are available to rate pain intensity (Figure 23.3). Each tool provides a continuum in some

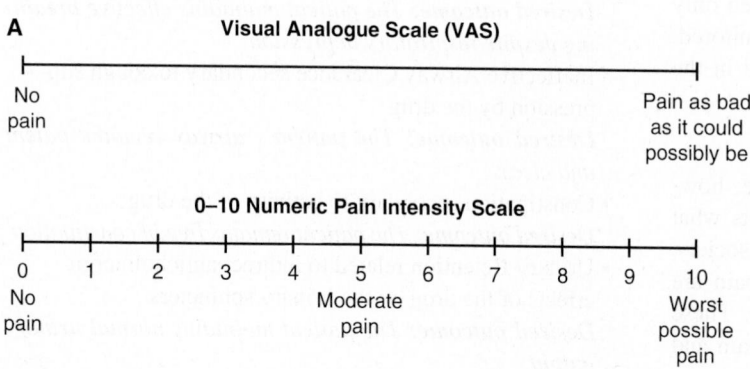

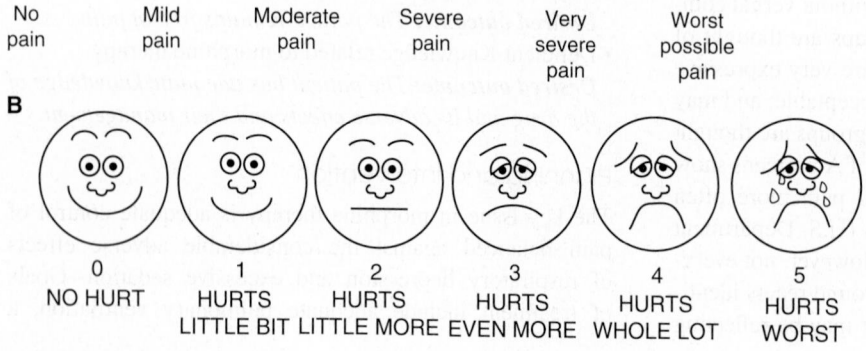

• FIGURE 23.3 Pain assessment tools. Many pain intensity scales are available for ranking the pain of children and adults alike. (**A**) Such scales as the visual analogue, numeric pain intensity, and simple descriptive pain intensity rank pain from no pain to worst pain possible. (**B**) Scales such as the Wong-Baker FACES Pain Rating Scale are ideal for children and others who have difficulty with numeric concepts. To assist children with the FACES scale, the nurse explains that each face represents a person who feels happy because the person has no pain or a person who feels sad because the person has a lot of pain. FACE 0: no hurt; FACE 1: hurts little bit; FACE 2: hurts little more; FACE 3: hurts even more; FACE 4: hurts whole lot; FACE 5: hurts worst. Then, the nurse asks the child to choose the face that best describes his or her own pain and documents the selection. (**Part B:** From Hockenberry, M. J., Wilson D., & Winkelstein, M. L. [2005]. **Wong's essentials of pediatric nursing** (7th ed). St. Louis: Mosby, p. 1259. Used with permission.)

form to represent a range from "no pain" to the "worst pain imaginable." Asking the patient to rate pain using an imaginary scale in his or her head is *not* considered a tool. One of the most widely recognized pain assessment tools for reliability and ease of use is the visual analogue scale, which is numeric. It may be a scale from 0 to 5 or 0 to 10, but both ranges allow patients to rate their pain by assigning a number that demonstrates greater pain as they move up the scale. The visual analogue scale may be printed, with the patient pointing to the appropriate number; or the scale may be on a hand-held device with a sliding pointer; with the patient sliding the pointer to the appropriate number to demonstrate his or her pain.

Because research findings indicate that approximately 7% to 11% of adults cannot conceptualize well enough to use the visual analogue pain scale, other pain assessment tools may be helpful. One alternative is a descriptive pain-intensity tool in which words replace the numbers 0 to 5, again with the two extremes being no pain or the worst imaginable pain. The FACES scale, used frequently with children, cognitively impaired adults, and those who do not speak English, shows a series of facial expressions ranging from very unhappy and crying to very happy and smiling (Hockenberry 2009; Wong & Baker, 1998). The patient is then asked to pick the face that most resembles how he or she feels. In the poker chip tool, four poker chips are placed in front of the patient. Each one is a "piece of hurt," with one piece being "just a little hurt" and four pieces being "the most hurt." Patients are asked to show how many pieces of hurt they have. This tool is also frequently used with children.

Each patient may interpret the extremes of any of the scales differently based on his or her past experiences. However, with consistent use, the pain assessment tool gives the patient and the provider a common ground on which to plan treatment and understand the degree of relief from the treatments provided.

Intensity of pain is only one aspect of pain that should be assessed; pain quality and character (affective descriptions) should also be measured. Not all pain assessment tools currently available assess for all these parameters. Some of the well-tested tools include the Brief Pain Inventory, the McGill Pain Questionnaire, and the Memorial Pain Assessment Card (Melzack, 1975; Daut, Cleeland, & Flanery, 1983; Cleeland & Ryan, 1994; Fishman, Pasternak, Wallenstein, et al., 1987).

Of these, the McGill Pain Questionnaire is the only one that is not a visual tool. Instead, it is a set series of questions to ask the patient, after which you record the patient's answers. This tool has long and short forms; the long form takes 5 to 15 minutes to complete, and the short form can be completed in 2 to 3 minutes, making it preferable in an acute care setting. Assessment of pain intensity and all aspects of pain is an important part of treating pain effectively, especially for patients who are stoic, who use coping mechanisms to deal with pain, or whose pain may be undertreated if you offer drug therapy only to those who state that they are in pain.

PROVIDING ANALGESIA

Morphine, like other drugs that relieve pain, is more effective when it is administered before the level of pain becomes severe. This is another reason why it is important to assess the patient's pain level frequently. When pain exists, analgesic dosages are best administered around the clock rather than as needed. Continual administration promotes a steady blood level of the drug, which prevents drug troughs that allow pain to escalate. In around-the-clock dosing, a baseline amount of the drug is administered over the 24-hour period when acute pain is expected or when severe, chronic pain occurs. Patients should be awakened for the analgesic if receiving it orally; however, they may refuse the drug at any time.

The appropriate dose of morphine must be given to control the patient's pain. No one dose is appropriate for every patient. Titration of dosage is usually required when therapy begins and continues for as long as the patient receives care. To titrate the morphine dose means to increase it incrementally. Aggressiveness of titration depends on pain intensity and response. Remember that patients with a history of substance abuse or drug tolerance need higher dosages of analgesics. Morphine is titrated until the desired therapeutic response, or efficacy, is achieved or until adverse effects occur. Efficacy is usually defined as a pain level below 4 out of 10 or a level determined by both the patient and health care provider. Nonopioids, such as NSAIDs, may be used in conjunction with morphine. Other adjunct drugs may be added to morphine if necessary for pain control.

A review of the literature by Hudcova et al. in 2009 found that patient controlled analgesia (PCA) had better pain control and greater satisfaction than those whose pain was managed with PRN doses of medication administered by the nurse. Those receiving PCA may use more milligrams of opioids than those who are not on PCA, and they may incur more problems with itching. Other adverse effects profiles are similar regardless if the drug is administered via PCA or from the nurse administering the medication on a PRN basis.

Finally, in addition to pharmacologic interventions, nonpharmacologic methods may be used in conjunction with morphine. These methods are not substitutes for morphine, but they are valuable adjuncts to therapy (see Table 23.1).

For patients with chronic pain, the use of a long-acting form of morphine may better manage the patient's pain. Recognizing the need for long-term control and facilitating the conversion from short-acting to long-acting morphine, or other opioid, is important. A thorough assessment is needed to best determine which particular drug and route would best meet the individual patient's needs. Make sure that a fast-acting rescue drug (see Minimizing Adverse Effects) is also prescribed to treat breakthrough pain.

Minimizing Adverse Effects

Minimizing the adverse effects of morphine requires frequent and astute assessment and implementation of basic nursing care (Box 23.4). Dosing the drug carefully to meet the needs posed by core patient variables can minimize adverse effects. In general, dosages need to be lower for children, older adults, and patients with renal or hepatic impairment. Morphine should be administered before pain becomes severe. Because this dosing schedule is more effective, a smaller dose of the drug can be given, which helps prevent or minimize adverse effects.

Breakthrough pain and incidental pain may occur during pain management with drug therapy. Clinicians use the term **breakthrough pain** to describe transitory flare-ups of pain over baseline in a patient receiving opioid therapy. Breakthrough pain is generally graded as moderate to severe in intensity. It may last from a few seconds to a few hours. It may or may not have a precipitating event. Spontaneous, or activity-related, pain is called incidental pain. An incident may be related to a specific movement or to all movements.

Factors to consider when assessing and treating breakthrough and incidental pain are those that relate to cause. When pain does occur, is it related to a specific time during the dosing schedule? If so, a change in the dosing interval or an increase in the drug dose may be beneficial. Does a certain movement cause pain, or is the pain unpredictable? Patients often have incidental or breakthrough pain associated with movement or activity. How long does the pain last? Although morphine has a fairly rapid onset, some severe pain may persist for less time than it takes for the analgesic to take effect.

All patients being treated for pain need access to **rescue doses** for breakthrough pain. The rescue dose should

---

Box 23.4 MINIMIZING ADVERSE EFFECTS OF MORPHINE

For All

- Consult with the physician and pharmacist to individualize dosage and dosing intervals based on the patient's weight, age, pain intensity, diagnosis, concurrent medical status, and use of other CNS depressants.
- Because ambulation may increase occurrence of the frequent adverse effects, have patient lie down after the dose has been taken.
- Because low pain levels may increase occurrence of the frequent adverse effects, consider a nonnarcotic analgesic for patients with mild to moderate pain.

Respiratory Depression

- Assess vital signs, especially respiratory function, on a regular, frequent basis.
- Measure the oxygen concentration of the blood with a pulse oximeter on a regular and as-needed basis.
- Have the patient perform turning, coughing, and deep breathing, and reposition the patient to remove secretions and maintain adequate pulmonary ventilation.
- Place the patient on the side, not flat on the back, to maintain an open airway until condition stabilizes. If the patient must be placed on the back, remove pillow, and tilt the patient's head back slightly to prevent the tongue from occluding the airway. Use an oral airway if necessary.
- Withhold the next dose and notify the physician if the patient is bradypneic.
- Administer oxygen as needed.
- Have emergency respiratory equipment available.
- Keep naloxone, the narcotic antidote, on hand. Administer as needed.

Hypotension

- Monitor blood pressure carefully in postoperative patients, patients who have low circulating blood volume, or patients who are simultaneously receiving a CNS depressant (e.g., phenothiazine) or general anesthetics. These conditions make such patients more prone to hypotension.
- Monitor for orthostatic hypotension, especially during transport, for patients with decreased circulating blood levels or impaired cardiac

function and for those receiving sympatholytic (blocking the action of the sympathetic nervous system) drugs.
- Monitor intake and output and replace fluids for patients who are hypovolemic.
- Assess ambulatory patients carefully for orthostatic hypotension.

Constipation

- Encourage dietary fiber when taking morphine orally.
- Encourage oral fluids when tolerated; keep patient well hydrated with IV fluids if NPO.
- Promote ambulation (assisted as necessary) as much as possible.
- Administer stool softeners or laxatives PRN.

Urinary Retention and Decreased Urinary Output

- Monitor intake and output at least every work shift.
- Question to determine whether the patient self-reports difficulty voiding, lack of voiding, frequent voiding of very small amounts, or feelings of bladder fullness or tenderness.
- Palpate the bladder to differentiate urinary retention from oliguria.
- Encourage oral fluids if allowed; provide adequate hydration with IV fluids if NPO.
- Use noninvasive means to promote voiding (ensure female patient sits upright, ensure male patient stands, run water in sink, pour water over perineum, use sitz baths).
- Obtain order and perform urethral catheterization if needed.

Light-headedness, Dizziness, and Sedation

- Assist the patient who is ambulating and getting out of bed.
- Ensure the use of side rails when the patient is in bed.

Nausea and Vomiting

- Keep the patient NPO during acute episodes; maintain the patient on IV fluids for hydration.
- Offer ice chips and clear liquids as symptoms diminish.
- Obtain order and administer antiemetics if indicated.

be equianalgesic to 10% to 30% of the dose the patient receives in 24 hours and is added to the established pain management. Patients who require more than three rescue doses in a day should have their analgesic dosage adjusted either by increasing the baseline dose or maximizing the co-analgesics. A thorough assessment helps the health care provider decide whether the best option is to increase the dosage or to incorporate other therapies. Rescue doses, sometimes referred to as "PRN" or bolus doses, may be administered by a PCA device if the patient is receiving IV or epidural analgesia. Program into the IV pump the dose that has been ordered for the rescue or bolus dose and the frequency that the patient may receive a dose. When patients experience pain, they press a button, similar to a call light, and the pump administers the correct dose if it is time. Some institutions, especially with older adults or others who are at risk for experiencing adverse effects from around-the-clock dosing, may use PCA without a basal rate. In other words, the pump administers medication only when patients request it. When the pump is used in this manner, patients need to request a dose as soon as they begin to experience pain.

Providing Patient and Family Education

- Patients being treated for pain need to know what the treatment plan will be for managing their pain and that they are not expected to suffer. Ensure patients that health care providers will listen to them and act when they report that they have pain.
- Patients need to know that they have an important role to play in managing their pain. Review the following points with them:
  - Know how to use the pain assessment tools.
  - Report honestly how they feel during assessment.
  - Establish (with the health care team) what pain level will trigger automatic re-evaluation of the pain management plan. Ideally, re-evaluation should happen before pain develops or increases (e.g., in the preoperative period or early in the course of a disease).
- Teach patients who are receiving PCA how to appropriately use it. Patients should be instructed to request a dose whenever they have pain; waiting for the pain to become severe before seeking a dose makes it more difficult for the drug to be effective and may require larger doses of the morphine. Emphasize to patients that they cannot overdose themselves because the computer in the pump is programmed to administer only a prescribed dose at a prescribed interval.
- Correct any fears or misconceptions, including the following:
  - Pain is inevitable.
  - Pain must be endured.
  - Patients will "lose control" of themselves if they take drugs for pain.
  - Patients will become addicted.

- Teach patients that drug therapy with morphine over a prolonged period (as in chronic or cancer pain) may produce physical dependence on the drug. Explain that physical dependence is neither the same as addiction nor a reason to withhold pain treatment. If the pain resolves, the patient can be weaned from the drug to prevent withdrawal. Weaning is not appropriate with cancer pain because the pain will not resolve on its own.
- If patients are discharged home on morphine, teach the following:
  - Administration
  - Effects (adverse and otherwise)
  - Avoidance of driving and other hazardous activities during drug therapy
  - Avoidance of alcohol and concurrent CNS depressant therapy, unless a health care provider is managing the concurrent therapy
  - Placement of drug securely away from children and anyone likely to abuse it

Ongoing Assessment and Evaluation

Documentation of pain management with morphine should include the following:

- The pain scale used by the patient
- The rating given by the patient
- The components, sensory and affective, of pain
- The amount of morphine, route, and the time each dose is administered
- The degree of pain relief obtained from morphine therapy
- The effectiveness of adjunct drug therapy and nonpharmacologic interventions used
- Any morphine-induced adverse effects

Increasing pain in a patient previously stabilized on a certain dose of morphine should not be automatically attributed to tolerance without investigating for evidence of disease progression or complications. Cancer pain, for example, changes constantly. It may increase or decrease secondary to anticancer treatment, infectious processes, spreading tumors, or natural degenerative body changes (arthritis). Postoperative pain that morphine does not relieve may indicate postoperative complications, such as compartment syndrome.

The patient should have adequate pain control with minimal adverse effects. Breakthrough pain should be minimal if the pain is adequately controlled. The patient should remain free from injury from orthostatic hypotension or sedation. The patient and family should show an understanding of adverse effects if the patient is discharged on morphine and should be able to describe how to manage those effects should they occur.

MEMORY CHIP

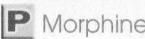 Morphine

- Narcotic analgesic used in moderate to severe pain
- Standard against which all other narcotic analgesics are measured for effectiveness
- Major contraindications: significant respiratory depression, increased intracranial pressure, and CNS depression
- Most common adverse effects: light-headedness, dizziness, sedation, nausea, and vomiting
- Most serious adverse effect: respiratory depression
- **Life span alert: Avoid use in premature infants or during labor when delivery of premature infant is expected.**
- Maximizing therapeutic effects: Assess pain thoroughly before and during therapy and titrate the dose until the desired pain-relieving effect is achieved.
- Minimizing adverse effects: Individualize dose based on patient-related variables; monitor vital signs, especially respiratory rate, frequently; and have the antidote, naloxone, on hand.
- Most important patient education: For long-term use in cancer pain, physical dependency will develop. This is not the same as addiction and not an appropriate reason to withhold the drug.
- **Patient safety alert: Check dose and patient status carefully; adverse effects and medication errors are common with this drug. Monitor patient closely, because fall risk is increased.**

Drugs Closely Related to P Morphine

Hydromorphone

Hydromorphone (Dilaudid) is a semisynthetic analogue of opium and is used to treat acute and chronic pain (Quigley, 2009). Its effects on the body are almost identical to those of morphine. As an analgesic, hydromorphone is equally effective as morphine, although more potent (Quigley, 2009). Between 1 and 1.5 (1 to 1.50) mg of SC or IM hydromorphone is equal to 10 mg of morphine given through the same routes. Hydromorphone is available in oral, parenteral, and rectal forms. Hydromorphone also has equal antitussive (cough suppression) effects; however, its ability to cause respiratory depression and physical dependency is less than that of morphine. Hydromorphone's ability to cause constipation, sedation, and emesis is unknown; thus, comparisons with morphine cannot be made. Unlike morphine, hydromorphone can cause transient hyperglycemia.

Levorphanol

Levorphanol (Levo-Dromoran), a synthetic compound, can be used to manage pain and as a preoperative agent. It has analgesic, constipating, respiratory-depressive, sedating, and physical dependency qualities similar to those of morphine. It has fewer antitussive and emetic effects. Like hydromorphone, levorphanol is more potent than morphine, with an SC dose of 2 mg equal to 10 mg of morphine.

Oxycodone

Oxycodone is a semisynthetic analogue of opium. Oxycodone is metabolized by the 2D6 isoenzyme. Unlike morphine, it is available only as an oral preparation. It is available in regular-release (Roxicodone), timed-release (OxyContin), and rapid-release formulas (OxyIR). Oxycodone has analgesic, antitussive, constipating, respiratory-depressive, sedating, emetic, and physical dependency effects similar to those of morphine.

The long-acting, timed-release forms are very helpful in managing severe chronic pain, either cancer pain or noncancer chronic pain.

Although oxycodone has been a safe and effective therapy for patients with severe chronic pain, unfortunately, it has also been abused as a street drug. When abused, the drug is crushed before being taken, so that an extremely high dose of the narcotic is available all at once, instead of being released slowly over time. Severe adverse effects are possible when it is used in this manner. Those who abuse it are most probably addicted to the drug.

Oxycodone is often administered as a combination drug with either aspirin (Percodan, Roxiprin) or acetaminophen (Tylox, Percocet, Roxicet). One problem with using combination drugs is that the amount of these other drugs that can be administered daily is limited. When increasing the dosage to provide for adequate pain control, calculate the total daily intake of aspirin or acetaminophen, because overdosage of either of these drugs can cause serious adverse effects (see Chapter 24 for more information).

Oxymorphone

Oxymorphone (Numorphan) is a semisynthetic analogue of opium. It is used in pain control, as a preoperative medication, to support anesthesia, as an obstetric analgesic, and for the relief of anxiety in patients with dyspnea associated with pulmonary edema secondary to acute left ventricular dysfunction. Oxymorphone is available in injection and rectal forms. It has analgesic and constipating effects similar to those of morphine; however, it causes more respiratory depression, emesis, and physical dependence. Oxymorphone has fewer antitussive effects than morphine; its sedating effects are unknown.

Meperidine

Meperidine (Demerol) is a synthetic compound used to treat pain as a preoperative medication, to support anesthesia, and during labor. Meperidine has similar analgesic and respiratory depressive effects and abilities to cause physical dependence as morphine. Meperidine has fewer sedative and constipating effects and substantially fewer antitussive effects than morphine. Meperidine has a longer half-life and is less potent than morphine, requiring 75 mg IM or SC to have an analgesic effect equal to that of 10 mg of morphine. A unique drug interaction occurs between meperidine and the hydantoins (antiepileptics), which decreases the effectiveness of meperidine. This effect may result from an increased hepatic metabolism of meperidine.

The most important difference between morphine and meperidine is related to the pharmacokinetics of meperidine. Meperidine is metabolized to an active metabolite, normeperidine. Normeperidine has a long half-life (15 to 30 hours) and accumulates in the body with chronic dosing. Half-life is further extended in patients with renal impairment, which slows excretion of normeperidine. Normeperidine is a CNS toxin. Accumulated doses in the body can cause tremors, seizures, and changes in level of consciousness. Older adults are especially sensitive to the adverse effects of normeperidine, which may be the result of impaired renal function. For these reasons, meperidine should normally be avoided in pain management when multiple doses will be given. The exception would be if the patient were allergic to morphine; however, the patient must have normal renal function.

Fentanyl

Fentanyl is a synthetic compound. Its major uses are as a preanesthetic, anesthetic, and analgesic. Fentanyl's analgesic properties are equal to those of morphine. It produces fewer respiratory and emetic effects. Its antitussive, constipating, sedating, and physical dependency effects are unknown in comparison with those of morphine. Fentanyl is much more potent than morphine, with 0.1 mg producing equianalgesia to that of 10 mg of morphine.

Fentanyl is available in various forms. Fentanyl as a liquid for injection (Sublimaze) is used as an anesthetic, an analgesic of short duration during anesthesia, and a supplement to general or regional anesthesia. An off-label use is pain control through epidural PCA, usually after surgery.

Fentanyl is also available in a transdermal system (Duragesic). This formulation is used in persistent, moderate to severe chronic pain, usually related to cancer but also in other chronic pain conditions, when continuous opioid analgesia is necessary for pain that cannot be controlled by other methods. When the transdermal system is first used, the full pain-relieving effect is not achieved for approximately 24 hours. Patients should be treated with short-acting opioids during this period. Short-acting opioids are not needed when changing the patch after 72 hours, except for rescue doses for breakthrough pain.

The fentanyl transdermal system contains several Black Box warnings. The drug preparation should be used only in patients who have been taking opioids and have a demonstrated opioid tolerance, never to those who have not been receiving opioids (i.e., those who are opioid naive), because fatal respiratory depression may result. It should never be used in patients who require only short-term opioid treatment (e.g., after a surgical procedure). Another Black Box warning concerns a significant drug interaction. Transdermal fentanyl has a drug interaction with potent cytochrome P-450 3A4 inhibitors (ritonavir, ketoconazole, itraconazole, troleandomycin, clarithromycin, nelfinavir, and nefazodone). Because fentanyl is metabolized by this pathway, inhibition may result in significant increases in plasma concentrations of fentanyl, which could increase or prolong the adverse effects, possibly causing respiratory depression. Patients receiving both fentanyl transdermal and one of the P-450 3A4 inhibitors

should be monitored closely for adverse effects; a decreased dose of fentanyl may be warranted. The label for transdermal fentanyl also warns that, due to its potency, transdermal fentanyl may be abused or illegally diverted.

A final Black Box warning is that fentanyl transdermal systems may only be used in children if they are 2 years of age or older and they are opioid tolerant. For information on patient and family education for transdermal fentanyl, see Box 23.5.

BOX 23.5 COMMUNITY BASED CONCERNS

Teaching About Transdermal Fentanyl

As more and more patients learn to manage their own health care and drug therapy at home, the nurse assumes an even greater role in teaching patients and their caregivers about safe self-care and drug administration. For a patient who will be discharged while receiving transdermal fentanyl, some important drug administration teaching points for the patient or the caregiver follow:

1. Caregivers who administer or remove a transdermal fentanyl patch should first put on gloves to avoid absorbing any of the drug themselves.
2. Tear open a new patch packet carefully; never cut the patch with scissors. Transdermal systems that have been cut may increase the amount of drug that is absorbed, which increases the risk of developing hypoventilation and respiratory depression.
3. Remove the liner on the sticky side of the patch.
4. Apply the fentanyl patch to nonirritated, smooth, hairless skin (clip hair; avoid shaving to avoid breaking the skin) on the chest, back, flank, or upper arm right after opening the patch package. If necessary, wash the skin with clear water and dry completely before applying the patch. Do not use soaps, creams, alcohol, oils, lotions, or anything else that might irritate the skin or alter its characteristics.
5. Hold the patch in place for 30 seconds to ensure firm adherence.
6. Wear the system continually for 72 hours and then replace with a new patch, placed in a different location.
7. Avoid exposing the transdermal patch site to sources of heat such as heating pads, sun lamps, electric blankets, heated water beds, hot tubs, or saunas. Vasodilation occurs in these situations, which may result in increased absorption of fentanyl, resulting in possible adverse effects or overdose. Contact the prescriber if the patient develops a fever while using the transdermal systems, because this can also increase the absorption rate.
8. If the gel from the drug pad accidentally comes in contact with the skin, clean the area with plain water only. The use of soaps, alcohol, or other chemicals may actually increase the drug absorption through the skin.
9. To discard a used patch, fold it in half with the sticky sides together (to prevent any residual drug from touching the skin) and flush the patch down the toilet, because active drug remains in the patch. (Patches discarded in the trash may be attractive to and accidentally come in contact with children or pets.)
10. Use the short-acting drug prescribed as a rescue dose for any breakthrough pain. Keep a log of how often rescue doses are needed, and bring this information with you to your next appointment. This log provides valuable information about how well the prescribed drug and dose are controlling your pain. Do not adjust the dose of fentanyl except under the direction of the physician.

The newest form of fentanyl transdermal administration is the fentanyl iontophoretic transdermal system (IONSYS). It is used as a transdermal route of PCA for hospitalized patients. Unlike other transdermal delivery systems of fentanyl, it is used to treat acute postoperative pain in adults. It is not intended for home use, and the system must be removed prior to discharge. Patients must be alert and able to control the device on their own; overdose is possible if someone other than the patient administers a dose. The patient should have received sufficient other opioids to provide comfort prior to starting this system. Each activation of the unit provides 40 mcg of fentanyl over a 10-minute period. To activate the system and release a dose, the patient presses the button on the top of the unit twice firmly within 3 seconds; an audible beep sounds and a red light comes on, indicating that the system is releasing a dose. The red light remains lit during the entire 10-minute dosing period. The system is designed to deliver a maximum of six 40-mcg doses per hour. Each system works for either 24 hours or to deliver 80 doses, whichever comes first. Up to three consecutive systems may be used (one per day). Site-selection criteria for this system are similar to those for transdermal fentanyl patches. A sticker on the back of the system is designed for the nurse to record the date and time the system was applied to the patient; this alerts nurses on subsequent shifts when the system will need to be changed. Pharmacodynamics, adverse effects, and actions for accidental contact and disposal are similar to transdermal fentanyl patches.

Finally, fentanyl is available in a transmucosal and a buccal tablet form—as fentanyl citrate. Both the transmucosal form (Actiq) and the buccal tablet form (Fentora) are used only for the management of breakthrough pain in patients with cancer who are already receiving and are already tolerant of opioid therapy. Only oncologists and pain specialists who are familiar with opioids should prescribe it to treat cancer pain. If it is used in the home, storage of the drug in a safe place is critical, because the dose found in this form may be fatal to children.

Alfentanil

Alfentanil (Alfenta) is used in the operating room as an analgesic during anesthesia, to induce anesthesia when intubation and mechanical ventilation are required, and as the analgesic component of MAC. Its analgesic effects are similar to those of morphine. Its onset of action is immediate.

Sufentanil

Sufentanil (Sufenta) produces a greater analgesic effect than morphine. It is used as an anesthetic and analgesic adjunct to maintain balanced anesthesia when patients are intubated and on a ventilator. It is also used as an epidural analgesic during labor and vaginal delivery (when combined with low-dose bupivacaine).

Methadone

Methadone (Methadose, Dolophine) can be used for pain, to prevent withdrawal symptoms from heroin (detoxification), and as a maintenance treatment for narcotic abuse. Although

its ability to produce analgesia and the duration of its analgesic effect (4 to 6 hours, compared with 3 to 7 hours) are similar to those of morphine, its half-life is much longer. The half-life of methadone is 15 to 30 hours, compared with 1.5 to 2 hours for morphine. Adverse effects and signs of overdose may occur when methadone is used as pain management, because of these pharmacokinetic properties. Methadone may be initiated in a hospital setting only for prevention of withdrawal. Only approved treatment programs for narcotic abuse may initiate treatment with methadone for maintenance treatment of addiction. If a patient is already in a maintenance treatment program with methadone and requires hospitalization, the hospital may provide the methadone, after personnel confirm the dose with the treatment center that normally observes the patient.

Remifentanil

Remifentanil (Ultiva), although classified as a narcotic agonist-analgesic, is used as a general anesthetic and as part of MAC. Remifentanil has more analgesic effects than morphine but similar respiratory depressive and emetic effects. Physical dependence and constipation occur less often than with morphine.

Tramadol

Like morphine, tramadol (Ultram) is an opioid analgesic, with many similarities and a few differences. This opioid does not act primarily at the mu receptors; instead, it exerts its effect by inhibiting norepinephrine and serotonin reuptake. It is used in the treatment of cancer pain, moderate to moderately severe chronic pain, and moderate to moderately severe acute pain. Unlike morphine, its safety and efficacy in patients younger than 16 years of age have not been established. The drug should not be used in patients with severe renal or hepatic impairment.

In addition, unlike morphine, tramadol is available only in oral forms (immediate and extended release). It has a much longer half-life than morphine: in its immediate-onset form, the half-life is 6.3 ± 1.4 hours; and in its extended-release form, the half-life is almost 8 hours. Unlike morphine, tramadol does not commonly cause respiratory depression, light-headedness, or urinary retention. It only rarely causes hypotension, and then only orthostatic hypotension. However, unlike morphine, it can cause seizures and hallucinations. If naloxone is given to treat tramadol overdose, it may increase the risk of seizures.

Drug Significantly Different From P Morphine

Naloxone (Narcan) is a narcotic antagonist. It is believed to antagonize the effects of narcotics by competing for opioid receptor sites. It is used to reverse the effects of opiates (e.g., respiratory depression) and to treat opioid overdose. Naloxone is not effective for respiratory depression caused by anything other than narcotic agonist analgesics. Because naloxone competes for opioid receptors it may be combined with preparations of morphine or fentanyl for use in patient controlled analgesia to minimize adverse effects. Naloxone can be used in adults, children, and neonates.

Although naloxone can be given by the IM, SC, or IV route, the most rapid onset is achieved with IV use, and this route is recommended in emergencies. IV onset is within 2 minutes; duration of action depends on the dose given and the route used, although it is quite short. Careful monitoring of the patient beyond initial response is warranted because the duration of action of the narcotic agonist may be longer than the duration of naloxone. Thus, the patient may relapse into respiratory arrest or depression. Repeated doses may be necessary to maintain reversal of the opiate's effects. Abrupt reversal of narcotic depression may result in the adverse effects of nausea, vomiting, sweating, tachycardia, increased blood pressure, and tremors. Administration of naloxone precipitates withdrawal in people who are physically dependent on narcotics. It also reverses all the analgesic effects in those receiving morphine or other narcotic agonists for pain control if the dose is sufficient.

Naloxone's reversal of respiratory depression from buprenorphine (a mixed agonist and antagonist) may be incomplete, necessitating mechanical assistance for respiration. Naloxone may be combined with sublinguinal preparations of buprenorphine to treat drug addiction. (For further information on buprenorphine, see Drugs Closely Related to Pentazocine, below.)

C MILD NARCOTIC AGONISTS

The mild narcotic agonists include codeine, hydrocodone, and propoxyphene. Codeine is the prototype for the mild narcotic agonists.

Nursing Management of the Patient Receiving P Codeine

Core Drug Knowledge

Pharmacotherapeutics

Codeine is used to control mild to moderate pain in adults and children. For this purpose, it is available in oral tablets and an injectable form for parenteral use. Orally, it may be combined with acetaminophen or with nonsteroidal anti-inflammatory drugs. A review of the literature indicates that a standard dose of 60 mg of codeine, used without other analgesics, provides unsatisfactory post-operative pain control (most trials looked at dental surgery) for most patients. Thus codeine combined with a nonsteroidal anti-inflammatory would be the best option to control post-operative pain, especially after dental surgery (Derry et al., 2010). Codeine is also used for cough suppression. The dose needed to achieve an antitussive effect is less than the dose required for analgesia. Although codeine has fewer antitussive effects than morphine (when comparing similar weights of the drugs), it is more widely used to suppress coughs because it has low adverse effects at the antitussive doses.

Codeine may be used alone, in the form of oral tablets, or in combination with other drugs that are expectorants (in a liquid or syrup form) to suppress coughs.

Pharmacokinetics

Codeine is well absorbed from the GI tract. Its peak effect occurs in 1 to 2 hours. (Other pharmacokinetic parameters are identified in Table 23.3.) Codeine is metabolized in the liver by oxidative reactions through the P-450 isoenzyme system. Whether codeine is actually a prodrug, which requires changing by the P-450 system to be active, is the subject of some debate. Codeine is excreted in the urine. It crosses the placenta and is secreted in breast milk.

Pharmacodynamics

Codeine has pharmacologic effects similar to those of morphine, but its actions are milder. Codeine acts at specific opioid receptors in the CNS to produce analgesia, euphoria, and sedation. Codeine also acts directly on the medullary cough center to depress the cough reflex. It has a drying effect on mucous membranes and can increase the viscosity of respiratory tract secretions.

Contraindications and Precautions

Codeine should not be administered to patients receiving other narcotic analgesics for pain relief; such a combination can cause serious respiratory depression and sedation. Codeine should be used with caution in patients who need to cough to maintain the airways (postoperative patients and patients who have undergone major abdominal or thoracic surgery). Careful use is recommended for patients with asthma and emphysema because cough suppression in these patients can lead to accumulation of secretions and a loss of respiratory reserve. Codeine is used with caution in patients with pre-existing cardiac disease because of its potential to induce bradycardia and peripheral vasodilation.

Codeine is assigned to pregnancy category C. Like other opiate narcotics, it crosses the placenta, is secreted in breast milk, and can cause sedation and respiratory depression in the fetus or infant. Therefore, it should be used with caution during pregnancy and lactation. The closer it is given to delivery, the more likely it is for respiratory depression to occur in the newborn. Resuscitation equipment should be on hand if the mother has received codeine or other opiates during labor. Codeine should be avoided if the delivery of a premature infant is expected. Caution should also be used with patients who are hypersensitive to or have a history of addiction to narcotics; codeine is a narcotic and has a potential for addiction. Patients who need to drive or be alert should use codeine with extreme caution because it can cause sedation and drowsiness. Caution is important when codeine is used for patients who have experienced a head injury or undergone a craniotomy. Codeine can increase intracranial pressure, which can be detrimental to these patients.

Adverse Effects

As already stated, codeine has a low incidence of adverse effects when used at the appropriate dosage level as an antitussive. The most frequent adverse effects observed with the use of codeine as a cough suppressant include drowsiness, sedation, dry mouth, nausea and vomiting, and constipation. When dosed as an analgesic, the adverse effects are similar to those of morphine, although they are less severe. Allergic reactions, including rashes and urticaria, have been noted in highly sensitive people. Respiratory depression and cardiovascular effects have occurred with higher doses.

Drug Interactions

An increased likelihood of respiratory depression, hypotension, or profound sedation exists when codeine is given with any other drugs that cause CNS depression, such as antihistamines, phenothiazines, barbiturates, sedative-hypnotics, tricyclic antidepressants, and alcohol. Codeine may also interact with histamine-2 antagonists, such as cimetidine. Table 23.5 lists drugs that interact with codeine.

Assessment of Relevant Core Patient Variables

Health Status

Assess whether the patient needs to cough to maintain a patent airway. Such patients (e.g., postoperative patients) should not receive codeine. In this situation, the cough is a protective mechanism to rid the airways of potentially harmful substances that may lead to pneumonia. The same rationale is used when treating patients with asthma or emphysema. If they do not cough, they have the potential to retain secretions that may exacerbate their disease.

Before therapy, perform a physical examination to establish a baseline to monitor the effects of the drug. Parameters to evaluate include orientation, affect, respiratory rate, adventitious sounds, and character of bowel sounds. If prolonged use is anticipated or the patient has a history of hepatic dysfunction, ensure that liver function tests are performed, because codeine is metabolized in the liver.

Life Span and Gender

Consider the patient's age before administering codeine. Older adult patients are especially sensitive to respiratory depression with the use of narcotics. Therefore, a reduced dosage of codeine is advised. Codeine use is contraindicated in premature infants because of their sensitivity to respiratory depression. In addition, carefully assess whether female patients are pregnant before administering codeine. The drug should not be given to women in labor unless absolutely necessary.

Lifestyle, Diet, and Habits

Codeine has less potential for causing physical dependence than morphine. Withdrawal symptoms from codeine dependency are similar to those seen in withdrawal from morphine, although the symptoms are less severe. Assess patients for a history of drug abuse and administer codeine cautiously in such patients.

Environment

If patients will be taking codeine as an outpatient, assess their need to drive or operate potentially dangerous equipment. Patients must refrain from these activities until the drug's sedative effects are assessed.

Nursing Diagnoses and Outcomes

- Disturbed Sensory Perception related to drowsiness and sedation
  Desired outcome: *The patient will be protected from injury related to sedation and drowsiness.*
- Risk for Ineffective Airway Clearance related to suppression of cough reflex
  Desired outcome: *The patient will maintain baseline respiratory function.*
- Constipation secondary to activity of the drug
  Desired outcome: *The patient remains free of constipation.*

Planning and Intervention

Maximizing Therapeutic Effects

Actions are similar to those for morphine.

TABLE 23.5	Agents That Interact with P Codeine	
Interactants	**Effect and Significance**	**Nursing Management**
antihistamines	Additive effects when given simultaneously, resulting in CNS depression	Monitor closely for CNS depression. Avoid coadministration if possible.
barbiturates	Additive effects when given simultaneously, resulting in CNS depression	Monitor closely for CNS depression. Avoid coadministration if possible.
histamine-2 receptor antagonists	Actions of narcotic analgesics enhanced, resulting in toxicity and increased risk for respiratory depression	Monitor for respiratory depression. Decrease dosage of narcotic analgesic as needed. Avoid coadministration if possible.
phenothiazines	Additive effects when given simultaneously, resulting in CNS depression	Monitor closely for CNS depression. Avoid coadministration if possible.

Minimizing Adverse Effects

During therapy, ensure the use of safety precautions, such as raising side rails and assisting to walk if the patient is having CNS adverse effects. Monitor movement of air and respiratory status periodically during drug use. The use of codeine should be avoided in patients who need a strong cough reflex. Other actions are similar to those of morphine.

Providing Patient and Family Education

• Remind patients that drowsiness and impaired orientation can occur. Thus, patients should not drive or perform other tasks requiring alertness until the effects of the drug are known.

• Teach patients to avoid combining use of codeine with alcohol or other CNS depressants.

• Instruct patients and their families to report respiratory difficulty at once to you or the prescriber.

• Provide general pain control information, similar to that given for morphine.

Ongoing Assessment and Evaluation

Monitor codeine's effect on motor control and sedation, and the patient's respiratory status. By the end of therapy, the patient should be free from injury related to sedation and have open and functioning airways manifested by breathing without difficulty. Assessment and evaluation of pain control are the same as for morphine.

Drugs Closely Related to **P** Codeine

A drug similar to codeine is hydrocodone.

Hydrocodone

Hydrocodone, classified as a narcotic agonist, has an action similar to codeine and is administered orally. It is available as combination drug therapy only. When combined with acetaminophen (Lorcet, Lortab, Vicodin, among other trade names), it is used for moderate to severe pain. Hydrocodone can also be combined with ibuprofen (Vicoprofen) as an analgesic that acts via both opioid and NSAID pathways; like codeine, it also has antitussive effects. When hydrocodone is combined with homatropine (Hycodan, Hydromet, Tussigon), it is an antimuscarinic/antitussive. It is available in tablet and syrup forms.

• **C** NARCOTIC AGONIST-ANTAGONISTS

Some narcotic analgesics have mixed opioid effects, being agonists at some receptors and antagonists at others. Pentazocine (Talwin) is an example of a mixed narcotic agonist-antagonist and is also the prototype narcotic agonist-antagonist. Drugs similar to pentazocine include buprenorphine, butorphanol, and nalbuphine.

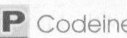

MEMORY CHIP

P Codeine

• Used to treat mild to moderate pain and as a cough suppressant
• Major contraindications: same as for all narcotics (e.g., respiratory depression, use of other CNS depressants)
• Most common adverse effects: as a cough suppressant—drowsiness, sedation, dry mouth, nausea and vomiting, and constipation (all incidence is low at this dose); as an analgesic— similar to those of morphine, although less severe
• Most serious adverse effect: respiratory depression (in overdoses)
• **Life span alert: same as for morphine**
• Maximizing therapeutic effects: same as for morphine
• Minimizing adverse effects: Avoid use if patient's health status requires a strong cough; other considerations are the same as for morphine.
• Most important patient education: Provide general information on pain management, as for all other narcotics.
• **Patient safety alert: Monitor patient closely, because fall risk is increased.**

Nursing Management of the Patient Receiving **P** Pentazocine

Core Drug Knowledge

Pharmacotherapeutics

In patients not previously exposed to opioids, pentazocine can be used as an agonist to control pain. In normal doses, pentazocine is effective for moderate to severe pain, such as postoperative pain or pain during labor. It is also used as premedication for anesthesia and as a supplement to surgical anesthetics.

Pharmacokinetics

Pentazocine is well absorbed orally and from SC and IM sites. When given orally, it undergoes a substantial first-pass effect of hepatic metabolism, and bioavailability is less than 20% of the dose given. The peak serum levels from oral doses occur within 1 to 3 hours, with a duration of action of 3 hours (see Table 23.3). Pentazocine's metabolites and the small proportion of drug not metabolized are excreted in urine. Pentazocine crosses the placenta.

Pharmacodynamics

Pentazocine is a mixed agonist-antagonist. It stimulates kappa receptors much as morphine does but also exhibits weak antagonist effects at the mu receptors, the primary morphine receptors. In patients who abuse opioids or are receiving narcotic agonists, such as morphine, for pain control, this drug may precipitate a withdrawal syndrome because of its antagonistic effects. Pentazocine may increase intracranial pressure. When pentazocine is given intravenously, it elevates systemic and pulmonary arterial pressure, systemic vascular resistance, and left ventricular end-diastolic pressure. These effects increase the workload of the heart.

Contraindications and Precautions

Pentazocine is contraindicated for patients with known hypersensitivity to it. Caution and low doses should be used if the drug is administered to patients with respiratory depression, severely limited respiratory reserves, severe bronchial asthma, obstructive respiratory conditions, and cyanosis. Pentazocine may cause allergic reactions in patients sensitive to sulfites. This event is uncommon in the general population but more likely in patients with asthma.

Adverse Effects

The most common adverse effects of pentazocine are nausea, vomiting, dizziness or light-headedness, and euphoria. Pentazocine causes little respiratory depression because of its antagonist action at the mu receptors. Areas that may experience other possible adverse effects include cardiovascular (hypotension, hypertension, tachycardia, circulatory depression, and shock), CNS (sedation, headache, weakness, depression, disturbed dreams, insomnia, syncope, hallucinations, tremor, irritability, excitement, tinnitus, disorientation, and confusion), and dermatologic (soft-tissue induration, nodules, cutaneous depression, ulceration with sloughing, sclerosis of the skin and subcutaneous tissues at site of injection, diaphoresis, stinging during injection, flushed skin, pruritus, and toxic epidermal necrolysis).

Drug Interactions

Pentazocine increases the action of alcohol and subsequently its accompanying CNS-depressant effects. Barbiturate anesthetics increase the effect of respiratory and CNS depression from pentazocine because of additive pharmacologic activity. Table 23.6 lists drugs that interact with pentazocine.

Assessment of Relevant Core Patient Variables

Health Status

Assess the patient for conditions that are contraindications or precautions to drug therapy as well as for hepatic disease,

because decreased metabolism of the drug occurs, which predisposes the patient to greater adverse effects.

Because of the effect of increasing intracranial pressure, pentazocine may compound the clinical course of patients with head injuries. Its use in these patients should be avoided if at all possible; if pentazocine must be used, it should be done very cautiously and the patient carefully monitored. Because of the cardiac effects, IV pentazocine should not be given to patients with an MI. If oral forms are given, they must be administered cautiously, with the patient monitored carefully.

Life Span and Gender

Assess female patients for pregnancy before administration. Pentazocine is a pregnancy category C drug. Infants born to mothers who abuse pentazocine exhibit neonatal withdrawal and have lower birth weights than normal. The safety and efficacy of pentazocine in children younger than 12 years have not been established; therefore, clarify that the pediatric patient is age 12 years or older before administration.

Lifestyle, Diet, and Habits

A common form of pentazocine abuse is called "T's and Blues." The "T's" refers to oral doses of pentazocine (under its trade name Talwin), and the "Blues" refers to tripelennamine (trade name, PBZ), a histamine-1 antihistamine. In this abused form, tablets are dissolved in tap water, filtered, and then injected intravenously as a substitute for heroin. The most frequent and serious complication of this form of addiction is pulmonary disease. Pulmonary disease results from blocking the pulmonary arteries and arterioles with unsterile particles of cellulose and talc from the tablets. Neurologic complications from "T's and Blues" may also occur, including seizures, strokes, and CNS infections. Pentazocine with naloxone (Talwin NX) has been produced in an effort to decrease the prevalence of this abuse. Giving

TABLE 23.6 Agents That Interact with P Pentazocine

Interactants	Effect and Significance	Nursing Management
alcohol	Increased sedation	Avoid concurrent use. Caution against operating hazardous machinery or driving a motor vehicle.
thiopental	Increased CNS depression	Caution patient not to drive until effects subside completely. Avoid concurrent usage.
fluoxetine	Hypertension, diaphoresis, ataxia, flushing, nausea, dizziness, and anxiety	Monitor patient with caution if both drugs are used concurrently.
Methohexital	Increased CNS depression	Consult prescriber about possible dosage adjustment.
zotepine	Increased risk of pentazocine-induced respiratory depression; enhanced sedation	Reduce dosage of pentazocine if necessary. Monitor for respiratory depression.
Tobacco	Metabolism of pentazocine about 40% higher in smokers	Consult prescriber about increasing pentazocine dosage.

pentazocine to patients who are dependent on opiates may induce withdrawal symptoms.

Environment

Pentazocine in parenteral form is administered in a hospital setting; oral forms may be administered in any setting by physicians, nurses, or patients themselves. Discuss any possible risks in the home or living environment with the patient.

Nursing Diagnoses and Outcomes

- Disturbed Sensory Perception related to dizziness and light-headedness
  Desired outcome: The patient will not be injured from falls while taking pentazocine.
- Imbalanced Nutrition secondary to nausea and vomiting
  Desired outcome: The patient's nutrition will not be compromised while he or she is on pentazocine.
- Ineffective Health Maintenance related to abuse of pentazocine
  Desired outcome: The patient will use drug therapy appropriately.
- Deficient Knowledge related to pentazocine therapy
  Desired outcome: The patient has adequate knowledge of the drug and its adverse effects and their management.

Planning and Intervention

Maximizing Therapeutic Effects

Be sure to provide environmental controls to reduce sensory stimuli and aid relaxation. For example, dim lights, reduce noise, and adjust room temperature for greatest comfort. General actions for pain control are similar to those described for morphine.

Minimizing Adverse Effects

During therapy, ensure that safety precautions are used, such as raising side rails and assisting with ambulation. In cases of overdosage, naloxone is indicated. General principles for pain control are the same as those followed for morphine.

Providing Patient and Family Education

- Teach patients that pentazocine may cause drowsiness. They must use it with caution while driving or performing tasks that require mental alertness, physical dexterity, or coordination.
- Emphasize that patients must avoid concurrent use of pentazocine with alcohol and other CNS depressants.
- Instruct patients to notify their physician if skin rash, confusion, or disorientation develops.

Ongoing Assessment and Evaluation

Monitor the effect of pentazocine on motor control, sedation, and pain. Adequate pain control should be achieved without adverse effects. Effectiveness of pain control is assessed similarly to that of morphine.

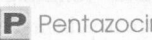 MEMORY CHIP

P Pentazocine

- Used for moderate to severe pain
- Is an agonist at some opioid receptors and a weak antagonist at others
- May precipitate withdrawal in patients physically dependent on narcotics
- Abused on the street (known as "T's and Blues")
- Most common adverse effects: nausea, vomiting, dizziness, light-headedness, and euphoria
- Most serious adverse effects: respiratory depression and circulatory depression
- Maximizing therapeutic effects: same as for all narcotics
- Minimizing adverse effects: same as for all narcotics
- Most important patient education: Avoid alcohol and CNS depressants while taking drug.
- **Patient safety alert: Monitor patient closely, because fall risk is increased.**

Drugs Closely Related to P Pentazocine

Buprenorphine

Buprenorphine (Buprenex), used in the treatment of moderate to severe pain, has a high affinity at the mu receptors and disassociates from these sites slowly. This characteristic may explain its long duration of action (6 hours, versus 3 hours for pentazocine) and its low ability to cause physical dependence. When used as an analgesic, it is administered either by the IV or the IM route. It also possesses very strong antagonist tendencies at opioid receptors, similar to the action of naloxone. Because of this, buprenorphine (either alone [Subutex] or combined with naloxone [Suboxone]) has been approved for use in the initial treatment of drug dependency. Naloxone is added to prevent against IV misuse of buprenorphine. This combination drug is used for maintenance treatment for drug abuse. Initiation of withdrawal symptoms, which could occur if the combination drug were administered parenterally, does not occur if it is used as intended. Buprenorphine and buprenorphine with naloxone are supplied in subinguinal tablets, prescribed only by physicians who have a special United States Drug Enforcement Agency (DEA) registration and have participated in the required education.

How buprenorphine, a narcotic analgesic with strong receptor antagonist action, produces pain relief is not specifically known.

Buprenorphine is metabolized by the hepatic enzyme CYP3A4. Drugs that inhibit this pathway, such as antifungals (e.g., ketoconazole), macrolide antibiotics (e.g., erythromycin), and human immunodeficiency virus (HIV) protease inhibitors (e.g., ritonavir, indinavir, and saquinavir), increase the circulating volume of buprenorphine. Lower doses of Subutex or Suboxone will be required.

Sedation is the most frequently occurring adverse effect of buprenorphine, affecting more than half of the patients. The next most common adverse effects, although their prevalence is much lower than sedation, are dizziness and vertigo, hypotension, headache, sweating, nausea and vomiting, miosis, and hypoventilation. When given to treat substance abuse, the most common adverse effects from buprenorphine and buprenorphine with naloxone are cold or flu-like symptoms, headaches, sweating, sleeping difficulties, nausea, and mood swings. Adverse effects are most severe in the beginning of treatment and may last several weeks. Strong respiratory depression can occur with buprenorphine, especially if the drug is crushed and given intravenously. Several deaths have occurred with this type of drug abuse; these drugs are especially dangerous if taken concurrently with benzodiazepines, because this combination increases CNS depression. Other CNS depressants, such as other narcotic analgesics, tranquilizers, or alcohol, also potentiate the CNS depression that can occur, possibly with fatal results. Buprenorphine may also produce cytolytic hepatitis and hepatitis with jaundice. The amount of liver damage ranges from a transient asymptomatic elevation in liver enzymes to hepatic failure. It is unclear at this time whether the liver complications are related to the drug or to pre-existing liver problems secondary to IV drug abuse.

Because of these adverse effects, buprenorphine should be used cautiously in patients with compromised respiratory status and those receiving additional drugs that cause respiratory depression. Likewise, it should be used cautiously in those with hepatic disease. Like pentazocine, it is a pregnancy category C drug, and the safety of its use in children under the age of 16 years and during breast-feeding has not been established. Buprenorphine may have some advantages as an analgesic for older adults. This is because the half life of the drug and active metabolites is not lengthened in older adults or in those with renal disease, unlike other opioids. It therefore does not require a reduced dose, or longer interval between doses like other opioids (Pergolizzi et al., 2008). Like pentazocine, if buprenorphine is given to a patient who is opioid dependent, withdrawal occurs. The likelihood of withdrawal is greater with buprenorphine than with pentazocine because buprenorphine has strong antagonist action, whereas pentazocine has only weak antagonist properties. Neonatal withdrawal occurs in those neonates whose mothers received buprenorphine during pregnancy.

When using buprenorphine to treat drug addiction, teach patients to place the tablet under their tongue and allow the tablet to dissolve, which will take 2 to 10 minutes. Tablets should not be swallowed because the medication is not effective this way, and opioid withdrawal may occur. If more than two tablets are prescribed and patients cannot get them all under the tongue at one time, they should place two under the tongue, and as soon as the tablets dissolve, place the additional tablets under the tongue. This medication must be taken regularly to be effective; it cannot be taken on an as-needed basis.

Patient education for those prescribed buprenorphine or buprenorphine with naloxone should include warnings about the serious, and potentially fatal, adverse effects that can occur if the drug is intravenously abused. In addition, if buprenorphine with naloxone is used intravenously in the presence of other narcotics, it induces severe withdrawal symptoms. Buprenorphine, both in Subutex and Suboxone, causes dependency. The drug should not be stopped suddenly because withdrawal occurs.

Assess the patient for concurrent use of benzodiazepines, alcohol, and other CNS depressants that may increase the risk of serious CNS depression from buprenorphine. Patients should be instructed not to take any of these substances while on buprenorphine. Patients should not drive or operate heavy machinery or perform any other dangerous activity until they know whether they experience sedation from the buprenorphine. They should be cautioned about this possibility at the start of therapy and at each dose increase. Assess also for the use of drugs that are inhibitors of the CYP3A4 enzymatic pathway, because these drugs will interact with buprenorphine.

Determine that liver function has been assessed before the beginning of therapy. Additionally, the patient needs to know that re-evaluation of liver function will be important throughout therapy.

Advise patients that they should keep the buprenorphine or buprenorphine with naloxone in a safe place and protect it from theft because it contains a narcotic painkiller, and that selling or giving this medication to another person is against the law. Finally, educate the patient's family that in case of an emergency, such as a drug overdose, emergency department personnel need to be told that the patient is receiving buprenorphine.

Butorphanol

Butorphanol (Stadol) is used as an analgesic, preoperative medication, supplement to balanced anesthesia, and pain reliever during labor. An intranasal form was shown effective in clinical trials in treating the pain of migraine headaches. The analgesic potency of butorphanol, compared by weight, is 20 times that of pentazocine and 3.5 to 7 times that of morphine. Like pentazocine, butorphanol has both narcotic agonist and antagonist effects. Its antagonist activity is approximately 30 times that of pentazocine but only one fortieth that of naloxone. Its mechanism for pain relief is not completely understood. Like pentazocine, it produces the same cardiovascular effects when given intravenously, increases intracranial pressure, is metabolized in the liver (by the 3A4 isoenzyme), is a pregnancy category C drug, and has no known safety data relevant to its use in children. It may induce withdrawal in patients who abuse opiates, although whether it is an antagonist at the mu receptors is not definitely known. Unlike pentazocine, its most common adverse effect is somnolence. Common adverse effects similar to pentazocine include nausea and vomiting and dizziness. Other adverse effects that occur with regularity include confusion, sweating, dry mouth, headache, vasodilation, insomnia, constipation, and an unpleasant taste.

Nalbuphine

Nalbuphine (Nubain) is a potent analgesic with agonist and antagonist effects. Its analgesic potency is essentially the same as that of morphine and about three times greater than that of pentazocine. Its antagonist activity is approximately 10 times that of pentazocine. Nalbuphine is used for moderate to severe pain, as a preoperative analgesic, as a supplement to balanced anesthesia, and as an obstetric analgesic during labor and delivery. Unlike pentazocine, nalbuphine does not increase pulmonary artery pressure, systemic vascular resistance, or cardiac work. Nalbuphine produces respiratory depression similar to morphine. Unlike morphine, the depressive effects seem to have a ceiling effect, with increases beyond 30 mg of nalbuphine producing no further respiratory depression. Like pentazocine, nalbuphine can produce an allergic response in patients with sulfite sensitivity and also trigger withdrawal in patients dependent on narcotics. The most common adverse effect is sedation, which occurs in about one third of the patients who use the drug. Other fairly common adverse effects are sweating, nausea and vomiting, dizziness and vertigo, dry mouth, and headache.

CHAPTER SUMMARY

- Pain is a subjective experience. Objective signs may or may not accompany pain. Lack of objective data does not mean that the pain is not present.
- Pain, a complex physiologic phenomenon, is not clearly or completely understood at this time.
- Pain is mediated through the CNS by nociceptors and perceived by the opiate receptors. When the opiate receptors are stimulated, perception of pain decreases.
- Pain has many types or classifications, which are based on the pathophysiologic origin of the pain (nociceptive versus neuropathic), whether the pain reflects a current injury or period of healing or extends beyond this time (acute versus chronic), or a subgroup of one of these classifications (visceral, somatic, cancer, or noncancer chronic).
- Pain, to be treated appropriately, must be assessed with a pain assessment tool. Simply asking patients to rate their pain on a scale in their head is not the same as using an assessment tool.
- Pain is best controlled when patients take analgesics before pain becomes severe and when doses are administered around the clock.
- Doses of analgesics should be titrated to obtain maximum efficacy with minimal adverse effects.
- Nonanalgesics and nonpharmacologic methods of pain management may be used to supplement drug therapy.
- Patients who have been receiving opioids for an extended period develop tolerance to the pain relief from the analgesics and need increased doses. Patients who abuse substances have cross-tolerance and need higher than expected doses to receive analgesia from drug therapy.

- Morphine is the standard narcotic analgesic. It is an agonist at the opioid receptors. All other narcotics are compared with morphine to measure their efficacy. Morphine is indicated in the treatment of moderate to severe pain.
- In addition to analgesia, morphine, like all narcotics, produces a wide variety of other effects on the body. The most serious of these is respiratory depression, which if severe, can be life threatening.
- The antidote to morphine overdosage and respiratory depression caused by any narcotic is naloxone, a narcotic antagonist.
- Morphine, like all narcotics, is a controlled substance. By law, every dose must be properly accounted for and documented. This rule includes partial doses that may be wasted.
- Relevant core patient variables are important to consider when providing morphine or other narcotics for pain control. The variables may alter the drug chosen, dose, frequency, route, patient's emotional response to pain, or frequency and depth of assessment made while the patient receives morphine or other narcotics.
- Codeine is another narcotic analgesic used for mild to moderate pain. It is also used to suppress coughs. Its effects are similar to those of morphine, but usually milder.
- Pentazocine, a different type of narcotic, is a combination of opioid agonists and opioid antagonists. Because of the antagonist effects at some receptors, it generally causes less respiratory depression than morphine and has less risk for inducing physical dependence. If given to a patient physically dependent on a narcotic, pentazocine may induce withdrawal.
- Patients and their families need education about the importance of pain control and what will be done when they report pain. Moreover, they need to know that they are not expected to suffer. Discuss with them any fears or misconceptions about analgesic use and dispel such mistaken beliefs with facts.
- Reassess patients for pain following changes in drug therapy, after every dose until a set dose controls pain, and periodically during the course of therapy.

QUESTIONS FOR STUDY AND REVIEW

1. Why should morphine not be administered to treat acute pain in an opioid-naive person with respiratory depression?
2. Can morphine be administered to treat chronic pain if the patient's respiratory rate is between 8 and 12 breaths/minute? Why?
3. Your patient has a history of opioid abuse, just came from surgery, and has a chest tube. Explain why this patient might need a larger dose of morphine to control postoperative pain than other patients require.
4. What is a "rescue dose"?

5. Why might more than one dose of naloxone, a narcotic antagonist, be needed when a patient has severe respiratory depression from opiate overdose?

6. Why should codeine not be administered to anyone who needs to be able to cough to clear his or her airway?

NEED MORE HELP?

Chapter 23 of the Study Guide to Accompany *Drug Therapy in Nursing,* 4th Edition, contains NCLEX-style questions and other learning activities to reinforce your understanding of the concepts presented in this chapter. For additional information or to purchase the study guide, visit thePoint.

REFERENCES

American Academy of Pain Medicine, American Pain Society, and the American Society of Addiction Medicine. (2006). Consensus document: Definitions related to the use of opioids for the treatment of pain. Retrieved from *http://www.asam.org/ppol/Opoid%20 Definition%20C%2002.htm.*

Cleeland, C. S. & Ryan K. M. (1994). Pain assessment: Global use of the Brief Pain Inventory. *Annals of Academic Medicine Singapore,* 23(2):129–138.

Daut, R. L., Cleeland, C. S., & Flanery, R. C. (1983). Development of the Wisconsin Brief Pain Questionnaire to assess pain in cancer and other diseases. *Cancer,* 17(2): 197–210.

Derry, S., Moore, R. A., & McQuay, H. J. Single dose oral codeine, as a single agent, for acute postoperative pain in adults. *Cochrane Database of Systematic Reviews* 2010, Issue 4. Art. No.: CD008099. DOI: 10.1002/14651858. CD008099.pub2.

Fishman, B., Pasternak, S., Wallenstein, S. L., et al. (1987). The Memorial Pain Assessment Card: A valid instrument for the evaluation of cancer pain. *Cancer,* 60(5):1151–1158.

Hockenberry, M. J. (2009). *Wong's essentials of pediatric nursing* (8th ed.). St. Louis: Mosby.

Hudcova, J., McNicol, E. D., Quah, C. S., et al. (2006). Patient controlled opioid analgesia versus conventional opioid analgesia for postoperative pain. *Cochrane Database of Systematic Reviews,* Issue 4. Art. No.: CD003348. DOI: 10.1002/14651858.CD003348.pub2. Edited (no change to conclusions), published in Issue 1, 2009.

International Association for the Study of Pain. Pain terminology. Retrieved from *http://www.iasp-pain.org/Content/NavigationMenu/GeneralResourceLinks/PainDefinitions/default.htm.* Accessed on May 23, 2011.

McCaffery, M. (1968). *Nursing practice theories related to cognition, bodily pain and man-environmental interactions.* Los Angeles: UCLA Students Store.

Melzack, R. (1975). The McGill Pain Questionnaire: Major properties and scoring methods. *Pain,* 1(3):277–299.

Pergolizzi, J., Böger, R. H., Budd, K., et al. (2008). Opioids and the management of chronic severe pain in the elderly: consensus statement of an International Expert Panel with focus on the six clinically most often used World Health Organization Step III opioids (buprenorphine, fentanyl, hydromorphone, methadone, morphine, oxycodone). *Pain Practice:The official journal of the World Institute of Pain,* 8(4):287–313.

Quigley C. (2002). Hydromorphone for acute and chronic pain. *Cochrane Database of Systematic Reviews,* Issue 1. Art. No.: CD003447. DOI: 10.1002/14651858.CD003447. (no change to conclusions), published in Issue 1, 2009.

Seidel, S., Aigner, M., Ossege, M., et al. (2008). Antipsychotics for acute and chronic pain in adults. *Cochrane Database of Systematic Reviews* -, Issue 4. Art. No.: CD004844. DOI: 10.1002/14651858.CD004844.pub2.

U.S. Department of Health and Human Services, Centers for Disease Control and Prevention, National Center for Health Statistics. (2006). Health, United States, 2006 with chartbook on trends in the health of Americans. Retrieved from *http://www.cdc.gov/ nchs/data/hus/hus06.pdf#executive summary.*

Wong, D. & Baker, C. (1998). Pain in children: Comparison of assessment scales. *Pediatric Nursing,* 14(1):9–17.

Drugs Treating Mild to Moderate Pain, Fever, Inflammation, and Migraine Headache

Learning Objectives

At the completion of this chapter the student will:

1. Correlate the processes of inflammation, fever, and pain with the actions of salicylates, nonsteroidal anti-inflammatory drugs (NSAIDs), para-aminophenol derivative drugs, and antimigraine drugs.

2. Identify core drug knowledge pertaining to salicylates, NSAIDs, para-aminophenol derivative drugs, and antimigraine drugs.

3. Identify the core patient variables pertaining to salicylates, NSAIDs, para-aminophenol derivative drugs, and antimigraine drugs.

4. Relate the interaction of core drug knowledge to core patient variables for salicylates, NSAIDs, para-aminophenol derivative drugs, and antimigraine drugs.

5. Generate a nursing plan of care from the interactions between core drug knowledge and core patient variables for salicylates, NSAIDs, para-aminophenol derivative drugs, and antimigraine drugs.

6. Describe nursing interventions to maximize therapeutic and minimize adverse effects for salicylates, NSAIDs, para-aminophenol derivative drugs, and antimigraine drugs.

7. Determine key points for patient and family education for salicylates, NSAIDs, para-aminophenol derivative drugs, and antimigraine drugs.

Key Terms

cyclooxygenase	prostaglandin synthetase inhibitors	salicylates
nonsteroidal anti-inflammatory drug (NSAID)	Reye syndrome	salicylism
para-aminophenol derivative	salicylate poisoning	triptans

Drugs Treating Mild to Moderate Pain, Fever, Inflammation, and Migraine Headache

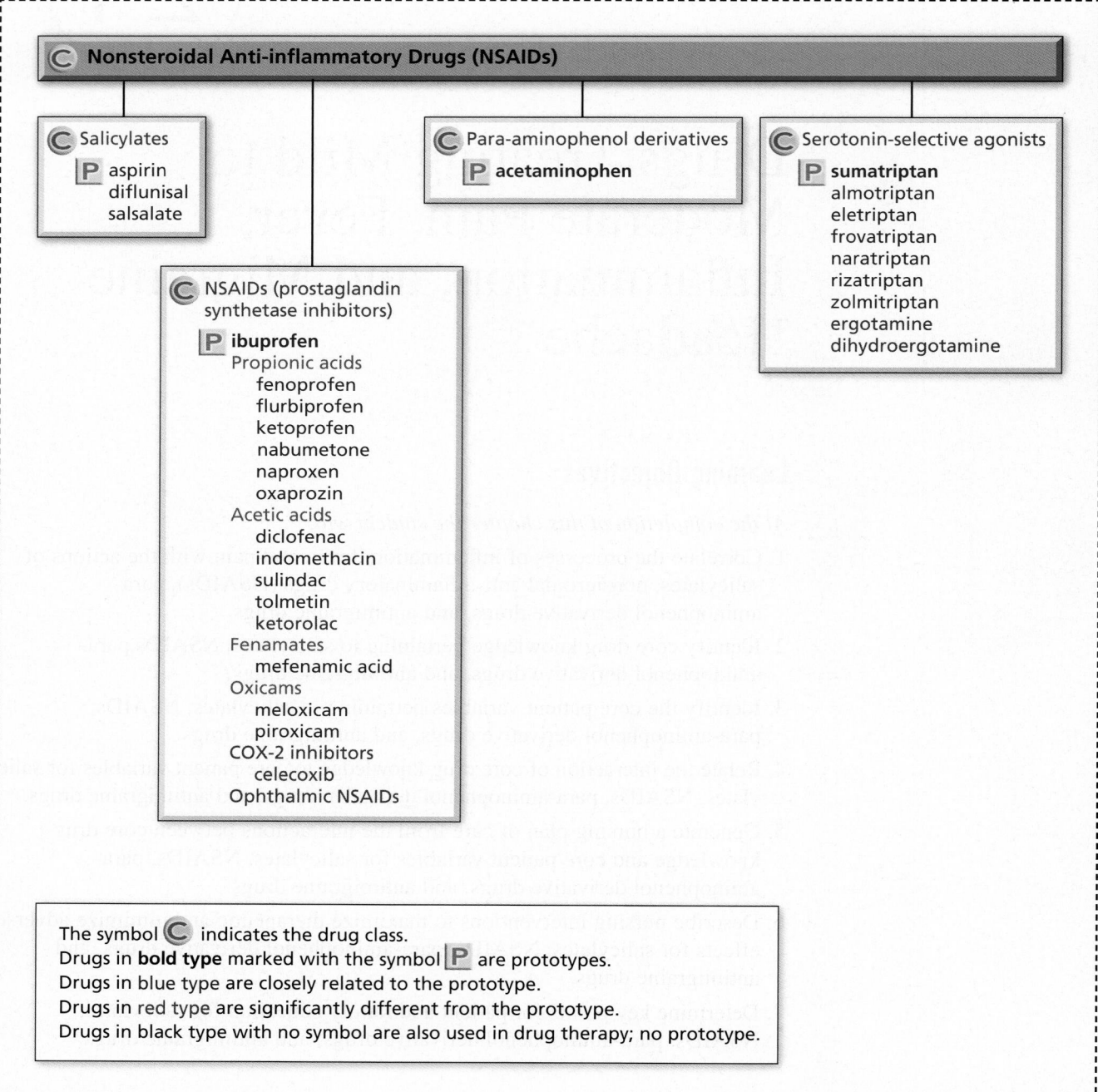

© **Nonsteroidal Anti-inflammatory Drugs (NSAIDs)**

© Salicylates
P aspirin
diflunisal
salsalate

© Para-aminophenol derivatives
P **acetaminophen**

© Serotonin-selective agonists
P **sumatriptan**
almotriptan
eletriptan
frovatriptan
naratriptan
rizatriptan
zolmitriptan
ergotamine
dihydroergotamine

© NSAIDs (prostaglandin synthetase inhibitors)
P **ibuprofen**
Propionic acids
fenoprofen
flurbiprofen
ketoprofen
nabumetone
naproxen
oxaprozin
Acetic acids
diclofenac
indomethacin
sulindac
tolmetin
ketorolac
Fenamates
mefenamic acid
Oxicams
meloxicam
piroxicam
COX-2 inhibitors
celecoxib
Ophthalmic NSAIDs

The symbol © indicates the drug class.
Drugs in **bold type** marked with the symbol P are prototypes.
Drugs in blue type are closely related to the prototype.
Drugs in red type are significantly different from the prototype.
Drugs in black type with no symbol are also used in drug therapy; no prototype.

Fever, inflammation, and pain are symptoms of acute illness and frequently coexist. Inflammation and pain also can be symptoms of chronic diseases, such as arthritis and gout. Inflammation may also induce intense pain called migraine headache. Fever, inflammation, and pain commonly are treated with salicylates, nonsteroidal anti-inflammatory drugs (NSAIDs, also known as prostaglandin synthetase inhibitors), or para-aminophenol derivative drugs. Migraine headaches are commonly treated with serotonin-selective drugs called **triptans** or antimigraine agents.

This chapter discusses the therapeutic classes of drugs used for fever, inflammation, pain, and migraine headache. It also addresses the core drug knowledge, core patient variables, nursing management, potential nursing diagnoses, and patient education related to the use of these drugs.

PHYSIOLOGY

Fever

Temperature regulation is a function of the hypothalamus. Normally, a homeostatic balance exists between body heat generated and body heat lost. When heat is excessive, the regulatory mechanism is activated, and the body responds with integumentary vasodilation, leading to perspiration and a net heat loss.

Fever is the result of fever-inducing substances called pyrogens, which activate certain monocytes/macrophages, which in turn secrete cytokines. Cytokines increase the synthesis and secretion of prostaglandin E_2 (PGE_2) in the hypothalamus, and PGE_2 stimulates the hypothalamus to reset the regulating mechanism to tolerate a higher body temperature.

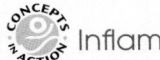

Inflammation

Numerous types of stimuli, such as trauma, surgery, infection, and ischemia, evoke the inflammatory response. The classic signs of local inflammation are swelling (tumor), heat (calor), redness (rubor), pain (dolor), and loss of function (functio laesa). Regardless of the etiology, the sequence of physiologic effects is similar.

Acute inflammation is divided into vascular and cellular responses. The vascular response occurs almost immediately after the injury. Initially, vasoconstriction occurs in the surrounding vessels, quickly followed by vasodilation of both the arterioles and venules in the area. The vasodilation allows increased blood flow to the area, which accounts for the signs of redness and warmth. At the same time, capillary permeability increases, allowing fluid to accumulate in the surrounding tissues, causing swelling. With the swelling of the surrounding tissues and the release of chemical mediators from the injured tissues, pain and impaired function occur.

The cellular response is divided into four phases:

1. Margination of white blood cells (WBCs)—WBCs move to the periphery of the blood vessels to prepare for emigration.
2. Emigration of WBCs—The WBCs pass through the capillary walls and migrate into the tissue spaces.
3. Chemotaxis—Cellular debris or bacteria become more "attractive" to the WBCs.
4. Phagocytosis—Neutrophils and monocytes engulf and degrade the cellular debris.

Rupture of the mast cells, which release biochemical mediators, such as histamine, prostaglandins, and leukotrienes, also contribute to inflammation. Prostaglandins are thought to be pivotal in the inflammatory response by potentiating pain and edema caused by other chemical mediators.

Prostaglandin Synthesis

Prostaglandins modulate some components of inflammation, body temperature, pain transmission, platelet aggregation, and many other body actions. They are derived from arachidonic acid, which is liberated from the cell membrane in response to physical, chemical, hormonal, bacterial, or other stimuli (Figure 24.1). They are converted from arachidonic acid to prostaglandins by the enzyme **cyclooxygenase** (COX). There are two forms of the COX enzyme: COX-1 and COX-2. COX-1 synthesizes prostaglandins that are involved in the regulation of normal cell activity, whereas COX-2 appears to produce prostaglandins mainly at sites of inflammation. For instance, in the gastrointestinal (GI) tract, COX-1 is responsible for secretion of cytoprotective mucus and bicarbonate, suppression of the output of gastric acid, and support for submucosal blood flow. In the renal system, COX-1 promotes vasodilation, resulting in increased blood flow to the kidneys. COX-2 is activated by arthritis and other stimuli and produces the prostaglandins that lead to inflammation, swelling, and joint pain. Most NSAIDs indiscriminately target both COX-1 and COX-2, thereby depleting the prostaglandins needed for normal cell function and protection. This lack of discrimination explains the etiology of many of these drugs' adverse effects.

Pain

The physiologic mechanisms involved in the pain response are complex (see Chapter 23). The sensation of peripheral pain begins in afferent neurons called nociceptors, which are found in skin, muscle, connective tissue, the circulatory system, and abdominal, pelvic, and thoracic viscera. Although these receptors may be activated by mechanical, chemical, or thermal stimuli, they also are activated by chemical mediators, such as prostaglandins, histamine, bradykinin, and serotonin, which are released during cellular destruction. It is theorized that the inhibition of prostaglandins may diminish activation of peripheral pain sensors, resulting in decreased pain.

Platelet Aggregation

Simply speaking, platelet aggregation is the clumping together of platelets in the blood. Platelet aggregation can be a beneficial process. In fact, it is one of the body's protective mechanisms. For instance, when bleeding from a wound suddenly occurs, the platelets gather at the wound and attempt to block the blood flow. However, platelet aggregation can also be harmful. It is the first step in a sequence of events that leads to the formation of a thrombus.

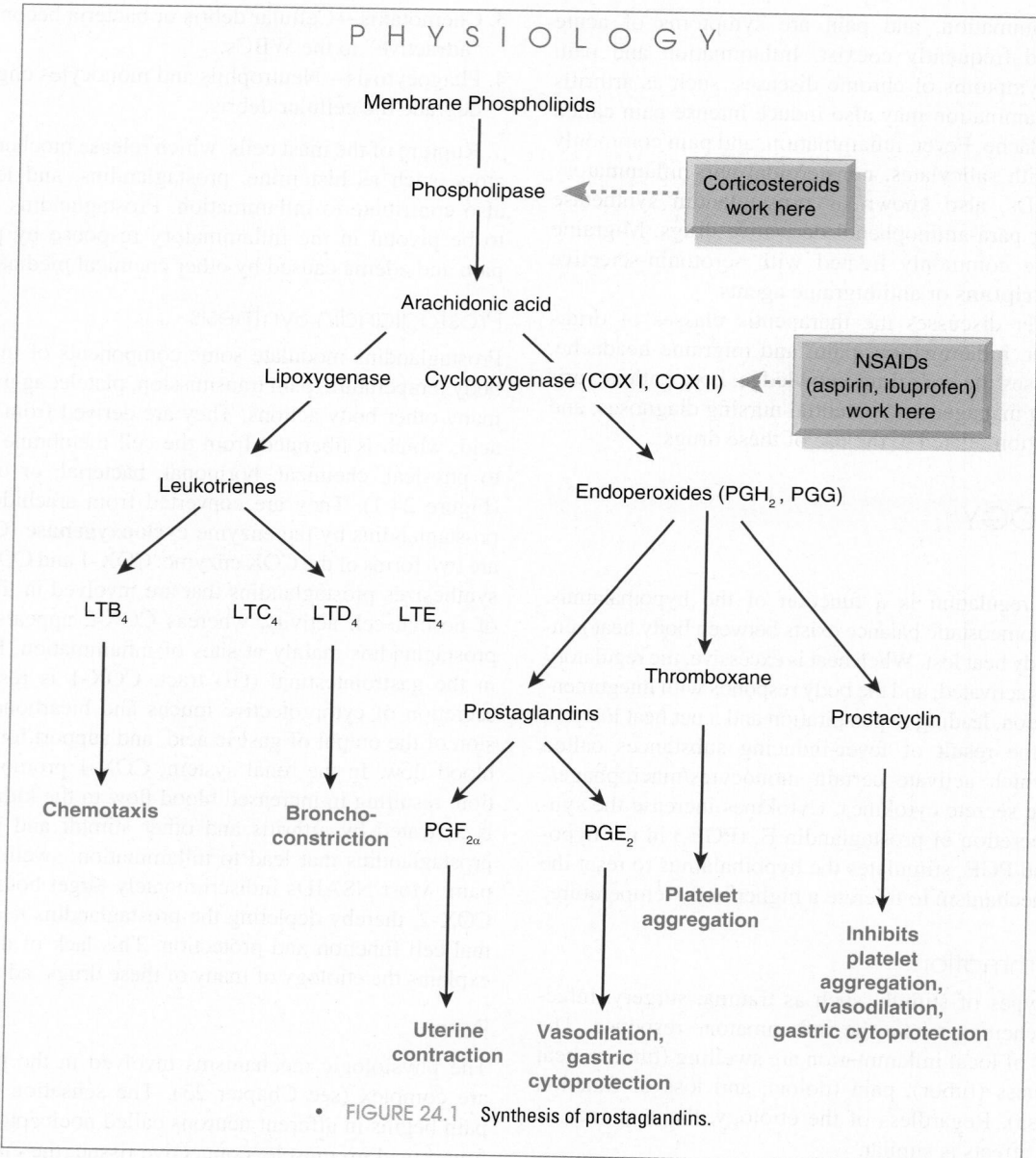

PHYSIOLOGY

Membrane Phospholipids

Phospholipase ◄╌╌╌╌╌╌ Corticosteroids work here

Arachidonic acid

Lipoxygenase   Cyclooxygenase (COX I, COX II) ◄╌╌╌ NSAIDs (aspirin, ibuprofen) work here

Leukotrienes   Endoperoxides (PGH_2, PGG)

LTB_4 LTC_4 LTD_4 LTE_4

Thromboxane

Prostaglandins   Prostacyclin

Chemotaxis   Broncho-constriction $PGF_{2\alpha}$ PGE_2

Platelet aggregation

Inhibits platelet aggregation, vasodilation, gastric cytoprotection

Uterine contraction   Vasodilation, gastric cytoprotection

• FIGURE 24.1 Synthesis of prostaglandins.

When blood vessels are damaged, fibrils of collagen are exposed. Collagen acts as a potent activator of platelets, changing the platelet from a smooth discoid shape to a spiculated (spiky) form that allows platelets to bind together. The bound platelets release adenosine triphosphate and thromboxane A_2 (TXA_2), which recruit and activate still more platelets circulating in the blood. The risk of platelet aggregation and its associated blood vessel damage is increased in patients who smoke cigarettes and in those who have hypercholesterolemia.

PATHOPHYSIOLOGY

Migraine Headache

Many patients believe that any severe headache is a migraine headache. Actually, migraine headache is much more than just severe pain. In the United States, it affects almost 30 million people, many of whom are undiagnosed. Migraine affects women more frequently than men, possibly because of the interaction between hormones and migraine.

Migraine headache is one of the four types of primary headaches (Box 24.1). The two major subtypes of migraine headache are migraine with aura (previously classic migraine) and migraine without aura (previously common migraine). Migraine headaches are divided into four phases: prodrome, aura, headache, and postheadache. The characteristic symptoms of each phase are listed in Box 24.2. The prodromal phase occurs initially. In the 20% to 60% of patients who experience this phase, symptoms may ease as the headache begins. The aura phase is a group of neurologic symptoms that develop in 15 to 20 minutes and last for up to an hour; 15% to 20% of patients experience this phase. The headache phase develops within 60 minutes after the cessation of the aura and can last from hours to days. The postheadache phase begins after the symptoms of the headache cease.

Box 24.1 INTERNATIONAL CLASSIFICATION OF HEADACHES

The Primary Headaches

1. Migraine
2. Tension-type headache
3. Cluster headache and other trigeminal autonomic cephalalgias
4. Other primary headache

The Secondary Headaches

5. Headache attributed to head and/or neck trauma
6. Headache attributed to cranial or cervical vascular disorder
7. Headache attributed to non-vascular intracranial disorder
8. Headache attributed to a substance or its withdrawal
9. Headache attributed to infection
10. Headache attributed to disorder of homoeostasis
11. Headache or facial pain attributed to disorder of cranium, neck, eyes, ears, nose, sinuses, teeth, mouth or other facial or cranial structures
12. Headache attributed to psychiatric disorders

Cranial Neuralgias Central and Primary Facial Pain and Other Headaches

13. Cranial neuralgias and central causes of facial pain
14. Other headache, cranial neuralgia, central or primary facial pain

The understanding of the etiology of migraine headache has been evolving for years. In the past migraine was classified as a vascular event; however, migraine is now classified as a neurovascular disorder. It is postulated that migraine begins when intracranial blood vessels dilate. This dilation stimulates the trigeminovascular system, resulting in abnormally excitable neurons that send pain impulses to the brain's pain receptors. Stimulation of the trigeminovascular system also causes release of brain chemicals called neuropeptides (substance P, calcitonin gene–related peptide [CGRP], neurokinin A, serotonin, and noradrenalin). The release of these chemicals causes inflammation, with resultant increased perception of pain. As the pain increases, activation and sensitization of sensory neurons of the trigeminal nuclei in the caudal brainstem and upper cervical spinal tract occur. This produces a lowered pain threshold, and sensations that are not normally painful (light, touch, noise, movement) are perceived as painful.

DRUGS TO TREAT INFLAMMATION AND FEVER

Salicylates, NSAIDs, and para-aminophenol derivative drugs are used to treat inflammation and fever in a variety of conditions. Salicylates are used in managing conditions ranging from a simple headache to acute myocardial infarction (MI). NSAIDs are used primarily as anti-inflammatory drugs but are also used extensively as analgesics. The newest NSAIDs have been approved for other conditions such as familial adenomatous polyposis (FAP) and are undergoing extensive research into their viability to affect disorders such as Alzheimer and kidney disease.

Ⓒ NONSTEROIDAL ANTI-INFLAMMATORY AGENTS

This class of drugs is conventionally categorized as **salicylates,** nonsteroidal anti-inflammatory drugs (NSAIDs), and para-aminophenol derivatives. The literature sometimes refers to NSAIDs as **prostaglandin synthetase inhibitors.** Both salicylates and NSAIDs work by inhibiting COX and decreasing prostaglandins and thromboxane. A major

Box 24.2 PHASES OF MIGRAINE HEADACHE

Prodromal Phase (symptoms vary)

- Depression/moodiness
- Food cravings/thirst
- Difficulty concentrating
- Fatigue
- Shivering
- Stiff neck

Aura Phase

Visual Symptoms:
- Specks
- Flashing
- Shimmering
- Geometric forms
- Telescoping vision

Motor Symptoms:
- Weakness
- Language difficulty

Sensory Symptoms:
- Numbness

Headache Phase

Head Pain:
- Gradual onset
- Unilateral (bilateral in 40%)
- Throbbing, moderate to severe pain
- Aggravated by movement

Associated Symptoms:
- Nausea and vomiting
- Photophobia and phonophobia
- Anorexia
- Blurred vision

Postheadache Phase

- Fatigue
- Irritability
- Impaired concentration
- Scalp tenderness
- Mood changes
- Euphoria or depression

TABLE 24.1   Summary of Selected ⓒ Salicylates

Drug (Trade) Name	Selected Indications	Route and Dosage Range	Pharmacokinetics
ⓒ Salicylates			
Ⓟ acetylsalicylic acid (aspirin, Bayer Aspirin)	Minor aches, pains, or temperature Anti-inflammatory Acute rheumatic fever Prevention of transient ischemic attacks Prevention of myocardial infarction	*Adult:* PO, dependent on indication, in order of indications listed to the left: 325–1,000 mg q4h; 2.6–5.2 g/d in divided doses; 7.8 g/d in divided doses; 325 mg–1.3 g/d in two to four divided doses; 325 mg/d *Child:* PO, <25 kg; 60–90 mg/kg/d; >25 kg, 2.4–3.6 g/d in divided doses	*Onset:* 15–30 min *Duration:* 3–6 h $t_{1/2}$: 2–3 h
diflunisal (Dolobid)	Arthritis Mild to moderate pain Headache	*Adult:* PO, 250–500 mg bid not to exceed 1.5 g/d *Adult:* PO, 1 g initially followed by 500 mg q12h (under 50 kg or elderly, 500 mg initially followed by 250 mg q12h) *Adult:* PO, 500 mg q12h *Child:* Safe dosage not established	*Onset:* 30–60 min *Duration:* 12 h $t_{1/2}$: 8–12 h
salsalate (Disalcid)	Arthritis Musculoskeletal inflammation	*Adult:* PO, initially 500 mg–1 g bid or tid; maintenance, 2–4 g in divided doses *Child:* Safe dosage not established	*Onset:* 10–30 min *Duration:* 3–6 h $t_{1/2}$: 2–3 h

difference is that the inhibition of COX by salicylates is *irreversible*, whereas the action of the NSAIDs is *reversible*. Salicylates are discussed first, followed by NSAIDs.

• ⓒ SALICYLATES

Since salicylates were isolated from the bark of the willow tree in 1829, they have become one of the mainstays of drug therapy in a variety of diseases and disorders. The therapeutic uses of salicylates continue to be researched in all areas of medicine. The prototype salicylate is acetylsalicylic acid, commonly known as aspirin. Table 24.1 presents a summary of selected salicylates.

Nursing Management of the Patient Receiving Ⓟ Aspirin

Core Drug Knowledge

Pharmacotherapeutics

Aspirin has a variety of therapeutic uses. It is indicated for mild to moderate pain, especially pain resulting from inflammation. It is used frequently to relieve headache, neuralgia, myalgia, arthralgia, postpartum pain, dental or oral surgery pain, and dysmenorrhea (painful menstruation). The preferred agent for treating pain and inflammation associated with juvenile arthritis, rheumatoid arthritis, and osteoarthritis, it also is the favored drug in treating fever (in adults), pleurisy, and arthritis. Other inflammatory conditions, such as tendonitis and bursitis, respond well to aspirin. In addition, it is used for treating pericarditis in patients with systemic lupus erythematosus (SLE).

Because of its antiplatelet and anti-inflammatory effects, low-dose aspirin (81 mg daily) is useful in preventing or reducing the risk of transient ischemic attacks (TIAs), MI, and ischemic cerebral vascular accident (stroke or brain attack). It is also indicated for patients with a previous MI, patients with chronic or unstable angina, and those undergoing angioplasty or other revascularization procedures Interestingly, low-dose aspirin therapy affects men and women differently. The maximum recommended daily dose is 4 grams.

Pharmacokinetics

Aspirin absorption usually occurs within 30 minutes, depending on the dosage form, gastric pH, and the presence of food or antacids in the stomach. Although some aspirin is absorbed in the stomach, most is absorbed in the small intestine. Aspirin suppositories are slowly and variably absorbed, resulting in a lower blood concentration than with oral forms. Buffered aspirin does not delay absorption; however, enteric-coated and extended-action preparations do delay absorption.

Aspirin is 99% metabolized into salicylate and other metabolites by the liver. Aspirin and its metabolites are highly bound to plasma albumin and widely distributed throughout the body and body fluids, including breast milk. Additionally, they cross the placental barrier. Peak plasma levels occur within 2 hours. The half-life of aspirin is 15 minutes, whereas the half-life of salicylate is 2 hours. Aspirin and its metabolites are excreted by the kidneys (see Table 24.1).

Pharmacodynamics

Aspirin is used for its antipyretic, anti-inflammatory, analgesic, and antiplatelet effects. The antipyretic effects are a result of inhibited PGE_2 synthesis in the hypothalamus, the body's temperature regulator. Aspirin may enhance peripheral vasodilation and sweating. The anti-inflammatory action is believed to be caused by peripheral inhibition of prostaglandin synthesis, but aspirin also may inhibit the action and synthesis of other mediators of inflammation. Pain is mediated by prostaglandins in the periphery that sensitize pain receptors. The analgesic effects result from the ability to inhibit COX-2, resulting in decreased production of prostaglandins. The antiplatelet action results from the *irreversible* inhibition of thromboxane A_2, a prostaglandin that induces platelet aggregation.

Contraindications and Precautions

Aspirin is contraindicated in patients with salicylate hypersensitivity. It also is contraindicated in patients with peptic ulcer disease or bleeding disorders. Aspirin should not be given to patients on anticoagulation therapy because of its antiplatelet activity. Additionally, aspirin is contraindicated in patients with gout and for those with renal or liver impairment. Aspirin is contraindicated in children with varicella or flu-like illness because it is associated with the occurrence of **Reye syndrome,** a potentially fatal disease characterized by swelling in the brain, increased intracranial pressure, and seizures.

Aspirin is assigned to pregnancy category D and should be avoided by pregnant women because it can interfere with the prostaglandins that mediate uterine contraction, resulting in delayed or prolonged labor. In addition, aspirin's antiplatelet activity increases the risk of maternal or neonatal hemorrhage. Aspirin also should be avoided by lactating women because it is secreted in breast milk and may exert its antiplatelet action in infants.

Aspirin should be avoided by patients who smoke cigarettes and by patients with a history of alcohol abuse; both agents are known to be ulcerogenic. Aspirin should be given with caution to patients with asthma, nasal polyps, and hyperuricemia. Patients older than 60 years and those taking corticosteroids have a higher risk for aspirin's adverse effects.

Adverse Effects

Two adverse effects specific to aspirin therapy are salicylism and salicylate poisoning. **Salicylism** is mild aspirin toxicity, which may occur with long-term or high-dose aspirin therapy. Typical symptoms include headache, tinnitus, GI distress, paresthesias, and respiratory stimulation (i.e., increased respiratory rate secondary to stimulation in the central nervous system [CNS]). Patients may appear drowsy or confused. The only intervention needed for salicylism is to reduce the dose of aspirin or stop aspirin therapy.

Salicylate poisoning is a life-threatening event. The lethal dose of aspirin is 5 to 8 g for a child and 10 to 30 g for an adult. There is no antidote for salicylate poisoning. Treatment of salicylate poisoning includes gastric lavage; administration of activated charcoal; and life support, if indicated. Consequences of salicylate poisoning include respiratory alterations; fluid, electrolyte, and acid-base imbalances; seizures; high temperature; and shock leading to coma and death. Patients with suspected salicylate poisoning should be taken to an emergency department rather than a clinic or doctor's office for treatment. Children's

aspirin has a pleasant flavor and may not be recognized as a drug by children. Therefore, it is important to keep aspirin in a safe place.

Common adverse effects related to aspirin are the result of prostaglandin inhibition. It is important to remember that prostaglandins are found in most body tissues and organs and frequently have opposing effects on the body. Adverse effects occur because of the inhibition of a particular prostaglandin necessary for normal cell function by inhibiting COX-1.

The most common adverse effects of aspirin are related to the GI system. Aspirin may irritate the gastric mucosa, resulting in nausea, vomiting, abdominal pain, ulcerations, perforation, and bleeding. These effects occur because of a direct irritating action to the mucosa of the GI tract and the inhibition of PGE_2, which has a cytoprotective mechanism to the mucosa. Aspirin can be given with antacids to decrease its GI effects; however, antacids also decrease the absorption of aspirin. Severe gastropathies occur most frequently in patients older than 60 years, those with a history of peptic ulcer disease, cigarette smokers, those who concomitantly use alcohol or corticosteroids, and those with dyspepsia during aspirin therapy.

Aspirin may cause hypersensitivity reactions, such as rashes, hives, or bronchoconstriction, and possibly respiratory distress and anaphylaxis. Patients prone to these reactions usually have severe corticosteroid-dependent asthma, nasal polyps, or chronic urticaria. High aspirin levels may induce ototoxicity manifested by tinnitus.

Another potentially serious adverse effect of aspirin is excessive or abnormal bleeding, especially in patients with hemophilia, anemias, or severe liver disease. Aspirin inhibits platelet aggregation by the inhibition of the prostaglandin thromboxane. Aspirin's antithrombotic action lasts for the life of the platelet (8 days). Other hematopoietic problems, such as agranulocytosis and aplastic anemia, have been reported infrequently.

Aspirin has been associated with hepatotoxicity in patients with juvenile arthritis, active SLE, rheumatic fever, or pre-existing hepatic impairment. The hepatotoxicity is thought to be a direct toxicity to the liver and is associated with high-dose therapy.

In the renal system, acute renal failure may occur in susceptible patients. Patients with conditions associated with diminished renal blood flow, such as chronic heart failure (CHF), cirrhosis, renal insufficiency, and advanced age, are at the highest risk. Prostaglandins play a role in opposing potent renal vasoconstrictors. Therefore, when the action of these prostaglandins is inhibited, vasoconstriction occurs, and blood flow is diminished to the renal system, resulting in acute renal failure. Another problem that occurs when renal prostaglandins are inhibited is sodium and water retention. This inhibition is especially problematic for patients with conditions such as hypertension and CHF. Less common renal toxicities include interstitial nephritis and nephrotic syndrome. In addition to increased blood urea nitrogen (BUN) and creatinine levels, protein- uria occurs. Acute renal failure, water retention, intersti- tial nephritis, and nephrotic syndrome usually occur early in aspirin therapy and are reversible by stopping aspirin treatment.

Additionally, aspirin decreases uric acid excretion by the kidneys; therefore, aspirin may potentiate gout.

Drug Interactions

Aspirin is a highly protein-bound drug and may interact with other drugs that are also highly protein-bound. Because aspirin displaces the other active drugs into the serum, the pharmacologic effects of the displaced drug are enhanced. Drugs such as anticoagulants, oral hypoglycemics, insu- lin, methotrexate, and alcohol may be enhanced enough to cause toxicity. Conversely, drugs such as antacids, proben- ecid, and corticosteroids may decrease the effectiveness of salicylates. Ibuprofen may block aspirin's antiplatelet activ- ity, diminishing its protective effects against cardiovascular and cerebrovascular events.

In addition, aspirin can cause false-negative results on the glucose oxidase test (Tes-Tape) and a false-positive result on the copper reduction test (Clinitest). These false-positive results have become less important since use of home blood glucose monitoring systems has become widespread. A summary of drug–drug interactions for aspirin is provided in Table 24.2.

Assessment of Relevant Core Patient Variables

Health Status

Assess the patient for potential medical conditions or drugs that contraindicate the use of aspirin or require close patient monitoring. It is important to assess for potential hypersen- sitivities to salicylates or other NSAIDs and for a history of asthma or nasal polyps because patients with these condi- tions are prone to bronchospasm. Also, assess gross hearing as a baseline for possible ototoxicity.

For patients on long-term therapy, obtain a history of GI complaints because of the possibility of *Helicobacter pylori* infection. Patients with *H. pylori* have an increased risk of GI complications with aspirin therapy. Assess a baseline complete blood count (CBC), platelet count, and test results for renal and hepatic function. It is important to assess the patient's knowledge concerning the potential adverse effects and drug interactions associated with aspirin and to assess the patient for efficacy of the therapy.

Life Span and Gender

Determine whether female patients are pregnant. Aspirin should not be given to women in the last trimester of preg- nancy because of an increased risk of maternal hemor- rhage. In addition, taking aspirin during late pregnancy can result in adverse fetal effects, including low birth weight, increased intracranial hemorrhage, stillbirth, and neonatal death. Determine the patient's age before administering aspirin. Aspirin should not be given to children younger

than 16 years with flu-like symptoms because of its associa- tion with Reye syndrome. Aspirin should be given with cau- tion to patients older than 60 years because of an increased risk of adverse effects, especially gastropathies.

Lifestyle, Diet, and Habits

It is important to inquire about the patient's use of over-the- counter (OTC) drugs because many OTCs contain aspirin as an ingredient. Concomitant use increases the risk of hepatic and renal toxicity. Assess for alcohol or drug abuse because the patient may have undiagnosed pre-existing hepatic dys- function. Assessing for cigarette smoking also is important because smoking increases gastric acid production. With the loss of the cytoprotective mechanisms in the stomach from aspirin therapy, the risk of GI bleeding is increased.

Environment

Assess the patient's understanding of aspirin therapy. Aspirin is the least expensive and the most common of all household remedies. Because of its OTC availability and low cost, many people do not understand the potentially life-threatening effects it may cause. They do not believe that aspirin is an important therapeutic intervention and are offended by receiving instructions to take it. For these rea- sons, patient education is vital.

Nursing Diagnoses and Outcomes

- Acute or Chronic Pain related to ineffectiveness of aspirin
  Desired outcome: *The patient will contact the prescriber if pain persists.*
- Risk for Injury: GI Bleeding, Hepatic or Renal Toxicity related to aspirin therapy
  Desired outcome: *The patient will avoid injury by contacting the prescriber if any signs of toxicity occur.*
- Ineffective Protection related to blood dyscrasias or rash

CRITICAL THINKING SCENARIO

ASPIRIN THERAPY FOR ARTHRITIS

Mrs. Tyler, age 55, has been a patient at your clinic for the past 5 years. She has severe persistent asthma and takes oral prednisone as well as beta-adrenergic agonists as needed. She intermittently has an elevated glucose and follows a 2,400-calorie diet. She was diagnosed with degenerative arthritis of her back today. The health care provider advised Mrs. Tyler to take 2 aspirin every 6 hours to relieve her discomfort and to increase the dose to 3 tablets every 6 hours if the pain continues. As Mrs. Tyler leaves, she turns to you and states, "Aspirin—what a joke— I could have gotten that advice from a website on my computer."

1. How would you respond to Mrs. Tyler?
2. What patient education would you do?
3. Does Mrs. Tyler's medical history predispose her to any problems with aspirin?

TABLE 24.2	Agents That Interact with P Aspirin	
Interactants	**Effect and Significance**	**Nursing Management**
ACE inhibitors	Aspirin decreases the hypotensive and vasodilator effects of ACE inhibitors	Monitor BP and hemodynamic parameters.
antacids	Antacids increase urinary pH, thus reducing renal reabsorption of aspirin and increasing aspirin clearance. As more aspirin is cleared from the body, a potentially subtherapeutic aspirin level may result.	Monitor serum aspirin level when initiating or discontinuing antacid therapy.
Anticoagulants, oral	Aspirins inhibit platelet function, thus prolonging bleeding time. Aspirins displace anticoagulants from protein binding sites, thus increasing their effects. Both actions may result in hemorrhage.	Avoid administering aspirin or other salicylates if possible. Monitor PT, PTT, and INR.
Beta blockers	Salicylates may decrease the antihypertensive effects of beta blockers as well as decrease the beneficial effects on left ventricular ejection fraction (LVEF) in patients with chronic heart failure.	Monitor BP. Monitor for signs of CHF.
Carbonic anhydrase inhibitors (CAIs)	Aspirins displace CAI from protein binding sites and inhibit renal clearance. CAI accumulation and toxicity may result in central nervous system (CNS) depression and metabolic acidosis.	Coadministration should be avoided. When a CAI is required, monitor plasma aspirin level and arterial blood gas (ABG) values. Monitor neurologic status.
clopidogrel	Clopidogrel in combination with salicylates increases the risk of life-threatening bleeding (e.g., intracranial and GI hemorrhage) in patients with transient ischemic attack or ischemic stroke.	Monitor for bruising or bleeding. Monitor neurologic status. Discuss alternative therapy with the health care provider
Corticosteroids	Corticosteroids stimulate metabolism of aspirins and increase renal elimination. Aspirin levels may become subtherapeutic. Discontinuation of corticosteroids may increase aspirin level.	Monitor aspirin concentrations when adding or withdrawing corticosteroids. Monitor for bruising or bleeding. Monitor platelet count.
ethanol (alcohol)	Both aspirin and alcohol damage the gastric mucosal barrier. The production of gastric acid stimulated by alcohol promotes the damage. Aspirin decreases the activity of gastric alcohol dehydrogenase, increasing bioavailability. Alcohol may potentiate aspirin-induced GI blood loss and prolong bleeding time.	Separate aspirin and alcohol intake by 12 h. Use buffered aqueous solutions or enteric-coated or extended-release aspirins.
Heparin	Administration of heparin and aspirin together has an additive effect resulting in an increased risk for adverse effects.	Teach the patient to avoid taking these two drugs together. Monitor for signs of bleeding.
insulin	Basal insulin concentrations are increased, and the acute insulin response to a glucose load is enhanced. This potentiates the serum glucose–lowering action of insulin and results in hypoglycemia.	Monitor blood glucose concentration, and discuss insulin dosage changes with the health care provider.
ketorolac	Aspirin may displace the ability of ketorolac to bind to protein, resulting in an increased ketorolac serum concentration.	Discuss alternate therapy with the health care provider. Teach the patient to avoid this combination.
methotrexate	Aspirins may decrease renal clearance and plasma protein binding of methotrexate, leading to methotrexate toxicity.	Monitor for myelosuppression. Monitor CBC. Monitor methotrexate plasma level.
NSAIDS	NSAIDS decrease the cardioprotective and cerebroprotective effects of low-dose uncoated aspirin. The pharmacologic effect of NSAIDS may be decreased. Both drugs are gastric irritants and may increase the risk for GI distress.	Teach the patient to avoid taking these two drugs together. Monitor for cardiovascular adverse effects. Monitor for efficacy of NSAIDS Monitor for GI distress or bleeding.

(Continued)

TABLE 24.2	Agents That Interact with P Aspirin *(continued)*	
Interactants	**Effect and Significance**	**Nursing Management**
probenecid	Renal filtration of uric acid may be altered, leading to the inhibition of uricosuric action of either drug.	Avoid coadministration.
sulfinpyrazone	Salicylates and sulfinpyrazone impair each other's uricosuric activity.	Teach the patient taking sulfinpyrazone to avoid extended use of aspirin.
Sulfonylureas	Hypoglycemic effect of sulfonylureas may be increased, but the mechanism of this action is not known.	Monitor blood glucose. If hypoglycemia occurs, discuss alternative therapy with the health care provider.
valproic acid	Aspirin displaces valproic acid from protein binding sites. Coadministration may cause valproic acid toxicity.	Monitor serum valproic acid concentrations and liver enzyme levels.

Desired outcome: The patient will contact the prescriber if any signs of blood dyscrasias or rash occur.
- Deficient Fluid Volume related to nausea and vomiting
Desired outcome: The patient will avoid dehydration by contacting the prescriber if persistent nausea or vomiting occurs.
- Disturbed Sensory Perception (visual and auditory) related to blurred vision or tinnitus
Desired outcome: The patient will contact the prescriber if blurred vision or tinnitus occurs.
- Risk for Injury related to self-medication
Desired outcome: The patient will avoid injury by taking aspirin as prescribed.

Planning and Intervention

Maximizing Therapeutic Effects
Give aspirin with milk or food to decrease gastric distress, as needed. When giving aspirin for its cardiovascular properties, use uncoated aspirin, because compared with enteric-coated aspirin, its bioavailability and antiplatelet activity are greater.

Minimizing Adverse Effects
Do not administer aspirin to a patient with a medical condition that contraindicates its use. It is important to monitor closely patients with pre-existing medical conditions or those on drug therapy that may interact with aspirin. Anticipate the use of proton pump inhibitors or misoprostol in combination with aspirin to decrease the potential for adverse effects. For patients on long-term aspirin therapy, arrange for periodic laboratory testing, including a CBC, platelet count, and liver and renal function tests.

Providing Patient and Family Education
- Encourage patients to take the drug exactly as prescribed to avoid adverse effects or overdose of aspirin.
- Advise patients to take uncoated aspirin rather than enteric-coated aspirin if they are taking it for its cardiovascular properties.
- Caution patients not to take aspirin if they have problems with their kidney or liver, are asthmatic and have nasal polyps (aspirin can cause an asthma attack), or are in

their last trimester of pregnancy (aspirin may cause hemorrhage during delivery and adverse fetal effects).
- Teach patients about potential adverse effects of aspirin and the importance of contacting the prescriber if any occur. Advise the patient to contact the health care provider if any of the following serious adverse effects occur:
- Confusion, dizziness, drowsiness
- Seizures (convulsions)
- Difficulty breathing, wheezing
- Tinnitus (ringing in the ears)
- Blurred vision
- Black, tarry stools; unusual bleeding or bruising; red or purple spots on the skin; dark urine; prolonged bleeding from a cut; vomiting blood or what looks like coffee grounds
- Caution patients that if aspirin is taken for a long time or in high doses, it can cause problems with the blood, kidneys, or liver.
- Advise patients to avoid drinking alcohol and smoking when taking aspirin because these activities can increase the risk of gastric irritation and bleeding.
- Explain the importance of taking the drug exactly as prescribed to avoid potential GI distress or bleeding. For example, it is best to adhere to the following directions when taking different types of aspirin:
- Chewable tablets can be chewed before swallowing, crushed and taken with food, or mixed in a drink.
- Extended-release tablets should be swallowed whole, never crushed or chewed.
- Tablets, caplets, or gel-caps should be swallowed with a full glass of water.
- Suppositories should be removed from the foil, the tip moistened, and then placed in the rectum.
- Caution patients to contact the prescriber in the event of persistent nausea or vomiting to avoid fluid loss.
- Tell patients to take aspirin with food, milk, or antacid to prevent GI upset, and that if they miss a dose, the dose should be taken as soon as possible. If it is time for the next dose, only that dose should be taken; double or extra doses should never be taken.

MEMORY CHIP

 Aspirin

- Used for its analgesic, antipyretic, anti-inflammatory, and antiplatelet effects; irreversibly inhibits cyclooxygenase (COX)
- Major contraindications: peptic ulcer disease, gout, renal or hepatic impairment, bleeding disorders, and patients already on anticoagulation therapy
- Most common adverse effect: GI distress
- Most serious adverse effects: renal impairment, gastric ulceration, and GI bleeding
- **Life span alerts: Aspirin should not be given to children with varicella- or flu-like illness; it should not be given during pregnancy, especially during the third trimester; *monitor patients older than 60 years carefully*. Low-dose aspirin therapy is routinely given to healthy adults older than 40 years age to prevent MI and stroke.**

- Encourage patients to read all OTC drug labels to avoid taking any drugs with aspirin or ibuprofen as an ingredient.
- Encourage patients with diabetes to use blood glucose monitoring rather than urine testing.
- Inform patients never to give aspirin to children younger than 16 years, unless directed to do so by the prescriber, and to keep aspirin out of the reach of children.
- Tell patients to keep aspirin in a cool, dry place to maintain its potency and to discard any aspirin that smells like vinegar.
- Explain to patients that if the fever does not resolve in 3 days or pain does not go away in 10 days, they should see their health care provider.
- Instruct patients on long-term aspirin therapy to see their health care provider every 6 months for blood work to avoid serious adverse effects. Depending on the health care provider, this may not be necessary for the patient taking low-dose therapy.

Ongoing Assessment and Evaluation

Monitor the patient who is taking aspirin for signs and symptoms of GI distress or bleeding, anemia, hepatotoxicity, and renal failure. It is important to discontinue aspirin if the patient develops a rash, unexplained fever, or angioedema. Monitor for tinnitus and contact the prescriber immediately if this symptom occurs. Also, monitor the patient for efficacy of aspirin therapy.

Therapy is considered effective if the patient is free of fever, pain, or inflammation and does not develop serious adverse effects. In addition, the patient realizes and can explain the importance of contacting the health care provider immediately if any adverse reactions occur.

Drugs Closely Related to P Aspirin

Diflunisal

Diflunisal (Dolobid) is similar to aspirin, but it does not metabolize into salicylic acid. It is used for acute or long-term relief of mild to moderate pain, acute and chronic rheumatoid arthritis, and osteoarthritis. It is not recommended for use as an antipyretic. Diflunisal has an onset of 1 hour, and peak action occurs in 2 to 3 hours. The half-life is 8 to 12 hours. Potential adverse effects are the same as for aspirin. The main advantage of diflunisal is its twice-a-day dosing schedule. The main disadvantage of diflunisal is its cost. Its efficacy for children has not been established.

Salsalate

Salsalate (Disalcid) is the ester of salicylic acid. Salsalate is absorbed completely from the GI tract. Absorption occurs in the small intestine because salsalate acid is practically insoluble in acidic gastric fluids. As an anti-inflammatory and analgesic drug, salsalate acid has the same efficacy as aspirin; however, it does not have antiplatelet or antipyretic effects. Salsalate is useful particularly for patients who cannot tolerate aspirin's GI effects or for patients at risk for anticoagulation. Peak action of salsalate occurs in 2 to 4 hours, and therapeutic levels may be maintained for up to 16 hours with twice-a-day dosing. Salsalate is not recommended for children.

• C NONSTEROIDAL ANTI-INFLAMMATORY DRUGS

The NSAIDs are grouped by chemical classes—propionic acids, acetic acids, fenamates, oxicams, and COX-2 inhibitors. Despite the chemical differences among NSAIDs, they all inhibit COX and prostaglandin synthesis. Different NSAIDs may inhibit specific isoenzymes of the COX group, which may explain the differences in efficacy and adverse effects among the NSAIDs when used in specific disease states. The therapeutic efficacy of an NSAID in a particular patient is based on clinical response and usually cannot be predicted before its use. As previously mentioned, there are two distinct forms of COX. It is proposed that NSAIDS should be classified as either COX-1 specific, COX nonspecific, COX-2 preferential, or COX-2 specific (Box 24.3). All NSAIDs, regardless of their preference for COX-1 or COX-2, carry a Black Box warning stating that it increases the risk of MI and stroke, and that the risk increases with the duration of therapy.

Ibuprofen has had Food and Drug Administration (FDA) approval since the mid-1970s and currently is available in prescription and nonprescription dosages. Ibuprofen (Motrin, multiple other trade names) is the prototype for NSAIDs. Table 24.3 presents a summary of selected NSAIDs.

Box 24.3 SELECTIVITY OF NSAIDS

COX-1 Selective	COX-1 Slightly Selective	COX-2 Selective	COX-2 Slightly Selective
aspirin	**diclofenac**	**celecoxib**	**etodolac**
indomethacin	**ibuprofen**		**meloxicam**
ketoprofen	**naprosyn**		**nabumetone**
piroxicam			
sulindac			

TABLE 24.3 Summary of Selected ⓒ Nonsteroidal Anti-Inflammatory Drugs

Drug (Trade) Name	Route and Dosage Range	Pharmacokinetics
ⓒ Nonsteroidal Anti-Inflammatory Drugs		
ⓟ ibuprofen (Motrin, Advil)	Adult: PO, 200–800 mg tid–qid, not to exceed 3,200 mg/d Child: PO, 20–40 mg/kg/d in three to four divided doses	Onset: Rapid Duration: 24 h t1/2: 1.8–2 h
ibuprofen lysine (NeoProfen)	Premies <32 wk gestation: IV, 10 mg/kg IV ×1, then 5 mg/kg IV q24h ×2; wait 24 h between 1st and 2nd dose; may repeat course ×1 if treatment is unsuccessful; all doses based on birthweight	
bromfenac (Xibrom)	Adult: Topical, 1 drop 2×/d for 14 d	Onset: Rapid Duration: Unknown $t_{1/2}$: Unknown
diclofenac sodium (Voltaren, Flector)	Adult: PO, 100–200 mg/d in two to four divided doses Adult: Transdermal (Flector), 1 patch to the most painful area 2×/d Child: Safety and efficacy not established	Onset: 1 h Duration: 4–6 h $t_{1/2}$: 2 h
fenoprofen (Nalfon)	Adult: PO, 300–600 mg tid–qid, not to exceed 3,200 mg/d Child: Safety and efficacy not established	Onset: 30 min Duration: 4–6 h $t_{1/2}$: 3 h
flurbiprofen (Ansaid)	Adult: PO, 50–100 mg bid–tid; maximum dose, 300 mg/d Child: Safety and efficacy not established	Onset: 1 h Duration: 4–8 h $t_{1/2}$: 5.7 h
indomethacin (Indocin)	Adult: PO, 25 mg bid or tid up to total 150–200 mg/d Child: IV, 0.1–0.25 mg/kg/d (patent ductus arteriosus) Child: PO; 1–2 mg/kg/d (rheumatoid arthritis)	Onset: PO, 30 min; IV, immediate Duration: PO, 4–6 h; IV, 15–20 min $t_{1/2}$: 2.6–11 h
ketoprofen (Orudis)	Adult: PO, 150–300 mg/d single or divided doses; maximum 300 mg/d Child: Safety and efficacy not established	Onset: 30 min Duration: 4–8 h $t_{1/2}$: 2–4 h
ketorolac (Toradol, Acular)	Adult: PO, 10 mg q4–6h for maximum of 5 d; IM/IV, 30–60 mg, followed by 15–30 mg q6h for a maximum of 5 d Child: IM/IV, 0.5 mg/kg q6h to a maximum of 72 h	Onset: PO, varies; IM/IV, 30 min Duration: PO, IM/IV, 6 h $t_{1/2}$: 2.4–8.6 h
mefenamic acid (Ponstel)	Adult: PO, initially 500 mg q6h, then decrease to 250 mg q6h; maximum dose, 1,000 mg/d, not to exceed 5–7 d Child: Not indicated for age <14 y	Onset: 1–2 h Duration: 6 h $t_{1/2}$: 2–4 h
meloxicam (Mobic)	Adult: 7.5 mg once daily Child: 2–17 y; PO, 0.125 mg/kg/d, not to exceed 7.5 mg daily	Onset: Rapid Duration: Unknown $t_{1/2}$: 15–20 h
nabumetone (Relafen)	Adult: PO, 1,000 mg/d, not to exceed 2,000 mg/d Child: Safety and efficacy not established	Onset: 1–2 h Duration: 24–48 h $t_{1/2}$: 24 h
naproxen (Naprosyn)	Adult: PO, 250–750 mg bid, not to exceed 1,500 mg/d; acute gout, 750–825 mg initially, followed by 250–275 mg qid; moderate pain or dysmenorrhea, 500–550 mg, followed by 250–275 mg Child: PO, 10 mg/kg in 2 doses	Onset: 1–2 h Duration: 7–12 h $t_{1/2}$: 12–15 h
nepafenac (Nevanac)	Adult and Child >10 y: Topical, 1 drop 3x/d for 15 d; start 1 d post cataract surgery	Onset: Rapid Duration: Unknown $t_{1/2}$: Unknown
oxaprozin (Daypro)	Adult: PO, 600–1,200 mg once daily Child 6–16 y: PO, 10–20 mg/kg daily, not to exceed 1200 mg/d	Onset: 1 h Duration: 24–48 h $t_{1/2}$: 42–50 h
piroxicam (Feldene)	Adult: PO, 10–20 mg/d or in divided dose Child: Safety and efficacy not established	Onset: 15–30 min Duration: 24–48 h $t_{1/2}$: 30–86 h
sulindac (Clinoril)	Adult: PO, 150–200 mg bid, not to exceed 400 mg/d Child: Safety and efficacy not established	Onset: 1 h Duration: 7–16 h $t_{1/2}$: 7–8 h

TABLE 24.3 Summary of Selected C Nonsteroidal Anti-Inflammatory Drugs *(continued)*

Drug (Trade) Name	Route and Dosage Range	Pharmacokinetics
tolmetin (Tolectin)	*Adult:* PO, initial 200–400 mg tid–qid; maintenance, 600–1,800 mg in divided doses, not to exceed 1,800 mg *Child:* PO, initial 20 mg/kg/d in three to four divided doses; maintenance, 15–30 mg/kg/d in three to four divided doses	*Onset:* Rapid *Duration:* 6–8 h $t_{1/2}$: 2–7 h
COX-2 Inhibitors		
celecoxib (Celebrex)	*Adult:* PO, 100–200 mg bid	*Onset:* <1 h *Duration:* Unknown $t_{1/2}$: 11 h

Nursing Management of the Patient Receiving P Ibuprofen

Core Drug Knowledge

Pharmacotherapeutics

Labeled uses for ibuprofen include rheumatoid arthritis, juvenile rheumatoid arthritis, osteoarthritis, mild to moderate pain, primary dysmenorrhea, migraine headache, and fever. Ibuprofen lysine (NeoProfen) is an intravenous (IV) formulation used for closure of patent ductus arteriosus in premature infants. Table 24.4 presents labeled and unlabeled indications for selected NSAIDs. The maximum dose is 3.2 g/d.

Pharmacokinetics

Approximately 80% of ibuprofen is absorbed from the GI system after oral administration. Absorption is slower if the drug is taken with food; however, the extent of absorption is not affected. Peak serum concentrations occur in

TABLE 24.4 Indications for Nonsteroidal Anti-Inflammatory Drugs

	Rheumatoid Arthritis	Osteoarthritis	Juvenile RA	Ankylosing Spondylitis	Mild to Moderate Pain	Severe Pain	Migraine	Headaches	Dysmenorrhea	Acute Gout	Tendonitis	Bursitis	Fever	Premenstrual Syndrome	Polyhydramnios	Eye Inflammation	Dental Pain	GYN Postoperative Pain
celecoxib	A	A		A		A		U	A									
diclofenac potassium	A	A			A				A	A								A
diclofenac sodium	A	A		A	U			U	U	U			U				A	U
etodolac	A	A																
fenoprofen	A	A	U		A			U									A	A
flubiprofen	A	A		U				U	U							U	U	U
ibuprofen	A	A	A		A			A	A				A					
indomethacin	A	A	A	A		A	U		A	U	U				U			
ketoprofen	A	A			A				A									
ketorolac					A	A	U										A	
mefenamic acid					A				A					U	U			
meloxicam	A	A	A															
nabumetone	A	A																
naproxen	A	A	A	A				U	A	A	A	A	A	U				
oxaprozin	A	A	A											U				U
piroxicam	A	A					U	U		U							U	U
sulindac	A	A	U	A	A					A							U	
tolelmetin	A	A	A															

A, approved use; U, unlabeled use

Health care providers may prescribe any of these drugs for other conditions not represented.

1 to 2 hours. Analgesic and antipyretic effects occur in 2 to 4 hours, whereas a therapeutic inflammatory response takes a few days to 2 weeks. Ibuprofen is highly protein bound and is metabolized in the liver. Plasma half-life is 1.8 to 2 hours, with urinary excretion within 24 hours.

Pharmacodynamics

Ibuprofen's effects are believed to be secondary to inhibited synthesis or release of prostaglandins. Ibuprofen probably has a peripheral rather than a central action as an analgesic. Higher doses are required for an anti-inflammatory effect than for analgesia. Antipyretic activity may be the result of action on the hypothalamus, leading to increased peripheral blood flow, vasodilation, and subsequent heat dissipation.

Contraindications and Precautions

Because chronic use of ibuprofen can result in gastritis, ulceration with or without perforation, or GI bleeding, ibuprofen is contraindicated in patients with a history of or active GI disease, including peptic ulcer disease, ulcerative colitis, or GI bleeding. Other patients at high risk for GI adverse effects are those who routinely consume alcohol or smoke tobacco products because these behaviors are also conducive to ulcer development. Ibuprofen is contraindicated for use before or after a coronary artery bypass graft procedure. It is given with great caution to patients with pre-existing cardiovascular or cerebrovascular disorders because of the associated risk of induction of MI or stroke.

Ibuprofen should be used cautiously in patients with pre-existing hepatic, renal, or hemopoietic dysfunction and in patients older than 60 years. Liver dysfunction can occur during therapy with NSAIDs, resulting in jaundice and fatal hepatitis. Ibuprofen is metabolized in the liver, and accumulation can occur with liver dysfunction, increasing the risk of toxicity. Ibuprofen and its metabolites are excreted renally. Again, accumulation may occur in patients with renal impairment, increasing the risk of toxicity. Additionally, reduced renal blood flow caused by inhibition of prostaglandin synthesis can result in overt renal decompensation. Patients with the highest risk of renal decompensation are those with renal disease, hepatic disease, CHF, diabetes mellitus, SLE, edema, or extracellular volume depletion; those taking diuretics or nephrotoxic drugs; and elderly patients.

Ibuprofen should be used cautiously in patients with pre-existing coagulopathy or hemophilia, because of the effect of the drug on platelet function and vascular response to bleeding. Ibuprofen can prolong bleeding time. Anemia may be exacerbated with the use of ibuprofen.

Conditions associated with fluid retention, such as CHF, can be exacerbated with ibuprofen therapy. Hypertension may be exacerbated by ibuprofen-induced fluid retention.

Ibuprofen is classified as a pregnancy category B drug until the third trimester, when ibuprofen enters pregnancy category D because of the potential for NSAIDs to cause premature closure of the ductus arteriosus in utero.

Additionally, persistent pulmonary hypertension arising from ductus arteriosus constriction is a potential complication. NSAIDs also have the potential to prolong pregnancy and inhibit labor if taken during the third trimester.

Adverse Effects

Ibuprofen, like salicylates, inhibits COX-1 and COX-2, resulting in adverse effects. Ibuprofen and all other NSAIDS have a Black Box warning that they may increase the risk of serious and potentially fatal cardiovascular thrombotic events such as MI and stroke. This risk increases with duration of use.

Serious GI events are also listed as a Black Box warning. Nausea, vomiting, diarrhea, constipation, flatulence, and abdominal pain may be representative of minor adverse effects in some patients or serious GI toxicity in others. During long-term administration, the most serious effects are peptic ulcer disease or gastritis that leads to GI bleeding or even perforation. These events can occur at any time, with or without warning. Within the NSAID group, ibuprofen is rated as a low GI risk (Prescriber's Letter, 2010)

Ibuprofen also can induce blurred vision, decreased visual acuity, and corneal deposits. The mechanism for visual disturbances is unclear. Vision generally improves after the drug is discontinued. In addition, like aspirin, ibuprofen may induce tinnitus.

In the renal system, acute renal failure may occur in susceptible patients. Patients with conditions associated with diminished renal blood flow, such as CHF, cirrhosis, renal insufficiency, and advanced age, are at the highest risk. Vasodilatory renal prostaglandins and the potent vasoconstrictor angiotensin II work in concert to maintain renal blood flow. Inhibition of renal prostaglandins diminishes renal blood flow, leading to acute renal failure. Less common renal toxicities include interstitial nephritis and nephrotic syndrome. In addition to increased BUN and creatinine levels, proteinuria occurs. Another problem resulting from the inhibition of the renal prostaglandins is sodium and water retention. This effect is especially problematic for patients with conditions such as hypertension and CHF. Acute renal failure, water retention, interstitial nephritis, and nephrotic syndrome usually occur early in ibuprofen therapy and are reversible by stopping drug therapy.

Ibuprofen may cause excessive or abnormal bleeding, especially in patients with hemophilia, anemias, or severe liver disease. Ibuprofen diminishes platelet aggregation by inhibiting the prostaglandin thromboxane. This effect is transient and reversible. Other blood dyscrasias, such as agranulocytosis and aplastic anemia, have been infrequently reported.

Ibuprofen has been associated with hepatotoxicity, such as hepatitis or jaundice. Hepatotoxicity is uncommon, but patients should be monitored closely if on prolonged therapy.

Some patients taking ibuprofen may experience cross-sensitivity to aspirin or other NSAIDs, including those in a different chemical class. However, cross-sensitivities are not always complete, and patients may be able to take other NSAIDs, even those in the same chemical class.

TABLE 24.5	Agents That Interact with P Ibuprofen	
Interactants	**Effect and Significance**	**Nursing Management**
aminoglycoside antibiotics	Ibuprofen may cause an accumulation of aminoglycoside antibiotics by reducing the glomerular filtration rate.	Monitor BUN and creatinine. Monitor I and O. Monitor hearing. Monitor neurologic status.
Anticoagulants, oral	Ibuprofen inhibits platelet function and possibly produces gastric erosion. Anticoagulation effect is increased; hemorrhage may develop.	Avoid coadministering salicylates if possible. Monitor PT, PTT, and INR. Monitor for bruising or bleeding.
Aspirin/Salicylates	The pharmacologic effects of NSAIDS may be decreased. The cardioprotective effect of low-dose uncoated aspirin may be reduced. Both drugs are gastric irritants and may increase risk for GI distress.	Teach the patient to avoid taking these two drugs together. Monitor for cardiovascular adverse effects. Monitor for efficacy of NSAIDS Monitor for GI distress or bleeding.
Azole antifungal agents	Azole antifungal agents such as fluconazole and voriconazole inhibit NSAID metabolism. This increases NSAID plasma concentrations which increases the risk for pharmacologic and adverse effects.	Teach the patient to avoid this combination. Monitor for adverse effects and toxicity related to NSAIDS.
beta blockers	Ibuprofen inhibits renal prostaglandin synthesis, allowing unopposed pressor systems to produce hypertension. It also impairs antihypertensive effect of beta blockers.	Avoid coadministering if possible. Monitor blood pressure. Discuss alteration of beta blocker dose with health care provider.
Charcoal, activated	Charcoal inhibits the absorption of NSAIDS which decreases its systemic circulation.	Monitor for efficacy of NSAID therapy.
Heparin	Both heparin and NSAIDS inhibit the clotting cascade and platelet hemostasis. This increases the risk for hemorrhage or other adverse effects.	Monitor for signs of bleeding Monitor aPTT and bleeding time.
lithium	Ibuprofen is suspected to reduce renal elimination of lithium. Interaction may cause lithium toxicity.	Monitor lithium levels every 4–5 d until they stabilize after ibuprofen is added or withdrawn from treatment. Discuss lithium dose adjustment with the health care provider.
loop diuretics	Ibuprofen reduces natriuresis and antihypertensive response, resulting in decreased diuretic effect.	Discuss administration of a salicylate instead of ibuprofen with the health care provider.
methotrexate	Ibuprofen is suspected to reduce renal elimination of methotrexate and may cause methotrexate toxicity. Toxicity is less likely to occur with doses given for rheumatoid arthritis.	Monitor methotrexate levels. Monitor CBC, platelets. Anticipate longer leucovorin rescue therapy in patients receiving ibuprofen if leucovorin is administered at antineoplastic doses.
selective serotonin reuptake inhibitors	Coadministration increases the risk for upper GI bleeding.	Monitor for nausea or vomiting. Monitor for abdominal pain. Monitor for hematemesis or melena.

Drug Interactions

Ibuprofen is highly protein bound and has many interactions similar to those produced by salicylates. Table 24.5 lists drug interactions with ibuprofen. In addition to the drugs listed in the table, ibuprofen should not be given along with salicylates. Giving these drugs together does not increase efficacy but does increase the risk of adverse effects. Ibuprofen should be discontinued 72 hours before

adrenal function tests are performed. Ibuprofen also may elevate sodium and chloride levels.

Assessment of Relevant Core Patient Variables

Health Status

Assess the patient for potential contraindications to ibuprofen therapy. It is important to obtain a drug history to identify potential drug–drug interactions and to assess for potential hypersensitivities to salicylates or other NSAIDs. Assess for a history of MI or stroke, because patients who take ibuprofen have an increased risk of cardiovascular or cerebrovascular events. Assess for a history of gastric ulcers or GI bleeding. Assess for a history of asthma or nasal polyps, because patients with these conditions are prone to bronchospasm.

In addition, it is important to assess a patient's baseline gross hearing because of the potential for ototoxicity from ibuprofen use. For patients on long-term therapy, obtain a baseline CBC, platelet count, and test results of renal and hepatic function. Assess the patient for efficacy of ibuprofen therapy; severe or visceral pain may not be affected by ibuprofen.

Life Span and Gender

Determine whether female patients are pregnant. Ibuprofen should not be given to women in the last trimester of pregnancy because it may cause premature closure of the ductus arteriosus. Determine the patient's age before administering ibuprofen. Although ibuprofen is considered safe for children, some of the other NSAIDs are contraindicated. Ibuprofen should be given with caution to patients older than 60 years because these patients have an increased risk of adverse effects, especially GI bleeding. Ibuprofen, like aspirin, is thought to be metabolized faster in men, which may result in a shorter duration of action than in women.

Lifestyle, Diet, and Habits

As with aspirin, it is important to inquire about the patient's use of OTC drugs because many OTCs contain ibuprofen or aspirin. Concomitant use of either or both increases the risk of hepatic and renal toxicity.

Assess for alcohol or drug abuse because the patient may have undiagnosed pre-existing hepatic dysfunction. In addition, assess the patient for a history of cigarette smoking because ibuprofen, like aspirin, decreases the cytoprotective mechanisms of the stomach.

Environment

Ascertain the setting in which ibuprofen will be administered. Ibuprofen may be self-administered at home or given in any health care setting. Because this drug first appeared on the market as a prescription drug, the lay public often believes that it is more effective than aspirin or acetaminophen. Because of ibuprofen's reasonable cost and high efficacy, some patients may take the drug at a higher dose than the labeling suggests or for a much longer duration without seeing a medical provider. This practice places patients at a higher risk for adverse effects, or other problems, if the etiology of their symptoms is not addressed.

Nursing Diagnoses and Outcomes

- Acute or Chronic Pain related to ineffectiveness of ibuprofen
  Desired outcome: The patient will contact the prescriber if pain persists.

- Increased Risk for Injury related to incorrect self-administration or to drug-induced GI bleeding or hepatic and renal toxicity
  Desired outcome: The patient will remain free of injury by taking the drug only as directed. In addition, the patient will be able to explain the importance of contacting the health care provider immediately if any adverse effects occur.
- Increased Risk for Deficient Fluid Volume related to nausea and vomiting
  Desired outcome: The patient will contact the prescriber immediately if intractable nausea or vomiting occurs.
- Ineffective Protection related to blood dyscrasias
  Desired outcome: The patient will contact the prescriber immediately if any signs and symptoms of blood dyscrasias occur.
- Disturbed Sensory Perception (visual) related to blurred vision
  Desired outcome: The patient will discontinue ibuprofen immediately and contact the health care provider if vision is affected.

Planning and Intervention
Maximizing Therapeutic Effects
Give ibuprofen with milk or food to decrease gastric distress, if needed.

Minimizing Adverse Effects
Closely monitor patients with pre-existing medical conditions or drug therapy that may interact with ibuprofen. It is important to administer misoprostol to patients at high risk for developing gastropathies with ibuprofen (Box 24.4). Periodic CBC, platelet count, and liver and renal function tests should be obtained for patients on long-term ibuprofen therapy. Limit 24 hours intake to 3.2 grams.

Providing Patient and Family Education
- Instruct patients to take the drug exactly as directed by the prescriber to avoid adverse effects or overdose with ibuprofen. Daily intake should not exceed 3.2 grams.
- Tell patients not to take ibuprofen if they have problems with their kidneys or liver, to use ibuprofen cautiously

 Box 24.4 USING MISOPROSTOL TO REDUCE NSAID ADVERSE EFFECTS

Misoprostol (Cytotec) increases bicarbonate and mucous production in the gastrointestinal tract. It may also inhibit gastric acid secretion. To minimize possible gastropathies in patients on long-term nonsteroidal anti-inflammatory drug (NSAID) therapy, consider prophylactic therapy with misoprostol for patients with any of the following characteristics:

- Age >60 years
- History of peptic ulcer disease
- Cigarette smoker
- Concomitant use of alcohol
- Concomitant use of corticosteroids
- Dyspepsia during salicylate or NSAID use
- Poor surgical risk if ulcer complications occur

during the first two trimesters of pregnancy, and not to take it at all during the third trimester of pregnancy. In addition, patients should not take ibuprofen if they are asthmatic and have nasal polyps, because ibuprofen could cause an asthma attack.

- Advise patients that ibuprofen increases the risk of cardiovascular and cerebrovascular events, especially when taken for a long duration or in patients with a previous history of cardiovascular or cerebrovascular disorders.
- Advise patients to take ibuprofen with food, milk, or possibly an antacid to prevent GI upset.
- Instruct patients that if a dose is missed, it should be taken as soon as possible. If it is almost time for the next dose, only that dose should be taken; double or extra doses should never be taken.
- Caution patients that drinking alcohol and smoking while taking ibuprofen can increase the risk for GI irritation and bleeding.
- Advise patients to contact their health care provider if minor adverse effects such as diarrhea, dizziness, drowsiness, heartburn, nausea, and vomiting do not subside or if they are bothersome.
- Warn patients about serious adverse effects of ibuprofen and to advise them to seek medical attention immediately if they occur. Adverse effects include the following:
  - Black, tarry stools; blood in urine; dark yellow or brown urine
  - Difficulty breathing, wheezing; skin rash, redness, blistering, peeling, or itching; swelling of eyelids, throat, lips, or feet
  - Rapid heartbeat
  - Blurred vision
  - Muscle aches and pains, fever, chills
  - Weight change
  - Unusual bleeding or bruising, unusual tiredness or weakness, prolonged bleeding from a cut, vomiting blood or what looks like coffee grounds
- Instruct patients to change position slowly to avoid dizziness. If dizziness occurs, the patient should refrain from driving a car or operating machinery.
- Tell patients to read the labels of all OTC drugs and to avoid any with aspirin or other NSAIDs as an ingredient.
- Warn patients to seek immediate medical assistance if they accidentally take too many tablets.
- Advise patients with diabetes to monitor their blood glucose levels rather than testing their urine.
- Instruct patients to keep ibuprofen in a cool, dry place to preserve its potency.
- Tell patients to see their health care provider if their fever does not resolve in 3 days or their pain does not go away in 10 days.
- Advise patients on long-term ibuprofen therapy to see their health care provider every 6 months for blood testing to make sure they are not having adverse effects from the drug.

MEMORY CHIP

P Ibuprofen

- Used for its antiinflammatory, analgesic, and antipyretic effects; reversibly inhibits cyclooxygenase (COX)
- Major contraindications: active GI diseases; used with caution in patients with renal or hepatic impairment, hemopoietic dysfunction, pre-existing coagulopathy, cardiac impairment, and age greater than 60 years
- Most common adverse effects: GI related
- Most serious adverse effects: hepatic and renal toxicity
- **Life span alert: Ibuprofen is in pregnancy category D in the third trimester; monitor patients over the age of 60 years carefully.**
- **Black box warning: All NSAIDs, including ibuprofen, have an increased risk of inducing MI or stroke. The risk escalates the longer the duration of therapy. Monitor patients for signs of MI and stroke.**

Ongoing Assessment and Evaluation

The patient who is taking ibuprofen requires monitoring for signs and symptoms of cardiovascular or cerebrovascular symptoms, GI distress or bleeding, anemia, tinnitus, hepatotoxicity, and renal failure. Monitor patients older than 60 years closely for these adverse effects. Arrange periodic laboratory tests for patients on long-term therapy or those at high risk for adverse effects. Monitor the patient for relief of pain and inflammation.

Therapy is considered effective if the patient is free of fever, pain, or inflammation and is free from adverse effects.

Drugs Closely Related to P Ibuprofen
Propionic Acids

In addition to ibuprofen, the following drugs are in the propionic class of NSAIDs: fenoprofen (Nalfon), flurbiprofen (Ansaid), ketoprofen (Orudis), naproxen (Naprosyn, Anaprox), and oxaprozin (Daypro). These drugs are similar to ibuprofen in action, indications, nursing management, and patient education. They differ in their onset, peak, and duration of action. Although these drugs are chemically similar, patients may have relief of symptoms from one drug in this group but not another. Naproxen is also available in a combination formulation with lansoprazole (a proton pump inhibitor) by the trade name Prevacid NapraPAC. Naproxen and ketoprofen, like ibuprofen, may be purchased OTC. Adverse effects are most frequently GI in nature, and flurbiprofen causes GI symptoms more frequently than ibuprofen. Naproxen is better tolerated than other NSAIDs and has the lowest cardiovascular risk (Prescriber's Letter, 2010).

Acetic Acids

The acetic acids include diclofenac (Voltaren), etodolac (Lodine), indomethacin (Indocin), ketorolac (Toradol), nabumetone (Relafen) sulindac (Clinoril), and tolmetin (Tolectin). These agents are potent NSAIDs, highly protein bound, and may displace other protein-bound drugs, which may cause toxicities. They are associated with a high incidence of GI distress and should be given with meals or milk. They also may increase blood pressure or cause sodium and water retention. This group of NSAIDs also has an increased risk for causing liver dysfunction. Patients should have periodic liver function tests evaluated.

Diclofenac is available as a transdermal patch (Flector), an oral solution (Cambia), and a topical formulation (Pennsaid, VoltarenGel). It is approved for acute pain due to migraine headache, strains, sprains, and contusions. The patch or topical formulation should be placed on the most painful area two to four times a day. Diclofenac has the highest cardiovascular risk (Prescriber's Letter, 2010).

Patients taking indomethacin have an increased risk of additional adverse effects. It may aggravate depression, other psychiatric disturbances, epilepsy, and parkinsonism. Indomethacin is also associated with a high incidence of severe frontal headaches. Indomethacin is available in both oral and IV forms, and the other acetic acids are all oral drugs.

Nabumetone (Relafen) is a new type of NSAID indicated for osteoarthritis and rheumatoid arthritis. Despite its high efficacy, it has a relatively low incidence of side effects. It appears to cause less gastric damage than other NSAIDs. It is assumed that its decreased GI effects are related to its partial selectivity to COX-2. Because nabumetone has a long half-life, it can be administered once a day. Again, the disadvantage of this drug is its high cost. Ketorolac (Toradol) is only NSAID that is administered by the intramuscular (IM) or intravenous (IV). It is also available orally. IM, and IV ketorolac is used only for the management of severe pain, most frequently postsurgical pain. The efficacy of its IM and IV administration is similar to that of morphine and opioid analgesics. Despite its parenteral administration, ketorolac may induce the same severe adverse effects, especially GI events, as the other oral NSAIDs and carries the same Black Box warnings. Topical ketorolac (Acular) is an ophthalmic drug used for allergic conjunctivitis and postcataract extraction or laser procedures. Because of its limited systemic absorption, topical ketorolac does not carry the Black Box warnings.

An advantage of acetic acids is their long-half life, with resultant once-daily or twice-daily dosing. A major disadvantage is their high cost.

Fenamates

Mefenamic acid (Ponstel) and meclofenamate (generic) are the only fenamate drugs used in the United States. Both are approved to treat mild to moderate pain and dysmenorrhea. Meclofenamate is also used in the management of osteoarthritis and rheumatoid arthritis. They have no clear advantage over other NSAIDs and have an increased risk of adverse effects, especially diarrhea.

Oxicams

Meloxicam (Mobic) and piroxicam (Feldene) are the only oxicams currently available in the United States. They are equivalent to aspirin, indomethacin, and naproxen in treating osteoarthritis and rheumatoid arthritis. Generally, they are better tolerated because they have some COX-2 selectivity; however, severe adverse effects may still occur. Piroxicam has one of the highest GI risks. The advantage of oxicams is their once-daily dosing. The high cost is a disadvantage.

Ophthalmic NSAIDs

Nepafenac (Nevanac) and bromfenac (Xibrom), which are available only as ophthalmic solutions, are used specifically for pain and inflammation from cataract surgery. Ophthalmic NSAIDs can cause corneal ulceration if administered too long. Ophthalmic NSAIDs may delay healing, so they should not be used concurrently with topical steroids. Bromfenac is contraindicated for patients with sulfite hypersensitivity because the solution contains sodium sulfite. Adverse effects associated with bromfenac include headache, a burning sensation in the eye, conjunctival hyperemia, eye irritation, iritis, and rarely, corneal ulceration. Adverse effects associated with nepafenac include conjunctival edema, dry eyes, a foreign body sensation, light intolerance, reduced visual acuity, and an itching sensation is the eye. A serious, but rare, complication is vitreous detachment.

Emphasize to patients that they should begin therapy 24 hours after surgery and take the drug for only 14 days. Ophthalmic NSAIDs may induce bleeding in the eye tissues; tell patients to contact their health care provider if bleeding occurs. In addition, instruct patients in the correct administration of eye drops, focusing on aseptic technique, and inform them to shake the bottle before use and remove contacts prior to administration.

COX-2 Inhibitors

The discovery of COX-2 has made possible the design of drugs that reduce inflammation without removing the protective prostaglandins in the stomach and kidney made by COX-1. Currently, only the COX-2 inhibitor celecoxib is available in the United States. This drug exhibits anti-inflammatory and analgesic activities by selectively inhibiting COX-2 prostaglandin synthesis but not platelet aggregation. This highly selective drug may be useful not only in conditions such as rheumatic and osteoarthritis but also in colon cancer, Alzheimer disease, and kidney disease.

Rofecoxib (Vioxx) and valdecoxib (Bextra), other COX-2 inhibitors, have been taken off the market in the United States because of an unreasonable risk of cardiovascular and cerebral events. They may be available in other countries and through Internet pharmacies based in those countries.

Celecoxib

Celecoxib (Celebrex), the first COX-2 inhibitor on the market, has pharmacotherapeutics that are similar to those of other NSAIDs. In addition, celecoxib also is approved to reduce the number of adenomatous colorectal polyps in patients with the rare genetic disease called Familial Multiple Polyposis Syndrome. It is given orally.

Celecoxib should not be given to patients who have had salicylate hypersensitivity evidenced by asthma, urticaria, or allergic-type reactions after taking aspirin or other NSAIDs. It is also contraindicated in patients with known sulfonamide hypersensitivity because it is structurally related to sulfonamides. Precautions are similar to those of ibuprofen, with the exception of hemophilia, because celecoxib does not inhibit platelet aggregation. Celecoxib is not approved for use in adolescents or children.

Potential adverse effects of celecoxib also are similar to ibuprofen. Like other NSAIDs, it carries the same Black Box warning. Theoretically, because of the specificity of celecoxib for the COX-2 pathway, it has the potential to cause less gastropathy and risk for GI bleeding. However, despite its cytoprotective properties, serious GI bleeding or obstruction has been reported.

Celecoxib may interact with multiple drugs. It can decrease the effectiveness of loop or thiazide diuretics and angiotensin-converting enzyme inhibitors. Celecoxib decreases the excretion of methotrexate, vancomycin, and aminoglycosides, resulting in an increased risk of toxicity or adverse effects from these drugs. Celecoxib may increase the serum drug levels of warfarin and lithium, again placing the patient at risk for toxicity or adverse effects. When given with fluconazole, the serum concentration of celecoxib is increased. Celecoxib is in pregnancy category C drug. Like other NSAIDs, it should not be given during the last trimester of pregnancy because it may cause premature closure of the ductus arteriosus.

● Ⓒ PARA-AMINOPHENOL DERIVATIVES

Acetaminophen (Tylenol), a widely used analgesic and antipyretic, is the only **para-aminophenol derivative** available in the United States. It was first used in clinical medicine in 1893, but widespread use began after it received FDA approval in 1950. It is available without a prescription as an individual agent and in combination with a variety of other drugs. Table 24.6 presents a summary of acetaminophen's pharmacokinetics.

Nursing Management of the Patient Receiving Ⓟ Acetaminophen

Core Drug Knowledge

Pharmacotherapeutics

Oral acetaminophen is indicated for treating fever or mild pain. It is used for patients with a hypersensitivity to aspirin or NSAIDs or intolerance to their GI effects and for patients who are receiving anticoagulant therapy. The maximum recommended dose in 24 hours is 4 gram in adults and 200 mg/kg or 10 g/d whichever is less in children. In addition to fever or mild pain in patients who cannot tolerate oral or rectal medications, intravenous acetaminophen (Ofirmev) is indicated for the management of moderate to severe pain with adjunctive opioid analgesics.

Pharmacokinetics

Acetaminophen is administered by oral, rectal, and intravenous routes. When administered enterally, it is absorbed rapidly and completely from the GI tract or rectal mucosa. The drug is predominately metabolized in the liver into nontoxic substances and eliminated by the kidneys. A small amount is metabolized in a different pathway, resulting in a toxic metabolite that is converted by glutathione into a nontoxic form. Acetaminophen crosses the placenta and is secreted in breast milk. Children metabolize less of the drug via the pathway that produces the metabolite than adults. this is why the dose that produces toxicity is higher in children than adults.

Pharmacodynamics

Acetaminophen is primarily centrally acting, has no effects on platelet aggregation, and is a reversible weak inhibitor of COX in the periphery. Its analgesic effect is believed to result from inhibiting prostaglandin synthesis in the CNS and possibly from blocking the generation of pain impulses in the periphery. Its antipyretic activity results from inhibiting prostaglandin synthesis in the CNS. Blocking prostaglandin synthesis in the CNS allows the hypothalamic heat-regulating center to produce peripheral vasodilation, causing increased blood flow through the skin, sweating, and heat loss.

Contraindications and Precautions

Acetaminophen is contraindicated in patients with active hepatic disease, viral hepatitis, chronic malnutrition, severe hypovolemia, or alcoholism. In these diseases, metabolism of the drug may be decreased, resulting in a risk of hepatotoxicity. Because acetaminophen is excreted primarily by the kidneys, serum concentrations may increase in patients with renal impairment, again resulting in an increased risk of toxicity.

TABLE 24.6	Summary of Selected Ⓒ Para-Aminophenol Derivatives		
Drug (Trade) Name	**Selected Indications**	**Route and Dosage Range**	**Pharmacokinetics**
Ⓒ Para-Aminophenol Derivatives			
Ⓟ acetaminophen (Tylenol)	Fever, analgesia	*Adult:* PO, 325–1000 mg q4–6 h, not to exceed 4 g/d IV <50 kg: 15 mg/kg every 6 h IV >50 kg: 1 g every 6 h *Child:* PO, 10 mg/kg q4–6 h IV 2–12 y: 15 mg/kg every 6 h IV >13 y <50 kg: 15 mg/kg every 6 h IV >13 >50 kg: 1 gram every 6 h	*Onset:* 10–30 min orally; 15 min IV *Duration:* 3–5 h $t_{1/2}$: 2–4 h

Acetaminophen is also used with caution in patients with pre-existing anemia because acetaminophen may exacerbate anemias. It is also used carefully in patients who take warfarin. Patients who have phenylketonuria or who must restrict intake of phenylalanine should avoid acetaminophen products containing aspartame (NutraSweet), such as Tempra chewable tablets, Alka-Seltzer Advanced Formula, Children's Anacin-3, Junior Strength Tylenol, Children's Tylenol, and Double-Strength Tempra.

Acetaminophen is assigned to pregnancy category B and therefore should be used cautiously in patients who are pregnant or lactating. However, it is the safest antipyretic or analgesic drug to use, if necessary, during pregnancy or lactation.

Adverse Effects

Acetaminophen is generally well tolerated. Most adverse effects occur when the drug is taken in high doses or for prolonged periods. However, acetaminophen overdose is potentially fatal. As previously mentioned, acetaminophen is partially metabolized into a toxic metabolite that glutathione normally converts to a nontoxic form. In an overdose, glutathione stores are quickly depleted in an attempt to convert the toxic metabolite. Because the glutathione supply is depleted, accumulation of the toxic metabolite occurs, resulting in liver damage.

Symptoms of acute toxicity reflect liver damage and include anorexia, nausea, vomiting, pallor, and abdominal discomfort. During the intermediate stage (days 1 to 3), the patient may complain of right-upper-quadrant pain and experience decreased urine output. The late stage (days 3–5) is characterized by jaundice, elevated aspartate transaminase and alanine transaminase levels, and a dramatic rise in prothrombin time, indicating hepatic necrosis. During this stage, the patient also may experience CNS stimulation followed by CNS depression. Early administration of acetylcysteine, which replaces glutathione reserves, is the antidote for overdose. Acetaminophen overdose is an emergency that must be treated in the hospital as it is the leading cause of acute liver disease in the United States. Liver failure may result.

Acetaminophen may cause adverse effects in the hepatic, renal, hematologic, and GI systems. Hepatotoxicity and hepatic necrosis may occur in patients who are on overdose or high-dose or long-term therapy. Other potential adverse effects in patients with high-dose or long-term therapy are acute renal failure, renal papillary necrosis, or renal tubular necrosis. In the hematologic system, acetaminophen may cause anemia, leukopenia, thrombocytopenia, or pancytopenia. In the GI system, acetaminophen may cause GI bleeding. Bleeding occurs secondarily to low prothrombin levels.

Drug Interactions

Acetaminophen may interact with activated charcoal, antacids, ethanol, hydantoins, warfarin, and sulfinpyrazone. In rats, S-adenosyl-L-methionine (SAMe), an herbal product, decreases acetaminophen binding to hepatic microsomal proteins and has been shown to improve survival after acetaminophen overdose. The utility of these findings in preventing acetaminophen hepatotoxicity is uncertain; more studies to evaluate the role of SAMe in human acetaminophen toxicity are necessary. Table 24.7 presents additional information about drug interactions with acetaminophen.

TABLE 24.7	Agents That Interact with P Acetaminophen	
Interactants	Effect and Significance	Nursing Management
charcoal, activated	Charcoal reduces gastrointestinal (GI) absorption of ingested drugs and adsorbs enterohepatically circulated drugs. Charcoal may actually remove drugs from the systemic circulation. Depending on the clinical situation, this will reduce the effectiveness or toxicity of a given agent.	Administer activated charcoal as soon as possible in a situation involving toxicity of acetaminophen. Do not administer activated charcoal within 2–3 h of acetaminophen administration if acetaminophen is being used therapeutically.
ethanol (alcohol)	Induction of hepatic microsomal enzymes by chronic ethanol consumption may be associated with acetaminophen-induced hepatotoxicity. Chronic consumption of ethanol may increase the risk of acetaminophen-induced liver damage.	Caution patient who consumes ethanol chronically and in excess about the potential interaction. Advise patients to avoid ethanol ingestion while taking acetaminophen. Monitor suspected ethanol abusers closely for hepatotoxicity.
Hydantoins, sulfinpyrazone	Hydantoins and sulfinpyrazone may induce hepatic microsomal enzymes, which accelerate the metabolism of acetaminophen. An unusually high rate of acetaminophen metabolism could lead to abnormally high levels of hepatotoxic metabolites. The potential hepatotoxicity of acetaminophen may be increased and the therapeutic effects of acetaminophen may be decreased when administered with chronic doses of hydantoins or sulfinpyrazone.	At usual therapeutic doses of acetaminophen and hydantoins or sulfinpyrazone, no special dosage adjustment is required. Risk is greatest when acetaminophen overdose accompanies chronic use of hydantoins or sulfinpyrazone. Monitor for hepatoxicity.
warfarin	Acetaminophen inhibits the metabolism of warfarin, resulting in an elevated serum warfarin concentration, and possibly antagonizes the production of vitamin K.	Monitor PT and INR. Monitor for bruising or bleeding.

Assessment of Relevant Core Patient Variables

Health Status

Assess the patient's pain level. Acetaminophen is effective for mild to moderate pain. Assess for pre-existing medical conditions or drug therapy that contraindicates using acetaminophen or necessitates close monitoring of the patient. For patients expected to be on long-term therapy, obtain and document baseline CBC, platelet count, and renal and hepatic function values.

Life Span and Gender

Acetaminophen is an excellent drug for treating children's fever and pain. Unlike aspirin, it is not associated with Reye syndrome. Elderly patients are more likely to develop hepatic and renal toxicity because of age-related decreases in hepatic and renal function. Acetaminophen is the drug of choice for pregnant women because it does not have any antiplatelet activity.

Lifestyle, Diet, and Habits

Inquire about the patient's use of OTC drugs because many of these products contain acetaminophen as an ingredient. Concomitant use increases the risk of hepatotoxicity. Assess for alcohol or drug abuse because the patient may have undiagnosed pre-existing hepatic dysfunction.

Environment

Determine the patient's understanding of acetaminophen therapy. Acetaminophen is self-administered easily at home without medical supervision. Because of its low cost and availability, many people do not understand acetaminophen's potentially life-threatening adverse effects. Patient education is important to avoid unintentional overdose or long-term complications.

Nursing Diagnoses and Outcomes

- Acute or Chronic Pain related to ineffectiveness of acetaminophen
  Desired outcome: The patient will contact the health care provider if pain persists.
- Risk for Injury related to drug-induced hepatic and renal toxicity or to improper self-medication
  Desired outcome: The patient will take drug as directed and contact the health care provider if any signs of toxicity occur.
- Ineffective Protection related to potential blood dyscrasias
  Desired outcome: The patient will contact the health care provider if any signs of blood dyscrasias occur.

Planning and Intervention

Maximizing Therapeutic Effects

Acetaminophen can be administered without regard to meals. Monitor the patient for therapeutic effect of acetaminophen and relief of symptoms.

Minimizing Adverse Effects

Assess patients for medical conditions that contradict the use of acetaminophen. Carefully monitor patients with pre-existing medical conditions or drug therapy that may interact with acetaminophen. Coordinate periodic CBC, platelet count, and liver and renal function tests for patients on long-term therapy. Overdosage is treated with the antidote, acetylcysteine orally or IV. Administer intravenous acetaminophen as a 15 minute infusion.

Providing Patient and Family Education

- Tell patients to take the drug exactly as prescribed by the health care provider to avoid adverse effects or overdose.
- Remind patients that the maximum adult dose is 4 g/d and that exceeding this dose may cause acute liver disease or kidney disease.
- Warn patients not to take this drug if they have kidney or liver dysfunction, or consume more than 3 alcoholic beverages per day.
- Teach patients exact directions for correct administration, because acetaminophen is manufactured in a variety of formulations.
- Teach patients with diabetes to monitor their blood glucose level for signs of hypoglycemia.
- Teach patients who take warfarin to refrain from consistent use of acetaminophen. An occasional dose is acceptable.
- Instruct patients to read all OTC drug labels and to avoid any with acetaminophen as an ingredient.
- Stress the potential for acetaminophen overdose and the importance of seeking medical attention should the patient accidentally take too many tablets.
- Advise patients to keep acetaminophen in a light-resistant container out of the reach of children.
- Encourage patients to contact the health care provider immediately if they have any adverse effects (e.g., signs of blood dyscrasias and signs of hepatic or renal toxicity), if fever does not subside within 3 days, or if pain is not relieved within 10 days.

Ongoing Assessment and Evaluation

Monitor the patient who is taking acetaminophen for sore throat, chills, easy bruising, and unusual bleeding because

MEMORY CHIP

P Acetaminophen

- Used for mild to moderate pain and fever; usually well tolerated; has no anti-inflammatory effect
- Major contraindications: hepatic disease, viral hepatitis, and alcoholism
- Most common adverse effects: rash, urticaria, and nausea
- Most serious adverse effects: Acetaminophen may cause hepatic or renal toxicity in susceptible patients.
- **Life span alert: Acetaminophen is the drug of choice for infants and children with flu or flu-like symptoms; analgesic of choice during pregnancy or lactation.**
- **Patient safety alert: Acetaminophen overdose is potentially fatal. The patient must receive treatment in an acute care facility. Anticipate the use of acetylcysteine as an antidote.**

these signs may indicate blood dyscrasias. It also is important to monitor the patient for any signs and symptoms of hepatotoxicity and renal failure. Do not give acetaminophen if the patient develops a rash, unexplained fever, or angioedema. The patient needs to contact the health care provider immediately if any of these symptoms occur.

Therapy is considered effective if the patient is free of fever and pain. In addition, the patient should remain free of adverse effects and should be able to explain the importance of contacting the health care provider immediately if any adverse effects occur.

• Ⓒ Serotonin-Selective Drugs

Serotonin-selective drugs are used to relieve pain and inflammation related to migraine headache. These drugs are also known as "triptans" because the generic name of these drugs ends as such. At the moment, triptans are considered first-line drugs for the treatment of acute migraine headache. Sumatriptan (Imitrex), the first 5-HT$_{1B/1D}$ agonist approved for use in the United States, is the prototype for this class of drugs. While sumatriptan and the other triptans are excellent drugs, many patients with migraine cannot take them because of their vasoconstrictive effects that might exacerbate cardio or cerebral pathologies. Another promising class of drugs migraine is the neuropeptide calcitonin gene-related peptide antagonist (Box 24.5). Table 24.8 presents a summary of selected serotonin receptor agonists.

Nursing Management of the Patient Receiving Ⓟ Sumatriptan
Core Drug Knowledge
Pharmacotherapeutics
Sumatriptan is used to treat acute migraine headache with or without aura and to manage cluster headache. Because of its serotonin agonist properties, it is currently being studied for the treatment of irritable bowel syndrome when constipation is the primary symptom.

Pharmacokinetics
Sumatriptan may be administered orally, intranasally, or subcutaneously. It's newest formulation is a needleless injection (Sumavel DosePro). It is also available as an oral combination with Naprosyn (Treximet). When administered orally, pain relief begins within 1 hour and complete pain relief occurs within 4 hours in 50% to 60% of patients. When administered intranasally, absorption is rapid; the onset of action is 15 minutes. The most effective route of administration is subcutaneous. When administered subcutaneously, onset of pain relief occurs within 10 minutes, and approximately 75% of patients have complete pain relief within 2 hours. The bioavailability of subcutaneous sumatriptan is 97%, that of the oral drug is approximately 15%, and that of the intranasal drug is approximately 17%. Sumatriptan is metabolized in the liver and excreted by the kidneys.

Pharmacodynamics
Sumatriptan is selective for 5-HT$_{1B/1D}$ receptors located on cranial blood vessels and sensory nerves of the trigeminovascular system. Stimulation of these receptors results in vasoconstriction and inhibition of the release of proinflammatory neuropeptides such as CGRP. The end result is a decrease in the vasodilation-caused throbbing sensation in the head and a decrease in vascular inflammation.

Contraindications and Precautions
Sumatriptan is contraindicated in patients with coronary artery disease (CAD), arteriosclerosis, and ischemic cardiac diseases such as uncontrolled hypertension, angina pectoris—especially vasospastic angina—and acute MI or

BOX 24.5 FOCUS ON RESEARCH

TELCAGEPANT FOR THE ACUTE TREATMENT OF MIGRAINE

Connor K.M., Shapiro, R.E., Diener, H.C., Lucas, S., Kos,t J., Fan, X., Fei, K., Assaid, C., Lines, C., Ho, T.W., (2009), Randomized, controlled trial of telcagepant for the acute treatment of migraine, Neurology, Sep 22;73(12):970–7.

The Study
Researchers are evaluating other classes of drugs that will be as efficacious as the triptans without causing vasoconstriction. Neuropeptide calcitonin gene-related peptide (CGRP) plays a key role in migraine pathophysiology, thus blocking this action should be helpful in the management of migraine. The study researchers wanted to confirm the efficacy of telcagepant, the first orally bioavailable CGRP receptor antagonist. Adults with moderate or severe migraine with or without aura were treated with oral telcagepant 50 mg (n = 177), 150 mg (n = 381), 300 mg (n = 371), or placebo (n = 365) in a randomized, double-blind trial. The goal endpoints were pain freedom, pain relief, and absence of photophobia, absence of phonophobia, and absence of nausea, all at 2 hours postdose. The key secondary endpoint was 2 to 24 hour sustained pain freedom. Telcagepant 300 mg was more effective than placebo on all primary endpoints and the key secondary endpoint, as was telcagepant 150 mg. Telcagepant 300 mg showed a slight numeric advantage over telcagepant 150 mg on most measures. Telcagepant 50 mg values were numerically intermediate between placebo and telcagepant 150 mg and 300 mg. This study confirmed previous findings that telcagepant 300 mg was effective at relieving pain and other migraine symptoms at 2 hours and providing sustained pain freedom up to 24 hours.

Nursing Implications
Acute migraine headache is a debilitating event. It is estimated that more than 3 million people will experience a migraine headache within their lifetime. While the triptans are the number 1 class of drugs for migraine, many patients cannot take these drugs because of comorbid disorders that would be exacerbated by the vasoconstrictive effects of these drugs. The nurse must keep abreast of new drugs for old disorders. Telcagepant is a promising new drug, although not yet FDA approved in the U.S. It offers hope to many migraineurs.

TABLE 24.8	Summary of ⊖ Serotonin Receptor Agonists		
Drug (Trade) Name	**Selected Indications**	**Route and Dosage Range**	**Pharmacokinetics**
P sumatriptan (Imitrex)	Migraine and cluster headache	*Adult:* PO, 25–100 mg; may repeat once after 2 h *Adult:* nasal spray, 5–20 mg; may repeat once after 2 h *Adult:* SC, 4 or 6 mg; may repeat after 1 h *Adult:* PO (85mg sumatriptan and 500 mg naproxen) 1 tablet; may repeat after 2 h	*Onset:* PO, 30–60 min INH, 15–20 min SC, 10–15 min *Duration:* Short $t_{1/2}$: PO, 2.5 h INH, 2 h SC, 115 min
almotriptan (Axert)	Migraine and cluster headache	*Adult:* PO, 6.25–12.5 mg	*Onset:* 30 min–2 h *Duration:* Short $t_{1/2}$: 3.1 h
eletriptan (Relpax)	Migraine and cluster headache	*Adult:* PO, 20–40 mg	*Onset:* 1 h *Duration:* Long $t_{1/2}$: 4 h
frovatriptan (Frova)	Migraine and cluster headache	*Adult:* PO, 2.5 mg; may repeat in 2 h	*Onset:* 2–3 h *Duration:* Long $t_{1/2}$: 26 h
naratriptan (Amerge)	Migraine and cluster headache	*Adult:* PO, 2.5 mg; may repeat once in >4 h	*Onset:* 1–3 h *Duration:* Long $t_{1/2}$: 6 h
rizatriptan (Maxalt, Maxalt MLT)	Migraine and cluster headache	*Adult:* PO, 5 or 10 mg; may repeat in 2 h	*Onset:* 30 min–2 h *Duration:* Short $t_{1/2}$: 2–3 h
zolmitriptan (Zomig, Zomig ZMT)	Migraine and cluster headache	*Adult:* PO, 2.5 mg; may repeat in >2 h *Adult:* nasal spray, 5 mg; may repeat in 2 h	*Onset:* 15 min *Duration:* Short $t_{1/2}$: 3 h

a history of MI. In addition, it is contraindicated in patients with cerebrovascular diseases, such as stroke, intracranial bleeding, and TIAs, and in peripheral vascular diseases, such as Raynaud disease. It is strongly recommended that sumatriptan not be given to patients with chronic diseases that increase the risk of CAD until those patients have had a cardiac workup. Those diseases include diabetes mellitus, hypertension, hypercholesterolemia, and obesity. Patients with a family history of CAD, those who smoke tobacco, postmenopausal women, and men older than 40 years of age should also have a cardiovascular workup before using sumatriptan.

Because sumatriptan is metabolized by the liver and excreted by the kidneys, it should be used cautiously in patients with hepatic or renal impairment, or in those patients at risk for hepatic or renal dysfunction, such as the elderly. Sumatriptan should also be used with care in patients with a history of seizures because it may induce them.

Studies have shown that sumatriptan is embryolethal in rabbits at dosages that are similar to the maximum recommended dose for humans. No studies indicate that sumatriptan is a human teratogen; however, it should be used during pregnancy only if the benefits outweigh the risk to the fetus.

Adverse Effects
Adverse reactions are less likely to occur when sumatriptan is administered orally or intranasally. The most serious adverse effects of sumatriptan are cardiac events; however, they rarely occur. These events include coronary artery vasospasm, cardiac dysrhythmias such as ventricular tachycardia, or ventricular fibrillation, angina, myocardial ischemia (including MI), and cardiac arrest. These events occur more frequently in patients with risk factors for CAD, especially if they had taken ergotamine within the previous 24 hours.

More frequently, cardiovascular adverse effects include hypotension or hypertension, palpitations, or syncope. Chest pressure syndrome also occurs frequently. This syndrome includes sensations of chest tightness or heaviness, jaw pain or tightness, and regional pain or pressure.

Sumatriptan can also induce cerebrovascular events such as cerebral vasospasm, resulting in intracranial bleeding, subarachnoid hemorrhage, stroke, or seizures. Again, these events are rare and generally occur in patients with risk factors for, or a history of, cerebral vascular disorders.

More commonly, patients may feel weak, dizzy, or lightheaded. They may also experience myalgias, muscle cramps, and stiffness.

Patients receiving intranasal sumatriptan may experience atypical burning sensations in the ear, nose, throat, nasal cavity, or sinus. They may also experience throat discomfort or dysgeusia (a distortion of the sense of taste). Subcutaneous sumatriptan may induce flushing or a sensation of warmth, burning, or heat.

Drug Interactions

Sumatriptan interacts with drugs that contain ergotamine, other 5-HT$_1$ agonists, sibutramine, and antidepressants such as selective serotonin reuptake inhibitors and monoamine oxidase inhibitors (MAOIs). Table 24.9 highlights these interactions.

Assessment of Relevant Core Patient Variables

Health Status

Assess the characteristics of the headache, including location, quality, intensity, and presence or absence of an aura. Assess also for trigger factors that may have caused or may continue the headache (Box 24.6). Sumatriptan is ineffective for other types of headaches.

Take a careful patient history, focusing on cardiovascular and cerebrovascular disorders or diseases. Question patients with diabetes mellitus, hypertension, hypercholesterolemia, or obesity for signs and symptoms that may suggest CAD. Evaluate available laboratory tests, especially liver and renal function tests, because dysfunction of the liver and kidneys may contribute to accumulation of sumatriptan, resulting in increased risk for adverse effects and toxicity. Communicate any positive findings to the health care provider before administering sumatriptan.

Life Span and Gender

Evaluate female patients for pregnancy, breast-feeding, or menopausal symptoms. As previously stated, there is no evidence that establishes that sumatriptan is a human teratogen. Although sumatriptan is a pregnancy category C drug, it should not be given during pregnancy unless the benefits outweigh the risk to the fetus. It is unclear whether sumatriptan is secreted in breast milk; therefore, it should not be taken by nursing mothers. Postmenopausal women and men older than 40 years should have a cardiovascular workup before receiving sumatriptan, to rule out the potential for CAD.

Lifestyle, Diet, and Habits

Identify trigger factors that may be part of the patient's lifestyle. Evaluate the patient for a history of smoking tobacco because smoking is a risk factor for the development of CAD.

Environment

Sumatriptan is routinely given in the outpatient area.

Nursing Diagnosis and Outcome

- Risk for Tissue Perfusion, Impaired, related to cardiovascular or cerebrovascular events
  Desired Outcome: *The patient will recognize the signs and symptoms of cardiovascular or cerebrovascular events and seek medical assistance immediately.*
- Risk for Injury related to weakness, dizziness or syncope, or light-headedness
  Desired Outcome: *The patient will remain free of injury while taking sumatriptan.*

Planning and Intervention

Maximizing Therapeutic Effects

Administer sumatriptan as soon as the headache begins. Sumatriptan is more efficacious when given before the headache escalates. Decrease the environmental stimuli

TABLE 24.9 Agents That Interact with P Sumatriptan

Interactants	Effect and Significance	Nursing Management
ergotamine-containing drugs ergotamine dihydroergotamine methysergide	Coadministration with ergotamine-containing drugs within 24 h may have additive vasospastic effects.	Do not administer sumatriptan within 24 h of ergotamine-containing drugs.
Monoamine oxidase inhibitors (MAOIs)	MAOIs inhibit the metabolism of oral sumatriptan.	Do not administer sumatriptan within 14 d of MAOI use.
Serotonin receptor agonists	Coadministration with other serotonin receptor agonists increases the risk for vasospastic effects and serotonin syndrome.	Do not administer sumatriptan with other serotonin receptor agonists.
selective serotonin reuptake inhibitors (SSRIs)	Coadministering sumatriptan with SSRIs may cause rapid accumulation of serotonin in the CNS.	Monitor for signs of serotonin syndrome.
sibutramine	Coadministering sumatriptan with sibutramine may have additive effects.	Monitor for signs of serotonin syndrome.

Migraine Headache Triggers

Migraines sometimes can be prevented, which eliminates the need to treat them. Exactly what triggers a migraine differs from patient to patient, and many patients' migraines can be triggered by multiple factors. You can help patients to track and identify their personal triggers so that they can avoid them and, perhaps, forestall migraine headaches. Common migraine triggers include:

Physiologic Triggers
- Hormonal fluctuations (before or during monthly menstrual period, or during treatment with hormone therapy such as birth control pills or estrogen replacement)
- Sleep deprivation, fatigue, or excessive sleep
- Head trauma

Dietary Triggers
- Alcohol, especially red wine
- Tyramine (aged cheese, marinated foods, fresh-baked yeast products)
- Aspartame (artificial sweetener)
- Monosodium glutamate (MSG)
- Phenylethylamine (present in some OTC drugs and chocolate)
- Nitrates (preservatives used in sausage, bacon, and lunch meats)
- Caffeine (either having more or withdrawal from use)

Psychological Triggers
- Stress, worry, or anxiety (especially after stressful situations; headache occurs over the weekend)
- Depression
- Fear
- Anger

Environmental Triggers
- Light (strong or glaring light, such as flickering lights from TV or computer screen, strobe or laser lights, or reflections)
- Weather changes (high humidity, atmospheric pressure changes, rapid temperature fluctuations, exposure to extreme heat or cold)
- Noises
- Smells, odors (intense, specific food odors, cigarette or other smoke, perfumes, cleaning products)

Pharmacologic Triggers
- Oral contraceptives
- Glyceryl trinitrate
- Theophylline
- Reserpine
- Nifedipine
- Indomethacin
- Cimetidine

during the migraine attack by closing the curtains over the windows and turning the lights off or down. Close the door to the patient's room unless contraindicated.

Minimizing Adverse Effects
Assess the patient for a history of cardiovascular or cerebrovascular disorder that might induce adverse effects during sumatriptan therapy. After administering sumatriptan, monitor for signs and symptoms of vasospasm and allergy.

Administer sumatriptan as ordered—orally, intranasally, or subcutaneously. Use aseptic technique when administering subcutaneously.

Providing Patient and Family Education
- Teach patients to take sumatriptan for migraine or cluster headache only. Emphasize that they should avoid the use of sumatriptan if the headache pain is not the same as their usual pain pattern.
- Explain the importance of avoiding sumatriptan if patients have cardiovascular or cerebrovascular disorders or chronic medical conditions that increase the risk of CAD.
- Teach patients the signs and symptoms of vasospastic events and the importance of seeking medical care immediately if they occur.
- Instruct patients to take the sumatriptan exactly as directed by the health care provider to avoid adverse effects or toxicity. If the pain is not relieved with the first dose of sumatriptan, patients should follow the instructions of the health care provider for subsequent dosing.
- Teach patients that the headache may recur. It is important to take only the prescribed dose and not to exceed 200 mg of sumatriptan in a 24-hour period.
- Teach patients the importance of avoiding smoking cigarettes.
- Teach patients the correct way to take sumatriptan. The oral medication should be taken with a full glass of water and not crushed or chewed. The intranasal inhaler should be used with the head upright. Also, teach patients aseptic technique to administer sumatriptan subcutaneously.
- Teach patients to identify trigger factors that induce migraine. Once they are identified, help the patients develop a plan to avoid or eliminate the trigger factor from their lifestyle.
- Teach patients complementary interventions when taking sumatriptan. They should decrease environmental stimuli, rest in a darkened room, and place an ice bag at the back of the neck.

Ongoing Assessment and Evaluation

Evaluate patients taking sumatriptan for the cessation of headache and for signs and symptoms of vasospastic events. Monitor the patient's blood pressure after administering the drug. Evaluate the frequency of migraine attacks and refer the patient to the health care provider for prophylaxis as needed. The patient should be pain free after sumatriptan is administered. The patient should remain free of symptoms of vasospastic events and serotonin syndrome. Box 24.7 discusses serotonin syndrome.

Drugs Closely Related to P Sumatriptan

The other serotonin receptor agonists, also called triptans, which are used in managing migraine, are all very similar to sumatriptan. They have the same pharmacotherapeutics,

---

Box 24.7 SEROTONIN SYNDROME

Symptoms of serotonin syndrome include:

- excitement
- hypomania
- restlessness
- loss of consciousness
- confusion
- disorientation
- anxiety
- agitation
- motor weakness
- myoclonus
- tremor
- hemiballismus
- hyperreflexia
- ataxia
- dysarthria
- incoordination
- hyperthermia
- shivering
- pupillary dilation
- diaphoresis
- emesis
- tachycardia

pharmacodynamics, and adverse effects. They have very similar contraindications and precautions and drug–drug interactions (see Table 24.9). The major difference among the triptans is the pharmacokinetics. All of the triptans are pregnancy category C drugs and should be used only when the benefits outweigh the risks.

Almotriptan

Almotriptan (Axert) has a rapid onset, short duration, and 70% to 80% bioavailability. It is available as an oral tablet. Almotriptan may be better tolerated than sumatriptan and may have a lower incidence of chest pain, tightness, or pressure. It may be given with MAOIs.

Eletriptan

Eletriptan (Relpax) has a slower onset than almotriptan and a longer duration, with a 50% bioavailability. It, too, is available as an oral tablet. Its bioavailability is increased when taken with a high-fat meal. Like almotriptan, eletriptan may be taken with MAOIs but should be avoided with CYP3A4 inhibitors such as ritonavir, nelfinavir, indinavir, erythromycin, clarithromycin, ketoconazole, and itraconazole.

Frovatriptan

Frovatriptan (Frova) has a very slow onset and a very long duration, and it is only 20% to 30% bioavailable. It is available as an oral tablet. Frovatriptan has the longest half-life of all the triptans; thus, rebound headaches may occur less frequently. Like almotriptan and eletriptan, it may be given with MAOIs.

Naratriptan

Naratriptan (Amerge) has an onset similar to sumatriptan, a longer duration, and 70% bioavailability. It is available as an oral tablet. Naratriptan has less headache recurrence than sumatriptan and may be given with MAOIs.

Rizatriptan

Rizatriptan (Maxalt) has a rapid onset and duration, with a bioavailability of 45%. It is available as an oral tablet or a dissolving tablet. Rizatriptan requires a dosage adjustment if taken with propranolol (Inderal). It may not be used in combination with MAOIs.

Zolmitriptan

Zolmitriptan (Zomig) has the fastest onset of action, a short duration, and a bioavailability of 40%. It is available as an oral tablet, dissolving tablet, or nasal spray. Like rizatriptan, it may not be used with MAOIs.

Drugs Significantly Different From 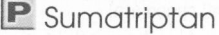 Sumatriptan

Ergotamine

Ergotamine (Ergomar, Cafergot, Migergot) is another type of drug used to abort an acute migraine or cluster headache. It has a complex mechanism of action that is very different from sumatriptan. Like sumatriptan, ergotamine stimulates 5-HT$_{1B/1D}$ receptors. It also affects serotonergic, dopaminergic, and alpha-adrenergic receptors. In addition, it stimulates uterine contractions and has emetic properties.

MEMORY CHIP

Sumatriptan

- Used for treatment of acute migraine or cluster headache
- Major contraindications: cardiovascular and cerebrovascular disorders
- Most common adverse effects: flushing, dizziness, weakness, nausea, drowsiness, stiffness, or feelings of tingling, heat, fatigue
- Most serious adverse effects: vasospasm resulting in ischemic events to the cardiovascular and cerebrovascular systems
- Maximizing therapeutic effects: Administer only to patients with documented migraine or cluster headaches.
- Minimizing adverse effects: Avoid administration to patients with cardiovascular or cerebrovascular disorders. Do not administer to patients with atypical headaches.
- Most important patient education: signs and symptoms of ischemic events and importance of seeking medical care should any occur
- **Life span alert: Sumatriptan is embryolethal in rabbits. Do not administer to pregnant women unless the benefit to the fetus outweighs the risk.**

Ergotamine has several routes of administration. It can be given orally, sublingually, rectally, or by inhalation. When given orally or rectally, it is often combined with caffeine, which increases its absorption. Although pain relief occurs within 0.5 to 2 hours of administration, vasoconstriction may persist for up to 48 hours. Ergotamine is metabolized in the liver, and its major metabolites are excreted in bile.

Contraindications for the use of ergotamine include alkaloid hypersensitivity, history of cardiovascular or cerebrovascular disorders, and pre-existing hepatic dysfunction. Ergotamine is a pregnancy category X drug because it stimulates uterine contractions. It is also contraindicated for use when breast-feeding because it may cause ergotism (vomiting, diarrhea, weak pulse, and unstable blood pressure) in nursing infants. Ergotamine is used with caution in patients with chronic diseases that increase the risk of cardiovascular disorders.

The most serious adverse effect of ergotamine is overdose or ergotism. Overdose can cause ischemia to peripheral arteries and arterioles, with resultant hypoxia to the extremities. As hypoxia continues, the extremities become cold, mottled, or numb. Untreated, gangrene may develop, and amputation may be necessary.

More common adverse effects include abdominal pain, nausea or vomiting, myalgias, leg weakness, and numbness or tingling in the extremities. Daily or frequent use of ergotamine may cause physical dependence.

Drug–drug interactions may occur with CYP3A4 inhibitors such as ritonavir, nelfinavir, indinavir, erythromycin, clarithromycin, ketoconazole, and itraconazole. Concurrent use of these drugs may cause vasospasm and cerebral or peripheral ischemia. Concurrent use of beta-blocking agents, hormonal contraceptives, vasoconstrictors, or nicotine increases the risk of peripheral vasoconstriction. The use of ergotamine and triptans should occur at least 24 hours apart.

Dihydroergotamine

Dihydroergotamine is a semisynthetic ergot alkaloid administered parenterally or intranasally to treat migraine. Dihydroergotamine is generally reserved for treating severe migraine because less toxic agents are available for mild to moderate migraine and cluster headache relief. Its pharmacodynamics are similar to those of ergotamine; however, it causes less peripheral vasoconstriction, nausea, and vomiting.

Contraindications and drug–drug interactions are also similar to those of ergotamine. Dihydroergotamine is a pregnancy category X drug because it induces uterine contractions. Although it is not known whether dihydroergotamine is secreted in breast milk, it should not be used by nursing mothers because of its structural similarity to ergotamine.

Analgesics

Several analgesic agents may be used to abort a migraine headache, although the triptans are generally more efficacious.

Acetaminophen or acetaminophen combinations (Excedrin, Excedrin Migraine) have been very successful. One small study found them to be as efficacious as triptans.

More powerful analgesics such as codeine combinations (usually combined with acetaminophen) and oxycodone have also been used. Of course, the problem with these drugs is the potential for abuse or tolerance.

Nonsteroidal Anti-inflammatory Drugs

Several NSAIDs have been approved by the FDA for migraine headaches. They include aspirin, indomethacin, naproxen, and ibuprofen. Although not approved by the FDA, fenoprofen, flurbiprofen, ketoprofen, ketorolac, and mefenamic acid are also used to abort migraine headache.

DRUGS USED AS PROPHYLAXIS FOR MIGRAINE HEADACHE

Drugs for migraine prophylaxis may be prescribed for patients with frequent migraine to decrease the frequency and severity of acute migraine. These drugs are not useful in treatment of an acute migraine headache.

Antiepileptics

Antiepileptics are increasingly recommended for migraine prevention. The exact mechanism of action is unclear; however, antiepileptics are thought to prevent migraines by blocking sodium or calcium channels or by enhancing the activity of gamma-aminobutyrate. Divalproex sodium (Depakote) and sodium valproate (Depakene) are the only antiepileptics with FDA approval for migraine prophylaxis. Nausea, vomiting, and GI distress are the most common side effects and are generally self-limiting. Additional adverse effects include weight gain, hair loss, tremor or shakiness, and fetal neural tube defects during pregnancy. Rare but severe adverse effects include fatal pancreatitis and hepatitis.

Several studies have shown the efficacy of gabapentin (Neurontin) as well, although it is not FDA approved for this therapeutic use. The most common adverse events with gabapentin are dizziness or giddiness and drowsiness.

Two other antiepileptics, tiagabine (Gabitril) and topiramate (Topamax), have been efficacious in small studies. However, the sample size in these studies was too small to generalize the conclusions of these studies. For a more thorough discussion of these antiepileptics, see Chapter 21.

Antidepressants

Antidepressants are useful in treating many chronic pain states, including migraine headache. Although the actual mechanism of action is unknown, the pain response occurs sooner than the expected antidepressant effect. Amitriptyline (Elavil) is the most common antidepressant used for migraine prophylaxis. Although other antidepressants have been prescribed, only amitriptyline has been studied in clinical trials.

Common adverse effects to amitriptyline include dry mouth, constipation, blurred vision, urinary retention, weight gain, and orthostatic hypotension. Amitriptyline is discussed in Chapter 19.

Beta-Adrenergic Blocking Agents

Beta blockers are used to prevent migraine headache because of their ability to relax blood vessels. The drug of choice is propranolol (Inderal), although nadolol (Corgard), atenolol (Tenormin), timolol (Blocadren), and metoprolol (Lopressor, Toprol) are also effective. Long-term therapy may induce sleep problems and vivid dreams, memory problems, fatigue, depression, and impotence. Beta blockers require close monitoring in patients with asthma, chronic obstructive pulmonary disease, diabetes, or high cholesterol because they may worsen symptoms of lung disease and asthma, may affect cholesterol levels, and may also affect how the body responds to low blood sugar. Beta-adrenergic blocking agents are discussed in Chapter 13.

Calcium Channel Blockers

Several calcium channel blockers are used as migraine prophylaxis. They include diltiazem (Cardizem), nifedipine (Procardia, Adalat), nimodipine (Nimotop), and verapamil (Calan). Calcium channel blockers are used to prevent migraine headache because of their ability to prevent vasoconstriction.

Constipation is the most frequent adverse effect of calcium channel blockers. Other adverse effects include dizziness, headache, facial flushing, and edema. Additional information regarding calcium channel blockers can be found in Chapter 29.

CHAPTER SUMMARY

- Drugs for fever, inflammation, and pain include salicylates (aspirin), prostaglandin synthetase inhibitors (NSAIDs, e.g., ibuprofen), and para-aminophenol derivatives (acetaminophen). These drugs work by inhibiting the synthesis of prostaglandins.
- Prostaglandins are found in almost all body tissues and affect the body in a multitude of ways. They are subdivided into COX-1 and COX-2 prostaglandins. COX-1 are involved in cell maintenance, whereas COX-2 are generally found at the site of inflammation.
- Salicylates and most NSAIDs block both COX-1 and COX-2. Inhibition of COX-1 is responsible for many of the adverse effects associated with these drugs.
- Aspirin has analgesic, anti-inflammatory, antipyretic, and antiplatelet activity.
- Low-dose aspirin therapy is used in healthy people to decrease the risk of cardiovascular or cerebrovascular events.
- Aspirin is a highly protein-bound drug and may interact with other highly protein-bound drugs.
- Aspirin and acetaminophen overdoses are common. Patients do not realize the potentially serious consequences

of ingesting these drugs because they are easily obtained without a prescription.
- The most common adverse effects of aspirin and ibuprofen are GI in nature.
- Serious adverse effects related to aspirin and NSAIDs are renal impairment, gastric ulceration, and GI bleeding.
- The major difference between aspirin and NSAIDs is related to antiplatelet activity. Inhibition of cyclooxygenase by aspirin is *irreversible,* whereas inhibition of cyclooxygenase by NSAIDs is *reversible.*
- Although NSAIDs have antiplatelet activity, they are not used to prevent MI or stroke.
- All NSAIDs, including COX-2 inhibitors, have a Black Box warning regarding the increase in risk of serious and potentially fatal MI and stroke. This risk increases with the duration of use.
- COX-2 inhibitors decrease the potential for GI bleeding, although it may still occur in some patients. These agents do not inhibit platelet aggregation.
- Acetaminophen is an analgesic and antipyretic. It does not have antiplatelet effects.
- The anti-inflammatory effects of acetaminophen occur only in the CNS; therefore, it cannot be used for inflammation in the periphery of the body.
- Because acetaminophen does not affect prostaglandins in the periphery of the body, it does not cause renal impairment or gastric distress.
- The most serious adverse effect of acetaminophen is hepatic dysfunction.
- Migraine headache has a complex etiology. Pain occurs because of both vasodilation and inflammation.
- The drugs used for prophylaxis of migraine headaches include beta-blocking agents, antiepileptics, antidepressants, and calcium channel blocking agents.
- The drugs of choice for managing acute migraine headaches are selective serotonin agonists, also known as "triptans" or antimigraine agents.
- The triptans are generally well tolerated and rarely cause coronary vasospasm.

QUESTIONS FOR STUDY AND REVIEW

1. How do prostaglandins affect the processes of inflammation, pain, and fever?
2. How does prostaglandin inhibition induce adverse effects of salicylates, NSAIDs, and acetaminophen?
3. What are the most potentially serious adverse effects of salicylates, NSAIDs, and acetaminophen, and how might you decrease their occurrence?
4. Describe the major differences between aspirin and NSAIDs.
5. Identify two major differences between nonselective NSAIDs and COX-2 inhibitors.
6. How do the triptans decrease migraine headache pain?
7. What is the key difference between serotonin receptor agonists and ergotamine-containing drugs in the management of migraine headache?

NEED MORE HELP?

Chapter 24 of the Study Guide to Accompany *Drug Therapy in Nursing*, 4th Edition, contains NCLEX-style questions and other learning activities to reinforce your understanding of the concepts presented in this chapter. For additional information or to purchase the study guide, visit thePoint.

REFERENCES

Amer, M., Bead, V. R., Bathon, J., et al. (2010). Use of nonsteroidal anti-inflammatory drugs in patients with cardiovascular disease: a cautionary tale, *Cardiology in Review*, 18(4):204–212.

Bartleson, J. D. & Cutrer, F. M. (2010). Migraine Headache: Diagnosis and Treatment, *Minnesota Medicine*, 93(5):36–41.

Bajwa, Z. H. & Sabahar, A. (2010). Pathophysiology, clinical manifestations, and diagnosis of migraine in adults, Up to Date. Retrieved from http://www.uptodate.com/online/content/topic.do?topicKey=headache/4701&selectedTitle=1~150&source=search_result on August 1, 2010.

Facts and Comparisons. (2010). *Drug facts and comparisons*. Philadelphia, PA: Lippincott Williams & Wilkins.

Karch, A. M. (2010). *Nursing drug guide*, Philadelphia, PA: Lippincott, Williams, and Wilkins.

Koda-Kimbal, M. A., Young, L. Y., Kradian, W. A., et al. (2008). *Applied therapeutics: the clinical use of drugs (9th Ed)*, Philadelphia, PA: Lippincott, Williams, and Wilkins.

International Headache Society. *Classifications of Headache*. Retrieved from http://www.ihs-classification.org/en/02_klassifikation on August 1, 2010.

Masso-Gonzalez, E. L., Patrignani, P., Tacconelli, S., et al. (2010). Variability among nonsteroidal antiinflammatory drugs in risk of upper gastrointestinal bleeding, *Arthritis and Rheumatism*, 62:1592–1601.

Micromedex Healthcare Series. Retrieved from *http://thomsonhc.com*.

Pierce, M. W. (2010). Transdermal delivery of sumatriptan for the treatment of acute migraine, *Neurotherapeutics*, 7(2):159–163.

Porth, C. M. (2008). Pathophysiology: *Concepts of Altered Health States (8th Ed)*, Philadelphia: Lippincott Williams & Wilkins.

Prescriber's Letter (2010). Managing NSAID Risk, 17(8):260810. Retrieved from http://www.prescribersletter.com/%28S%28fs15wsq1bbbhzl45tti4yc3u%29%29/pl/detaildocuments/260810.pdf?cs=&s=PRL on August 1, 2010.

Solomon, D. H. (2010). Nonselective NSAIDs: Overview of adverse effects, Up To Date. Retrieved from http://www.uptodate.com/online/content/topic.do?topicKey=treatme/7262&selectedTitle=2~150&source=search_result on August 1, 2010.

Solomon, D. H. (2010). COX-2 selective inhibitors: Adverse cardiovascular effects, Up to Date. Retrieved from http://www.uptodate.com/online/content/topic.do?topicKey=treatme/4488&source=see_link on August 1, 2010.

Tatro, D. S. (2011). *Drug Interaction Facts: The Authority on Drug Interactions*. Philadelphia, PA: Lippincott Williams & Wilkins.

25

Drugs Treating Rheumatoid Arthritis and Gout

Learning Objectives

At the completion of this chapter the student will:

1. Correlate the processes of inflammation and pain with antirheumatic drugs, antigout drugs, and uricosuric drugs.

2. Identify core drug knowledge pertaining to antirheumatic drugs, antigout drugs, and uricosuric drugs.

3. Identify core patient variables pertaining to antirheumatic drugs, antigout drugs, and uricosuric drugs.

4. Relate the interaction of core drug knowledge to core patient variables for antirheumatic drugs, antigout drugs, and uricosuric drugs.

5. Generate a nursing plan of care from the interactions between core drug knowledge and core patient variables for antirheumatic drugs, antigout drugs, and uricosuric drugs.

6. Describe nursing interventions to maximize therapeutic and minimize adverse effects for antirheumatic drugs, antigout drugs, and uricosuric drugs.

7. Determine key points for patient and family education for antirheumatic drugs, antigout drugs, and uricosuric drugs.

Key Terms

ankylosis
antigout drugs
chrysotherapy
cytokine

disease-modifying
antirheumatic drug (DMARD)
monoclonal antibody
nitritoid crisis

pannus
tophi
uricosuric drugs

Drugs Treating Rheumatoid Arthritis and Gout

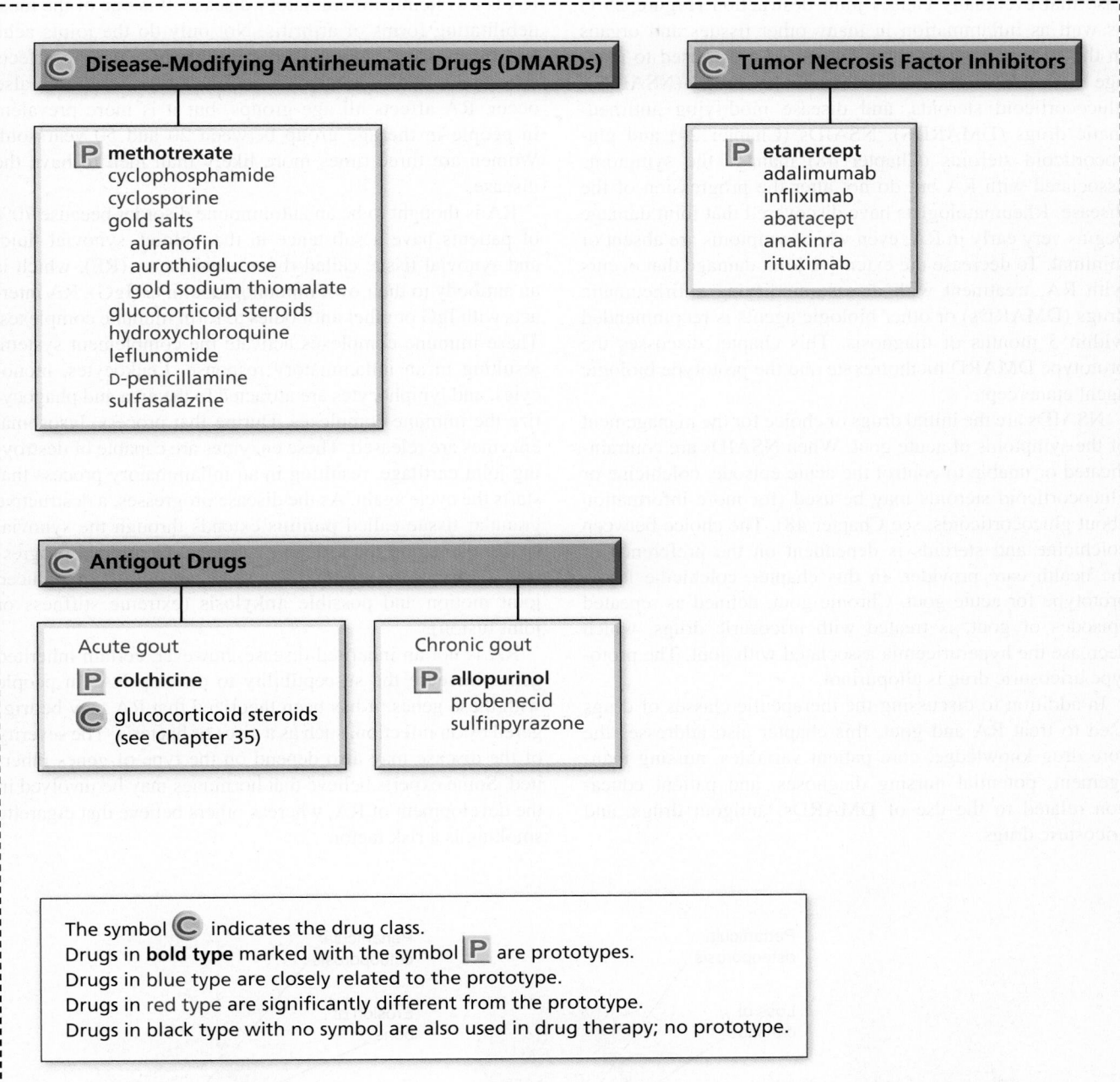

C Disease-Modifying Antirheumatic Drugs (DMARDs)

P **methotrexate**
cyclophosphamide
cyclosporine
gold salts
    auranofin
    aurothioglucose
    gold sodium thiomalate
glucocorticoid steroids
hydroxychloroquine
leflunomide
D-penicillamine
sulfasalazine

C Tumor Necrosis Factor Inhibitors

P **etanercept**
adalimumab
infliximab
abatacept
anakinra
rituximab

C Antigout Drugs

Acute gout

P **colchicine**

C glucocorticoid steroids
(see Chapter 35)

Chronic gout

P **allopurinol**
probenecid
sulfinpyrazone

The symbol **C** indicates the drug class.
Drugs in **bold type** marked with the symbol **P** are prototypes.
Drugs in blue type are closely related to the prototype.
Drugs in red type are significantly different from the prototype.
Drugs in black type with no symbol are also used in drug therapy; no prototype.

This chapter focuses on two inflammatory conditions, rheumatoid arthritis (RA) and gout. RA is not a wear-and-tear disease like osteoarthritis; it is an autoimmune disease that eventually causes joint destruction (Figure 25.1) as well as inflammation in many other tissues and organs in the body. There are three classes of drugs used to manage RA: nonsteroidal antiinflammatory drugs (NSAIDS), glucocorticoid steroids, and disease modifying antirheumatic drugs (DMARDS). NSAIDs (Chapter 24) and glucocorticoid steroids (Chapter 48) manage the symptoms associated with RA but do not alter the progression of the disease. Rheumatologists have discovered that joint damage begins very early in RA, even when symptoms are absent or minimal. To decrease the extensive joint damage that occurs with RA, treatment with disease-modifying antirheumatic drugs (DMARDs) or other biologic agents is recommended within 3 months of diagnosis. This chapter discusses the prototype DMARD methotrexate and the prototype biologic agent etanercept.

NSAIDs are the initial drugs of choice for the management of the symptoms of acute gout. When NSAIDs are contraindicated or unable to control the acute episode, colchicine or glucocorticoid steroids may be used (for more information about glucocorticoids, see Chapter 48). The choice between colchicine and steroids is dependent on the preference of the health care provider. In this chapter, colchicine is the prototype for acute gout. Chronic gout, defined as repeated episodes of gout, is treated with uricosuric drugs, which decrease the hyperuricemia associated with gout. The prototype uricosuric drug is allopurinol.

In addition to discussing the therapeutic classes of drugs used to treat RA and gout, this chapter also addresses the core drug knowledge, core patient variables, nursing management, potential nursing diagnoses, and patient education related to the use of DMARDs, antigout drugs, and uricosuric drugs.

PATHOPHYSIOLOGY
Rheumatoid Arthritis

RA is a systemic inflammatory disease. It is one of the most debilitating forms of arthritis. Not only do the joints ache and throb, they eventually become deformed. The effects are not limited to joint destruction; systemic effects also occur. RA affects all age groups, but it is more prevalent in people in the age group between 20 and 50 years old. Women are three times more likely than men to have the disease.

RA is thought to be an autoimmune disorder because 70% of patients have a substance in their blood, synovial fluid, and synovial tissue called rheumatoid factor (RF), which is an antibody to their own immunoglobulin G (IgG). RA interacts with IgG or other antibodies to form immune complexes. These immune complexes activate the complement system, resulting in an inflammatory response. Leukocytes, monocytes, and lymphocytes are attracted to the area and phagocytize the immune complexes. During that process, lysosomal enzymes are released. These enzymes are capable of destroying joint cartilage, resulting in an inflammatory process that starts the cycle again. As the disease progresses, a destructive granular tissue called **pannus** extends through the synovial space, damaging the articular cartilage. Continued progression destroys the entire joint space, resulting in reduced joint motion and possible **ankylosis** (extreme stiffness or joint fusion).

RA is not an inherited disease; however, certain inherited genes increase the susceptibility to develop RA. In people with these genes, it has been theorized that RA may be triggered by an infection, such as a virus or bacteria. The severity of the disease may also depend on the type of genes inherited. Some experts believe that hormones may be involved in the development of RA, whereas others believe that cigarette smoking is a risk factor.

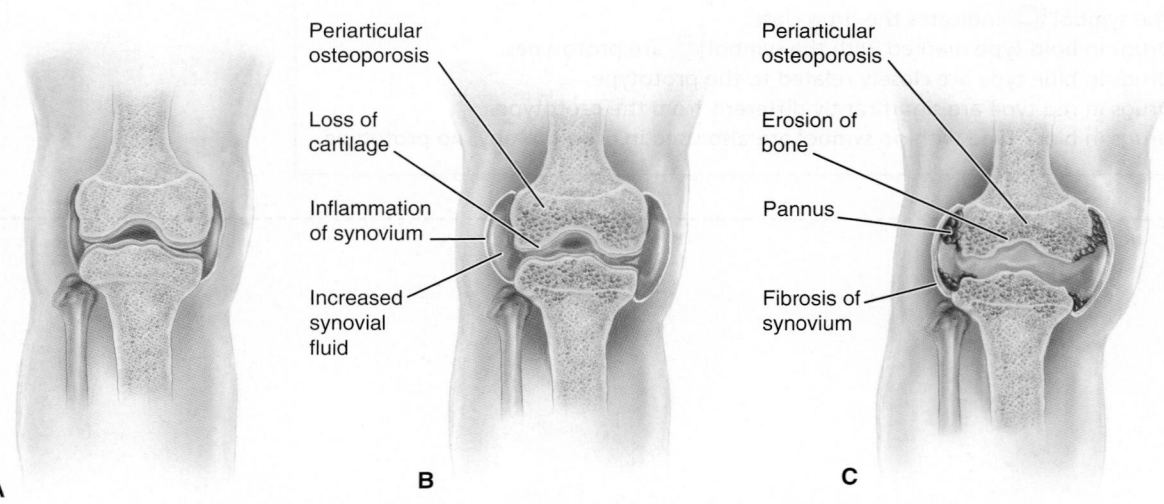

A B C

• FIGURE 25.1 (**A**) Normal joint; (**B**) early rheumatoid arthritis with fluid accumulation and synovial swelling; (**C**) late rheumatoid arthritis with pannus formation, eroded articular cartilage, and joint space narrowing.

The primary characteristic of RA is symmetric polyarticular inflammation, especially in the small joints of the hands and feet. Additional symptoms of RA include:

- Generalized aching or stiffness of the joints and muscles, especially in the morning or after a period of rest
- Loss of motion of the affected joints
- Loss of strength in muscles attached to the affected joints
- Fatigue, especially during an exacerbation
- Low-grade fever
- Malaise

Small lumps, called rheumatoid nodules, may form under the skin at pressure points such as the elbows, hands, feet, and Achilles tendons. In addition to pressure points, rheumatoid nodules may occur anywhere in the body, including the back of the scalp, over the knees, or even in the lungs. Rheumatoid nodules are usually painless and range in size—from as small as a pea to as large as a walnut.

In contrast to osteoarthritis, which affects only the bones and joints, RA can cause inflammation of glands such as tear and salivary glands, the linings of the heart and lungs, the lungs themselves and, in rare cases, the vascular system. Patients with RA have an increased risk of heart attack and stroke (Box 25.1).

The clinical course of RA is highly variable. It tends to vary in severity and may even come and go. Exacerbations of RA (called flare-ups or flares) alternate with periods of relative remission, during which the symptoms of RA fade or disappear.

RA has a substantial effect on quality of life because of the associated pain, fatigue, and depression, and the increased risk of heart disease. Because of these issues, RA can reduce the life span of people who have it.

Gout

Gout is a disease of purine metabolism. It occurs more frequently in men greater than 30 years and women greater than 50 years. The risk of gout increases in women after menopause because uric acid levels rise in women at that time. Hyperuricemia, defined as a uric acid level greater than 6.8 mg/dL, may result from overproduction or underexcretion of uric acid. Gout occurs when the hyperuricemia forms monosodium urate crystals, which precipitate into the synovial fluid and initiate an inflammatory response.

Hyperuricemia is clearly a risk factor for the development of gout, and the risk increases as the urate concentration increases. However, many years of asymptomatic hyperuricemia have usually elapsed before the development of acute gouty arthritis, and in some patients with asymptomatic hyperuricemia, gout never develops. Other risk factors for gout include lifestyle factors such as alcohol consumption (especially beer); obesity; high meat and seafood consumption (especially red organ meat and shellfish) ; medical conditions such as hypertension, hyperlipidemia, chronic renal impairment, cardiovascular disease, insulin resistance, diabetes mellitus, or metabolic syndrome; drugs such as thiazide and loop diuretics, aspirin (low-dose), some antituberculosis drugs, and nicotinic acid or antirejection drugs; and a family history of gout. Transplant patients receiving cyclosporine develop gout because cyclosporine decreases the renal excretion of uric acid.

Gout has four distinct phases: asymptomatic hyperuricemia, acute gouty arthritis (flare), intercritical gout (interval between flares), and chronic advanced gout (uncontrolled hyperuricemia with chronic arthritis tophi). The onset of acute gouty arthritis is rapid. The pain frequently starts during the night and is often described as throbbing, crushing, or excruciating. The affected joints show signs of warmth, redness, and tenderness (Figure 25.2). In more than half of the initial attacks, the onset is in the first metatarsophalangeal joint (MTP), and overall, 90% of patients have the MTP affected at some point. Chronic gout may cause joint deformity and limited motion in affected joints. Uric acid deposits called **tophi** can be found in bursae, synovium, and tendons and along the extensor surface of the forearm. Tophi can also deposit in the kidney, leading to chronic

---

BOX 25.1 FOCUS ON RESEARCH

Therapeutic Alternative for Chronic Gout

Becker, M. A., Schumacher, H. R., Espinoza, L. R., Wells, A. F., MacDonald, P., Lloyd, E., vLademacher, C. (2010). The urate-lowering efficacy and safety of febuxostat in the treatment of the hyperuricemia of gout: the CONFIRMS trial, *Arthritis Research and Therapy*, 12(2):R63.

The Study

The researchers studied the safety and efficacy of daily febuxostat and allopurinol in subjects with gout and serum urate (sUA) > or = 8.0 mg/dL. The goal was to reach and maintain a sUA < 6 mg/dL. 2,269 patients were randomized to febuxostat 40 mg or 80 mg, or allopurinol 300 mg (200 mg in moderate renal impairment). Safety assessments included blinded adjudication of each cardiovascular (CV) adverse event (AE) and death. In the febuxostat 40 mg group 45% met the end goal; febuxostat 80 mg 67%; and in the allopurinol groups 42%. Achievement of target sUA in subjects with renal impairment was also superior with febuxostat 80 mg (72%) compared with febuxostat 40 mg (50%) or allopurinol (42%). Rates of

AEs did not differ across treatment groups. CV event rates were 0.0% for febuxostat 40 mg and 0.4% for both febuxostat 80 mg and allopurinol. One death occurred in each febuxostat group and three in the allopurinol group. Urate-lowering efficacy of febuxostat 80 mg exceeded that of febuxostat 40 mg and allopurinol (300/200 mg), which were comparable. In subjects with mild/moderate renal impairment, both febuxostat doses were more efficacious than allopurinol and equally safe.

Nursing Implications

It is important for nurses to remain knowledgeable regarding treatment options for patients with gout. For approximately 40 years allopurinol was the main therapy in lowering urate production until the FDA approval of febuxostat (Uloric). Become familiar with the action and potential adverse effects of febuxostat. Monitor the patient for diarrhea, headache, and rash. Remember that febuxostat is associated with an increased risk for cardiovascular events and monitor for these potential complications.

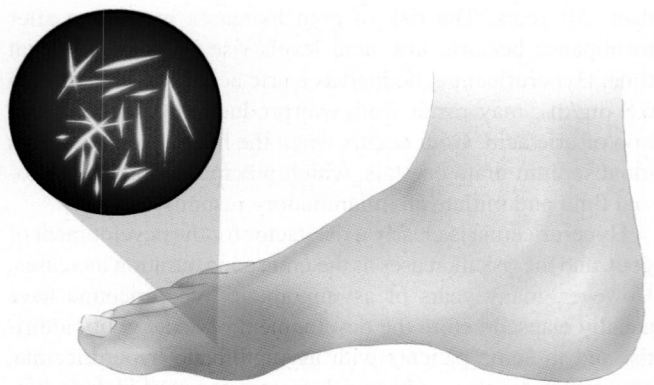

• FIGURE 25.2   Gout in the first metatarsal phalangeal joint of the right foot.

kidney failure. Fortunately, chronic advanced gout is a rare occurrence today because of the prevalence of appropriate pharmacotherapy.

The diagnosis of gout is made by identification of uric acid crystals in joints, tissues, or body fluids.

© DISEASE-MODIFYING ANTIRHEUMATIC DRUGS

Disease-modifying antirheumatic drugs (DMARDS) are drugs that are capable of arresting the progression of RA and can induce remission in some patients. They are used in conjunction with salicylates and NSAIDs, or as monotherapy when salicylates and NSAIDs are ineffective or not tolerated. The therapeutic class of DMARDs is subdivided into non-biological DMARDS and biological DEMARDS. These drugs include alkylating agents, antimetabolites, antimalarials, gold salts, sulfonamide antibiotics, TNF inhibitors, monoclonal antibodies, interleukin antagonists, and immune response modifiers. Although the mechanism of action is different for each of these drugs, they are all similar in the fact that they slow the progression of RA.

Non-Biologic AI Demards

Methotrexate (Rheumatrex, Trexall, MTX) is the prototype non-biological-DMARD (Table 25.1). Although there are many treatment options for RA, most rheumatologists concur that methotrexate is the drug of choice, either as monotherapy or in combination with tumor necrosis factor (TNF) drugs or other biologic agents. Anti-TNF monotherapy is similar in efficacy to treatment with methotrexate alone, while the combination of an anti-TNF agent with methotrexate reduces disease activity more and slows radiographic progression to a greater extent than monotherapy with methotrexate or anti-TNF drugs.

Because the onset of action of all DMARDs is slow, salicylates or NSAIDs are given to control the symptoms of RA until the DMARD action begins. Depending on the rheumatologist, when the DMARD begins to work, NSAID therapy may be continued with the DMARD or discontinued.

Nursing Management of the Patient Receiving P Methotrexate

Core Drug Knowledge

Pharmacotherapeutics

MTX is a folate antimetabolite used in treating various malignancies, including osteosarcoma, non-Hodgkin's lymphoma, Hodgkin's disease, cutaneous T-cell lymphoma, head and neck cancer, lung cancer, and breast cancer. Because it also has immunosuppressive effects, it is used to treat adult and juvenile RA and psoriasis.

Pharmacokinetics

MTX is given orally to manage RA. Its absorption may be decreased in the presence of food. A small portion is metabolized in the liver; the drug is excreted in the urine mostly as unchanged drug Relief of symptoms occurs in 3 to 6 weeks.

Pharmacodynamics

MTX exerts immunosuppressive effects by inhibiting the replication and function of T lymphocytes that stimulate the production of cytokines, in particular interleukin-1 (IL-1), IL-6, and IL-8, as well as TNF-alpha. MTX also induces folate depletion, which leads to inhibition of purine synthesis and results in the arrest of deoxyribonucleic acid (DNA), ribonucleic acid (RNA), and protein synthesis. Because MTX targets rapidly proliferating cells, such as epithelial cells, it slows progression of psoriasis.

Contraindications and Precautions

MTX is contraindicated in patients with immunosuppression, pre-existing blood dyscrasia, or impaired bone marrow function, and during pregnancy and lactation. It is also contraindicated for patients with psoriasis or RA in patients with alcoholism, alcoholic liver disease, or other chronic liver disease. It is given cautiously to patients with pre-existing hepatic or renal dysfunction, malnutrition, or ulcerative colitis. MTX is a pregnancy category X drug because fetal abnormality has been documented. MTX therapy used for cancer has additional precautions, including significant Black Box warnings (Box 25.2).

Adverse Effects

Stomatitis and oral ulcers, mild alopecia and hair thinning, and GI upset may occur and are related to folic acid antagonism. Headache, fatigue, and feeling "wiped out" may occur and is referred to as "methotrexate fog". The most serious adverse effects to methotrexate therapy include hepatic cirrhosis, interstitial pneumonitis, and severe myelosuppression. Because relatively low doses are used to manage RA, the risk of these severe adverse effects is greatly reduced. However, this reduction does not change the need to monitor closely for these potential adverse effects. Lastly, lymphoma has rarely been reported with MTX therapy. It is important to remember that patients with RA have an increased risk of developing lymphoma as a consequence of their autoimmune disease, and may not be related to the MTX therapy.

TABLE 25.1 Summary of Selected Disease-Modifying Ⓒ Antirheumatic Drugs

Drug (Trade) Name	Selected Indications	Route and Dosage Range	Pharmacokinetics
P methotrexate (Rheumatrex, TREXALL, MTX)	RA, psoriasis	*Adult:* PO/IM, 7.5–25 mg/wk in a single dose; administer with folic acid 1 mg daily or leucovorin 5 mg/wk *Child 2–16 y:* PO/IM, 5–15 mg m²/wk; administer with folic acid 1 mg daily or leucovorin 5 mg/wk	*Onset:* Varies *Duration:* Unknown $t_{1/2}$: 2–4 h
P auranofin (Ridaura)	RA	*Adult:* PO, 5–9 mg/d in 1 or 2 doses *Child:* PO, 0.1 mg/kg/d initially, titrate up to 0.15 mg/kg/d; maximum dose, 0.2 mg/kg/d	*Onset:* Varies *Duration:* 6 mo $t_{1/2}$: 26 d
aurothioglucose (Solganal)	RA	*Adult:* IM, 10 mg initially, then 25 mg for the second and third doses, given at weekly intervals, followed by 50 mg weekly until a total dose of 0.8–1.0 g has been administered Maintenance dosage is 25–50 mg IM given at 3- to 4-wk intervals indefinitely *Child:* IM, 0.25 mg/kg the first week; increase dosage by 0.25 mg/kg weekly up to a maintenance dosage of 0.75–1 mg/kg once per week. Doses are given once per week for a total of 20 doses, then continued every 2–4 wk.	*Onset:* Slow *Duration:* 6 mo $t_{1/2}$: 26 d
azathioprine (Azasan, Imuran)	RA Crohn's disease Ulcerative Colitis	*Adult:* PO 1–2.5 mg/kg/d divided 1-2x/d *Adult:* PO 100–250 mg daily	*Onset:* unknown *Duration:* unknown $t_{1/2}$: 5 h
cyclophosphamide (Cytoxan)	RA	*Adult and child:* PO, 1.5–3 mg/kg/d	*Onset:* Rapid *Duration:* Unknown $t_{1/2}$: 4–6 h
cyclosporine (Neoral, Gengraf)	RA	*Adult:* PO, 2.5–4 mg/kg/d, divided, 2× d *Child:* not approved for this indication	*Onset:* Varies *Duration:* 24–36 h $t_{1/2}$: 17.9 h
hydroxychloroquine (Plaquenil)	RA	*Adult:* PO, 200–600 mg/d in 1 or 2 doses *Child:* not approved	*Onset:* Rapid *Duration:* Unknown $t_{1/2}$: 3–5 d
gold sodium thiomalate (Myochrysine)	RA	*Adult:* IM, 10 mg in a single injection the first week, 25 mg the following week, then 25–50 mg/wk thereafter	*Onset:* Slow *Duration:* 6 mo $t_{1/2}$: 3–27 d
leflunomide (Arava)	RA	*Adult:* PO, 10–20 mg/d in a single dose	*Onset:* Varies *Duration:* Unknown $t_{1/2}$: 14 d
minocycline	RA	*Adult:* PO 100 mg 2x/d *Child:* not approved for this non-FDA use	*Onset:* rapid *Duration:* unknown $t_{1/2}$: 11-18 h
penicillamine (Cuprimine)	RA	*Adult:* PO, 250–500 mg daily *Child:* PO, 10 mg/kg/d, divided, 1–2× d for 4 mo	*Onset:* Varies *Duration:* Unknown $t_{1/2}$: 1.7–3.2 h
sulfasalazine (Azulfidine EN-tabs)	RA, ulcerative colitis, Crohn's disease	*Adult and elderly:* PO, 2 g/d given in 2–3 divided doses *Child >6 y:* PO, 30–50 mg/kg/d in 2 divided doses	*Onset:* 1 h *Duration:* 6–12 h $t_{1/2}$: 5–10 h

Box 25.2 METHOTREXATE BLACK BOX WARNINGS

Methotrexate should be used only by physicians whose knowledge and experience include the use of antimetabolite therapy.

- Because of the possibility of **serious toxic reactions** (possibly fatal):
  1. Methotrexate (MTX) should be used only in life-threatening neoplastic diseases, or in patients with psoriasis or rheumatoid arthritis (RA) with severe, recalcitrant, disabling disease that is not adequately responsive to other forms of therapy.
  2. Deaths have been reported with the use of MTX in the treatment of malignancy, psoriasis, and RA.
  3. Patients should be closely monitored for bone marrow, liver, lung, and kidney toxicities.
  4. Patients should be informed by their physicians of the risks involved and be under a physician's care throughout therapy.
- The use of high-dose MTX regimens recommended for osteosarcoma requires meticulous care. High-dose regimens for other neoplastic diseases are investigational, and a therapeutic advantage has not been established.
- MTX formulations and diluents containing preservatives must not be used for intrathecal or high-dose MTX therapy.
  1. MTX has been reported to cause fetal death or congenital anomalies. Therefore, it is not recommended for women of childbearing potential unless there is clear medical evidence that the benefits can be expected to outweigh the considered risks. Pregnant women with psoriasis or RA should not receive the drug.
  2. MTX elimination is reduced in patients with impaired renal function, ascites, or pleural effusions. Such patients require especially careful monitoring for toxicity and require dose reduction or, in some cases, discontinuation of methotrexate administration.
  3. Unexpectedly severe (sometimes fatal) bone marrow suppression and gastrointestinal toxicity have been reported with concomitant administration of MTX (usually in high dosage) along with some nonsteroidal anti-inflammatory drugs (NSAIDs).
  4. MTX causes hepatotoxicity, fibrosis, and cirrhosis, but generally only after prolonged use. Acutely, liver enzyme elevations are

frequently seen. These are usually transient and asymptomatic and also do not appear predictive of subsequent hepatic disease. Liver biopsy after sustained use often shows histologic changes, and fibrosis and cirrhosis have been reported; these latter conditions may not be preceded by symptoms or abnormal liver function tests in the people with psoriasis. For this reason, periodic liver biopsies are usually recommended for patients with psoriasis who are under long-term treatment. Persistent abnormalities in liver function tests may precede appearance of fibrosis or cirrhosis in the RA population.
  5. MTX-induced lung disease is potentially dangerous and may occur acutely at any time during therapy. It has been reported at doses as low as 7.5 mg/wk and is not always completely reversible. Pulmonary symptoms (especially a dry, nonproductive cough) may require interruption of treatment and careful investigation.
  6. Diarrhea and ulcerative stomatitis require interruption of therapy; otherwise, hemorrhagic enteritis and death from intestinal perforation may occur.
  7. Malignant lymphomas, which may regress following withdrawal of MTX, may occur in patients receiving low-dose MTX therapy. They may not require cytotoxic treatment. Discontinue methotrexate first and, if the lymphoma does not regress, institute appropriate treatment.
  8. Like other cytotoxic drugs, MTX may induce "tumor lysis syndrome" in patients with rapidly growing tumors. Appropriate supportive and pharmacologic measures may prevent or alleviate this complication.
  9. Severe, occasionally fatal, skin reactions have been reported following single or multiple doses of MTX. Reactions have occurred within days of drug administration. Recovery has been reported with discontinuation of therapy.
  10. Potentially fatal opportunistic infections, especially *Pneumocystis carinii* pneumonia, may occur with MTX therapy.
  11. MTX given concomitantly with radiotherapy may increase the risk of soft-tissue necrosis and osteonecrosis.

Drug Interactions

MTX may interact with many drugs. In general, MTX should not be given concurrently with other drugs associated with the development of nephrotoxicity, hepatotoxicity, or suppressed bone marrow function. Table 25.2 presents potential drug interactions with MTX.

Assessment of Relevant Core Patient Variables

Health Status

Assess the patient for comorbid states or drugs that contradict the use of MTX. Complete a thorough physical examination, carefully evaluating for signs of hepatic or renal insufficiency, suppressed bone marrow function, or adventitious lung sounds. Document the severity of joint inflammation and any restriction in range of motion as a baseline for later comparison to assess the efficacy of MTX therapy.

Before beginning therapy, evaluate the results of a complete blood count (CBC); renal and hepatic function tests; hepatitis B and C serologies, and chest x-ray. Coordinate

serial laboratory testing. Routine monitoring includes a CBC, liver profile, serum albumin, and serum creatinine every 4 to 8 weeks. Assess the patient's willingness to adhere to this close monitoring. If the patient is female, evaluate for possible pregnancy and help the patient develop a plan for contraception during therapy.

Life Span and Gender

MTX is given cautiously to very young and elderly patients because these patients' livers and kidneys may not be able to adequately clear the drug, and they therefore risk accumulation. Because MTX is a pregnancy category X drug, planning pregnancy is essential: Women should discontinue methotrexate for at least one ovulatory cycle prior to attempting conception, while men should wait 3 months. MTX is secreted in breast milk and may be toxic to the infant.

Lifestyle, Diet, and Habits

Evaluate for the use of alcohol or illicit drugs because these substances may predispose the patient to hepatic dysfunction.

TABLE 25.2	Agents That Interact with P Methotrexate	
Interactants	**Effect and Significance**	**Nursing Management**
acitretin	Although the mechanism of action is unknown, acitretin increases the risk of hepatotoxicity when administered with MTX.	Monitor liver function tests. Monitor for signs of hepatotoxicity.
aspirin, salicylates	Salicylates decrease the renal clearance of MTX, resulting in an increased risk of MTX toxicity. Less likely to occur with weekly administration of MTX.	See amiodarone.
Charcoal, activated	Charcoal reduces the absorption of MTX.	Monitor for efficacy of MTX therapy.
cyclosporine	Cyclosporine blocks the oxidation of MTX to its relatively inactive metabolite, decreasing its efficacy	Monitor for increased symptoms of RA.
digoxin	MTX may reduce GI absorption of digoxin, resulting in decreased serum digoxin concentration.	Monitor for efficacy of digoxin therapy. Monitor serum digoxin levels frequently.
Hydantoins	MTX may decrease the absorption of Hydantoins resulting in decreased efficacy	Monitor drug levels levels. Monitor for seizure activity. Ensure safety.
NSAIDS	NSAIDS reduce the renal clearance of MTX resulting in toxicity. Less likely to occur with weekly administration of MTX.	Same as amiodarone
penicillins	Penicillins impair the renal excretion of MTX.	Obtain MTX serum concentration if penicillins are initiated. Same as amiodarone.
probenecid	Probenecid impairs the renal excretion of MTX.	Obtain MTX serum concentration if probenecid is initiated. Same as amiodarone
sulfonamides	Sulfonamides displace MTX from protein binding sites and decrease renal clearance of MTX resulting in an increased serum concentration of MTX. MTX may induce folate deficiency, which develops into acute megaloblastic anemia when administered with TMP-SMZ.	Same as amiodarone

Also, evaluate the nutritional status of the patient; malnourished patients are more likely than others to be immunosuppressed or have blood dyscrasias. Evaluate the patient's caffeine intake because caffeine may decrease the effectiveness of MTX. To minimize the potential for MTX photosensitivity, determine how frequently the patient must be in the sun.

Environment

MTX as an oral medication for RA is routinely taken by the patient at home. In some circumstances, MTX may be given by the intramuscular route. In such cases, teach the patient the correct aseptic technique for self-administering an intramuscular injection. If you, the nurse, administer the intramuscular injection, handle MTX according to the facility's protocol, because skin contact with MTX poses a risk for carcinogenicity, mutagenicity, or teratogenicity.

Nursing Diagnoses and Outcomes

• Comfort Impaired: Nausea related to drug therapy
  Desired outcome: The patient will eat small, frequent meals when nauseated to maintain nutritional balance.

• Risk for Infection related to potential depression of bone marrow function and blood dyscrasias
  Desired outcome: The patient will recognize signs of depressed bone marrow function and blood dyscrasias and contact the health care provider immediately for intervention if any appear.

• Imbalanced Nutrition: Less than Body Requirements, related to potential nausea, stomatitis, and gingivitis
  Desired outcome: The patient will maintain nutritional balance throughout therapy.

• Risk for Injury related to drug accumulation caused by hepatic or renal dysfunction
  Desired outcome: The patient will remain injury free throughout therapy.

Planning and Intervention

Maximizing Therapeutic Effects

Administer MTX weekly as ordered. Ensure that the patient drinks enough water to minimize the risk of nephrotoxicity. Encourage the patient to continue pharmacotherapy with MTX, even if the patient has not yet experienced any beneficial results.

Minimizing Adverse Effects

Vitamin B (folic acid), 1 mg every day, may decrease the potential for adverse effects of MTX. If the patient has mouth ulcers, consult with the prescriber to request an order for allopurinol, 300 mg. Dissolve the allopurinol in 50 mL of water. It is important to instruct the patient to use this solution to rinse the mouth but not to swallow the solution. Remind the patient that MTX can cause photosensitivity. Patients should take care to remain out of the sun, wear protective clothing, and use a lotion with skin protection factor (SPF) 45 if they cannot avoid being in the sun.

Providing Patient and Family Education

- Assist patients in preparing a schedule for MTX because this drug is not taken daily.
- Instruct patients to use puncture-resistant containers to dispose of the needles and syringes.
- Advise patients to contact the health care provider before starting other prescription drugs, or over-the-counter (OTC) medication such as vitamins, minerals, or herbs.
- Instruct patients to contact the prescriber immediately if they experience:
  - Symptoms of infection—fever or chills, cough, sore throat, pain, or difficulty passing urine
  - Symptoms of decreased platelets or bleeding—bruising, pinpoint red spots on the skin, black and tarry stools, blood in the urine
  - Symptoms of anemia—unusual weakness or tiredness, fainting spells, light-headedness
  - Diarrhea
  - Difficulty breathing, a nonproductive cough
  - Mouth or throat ulcers
  - Redness, blistering, peeling or loosened skin, including inside the mouth
  - Skin rash, hives, or itching
  - Changes in vision
  - Vomiting
- Teach patients the importance of adequate nutrition and hydration to minimize the risk of adverse effects.
- Stress the effects of alcohol and drugs in precipitating adverse effects on the liver.
- Encourage patients to limit their intake of caffeine.
- Instruct patients to keep out of the sun or to wear protective clothing outdoors and use a sunscreen. Emphasize that they must not use sun lamps or sun tanning beds or booths.
- Instruct patients on the importance of serial laboratory testing and coordinate dates for testing to occur.
- Explain the importance of self-care in addition to pharmacotherapy:
  - Range-of-motion exercises
  - Weight control
  - Daily exercise, especially walking

- Healthy diet
- Heat for aching joints
- Cold for acute flares
- Relaxation techniques
- Advise patients that the beneficial effects from MTX take 1 to 2 months and that it is important to continue therapy to allow the benefits to begin.

Ongoing Assessment and Evaluation

Monitor patients for signs of blood dyscrasias, suppressed bone marrow function, pulmonary changes, and hepatic or renal dysfunction at each visit. Assess the degree of joint pain, duration of morning stiffness, limitation of function, and degree of fatigue at each visit. Coordinate serial testing that includes CBC, urinalysis, and liver and renal function tests.

Effective treatment with MTX should decrease (1) subjective symptoms such as perceived pain level and (2) objective symptoms such as decreased joint inflammation and increased range of motion. The patient should be free of adverse effects or be receiving appropriate interventions focused on ameliorating adverse effects.

Drugs Similar to P Methotrexate

Azathioprine

Azathioprine (Azasan, Imuran) is an intravenously infused antimetabolite that splits into a precursor, mercaptopurine. It is a unique antimetabolite agent because it is exclusively an immunosuppressant and not an antineoplastic. Because of its action, it is highly mutagenic and has been associated with the development of secondary malignancies, both

CRITICAL THINKING SCENARIO

DMARD THERAPY

Ms. Ruben, a 50-year-old woman, was diagnosed with rheumatoid arthritis by her primary care physician, who referred her to the rheumatologist at your clinic. She has been taking indomethacin for the past month and has come to the clinic for her first visit. When asked how well the indomethacin is controlling her pain, Ms. Ruben replied, "I barely know it's there." She also denies experiencing any adverse effects. The rheumatologist orders MTX for Ms. Ruben in combination with indomethacin.

1. Why do you think the rheumatologist ordered MTX even though the patient is doing so well on her current medication?
2. What assessments should you document before administering MTX?
3. Consider which laboratory tests you anticipate will be performed before MTX is administered.
4. Prepare patient teaching about MTX for Ms. Ruben.
5. When do you anticipate Ms. Ruben will attain optimal response from MTX therapy?
6. What is the purpose of continuing indomethacin at this time?
7. Ms. Ruben asks, "What if this doesn't work? What then?" How would you respond?

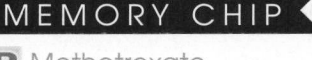

MEMORY CHIP

P Methotrexate

- Disease-modifying antirheumatic drug (DMARD) used as monotherapy or in combination with glucocorticoid steroids, NSAIDs, or other DMARDs to decrease the progression of RA
- Major contraindications: immunosuppression, blood dyscrasias, pregnancy
- Most common adverse effects: nausea, headache, stomatitis, gingivitis, alopecia
- Most serious adverse effect: depressed bone marrow function
- Maximizing therapeutic effects: remain hydrated
- Minimizing adverse effects: Take vitamin B, 5 mg every day.
- Most important patient education: Substantial adverse effects may occur. Be sure to contact the health care provider if they occur.
- **Black box warning: See Box 25.2**

---

listed as black box warnings. It is indicated as part of a multidrug regimen to prevent rejection in renal transplantation and to treat rheumatoid arthritis not responsive to conventional management. Unlabeled uses include treating Crohn disease and myasthenia gravis and preventing rejection after cardiac transplantation. Notable drug interactions occur with allopurinol, angiotensin-converting enzyme inhibitors, and anticoagulants. The most common and severe adverse event is infection, although GI distress may be great enough to warrant limiting the dose. Azathioprine is given cautiously with other immunosuppressants because of increased risk of infection, and dose reduction is necessary in hepatic dysfunction.

Gold Salts

The administration of gold salts is called **chrysotherapy**. Gold is an antiinflammatory agent that interferes with cells and substances in the immune system. There are two forms of IM gold salts: gold sodium thiomalate (Myochrysine) and aurothioglucose (Solganal). There is also an oral tablet that contains gold, auranofin (Ridaura); however, this preparation is distinct from the injectable forms and much less effective. Gold has been used for RA for over 70 years, but its relatively modest efficacy and high side-effect profile, coupled with the increased use of methotrexate and biologicals, have led to a dramatic decrease in its use.

Hydroxychloroquine

Hydroxychloroquine (Plaquenil) is an antimalarial drug also used in managing RA and discoid lupus erythematosus. In treating malaria, the mechanism of action is the same as for chloroquine. In managing RA and discoid lupus erythematosus, the mechanism of action is unclear. Optimal benefits may take between 2 and 6 months.

Hydroxychloroquine is generally well tolerated. For patients on long-term therapy, those over the age of 60, and patients with significant kidney disease, hydroxychloroquine may cause visual changes or loss of vision.

Drug–drug interactions, adverse effects, nursing management, and patient education are the same as for patients taking chloroquine (see Chapter 47).

Leflunomide

Leflunomide (Arava) is an innovative DMARD that was designed specifically for RA. The pharmacologic activity of leflunomide is accomplished through its active primary metabolite, A77 1725, also known as M1. M1 inhibits dihydro-orotate dehydrogenase, an enzyme involved in the autoimmune process, which inhibits a key step in pyrimidine synthesis. Suppression of pyrimidine synthesis within T and B lymphocytes interferes with RNA and protein synthesis within the cells and prevents further cell-cycle progression. Reduced lymphocyte activity leads to reduced cytokine and antibody-mediated destruction of the synovial joints and decreases the inflammatory process. Symptoms may abate in as little as 4 to 12 weeks. Additionally, because of its unique mechanism of action, leflunomide may be used in conjunction with other drugs such as NSAIDs and other DMARDs.

Leflunomide is contraindicated in patients with severe hepatic insufficiency and in patients with diagnosed hepatitis B or hepatitis C. Leflunomide may increase concentrations of liver enzymes such as aspartate aminotransferase (AST) and alanine aminotransferase (ALT) and has been associated with inducing hepatotoxicity. Leflunomide also is contraindicated for use during pregnancy or breast-feeding. Leflunomide is a category X drug because it has been shown to induce fetal deformity. Women who have received leflunomide and wish to become pregnant must undergo a drug elimination process before conception. Cholestyramine (8 g) is administered three times a day for 11 days. The days do not have to be consecutive, but they must total 11 days. Plasma leflunomide levels are then evaluated twice, at least 14 days apart. The plasma drug level should be less than 0.02 mcg/mL before conception is attempted. Without this procedure, blood levels greater than 0.02 mcg/mL may persist for up to 2 years, depending on individual variations in clearance.

Patients with bone marrow dysplasia, immunodeficiency, or severe uncontrolled infections are poor candidates for leflunomide therapy. Vaccinations with live vaccines are not recommended during therapy.

Common adverse effects include nausea, diarrhea, increased AST and ALT levels, alopecia, rash, headache, and increased risk for immunosuppression and infections.

Potential drug interactions include cholestyramine, charcoal, rifampin, and drugs that induce hepatotoxicity. Women of childbearing age must take a reliable contraceptive agent while taking leflunomide therapy, because it is a pregnancy category X drug. Fortunately, it does not interact with triphasic oral contraceptives.

Minocycline

Minocycline (Minocin, Dynacin) is a tetracycline antibiotic. It is unclear exactly how minocycline exerts an effect on RA. One theory is that RA has a mycoplasma component to it, thus minocycline affects the mycoplasma. A second theory is that RA may reduce certain proteins that erode cartilage. It is used only for patients with mild RA symptoms. Adverse effects include nausea, dizziness, skin color changes, and rash (especially with sun exposure).

D-Penicillamine

Penicillamine (Cuprimine) is used in treating patients with early, mild, and nonerosive RA. Its antirheumatic action may result from its ability to inhibit the formation of collagen. Penicillamine also appears to depress circulating levels of IgM rheumatoid factor and immune complexes in serum and synovial fluid. It also may decrease cell-mediated immune response by selectively inhibiting T-lymphocyte function. In addition to its use as an antirheumatic drug, penicillamine is used as a chelating agent for removing excess copper from the blood of patients with Wilson disease and in reducing cystine excretion in patients with cystinuria. Optimal benefits may take 3 to 6 months.

Although penicillamine is a by-product of penicillin, it has no antibiotic activity. However, the possibility of cross-sensitization between penicillin and penicillamine exists; therefore, penicillamine should not be given to patients who are allergic to penicillin.

Penicillamine has potentially toxic adverse effects, including cutaneous lesions, blood dyscrasias, and a number of autoimmune disorders. Penicillamine is associated with a high incidence of potentially life-threatening adverse hematologic reactions because it depresses bone marrow function. Patients with a history of hematologic disorders or previous penicillamine-induced dyscrasias could experience these adverse reactions, which include leukopenia, thrombocytopenia, aplastic anemia, pancytopenia, sideroblastic anemia, agranulocytosis, and leukopenia. Penicillamine should be discontinued when the platelet count decreases to less than 100,000/mm^3, the leukocyte count decreases to less than 3,000/mm^3, or neutropenia occurs.

Rare but serious adverse effects are myasthenia gravis (MG) syndrome and obliterative bronchiolitis. Penicillamine should be discontinued at the first sign of ptosis or diplopia (signifying MG syndrome) or exertional dyspnea, cough, or wheezing (signifying obliterative bronchiolitis). These symptoms should be reported immediately.

In the renal system, penicillamine can induce hematuria and proteinuria, which may indicate an impending immune complex membranous glomerulonephritis. This condition can degenerate into nephrotic syndrome. Penicillamine should be discontinued when proteinuria values exceed 1 g per 24 hours.

The most common adverse effects involve the integumentary system. Rash and pruritus occurring in the first few months (early rash) are generally typical of drug hypersensitivity. Early rash usually disappears when the drug is discontinued. Late rash during therapy may be accompanied by intense pruritus, fever, arthralgia, or lymphadenopathy. This rash may take weeks to disappear. Patients may also develop exfoliative dermatitis, increased skin friability, vesicular ecchymoses, and pemphigus.

Penicillamine also can cause GI upset such as nausea, vomiting, anorexia, abdominal pain, and diarrhea. Patients with a history of peptic ulcer, hepatic dysfunction, and pancreatitis may experience reactivation of the disorder.

Because of the potential for adverse effects from penicillamine, patients should be taught carefully about this drug, including the signs and symptoms of potentially serious consequences. Inform female patients that this drug should not be taken if they are pregnant or breast-feeding. It also should not be taken by patients who have severe renal dysfunction or severe anemia; have taken penicillamine before and developed a high fever; or are taking gold salts by mouth or injection. Moreover, patients allergic to penicillin should not take penicillamine.

Explain minor side effects, such as change in taste, diarrhea, loss of appetite, nausea, vomiting, and stomach pain, and advise patients to discuss these effects with the health care team if the effects do not subside or are particularly annoying. Patients should learn to take penicillamine at least 1 hour before or 2 hours after eating food. Patients taking penicillamine for Wilson disease must avoid foods that contain copper, such as chocolate, nuts, liver, and broccoli. In addition, patients should drink plenty of water to prevent kidney stones from forming. Patients should avoid taking antacids and iron preparations because they may prevent the drug from working properly.

A missed dose should be taken as soon as possible, but if it is almost time for the next dose, only that dose should be taken (double or extra doses should never be taken). Instruct patients to continue to take penicillamine even if it appears that it is not working. Penicillamine should be stored away from moisture (particularly away from a bathroom) and out of the reach of children. Urge patients to schedule monthly blood and urine tests to make sure they are not having any adverse reactions to penicillamine.

Sulfasalazine

Sulfasalazine (Azulfidine) is a sulfonamide antibiotic that is considered a first-line treatment for both adult and juvenile RA. Sulfasalazine is a prodrug of sulfapyridine and mesalamine. Mesalamine inhibits cyclooxygenase, resulting in decreased production of arachidonic acid metabolites and reducing inflammation. Benefits occur in 1 to 3 months.

Sulfasalazine is contraindicated in patients with salicylate hypersensitivity, sulfonamide hypersensitivity, furosemide hypersensitivity, thiazide diuretic hypersensitivity, sulfonylurea hypersensitivity, or carbonic anhydrase inhibitor hypersensitivity, because it is broken down to a salicylate component and a sulfonamide component. It is also contraindicated for patients with intestinal or urinary obstruction and porphyria. It is given cautiously to patients with pre-existing megaloblastic anemia or glucose-6-phosphate dehydrogenase (G6PD) insufficiency because, as a sulfonamide, it decreases folate absorption.

The most common adverse reactions associated with Azulfidine EN-tabs are rash, anorexia, headache, nausea, vomiting, gastric distress, and reversible low sperm count. Serious adverse effects include suppressed bone marrow function and hepatitis. These potentially serious adverse effects require that a baseline CBC, renal function tests, and liver function tests be completed before initiation of therapy and repeated periodically throughout therapy.

Sulfasalazine is a pregnancy category B drug. Although sulfasalazine is not secreted in breast milk, one of its metabolites, sulfapyridine, does enter the milk. Sulfapyridine is generally considered safe except in stressed or ill infants, those with G6PD deficiency, and premature infants.

Drugs Significantly Different From P Methotrexate

Cyclophosphamide

Cyclophosphamide (Cytoxan) is an alkylating agent used primarily for its antitumor activity. Because of the oncogenicity associated with alkylating agents, cyclophosphamide is used primarily in severe, refractory RA and RA vasculitis. Cyclophosphamide is presented as the prototype alkylating agent in Chapter 57.

Cyclosporine

Cyclosporine (Neoral, Sandimmune, Gengraf) is an oral and parenteral immunosuppressive agent used most frequently to prevent organ transplant rejection. It is also approved to treat severe RA in patients unresponsive to conventional therapy, alone or in combination with MTX when the disease has not adequately responded to MTX. It is not generally used as monotherapy in RA because when used alone there is an 80% increase in the likelihood of myocardial infarction and stroke. The immunosuppressive effects of cyclosporine result from inhibiting proliferation of T lymphocytes, production and release of lymphokines, and release of IL-2. Optimal benefits may take 2 to 4 months. As the prototype immune modulator, cyclosporine is presented in depth in Chapter 54.

Glucocorticoid Steroids

Glucocorticoid steroids such as prednisone and prednisolone can be administered as oral or intravenous preparations for systemic effects and as an intra-articular injection for a local effect. They are generally given as "pulse therapy" for an acute exacerbation of RA. This approach allows a "resetting" of the inflammatory thermostat, improves the patient's symptoms, and allows other DMARDs to become active in suppressing joint destruction. Intermittent therapy also decreases the potential for serious adverse effects associated with steroids. Long-term steroid therapy, even at low doses, increases the risk for pneumonia in RA patients. Glucocorticoid steroids are discussed in depth in Chapter 48.

Ⓒ BIOLOGICAL DMARDS

Etanercept (Enbrel) is the first Tumor Necrosis Factor (TNF) inhibitor developed and the prototype TNF drug. It was produced by recombinant DNA technology. In the past, TNF inhibitors were used in patients who did not respond to MTX. Combination therapy with TNF inhibitors and MTX has exceptional results and is now considered the "gold standard" of RA treatment. Table 23.3 presents a summary of TNF and other biological drugs.

Nursing Management of the Patient Receiving Ⓟ Etanercept
Core Drug Knowledge
Pharmacotherapeutics

Etanercept is used in managing RA—to reduce signs and symptoms of the disease and to delay structural damage in patients with moderately to severely active RA. The drug is also indicated for reducing signs and symptoms of moderately to severely active polyarticular-course juvenile idiopathic RA (JIA), psoriatic arthritis, ankylosing spondylitis, and moderate to severe active plaque psoriasis..

Pharmacokinetics

Etanercept is a weekly subcutaneous injection. Its onset is slow and duration is uncertain. The pharmacokinetic profile is not affected by age or gender. Benefits from therapy can begin in a few days or may take up to 12 weeks.

Pharmacodynamics

In RA, activated T cells release inflammatory mediators called **cytokines,** including interleukins and tumor necrosis factor. TNF binds to TNF receptors on cellular membranes and triggers a cascade of inflammatory events that results in increased inflammation of the synovial membrane, the release of destructive lysosomal enzymes, and further joint destruction. Etanercept binds specifically to circulating TNF, prevents it from binding to TNF receptors on the cell membranes, and prevents the TNF-mediated cellular response.

Contraindications and Precautions

The only absolute contraindications to etanercept are hypersensitivity and current active infections. However, several cautions must be considered before using this drug. Etanercept has been associated with inducing sepsis and fatal infections in patients with predisposing diseases, such as advanced or poorly controlled diabetes. In addition, etanercept may induce demyelinating disorders such as multiple sclerosis, myelitis, and optic neuritis and should be used cautiously in patients with these disorders.

Because etanercept blocks the biological activity of TNF, it could potentially affect host defenses against infections and malignancy. The safety and efficacy of etanercept in patients with suppressed bone marrow function or other types of immunosuppression are not known. Live vaccines should be avoided during etanercept therapy because definitive clinical data on potential effects are not yet available.

Adverse Effects

Common adverse reactions to etanercept include injection-site reactions, upper respiratory infections, especially sinusitis, headache, nausea, and rhinitis. Less common but very

TABLE 25.3 Summary of Selected ⓖ Biological Drugs

Drug (Trade) Name	Selected Indications	Route and Dosage Range	Pharmacokinetics
Ⓟ etanercept (Enbrel)	RA	*Adult or child >62 kg:* SC, 50 mg/wk or 25 mg 2×/wk, 72–96 h apart *Child 4–17 y:* SC, <31 kg: 0.8 mg/kg weekly 31–62 kg: 0.8 mg/kg weekly given as 0.4 mg/kg ×2 in separate sites on the same day or 72–96 h apart	*Onset:* 2–4 wk *Duration:* Unknown $t_{1/2}$: 115 h
adalimumab (Humira)	RA, psoriasis, ankylosing spondylitis	*Adult:* SC, 40 mg every other week *Child >4y:* SC 20 mg every other week	*Onset:* 1–7 d *Duration:* Unknown $t_{1/2}$: 14 d
abatacept (Orencia)	RA	*Adult and Child >17y:* IV <60 kg: 500 mg initially, repeat dose at 2 and 4 wk then monthly 60–100 kg: 750 mg initially, repeat dose at 2 wk and 4 wk then monthly >100 kg: 1000 mg initially, repeat dose at 2 and 4 wk then monthly	*Onset:* unknown *Duration:* unknown $t_{1/2}$: 13 days
anakinra (Kineret)	RA	*Adult:* SC, 100 mg daily *Child:* not approved	*Onset:* Slow *Duration:* Unknown $t_{1/2}$: 4–6 h
certolizumab pegol (Cimzia)	RA Crohn's Diesease	*Adult:* SC 200 mg wk 2 and 4; maintenance 200 mg every other week *Adult:* SC 400 mg every other week	*Onset:* unknown *Duration:* unknown $t_{1/2}$: 14 d
golimumab (Simponi)	RA Psoriatic arthritis Ankylosing Spondylitis	*Adult:* SC 50 mg monthly *Child:* not approved	
infliximab (Remicade)	RA Psoriasis, Crohn's disease, ankylosing spondylitis	*Adult:* IV, 3 mg/kg every 8 wk *Adult:* IV, 5 mg/kg every 6–8 wk	*Onset:* 3–7 d *Duration:* 6–12 wk $t_{1/2}$: 9.5 d
Rituximab (Rituxan)	RA	*Adult IV:* 1000 mg, repeat in 2 wk	*Onset:* unknown *Duration:* 3–6 mo $t_{1/2}$: 59.8 h
tocilizumab (Actemra)	RA	*Adult:* IV 4 mg/kg over 1 h every 4-wk; increase to 8 mg/kg based on clinical response *Child:* not approved	*Onset:* unknown *Duration:* unknown $t_{1/2}$: 11–13 d

serious adverse effects include severe infections; induction of multiple sclerosis; seizure activity; optic neuritis; blood dyscrasias; new or recurrent heart failure; psoriasis; lupus-like syndrome; and hepatitis..

There are three important black box warnings for all TNF inhibitors, including etanercept. The first is a reminder to weigh the treatment benefits and risk in patients with chronic or recurrent infections; pulmonary and extrapulmonary TB, invasive fungal infections (i.e., histoplasmosis, coccidiomycosis, and blastomycosis), and other opportunistic infections. The second is an increased risk for lymphoma and other malignancies, especially in children and adolescents. In addition, all TNF inhibitors, including etanercept, may induce hepatosplenic T-cell lymphoma (HSTCL), a rare type of cancer. HSTCL has occurred most frequently in teenagers or young adults, who also have either Crohn disease or ulcerative colitis and concurrently receiving azathioprine or 6-mercaptopurine.

Drug Interactions

Etanercept interacts with many of the other drugs used to treat RA and psoriasis, especially other biologic DMARDS. Coadministration with other TNF inhibitors does not increase the effectiveness of treatment but substantially increases the risk for severe infections. Table 25.4 presents potential drug interactions with etanercept.

Assessment of Relevant Core Patient Variables

Health Status

Assess the patient for comorbid states or drugs that contradict the use of etanercept or require close monitoring.

TABLE 25.4	Agents That Interact with [P] Etanercept	
Interactants	**Effect and Significance**	**Nursing Management**
abatacept	Coadministration increases the risk for serious infections.	Monitor CBC. Monitor for signs of myelosuppression. Assess lung sounds daily. Use aseptic technique consistently. Caution patient to refrain from contact with people who are ill.
anakinra	Coadministration increases the risk of serious infections and neutropenia.	Same as abatacept
cyclophosphamide	Coadministration increases the risk of noncutaneous solid malignancy.	Monitor CBC. Monitor ESR.
imatinib	Coadministration increases the risk of myelosuppression.	Same as abatacept
natalizumab	Coadministration increases the risk of serious infections, including PML.	Monitor for clumsiness, progressive weakness, visual or speech changes, and personality changes.
TNF Inhibitors	Coadministration increases the risk of serious infections.	Same as abatacept
sulfasalazine	Coadministration may decrease neutrophil count.	Same as abatacept
Live-vaccines	Coadministration decreases immunologic response and increases risk of disseminated infections.	Do not administer

Assess for rubber or latex allergy because the needle covers of the syringe contain dry natural rubber. Assess for a history of recurrent infections, pulmonary or extrapulmonary TB, invasive fungal infections or malignancies. Convey any positive response to the healthcare provider immediately.

Complete a thorough physical examination, carefully evaluating for signs of infection, suppressed bone marrow function, and adventitious lung sounds. Complete a baseline neurologic examination. Document the severity of joint inflammation and any restriction in range of motion as a baseline for later comparison to assess the efficacy of etanercept therapy.

Before beginning therapy, document the results of a TB skin test (PPD), complete blood count (CBC), urinalysis, tests for C-reactive protein level and ESR, hepatitis screen, and chest x-ray. Coordinate serial laboratory testing. Assess the patient's willingness to adhere to close monitoring.

Lifespan and Gender
Etanercept is a pregnancy category B drug. Whether it is excreted into breast milk or has potential risks to the infant is unknown. Etanercept is not approved for use in children under the age of 4 years. Assess the immunization status of children; vaccinations should be avoided during therapy.

Lifestyle, Diet, and Habits
As with MTX, evaluate the nutritional status of the patient; malnourished patients are more likely than others to be immunosuppressed or have blood dyscrasias.

Environment
Etanercept is generally administered in the home environment. Assess if the patient lives with or has close contact with anyone with active tuberculosis.

Nursing Diagnoses and Outcomes
• Risk for Infection related to potential depression of bone marrow function and blood dyscrasias
  Desired outcome: The patient will recognize signs of depressed bone marrow function and blood dyscrasias and contact the health care provider immediately for intervention if any appear.
• Comfort Impaired: Nausea related to drug therapy
  Desired outcome: The patient will eat small, frequent meals when nauseated to maintain nutritional balance.

Planning and Intervention
Maximizing Therapeutic Effects
Administer etanercept weekly as prescribed. Rotate the injection site between the middle of the thigh, on the abdomen except around the navel, and the back outer area of the upper arm. Do not inject within one inch of the previous injection. Avoid areas that are tender, red, or hard. Keep the medication refrigerated.

Minimizing Adverse Effects
Use aseptic technique when administering etanercept. Do not administer if the drug solution is discolored, cloudy, or contains particles. Avoid placing hospitalized patients taking etanercept in the same room with other patients who

have colds, the flu, or other contagious illnesses. Do not administer live-virus vaccines.

Providing Patient and Family Education

- Advise the patient to read the accompanying Medication Guide with each administration of etanercept.
- Teach the patient to report symptoms of possible adverse effects to the healthcare provider:
  - CNS symptoms: numbness or tingling to extremities, vision changes, weakness in arms or legs dizziness
  - Infection: fever, sweat, or chills; muscle aches; red, warm or painful skin or abscess formation; diarrhea; dysuria, fatigue
  - Blood dyscrasias: fever, bruising, bleeding easily, or looking pale.
  - Heart failure: shortness of breath, swelling in lower legs and feet
  - Psoriasis: red scaly patches or hard raised bumps
  - Lupus-like syndrome: rash to face and arms that intensifies in sunlight
  - Hepatitis B infection: fatigue, jaundice, anorexia, vomiting, right upper quadrant pain, muscle aches, dark urine, clay-colored feces, fever or chills.
  - TB: anorexia, weight loss, night sweats, cough, fatigue, chest pain, shortness of breath
- Teach aseptic technique to patients for the subcutaneous injection. Instruct the patient how to use SureClick auto injector if ordered.
- For patients using the multi-dose vial, teach patients to roll the vial, rather than shake it, when administering the drug.
- Instruct patients to use puncture-resistant containers to dispose of needles and syringes.
- Assist the patient to prepare a chart of injection sites to ensure regular rotation of sites.
- Explain the potential for an injection site reaction such as redness, rash, swelling, itching, or bruising. Assure patients that these reactions usually disappear within 3 to 5 days. If they do not, patients should contact their health care provider.
- Teach patients the importance of contacting their health care provider before taking any other prescription medication, or OTC medicines, including vitamins, minerals, and herbal products.
- Stress the importance of avoiding others with coughs, colds, or flu.
- Urge patients to refrain from receiving live-vaccinations while taking etanercept.
- Explain the importance of follow-up with the health care provider to evaluate the efficacy of therapy and monitor for adverse effects.

Ongoing Assessment and Evaluation

Assess patients taking etanercept for improved range of motion, decreased early morning stiffness, and painful or swollen joints. Assess patients each visit for potential

adverse effects to etanercept, especially for signs infection, TB or malignancies. Coordinate laboratory testing for CBC, C-reactive protein levels, and ESR. Review aseptic technique at each visit. Evaluate the efficacy of etanercept therapy; successful etanercept therapy is demonstrated by decreased RA symptoms and an absence of adverse effects.

Drugs Closely Related to P Etanercept
Adalimumab

Adalimumab (Humira) is a TNF inhibitor approved for the management of RA, idiopathic juvenile arthritis, psoriatic arthritis, plaque psoriasis, ankylosing spondylitis, and Crohn's disease. Adalimumab differs from etanercept because it is a **monoclonal antibody** (a cell that is produced with the ability to recognize and bind to a specific antigen) that specifically inhibits the activity of TNF-alpha. It may be given as monotherapy or in combination with other DMARDS. Adalimumab is administered biweekly. Assessment (including baseline labs), contraindications and precautions, adverse effects and patient teaching are the same as etanercept and it carries the same Black Box warnings. The most common adverse effects associated with adalimumab are injection site reactions, upper respiratory infections such as sinusitis, headaches, rash, and nausea. Risk for hepatosplenic T-cell lymphoma. It is available in a prefilled syringe or pen. Advise the patient to return the syringe to the pharmacy if the solution is cloudy or contains large particles. Advise the patient not to use adalimumab if the syringe or pen was frozen or left in direct sunlight. Adalimumab is a pregnancy category B.

Certolizumab Pegol

Certolizumab pegol (Cimzia) is another TNF inhibitor that is a monoclonal antibody. It approved for the management of RA and Crohn's disease. Certolizumab is the only PEGlyated

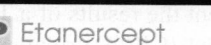

MEMORY CHIP

P Etanercept

- Disease-modifying antirheumatic drug (DMARD) used in combination with methotrexate to decrease the progression of RA
- Major contraindications: immunosuppression, blood dyscrasias, infections
- Most common adverse effects: nausea, headache, upper respiratory infections, injection site reactions
- Most serious adverse effects: severe infections, blood dyscrasias
- Maximizing therapeutic effects: rotate site of injection
- Minimizing adverse effects: Use aseptic technique for injections.
- Most important patient education: high risk for severe infection. Be sure to contact the health care provider if they occur.
- **Black box warning: Risk/benefit ratio due to serious infections and malignancies. Increased risk for lymphoma with children and adolescents**

TNF inhibitor currently on the market. PEGylation provides a protective barrier around part of the medication that allows it to remain in the body longer. After initial administration of certolizumab, it is repeated at weeks 2 and 4. Maintenance is then monthly thereafter. Like adalimumab, assessment, contraindications and precautions, adverse effects and patient teaching are the same as etanercept and it carries the same Black Box warnings. The most common adverse effects with certolizumab are upper respiratory infections such as flu or colds, urinary tract infections, and rash. It is available in a prefilled syringe that should be kept refrigerated. Advise the patient to return the syringe to the pharmacy if the solution is cloudy or contains visible particles. Teach the patient to allow certolizumab to reach room temperature before self-administration. Advise the patient not to use certolizumab if the syringe was frozen or left in direct sunlight. Certolizumab is a pregnancy category B.

Golimumab

Golimumab (Simponi) is the newest monoclonal antibody TNF inhibitor on the market. It is approved for the treatment of RA (in combination with MTX), active psoriatic arthritis, and active ankylosing spondylitis. Golimumab is administered monthly. Like other TNF inhibitors, assessment, contraindications and precautions, adverse effects and patient teaching are the same as etanercept and it carries the same Black Box warnings. The most common adverse effects associated with golimumab are upper respiratory infections, colds/flu, sinusitis, rhinitis, bronchitis, hypertension, injection site reactions, abnormal liver function tests, nausea, and paresthesias. Golimumab is available in a prefilled syringe or SmartJect autoinjector. Teach the patient to remove the prefilled syringe or SmartJect autoinjector from the refrigerator 30 minutes before administration. Advise the patient that it is normal to see tiny particles in the solution but not to use if the solution is cloudy or contains large particles. Golimumab is a pregnancy category B

Infliximab

Infliximab (Remicade) is another monoclonal antibody TNF inhibitor approved for the management of moderate to severe active RA, ankylosing spondylitis, psoriatic arthritis, plaque psoriasis, and Crohn's disease or ulcerative colitis, in patients unresponsive to other therapy. In patients with RA, it is given concurrently with MTX. Infliximab is administered intravenously at weeks 0, 2, and 6, then every 6 to 8 weeks as maintenance. Like other TNF inhibitors, assessment, contraindications and precautions, adverse effects and patient teaching are the same as etanercept and it carries the same Black Box warnings. The most common adverse effects associated with infliximab are respiratory infections such as sinus infections and sore throat, headache, rash, cough, and abdominal pain. Children with Crohn's disease on infliximab therapy frequently experienced anemia, neutropenia, leukopenia, viral and bacterial infections, flushing, bone fractures, and melena.

Infuse infliximab over at least 2 hours. Infliximab is a pregnancy category B.

Drugs Significantly Different From [P] Etanercept

Abatacept

Abatacept (Orencia) is a T cell costimulation blocking agent. It is given by intravenous infusion over 30 minutes; this is repeated 2 and 4 weeks after the first infusion and every 4 weeks thereafter. It was developed specifically to manage moderate to severe RA as monotherapy or in combination with other DMARDs, although it should not be given with TNF inhibitors or anakinra. Fully activated T-lymphocytes are implicated in the pathogenesis of RA and are found in the synovium of patients with RA. Abatacept binds to specific receptors on the antigen-presenting cell and prevents optimal T-cell activation.

Contraindications and precautions of abatacept are similar to those of etanercept, with the addition of cautious administration to elderly patients because, due to their age, they have a higher risk of infection and malignancy. Infusion-related adverse effects include hypotension, hypertension, dyspnea, nausea, flushing, urticaria, cough, hypersensitivity, pruritus, rash, and wheezing. Like other biologicals, abatacept may cause serious infections and malignancy.

Abatacept is a pregnancy category C drug and not recommended for use in women who are breast-feeding. It is not approved for use in children.

Anakinra

Anakinra (Kineret), a recombinant form of the human interleukin-1 receptor antagonist (IL-1Ra), is produced by recombinant DNA technology. It is approved for use in patients with moderate to severe active RA who have unsuccessfully tried therapy with one or more DMARDs. It is administered as a subcutaneous injection. Therapeutic response occurs in 1 to 3 weeks.

Anakinra acts similarly to the native IL-1Ra. IL-1 and TNF are the primary proinflammatory cytokines associated with RA. IL-1 plays a dominant role in cartilage damage and bone resorption in rheumatoid arthritis, whereas TNF-alpha is more responsible for inflammation. By antagonizing IL-1, stimulation of osteoclasts is decreased, resulting in decreased bone resorption and joint destruction.

Anakinra is contraindicated in patients with hypersensitivity to Escherichia coli protein. It is also contraindicated in immunocompromised patients because it further decreases the immune response. The drug is administered as a subcutaneous injection, and the needle cover of the syringe contains latex, which may cause reactions in patients (and health care workers) with latex hypersensitivity. Anakinra should not be given to patients with an active infection, because the risk of infection is increased during therapy. It should be given cautiously to patients with pre-existing renal dysfunction because it is renally excreted. Live-virus vaccines should not be administered during anakinra therapy because of the drug's effects on the immune response.

Common adverse effects include headache, sinusitis, abdominal pain, diarrhea, upper respiratory infection, and injection site reactions. More serious adverse effects include neutropenia and severe infections.

Anakinra is a pregnancy category B drug. It is unclear whether it is secreted in breast milk. Safety and efficacy have not been established for children.

Rituximab

Rituximab (Rituxan) is a monoclonal antibody B cell depleting agent. The depletion of B cells has been shown to be effective in reducing signs and symptoms of RA and in slowing radiographic progression. It is approved for use in patients with RA who have not responded to TNF inhibitors and those with non-Hodgkin's lymphoma. Effects from rituximab are not seen for up to 3 months after an infusion, however, may last between 6 months and 2 years following a single infusion course. It is used off-label for chronic lymphoid leukemia, thrombocytopenic purpura, and Waldenström's macroglobulinemia (a type of cancer of the blood).

Rituximab has many severe adverse effects. It has Black Box warnings regarding fatal infusion reactions, tumor lysis syndrome, and severe mucocutaneous reactions, as well as progressive multifocal leukoencephalopathy, a viral infection of the brain caused by reactivated JC virus, which is present in about 80% of adults. Rituximab is a prototype monoclonal antibody presented in Chapter 55.

Tocilizumab

Tocilizumab (Actemra) is a monoclonal antibody interleukin-6 receptor antagonist specifically developed for the treatment of RA. IL-6 has been identified as having a fundamental role in the inflammation process in RA. Tocilizumab is used for the management of adult patients with moderate to severe RA who are unable to take or have had an inadequate response to MTX or other DMARDS. Studies of tocilizumab have been promising. The AMBITION trial demonstrated that monotherapy with tocilizumab is more efficacious than monotherapy with MTX (Jones, 2010). In addition the OPTION study concluded that combination therapy with tocilizumab and MTX is more effective than MTX monotherapy in inhibiting the progression of structural joint damage in rheumatoid arthritis (Garnero, Thompson, Woodworth, et al., 2010). The RADIATE trial concluded that tocilizumab, in combination with MTX, was able to achieve and maintain improvement in RA symptoms in patients with an inadequate response to TNF-inhibitors

(Emery, Keystone, Tony, 2008). Because tocilizumab is a monoclonal antibody, assessment, contraindications and precautions, adverse effects and patient teaching are the same as etanercept and it carries the same Black Box warnings. The most common adverse effects to tocilizumab include upper respiratory tract infection, nasopharyngitis, headache, increased AST/ALT, and hypertension. Tocilizumab is given intravenously every 4 weeks. It is a pregnancy category C.

ANTIGOUT DRUGS

Antigout drugs are used to treat an acute attack of gout, prevent or decrease the frequency of flares, and prevent complications associated with the development of tophi. As previously explained, gout is associated with hyperuricemia, although it may occur in patients with normal uric acid levels. Hyperuricemia occurs either because of increased uric acid production or by accumulation of uric acid because of decreased renal excretion. Antigout drug therapy focuses on either decreasing the inflammatory response caused by hyperuricemia or on reducing hyperuricemia itself.

DRUGS FOR TREATING ACUTE GOUT

As previously mentioned, the first-line drugs for acute gouty arthritis are NSAIDs. The most common NSAID used is indomethacin, however, ibuprofen, naproxen, piroxicam, sulindac, and ketoprofen are also effective. NSAIDS are continued for at least 24 hours after the resolution of the acute attack and then taped over 2 to 3 days. For patients who are unable to take NSAIDs or those who respond inadequately, second-line drugs are colchicine and glucocorticosteroids. Colchicine (Colcrys) is the prototype for the management of acute gout (Table 25.5)

Nursing Management of the Patient Receiving P Colchicine
Core Drug Knowledge
Pharmacotherapeutics
The most common use of colchicine is for treating acute gouty arthritis and as presurgical prophylaxis to prevent gout. A short course of colchicine may be given when uricosuric drug therapy is initiated to prevent a flare-up of gout symptoms. It is occasionally effective for other types of arthritis. Non–FDA-approved uses of colchicine include

TABLE 25.5	Summary of Selected Antigout Drugs			
Drug (Trade) Name	Selected Indications	Route and Dosage Range	Pharmacokinetics
colchicine (Colcrys)	Acute gouty arthritis	*Adult PO:* 1.2 mg initially, then 0.6 1 h later max: 1.8 mg per attack	*Onset:* PO, 0.5–2 h *Duration:* PO, unknown; $t_{1/2}$: PO, 20 min
	Gout prophylaxis	*Adult:* PO, 0.6 2x/d *Child:* Safety and efficacy not established	

treatment of amyloidosis, Behçet syndrome, biliary cirrhosis, hepatic cirrhosis, Mediterranean fever, and scleroderma, as well as prophylaxis for recurrent pericarditis.

Pharmacokinetics

Colchicine can be given either orally or intravenously. However, parenteral use is avoided because of potential toxicity. Colchicine should never be injected subcutaneously or intramuscularly because such injections cause severe local irritation. Oral colchicine is rapidly absorbed, metabolized in the liver, and excreted primarily in the feces, with 10% to 20% eliminated unchanged in the urine. Patients with hepatic disease may have increased renal elimination. Enterohepatic recirculation occurs to a large extent and can lead to adverse GI effects with larger dosages. Colchicine distributes to the kidney, liver, spleen, and intestinal tissues and concentrates primarily in the leukocytes. It can be found in leukocytes for 10 days after administration.

Pharmacodynamics

Colchicine possesses anti-inflammatory properties. Although it is highly effective in treating acute gouty arthritis, it is not an effective analgesic for other types of pain, nor does it affect uric acid clearance. Colchicine inhibits the activity of leukocytes by decreasing their migration into the affected area, resulting in an interruption of the cyclic inflammatory response. Another action of colchicine is to prevent the release of an inflammatory glycoprotein from phagocytes, although it does not inhibit phagocytosis of uric acid crystals. Additional pharmacologic actions of colchicine include lowering body temperature, suppressing the respiratory center, and vasomotor stimulation, leading to hypertension. These actions can be extremely serious in cases of overdose.

Contraindications and Precautions

Colchicine is contraindicated in patients with severe cardiac disease, hepatic disease, and renal disease because these patients are at risk for developing cumulative toxicity. Other patients at risk for cumulative toxicity are elderly or debilitated patients. These patients should be monitored closely.

Patients with renal impairment or elevated plasma levels of colchicine because of renal disease can develop a myoneuropathy characterized by proximal weakness and elevated serum creatine kinase levels. This reaction usually occurs in patients who have been taking colchicine for several years; however, it is prudent to monitor all patients with renal insufficiency for this reaction.

Colchicine is eliminated primarily through the biliary pathway. Patients with hepatic disease should be monitored closely during treatment with colchicine. Additionally, patients at risk for hepatic disease, such as those with alcoholism, should be monitored closely.

Colchicine should be used cautiously in patients with pre-existing GI disease or depressed bone marrow function. These patients are at a higher risk for adverse effects of colchicine.

Patients with myelosuppression are at risk for infections or bleeding. Dental work should be performed before initiating colchicine therapy or deferred until blood counts return to normal.

Oral colchicine is classified as a pregnancy category C drug, and parenteral colchicine is in pregnancy category D.

Adverse Effects

The most common adverse effects of colchicine affect the GI tract. Up to 80% of patients taking colchicine may experience nausea, vomiting, diarrhea, abdominal pain, and paralytic ileus. These reactions can indicate toxicity, and the drug should be discontinued until the symptoms resolve.

Long-term therapy with colchicine may depress bone marrow function, inducing aplastic anemia, pancytopenia, thrombocytopenia, leukopenia, or agranulocytosis. Patients receiving parenteral colchicine experience depressed bone marrow function more frequently than do patients receiving the drug orally. Signs and symptoms of serious adverse reactions that must be reported to the prescriber include fever, chills, or sore throat; wheezing or difficulty breathing; muscle weakness; numbness or tingling in hands and feet; skin rash, itching; stomach pain; swelling of face or mouth; unusual bleeding, bruising, and pinpoint red spots on skin; and unusual tiredness or weakness.

Other adverse effects include renal, integumentary, hematologic, and endocrinologic effects. In the renal system, potential adverse effects are bladder spasms, nephrotoxicity, proteinuria, hematuria, anuria, and acute renal failure. Integumentary effects include angioedema, urticaria, injection-site reaction, skin necrosis, tissue necrosis, and median nerve neuritis. Effects on the endocrine system can include hypothyroidism.

Acute colchicine poisoning is a rare adverse effect. Symptoms include gastroenteritis, hypotension, lactic acidosis, and prerenal azotemia.

Drug Interactions

Colchicine can enhance the effects of radiation therapy or drugs that depress bone marrow function. Colchicine also may interact with cyanocobalamin (vitamin B_{12}), cyclosporine, erythromycin, and NSAIDs. Colchicine use may interfere with certain test results, yielding a false-positive finding when assessing for hemoglobin in urine. Table 25.6 presents potential drug interactions with colchicine.

Assessment of Relevant Core Patient Variables

Health Status

Assess the patient for potential medical conditions or drugs that contradict the use of colchicine or require close patient monitoring. Assess the joints for edema, erythema, or increased warmth. In addition, assess for signs of hypothyroidism. Obtain a baseline CBC, platelet count, and tests for renal and hepatic function.

Life Span and Gender

Determine whether a female patient is pregnant or breastfeeding. Because oral colchicine is classified as a pregnancy

TABLE 25.6	Agents That Interact with 🅿 Colchicine	
Interactants	**Effect and Significance**	**Nursing Management**
agents that cause bone marrow suppression	Drugs possessing hematoxic properties similar to those of gold salts may potentiate the action of both agents, resulting in bone marrow suppression.	Avoid coadministration if possible. Monitor complete blood count (CBC) and platelet count frequently. Monitor patient for sore throat, chills, easy bruising, or bleeding tendencies.
cyclosporine	Cyclosporine may cause hyperuricemia. Concomitant use of cyclosporine and colchicine may also increase cyclosporine concentrations, resulting in a high risk of nephrotoxicity.	Avoid coadministration, if possible. Monitor blood urea nitrogen, creatinine, and cyclosporine levels. Monitor intake and output.
macrolide antibiotics	The addition of macrolide antibiotics to colchicine therapy may lead to colchicine toxicity.	Monitor for fever, gastrointestinal (GI) symptoms, myalgia, and leukopenia.
ethanol (alcohol)	Ethanol ingestion increases the risk of adverse GI effects and can increase serum urate concentration, thus decreasing the antigout effects of colchicine.	Avoid alcohol ingestion during therapy. Monitor for effectiveness of colchicine.
nonsteroidal anti-inflammatory drugs (NSAIDs)	Concomitant use of NSAIDs and colchicine increases the likelihood of developing adverse GI effects, especially ulceration or hemorrhage.	Avoid coadministration. Monitor for adverse GI effects. Monitor for easy bruising or bleeding.

category C drug, it should be avoided by pregnant or breast-feeding women. Parenteral colchicine, in pregnancy category D, should never be administered to pregnant or breast-feeding women.

Lifestyle, Diet, and Habits

Evaluate the patient's diet. High consumption of red meat products and seafood confers a high risk of hyperuricemia and resultant gout. Dairy products, vegetables, nuts, legumes, fruits (with minimal sugar), and whole grains may help prevent gout by reducing insulin resistance. (Choi, 2010). Also, evaluate the patient's intake of alcohol and beer. Alcohol can cause both overproduction and underexcretion of uric acid. Beer contains a high content of the purine guanosine, which increases the uric acid level. Assess the patient's fluid intake, because dehydration can trigger acute gout attacks. It is important to ensure that the patient consumes adequate amounts of fluids. Plasma uric acid levels rise during starvation. Therefore, ensure that the patient eats at regular intervals throughout the day.

Environment

Be aware that colchicine is self-administered most frequently by patients in the home environment. Patients are advised to take the drug three to four times a day unless nausea, vomiting, or diarrhea occurs, or the maximum dose for one day is reached. In special circumstances, colchicine can be given intravenously in an acute care setting. However, this is rarely done because of colchicine's narrow therapeutic margin and because the drug has been associated with induction of aplastic anemia, which can result in death.

Nursing Diagnoses and Outcomes

- Acute Pain related to drug-induced abdominal cramps or paralytic ileus
  Desired outcome: The patient will contact the prescriber if abdominal pain occurs.
- Risk for Injury related to drug-induced renal toxicity or possible extravasation of IV colchicine
  Desired outcome: The patient administering colchicine at home will contact the prescriber if urinary changes occur. The hospitalized patient will remain free of extravasation of IV colchicine.
- Risk for Deficient Fluid Volume related to drug-induced nausea, vomiting, and diarrhea
  Desired outcome: The patient will contact the prescriber if GI symptoms occur.
- Ineffective Protection related to possible blood dyscrasias
  Desired outcome: The patient will contact the prescriber if sore throat, easy bruising, or lethargy occurs.

Planning and Intervention

Maximizing Therapeutic Effects

In an acute care setting, administer colchicine with a full glass of water at evenly spaced intervals throughout the day. Patients who self-administer the drug should follow the regimen prescribed by the health care provider. Generally, patients who have less than one attack per year take low-dose colchicine 3 or 4 days a week. For patients with more frequent attacks, colchicine is taken daily. Adherence to diet and alcohol restrictions decreases hyperuricemia, thus allowing colchicine to achieve its maximum effect.

Minimizing Adverse Effects

Closely monitor patients with pre-existing medical conditions or those on drug therapy that may interact with colchicine. For an acute attack, the patient needs to take colchicine at the first sign of an acute gout attack.

It is important to question the female patient about the possibility of pregnancy before administering intravenous colchicine. Administer intravenous colchicine cautiously and monitor frequently for signs of extravasation.

Providing Patient and Family Education

- Advise patients not to take colchicine if they have severe cardiac disease, hepatic disease, or renal disease.
- Make sure that pregnant or breast-feeding patients are not given intravenous colchicine.
- Advise patients to take colchicine at the first sign of a gout attack and to follow the directions on the drug container.
- Tell patients that if they miss a dose, they should take it as soon as they can. If it is almost time for the next dose, only that dose should be taken; patients should not take double or extra doses.
- Emphasize that colchicine can cause minor side effects, such as loss of appetite and hair loss, and that patients should tell their health care teams if the adverse effects do not go away or if they are particularly annoying.
- Caution patients to report GI adverse effects (e.g., nausea, vomiting, diarrhea, and abdominal pain) because these symptoms could indicate drug toxicity or lead to fluid loss over time.
- Stress to patients that colchicine can cause serious adverse effects and that they should call their prescribers immediately if any signs and symptoms occur, including sore throat, easy bruising, lethargy, or signs of renal toxicity.
- Advise patients to avoid alcohol because it can cause stomach problems and increase uric acid concentrations in the blood, making a gouty attack more likely. Review foods that are high in purines to decrease dietary intake of uric acid.
- Inform patients that colchicine may produce severe adverse effects when coadministered with many prescription and OTC drugs and advise them never to take any other drugs without consulting their prescribers.
- Tell patients to keep colchicine away from light and out of the reach of children.
- Stress that patients must see their health care teams every month for blood and urine tests to make sure that they are not experiencing adverse effects from colchicine.

Ongoing Assessment and Evaluation

Monitor for hematopoietic and renal toxicity, joint involvement, deformity, and range of motion. The patient needs to be monitored for efficacy of colchicine therapy.

Therapy is considered effective if the patient reports decreased frequency of acute gout attacks and remains free of adverse effects. The patient should understand and be able

MEMORY CHIP

P Colchicine

- Decreases the inflammatory reaction of **acute** gout
- Major contraindications: severe cardiac, hepatic, or renal diseases
- Most common adverse effects: related to gastrointestinal system
- Most serious adverse effects: blood dyscrasias, including bone marrow suppression
- Maximizing therapeutic effects: adherence to diet and alcohol restrictions to reduce hyperuricemia
- Minimizing adverse effects: Take colchicine at the first sign of an attack, then only until the symptoms start to resolve.
- Most important patient education: related to diet and alcohol restrictions

to explain the importance of contacting the health care team immediately if any adverse effects occur, of scheduling periodic hematologic and renal testing, and of contacting the prescriber before taking any other prescription or OTC drugs.

Drugs Significantly Different From P Colchicine

Glucocorticoid steroids are also prescribed for acute gout. They may be given orally or as an intra-articular injection. Teach patients taking oral steroids to follow the health care provider's instructions carefully and never abruptly stop the medication. Explain the process of tapering the drug to avoid complications. For patients receiving an intra-articular injection, teach them to avoid overuse of the joint until the acute attack is resolved. For in-depth coverage of glucocorticoid steroids, see Chapter 48.

• DRUGS FOR GOUT PROPHYLAXIS

Uricosuric drugs balance urate concentration. Because they have no anti-inflammatory or analgesic activity, they are not useful in treating acute gout attacks. In fact, when first initiated, they can exacerbate an acute attack of gout. Uricosuric drugs include allopurinol, probenecid, and sulfinpyrazone. Allopurinol (Zyloprim, Lopurin) is the prototype uricosuric drug. Table 25.7 presents a summary of uricosuric drugs.

Nursing Management of the Patient Receiving P Allopurinol

Core Drug Knowledge

Pharmacotherapeutics

Allopurinol is indicated for the management of chronic gout, recurrent calcium renal stones, and hyperuricemia related to cancer or tumor lysis syndrome. Off-label uses include prevention of ischemic reperfusion tissue damage and arrhythmias in patients who have undergone

TABLE 25.7	Summary of Selected Ⓒ Uricosuric Drugs		
Ⓟ allopurinol (Zyloprim)	Gout Prophylaxis	Adult: PO, 200–600 mg/d divided 2–4× d Child: Not approved	Onset: 30 min–1 h Duration: 18–30 h $t_{1/2}$: 1–2 h; metabolite, 18–30 h
febuxostat	Gout Prophylaxis	Adult: PO 40–80 mg daily Child: Not approved	Onset: rapid Duration: unknown T1/2: 5–8 h
probenecid (Benemid;	Gout Prophylaxis	Adult: PO, 500 mg 2× d Child: Not approved	Onset: 30 min Duration: 3–8 h $t_{1/2}$: 4–7 h
sulfinpyrazone (Anturane)	Chronic gout, inhibition of platelet aggregation	Adult: PO 100–400 mg 2× d Child: Safety and efficacy not established	Onset: 30 min Duration: 4–6 h $t_{1/2}$: 3 h
Combination Drugs			
probenecid and colchicine (ColBenemid, Col-Probenecid, Proben-C)	Chronic gout	Adult: PO, 1 tablet 2×/d (500 mg probenecid and 0.5 mg colchicine)	See individual drugs

coronary artery bypass surgery; decrease in Helicobacter pylori–induced duodenal ulcer recurrence rates; treatment of hematemesis from NSAID-induced erosive gastritis; decrease in pain in patients with acute pancreatitis; and reduction of renal transplant rejection in patients receiving triple immunosuppressive therapy.

Pharmacokinetics

Allopurinol may be administered orally or intravenously. When given orally, approximately 90% is absorbed. It is widely distributed except to the central nervous system. It undergoes hepatic metabolism and is rapidly oxidized to oxypurinol. Both the parent drug and oxypurinol have renal elimination.

Pharmacodynamics

Allopurinol decreases the production of uric acid by inhibiting the action of xanthine oxidase, an enzyme that converts hypoxanthine to xanthine and xanthine to uric acid. Because of the decrease in uric acid concentration, there are fewer urate deposits, a circumstance which prevents or decreases tophi formation, chronic joint changes, and the formation of uric acid or calcium oxalate calculi.

Contraindications and Precautions

The only contraindication to allopurinol is hypersensitivity. The drug should be given cautiously to patients who cannot sustain a fluid intake of 2 L/d (e.g., those with CHF), because increased fluid intake is required to avoid complications such as formation of xanthine calculi or renal precipitation of urates. Other precautions include decreased renal or liver function. Care should be used in patients taking thiazide diuretics or drugs that may induce myelosuppression such as azathioprine.

Adverse Effects

Therapeutic dosages of allopurinol are generally well tolerated, with few adverse effects. The most common adverse effects include pruritus, maculopapular rash, nausea and vomiting, elevated liver function tests, and acute gout symptoms. Serious adverse effects include blood dyscrasias, myelosuppression, hepatic or renal toxicity, exfoliative dermatitis, and Stevens-Johnson syndrome.

Drug Interactions

Allopurinol interacts with many drugs that increase the potential for a hypersensitivity reaction to allopurinol. Allopurinol interacts with many immunosuppressive and cytotoxic drugs, resulting in an increased risk of myelosuppression. Table 25.8 presents potential drug interactions.

Assessment of Relevant Core Patient Variables

Health Status

Assess the patient for potential medical conditions or drug therapies that contraindicate the use of allopurinol or require close patient monitoring. Obtain baseline CBC, uric acid level, liver function tests, and metabolic profile. Document baseline joint stiffness and range of motion and patient's pain level.

Life Span and Gender

Determine whether a female patient is pregnant or breastfeeding. Allopurinol is a pregnancy category C drug. There are no human clinical trials to ensure its safety during pregnancy. Fortunately, gout is very rare in women during their reproductive years. The potential effect to an infant who receives breast milk is unknown.

Dosage adjustment is necessary for elderly patients with impaired renal function.

Lifestyle, Diet, and Habits

Administer allopurinol after a meal to decrease the potential for nausea or vomiting. Encourage the patient to follow the same diet plan for patients taking colchicine to avoid

TABLE 25.8	Agents That Interact with P Allopurinol	
Interactants	**Effect and Significance**	**Nursing Management**
ampicillin/amoxicillin	Although the mechanism of action is not understood, allopurinol may increase the frequency of ampicillin-induced rash.	Monitor for rash; contact the health care provider should rash appear. Do not assume ampicillin-induced rash; hypersensitivity to allopurinol must be considered.
antacids, aluminum salts	Antacids and aluminum salts decrease the absorption of allopurinol, decreasing its efficacy	Monitor for signs of acute gouty arthritis.
azathioprine/mercaptopurine	Azathioprine converts to mercaptopurine. Allopurinol inhibits the first-pass metabolism of mercaptopurine, resulting in an increased risk of toxicity.	Discuss the need for dosage adjustment of azathioprine with the health care provider (dosage should be decreased 25%–33%). Monitor for immunosuppression.
captopril	Captopril is associated with an increased risk of hypersensitivity to allopurinol.	Monitor for rash. Monitor CBC. Monitor renal/hepatic status.
cyclophosphamide	Allopurinol may increase the myelosuppressive effects of cyclophosphamide.	Monitor CBC. Monitor for bruising and bleeding. Monitor for signs of infection.
hydantoins	Allopurinol inhibits the metabolism of hydantoins, resulting in an increased risk of adverse effects and toxicity.	Monitor hydantoin levels. Monitor CBC, liver function tests. Monitor for changes in speech, thought process, and gait.
theophylline/aminophylline	Allopurinol decreases the renal clearance of theophylline, resulting in an increased risk of adverse effects and toxicity.	Monitor for signs of toxicity, such as nausea, tachycardia, and nervousness.
warfarin	Allopurinol may inhibit the hepatic metabolism of warfarin. This interaction is unpredictable.	Monitor PT/INR Monitor for signs of bleeding.

decreasing the efficacy of drug therapy. Teach the patient to ingest 2.5 to 3 L of fluid daily to avoid renal calculi.

Nursing Diagnoses and Outcomes

- Increased Risk for Injury related to allopurinol-induced renal toxicity
  Desired outcome: The patient will contact the prescriber if any urinary changes occur.
- Deficient Fluid Volume related to nausea and vomiting
  Desired outcome: The patient will contact the prescriber if nausea and vomiting persist.
- Ineffective Protection related to drug-induced blood dyscrasias
  Desired outcome: The patient will contact the prescriber if sore throat, easy bruising, or lethargy occurs.

Planning and Intervention

Maximizing Therapeutic Effects

Administer allopurinol in conjunction with colchicine to decrease the potential for a gout flare-up in the initial stages of therapy. Assist the patient to develop meal plans that limit uric acid production.

Minimizing Adverse Effects

Administer after meals to decrease nausea or vomiting. Fluid intake should range between 2.5 and 3 L/d (unless contraindicated) to minimize potential for renal stone formation. Review the allopurinol order. Allopurinol therapy is generally started at 100 mg daily, then increases 100 mg at weekly intervals until the uric acid level is less than 6 mg/dL or the maximum dose is reached. Teach the patient the importance of following this schedule to avoid an acute gout flare.

Providing Patient and Family Education

- Emphasize the need to follow the health care provider's dosage instructions. Advise patients not to hasten the schedule or double the dose, even if a dose is missed.
- Advise patients that allopurinol can cause minor adverse effects, such as nausea, vomiting, and pruritus. Teach patients to contact the health care provider if they do not go away or if they are particularly annoying.
- Advise patients that any rash needs to be evaluated by the health care provider.
- Be sure patients understand that allopurinol can cause serious adverse effects and that they should call their health care teams immediately if they observe signs of

renal toxicity (urinary changes) or signs of blood abnormalities (e.g., sore throat, easy bruising, or lethargy).

- Advise patients that optimal benefits from allopurinol therapy may take 2 to 6 weeks.
- Stress to patients that they should avoid alcohol because it can cause stomach problems and increase uric acid levels in the blood, which makes a gouty attack more likely.
- Inform patients of foods that decrease uric acid production.
- Tell patients to drink at least 2.5 to 3 L of water a day to prevent renal stones.
- Explain the importance of routine follow-up to assess efficacy of drug therapy and to monitor for potential adverse effects.
- Advise patients to never start or stop allopurinol therapy during an acute flare.

Ongoing Assessment and Evaluation

Coordinate serial laboratory tests, including uric acid level, CBC, and liver and renal function tests. The goal of therapy is to lower the uric acid level to less than 6 mg/dL. Consistently monitor for rash at each visit. Ask the patient to describe joint stiffness or pain and any limitation of movement.

Therapy is considered effective when the patient reports reduced pain and inflammation and remains free of adverse effects. In addition, the patient should express an understanding of the need to contact the health care provider immediately if a rash occurs, and of the advantages of increasing fluid intake, refraining from alcohol, and making appropriate diet choices.

Drugs Similar to Allopurinol
Febuxostat

Febuxostat (Uloric) is a xanthine oxidase inhibitor approved for the management of hyperuricemia in patients with gout. It

---

MEMORY CHIP

P Allopurinol

- Used for the management of **chronic** gout
- Major contraindications: coadministration with drugs that induce myelosuppression.
- Most common adverse effects: pruritus, maculopapular rash, nausea and vomiting, elevated liver function test values, and acute gout symptoms
- Most serious adverse effects: blood dyscrasias, severe dermatologic disorders
- Maximizing therapeutic effects: adhere to diet that limits uric acid production
- Minimizing adverse effects: Ingest 2.5 to 3 L of fluid daily.
- Most important patient education: Any rash must be evaluated by the health care provider.
- Nursing alert: Many drugs increase the incidence of hypersensitivity that is potentially fatal.

---

differs from allopurinol because it is not a purine base analogue. In a recent study febuxostat outperformed allopurinol in its ability to achieve and maintain a uric acid level less than 6 mg/dL (Becker, Schumacher, MacDonald, 2009).

Febuxostat should not be used in patient taking theophylline, azathioprine, or mercaptopurine. It raises the serum levels of these drugs and increases the risk for toxicity of these drugs.

A gout flare may occur with the initiation of febuxostat. Encourage patients to continue the drug despite the flare. NSAIDS or colchicine may be given to control the flare. Common adverse effects include nausea, arthralgias, rash and liver function abnormalities. Febuxostat is also associated with an increased risk for thromboembolic events such as heart or brain attacks (MI and CVA, respectively). Monitor carefully for these potential adverse effects. Febuxostat is a pregnancy category C.

Drugs Significantly Different From **P** Allopurinol

Probenecid (Benemid, Probalan) and sulfinpyrazone (Anturane) are also uricosuric drugs, which differ from allopurinol by their mechanism of action. Allopurinol works by inhibiting uric acid formation, whereas probenecid and sulfinpyrazone work by increasing uric acid excretion.

Probenecid

Probenecid is an oral drug that interferes with tubular handling of organic acids within the nephron. It inhibits the active resorption of uric acid at the proximal convoluted tubules, resulting in increased excretion of uric acid. It also reduces the renal tubular secretion of some antibiotics. Because the antibiotics are not excreted, serum concentrations are elevated, and their activity is prolonged.

Probenecid is contraindicated in patients with blood dyscrasias or uric acid kidney stones because the drug can exacerbate these conditions. It should not be administered to patients with severe renal impairment (glomerular filtration rate less than 50 mL/min) or to patients with medical conditions in which uric acid production can increase acutely, such as those undergoing cancer chemotherapy or radiation therapy.

Therapeutic dosages of probenecid are generally well tolerated, with few adverse effects. The most common adverse effects are similar to those of allopurinol. Some patients with gout can experience an increased incidence of uric acid stones or of acute gouty attacks during the first 6 to 12 months of therapy. These increases occur because of increased renal clearance of uric acid. Probenecid interferes with the copper sulfate urine glucose tests that may be used by patients with diabetes. Advise patients with diabetes who are taking the drug to use capillary blood glucose monitoring.

In addition to the dietary considerations for allopurinol, teach patients to avoid cranberry juice and vitamin C. These substances tend to acidify the urine, which decreases probenecid excretion; thus, there is an increased risk of adverse effects and toxicity. Nursing management and ongoing assessment are similar to those with allopurinol.

Sulfinpyrazone

Sulfinpyrazone is an active metabolite of the NSAID phenylbutazone, so it has some anti-inflammatory effects. Its action is the same as that of probenecid; however, it is longer acting and more potent. In addition to increasing uric acid excretion, sulfinpyrazone inhibits platelet aggregation and thus can be used in the prophylaxis of myocardial infarction. Because of its antiplatelet action, monitor the patient for signs of bleeding and do not administer sulfinpyrazone with other drugs, such as salicylates or anticoagulants (warfarin), which affect platelet aggregation. Sulfinpyrazone may induce GI distress; thus, administering the drug with meals or milk may be helpful.

CHAPTER SUMMARY

- Arthritic inflammatory diseases are initially treated with salicylates and NSAIDs.
- Disease-modifying antirheumatic drugs (DMARDs) delay joint destruction and should be initiated within 3 months of diagnosis of rheumatoid arthritis.
- DMARDs have a common goal of reducing the progression of rheumatoid arthritis but have different mechanisms of action to achieve that goal.
- There are two types of DMARDS: non-biological and biological. Pharmacologic classes of DMARDs include alkylating agents, antimetabolites, antimalarials, gold salts, sulfonamide antibiotics, tumor necrosis factor (TNF) inhibitors, monoclonal antibodies, interleukin antagonists, and immune response modifiers.
- Methotrexate is the DMARD of choice for most rheumatologists. Its efficacy is enhanced when given in combination with TNF inhibitors or other biological DMARDS.
- TNF inhibitors and other biologic DMARDs may induce serious infections or malignancies.
- Patients receiving biological DEMARDS must be evaluated for systemic infections including bacteria, virus, fungi, or TB prior to initiation of therapy and throughout therapy.
- Gout is a disease of altered purine metabolism resulting in hyperuricemia. However, hyperuricemia alone does not always result in gout.
- Antigout drugs resolve symptoms in two different ways: colchicine opposes leukocyte phagocytosis, which inhibits further urate deposits, whereas uricosuric agents reduce hyperuricemia.

QUESTIONS FOR STUDY AND REVIEW

1. What advantage do DMARDs have over salicylates, NSAIDs, and acetaminophen?
2. What is the major disadvantage of using DMARDs?
3. What is the advantage of using DMARDs within 3 months of diagnosis of RA?
4. Why are so many different classes of medications under the umbrella term DMARD?
5. What is TNF?
6. What contraindication and potential adverse effect is common to all TNF inhibitors? Why?
7. Why are biologic drugs such as etanercept, abatacept, and anakinra not given as combination therapy with each other?
8. Compare colchicine and allopurinol.

NEED MORE HELP?

Chapter 25 of the Study Guide to Accompany *Drug Therapy in Nursing*, 4th Edition, contains NCLEX-style questions and other learning activities to reinforce your understanding of the concepts presented in this chapter. For additional information or to purchase the study guide, visit thePoint.

REFERENCES

Becker, M. A., & Ruoff, G. E. (2010). What do I need to know about gout? *The Journal of Family Practice*, 59(6 Suppl):S1–S8.

Becker, M. A., Schumacher, H. R., MacDonald. P. A., et al. (2009). Clinical efficacy and safety of successful long term urate lowering with febuxostat or allopurinol in subjects with gout. *The Journal of Rheumatology*, 36(6):1273–1282.

Choi, H. K. (2010). A prescription for lifestyle change in patients with hyperuricemia and gout. *Current Opinion in Rheumatology*, 22(2):165–172.

Emery, P., Keystone, E., Tony, H. P., et al. (2008). IL-6 receptor inhibition with tocilizumab improves treatment outcomes in patients with rheumatoid arthritis refractory to anti-tumour necrosis factor biologicals: results from a 24-week multicentre randomized placebo-controlled trial. *Annals of the Rheumatic Diseases*, 67(11):1516–1523.

Facts and Comparisons. (2010). *Drug facts and comparisons*. Philadelphia, PA: Lippincott Williams & Wilkins.

Finkelstein, Y., Aks, S. E., Hutson, J. R., et al. (2010). Colchicine poisoning: the dark side of an ancient drug. *Clinical Toxicology*, 48(5):407–414.

Garnero, P., Thompson, E., Woodworth, T., et al. (2010). Rapid and sustained improvement in bone and cartilage turnover markers with the anti-interleukin-6 receptor inhibitor tocilizumab plus methotrexate in rheumatoid arthritis patients with an inadequate response to methotrexate: results from a substudy of the multicenter double-blind, placebo-controlled trial of tocilizumab in inadequate responders to methotrexate alone. *Arthritis and Rheumatism*, 62(1):33–43.

Hutus, G. (2010). Golimumab as the first monthly subcutaneous fully human anti-TNF-alpha antibody in the treatment of inflammatory arthropathies. *Immunotherapy*, 2(4):453–460.

Jones, G. (2010). The AMBITION trial: tocilizumab monotherapy for rheumatoid arthritis. *Expert Review of Clinical Immunology*, 6(2):189–195.

Karch, A. M. (2010). *Nursing Drug Guide*. Philadelphia, PA: Lippincott Williams & Wilkins.

Koda-Kimbal, M. A, Young, L. Y., Kradian, W. A., et al. (2008). *Applied therapeutics: the clinical use of drugs* (9th Ed). Philadelphia, PA: Lippincott Williams & Wilkins.

Micromedex Healthcare Series. Retrieved from *http://thomsonhc.com*.

Porth, C. M. (2008). *Pathophysiology: concepts of altered health states* (8th Ed). Philadelphia, PA: Lippincott Williams & Wilkins.

Schumacher, H. R., Becker, M. A., Lloyd, E., et al. (2009). Febuxostat in the treatment of gout: 5-yr findings of the FOCUS efficacy and safety study, *Rheumatology (Oxford)*, 48(2):188–194.

Schumacher, H. R., Becker, M. A., Lloyd, E., et al. (2009). Febuxostat in the treatment of gout: 5-yr findings of the FOCUS efficacy and safety study, *Rheumatology (Oxford)*, 48(2):188–194.

Rantalaiho, V., Korpela, M., Laasonen, L., et al. (2010). Early combination disease-modifying antirheumatic drug therapy and tight disease control improve long-term radiologic outcome in patients with early rheumatoid arthritis: the 11-year results of the Finnish Rheumatoid Arthritis Combination Therapy trial, *Arthritis Research and Therapy*, 12(3):R122.

Schur, P. H. (2010). Treatment of persistently active rheumatoid arthritis in adults, *Up To Date*. Retrieved from http://www.uptodate.com/online/content/topic.do?topicKey=rheumart/15251&selectedTitle=6~150&source=search_result on July 30, 2010.

Seo, P., & Stone, J. H. (2010). Overview of the use of immunosuppressive and disease modifying drugs in the rheumatic disease, *Up To Date*. Retrieved from http://www.uptodate.com/online/content/topic.do?topicKey=treatme/8797&selectedTitle=1~84&source=search_result on July 30, 2010.

Stone, J. H. (2010). Overview of biologic agents in the rheumatic diseases, *Up To Date*. Retrieved at http://www.uptodate.com/online/content/topic.do?topicKey=treatme/11280&selectedTitle=1~150&source=search_result on July 30, 2010.

Tatro, D. S. (2011). *Drug interaction facts: the authority on drug interactions*. Philadelphia, PA: Lippincott Williams & Wilkins.

Vaz, A., Lisse, J., Rizzo, W., et al. (2009). Discussion: DMARDs and biologic therapies in the management of inflammatory joint diseases, *Expert Review of Clinical Immunology*, 5(3):291–299.

UNIT 7
Hematopoietic, Cardiovascular, and Renal System Drugs

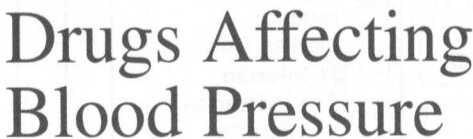

Drugs Affecting Blood Pressure

Learning Objectives

At the completion of this chapter the student will:

1. Describe therapy appropriate for prehypertension, stage 1 hypertension, and stage 2 hypertension.
2. Identify the core drug knowledge for drugs that affect blood pressure.
3. Differentiate the antihypertensive drug classes.
4. Identify core patient variables relevant to drugs that affect blood pressure.
5. Relate the interaction of core drug knowledge to core patient variables for drugs that affect blood pressure.
6. Generate a nursing plan of care from the interaction between core drug knowledge and core patient variables for drugs that affect blood pressure.
7. Describe nursing interventions to maximize therapeutic effects and minimize adverse effects for drugs that affect blood pressure.
8. Determine key points for patient and family education for drugs that affect blood pressure.

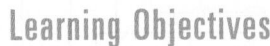

Key Terms

cardiac cycle	hypertensive crisis	sympatholytic
diastole	primary hypertension	sympathomimetic
diastolic blood pressure	renin-angiotensin-aldosterone system	systole
essential hypertension	secondary hypertension	systolic blood pressure
hypertension	shock	

Drugs Affecting Blood Pressure

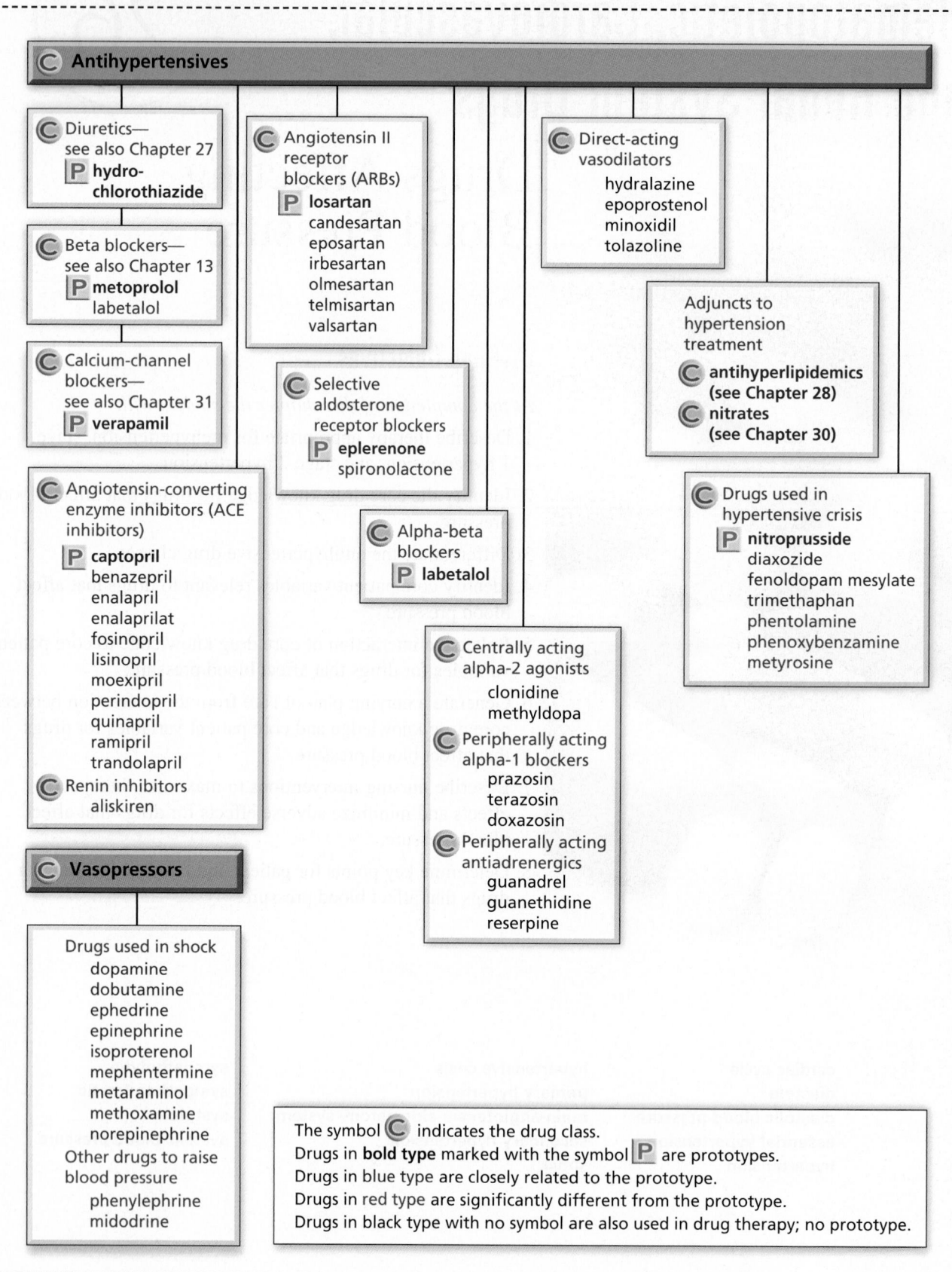

Antihypertensives

Diuretics—
see also Chapter 27
hydro-
chlorothiazide

Beta blockers—
see also Chapter 13
metoprolol
labetalol

Calcium-channel
blockers—
see also Chapter 31
verapamil

Angiotensin-converting
enzyme inhibitors (ACE
inhibitors)
captopril
benazepril
enalapril
enalaprilat
fosinopril
lisinopril
moexipril
perindopril
quinapril
ramipril
trandolapril

Renin inhibitors
aliskiren

Angiotensin II
receptor
blockers (ARBs)
losartan
candesartan
eposartan
irbesartan
olmesartan
telmisartan
valsartan

Selective
aldosterone
receptor blockers
eplerenone
spironolactone

Alpha-beta
blockers
labetalol

Centrally acting
alpha-2 agonists
clonidine
methyldopa

Peripherally acting
alpha-1 blockers
prazosin
terazosin
doxazosin

Peripherally acting
antiadrenergics
guanadrel
guanethidine
reserpine

Direct-acting
vasodilators
hydralazine
epoprostenol
minoxidil
tolazoline

Adjuncts to
hypertension
treatment
antihyperlipidemics
(see Chapter 28)
nitrates
(see Chapter 30)

Drugs used in
hypertensive crisis
nitroprusside
diaxozide
fenoldopam mesylate
trimethaphan
phentolamine
phenoxybenzamine
metyrosine

Vasopressors

Drugs used in shock
dopamine
dobutamine
ephedrine
epinephrine
isoproterenol
mephentermine
metaraminol
methoxamine
norepinephrine

Other drugs to raise
blood pressure
phenylephrine
midodrine

The symbol **C** indicates the drug class.
Drugs in **bold type** marked with the symbol **P** are prototypes.
Drugs in blue type are closely related to the prototype.
Drugs in red type are significantly different from the prototype.
Drugs in black type with no symbol are also used in drug therapy; no prototype.

Hypertension occurs when systolic or diastolic blood pressure is elevated beyond normal ranges over time. Lifestyle changes and antihypertensive drugs may be used to restore blood pressure to normal levels and to prevent the adverse effects of hypertension. The main drug classes used as first-line treatment for hypertension are diuretics, beta blockers, calcium channel blockers, angiotensin-converting enzyme (ACE) inhibitors, angiotensin II receptor blockers (ARBs), and selective aldosterone blockers. The drug classes used as second-line treatment for hypertension are direct vasodilators, alpha-2 stimulators, alpha-1 blockers, and anti-adrenergics. These drugs are discussed briefly in this chapter.

Although many of these drug classes have multiple therapeutic indications, this chapter focuses on their capacity as antihypertensives. Diuretics, beta blockers, and calcium channel blockers and their prototypes are discussed in greater depth elsewhere in the text. The prototype ACE inhibitor is captopril (Capoten). A drug significantly different is the novel renin inhibitor, aliskiren (Tekturna). The prototype ARB is losartan (Cozaar). The prototype selective aldosterone receptor blocker is eplerenone (Inspra). The prototype beta blocker is metoprolol (Lopressor), and a drug significantly different from metoprolol is labetalol an alpha-beta blocker. Another alpha-beta blocker, carvedilol (Coreg), is also used in the treatment of chronic heart failure (HF); this is discussed further in Chapter 29.

This chapter also examines drugs used to treat hypertensive crises and drugs used to increase blood pressure. The prototype drug used to treat hypertensive crises is nitroprusside. The prototype vasopressor is dopamine. The use of dopamine in shock is discussed in this chapter, and the full discussion of dopamine as a prototype is in Chapter 13. Treatment of hypotension from other conditions is also presented briefly.

PHYSIOLOGY

The heart is composed of four chambers: the left atrium, the right atrium, the left ventricle, and the right ventricle. Blood is returned from the body to the right atrium and then progresses to the right ventricle and on to the lungs, where it is reoxygenated and carbon dioxide is removed. The reoxygenated blood returns to the left atrium and then to the left ventricle. The contraction of the left ventricle pushes the blood into the aorta; thus, it returns to systemic circulation.

Blood is circulated throughout the body by a coordinated sequence of chamber contractions and valve openings and closings known as the **cardiac cycle.** The two phases of the cardiac cycle are systole and diastole. Together they describe the timeframe from the beginning of one heartbeat to the beginning of another. During **systole,** the ventricles contract, and the aortic and pulmonic valves open, allowing blood to be ejected into the aorta and pulmonary artery. During **diastole,** the ventricles relax, and the mitral and tricuspid valves open; at the same time, blood flows into the atria. This blood is propelled into the ventricles by atrial contraction, which occurs at the end of diastole. As systole begins again, the increased pressure from ventricular contraction causes the mitral and tricuspid valves to shut.

Contractions of the heart propel blood through the vascular system. Each contraction increases outflow from the heart and pushes along the volume of blood already in the systemic circulation. As the blood moves through the circulatory system, the tightness or constriction (tension) of the vessels provides resistance. Arterial pressure, which results from these forces, is measured as blood pressure. The highest pressure is achieved during systole (when the heart contracts and ejects blood into the circulation) and is known as **systolic blood pressure.** The lowest pressure that can be measured is achieved during diastole (when the heart relaxes and fills with blood and the vessels propel the blood already in circulation) and is known as **diastolic blood pressure.**

Blood pressure is measured in millimeters of mercury (mm Hg) and is calculated by measuring the amount of blood leaving the heart multiplied by the amount of resistance in the peripheral vessels. The formula for measuring blood pressure is blood pressure = cardiac output × peripheral resistance, or BP = CO × PR. Figure 26.1 depicts the mechanisms involved in regulating blood pressure.

When cardiac output or peripheral resistance increases, blood pressure increases. When cardiac output or peripheral resistance decreases, blood pressure decreases. When cardiac output and peripheral resistance move in opposite directions, the effect on blood pressure is related to the net difference between the two (example: if cardiac output decreases more than peripheral resistance increases, then the net effect will be to decrease the blood pressure). Several innate mechanisms regulate blood pressure by affecting either cardiac output or peripheral resistance. If you think of blood pressure as a math equation, then it makes sense that drug therapy to change blood pressure (the product) must either effect cardiac output or peripheral resistance (the two factors) in some way.

Role of Adrenergic Receptors

Adrenergic receptors in the nervous system have a role in blood pressure management. Adrenergic receptors are grouped into receptor sites—alpha-1, alpha-2, beta-1, and beta-2. When alpha-1 receptors are stimulated, they cause peripheral constriction, and blood pressure increases as a result. This effect, which is similar to stimulation of the sympathetic nerves, is called a **sympathomimetic** effect (one that mimics the effect of the sympathetic system). Conversely, blockage of these receptor sites dilates resistance vessels (arterioles) and capacitance vessels (veins), thereby decreasing pressure.

Alpha-2 receptor sites are located on the presynaptic side of the neural synapse within the brain. Stimulation of these receptors inhibits the sympathetic system, causing a **sympatholytic** effect (one that stops the effect of the sympathetic system). The resulting reduction in sympathetic outflow from the central nervous system (CNS) has two effects. It decreases the heart rate and, therefore, cardiac output. It also decreases vasoconstriction, which reduces peripheral resistance. The effect from both of these actions is a decrease in blood pressure.

Beta-1 receptor sites are located primarily in the heart. Stimulation of beta-1 receptor sites increases the heart rate, the speed

PHYSIOLOGY

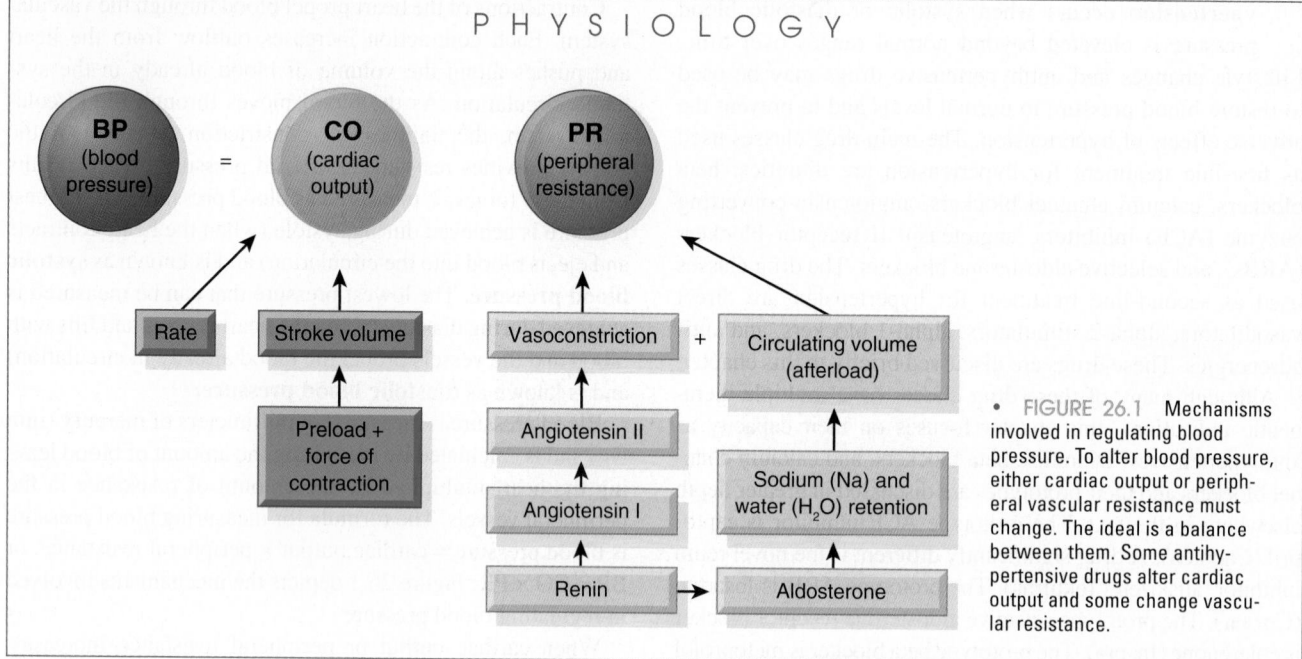

• FIGURE 26.1 Mechanisms involved in regulating blood pressure. To alter blood pressure, either cardiac output or peripheral vascular resistance must change. The ideal is a balance between them. Some antihypertensive drugs alter cardiac output and some change vascular resistance.

of cardiac conduction, and the force of cardiac contraction. Cardiac output is increased, thereby increasing blood pressure.

Beta-2 receptor sites are located primarily in the bronchial and vascular musculature. Stimulation of these sites induces bronchial and peripheral dilation. The peripheral dilation contributes to decreased blood pressure by decreasing peripheral resistance. If beta-1 and beta-2 receptors are stimulated at different rates, the one with the greatest stimulation will show its effect on blood pressure. If both beta-1 and beta-2 receptor sites are stimulated equally and simultaneously, the effect on blood pressure is negligible. (See Chapter 13 for more information about adrenergic receptors.)

Role of Renin-Angiotensin-Aldosterone System

Another mechanism involved in blood pressure regulation is the **renin-angiotensin-aldosterone system.** Renin, which is synthesized by the kidneys, produces angiotensin I. Angiotensin I is a basically inactive substance until it is converted to the active angiotensin II by a special enzyme, angiotensin-converting enzyme (ACE). Angiotensin II is formed from various alternative pathways and is also formed at the cellular level. Angiotensin II is a potent vasoconstrictor. It also stimulates secretion of aldosterone from the adrenal medulla. Aldosterone increases retention of sodium and water in the body, which, in turn, increases circulating volume. The resulting vasoconstriction and increased circulating volume raise blood pressure by increasing peripheral resistance and cardiac output. The effects on vasoconstriction and circulating volume have traditionally been viewed as the total effects of aldosterone and angiotensin II on hypertension. Additional effects from angiotensin II and aldosterone are now recognized that contribute to the pathologies seen with hypertension. These hormones also promote the growth of certain

cells and stimulate increased mass in both the arterial wall and the left ventricle. Angiotensin II and aldosterone make the following more likely to occur: inflammation of the vessels, thrombosis, oxidative stress, chronic heart failure (CHF), cardiac arrhythmias, reduced fibrinolysis, and sudden cardiac death. Aldosterone is also believed to play a role in structural renal injury, proteinuria, collagen synthesis, and myocardial fibrosis. When released by the adrenals into the circulation, aldosterone appears to be taken up by cardiac tissue, resulting in cardiac damage (Fiebeler, Nussberger, Shagdarsuren, et al., 2005). Although the interruption of the renin-angiotensin-aldosterone system is target-organ protective, complete blockade is difficult to achieve because the body has some escape mechanisms; aldosterone levels remain elevated even though angiotensin II production is inhibited or its action is blocked. These escape mechanisms are not completely understood, but aldosterone has been identified as an important escape mediator (Fiebeler, Nussberger, Shagdarsuren, et al., 2005).

PATHOPHYSIOLOGY

Hypertension is a chronic disorder. Why is hypertension a problem? The answer to this is clear from these statistics about adults with hypertension from the American Heart Association (statistics are from the most current year available as of 2009).

"In the United States, hypertension affects an estimated 73.6 million people aged 20 years and older, or approximately 1 in 3 adult Americans Twenty-one percent of these people do not realize that they have high blood pressure. High blood pressure was listed on death certificates as the primary cause of death of 57,356 Americans in 2005. High blood pressure was listed as a primary or contributing cause of death in about 319,000 of the more than 2.4 million U.S. deaths in 2005. The 2005 overall death rate from HBP (per 100,000 people) was 18.4. From 1995 to 2005 the death rate from HBP increased 25.2 percent, and the actual number of deaths rose 56.4 percent." (American Heart Association, 2009a).

Hypertension is common in all racial groups, although some groups are more prone to hypertension than others. In the United States, Native Americans have about the same, or a somewhat higher, incidence of hypertension than the general population. Hispanics have generally the same, or a lower, rate than non-Hispanic whites, but African Americans have the highest rate. About 40% of African Americans have hypertension (American Heart Association, 2009b). Compared with white Americans, African Americans have an earlier onset, higher prevalence, and greater rate of stage 2 hypertension. This explains why African Americans also have a greater rate of nonfatal stroke, fatal stroke, death from heart disease, and end-stage kidney disease. Rates of hypertension do vary within the African American population. Those African Americans with the highest rates are more likely to be middle aged or older, less educated, overweight or obese, physically inactive, and diabetic. Death rates from hypertension are higher for African Americans than for whites and are higher for black males than black females (American Heart Association, 2009a).

Part of the explanation for the variation in hypertension among races may be the variation of obesity, a known risk factor for hypertension. Obesity and being overweight are defined by an elevated body mass index (determined by dividing the weight in kilograms by the height in meters squared), an indicator of how much body fat is present. For adults, a BMI score of 30 or greater indicates obesity (Box 26.1). According to the Centers for Disease Control, adult "blacks had 51% higher prevalence of obesity, and Hispanics had 21% higher obesity prevalence compared with whites. Greater prevalences of obesity for blacks and whites were found in the South and Midwest than in the West and Northeast. Hispanics in the Northeast had lower obesity prevalence than Hispanics in the Midwest, South or West" (CDC, 2009b).

Minority (Mexican American, African American, Native American) children are also more likely to be overweight or obese compared to nonminority (Caucasian American) children and thus are more likely to have hypertension (Flynn, 2009; Eichner, Moore, Perveen, et al., 2008; Moore, Stephens, Wilson, et al., 2006; Urrutia-Rojas, Egbuchunam, Bae, et al., 2006; Ogden, Carroll, Curtin, et al., 2006).

Women who take oral contraceptives have a small increase in both systolic and diastolic pressures, although the blood pressure usually continues to remain within the normal range. However, women who take oral contraceptives, smoke, are

overweight, and are older than 35 years do experience hypertension. It is three times more common in this group than in women without these risk factors. High blood pressure is extremely common in older adults. Depending on their race, between almost two thirds and nearly three fourths of older adult Americans have hypertension. Older adults often are responsive to lifestyle changes, which should be included as part of their treatment along with drug therapy.

Hypertension is also now a problem in children and adolescents because of high rates of childhood obesity, with accompanying lack of exercise and the increasing prevalence of type I diabetes. The incidence of hypertension has been steadily increasing since 1988 (Flynn, 2009; Din-Dzietham, Liu, Bielo, et al., 2007). Research has indicated that between approximately 5% and 20% of American school-age children and adolescents have hypertension; and the prevalence of obesity among children aged 6 to 11 more than doubled in the past 20 years, going from 6.5% in 1980 to 17.0% in 2006. The rate among adolescents aged 12 to 19 more than tripled, increasing from 5% to 17.6% (Centers for Disease Control, 2009a). Overweight and obesity as determined by high BMI has been consistently shown to be an important risk factor for hypertension in school-aged children and adolescents (Eichner, Moore, Perveen, et al., 2008; Urrutia-Rojas, Egbuchunam, Bae, et al., 2006; Moore, Stephens, Wilson, et al., 2006; Ogden, Carroll, Curtin, et al., 2006; Sorof, Lai, Turner, et al., 2004). The likelihood of hypertension is more than three times higher in overweight children (Urrutia-Rojas, Egbuchunam, Bae, et al., 2006; Box 26.2). The long-term consequences of hypertension in children and adolescents cannot be predicted at this time, as there is no research yet on this topic (Flynn, 2008).

The American Heart Association defines adult hypertension as persistent elevation of systolic pressure equal to or greater than 140 mm Hg or diastolic pressure equal to or greater than 90 mm Hg. The diastolic pressure for all age groups is based on the fifth Korotkov sound, which is the disappearance of sound. Many factors, ranging from exercise to stress to a variation in normal sodium intake, may increase blood pressure temporarily. Therefore, a definitive diagnosis of hypertension is not made until the average of two or more readings, each recorded at two or more visits, reveals persistent elevations (Joint National Committee on Detection, Evaluation and Treatment of High Blood Pressure— 7th report, 2003). Diagnosis of hypertension in children requires more than knowledge of the systolic and diastolic pressure because children vary widely in their body size based on age, height, and gender. The blood pressure reading is compared to standardized charts to determine if the child has normal blood pressure, pre-hypertension, or hypertension.

There are two main categories of hypertension: primary hypertension and secondary hypertension. **Primary hypertension,** also known as **essential hypertension,** is responsible for 90% to 95% of all hypertension; secondary hypertension accounts for the remaining percentage. Primary hypertension has no identified cause. However, it can be managed successfully with lifestyle changes and drug therapy to prevent the adverse effects of hypertension. Risk factors associated

---

Box 26.1	UNDERSTANDING BMI
When the BMI is …..	It is considered this…
Below 18.5	Underweight
18.5–24.9	Normal
25.0–29.9	Overweight
30.0 and Above	Obese

The Basal Metabolic Index (BMI) is considered an obesity index. It is the relationship of weight to height.

BOX 26.2 FOCUS ON RESEARCH

Obesity, High Blood Pressure, and School-Aged Children

Urrutia-Rojas, X., Egbuchunam, C. U., Bae, S., et al. (2006). High blood pressure in school children: Prevalence and risk factors. Retrieved from http://www.biomedcentral. com/1471-2431/6/32.

The Study

Children from 17 elementary schools in Fort Worth, Texas, chosen to represent the ethnic and geographical profile of the school district's student population, were studied to determine the prevalence of hypertension and its risk factors in children. The 1,066 children were fifth-graders and ranged in age from 8 to 13 years, with the overwhelming majority being between 10 and 12 years. By race, there were 58.7% Hispanic, 24.6% African American, and 16.7% Caucasian children. (Although there was a very small percentage of Asian students and other races, the numbers were too small to include.) Approximately one third of the children were overweight (defined as a body mass index of greater than or equal to the 85th percentile). About one third (32.8%) of the African American children were overweight, nearly one third (31.9%) of the Hispanic children were overweight, and less than one fourth (23.5%) of the Caucasian children were overweight. Overall, about one in five children had hypertension (20.6%) (defined as a blood pressure greater than or equal to the 95th percentile; either systolic alone was elevated or both systolic and diastolic were elevated). Overweight children were at least three times more likely

to have hypertension. The Hispanic children were much more likely to have hypertension in comparison to African American and Caucasian children, and the African American children were more likely than Caucasian children to have hypertension. These findings conflict somewhat with previous studies, where it was found that African American children had the highest risk of hypertension.

Nursing Implications

This study highlights some important public health concerns. Overweight and obese children are more common now than 30 or 40 years ago. In this study, being overweight was the most significant risk factor for childhood hypertension. Without correction of this significant risk factor, children will develop long-term complications related to hypertension, such as MI, stroke, heart failure, and renal disease, which have been historically associated with adults, at an earlier and earlier age. Minority children are more at risk of obesity and hypertension. The finding that Hispanic children had the highest risk for hypertension appears to contradict the conclusion drawn from previous studies that African American children were at most risk. A likely explanation is that unlike other studies that compared only two races, this study compared all three races together; thus, it is the first study to identify risk for hypertension by race truly. Nurses have an important role in teaching children and their parents about the risk of obesity and hypertension to help prevent long-term morbidity and mortality.

---

with the development of primary hypertension include elevated blood lipid levels, obesity, smoking, diabetes, age older than 60 years, gender (male and postmenopausal women), and family history of cardiovascular (CV) disease (women younger than 65 years or men younger than 55 years).

Secondary hypertension occurs secondary to another condition, such as renal stenosis or renal tumor. Therapy aims to correct or remove the underlying cause. If this therapy is successful, the secondary hypertension will be eliminated. However, when the cause cannot be treated successfully, antihypertensive agents are used to control the blood pressure.

Hypertension, if untreated, can lead to stroke, myocardial infarction (MI), kidney disease, CHF, and even death. These diseases and disorders result from several physiologic changes. Persistently elevated pressure constricts the arterioles, which increases peripheral vascular resistance. The increased peripheral vascular resistance in turn increases the workload of the left ventricle, which results in ventricular hypertrophy. The myocardium must work ever harder to overcome the increased resistance to outflow. Hence, the demand for oxygen increases. Eventually, the heart can compensate no longer, and CHF results. Hypertension is the most common risk factor for CHF. At least 90% of the time, hypertension precedes CHF. A recent study of Native Americans aged 14 to 39 found that ventricular hypertrophy begins at an early age if the patient has hypertension or prehypertension; compared to individuals without hypertension, left ventricular hypertrophy was three times higher among those with hypertension and two times higher in those with prehypertension (Drukteinis, Roman, Fabsitz, et al., 2007). Yet, as previously stated, many people do not realize that they have high blood pressure and therefore do not seek medical attention; thus, their hypertension remains uncontrolled, increasing the risk of heart failure and other complications.

Another change resulting from persistent hypertension is a sclerosing (thickening and hardening) of the blood vessel wall, which narrows the blood vessel's lumen. The narrowed lumen inhibits blood flow, leading to decreased organ perfusion and, possibly, arterial thrombosis and tissue ischemia. Tissues at the greatest risk for damage include the brain, heart, eyes, and kidneys. As mentioned earlier, angiotensin II and aldosterone are now believed to be associated with inflammation of the arteries and cell growth in the arteries and heart; these effects may contribute to narrowed arteries, increased ventricular size, and stiffening of the ventricle. Aldosterone's proposed effects on the kidney (structural renal injury, proteinuria) may account for the renal damage seen with hypertension.

Chronic hypertension produces changes that may result in a stroke. However, hypertension can also develop after a stroke in patients who previously had normal blood pressure. Sudden and severe blood pressure increases after a stroke may indicate or cause intracerebral hemorrhage. This situation often warrants therapy to decrease blood pressure. To complicate matters somewhat, some degree of hypertension is physiologically necessary after a stroke to help maintain perfusion to the brain. Additionally, after a stroke, elevations in blood pressure may be related to other factors such as emotional stress, bladder distention, pain, or hypoxia.

Memory changes may be an outcome from narrowing of vessels that supply the brain. Research has shown that hypertension, likely due to related vessel wall changes in the brain, chronic brain hypoperfusion, or cerebrovascular disease, increases the risk for some aspects of Alzheimer disease (Cechetto, Hachinski, and Whitehead, 2008; Goldstein, Ashley, Endewshaw, et al., 2008; Skoog & Gustafson, 2006). Whether the treatment of hypertension will decrease the severity of Alzheimer disease is debatable, as there are conflicting findings in the literature (Poon, 2008; Johnson, Margolis, Espeland, et al., 2008; Peters, Beckett, Forette, et al., 2008; Launer, Ross, Petrovistch, et al., 2000). It has been postulated that the positive effects found in some of the major studies may be related to the types of antihypertensive drugs used in each study, with the use of angiotensin converting enzyme inhibitors, angiotensin receptor blockers, diuretics, and calcium channel blockers may be more effective in reducing dementia risk than other antihypertensives (Poon, 2008).

People with primary hypertension are relatively symptom free for a long time. Hypertension often is detected initially at an incidental blood pressure screening or during a routine physical examination. Because it is painless and symptom free, primary hypertension often remains undiagnosed until the symptoms of end-organ damage surface.

Hypertension is classified according to the degree of elevation. The risk of coronary vascular disease doubles with each increment of 20/10 mm Hg above 115/75 mm Hg. The treatment guidelines for hypertension from the *Seventh Report of the Joint National Committee on Prevention, Detection, Evaluation, and Treatment of High Blood Pressure* (JNC 7), released in 2003, created a new category of hypertension, prehypertension. Individuals with a systolic reading of 120 to 139 mm Hg or a diastolic blood pressure of 80 to 89 mm Hg are considered to have prehypertension, which means that they are at increased risk for hypertension later in life and should take steps to modify their lifestyles to minimize the risk of developing coronary vascular disease. Stage 1 hypertension occurs when the systolic pressure is 140 to 159 mm Hg or the diastolic pressure is 90 to 99 mm Hg. Stage 2 hypertension occurs when the systolic pressure is equal to or greater than 160 mm Hg or the diastolic pressure is equal to or greater than 100 mm Hg. *The eighth report of the Joint National Committee is due to be available after the text is published. Please refer to the revised report for any updates.*

Table 26.1 shows the classifications of blood pressure for individuals 18 years and older. If the systolic and diastolic blood pressure readings are in different categories, then the classification is based on the higher values.

Hypertension in children is defined as an average systolic or a diastolic blood pressure greater than or equal to the 95th percentile when the child is compared to others of the same sex, age, and height. Prehypertension in children

is defined as an average systolic or diastolic blood pressure level greater than or equal to the 90th percentile; average readings less than the 90th percentile are considered normal. Adolescents should be considered to have prehypertension if their blood pressure readings are equal to or greater than 120/80 mm Hg. Children older than 3 years of age should have their blood pressure checked when they are in a medical setting, preferably by the auscultation method with a cuff of the appropriate size. Elevated readings should be confirmed on repeated visits before the diagnosis of hypertension is made (National High Blood Pressure Education Program Working Group on Adolescents and Children, 2004). For information on home blood pressure assessment, see Box 26.3.

Hypertensive Crisis

When the patient's blood pressure is elevated acutely, the condition is termed a **hypertensive crisis.** This situation is defined as systolic blood pressure exceeding 210 mm Hg and diastolic blood pressure exceeding 120 mm Hg. When hypertensive crisis occurs, the patient is in danger of rapidly developing damage to one of the vital organs, such as the brain, heart, or kidneys, and it is considered an emergency. The situation requires immediate assessment and intervention. The priority is to reduce the blood pressure as quickly as can be managed safely to prevent injury. However, blood pressure does not need to be reduced to a normal level immediately. Although it must be reduced, it must stay high enough to maintain perfusion of vital organs. The initial goal of treatment in hypertensive emergencies is to reduce the blood pressure by no more than 25% within minutes and up to 2 hours. It should then be reduced toward 160/100 mm Hg within 2 to 6 hours. The purpose of the gradual reduction is to avoid excessive falls in pressure that could induce renal, cerebral, or coronary ischemia. The exact level of pressure reduction depends on patient-related variables.

Hypertensive crisis may be caused by an ongoing condition, such as hypertensive encephalopathy, cerebral hemorrhage, eclampsia, pheochromocytoma (a tumor of the adrenal medulla), dissecting aortic aneurysm, unstable angina pectoris, acute MI, or acute left ventricular failure with pulmonary edema. It also could be induced from a drug–food interaction, for example, when monoamine oxidase inhibitors (MAOIs) are prescribed as drug therapy and tyramine-rich food is eaten. The symptoms manifested are acute and include decreased level of consciousness, neurologic deficits, decreased renal output, vomiting, and severe headache (cephalalgia). Emergencies initially are treated with intravenous (IV) administration of an appropriate agent for rapid onset.

A hypertensive crisis that is less serious occurs when it is desirable to reduce the blood pressure within a few hours, but risk of target organ damage is not imminent. This situation is called hypertensive urgency. Examples of hypertensive urgency are upper levels of stage 2 hypertension, hypertension with optic disc edema, and severe perioperative hypertension. Urgent situations may be treated with oral doses of drugs with relatively fast onset of action, including loop diuretics, beta blockers, ACE inhibitors, alpha-2 agonists, or calcium channel blockers.

TABLE 26.1	Blood Pressure and Hypertension Categories*	
Category	Systolic	Diastolic
Normal	<120 mm Hg	<80 mm Hg
Prehypertension	120–139 mm Hg	80–89 mm Hg
Stage 1 hypertension	140–159 mm Hg	90–99 mm Hg
Stage 2 hypertension	≥160 mm Hg	≥100 mm Hg
Hypertensive crisis	>210 mm Hg	>120 mm Hg

*In the categories of prehypertension, stage 1 hypertension, and stage 2 hypertension, diagnosis is made based on either the systolic or the diastolic reading being at the specified level.

BOX 26.3 COMMUNITY BASED CONCERNS

How do we determine if the antihypertensive drug therapy is effective? The answer is by monitoring the blood pressure to confirm that the reading is moving toward, or has achieved, the targeted blood pressure goal. More frequent monitoring provides better data as it is not a single snapshot of the blood pressure at a particular time, but a pattern of readings that can show the average reading over 1 day or several days. The most common method for checking a patient's blood pressure is to have them return to the health care provider's office or clinic periodically. However, it is not reasonable to expect that patients will return daily or even weekly to have their blood pressure assessed. And it is well known that the blood pressure can be be elevated during office visits due to "white coat effect" (temporary elevation of blood pressure due to stress of having a health care provider take your blood pressure). If the patient measured their blood pressure at home, these problems could be resolved. However, it can be difficult for many patients to learn how to measure their blood pressure with a cuff and stethoscope. A joint scientific statement of the American Heart Association, the American Society of Hypertension, and the Preventive Cardiovascular Nurses Association has called for wide-spread use of home blood pressure monitoring with oscillometric equipment. In oscillometric blood pressure monitoring, an electronic pressure sensor detects changes in the blood flow instead of using a stethoscope and one's ears to hear the Korotkoff sounds. The cuff, which fits around the patient's upper arm or sometimes the wrist, is automatically inflated and deflated; thus it is extremely easy to use. While these monitors are not quite as accurate as ambulatory home monitoring (where the patient wears sensors for 24 to 78 hours at home to obtain blood pressure readings throughout the day), they are easier to use and still accurate and reliable. Home readings have been found to be more reproducible than those taken periodically in the provider's office and appear to better predict risk for cardiovascular complications. Additionally, readings from home blood pressure monitoring with oscillometric equipment are closer to the average readings from the ambulatory home monitor (which is the blood pressure that best predicts cardiovascular risk), and home readings show better correlation with the measures of target organ damage. Home blood pressure readings eliminate the risk of falsely elevated readings from white coat effect. Another advantage is that with home blood pressure monitoring, the patient can take multiple readings easily, the larger data base helps to identify the true blood pressure throughout the patient's day. Oscillometric equipment is not excessively expensive (about $100), however, some patients cannot afford them. The position of these three organizations was that this cost should be reimbursed to patients or covered by insurance policies as it is an evidenced-based practice of effective monitoring. Although hypothesized, it is not yet known whether frequent home monitoring will improve adherence with therapy or decrease the long-term cost of drug therapy by controlling blood pressure sooner. Additional research is still needed in this area. In the meantime, nurses should teach patients to monitor their blood pressure and encourage them to monitor it at home frequently via the oscillometric method. As patients take a more active role in their own health, hopefully they will have more therapeutic and less adverse effects from their blood pressure medication.

should be continued if the patient becomes hypertensive and is treated with drug therapy. The American Heart Association suggests the following:

- Lose weight or maintain a healthy body weight.
- Exercise.
- Eat a diet rich in vegetables and fruits.
- Eat whole-grain, high-fiber foods.
- Eat fish, especially oily fish, at least twice a week.
- Limit your intake of saturated fat to 7% of energy, *trans* fat to 1% of energy, and cholesterol to 300 mg/d by
  - choosing lean meats and vegetable alternatives;
  - selecting fat-free (skim), 1%-fat, and low-fat dairy products; and
  - minimizing intake of partially hydrogenated fats.
- Increase intake of potassium.
- Decrease salt intake.
- Minimize your intake of beverages and foods with added sugars.
- Consume alcohol in moderation.
- Don't smoke.

(Lichtenstein, Appel, and Brands, et al., 2006; Appel, Brands, and Daniels, et al., 2006).

Two examples of diets that meet these recommendations are the DASH diet (Dietary Approaches to Stop Hypertension) and the TLC diet (Therapeutic Lifestyle Changes). See Table 26.2 for examples of these diets.

Research indicates that following a diet such as the DASH diet promotes salt excretion and increases urine production, similar to the effects seen with diuretic drugs. These effects appear to be most prominent in those whose blood pressure is sensitive to the effects of sodium (e.g., African Americans or older adults). About half of the population with hypertension is salt sensitive. It is not known whether these effects are from specific foods in the diet or the combination of foods. African Americans who adhere to a low-sodium diet in addition to the DASH diet achieve a greater lowering of blood pressure than with the DASH diet alone; this effect is more pronounced in African American than other races (Douglas, Bakris, Epstein, et al., 2003). Potassium and calcium cause natural sodium loss and are found in high levels in this diet, but the effects on salt excretion seem greater than accounted for by either of these dietary sources of electrolytes, suggesting that a combination of factors is likely to be involved (American Heart Association, 2007).

Lifestyle modification remains an important aspect of therapy for patients in stage 1 or stage 2 hypertension. Lifestyle modifications may decrease the required drug therapy dosage.

LIFESTYLE MODIFICATION AND HYPERTENSION

In prehypertension, therapy usually consists of lifestyle changes, which include reducing weight and adopting a healthy diet and life style. Dietary and life style changes

OVERVIEW OF DRUG THERAPY AND HYPERTENSION

Drug therapy is now recommended to be started with every patient who has been diagnosed as having hypertension, whether it is stage 1 or stage 2. Drug therapy is also

TABLE 26.2	Two Examples of Daily Dietary Patterns That Are Consistent With AHA-Recommended Dietary Goals at 2000 Calories		
Eating Pattern	DASH (Dietary Approaches to Stop Hypertension)	TLC (Therapeutic Lifestyle Changes)	Serving Sizes
Grains	6 to 8 servings per day	7 servings per day	1 slice bread; 1 oz dry cereal; 1/2 cup cooked rice, pasta, or cereal
Vegetables	4 to 5 servings per day	5 servings per day	1 cup raw leafy vegetable, 1/2 cup cut-up raw or cooked vegetable, 1/2 cup vegetable juice
Fruits	4 to 5 servings per day	4 servings per day	1 medium fruit; 1/4 cup dried fruit; 1/2 cup fresh, frozen, or canned fruit; 1/2 cup fruit juice
Fat-free or low-fat milk and milk products	2 to 3 servings per day	2 to 3 servings per day	1 cup milk, 1 cup yogurt, 1 1/2 oz cheese
Lean meats, poultry, and fish	6 oz per day	5 oz per day	Lean cuts include sirloin tip, round steak, and rump roast; extra lean hamburger; and cold cuts made with lean meat or soy protein. Lean cuts of pork are center-cut ham, loin chops, and pork tenderloin
Nuts, seeds, and legumes	4 to 5 servings per week	Counted in vegetable servings.	1/3 cup (11/2 oz), 2 Tbsp peanut butter, 2 Tbsp or 1/2 oz seeds, 1/2 cup dry beans or peas
Fats and oils	2 to 3 servings per day	Amount depends on daily calorie level	1 tsp soft margarine, 1 Tbsp mayonnaise, 2 Tbsp salad dressing, 1 tsp vegetable oil
Sweets and added sugars	5 or fewer servings per week	No recommendation	1 Tbsp sugar, 1 Tbsp jelly or jam, 1/2 cup sorbet and ices, 1 cup lemonade

Reprinted with permission from Lichtenstein, A.H.; Appel, L.J.; Brands, M., et al. (2006). Diet and Lifestyle Recommendations Revision 2006. A Scientific Statement From the American Heart Association Nutrition Committee. *Circulation : Journal of the American Heart Association*. Retrieved from http://circ.ahajournals.org/cgi/reprint/CIRCULATIONAHA.106.176158v2

recommended in prehypertension if the patient has compelling indications, such as type 1 diabetes with proteinuria, heart failure, isolated systolic hypertension (older adults), or MI. Drug therapy for treating hypertension has proven efficacy in decreasing CV morbidity and mortality. Additionally, the use of drug therapy has been found to be protective against stroke, coronary events, heart failure, progression of renal disease, progression to more severe hypertension, and deaths from all causes.

Drugs used to manage blood pressure primarily include those classified as diuretics, beta blockers, calcium channel blockers, ACE inhibitors, and angiotensin II receptor blockers. Combination therapy, where more than one drug is prescribed, is common. Figure 26.2 provides an overview of how the various drug classes work to decrease blood pressure.

Additional therapy, which may be added when hypertension cannot be adequately controlled with combinations of first-line therapy, includes the selective aldosterone blockers, renin inhibitors, alpha-2 stimulators, alpha-beta blockers, and direct vasodilators. The renin inhibitor aliskiren is discussed in the section on Drugs Significantly Different from Captopril. The other second line drugs are discussed later in the chapter.

Adjunctive treatment includes the lipid-lowering agents to help, decrease the narrowing of the blood vessels from fat deposits and nitrates for vasodilation.

A thiazide diuretic should be used in drug treatment for most patients with uncomplicated hypertension, either alone or with drugs from other classes. Thiazide diuretics have been shown to be as effective as, but less expensive than, other drug classes (ALLHAT Officers and Coordinators, 2002). First-line treatment with dose doses of a thiazide have been found to reduce morbidiy and mortality from hypertension (Wright & Musini, 2009). Sometimes, hypertension occurs in conditions in which another complicating physiologic condition is present. These other conditions may respond best to other agents and are considered compelling reasons for starting single-agent drug therapy with a drug class other than a thiazide. Single-agent therapy is usually tried in stage 1 hypertension, although combination therapy (two or more drugs) may be used. Monotherapy may be effective when the blood pressure is not significantly elevated over the target blood pressure.

Combination therapy is indicated for stage 2 hypertension. Most patients with hypertension require two or more antihypertensive drugs to achieve a target blood pressure of less than 140/90 mm Hg or a target of less than 130/80 mm Hg if they have diabetes or chronic kidney disease. Two drugs as initial therapy should be considered in patients with blood pressures that are more than 20/10 mm Hg above their goal blood pressure (JNC 7, 2003).

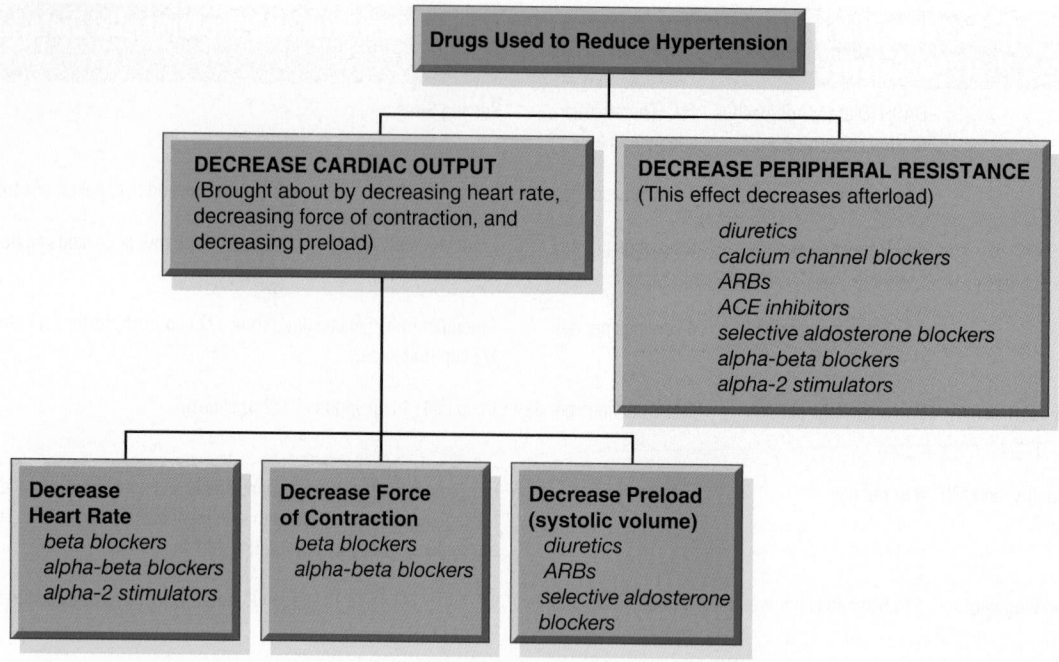

• FIGURE 26.2 Focus of drug therapy in reducing hypertension.

The exact combinations of drugs used to treat hypertension will vary, based on whether the hypertensive patient has comorbidities. As new information is acquired regarding pharmacodynamic effects of antihypertensives, the clinical guidelines concerning drug therapy choices are likely to change. These recommendations are from the JNC 7, which were current at time of publication. The reader should check for updates to these recommendations when the JNC 8 is released.

The drug dosage should be started low and titrated up to what is considered an adequate dose for efficacy. Ideally, the drug should have a therapeutic effect for 24 hours, requiring a dose to be taken only once daily. If some therapeutic response occurs from one drug given at a moderate dose, but the target blood pressure has not been achieved, then a second may be added. Adding a drug at this point, rather than after raising the first drug to an ultimate maximum, has two advantages. First, therapeutic response is frequently achieved with a relatively low dose; adding a second drug also at a low dose may increase efficacy not seen by merely maximizing the dose of the first drug. Second, using lower doses of a drug or drugs usually decreases the risk of adverse effects, so the therapy is better tolerated and adherence is improved. Many antihypertensives are now available from drug manufacturers as a combination of more than one drug in the same tablet. Combination antihypertensives provide the patient with the benefits of both types of therapy and the added advantage of needing to take only one pill, thereby improving adherence. Table 26.3 lists health status considerations for selecting drugs as first-line therapy for hypertension. Table 26.4 provides a summary of selected antihypertensives.

FIRST-LINE DRUGS TO TREAT HYPERTENSION

• 🅒 DIURETICS

Diuretics exert their effect in different areas of the renal tubules to promote excretion of sodium and water from the body. Because water is not reabsorbed to as great an extent as usual from the kidneys, the volume of circulating fluid decreases. Although the exact mechanism of how diuretics reduce blood pressure is not known, it is generally accepted that the resulting decrease in peripheral resistance, from decreased circulating volume, is what lowers blood pressure. Findings from the landmark Antihypertensive and Lipid-Lowering Treatment to Prevent Heart Attack Trial (ALLHAT), a study of more than 33,000 North American hypertensive patients with at least one other coronary heart disease (CHD) risk factor, showed that thiazide-type diuretics are superior to ACE inhibitors or calcium channel blockers in preventing one or more major forms of CV disease (ALLHAT Officers and Coordinators, 2002). Meta-analysis of 57 clinical trials (58,040 patients in all) also showed that low-dose diuretics were effective in reducing the incidence of CHD, CV disease events, stroke, and mortality, however high-dose thiazide treatment does not decrease CHD. (Wright & Musini, 2009). This confirms findings from a previous meta-analysis of 42 clinical trials (192,478 patients in all) from 2003 (Psaty, Lumley, Furberg, et al., 2003). First-line ACE inhibitors and calcium channel blockers may be similarly effective as low-dose thiazides, but the evidence is not as strong (Wright & Musini, 2009). Low-dose thiazides have been found to be effective, so if a patient is not achieving the desired therapeutic response from

TABLE 26.3	Health Status Considerations for Selecting Drugs as First-Line Therapy for Hypertension
Health Status	**Drug Class**
Compelling Indications (Unless Contraindicated by Comorbidity)	
Diabetes mellitus (type 1)	ACE inhibitors, beta blockers, calcium channel blockers
Heart failure (asymptomatic)	ACE inhibitors, diuretics, beta blockers
Isolated systolic hypertension (older adults)	Diuretics (preferred), calcium channel blockers (long-acting dihydropyridine)
Myocardial infarction	Beta blockers (nonintrinsic sympathomimetic activity), ACE inhibitors (with systolic dysfunction)
Possible Indications	
Angina	Beta blockers, calcium channel blockers
Atrial tachycardia and fibrillation	Beta blockers, calcium channel blockers (nondihydropyridine)
Cyclosporine-induced hypertension (caution with the dose of cyclosporine)	Calcium channel blockers
Diabetes mellitus (types 1 and 2) with proteinuria	ACE inhibitors (preferred), angiotensin II receptor blockers
Diabetes mellitus (type 2)	Low-dose diuretics
Dyslipidemia	Alpha blockers
Essential tremor	Beta blockers (noncardioselective)
Heart failure (symptomatic)	Angiotensin II receptor blockers, aldosterone receptor blockers
Hyperthyroidism	Beta blockers
Migraine	Beta blockers (noncardioselective), calcium channel blockers (nondihydropyridine)
Myocardial infarction	Diltiazem, verapamil
Osteoporosis	Thiazides
Preoperative hypertension	Beta blockers
Benign prostatic hypertrophy (BPH)	Alpha blockers
Chronic kidney disease	ACE inhibitors, angiotensin II receptor blockers, loop diuretics
Possible Precautions (Needs Special Monitoring) and Contraindications	
Bronchospastic disease	Beta blockers (contraindicated)
Depression	Beta blockers, central alpha stimulants, reserpine (contraindicated)
Diabetes mellitus (types 1 and 2)	Beta blockers, high-dose diuretics (precaution)
Dyslipidemia	Beta blockers (nonintrinsic sympathomimetic activity), diuretics (high dose) (precaution)
Gout	Diuretics (precaution)
Second- or third-degree heart block	Beta blockers (contraindicated), calcium channel blockers (nondihydropyridine) (contraindicated)
Heart failure	Beta blockers (except carvedilol), calcium channel blockers (except amlodipine, felodipine) (precaution)
Liver disease	Metoprolol, methyldopa (contraindicated)
Peripheral vascular disease	Beta blockers (precaution)
Pregnancy	ACE inhibitors (contraindicated), angiotensin II receptor blockers (contraindicated)
Renal insufficiency	Potassium-sparing diuretics (precaution)
Renovascular disease	ACE inhibitors, angiotensin II receptor blockers (precaution)

From the Joint National Committee on Detection, Evaluation and Treatment of High Blood Pressure. (2003). Seventh report of the Joint National Committee on Prevention, Detection, Evaluation, and Treatment of High Blood Pressure. *Journal of the American Medical Association,* 289 (19), 2560–2571.

thiazide therapy, increasing the dose generally does not bring additional efficacy. In this situation, a second drug should be added.

When polypharmacy is indicated to achieve blood pressure control, thiazide diuretics can be combined with beta blockers, ACE inhibitors, ARBs, or calcium channel blockers. Because of their ability to minimize the circulating volume, diuretics increase the efficacy of all other antihypertensives.

The combination of a thiazide with an ACE inhibitor or an ARB also helps minimize hypokalemia, hyperuricemia, and hyperlipidemia that can be adverse effects when thiazides are used in monotherapy.

Although thiazide diuretics are recommended as the first drug therapy for most hypertensive patients, loop diuretics might be used if the patient had pre-exisiting renal disease as thiazides decrease the glomerular filtration rate.

TABLE 26.4	Summary of Selected Ⓒ Antihypertensives		
Drug (Trade) Name	**Selected Indications**	**Route and Dosage Range**	**Pharmacokinetics**
Ⓒ Angiotensin-Converting Enzyme (ACE) Inhibitors			
Ⓟ captopril (Capoten)	Hypertension	*Adult:* PO, 25–150 mg bid or tid *Child (off-label):* 0.05–0.5 mg/kg PO q 12 h	*Onset:* 15 min *Duration:* Dose related $t_{1/2}$: <2 h
	Heart failure LVD after MI Diabetic neuropathy	*Adult:* PO, 25–100 mg tid *Adult:* PO, 50 mg tid *Adult:* PO, 25 mg tid	
benazepril (Lotensin)	Hypertension	*Adult:* PO, 20–40 mg/d	*Onset:* 1 h *Duration:* 24 h $t_{1/2}$: 10–11 h
enalapril (Vasotec)	Hypertension	*Adult:* PO, 10–40 mg/d *Adult:* IV, 1.25 mg over 5 min every 6 h	*Onset:* 1 h *Duration:* 24 h $t_{1/2}$: 1.3 h *Onset:* 15 min *Duration:* 6 h $t_{1/2}$: 1.3 h
fosinopril (Monopril)	Hypertension CHF	*Adult:* PO, maintenance: 20–40 mg/d *Adult:* PO, 20–40 mg/d	*Onset:* 1 h *Duration:* 24 h $t_{1/2}$: 12 h
lisinopril (Prinivil, Zestril)	Hypertension CHF Acute MI	*Adult:* PO, maintenance: 20–40 mg/d *Adult:* PO, 5 mg/d with diuretics and digitalis *Adult:* PO, maintenance: 10 mg/d	*Onset:* 1 h *Duration:* 24 h $t_{1/2}$: 12 h
moexipril (Univasc)	Hypertension	*Adult:* PO, maintenance: 7.5–30 mg/d	*Onset:* 1 h *Duration:* 24 h $t_{1/2}$: 2–9 h
ramipril (Altace)	Hypertension	*Adult:* PO, 2.5–20 mg/d	*Onset:* 1–2 h *Duration:* 24 h $t_{1/2}$: 13–17 h
quinapril (Accupril)	Hypertension CHF	Adult: PO, 20–40 mg/d Adult: PO, 20–80 mg/d with diuretics and digitalis	Onset: 1 h Duration: 24 h t1/2: 2 h
Ⓒ Angiotensin II Receptor Antagonists			
Ⓟ losartan (Cozaar)	Hypertension	*Adult:* PO, 25–100 mg/d	*Onset:* 1 wk (therapeutic effect) *Duration:* Unknown $t_{1/2}$: 2 h
Ⓒ Selective Aldosterone Receptor Blockers			
Ⓟ eplerenone (Inspra)	Hypertension	*Adult:* PO, 50–100 mg/d	*Onset:* 4 wk (full therapeutic) *Duration:* Unknown $t_{1/2}$: 4–6 h
Ⓒ Centrally Acting Alpha-2 Stimulators and Others			
clonidine (Catapres)	Hypertension	*Adult:* PO, 0.2–0.6 mg/d in divided doses not to exceed 2.4 mg/d; transdermal, one 0.1-mg to two 0.3-mg patches q7d *Child:* PO, 0.05–0.4 mg bid	*Onset:* 30–60 min *Duration:* 12–24 h $t_{1/2}$: 12–16 h *Onset (transdermal):* Slow *Duration:* 7 d $t_{1/2}$: Unknown
prazosin (Minipress)	Hypertension	*Adult:* PO, maintenance, 6–15 mg/d in divided doses *Child:* PO, 0.5–7 mg tid	*Onset:* 2 h *Duration:* 6–12 h $t_{1/2}$: 2–3 h

TABLE 26.4	Summary of Selected ⓒ Antihypertensives *(continued)*		
Drug (Trade) Name	**Selected Indications**	**Route and Dosage Range**	**Pharmacokinetics**
terazosin (Hytrin)	Hypertension Benign prostatic hypertrophy	*Adult:* PO, maintenance, 1–5 mg/d up to 20 mg/d *Adult:* PO, 10 mg/d	*Onset:* Up to 15 min *Duration:* 12–24 h $t_{1/2}$: 9–12 h
doxazosin (Cardura)	Hypertension Benign prostatic hypertrophy	*Adult:* PO, initially 1 mg/d, increasing to maximum of 16 mg/d, if needed *Adult:* PO, 1–8 mg/d	*Onset:* Unknown *Duration:* Unknown $t_{1/2}$: 22 h
ⓒ Direct-Acting Vasodilators			
hydralazine	Hypertension Hypertension in eclampsia	*Adult:* PO, 50 mg qid *Child:* PO, 7.5 mg/kg/d or 200 mg/d *Adult:* IV or IM, 20–40 mg, repeat as needed *Child:* IV or IM, 0.1–0.2 mg/kg/dose every 4 to 6 h as needed *Adult:* IV, 5–10 mg bolus every 20 min; after 20 mg, try another drug	*Onset:* Unknown *Duration:* 6–8 h $t_{1/2}$: 3–7 h *Onset:* 10–20 min *Duration:* 2–4 h

Hydrochlorothiazide is the prototype thiazide diuretic. A brief description of its use in hypertension is presented here.

Nursing Management of the Patient Receiving ⓟ Hydrochlorothiazide

Hydrochlorothiazide is normally administered orally once or twice a day in low doses. Twelve and a half milligrams provides the full antihypertensive effect, althouqh increased urine production can be achieved with larger doses. The full reduction in blood pressure can be measured after 4 weeks on drug therapy. Hydrochlorothiazide, like other thiazide diuretics, is equally effective as monotherapy in African Americas as European Americans. Monotherapy with hydrochlorothiazie is more effective in African American than monotherapy with beta blockers, ACE inhibitors, and ARBs. Adding a thiazide diuretic to those drug classes improves their ability to lower blood pressure in African Americans (Ferdinand & Armani, 2007; Douglas, Bakris, Epstein, et al., 2003). For a listing of some practice tips for assisting the African American with hypertension (see Box 26.4).

The common adverse effects from hydrochlorothiazide are related to fluid and electrolyte imbalances (i.e., hypovolemia, low potassium, magnesium, and sodium levels, and elevated uric acid and elevated blood glucose levels). Patients receiving too great a dose for their needs may demonstrate hypotension. The nurse should monitor the patient's intake and output, weight changes, and electrolyte levels while they receive hydrochlorothiazide. Because patients with hypertension will normally require more than one drug to control their hypertension, hydrochlorothiazide is also found in many combination antihypertensive drugs. Diuretics are discussed in detail in Chapter 27.

Box 26.4 TIPS FOR HELPING AFRICAN- AMERICANS WITH HYPERTENSION

- Across the lifespan and in all primary care settings, African Americans need to have their blood pressure checked regularly
- Across the lifespan and in all primary care settings, African Americans need assessment for risks for cardiovascular disease.
  i. Assess for inactivity and obesity. Provide patient education and encouragement on diet and exercise to maintain a normal weight.
  ii. Assess for high salt intake. Provide patient education about the Dietary Approaches to Stop Hypertension (DASH diet) to help mange their hypertension and assist the patient to make dietary changes.
  iii. Monitor lipid levels. African Americans should receive anti-lipid therapy to achieve or maintain a low-density lipoprotein cholesterol goal of less than 100 mg/dL to help decrease their risk for CHD.

- Patient education for African Americans should emphasis the link between hypertension, lifestyle choices, and cardiovascular and renal outcomes.
- African Americans may use all types of antihypertensive drug therapies. Monotherapy is most effective with low dose thiazide diuretics and calcium channel blockers. Combination therapy is frequently warranted to treat hypertension, however.
- If clinical guidelines indicate that there are compelling reasons to start hypertensive therapy with a specific class of antihypertensive other than a thiazide, these guidelines should also be applied to African American patients.
- If African Americans are prescribed an ACE inhibitor, monitor them closely for the adverse effects of angiodema and/or cough, as they are more at risk for these adverse effects.

Based on Table 11 Treatment Pearls: management of High Blood pressure in African Americans from: Douglas, J. G., Bakris, G. L., Epstein, M., et al. (2003). Management of high blood pressure in African Americans: Consensus statement of the Hypertension in African Americans Working Group of the International Society on Hypertension in Blacks. *Archives of Internal Medicine, 163*(5), 525–541. Retrieved from: http://ishib.org/supportfiles/Mgt_of_Hypertension_in_African_Americans.pdf

• C BETA BLOCKERS

How beta blockers work is arguable, and several mechanisms of action have been proposed to explain how they reduce hypertension. Clinically, they have been proven to slow heart rate, decrease cardiac output, and lower blood pressure. Although beta blockers (at beta-2 receptor sites) increase peripheral resistance through vasoconstriction, this effect is outweighed by the substantial decrease in cardiac output, thereby lowering blood pressure. The peripheral vasoconstriction appears to be temporary, with resistance returning to baseline or lower levels with prolonged therapy. It is also believed that beta blockers have a central effect, which may decrease sympathetic outflow to the peripheral nervous system. Additionally, beta-adrenergic receptors are responsible for the release of renin from the kidneys. This release is prevented by using beta blockers.

Beta blockers may be selected as primary therapy for patients with hypertension and the following comorbidities: MI, stable heart failure, asymptomatic left ventricular dysfunction, atrial fibrillation, and angina. If these comorbidities are not present, the use of beta blockers as primary therapy for hypertension should be avoided, because, while they reduce stroke and cardiovascular events, they do not decrease CHD or mortality. First-line use of beta blockers appears to be inferior to low-dose thiazides (Wright & Musini, 2009). Beta blockers only weakly reduce the risk of stroke and may not have any effect on coronary heart disease; additionally, beta blockers seem to create worse outcomes in comparison to calcium channel blockers, renin-angiotensin system inhibitors, and thiazides (Wiysonge, Bradley, Mayosi, et al., 2007).

Metoprolol is the prototype beta blocker. A full discussion of metoprolol is in Chapter 13. Here are a few key points related to its use in treating hypertension.

Nursing Management of the Patient Receiving P Metoprolol

Metoprolol is used to treat hypertension, as well as the cardiac problems angina and congestive heart failure. It is usually administered as a sustained-release oral tablet for blood pressure control, although a rapid release formula is also available. A full week of therapy should be used to determine the effectiveness of a particular dose before increasing the daily dose. Metoprolol may be used in monotherapy or in combination with other antihypertensives. Use of a beta blocker as monotherapy to treat hypertension in African Americans will produce less therapeutic effect than when used to treat European Americans with hypertension (Ferdinand & Armani, 2007; Douglas, Bakris, Epstein, et al., 2003).

Because of its effects on blocking beta-1 receptors, metoprolol slows heart rate, the speed of conduction, and decreases the force of contraction, thus cardiac output is decreased, decreasing blood pressure. Metoprolol is a relatively selective beta-1 blocker, meaning that there is little stimulation of beta-2, alpha-1, or alpha-2 receptors. This helps to minimize adverse effects to drug therapy. As the dose increases, however, metoprolol becomes less selective for beta-2 receptors, and so the patient may begin to experience adverse effects from having the other adrenergic recetors blocked (such as bronchospasm, wheezing, or dyspnea). One adverse effect common to metoproplol and all beta blocker is depression (nurses sometimes use the expression "beta blocker blues" to remember this adverse effect). Assess patients carefully for a history of depression, suicidal ideation, or attempted suicide as metoprolol, like all beta blockers need to be used very cautiously in these patients; depending on the patient history, this class of drugs may not be suitable. Sudden discontinuation of the drug may create rebound hypertension. If the patient also has angina it can also create rebound angina, possibly precipitating an MI. It is important to consult with the surgeon and anesthetist before major surgery because metropolol may or may not be discontinued. The physician may wish for the patient to receive the drug for blood pressure control on the morning of surgery. Withdrawal of beta-blocking drug therapy before major surgery is controversial because hypersensitivity to catecholamines has been noted in patients after withdrawal. Because reflex hypertension or angina can occur with sudden stoppage of a beta blocker, the dose of metoprolol is recommended to be slowly tapered downwards over 2 weeks if the drug is to be discontinued. Teach your patients not to stop taking their medication on their own and to be certain not to allow their prescriptions to run out. As metoprolol decreases both pulse rate and blood pressure, be sure to assess both of these before administering the drug. Do not administer the dose if the patient is bradycardic or hypotensive. Let the physician know of these findings. Teach your patients or their families how to check their pulse and blood pressure at home, and what to do if there is a problem.

Drugs significantly different from metoprolol
Labetalol

Labetalol is an adrenergic blocking agent that has a non-specific beta-blocking action at both the beta-1 and beta-2 receptor sites, and a selective alpha-1-blocking action, unlike metoprolol, which blocks beta 2 receptors selectively. The ratio of alpha-beta-blocking action is 1:3 with oral use and 1:7 with IV use. The alpha-blocking actions cause peripheral vasodilation. Because the alpha-blocking action decreases standing blood pressure more than it decreases supine blood pressure, orthostatic hypotension may occur (in about 2% of patients), although it is transient. The beta-1 and -2 blocking action prevents reflex tachycardia. It also prevents exercise-induced tachycardia and elevations in blood pressure; however, it has no effect on respiratory rate. The beta-blocking effect also results in a decrease in the plasma renin level.

Labetalol is used for treating hypertension, usually with other agents, especially thiazide and loop diuretics, although it may be used alone. Labetalol reduces blood pressure while maintaining glomerular filtration rate and renal blood flow. The parenteral form is used for managing severe hypertension and is given only in the hospital. Labetalol is often used to manage acute, severe hypertension that occurs after an acute ischemic stroke. Unlabeled uses include lowering hypertension associated with encephalopathy. Labetalol also has been used in clonidine-withdrawal hypertension. Labetalol has similar contraindications and precautions, and adverse effects as the prototype, metoprolol.

When labetalol is administered orally, it is completely absorbed and the peak action occurs in 2 to 4 hours. Maximum steady-state blood pressure response occurs within 24 to 72 hours. Labetalol has an extensive first-pass effect and is metabolized rapidly by the liver. It is excreted in the stool and urine. Labetalol penetrates the CNS, crosses the placenta, and appears in breast milk in minimal amounts. Verify that orthostatic blood pressure remains stable after an initial oral dose or after a dosage increase.

The drug also can be administered parenterally, with the onset occurring rapidly and peaking in 5 minutes. Although labetalol can be parenterally administered as either repeated IV boluses or a continuous IV infusion, IV infusion has certain benefits, including greater control of antihypertensive action and a decrease in the severity and rate of adverse effects. IV labetalol is administered only in the hospital. Prepare IV infusions of labetalol carefully. Multiple concentrations may be ordered, and the required diluent varies depending on the desired concentration. Different manufacturers make different concentrations of labetalol, which also influences how much drug volume needs to be added to the diluent. Carefully read the labels and follow the manufacturer's instructions when preparing IV infusions of labetalol.

Monitor closely the blood pressure of patients receiving IV infusions of labetalol. The blood pressure should be assessed every 5 to 10 minutes during the infusion. In addition, assess orthostatic blood pressures. Keep patients who

receive IV labetalol flat during infusion to prevent orthostatic hypotension, and assess patients' tolerance to an upright position before allowing them to ambulate. When labetalol infusion is used to treat hypertension after acute ischemic stroke, it is imperative to reduce blood pressure gradually to reduce the risk of intracerebral hemorrhage while maintaining sufficient cerebral perfusion. After IV infusions of labetalol have been stopped, assess blood pressure (including orthostatics) carefully and frequently to confirm that the blood pressure remains stable. After IV therapy is discontinued, blood pressure returns gradually to near-baseline levels in 16 to 18 hours. For information on managing complications of labetalol see Box 26.3. More information about beta blockers is found in Chapter 13.

CALCIUM CHANNEL BLOCKERS

Calcium channel blockers inhibit the movement of calcium ions across cell membranes, which decreases the mechanical contraction of the heart, reduces impulse formation (automaticity), and lessens conduction velocity. Calcium channel blockers also dilate coronary vessels and peripheral arteries, thereby decreasing peripheral resistance and blood pressure. Although decreased contractions of the heart usually result in decreased cardiac output, cardiac output is not decreased by calcium channel blocker therapy, most likely because of the reflex tachycardia that occurs secondary to vasodilation.

Use of calcium channel blockers as primary therapy in hypertension appear to be effective (Law, Morris, & Wald, 2009), although the literature that supports this is not considered robust (Wright & Musini, 2009). Calcium channel blockers provide some additional protection from stroke than other classes of hypertensives (Law, Morris, & Wald, 2009). Patients with comorbid atrial fibrillation or angina are prescribed a calcium channel blocker as the initial antihypertensive agent. African Americans respond equally as white Americans to monotherapy with calcium channel blockers (Douglas, Bakris, Epstein, et al., 2003). The prototype calcium channel blocker is verapamil. A full discussion of verapamil is in Chapter 31. Here are a few key points related to its use in treating hypertension.

Nursing Management of the Patient Receiving P Verapamil

Verapamil is used to treat hypertension as well as angina and cardiac arrhythmias. When used as an antihypertensive, it is administered orally. Calcium channel blockers, like verapamil, are effective as monotherapy or combination therapy when used in African Americans (Ferdinand & Armani, 2007; Douglas, Bakris, Epstein, et al., 2003).

Verapamil selectively blocks the movement of calcium ions into arterial smooth muscles of all tissue, including conductile and contractile myocardial cells, without affecting the concentration of serum calcium. Its hypertensive effect is attributed to the reduction of systemic vascular

CRITICAL THINKING SCENARIO

MANAGING COMPLICATIONS OF LABETALOL THERAPY

Your patient, Mr. Parker, is receiving labetalol IV for hypertension. Today, for the first time, he has rales (crackles) in the mid and lower lobes of both lungs. He has gained 3 lb since he was last weighed 2 days ago. On checking, you note that his urinary output has decreased in the last 2 days also.

1. What do you conclude from these findings? And what is the rationale for your conclusions?
2. Based on your assessment, which type of orders might you seek from the physician or nurse practitioner?
3. Which nursing actions would you propose implementing independently?

resistance and selective vasodilation of peripheral arteries, thus it decreases afterload. One of the main adverse effects is hypotension. Because it can alter the rhythm of the heart and decrease the rate and force of contraction, verapamil may cause cardiac adverse effects such as new or worsening arrhythmias, bradycardia, angina, and worsening of congestive heart failure. A unique adverse effect of verapamil is that it can cause significant constipation; this adverse effect is less with other calcium channel blockers.

Assess the patient's blood pressure and pulse before administering a calcium channel blocker such as verapamil. Withhold the dose of the drug if the patient is hypotensive or bradycardic and notify the physician. Teach your patient and their family how to assess the pulse and blood pressure and when they should notify the physician. Encourage fluid intake of at least 2000 cc/d and a diet rich in fruits and vegetables to help prevent constipation.

C ANGIOTENSIN-CONVERTING ENZYME INHIBITORS

In the renin-angiotensin-aldosterone sequence, a special enzyme is needed to convert the inactive angiotensin I to the active angiotensin II. Angiotensin II is a potent vasoconstrictor. Its presence increases secretion of aldosterone. When aldosterone levels rise, sodium and water are retained, and other effects are exerted on the heart, vessels, and kidneys. The ACE inhibitors prevent the conversion of angiotensin I to angiotensin II, which in turn decreases peripheral arterial resistance and sodium and water retention. ACE inhibitors are also likely to decrease the other negative effects from angiotensin and aldosterone.

ACE inhibitors are used as first-line antihypertensives if the patient has any of the following comorbidities: heart failure, asymptomatic left ventricular dysfunction, history of ST-elevation MI, history of non-ST elevation MI with an anterior infarct, diabetes, systolic dysfunction, or proteinuric chronic renal failure. Combination therapy with an ARB may be especially beneficial in patients with heart failure or proteinuric chronic renal failure. Combination therapy with an ARB may provide more antihypertensive effect and help to prevent end-organ damage more than use of either of these classes alone (Weir, 2007). Reviews of the literature indicate that there are no clinically significant differences in the blood pressure lowering abilities of different ACE inhibitors, they all create a modest effect (Heran, Wong, Heran, & Wright, 2008a). African Americans do not have as great a response as white Americans to monotherapy with ACE inhibitors; adding a thiazide diuretic or a calcium channel blocker to an ACE inhibitor greatly improves its effectiveness (Ferdinande & Armani, 2007; Douglas, Bakris, Epstein, et al., 2003).

Captopril (Capoten) is the prototype angiotensin-converting enzyme (ACE) inhibitor.

Nursing Management of the Patient Receiving P Captopril

Core Drug Knowledge

Pharmacotherapeutics

Captopril, like other ACE inhibitors, is administered orally to lower blood pressure in hypertensive patients. Captopril is also used in treating CHF (usually in combination with diuretics, beta blockers, and digitalis, although digitalis is not required for captopril to be effective). In addition, captopril is useful in treating diabetic nephropathy and left ventricular dysfunction after MI. Unlabeled uses include treating hypertensive crisis, neonatal and childhood hypertension, non-diabetic kidney disease, kidney imaging in renovascular hypertension; as an adjunct in treating acute pulmonary edema; renovascular hypertension hypertension related to scleroderma, renal crisis; captopril is also used to diagnose anatomic renal artery stenosis (captopril test) and primary aldosteronism.

Pharmacokinetics

Captopril is absorbed rapidly after oral ingestion. Food decreases absorption. Captopril has a rapid onset of action. The drug is metabolized (50%) by the liver. It crosses the placenta and also appears in breast milk. It is in pregnancy category C in the first trimester and category D in the second and third trimesters. Captopril does not cross the blood–brain barrier. It is eliminated unchanged (50%) by the kidneys. Its half-life is less than 2 hours in normal renal function and 3.5 to 32 hours in renal impairment (Table 26.4).

Pharmacodynamics

Captopril inhibits the ACE needed to change the inactive angiotensin I to the active form angiotensin II. This reduction of angiotensin II decreases the secretion of aldosterone, thus preventing sodium and water retention. Captopril therefore decreases peripheral vascular resistance and lowers blood pressure. Cardiac output increases, but the heart rate does not. However, peripheral vascular resistance is lowered more than cardiac output is increased, resulting in a substantial decrease in blood pressure. Captopril also increases renal blood flow but has no effect on the glomerular filtration rate. The serum potassium level may increase slightly as a result of decreased aldosterone levels.

ACE is similar to bradykinase (kinase II). Therefore, ACE inhibitors increase the levels of bradykinin, and bradykinin stimulates the synthesis of prostaglandins. It has been hypothesized that the prostaglandins contribute to the antihypertensive effect of the ACE inhibitors.

Contraindications and Precautions

Captopril (and all other ACE inhibitors) can cause injury and death to a developing fetus during the second and third trimesters and carry a Black Box warning for this effect. It is contraindicated in patients with a history of angioedema and in patients with a hypersensitivity to the drug, and there may be a cross-sensitivity to other ACE inhibitors. Captopril should be administered cautiously to patients with hypovolemia (from aggressive diuretic use or dialysis), aortic stenosis (theoretically, patients treated with vasodilators are at risk for decreased coronary perfusion because they do not develop the afterload reduction as other patients do), hepatic dysfunction, hyperkalemia greater than 5.5 mEq mL, neutropenia, proteinuria, and renal insufficiency. Care should also be used with children (safety and efficacy are not established), pregnant women (pregnancy category C for first trimester, D for second and third trimesters) and breast-feeding women (concentrations of captopril in breast milk equal about 1% of maternal concentrations, although are usually compatible with breast-feeding). In addition, caution is also necessary if the patient is undergoing surgery or anesthesia, because this may increase the risk of hypotension.

Adverse Effects

Chronic cough can occur with captopril and all ACE inhibitors, presumably because the drug inhibits the degradation of endogenous bradykinin. The cough is nonproductive and persistent. It resolves within 1 to 4 days after therapy stops but is a major reason for nonadherence to therapy. The next most common adverse effect is rash. Other adverse effects that may occur are first-dose hypotension (especially in severely salt- or volume-depleted patients, i.e., those treated aggressively with diuretics), and hypotension, although this effect usually is limited to patients with CHF and is transient. Although the risk is uncommon, captopril, like other ACE inhibitors, carries the risk for two serious life-threatening effects—angioedema and neutropenia. Angioedema can occur after the first dose of captopril, or at any other time during therapy. Angioedema confined to the face and lips may resolve untreated. Angioedema associated with laryngoedema can be fatal and needs immediate emergency care. The risk for neutropenia depends on the patient's clinical status. Most at risk are patients with collagen vascular diseases, such as systemic lupus erythematosus (SLE), and impaired renal function. Also at risk are patients with heart failure. Neutropenia generally resolves quickly after captopril is discontinued. Fatalities have occurred, mostly in patients ill with the above-mentioned diseases.

Allergic reactions and anaphylaxis also are possible with captopril. Other adverse effects, which are not common, include:

- Proteinuria
- CV: chest pain, angina, MI, palpitations, orthostatic hypotension, tachycardia, and rhythm disturbances
- CNS: insomnia, paresthesia, dizziness, headache, fatigue, drowsiness, ataxia, confusion, depression, malaise, and nervousness
- Gastrointestinal (GI) and genitourinary (GU): abdominal pain, nausea and vomiting, diarrhea, constipation, anorexia, oliguria, dry mouth, dyspepsia, pancreatitis, and hepatitis
- Respiratory: asthma, bronchospasm, and dyspnea
- Dermatologic: alopecia, pruritus, flushing, photosensitivity, erythema multiforme, and exfoliative dermatitis

- Miscellaneous: impotence, syncope, asthenia, anemia, blurred vision, fever, myalgia, arthralgia, eosinophilia, and vasculitis

Overdosage of captopril most frequently results in hypotension. Vascular re-expansion with IV normal saline solution is the treatment of choice.

Drug Interactions

Captopril interacts with several other drugs, as presented in Table 26.5. Captopril may cause a false-positive test result with urine acetone. Food greatly decreases the bioavailability of captopril (by 30% to 40%), but it remains unknown whether the therapeutic effects of captopril are affected to a similar degree.

Assessment of Relevant Core Patient Variables

Health Status

Blood pressure should be determined before captopril therapy begins. Patients receiving captopril to treat CHF are likely to be receiving concurrent diuretics. If the drug history reveals that the patient has received diuretics, especially high doses of diuretics, assess for signs of hypovolemia, which places the patient at increased risk for hypotension. Other factors that may cause hypovolemia include excessive perspiration, vomiting, and diarrhea. Watch for signs of dehydration and determine whether the patient has renal impairment, because some patients have developed increases in blood urea nitrogen (BUN) and serum creatinine levels after blood pressure is reduced.

Patients with CHD may develop stable elevations of the BUN and serum creatinine with long-term captopril use, although discontinuation of treatment is not usually required. Electrolytes, especially potassium and sodium, should be in normal ranges to start therapy because hyperkalemia and hyponatremia may result from therapy.

Life Span and Gender

Determine whether the patient is pregnant. Patients who are pregnant should not receive captopril or other ACE inhibitors. If the patient becomes pregnant while taking captopril, therapy should be discontinued as soon as possible. Also, determine whether the patient is breast-feeding because captopril crosses into breast milk; the American Academy of Pediatrics has reported that captopril and breast-feeding are compatible.

Note that the adverse effect of cough appears to affect women more than men.

Lifestyle, Diet, and Habits

Assess the patient's normal dietary habits before administering captopril. Poor oral intake and decreased sodium intake may predispose the patient to adverse effects of captopril. If the patient normally uses a salt substitute containing potassium or potassium supplements, these substances may need to be discontinued to avoid possible hyperkalemia. Also, explore with the patient lifestyle changes intended to decrease blood pressure, such as weight loss, smoking cessation, increased exercise, and limited salt intake.

TABLE 26.5 Agents That Interact with P Captopril

Interactants	Effect and Significance	Nursing Management
antacids	Decreases bioavailability of captopril	Stagger drug administration by at least 2-h intervals.
azathioprine	Myelosuppression (anemia or leukopenia) can be induced by this combination, although the exact mechanism is unknown.	Avoid this combination. If coadministration cannot be avoided, monitor carefully for myelosuppression.
bupivacaine	Suppression of the renin-angiotensin system may increase the risk of bradycardia and hypotension from spinal anesthesia.	Monitor patients closely during surgery, and treat any hemodynamic instability appropriately.
loop diuretics and other diuretics	First-dose postural hypotension can be severe when ACE inhibitors are added to loop diuretics if patient is sodium depleted or hypovolemic. Effect is transient. Other types of diuretics increase this risk also.	Titrate dose of ACE inhibitors to minimize first-dose hypotension. Monitor blood pressure closely for 4 h after first dose. If possible, administer at bedtime.
capsaicin	Increases effect of captopril and may exacerbate coughing	Inform patient that coughing may attend coadministration, and suggest cough-control measures. Assess for adherence to therapy.
cyclosporine	Potential to induce acute renal dysfunction	Monitor patients for renal dysfunction.
interferon alfa-2a	Possible increased risk of hematologic abnormalities (granulocytopenia, thrombocytopenia)	Monitor CBCs closely during combined therapy.
phenothiazine antipsychotics	Increases pharmacologic effects of captopril via synergistic action	Monitor blood pressure for hypotension.
probenecid	Increases effect of captopril, possibly raising serum levels and decreasing total clearance	Monitor blood pressure for hypotension.
allopurinol	Possibility for cross-sensitivity	Avoid concurrent administration. Monitor for signs of allergic reaction.
digoxin	Increases plasma digoxin levels	Monitor for possible bradycardia and other adverse effects.
epoetin alfa	Patients receiving hemodialysis may need higher doses of epoetin alfa to achieve therapeutic effect if receiving an ACE inhibitor.	Monitor red blood cell count. Seek orders to adjust dose if needed.
lithium	Increases serum lithium levels	Monitor laboratory data for evidence of lithium level elevation and patient for symptoms of lithium toxicity.
potassium preparations or potassium-sparing diuretics, aldosterone blockers	Increases serum potassium levels	Monitor electrolyte values. Observe patient for signs of hyperkalemia.
NSAIDs	May decrease the antihypertensive effect and loss of sodium in the urine	Caution is advised if an NSAID is coadministered with an ACE inhibitor, especially in patients predisposed to or with preexisting nephropathy. Monitor blood pressure and cardiovascular function for a reduction in the efficacy of the ACE inhibitor. Also monitor patient for hyperkalemia or acute renal failure.
aspirin	Aspirin when used in anti-inflammatory doses can decrease the antihypertensive effect of captopril, especially in low-renin hypertensives, possibly related to an inhibition of prostaglandin synthesis. However, aspirin did not alter captopril's positive effects post-MI.	Although studies have suggested an interaction between ACE inhibitors and aspirin, the clinician should weigh the benefits against the risks of combining these two agents. A dose adjustment may be necessary if the antihypertensive effect is not achieved.

TABLE 26.5	Agents That Interact with ℗ Captopril (continued)	
Interactants	Effect and Significance	Nursing Management
ma huang (Ephedra)	May decrease the antihypertensive effectiveness through antagonist effects	Avoid this combination.
vasodilators	Additive hypotensive response	Monitor blood pressure carefully during combined therapy.
yohimbine	Increased norepinephrine release by yohimbine may counteract the hypotensive effect of ACE inhibitors.	Avoid concomitant use.

Environment

Although captopril may be given in any environment, it is important to assess the safety of the patient's environment before taking the first dose because of the possibility of first-dose hypotension.

Culture and Inherited Traits

Note the patient's ethnic and cultural background before administering captopril. When captopril is used as monotherapy in African Americans who are "low-renin hypertensive," a smaller antihypertensive response occurs than that seen in the general population, although the drug is still effective. Adding a thiazide diuretic will increase its effectiveness.

Nursing Diagnoses and Outcomes

- Risk for Injury from first-dose hypotension related to effect of drug therapy and from drug-induced neutropenia
  Desired outcome: The patient will not sustain injury from a hypotensive event or neutropenia.
- Ineffective Therapeutic Regimen Management, Nonadherence, related to persistent dry cough secondary to drug therapy
  Desired outcome: Adherence to drug therapy will be unaffected by chronic cough.
- Disturbed Sensory Perception related to possible electrolyte imbalance, hyperkalemia, and hyponatremia, related to effects of captopril
  Desired outcome: The patient's electrolyte levels will remain within normal ranges.
- Risk for Impaired Skin Integrity related to drug-induced rash and pruritus
  Desired outcome: Skin integrity will not be impaired.

Planning and Intervention

Maximizing Therapeutic Effects

Administer captopril 1 hour before meals because food decreases absorption.

Minimizing Adverse Effects

FIRST-DOSE HYPOTENSION

Monitor the patient for at least 2 hours after the initial dose and until blood pressure stabilizes. Transient hypotension does not indicate that captopril should be discontinued; the dose can be restarted after blood pressure stabilizes. It is important to assist the patient to a supine position and give

normal saline solution IV if severe hypotension occurs. Assess patients receiving diuretic therapy, especially when the diuretic dose increases, because salt deficiency or volume depletion increases risk.

HYPOTENSION

Assess patients with CHF very carefully. It is important to start therapy with low doses, to decrease the diuretic before starting captopril therapy, or to increase salt intake about 1 week before starting captopril therapy.

Altered Laboratory Results

Assess blood reports for hyperkalemia, hyponatremia, and neutropenia, and assess urine for proteinuria.

Allergic Reactions

If a polyacrylonitrile dialyzer is used, extreme care is needed during dialysis of a patient on captopril. Allergic reactions may occur suddenly, with severe or fatal effects. Make sure that dialysis stops at the first sign of nausea, abdominal cramping, burning, angioedema, or shortness of breath leading to severe hypotension. Be prepared to intervene if the patient experiences anaphylactic reactions.

Providing Patient and Family Education

- Explain the purpose of the drug therapy and its possible adverse effects. If patients are to start on captopril at home, advise them to take the first dose at bedtime to minimize the possibilities of injury from first-dose hypotension.
- Tell patients to arise slowly from a lying or seated position in case of orthostatic hypotension and dizziness.
- Explain that the drug may produce a persistent dry cough, but that it is not serious. It is a good idea to encourage patients to continue therapy and to provide ideas for minimizing the cough. However, tell patients to consult the prescriber if the cough becomes intolerable.
- Advise patients to notify the prescriber promptly about the following adverse effects: sore throat; fever; swollen hands or feet; irregular heartbeat; chest pain; swollen face, eyes, lips, and tongue; difficulty breathing; or hoarseness. A rash may also appear and should be reported, although this finding is not as urgent as the others.
- Tell patients not to use potassium supplements or salt substitutes containing potassium, because of the risk of hyperkalemia.

• Explain the importance of adhering to schedules for follow-up blood tests.
• Counsel patients to make lifestyle changes (e.g., diet, weight loss, and exercise) to reduce blood pressure. Offer positive reinforcement for changes made, and encourage patients to sustain these changes.
• Teach patients how to self-monitor blood pressure to assess drug effectiveness.

Ongoing Assessment and Evaluation

Monitor blood pressure throughout captopril therapy. Blood pressure that decreases to a normal range is indicative of successful drug therapy. Monitor white blood cell counts, potassium and sodium levels, and urine protein values throughout therapy as well. Levels that remain in the normal range demonstrate that adverse effects have not occurred. In patients with CHF, cardiac output increases because of decreased peripheral resistance, and the patient's exercise tolerance time increases. These findings also indicate effective drug therapy. The decreased peripheral resistance (afterload) improves ejection fraction in patients who have left ventricular dysfunction resulting from MI, reducing the incidence of overt heart failure that requires hospitalization.

Monitor for evidence of renal insufficiency in patients receiving captopril for diabetic nephropathy. Progressing renal insufficiency and serious clinical outcomes (need for dialysis, need for kidney transplantation, and death) should be slowed. Also, monitor these patients for proteinuria, even though captopril should decrease proteinuria.

MEMORY CHIP

 Captopril

• Inhibits the angiotensin-converting enzyme (ACE) needed to change angiotensin I (inactive) to angiotensin II (active). Angiotensin II is a potent vasoconstrictor, so that less angiotensin II means less vasoconstriction.
• Decreased angiotensin II also decreases secretion of aldosterone, which thus prevents retention of sodium and water
• Lowers blood pressure by decreasing peripheral vascular resistance; smaller antihypertensive response (monotherapy) in African Americans than whites
• Most common adverse effect: chronic cough
• Most serious adverse effects: angioedema and neutropenia
• **Life span alert: avoid use during second and third trimesters of pregnancy.**
• Minimizing adverse effects: Monitor blood pressure for 2 hours after initial dose until stabilized, and monitor patient's blood pressure throughout therapy.
• Most important patient education: Urge continuation of lifestyle changes while on drug therapy, and teach the signs and symptoms of hypotension.
• **Black box warning: Captopril can cause injury and death to a developing fetus during the second and third trimesters.**

Drugs Closely Related to [P] Captopril

The other ACE inhibitors that are closely related to captopril are benazepril (Lotensin), enalaprilat (Vasotec IV; IV form of enalapril), enalapril (Vasotec), fosinopril (Monopril), lisinopril (Prinivil, Zestril), moexipril (Univasc), perindopril (Aceon), quinapril (Accupril), ramipril (Altace), and trandolapril (Mavik). The differences between these drugs and captopril relate to labeled indication, being a prodrug for the active ACE inhibition, half-life, or the route of administration. The following drugs have different labeled indications from captopril: benazepril (labeled for hypertension only, but used off-label for CHF); enalaprilat (labeled for hypertension only); enalapril (labeled for hypertension, heart failure, and renal disease for patients without diabetes); fosinopril (labeled for CHF and hypertension only); lisinopril (labeled for hypertension, CHF, and acute MI); moexipril (labeled for hypertension only); perindopril (labeled for hypertension and as prophylaxis in patients with risk of CV events or stable coronary artery disease); quinapril (labeled for use in CHF or hypertension only); and ramipril (labeled for use in CHF, hypertension, and reduction of CV events). The following drugs, unlike captopril, are actually prodrugs that are converted into the active form: benazepril; perindopril; quinapril; ramipril; and trandolapril. All of the other ACE inhibitors, except enalapril, have longer half-lives (some of them extremely longer) than captopril. Enalaprilat is the intravenous form of enalapril.

Drugs Significantly Different From [P] Captopril

Aliskiren (Tekturna) is the first drug in a new class of antihypertensives, the renin inhibitors. Unlike captopril, which prevents the conversion of angiotensin I to angiotensin II, aliskiren directly inhibits renin, thus decreasing plasma renin activity and preventing the formation of angiotensin I. Even though the negative feedback loop in the renin-angiotensin-aldosterone loop is altered, additional renin is not released due to the action of aliskiren. This makes aliskiren also different from the actions of ARBs and selective aldosterone inhibitors (further discussed in later sections), where the circulating plasma levels of renin increase because there is not a high enough level of angiotensin II and aldosterone to shut off the renin production. The long-term effect (positive or negative) of reducing renin levels is not yet known. For this reason, aliskiren is not currently used as initial therapy in treating hypertension, however with additional research it may become a first-line drug.

Aliskiren was tested and found effective in treating mild to moderate hypertension, either alone or in combination therapy with other antihypertensives. Its therapeutic effectiveness was evident after 2 weeks of therapy. Clinical trials showed aliskiren to be at least as effective as an ARB or an ACE inhibitor, such as captopril (Musini, Fortin, Bassett, Wright, 2009; Andersen, Weinberger, Egan, et al, 2008; Strasser, Puig, Farsang, et al., 2007). Although aliskiren lowers blood pressure, no long-term studies have yet demonstrated that morbidity or mortality from hypertension is decreased. Similar to other drugs that alter the renin-angiotensin-aldosterone system, monotherapy with aliskiren produced fewer antihypertensive effects in African Americans than in Caucasians or Asians, probably because most African Americans are "low-renin hypertensives."

Aliskiren may be helpful in treating diabetic nephropathy from hypertension based on the findings of the Aliskiren in the Evaluation of Proteinuria in Diabetes (AVOID) trial. This clinical trial found that treatment with aliskiren led to a greater reduction in albuminuria at 6 months compared to placebo in patients with hypertension, type 2 diabetes and nephropathy receiving losartan and additional optimal antihypertensive therapy concomitantly (Parving, Persson, Lewis, et al., 2008). Use of aliskiren for diabetic nephropathy is an off-label use.

Like ACE inhibitors, such as captopril, and ARBs, aliskiren carries a Black Box warning that it should not be used in the second or third trimester of pregnancy because it can cause fetal injury and death. It is a pregnancy category D drug (second and third trimesters).

Aliskiren is metabolized by the P-450 isoenzyme system, specifically 3A4. It does not induce or inhibit any part of the P-450 system. Some drugs can alter the levels of aliskiren when used in combination. Irbesartan, one of the ARBs, decreases the availability of aliskiren. Atorvastatin, an antilipid statin drug, and ketoconazole, an antifungal agent, significantly increase the availability of aliskiren. When given with furosemide, the loop diuretic, aliskiren significantly reduces the available amount of furosemide. Changes in the dosage may be indicated if the patient is receiving any of the drugs that interact with aliskiren.

Aliskiren is usually well tolerated. Patients tolerate aliskiren similarly to how they tolerate ACE inhibitors (Strasser, Puig, Farsang, et al., 2007). Hypotension is unlikely, although it may occur if patients are already salt and volume depleted from aggressive diuretic therapy. These conditions should be corrected before starting treatment with aliskiren. If hypotension does occur, treatment with IV infusions of a normal saline solution is necessary. Hyperkalemia can occur when aliskiren is administered to patients with diabetes who are also receiving an ACE inhibitor, such as captopril, but this condition is rare otherwise. Serum levels in these patients should be monitored closely. GI adverse effects, such as diarrhea, may occur, although these adverse effects are usually mild; they occur more frequently when larger doses of aliskiren are administered. Cough can occur in patients taking aliskiren, similar to captopril and other ACE inhibitors; however, the incidence of cough from aliskiren is much less. At this time, it is not known whether a patient who has been taken off captopril or any other ACE inhibitor because of cough would be more likely to develop a cough from aliskiren.

ANGIOTENSIN II RECEPTOR BLOCKERS

Angiotensin II receptor blockers, or ARBs (sometimes referred to as angiotensin II receptor antagonists, or AIIRAs), block the action of angiotensin II from all the different pathways where it is formed, not just the single substrate altered by ACE inhibitors. These drugs are effective in lowering blood pressure modestly and are similar in effectiveness to ACE inhibitors as a class (Heran, Wong, Heran, and Wright, 2008b). In addition, they seem to block deleterious effects from angiotensin II at the end-organ stage, which is where serious complications of sustained hypertension occur (Weir, 2007). This effect seems to be independent of the antihypertensive effect produced by the drugs. Combining an ACE inhibitor and an ARB such as losartan may provide greater antihypertensive effect and end-organ protection than use of either drug class alone (Weir, 2007). For patients with diabetic renal disease, ARBs have been shown to reduce the rate of end-stage renal disease (Igarashi, Hirata, Kadomoto, et al., 2006; Osawa, Nakamura, Shirato, et al., 2006; Prisant, 2003). Combination of an ACE inhibitor with an ARB has been found to help remodel the left ventricle to improve its function again after hypertension has caused deleterious effects; it is more effective than the combination of an ACE inhibitor with a calcium channel blocker (Grandi, Solbiati, Laurita, et al., 2008).

The indications for ARBs and their efficacy are similar to those of ACE inhibitors. An ARB is used if a patient cannot tolerate the adverse effects from an ACE inhibitor. Patients can be safely switched from an ACE inhibitor to an ARB with similar effects on blood pressure control occurring from either drug (Spinar, Vitovec, Soucek, et al., 2009). A unique comorbidity in which an ARB appears to be preferred as first-line therapy is severe hypertension with electrocardiographic (ECG) evidence of left ventricular hypertrophy. Like ACE inhibitors, ARBs do not create the same efficacy in African American as in white Americans if they are used as monotherapy (Douglas, Bakris, Epstein, et al., 2003). Losartan (Cozaar) is the prototype angiotensin II receptor blocker (ARB).

Nursing Management of the Patient Receiving P Losartan
Core Drug Knowledge
Pharmacotherapeutics

Losartan, a monopotassium salt, is used to treat hypertension. Clinical trials have shown that if a patient was receiving an ACE inhibitor for hypertension, he or she could be safely switched to the ARB losartan while maintaining effective blood pressure control (Spinar, Vitovec, Soucek, et al., 2009). Losartan is also used to treat diabetic nephropathy. For these patients, losartan reduces the rate of progression of nephropathy, determined by the doubling of serum creatinine or end-stage renal disease requiring dialysis or renal transplantation. Losartan has been found to decrease the risk of fatal and nonfatal stroke in patients with hypertension and left ventricular hypertrophy, but there is evidence that this benefit does not apply to African American patients. Losartan can be used in treating heart failure, but this use is currently unlabeled. (See Chapter 29 for more about the use of ARBs in heart failure.) Another off-label use is the treatment of erythrocytosis.

Pharmacokinetics

Losartan undergoes a substantial first-pass metabolism and is converted to an active metabolite, which performs most of the antagonism at the angiotensin II receptors. Cytochrome P-450 2C9 and 3A4 isoenzymes are involved in the metabolism of losartan. Both the drug and the active metabolite (which produces the therapeutic effect) are highly protein bound. The peak concentration occurs in 1 hour for losartan and in 3 to 4 hours for its metabolite. The half-life is about 2 hours for the drug and 6 to 9 hours for the metabolite. Excretion occurs in the urine and stool.

Pharmacodynamics

Angiotensin II receptor blockers do not inhibit ACE. Instead, they block the vasoconstricting and aldosterone-secreting effects of angiotensin II by selectively blocking the binding of angiotensin II to the angiotensin I receptors in many tissues, especially in the vascular smooth muscle and adrenal gland tissues. Although an angiotensin II receptor exists, it does not seem to have an effect on the CV system. ARBs have a much greater affinity for angiotensin I than angiotensin II receptors. Losartan has about a 1,000-fold increase in affinity for angiotensin I. Losartan is a reversible, competitive inhibitor of the angiotensin I receptor. The active metabolite appears 10 to 40 times more potent by weight than losartan. It appears to be a reversible but not competitive inhibitor of the angiotensin I receptor.

Losartan, like other ARBs, inhibits the pressor effect of angiotensin II, removing the negative feedback that occurs normally. This effect causes a twofold to threefold increase in plasma renin activity and a rise in angiotensin II plasma levels. These increases are not enough to offset the positive effects that ARBs have on hypertension. Although aldosterone secretion decreases, potassium levels do not seem to be affected by losartan. There is a minimal decrease in serum uric acid when oral losartan is administered long-term.

Research indicates that losartan contributes to the regression of left ventricular hypertrophy that is associated with chronic hypertension. Additionally, losartan appears to increase exercise capacity in patients with either asymptomatic or symptomatic heart failure.

Contraindications and Precautions

Like ACE inhibitors and renin inhibitors, ARBs such as losartan carry a black box warning that it may cause fetal injury or death if used in the second or third trimesters. Losartan is a pregnancy category C for the first trimester and category D for the second and third trimesters. The only other contraindication to losartan is hypersensitivity to any component of the drug.

Adverse Effects

A major advantage of losartan and other ARBs is that it does not cause the dry cough that occurs so frequently with ACE inhibitors. Overall, ARBs are well tolerated, with only about 2% of patients receiving losartan experiencing adverse effects bothersome enough to warrant discontinuing the drug. Of the adverse effects that do occur, the most frequent are hypotension, diarrhea, asthenia, dizziness, and fatigue. The most serious adverse effects are all rare: thrombocytopenia, rhabdomyolysis, and angioedema. Other effects that may occur, but are not common, include anxiety and nervousness; musculoskeletal pain, cramps, and myalgia; nasal congestion, sinus disorder, and sinusitis; rash; tachycardia; and urinary tract infection.

Overdosage of losartan may produce hypotension, dizziness, and tachycardia. Bradycardia may be produced from parasympathetic (vagal) stimulation. Hypotension should be treated with supportive therapy. Valsartan cannot be removed by dialysis.

Drug Interactions

Losartan is known to interact with lithium, increasing the resorption of lithium and the risk of lithium toxicity. Fluconazole, indomethacin, and rifampin can also interact with losartan. Food slows the absorption of losartan but has minimal effects on the activity of the drug. Losartan, when taken with either potassium supplements or drugs that spare potassium loss (e.g., triamterene), may lead to elevated serum potassium levels. Grapefruit juice will slow the metabolism of losartan to its active form and thus may decrease the effectiveness of losartan. Table 26.6 presents a summary of agents that interact with losartan.

Assessment of Relevant Core Patient Variables

Health Status

Patients who have pathologies that are dependent on the renin-angiotensin-aldosterone system (e.g., patients with severe CHF) should not use ARBs because oliguria, progressive azotemia, or (rarely) acute renal failure or death may result. Patients receiving ACE inhibitors who have renal artery stenosis have shown elevated serum creatinine or BUN, and it is hypothesized that ARBs would have the same effect. Assess patients for these conditions and monitor them for possible effects. Elevations in serum creatinine or BUN also may occur in other patients taking losartan. Of all patients who use losartan for hypertension, minor elevations in BUN and creatinine occur in fewer than 1%. Although elevated serum levels of losartan have been found in patients with decreased creatinine clearance, the active metabolite is not affected. Therefore, no dose adjustment is required for these patients.

Determine whether the patient is taking a prescribed potassium supplement or a potassium-sparing diuretic, either of which can produce hyperkalemia when taken with losartan, because of the potassium in its chemical formulations.

Patients who have impaired hepatic impairment do have increased bioavailability of losartan because metabolism is impaired. They should be given a lower starting dose of the drug and be monitored for therapeutic and adverse effects. Small decreases in hemoglobin and hematocrit occur in patients taking losartan. Although the effect is normally not clinically important, monitor these patients.

TABLE 26.6	Agents That Interact with P Losartan	
Interactants	**Effect and Significance**	**Nursing Management**
lithium	Increased renal resorption of lithium may produce lithium toxicity. .	Monitor lithium levels.
fluconazole	Metabolism of losartan via CYP2C9 may be inhibited; possibility of hypotension or adverse effects	Monitor blood pressure and assess for adverse effects if coadministered.
indomethacin	May decrease the effectiveness of losartan; blood pressure may not be as well controlled	Monitor blood pressure closely if coadministered; contact prescriber if loss of blood pressure control.
rifampin	Increases the metabolism of losartan; blood pressure may not be as well controlled	Monitor blood pressure closely if coadministered; contact prescriber if loss of blood pressure control.
potassium-sparing diuretics; other potassium-sparing drugs; potassium supplements; salt substitutes containing potassium	Additive effects to increase potassium levels; serious elevations of serum potassium may occur	Avoid coadministration with losartan.
grapefruit juice	Decreases the metabolism of losartan, which decreases the conversion to its active form. Decreased active drug can decrease the antihypertensive effect achieved.	Monitor for therapeutic effect.
ma huang (Ephedra)	May decrease the antihypertensive effectiveness through antagonist effects.	Avoid this combination
yohimbine	Increased norepinephrine release by yohimbine may counteract the hypotensive effect of ACE inhibitors.	Avoid concomitant use

Hypovolemia and salt depletion (usually from diuretic therapy) pose the same risk for hypotension to patients receiving losartan as to patients receiving captopril. It is important to correct these conditions before giving losartan.

Life Span and Gender

Determine whether the patient is pregnant or breast-feeding before administering losartan. Because of adverse effects on the fetus and neonate, losartan should not be used during pregnancy. Animal studies indicate that losartan passes into breast milk; it is not known whether losartan also passes into human milk. However, because of the serious effects that may occur, patients should not breast-feed while taking losartan. Additional concerns for women taking losartan come from other animal studies showing that female rats receiving the drug have a slightly higher rate of pancreatic cancer and impaired fertility. Again, the effects in humans are not known. The safety and efficacy of losartan and other ARBs in children younger than 18 years is not known. No dosage adjustments seem to be necessary for older adults, because losartan is equally safe and effective in this group compared with younger adults. Older adults generally tolerate ARB therapy better than therapy with other antihypertensive drug classes. Because losartan has essentially no contraindications, older adults with hypertension and other comorbidities can still take losartan at standard doses.

Lifestyle, Diet, and Habits

Assess the patient's usual lifestyle. Lifestyle modifications that are general for all patients requiring hypertensive therapy should be followed for patients taking losartan. Assess whether the patient is taking an over-the-counter (OTC) potassium supplement or uses a salt substitute containing potassium, because either one in combination with losartan may produce hyperkalemia. Assess for use of grapefruit juice because it may decrease the effectiveness of the drug.

Environment

Losartan may be administered in any setting.

Culture and Inherited Traits

It is a good idea to note the patient's racial background before administering losartan. Like captopril, losartan is less effective when used as monotherapy in hypertensive African Americans than in other racial groups. This effect may be because this racial group usually carries a low renin level. Again, adding a thiazide diuretic to the therapy will increase its effectiveness (Ferdinand & Armani, 2007; International Society of Hypertension in Blacks Guidelines, 2003).

Nursing Diagnoses and Outcomes

• Risk for Injury related to adverse effects on fetus and neonate. ***Desired outcome:*** *The patient receiving losartan will report pregnancy to prescriber as soon as possible.*

- Risk for Injury related to fall secondary to adverse effect of dizziness.
  Desired outcome: *The patient will not fall.*
- Risk for Infection (upper respiratory) related to adverse effects of drug therapy.
  Desired outcome: *The patient will not develop an upper respiratory infection, or if one develops, it will be managed appropriately to minimize complications.*

Planning and Intervention

Maximizing Therapeutic Effects

Like all drug therapy for hypertension, the use of losartan should be accompanied by the recommended lifestyle changes. Determine whether the patient has made these changes and provide encouragement to continue with them throughout drug therapy.

If losartan is ineffective alone, add a diuretic. Hydrochlorothiazide has been found to have an additive effect. A combination of losartan and hydrochlorothiazide is available. Consult with the physician or nurse practitioner for additional drug orders if indicated. Avoid giving losartan with grapefruit juice.

Minimizing Adverse Effects

Help the patient out of bed when he or she is first started on losartan therapy, in case dizziness occurs. It is important to treat the patient symptomatically for upper respiratory tract infections and diarrhea, if they are present. Monitor creatinine, BUN, hemoglobin, and hematocrit levels to verify that changes are not clinically meaningful. If the patient is currently prescribed a potassium supplement or a drug that increases potassium levels indirectly, consult with the prescriber about changing this therapy before starting losartan.

Providing Patient and Family Education

- If female patients are of childbearing age, caution them about the adverse effects that losartan can have on the fetus and neonate. Teach women to notify their prescriber immediately if they become pregnant.
- Explain the importance of arising slowly until the effects of the drug are known or if dizziness is present.
- Teach patients to avoid hazardous activities until effects of the drug are known.
- Teach patients not to take OTC potassium supplements or use a salt substitute that contains potassium.
- Tell patients to notify the prescriber if upper respiratory infection occurs.
- Provide general teaching about hypertension, lifestyle changes, and losartan core drug knowledge.

Ongoing Assessment and Evaluation

Monitor blood pressure throughout losartan therapy and determine whether the desired blood pressure goal has been achieved. Consider adding a diuretic if losartan is not effective in monotherapy. Verify that the patient continues with lifestyle changes. Treatment is effective if the desired reduction in blood pressure occurs in either monotherapy or multidrug therapy without the patient having serious adverse effects.

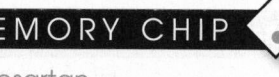

MEMORY CHIP

P Losartan

- Used to treat hypertension and kidney damage in people with type 2 diabetes
- Blocks vasoconstricting and aldosterone-secreting effects of angiotensin II by preventing angiotensin II from binding to receptor sites
- Does not produce ACE cough
- Most frequent adverse effects: upper respiratory infections, dizziness, and diarrhea
- No serious adverse effects in normal dosing
- **Life span alert: Do not give to women who are pregnant or breast-feeding.**
- Maximizing therapeutic effect: Continue with lifestyle changes.
- Minimizing adverse effects: Assist patient out of bed and with ambulation.
- Most important patient education: Use caution until it is known whether drug will cause dizziness; avoid OTC potassium supplements and salt substitutes containing potassium.
- **Black box warning: Can cause injury and death to a developing fetus during the second and third trimesters.**

Drugs Closely Related to **P** Losartan

ARBs that are closely related to losartan are candesartan (Atacand), eprosartan (Teveten), irbesartan (Avapro), olmesartan (Benicar), telmisartan (Micardis), and valsartan (Diovan). Major differences from losartan relate to labeled indication, half-life, and means of metabolism. The following drugs have differences in labeled indications: candesartan (heart failure and hypertension only); eprosartan (hypertension only); irbesartan (diabetic nephropathy and hypertension only); olmesartan (hypertension only); telmisartan (hypertension only); and valsartan (hypertension; additionally labeled for use in MI but not for diabetic nephropathy). The following drugs have a longer half-life than losartan: candesartan, eprosartan, irbesartan, olmesartan, and valsartan. Unlike losartan, olmesartan, telmisartan, and valsartan do not rely on the P-450 system for metabolism.

DRUGS USED AS SECOND-LINE ANTIHYPERTENSIVES

Second-line antihypertensives are added, usually as fourth or fifth drugs in a patient's drug therapy, when it is difficult to control the blood pressure with combinations of the first-line antihypertensives.

C SELECTIVE ALDOSTERONE BLOCKERS

Selective aldosterone blockers are approved for use in treating hypertension. These drugs block the mineralocorticoid receptors while having little interaction with androgen and progesterone receptors (thus the term *selective aldosterone blocker*). Blockade of these selective aldosterone receptors lowers blood pressure and reduces the end-organ damage that occurs with hypertension. The use of ACE inhibitors and ARBs alone does not protect organs from damage completely because the body uses renin-angiotensin-aldosterone system escape mechanisms. Aldosterone blockers, when added to either ACE inhibitor therapy or ARB therapy, provide added benefit, which may be attributable to preventing the deleterious effects from renin-angiotensin-aldosterone system escape mechanisms. One study showed that the addition of the aldosterone blocker spironolactone to therapy with an ARB helped reduce the left ventricular mass index and had beneficial effects on CV remodeling (Taniguchi, Kawai, Date, et al., 2006). Aldosterone blockers, like spironolactone, when added to other antihypertensive therapy, may help decrease albuminuria in patients with diabetic nephropathy (Schjoedt, Rossing, Juhl, et al., 2005).

Although JNC 7 guidelines do not list aldosterone blockers as part of primary therapy for hypertension, eplerenone is labeled for use as monotherapy or combination therapy and spironolactone is labeled for combination therapy in primary hypertension. As more research is completed with these drugs, it is likely that they may become part of primary therapy. These drugs are also indicated in the treatment of CHF (see Chapter 29). Eplerenone (Inspra) is the prototype selective aldosterone blocker.

Nursing Management of the Patient Receiving P Eplerenone

Core Drug Knowledge

Pharmacotherapeutics

Eplerenone is used to treat hypertension, either alone or with other antihypertensives. Eplerenone has been shown to lower blood pressure and reduce end-organ damage that can occur in hypertension. The full therapeutic effect of eplerenone takes 4 weeks to be evident. When given after MI to patients with evidence of systolic left ventricular dysfunction and symptoms of heart failure, eplerenone reduced hospitalizations for CV problems and deaths from CV disease (Stier, 2003). Eplerenone has been approved for treatment of heart failure after an MI.

Pharmacokinetics

Eplerenone is well absorbed from the GI system and reaches mean peak plasma concentrations within 1.5 hours after administration. Absorption is not affected by food. Eplerenone is about 50% protein bound and is bound primarily to alpha-1 acid glycoproteins. Metabolism of eplerenone is through the liver and CYP3A4 is the primary isoenzyme involved in its metabolism. Metabolism produces inactive metabolites. Elimination half-life is about 4 to 6 hours. Steady state is achieved within 2 days. Less than 5% of eplerenone is excreted unchanged. About two thirds of the drug is excreted by the kidneys through the urine, and about one third is excreted through the GI tract through stool.

Pharmacodynamics

Eplerenone binds selectively to the mineralocorticoid receptors, thereby blocking aldosterone from binding to these receptors. Eplerenone does not bind significantly to the glucocorticoid receptors, or to the progesterone or androgen receptors, which are also stimulated by aldosterone. By preventing aldosterone from binding to its receptor sites in the kidney, heart, blood vessels, and brain, eplerenone inhibits sodium and water retention as well as the other effects of aldosterone, which cause hypertension. For this reason, eplerenone can also be considered a potassium-sparing diuretic. By inhibiting aldosterone from attaching to its receptors, eplerenone also impairs the negative regulatory feedback mechanism of the renin-angiotensin-aldosterone system. Because the body does not receive the feedback message that aldosterone levels are sufficiently high, the body produces extra renin and aldosterone. However, increasing renin activity and elevated plasma levels of aldosterone do not offset the beneficial effects on blood pressure exerted by eplerenone.

Contraindications and Precautions

Eplerenone is contraindicated if patients have a serum potassium level greater than 5.5 mEq/L; type 2 diabetes with microalbuminuria; serum creatinine greater than 2 mg/dL in men or greater than 1.8 mg/dL in women; or a creatinine clearance less than 50 mL/min. Eplerenone is also contraindicated if patients are currently taking any of the following medications: potassium supplements; potassium-sparing diuretics (amiloride, spironolactone, triamterene); or a strong inhibitor of CYP3A4 (e.g., ketoconazole or itraconazole). All of these conditions increase the risk of developing hyperkalemia. Weak inhibitors of CYP3A4 (e.g., erythromycin, saquinavir, verapamil, fluconazole) may potentially also cause this, so precaution must be used. No adequate and well-controlled studies have been conducted for eplerenone in pregnant women, although animal studies have not shown potential complications; it is considered a pregnancy category B drug.

Adverse Effects

Generally, eplerenone is well tolerated, and adverse effects are mild. Hyperkalemia is the primary adverse effect. This is a potentially serious adverse effect, because the potassium levels may be high enough to cause serious or fatal arrhythmias. Another electrolyte imbalance that can occur, although not as frequently as hyperkalemia, is hyponatremia. Elevated triglyceride levels are also possible. Dizziness is another fairly common adverse effect, although its incidence is less than half that of hyperkalemia. Other possible serious adverse effects include angina and MI.

Other adverse effects that can occur, but are rare or infrequent, include:

- GI: diarrhea, abdominal pain
- GU: albuminuria, painful breasts and gynecomastia (in men), abnormal vaginal bleeding
- Metabolic: hypercholesterolemia, increased BUN, increased uric acid, increased serum creatinine, and increased ALT
- Miscellaneous: coughing, fatigue, flu-like symptoms

Drug Interactions

Eplerenone interacts with a few other drugs, mostly those that are ACE inhibitors, ARBs, or CYP3A4 potent inhibitors. Drugs that increase potassium levels, either directly or indirectly, can also have an additive effect with eplerenone. Administration with St. John's wort decreases the availability of eplerenone by about 30%. Grapefruit juice increases the availability of eplerenone by about 25%. Both of these changes are related to interactions involving the P-450 system. Table 26.7 presents a summary of drugs that interact with eplerenone.

Assessment of Relevant Core Patient Variables

Health Status

Before administering eplerenone, verify that the patient has hypertension. Assess serum potassium, serum creatinine, and creatinine clearance for alterations that indicate a contraindication to the drug. Also, assess whether the patient is receiving any concurrent drug therapy that is considered a contraindication to eplerenone therapy. The safety and efficacy of eplerenone in severe liver disease have not been established.

Life Span and Gender

Assess the life span status of the patient. Because the exact effect of eplerenone on pregnancy is not known, assess whether the patient is pregnant. The drug should be used only if potential benefits outweigh potential risks. Eplerenone passes into breast milk, but the exact concentration of the drug is unknown. The effects on the breast-fed infant are unknown at this time. Nursing mothers should most likely either discontinue the drug or discontinue nursing. The efficacy and safety of eplerenone are not known for children. Older adults may safely take eplerenone unless they have severe renal impairment.

Lifestyle, Diet, and Habits

Assess whether the patient uses an OTC potassium supplement or a salt substitute containing potassium; both are contraindications to drug therapy with eplerenone. Determine whether the patient uses St. John's wort or drinks grapefruit juice, both of which change the amount of drug available.

Environment

Eplerenone can be administered in any environmental setting and does not require special assessment of the environment.

TABLE 26.7 Agents That Interact with P Eplerenone

Interactants	Effect and Significance	Nursing Management
ACE inhibitors, ARBs	Increased risk of hyperkalemia; may cause arrhythmias	Avoid coadministration if possible; monitor serum potassium levels closely if coadministered.
potent CYP3A4 inhibitors (e.g., ketoconazole, itraconazole); weak CYP3A4 inhibitors (e.g., erythromycin, saquinavir, verapamil, fluconazole)	Potent inhibitors increase circulating levels of eplerenone fivefold; weak inhibitors increase them twofold. This increases risk of adverse effects, especially hyperkalemia.	Avoid coadministration of potent CYP3A4 inhibitors. Give lower initial dose of eplerenone if weak inhibitors are coadministered; titrate slowly while monitoring serum potassium levels.
ma huang (Ephedra)	May decrease the antihypertensive effectiveness through antagonist effects	Avoid this combination.
NSAIDs	Theoretical interaction; NSAIDs given with other potassium-sparing antihypertensives decrease antihypertensive effect and produce severe hyperkalemia in patients with impaired renal function. This interaction may possibly also occur with eplerenone.	Monitor blood pressure and potassium levels closely if these drugs are coadministered.
St. John's wort	Decreases available eplerenone by 30%	Avoid starting St. John's wort after dosage has been titrated to achieve therapeutic effect from eplerenone; alternately, monitor for therapeutic effect if herb is to be started. Increase dose of eplerenone if needed.
lithium	Theoretical interaction; coadministration of lithium and diuretics or ACE inhibitors has led to lithium toxicity	Monitor lithium levels if coadministered with eplerenone.
yohimbine	Increased norepinephrine release by yohimbine may counteract the hypotensive effect of ACE inhibitors.	Avoid concomitant use.

Nursing Diagnoses and Outcomes

- Risk for Injury related to the adverse effect of dizziness
  Desired outcome: The patient will not become injured from a fall caused by dizziness while on eplerenone therapy.
- Potential Complication: Hyperkalemia related to eplerenone therapy
  Desired outcome: The patient will maintain normal potassium levels while taking eplerenone therapy.
- Deficient Knowledge related to avoiding potassium supplements and potassium-based salt substitutes
  Desired outcome: Patient will have adequate knowledge to make informed decisions when choosing OTC supplements and salt substitutes while taking eplerenone.

Planning and Intervention

Maximizing Therapeutic Effects

The nursing actions to maximize the therapeutic effects of eplerenone therapy are discussed under Patient and Family Education.

Minimizing Adverse Effects

Monitor the patient's serum potassium level periodically during eplerenone therapy. Monthly assessments throughout therapy are indicated for those at risk for hyperkalemia (including those on ACE inhibitors and ARBs); however, more frequent assessment (every other week) is warranted initially until the effects of the drug on the patient are known. Hyperkalemia occurs more frequently as renal function decreases, so that patients with deteriorating renal function need to be assessed carefully. If the patient is receiving drugs that are weak CYP3A4 inhibitors (e.g., erythromycin, saquinavir, verapamil, fluconazole), the initial dose should be half of what is normally given until the effect on the potassium level is known. Patients who are experiencing dizziness while on eplerenone therapy should be assisted in ambulation and protected from falls.

Providing Patient and Family Education

- Teach patients to take eplerenone daily, as it is most effective if taken as directed.
- Encourage patients to make lifestyle changes that are known to decrease hypertension, including following a DASH diet (with the exception of adding potassium-rich food).
- Teach patients and their families to avoid foods very high in potassium, such as bananas.
- Teach patients to avoid salt substitutes that contain potassium. This advisory is especially important because many patients use a salt substitute when they are limiting sodium intake as part of implementing the lifestyle changes recommended for hypertension.
- Teach patients to avoid potassium supplements and the contraindicated drugs while taking eplerenone.
- Teach patients and families the rationale for and importance of periodic blood tests to check potassium levels.

- Teach patients that eplerenone may be taken either with or without food.
- Teach patients and families to avoid using St. John's wort or drinking grapefruit juice without first contacting the patient's physician or nurse practitioner because these substances change the amount of eplerenone available in the bloodstream. For patients who use these substances, the dosage of eplerenone may need to be adjusted downward with grapefruit juice consumption and upward with the start of St. John's wort.
- Teach patients who experience dizziness to use handrails when going up and down stairs, to stand slowly from a sitting or a lying position, and to obtain assistance when walking to prevent falls.

Ongoing Assessment and Evaluation

Potassium levels and renal function should be assessed throughout therapy. Drug therapy with eplerenone is successful if the patient has a decrease in blood pressure and does not experience substantial adverse effects.

Drug Significantly Different From
P Eplerenone

Spironolactone

Spironolactone (Aldactone) is a nonspecific aldosterone blocker and a potassium-sparing diuretic. Like eplerenone, it can block the mineralocorticoid receptors for aldosterone, preventing sodium and fluid retention that contributes to hypertension. Hyperkalemia is possible with both spironolactone and eplerenone. However, unlike eplerenone, spironolactone also equally stimulates androgen and progesterone receptors, which is likely the cause of the frequent endocrine adverse effects, such as inability to achieve an erection, gynecomastia (in men), irregular bleeding or postmenopausal bleeding (in women), hirsutism, and deepening of the voice.

 MEMORY CHIP

P Eplerenone

- Used in treating hypertension
- Works by selectively blocking aldosterone receptors
- Major contraindications: elevated potassium levels, severe renal failure, type 2 diabetes with microalbuminuria, concurrent administration of drugs that increase potassium levels either directly or indirectly
- Most common adverse effects: hyperkalemia, dizziness, hyponatremia
- Most serious adverse effect: hyperkalemia
- Maximizing therapeutic effect: Take regularly, implement or continue lifestyle changes along with drug therapy.
- Minimizing adverse effects: Monitor potassium levels and renal function.
- Most important patient education: Avoid potassium-based salt substitutes; avoid potassium supplements.

The frequency of these adverse effects (compared with their rarity with eplerenone) makes spironolactone less desirable as an antihypertensive agent.

Like eplerenone, spironolactone is labeled for used in hypertension and CHF. Unlike eplerenone, spironolactone is also labeled for use in ascites, nephritic syndrome, edema, hypokalemia, and primary aldosteronism. More information about spironolactone is provided in Chapter 27.

Direct-Acting Vasodilators

Hydralazine, minoxidil, epoprostenol, and tolazoline are all direct-acting vasodilators. Hydralazine and minoxidil are second-line drugs for hypertension; epoprostenol and tolazoline are used solely for treating pulmonary hypertension.

Hydralazine (Apresoline), a direct-acting vasodilator, is normally used as an adjunct to other antihypertensives, perhaps as the third or fourth drug in a therapeutic regimen. Parenteral hydralazine is used for severe hypertension when the need to reduce the blood pressure is urgent or the patient cannot take oral drugs. It may also be given alone. In unlabeled use, hydralazine is used following valve replacement, for treating severe aortic insufficiency, and for reducing afterload to manage CHF.

Hydralazine produces direct smooth muscle relaxation of the arterioles. Hydralazine alters cellular calcium metabolism, thereby interfering with calcium movement within the vascular smooth muscles responsible for venous contraction and dilation. Peripheral vasodilation results, promoting a decrease in arterial blood pressure and decreased peripheral resistance. As a reflexive action to the peripheral vasodilation, the body increases heart rate, stroke volume, and cardiac output. The reflex mechanism is caused by an increase in sympathetic stimulation. Because hydralazine preferentially dilates arterioles rather than veins, orthostatic hypotension does not occur as frequently as with other antihypertensives. However, this effect promotes an increase in cardiac output. Hydralazine also increases plasma renin activity, leading to production of angiotensin II. Angiotensin II increases aldosterone production, which increases sodium and water retention. Because of the reflexive increases in cardiac function, hydralazine is commonly given with drugs that decrease sympathetic activity, such as beta blockers or the alpha-2 stimulant clonidine. Because of the increases in sodium and water retention, hydralazine is coadministered frequently with a diuretic. Consult with the physician or nurse practitioner if these drugs are not currently ordered.

Hydralazine is a pregnancy category C drug. It crosses the placenta and may enter breast milk. It is compatible with breast-feeding, according to the American Academy of Pediatrics.

The drug is contraindicated with coronary artery disease, and mitral valvular rheumatic disease. It should be administered cautiously to patients with advanced renal damage, cerebral vascular accidents, suspected coronary artery disease, pulmonary hypertension, and sensitivity to tartrazine (FDC yellow dye #5) because some of the products contain this substance. The adverse effects of hydralazine usually resolve when the dose is reduced. Occasionally, the drug needs to be discontinued because of adverse effects. Many of the adverse effects are related to increased cardiac output. The most common adverse effects include palpitations, tachycardia, angina, anorexia, nausea, and vomiting.

A serious adverse effect that may occur while taking hydralazine is the development of symptoms of systemic lupus erythematosus (SLE), an autoimmune disease, such as arthralgia, dermatoses, fever, splenomegaly, and glomerular nephritis. The syndrome usually occurs after 6 months of drug therapy or more, and the likelihood of occurrence increases with larger doses and longer duration of therapy. Complete blood counts (CBCs) and antinuclear antibody titer are affected. Monitor these lab result s to assess for adverse effects from the drug.

Assess for signs of peripheral neuritis (numbness, tingling in hands and feet). If these signs are present, seek an order to administer pyridoxine (a B vitamin) because the neuritis may be caused by the antipyridoxine effect of drug therapy. If hydralazine is given parenterally, administer it as soon as possible after drawing it into a syringe to promote stability of the drug. (Note: hydralazine changes color after contact with a metal filter.)

Minoxidil (Loniten), like hydralazine, is a direct-acting vasodilator. It also does not create orthostatic hypotension because it does not affect vasomotor reflexes. It appears to block calcium uptake through the cell membrane. Like hydralazine, it is used with beta blockers to control reflex tachycardia and with a diuretic—preferably one acting in the ascending loop of Henle—to prevent substantial fluid accumulation.

Minoxidil differs in its serious adverse effects. It can cause pericardial effusion, occasionally progressing to cardiac tamponade, and it can worsen angina pectoris. Fluid retention and several hundred milliequivalents of salt accumulation can occur in a few days of use if the drug is not prescribed with a loop diuretic.

Hypertrichosis (excess hair growth) occurs in 3 to 6 weeks after starting therapy in 80% of patients receiving minoxidil. Elongation, thickening, and enhanced pigmentation of fine body hair develops. It is usually noticed first on the temples, between eyebrows, at the hairline, and in the eyebrows or sideburn area of the upper lateral cheek. It will progress down the back, arms, legs, and scalp. New hair growth stops when minoxidil use is discontinued, although it will take 1 to 6 months for appearance to return to normal. This adverse effect of hypertrichosis spawned a new therapeutic use for minoxidil—treating male pattern baldness and female hair loss or thinning of hair in the frontoparietal area. For growing hair, topical minoxidil (Rogaine) is the drug of choice. (See Chapter 51 for more information.)

Epoprostenol (Flolan), like hydralazine, also directly dilates peripheral vessels. Unlike hydralazine, epoprostenol also directly dilates pulmonary vascular beds and inhibits platelet aggravation. For these reasons, the sole clinical indication for epoprostenol is to treat primary pulmonary hypertension. It is administered via IV infusions through a central venous catheter with the rate regulated by an infusion pump.The correct dose is determined by increasing the amount infused until the desired effect on the pulmonary arteries is achieved. This dose is then continued as the maintainence dose. Abrupt withdrawal, including interruptions in the drug delivery (e.g., temporarily running out of drug), or sudden large dose reductions, may result in rebound pulmonary hypertension. Treatment of primary pulmonary hypertension is chronic. Patients are discharged with the drug and the infusion pump. Treatment may last up to several years. Patients should be aware of this fact before instituting therapy. Patients who will receive epoprostenol at home (and their families) need teaching regarding drug reconstitution, administration, and central catheter care in addition to information about the drug. A firm commitment to this treatment on the part of patient and families is required for the drug therapy to be effective.

Epoprostenol is contraindicated in patients who have CHF with severe left ventricular systolic dysfunction. The drug is in pregnancy category B; whether it is excreted in breast milk is unknown.

Adverse effects of epoprostenol are mostly cardiovascular and include: chest pain, hypotension, bradycardia or tachycardia, arrythmias, palpitations, MI, right-sided heart failure, edema, and shock. Other adverse effects include facial flushing, sweating, and muscular aches and pains.

Tolazoline (Priscoline) is a peripheral vasodilator and an alpha blocker. Administered via the IV route, it is used to treat pulmonary hypertension. CV adverse effects such as palpitations, hypertension, hypotension, and tachyarrhythmias are common; headache and vertigo also occur frequently. Serious adverse effects such as leukopenia, thrombocytopenia, hepatitis, or renal failure are rare. Tolazoline is a pregnancy category C drug.

Centrally Acting Alpha-2 Agonists

Clonidine (Catapres) and metheldopa are the two centrally acting alpha-2 agonists used to lower blood pressure. Clonidine's alpha-2 stimulation results in decreased heart rate, decreased blood pressure, decreased vasoconstriction, and decreased renal vascular resistance. However, renal blood flow and glomerular filtration rate remain unchanged essentially. Clonidine is considered a secondary or supplemental antihypertensive. It is used in step 2 antihypertensive therapy. Clonidine may be administered orally, parenterally, or, most frequently, transdermally. When administered transdermally, the drug is released at a constant rate for 7 days.

Some adverse effects of clonidine, such as dry mouth, drowsiness, dizziness, sedation, and constipation, are fairly common. Dry mouth and drowsiness also occur frequently when clonidine is administered transdermally. Rebound hypertension may occur if the drug is discontinued abruptly. Erythema is a common adverse effect.

Before the initiation of therapy, the nurse should confirm that the patient does not have severe coronary insufficiency, recent MI, or cerebrovascular disease, which may be affected adversely by decreased sympathetic outflow from the CNS. Assess for chronic renal failure because this condition increases the drug half-life, and a decreased dose may be needed.

In the hospital before surgery, drug administration with clonidine may continue for up to 4 hours before the procedure and be resumed as soon as possible thereafter to prevent hypertensive rebound from withdrawal. When clonidine is self-administered in the home setting with a transdermal patch, teach patients to discard used patches with care so that children cannot find the patch, play with it, or suck on it and sustain severe hypotension. Because clonidine can be used to prevent the symptoms of narcotic withdrawal, a black market exists for clonidine in some communities, and the patient may be tempted to sell the prescription. Nurses and other health care providers should be alert to patients returning for a duplicate prescription of clonidine, claiming to have lost the original shortly after it was prescribed. This may indicate the patient has sold or stored the prescription. In such cases, the prescriber may be notified and consulted about a change in the prescription, particularly if it appears that the patient is not taking the clonidine. Because of these concerns and the risk for adverse effects clonidine's use as an antihypertensive is currently limited. A discussion of clonidine's off-label uses is presented in Chapter 13.

Methyldopa (Aldomet) is similar to clonidine except that it stimulates both alpha-1 and alpha-2 receptors to lower blood pressure. This drug also works centrally to achieve its effects. It is contraindicated if the patient is currently receiving any monoamine oxidase inhibitor (MAOI). Adverse effects are fairly common and affect the following systems: CV (angina, bradycardia, hypotension); GI; neurologic (asthenia, dizziness, headache, sedation); and psychiatric (anxiety, depression, dream anxiety disorder). Because of its many adverse effects, methyldopa is not widely used at this time.

Peripherally Acting Alpha-1 Blockers

The alpha-1 blockers are also secondary hypertensive drugs; they are composed of prazosin (Minipress), terazosin (Hytrin), and doxazosin (Cardura). These drugs block postsynaptic alpha-1 adrenergic receptors, producing vasodilation of resistance vessels (arterioles) and capacitance vessels (veins) and thereby decreasing blood pressure. Both standing and lying blood pressures are reduced, particularly the diastolic blood pressure. A substantial first-dose effect of hypotension, especially orthostatic hypotension, can occur with these drugs. Prazosin has the unique disadvantage of causing sodium and water retention and increasing plasma volume. For these reasons these drugs are used infrequently in treating hypertension.

These drugs differ from metoprolol in that they have unique therapeutic actions. Terazosin and doxazosin also are used in treating benign prostatic hypertrophy. The reduction of symptoms and increase in urine flow rate are attributed to relaxation of smooth muscle from the alpha-1 blockade in the bladder neck and prostate gland. Bladder contractility is not affected because there are few alpha receptors in the bladder body.

Unlabeled uses of these drugs include treating refractory CHF, managing Raynaud vasospasm, treating benign prostatic hyperplasia (prazosin and terazosin), and treating CHF with concurrent digoxin and diuretics (doxazosin). Frequent adverse effects of these drugs are dizziness, hypotension, somnolence, asthenia, headache, palpitations, and nausea. These drugs are in pregnancy category C.

Peripherally Acting Antiadrenergics

Reserpine, guanethidine, and guanadrel are peripherally acting antiadrenergics and are secondary antihypertensives.

Unlike metoprolol, reserpine (Resa, Serpalan) is also used to relieve symptoms in agitated psychotic states, such as schizophrenia, primarily if the patient cannot tolerate phenothiazides. Reserpine as a peripherally acting antiadrenergics has a different mechanism of action than metoprolol. Reserpine depletes the stores of norepinephrine. Therefore, less norepinephrine is available for release into the synaptic cleft, which causes depression of sympathetic nerve function and also decreases heart rate and blood pressure. Reserpine also has sedative and tranquilizing effects believed to result from depletion of catecholamine and 5-hydroxytryptamine.

Adverse effects associated with reserpine are serious. This drug can cause severe depression— severe enough to result in suicide—and therefore is contraindicated if the patient's emotional health record shows a history of depression. The drug should be discontinued at the first sign of depression. This drug is used only if other drug therapies have been unsuccessful in controlling hypertension.

Both guanethidine (Ismelin) and guanadrel (Hylorel) are used to treat hypertension as adjuncts to other therapy. Guanethidine can also be used in treating renal hypertension. Guanethidine and guanadrel inhibit or interfere with the release and distribution of norepinephrine at the sympathetic neuroeffector junction, which leads to decreased sympathetic function and results in decreased heart rate and blood pressure.

Contraindications for both drugs are pheochromocytoma (rare adrenal tumor), uncontrolled CHF, and use of MAOIs. A major adverse effect is orthostatic hypotension, which can occur frequently with these drugs because they decrease the reflexive vasoconstriction that occurs when arising from a lying position.

ADJUNCT THERAPY IN HYPERTENSION

Antihyperlipidemic Drugs

Antihyperlipidemic drugs reduce blood lipid levels. They are used as adjuncts to hypertensive drug therapy. Because hypertension can be caused or aggravated by the narrowed arterial passages when fat is deposited on the wall of the vessel, decreasing fat levels circulating in the blood is advantageous. Dietary modifications are a common first step for both hypertension and elevated cholesterol levels. Therefore, patient education should stress dietary modifications heavily for patients who are hypertensive and have elevated serum lipid levels. Antihyperlipidemic drugs are discussed in more detail in Chapter 28.

Nitrates

Nitroglycerin is a nitrate that is sometimes used as an adjunct therapy in treating hypertension. Nitroglycerin is a vasodilator and has most of its effect on the venous side, causing venous dilation, peripheral pooling of blood, and decreased return to the heart. These factors decrease peripheral resistance and cardiac output, thus lowering blood pressure. IV nitroglycerin is used to treat severe hypertension. Nitroglycerin is discussed fully in Chapter 30.

DRUGS USED IN HYPERTENSIVE CRISIS

As described earlier in the chapter, a hypertensive crisis is an acute event and is defined as systolic blood pressure exceeding 210 mm Hg and diastolic blood pressure exceeding 120 mm Hg. When hypertensive crisis occurs, the patient is in danger of rapidly developing damage to one of the vital organs. The goal is to reduce the blood pressure by no more than 25% in the initial period of drug therapy (within minutes of starting therapy and up to 2 hours after the start of the infusion). Further blood pressure reductions toward 160/100 mm Hg should then be the goal within 2 to 6 hours after starting drug infusion. A recent meta-analysis found that there is insufficient evidence from randomized controlled clinical trials to determine which drug or drug class is the most effective in reducing mortality and morbitiy form hypertensive crisis (Perez & Musini, 2008). The prototype drug chosen for use in hypertensive crisis is nitroprusside (Nitropress; Table 26.8).

Nursing Management of the Patient Receiving P Nitroprusside

Core Drug Knowledge

Pharmacotherapeutics

Nitroprusside is the drug of choice when an immediate reduction of blood pressure is indicated in hypertensive crisis. It should be administered concurrently with longer-acting antihypertensives to minimize the duration of treatment. Other uses include reducing bleeding during surgery

TABLE 26.8 Summary of Selected Drugs for ⓒ Hypertensive Crisis

Drug (Trade) Name	Selected Indications	Route and Dosage Range	Pharmacokinetics
ℙ nitroprusside (Nitropress)	Hypertensive crisis	*Adult:* IV, 0.3 mcg/kg/min with gradual upward titration until desired effect or maximum rate of 10 mcg/kg/ min occurs	*Onset:* 1–2 min *Duration:* 3–5 min $t_{1/2}$: 2 min
diazoxide (Hyperstat IV)	Hypertensive crisis	*Adult:* direct IV, 1–3 mg/kg to a maximum of 150 mg in a single injection; repeat every 5–15 min until blood pressure drops, then repeat at 4- to 24-h intervals to maintain blood pressure until oral drug can begin	*Onset:* 1–2 min *Duration:* <12 h $t_{1/2}$: 28 ± 8.3 h
phentolamine (Regitine)	Preoperatively to prevent or control hypertension with pheochromocytoma Prevent or treat dermal necrosis and sloughing resulting from administration or extravasation of IV norepinephrine Diagnosis of pheochromocytoma	*Adult:* IV/IM, 5 mg 1 or 2 h before surgery, repeated if needed; 5 mg as needed during surgery *Child:* IV/IM, 1 mg *Adult:* IV (prophylactic), 10 mg/L of norepinephrine solution; SC (treatment), 5–10 mg in 10 mL of saline solution into area of extravasation within 12 h *Child:* 0.1–0.2 mg/kg to maximum 10 mg *Adult:* IV, 2.5 mg dissolved in 1 mL sterile water, injected directly by syringe into vein *Child:* 1 mg as above	*Onset:* Immediate *Duration:* 3–10 min $t_{1/2}$: Unknown

through the production of a controlled hypotensive state. It is also used for treating acute HF.

Pharmacokinetics

Nitroprusside is administered intravenously for immediate onset. Maximum effects are observed in 1 to 2 minutes. Resting circulating half-life is about 2 minutes. When the drug is discontinued, the blood pressure may return to its previous level within minutes. The metabolism of nitroprusside is important to understand because it has bearing on dosing and adverse effects. Nitroprusside is metabolized rapidly to cyanide through a reaction with hemoglobin. Cyanide is poisonous. Thiosulfate, an endogenous sulfate derivative created through normal physiologic mechanisms, reacts with the cyanide to produce another element, thiocyanate. The thiocyanate is processed by the liver and then excreted in the urine. Cyanide that becomes thiocyanate and is excreted is prevented from producing poisonous effects in the patient. Cyanide that does not become thiocyanate will bind with cytochromes. This binding prevents the cytochromes from participating in oxidative metabolism. Without oxidative metabolism, the cells cannot provide for their energy needs. Lactic acid is created, and eventually the cells die from hypoxia. Conversion of cyanide to thiocyanate occurs at a rate of 1 mcg/kg per minute. This rate of cyanide clearance corresponds to steady-state processing when nitroprusside is infused at slightly more than 2 mcg/kg per minute. If this rate is exceeded, cyanide builds up and poisons the patient. The half-life of thiocyanate increases from about 3 days to double or triple this time in patients with renal failure.

Pharmacodynamics

Nitroprusside directly relaxes vascular smooth muscle, allowing dilation of peripheral arteries and veins. It is more active on veins than on arteries, thereby promoting peripheral pooling of blood. This effect decreases venous return to the heart, reducing left ventricular end-diastolic pressure and pulmonary capillary wedge pressure (preload). The arteriolar dilation that occurs reduces systemic resistance and decreases mean arterial pressure (afterload). Dilation of coronary vessels also occurs. These processes produce a marked reduction in blood pressure, a slight increase in pulse rate, a slight decrease in cardiac output, and an increased production of renin. The ability to decrease the blood pressure is seemingly unlimited.

Contraindications and Precautions

Nitroprusside is contraindicated for compensatory hypertension in which the primary hemodynamic lesion is aortic coarctation or arteriovenous shunting. Nitroprusside also is contraindicated for providing surgical hypotension in patients with known inadequate cerebral circulation or in moribund patients undergoing emergency surgery. Another contraindication is acute HF associated with reduced peripheral vascular resistance, such as high-output heart failure, which may be seen in endotoxic sepsis. Additionally, the drug is contraindicated in patients with the rare condition of congenital optic atrophy or tobacco amblyopia; these patients have unusually high cyanide-to-thiocyanate ratios.

Nitroprusside is used cautiously in older adults and in patients with renal and hepatic impairment, hypovolemia, and anemia. Nitroprusside given for its hypotensive effect during surgery may decrease the patient's ability to compensate for hypovolemia and anemia. Nitroprusside is a pregnancy category C drug.

Nitroprusside carries the following Black Box warnings: (1) after reconstitution it must be further diluted;

(2) severe drop in blood pressure is possible which can lead to irreversible ischemic injuries or deaths; monitor blood pressure continuously; and (3) cyanide poisoning is possible with high doses.

Adverse Effects

Small, transient excesses in the rate of nitroprusside infusion can result in excessive hypotension, sometimes compromising perfusion of vital organs. This hypotension is self-limiting after discontinuation of the drug. A too-rapid reduction of blood pressure can result in abdominal pain, apprehension, diaphoresis, dizziness, headache, muscle twitching, nausea, palpitations, restlessness, retching, and retrosternal discomfort. Symptoms quickly subside when the nitroprusside infusion slows or stops; they do not return when the infusion resumes at a slower rate.

A life-threatening and unique adverse effect from nitroprusside is cyanide toxicity. Cyanide toxicity can occur when the nitroprusside infusion rate exceeds the rate of cyanide excretion. Cyanide toxicity may manifest as venous hyperoxemia (in which venous blood appears bright-red, similar to arterial blood, as the cells become unable to extract the oxygen delivered to them), metabolic (lactic) acidosis, air hunger, confusion, and death.

Elimination of cyanide increases with the administration of thiosulfate. Coadministration with thiosulfate prevents most cases of nitroprusside induced cyanoide poisoning except when the dose is extremely large. However, this action also has risks. Thiosulfate increases the production of thiocyanate. Thiocyanate is mildly neurotoxic; neurotoxicity is signaled by tinnitus, miosis, and hyperreflexia at serum levels of 1 mmol/L (60 mg/L). Thiocyanate toxicity is life threatening when levels are three or four times higher (200 mg/L). Thiocyanate also interferes with iodine uptake by the thyroid.

Methemoglobin, derived from hemoglobin, can hide cyanide. After nitroprusside is administered, hemoglobin can convert to methemoglobin, leading to methemoglobinemia. This adverse effect is rare, occurring when a patient receives the maximum rate of nitroprusside infusion for a prolonged period (greater than 16 hours). Methemoglobinemia is characterized by blood that appears chocolate brown and that does not change color after exposure to air.

Like other vasodilators, nitroprusside may increase intracranial pressure and cause adverse CV effects, such as bradycardia or tachycardia, and ECG changes. Platelet aggregation may be decreased, and flushing, venous streaking, irritation at the infusion site, rash, hypothyroidism, and ileus may be detected.

Drug Interactions

Additional vasodilation will occur if co-administered with PDE5 inhibitors used to treat erectile dysfunction (Table 26.9).

Assessment of Relevant Core Patient Variables

Health Status

Initially, assess the patient's blood pressure and check for physical states that are contraindications for nitroprusside use, such as compensatory hypertension, acute HF associated with reduced peripheral vascular resistance, inadequate cerebral circulation before anesthesia, moribundity before emergency surgery, congenital optic atrophy, or tobacco amblyopia. Also, determine whether intracranial pressure is elevated. Determine if the patient is at risk of having deficient entrinsic stores of thiosulfate. Patients with relative deficiencies of thiosulfate can include those who are malnourished, have had recent surgery, or are taking diuretics; these patients would be more at risk of cyanonide poisoning from nitroprusside, as they would not clear the cyanonide at the normal rate.

Life Span and Gender

Determine the patient's age before administering nitroprusside. Nitroprusside is given with caution to children and the elderly, who may be more sensitive to the hypotensive effects of the drug. Determine whether the patient is pregnant before administering nitroprusside. In patients who are pregnant, nitroprusside is given only if clearly indicated because it is a pregnancy category C drug.

Environment

Be aware of the setting in which nitroprusside may be administered. Nitroprusside is administered in a hospital setting, where blood pressure can be monitored continuously by a continually reinflated sphygmomanometer (automatic blood pressure cuff) or preferably by an intra-arterial pressure sensor. Once diluted, nitroprusside is sensitive to light and will lose some of its efficacy.

Culture and Inherited Traits

Nitroprusside has a prompt hypotensive effect on all populations.

TABLE 26.9	Agents That Interact with P Nitroprusside	
Interactants	**Effect and Significance**	**Nursing Management**
PDE5 inhibitors: sildenafil, vardenafil, tadalafil	Additional vasodilation effects and hypotensive effects. Whether a nitrate can be administered after sildenafil treatment is unknown.	These drugs are contraindicated to be given together. However, if the patient develops a sudden pathology where nitroprusside is warranted, the blood pressure should be monitored carefully and the nitroprusside dose should be slowly increased.

Nursing Diagnoses and Outcomes

- Decreased Cardiac Output related to venous dilation, diminished preload, and severe hypotension secondary to therapeutic and adverse effects of drug therapy
  Desired outcome: Hypotension will not occur to an extent that cardiac output cannot meet the perfusion needs of the vital organs.
- Acute Pain related to decreased comfort from rapid blood pressure reduction secondary to too-rapid drug infusion
  Desired outcome: The patient's blood pressure will not drop so quickly that adverse effects result.
- Risk for Injury related to increased intracranial pressure, cyanide poisoning, or thiocyanate toxicity secondary to adverse effects of drug therapy.
  Desired outcome: The patient will not suffer injury while on drug therapy.

Planning and Intervention

Maximizing Therapeutic Effects

The infusion rate for nitroprusside must be titrated to reduce blood pressure without compromising organ perfusion. When it is given for CHF, titrate the nitroprusside infusion so that measured cardiac output does not increase and systemic blood pressure remains as low as possible without compromising organ perfusion or the maximum infusion rate has been reached—whichever comes first.

Nitroprusside can be inactivated by reactions with trace contaminants. If these reactions have occurred, the nitroprusside will appear blue, green, or red; it will be much brighter than its normal faint brownish color. If the solution appears discolored or if particulate appears, the solution should not be used.

After reconstituting nitroprusside in 2 to 3 mL of dextrose in water or sterile water, dilute it in 250 to 1,000 mL of 5% dextrose in water (D_5W). Reconstituted nitroprusside should not be injected directly. Protect the container of diluted solution from light by placing it in an opaque sleeve or wrapping it in aluminum foil for stability of the solution. It is not necessary to cover the drip chamber or the IV tubing.

Minimizing Adverse Effects

To avoid extreme hypotensive effect, start nitroprusside at a low infusion rate (0.3 mcg/kg/min) and increase it gradually until the desired effect has been achieved or the maximum infusion rate (10 mcg/kg/min) is attained. Each 100 mg of sodium nitroprusside should be mixed with 1 g of sodium thiosulfate to maintain an adequate level of thiosulfate to promote cyanide elimination and prevent nitroprusside-induced cyanide poisoning in the majority of patients.

Do not adjust the infusion rate by gravity because slight variations in infusion rate can lead to substantial variations in blood pressure. Always use an infusion pump, preferably a volumetric infusion pump. It is important to monitor the patient's blood pressure constantly during the infusion, either with a continually inflating sphygmomanometer or (preferably) with an intra-arterial pressure sensor. Excessive or too-rapid reduction in arterial blood pressure may produce nausea, diaphoresis, anxiety, restlessness, and muscle twitching. If these occur, then the infusion rate should be slowed. The purpose of the gradual reduction in blood pressure is to avoid excessive falls in pressure that could induce renal, cerebral, or coronary ischemia.

The usual dosage rate is 0.3 to 10 mcg/kg/min. However, cyanide clearance occurs when the dosage rate is less than 2 mcg/kg/min. To prevent dangerous, possibly lethal, buildup of cyanide, the maximum infusion should never exceed 10 minutes.

If the blood pressure remains uncontrolled after 10 minutes at the maximum infusion rate, stop the infusion immediately. Cyanide level assay is technically difficult to perform, and cyanide levels in body fluids other than packed red blood cells are difficult to interpret. Therefore, it is difficult to determine cyanide toxicity directly from laboratory findings.

Monitoring the acid-base balance and venous oxygen concentrations may help indicate cyanide toxicity. However, these tests do not always accurately reflect cyanide levels. Clinical studies show that metabolic acidosis, although normally occurring with elevated cyanide levels, may lag behind peak cyanide levels by an hour or more. Therefore, monitor also for other signs of cyanide toxicity, such as red venous blood, dyspnea, or confusion. It is also important to monitor for signs of thiocyanate toxicity (tinnitus, miosis, hyperreflexia) and methemoglobinemia (chocolate-brown blood).

Toxicity to nitroprusside can occur even if the dose is well within recommended limits. Toxicity may be evident by excessive hypotension, cyanide toxicity, or thiocyanate toxicity. Closely monitoring the patient throughout therapy is the key to safety. The development of nausea, vomiting, or altered mental function should be considered signs of potential cyanide toxicity unless proven otherwise. Symptoms of thiocyanate toxicity include fatigue, tinnitus, mental confusion, skin rash, psychosis, and anorexia.

Administer other longer-acting antihypertensives as needed during nitroprusside therapy to limit the dosage of nitroprusside as necessary. It is important to monitor for signs that blood pressure has been reduced too rapidly (e.g., abdominal pain, apprehension, diaphoresis, dizziness, headache, muscle twitching, nausea, palpitations, restlessness, retching, or retrosternal discomfort). Slow or discontinue the infusion until symptoms diminish. The infusion may then resume at a slower rate.

Also, assess for signs of increased intracranial pressure and other adverse effects; correct pre-existing anemia and hypovolemia before administration with anesthesia, if appropriate. Administer to a pregnant patient only if clearly indicated.

Providing Patient and Family Education

- Explain to patient and families that the drug is being given to lower blood pressure quickly and that blood pressure will be monitored constantly to prevent it from dropping too low.
- Urge patients to report adverse effects (such as abdominal pain, apprehension, diaphoresis, dizziness, headache, muscle twitching, nausea, palpitations, restlessness, retching, or retrosternal discomfort) immediately to the nurse.

Ongoing Assessment and Evaluation

Monitor blood pressure throughout nitroprusside therapy so that it is reduced without sacrifice to vital organs. Signs of increasing intracranial pressure and other adverse effects should be assessed as well. Drug therapy is effective when blood pressure falls to a safe level, organ damage is averted, and severe hypotension, cyanide toxicity, or thiocyanate toxicity does not develop.

Drugs Closely Related to P Nitroprusside
Fenoldopam

Fenoldopam (Corlopam) is a newer drug for treating hypertensive emergencies. A rapid vasodilator, fenoldopam works differently than nitroprusside; it stimulates dopamine receptors and moderately binds to alpha-2 receptors. Because of its dopaminergic effects, it increases renal blood flow. Fenoldopam is administered only as a continuous IV infusion, never as a bolus dose. The dose should be titrated up or down every 15 minutes until the desired blood pressure has been achieved.

MEMORY CHIP

P Nitroprusside

- Drug of choice for hypertensive crisis when blood pressure must be reduced immediately
- Major contraindications: compensatory hypertension resulting from aortic coarctation or arteriovenous shunting, and surgical procedures on patients with inadequate cerebral circulation
- Most common adverse effect: hypotension from too-rapid infusion
- Most serious adverse effects: severe hypotension and cyanide poisoning
- Maximizing therapeutic effects: Wrap diluted bag of drug in an opaque sleeve or aluminum foil to protect from light.
- Minimizing adverse effects: Always use an IV pump to regulate infusion; start the infusion at a low dose and slowly increase; once the maximum infusion rate has been achieved, do not continue for more than 10 minutes; and monitor blood pressure throughout therapy.
- **Black box warning: Nitroprusside is not suitable for direct injection after initial reconstitution but must be further diluted. Nitroprusside can cause sudden substantial decreases in blood pressure. Nitroprusside can cause cyanide toxicity, which can be lethal.**

Unlike nitroprusside, fenoldopam does not carry Black Box warnings. It is a pregnancy category B drug. The most common adverse effects are flushing, GI disturbances; dizziness, headache, and dose-related tachycardia. Hypotension may also occur.

Trimethaphan

Trimethaphan (Arfonad) differs slightly from nitroprusside in its therapeutic action. It is used to treat hypertensive crisis when there is aortic dissection when nitroprusside is ineffective or cannot be used. It is labeled for use in treating intraoperative hypertension and malignant hypertension. Like nitroprusside, it is a direct vasodilator, but only when given in high doses. Unlike nitroprusside, trimethaphan is also a short-acting ganglionic blocker. It blocks the transmission in autonomic ganglia (both sympsathetic and parasympathetic) without producing a change in the membrane potential. It does not modify impulse conduction in the preganglionic or postganglionic neurons, or prevent acetylcholine release by preganglionic impulses. It occupies ganglionic receptors and stabilizes postsynaptic membranes from the action of acetylcholine, which is released by the presynaptic nerve endings.

Trimethaphan shows a fall in cardiac output, whereas nitroprusside exhibits no change or a slight increase. Nitroprusside increases heart rate and decreases central venous pressure. Early tachyphylaxis seen with trimethaphan is not seen with nitroprusside. Recovery of arterial blood pressure after nitroprusside is rapid (2 to 6 minutes) compared with trimethaphan (10 to 15 minutes). Trimethaphan, unlike nitroprusside, does not carry Black Box warnings.

Only physicians properly trained to use and monitor this drug therapy should attempt surgical hypotension with trimethaphan. The nurse assists in monitoring the patient closely during surgery for signs of complications; severe hypotension, with its ramifications, may occur.

Drugs Significantly Different From P Nitroprusside

Phentolamine (generic only), phenoxybenzamine (Dibenzyline), and metyrosine (Demser) are used only to treat the marked elevations in blood pressure associated with pheochromocytoma, a catecholamine-secreting tumor of the adrenal medulla. Phentolamine is also used in preventing and treating dermal necrosis and sloughing after IV extravasation of norepinephrine.

Phentolamine and phenoxybenzamine are both alpha-adrenergic blockers. They lower peripheral vascular resistance and therefore decrease blood pressure. Metyrosine inhibits tyrosine hydroxylase, which is the catalyst for the first transformation in catecholamine biosynthesis. Because of this blockade, endogenous levels of catecholamine decrease. Most patients receiving this drug experience decreased frequency and severity of hypertensive attacks. Patients who respond to therapy normally experience a decrease in blood pressure within the first 2 days of therapy. Metyrosine is administered orally as chronic therapy, unlike nitroprusside.

Cardiac stimulation occurs with phentolamine. The concomitant use of a beta blocker may be needed to control tachycardia. Tachycardia may occur with phenoxybenzamine but to a lesser extent. Cardiac responses do not occur with metyrosine. Orthostatic hypotension may occur with both phentolamine and phenoxybenzamine. Sedation, galactorrhea, sexual dysfunction, nasal sinus congestion, and diarrhea are adverse effects unique to metyrosine. Extrapyramidal effects and hallucinations are possible serious adverse effects from metyrosine.

PATHOPHYSIOLOGY OF SHOCK

Shock is the result of inadequate tissue perfusion, leaving the cells without the necessary oxygen and nutrients they need to have normal function and survive. When cell dysfunction is widespread, the result can be death for the patient. Shock has multiple causes. Hypovolemic shock results from a decrease in circulating blood volume from bleeding or hemorrhage. It occurs when intravascular volume decreases more than 15% to 25%. Cardiogenic shock is caused by the heart's inability to pump enough blood to adequately perfuse the vital organs, which may itself be caused by MI, ventricular arrhythmias, severe cardiomyopathy, or CHF. Septic shock occurs when a severe infection brings about circulatory insufficiency. Obstructive shock is caused by a massive blockage in blood flow and results in inadequate tissue perfusion. This event could be caused by a large pulmonary embolus, cardiac tamponade, restrictive pericarditis, or severe cardiac valve dysfunction. Neurogenic shock is uncommon. It occurs as a result of blockade of neurohormonal outflow. This event may be induced by drugs (e.g., spinal anesthesia) or trauma to the spinal cord.

Shock has two phases—early (or compensated) and late (or noncompensated). In early shock, the body tries to compensate for the decreased perfusion. The heart and respiratory rates increase, and blood pressure is generally maintained, or it may be low to normal. The body begins to shunt some blood flow away from the skin, although the skin is still perfused. Urine output decreases slightly as renal blood flow is reduced. Emotionally, the patient may be anxious or confused. When the body is no longer able to make up for changes brought on by shock, the patient develops late, or uncompensated, shock. Tachycardia persists, but the blood pressure falls dramatically, and respiration rates decrease. Venous constriction occurs; with the circulation shut off, the skin becomes cold and clammy. Urine output declines dramatically and may cease as the kidneys are no longer perfused. The patient becomes nonresponsive and unconscious.

DRUGS TO TREAT HYPOTENSION RESULTING FROM SHOCK

Vasopressors

Drug therapy in shock is directed toward increasing blood pressure to help support tissue perfusion. Drugs are given in addition to fluid volume. Vasopressors, drugs to increase the blood pressure, are sympathomimetic. They increase cardiac contractility and heart rate, constrict veins (vasoconstriction), and dilate arteries. See Table 26.10 for a summary of selected vasopressors.

Dopamine

Dopamine (Intropin) is used to correct the hemodynamic imbalances present in shock caused by MI, trauma, endotoxic septicemia, open heart surgery, renal failure, and chronic cardiac decompensation (CHF). For the treatment to be most effective, the patient should not be experiencing severe disruptions in urine production, myocardial function, and blood pressure. In other words, the earlier the signs of shock are recognized and treatment is started with fluids and dopamine, the more successful the therapy. The onset of action of IV dopamine is less than 5 minutes, and duration of action is less than 10 minutes. The drug is distributed widely in the body but does not cross the blood–brain barrier.

Dopamine is a naturally occurring catecholamine and a precursor to norepinephrine. It stimulates alpha-1 and beta-1 receptors through direct and indirect (by releasing the stored epinephrine) methods. It also has dopaminergic effects. Beta-1 stimulation produces increased cardiac output by increasing the force of contraction and heart rate. Although there is an increase in the oxygen needs of the myocardium from dopamine, this effect is less pronounced than when isoproterenol is administered. Tachyarrhythmias usually do not occur. Systolic blood pressure increases, whereas diastolic pressure usually does not. Minimal increases in the diastolic pressure may occur. Total peripheral resistance (from alpha effects) is not changed substantially if dopamine is given at low or intermediate levels of dosing. Although blood flow to the peripheral beds may decrease, blood flow to the mesenteric beds increases. Dopamine dilates renal and mesenteric vasculature as well as cerebral and cardiac beds; this effect is believed to be caused by stimulation of dopaminergic receptors. An increase in renal blood flow, glomerular filtration rate, and urinary output is then seen. The dopaminergic effect of no change in the peripheral resistance is lost as the dose becomes high, with the alpha stimulation taking precedence. The alpha stimulation brings about increased peripheral resistance, raising blood pressure at higher doses of dopamine. The drug's dosage should be titrated upward until adequate perfusion of vital organs is achieved.

Dopamine is discussed fully as a prototype drug in Chapter 13.

Dobutamine

Dobutamine is another vasopressive drug that is chemically similar to dopamine. Like dopamine, its primary influence is on beta-1 receptors, with similar effects on the force of contraction. Dobutamine is somewhat less effective than dopamine at increasing the rate at the sinoatrial (SA) node. Also like dopamine, dobutamine's beta-2 effects on vasodilation are minimal. Unlike dopamine, dobutamine has almost no effect on alpha receptors to cause vasoconstriction. Although cardiac output and blood pressure are similarly increased with both drugs,

TABLE 22.10	Summary of Selected Vasopressors		
Drug (Trade) Name	Selected Indications	Route and Dosage Range	Pharmacokinetics
dopamine (Intropin)	Hemodynamic imbalances	*Adult:* IV, 2–5 mcg/kg/min *Seriously ill adult:* IV, 5 mcg/kg/min; increase in increments of 5–10 mcg/kg/min up to a rate of 20–50 mcg/kg/min *Child:* Safety and efficacy not established	*Onset:* IV, 1–2 min *Duration:* IV, length of infusion $t_{1/2}$: 2 min
dobutamine (Dobutrex)	Cardiac decompensation due to decreased contractility	*Adult:* IV infusion, 2.5–10 mcg/kg/min	*Onset:* 1–2 min Duration: Unknown $t_{1/2}$: 2 min
epinephrine (Adrenaline)	Cardiac arrest	*Adult:* IV, 0.5–1.0 mg *Child:* Injection, 1:1,000 solution, 0.01 mg/kg or 0.3 mg/m² SC q4 h	*Onset:* SC, IM, 5–10 min; IV, instant; inhalation, 3–5 min *Duration:* SC, IM, IV, short-acting inhalation, 1–3 h
	Respiratory distress	*Adult:* SC, 0.3–0.5 mg of 1:1,000 solution; inhalation, individualize dosage; wait 1–5 min between doses. *Child:* SC, 0.01 mg/kg; topical nasal solution, same as adult	
isoproterenol (Isuprel)	Bronchospasm (during anesthesia)	*Adult:* IV, 0.01–0.02 mg of diluted solution	*Onset:* IV, immediate *Duration:* IV, 1–2 min $t_{1/2}$: Unknown
	Shock or cardiac standstill and arrhythmias	*Adult:* IV infusion, 5 mcg/min of diluted solution; IV push, 0.02–0.10 mg of diluted solution; IM/SC, 0.2 mg of undiluted 1:5,000 solution	
mephentermine (Wyamine)	Hypotension attendant to spinal anesthesia	*Adult:* IM, 30–45 mg 10–20 min prior to procedure	*Onset:* IM, 10–15 min; IV, immediate *Duration:* IM, 1–2 h $t_{1/2}$: 15–20 min
	Hypotension following spinal anesthesia	*Adult:* IV, 30–45 mg as a single injection	
	Shock following hemorrhage	*Adult:* IV, 0.1% solution in 5% dextrose in water just until blood replacement achieved	
norepinephrine (levarterenol, Levophed)	Acute hypotension, shock Cardiac arrest	*Adult:* IV, 8–12 mcg/min; maintenance rate, 2–4 mcg/min *Adult:* IV, administer during cardiac resuscitation to restore and maintain blood pressure after effective heartbeat and ventilation established	*Onset:* IV, rapid *Duration:* 1–2 min after discontinuation of infusion $t_{1/2}$: Unknown
phenylephrine (Neo-Synephrine)	Mild/moderate hypotension	*Adult:* SC or IM, 2–5 mg; IV, 0.2 mg, do not repeat injections more often than every 10–15 min	*Onset:* IV, immediate; IM/SC, 10–15 min *Duration:* IV, 15–20 min; SC/IM, 1–2 h $t_{1/2}$: Unknown
	Severe hypotension/shock	*Adult:* IV, add 10 mg to 250 or 500 mL of dextrose injection; start at 100–180 mcg/min; maintenance, 40–60 mcg/min	
	Pediatric hypotension	*Child:* SC or IM, 0.5–1 mg/11.3 kg	

dobutamine does not produce the increased renal output that dopamine does. Furthermore, its effect on peripheral resistance is always to decrease it, whereas dopamine may increase or decrease peripheral resistance. Dobutamine does not cause the release of endogenous norepinephrine that dopamine causes.

The pharmacotherapeutic uses of dobutamine differ from those of dopamine. Dobutamine is indicated in the short-term treatment and support of patients experiencing cardiac decompression caused by depressed contractility. The decreased contractility may be secondary to either organic heart disease or cardiac surgery. Patients with atrial fibrillation and a rapid ventricular rate should be treated first with digoxin, before dobutamine treatment, to protect the ventricles. Onset of action is 1 to 2 minutes, but it may take as long as 10 minutes to reach peak effect.

A contraindication unique to dobutamine is the presence of idiopathic hypertrophic subaortic stenosis. Although elevated pulse usually does not occur when using dobutamine, tachycardia can occur, with increases of 30 bpm or more. Accompanying the tachycardia is a rapid and substantial increase in blood pressure, with the systolic pressure rising 50% or greater. These adverse effects are usually dose related, and reducing the dose promptly corrects the problem. Interestingly, dobutamine also can cause substantial hypotension if given in excessive amounts; again, decreasing the dose usually corrects the problem. Dobutamine may cause or exacerbate ventricular ectopic beats, although ventricular tachycardia is rare. Other rare adverse effects include nausea, headache, anginal pain, nonspecific chest pain, palpitations, and shortness of breath. Phlebitis and local inflammation at the IV site may occur; a large vein should be chosen to administer the drug to minimize this possibility.

Patients receiving dobutamine, like dopamine, need to be monitored continuously on a cardiac monitor while receiving the drug. Blood pressures should be checked frequently. Pulmonary wedge pressure and cardiac output should be checked whenever possible.

Isoproterenol

Like dopamine, isoproterenol (Isuprel) has a strong effect on beta-1 receptors, producing similar increases in contractility. However, isoproterenol's effect on the heart rate and vasodilation is much greater than dopamine's. Isoproterenol does not stimulate the alpha receptors for vasoconstriction. Isoproterenol increases cardiac output like dopamine. Renal perfusion is also affected, although unlike dopamine, it can increase or decrease it. Peripheral resistance is always decreased, but blood pressure may be increased or decreased by isoproterenol. Although isoproterenol may be used to treat shock, this practice is not common because it can cause tachycardia. The other uses of isoproterenol and more complete information about it are found in Chapter 13.

Epinephrine

Epinephrine is also a vasopressor, as is dopamine. Epinephrine stimulates both alpha and beta receptors. Its effect on the contractility of the heart (beta-1) is similar to dopamine's effect, whereas its effects on SA node rate (beta-1), vasodilation (beta-2), and vasoconstriction (alpha-1) are stronger than dopamine's effects. Although epinephrine increases the cardiac output, its other pharmacodynamic effects differ from those of dopamine. It decreases renal perfusion, decreases total peripheral resistance, and elevates systolic blood pressure, while lowering diastolic blood pressure. Epinephrine is indicated in the treatment and prophylaxis of cardiac arrest and attacks of transitory atrioventricular heart block with syncopal seizures (Stokes-Adams syndrome). Epinephrine is discussed completely in Chapter 13.

Norepinephrine

Norepinephrine (Levophed) is another vasopressor that stimulates the adrenergic system. Its beta-1 effects on contractility are less than the effects of dopamine, whereas its effect on the SA node rate is similar. Similar to dopamine, norepinephrine has strong alpha-receptor stimulation, producing vasoconstriction, but no effect on vasodilation from beta-2 receptors. Although peripheral resistance and blood pressure are raised, norepinephrine decreases renal perfusion and either has no effect on, or decreases, cardiac output. Norepinephrine is used to restore blood pressure when hypotension is caused by one of the following conditions: pheochromocytomectomy, sympathectomy, poliomyelitis, spinal anesthesia, MI, blood transfusion, and drug reactions. It also is used as an adjunct in treating cardiac arrest and severe hypotension. More information about norepinephrine is also found in Chapter 13.

Ephedrine

Ephedrine has less effect on contractility (beta-1 receptors) and less effect on vasoconstriction (alpha-1) than dopamine. Its effect on heart rate (beta-1) and vasodilation (beta-2) is similar to the effect of dopamine. Ephedrine's pharmacodynamic effects of increasing blood pressure, increasing cardiac output, and increasing or decreasing peripheral resistance are similar to those of dopamine. Unlike dopamine, ephedrine decreases renal perfusion. Ephedrine, administered parenterally (most commonly via the IV route), is used clinically in acute hypotension, especially that caused by spinal anesthesia, Stokes-Adams syndrome with complete heart block, use of a CNS stimulant in narcolepsy and depressive states, and acute bronchospasm (occasionally). It is also used as a vasopressor following sympathectomy or drug overdosage (from ganglionic blocking drugs, antiadrenergic drugs, *Veratrum* alkaloids, or other drugs used to lower blood pressure during treatment of hypertension). Ephedrine is also used in enuresis and myasthenia gravis. Oral ephedrine is included in some nasal decongestants.

Metaraminol

Metaraminol is used to prevent and treat acute hypotensive states that occur with spinal anesthesia. It is an adjunct treatment for hypotension caused by hypovolemia, reactions to drug therapy, surgical complications, and shock associated with brain damage caused by trauma or tumor. Metaraminol has only minor effects on beta-1 receptors, creating mild increases in contractility and heart rate. It has more effect on vasoconstriction from alpha-1 stimulation than mephentermine, but less than dopamine. It has no effect on vasodilation from beta-2 stimulation. It primarily increases blood pressure by increasing peripheral resistance. Unlike dopamine, it lowers cardiac output and renal perfusion. Although the SA node is stimulated somewhat (which theoretically should increase the heart rate), the net effect on the heart is bradycardia, resulting from a strong reflexive response to the substantial vasoconstriction this drug achieves. Unlike dopamine, it can be given intramuscularly or subcutaneously as well as by IV infusion.

DRUGS TO TREAT HYPOTENSION RESULTING FROM VARIOUS MECHANISMS

Vasopressors also treat hypotension resulting from mechanisms other than shock.

Phenylephrine

Unlike dopamine, the effects of phenylephrine are solely on alpha-1 receptors, producing strong vasoconstriction effects. Renal perfusion and cardiac output are decreased. Blood pressure is increased by the increase in peripheral resistance.

Phenylephrine is used to treat vascular failure in shock-like states, drug-induced hypotension, or hypersensitivity. It is also used to overcome paroxysmal supraventricular tachycardia, to prolong spinal anesthesia, as a vasoconstrictor in regional analgesia, and to maintain an adequate blood pressure during spinal and inhalation anesthesia. Phenylephrine is discussed completely in Chapter 13.

Midodrine

Midodrine (ProAmatine) raises blood pressure, but it is not used as a vasopressor in shock. Instead, it is used for symptomatic treatment of orthostatic hypotension in patients whose lives are impaired substantially by this condition, despite standard clinical treatment. It carries a Black Box warning that its use should be so limited. Midodrine is administered orally. It is a prodrug that becomes active when it changes into the metabolite desglymidodrine. The metabolite is an alpha-1 agonist that increases the tone of the arteriolar and venous vasculature, increasing peripheral resistance. It results in increased standing, sitting, and lying blood pressures. Because supine systolic blood pressure can rise to 200 mm Hg or greater, midodrine should not be given less than 4 hours before bedtime. Suggested dosing times are shortly before or just after arising in the morning, midday, and late afternoon. This dosing schedule should assist the patient to maintain his or her normal daytime activities and prevent supine hypertension during the night. If supine hypertension does occur, it may be controlled by preventing the patient from lying completely flat (e.g., lying with the head of the bed elevated). Midodrine is a pregnancy category C drug.

CHAPTER SUMMARY

- Blood pressure is derived from the amount of blood leaving the heart times the resistance in the peripheries (blood pressure = cardiac output × peripheral resistance). When either cardiac output or peripheral resistance increases, the blood pressure rises. Drug therapy to reduce hypertension is designed to decrease either cardiac output or peripheral resistance or both. Drug therapy to increase blood pressure increases cardiac output, peripheral resistance, or both.
- Hypertension is classified in 3 stages (from prehypertension to stage 2), according to the degree of blood pressure elevation.
- In prehypertension, blood pressure is usually managed by lifestyle changes alone. These changes include weight reduction, dietary restriction of saturated fat, moderation of alcohol intake, regular physical activity, reduction of sodium intake, increased intake of potassium- and calcium-rich foods, and smoking cessation. Lifestyle modifications continue even if the patient advances to stage 1 or 2 hypertension.
- Drug therapy may be initiated in prehypertension if the patient has certain other comorbidities. Drug therapy is always initiated in stage 1 or 2 hypertension.

Most patients require the use of at least two types of antihypertensives to achieve full therapeutic effect. Patients whose blood pressure is difficult to control may be on three or more first-line drugs as well as some second-line drugs.

- Drug classes used as first-line therapy include: thiazide diuretics, beta blockers, ACE inhibitors, ARBs, calcium channel blockers (for some patients), and occasionally aldosterone blockers.
- Drug classes used as second-line therapy include: vasodilators, alpha-2 stimulants, alpha-1 blockers, peripheral antiadrenergics.
- Thiazide diuretics (such as hydrochlorothiazide) are effective and less expensive than other antihypertensives. A thiazide diuretic is usually used as the drug of first choice in monotherapy. Other classes of first-line drugs may be added if necessary. Thiazides are effective in monotherapy in African Americans unlike most of the first-line drugs. The most common adverse effects are related to electrolyte changes and fluid volume loss (i.e., hypovolemia, low potassium, magnesium, and sodium levels, and elevated uric acid and blood glucose levels).
- Beta blockers (such as metoprolol) slow heart rate, speed conduction, and decrease force of contraction and thus decrease cardiac output. This decreases the blood pressure. Although beta blockers (at beta-2 receptor sites) increase peripheral resistance through vasoconstriction, this effect is outweighed by the substantial decrease in cardiac output, thereby lowering blood pressure. Beta blockers also decrease the release of renin from the kidneys so the renin-angiotensin-aldosterone system is not activated, so vasoconstriction does not occur. Beta blockers are used as the initial therapy for patients with certain comorbidities; they are not as effective as monotherapy in African Americans.
- Captopril, an ACE inhibitor, inhibits the angiotensin-converting enzyme needed to change the inactive angiotensin I to the active form angiotensin II, thereby preventing sodium and water retention, decreasing peripheral vascular resistance, and lowering blood pressure. A major adverse effect is a chronic cough, which may be so severe that the patient cannot tolerate or continue drug therapy. First-dose hypotension may occur. As monotherapy it does not achieve the same therapeutic effects in African Americans as in other races.
- Aliskaren is a renin inhibitor. Similar to other drugs that alter the renin-angiotensin-aldosterone system, monotherapy with aliskaren produced fewer antihypertensive effects in African Americans, probably because most African Americans are "low-renin hypertensives."
- Losartan is an ARB; it does not inhibit ACE. Instead, it blocks the vasoconstricting and aldosterone-secreting effects of angiotensin II by selectively blocking the binding of angiotensin II to the angiotensin receptors in many tissues, especially in the vascular smooth muscle and adrenal gland tissues.

- Eplerenone is a selective aldosterone receptor blocker. It interferes with the renin-angiotensin-aldosterone system. By blocking the mineralocorticoid aldosterone receptors, it prevents sodium and fluid reabsorption that leads to hypertension.
- Nitroprusside, an agent used in hypertensive crisis, directly relaxes vascular smooth muscle. It is more active on veins than arteries, thereby promoting peripheral pooling of blood. This effect decreases venous return to the heart, reducing left ventricular end-diastolic pressure and pulmonary capillary wedge pressure (preload). The resultant arteriolar dilation reduces systemic resistance and decreases mean arterial pressure (afterload). The result is markedly reduced blood pressure. The ability to decrease the blood pressure is seemingly unlimited. Nitroprusside is rapidly metabolized to cyanide through a reaction with hemoglobin. Cyanide poisoning may occur during its use. If blood pressure remains uncontrolled after 10 minutes at the maximum infusion rate, stop the infusion immediately. The nitroprusside infusion should be controlled by an administration pump, and the blood pressure must be monitored constantly.
- Dopamine, a vasopressor, is used to correct the hemodynamic imbalances present in shock. Dopamine is a naturally occurring catecholamine and a precursor to norepinephrine. It stimulates alpha-1 and beta-1 receptors through direct and indirect (releasing the stored epinephrine) methods. It has either no or only a minimal effect on beta-2 receptors. It also has dopaminergic effects. The effects from dopamine are increased renal perfusion, increased cardiac output, increased or decreased peripheral resistance (depending on the dose), and increases in blood pressure. Dopamine is administered by IV continuous infusion. The patient must be monitored closely and continuously while on dopamine infusion.

QUESTIONS FOR STUDY AND REVIEW

1. What lifestyle changes constitute Step 1 in antihypertensive therapy?
2. Why are thiazide diuretics now the agents of first choice for most patients with hypertension?
3. How do ACE inhibitors such as captopril lower the blood pressure?
4. Describe how an ARB works differently than an ACE inhibitor. What are the advantages of ARB therapy over ACE inhibitor therapy?
5. What is the black box warning that is carried by ACE inhibitors, ARBs, and renin inhibitors?
6. Which electrolyte imbalance is most likely to occur when the selective aldosterone receptor blocker eplerenone is administered?
7. Describe nursing actions that promote safety for the patient receiving nitroprusside.
8. Why is dopamine dosage determined by urinary output and CV response?

NEED MORE HELP?

Chapter 26 of the Study Guide to Accompany *Drug Therapy in Nursing*, 4th Edition, contains NCLEX-style questions and other learning activities to reinforce your understanding of the concepts presented in this chapter. For additional information or to purchase the study guide, visit the**Point**.

REFERENCES

ALLHAT Officers and Coordinators for the ALLHAT Collaborative Research Group. (2002). Major outcomes in high-risk hypertensive patients randomized to angiotensin-converting enzyme inhibitor or calcium channel blocker vs diuretic: The Antihypertensive and Lipid-Lowering Treatment to Prevent Heart Attack Trial (ALLHAT). *Journal of the American Medical Association,* 288(23):2981–2997.

Anderson, K., Weinberger, M. H., Egan, B. et al. (2008). Comparative efficacy and safety of aliskiren, an oral direct renin inhibitor, and remipril in hypertension: a 6 mopnth, randomized, double-blind trial. *Journal of Hypertension,* 26(3):589–599.

Appel, L. J., Brands, M., & Daniels, S. (2006). Dietary approaches to prevent and treat hypertension. A Scientific Statement From the American Heart Association. *Hypertension.*47:296. Retrieved from http://hyper.ahajournals.org/cgi/content/full/47/2/296#SEC1

American Heart Association. Last updated 3/23/09 (2009a). High blood pressure statistics. Retrieved from http://www.americanheart.org/presenter.jhtml?identifier=2139.

American Heart Association. Last updated 4/09/09. (2009b). A special high blood pressure message for African Americans. Retrieved from http://www.americanheart.org/presenter.jhtml?identifier=2150

Antihypertensive and Lipid-Lowering Treatment to Prevent Heart Attack Trial Collaborative Research Group. (2003). Diuretic versus alpha-blocker as first-step antihypertensive therapy: Final results from the Antihypertensive and Lipid-Lowering Treatment to Prevent Heart Attack Trial (ALLHAT). *Hypertension,* 42(3):239–246.

Cechetto, D. F., Hachinski, V., & Whitehead, S. N. (2008). Vascular risk factors and alzheimer's disease. *Expert Review of Neurotherapeutics,* 8(5):743–750.

Centers for Disease Control website. Healthy Youths. http://www.cdc.gov/HealthyYouth/obesity/#1; (2009a). Accessed on August 13, 2009.

Centers for Disease. Obesity by Race/Ethnicity 2006–2008 (updated 2009b) http://www.cdc.gov/obesity/data/trends.html#Race Accessed August 14, 2009.

Din-Dzietham, R., Liu, Y., Bielo, M.V., et al. (2007). High blood pressure trends in children and adolescents in national surveys, 1963-2002. *Circulation,* 116(13):1488–1496.

Douglas, J. G., Bakris, G. L., Epstein, M., et al. (2003). Management of high blood pressure in African Americans: Consensus statement of the Hypertension in African Americans Working Group of the International Society on Hypertension in Blacks. *Archives of Internal Medicine,* 163(5):525–541. Retreived from: http://ishib.org/supportfiles/Mgt_of_Hypertension_in_African_Americans.pdf

Eichner, J. E., Moore, W. E., Perveen, G., et al. (2008). Overweight and obesity in an ethnically diverse rural school district: the Healthy Kids Project. *Obesity (Silver Spring),* 16(2):501–504.

Fiebeler, A., Nussberger, J., Shagdarsuren, E., et al. (2005). Aldosterone synthase inhibitor ameliorates angiotensin II–induced organ damage. *Circulation,* 111:3087–3094.

Ferdinand, K. C., & Armani, A. M. (2007). The management of hypertension in African Americans. *Critical Pathways in Cardiology*, 6(2):67–71.

Flynn, J. T. (2009). Hypertension in the young: epidemiology, sequelae, and therapy. *Nephrology Dialysis Transplantation*, 24(2):370–375.

Goldstein, F. C., Ashley, A. V., Endeshaw, Y. M., et al. (2008). Effects of hypertension and hypercholesterolemia on cognitive functioning in patients with alzheimer disease. *Alzheimer Disease and Associated Disorders*, 22(4):336–342.

Grandi, A. M., Solbiati, F., Laurita, E., et al. (2008). Effects of dual blockade of Renin-angiotensin system on concentric left ventricular hypertrophy in essential hypertension: a randomized, controlled pilot study. *American Journal of Hypertension*, 21(2):231–237.

Heran, B. S., Wong, M. M., Heran, I. K., & Wright, J. M. (2008a). Blood pressure lowering efficacy of angiotensin converting enzyme (ACE) inhibitors for primary hypertension. *Cochrane Database Systematic Reviews*, (4):CD003823.

Heran, B. S., Wong, M. M., Heran, I. K., & Wright, J. M. (2008b). Blood pressure lowering efficacy of angiotensin receptor blockers for primary hypertension. *Cochrane Database Systematic Reviews*, (4):CD003822.

Igarashi, M., Hirata, A., Kadomoto, Y. (2006). Dual blockade of angiotensin II with enalapril and losartan reduces proteinuria in hypertensive patients with type 2 diabetes. *Endocrine Journal*, 53(4):493–501.

Joint National Committee on Detection, Evaluation and Treatment of High Blood Pressure. The seventh report of the Joint National Committee on Detection, Evaluation and Treatment of High Blood Pressure (JNC 7). (2003). Retrieved from *http://www.nhlbi.nih.gov/health/ prof/heart/hbp/hbp_ped.pdf*.

Johnson, K. C., Margolis, K. L., Espeland, M. A., et al.; Women's Health Initiative Memory Study and Women's Health Initiative Investigators. (2008). A prospectice study of the effect of hypertension and baseline blood pressure on cognitive decine and dementia in postmenopausal women: the Women's Health Initiative Memory Study.

Law, M. R., Morris, J. K., Wald, N. J. (2009). Use of blood pressure lowering drugs in the prevention of cardiovascular disease: meta-analysis of 147 randomised trials in the context of expectations from prospective epidemiological studies. *British Medical Journal*, 338:b1655

Lichtenstein, A. H., Appel, L. J., Brands, M., et al. (2006). Diet and Lifestyle Recommendations Revision 2006. A Scientific Statement From the American Heart Association

Nutrition Committee. *Circulation : Journal of the American Heart Association*. Retrieved from http://circ.ahajournals.org/cgi/reprint/CIRCULATIONAHA.106.176158v2

Launer, L. J., Ross, G. W., Petrovistch, H., et al. (2000). Midlife blood pressure and dementia: The Honolulu–Asia aging study. *Neurobiological Aging*, 21(1):49–55.

Moore, W. E., Stephens, A., Wilson, T., et al. (2006). Body mass index and blood pressure screening in a rural public school system: the Healthy Kids Project. *Preventing Chronic Disease*, 3(4):A114.

Musini, V. M., Fortin, P. M., Bassett, K., & Wright, J. M. (2009). Blood pressure lowering efficacy of renin inhibitors for primary hypertension: a Cochrane systematic review. *Journal of Human Hypertension*, 34(8):495–502.

National High Blood Pressure Education Program Working Group on Adolescents and Children. (2004). The fourth report on the diagnosis, evaluation, and treatment of high blood pressure in children and adolescents. *Pediatrics*, 114(2):555–576.

Ogden, C. L., Carroll, M. D., Curtin, L.R., et al. (2006). Prevalence of overweight and obesity in the United States 1999–2004. *Journal of the American Medical Association*, 295(13):1549.

Parving H. H., Persson, F., Lewis, J. B., et al. AVOID Study Investigators, (2008). Aliskiren combined with losartan in type 2 diabetes and nephropathy. *New England Journal of Medicine*, 358(23):2433–2446.

Poon, I. Q. (2008). Effects of antihypertensive drug treatment on the risk of dementia and cognitive impairment. *Pharmacotherapy*, 28(3):366–375.

Perez, M. I., & Musini, V. M. (2008). Pharmacological interventions for hypertensive emergencies. *Cochrane Database of Systematic Reviews*, 1:CD003653.

Peters, Beckett, Forette, et al. HYVET Investigators. (2008). Incident dementia and blood pressure lowering in the Hypertension in the Very eldery Trial conginitve function assessment (HYVET-COG): a double-blind, placebo controlled trial. *Lancet Neurolog*, 7(8):683–689.

Psaty, B. M., Lumley, T., Furberg, C. D., et al. (2003). Health outcomes associated with various antihypertensive therapies used as first-line agents: A network meta-analysis. *Journal of the American Medical Association*, 289(19):2534–2544.

Schjoedt, K. J., Rossing, K., Juhl, T. R., et al. (2005). Beneficial impact of spironolactone in diabetic nephropathy. *Kidney International*, 68(6):2829–2836.

Skoog, I., & Gustafson, D. (2006). Update on hypertension and Alzheimer's disease. *Neurological Research*, 28(6):605–611.

Sorof, J. M., Lai, D., Turner, J., et al. (2004). Overweight, ethnicity, and the prevalence of hypertension in school-aged children. *Pediatrics*, 113(3 Pt 1):475–482.

Spinar, J., Vitovec, J., Soucek, M., Dusek, L., Pavlik, T.; CORD Investigators. (2009). CORD: Comparison of Reccomended Doses of ACE Inhibitors and angiotensin II receptor blockers. *Vnitřní lékařství* (in Czech), 55(5):481–488.

Strasser, R. H., Puig, J. G., Farsnag, C., et al. (2007). A comparison of the tolerability of the direct renin inhibitor aliskiren and lisinopril in patients with severe hypertension. *Journal of Human Hypertension*, 21(10):780–787.

Taniguchi, I., Kawai, M., Date, T., et al. (2006). Effects of spironolactone during an angiotensin II receptor blocker treatment on the left ventricular mass reduction in hypertensive patients with concentric left ventricular hypertrophy. *Circulation*, 70(8):995–1000.

Urrutia-Rojas, X., Egbuchunam, C. U., Bae, S., et al. (2006). High blood pressure in school children: Prevalence and risk factors. *BioMed Central Pediatrics*, 6:32.

Weir, M. R. (2007). Effects of renin-angiotensin system inhibiton on end-organ protection: can we do better? *Clinical Therapeutics*, 29(9):1803–1824.

Wiysonge, C. S., Bradley, H., Mayosi, B. M., et al. (2007). Beta –blockers for hypertension. *Cochrane Database of Systematic Reviews*, 1:CD002003.

Wright, J. M., & Musini, V. M. (2009). First-line drugs for hypertension. *Cochrane Database of Systematic Reviews*, (3):CD001841.

Drugs Affecting Urinary Output

Learning Objectives

At the completion of this chapter the student will:

1. Describe normal kidney function and explain how diuretics work in the kidney.
2. Identify core drug knowledge about drugs that affect diuresis.
3. Identify core patient variables related to drugs that affect diuresis.
4. Relate the interaction of core drug knowledge to core patient variables for drugs that affect diuresis.
5. Generate a nursing plan of care from the interactions between core drug knowledge and core patient variables for drugs that affect diuresis.
6. Describe nursing interventions to maximize therapeutic and minimize adverse effects for drugs that affect diuresis.
7. Determine key points for patient and family education for drugs that affect diuresis.

Key Terms

diuresis
diuretic
edema
glomerular filtration

hyperkalemia
hypertension
hypervolemia
hypokalemia

osmolality
renal tubular
reabsorption
renal tubular secretion

Drugs Affecting Urinary Output

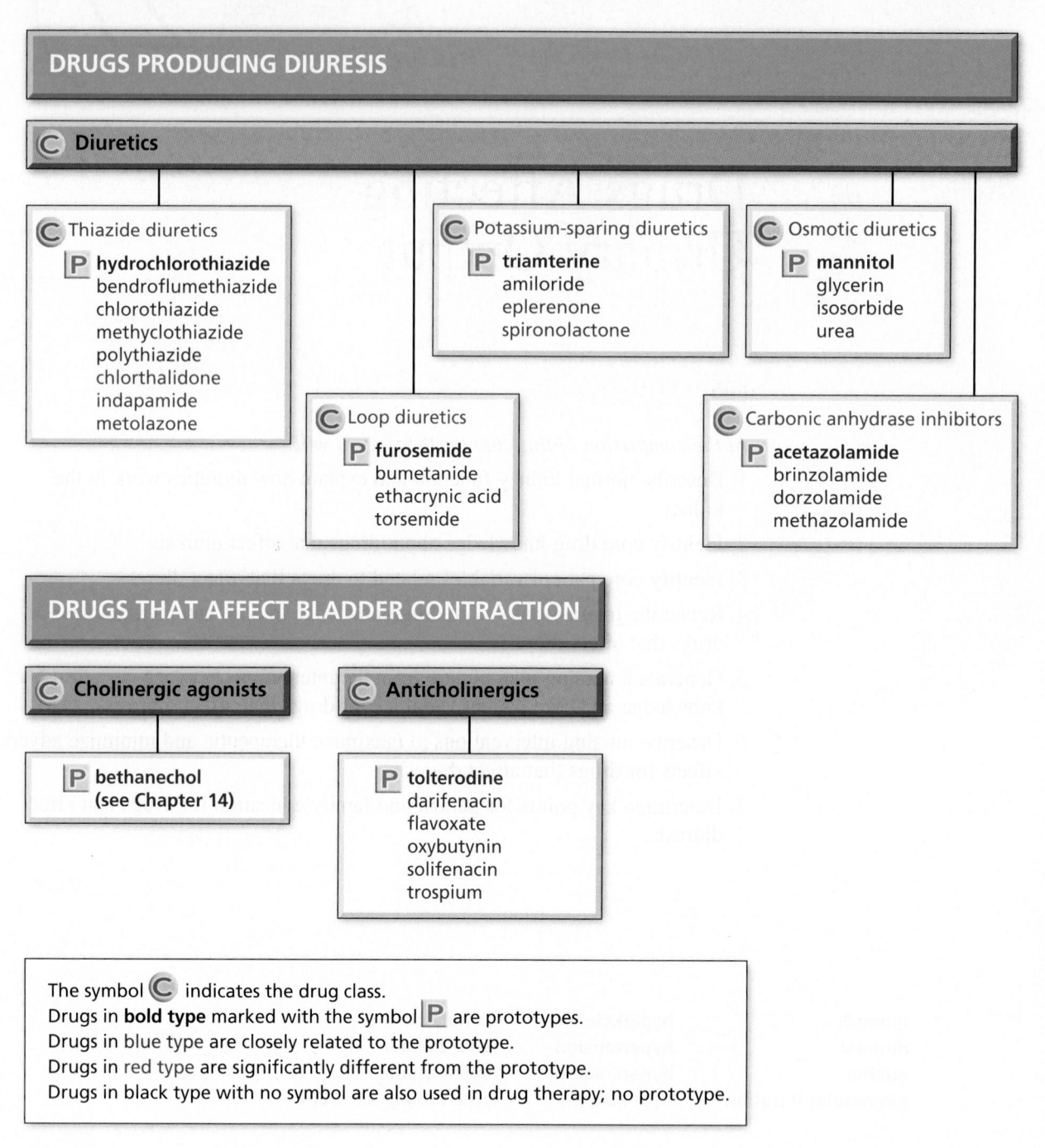

DRUGS PRODUCING DIURESIS

C **Diuretics**

C Thiazide diuretics
P **hydrochlorothiazide**
bendroflumethiazide
chlorothiazide
methyclothiazide
polythiazide
chlorthalidone
indapamide
metolazone

C Loop diuretics
P **furosemide**
bumetanide
ethacrynic acid
torsemide

C Potassium-sparing diuretics
P **triamterine**
amiloride
eplerenone
spironolactone

C Osmotic diuretics
P **mannitol**
glycerin
isosorbide
urea

C Carbonic anhydrase inhibitors
P **acetazolamide**
brinzolamide
dorzolamide
methazolamide

DRUGS THAT AFFECT BLADDER CONTRACTION

C **Cholinergic agonists**

P **bethanechol**
(see Chapter 14)

C **Anticholinergics**

P **tolterodine**
darifenacin
flavoxate
oxybutynin
solifenacin
trospium

The symbol C indicates the drug class.
Drugs in **bold type** marked with the symbol P are prototypes.
Drugs in blue type are closely related to the prototype.
Drugs in red type are significantly different from the prototype.
Drugs in black type with no symbol are also used in drug therapy; no prototype.

Diuresis is the process of ridding the body of fluids by increasing production of urine and excretion of water and electrolytes, such as sodium, by the kidneys. Diuresis occurs naturally if fluid intake has exceeded the body's normal requirements. This self-regulating or homeostatic mechanism keeps the body's fluid volume in balance.

A **diuretic** is a substance that causes diuresis. Drugs that are diuretics are used to decrease fluid volume in pathologic conditions in which the body cannot regulate fluid volume effectively. Diuretics decrease renal reabsorption of sodium and promote its excretion in water. The greater the sodium excretion, the greater the water excretion will be. During this process, reabsorption of other electrolytes (e.g., potassium) may also decrease, thereby promoting their excretion as well.

The various types of diuretics work differently in the body. Which diuretic is prescribed for a patient depends on the patient's underlying pathologies and the desired therapeutic effects. This chapter discusses five classes of diuretics: thiazide, loop, potassium-sparing, osmotic, and carbonic anhydrase inhibitors. The thiazide, loop, and potassium-sparing classes all are used to decrease circulating volume and complications related to excess volume. Thiazide diuretics work in the distal tubule of the kidney, whereas loop diuretics work in the loop of Henle. Potassium-sparing diuretics are used commonly in combination with other diuretics, and they work in the distal tubule. Prototype drugs for thiazide, loop, and potassium-sparing classes are hydrochlorothiazide, furosemide, and triamterene, respectively.

The osmotic diuretics, for which mannitol is the prototype, are used to decrease intraocular and intracranial pressure and to treat or prevent acute renal failure (ARF). The osmotic diuretics are filtered by the kidneys but poorly reabsorbed in the tubule. Acetazolamide, which is the prototype for the carbonic anhydrase inhibitors, induces diuresis by decreasing hydrogen ion secretion by the tubules and increasing excretion of sodium and water. Although the diuretic effect is limited, aqueous humor formation is reduced, thereby making these drugs useful for reducing intraocular pressure in glaucoma.

Urinary output can also be modified by drugs that bind to cholinergic receptors in the bladder. Cholinergic stimulation of these receptors stimulates bladder contraction. Bethanechol, a cholinergic drug used for this therapeutic effect, is discussed in Chapter 14. Drugs that have an anticholinergic effect on these receptors decrease bladder contraction and are used to treat overactive bladder. The prototype for this class, tolterodine, is discussed in this chapter.

PHYSIOLOGY

The renal system is a complex mechanism that has several important functions in maintaining health. It is the body's filtering and purifying center, ridding the body of impurities and waste by producing urine and excreting water, electrolytes, and other substances. Other functions of the renal system include regulating the body's acid-base balance, maintaining blood pressure, influencing circulating fluid volume, assisting in the production of red blood cells, and contributing to calcium metabolism (Figure 27.1).

The renal system consists of the kidneys, ureters, and bladder. The kidneys are a pair of intricate, bean-shaped organs located behind the upper abdomen outside the peritoneal cavity. They are active in filtering, reabsorbing, and excreting fluid, electrolytes, and waste products. The ureters are tubes that transport waste products and excess fluid from the kidneys to the bladder, a balloon-like receptacle, for later excretion.

Urine formation, which occurs as a result of kidney function, involves three complex processes: glomerular filtration, renal tubular reabsorption, and renal tubular secretion. These mechanisms, which are discussed individually below, work together in a part of the kidney called the nephron, which processes blood plasma into urine.

The nephron has many parts, including the glomerulus, Bowman capsule, and various tubules and membranes. In the nephron, water and solutes move from the blood plasma across a glomerular capsular membrane into an area known as a Bowman capsule. This movement across the capsular membrane is called **glomerular filtration.**

As the blood flows through the kidney capillaries, pressure in the capillaries causes fluid to filter into the Bowman capsule. The glomerular capsular membrane (the basement membrane), which lies between the glomerulus and the Bowman capsule, allows fluid and electrolytes but not blood cells and plasma proteins to pass into the Bowman capsule. The average glomerular filtration rate is 125 mL/min (or about 180 L of plasma in 24 hours). More than 99% of the plasma filtered is reabsorbed in the tubules.

Usually, the kidneys produce less than 2 L of urine daily. However, changes in colloid osmotic pressure or capsular hydrostatic pressure can alter glomerular filtration. For example, a decrease in colloid osmotic pressure may increase filtration. Conversely, an increase in capsular hydrostatic pressure, which occurs in obstructive disease, may decrease filtration.

The conversion of the filtrate into urine occurs in the renal tubule by processes known as renal tubular reabsorption and renal tubular secretion. In **renal tubular reabsorption,** molecules move from the renal tubule across a semipermeable membrane into the peritubular blood (the blood surrounding the renal tubule). In **renal tubular secretion,** molecules move from the blood surrounding the renal tubule into the tubule. In both reabsorption and secretion, diffusion and active transport are key mechanisms.

The strength, or concentration, of the urine produced is known as **osmolality,** which is the density of active particles in solution or the osmotic concentration, determined by the ionic concentration of dissolved substances per unit of solution. Urine osmolality depends on the volume and composition of extracellular fluids. It also depends on a countercurrent mechanism in the renal medulla (a part of the kidney), which controls the flow of water and solute so that water is kept out of the area around the tubule and so that sodium and urea are retained. An important contributor to this process

PHYSIOLOGY

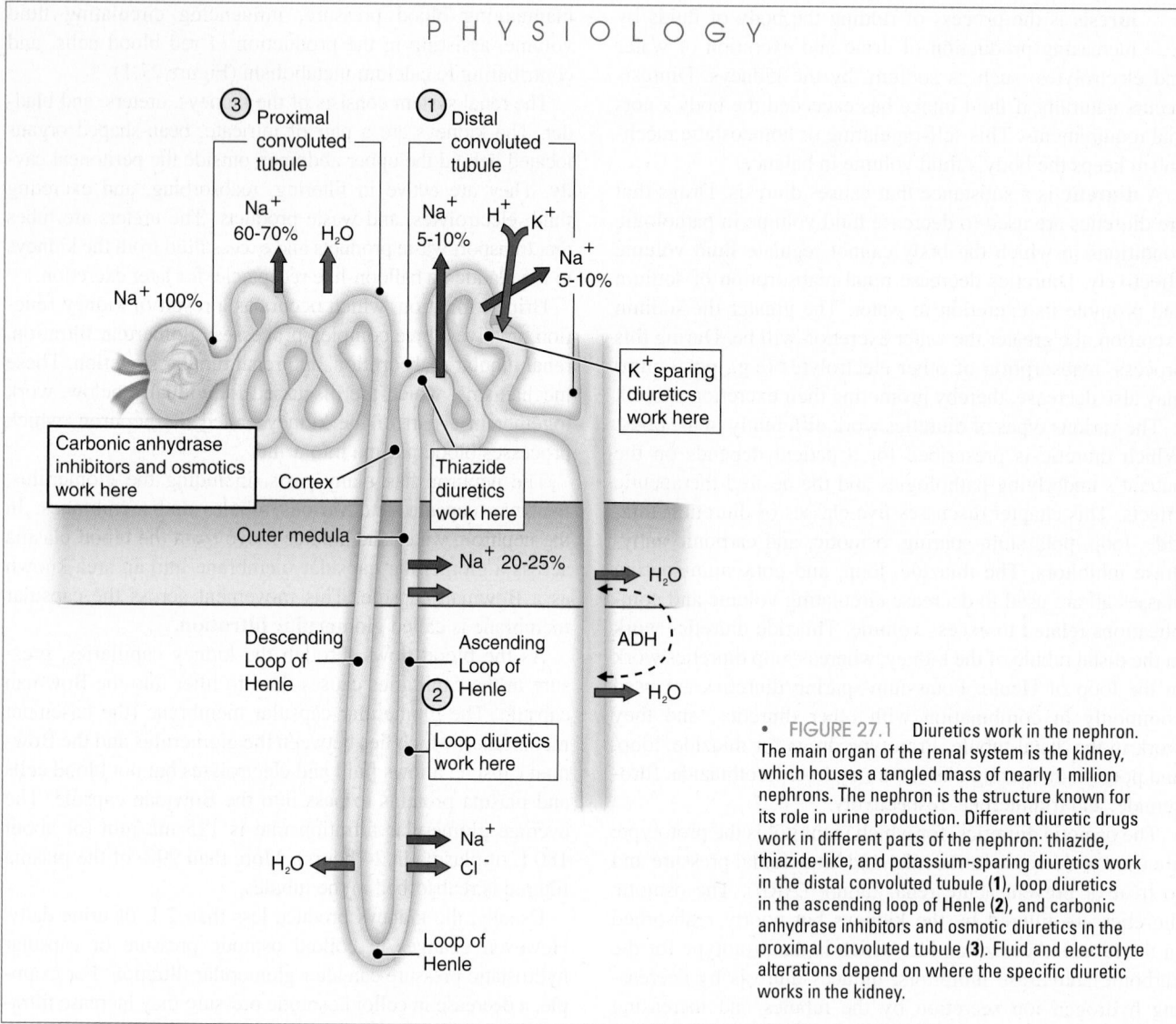

• FIGURE 27.1 Diuretics work in the nephron. The main organ of the renal system is the kidney, which houses a tangled mass of nearly 1 million nephrons. The nephron is the structure known for its role in urine production. Different diuretic drugs work in different parts of the nephron: thiazide, thiazide-like, and potassium-sparing diuretics work in the distal convoluted tubule (**1**), loop diuretics in the ascending loop of Henle (**2**), and carbonic anhydrase inhibitors and osmotic diuretics in the proximal convoluted tubule (**3**). Fluid and electrolyte alterations depend on where the specific diuretic works in the kidney.

is antidiuretic hormone (ADH), which is released when the osmolality of the extracellular fluid increases.

To enable water to move out of the tubule and into the surrounding capillaries, ADH increases the permeability of the collecting tubule to water; from the capillaries, it returns to the vascular system for circulation. As a result of increased water reabsorption, urine osmolality (concentration) increases. Without ADH, the renal tubules are impermeable to water, water is not reabsorbed, and dilute urine is produced.

The kidneys play a major role in regulating acid-base balance and maintaining a normal blood pH (7.35–7.45) by excreting hydrogen ions or reabsorbing bicarbonate. The kidneys regulate hydrogen ion secretion so that bicarbonate levels remain within normal limits. Most of the hydrogen ions excreted in the urine are secreted into the tubular fluid. Tubular fluid pH is acidic, and the kidney depends on buffers in the urine to combine with the hydrogen ion for excretion. The three buffers are bicarbonate (HCO_3), phosphate (HPO_4), and ammonia (NH_3).

The first step in bicarbonate reabsorption is the movement of carbon dioxide (CO_2) into a tubular cell, where the CO_2 combines with water to form a hydrogen ion and a bicarbonate ion. The hydrogen ion is then secreted into the tubular fluid, and a sodium ion is reabsorbed. The sodium ion and bicarbonate ion pass into the extracellular fluid. The free hydrogen ion then combines with a filtered bicarbonate ion to form carbon dioxide and water. The water is eliminated in the urine, and the CO_2 diffuses into the tubular cell to combine with water, thereby forming a hydrogen ion and a bicarbonate ion to begin the process again.

Additional hydrogen ions are excreted in the urine in combination with a phosphate or ammonium buffer. The phosphate ion is filtered into the tubular fluid, where it combines with a free hydrogen ion and is excreted. Ammonia is synthesized in the tubular cells and diffuses into the tubular fluid, where it combines with a hydrogen ion to form an ammonium ion (NH_4), which is excreted.

Normally, the number of hydrogen ions secreted by the tubules is about equal to the number of bicarbonate ions filtered in the glomerulus. However, in metabolic acidosis, the number of hydrogen ions secreted exceeds bicarbonate filtration, and the urine becomes acidic. In metabolic alkalosis, bicarbonate filtration exceeds hydrogen ion secretion, and the urine becomes alkaline.

The kidneys also play a role in the reabsorption and secretion of electrolytes. Vast quantities of sodium and chloride are filtered through the glomerulus. Most of the filtered sodium and chloride (60% to 65%) is reabsorbed in the proximal tubule, and about 20% is reabsorbed in the loop of Henle. Smaller amounts are reabsorbed in the distal tubule and the collecting tubule. Sodium reabsorption occurs primarily through active transport. Filtered potassium is then mostly reabsorbed, much of this occurring in the loop of Henle. Coupled with the sodium transport, potassium moves by active transport into the proximal tubule from cells. (Remember, potassium moves opposite to sodium.) This transport moves some potassium into the urine in the distal and collecting tubule. Again, most of it is reabsorbed, but some of it is excreted in the urine.

Additional work of the kidneys includes endocrine functions, whereby chemicals are produced to exert action elsewhere in the body. In this regard, the kidneys help maintain and regulate blood pressure and vascular resistance, red blood cell production, and calcium metabolism.

Blood pressure is also affected by the kidneys' role in the renin-angiotensin-aldosterone mechanism. Renin, an enzyme, is synthesized and stored in the kidney and released in response to decreased blood flow or a change in the composition of fluid in the distal tubule. The release of renin plays a role in converting angiotensin I, a substance in the blood, into the powerful vasoconstrictor angiotensin II. The vasoconstriction increases peripheral resistance, resulting in an increase in blood pressure. Angiotensin II also stimulates the adrenal cortex to secrete the hormone aldosterone. Aldosterone has an effect in the distal tubule and the collecting tubule, where it promotes sodium and water reabsorption as well as potassium loss. Only about 3% of the original filtered sodium remains in the distal and collecting tubule; the body varies its reabsorption based on signals it receives related to fluid status. Higher amounts of aldosterone cause the body to reabsorb more sodium and water. This in turn increases blood pressure.

The kidney produces erythropoietin, which stimulates the bone marrow to produce and release red blood cells, particularly in response to hypoxia (oxygen deprivation). The kidneys play a vital role in the chemical transformation of compounds that are precursors to the active form of vitamin D, which is needed to absorb calcium from the gastrointestinal (GI) tract. Vitamin D also helps to regulate calcium deposition in the bones.

Stimulation of the adrenergic and cholinergic receptors in the genitourinary (GU) tract has a role in urinary production and bladder emptying.

- Alpha-1 receptor stimulation causes the muscles of the bladder neck to contract, preventing bladder emptying; blockade of these receptors has the opposite effect.

- Beta-1 stimulation causes the release of renin, setting off the renin-angiotensin-aldosterone system, which ultimately has an effect on the reabsorption of sodium and water.
- Adrenergic dopamine-1 receptor stimulation in the proximal tubule maintains or increases the glomerular filtration rate (GFR), whereas in the distal tubules this stimulation increases sodium loss in the urine (natriuresis) and diuresis. A consequence of this is an increase in aldosterone production.
- Adrenergic dopamine-2 receptor stimulation has the opposite effect: decreased renal blood flow, decreased GFR, decreased sodium and water loss, and thus less aldosterone production.
- Cholinergic receptor stimulation in the bladder results in contraction of the detrusor muscle, producing micturition; blockade of these receptors has the opposite effect.

PATHOPHYSIOLOGY

When the body cannot maintain a balance of body fluid levels, fluid overload or volume depletion occurs. **Hypervolemia** (an abnormal increase in circulating blood volume) may result from excessive sodium and water retention. Shifting of fluid into the interstitial spaces (**edema**) may occur with fluid volume excess. Peripheral edema increases the cardiac workload and decreases tissue perfusion. Moreover, other organ systems may be affected adversely by the congestion associated with edema. When systemic edema is severe, the congestion backs up into the lungs, affecting breathing and gas exchange.

Diuretic drugs are used in treating pathologic conditions in which fluid overload and, frequently, edema have occurred. These conditions include chronic heart failure (CHF), pulmonary edema, hypertension, cirrhosis, nephrotic syndrome, and kidney failure. Additionally, diuretics are used for treating adverse effects from long-term steroid or antiepileptic drug therapy and symptoms of fluid overload such as increased intracranial and intraocular pressure and premenstrual syndrome.

Ineffective pumping of the heart can result in CHF because the heart does not empty well, and cardiac output is diminished. Increased demands placed on the heart by other systemic problems can also cause the heart to fail. When the heart chambers do not empty well with each contraction, blood backs up into the body, and congestion occurs in the body tissues. Edema in CHF usually results from increased sodium and water retention and venous congestion, which increases capillary pressure in the peripheral and pulmonary circulation. As a result of the ineffective pumping ability of the heart, the kidneys receive a diminished blood supply. Impaired glomerular filtration and reduced blood flow to the renal tubules then occur. The kidney interprets these occurrences as signs of hypovolemia (insufficient circulating fluid or volume depletion) and activates mechanisms to retain sodium and water and increase circulating volume. Thus, volume is increased in an already congested system, and CHF actually worsens.

Drug therapy for CHF is now focused on improving survival. Drugs proven to reduce morbidity and mortality in CHF are angiotensin-converting enzyme (ACE) inhibitors, diuretics, and beta blockers. Diuretics have been found in small clinical studies to reduce the risk of death and worsening of heart failure. Compared to other drug classes used in treating CHF, diuretics appear to improve exercise capacity (Faris, Flather, Purcell, et al., 2006). In large clinical trials and meta-analysis of trials, thiazides have been found to be superior to other drug therapies used in treating hypertension to prevent heart failure (Wright, J.T. Jr, Probstfield, J.L., Cushman, W.C., et al., 2009).

For a complete discussion of CHF and its treatment, see Chapter 29.

The increased urinary output resulting from diuretic therapy is useful in CHF because it reduces edema and circulating volume and prevents further fluid retention by the kidneys. These actions have a net effect of decreasing preload (volume returned to the heart) and afterload (resistance exerted by the vessels to blood pumped by the heart) and easing the heart's workload. Pulmonary edema, characterized by fluid-filled lungs, is a life-threatening condition. It commonly results from CHF, but it also can result from infections, exposure to toxic gases, and reactions to drugs. However, the pulmonary edema associated with CHF occurs because pulmonary capillary pressure is greater than capillary osmotic pressure (because of increased left ventricular end-diastolic pressure). In addition, the capillary permeability of the pulmonary capillary membrane increases, thereby allowing fluid to leak into the lungs' interstitial spaces and the alveoli. This leakage impairs gas exchange, which stiffens the lungs and impairs expansion. Diuretics return fluid to the vascular space and increase fluid excretion, which eases breathing. Loop diuretics are now most commonly used in treatment of CHF.

Nephrotic syndrome is a kidney disorder characterized by generalized edema. This condition alters glomerular permeability to protein, allowing massive proteinuria, because plasma proteins are lost by way of the kidney. This loss causes hypoalbuminemia (a lower-than-normal blood level of the protein albumin). Low albumin levels decrease colloid osmotic pressure, which allows fluid to move out of the vascular system, resulting in edema and decreased circulating volume. The kidneys attempt to compensate for the decreased blood volume by retaining sodium and water, which contributes to additional edema. Diuretics promote excretion of sodium and water, and therefore decrease the circulating blood volume.

A potentially reversible condition, acute renal failure results from acutely reduced kidney function. Chronic kidney disease (CKD), an irreversible and progressive reduction of kidney function, is caused by various conditions, although hypertension and diabetes mellitus are responsible for two-thirds of the incidence (other conditions that may lead to CKD include: systemic lupus erythematosus (SLE); glomerulonephritis; inherited diseases, such as polycystic kidney disease; recurrent urinary tract infections; obstruction; and

congenital malformation). Chronic kidney disease leads to renal failure. Chronic kidney disease is defined as structural or functional kidney abnormalities (most commonly persistent albuminuria or microalbuminuria) that last for at least 3 months, with or without a decreased GFR or a decreased GFR with or without evidence of kidney damage. Twenty-six million American adults have chronic kidney disease (National Kidney Foundation, 2009). Chronic kidney disease is classified into five stages (Levy, Coresh, Balk, et al., 2003) (Box 27.1). As renal failure becomes more severe, the following may be observed: hypervolemia, hyperkalemia, metabolic acidosis, hypertension, anemia, and bone disease. With end-stage renal failure, uremia is present; signs and symptoms include anorexia, nausea, vomiting, pericarditis, peripheral neuropathy, and central nervous system abnormalities ranging from loss of concentration or lethargy to seizure to coma and death.

In pathologic conditions in which sodium and water reabsorption cause hypervolemia, diuretics are used to promote sodium loss. Sodium loss from a diuretic is related to the dose of the diuretic. Natriuresis is not seen until a threshold rate of drug excretion is attained. A patient who does not respond to a particular dose of a diuretic may not be reaching this threshold. Thus, the single dose should be increased, rather than two equal doses administered twice as often. In end-stage renal failure (where anuria is present), diuretics are generally of little value, and increasing the dose does not increase the therapeutic response.

In kidney failure, loss of the ability to produce erythropoietin contributes to anemia. Exogenous erythropoietin can be given as a replacement when this occurs. Chapter 33 discusses erythropoietin.

Hypertension (blood pressure that is chronically elevated above normal), one of the most common cardiovascular disorders in the United States, is closely associated with kidney function. Renin is released by the kidneys. The outflow of renin activates several mechanisms that lead to activation of angiotensin II, a potent vasoconstrictor. Angiotensin II stimulates secretion of aldosterone, which promotes sodium retention. Sodium retention promotes water retention. The resulting increased vascular resistance and the increased fluid volume elevate blood pressure.

Although hypervolemia is not necessarily present in the hypertensive patient, the action of diuretics effectively

Box 27.1	STAGES OF CHRONIC KIDNEY DISEASE
STAGE 1	Normal GFR (>90 mL/min per 1.73 m^2) and persistent albuminuria
STAGE 2	GFR between 60 and 89 mL/min per 1.73 m^2 and persistent albuminuria
STAGE 3	GFR between 30 and 59 mL/min per 1.73 m^2
STAGE 4	GFR between 15 and 29 mL/min per 1.73 m^2
STAGE 5	GFR of less than 15 mL/min per 1.73 m^2 (end-stage renal disease)

lowers the blood pressure. Blood pressure (BP) is cardiac output (CO) multiplied by peripheral resistance (PR): BP = CO × PR. By reducing circulating volume, diuretics decrease cardiac output and reduce blood pressure. In reducing circulating volume, fluid is pulled back into the vascular space, reducing edema and the symptoms associated with it. Peripheral vascular resistance is thus decreased, further promoting reduction in blood pressure and decreasing the workload on the heart. Diuretics have been found to be at least as effective as other antihypertensives, and findings from the Antihypertensive and Lipid-Lowering Treatment to Prevent Heart Attack Trial (ALLHAT) indicate that they, and specifically the thiazides, should be used as first-line therapy in hypertension. In fact, findings from ALLHAT, in a study of more than 33,000 North American hypertensive patients with at least one other CHF risk factor, showed that thiazide-type diuretics are as good if not superior to ACE inhibitors or calcium channel blockers in preventing one or more major forms of cardiovascular disease (CVD) (ALLHAT Officers and Coordinators, 2002). Evidence from subsequent analyses of ALLHAT and other clinical outcome trials have confirmed that no other drug therapy for hypertension is superior to thiazide-type diuretics as initial therapy for reduction of cardiovascular or renal risk from hypertension (Wright, J.T. Jr., Probstfield, J.L., Cushman, W.C., et al., 2009).

Diuretics may be used alone or with antihypertensive drugs to lower blood pressure. The kind of diuretic drug prescribed depends on the patient's condition and the severity of the hypertension. For more information on hypertension and its treatment, refer to Chapter 26.

A completely different problem with urinary output arises from alterations in the stimulation of adrenergic or cholinergic receptors in the bladder. When there is excessive cholinergic stimulation, an overactive bladder can result. An overactive bladder is a condition that results from sudden, involuntary contraction of the muscle in the wall of the urinary bladder. Overactive bladder causes an immediate need to urinate (urinary urgency). This condition is also referred to as urge incontinence and is a form of urinary incontinence (unintentional loss of urine).

C THIAZIDE DIURETICS

The thiazides comprise the largest group of diuretics. They are related structurally to the antibacterial sulfonamides. Thiazide diuretics include hydrochlorothiazide, chlorothiazide, bendroflumethiazide, hydroflumethiazide, polythiazide, and methyclothiazide. A few thiazides differ slightly in chemical structure. These drugs are called thiazide-related diuretics and include indapamide, chlorthalidone, and metolazone. They exhibit the same diuretic mechanism of action, efficacy, and adverse reactions as the thiazides. The prototype thiazide diuretic is hydrochlorothiazide (HydroDIURIL). Table 27.1 presents a summary of selected diuretic drugs.

Nursing Management of the Patient Receiving P Hydrochlorothiazide
Core Drug Knowledge
Pharmacotherapeutics

Hydrochlorothiazide is used widely in managing hypertension, either alone or with other drugs. Several days are required to see the antihypertensive effects, and full therapeutic effects may not occur for 2 to 4 weeks. Hydrochlorothiazide or other thiazide diuretics have long been recommended by clinical guidelines to be the first drug prescribed to treat hypertension. Only about one-third of practitioners actually prescribe a thiazide diuretic as first-line treatment for hypertension, however (Bonds, D.E., Hogan, P.E., Bertoni, A.G., 2009). Sometimes hydrochlorothiazide is also used in treating edema resulting from CHF, hepatic cirrhosis, and long-term steroid or estrogen therapy. Paradoxically, hydrochlorothiazide is used in diabetes insipidus as an antidiuretic, possibly because it enhances the action of ADH as a consequence of sodium depletion. Hydrochlorothiazide is only administered orally.

Hydrochlorothiazide appears to prevent recurrence of calcium kidney stones in individuals who have unexplainable elevations of calcium in the urine and have experienced kidney stones (Escribano J., Balaguer A., Pagone F., et al., 2009; Arrabal-Martin, Fernandez-Rodriguez, Arrabal-Polo, et al., 2006; Fernandez-Rodriguez, Arrabal-Martin, Garcia-Ruiz, et al., 2006). Thiazides appear to produce this effect this by promoting reabsorption of calcium.

Pharmacokinetics

Administered orally, hydrochlorothiazide is absorbed rapidly from the GI tract, and more than 50% of the circulating drug is bound to plasma proteins. Action begins within a few hours. The drug crosses the placental barrier and is secreted in breast milk. Hydrochlorothiazide is metabolized by the liver and excreted in the urine.

Pharmacodynamics

Hydrochlorothiazide acts in the distal tubule and possibly in the diluting segment of the ascending loop of Henle. It increases excretion of sodium and chloride in the distal convoluted tubule by slightly inhibiting the ion pumps that work in sodium and chloride reabsorption. This action also inhibits water reabsorption. Because most of the sodium is reabsorbed before the distal tubule, hydrochlorothiazide has a weak diuretic effect. It also increases the excretion of potassium, bicarbonate, and magnesium and decreases the urinary excretion of calcium. The effects on electrolytes occur early in therapy. With long-term treatment at the same dose (and assuming that sodium intake remains constant), the kidney undergoes some compensatory changes to maintain homeostasis.

The initial volume depletion from the thiazide leads to increases in a variety of sodium-retaining factors, such as angiotensin II and aldosterone. These sodium-retaining forces eventually equal the sodium-losing activity of the

TABLE 27.1 Summary of Selected Diuretic Drugs

Drug (Trade) Name	Selected Indications	Route and Dosage Range	Pharmacokinetics
C Thiazide Diuretics			
P hydrochlorothiazide (Esidrix, HydroDIURIL, Oretic)	Hypertension	*Adult:* PO, 12.5–50 mg/d; increase to 25–100 mg/d as a single or two divided doses *Child:* PO, 1–2 mg/kg/d in single or two divided doses; infants <6 mo may require 3 mg/kg/d in two doses	*Onset:* 2 h *Duration:* 6–12 h $t_{1/2}$: 5.6–14.8 h
	Edema	*Adult:* PO, 25–200 mg/d initially, then 25–100 mg/d *Child:* PO, 1–2 mg/kg/d in two doses; infants <6 mo may require 3 mg/kg/d in two doses	
C Loop Diuretics			
P furosemide (Lasix;)	Edema	*Adult:* PO, 20–80 mg/d in a single dose, may repeat 6 to 8 h later; titrate up to 600 mg/d in severe edema *Adult:* IM, IV, 20–40 mg, may repeat 2 h later	*Onset:* PO, within 1 h; IV, within 5 min *Duration:* PO, 6–8 h; IV, 2 h $t_{1/2}$: 2 h
	Hypertension	*Adult:* PO, 40 mg bid *Child:* PO, 2 mg/kg; may increase by 1–2 mg/kg, not to exceed 6 mg/kg	
	CHF, CRF Pulmonary edema	*Adult:* PO, IV, 2–2.5 g/d *Adult:* IV, 40 mg over 1–2 min; may increase to 80 mg *Child:* IV, 1 mg/kg; may increase by 1 mg/kg but not more than 6 mg/kg	
C Potassium-Sparing Diuretics			
P triamterene (Dyrenium)	Hypertension	*Adult:* PO, 100 mg bid when used alone; decrease starting dose when given with other diuretics; decrease dose of each, adjust to need; not to exceed 300 mg/d	*Onset:* PO, 2–4 h *Duration:* 12–16 h $t_{1/2}$: 3 h
amiloride (Midamor)	Hypertension	*Adult:* PO, add 5 mg/d to usual antihypertensive or other diuretic therapy; increase up to 10 mg/d	*Onset:* 2 h *Duration:* 24 h $t_{1/2}$: 6–9 h
spironolactone (Aldactone;	Hyperaldosteronism Edema Hypertension Diuretic-induced hypokalemia	*Adult:* PO, 100–400 mg/d *Adult:* PO, 100 mg/d (range: 25–200 mg/d) *Child:* PO, 3.3 mg/kg/d in single or divided doses *Adult:* PO, 50–100 mg/d, single or divided doses *Child:* PO, 1–2 mg/kg bid *Adult:* PO, 25–100 mg/d	*Onset:* 24–48 h *Duration:* 48–72 h $t_{1/2}$: 20 h
C Osmotic Diuretics			
P mannitol (Osmitrol)	Acute renal failure Intracranial pressure Intraocular pressure Diuresis in intoxications Urologic irrigation	*Adult:* IV, 50–100 g of 5%–25% solution (preventive) or 50–100 g of 15%–25% solution (treatment) *Adult:* IV, 1.5–2 g/kg as 15%–25% solution infused over 30–60 min *Adult:* IV, 1.5–2 g/kg as 15%–20% solution infused over 30 min *Adult:* IV, up to 200 g *Adult:* Bladder catheter, 2.5% solution; add two 50-mL vials (25% mannitol) to 900-mL sterile water	*Onset:* 0.5–1 h *Duration:* 6–8 h $t_{1/2}$: 15–100 min
C Carbonic Anhydrase Inhibitors			
P acetazolamide (Diamox)	Chronic open-angle glaucoma Secondary glaucoma/ preoperative acute congestive closed-angle glaucoma CHF Drug-induced edema Epilepsy Mountain sickness	*Adult:* PO, 250 mg–1 g daily in divided doses *Adult:* PO, IV, 250 mg q4h or 250 mg bid, or 500 mg followed by 125 or 250 mg q4h *Child:* IM, IV, 5–10 mg/kg/dose q6h; PO, 10–15 mg/kg/d in divided doses *Adult:* PO, 250–375 mg (5 mg/kg)/d *Adult:* PO, 250–375 mg daily; give every other day, or 2 d on then 1 d off *Child:* PO, IV 5 mg/kg/dose *Adult and child:* PO, IV, 8–30 mg/kg/d in divided doses *Adult:* PO, 500–1,000 mg/d in divided doses; may use sustained-release preparation	*Onset:* PO, 1–1.5 h; IV, 2 min *Duration:* PO, 8–12 h; IV, 4–5 h $t_{1/2}$: Unknown
C Anticholinergic Agents			
P tolterodine (Detrol)	Overactive bladder	*Adult:* IR, 2 mg 2×/d ER, 4 mg 2×/d	*Onset:* 1 wk *Duration:* Unknown $t_{1/2}$: 1.9–3.7 h (parent compound)

diuretic; the net effect is a new steady state in which the extracellular fluid volume is reduced by the amount of sodium lost from initial therapy. Structural adaptations in the distal and collecting tubules are also likely to increase the compensatory sodium retention. Blood pressure is then maintained at the new, lower level in response to the diuretic. The same process occurs when hydrochlorothiazide or other diuretics are given to treat edema, such as from heart failure. The compensatory mechanisms are not activated until the fluid volume has been returned to a normal level. To state that there is a new steady state of sodium balance does not mean that no effect is achieved from hydrochlorothiazide or other diuretics. Sodium is lost while the diuretic is acting, but sodium loss will be very low for the remainder of the day due to increased activity of the sodium-retaining forces.

Water-soluble vitamins also are lost with the increased urine elimination from hydrochlorothiazide, as well as other diuretics. Hydrochlorothiazide decreases GFR and increases blood urea nitrogen (BUN).

Long-term thiazide use appears to increase bone density and decrease the risk of fracture, but these effects are modest, and thiazide treatment is not recommended routinely for its effects on bone density. However, if patients with osteoporosis also have hypertension or nephrolithiasis, then they would receive some additional benefit from using the thiazide to treat their condition.

Contraindications and Precautions

Important contraindications to hydrochlorothiazide therapy include severe renal impairment or anuria (urine output greater than 250 mL daily), hepatic coma, and hypersensitivity to the drug or to sulfonamide antibiotics, which are similar chemically to hydrochlorothiazide and therefore increase the risk for cross-sensitivity. Thiazides should be used with caution in patients with renal disease, lupus erythematosus, liver disease, fluid and electrolyte imbalances, diabetes, gout, elevated cholesterol levels, elevated triglycerides, bronchial asthma, advanced arteriosclerosis, and heart disease. Hydrochlorothiazide is a pregnancy category B drug.

Adverse Effects

Adverse effects are due mostly to the effects of fluid loss or imbalance or from the effects of electrolyte imbalances, which may include hypokalemia, hyponatremia, hypochloremia, and hypercalcemia. Variation in electrolyte levels, which is largest within the first 2 weeks of therapy, is most problematic with larger doses of hydrochlorothiazide; small doses that are now frequently used in treating hypertension (e.g., 12.5 mg) have only a small risk of causing electrolyte imbalance. Thus, fear of electrolyte imbalance should not be a reason to avoid using thiazide diuretics to treat hypertension (Jiang JY, Wong MC, Ali MK, et al., 2009).The most common adverse effects occur in various systems, as follows: cardiovascular (hypotension), central nervous system (CNS; dizziness, light-headedness, and vertigo), GI (anorexia, nausea, and vomiting), and GU (polyuria and nocturia).

Other adverse effects related to fluid and electrolyte imbalances include CNS effects, such as paresthesia (numbness and tingling), headache, and drowsiness. Cardiovascular effects include orthostatic hypotension, volume depletion, cardiac arrhythmias, and chest pain. GI disturbances include diarrhea, constipation, jaundice, and pancreatitis. Dermatologic effects include poor skin turgor and dry mucous membranes. Finally, the musculoskeletal system may be prone to weakness and muscle cramps or spasms resulting from potassium loss, and possibly gout resulting from increased uric acid levels.

Drug Interactions

Hydrochlorothiazide and other thiazide diuretics interact with many drugs and drug classes. Table 27.2 provides the complete list of agents that interact with hydrochlorothiazide. The one drug that should not be used with hydrochlorothiazide is dofetilide, because severe cardiac effects, including lethal arrhythmias, are possible. High-sodium food decreases the effectiveness of hydrochlorothiazide. With large doses of hydrochlorothiazide, the measurement of acetaminophen levels in the blood may be altered.

Assessment of Relevant Core Patient Variables

Health Status

Determine whether the patient is allergic to sulfa or to other thiazides, because these allergies are contraindications for use. Renal status must be assessed because severe renal impairment is a contraindication for hydrochlorothiazide use. Patients who have pre-existing renal disease, a creatinine clearance rate of 40 to 50 mL/min, a GFR of 25 mL/min, or a history of nonresponsiveness to thiazides most likely should be treated with loop diuretics instead of hydrochlorothiazide. If used, hydrochlorothiazide therapy in these patients must be monitored carefully.

Assess hepatic status because hepatic coma is a contraindication, and hepatic disease warrants cautious use. Other problems include a history of systemic lupus erythematosus, diabetes, gout, bronchial asthma, arteriosclerosis, heart disease, or elevated triglyceride or cholesterol levels. In patients with diabetes, blood glucose levels must be assessed; in patients with gout, uric acid levels must be assessed; and in patients with kidney disease or kidney failure, creatinine levels must be assessed, because hydrochlorothiazide elevates blood glucose, lipid, and uric acid levels. The elevation of blood glucose from thiazides also can create new onset of diabetes, however research does not show that it increases the incidence of cardiovascular disease as endogenous diabetes does (Wright, J.T. Jr, Probstfield, J.L, Cushman, W.C., et al., 2009).

Before therapy begins, it is important to assess fluid and electrolyte status because hydrochlorothiazide causes fluid

TABLE 27.2 Agents That Interact with P Hydrochlorothiazide

Interactants	Effect and Significance	Nursing Management
ACE inhibitors	Increased risk of first-dose orthostatic hypotension when the ACE I is started	Start with low doses of ACE inhibitors and then titrate upwards. Monitor blood pressure carefully for 4 h after first dose.
allopurinol	May increase the incidence of hypersensitivity reactions to allopurinol	Monitor for allergic effects.
anesthetics	More anesthetic effect	Dosage may need to be decreased. Monitor/correct fluid imbalance prior to surgery if possible.
anticoagulants	Decreased anticoagulant effect	Monitor prothrombin time, partial thromboplastin time; dose may need adjustment.
antidiabetic agents	Increased blood glucose	Dose may need adjusting.
antigout agents	Decreased effect with thiazides; increased uric acid levels	Monitor uric acid levels; dose may need to be adjusted.
antineoplastics	Enhanced myelosuppression may result in granulocytopenia.	Monitor white blood cell count.
calcium salts	Hypercalcemia because thiazides promote calcium retention	Monitor calcium levels.
carbamazepine	Hyponatremia from additive effects	Monitor calcium levels during therapy.
corticosteroids	Additive potassium loss may result in hypokalemia.	Monitor potassium level during therapy.
diazoxide	Hyperglycemia possible	Monitor blood glucose level.
digitalis glycosides	Hypokalemia from thiazides, which may induce digitalis toxicity	Monitor potassium level. Monitor for digitalis toxicity. Provide potassium in diet or supplements.
dofetilide	Increased plasma concentration of dofetilide, leading to increased risk of cardiotoxicity	Coadministration of these drugs is contraindicated. After stopping dofetilide, a washout period of at least 2 d should be allowed before starting hydrochlorothiazide.
droperidol	Possible additive cardiac effects related to potassium loss may increase risk of cardiotoxicity.	Administer droperidol with extreme caution if coadministration required.
ginkgo	May possibly increase blood pressure	Assess for use of this herb. Monitor carefully if coadministered; ginkgo may need to be stopped.
levomethadyl	Additive hypokalemia or hypomagnesemia effects may increase risk of QT prolongation.	Coadminister with extreme caution.
licorice	Pseudoaldosteronism from licorice can increase the risk of hypokalemia or reduce the effectiveness of hydrochlorothiazide.	Avoid coadministration.
lithium	Sodium possibly lost instead of lithium ions, inducing lithium toxicity	Monitor blood lithium levels.
loop diuretics	Profound diuresis and serious electrolyte imbalance	Monitor electrolyte levels.
ma huang	Oppositional effects many reduce the hypotensive effect from hydrochlorothiazide.	Avoid coadministration.
mermantine	Altered plasma levels of either drug may result	Monitor for effectiveness of each drug if coadministration is required.

TABLE 27.2	Agents That Interact with P Hydrochlorothiazide *(continued)*	
Interactants	**Effect and Significance**	**Nursing Management**
methyldopa	Rare occurrences of hemolytic anemia with concurrent use	Monitor complete blood chemistry.
nondepolarizing muscle relaxants	Possible prolonged neuromuscular blocking effects and respiratory depression	Assess respiratory status.
porfimer	Additive photosensitizing effects may lead to excessive tissue damage.	Advise patients to avoid exposure of skin and eyes to direct sunlight or bright indoor light if taking both drugs; sunscreens do not protect against the photosensitivity reactions.
propranolol	Hyperglycemia and hypertriglyceridemia may result, as propranolol may potentiate these effects.	Avoid coadministration in patients with diabetes or hyperglycemia. Monitor glucose and lipid levels if coadministration required.
vitamin D	Biologic actions of vitamin D enhanced; hypercalcemia may have role	Monitor calcium levels.
amphotericin B, corticosteroids	Electrolyte depletion intensified	Monitor electrolyte levels, particularly potassium.
anticholinergics	Increased absorption of thiazides	Monitor blood pressure, electrolyte levels.
bile acid sequestrants (cholestyramine, colestipol)	Bind thiazides, reduce absorption	Give thiazides at least 2 h before resin.
methenamines	Possible decreased effect of thiazides due to alkalinization of urine	Monitor blood pressure, electrolyte levels; may need to adjust dosage.
nonsteroidal anti-inflammatory drugs	Reduced diuretic, natriuretic, and antihypertensive effects	Observe for therapeutic effect.
sotalol	Additive potassium and magnesium loss increases the risk of cardiotoxicity.	Correct potassium and magnesium imbalance prior to starting sotalol therapy. Monitor for complications.
topiramate	Increased levels of topiramate	Assess for adverse effects of topiramate; adjust dose if necessary.
yohimbine	Increased blood pressure; yohimbine increases norepinephrine release; reduced effectiveness of hydrochlorothiazide	Avoid use of yohimbine.

and electrolyte losses. If the patient has fluid and electrolyte deficiencies before therapy, additional losses increase the risk of serious adverse effects. If the patient receives large doses of hydrochlorothiazide, it is more likely that he or she will experience hyponatremia or **hypokalemia** (low levels of potassium in the blood). However, electrolyte imbalances are rarely significant when low-dose therapy is used. Additional baseline measurements should include blood pressure and other vital signs; body weight; edema in the ankles, sacrum, and abdomen; and urinary elimination patterns and output volume. Because many drugs interact with hydrochlorothiazide, assess the patient's drug history, particularly the current drug regimen. Drug therapy that also causes electrolyte loss or that may be affected adversely by the electrolyte loss induced from hydrochlorothiazide therapy should be most closely assessed. For example, hydrochlorothiazide

causes hypokalemia. Hypokalemia increases the effect of the drug digoxin. Therefore, patients receiving digoxin for CHF have an increased risk for digoxin toxicity if they become hypokalemic during hydrochlorothiazide therapy.

Life Span and Gender

It is important to determine whether the patient is pregnant or breast-feeding. Although hydrochlorothiazide is a pregnancy category B drug, it can be present in breast milk, and the drug must be used with caution by pregnant or breast-feeding women.

Determine the patient's age before administering hydrochlorothiazide therapy. Hyponatremia is more likely to occur in older adults (> 65 years), especially women (Clayton, Rodgers, Blakey, et al., 2006). Larger doses of thiazide diuretics greatly increase the risk of hyponatremia in older adults.

Such individuals also tend to have more risk factors (e.g., decreased dietary potassium intake, diminished renal reserve, concurrent disease, and concomitant therapy with drugs such as glucocorticoids) for hypokalemia. As previously stated, electrolyte imbalances are most likely to occur within the first 2 weeks of therapy. Sodium deficiency may develop at a later time, but only if there was a physiological change (e.g., heart failure) or an increase in the dose of hydrochlorothiazide. Later development of hypokalemia can occur if the diuretic dose is increased, extrarenal potassium losses increase, or dietary potassium intake is reduced. One small study found that older adults also appear to be at increased risk for vitamin B_1 deficiency while taking hydrochlorothiazide or other diuretics. This deficiency is caused by vitamin loss with increased urination. In addition, the diets of older adults receiving hydrochlorothiazide may contain less thiamine than recommended (McCabe-Sellers, Sharkey, & Browne, 2005).

Lifestyle, Diet, and Habits

Assess the patient's dietary sodium intake, because a high sodium intake can prevent a net fluid loss from the hydrochlorothiazide. Assess the patient's normal fluid intake and dietary sources of electrolytes, particularly potassium, to evaluate whether the patient's nutritional intake can compensate adequately for electrolytes lost during drug therapy.

Environment

Assess whether the patient can get easily to a toilet, especially at the beginning of therapy, when urine output increases. The patient's home must be set up for safety because falls may occur as a result of adverse effects of therapy. Hydrochlorothiazide can be self-administered at home or administered in acute care, long-term care, or subacute care settings.

Culture and Inherited Traits

Note the patient's ethnic background. In African Americans, hydrochlorothiazide therapy is somewhat more effective than in patients who are of European descent. It is believed that hypertensive African Americans have features that are consistent with a theory of corrected volume status where the sodium and potassium pump is inhibited. Because hydrochlorothiazide stimulates excretion of sodium and potassium, it exerts an additional effect in hypertensive African Americans.

Nursing Diagnoses and Outcomes

- Risk for Deficient Fluid Volume related to action and adverse effects of hydrochlorothiazide
 Desired outcome: The patient will not experience fluid imbalance while on hydrochlorothiazide therapy.
- Risk for Injury, Falls, related to adverse effects of hydrochlorothiazide
 Desired outcome: The patient will not suffer injury from falls while taking hydrochlorothiazide.
- Risk for Injury, Drug Interactions, related to multiple drug therapies
 Desired outcome: The patient will not have adverse effects from drug interactions while taking hydrochlorothiazide.

Planning and Intervention
Maximizing Therapeutic Effects

Administer hydrochlorothiazide in the morning so that the maximum diuretic effect does not disturb sleep (assuming the patient is awake days and sleeps nights). It is important to provide ready access to a bathroom (or bedside urinal, bedpan, or commode) to ensure comfort during peak drug action.

Monitor fluid intake, urine output, and body weight for changes. It is important to encourage the patient to avoid foods high in sodium content and not to increase sodium intake after hydrochlorothiazide dosage has been regulated, because that increase could counteract the effect of drug therapy. Encourage continued efforts at lifestyle changes that lower blood pressure (when used to treat hypertension). Work with the patient to identify and correct lifestyle factors that can affect adherence, as described in Box 27.2.

BOX 27.2 COMMUNITY BASED CONCERNS

Factors That Can Decrease Adherence to Diuretic Therapy

Older adults are often prescribed diuretic therapy as part of their drug regimen to treat hypertension or chronic heart failure. Sometimes, therapeutic or adverse effects from the drug therapy cause older adults to choose not to take their prescribed diuretic regularly. Here are some common reasons patients give for not wanting to take a diuretic, and some suggestions for how you can help the patient minimize these problems.

- *I have to get up and go to the bathroom several times during the night.* Encourage the patient to take the drug early in the morning. If he is to take it twice a day, have him take the second dose before 6 PM. If timing the dose this way still does not minimize the problem, consult with the prescriber to see if the dose can be given as one daily dose instead of two daily doses.
- *I can't get to the bathroom quick enough, and I wet myself.* The problem may not be the diuretic itself, but impaired mobility or fine motor skills required to unzip pants or manipulate clothing. If the patient has difficulty moving quickly, suggest that he empty his bladder routinely throughout the day so that he doesn't ever get an extremely full bladder, which may contribute to feelings of urgency. A bedside commode might be helpful if the patient is having trouble getting to the bathroom in the middle of the night. Clothing modifications, such as Velcro closures, might make manipulating clothing easier. A consultation with an occupational therapist may be helpful.
- *I can't go anywhere, because if I can't find a bathroom right away, I might have an accident.* Time the dosing of the diuretic so that it will have had a chance to reach full effect before the patient wants to go out. For example, if the patient wishes to go out at 10 AM, he might want to vary the time he takes his medication, taking it earlier in the morning that day. If he takes the drug at 6 AM and the drug's peak effect occurs in 2 hours, then by 10 AM, the effect on urinary output would be less. Explore the patient's feelings regarding the use of absorbent pads or briefs. Some patients find these provide a feeling of security, knowing that they cannot accidentally wet their clothing, and others find the use of these items humiliating and refuse to wear them.

Minimizing Adverse Effects

Correct any electrolyte imbalance prior to starting hydrochlorothiazide therapy. Monitor serum electrolyte levels for hypokalemia, hyponatremia, hypomagnesemia, and hypercalcemia after the first 2 weeks of therapy. Decreasing the dose of the hydrochlorothiazide usually corrects any electrolyte loss. Potassium supplements are given if serum potassium levels fall below 3.0 mEq/L or if levels are less than 3.5 mEq/L in patients who are receiving digitalis, have ischemic heart disease, or have ectopic rhythms. Monitor for hyperglycemia, hyperuricemia, serum triglyceride, cholesterol, and creatinine levels throughout therapy. Also, closely monitor older adults for hyponatremia. In addition, assess older adults for signs of water-soluble vitamin deficiencies; a multivitamin may be indicated, especially if patients do not eat a nutrient-rich diet.

It is important to assess the complete blood count (CBC) to detect blood abnormalities, and to inspect the skin for rashes or hives to detect sensitivity responses. Observe patients for related signs and symptoms of fluid and electrolyte abnormalities. It also is important to weigh patients regularly to determine extraordinary fluid loss (reflected in weight loss) and complications (reflected in weight gain). They may be weighed daily during the initial period of therapy and then weekly or biweekly once therapy is stabilized. A weight gain exceeding 3 lb in 1 day—a sign of fluid retention and complications—should be reported to the prescriber.

Caution patients to avoid rapid position changes that may intensify orthostatic hypotension and precipitate falls. As needed, elderly or debilitated patients should be assisted with walking to the bathroom to prevent injury. Hydrochlorothiazide can be administered with meals or milk to prevent or minimize GI upset. It is important to assess for signs of drug interactions if patients are currently receiving other drug therapies known to interact with hydrochlorothiazide.

Providing Patient and Family Education

- Explain the importance of follow-up blood work to monitor electrolyte levels.
- Urge patients to report signs and symptoms of hypokalemia (irregular pulse rate, muscle weakness or cramps, constipation, or abdominal pain).
- Tell patients to take their pulse and compare the rate with former or normal rates. (You may need to teach them how to take a pulse.)
- Encourage patients to consume potassium-rich foods, such as bananas, apricots, and orange juice, and other electrolyte-rich beverages and food to counter electrolyte losses, especially potassium.
- Teach older adults and their family members to report signs and symptoms of hyponatremia (weakness, nerve disorders, loss of weight, "salt hunger," cramps, problems with digestion).
- Teach patients to avoid injury from falls by rising slowly and balancing carefully to counter orthostatic hypotension.

- Instruct patients to take hydrochlorothiazide with food if they have problems with GI discomfort.
- Explain the importance of wearing sunglasses, sunscreen, wide-brimmed hats, and cover-up clothing to avoid a possible photosensitivity reaction.
- Store hydrochlorothiazide safely to prevent accidental poisoning of children, forgetful adults, or others.

Ongoing Assessment and Evaluation

Evaluate the effects of therapy and the degree to which expected outcomes have been achieved. Most patients receiving hydrochlorothiazide can expect to have a reduction in fluid retention, edema, and blood pressure. To that end, edema and blood pressure may be compared with baseline values. Fluid balance may be evaluated by weighing the patient at the same time of day on the same scale, ideally with the patient wearing the same weight of clothing. Laboratory tests may be reviewed regularly to detect electrolyte imbalances and blood abnormalities.

Patients who appear resistant to therapy should have a 24-hour urine specimen collected to assess sodium excretion. Because daily sodium excretion is approximately equal to intake, high levels of sodium in a 24-hour urine specimen indicate that the patient has not been adherent with dietary sodium restrictions. A value greater than 100 mEq/d in a patient whose daily weight is stable indicates that there has been an adequate diuretic response but the dietary intake of sodium is too great to see the whole therapeutic response. Random single voided specimens are often misleading about the patient's total sodium intake, depending on when the specimen is obtained in relation to when the drug was administered.

Drugs Closely Related to P Hydrochlorothiazide

Bendroflumethiazide (Naturetin), chlorothiazide (Diuril), methyclothiazide (Enduron), and polythiazide (Renese) are all thiazide diuretics. They are all extremely similar to hydrochlorothiazide, with a few minor differences. Bendroflumethiazide is not approved for use in children; it is a pregnancy category C drug. Chlorothiazide can be given either orally or intravenously to adults, it has a much shorter half-life than hydrochlorothiazide, and it is a pregnancy category C drug. Methyclothiazide is not approved for use in children. Polythiazide is not labeled for use in children and has an unknown pregnancy category: Infant risk from breast milk cannot be ruled out.

Drugs Significantly Different From P Hydrochlorothiazide

The thiazide-related drugs chlorthalidone (Hygroton), indapamide (Lozol), and metolazone (Zaroxolyn) have a slightly different chemical structure than hydrochlorothiazide and other thiazides. Other differences are related to labeled indications and pharmacokinetics. Chlorthalidone is not

MEMORY CHIP

 Hydrochlorothiazide

- Widely used alone or with other agents to reduce blood pressure; also used to treat edema from CHF, from hepatic or renal disease, or secondary to drug use
- Works in the distal tubule to promote excretion of sodium, chloride, potassium, and water
- Major contraindication: severe renal disease
- Most common adverse effects: from fluid and electrolyte loss (dizziness, light-headedness, vertigo, nausea, and vomiting)
- Most serious adverse effects: aplastic anemia and thrombocytopenia (although not normally life-threatening)
- Minimizing adverse effects: Monitor blood pressure, weight, intake and output, and serum electrolyte levels during therapy with this drug.
- Most important patient education: Explain the importance of periodic blood work to monitor electrolytes.

approved for use in children and has a much longer half-life. Indapamide is specifically used for edema in CHF as opposed to other causes of edema, is not approved for use in children, and is extensively metabolized in the liver. Dosage adjustments are required in liver disease. Metolazone is not approved for use in children.

ⓒ LOOP DIURETICS

The loop diuretics work in the loop of Henle to inhibit reabsorption of sodium and chloride. They exert a powerful effect on fluid and electrolyte balance. Loop diuretics are sometimes referred to as high-ceiling diuretics because the maximum diuretic effect that can be achieved is higher than with other diuretics. Loop diuretics include furosemide, bumetanide, ethacrynic acid, and torsemide. The prototype drug in this class is furosemide (Lasix).

Nursing Management of the Patient Receiving P Furosemide

Core Drug Knowledge

Pharmacotherapeutics

Furosemide is a potent diuretic that is effective in reducing peripheral edema from CHF and hepatic and renal diseases, including nephrotic disease. It is highly effective in treating pulmonary edema. It also is effective in treating hypertension and is the first choice over thiazides in patients with pre-existing renal disease because, unlike thiazides, it does not decrease GFR. Furosemide can be given either orally or intravenously.

Pharmacokinetics

After oral administration, furosemide is absorbed rapidly and well from the GI tract. However, after intravenous (IV) administration, furosemide acts even more rapidly—within 10 minutes. Duration of action is 2 hours. The drug is about

95% bound to plasma proteins. Furosemide is metabolized in the liver and excreted by the kidneys. It crosses the placenta and may be excreted in breast milk (Table 27.3).

Pharmacodynamics

Furosemide inhibits the reabsorption of sodium, chloride, and water in the ascending loop of Henle. It also has some effect in the proximal and distal tubules. As a result, excretion of sodium, chloride, potassium, and water increases. Excretion of filtered sodium is between 20% and 25%. Excretion of magnesium and calcium occurs as well. The negative calcium balance created by furosemide and other loop diuretics may increase the risk of hip fracture. As with thiazide diuretics, most of the electrolyte loss occurs in the first 2 weeks of therapy, as long as the dose remains constant. Electrolytes, especially sodium and potassium, will level off with continued therapy as compensatory mechanisms for sodium retention occur, creating a new steady state for sodium. For a complete discussion of this process, see the Pharmacodynamics section for hydrochlorothiazide.

Furosemide can increase blood glucose, low-density lipoprotein, total cholesterol, and triglyceride levels. In addition, it decreases excretion of uric acid, which may raise uric acid levels.

Contraindications and Precautions

Furosemide should not be used in anuria or if hypersensitivity to the compounds or allergy to sulfa drugs exists. Cautious use must be exercised in patients with poor renal function and lupus erythematosus. Furosemide is a pregnancy category C drug.

Adverse Effects

Most of furosemide's adverse effects relate to fluid or electrolyte imbalance. Electrolyte imbalances, which are most likely to occur within the first 2 weeks of therapy, include hyponatremia, hypokalemia, hypochloridemia, and hypocalcemia. Loss of hydrogen ions can also lead to metabolic alkalosis. A marked diuretic effect (from large doses) decreases the volume returning to the heart and can lead to a decrease in cardiac output of as much as 20%. Hypotension, especially orthostatic hypotension, dizziness, and vertigo, may result.

Excessive diuresis from furosemide can result in dehydration, reduction in blood volume with circulatory collapse, and the possibility of vascular thrombosis and embolism, particularly in the elderly. Warning signs of dehydration and significant electrolyte imbalance are dry mouth, thirst, anorexia, weakness, lethargy, drowsiness, restlessness, muscle pains or cramps, muscle fatigue, tetany (rarely), hypotension, oliguria, tachycardia, arrhythmia, and GI disturbances (e.g., nausea/vomiting). BUN levels and serum creatinine levels may rise after aggressive diuresis from furosemide due to poor renal perfusion if cardiac output falls significantly. Patients with hepatic cirrhosis and ascites must be monitored carefully because rapid electrolyte shifts

TABLE 27.3 Agents That Interact with P Furosemide

Interactants	Effect and Significance	Nursing Management
ACE inhibitors	First-dose postural hypotension when ACE inhibitor is added to diuretic therapy	Start therapy first with ACE inhibitors if possible; otherwise, start with small doses of ACE inhibitors and titrate upwards. Monitor blood pressure closely for first 4 h after dose of ACE inhibitors.
aminoglycosides	Increased ototoxicity; possible hearing loss	Avoid coadministration if at all possible. Monitor BUN and creatinine; adverse effects will increase if drugs are not excreted well. Assess for hearing problems; stop drug therapy at first indication of ototoxicity if coadministered.
anticoagulants	Enhanced anticoagulant action possible	Monitor PT, PTT.
beta blockers (propranolol)	Increased plasma levels of propranolol	Monitor therapeutic effect and adverse effects of propranolol.
corticosteroids	Increased potassium loss; hypokalemia	Monitor potassium levels.
chloral hydrate	Rare transient diaphoresis, hot flashes, hypertension, tachycardia, weakness, and nausea	Consider drug interaction if these effects occur.
Class III antiarrhythmics	Hypokalemia from furosemide increases the risk of serious, potentially life-threatening cardiotoxicity.	Use extreme caution if coadministered. Monitor serum potassium levels and maintain in normal range.
digitalis glycosides	Furosemide-induced hypokalemia, increasing digitalis toxicity	Monitor serum potassium level. Supply potassium in diet or as supplement. Monitor for signs of digitalis toxicity.
droperidol	Additive cardiac effects increasing risk of cardiotoxicity	Coadminister with extreme caution.
germanium, ginseng	May increase blood pressure and decrease effectiveness of diuretics	Avoid coadministration.
hydralazine	Increased plasma clearance of furosemide, creating an enhanced diuretic response	Monitor for diuretic response; dose adjustments may be needed.
licorice	Increased risk of hypokalemia and/or reduced diuretic effect	Avoid coadministration.
lithium	Possible increased plasma lithium levels and toxicity	Monitor lithium levels.
ma huang, yohimbine	Increase in blood pressure and reduced hypotensive effect of furosemide	Avoid coadministration.
nondepolarizing muscle relaxants	Antagonized or potentiated action of muscle relaxants, perhaps depending on furosemide dose	Monitor for therapeutic effect.
sulfonylureas	Loss of sulfonylureas' effect, resulting in hyperglycemia	Sulfonylureas dosage may need adjustment.
theophylline	Theophylline effect enhanced or inhibited	Monitor for therapeutic effect of theophylline.
charcoal	Decreased absorption of furosemide	Monitor for therapeutic effect. May be antidote in case of furosemide overdose.
cisplatin	Additive ototoxicity	Avoid coadministration if at all possible. Monitor BUN and creatinine; adverse effects will increase if drugs are not excreted well. Assess for hearing problems; stop furosemide therapy at first indication of ototoxicity if coadministered.

(Continued)

TABLE 27.3	Agents That Interact with P Furosemide (continued)	
Interactants	Effect and Significance	Nursing Management
clofibrate	Exaggerated diuretic response	Monitor intake and output, blood pressure, edema, and fluid and electrolyte levels.
phenytoin and other hydantoins	Decreased diuretic response	Monitor for therapeutic response.
NSAIDs	Decreased diuretic response	Monitor for therapeutic response.
probenecid	Decreased diuretic response	Monitor for therapeutic response.
salicylates	Diuretic response impaired in patients with cirrhosis and ascites	Monitor for therapeutic response.
thiazides	Profound diuresis and serious electrolyte levels	Monitor blood pressure, edema, and fluid and electrolyte levels.

resulting from furosemide therapy may induce hepatic encephalopathy and coma. Because hyperuricemia is also possible from furosemide therapy, patients with a history of gout may find its use problematic.

A common and serious adverse effect is ototoxicity. Ototoxicity can occur with rapid IV therapy, especially in patients with poor renal function, and in those patients receiving high doses of oral of IV furosemide. Signs of ototoxicity include tinnitus, vertigo, a feeling of fullness in the ear, and medium- and high-frequency hearing loss. Although usually transient (lasting 1 to 24 hours), ototoxicity may result in permanent damage, including deafness. Ototoxicity is believed to be due to furosemide's inhibition of the Na-K-Cl active cotransport system. An isoform of this transporter is present in the inner ear, and it appears that when the transport system is inhibited in the kidney, it is also inhibited in the inner ear, causing deafness, imbalance, or structural damage to the inner ear.

Another major problem from furosemide is related to hypersensitivity and allergic responses. Hypersensitivity reactions include rash or acute interstitial nephritis (rare); these reactions are similar to those produced by other sulfonamide drugs. Allergic responses from those with a known sulfonamide antibiotic allergy include asthma, eczema, urticaria, dermatitis, Stevens-Johnson syndrome, and anaphylaxis.

Other adverse effects occur in various systems, as follows: CNS (paresthesias, xanthopsia, blurred vision, and fever); cardiovascular (chronic aortitis), GI (constipation, diarrhea, cramping, pancreatitis, jaundice, ischemic hepatitis); hematologic (leukopenia, anemia, thrombocytopenia, and agranulocytosis); GU (urinary bladder spasm); dermatologic (photosensitivity); and metabolic (increases in blood glucose and alterations in glucose tolerance tests; increases in low-density lipoprotein, total cholesterol, and triglycerides; and minor decreases in high-density lipoprotein).

Patients with SLE may have exacerbations of the illness when receiving furosemide.

Drug Interactions

Furosemide and aminoglycoside antibiotics should not be coadministered because they both can cause ototoxicity. The hypokalemia that may result from furosemide increases the risk of digoxin toxicity without increasing digoxin levels. Furosemide interacts with many other drugs. Bioavailability and degree of diuresis are reduced when furosemide is administered with food. Table 27.3 lists agents that interact with furosemide.

Assessment of Relevant Core Patient Variables

Health Status

Initially, assess for allergies to furosemide or other contraindications. A baseline assessment is then performed. This assessment is much like the one for a patient receiving hydrochlorothiazide. Begin by taking blood pressure and vital signs and reviewing relevant blood test results and electrolyte levels. Patients who receive digoxin or have a history of arrhythmias or other cardiac abnormalities may be especially prone to complications from the hypokalemia that can result from furosemide. Potassium levels should generally be greater than 4.0 mEq/L prior to starting furosemide. To assess fluid status and obtain baseline data for therapy, weigh the patient. Apparent edema is inspected and palpated. It is important to auscultate breath sounds, particularly in patients with CHF or pulmonary edema. Assess skin turgor and mucous membranes and measure fluid intake and urinary output.

During assessment, keep the proposed route of administration in mind because IV furosemide may have a substantially more potent effect than oral furosemide on blood pressure and vital signs (cardiac arrest has been reported). As with hydrochlorothiazide, also assess for gout, diabetes, and high serum cholesterol and triglyceride levels.

Life Span and Gender

Determine whether the female patient is pregnant. Furosemide, a pregnancy category C drug, should be used during pregnancy only if necessary and then with great caution. It also is important to determine the patient's age before administering furosemide. Furosemide may increase the risk for developing patent ductus arteriosus when given during the first few weeks of life to premature infants with respiratory distress syndrome. Development of renal calcifications (kidney stones) also has been reported when furosemide is used in severely premature infants. Premature infants have a greater risk of ototoxicity. Furosemide can be used safely in children, but doses should not exceed 6 mg/kg of body weight.

If severe diuresis occurs from use of the drug, acute hypotensive episodes may occur, especially in elderly people. Elderly patients are at increased risk for rapid changes in fluid volume, which can lead to circulatory collapse. Moreover, elderly adults also are less tolerant of the rapid changes in blood pressure that may occur with furosemide therapy. In older adults, the rapid loss of plasma volume and the resulting hemoconcentration are likely to cause thromboembolic episodes, such as cerebral vascular thromboses and pulmonary embolism.

In postmenopausal women, who are already at risk of osteoporosis and hip fracture, the additional calcium loss from furosemide and other loop diuretics can increase the risk of hip fracture.

Lifestyle, Diet, and Habits

Assess the patient's dietary sodium intake, because a high sodium intake can prevent a net fluid loss from the diuretic

Exactly how much sodium should be consumed daily in relationship to how much furosemide is still under debate for patients who have heart failure. One recent research study of patients with class 2 to 4 chronic, compensated heart failure found that a normal sodium intake with fluid restrictions of 1,000 cc/d and oral furosemide in high doses (250 mg twice a day) significantly reduced the need for readmission compared to lower sodium levels and conventional (for heart failure) doses of furosemide (Paterna, Parrinello, Cannizzaro et al., 2009). However, when the patient has acute decompensated heart failure, higher doses of furosemide IV seem to be deleterious (see Maximizing Therapeutic Effects below, and the Focus on Research Box 27.3.). Furosemide may promote severe electrolyte imbalances, especially in patients who have high dosages and who are on sodium-restricted diets. Therefore, normal fluid intake and dietary preferences should be determined and evaluated for the adequacy of electrolyte content, especially potassium.

Environment

Assess whether the patient can get to a toilet easily when needed, especially at the beginning of therapy, when urine output increases. The patient's home should be assessed for risk factors that may contribute to injuries (falls) resulting from adverse effects of drug therapy. Oral furosemide can be self-administered at home or administered by others in acute care, long-term care, or subacute care environments. Parenteral dosing is generally restricted to an acute care environment.

BOX 27.3 FOCUS ON RESEARCH

What Is the Proper Dose of Furosemide for Treating Acute Decompensated Heart Failure?

Peacock, W. F., Costanzo, M. R., De Marco, T., et al., for the ADHERE Scientific Advisory Committee and Investigators. Impact of Intravenous Loop Diuretics on Outcomes of Patients Hospitalized with Acute Decompensated Heart Failure: Insights from the ADHERE Registry. Cardiology, 113:12–19.

The Study

The ADHERE registry (**A**cute **D**ecompensated **He**art Failure National **Re**gistry) is the largest database on acute heart failure in the world with over 100,000 patients enrolled in the United States.

Findings of the retrospective analysis of hospitalized patients with acute decompensated heart failure suggest that treatment with high doses of fuosemide (160 mg/d or greater IV) is associated with poorer renal function, the need for more hospital resources, and increased mortality, compared to patients with acute heart failure who received lower IV doses of furosemide (less than 160 mg/d IV). Other observational data from the ADHERE registry shows that renal dysfunction is associated with poorer outcomes for patients with acute decompensated heart failure.

As heart failure progresses, resistance develops to furosemide; most commonly in practice this is addressed by administering larger doses or more frequent doses of furosemide to bring about the same diuretic effect. This review questions that practice and indicates that for this may worsen the condition of patients already seriously ill.

Nursing Implications

There are some problems with this study, as the authors point out that limit the interpretation of the data. Because the data from the ADHERE registry analysis was retroactive and observational, none of the findings can be considered to demonstrate a direct cause and effect. One can only draw the conclusion of an apparent association between factors in this type of study. And because medical chart reviews are dependent on what is written into the record, and medical records are not always completely accurate or complete, data could have been lost or misinterpreted. The study also could not differentiate between giving the furosemide via IV bolus or continuous infusion.

Despite these limitations, this study gives the nurse some important information to consider. The evidence seems to show that the current practice of continually increasing the dose of furosemide to treat worsening acute decompensated heart failure may not be the best practice to improve patient outcomes. While urine output may increase, this does not appear to be clinically important in improving renal function, and renal function is the more important issue for decreased mortality. Nurses should be aware that as research continues on furosemide use in acute decompensated heart failure, the standards of care may evolve from where they are today. It is important that more research be done to determine the best dose of furosemide in treatment for both acute and chronic heart failure and that nurses stay abreast of the research findings.

Nursing Diagnoses and Outcomes

- Risk for Deficient Fluid Volume related to action and adverse effects of furosemide
  Desired outcome: The patient will not experience fluid and electrolyte imbalance while taking furosemide.
- Risk for Injury, Falls, related to adverse effects of furosemide
  Desired outcome: The patient will not suffer injury while taking furosemide.
- Risk for Injury, Drug Interactions, related to multiple drug therapies
  Desired outcome: The patient will not have adverse effects from drug interactions while taking furosemide.

Planning and Intervention

Maximizing Therapeutic Effects

If therapy begins in the hospital, the patient receives small doses that may increase gradually and incrementally. If the response to a daily dose is not adequate in relieving edema, then the daily dose should be increased, rather than a second equal dose being administered later in the day. In patients with severe CHF, a continuous infusion is more effective than an equal dose given as an IV bolus in decreasing edema. However, the best IV dose of furosemide given for acute decompensated heart failure is not completely known. A recent review of American patients enrolled in the Acute Decompensated Heart Failure National Registry (ADHERE), the largest database on acute heart failure in the world with over 100,000 patients enrolled, examined 62,866 patients receiving less than 160 mg IV of furosemide and 19,674 patients greater than or equal to 160 mg IV of furosemide. The patients receiving the lower doses had a lower risk for in-hospital mortality, ICU stay, prolonged hospitalization, or adverse renal effect (Peacock, Costanzo, De Marco, et al., 2009). Other interventions are the same as for hydrochlorothiazide.

Minimizing Adverse Effects

When giving furosemide, follow the same procedures used for minimizing adverse effects of hydrochlorothiazide therapy. Hypokalemia is a greater risk from furosemide than from hydrochlorothiazide; closely monitor potassium levels during the first 2 weeks of chronic therapy and whenever an increase in the daily dosage occurs. The drug administration route must be considered carefully because furosemide may be given intravenously or orally.

Several interventions help minimize the risk of ototoxicity. Administer 20 to 40 mg of IV-push furosemide slowly over at least 1 to 2 minutes. Dilute high-dose infusions of furosemide into normal saline, Ringer's lactate, or D_5W and then administer no faster than 4 mg/minute. Slow, continuous infusions as opposed to bolus doses are believed to prevent high peaks in blood levels, which are associated with ototoxicity. However, the data are still somewhat inconclusive (Salvador, Rey, Ramos, et al., 2005). Although there is no set serum level for therapeutic efficacy, it may be necessary to obtain serum levels of furosemide to identify patients at high risk for ototoxicity; blood levels greater than 50 mcg/mL are associated with hearing problems. Consider a divided daily dose, which decreases the peak level of the drug and may help prevent hearing problems. Finally, avoid giving aminoglycoside antibiotics with furosemide, because the additive adverse effects on hearing greatly increase the risk of hearing damage. If increasing azotemia, oliguria, or BUN or creatinine levels occur in patients with renal impairment, discontinue furosemide therapy.

It is a good idea to give oral furosemide with food or milk to minimize possible GI upset. Report the adverse effects of rapid onset or worsening of edema and deterioration in breath sounds to the prescriber. These signs indicate that dosage may need to be adjusted or that a complication is developing.

Providing Patient and Family Education

The patient's and family's educational needs are similar to the needs of patients taking hydrochlorothiazide.

Ongoing Assessment and Evaluation

To judge an identified therapeutic outcome of furosemide, such as a reduction in edema and blood pressure, ongoing assessments of the following parameters are obtained: CBC, serum electrolyte and uric acid levels, and other test values are compared with baseline values to measure progress or complications. For example, in a patient with diabetes mellitus, it is important to monitor regularly serum glucose levels because furosemide therapy may alter the amount of insulin or oral antidiabetic needed. Patients who appear to be resistant to therapy should have a 24-hour urine specimen collected to assess sodium excretion. A value greater than 100 mEq/d in a patient whose daily weight is stable indicates that there has been an adequate diuretic response but the dietary intake of sodium is too great to see the whole therapeutic response.

Drugs Closely Related to P Furosemide

There are three other loop diuretics: bumetanide (Bumex), ethacrynic acid (Edecrin), and torsemide (Demadex). They resemble furosemide in action and adverse effects with the following exceptions. Bumetanide is more potent than furosemide and carries a Black Box warning that it can cause profound diuresis, water loss, and electrolyte loss if given in too large a dose. Unlike furosemide, bumetanide is used to treat only edema, not hypertension; bumetanide is not approved for use in children. Ethacrynic acid differs from furosemide in several ways. It is not a sulfonamide and is used primarily in people who are allergic to other sulfa-based drugs. It is given only to treat edema. A pregnancy category B drug, it is not approved for use in children. Torsemide is metabolized by the P-450 system to active and inactive metabolites.

P Furosemide

- A potent diuretic used to treat edema from CHF, pulmonary edema, and in hepatic and renal disease; may be used as an antihypertensive
- First-choice diuretic for treating hypertension with preexisting renal disease
- Works in the loop of Henle to promote excretion of large amounts of sodium, chloride, potassium, and water
- Most important contraindication: anuria in CRF
- Most common adverse effects: related to fluid and electrolyte loss, especially potassium loss
- Most serious adverse effects: significant hypokalemia, permanent deafness, and activation or exacerbation of SLE
- **Life span alert: Older adults are more sensitive to effects of rapid fluid loss.**
- Minimizing adverse effects: Administer IV push slowly, and monitor blood pressure, edema, breath sounds, weight, intake and output, and serum electrolyte levels while therapy continues.

C POTASSIUM-SPARING DIURETICS

The potassium-sparing diuretics promote sodium and water excretion in the distal tubule. At the same time, potassium is not excreted; rather, it is reabsorbed. This group of drugs produces weak diuresis and antihypertensive effects when used alone. However, the drugs are used more frequently in combination with loop and thiazide diuretics to minimize potassium loss because they work synergistically with other diuretics. Patients taking potassium-sparing diuretics are at risk for developing hyperkalemia. Potassium-sparing diuretics include triamterene, amiloride, eplerenone, and spironolactone (Table 27.1). Eplerenone and spironolactone work differently compared with the other two drugs and block aldosterone receptors. They are used in treating CHF and hypertension and are fully discussed in Chapter 26. The prototype of the potassium-sparing diuretics is triamterene (Dyrenium).

Nursing Management of the Patient Receiving **P** Triamterene

Core Drug Knowledge

Pharmacotherapeutics

Like furosemide, triamterene is used as an adjunct to manage edema and hypertension. The edema may be associated with CHF, cirrhosis, nephrotic syndrome, steroid use, or secondary hypoaldosteronism. It typically is used with other diuretics because it allows potassium to be reabsorbed and sodium to be excreted. Triamterene is given orally.

Pharmacokinetics

Triamterene is absorbed incompletely after oral administration. The drug is metabolized in the liver and excreted by the kidneys. Triamterene crosses the placenta and is excreted in small amounts in breast milk.

Pharmacodynamics

Triamterene achieves its diuretic effect by inhibiting transport of sodium in the distal tubules independent of aldosterone. This mechanism causes increased loss of sodium, chloride, water, bicarbonate, and calcium. However, the drug causes only 1% to 2% of filtered sodium to be excreted; thus, it has a small diuretic effect. The drug promotes retention of potassium and magnesium. Triamterene does not inhibit uric acid excretion and thereby elevates serum uric acid levels, as do the loop diuretics.

Contraindications and Precautions

Contraindications to triamterene include known hypersensitivity, use of other potassium-sparing diuretics, pre-existing **hyperkalemia** (serum potassium level >5.5 mEq/L), anuria, severe or progressive renal disease (except nephrosis), severe liver disease, and hepatic coma.

Precautions to its use include electrolyte imbalance, history of renal stone formation (it has been found in some renal calculi), diabetes (it can raise blood glucose), and when folic acid stores have been depleted (it is a weak folic acid antagonist). It is in pregnancy category C, and safety and efficacy have not been established in children.

Triamterene carries a Black Box warning that it can raise serum potassium levels to greater than or equal to 5.5 mEq/L. Hyperkalemia is more likely to occur in patients with renal impairment and diabetes (even without evidence of renal impairment) and in the elderly or severely ill.

Adverse Effects

Serious adverse effects include hyperkalemia (potentially fatal), electrolyte imbalance, and signs of fluid and electrolyte loss (weakness, nausea, anorexia, vomiting, and dry mouth). Triamterene is potentially nephrotoxic, possibly leading to crystalluria and cast formation (in up to 50% of the patients treated) and (very rarely) to triamterene stones or ARF.

Other adverse effects occur in various systems, as follows: GI (diarrhea, jaundice, and liver enzyme abnormalities); renal (azotemia, elevated BUN and creatinine levels); hematologic (thrombocytopenia and megaloblastic anemia); CNS (fatigue, dizziness, and headache); and miscellaneous (anaphylaxis, photosensitivity, and rash).

Drug Interactions

Triamterene increases the effect of amantadine and potassium preparations. ACE inhibitors, cimetidine, and indomethacin all increase the effect of triamterene. Triamterene interferes with the fluorescent measurement of serum quinidine levels. Table 27.4 lists agents that interact with triamterene.

Assessment of Relevant Core Patient Variables

Health Status

Assessment activities include determining whether the patient has any known hypersensitivity to triamterene and carefully examining electrolyte values, especially potassium

TABLE 27.4	Agents That Interact with P Triamterene	
Interactants	**Effect and Significance**	**Nursing Management**
amantadine	Increased amantadine plasma levels and decreased urinary excretion; more risk for adverse effects	Monitor for adverse effects.
potassium preparations and drugs that increase potassium levels	Severe hyperkalemia; possible cardiac arrhythmias or cardiac arrest	Avoid concurrent use.
ACE inhibitors	Elevated serum potassium from ACE inhibitors; hyperkalemia	Monitor serum potassium level.
cimetidine	Increased bioavailability and decreased renal clearance of triamterene	Monitor for increased therapeutic effect.
indomethacin	Rapid progress into acute renal failure with concurrent use	Use together only if truly necessary.

levels. As for other diuretic drugs, additional assessments include measuring blood pressure, edema, weight, and urine output; examining serum glucose and creatinine levels; and identifying pre-existing conditions, such as diabetes mellitus, that may affect triamterene therapy. Assess for drug therapy that also increases potassium levels, because this increases the risk of hyperkalemia.

Life Span and Gender
Triamterene must be used cautiously in pregnancy; it is in risk category C. Triamterene crosses into breast milk, and because safety has not been established in children, the drug should not be used in breast-feeding women.

Glomerular filtration decreases with age; consequently, elderly patients do not excrete as much potassium as younger adults. Therefore, triamterene should be given cautiously to older adults because of the increased risk for hyperkalemia.

Lifestyle, Diet, and Habits
Determine whether the patient normally eats a diet high in potassium, takes a potassium supplement, or uses a potassium chloride salt substitute.

Environment
Assess whether the patient can get to a toilet easily when needed, especially at the beginning of therapy, when urine output increases. The patient's home should be assessed for risk factors that may contribute to injuries (falls) resulting from adverse effects of drug therapy. Triamterene can be self-administered at home or administered by others in acute care, long-term care, or subacute care environments.

Nursing Diagnoses and Outcomes

• Risk for Deficient Fluid Volume related to action and adverse effects of triamterene
  Desired outcome: *The patient will not experience fluid and electrolyte imbalance while taking triamterene.*
• Risk for Injury related to adverse effects of triamterene, including risk for hyperkalemia

Desired outcome: *The patient will not suffer injury, and potassium levels will remain within normal limits while patient is on triamterene therapy.*
• Risk for Injury, Drug Interactions, related to multiple drug therapies
  Desired outcome: *The patient will not have adverse effects from drug interactions while taking triamterene.*

Planning and Intervention
Maximizing Therapeutic Effects
As with other diuretics, triamterene should be administered in the morning so that increased diuretic effect occurs during waking hours.

Minimizing Adverse Effects
Monitor blood potassium levels and assess for signs of hyperkalemia (nausea, diarrhea, muscle weakness or cramping, oliguria, weak pulse, and cardiac arrhythmias). The greatest risk of electrolyte imbalance with triamterene, as with all diuretics, occurs within the first 2 weeks of therapy. It is important to limit the patient's intake of potassium-rich foods and avoid potassium supplements. Monitor for signs of fluid and electrolyte imbalance. Give oral triamterene with food or milk to prevent GI upset. It is a good idea to have the patient get out of bed slowly; assist with ambulation to prevent falls from dizziness.

Providing Patient and Family Education
The main distinction between triamterene and other diuretics is the hyperkalemia that may develop with drug use. Because triamterene is usually added to therapy with other types of diuretics, patients may become accustomed to being at risk for hypokalemia. The patient needs to learn to cope with the different risks associated with triamterene. Other patient and family education points are similar to those points provided for the other diuretics.

• Teach patients to avoid potassium-rich foods, supplements, and potassium chloride salt substitutes.
• Teach patients the signs and symptoms of hyperkalemia.

ADDING TRIAMTERENE TO HYPERTENSION THERAPY

Mr. Nixon is a 53-year-old white man being treated for hypertension with hydrochlorothiazide. After 2 weeks of therapy, his potassium level is 2.9 (N=3.5-5). He is started on 20 mEq of potassium as a daily supplement. His potassium levels continue to be low (3.1). Mr. Nixon's prescriber writes an order to add triamterene to his drug regimen.

1. Identify the major electrolyte imbalance that Mr. Nixon may now experience.
2. Suggest actions that you can take to prevent this electrolyte imbalance.

Ongoing Assessment and Evaluation

Monitor the patient's potassium and other electrolyte levels, blood pressure, edema, weight, and urine output. Drug therapy with triamterene is effective when blood pressure is reduced to therapeutic levels or edema is reduced without the patient developing hyperkalemia.

Drug Closely Related to P Triamterene

Amiloride (Midamor), which has the same mechanism of action, efficacy, and adverse reactions as triamterene, has two unique uses. It is approved for use specifically in CHF. In addition, in patients taking lithium, amiloride can reduce lithium-induced polyuria without increasing lithium levels; this is an off-label use of amiloride. Compared with triamterene, amiloride is different in the following ways: it is generally better tolerated, it is not metabolized similarly, it does not cause crystalluria or cast formation, it is a pregnancy category B drug, and it is not approved for use in children.

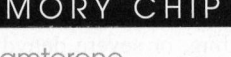

MEMORY CHIP

P Triamterene

- Potassium-sparing diuretic used to manage edema and hypertension
- Major contraindication: the patient is already receiving a potassium-sparing diuretic
- Most common adverse effects: nausea, vomiting, anorexia, dry mouth, and headache
- Most serious adverse effect: hyperkalemia (electrolyte imbalance)
- **Life span alert: Older adults are especially at risk for hyperkalemia.**
- **Patient safety alert: Life-threatening hyperkalemia may result when combined with potassium supplements or drugs that increase potassium levels indirectly.**
- Most important patient education: Tell the patient to avoid eating potassium-rich food, taking potassium supplements, or using a salt substitute containing potassium chloride.

Drugs Significantly Different From P Triamterene

Spironolactone

Like triamterene, spironolactone (Aldactone) works in the distal tubule to increase sodium and water loss and to retain potassium. Unlike triamterene, spironolactone is an aldosterone antagonist. It blocks all aldosterone receptors: mineralocorticoid, glucocorticoid, progesterone, and androgen receptors. This accounts for its positive effects as well as its adverse effects. It interferes with testosterone synthesis, which leads to altered estrogenic and androgenic activity. Like other potassium-sparing diuretics, spironolactone can be used as an adjunct therapy to treat hypertension and edema associated with CHF, nephrosis, and cirrhosis. Its benefits in CHF are believed to extend beyond merely decreasing edema. It has been found to have marked and sustained antiproteinuric effect when combined with an ACE inhibitor and an angiotensin-receptor blocker in patients with type 2 diabetic nephropathy (Box 27.3). In addition, it is used in preventing or treating hypokalemia in high-risk patients, particularly those patients also taking digitoxin for cardiac disease or those patients with cardiac arrhythmias. Because of its antialdosterone effects, a major use is in diagnosing and treating primary hyperaldosteronism. Unlabeled uses of spironolactone include treatment of hirsutism, familial male precocious puberty, symptoms of premenstrual syndrome, and acne vulgaris (short-term use).

The effect of spironolactone is delayed. Onset of action may not occur for 24 to 48 hours. This delayed onset occurs because the drug blocks the effect of aldosterone, which then blocks the synthesis of the proteins required for sodium and potassium transport. The existing proteins continue to do their job, and diuretic effect does not occur until the existing proteins are inactive. Spironolactone carries a Black Box warning that it has been found to be tumorigenic in chronic toxicity studies in rats. Unnecessary use should be avoided.

Nursing management unique to spironolactone therapy involves helping the patient understand and cope with such adverse effects as impotence, menstrual irregularities, and gynecomastia. Additionally, it is important to teach the patient about the drug interaction between spironolactone and salicylates, such as aspirin, which decreases the diuretic effect of therapy.

Eplerenone

Eplerenone (Inspra) also is an aldosterone blocker and potassium-sparing diuretic. Unlike spironolactone, it is specific for the mineralocorticoid aldosterone receptors. It is used in CHF and hypertension and discussed as the prototype in Chapter 26.

C OSMOTIC DIURETICS

Osmotic diuretics are filterable freely in the glomerulus and not reabsorbed by the tubules. They increase osmotic pressure and pull fluid into the vascular space. Because they are not reabsorbed by the tubules, they prevent water reabsorption as well. They also prevent reabsorption of sodium and chloride. Osmotic diuretics include mannitol glycerin, isosorbide, and urea (Table 27.1). The prototype osmotic diuretic is mannitol (Osmitrol).

Nursing Management of the Patient Receiving Mannitol

Core Drug Knowledge

Pharmacotherapeutics
Mannitol is not used to treat hypertension or peripheral edema. Instead, it is used more in acute situations. Major uses include preventing and treating ARF, reducing intracranial pressure in cerebral edema, reducing intraocular pressure when other drugs have not worked, and promoting excretion of toxic substances in urine. In addition, mannitol is used diagnostically to measure GFR and postoperatively as an irrigant after transurethral procedures. It is sometimes used as an adjunct to promote renal excretion of drugs that are at toxic levels.

Pharmacokinetics
Mannitol, a sugar, usually is administered as an IV solution because it does not diffuse across the GI epithelium and is not distributed like other sugars. It can be administered as a urinary irrigant but only in transurethral prostatic resections or other transurethral surgical procedures. It is metabolized poorly, and most of it is excreted in the urine. When used as an irrigant, mannitol has a rapid onset and a short duration of action. Mannitol crosses the placenta and may enter breast milk.

Pharmacodynamics
As a systemic agent, mannitol elevates blood plasma osmolarity that draws fluid from tissues, including the brain, cerebrospinal fluid, and the eye into the vascular space. As a result, cerebral edema, elevated intracranial pressure, cerebrospinal fluid volume, and intraocular pressure may be reduced. As a diuretic, mannitol increases the concentration of molecules in the glomerular filtrate because it is not reabsorbed in the renal tubule. This increased osmolality causes the osmotic pressure to rise, and the increased pressure inhibits water reabsorption, which leads to an increased and faster flow of water in the tubules and therefore water loss. Mannitol also decreases reabsorption of sodium and chloride.

Contraindications and Precautions
Mannitol is contraindicated in severe renal disease, severe pulmonary congestion or frank pulmonary edema, active intracranial bleeding (except during craniotomy), severe dehydration, progressive renal damage or dysfunction after mannitol therapy, and progressive heart failure or pulmonary congestion after mannitol therapy.

Mannitol must be used very cautiously in CHF, renal disease, electrolyte imbalance, pseudoagglutination, and hemoconcentration. Mannitol is a pregnancy category C drug. Safety and efficacy for children 12 years and younger have not been established.

Adverse Effects
Several adverse effects result from mannitol use. They are related mostly to the fluid changes induced by its use. Problems with volume overload or volume depletion are both possible. When very high doses of mannitol are given or if the kidney is not able to excrete the mannitol, fluid volume expansion occurs. Sodium levels are diluted by the excessive fluid volume, so hyponatremia is possible. The most serious adverse effect is acute CHF or pulmonary edema in susceptible patients, resulting from the sudden expansion of the extracellular fluid.

Fluid and electrolyte alterations may occur suddenly with the rapid expansion of extracellular fluid. Therefore, monitor for possible water intoxication and advise the patient to report chest pain or shortness of breath. These symptoms may occur when fluid or electrolyte losses induce hypotension or tachycardia.

Volume depletion, resulting mostly from free water loss, can result in hypernatremia when significant diuresis occurs from mannitol. The patient may show signs of dehydration. The most common indications of this are CNS related (dizziness) and GI related (nausea, anorexia, dry mouth, and thirst). Overdosage from larger than recommended doses may result in increased loss of electrolytes, particularly sodium, chloride, and potassium. Electrolyte depletions may be severe enough to cause hypotension and cardiac irregularities.

Drug Interactions
Mannitol does not interact with any foods, interfere with any laboratory test results, or create any major drug–drug interactions.

Assessment of Relevant Core Patient Variables

Health Status
Initially determine any contraindications to mannitol therapy, including anuria resulting from severe renal disease, pulmonary congestion, impaired cardiac function or CHF, active intracranial bleeding, or severe dehydration. These conditions contraindicate therapy because they may worsen with mannitol, which increases extracellular fluid volume. If urine output does not range between 30 and 50 mL/h after two test doses of mannitol, the drug should not be used.

Assess blood pressure, pulse rate and character, respiratory rate and character, and breath sounds. Other general assessments include checking skin color and edema, hydration status, level of consciousness, reflexes, and muscle strength before and during the mannitol infusion to detect adverse effects.

Life Span and Gender
Assess the patient for pregnancy and breast-feeding. Pregnant patients should only receive mannitol, which is a pregnancy category C drug, if therapy is clearly warranted and the benefits outweigh potential fetal harm. Explain

to breast-feeding patients that mannitol may or may not be secreted in breast milk. It also is important to note the patient's age before administering mannitol. Mannitol's effect on children younger than 12 years remains unknown. Elderly patients are at increased risk for developing dizziness, disorientation, and confusion caused by rapid fluid loss when receiving mannitol.

Environment

Note that mannitol is administered only in an acute-care setting.

Nursing Diagnosis and Outcome

- Risk for Deficient Fluid Volume or excessive fluid volume related to the action of mannitol

  Desired outcome: *The patient's fluid and electrolyte levels will remain within normal limits after the therapeutic effect has been achieved.*

Planning and Intervention

Maximizing Therapeutic Effects

Concentrations of mannitol that exceed 15% have a tendency to crystallize. This crystallizing is a characteristic of the drug because it is a sugar; it is not a sign that the drug is old and should be discarded. Therefore, the drug vial should be warmed to no more than body temperature before administration to eliminate crystals. An in-line filter should be used for the infusion.

Minimizing Adverse Effects

Monitor the patient's hourly urine output. Accuracy is essential; therefore, an indwelling catheter normally is required. It is important to adjust the drug infusion rate to maintain the patient's urine output between 30 and 50 mL/h.

Adequacy of renal function is determined in patients with renal impairment by administering one or two test doses of 0.2 g/kg over 3 to 5 minutes before beginning an infusion. If urine output is less than 30 mL/h after the test doses, mannitol is usually withheld.

Monitor blood pressure, pulse rate, electrocardiographic tracings, intake-to-output ratios, renal function test results, and serum electrolyte levels to monitor for rapid fluid and electrolyte alterations. It is important to assess for water intoxication as evidenced by nausea, chest pain, and shortness of breath. Breath sounds and respiratory rate and character should be assessed regularly to detect complications, such as pulmonary congestion.

Provide mouth care and ice chips for dry mouth or thirst. It also is important to assess for hives, itching, or pain at the IV site, and to provide comfort and corrective measures as needed. It is a good idea to assist patients in rising slowly from bed and provide assistance when they walk if they must get out of bed. Treatment of overdosage includes discontinuing infusion therapy at once and institution of measures to normalize electrolyte levels. Hemodialysis may be needed to eliminate mannitol and reduce serum osmolarity.

Providing Patient and Family Education

- Explain the purpose of mannitol therapy.
- Urge patients to report any difficulty breathing, chest pain, or peripheral swelling (edema).
- Tell patients that blurred vision or a runny nose (if these findings occur) should subside when therapy is discontinued.

Ongoing Assessment and Evaluation

Monitoring is ongoing throughout therapy with mannitol and includes measuring urine output and checking for signs of fluid or electrolyte imbalance. Therapy is effective when urine output increases and intracranial or intraocular pressure is decreased without complications to the patient.

Drugs Closely Related to 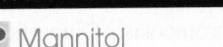 Mannitol

Glycerin (Glycerol)

Glycerin is an osmotic agent given orally to reduce intraocular pressure before ophthalmic surgery and during acute glaucoma attacks. It is metabolized and eliminated by the kidneys. Peak reduction of intraocular pressure occurs 1 hour after administration. Duration of action is about 5 hours. Contraindications are similar to those for mannitol and include well-established anuria, severe dehydration, frank or impending acute pulmonary edema, severe cardiac decompensation, and hypersensitivity to any ingredient. Caution should be used if the patient has acute urinary retention, hypervolemia, chronic heart disease, diabetes, or cardiac, renal, or hepatic disease. It can cause adverse reactions similar to those reactions caused by mannitol (e.g., nausea, vomiting, headache, confusion, and disorientation). Serious complications of severe dehydration, cardiac arrhythmias,

---

MEMORY CHIP

P Mannitol

- Treats acute renal failure, increased intracranial pressure, and increased intraocular pressure
- A sugar that draws water into the vascular space through osmosis. Freely filtered but not reabsorbed; thereby causes diuresis
- Major contraindications: anuria due to severe renal disease, pulmonary edema, and intracranial bleeding
- Most common adverse effects: dizziness and GI problems
- Most serious adverse effects: worsening of CHF; serious imbalances of fluid and electrolytes; and obscure or worsened hypovolemia
- Maximizing therapeutic effects: Warm the drug vial in water before using if crystals are seen, and administer no warmer than body temperature, using an in-line filter.
- Minimizing adverse effects: Give a test dose for patients with marked oliguria or inadequate renal function. If urine output does not increase after two test doses, discontinue use.

and hyperosmolar nonketotic coma are possible and may be fatal. Glycerin is a pregnancy category C drug.

A suppository form (glycerin suppositories, Fleet Babylax, Sani-Sipp) also is available and is used as a hyperosmolar laxative for temporary relief of constipation.

Isosorbide

Isosorbide (Ismotic) also is used to provide short-term reduction of intraocular pressure before and after intraocular surgery and to interrupt acute attacks of glaucoma. Isosorbide causes less risk for nausea and vomiting, and it should be used in place of other osmotics when these adverse effects are undesirable for the patient. Isosorbide has a much longer half-life than mannitol. Like glycerin, it is given only orally. It is a good idea to pour the drug over cracked iced and have the patient sip the drug to improve its taste and acceptance. Contraindications and adverse effects are similar to those of mannitol. Isosorbide is a pregnancy category B drug.

Urea

Urea (Ureaphil), like mannitol, is administered by IV infusion and is used to decrease intracranial pressure (in the control of cerebral edema) and intraocular pressure. An unlabeled use has been to induce abortion. Contraindications are severely impaired renal function, active intracranial bleeding, marked dehydration, and frank liver failure. Urea is a pregnancy category C drug.

No serious adverse effects occur if urea is infused slowly, if renal function is adequate, and if intracranial bleeding is not present. Adverse effects that occur are similar to those effects seen with mannitol and include headache, nausea, vomiting, syncope, and disorientation.

Urea should be mixed with 5% or 10% dextrose solution to prevent the hemolysis produced by pure solutions of urea. Infusions should be slow, because rapid infusion may be associated with hemolysis and a direct effect on the cerebral vasomotor centers, causing increased capillary bleeding. It is important to avoid using veins in lower extremities of older adults because phlebitis and thrombosis of superficial and deep veins may occur. Monitor the infusion site carefully because extravasation may cause mild irritation to tissue necrosis.

© CARBONIC ANHYDRASE INHIBITORS

Carbonic anhydrase is an enzyme that plays a role in renal excretion of acid urine and reabsorption of sodium and potassium in the proximal tubule. However, an agent that inhibits carbonic anhydrase promotes the excretion of sodium, potassium, bicarbonate, and water, resulting in an alkaline diuresis. However, carbonic anhydrase inhibitors are not used in the treatment of CHF, hypertension, or CKD. Inhibition of carbonic anhydrase decreases aqueous humor formation and consequently decreases intraocular pressure; this is the primary use of these drugs. Carbonic anhydrase inhibitors include acetazolamide, methazolamide, brinzolamide, and

dichlorphenamide (Table 27.1). The prototype carbonic anhydrase inhibitor is acetazolamide (Diamox Sequels).

Nursing Management of the Patient Receiving Ⓟ Acetazolamide
Core Drug Knowledge
Pharmacotherapeutics

Acetazolamide is used to treat chronic open-angle glaucoma. It also can be used in acute closed-angle glaucoma when delay of surgery is desired to reduce intraocular pressure; as an adjunct in treating edema resulting from CHF or use of drugs; as an adjunct in treating epilepsy; and in preventing and treating acute mountain sickness. It can be administered orally or intravenously.

Pharmacokinetics

Acetazolamide is well absorbed from the GI tract and excreted unchanged by the kidneys.

Pharmacodynamics

Acetazolamide is a nonbacteriostatic sulfonamide that blocks the action of carbonic anhydrase, which is needed for active transport of ions across the proximal tubule. Inhibition of carbonic anhydrase results in decreased hydrogen ion secretion by the tubules and increased sodium, potassium, bicarbonate, and water excretion. Increased excretion of these electrolytes reduces the pH of body fluids. Another effect of carbonic anhydrase inhibition is decreased formation of aqueous humor, which thereby lowers intraocular pressure. It also delays abnormal, paroxysmal excessive discharge from CNS neurons.

Contraindications and Precautions

Contraindications to acetazolamide therapy are hypersensitivity, depressed sodium or potassium serum levels, marked kidney and liver disease or dysfunction, suprarenal gland failure, hyperchloremic acidosis, adrenocortical insufficiency, severe pulmonary obstruction, cirrhosis, and long-term use in chronic noncongestive closed-angle glaucoma.

Acetazolamide should be administered cautiously to patients with adrenocortical insufficiency because patients with this disorder are susceptible to electrolyte imbalances. Acetazolamide is a pregnancy category C drug. It is secreted in breast milk, although dosage received by the infant is minute. However, safety and efficacy in children have not been established.

Adverse Effects

Sulfonamide-type adverse reactions may occur because of cross-sensitivity. Adverse effects are varied. The most common are GI related and include anorexia, nausea, vomiting, and constipation. Symptoms of overdose include drowsiness, anorexia, nausea, vomiting, dizziness, paresthesia, ataxia, tremor, and tinnitus. The electrolyte disturbance most likely to occur from overdosage is hyperchloremic acidosis. Treatment involves inducing vomiting or performing gastric lavage. Hyperchloremic acidosis may respond to bicarbonate administration. Potassium supplements may be required.

Drug Interactions

Acetazolamide interacts with a few other drugs. Because acetazolamide promotes excretion of bicarbonate ions, the patient's urine will become alkaline, which may cause some laboratory test results to be false positive for urinary protein. Table 27.5 lists agents that interact with acetazolamide.

Assessment of Relevant Core Patient Variables

Health Status

Assessment should focus on whether the patient is allergic to acetazolamide or to the chemically similar sulfonamide antibiotics and thiazide diuretics. Investigate any history of chronic closed-angle glaucoma, renal or hepatic disease, respiratory acidosis, and chronic obstructive pulmonary disease.

Review blood tests for electrolyte and fluid disturbances, because the drug should be used cautiously in patients with fluid and electrolyte imbalances, especially hyponatremia, hypokalemia, and hyperchloremic acidosis; hepatic disease; adrenocortical insufficiency; respiratory acidosis; or chronic obstructive pulmonary disease.

Life Span and Gender

Determine the patient's breast-feeding status and age before administering acetazolamide. Safety has not been established for breast-feeding women because safety and efficacy have not been established in children. Elderly patients do not tolerate excessive diuresis and may experience hypotension and orthostatic changes. In these patients, dosage may need to be reduced.

Environment

Note the setting in which acetazolamide may be administered. Acetazolamide may be administered in any environmental setting. However, IV administration is performed only in the hospital.

Nursing Diagnoses and Outcomes

• Risk for Deficient Fluid Volume related to therapeutic action of acetazolamide

Desired outcome: The patient will have desired fluid volume changes without experiencing complications from these changes.

• Risk for Injury related to adverse effects of acetazolamide (blood dyscrasias, metabolic acidosis, paresthesia)

Desired outcome: The patient will not suffer injury while taking acetazolamide.

Planning and Intervention

Maximizing Therapeutic Effects

Use acetazolamide with miotics or mydriatics for complementary effect when treating open-angle glaucoma. The best diuretic effects in CHF and drug-induced edema occur when the drug is given every other day or daily for 2 days, with the third day off. Palatability may be enhanced with honey or other sweet syrup for crushed oral tablets.

Minimizing Adverse Effects

It is important to allow the kidneys to recover and prevent overdosage when acetazolamide is used as a diuretic to reduce edema. If reduction in edema ceases after first dose, do not increase the dose; instead, a day of medication should be skipped. Overdosage can be treated by gastric lavage or by inducing vomiting.

Monitor CBC and platelet counts during therapy; bone marrow suppression is rare but may occur. It also is important to monitor serum potassium levels (especially if severe cirrhosis is present or there is concurrent use of steroids or adrenocorticotropic hormones).

Administer orally or by IV injection; intramuscular administration is painful. Do not add to syrups containing glycerin or alcohol if the drug must be crushed.

Providing Patient and Family Education

• Explain the importance of returning for follow-up blood work to check CBC and electrolyte levels.
• Urge patients to notify the prescriber if sore throat, easy bruising, petechiae, and mucosal ulcerations develop (signs of blood abnormalities).

TABLE 27.5	Agents That Interact with P Acetazolamide	
Interactants	**Effect and Significance**	**Nursing Management**
cyclosporine	Increased trough levels of cyclosporine; possible nephrotoxicity and neurotoxicity	Monitor for signs of nephrotoxicity and neurotoxicity.
primidone	Decreased concentrations of primidone in blood and urine	Monitor for therapeutic effect.
salicylates	Accumulation and toxicity of acetazolamide, including CNS depression and metabolic acidosis; CAI-induced acidosis may allow increased CNS penetration by salicylates	Monitor for therapeutic effects.
diflunisal	Significant decrease in intraocular pressure; increased adverse effects possible	Monitor for therapeutic response. Monitor for adverse effects.

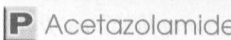

MEMORY CHIP

P Acetazolamide

- Used primarily in treating chronic, open-angle glaucoma because it prevents formation of aqueous humor and decreases intraocular pressure
- Inhibits hydrogen ion secretion in renal tubule, and therefore increases loss of sodium, potassium, bicarbonate, and water
- Major contraindications: severe renal or hepatic disease
- Most common adverse effects: related to gastrointestinal system
- Most serious (although rare) adverse effect: bone marrow suppression
- **Life span alert: Older adults may have hypotension and orthostatic changes; dosage may need to be reduced.**
- Maximizing therapeutic effects (of CHF diuresis): Give every other day or every 2 days, with the next day off.
- Minimizing adverse effects: Allow kidney to recover, and prevent overdosage when used to reduce edema.
- Most important patient education: Explain the importance of follow-up blood work.

- Tell patients to notify the prescriber if nausea, fatigue, abdominal pain, tinnitus, hyperpnea, and numbness in extremities occur (signs of metabolic acidosis).
- Encourage patients to take acetazolamide with food if GI upset occurs.
- Caution patients to avoid prolonged sunlight exposure.
- Tell patients to use caution when performing activities requiring alertness until effects of the drug are known.

Ongoing Assessment and Evaluation

Throughout acetazolamide therapy, the patient should be alert for unusual vision problems and should maintain the follow-up schedule previously established. Drug therapy and nursing care are considered successful if ocular pressure remains controlled and the patient's fluid and electrolyte values stay within normal ranges.

Drugs Closely Related to P Acetazolamide

The other carbonic anhydrase inhibitors are methazolamide (Neptazane), brinzolamide (Azopt), and dorzolamide (Trusopt Ocumeter). Like acetazolamide, methazolamide is used in the treatment of glaucoma but not as often as the prototype, as it has lesser efficacy. It is sometimes used off-label in the prophylactic treatment of acute mountain sickness. It is administered orally to adults. Brinzolamide and dorzolamide differ from the prototype in that they are ophthalmic drops.

C ANTICHOLINERGIC AGENTS

Anticholinergic drugs affect bladder contraction because receptors for these agents are found in the bladder. When the receptors are blocked, bladder contraction cannot occur, and urinary output decreases. Anticholinergics are used to treat overactive bladder. The prototype is tolterodine (Detrol). Drugs closely related to tolterodine are oxybutynin, darifenacin, solifenacin, trospium, and flavoxate (Table 27.1).

Nursing Management of the Patient Receiving P Tolterodine

Core Drug Knowledge

Pharmacotherapeutics

Tolterodine is used in treating overactive bladder, to help manage the symptoms of urinary frequency, urgency, and urge incontinence. It is administered orally twice a day and is available in regular and extended-release forms.

Pharmacokinetics

Oral absorption of tolterodine is rapid, although the absolute bioavailability can vary a great deal. Maximum steady-state serum levels usually occur within 1 to 2 hours. Tolterodine is a highly protein-bound drug, although its active metabolite is not. Extensive, although variable, first-pass metabolism occurs after an oral dose. Several metabolites are formed, including an active one. This metabolite is formed from oxidation through the P-450 2D6 isoenzyme. Most hepatic metabolism is through P-450 3A4. Excretion of drug and metabolites is in the urine, primarily, and in the stool.

Pharmacodynamics

Tolterodine is a competitive anti-cholinergic. Although cholinergic (specifically the muscarinic) receptors exist in both the bladder and the salivary glands, tolterodine has relative selective preference for the cholinergic receptors in the bladder. Blockade of these cholinergic receptors decreases the ability of the bladder to contract. Tolterodine and its active metabolite do not have affinity for other neurotransmitter receptors or other potential cellular targets, such as the special channels for calcium ions. Tolterodine produces a pronounced effect on the bladder function. It can cause an increase in residual urine and a decrease in detrusor pressure.

Contraindications and Precautions

Tolterodine is contraindicated if the patient has urinary retention, gastric retention, uncontrolled narrow-angle glaucoma, or hypersensitivity to the drug. Patients with renal or hepatic impairment should receive doses that are half of what is normally prescribed. Use cautiously if the patient has bladder outflow obstruction or GI obstructive disorders (e.g., pyloric stenosis), as urinary retention or gastric retention may occur. Tolterodine is a pregnancy category class C drug.

Adverse Effects

The most frequent adverse effect of tolterodine is dry mouth, which is related to the anticholinergic effects from the drug. Headache is another fairly common adverse effect. Other adverse effects that are related to the antimuscarinic (anticholinergic) effects of the drug are constipation, abnormal vision (accommodation abnormalities), urinary retention, and xerophthalmia (conjunctival dryness).

TABLE 27.6 Agents That Interact with P Tolterodine		
Interactants	**Effect and Significance**	**Nursing Management**
Cytochrome 3A4 inhibitors (erythromycin, clarithromycin, ketoconazole, itraconazole, miconazole)	Inhibition of this metabolic pathway may make hepatic function suboptimal and place the patient at increased risk for adverse effects.	Dosage should be limited to 1 mg/d (half usually prescribed).

Drug Interactions

A few drug interactions are known to occur with tolterodine; most are not clinically important. Fluoxetine, a potent inhibitor of P-450 2D6, interacts with tolterodine and increases unbound tolterodine drug concentrations, but no dosage changes are needed. Drugs that inhibit P-450 3A4 (e.g., macrolide antibiotics such as erythromycin and clarithromycin, and antifungal agents such as ketoconazole, itraconazole, and miconazole) increase levels of tolterodine and require smaller doses. Food increases the bioavailability of tolterodine, although not the levels of active metabolite. Dosage changes are not needed. Interactions that require nursing management are listed in Table 27.6.

Assessment of Relevant Core Patient Variables

Health Status

Assess for urinary retention, bladder outlet obstruction, gastric retention, GI obstructive disorders, renal impairment, hepatic impairment, and uncontrolled narrow-angle glaucoma, which are contraindications or precautions to using the drug.

Life Span and Gender

The safety and efficacy of tolterodine have not been established in children. The drug is in pregnancy category C, meaning that animal studies produced teratogenic effects. If the woman is pregnant or might become pregnant, the drug should be used only if the benefit to the mother is believed to outweigh the potential risk to the infant. It is not known whether tolterodine is excreted in human breast milk; hence, breast-feeding should be avoided.

Although older adults have higher serum levels of tolterodine, adjustments are not needed. However, older adults may have decreased renal function or hepatic impairment and should be checked for these problems. Men and women can achieve equal therapeutic effects from drug therapy.

For men, a combination treatment of tolterodine with tamsulosin (an alpha-1 receptor blocker used in benign prostatic hypertrophy) has been found to provide more benefit than either drug alone in decreasing urinary frequency and incontinence in men with overactive bladder and other lower urinary tract symptoms (Kaplan, Roehrborn, Chancellor, et al., 2008).

Environment

Tolterodine is usually administered in the home environment.

Nursing Diagnosis and Outcomes

- Altered Urinary Elimination related to overactive bladder
  Desired outcome: *Urinary elimination will be normal with tolterodine drug therapy.*
- Risk for Urinary Retention related to adverse effects of tolterodine
  Desired outcome: *Urinary retention will not occur while taking tolterodine.*

Planning and Intervention

Maximizing Therapeutic Effect

Administer the drug on a regular prescribed basis.

Minimizing Adverse Effects

If the patient has renal or hepatic dysfunction, or is receiving drugs that are P-450 3A4 inhibitors, administer a dose of tolterodine that is no more than half of what is commonly administered daily.

Providing Patient and Family Education

- Teach patients and family to be alert for problems with urinary retention, GI retention, or visual changes such as blurred vision, and to report these adverse effects to the prescriber.
- Suggest that patients keep a diary that records the episodes of incontinence and frequency of urination, which may be helpful in determining whether drug therapy is effective.
- Tell patients for whom dry mouth is a problem to suck on hard candies or ice chips to relieve the dryness.

Ongoing Assessment and Evaluation

Treatment with tolterodine is effective if urinary incontinence and frequency are decreased and the patient does not develop serious adverse effects.

MEMORY CHIP

P Tolterodine

- Blocks cholinergic muscarinic receptors in the bladder, decreasing bladder function
- Used to treat overactive bladder, controlling symptoms of urinary frequency, urgency, or urge incontinence
- Major contraindications: urinary retention, gastric retention, and uncontrolled narrow-angle glaucoma
- Most common adverse effects: dry mouth and headache
- Minimizing adverse effects: Decrease the dose if patient has renal or liver disease.
- Most important patient education: Urinary retention, GI retention, or visual changes such as blurred vision may occur and need to be reported.

Drugs Closely Related to P Tolterodine

Drugs closely related to tolterodine are oxybutynin (Oxytrol), darifenacin (Enablex), solifenacin (Vesicare), trospium (Sanctura), and flavoxate (Urispas). These drugs have similar actions and indications to tolterodine. Oxybutynin is a transdermal system instead of an oral drug like tolterodine and is a pregnancy category B drug. Darifenacin, solifenacin, and trospium have longer half-lives than tolterodine, so they can be given once daily. Unlike the prototype tolterodine, flavoxate is not used for overactive bladder but is prescribed for symptomatic relief of cystitis, urethritis, prostatitis, urethritis, or urethrocystitis/urethrotrigonitis.

CHAPTER SUMMARY

- Diuretics are used widely to treat conditions in which increased extracellular fluid and edema are problems. Examples include hypertension, CHF, cirrhosis, renal disorders, intracranial pressure, and intraocular pressure.
- Diuretics work along the renal tubule and inhibit sodium and water reabsorption to increase water loss. The degree of diuretic effect depends on the section of the tubule in which the drug works.
- Diuretic drugs affect the excretion and reabsorption of other electrolytes, especially potassium, leading to one of the major adverse effects of diuretic therapy, an electrolyte imbalance.
- Thiazide and loop diuretics are the two classes of diuretics most frequently used.
- To prevent hypokalemia, patients taking non–potassium-sparing diuretics may need to increase their dietary intake of potassium or take supplements. Conversely, patients taking potassium-sparing diuretics are at risk for hyperkalemia and need to avoid excess potassium intake.
- Osmotic diuretics work by increasing the osmotic pressure within the vascular space. They are used primarily in ARF, in increased intracranial pressure, in increased intraocular pressure, and to promote excretion in the urine of toxic substances.
- Carbonic anhydrase inhibitors work by a different mechanism to cause a mild diuresis. They are used in treating open-angle glaucoma.
- Tolterodine is an antimuscarinic used to treat overactive bladder disease. Tolterodine selectively blocks muscarinic receptors in the bladder to produce its effects.

QUESTIONS FOR STUDY AND REVIEW

1. Identify the physical assessments for health status that should be completed before a patient starts thiazide therapy for hypertension.
2. Identify at least three conditions treated by diuretic therapy.
3. Discuss at least three fluid and electrolyte problems likely to occur in patients receiving thiazide or loop diuretics.
4. Why is a patient more likely to develop hypokalemia when on loop diuretics than on thiazide diuretics?
5. How are osmotic diuretics different from thiazide or loop diuretics?
6. What is the primary therapeutic use of carbonic anhydrase inhibitors?
7. What is the effect on the bladder from excessive blockade of muscarinic receptors?

NEED MORE HELP?

Chapter 27 of the Study Guide to Accompany *Drug Therapy in Nursing*, 4th Edition, contains NCLEX-style questions and other learning activities to reinforce your understanding of the concepts presented in this chapter. For additional information or to purchase the study guide, visit thePoint.

REFERENCES

ALLHAT Officers and Coordinators for the ALLHAT Collaborative Research Group. (2002). Major outcomes in high-risk hypertensive patients randomized to angiotensin-converting enzyme inhibitor or calcium channel blocker vs diuretic: The Antihypertensive and Lipid-Lowering Treatment to Prevent Heart Attack Trial (ALLHAT). *Journal of the American Medical Association*, 288(23):2981–2997.

Arrabal-Martin, M., Fernandez-Rodriguez, A., Arrabal-Polo, M. A., et al. (2006). Extracorporeal renal lithotripsy: Evolution of residual lithiasis treated with thiazides. *Urology*, 68(5): 956–959.

Bonds, D. E., Hogan, P. E., Bertoni, A. G., et al. (2009). A multifaceted intervention to improve blood pressure control: The Guideline Adherence for Heart Health (GLAD) study, *American Heart Journal*,157(2):278–284.

Clayton, J. A., Rodgers, S., Blakey, J., et al. (2006). Thiazide diuretic prescription and electrolyte abnormalities in primary care. *British Journal of Clinical Pharmacology*, 61(1): 87–95.

Escribano, J., Balaguer, A., Pagone, F., et al. (2009). Pharmacological interventions for preventing complications in idiopathic hypercalciuria. *Cochrane Database of Systematic Review*, 1:CD004754.

Faris, R., Flather, M. D., Purcell, H., et al. (2006). Diuretics for heart failure. Cochrane Database of Systematic Review.(1): CD003838.

Fernandez-Rodriguez, A., Arrabal-Martin, M., Garcia-Ruiz, M. J., et al. (2006). The role of thiazides in the prophylaxis of recurrent calcium lithiasis. *Actas Urologicas Españolas*, 30(3):305–309.

Jiang, J. Y., Wong, M. C., Ali, M. K., et al. (2009). Association of antihypertensive monotherapy with serum sodium and potassium levels in Chinese patients. *American Journal of Hypertension*, 22(3):243–249.

Kaplan, S. A., Roehrborn, C. G., Chancellor, M., et al. (2008). Extended-release tolterodine with or without tamsulosin in men with lower urinary tract symptoms and overactive bladder: effects on urinary symptoms assessed by the International Prostate Symptom Score. *BJU International*;102(9):1133–1139.

McCabe-Sellers, B. J., Sharkey, J. R., & Browne, B. A. (2005). Diuretic medication therapy use and low thiamin intake in homebound older adults. *Journal of Nutrition for the Elderly*, 24(4):57–71.

Levy, A. S., Coresh, J., Balk, E. et al. (2003). National Kidney Foundation Practice Guidelines for Chronic Kidney Disease: Evaluation, Classification, and Stratification. *Annals of Internal Medicine*, 139(2):137–147. Retrieved from *http://www.annals. org/cgi/content/full/139/2/137#otherarticles. Accessed October 16,2009.*

National Kidney Foundation. The Facts about Chronic Kidney Disease. Retrieved from: http://www.kidney.org/kidneydisease/ckd/index.cfm#facts Accessed October 18, 2009.

Paterna, S., Parrinello, G., Cannizzaro, S., et al. (2009). Medium term effects of different dosage of diuretic, sodium, and fluid administration on neurohormonal and clinical outcome in patients with recently compensated heart failure. *American Journal of Cardiology*, 103(1):93–102.

Peacock, W. F., Costanzo, M. R., De Marco, T., et al., for the ADHERE Scientific Advisory Committee and Investigators. Impact of Intravenous Loop Diuretics on Outcomes of Patients Hospitalized with Acute Decompensated Heart Failure: Insights from the ADHERE Registry. *Cardiology*,113,12ogyr

Salvador, D. R., Rey, N. R., Ramos, G. C., et al. (2005). Continuous infusion versus bolus injection of loop diuretics in congestive heart failure. *Cochrane Database Systemic Reviews,* 3:CD003178.

Wright, J. T., Jr, Probstfield, J. L., Cushman, W. C. et al. (2009). ALLHAT findings revisited in the context of subsequent analyses, other trials, and meta-analyses. *Archives of Internal Medicine,* 169(9):832–842.

28

Drugs Affecting Lipid Levels

Learning Objectives

At the completion of this chapter the student will:

1. Identify the core drug knowledge for drugs that affect lipid levels.

2. Differentiate the drug classes that affect lipid levels.

3. Identify core patient variables relevant to drugs that affect lipid levels.

4. Relate the interaction of core drug knowledge to core patient variables for drugs that affect lipid levels.

5. Generate a nursing plan of care from the interaction between core drug knowledge and core patient variables for drugs that affect lipid levels.

6. Describe nursing interventions to maximize therapeutic effects and minimize adverse effects for drugs that affect lipid levels.

7. Determine key points for patient and family education for drugs that affect lipid levels.

Key Terms   arteriosclerosis   hyperlipidemia
                 atherosclerosis   lipids

Drugs Affecting Lipid Levels

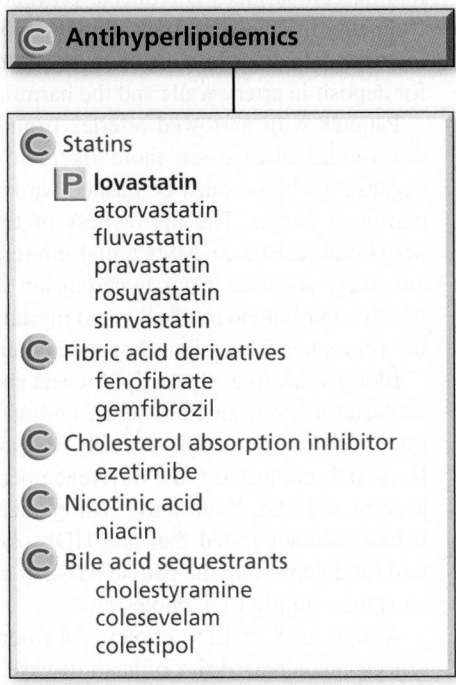

C Antihyperlipidemics

C Statins
P lovastatin
atorvastatin
fluvastatin
pravastatin
rosuvastatin
simvastatin

C Fibric acid derivatives
fenofibrate
gemfibrozil

C Cholesterol absorption inhibitor
ezetimibe

C Nicotinic acid
niacin

C Bile acid sequestrants
cholestyramine
colesevelam
colestipol

The symbol **C** indicates the drug class.
Drugs in **bold type** marked with the symbol **P** are prototypes.
Drugs in blue type are closely related to the prototype.
Drugs in red type are significantly different from the prototype.
Drugs in black type with no symbol are also used in drug therapy; no prototype.

lipids are fats or fat-like substances that are composed largely of carbon and hydrogen. They are generally insoluble in water. Involved mainly with long-term energy storage, they also function as structural components (as in the case of phospholipids, which are the major building blocks in cell membranes) and as "messengers" (hormones) that play roles in communications within and between cells. However, when serum lipid levels are too high, harmful effects on the body can result. High serum lipid levels are associated with hypertension, coronary artery disease, coronary heart disease, and other cardiovascular disorders. To decrease the risk of morbidity and mortality from lipid-induced pathologies, drug therapy to lower lipid levels is prescribed. This chapter discusses drugs used to lower serum lipid levels. The prototype drug is lovastatin (Mevacor).

PHYSIOLOGY

Serum **lipids** are fats found in the bloodstream. These lipids include cholesterol, cholesterol esters (compounds), phospholipids, and triglycerides. They are transported in the blood as part of large molecules called lipoproteins. The five major families of blood (plasma) lipoproteins are:

Chylomicrons
Very-low-density lipoproteins (VLDLs)
Intermediate-density lipoproteins (IDLs)
Low-density lipoproteins (LDLs)
High-density lipoproteins (HDLs)

Cholesterol is a soft, waxy substance found among the lipids in the bloodstream and in all of the body's cells. The body, mostly in the liver, produces essentially all of the cholesterol needed for normal functioning—about 1,000 mg a day. Cholesterol plays a role in forming cell membranes, some hormones, and other needed tissues. LDL is the major cholesterol carrier in the blood; about two thirds to three quarters of blood cholesterol is carried by LDL. LDL has a structure that can vary, based on its size and density. LDL includes VLDL and IDL. (IDL is considered an abnormal lipoprotein.) Lipoprotein a (Lp[a]) is a type of LDL and is considered a genetic variation. About one third to one fourth of blood cholesterol is carried by HDL. Chylomicrons are the largest and least dense of the lipoproteins. Triglycerides are transported primarily by the chylomicrons and VLDL, a subgroup of LDL.

PATHOPHYSIOLOGY

Hyperlipidemia is an elevation of blood lipid levels. Hyperlipidemia is considered a risk factor for the following disorders: **atherosclerosis** (also called **arteriosclerosis**), a narrowing of the arterial interior caused by buildup of hard, thick deposits, and a hardening and loss of elasticity of the arterial wall; coronary artery disease (CAD); and production of thromboses. How can cholesterol be both beneficial and potentially harmful? The receptors for LDL on the cell surface normally bind LDL circulating through the bloodstream, allowing the LDL and its cholesterol to enter cells and create its beneficial effects. When the amount of cholesterol within cells builds up, the number of these receptors on cell surfaces is reduced, preventing all of the lipids from entering the cells, thus allowing blood levels of LDL to increase. This can lead to more cholesterol being available for deposit in artery walls and the harmful effects.

Patients with narrowed arteries from atherosclerotic cardiovascular disease are more likely to have hypertension because the blood must be pushed harder to get through the narrowed lumen. The narrowness of the vessels increases peripheral resistance. Myocardial infarction (MI) and stroke are likely sequelae from hypertension and atherosclerosis, which contribute to morbidity and mortality. (See Chapter 26 for a complete discussion of hypertension and its treatments.)

Blood work to evaluate lipid levels should include a total cholesterol level, an LDL level, and an HDL level. Sometimes, the ratio of HDL to LDL is also given (Box 28.1). Non-HDL cholesterol, the difference between the total cholesterol and HDL cholesterol, is often measured and reported. It has been suggested that non-HDL cholesterol is a better tool for determining the patient's risk of cardiovascular problems than simply LDL cholesterol.

A high level of LDL cholesterol (more than 130 mg/dL) reflects an increased risk of heart disease, which is why LDL cholesterol is often called "bad" cholesterol. Lower levels of LDL cholesterol reflect a lower risk of heart disease. A high level of Lp(a) is an important risk factor for developing atherosclerosis prematurely. The way an increased Lp(a) level contributes to disease is not understood. The lesions in artery walls contain substances that may interact with Lp(a), leading to the buildup of lipids in atherosclerotic plaques.

Box 28.1 INTERPRETING BLOOD LIPID LEVELS

Total Cholesterol

- Less than 200 mg/dL: desirable blood cholesterol level
- 200 to 239 mg/dL: borderline-high blood cholesterol level
- 240 mg/dL and over: high blood cholesterol level

High-Density Lipoprotein (HDL) Cholesterol

- 40 to 59 mg/dL: desired HDL level
- Less than 35 mg/dL: low HDL level

Low-Density Lipoprotein (LDL) Cholesterol

- Less than 100 mg/dL: optimum desired LDL level
- Less than 70 mg/dL: reasonable goal if patient already has coronary or other atherosclerotic vascular disease
- More than 130 mg/dL: elevated LDL level

Non-HDL Concentration (recommended as second target of therapy if triglycerides greater than or equal to 200 mg/dL)

- Less than 130 mg/dL: desired goal

Medical experts think HDL tends to carry cholesterol away from the arteries and back to the liver, where it is passed from the body. Some experts believe HDL removes excess cholesterol from atherosclerotic plaques and thus slows their growth. HDL cholesterol is known as "good" cholesterol because a high level of HDL seems to protect against heart attack. The opposite is also true: a low HDL level (less than 35 mg/dL) indicates a greater risk of heart disease.

In most patients with cardiovascular disease, the underlying disorder is atherosclerosis, for which LDL is known to be a major risk factor. Elevated lipid levels are also a risk factor for CAD included in a group of atherosclerotic risk factors, known collectively as metabolic syndrome. The other risk factors include insulin resistance, obesity, and hypertension. Approximately 34% of American adults have metabolic syndrome. As age increases, it is more likely that the person will have metabolic syndrome, as men and women ages 40 to 59 years of age are about three times as likely as those 20 to 39 years of age to have metabolic syndrome, while men 60 years of age and over are more than four times as likely and women 60 years of age and over are more than six times as likely as the youngest age group to have metabolic syndrome. (Ervine, National Health statistics Reports, 2009). It is more difficult to describe the state of the problem in children and adolescents. At this time, there are limited studies examining how these risk factors (elevated lipid levels, insulin resistance, obesity, and hypertension) in children may relate to adult cardiovascular disease. A further complications is the fact that "there is still no universally accepted definition of metabolic syndrome in children and adolescents, the criteria used in pediatric studies have been variably adapted from adult standards with the use of gender- and age-dependent normal values" (AHA scientific statement, 2009). Despite the lack of a research-based definition, there is agreement that known adult cardiovascular-metabolic risk factors should be assessed in youth, and that early detection and preventive measures for these risk factors in children and adolescents is important. The current state of the science encourages assessing children and adolescents for these risk factors for metabolic syndrome: obesity, inflammation, insulin resistance, dyslipidemia, and hypertension, as long term in adulthood these increase morbidity. The best recommendation at the present time for the treatment of children with these cardiovascular-metabolic risk factors is to reduce obesity, encourage an increase in physical activity, and to treat the various components of the metabolic syndrome (e.g., hypertension or hyperlipidemia; AHA scientific statement, 2009).

Data from epidemiologic studies and from clinical trials have shown that lowering cholesterol levels is associated with a lower overall risk for morbidity and mortality because of coronary heart disease. Additionally, aggressive reduction of cholesterol can yield more clinical benefits than can be achieved with less aggressive therapy even after acute coronary syndrome (Murphy, Cannon, Wiviott, et al., 2007; Wiviott, de Lemos, Cannon, et al., 2006; Grundy, Cleeman, Bairey Merz, et al., 2004). Left ventricular mass is also a powerful predictor for future cardiovascular events; hyperlipidemia is associated with higher left ventricular mass. The healthy endothelium usually provides an anticoagulant, vasodilatory, and anti-inflammatory array of functions, which are basic to vascular homeostasis. Dysfunction of the endothelium is a common pathologic feature evident in all phases of atherosclerosis. Hypercholesterolemia (elevated LDL levels) provokes many aspects of endothelial dysfunction, both before and during the thickening of the walls of the larger arteries in atherosclerosis.

Guidelines from the Third Report of the National Cholesterol Education Program (NCEP), Adult Treatment Panel (ATP III) (Grundy et al., 2004) (NOTE TO EDITOR: the fourth report is due out summer 2010) recommend that total cholesterol levels be less than 200 mg/dL; LDL cholesterol levels optimally should be less than 100 mg/dL, and HDL levels should be between 40 and 59 mg/dL. The recommended LDL levels have been shifted downward considerably from previous recommendations, as studies continue to show that lower LDL levels decrease risk of coronary heart disease (CHD). Many Americans have cholesterol levels that greatly exceed these recommendations. About 17% of adult Americans aged 20 years and older have high total cholesterol (240 mg/dL or above). The average blood cholesterol level in adult Americans is about 203 mg/dL (CDC website). Put another way, over 106 million American adults (age 20 and older) have total blood cholesterol values of 200 mg/dL and higher, and about 37 million American adults have levels of 240 or higher. Elevations of LDL cholesterol (130mg/dL or higher), the "bad" cholesterol, occurs in about 30% to 40% of the populations, with variations by sex and race. The highest occurrence is in Mexican-American men (39%) and the lowest is in black women (29.8%; American Heart Association cholesterol statistics, 2008). Unfortunately, several studies and literature analyses have shown that practitioners undertreat elevated cholesterol levels, either by not prescribing drug therapy or by not prescribing a dose high enough to aggressively and effectively bring the total cholesterol and LDL levels down to recommended levels. In these studies, only 6% to 38% of patients had their lipid levels lowered to the level recommended in current clinical guidelines (Smith, Allen, Blair, et al., 2006).

Triglyceride levels have also been shown to be an independent risk factor for CHD. It has been hypothesized that triglyceride-rich lipoproteins move into macrophages in the bloodstream and then interact with small, dense LDL and HDL particles to form arterial thromboses. However, so far, clinical studies have not been able to demonstrate that lowering triglycerides alone will decrease the rate of MIs. The effect of lowering triglyceride levels may therefore be linked to lowering cholesterol, or to some other, unknown, process.

Patients who have combined hyperlipidemia (elevation of more than one lipid) exhibit a set lipid profile; it is hypothesized that such patients have an atherogenic lipoprotein phenotype. This phenotype is associated with elevated triglyceride levels, low levels of HDL, and a preponderance of small, dense, atherogenic LDL particles. These patients are at an increased risk of CHD, regardless of their total LDL. Research suggests that when plasma triglycerides exceed a critical level, approximately 133 mg/dL, the formation of small, dense LDL from larger, less dense LDL particles is more likely to occur. Lipid-lowering drugs that are also capable of lowering triglyceride levels below this critical level thus cause a shift to a less dense, and therefore less athero-genic, LDL profile.

Patients with diabetes are considered to be at high risk from elevated lipid levels because a link has been established between elevated cholesterol levels and diabetic nephropathy. High serum cholesterol levels seem to have the same effect on glomerular mesangial cells as on the endothelial cells in the vasculature. Thus, an atherosclerotic-like process appears to occur in the cells of the kidneys because the mesangial cells possess binding sites for LDL and oxidized LDL. Cho-lesterol lowering has been shown to have a beneficial effect on renal function in patients with diabetes.

Lifestyle and Reduction of Low-Density Lipoprotein Levels

The NCEP ATP III recommends a multipronged approach in reducing LDL levels. They title this approach *therapeutic lifestyle changes*. These lifestyle changes include reduced intake of saturated fats, trans fats, and cholesterol; minimum intake of fatty acids; weight reduction; increased physi-cal activity; increased intake of soluble fiber; and possibly increased intake of plant stanols and sterols (Table 28.1). Drug therapy is added if lipid levels are substantially ele-vated, if the patient has major risk factors for CHD even if lipid levels are not elevated (Box 28.2), or if the patient

TABLE 28.1	Daily Recommendations in Therapeutic Lifestyle Changes Die
Food Element	**Recommended Daily Intake**
Saturated fat	Less than 7% of total calories
Trans fatty acids	No percentage established; should be kept low
Polyunsaturated fat	Up to 10% of total calories
Monounsaturated fat	Up to 20% of total calories
Cholesterol	Less than 200 mg
Carbohydrate (predominantly complex sources including whole grains, fruit, and vegetables)	50%–60% of total calories
Fiber	20–39 g
Protein	Approximately 15% of total calories
Total calories	Balance intake with expenditure to maintain desirable body weight and prevent weight gain

From: Third Report of the National Cholesterol Education Program (NCEP) Expert Panel on Detection, Evaluation, and Treatment of High Blood Cholesterol in Adults (Adult Treatment Panel III). (2004). Executive Summary [O nline]. Available: *http:// www.nhlbi.nih.gov/ guidelines/cholesterol/atp3xsum.pdf.*

Box 28.2 CORONARY HEART DISEASE (CHD) EQUIVALENTS AND MAJOR RISK FACTORS FOR CHD

CHD equivalents are those risk factors that place the patient at similar risk for CHD events as a history of actual CHD.

- Diabetes mellitus
- Symptoms of carotid artery disease
- Peripheral arterial disease
- Abdominal aortic aneurysm
- Multiple risk factors (listed below)

Major CHD risk factors increase the risk of CHD. When two or more of them are present in a patient without CHD or CHD equivalent, they should be treated as if they have diagnosed CHD.

- Cigarette smoking
- Hypertension (blood pressure greater than 140/90 mm Hg or use of antihypertensive medication)
- Low HDL cholesterol (<40 mg/dL)
- Family history of premature CHD
- Age (men = 45 years, women = 55 years)

Although other risk factors for CHD have been suggested, there is no evidence from controlled trials that targeting these risk factors will improve patient outcomes. Thus, their presence does not influence current guidelines for cholesterol lowering. These other possible risk factors include obesity; physical inactivity; impaired fasting glucose; markers for inflammation, homocysteine, and abnormalities of throm-bosis; and endothelial dysfunction.

has been diagnosed with CHD. Please consult online for updates, to be published as NCEP ATP IV.

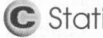 ANTIHYPERLIPIDEMICS

Lowering serum lipid levels decreases the risk of atheroscle-rosis, hypertension, and CHD. Lowering cholesterol levels can stop or reverse atherosclerosis in all vascular beds. Each 10% reduction in cholesterol levels is associated with a reduc-tion of approximately 20% to 30% in the incidence of CHD. Because most cholesterol is carried by the LDL and VLDL, it is important to target these lipoproteins, especially in drug therapy. The antihyperlipidemics are composed of the statins (also referred to as 3-hydroxy-3-methyl-glutaryl coenzyme A [HMG-CoA] reductase inhibitors), the fibric acid derivatives, cholesterol absorption inhibitors, nicotinic acid, the bile acid sequestrants, and dextrothyroxine sodium. Although these types of antihyperlipidemics work in slightly different ways, they all decrease cholesterol levels; most decrease triglycer-ide levels, most decrease LDL and VLDL levels, and most also increase HDL levels.

Statins

Statins lower blood cholesterol levels and thus decrease the uptake of modified lipoproteins by vascular cells. Statin therapy can lower LDL cholesterol by approximately 20% to 55% when given at the maximum recommended dose. Statins also raise HDL levels between 5% and 15% and lower triglycerides between 7% and 30%. (ATP III, 2004). In addition, evidence exists that statins work in other ways besides lowering cholesterol levels to decrease the occurrence of cardiovascular events. The drugs appear to have a positive effect on the vascular endothelium, by restoring it or improving its function. Statins seem to exert this effect by increasing the bioavailability of nitric oxide, which promotes vasodilation, promoting re-endothelialization, reducing oxidative stress (antioxidant effect), and inhibiting the inflammatory response (levels of C-reactive protein, an inflammatory marker, fall with statin therapy). Statins are also known to stabilize plaque in blood vessels (ruptured plaque is a central component of acute coronary syndrome) and to decrease thrombogenicity of blood (i.e., the likelihood that blood clots).

Statins are the only class of antilipid drugs identified in clinical trials to decrease overall mortality in both primary (before the patient has clinical evidence of CAD) and secondary (established CAD) prevention. Statins have also been found to decrease the risk of stroke in both primary and secondary prevention studies. Long-term statin use has been found to decrease mortality by 24% to 42% in patients with CAD. They provide additional effectiveness when used jointly with other therapies for heart disease, such as angiotensin converting enzyme inhibitors (ACE inhibitors), angiotensin receptor blockers (ARBs), and beta blockers. Unfortunately, many patients are not prescribed statins as often as recommended. (See Focus on Research Box 28.3: Statins Are Underprescribed.) The Heart Protection Study showed statin therapy to be effective in preventing CAD in patients at high risk (those with cerebrovascular disease, peripheral arterial disease, or diabetes), even if their blood lipid levels were not elevated when therapy began. In fact, this study suggests that the target level of less than 100 mg/dL, recommended by the Third Report of the NCEP Expert Panel, should be even lower (i.e., below 70 mg/dL), and that continued benefit may be derived from decreasing lipids to such levels. Those with acute coronary syndrome or at very high risk for CHD events may benefit the most from intensive lipid-lowering therapy. Two large-scale clinical trials, the Aggrastat to Zocor (A to Z) trial and the Pravastatin or Atorvastatin Evaluation and Infection Therapy-Thrombolysis in Myocardial Infarction 22 (PROVE-IT-TIMI 22) trials, found that continued intensive therapy with statins to lower lipids significantly decreased mortality in patients after an MI (Murphy, Cannon, Wiviott, et al., 2007; Wiviott, de Lemos, Cannon, et al., 2006). Older adults, as well as middle-aged adults, benefit from aggressive statin use in hypercholesterolemia. Thus, aggressive use of statin therapy has been found to be effective in primary and secondary prevention of a variety of cardiac complications.

Not all researchers agree, however, with the conclusion that an LDL level below 70 mg/dL is likely to bring additional cardiovascular benefits (Hayward, Hofer, & Vijan, 2006). Patients may need large doses of a statin to decrease their LDL to this level. However, high doses of statins carry an increased risk of adverse effects. Therefore, a more moderate dosing approach is suggested by some experts as prudent for patients who do not have very high cardiovascular risks; the dose should be the lowest possible that can achieve an LDL below 100 mg/dL . Whether the absolute value of the LDL or the percentage that the LDL has been decreased is the best indication of potential benefit from statin therapy is still the subject of debate.

Because of the anti-inflammatory effects of statins, further research indicates that statins can decrease morbidity and mortality associated with peripheral arterial disease (Hankey, Norman, & Eikelboom, 2006). They may play a role in the treatment of rheumatoid arthritis, multiple sclerosis, other neuroinflammatory disorders, and chronic renal disease (Weber and Zamvil, 2009; Shaw, Fildes, Yonan, et al., 2009; Steffens & Mach, 2006). More research is needed on the potential future uses of statins.

Although all the statins are considered to act similarly, some pharmacologic differences exist among them. The most notable difference is metabolism by the P-450 3A4 isoenzyme. All of the statins, with the exception of pravastatin and fluvastatin, are primarily metabolized by this pathway. Coadministration of drugs that inhibit this pathway will therefore decrease the metabolism of these statins and increase their circulating blood levels. This increase may contribute to adverse effects, especially myalgia (muscle aches or weakness without creatine kinase [CK] elevations), myositis (muscle symptoms with elevated CK levels), and rhabdomyolysis (a potentially lethal event with muscle symptoms with high CK levels and creatinine elevations). Individual, innate differences in the amount of P-450 3A4 isoenzyme available are also a factor in the metabolism of these statins. These differences can account for why some patients can tolerate a particular dose of a statin, or tolerate a statin in combination with an inhibitor of P-450 3A4 without complications, whereas others cannot. There is no way to predict inherited variability to increases in drug concentration from drug–drug interactions. Thus, patients need to be assessed for individual response to therapy. Certain fibric acid derivatives (also called fibrates), another drug class used to alter lipid levels, which may be combined with statins, have been found to have their own independent adverse effect of myopathy. When combined with some statins, but again not with pravastatin, elevations of statin levels may occur in some individuals, increasing the risk of myopathies.

Because so much research has shown the superior effectiveness of the statins, they are the most used antihyperlipidemic agents. When a patient follows a low-fat diet, the benefits of statin therapy are greater than those achieved by drug therapy alone. Unfortunately, multiple research studies show that statins continue to be underutilized (Smith, Allen, Blair, et al., 2006), and patients are not being treated to achieve the levels recommended in clinical guidelines (see Box 28.3).

Lovastatin (Mevacor) is the prototype statin discussed in this chapter. The other classes of antihyperlipidemic drugs will be discussed as drugs significantly different from lovastatin. Table 28.2 displays a summary of selected antihyperlipidemics.

BOX 28.3 FOCUS ON RESEARCH

Statins Are Underprescribed

Lee, H. Y., Cooke, C. E., Robertson, T. A. (2008). Use of secondary prevention drug therapy in patients with acute coronary syndrome after hospital discharge. *Journal of managed care pharmacy*, 14(3):271–280.
Kristianson, K., Fyhrquist, F., Devereux, R. B., et al. (2003). An analysis of cholesterol control and statin use in the Losartan Intervention for Endpoint Reduction in Hypertension Study. *Clinical Therapeutics*, 25(4):1186–1199.

The Study

With the onset of a acute coronary syndrome (ACS, which includes unstable angina, non-Q-wave myocardial infarction, and Q-wave-myocardial infarction), clinical guidelines call for the use of an angiotensin converting enzyme (ACE) inhibitor (or an angiotensin receptor blocker, ARB), a beta blocker, and a statin as combination therapy to decrease the risk of complications and death from the acute coronary syndrome. Research was conducted over a 1-year period on patients from a Mid-Atlantic managed care insurance group with a prescription benefit; the selected patients had been hospitalized with a diagnosis of ACS. The purpose of the study was to determine whether patients were receiving the evidence-based drug therapy for their ACS.

Of the 1,135 members with ACS, less than one-third (only 29.9%) of them filled at least one prescription for all three drugs while a little more than half filled at least 1 prescription for 1 or more of the three drugs in the 3-month period after their hospitalization for ACS. Patients who were between the ages of 45 to 64 years were the most likely to receive statins, compared to other age groups ($p < 0.05$). Women were less likely than men to receive statins ($p = 0.004$) and all 3 drug classes ($p = 0.012$). The severity of their illness played a significant role in whether they received the evidence-based drug therapy, as patients with intermediate coronary syndrome were significantly less likely than those with acute MI to receive any of the recommended drugs ($p < 0.001$). Patients who received the recommended drug therapy before hospitalization for ACS were more likely to receive these drugs again after hospitalization, compared to those who did not receive these drugs pre-hospitalization.

What is especially distressing about this study is that the findings are nearly identical to the findings on statin use in a previous, large, multicenter research study, the Losartan Intervention for Endpoint Reduction in Hypertension Study, published in 2003, that was conducted with 9,193 patients aged 55 to 80 years with hypertension and left ventricular hypertrophy. The use of statin therapy was left to the discretion of the cardiologist who was the investigator at each trial center location. After the primary study on losartan use was completed, a secondary study examined the baseline and the end-of-study mean total cholesterol and high-density lipoprotein cholesterol levels and the use of statins.. At the end of the study, only approximately 22% of the patients had been started on statin therapy, and almost 60% of these patients still had cholesterol levels above guideline

recommendations. Of those not receiving statins by the end of the study, nearly 79% had cholesterol levels in excess of those recommended. In this large study, statins were not optimally administered, and cholesterol levels were poorly controlled.

Nursing Implications

Elevated cholesterol levels have been known for some time to be a risk factor for cardiovascular events in patients. It has also been known for some time that lipid levels are undertreated, even with effective drug therapy available. Although in the 5 years between the reporting of these 2 studies there was a slight increase in the prescribed use of statins, statins are still under-prescribed despite clinical guidelines that show they are evidence-based care for patients with ACS. Although it is possible that patients were not filling the prescriptions given to them by their health care provider, the results of these studies lead additional credence to the belief that even cardiologists, who work with patients known to have high cholesterol and high-risk factors for cardiovascular events, tend to undertreat patients. Clearly more aggressive therapy is warranted to help reduce morbidity and mortality from elevated lipid levels. Additionally, this newer research confirms that there is some prescribing bias for statin use, where women and older adults are less likely to receive statin therapy even when it would be clinically useful. Exactly why this occurs is not known.

So why are the clinical guidelines regarding statin use not being followed, and what can nurses do to help patients with elevated cholesterol levels? First, nurses need to be knowledgeable about current guidelines for lipid management. Nurse practitioners should aggressively treat lipid levels in their patients with elevated lipid profiles by prescribing statin therapy and making sure that the prescribed drug and dose effectively lower lipid levels. Nurses who do not prescribe drug therapy should monitor patients' lipid levels carefully and consult with either the physician or nurse practitioner when the levels are above guideline recommendations and indicate that drug therapy is warranted. Nurses should pay special attention to female patients and older adult patients, as these patients appear less likely to receive evidence-based drug therapy with statins than other groups of patients. Nurses in a hospital setting may also participate in hospital-wide, multidisciplinary committees or quality-improvement projects that are charged with setting drug protocols and standards to ensure that the institution is following the current clinical guidelines. To help minimize the risk that prescriptions are being written but not filled by patients, nurses in all practice settings need to be active in patient education to help patients and their families understand the importance of reducing blood cholesterol and lipid levels and the role that drug therapy can play in achieving this goal. Additionally, nurses should include diet modification information and stress the importance of exercise in their patient teaching about reducing blood lipid levels.

Nursing Management of the Patient Receiving Lovastatin

Core Drug Knowledge

Pharmacotherapeutics

Lovastatin is used in the treatment of primary hypercholesterolemia and combined hyperlipidemia (also referred to as mixed dyslipidemia). It is also used in the secondary prevention of coronary events (e.g., MI, stroke) from thrombus formation.

Off-label uses of lovastatin include the treatment of diabetic dyslipidemia, nephrotic hyperlipidemia, neck artery disease, familial dysbetalipoproteinemia (alterations of the beta or LDL lipoproteins in the blood), and familial combined hyperlipidemia.

Lovastatin is available in both rapid-release and extended-release forms. Unlike the other statins, it is now available as both a trade name and a generic drug.

TABLE 28.2 Summary of Selected Ⓒ Antihyperlipidemics

Drug (Trade) Name	Selected Indications	Route and Dosage Range	Pharmacokinetics
Ⓒ Statins			
Ⓟ lovastatin (Mevacor	Reduce serum cholesterol levels	*Adult:* PO, 20–80 mg/d in single or divided dose	*Onset:* 1–2 wk *Duration:* Length of therapy $t_{1/2}$: 3–4 h
simvastatin (Zocor)	Reduce serum cholesterol and triglyceride levels	*Adult:* PO, 5–40 mg/d as single dose in the evening	*Onset:* 1–2 wk *Duration:* Length of therapy $t_{1/2}$: 3 h
pravastatin (Pravachol)	Reduce serum cholesterol and triglyceride levels	*Adult:* PO, 10–40 mg/d at bedtime	*Onset:* 1–2 wk *Duration:* Length of therapy $t_{1/2}$: 1.8 h
fluvastatin (Lescol)	Reduce serum cholesterol and triglyceride levels	*Adult:* PO, 20–80 mg/d single dose in the evening	*Onset:* 1–2 wk *Duration:* Length of therapy $t_{1/2}$: 1.2 h
Other Antihyperlipidemics			
cholestyramine (Questran)	Lower serum cholesterol levels	*Adult:* PO, powder, 4 g, one to two times daily, mixed in 60–180 mL of water or noncarbonated drink	*Onset:* Unabsorbed *Duration:* 1 mo after therapy concludes $t_{1/2}$: Unknown
colestipol (Colestid)	Lower serum cholesterol levels	*Adult:* PO, granules, 5–30 g/d mixed in about 90 mL of liquid; tablets, 2–16 g/d; may be divided	*Onset:* Unabsorbed *Duration:* Same as above $t_{1/2}$: Unknown
clofibrate (Atromid-S)	Reduce serum cholesterol and triglyceride levels	*Adult:* PO, 2 g/d in divided doses	*Onset:* Unknown *Duration:* Length of therapy $t_{1/2}$: 15 h (up to 110 h in renal impaired)
nicotinic acid (niacin, vitamin B_3)	Reduce serum cholesterol and triglyceride levels	*Adult:* PO, 1–2 g tid with meals; maximum 8 g/d; dietary supplement, 100–500 mg/d	*Onset:* Up to several days *Duration:* Length of therapy $t_{1/2}$: Unknown
gemfibrozil (Lopid)	Reduce serum cholesterol and triglyceride levels	*Adult:* PO, 1,200 mg/d in two divided doses, 30 min before meals	*Onset:* Unknown *Duration:* Length of therapy $t_{1/2}$: 1.5 h (plasma)

Pharmacokinetics

Although about 35% of the drug is absorbed, lovastatin has a high first-pass effect because metabolism by the isoenzyme CYP3A4 (an important subset of the CYP-450 family) allows less than 5% of the oral dose to reach the general circulation. An active metabolite, lovastatin acid, is formed from metabolism. The drug is highly protein bound (more than 95%). It is excreted primarily through the gastrointestinal (GI) tract in the feces, but about 10% is eliminated in the urine. Severe renal disease increases plasma concentration of lovastatin. Immediate-release forms are best absorbed after a meal. In contrast, extended-release forms have their absorption impaired by food.

Pharmacodynamics

Lovastatin, as well as the other statins, competitively inhibits HMG-CoA reductase, which is the enzyme that catalyzes the early rate-limiting step in cholesterol biosynthesis. The effect is to increase HDL and to decrease LDL, total cholesterol, VLDL, and plasma triglycerides. The mechanism that lowers LDL may involve both reduction of VLDL concentrations and increased catabolism of LDL. In clinical trials, lovastatin reduced total cholesterol between 16% and 29%, decreased LDL levels between 21% and 40%, decreased triglyceride levels between 6% and 30%, and increased levels of HDL between 2% and 9.5%.

This drug, as well as the others in the class, is highly effective in reducing total cholesterol and the LDL level in heterozygous familial and nonfamilial forms of hypercholesterolemia. The lipid lowering that occurs with the statins, such as lovastatin, is known to reduce the progression of atherosclerosis, reduce blood thrombogenicity, prevent MI and stroke, and prolong survival in patients with atherosclerosis.

Contraindications and Precautions

Contraindications include active liver disease, unexplained persistently elevated results of liver function tests, pregnancy (lovastatin is pregnancy category X), and breast-feeding. Heavy alcohol use increases the risk of liver dysfunction. Precaution should be used if lovastatin is coadministered with drugs that inhibit the CYP3A4 hepatic pathway (such as erythromycin or protease inhibitors), with large intake (more than 1 quart daily) of grapefruit juice, or with drugs that also can produce myopathy, such as fibric acid derivatives. Older adults, especially if they have other complicated co-morbidities, are more at risk of myopathy or rhabodomyolosis and thus should be monitored closely if they receive lovastatin. High-dose therapy of lovastatin is also associated with more risk for myopathy and rhabdomyolysis (see discussion below under Adverse Effects).

Precaution should be used if the patient has preexisiting amyotrophic lateral sclerosis (ALS), as the rate of functional decline that occurs with ALS may accelerate if given statins. Caution is needed if the patient has a history of renal insufficiency, as there can be an increased risk of rhabdomyolysis, especially in larger doses. Patients who must stop taking lovastatin due to needing surgery or hospitalization for a major medical condition may be at increased risk of developing rhabdomyolysis and should be monitored closely. Finally, patients who have homozygous familial hypercholesterolemia are at risk for reduced efficacy of lovastatin and an increased risk of elevated liver enzymes.

Adverse Effects

Adverse effects of lovastatin are usually mild and transient; the drug is generally well tolerated. A fairly common complaint with all statins, including lovastatin, is nonspecific muscle aches or joint aches, weakness, and/or cramps (myalgias), which are not associated with any signs of muscle damage. Usually this adverse effect is tolerable, but occasionally it is bothersome enough that the drug needs to be discontinued.

One adverse effect with potentially serious consequences is muscle damage, the exact cause of which is not known. The most serious skeletal muscle effect that may result from lovastatin is rhabdomyolysis, although it is very rare (occurring in 0.1% of patients on statins as monotherapy). Rhabdomyolysis is an acute, sometimes fatal disease, in which direct injury to the plasma membrane of the skeletal muscle occurs (manifested by increased levels of CK, also known as creatine phosphokinase [CPK]). The damage to the muscle causes leakage of the skeletal muscle components (myoglobin) into the blood or the urine. Brown urine usually occurs. Rhabdomyolysis can lead to acute renal failure and death. Diagnosis of rhabdomyolysis is made when the CK (1) is greater than 10,000 U/L regardless of whether there is any change in renal function or (2) is greater than 10 times the upper normal limit with worsening renal function and/or a medical requirement for intravenous hydration therapy. The risk of renal failure from rhabdomyolysis is increased if the patient is also taking drugs that share the same common metabolic path, such as cyclosporine or nicotinic acid.

Less serious muscle damage can also occur from statin therapy, and this is called myopathy. Myopathy should be considered in any patient who receives lovastatin and who shows diffuse myalgia, muscle tenderness or weakness, *and* has CK levels 10 times above the upper limit of normal. According to some sources, CK laboratory tests greater than 10 times the upper limit of normal should be repeated to confirm them prior to making a final diagnosis. The rate of serious myopathy appears to be equivalent among all the statins. Elevations of CK are believed to be dose dependent. If the myopathy is intolerable, then statin therapy should be discontinued. Stopping the drug should eliminate the symptoms (McKenney, Davidson, Jacobson, et al., 2006).

Transient, mildly elevated CK levels are common, especially in the first 3 months of therapy. These levels do not indicate a serious problem and should not be confused with myopathy or rhabdomyolysis. Drug therapy does not need to be stopped or modified so long as the patient is asymptomatic.

Lovastatin is likely to produce an elevation in the hepatic enzymes (measured by the laboratory tests alanine aminotransferase [ALT] and aspartate aminotransferase [AST]) to more than three times the upper limit of normal. This may occur fairly frequently and is usually dose related. The exact cause is not known. The increased levels of ALT and AST are usually transient, resolving spontaneously even if the specific statin and its dose are unchanged. Because of this, some sources believe that laboratory studies must indicate high enzyme levels on two consecutive occasions prior to making changes in the drug therapy. About 2% of patients taking lovastatin have marked persistent elevations of liver enzymes. There is still debate whether these greatly elevated liver enzymes can cause serious liver dysfunction or failure. Although some sources show that the rate of reported liver failure is the same whether or not a statin is used, the Food and Drug Administration (FDA) label on lovastatin and other statins states that liver failure is a rare adverse effect of the drug (McKenney, Davidson, Jacobson, et al., 2006).

Adverse effects that can occur but are not considered serious include effects in the central nervous system, such as headache, dizziness, and insomnia. GI complaints include nausea and vomiting, diarrhea, abdominal pain and cramps, constipation, flatulence, heartburn, dyspepsia, and altered taste. Other adverse effects are chest pain, rash, blurred vision, and alopecia. Statins such as lovastatin have not been found to cause renal failure (Kasiske, Wanner, & O'Neill, 2006; McKenney, Davidson, Jacobson, et al., 2006). Rarely, if ever, do the drugs cause peripheral neuropathy (Law & Rudnicka, 2006; McKenney, Davidson, Jacobson, et al., 2006).

Drug Interactions

Because lovastatin is metabolized through the hepatic enzyme CYP3A4, all inhibitors of this pathway have the potential to interact with the drug, decreasing its metabolism and elevating, sometimes dramatically, its level in the blood. Examples of CYP3A4 inhibitors are itraconazole (an antifungal), erythromycin (an antimicrobial), protease inhibitors (anti-HIV drugs) and grapefruit juice, which has been shown to substantially increase the serum levels of lovastatin and lovastatin acid (the active metabolite). Drugs that compete with lovastatin for metabolism by CYP3A4 also have the potential to interact with lovastatin. Rhabdomyolysis has been reported in heart transplant recipients who were treated with both lovastatin and cyclosporine (an antirejection drug used in the process of organ transplantation that is also metabolized by CYP3A4). Table 28.3 lists drugs that interact with lovastatin.

Food appears to increase drug absorption and elevate blood levels of lovastatin.

Laboratory tests that are altered by lovastatin use include increased serum transaminases AST, ALT, CPK, alkaline phosphatase, bilirubin, and γ-glutamyl transpeptidase, as well as thyroid function test abnormalities.

CRITICAL THINKING SCENARIO

MANAGING ADVERSE EFFECTS OF LOVASTATIN THERAPY

Janice Klinefelter, age 64 years, has been taking the lipid-lowering statin drug lovastatin for 9 months. She has tolerated the drug therapy well and up to this point has had no major adverse effects. Her cholesterol and LDL levels are close to reaching the desired goal. During an office follow-up visit, she complains that she must be getting old because she feels stiff and her leg muscles are cramping and painful, problems she has never complained of before. Her blood work, drawn the day before the office visit, shows that her liver function enzyme levels (AST and ALT) are mildly elevated, and her creatine kinase levels are four times upper normal levels. At baseline, both blood tests were within the normal range. She denies having started any new medication.

1. What questions would you ask Ms. Klinefelter as part of your assessment?
2. What course of action would you choose now?
3. What teaching would you provide to Ms. Klinefelter?

TABLE 28.3 Agents That Interact with P Lovastatin		
Interactants	**Effect and Significance**	**Nursing Management**
azole antifungals itraconazole ketoconazole	Increases lovastatin levels about 20-fold. May increase risk of adverse effects, including myopathy.	Consult with provider regarding temporarily stopping or reducing the dose of lovastatin while on the antifungal.
bile acid sequestrants	Decreases the bioavailability and effect of lovastatin and other statins.	Give the bile acid sequestrant 4 h after lovastatin.
cyclosporine	Increases circulating levels of lovastatin and increases risk of severe myopathy or rhabdomyolysis.	Consult with provider about stopping lovastatin or decreasing the dose. Monitor closely for adverse effects.
erythromycin	Increases circulating levels of lovastatin and increases risk of severe myopathy or rhabdomyolysis.	Consult with provider about stopping lovastatin or decreasing the dose. Monitor closely for adverse effects.
gemfibrozil	Increases circulating levels of lovastatin; severe myopathy or rhabdomyolysis reported.	Avoid this combination if at all possible.
isradipine	May increase clearance of lovastatin and its metabolites by increasing hepatic blood flow. This decreases the effect of lovastatin.	Increased dose for lovastatin may be needed; consult with provider if patient is not achieving desired cholesterol goals.
nicotinic acid	Increases circulating levels of lovastatin and increases risk of severe myopathy or rhabdomyolysis.	Consult with provider about stopping lovastatin or decreasing the dose. Monitor closely for adverse effects.
digoxin	Elevates digoxin levels slightly.	Monitor digoxin levels. Assess for signs of digoxin toxicity.
Warfarin	Increases prothrombin time. Bleeding has occurred in some patients receiving both drugs.	Monitor for bleeding. Consult with provider regarding adjusting dose of warfarin downward as needed to keep prothrombin time in therapeutic range.
grapefruit juice	Decreases metabolism of lovastatin via CYP3A4, so circulating levels of lovastatin will increase, placing the patient at increased risk of adverse effects.	Monitor for adverse effects. Assess labs for elevated liver enzymes and CPK levels.

Assessment of Relevant Core Patient Variables

Health Status

Before lovastatin therapy begins, the patient's serum cholesterol and lipid levels should be determined and a health history of diseases that contribute to increased blood cholesterol and LDL levels taken. These conditions include hypothyroidism, poorly controlled diabetes mellitus, nephrotic syndrome, dysproteinemia, obstructive liver disease, and alcoholism. These conditions should be investigated and treated before starting lovastatin. Assess for active liver disease because it is a contraindication for taking lovastatin. Also, determine liver function through liver enzyme measurements for baseline knowledge. Lovastatin, as well as other statins, should not be given if the patient has active liver disease or unexplained persistently elevated liver function test results (e.g., liver enzymes greater than three times the upper normal limit) because additional elevation of liver enzyme levels occurs during therapy with lovastatin and all statins. A baseline CK level should be drawn; many patients routinely have asymptomatic CK elevations, and knowing of such elevations at baseline assists in clinical decision making later in therapy.

Be aware that patients who have undergone organ transplantation and who require lifelong multidrug therapy are at increased risk for experiencing drug–drug interactions when also receiving lovastatin. Patients with chronic disease states such as diabetes and hypothyroidism are also at risk.

Determine whether the patient is receiving other drugs that are metabolized by (i.e., are substrates of) CYP3A4 or that inhibit metabolism by CYP3A4, because there may be potential drug interactions when starting lovastatin.

Assess the patient's body frame because a small body frame and frailty pose an increased risk for drug-related myopathy.

Assess for the presence of amyotrophic lateral sclerosis (ALS, also referred to as Lou Gehrig disease), as research has shown that these patients have a 63% increase in the rate of functional decline from their ALS when they take a statin drug.

Life Span and Gender

Determine whether the patient is pregnant or considering becoming pregnant because lovastatin is a pregnancy category X drug. Animal studies have shown skeletal malformations, but no such data exist for humans. However, fetal harm is likely because of the decrease in cholesterol synthesis and possibly other products in the cholesterol biosynthesis pathway. Lovastatin is excreted in breast milk; thus, breast-feeding should be avoided while taking this drug.

Older adults, because they are likely to have more drugs prescribed to them than younger people, are more at risk for drug interactions when receiving lovastatin. Adults older than 80 years, especially women, seem most at risk for statin-associated myopathy. However, information gleaned from clinical trials indicates that older adults benefit from lipid-lowering therapy as much as younger adults; therefore, treatment with lipid-lowering drugs is worthwhile in older adults and is recommended.

Safety and efficacy in patients younger than 18 years have not been determined. Treatment in this age group is not recommended at this time.

Lifestyle, Diet, and Habits

Before starting drug therapy, patients should be treated with nonpharmacologic methods of controlling cholesterol and lipids, including dieting to reduce cholesterol levels and LDL levels, exercising, and normalizing weight if needed. Diet therapy usually continues for 12 weeks before drug therapy starts and should be continued even after drug therapy is started.

Determine whether the patient has alcoholism, which may be a secondary cause of hyperlipidemia. High alcohol use also increases the risk of liver dysfunction. Determine whether the patient regularly drinks grapefruit juice and how much is usually consumed, because grapefruit juice is a major inhibitor of the CYP3A4 isoenzyme necessary for lovastatin metabolism. Patients should not consume more than a quart per day of grapefruit juice, as this amount is likely to produce alterations in metabolism of lovastatin and increase the risk for adverse effects.

Environment

Lovastatin may be started in any environment. Because therapy extends over a prolonged period, the drug is usually taken by the patient at home or in a long-term care facility.

Culture and Inherited Traits

Explore whether the patient observes cultural or religious dietary practices that promote high intake of fats and cholesterol.

Nursing Diagnoses and Outcomes

- Risk for Injury related to elevated blood lipid levels
  Desired outcome: The patient's blood lipid levels will be controlled without the patient's sustaining an injury.
- Risk for Injury to skeletal muscles related to adverse effects of drug therapy
  Desired outcome: The patient will not incur serious skeletal muscle injury while on drug therapy.
- Risk for Injury to liver function related to adverse effects of drug therapy
  Desired outcome: The patient will not incur serious liver injury while on drug therapy.
- Risk for Altered Nutrition: Less than Body Requirements, related to adverse effects of drug therapy
  Desired outcome: The patient will not have GI adverse effects serious enough to alter meeting the body's nutritional needs.

Planning and Intervention

Maximizing Therapeutic Effects

Lovastatin is most effective when administered in the evening, possibly because evening is also when most cholesterol synthesis occurs. Immediate-release lovastatin should be administered after the evening meal; extended-release lovastatin is administered at bedtime without food to be most effective. The patient should be advised to continue a cholesterol-reducing diet.

Minimizing Adverse Effects

Liver function test (AST and ALT) results should be monitored before starting therapy. The FDA label for lovastatin supports monitoring these enzymes at 12 weeks after starting therapy or after each dose adjustment, and then yearly or as indicated, but some experts do not believe this is necessary. Fractionated bilirubin may be monitored instead, because this is more likely to indicate significant liver injury (McKenney, Davidson, Jacobson, et al., 2006). Consult with the prescriber about reducing the dose or stopping the drug if the increased liver enzyme levels (more than three times the upper limits of normal) persist and other potential causes of this elevation have been ruled out.

Evaluate the patient carefully for muscle soreness, tenderness, or pain and CK levels before starting therapy. Reassess for muscle symptoms after 6 to 12 weeks of therapy and at each follow-up visit. CK levels may be monitored more frequently and on a regular basis depending on the patient's risk factors for myopathy and physician preference.

Rule out common causes of muscle aches, such as exercise or strenuous work, if the patient is experiencing muscle symptoms. Encourage the patient to avoid strenuous physical activity. Obtain a CK measurement when the patient has unexplained muscle symptoms and compare to baseline levels. If the CK levels are moderately elevated (3 to 10 times the upper limit of normal), continue with drug therapy but follow the patient's symptoms and CK levels weekly until either symptoms disappear or the CK levels return to within normal range. If CK levels reach above 10 times the upper limit of normal and the patient has symptoms, therapy should be stopped. This should eliminate the symptoms. Once the patient is asymptomatic, the same or different statin can be started at the same or a lower dose to test if the symptoms are reproduced. Recurrence of symptoms with multiple statins requires that a different type of antilipid drug be used than a statin (McKenney, Davidson, Jacobson, et al., 2006).

Monitor the older adult who receives polypharmacy carefully for drug interactions with lovastatin. Also, carefully monitor adults older than 80 years, especially women, who have small body frames and are frail, because they are more at risk for myopathies.

Providing Patient and Family Education

Stress the importance of following a low-cholesterol and low-saturated-fat diet while on drug therapy (Box 28.4).

Instruct patients to report any unexplained muscle pain, tenderness, or weakness at once.

Because of the risks of fetal harm, advise female patients to avoid taking lovastatin if they become pregnant.

In some patients taking lovastatin, photosensitivity may occur. Urge all patients to avoid prolonged exposure to sunlight and other ultraviolet light until their response to therapy is known.

Ongoing Assessment and Evaluation

The patient should have liver function tests and CK measurement performed periodically throughout drug therapy with lovastatin. Monitor the results of these tests for elevations. Assess the patient for muscle pain throughout therapy. Blood work that monitors the complete lipid profile should be obtained periodically throughout therapy. Therapy is considered effective when the total cholesterol level is below 200 mg/dL, LDL is lower than 100 mg/dL, and HDL is above 40 mg/dL and the patient has not incurred any serious adverse effects.

BOX 28.4 COMMUNITY BASED CONCERNS

Diet Teaching to Lower Cholesterol Levels

An important role of the nurse is to provide health education. Because heart disease is a leading cause of death in the United States, teaching the benefits of a low-cholesterol diet is an important nursing action—not just for patients with elevated cholesterol levels and their families, but also for the population at large.
Encourage a diet that is low in saturated fats, which would include the following foods:

- Fruits and vegetables
- Whole grains, such as cereal, rice, and pasta
- Lean red meats and poultry (no skin)
- Low-fat or skim milk dairy products
- Lean fish and shellfish
- Beans and peas

Unsaturated oils such as olive oil, corn oil, and safflower oil
Encourage a diet that limits foods that are high in saturated fat and cholesterol. This means avoiding or limiting the following foods:

- High-fat dairy products, such as whole milk, cream, ice cream, butter, and cheese
- Egg yolks
- Saturated oils such as coconut oil, palm oil, and palm kernel oil
- Solid fats such as shortening, soft margarine, and lard
- Organ meats such as liver, sweetbreads, kidneys, and brain
- High-fat processed meats such as hot dogs, sausage, bologna, and salami
- Fatty red meats that have not been trimmed
- Duck and goose meat
- Fried foods

Emphasize that patients should avoid not only highly saturated fats, but also foods that are made with them.

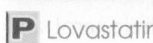

MEMORY CHIP

P Lovastatin

- Used to treat hyperlipidemia. It lowers LDL, triglycerides, and total cholesterol, and raises HDL.
- Major contraindications: active liver disease, unexplained persistently elevated liver function test results, and pregnancy
- Most common adverse effect: elevated liver enzyme levels
- Most serious adverse effects: rhabdomyolysis and myopathy
- **Life span alert: pregnancy category X; avoid lovastatin if the patient is breast-feeding. Older adults are more likely to have drug interactions.**
- Minimizing adverse effects: Monitor liver enzyme levels for at least first year of therapy.
- Most important patient education: Teach patients to continue on a low-fat diet and to report any unexplained muscle pain, tenderness, or weakness at once.

Drugs Closely Related to P Lovastatin

Atorvastatin (Lipitor), fluvastatin (Lescol), pravastatin (Pravachol), rosuvastatin (Crestor), and simvastatin (Zocor), and the newest statin, pitavastatin (Livalo), all work similarly to lower LDL cholesterol and have similar adverse effects. Pravastatin differs from the prototype lovastatin because it is not metabolized via the P-450 system and thus does not produce the drug interactions of lovastatin. Fluvastatin is primarily metabolized via a different isoenzyme pathway, 2D6, so is not as likely to have the same drug interactions. Unlike lovastatin, rosuvastatin does not raise digoxin levels but leads to other similar drug interactions. Asian subjects (including Filipino, Chinese, Japanese, Korean, Vietnamese or Asian-Indian origin) appear to be more sensitive to rosuvastatin; a twofold increase in drug levels can occur, so these patients should be started on the lowest dose possible. Pitavastatin is very similar to lovastatin, except that it is much more potent, requiring a daily dose of 1 to 4 mg as opposed to 10 to 80 mg daily for lovastatin. Pitavastatin carries additional warnings that if the patient has a moderate decrease in renal function, the dose should be decreased, and for severe renal impairment, pitavastatin is not recommended. A higher percentage of pitavastatin is renally eliminated than in lovastatin. See Table 28.4 for a comparison of statins.

Drugs Significantly Different From P Lovastatin

Fibric Acid Derivatives

Like lovastatin and the other statins, the fibric acid derivatives (also known as fibrates) fenofibrate (TriCor, Lipofen, and others) and gemfibrozil (Gemcor, Lopid), work to lower triglyceride levels and increase HDL cholesterol. These drugs can reduce triglyceride levels between 35% and 53%. However, unlike lovastatin and other statins, their effect on LDL cholesterol may be either to lower it between 6% and 20% or raise it slightly. These fibric acid derivatives are available as oral tablets or capsules.

Although in certain patients these drugs may be used alone, most frequently they are used in combination with statins. Some patients, such as those with diabetes or metabolic syndrome, need to lower triglycerides and increase HDL, and a combination of a fibric acid derivative and a statin may be the drug therapy of choice. The combined use of a fibrate and a moderate-dose statin carries a somewhat increased risk of myopathy, but the incidence is low, especially if used in populations without multisystem diseases or currently taking multiple medications. Gemfibrozil may substantially increase the circulating blood levels of some statins, such as lovastatin. Fenofibrate has not been linked as strongly, but the potential exists for a drug interaction with lovastatin or other statins. The fibric acid derivatives have similar common adverse effects: rash; gastrointestinal problems such as diarrhea, flatulence, and nausea and vomiting; and myalgia. These agents are pregnancy category C drugs. Safety and efficacy for children have not been established.

Fenofibrate

Fenofibrate (TriCor) reduces total cholesterol, LDL cholesterol, total triglycerides, and triglyceride-rich lipoprotein (VLDL) in treated patients while it increases HDL. (However, treatment of some patients with hyperlipoproteinemia may result in an increase in LDL cholesterol). Exactly how fenofibrate works has not been clearly established. The metabolite of fenofibrate, fenofibric acid, lowers plasma triglycerides apparently by inhibiting the synthesis of triglycerides, which reduces the amount of VLDL released into the circulation. It also stimulates the catabolism of triglyceride-rich VLDL. Fenofibrate reduces the serum uric acid levels in patients with

TABLE 28.4	Comparison of Statins					
Property	Lovastatin	Atorvastatin	Fluvastatin	Pravastatin	Rosuvastatin	Simvastatin
LDL reduction	29%–48%	38%–54%	17%–33%	19%–40%	52%–63%	28%–?
Protein binding	>95%	80%–90%	>99%	43%–55%	88%	95%
P-450 metabolism	3A4	3A4	2C9	None	Limited 2C9	3A4
Approximate monthly wholesale cost (U.S. dollars) based on usual dose	$90 (generic forms $30)	$96	$49	$122	$100	$122

Data derived from UpToDate. (2006). Overview of treatment of hypercholesterolemia. Retrieved January 11, 2007, from *www.uptodate.com* and from *www.CRBestBuyDrugs.org* (The statin drugs prescription and price trends November 2004 to October 2005. *Consumer Reports Best Buy Drugs*).

normal and elevated uric acid levels by increasing the urinary excretion of uric acid.

Fenofibrate is well absorbed from the GI tract; food increases absorption. Peak levels occur within 6 to 8 hours. Fenofibrate is highly protein bound (99%). It is rapidly hydrolyzed by esterases to the active metabolite, fenofibric acid, which is primarily conjugated with glucuronic acid and then excreted in the urine. Fenofibrate has a half-life of 20 hours. It is excreted, in the form of its metabolites, in the urine.

Fenofibrate is contraindicated in hepatic or severe renal dysfunction (including primary biliary cirrhosis and patients with unexplained persistent liver function abnormality), preexisting gallbladder disease, and hypersensitivity. Serious adverse effects of fenofibrate are rare and include pancreatitis, hepatotoxicity, and rhabdomyolysis.

Gemfibrozil

Gemfibrozil (Gemcor, Lopid) reduces plasma triglyceride (VLDL) concentrations and increases HDL concentrations. Its effect on LDL is varied; in some patients it may slightly reduce LDL cholesterol concentrations, in others it significantly increases them, and in still others it may have no significant effect. Exactly how gemfibrozil works is not known, but it may inhibit peripheral lipolysis and decrease the hepatic extraction of free fatty acids, thus reducing hepatic triglyceride production. In addition, the drug may reduce the incorporation of long-chain fatty acids into new triglycerides. It may also increase the turnover and removal of cholesterol from the liver and increase excretion of cholesterol in the feces.

Gemfibrozil is well absorbed from the GI tract. Peak levels occur 1 to 2 hours after administration of the dose. Gemfibrozil is primarily oxidized to hydroxymethyl and a carboxyl metabolite. Excretion is mostly renal.

Contraindications include hepatic or severe renal dysfunction, including primary biliary cirrhosis, preexisting gallbladder disease, or hypersensitivity.

Serious adverse effects of gemfibrozil include abnormal liver function tests and rhabdomyolysis. The drug causes a moderate hyperglycemic effect; special monitoring is necessary for patients with diabetes.

Cholesterol Absorption Inhibitor: Ezetimibe

Ezetimibe (Zetia) is an antilipid drug that is used to treat hypercholesterolemia. Its pediatric use is restricted to children older than 10 years of age with familial homozygous hypercholesterolemia. It is given orally once daily either as monotherapy or in combination therapy with a statin. Ezetimibe is available as a single-entity drug or as a combination drug with simvastatin (the combination has a trade name of Vytorin). Ezetimibe has a unique way of working compared with other antilipid drugs. The mechanism of action of ezetimibe is complementary to that of the statins, explaining why patients may receive both. It localizes and appears to act at the brush border of the small intestine, where it inhibits the absorption of cholesterol, leading to a decrease in the delivery of intestinal cholesterol to the liver. This causes a

reduction of hepatic cholesterol stores and an increase in the clearance of cholesterol from the blood. Ezetimibe decreases LDL about 17% but has no effect on HDL or triglycerides.

Food does not affect its bioavailability. Much of the drug is excreted in the feces unchanged, and the rest of it is metabolized in the liver.

Ezetimibe is contraindicated in active liver disease or if the patient has persistently elevated liver enzymes (when coadministered with a statin). It should be administered with caution to children under 10 years old because it is not labeled for this use. Other precautions are moderate to severe hepatic insufficiency as well as pregnancy and lactation (when coadministered with a statin).

Ezetimibe has some adverse effects; the most common are abdominal pain, diarrhea, arthralgia, back pain, myalgia, headache, and sinusitis. The potential serious adverse effects are all uncommon. They include hepatitis, increased liver function tests, hypersensitivity responses (anaphylaxis and angioedema), myopathy (very rare), and rhabdomyolysis (very rare).

Ezetimibe is a pregnancy category C drug, and the risk to the infant during breast-feeding cannot be ruled out.

Nicotinic Acid

Nicotinic acid (niacin or vitamin B_3) is used to treat hyperlipidemia. Like lovastatin, nicotinic acid reduces levels of triglycerides and LDL cholesterol levels and raises levels of HDL cholesterol. Triglycerides and VLDL levels are reduced by 25% to 30% in 1 to 4 days. LDL level reductions may be seen in 5 to 7 days, with the maximal effect seen in 3 to 5 weeks. The effect on LDL is dose dependent and ranges from 10% to 25%. The decrease would be greater if the patient is also receiving bile acid sequestrants (40% to 60% decrease). HDLs are increased between 15% and 35%. Although the exact mode of action is unknown, nicotinic acid is known to inhibit lipolysis in adipose tissue, to decrease esterification of triglyceride in the liver, and to increase lipoprotein lipase activity.

Nicotinic acid is rapidly absorbed from the intestine, with peak effects achieved 45 minutes after administration. It is excreted, mostly unchanged, in the urine. Contraindications to its use include hepatic dysfunction, active peptic ulcer, severe hypotension, and hemorrhaging.

The newer sustained-release forms of nicotinic acid have fewer adverse effects, making them more tolerable for patients and, therefore, excellent choices to elevate HDL levels. To achieve the lipid-lowering effects of nicotinic acid, doses that are larger than those used to treat niacin deficiency (pellagra) are needed. These larger doses produce peripheral vasodilation, mostly in the cutaneous vessels of the face, neck, and chest. Vasodilation results in flushing of the skin, which is usually transient. Vasodilation and increased blood flow from niacin administration are attributable to histamine release. Other common adverse effects, which include GI irritation, nausea, and vomiting, make niacin intolerable for many patients. Myalgias are possible when nicotinic acid is combined with statins, although they are uncommon. The most serious possible adverse effect is hepatotoxicity, but this is rare. An increase in uric acid levels can also occur.

Bile Acid Sequestrants

The bile acid sequestrants cholestyramine (LoCholest, Questran, Prevalite) and colestipol (Colestid) are used to reduce elevated serum cholesterol levels in patients with primary hypercholesterolemia who have not responded to other drug therapy A third, new bile acid sequestrant is colesevelam (WelChol). Cholestyramine and colestipol are also used to relieve pruritus associated with partial biliary obstruction.

Bile acid sequestrants are not absorbed orally but work in the GI tract. The reduction in LDLs is apparent in 4 to 7 days and ranges between 15% and 30%. A decline in serum cholesterol levels is usually apparent after 1 month of treatment. Once drug therapy is discontinued, cholesterol levels return to baseline within 1 month. These drugs do not increase HDL or change triglyceride levels (although an initial and transient elevation in triglycerides may occur).

A major difference between the bile acid sequestrants and lovastatin is how they achieve a decrease in the cholesterol levels. Unlike lovastatin, which works by decreasing the synthesis of cholesterol, the bile acid sequestrants promote the oxidation of cholesterol to bile acids. Cholesterol is the major, and perhaps the only, precursor to bile acids. Bile acids are secreted from the gallbladder and liver into the intestine during digestion. In the intestine, bile acids emulsify the fat and lipid particles from food, promoting absorption. Much of the bile acid that is secreted is reabsorbed and returned to the liver by hepatic circulation.

The bile acid sequestrants bind with the bile acids in the intestine to make them nonresorbable. The bile acids are then eliminated in the stool. The decrease in available bile acid causes the body to increase the oxidation of cholesterol to bile acids, which in turn decreases the LDL and serum cholesterol levels. Although hepatic synthesis of cholesterol rises, serum cholesterol levels fall because of an increased clearance of cholesterol-rich lipoproteins from the plasma. Because of their mechanism of action the bile acid sequestrants are all administered before a meal.

Patients with partial biliary obstruction have an increased bile acid concentration. Cholestyramine and colestipol, by decreasing circulating bile acid, reduce bile acid deposits in the skin tissues, with a resultant decrease in pruritus. Colesevelam is not noted to have this effect.

Cholestyramine and colestipol are extremely similar. Because of their adverse effects and frequent drug interactions, these agents are not frequently prescribed. The most common adverse effect is constipation, which can be severe and may lead to fecal impaction. Less frequently experienced adverse effects include abdominal pain, distention, and cramping; GI bleeding; belching; bloating; flatulence; nausea and vomiting; diarrhea and loose stools; indigestion and heartburn; anorexia; and steatorrhea. Chronic use of cholestyramine can result in prolonged bleeding resulting from

vitamin K deficiency. Headache can also occur with both cholestyramine and colestipol. In addition, dizziness, anxiety, vertigo, drowsiness, and fatigue have been noted with colestipol.

Absorption of fat-soluble vitamins such as A, D, E, and K may be impaired because cholestyramine interferes with the normal fat absorption and digestion. Because cholestyramine is a chloride anion exchange resin, prolonged use may cause hyperchloremic acidosis.

Cholestyramine and colestipol interact with many different drugs and may impair the absorption of those drugs. Consult a drug guide to determine whether a drug interaction is likely before giving these bile acid sequestrants with any other drug.

Before starting therapy with cholestyramine or colestipol, determine whether both the patient's serum cholesterol and triglyceride levels are elevated. If so, elevated triglyceride levels should be treated first with other drug therapy because triglycerides may rise initially from the treatment with cholestyramine.

Consideration should be given to the patient's life span before treatment with either of the bile acid sequestrants. Cholestyramine is a pregnancy category C drug, whereas colestipol is a pregnancy category B drug. Younger and smaller patients are more at risk for developing hyperchloremic acidosis. In adults older than 60 years, constipation is more likely to develop with ongoing cholestyramine therapy. Cholestyramine and colestipol come in a powdered form, which needs to be diluted with fluid. These preparations are considered unpalatable by some patients, and therefore, adherence with therapy may be limited. Both drugs also come in tablet form.

Colesevelam differs from cholestyramine and colestipol in some ways. Colesevelam is contraindicated in bowel obstruction. It is a pregnancy category B drug. Unlike the other bile acid sequestrants, it does not seem to reduce the absorption of fat-soluble vitamins, although a class effect is possible, so caution should be used if the patient has deficiency of one of these vitamins or is at risk of developing one of these deficiencies. It also does not seem to have the drug interactions that the other drugs in the class have. The GI adverse effects are much less frequent from colesevelam, so the drug is better tolerated than either cholestyramine or colestipol.

CHAPTER SUMMARY

- Hyperlipidemia is a known risk factor for atherosclerosis and the problems and complications associated with atherosclerosis. The blood lipids include the total cholesterol, HDL cholesterol, LDL cholesterol, VLDL cholesterol, and triglycerides.
- Use of statins decreases primary and secondary risks for cardiac disease and stroke. In addition to lowering lipid levels, statins appear to have protective and healing effects on the endothelium. Cardiovascular disease risk is decreased with statin use even if the LDL baseline is not considered elevated when therapy is started.

- Many patients being treated for elevated cholesterol levels do not achieve the recommended treatment goals of total cholesterol under 200 mg/dL, LDL under 100 mg/dL, and HDL above 40 mg/dL.
- Lovastatin, the prototype statin, lowers LDL, VLDL, triglyceride levels, and total cholesterol levels, and raises HDL levels. It has been shown to decrease mortality from cardiovascular complications associated with elevated cholesterol levels and LDL levels.
- Lovastatin is metabolized through the hepatic enzyme CYP3A4. All other drugs or agents that are inhibitors of this pathway may have a drug interaction with lovastatin, decreasing lovastatin metabolism and sometimes dramatically raising blood levels of lovastatin.
- All lipid-lowering drugs can elevate liver enzyme levels. This elevation is not normally serious, although the patient's liver enzyme levels should be monitored closely for up to the first year of therapy. Liver enzyme levels usually return to normal spontaneously while drug therapy continues; if this does not occur, then enzyme levels return to normal with either a dose reduction or discontinuation of the drug.
- Lipid-lowering drugs can produce myalgias and potentially serious myopathies. These occur most frequently with high doses of statins, or the combination of another antilipid with a statin. Some patients may be genetically predisposed to these adverse effects due to inherited differences in P-450 isoenzymes, because the statins are metabolized via these pathways.
- Dietary modifications to limit fat and cholesterol intake should be implemented before starting any drug to lower lipid levels. These modifications need to be continued once drug therapy has begun.
- The fibric acid derivatives gemfibrozil and fenofibrate lower triglyceride levels and increase HDL cholesterol. Their effect on LDL cholesterol can be either to lower it slightly or to increase it slightly. They are usually coprescribed with a statin. Gemfibrozil reduces hepatic triglyceride production. The mechanisms of fenofibrate are not clear.
- A cholesterol absorption inhibitor is ezetimibe, which decreases the absorption of cholesterol in the small intestine to lower serum LDL levels. It is also available in combination with the statin simvastatin.
- Nicotinic acid (niacin or vitamin B_3) reduces triglycerides, reduces LDL cholesterol, and increases HDL. Although the exact mode of action is unknown, nicotinic acid is known to inhibit lipolysis in adipose tissue, decrease esterification of triglyceride in the liver, and increase lipoprotein lipase activity.
- The bile acid sequestrants cholestyramine, colestipol, and colesevelam decrease LDL. They work differently than other lipid-lowering drugs by binding with the bile acids in the intestine so that the bile acids are nonresorbable and are eliminated in the stool. The decrease in available bile acid causes the body to convert cholesterol to bile acids.

QUESTIONS FOR STUDY AND REVIEW

1. Which of the forms of cholesterol is believed to provide some protective mechanism for the body and is termed "good" cholesterol?
2. How do elevated cholesterol levels contribute to hypertension?
3. Why is it important to determine whether other drugs received by a patient taking lovastatin are metabolized by CYP3A4 or are inhibitors of CYP3A4?
4. Why is it important to monitor liver enzymes while a patient is receiving lovastatin or other lipid-lowering drugs?
5. Why do CK levels greater than 10 times the upper limit of normal require that lovastatin therapy be discontinued?

NEED MORE HELP?

Chapter 28 of the Study Guide to Accompany *Drug Therapy in Nursing*, 4th Edition, contains NCLEX-style questions and other learning activities to reinforce your understanding of the concepts presented in this chapter. For additional information or to purchase the study guide, visit thePoint.

REFERENCES

ALLHAT Officers and Coordinators for the ALLHAT Collaborative Research Group. (2002). Major outcomes in moderately hypercholesterolemic hypertensive patients randomized to pravastatin vs usual care: The Antihypertensive and Lipid Lowering Treatment to Prevent Heart Attack Trial (ALLHAT-LLT). *Journal of the American Medical Association*, 288(23):2998–3007.

American Heart Association Cholesterol Statistics. Last updated April 2008. Retrieved from: http://www.americanheart.org/presenter.jhtml?identifier=536. Accessed on October 10, 2009.

American Heart Association. Cholesterol. (2009) *Circulation*;119:628–647. Retrieved, from *http://www. americanheart.org/presenter.jhtml?identifier=1516*. Accessed October 10, 2009

American Heart Association. Progress and Challenges in Metabolic Syndrome in Children and Adolescents. A Scientific Statement From the American Heart Association Atherosclerosis, Hypertension, and Obesity in the Young Committee of the Council on Cardiovascular Disease in the Young; Council on Cardiovascular Nursing; and Council on Nutrition, Physical Activity, and Metabolism. Retrieved from: http://circ.ahajournals.org/cgi/content/full/119/4/628#SEC12. Accessed October 10, 2009

Ervin, R. B. (2009). Prevalence of Metabolic Syndrome Among Adults 20 Years of Age and Over, by Sex, Age, Race and Ethnicity, and Body Mass Index: United States, 2003–2006. *National Health Statistics Reports*; Number 13 May 5, 2009. Retrieved from: http://www.cdc.gov/nchs/data/nhsr/nhsr013.pdf Accessed on October 10, 2009.

Centers for Disease Control and Prevention. Cholesterol Facts and Statistics webpage. http://www.cdc.gov/Cholesterol/facts.htm. Last modified November 2007. Accesssed October 10, 2009.

Cohen, D. E., Anania, F. A., & Chalasani, N. (2006). An assessment of statin safety by hepatologists. *American Journal of Cardiology*, 97(Suppl 8A):77C–81C.

Grundy, S. M., Cleeman, J. I., Bairey Merz, C. N., et al. (2004). National Cholesterol Education Program Report. Implications of recent clinical trials for National Cholesterol Education Program Adult Treatment Panel III guidelines. *Circulation*, 110(2):227–239.

Hankey, G. J., Norman, P. E., & Eikelboom, J. W. (2006). Medical treatment of peripheral arterial disease. *Journal of the American Medical Association*, 295(5):547–553.

Hayward, R. A., Hofer, T. P., & Vijan, S. (2006). Narrative review: Lack of evidence for recommended low density lipoprotein treatment targets: A solvable problem. *Annals of Internal Medicine*, 145(7):520–530.

Heart Protection Study Group. (2002). MRC/BHF Heart Protection Study of cholesterol lowering with simvastatin in 20,536 high-risk individuals: A randomized placebo-controlled trial. *Lancet*, 360(9326):7–22.

Kasiske, B. L., Wanner, C., & O'Neill, W. C. (2006). An assessment of statin safety by nephrologists. *American Journal of Cardiology*, 97(Suppl 8A):82C–85C.

Kristianson, K., Fyhrquist, F., Devereux, R. B., et al. (2003). An analysis of cholesterol control and statin use in the Losartan Intervention for Endpoint Reduction in Hypertension Study. *Clinical Therapeutics*, 25(4):1186–1199.

Law, M., & Rudnicka, A. R. (2006). Statin safety: Evidence from the published literature. *American Journal of Cardiology*, 97(Suppl 8A):52C–60C.

McKenney, J. M., Davidson, M. H., Jacobson, T. A., et al. (2006). Final conclusions and recommendations of the National Lipid Association Statin Safety Assessment Task Force. *American Journal of Cardiology*, 97(Suppl 8A):89C–94C.

Murphy, S. A., Cannon, C. P., Wiviott, S. D., et al, the TIMI Study Group. (2007). Effect of intensive lipid-lowering therapy on mortality after acute coronary syndrome (a patient-level analysis of the Aggrastat to Zocor and Pravastatin or Atorvastatin Evaluation and Infection Therapy-Thrombolysis in Myocardial Infarction 22 trials). *American Journal of Cardiology*, 100(7):1047–1051.

Shaw, S. M., Fildes, J. E., Yonan, N., et al. (2009). Pleiotropic Effects and Cholesterol-Lowering Therapy. *Cardiology*, 112(1):4–12.

Smith, S. C., Allen, J., Blair, S. N., et al. (2006). AHA/ACC guidelines for secondary prevention for patients with coronary and other atherosclerotic vascular disease: 2006 update. *Journal of the American College of Cardiology*, 47: 2130–2139.

Steffens, S., & Mach, F. (2006). Drug insight: Immunomodulatory effects of statins: Potential benefits for renal patients? *Nature Clinical Practice Nephrology*, 2(7):378–387.

Weber, M. S., Zamvil, S. S., (2008). Statins and demyelination. *Current Topics in Microbiology and Immunology*, 318: 313–324.

Wiviott, S. D., de Lemos, J. A., Cannon, C. P., et al., the TIMI Study Group. (2006). A tale of two trials: a comparison of the post-acute coronary syndrome lipid-lowering trials A to Z and PROVE IT-TIMI 22. *Circulation*, 113(11):1406–1414.

Drugs Treating Heart Failure

Learning Objectives

At the completion of this chapter the student will:

1. Understand the rationale for polypharmacy in treating heart failure.

2. Identify core drug knowledge about drugs used to treat heart failure.

3. Identify core patient variables relevant to drugs used to treat heart failure.

4. Relate the interaction of core drug knowledge to core patient variables for drugs that are used to treat heart failure.

5. Generate a nursing plan of care from the interactions between core drug knowledge and core patient variables for drugs that are used to treat heart failure.

6. Describe nursing interventions to maximize therapeutic effects and minimize adverse effects for drugs used to treat heart failure.

7. Determine key points for patient and family education for drugs used to treat heart failure.

Key Terms

afterload	contractility	inotropic
cardiac output	digitalization	peripheral resistance
cardiomyopathy	dromotropic	preload
chronotropic	ejection fraction	stroke volume

Drugs Treating Heart Failure

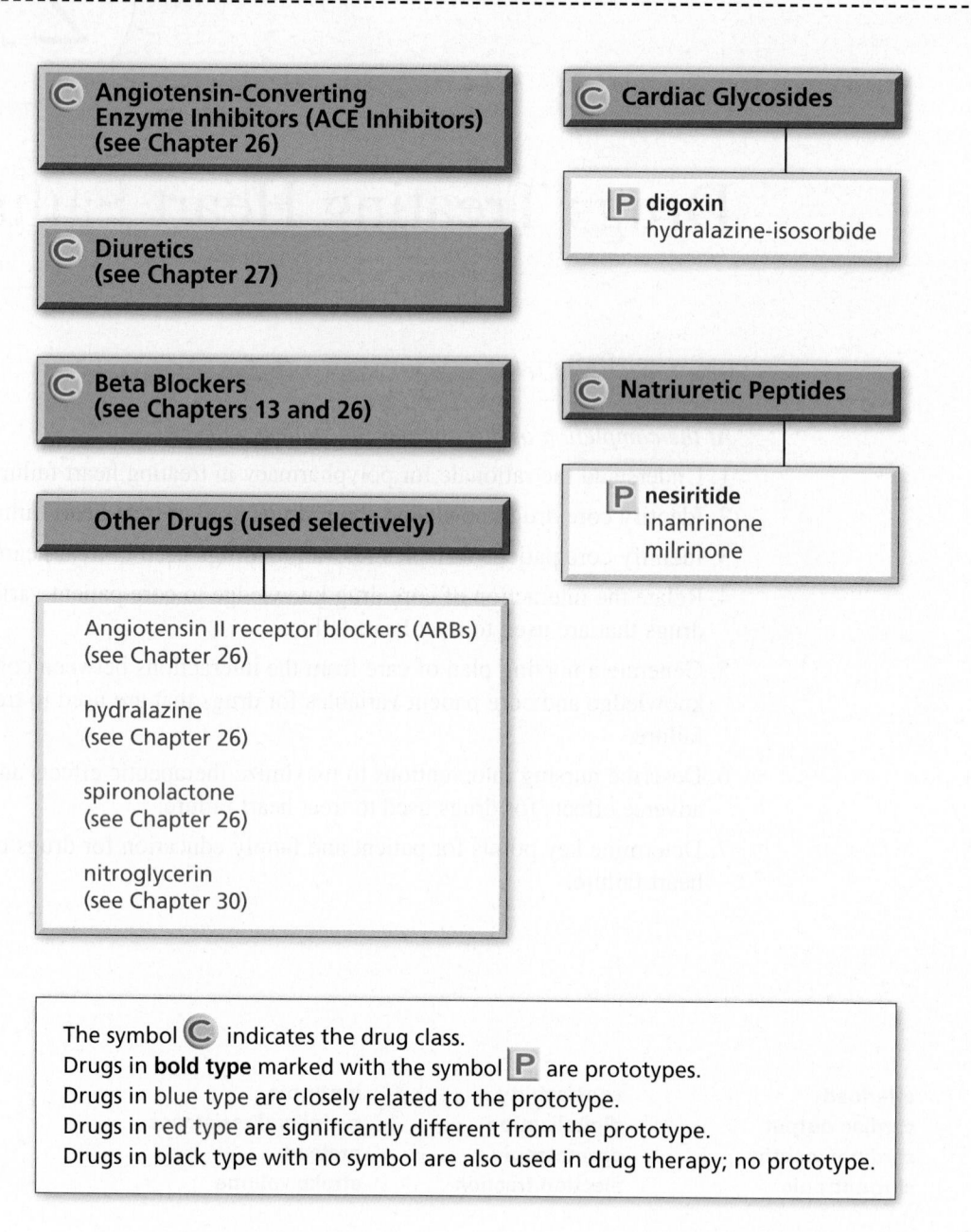

Angiotensin-Converting Enzyme Inhibitors (ACE Inhibitors)
(see Chapter 26)

Diuretics
(see Chapter 27)

Beta Blockers
(see Chapters 13 and 26)

Other Drugs (used selectively)

Angiotensin II receptor blockers (ARBs)
(see Chapter 26)

hydralazine
(see Chapter 26)

spironolactone
(see Chapter 26)

nitroglycerin
(see Chapter 30)

Cardiac Glycosides

P digoxin
hydralazine-isosorbide

Natriuretic Peptides

P nesiritide
inamrinone
milrinone

The symbol **C** indicates the drug class.
Drugs in **bold type** marked with the symbol **P** are prototypes.
Drugs in blue type are closely related to the prototype.
Drugs in red type are significantly different from the prototype.
Drugs in black type with no symbol are also used in drug therapy; no prototype.

The heart is the muscle responsible for pumping blood through the circulatory system. When disease processes interfere with the ability of the heart to pump blood effectively, the organs and tissues are affected and damage may occur. Heart failure (HF), historically referred to as congestive heart failure (CHF), is one such disease process. In HF, the heart does not pump effectively to meet the needs of the body.

The drug classes primarily used to treat chronic HF are angiotensin-converting enzyme (ACE) inhibitors, loop diuretics, and beta blockers. Additional drugs that have a selected place in therapy are the angiotensin II receptor blockers (ARBs), cardiac glycosides, aldosterone antagonists, and a combination of the vasodilator–antianginal drugs (hydralazine–isosorbide). The natriuretic peptides are a drug class used to treat decompensated acute HF. Except for the cardiac glycosides and the natriuretic peptides, which are discussed thoroughly in this chapter, these drug classes are described fully in other chapters. The prototype cardiac glycoside is digoxin (Lanoxin). The prototype natriuretic peptide is nesiritide (Natrecor).

PHYSIOLOGY

As stated in Chapter 26, the heart is composed of four chambers—the left atrium, the right atrium, the left ventricle, and the right ventricle. Blood is returned to the right atrium from the body. It progresses from the right atrium, moving to the right ventricle, and then to the lungs, where it is reoxygenated and has carbon dioxide removed. The reoxygenated blood returns to the left atrium and then to the left ventricle. The contraction of the left ventricle moves the blood back into systemic circulation, as is seen in Figure 29.1.

The volume of blood that leaves the left ventricle in 1 minute is the **cardiac output.** Cardiac output consists of two elements, stroke volume and heart rate, and is the product of these two elements (cardiac output = stroke volume × heart rate). **Stroke volume** is the amount of blood that leaves the left ventricle with each contraction. Stroke volume is normally about 75 mL. Heart rate is how fast the heart is beating, or the number of contractions per minute. The normal adult range is 70 to 80 bpm. Cardiac output is affected by factors that alter either stroke volume or heart rate.

Stroke volume is dependent on three factors: preload, contractility, and afterload. **Preload** is the passive stretching force exerted on the ventricular muscle created by the amount of blood that has filled the heart by the end of diastole. Preload is affected by the amount of blood that has returned to the heart (venous return), the ability of the atria to contract forcefully enough to move blood into the ventricles, and how much blood was left in the ventricle during the last contraction. **Contractility** is the force of the squeezing that the ventricle is able to achieve to eject the blood into the systemic circulation. **Afterload** is the amount of pressure the ventricular muscles must overcome

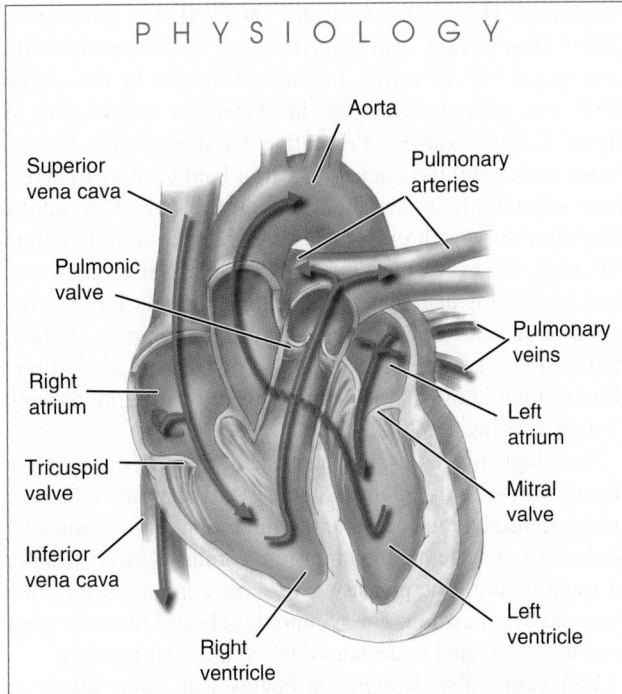

PHYSIOLOGY

• FIGURE 29.1. Cardiac circulation. The unoxygenated blood is returned through the superior and inferior vena cava to the right atrium, where it is removed to the right ventricle. Blood leaves the ventricle through the pulmonary artery to be reoxygenated in the lungs. The oxygenated blood returns to the left atrium via the pulmonary veins and then into the left ventricle. Blood is ejected from the ventricle to the body through the aorta.

to eject the blood into the systemic circulation. Contractility also is affected by the concentration of catecholamines in the heart muscle; that is, the more catecholamines, the greater the contractility. Afterload is controlled by the diameter of the vessel and the pressure within the vessel, which is known as **peripheral resistance** (PR = pressure × diameter of vessel).

Contractions of the heart are dependent on the unique electrical conduction system of the cardiac muscle. The physiology of the conduction system of the heart is described within the physiology section of Chapter 31, Drugs Affecting Cardiac Rhythm.

PATHOPHYSIOLOGY

Heart failure, a major pathologic problem in the United States, is associated with high morbidity and high mortality. Approximately 5 million people in the United States have HF; 550,000 people are diagnosed with the condition annually. More than three and a half million adults are hospitalized yearly in the United States with a primary or secondary diagnosis of HF. Heart failure is primarily a disease of older adults; about 80% of those admitted to the hospital with HF are older than 65 years of age. Total direct and indirect costs of HF are approximately $28 billion; the cost of drug therapy alone is almost $3 billion (American College of Cardiology/

American Heart Association [ACC/AHA] guidelines, 2009). Despite how common HF is, few Americans actually understand HF. A Harris Interactive Survey in December 2007 was commissioned by the American Association of Heart Failure Nurses, Preventive Cardiovascular Nurses Association, and the Society of Chest Pain Centers to determine what adults know about HF. Of the 4912 U.S. adults who were surveyed, only 47% were able to correctly define HF; only 4% were able to identify correctly all of the common symptoms of HF, nearly one third thought HF was the same as a heart attack, and nearly three fourths of them believed chest pain was a symptom of HF; and almost one third did not know that HF can be treated with drug therapy (Trupp & Wingate, 2008).

Pathologic processes that may cause HF occur either in the heart itself, such as an aortic stenosis, valvular heart disease, or myocardial deficiency after an infarction, or systemically, such as from systemic hypertension, coronary artery disease, or renal failure. The primary causes are coronary artery disease and hypertension. The symptoms of heart failure for most patients are related to decreased left ventricular function.

Left ventricular dysfunction begins with some injury to or stress on the heart and then is generally a progressive process. Cardiac output decreases when the left ventricle is unable to eject its normal volume of blood during systole; the **ejection fraction** (the amount leaving the ventricle with contraction compared with the total amount in the ventricle before contraction) is therefore decreased. For a while, the body attempts to compensate for the decreased cardiac output. The heart muscle enlarges (**cardiomyopathy**) to provide more contractile force to try to improve cardiac output. However, the heart eventually becomes less and less effective in contracting. As output becomes greatly diminished, the kidneys retain sodium and water to increase circulating volume. Unfortunately, this mechanism places more of a burden on the already overworked heart, increasing preload and afterload. The ventricles then eject less and less. As blood accumulates in the ventricles, the pressure in the vessels coming to the heart increases. Buildup of blood in the left ventricle causes pulmonary congestion or left-sided HF. The cardinal symptoms of heart failure are dyspnea (including rales, rhonchi, and shortness of breath) and fatigue (which may limit exercise tolerance), as well as fluid retention. Buildup of fluid in the right ventricle causes systemic congestion or right-sided heart failure. Symptoms include peripheral edema, positive jugular vein distention, and a third heart sound (S_3).

In HF, left-sided failure occurs first, then right-sided failure. This effect is sometimes called backward failure. In most patients, the compensatory hypertrophy of the heart muscle eventually leads to some degree of "stiffness," or loss of elasticity of the ventricle. This "stiffness" alters ventricular diastolic function and does not allow the ventricle to fill completely, further decreasing cardiac output. Although most patients develop systolic dysfunction first and then diastolic dysfunction, some patients do initially develop diastolic dysfunction. Diastolic dysfunction may also be caused by systemic hypertension and coronary artery disease. Additional causes of diastolic dysfunction are fibrosis from aging, infiltrative diseases (such as myocarditis), and constrictive pericarditis. Cardiac output is decreased with diastolic dysfunction, although the ejection fraction may be normal. The compensatory mechanisms of the body are identical in response to the diminished cardiac output. Initially with this type of failure, the body does not have a fluid overload; hence, the symptoms of fluid overload (e.g., S_3, jugular venous distention, and peripheral edema) are not present. For this reason, the term "heart failure" is now considered a more accurate description of the entire disease process than "congestive heart failure" (abbreviated CHF), although some practitioners still use the term "congestive heart failure" and the abbreviation CHF this way. Because of the chronicity of the disease, some authors and practitioners continue to refer to the pathology as the well-known abbreviation CHF but consider that the meaning of the "C" has changed and now represents "chronic" rather than "congestive." All of these terms—heart failure, congestive heart failure, and chronic heart failure—may be used in practice and should be considered synonyms. CHF (chronic heart failure) and HF are used interchangeably in this text.

Natriuretic peptides are endogenous cardiac hormones. Brain natriuretic peptide, working with atrial natriuretic peptide, regulates cardiovascular homeostasis and fluid volume. It is secreted primarily by the ventricular tissue in response to changes in wall tension. This hormone promotes natriuresis (sodium loss in the urine), diuresis, vasodilation, and smooth-muscle relaxation. It also inhibits the renin-aldosterone axis. The concentration of endogenous brain natriuretic peptides is elevated in CHF, acute myocardial infarction (MI), acute coronary syndrome, aortic stenosis, hypertension, end-stage renal failure, and cirrhosis with ascites. The presence of elevated natriuretic peptides may help to confirm the diagnosis of heart failure, although as these hormones may be elevated in some other situations (such as pulmonary embolism, chronic obstructive pulmonary disease, or in women over 60 years old who do not have heart failure); elevations of these natriuretic peptides without other symptoms or diagnostic findings should not be considered conclusive for the diagnosis of heart failure (ACC/AHA 2009; Anderson, 2008).

Because patients with CHF vary in the severity of their symptoms with progression of the pathologies, a classification system is used to group patients. Therapies are usually prescribed based on the classification. The most common classification historically used is the New York Heart Association (NYHA) groupings. Patients are placed into one of four classes depending on their functional abilities. More recently, the revised 2009 clinical guidelines from the American College of Cardiology and the American Heart Association have created four stages of heart failure with stages A and B representing patients at risk of developing HF. Patients with coronary artery disease, diabetes, and hypertension who are asymptomatic and who do not have left ventricular hypertrophy or dysfunction are in Stage A, while those who are asymptomatic but have left ventricular hypertrophy or dysfunction are grouped in Stage B. These new Stages of Heart Failure are not meant to replace the NYHA groupings,

Box 29.1 · NEW YORK HEART ASSOCIATION CLASSIFICATION FOR CHRONIC HEART FAILURE

- Class I: Patients are asymptomatic; patients have no limitation of their activities, and they do not have symptoms from ordinary activities.
- Class II: Patients are short of breath or fatigued with moderate activity such as climbing two flights of stairs; they are comfortable at rest or with mild exertion and have slight limitation of activity.
- Class III: Patients are short of breath or fatigued with very mild exertion activity, such as climbing one-half flight of stairs; are comfortable only with rest; and have marked limitation of their activity.
- Class IV: Patients are exhausted, short of breath, or fatigued at rest; any activity brings on discomfort and symptoms; they have severe limitations on their activity and are confined to bed or chair.

but to supplement them. The goal of the new stages is to help highlight for clinicians that there is a need for therapy before the patient develops complications of the left ventricle. Box 29.1 summarizes the NYHA classifications for CHF. Display 29.1 shows the ACC/AHA new classifications for HF and appropriate interventions.

DRUGS TO TREAT CHRONIC HEART FAILURE

When the heart cannot achieve the normal cardiac output for various reasons, a backlog of blood, or congestion, occurs, and heart failure develops. Several drug classes are used to treat CHF, and polypharmacy is considered the standard and most effective treatment. The *ACC/AHA 2009 Guideline Update for the Diagnosis and Management of Chronic Heart Failure in the Adult* suggest that drug therapy begin in the pre-HF stages of A and B. Initially, in stage A the underlying risk factor should be addressed with the goal to correct or minimize the risk (e.g., return the blood pressure readings to a normal level with drugs to treat the hypertension, control elevated glucose levels in those with diabetes, etc.). Additionally, other drug therapy may be started based on patient risk factors; these drugs include angiotensin converting enzyme inhibitors (ACE Is), angiotensin II receptor blockers (ARBs), and (occasionally) beta blockers. Drug therapy for Stage B is similar, with the emphasis that a beta blocker should be started on everyone who has had an MI. By Stage C when the patient now is diagnosed with heart failure, the guidelines state that the following therapies are

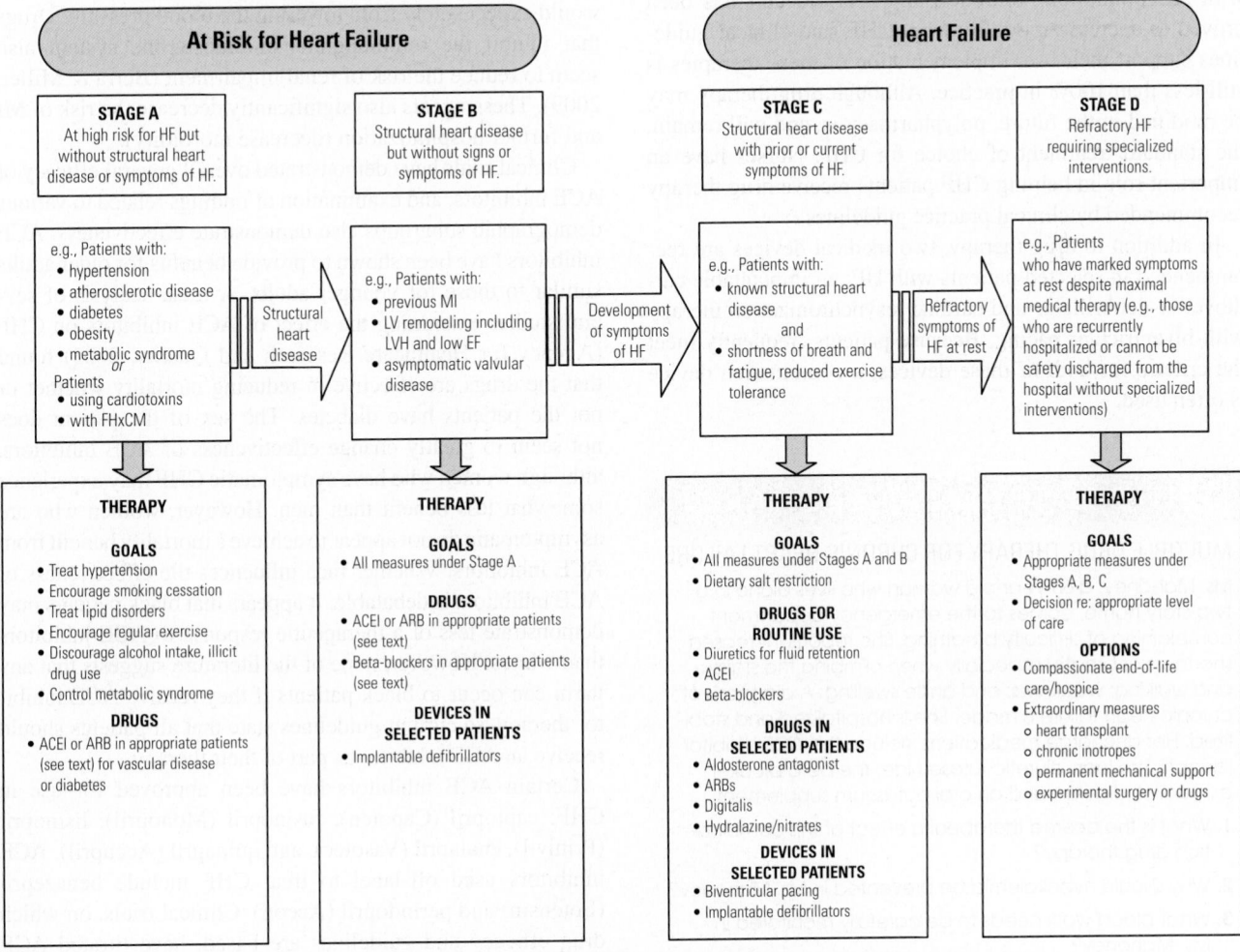

Display 29-1. Stages in the evolution of HF and recommended therapy by stage. FHx CM, family history of cardiomyopathy; IV, intravenous; LV, left ventricular; and MI, myocardial infarction.

appropriate for all patients with CHF (in the absence of contraindications): ACE inhibitors (or an ARB can be used if the patient cannot tolerate an ACE inhibitor), loop diuretics (with dietary salt restriction), and beta blockers. These drugs are to be considered the standard basis of care for CHF. Research suggests that the clinical benefits of ACE inhibitors and beta blockers are related to modifying the changes that occur in the left ventricle with CHF. ACE inhibitors seem to prevent progression of left ventricular dilation, and beta blockers such as carvedilol may reverse hypertrophy and improve systolic function.

Additionally, the following agents should be given to selected patients (in the absence of contraindications): aldosterone antagonists, ARBs, and a combination vasodilator–antianginal (hydralazine–isosorbide) for black patients. Cardiac glycosides (digoxin) may also be added to therapy as they have been found useful in the symptom management of CHF. Although digoxin, the prototype, does not decrease mortality, it has been shown to decrease the need for hospitalization.

Early diagnosis and treatment can improve quality of life expectancy for people who have heart failure (CDC, 2010). Drug therapy has been effective in increasing survival of individuals with CHF. Although the effective use of drug therapy with ACE inhibitors, diuretics, and beta blockers has been proved to decrease mortality from CHF, and clinical guidelines support their use, implementation of these therapies is still less than 100% in practice. Although drug therapy may be modified in the future, polypharmacy is, and will remain, the standard treatment of choice for CHF. Nurses have an important role in helping CHF patients receive drug therapy recommended by clinical practice guidelines.

In addition to drug therapy, two medical devices are recommended in selected patients with HF: an implantable cardioverter-defibrillator and cardiac resynchronization therapy with biventricular pacing. Because patients frequently meet the criteria for both of these devices, a combination device is often used.

CRITICAL THINKING SCENARIO

MULTIPLE DRUG THERAPY FOR CHRONIC HEART FAILURE

Ms. Mahoney, a 65-year-old woman who lives alone in a two-story home, comes to the emergency department complaining of difficulty breathing. She reports increased shortness of breath, especially when climbing the stairs and walking; weakness; and ankle swelling. A diagnosis of chronic heart failure is made. She is hospitalized and stabilized. Her discharge medications include the ACE inhibitor lisinopril, the loop diuretic furosemide, the beta blocker carvedilol, digoxin, and an oral potassium supplement.

1. What is the desired therapeutic effect of this combination drug therapy?
2. Why should hypokalemia be prevented in Ms. Mahoney?
3. What blood work needs to be carefully monitored in Ms. Mahoney?

Angiotensin-Converting Enzyme Inhibitors

As circulating volume to the kidneys decreases in CHF, the renin-angiotensin-aldosterone system is activated as the body attempts to "correct" for the low levels of circulating volume. Renin stimulates the production of angiotensin I, which is converted by a special enzyme, angiotensin-converting enzyme, into an extremely potent vasoconstrictor, angiotensin II. In turn, angiotensin II stimulates the production of aldosterone, which causes sodium and fluid retention, thereby increasing circulating blood volume. As a result, the already overworked heart must work harder. Vasoconstriction is designed to direct the diminished blood volume to vital organs. It also increases peripheral resistance, which decreases cardiac output and further increases the workload on the failing heart. ACE inhibitors stop the conversion of angiotensin to the active vasoconstrictor form, thereby preventing the deleterious effects from the renin-angiotensin-aldosterone system. These drugs are part of standard therapy for HF because they reduce mortality for all affected individuals regardless of whether their HF is symptomatic or whether it develops after an MI. Although it is known that hypertension is a risk factor for developing HF and its sequelae, the risk reduction achieved in HF from drug therapy with inhibitors of the renin-angiotensin-aldosterone system appears to be greater than one would expect solely from lowering the blood pressure. Drugs that inhibit the renin-angiotensin-aldosterone system also seem to reduce the risk of renal impairment (Berra & Miller, 2009). These agents also significantly decrease the risk of MI and further hospitalization (decrease morbidity).

Clinical trials have demonstrated overall general efficacy of ACE inhibitors, and examination of findings related to various demographic subgroups also demonstrate effectiveness. ACE inhibitors have been shown to provide benefits for older adults similar to those for younger adults. A meta-analysis of several studies examining the effect of ACE inhibitors on CHF (Agency for Healthcare Research and Quality, 2003) found that the drugs are effective in reducing mortality whether or not the patients have diabetes. The sex of the patient does not seem to greatly change effectiveness of ACE inhibitors, although women who have symptomatic CHF may experience somewhat less benefit than men. However, women who are asymptomatic do not appear to achieve a mortality benefit from ACE inhibitors. Whether race influences the effectiveness of ACE inhibitors is debatable. It appears that black patients may demonstrate less of a therapeutic response to ACE inhibitors than whites. However, none of the literature suggests that any harm can occur to black patients if they receive ACE inhibitor therapy, so current guidelines state that all patients should receive an ACE inhibitor as part of their therapy.

Certain ACE inhibitors have been approved for use in CHF: captopril (Capoten), fosinopril (Monopril), lisinopril (Prinivil), enalapril (Vasotec), and quinapril (Accupril). ACE inhibitors used off-label to treat CHF include benazepril (Lotensin) and perindopril (Aceon). Clinical trials, on which drug efficacy and guidelines are based, have titrated ACE inhibitor doses to a higher level than those frequently prescribed in practice. If the patient tolerates these higher doses, they should be used to maximize effectiveness of ACE inhibitor therapy. In addition, there also appears to be a cost benefit.

Adverse effects related to ACE inhibitors include cough (which often is severe enough that patients cannot tolerate using the drug), hypotension, worsening renal function, potassium retention, and angioedema. ACE inhibitors carry a Black Box warning that they should not be used in pregnant women.

More information about ACE inhibitors is found in Chapter 26.

Loop Diuretics

Loop diuretics are used to decrease fluid volume and edema present in CHF. Because loop diuretics increase the loss of sodium significantly and to a much greater extent than thiazide diuretics, loop diuretics are generally considered the diuretic of choice for treating HF. Other advantages of a loop diuretic over a thiazide include the enhancement of free water clearance and that the drugs do not lose effectiveness with kidney disease unless the kidney function is severely impaired. However, thiazide diuretics may be used in patients who also have hypertension and have limited fluid retention from HF. If the patient is admitted to the hospital, they should receive intravenous loop diuretics, regardless of their home therapy (ACC/AHA, 2009).

In general, diuretics act in the nephrons of the kidney to increase urinary output and electrolyte loss. This action decreases circulating volume and peripheral resistance, reducing the workload on the failing heart. Removal of fluid from the vascular space allows mobilization of edema from the interstitial spaces. With less volume in the vascular space, less blood is returned to the heart (decreased preload) and cardiac output is decreased. The drop in cardiac output is not usually clinically important unless the patient has been too aggressively treated with loop diuretics and overdiuresed. Cardiac output that is significant decreases tissue perfusion. To determine if this has occurred, assess the blood urea nitrogen (BUN) levels; a stable BUN implies adequate perfusion to the kidneys and other organs. If the patient remains edematous and the BUN is stable, it is safe to continue with diuretic therapy.

Appropriate diuretic therapy leads to the resolution of pulmonary and peripheral edema. The efficacy of the diuretic can be enhanced by concurrent therapy with an ACE inhibitor, which lowers the concentrations of both angiotensin II and aldosterone. In combination with loop diuretics, aldosterone antagonists also modestly enhance the diuresis and minimize the potassium loss; the combination has been found to improve survival. With loop diuretics, the maximum diuretic effect and loss of potassium occur within the first few days of daily therapy. After 2 weeks of continued use, the diuretic does not cause further fluid loss, but it does maintain the fluid loss that has been attained. Additional diuretic effect is seen only if the dose is increased or a second diuretic drug is added to the therapy.

The potential adverse effects of diuretics include loss of electrolytes, especially potassium and magnesium, which can predispose a patient to serious cardiac arrhythmias, particularly if the patient is also taking digoxin. Other adverse effects include hypotension and azotemia (increased urea in the blood).

Diuretics should be prescribed for all patients with fluid retention HF. They are used to treat fluid overload, and then as maintenance drugs to prevent reoccurrences of fluid imbalance. The dose of the diuretic should be large enough to correct the fluid volume excess, but not large as to cause significant adverse effects such as severe hypotension or significant electrolyte imbalances. As heart failure progresses, it is common that the patient will need a large dose of the diuretic to achieve the same therapeutic response.

Diuretics are discussed fully in Chapter 27.

Beta Blockers

Beta blockers have been shown to be highly effective in the treatment of all grades of HF that are attributable to left ventricular systolic dysfunction. Beta blockers, like ACE inhibitors, have been found to decrease mortality from CHF as well as decrease morbidity and enhance the patient's overall well-being. Although beta blockers can decrease contractility of the heart, thereby decreasing cardiac output (which is detrimental initially in CHF), they also block the effect of the sympathetic nervous system and cause vasodilation and decreased peripheral vascular resistance (which is helpful to patients with CHF). Clinical studies demonstrate that beta blockers actually reverse the remodeling process by reducing left ventricular volumes and improving systolic function (ACC/AHA, 2009). These changes can produce long-term clinical benefits to patients with CHF, even if coronary artery disease is the cause of heart failure. Beta blockers are known to suppress renin release in patients taking ACE inhibitors.

Because beta blockers improve survival and slow disease progression, treatment with a beta blocker should be started as soon as left ventricular dysfunction is diagnosed. Three beta blockers have been shown to be effective in reducing the risk of death in patients with CHF: bisoprolol (Zebeta) and sustained-release metoprolol (Lopressor), both of which selectively block beta-1 receptors, and carvedilol (Coreg), which blocks alpha-1, beta-1, and beta-2 receptors. Carvedilol, the first beta blocker approved for treating mild-to-moderate CHF, was the first new drug approved for treating CHF in many years.

Research on beta blocker effectiveness is limited to these three drugs, and use of other beta blockers is not currently recommended. Meta-analysis of many research studies (Agency for Healthcare Research and Quality, 2003) shows that beta blockers reduce mortality for men and women with symptomatic heart failure as well as for patients with and without diabetes. Black and white patients have the same risk reduction whether they receive bisoprolol, metoprolol, or carvedilol.

Beta blocker therapy is initiated once the HF is controlled, not during acute episodes of CHF. The patient should not have fluid overload from HF or hypovolemia from aggressive diuretic therapy; the patient should not be currently in the intensive care of a hospital for treatment of the HF. Beta blockers are recommended to be started, along with an ACE inhibitor, in patients who are asymptomatic (NYHA class I). In general, it is recommended that individuals start taking the ACE inhibitor prior to starting therapy with a beta blocker. Patients who are symptomatic (NYHA classes II–IV) should have normal fluid volume, or only minimal evidence of fluid retention, when they begin beta blocker treatment. Pretreatment with diuretics is important for these patients to prevent an acute exacerbation of CHF caused by the slowing of the heart rate and decrease in contractile force that occurs with beta blockers. Diuretic therapy should continue once other therapy has begun. The patient should be started on a small dose and monitored carefully for signs of hypotension and worsening CHF. Dosage is increased gradually over several weeks until the therapeutic dosage range is reached. Full therapeutic effects may not occur for 1 to 3 months, although some immediate response can be seen with carvedilol. Treatment is most effective if begun in the early stages of the disease. Patients who have been on long-term therapy with a beta blocker and develop an exacerbation of HF do not need to have the beta blocker therapy stopped immediately. This may in fact be detrimental to them, as it may increase the risk of further decompensation. Initially, the dose of the diuretic should be increased to offset fluid overload. If the worsening of their clinical status is accompanied by hypoperfusion of the organs, or requires intravenous drugs to increase the force of contraction, beta blocker therapy should either be decreased or halted temporarily. Once stabilized, the beta blocker should be reintroduced (ACC/AHA, 2009).

Potential adverse effects of beta blockers include fluid retention, worsening of heart failure, fatigue, bradycardia and heart block, and hypotension. With each new dose, the patient should be observed for dizziness or lightheadedness for 1 hour. Patients who have had initial difficulties with a beta blocker often have success when the drug is tried again. Although beta blocker use may worsen reactive airway disease, such as asthma, beta blockers may be considered for patients with HF who have reactive airway disease or asymptomatic bradycardia; however, they must be initiated very cautiously, because beta blockers may not be appropriate for patients with persistent symptoms of either condition.

For more information on beta blockers, see Chapters 13 and 31.

Angiotensin II Receptor Blockers

Like ACE inhibitors, angiotensin II receptor blockers (typically referred to as ARBs) work on the renin-angiotensin-aldosterone system. How ARBs achieve their effects is different from ACE inhibitors. Whereas ACE inhibitors block the formation of angiotensin II, ARBs block the binding of angiotensin II to its primary receptor. ARBs do not affect kinin metabolism; because the disturbance of kinin metabolism is what produces the adverse effect of cough in ACE inhibitors, this adverse effect does not occur with ARBs. Like ACE inhibitors, ARBs reduce sympathetic activation that occurs in HF and appear to prevent hypertrophy of the left ventricle after an MI. ARBs decrease the level of proinflammatory cytokines that are present in HF; it is not certain whether ACE inhibitors do this.

Current ACC/AHA guidelines recommend that ARBs be used in patients with current or prior symptoms of HF and reduced left ventricular ejection fraction who are ACE inhibitor intolerant. The three ARBs used in the treatment of CHF are valsartan (Diovan), losartan (Cozaar), and candesartan (Atacand). Clinical trials have shown that ARBs reduce mortality when given to patients who are not able to tolerate ACE inhibitors. Although the efficacy is less well established, it appears that when ARBs are coadministered with an ACE inhibitor, no changes in the mortality rate occur but the morbidity rate and need for hospitalization decrease significantly. Current recommendations therefore state that the combination of an ARB and an ACE inhibitor is reasonable, especially in patients who remain symptomatic on conventional drug therapy (ACE inhibitor, beta blocker, loop diuretic). In some patients, ARBs may be used as first-line therapy in place of an ACE inhibitor.

For more information on ARBs, see Chapter 26.

Aldosterone Antagonists

Aldosterone antagonists also work on the renin-angiotensin-aldosterone system. Aldosterone levels are elevated with HF. The heart has many mineralocorticoid receptors that are stimulated by aldosterone, so increased levels produce additional cardiac effects. Long-term elevation of aldosterone and stimulation of these cardiac mineralocorticoid receptors are believed to be responsible for some of the end-organ damage that can occur from HF. Aldosterone antagonists, when added to a standard regimen of HF drug therapy, improve survival in patients with moderately severe to severe symptoms of HF and reduced left ventricular ejection fraction. These drugs, spironolactone (Aldactone) and eplerenone (Inspra), are also potassium-sparing diuretics, so their use increases serum potassium levels. For this reason, they cannot be used if the patient has diminished renal function (because this causes potassium levels to increase).

Hyperkalemia is a potential serious adverse effect of aldosterone antagonists, and patients receiving these drugs need to be monitored carefully. Eplerenone differs from spironolactone in that it selectively blocks the mineralocorticoid receptors, whereas spironolactone blocks mineralocorticoid, glucocorticoid, androgen, and progesterone receptors. Endocrine adverse effects from eplerenone are thus much less common, but the drug cost is more expensive, leading to more frequent use of spironolactone.

For more information on aldosterone blockers, see Chapter 26.

Cardiac Glycosides

The cardiac glycosides also are known as digitalis preparations or digitalis glycosides. Currently, the only cardiac glycoside available in the United States is digoxin. Digoxin is used to maintain clinical stability and improve symptoms, quality of life, and exercise tolerance in patients with all phases of CHF; it does not decrease mortality from CHF. Current AHA/ACC guidelines recommend that digoxin can be added to reduce hospitalizations for HF or for rate control if patients also have atrial fibrillation. Digoxin is not used as the primary treatment for stabilizing patients with acute episodes of noncompensated heart failure; rather, it should be added after other drug therapy has stabilized the patient, as long as the patient is in normal sinus rhythm.

Digoxin increases the force of cardiac contraction, increasing cardiac output, which in turn increases perfusion to the kidneys. Higher renal perfusion increases the production of urine. Thus, the drug reduces preload and afterload. Although this effect historically has been considered the main pharmacodynamic action of digoxin, there is evidence that its primary benefit actually occurs through neurohormonal modulation. Digoxin has been shown to enhance vagal tone, slowing ventricular rate and reducing sympathetic tone when abnormally high (as in CHF). It also slows heart rate.

Combination Vasodilator–Antianginal Drugs

The combination vasodilator and antianginal drug hydralazine–isosorbide (BiDil) is recommended as an add-on therapy for black patients with a reduced left ventricular ejection fraction and persistent symptoms of CHF despite therapy with an ACE inhibitor and a beta blocker. Hydralazine–isosorbide is discussed in more depth in Drugs Significantly Different From Digoxin.

Drugs Under Investigation for Use in CHF

Natriuretic peptides such as nesiritide have been approved for use in the management of acute HF as in this setting it does improve symptoms. However, whether nesiritide will decrease mortality or morbidity is not known yet. Additionally, there are clinical trials underway that are trying to determine if nesiritide can be used as an adjunct therapy for intermittent intravenous administration in an outpatient setting for those with CHF. It is still unknown whether nesiritide will be useful when given to this patient population.

Vasopressin receptor antagonists are another new drug class that is under investigation for use in CHF. Early findings indicate that they reduce body weight and edema and normalize serum sodium in the presence of hyponatremia. However, the ramifications of these findings are not known at this time. One of these drugs is tolvaptan (Samsca), a vasopressin two (V_2) receptor antagonist approved in 2009 to treat hyponatremia that occurs with clinically significant hypervolemia (such as in heart failure). It is not established though if the drug provides symptomatic benefits to HF patients (FDA,

2009). More research is needed to know if drugs in this class may provide benefit in treating CHF.

Drugs to Be Avoided in Heart Failure

For most patients, there are three classes of drugs that can exacerbate the symptoms of HF and thus should be avoided. These agents are: antiarrhythmics, calcium channel blockers, and nonsteroidal anti-inflammatory drugs. The antiarrhythmics depress cardiac function and can induce other cardiac arrhythmias. The only two that have not been found to decrease survival for HF patients are amiodarone and dofetilide. Calcium channel blockers worsen HF and are associated with increasing the risk of cardiovascular events. The vasoselective ones are the exception to this finding. Nonsteroidal anti-inflamatory drugs produce peripheral vasoconstriction, increase sodium retention, and increase the risk for adverse effects from diuretics and ACE inhibitors.

Ⓒ CARDIAC GLYCOSIDES

The prototype cardiac glycoside drug is digoxin (Lanoxin).

Nursing Management of the Patient Receiving Ⓟ Digoxin

Core Drug Knowledge

Pharmacotherapeutics

Digoxin is used in treating symptomatic CHF. It is added to the standard therapy of ACE inhibitor, beta blocker, and loop diuretic. Digoxin is also used in treating chronic atrial fibrillation to maintain a satisfactory resting ventricular rate. Table 29.1 provides a summary of selected drugs used to treat heart failure. (A complete discussion of drugs used to treat arrhythmias can be found in Chapter 31.)

The therapeutic range for digoxin is generally considered to be 0.5 to 2 ng/mL. A lower range of 0.5 to 0.8 ng/mL has been suggested to minimize adverse effects without sacrificing efficacy. Digoxin has been shown to improve symptoms, increase the quality of life, and increase the exercise tolerance of patients with CHF. These benefits occur regardless of the underlying heart rhythm (normal sinus or atrial fibrillation), the etiology of the heart failure, or other drugs used in therapy (e.g., ACE inhibitors, beta blockers). Digoxin does not decrease mortality from HF.

Pharmacokinetics

Absorption of digoxin varies with the type of preparation. Tablet absorption is about 60% to 80%; elixirs, 70% to 85%; and solution-filled capsules, 90% to 100%. Taking digoxin with food slows down absorption, but total absorption usually is unchanged. The exception is when digoxin is taken with a meal that is very high in bran fiber, which may reduce absorption. Digoxin also may be administered intravenously. Digoxin is distributed widely in the tissues. High concentrations are found in the myocardium, skeletal muscle, liver, brain, and kidneys. Digoxin crosses the blood–brain barrier and the

TABLE 29.1	Summary of Selected Drugs Used to Treat Heart Failure		
Drug (Trade) Name	Selected Indications	Route and Dosage Range	Pharmacokinetics
P digoxin (Lanoxin)	Chronic heart failure (CHF), atrial fibrillation, atrial flutter	*Adult:* PO, loading dose, 0.75–1.25 mg in divided doses; maintenance of 0.125–0.25 mg/d; IV, loading, 0.4–1.0 mg in divided doses; maintenance, 0.063–0.25 mg *Child:* Dosage individualized	*Onset:* PO, 30–120 min; IV, 5–30 min *Duration:* PO, 6–8 d; IV, 4–5 d $t_{1/2}$: 30–40 h
hydralazine–isosorbide (BiDil)	CHF adjunct therapy for black patients	*Adult:* PO, one tablet (hydralazine, 37.5 mg/isosorbide, 20 mg) tid	*Onset:* Unknown *Duration:* Unknown $t_{1/2}$: Hydralazine, 4 h; isosorbide (parent compound), 2 h; metabolites, 2–5 h
P nesiritide (Natrecor)	HF, acutely decompensated	*Adult:* IV bolus, 2 mcg/kg, followed by IV infusion of 0.01 mcg/kg/min; may increase by 0.005 mcg/kg/min no more frequently than every 3 h, up to a maximum dose of 0.03 mcg/kg/min	*Onset:* hemodynamic improvement after bolus, 15 min; hemodynamic improvement after start infusion, 15–30 min; diuresis, natriuresis, 30–60 min after start infusion; plasma aldosterone reduction, 15–60 min after start infusion; dyspnea improvement, 3 h after start infusion (pharmacodynamic effects greater than pharmacokinetic half-life would indicate) *Duration:* about 3 h $t_{1/2}$: 18 min

placenta. Serum drug levels are not affected significantly by changes in fat tissue weight; thus, dosing is best calculated on lean (ideal) body weight rather than actual weight if the patient is obese. Metabolism takes place in the liver. However, much of the drug, 50% to 75%, is excreted unchanged by the kidneys. Digoxin is not removed by dialysis. Because of digoxin's long half-life, several days are required for a steady state to be achieved and for optimal clinical effects to be seen.

To speed the onset of therapeutic effects, a dose higher than normal, a loading dose, may be given to raise the blood level quickly to the desired range. This practice is known as **digitalization.** The total dose needed for digitalization is divided into several doses, with roughly half the loading dose given as the first dose. The remainder is divided and given at 6-hour to 8-hour intervals for oral (PO) dosage and 4-hour to 8-hour intervals for parenteral dosage. The dose is lower if the loading dose is given intravenously instead of orally. To avoid cumulative and toxic effects, dosage adjustments must be made when there is renal failure or suspected age-related deterioration of renal function.

Pharmacodynamics

The effect of digoxin on the heart is dose related. It exerts an indirect effect on the heart from stimulation of the autonomic nervous system and a direct action on both the cardiac muscle and the specialized electrical conduction system of the heart. The indirect effect of digoxin is to create a vagomimetic effect, one that mimics the action of stimulating the vagus nerve. The increase in the vagal tone is now believed to be the central effect of digoxin, which is primarily responsible for the therapeutic effects of the drug. Stimulating the vagus nerve depresses the sinoatrial (SA) node and prolongs conduction to the atrioventricular

(AV) node. This decrease in conduction is known as a negative **dromotropic** effect. Because of the prolonged conduction time, heart rate slows. This effect is termed a negative **chronotropic** effect. Cardiac output is increased as a result of these factors. The improved cardiac output results in an increase in renal perfusion, causing mild diuresis. Digoxin also inhibits sympathetic tone, especially when it is abnormally high, as it is in CHF. Inhibiting sympathetic tone decreases sympathetic stimulation of the heart rate and thereby slows the heart rate. This effect on sympathetic tone is partly from vagotonic action and is partly a direct effect.

The direct effect of digoxin is to strengthen the contractile force of the heart, which is called a positive **inotropic** effect. This effect is believed to be caused by digoxin increasing the movement of calcium ions across the myocardial cell membrane during depolarization discharge. Because calcium is needed for contraction, a stronger contraction can occur with more calcium. The way digoxin increases calcium in the cell is by directly blocking a special enzyme, Na^+-K^+-ATPase, on cell membranes. Because of the blockade, Na^+ concentration increases in the cell. The increased Na^+ concentration causes increases in intracellular Ca^{2+} levels because of the Na^+-Ca^{2+} exchanger. Digoxin competes with potassium to attach to Na^+-K^+-ATPase. When digoxin is attached, potassium cannot be attached at the same site. Digoxin also directly increases the refractory period at the AV node. During this time, the heart muscles cannot be stimulated into contracting again. Digoxin also is known to increase total peripheral resistance.

Contraindications and Precautions

Digoxin is contraindicated in heart block, ventricular fibrillation, certain cases of ventricular tachycardia, some cases of sick sinus syndrome, beriberi-related heart disease, hypersensitivity to digoxin, and allergies (although allergies are rare), and in the presence of digitalis toxicity. Caution must be used when administering digoxin over the long term to patients with CHF who are difficult to regulate or who have a greater than normal risk for developing toxicity (e.g., those with unstable renal function or a tendency toward hypokalemia). For these patients, the physician may consider a cautious withdrawal of digoxin. Monitor these patients very carefully for signs of returning or recurrent heart failure.

Also use caution when giving digoxin to patients with severe carditis, acute MI, severe pulmonary disease, and severe heart failure because these patients may be more sensitive to digoxin-induced arrhythmias. Patients with renal insufficiency are more likely to have adverse effects and develop digoxin toxicity. Use caution in patients who have thyroid disorders because plasma levels of digoxin are inversely proportional to thyroid status. In untreated hypothyroidism, digoxin requirements are reduced; in thyrotoxic patients, larger doses of digoxin may be necessary. Patient response to digoxin is unchanged in compensated thyroid disease. The electrolyte imbalances of hypokalemia, hypomagnesemia, and hypercalcemia potentiate the effect of digoxin, and the patient may develop signs of toxicity even with normal drug serum levels. Remember that digoxin competes with potassium for Na^+-K^+-ATPase receptor sites on cell membranes. Therefore, low potassium levels allow digoxin to occupy more receptors, increasing the risk for adverse effects. Hypocalcemia may nullify the effects of digoxin because digoxin creates its effect by increasing intracellular calcium to increase contraction. Serum calcium levels will need to be rectified to achieve therapeutic effects of digoxin.

Digoxin is a pregnancy category C drug, and its safety for use in breast-feeding women has not been established. Children may receive digoxin; however, premature and immature infants are very sensitive to its effects. Dosage must be titrated carefully in children, and they should be monitored closely for signs of toxicity.

Adverse Effects

Adverse effects are dose related and are signs of digoxin toxicity. Adverse effects occur in 5% to 20% of patients receiving digoxin, with between 1% and 4% experiencing serious reactions. The most common adverse effects are cardiac toxicity, followed by gastrointestinal (GI) disturbances and central nervous system (CNS) toxicity. The cardiac toxicities include bradycardia, AV block, complete heart block, ventricular tachycardia, premature ventricular contractions, ventricular fibrillation, paroxysmal and nonparoxysmal nodal rhythms, AV dissociation, accelerated junctional nodal rhythm, paroxysmal atrial tachycardia, and atrial fibrillation. Almost any type of arrhythmia can be stimulated by digoxin toxicity. It may seem paradoxical that digoxin slows the rate of the ventricles but can allow ventricular arrhythmias to occur. When digoxin slows down the normal pacemaker of the heart, ectopic pacemakers in the ventricle can take over, producing serious arrhythmias.

GI effects are anorexia, nausea, vomiting, diarrhea, and abdominal pain. CNS effects are headache, weakness, apathy, drowsiness, visual disturbances (e.g., blurred, yellow vision; halo effect in vision), confusion, restlessness, disorientation, seizures, electroencephalogram abnormalities, delirium, hallucinations, neuralgia, and psychosis.

When toxicity is suspected, an electrocardiogram (ECG) may help identify whether digoxin toxicity has occurred. Digoxin causes a normal slowing of heart rate, a narrower QRS complex, and a depressed T wave. However, toxicity results in a prolonged P-R interval and a shortened Q-T interval. In the event of toxicity, the drug must be discontinued until all signs of toxicity are gone. Occasionally, if severe arrhythmias have occurred, additional treatment may be necessary. Potassium chloride may be given to help correct the arrhythmia, especially if hypokalemia is present. It may be given orally or intravenously if the need is urgent. Women appear to achieve higher serum levels on the same dose compared with men, which may increase their risk for developing toxicity. Digoxin toxicity is usually associated with serum levels greater than 2 ng/mL; however, it can occur with lower serum levels if hypokalemia, hypomagnesemia, or hypothyroidism is also present. Evidence exists that higher doses of daily digoxin (>0.25 mg/d) or trough (the low point) serum levels greater than 1 ng/mL increase the risk of digoxin toxicity, including death. Digibind (digoxin immune Fab) is used as the antidote to digoxin toxicity.

Drug Interactions

Digoxin interacts with many drugs. The interactions usually relate to decreased or increased serum levels of digoxin or increased incidence of adverse effects, as can be seen in Table 29.2.

Assessment of Relevant Core Patient Variables
Health Status

Determine whether the patient has ventricular fibrillation, ventricular tachycardia, heart block, sick sinus syndrome, beriberi-associated heart disease, or hypersensitivity to digoxin, because these conditions are contraindications to its use. Obtain a baseline ECG for comparison in case digoxin toxicity is later suspected. Also, determine whether the patient is taking a drug that promotes the loss of potassium, such as a thiazide or loop diuretic, because hypokalemia increases the net effect of digoxin, placing the patient at increased risk for digoxin toxicity. Examine laboratory findings for indications of hypokalemia, hypomagnesemia, or hypercalcemia, all of which predispose to digoxin toxicity. Determine thyroid function, which can alter the dosage requirement of digoxin. In addition, determine whether the patient has renal impairment, because poor renal excretion may allow digoxin levels to build up to toxic levels.

TABLE 29.2	Agents That Interact with Digoxin	
Interactants	**Effect and Significance**	**Nursing Management**
amiodarone, anticholinergics, atorvastatin, beta blockers, benzodiazepines, calcium channel blockers, cimetidine, clarithromycin, cyclosporine, demeclocycline, diclofenac, diphenoxylate, dirithromycin, doxycycline, erythromycin, esomeprazole, etodolac, felodipine, flecainide, fluoxetine, frangula (buckthorn bark or berry), gatifloxacin, hydroxychloroquine, indomethacin, indecainide, itraconazole, lansoprazole, lenalidomide, lornoxicam, minocycline, neomycin, omeprazole, propafenone, propantheline, quinidine, quinine, quinupristin/dalfopristin, rifapentine, ritonavir, roxithromycin, simvastatin, telithromycin, tetracyclines, quercetin	Increased serum digoxin levels resulting from various mechanisms, such as altered GI flora, increased absorption, decreased clearance; may increase patient's risk for excessive levels and effects of digoxin	Monitor patient and blood tests for signs of digitalis toxicity.
activated charcoal, aminosalicylic acid, antacids, acarbose carbimazole, cholestyramine, colestipol, cyclophosphamide, kaolin/pectin, metoclopramide, penicillamine, rifampin, sucralfate, sulfasalazine, St. John's wort, vincristine	Decreased serum digitalis level, by various mechanisms, leads to decreased effectiveness.	Monitor patient to assess effects of drug therapy. Effect of digoxin may be reduced. Teach patient to take acarbose and digoxin daily at the same time interval to avoid fluctuations in digoxin levels after effective dose of digoxin is determined.
aloe, amphotericin B, thiazide and loop diuretics, cascara sagrada, ethacrynic acid, licorice, senna	Decreased potassium levels, which increase the risk for digoxin toxicity	
arbutamine	Altered heart rate from digoxin can lead to unreliable arbutamine test results.	
calcium IV	Additive or synergistic cardiac toxicity, resulting in arrhythmia and cardiovascular collapse	Avoid giving calcium IV if possible while patient is on digoxin. If calcium is needed in a digitalized patient, it should be infused over several hours or given orally.
canrenoate	Canrenoate displaces digoxin from the receptor sites, where digoxin exerts its therapeutic effect (Na-K-ATPase); enhances the cardiac contractility in digitalized patients	Monitor cardiac function closely in patients receiving both drugs.
carob seed powder	Increases digoxin concentrations by unknown mechanism, increasing risk of digoxin toxicity.	Teach patients to avoid use of carob seed flour.
chan su (an aphrodisiac), lily of the valley, oleander, pheasant's eye, sea cucumber	Additive digoxin effect increases risk of toxicity.	Teach to avoid concurrent use.
conivaptan	Decreased digoxin clearance by 30%, via unknown mechanism	Monitor digoxin concentrations when conivaptan is added to, changed during, or discontinued from concomitant treatment with digoxin. Also, monitor patients for signs and symptoms of digoxin toxicity. Adjust digoxin dose accordingly.
disopyramide	Altered pharmacologic effect of digoxin	Monitor for therapeutic effect of digoxin.
gossypol	Reduction of calcium release from the sarcoplasmic reticulum may decrease the effectiveness of digoxin or increase risk of digoxin toxicity	Teach patients to avoid coadministration.
khella	May antagonize the effects of digoxin, decreasing effectiveness	Teach patients to avoid coadministration.
kyushin (toad venom toxin)	Additive digoxin effects, increasing risk of toxicity	Teach patients to avoid coadministration.

TABLE 29.2	Agents That Interact with P Digoxin (continued)	
Interactants	**Effect and Significance**	**Nursing Management**
nondepolarizing muscle relaxants and succinylcholine	Increased potential for toxic levels of either digoxin or interactant	Monitor patient and laboratory test values for signs of toxicities.
metformin	Reduced metformin clearance leading to increased metformin levels, possible hypoglycemia	Monitor serum levels if both are administered, and be alert for altered glucose levels.
mibefradil, nefazodone, rabeprazole, ranolazine, sitagliptin, telmisartan, trazodone, trimethoprim, valspodar	Significant increases in digoxin serum concentrations, by unknown mechanism, increase risk of digoxin toxicity.	Monitor serum digoxin levels and assess for signs of digoxin toxicity. An initial digoxin dose reduction of 50% is recommended when treatment with valspodar is started.
spironolactone	Increased or decreased serum digoxin level	Monitor patient, electrolyte levels, and laboratory values to detect signs of toxicities and decreasing therapeutic drug effects.
sympathomimetics	Enhanced pacemaker activity, leading to increased risk for cardiac arrhythmias	Monitor pulse for arrhythmias, and evaluate ECG as indicated.
tramadol	Increased risk of digoxin toxicity, by unknown mechanism	Monitor serum digoxin levels.
antithyroid hormones	Increased serum levels of digoxin when patient first becomes euthyroid	Monitor digoxin levels when drug is first introduced.

Patients with renal impairment may require a lower dose of digoxin. Assess the patient's weight before beginning digoxin therapy, because along with renal function, weight is considered in determining dosage. Serum concentrations are not affected by large changes in fat tissue weight; therefore, to prevent potential overdose, calculate and use the obese patient's ideal body weight, instead of true weight, to determine proper dosage. Assess the patient for depression, as multiple studies have indicated that symptoms of depression in patients with HF is reported in 14% to 60% of the adults with HF (Delville & McDougall, 2008; see also the Focus on Research Box 29.2).

Life Span and Gender

Determine whether the patient is pregnant. Digoxin is administered with caution during pregnancy because 50% to 83% of the maternal serum concentration of digoxin affects the fetus. Also, determine whether the patient is breast-feeding because safety in infants has not been established. Carefully monitor women receiving digoxin because they may be at increased risk for toxicity.

Accidental poisoning of children in the home is common with digoxin. In these cases, digoxin usually had been prescribed for a parent or grandparent, not for a child.

Elderly patients must be given digoxin carefully because they tend to have low body mass and decreased renal functioning, making them more prone to adverse effects of the drug. A lower maintenance dosage (0.125 to 0.25 mg/d) should be used. Noncardiac signs of digoxin toxicity may be difficult to identify in older adults because the signs are

often vague. Also, the older adult may be confused because of adverse effects from other drug therapies or the confusion may be mistakenly believed to be caused by changes from aging. Additionally, some of the signs, such as nausea and weakness, can also occur with uncontrolled CHF.

Lifestyle, Diet, and Habits

Determine the patient's normal dietary intake of potassium, calcium, and magnesium because intake may have a bearing on the serum levels of these electrolytes. Low serum levels of potassium or magnesium increase the risk of toxicity, whereas low calcium decreases the effectiveness of digoxin.

Alternative medicines are a consideration with digoxin use. St. John's wort, an herbal preparation, should not be started after digoxin therapy is begun because it has been known to reduce the serum level of digoxin by about 25% and to decrease therapeutic activity. Patients already using St. John's wort who stop using it after digoxin therapy has been regulated are at risk for having adverse effects from the higher serum levels of digoxin.. Other complementary medicines can trigger digoxin toxicity. These substances include strophanthus and oleander, which contain cardiac glycosides. Senna and cascara may increase potassium loss, leading to digoxin toxicity (see Table 29.2).

Environment

Be aware of the environment in which digoxin will be administered. Digitalization of a patient most often occurs in the hospital where the patient can be monitored closely for adverse effects. In addition, intravenous (IV) doses of

---

BOX 29.2 FOCUS ON RESEARCH

Which patients are more likely to be involved in managing their Chronic Heart Failure?
Schnell-Hoehn, K., Naimark, B. J., Tate, R. B. (2009). Determinants of Self-care Behaviors in Community-Dwelling Patients with Heart Failure. *The Journal of Cardiovascular Nursing*, 24(1):40–47.

The Study

A convenience sample of 65 patients, 50 men and 15 women, ages 21 to 88 with HF were studied to determine what factors influenced their likelihood of engaging in the self-care strategies needed to manage their heart failure. Study participants were administered the Self-care of Heart Failure Index (SCHFI)-research version 3-22-01. This tool has 22 items with three subscales: self-care maintenance, self-confidence, and self-care management. The self-care maintenance subscale measures a person's ability to adopt seven therapeutic self-care behaviors: (1) weighing oneself daily; (2) keeping daily dietary salt intake less than 2 to 3 g; (3) exercising at least 3 times weekly; (4) taking medications as prescribed; (5) keeping within 10% of ideal weight; (6) seeking physician guidance; and (7) obtaining annual immunizations. The self-confidence subscale assesses the participant's belief of how effective they can be at performing self-care to manage their HF. The self-care management subscale measures the person's ability to recognize HF symptoms in themselves and implement self-therapy. Each subscale is scored out of 100, where a higher score indicates better self-care ability in that area. Patients were also assessed for the presence of anxiety or depressions with the General Well-being schedule designed for community-dwelling individuals; this 18-item scale measures 6 areas of mental well-being: anxiety, depresson, self-control, positive well-being, vitality, and general health. Participants were also assessed for the number and type of comorbdities they possessed.

The findings showed that the most common self-care behavior self reported by the participants was taking medications as ordered. The behaveiors of seeking advice from health care providers and following a low-sodium diet were the next most frequently reported self- care items. Participating in regular exercise was the least self reported self-care

activity; almost half of the participants reported difficulty meeting the recommendations for exercise. Neither age, marital status, sex, educational level, or socioeconomic status of the participant correlated to their self-care practices. Participants with five or more co-morbidities were less likely to participate in self-care activities. High levels of anxiety and stress were also found to decrease the amount of self-care that participants reported, compared to those with more positive feelings. Those participants who reported higher levels of self confidence in managing their HF were more likely to engage in self-care activities, and those with more confidence in recognizing symptoms of HF in themselves were significantly less likely to be admitted to the hospital. Thus, the authors concluded that "those with confidence in their abilities to manage self-care will likely achieve better symptom management."

Nursing Implications

Understanding that patients with HF are more likely to effectively self manage their disease if they feel confident in their knowledge of HF and can recognize symptoms of exacerbation is important for nurses working with this population. Nurses can focus their patient education to help provide this foundation. Additionally, nurses need to evaluate the effectiveness of their teaching to confirm that patients feel confident in their abilities before discharge. As patients with multiple co-morbidities are less likely to engage in self-care activities, nurses need to recognize these patients as being at high risk of recurrent hospitalization and disease progression from HF. Again, these patients need additional help in understanding what can be a complex pharmaceutical and medical management of their HF and co-morbidities so that they can develop feelings of confidence in their abilities for self-care. Finally, as patients with high anxiety and depression are less likely to engage in needed self-care activities to manage their HF, nurses should assess for these problems and, if identified, consult with the physicians for additional help for those patients.

---

digoxin are administered in the hospital. Once the patient is stabilized and on a PO maintenance dose, administration of digoxin may be performed in any setting, including self-administration at home.

Nursing Diagnoses and Outcomes

Decreased Cardiac Output related to altered cardiac function
***Desired outcome:** The patient's CHF will be well controlled.*
Risk for Injury related to drowsiness, confusion, disorientation, seizures, delirium, hallucinations, and psychosis secondary to adverse effects of drug therapy
***Desired outcome:** The patient will not sustain an injury related to adverse drug events while on drug therapy.*

Planning and Intervention

Maximizing Therapeutic Effects

To achieve rapid onset of therapeutic effects, the patient is digitalized with an IV or PO loading dose. Roughly half the loading dose is given in the first increment, and the remainder is given in divided doses at appropriate intervals. Assess for therapeutic and adverse effects before each dose.

Minimizing Adverse Effects

Digoxin has a narrow therapeutic index, which means that there is not much difference between the dosage needed to produce therapeutic effects and the dosage that produces toxic effects. It is important to monitor the serum levels of digoxin to help prevent serious drug toxicity. The safe therapeutic serum level is 0.5 to 2.0 ng/mL (some sources now state that the upper limit is 0.8 ng/mL). Unfortunately, some patients exhibit signs of digoxin toxicity even when their serum levels are within a "normal" range. Therefore, it is important to monitor for signs of digoxin toxicity. Box 29.3 provides guidelines for minimizing adverse effects of digoxin toxicity.

Providing Patient and Family Education

Explain the reason for taking digoxin and the adverse effects of the drug.

Teach patients how to check their own radial or carotid pulse. Instruct them to take the pulse for a full minute before taking digoxin. If the pulse is below 60 bpm (or another parameter set by the prescriber for the patient), patients should not take the drug without consulting with the prescriber.

Box 29.3 MINIMIZING ADVERSE EFFECTS FROM DIGOXIN TOXICITY

Monitor serum digoxin levels

- Measure levels at least 8 hours following the last oral dose and preferably 24 hours after the last dose if the patient is receiving maintenance therapy. Following this procedure will prevent reading falsely elevated digoxin blood levels.
- Monitor most closely when digoxin is first started, when the dose is changed, or when the patient has signs of toxicity.
- Periodic monitoring is needed when digoxin is used in long-term maintenance. The frequency of monitoring is based on patient response to drug therapy.

Assess for bradycardia

- Take the patient's apical pulse for 1 full minute to determine heart rate accurately before administering each dose of digoxin. If the pulse is below 60 beats/min, do not administer the dose without approval from the health care provider.

Correct electrolyte imbalances

- Monitor for low levels of potassium and magnesium and high levels of calcium, because these altered levels place the patient at risk of developing digoxin toxicity.
- If potassium and magnesium levels are low, seek an order for replacement of the electrolytes.
- Electrolytes should not be administered rapidly. Calcium and potassium, especially, may bring on serious arrhythmias when administered by IV.
- Encourage the patient to follow a diet of potassium-rich foods while taking digoxin to prevent hypokalemia and digoxin toxicity. However, potassium intake should just be normal if the patient is on a potassium-sparing diuretic, ACE inhibitor, or potassium chloride supplement.

Assess for other symptoms of digoxin toxicity

- Monitor for anorexia, nausea, vomiting, diarrhea, headache, blurred vision, confusion, and drowsiness.
- Anorexia, nausea, vomiting, and diarrhea may also be evident when CHF is uncontrolled. This makes the assessment for digoxin toxicity more difficult.

Treatment of digoxin-induced arrhythmias

- Oral or slow IV potassium often is used as a treatment. IV doses are for more urgent problems.
  - Divided oral doses for adults should total 3 to 6 g (40 to 80 mEq), as long as normal renal function exists.
  - When given to adults by IV, 40 to 80 mEq is diluted in 5% dextrose and water (D$_5$W) to a concentration not greater than 40 mEq/100 mL. The drug should be administered at a rate not exceeding 20 mEq/h and more slowly if the patient reports pain at the catheter insertion site.
  - For children, oral doses totaling 1 to 1.5 mEq/kg or about 0.5 mEq/kg/h IV are given, with careful ECG monitoring.
  - The ECG should be monitored for potassium toxicity (peaking of T waves). If the arrhythmia is corrected, the infusion should be stopped.
  - Potassium should not be used when renal failure exists or when complete heart block is secondary to digoxin toxicity and not related to tachycardia.
- Phenytoin, an antiepileptic, may be used to treat atrial and ventricular arrhythmias.
  - Give 50 to 100 mg of phenytoin every 5 minutes. Total dose should not exceed 600 mg.
  - Phenytoin is used when potassium is *not* effective.
- Lidocaine, an antiarrhythmic, is used to treat ventricular arrhythmias.
  - Give IV for a dose of 1 mg/kg over 5 minutes, then 15 to 50 mcg/kg/min to maintain rhythm.
  - Lidocaine is used when potassium is not effective.
- Atropine, an anticholinergic, may be used symptomatically to treat severe sinus bradycardia or slow ventricular rate due to secondary AV block.
  - Give 0.01 mg/kg IV.
- Cholestyramine, colestipol (both are antilipids), or activated charcoal may be used to bind with digoxin in the intestine and prevent enterohepatic recirculation.

Use of the digoxin antidote

- The drug digoxin immune Fab (Digibind) is considered the antidote to digoxin. This drug, used to treat potentially life-threatening toxicity, is given at approximately the same dosage as the digoxin in the patient's body. It combines with digoxin to make it unable to bind at its receptor site, therefore inactivating it.
- Improvement generally begins within 30 minutes of IV administration.
- Give digoxin immune Fab over 15 to 30 minutes through a 0.22-mm filter, although it may be given as a bolus when cardiac arrest is imminent. This may be given to children or adults.
- Serum digoxin levels will remain high after administration of digoxin immune Fab. Therefore, serum digoxin levels should not be used as a guideline for the antidote's effectiveness. Instead, the nurse should evaluate the patient's response to determine the antidote's effectiveness.

Miscellaneous

- Avoid administration of IM digoxin because it causes site pain.

Caution patients not to discontinue digoxin without approval from the prescriber.

Tell patients to avoid over-the-counter antacids and cough, cold, allergy, and diet drugs, except on the advice of the prescriber, because these drugs frequently contain antihistamines that may interact with digoxin.

Explain the importance of notifying the prescriber if any of the following occur while taking digoxin: loss of appetite, nausea, vomiting, diarrhea, stomach pain, unusual tiredness or weakness, drowsiness, headache, blurred or yellow vision, skin rash or hives, or mental depression.

It is important to instruct patients to return for requested laboratory work to check the serum digoxin level and electrolyte levels.

Caution patients to keep digoxin out of the reach of children (Box 29.4).

BOX 29.4 COMMUNITY BASED CONCERNS

Prevention of Digoxin Poisoning

Digoxin can cause fatal effects if taken accidentally by children. Adults prescribed digoxin should be aware of these risks and take the following precautions in their homes:

- Store digoxin out of the reach of children.
- Have a child-safety cap placed on the medication container.
- Do not leave loose pills out where children can see them.
- Do not tell children that digoxin is "candy."

Ongoing Assessment and Evaluation

Monitor the patient's pulse rate throughout therapy. Assess serum digoxin levels after the drug is first started and has reached a steady state, at each dosage change, and whenever signs of digoxin toxicity are present. Renal function is monitored periodically throughout therapy by measuring BUN, creatinine, and electrolyte levels (potassium, calcium, and magnesium). Again, blood work needs to be monitored when digoxin is first started; recurrent blood work will be done based on the individual's response to therapy.

Symptoms of CHF should improve, and the patient should have increased urinary output, less edema, less shortness of breath, and fewer rales. When digoxin is given for atrial fibrillation, the arrhythmia should be corrected. Assess for development of arrhythmias. Development of arrhythmias may be a sign of digoxin toxicity. When the patient's CHF or arrhythmia is controlled without injury to the patient from adverse effects or toxicity, the drug therapy is considered effective.

Drugs Significantly Different From P Digoxin
Vasodilator–Antianginal Combinations

Like digoxin, the new drug combination hydralazine–isosorbide (BiDil) has been found to prolong time to hospitalization for heart failure and to improve functional status. Unlike digoxin, it has also been found to improve survival. Vasodilators are occasionally used as adjuncts to CHF therapy. Hydralazine, a peripheral vasodilator and antihypertensive, relaxes arteries only. Nitrates provide coronary dilation that would be helpful to the patient with CHF; however, tolerance develops to nitrates when they are used continually. Isosorbide, an antianginal drug that dilates veins and arteries, apparently by releasing nitric oxide at the blood vessel wall, is a nitrate like nitroglycerine. Hydralazine–isosorbide provides the benefit of both of these therapies while avoiding the tolerance that can occur when isosorbide is used alone. How the two drugs work together is not known. Hydralazine–isosorbide is used as an adjunct to CHF drug therapy in black patients.

MEMORY CHIP

P Digoxin

- Used in treating CHF and atrial fibrillation
- Direct effect is to strengthen force of cardiac contraction (positive inotropic effect).
- Indirect effect is to depress the SA node and slow conduction to the AV node (negative dromotropic effect), thus slowing heart rate (negative chronotropic effect).
- Can cause the same arrhythmias it is used to treat
- Antidote for digoxin overdose is digoxin immune Fab.
- Major contraindications: heart block, ventricular fibrillation, certain cases of ventricular tachycardia, some cases of sick sinus syndrome, and digitalis toxicity
- Most common adverse effects: cardiac toxicity; hypokalemia, hypomagnesemia, and hypercalcemia increase the risk of toxicity
- Most serious adverse effect: ventricular fibrillation
- **Life span alert: Older adults tend to have increased risk for adverse effects due to decreased renal function. Children are often poisoned accidentally by digoxin.**
- Maximizing therapeutic effects: Achieve rapid onset of therapeutic effects with a loading dose ("digitalization").
- Minimizing adverse effects: Monitor serum digoxin levels, assess for bradycardia (take apical pulse for 1 minute before giving drug), monitor and correct electrolyte imbalances, and assess for noncardiac signs of digoxin toxicity.
- Most important patient education: Teach how to take pulse and to avoid taking the dose if pulse is below 60; keep digoxin out of the reach of children.

What truly sets hydralazine–isosorbide apart is that it is the first drug specifically labeled to be used to treat patients of a particular race. Initial clinical trials examining the effects of hydralazine–isosorbide in a general population (mixed races) with CHF found the drug noneffective, but retrospective analysis indicated that there was a positive benefit in the subgroup of patients who were black, indicating an apparent inherited response due to race to this combination therapy. An additional study of 1,050 self-identified black patients with stable symptomatic heart failure (more than 95% of them were NYHA class III) found a significant benefit from adding hydralazine–isosorbide to their standardized therapy. Those treated with hydralazine–isosorbide showed a 43% decrease in mortality and a 39% decrease in risk of first hospitalization for CHF. Blood pressure measurement also averaged 3/3 mm Hg lower than for patients who did not receive hydralazine–isosorbide in the study. Because most people with CHF have hypertension, this is an additional, although modest, benefit.

Major adverse effects from hydralazine–isosorbide are related to its arterial and venous dilatory effects. Patients are at increased risk of hypotension, especially if they are currently taking hypertensive drugs. Those who receive any potent parenteral antihypertensive require several hours of close monitoring, because significant hypotension may occur. A common adverse effect is headache, especially when starting to take the drug; this is usually transient and resolves with continued dosing. Light-headedness with standing is also possible, especially after standing from a seated or lying position. Patients should be taught to arise slowly to help prevent this. Patients should also remain well hydrated to help prevent hypotension and light-headedness. Patients should be cautioned about conditions that decrease fluid volume levels, such as vomiting, diarrhea, or excessive perspiration, and encourage them to drink extra fluids during these periods. Men should not take erectile dysfunction drugs that are phosphodiesterase-5 inhibitors, such as sildenafil, vardenafil, or tadalafil, because these drugs also produce vasodilation. Concurrent use of any of these agents in combination with hydralazine–isosorbide could produce an extreme drop in blood pressure significant enough to induce fainting, chest pain, or an MI. Because of a drug interaction, concurrent use of hydralazine–isosorbide with any monoamine-oxidase inhibitor may produce hypotension and should also be avoided.

Information related to each component of hydralazine–isosorbide is also relevant to use of this combination product. For more information on hydralazine, see Chapter 28. For more information on isosorbide, see Chapter 30.

C NATRIURETIC PEPTIDES

The natriuretic peptide is a new class of drugs used to treat CHF. Nesiritide (Natrecor), which is the only drug in the class, is the prototype.

Nursing Management of the Patient Receiving P Nesiritide

Core Drug Knowledge

Pharmacotherapeutics
Nesiritide is labeled for use in adults with acute, decompensated HF (congestive variety). It is used when some resistance to diuretics has occurred. Nesiritide has not been found to increase urinary output or sodium loss when used alone (Sica, Oren, Gottwald, et al., 2010). It is not used in chronic HF, although this use is being studied. Potential off-label uses include, cor pulmonale, hypertension, and diagnosis of MI, although there is inconclusive evidence that nesiritide is effective as treatment for any of these conditions (Table 29.1).

Pharmacokinetics
Onset of action of nesiritide is fairly rapid. Hemodynamic improvement is seen within 15 to 30 minutes, and peak hemodynamic improvement is within 1 hour of IV infusion. An IV bolus is generally used initially. The other effects of nesiritide take slightly longer to be evident: plasma aldosterone reduction takes 15 to 60 minutes, whereas diuresis and natriureses take 30 to 60 minutes after starting an infusion. The decrease in dyspnea is evident in 3 hours. Nesiritide is eliminated in the kidney, where it binds to special cell surface–clearing receptors and is then internalized into the cell and broken down. Two other processes are involved in the elimination of nesiritide, although they play less of a role than the cell surface–clearing receptors. The first is that a special enzyme, called an endopeptidase, found within the blood vessels breaks apart the peptide (a process called proteolytic cleavage). The second is renal filtration.

Pharmacodynamics
Nesiritide stimulates natriuretic peptide A/B receptors, promoting smooth-muscle cell relaxation and dilation of veins and arteries. This results in reduced pulmonary capillary wedge pressure, decreased vascular resistance, and decreased dyspnea and fatigue in patients with acute decompensated congestive heart failure. A recent review of the literature shows conflicting date as to whether nesiritide improves quality of life (Dontas, Xanthos, Dontas, et al., 2009).

Contraindications and Precautions
Nesiritide should not be used as the primary therapy to treat cardiogenic shock. It is contraindicated if there is hypersensitivity to nesiritide or if the systolic blood pressure is less than 90 mm Hg. Caution should also be used if any of these cardiovascular conditions are present: atrial arrhythmias, ventricular arrhythmias, or conduction defects; constrictive pericarditis; hypotension; pericardial tamponade; restrictive or obstructive cardiomyopathy; significant valvular stenosis; or suspected low cardiac filling pressures. Nesiritide should be used with caution in hepatic or renal insufficiency. Nesiritide is a pregnancy category C drug.

Adverse Effects
The most common adverse effect of nesiritide is hypotension, which occurs in 11% to 35% of patients. The effect on blood pressure is dose related. Hypotension may be significant enough that therapy needs to be discontinued. Less common adverse effects include headache and nausea. Other adverse effects include injection site reactions, rash, sweating, itching, leg cramps, anemia, confusion, light-headedness, dimmed vision, increased creatinine levels, cough, apnea, and hemoptysis.

The most serious adverse effects are all cardiac. They are ventricular tachycardia, atrial fibrillation, atrial-ventricular node conduction abnormalities, bradycardia, and angina. These cardiac abnormalities occur in about 1% of the patients. Some research indicates that an increased risk of mortality from renal impairment may accompany nesiritide use, and that it should be used after other therapies have failed (Sackner-Bernstein, Kowalski, Fox, et al., 2005). Yet other research finds that most clinical trials have not found nesiritide to decrease renal function or increase mortality

TABLE 29.3	Agents That Interact with Ⓟ Nesiritide	
Interactants	**Effect and Significance**	**Nursing Management**
ACE inhibitors	Increase in symptomatic hypotension due to an additive hypotensive response	Monitor blood pressure.
arsenic trioxide	Likely to induce hypokalemia or hypomagnesemia, increasing the risk of QT prolongation	Administer with extreme caution if they must be coadministered. Monitor ECG closely for QR changes; monitor serum potassium and magnesium levels.
heparin and heparin-coated central line catheters	Binds with heparin, decreasing amount of nesiritide delivered	Administer through a non–heparin-coated catheter. Administer heparin infusions via unique IV catheter if coadministration needed.
insulin, ethacrynate sodium, bumetanide, enalaprilat, hydralazine, furosemide, sodium metabisulfite (a preservative)	Physically or chemically incompatible if coadministered through same IV catheter	Administer these drugs through a separate IV catheter from that for nesiritide.

(Dontas, Xanthos, Dontas, et al., 2009). More research is needed to understand the adverse effects from nesiritide in relation to this drug's place in therapy.

Drug Interactions

Nesiritide is known to interact with some drugs (Table 29.3).

Assessment of Relevant Core Patient Variables

Health Status

Determine that patients are experiencing decompensated HF prior to starting nesiritide therapy. Assess their clinical symptoms of HF (e.g., shortness of breath). In addition, determine the patients' baseline hemodynamic measurements (e.g., pulmonary capillary wedge pressure, pulmonary arterial pressure, cardiac output), their baseline blood pressure and heart rate, and their baseline plasma brain natriuretic peptide concentrations and plasma aldosterone levels. Determine whether patients may have cirrhosis with ascites, because they may experience a significant blunting of hemodynamic/natriuretic response from nesiritide, possibly requiring a larger dose.

Life Span and Gender

Nesiritide is approved for use in adults. Determine the patient's age. In one open-label, retrospective study, nesiritide was well-tolerated in children with HF who were already receiving inotropic and diuretic therapy; it was associated with improved natriuresis and diuresis (Mahle, Cuadrado, Kirshbom, et al., 2005). Assess whether the patient could be pregnant or breast-feeding, as there is little clinical experience for using the drug under these conditions. It is not known whether nesiritide is excreted into breast milk, but risk to the infant cannot be ruled out.

Environment

Significant ECG or rhythm changes can occur from nesiritide therapy. Therefore, administer the drug only where patients can receive continuous cardiac monitoring, such as in an intensive care or cardiac care unit.

Nursing Diagnosis and Outcome

Decreased Cardiac Output related to altered stroke volume
Desired outcome: Drug *therapy with nesiritide will increase cardiac output.*

Maximizing Therapeutic Effects

Nesiritide must be reconstituted and then further diluted for infusion. Reconstitute one vial by adding 5-mL of diluent, which has been removed from a 250-mL plastic IV bag containing either 5% dextrose injection, 0.9% sodium chloride injection, 5% dextrose and 0.45% sodium chloride injection, or 5% dextrose and 0.2% sodium chloride. Do NOT shake the vial. Rock the vial gently so that all surfaces, including the stopper, are in contact with the diluent. When diluted, the solution should appear clear and essentially colorless. Add the entire contents of the reconstituted vial back to the 250-mL plastic IV bag, and invert the bag several times to ensure complete mixing. The resulting solution has a nesiritide concentration of approximately 6 mcg/mL.

Use the reconstituted nesiritide solution within 24 hours. The initial IV bolus must be drawn from the prepared infusion bag and administered over approximately 60 seconds through an IV port. Use an IV infusion pump to administer the infusion. Calculate the correct rate of infusion based on the patient's weight in kilograms and follow the guidelines for infusion that come with the medication.

Minimizing Adverse Effects

Monitor the patient's cardiac response to nesiritide therapy by keeping the patient on a continuous cardiac monitor during therapy. Assess for changes in QT intervals or for serious rhythm changes. Asses for renal changes. Stop the therapy if serious changes occur and notify the physician. Monitor the patient's blood pressure and pulse; if hypotension or bradycardia develops, slow the infusion rate or stop the infusion altogether. Nesiritide has a longer half-life than other drugs used to treat decompensated HF; thus, it is important not to increase the rate of infusion more frequently than every 3 hours, as needed (unlike other drugs, for which frequent titrations are common). Do not exceed the recommended dose, because this is likely to cause serious adverse effects.

Providing Patient and Family Education

Teach patients and families the purpose of nesiritide therapy and the rationale for frequent hemodynamic measurements and vital sign assessment.

Instruct patients to notify a nurse if the IV insertion site becomes sore or itches.

Ongoing Assessment and Evaluation

Monitor plasma brain natriuretic peptide concentrations and plasma aldosterone levels, both of which should decrease in response to the drug. Assess for improvement of clinical symptoms such as decreased shortness of breath and fatigue. In addition, monitor for signs of improvement in CHF by assessing hemodynamic measures (pulmonary artery wedge pressure, pulmonary arterial pressure, cardiac output). Monitor blood pressure and pulse throughout therapy. Nesiritide therapy is considered effective if the symptoms of CHF are controlled and the patient does not experience significant adverse effects.

Drugs Significantly Different From P Nesiritide

Inamrinone

Inamrinone (Inocor) was previously known as amrinone. The name was officially changed in the United States by the

---

MEMORY CHIP

P Nesiritide

- Used in the treatment of adults with acute, decompensated HF (congestive type)
- Administered by IV bolus and infusion
- Stimulates natriuretic peptide A/B receptors, promoting smooth-muscle cell relaxation and dilation of veins and arteries, resulting in reduced pulmonary capillary wedge pressure, decreased vascular resistance, and decreased dyspnea and fatigue
- Major contraindication: Avoid use as the primary therapy for cardiogenic shock.
- Most common adverse effect: hypotension
- Most serious adverse effects: cardiac arrhythmias (ventricular tachycardia, atrial fibrillation, AV node conduction abnormalities, bradycardia) and angina
- Maximizing therapeutic effect: Reconstitute via label instructions; use an infusion pump to administer.
- Minimizing adverse effects: Administer only if the patient can receive continuous cardiac monitoring (e.g., in ICU, CCU); monitor for ECG changes; monitor pulse and BP closely and slow or stop drug if bradycardia or hypotension occurs; avoid increasing infusion rate more frequently than every 3 hours.
- Most important patient education: Notify nurse if IV site becomes sore or itches.

U.S. Pharmacopeia (USP) and the United States Adopted Names Council in July 2000 because of several drug errors that occurred when the drug was confused with a similar sounding drug, amiodarone, which is an antiarrhythmic. This name change has not yet been adopted internationally. The International Nonproprietary Name (INN) is still amrinone. If this drug is purchased from a source outside of the United States, the label lists the ingredient as amrinone, not inamrinone. United States health care workers need to be very careful if faced with this situation to prevent making a drug error.

Like nesiritide, inamrinone is used in treating CHF. However, it is used only for short-term management of those patients who have not responded positively to treatment with digoxin, diuretics, and vasodilators. Unlike nesiritide, inamrinone is *not* a natriuretic peptide. Inamrinone has a positive inotropic effect like that of digoxin but a vasodilatory effect similar to that of nesiritide. However, inamrinone has a different structure and mode of action from nesiritide. Its mechanism of action is believed to be related to its ability to inhibit phosphodiesterase, which inactivates cyclic adenosine monophosphate (cyclic AMP) and alters calcium, resulting in the contraction of myocardial muscle cells. Afterload and preload are reduced by the direct relaxant effect of inamrinone on the vascular smooth muscle, creating vasodilation. These effects produce a prompt increase in cardiac output from the failing heart.

Like nesiritide, inamrinone is administered by IV infusion. The peak of action occurs within 10 minutes; duration of action varies with the size of the dose. Duration of action is about 2 hours when larger doses are given. The main route of elimination is in urine.

Some of the adverse effects of inamrinone are similar to those seen with nesiritide. Although hypotension and nausea can occur, they are not seen as frequently. Unlike nesiritide, inamrinone can also cause abdominal pain, diarrhea, loss of appetite, vomiting, and elevation of body temperature. Serious cardiac arrhythmias are possible and more likely than with nesiritide. In addition, inamrinone may cause two serious adverse effects—thrombocytopenia and hepatotoxicity. Thrombocytopenia occurs in about 2.5% of patients receiving the drug, although it is more common in patients receiving prolonged therapy. Hepatotoxicity is rare. Thrombocytopenia and hepatotoxicity may be fatal, which is why the drug is not considered first-line therapy and is limited to short-term use.

Milrinone

Milrinone (Primacor) is also used to treat CHF. It is indicated for short-term IV use in patients already receiving digoxin and diuretics. Unlike nesiritide, it is not a natriuretic peptide. Although it is not a cardiac glycoside it increases the force of contraction similarly to digoxin. Like nesiritide, milrinone is a vasodilator, although it works in the same way as inamrinone; it inhibits phosphodiesterase, which inactivates cyclic AMP and alters calcium, resulting in the contraction of myocardial muscle cells. Milrinone also has vasodilating effects. In addition to improving cardiac contractility, milrinone improves left ventricular diastolic relaxation. Milrinone produces a prompt increase in cardiac output and decreases pulmonary capillary wedge pressure and vascular resistance similar to nesiritide.

Like nesiritide, milrinone can have the adverse effect of hypotension or headache, although not as frequently. Serious ventricular arrhythmias are possible; this is the most common adverse effect of milrinone, occurring in about 12% of patients (much more often than with nesiritide). Milrinone can also cause thrombocytopenia, but much less frequently than inamrinone, and rarely hepatotoxicity. These serious and potentially fatal adverse effects limit the usefulness of milrinone in CHF therapy.

CHAPTER SUMMARY

- Heart failure (HF) occurs when the heart is unable to effectively contract and pump out the volume of blood in the left ventricle. The defining symptoms of heart failure are dyspnea (including rales, rhonchi, and shortness of breath), fatigue (which may limit exercise tolerance), as well as fluid retention.
- Chronic heart failure (CHF) is treated with combinations of drug therapy. Primary drug therapy includes the use of an ACE inhibitor, a beta blocker, and a diuretic. An ARB may be used if the patient cannot tolerate therapy with and ACE inhibitor. Digoxin may also be added.
- The combination of an ACE inhibitor and a diuretic has been shown to decrease mortality from CHF. The addition of a beta blocker also has been shown to decrease mortality. Digoxin does not decrease mortality from CHF, but it decreases symptoms and improves exercise tolerance, thereby improving the quality of life.
- Digoxin strengthens the force of contraction of the heart (positive inotropic effect), prolongs conduction to the AV node (negative dromotropic effect), and slows the heart rate (negative chronotropic effect).
- Adverse effects of digoxin are dose-related and are signs of digoxin toxicity. The most common adverse effects are cardiac toxicity, GI disturbances, and CNS toxicity.
- A low potassium level, low magnesium level, or high calcium level potentiates the effect of digoxin, and digoxin toxicity may occur. This effect can occur even if the serum level of digoxin is in "normal" range.
- Bradycardia is a clinical sign of excessive digoxin. Always check an apical pulse for 1 full minute to detect for bradycardia before administering digoxin. Notify the physician and do not give the drug if the pulse is less than 60 bpm, unless approved by the physician.
- Digoxin can be used to treat an arrhythmia, but it also may cause an arrhythmia.
- Nesiritide stimulates natriuretic peptide A/B receptors, promoting smooth-muscle cell relaxation, and dilation of veins and arteries. This results in reduced pulmonary

capillary wedge pressure, decreased vascular resistance, and decreased dyspnea and fatigue in patients with acute decompensated congestive heart failure when given intravenously. It is not used in CHF.

QUESTIONS FOR STUDY AND REVIEW

1. What are digoxin's primary effects on the heart?
2. Which classes of drugs used in treating HF decrease mortality? Which class decreases only morbidity (severity of symptoms and risk for hospitalization)?
3. What effect may occur if digoxin is given to someone with decreased renal function? What actions could be taken to minimize this effect?
4. How do beta blockers such as carvedilol or metoprolol assist patients with CHF?

NEED MORE HELP?

Chapter 29 of the Study Guide to Accompany *Drug Therapy in Nursing*, 4th Edition, contains NCLEX-style questions and other learning activities to reinforce your understanding of the concepts presented in this chapter. For additional information or to purchase the study guide, visit thePoint.

REFERENCES

ACC/AHA. 2009 Focused updates incorporated into the ACC/AHA 2005 guidelines for the diagnosis and management of heart failure in adults: A report of the American College of Cardiology Foundation/American Heart Association Task Force on Practice Guidelines: Developed in collaboraton with the International Society for Heart and Lung Transplantation. (2009). Retrieved from http://circ.ahajournals.org/cgi/reprint/CIRCULATIONAHA.109.192065

Agency for Healthcare Research and Quality. (2003). Pharmacologic management of heart failure and left ventricular systolic dysfunction: Effect in female, black, and diabetic patients, and cost-effectiveness. Summary: Evidence report/technology assessment number 82. Retrieved from *http://www.ahcpr.gov/clinic/epcsums/hrtfailsum.htm*.

Anderson, K. M. (2008). Clinical uses of brain natriuretic peptide in diagnosing and managing heart failure. *Journal of the American Academy of Nurse Practitioners*, 20(6):305–310.

Berra, K., & Miller, N. H. (2009). Inhibiting the rennin-angiotensin system: why and in which patients. *Journal fo the American Academy of Nurse Practitioners*, 21(1): 66–75.

Center for Disease Control (updated December 20, 2010). *Heart Failure Fact Sheet. http://www.cdc.gov/dhpsp/data_statistics/fact_sheet/fs_heart_failure.htm*

Delville, C. L., & McDougall, G. (2008). A systematic review of depression in adults with heart failure: instruments and incidence. *Issues in Mental Health Nursing*, 29(9): 1002–1017.

Dontas, I. D., Xanthos, T., Dontas, I., et al. (2009). Impact of nesiritide on renal function and mortality in patients suffering from heart failure. *Cardiovascular Drugs and Theraphy*, 23(3):221–233.

Feinglass, J., Martin, G. J., Lin, E., et al. (2003). Is heart failure survival improving? Evidence from 2323 elderly patients hospitalized between 1989–2000. *American Heart Journal*, 146(1):111–114.

Food and Drug Administration. Drug label for tolvaptin. Accessed at: http://www.accessdata.fda.gov/drugsatfda_docs/label/2009/022275lbl.pdf. Accessed on October 2, 2009.

Mahle, W. T., Cuadrado, A. R., Kirshbom, P. M., et al. (2005). Nesiritide in infants and children with congestive heart failure. *Pediatric Critical Care Medicine*, 6(5):543–546.

Roger, V. L., Weston, S. A., Redfield, M. M., et al. (2004). Trends in heart failure incidence and survival in a community-based population. *Journal of the American Medical Association*, 292(3):344–350.

Sackner-Bernstein, J. D., Kowalski, M., Fox, M., et al. (2005). Short-term risk of death after treatment with nesiritide for decompensated heart failure: a pooled analysis of randomized controlled trials. *Journal of the American Medical Association*, 293(15):1900–1905.

Sica, D., Oren, R. M., Gottwald, M. D., et al. (2010). Natriuretic and neurohormonal responses to nesiritide, furosemide, and combined nesiritide and furosemide in patients with stable systolic dysfunction. *Clinical Cardiology*, 33(6):330–336.

Trupp, R. J. & Wingate, S. (2008 Fall). Heart Failure: a call to action. *Progress in Cardiovascular Nursing*, 23(4):175–177.

30

Drugs Treating Angina

Learning Objectives

At the completion of this chapter the student will:

1. Differentiate drug therapy for chronic stable angina from unstable angina.
2. Identify core drug knowledge about drugs used to treat angina.
3. Identify core patient variables relevant to drugs used to treat angina.
4. Relate the interaction of core drug knowledge to core patient variables for drugs used to treat angina.
5. Generate a nursing plan of care based on interactions between core drug knowledge and core patient variables for drugs used to treat angina.
6. Describe nursing interventions to maximize therapeutic and minimize adverse effects for drugs used to treat angina.
7. Determine key points for patient and family education for drugs used to treat angina.

Key Terms

acute coronary syndrome
angina
microvascular angina

myocardial infarction
Prinzmetal angina
stable angina

unstable angina
variant angina

Drugs Treating Angina

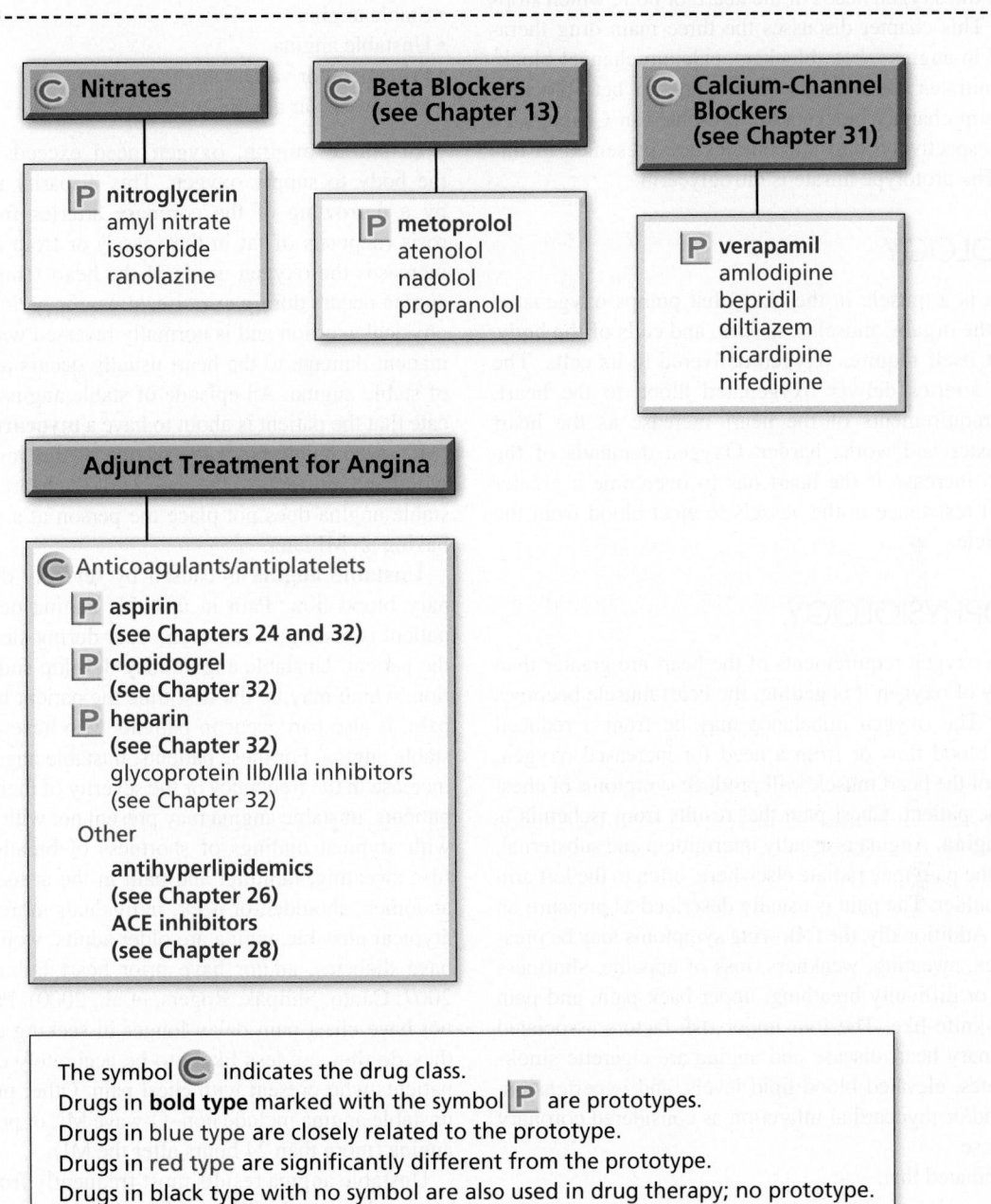

Nitrates

P nitroglycerin
amyl nitrate
isosorbide
ranolazine

**Beta Blockers
(see Chapter 13)**

P metoprolol
atenolol
nadolol
propranolol

**Calcium-Channel
Blockers
(see Chapter 31)**

P verapamil
amlodipine
bepridil
diltiazem
nicardipine
nifedipine

Adjunct Treatment for Angina

Anticoagulants/antiplatelets

P aspirin
(see Chapters 24 and 32)
P clopidogrel
(see Chapter 32)
P heparin
(see Chapter 32)
glycoprotein IIb/IIIa inhibitors
(see Chapter 32)
Other
**antihyperlipidemics
(see Chapter 26)
ACE inhibitors
(see Chapter 28)**

The symbol ⓒ indicates the drug class.
Drugs in **bold type** marked with the symbol Ⓟ are prototypes.
Drugs in blue type are closely related to the prototype.
Drugs in red type are significantly different from the prototype.
Drugs in black type with no symbol are also used in drug therapy; no prototype.

Angina is pain in the chest that occurs because the heart muscle is not receiving enough oxygen. Drug therapy to treat angina allows more oxygen to be delivered to the heart or decreases the oxygen needs of the heart, or both, which stops the pain. This chapter discusses the three main drug therapies used in angina—beta blockers, calcium channel blockers, and nitrates. Because the prototypes for beta blockers and calcium channel blockers are presented in Chapters 13 and 26, respectively, only the nitrates are presented in this chapter. The prototype nitrate is nitroglycerin.

PHYSIOLOGY

The heart is a muscle in the chest that pumps oxygenated blood to the organs, muscles, tissues, and cells of the body. The heart itself requires oxygen delivered to its cells. The coronary arteries deliver oxygenated blood to the heart. Oxygen requirements of the heart increase as the heart pumps faster and works harder. Oxygen demands of the heart also increase if the heart has to overcome a greater peripheral resistance in the vessels to eject blood from the left ventricle.

PATHOPHYSIOLOGY

When the oxygen requirements of the heart are greater than the supply of oxygen it is getting, the heart muscle becomes ischemic. The oxygen imbalance may be from a reduced coronary blood flow or from a need for increased oxygen. Ischemia of the heart muscle will produce symptoms of chest pain in the patient. Chest pain that results from ischemia is termed **angina.** Angina is usually intermittent and substernal, although the pain may radiate elsewhere, often to the left arm or left shoulder. The pain is usually described as pressure on the chest. Additionally, the following symptoms may be present: nausea, sweating, weakness, loss of appetite, shortness of breath or difficulty breathing, upper back pain, and pain that feels knife-like. The four major risk factors associated with coronary heart disease and angina are cigarette smoking, diabetes, elevated blood lipid levels, and hypertension. Angina and/or myocardial infarction as considered coronary heart disease

It is estimated that:

- 9,800,000 people in the United States currently have angina
- 500,000 new cases of stable angina occur each year.
- The age-adjusted prevalence of angina in women age 20 and older was 4.1% for non-Hispanic white women, 6.7% for non-Hispanic black women and 4.5% for Mexican-American women. Rates for men in these three groups were 4.1%, 4.4%, and 3.5%, respectively

(American Heart Association webpage)

The incidence of angina pectoris in those ages 45 to 74 is highest in black women. However, when only considering those over age 65, then men are more likely to have angina than women, and white men are more likely than black men (National Institute of Heart, Lung and Blood, 2006).

There are four types of angina:

- Stable angina
- Unstable angina
- Prinzmetal or variant angina
- Microvascular angina

In **stable angina,** oxygen need exceeds the ability of the body to supply oxygen. This disparity may be caused by a narrowing of the coronary arteries from atherosclerosis (deposits of fat in the vessel) or from an activity that increases the oxygen needs of the heart temporarily. Stable angina occurs during exercise, stress, or periods of increased physical exertion and is normally reversed with rest. No permanent damage to the heart usually occurs after an episode of stable angina. An episode of stable angina does not indicate that the patient is about to have a **myocardial infarction** (MI), a complete blockage of one of the vessels supplying blood and nutrients to the muscle of the heart. An episode of stable angina does not place the person at a greater risk for having an MI later.

Unstable angina is caused by severely decreased coronary blood flow. Pain in unstable angina occurs when the patient is resting; it can even occur during sleep and awaken the patient. Unstable angina may develop suddenly on exertion, which may be the first time the patient has had anginal pain. It also can occur in patients who have previously had stable angina. For these patients, unstable angina is a marked increase in the frequency or the severity of their pain. In some patients, unstable angina may present not with chest pain, but with atypical findings of shortness of breath, nausea, profuse sweating, fainting, and pain in the arms, upper middle abdomen, shoulder, or neck. Individuals more likely to have atypical unstable angina are older adults, women, those who have diabetes, and/or have prior heart failure (ACC/AHA 2007; Canto, Shlipak, Rogers, et al., 2000). Patients who do not have chest pain delay longer in seeking care and when they do they are less likely to be accurately diagnosed than patients who present with chest pain. Other presentations of unstable angina include non–Q-wave MI, or post-MI onset of angina (more than 24 hours after the MI).

Unstable angina results most frequently from plaque rupture in the vessel, followed by a local thrombus formation. Plaque rupture is caused by a complex sequence of events, including local inflammatory activity. *Because of this etiology, unstable angina is considered a critical phase of coronary heart disease and places the patient at high risk for having an MI.* For this reason anticoagulants, antiplatelets, and antilipids are used in treatment. The term **acute coronary syndrome (ACS)** is used to define a grouping of symptoms that are produced by acute myocardial ischemia; it represents a continuum of cardiovascular disease and vessel occlusion. ACS encompasses unstable angina, non-ST-segment elevation MI (NSTEMI), and ST-segment elevation MI (STEMI).

Special cardiac biomarkers, not normally found in the blood, have been found in patients with unstable angina and ACS. These regulatory contractile proteins are called cardiac troponin T and cardiac troponin In (jointly referred to as the "cardiac tropronins." As they are not normally found in the blood, their presence has been shown to be a sensitive and specific marker for ischemic myocardial cell damage. In addition, troponin T is a marker of thrombosis. Troponins T and I, which can be measured by a special blood test, appear to be better indicators of damage and early risk from unstable angina than the traditionally used creatine kinase myocardial band (isoenzyme M). Both fatal and nonfatal MIs were more frequent in patients with unstable angina who had elevations of one or both of these markers. There appears to be a direct relationship between the degree of troponin elevation and mortality even after revascularization procedures have occurred (ACC/AHA 2007; James, Lindbäck, Tilly, et al., 2006; Ohman, Armstrong, Christenson, et al., 1996; Antman, Tanasijevic, Thompson, et al., 1996).

The guidelines for American College of Cardiology/American Heart Association [ACC/AHA], 2007b) state that testing for biomarkers of cardiac injury should be performed in all patients who present with chest discomfort that is consistent with ACS; cardiac troponins T and I are the preferred markers. Cardiac tropronins wll begin to rise as early as 2 to 4 hours after the onset of symptoms. In some patients, the troponin level may not be elevated at the time they come to the emergency department but will rise within 12 hours of admission. Patients who are more likely to have a late rise in troponin levels are those who have ST-segment deviation; present to the emergency department less than 8 hours after the onset of symptoms; have had no prior percutaneous coronary intervention; have not used beta blockers; have unheralded angina; or have a history of previous MI (Januzzi, Newby, Murphy, et al., 2006).

Other cardiac markers of value are the natriuretic peptides, which are neurohormones produced mostly in the ventricular myocardium. Both B-type natriuretic peptide, as well as its less predominant relative N-terminal (NG) pro-B-type natriuretic peptide, have vasoactive properties and are markers of hemodynamic stress. They have been studied in relation to chronic heart failure (CHF) and ACS. Elevations of these peptides are associated with adverse outcomes, especially high mortality, in patients admitted with ACS (ACC/AHA 2007; James, Lindbäck, Tilly, et al., 2006). Measurement of B-type natriuretic peptide should be included in the assessment of risk factors for complications in ACS (James, Lindbäck, Tilly, et al., 2006; See & de Lemos, 2006; Wiviott, de Lemos, & Morrow, 2004). Heart failure can develop after ACS, and elevated B-type natriuretic peptide indicates an increased risk of developing heart failure after ACS (Scirica, Morrow, Cannon, et al., PROVE IT-TIMI 22 Investigators, 2006).

Another cardiac marker, C-reactive protein (a systemic sign of inflammation, associated with atherosclerosis), has been found to be important in unstable angina. Inflammation and atherosclerosis have both been associated with increased mortality and recurrent cardiac problems in patients with ACS. The higher the C-reactive protein level on admission to a hospital, the greater the likelihood of a cardiovascular event long-term (Tanaka, Tsurumi, & Kasanuki, 2006; Cannon & Turpie, 2003; Rosenson & Koenig, 2003; Lenderink, Boersma, Heeschen, et al., CAPTURE Investigators, 2003).

An additional risk factor for patients hospitalized for ACS is moderate to severe anemia. Patients with ACS who are discharged with moderate to severe anemia (i.e., a hematocrit of 33% or lower) have a 2.5 times greater risk of dying within 2 years after discharge than those with mild to no anemia (Vaglio, Safley, Rahman, et al., 2005).

Prinzmetal angina, also called **variant angina,** is caused by sudden coronary artery spasms that induce ischemia in the heart muscle. These spasms, if lengthy, can lead to sudden death. However, this type of angina is rare. Prinzmetal angina may be precipitated by emotional stress, medications, street drugs (e.g., cocaine), or exposure to cold temperatures.

Microvascular angina is a newly discovered form of angina. Patients with this type of angina experience chest pain but have no apparent coronary blockages. The pain results from impaired function of the tiny blood vessels that perfuse the heart, arms, and legs. Microvascular angina can be treated with some of the same drugs used to treat stable angina.

DRUGS TO TREAT ANGINA

Three main drug groups are used to treat angina—beta blockers, calcium channel blockers, and nitrates. Table 30.1 presents a summary of selected antianginal drugs. Some other drugs may be used as adjunct drug therapies.

Beta Blockers

Beta blockers prevent the beta-adrenergic receptors from being stimulated. These drugs have multiple effects on the heart and cardiovascular system, including slowing the heart rate, depressing atrioventricular (AV) conduction, decreasing cardiac output, and reducing systolic and diastolic blood pressure at rest and during exercise. These effects decrease the oxygen demands of the heart and thereby decrease angina. Beta blockers used commonly for treating angina are propranolol, atenolol, metoprolol, and nadolol. Other beta blockers that may be used in treating angina are bisoprolol (Zebeta), carteolol (Cartrol), and esmolol (Brevibloc), although this is an off-label use of these drugs. The beta blockers are discussed fully in Chapter 13.

Calcium Channel Blockers

Calcium is needed in the automatic and conducting cells of the heart to help create an action potential. In the cells of the heart that contract, calcium links excitation with contraction and controls energy storage and use. Calcium travels to these cells through special channels. Calcium channel blockers inhibit calcium from moving across cell membranes.

TABLE 30.1	Summary of Selected Ⓒ Antianginal Drugs		
Drug (Trade) Name	**Selected Indications**	**Route and Dosage Range**	**Pharmacokinetics**
Ⓒ Nitrates			
Ⓟ nitroglycerin (Nitrostat, Nitro-Bid IV, Nitrol, Nitro-Dur, Nitrolingual)	Acute angina Prophylaxis Hypertension	*Adult:* SL, 1 tablet under tongue, every 5 min; total of 3 tablets *Adult:* Topical (transdermal paste or patch), apply 12 inches q8 h; increase by 12 inches to achieve desired results; translingual spray, 0.4 mg/ metered dose into oral mucosa, not to exceed 3 doses/15 min *Adult:* IV, 5 mg/min by infusion pump; increase by 5-mg increments every 3–5 min as needed *Child:* Safety and efficacy not established	*Onset:* IV, 1–2 min; sublingual, 1–3 min; TL spray, 2 min; topical and transdermal, 30–60 min *Duration:* IV, 3–5 min; SL, 30–60 min; topical/ transdermal, up to 24 h $t_{1/2}$: IV, 1–4 min
isosorbide dinitrate (Isordil)	Treatment and prevention of angina pectoris	*Adult:* SL, 2.5–5 mg; PO, 5–40 mg tablets or capsules *Child:* Safety and efficacy not established	*Onset:* PO, 20–40 min; SL, 2–5 min *Duration:* PO, 4–6 h; SL, 1–2 h $t_{1/2}$: Unknown
Ⓒ Beta Blocker			
atenolol (Tenormin)	Hypertension Angina pectoris Acute myocardial infarction	*Adult:* PO, 50 mg/d; after 1–2 wk, dose may be increased to 100 mg *Child:* Dose has not been established *Adult:* PO, 50 mg daily; if optimal response not achieved in 1 wk, increase to 100 mg/d, up to 200 mg/d *Adult:* IV, 5 mg over 5 min; follow with 5 mg, 10 min later; switch to 50 mg PO 10 min after last IV dose; follow with 50 mg PO 12 h later; administer 100 mg PO daily or 50 mg PO bid for 6–9 d *Child:* Safety and efficacy not established	*Onset:* PO, varies, IV, immediate *Duration:* PO and IV, 24 h $t_{1/2}$: 6–9 h
Ⓒ Calcium Channel Blocker			
nifedipine (Adalat, Procardia; *Canadian:* Apo-Nifed)	Angina pectoris, stable angina, hypertension	*Adult:* PO, 10 mg tid, titrate over 7–14 d; SR: PO, 30–60 mg daily, titrate over 7–14 d *Child:* Safety and efficacy not established	*Onset:* PO and SR, 20 min *Duration:* 8–24 h $t_{1/2}$: 2–5 h
Ⓒ Other Antianginal			
ranolazine (Ranexa)	Chronic angina unresponsive to other treatment; used in combination with nitrates, beta blockers, or amlodipine	*Adult:* PO, 500 mg bid, may increase up to 1000 mg bid only	*Onset:* 2.5 h *Duration:* Unknown $t_{1/2}$: 8.9 h

The effects of this inhibition on the cardiovascular system are decreased contraction, depression of impulse formation (automaticity), and slowing of conduction velocity. These have the effect of decreasing the oxygen needs of the heart. Calcium channel blockers also cause arteriolar dilation, decreasing afterload. Calcium channel blockers are used in chronic stable angina when the patient cannot tolerate beta blockers, or if the symptoms are not adequately controlled while on this therapy (ACC/AHA, 2007b). The calcium channel blockers used for chronic stable angina are verapamil (Calan), amlodipine (Norvasc), bepridil (Vascor), diltiazem (Cardizem), nicardipine (Cardene), and nifedipine

(Procardia). The calcium channel blocker used in unstable angina is verapamil. Amlodipine, nifedipine, verapamil, and diltiazem are used in treating Prinzmetal angina. The calcium channel blockers are discussed more fully in Chapter 31.

Nitrates

Nitrates dilate vascular smooth muscle and both venous and arterial vessels (although more relaxation occurs on the venous side). Venous dilation decreases the returning flow of blood to the heart (preload). Arterial dilation reduces systemic vascular resistance and arterial pressure (afterload). These effects decrease the workload on the heart and its oxygen needs. Nitrates also improve the circulation to the heart itself by redistributing blood flow to the collateral vessels.

Adjunct Drug Therapies

Some other drugs are used as adjuncts to the main drug therapies for treating angina. These drug therapies are not designed to decrease oxygen demands on the heart. Rather, they are used to slow down the progression of coronary artery disease, prevent complications that may arise with angina, or minimize symptoms.

As mentioned earlier, thrombus formation is an important concern with unstable angina and some of these therapies specifically target this problem. Aspirin is one drug that is used in chronic stable angina and unstable angina. Per the 2007 Chronic Angina focused update of the ACC/AHA clinical guidelines, a patient with chronic angina should receive 75 to 162 mg of aspirin per day indefinitely, unless it is contraindicated. A patient with acute coronary syndrome should chew an aspirin tablet (325 mg) immediately. This anti-inflammatory agent has anticoagulant properties and antiplatelet properties, which are helpful in preventing thrombus formation and a potentially resulting MI. Aspirin's use as an antiplatelet agent is further discussed in Chapter 32, and aspirin is described as a prototype drug for mild to moderate pain in Chapter 24.

Clopidogrel, an antiplatelet drug, can be used in place of or in addition to aspirin in some patients with chronic or unstable angina. Other major uses of clopidogrel are when a patient has a cardiovascular event from a clot or is at risk for such an event; this use of clopidogrel is discussed in Chapter 32.

Another class of drugs is the glycoprotein IIb/IIIa receptor antagonists; these are monoclonal antibodies and a new class of platelet inhibitors that are more potent than aspirin. Glycoprotein IIb/IIIa receptor antagonists target the final common pathway of platelet aggregation. The glycoprotein IIb/IIIa complex is a membrane receptor for platelet aggregation. It binds platelets to fibrinogen and allows for the creation of interplatelet bridges. This receptor is the common end point of all platelet activities (Gabriel & Oliveira, 2006). Blocking this receptor therefore prevents platelet aggregation. Glycoprotein IIb/IIIa receptor antagonists include abciximab, tirofiban, and eptifibatide. Use of glycoprotein IIb/IIIa inhibitors is associated with lower rates of death, MI, and rehospitalization for acute coronary syndrome (Sabatine, Morrow, Guigliano, et al., 2004). Both clopidogrel and glycoprotein IIb/IIIa receptor antagonists are discussed in Chapter 32. One of these drugs should be added to aspirin and heparin therapies if the patient with unstable angina is to have percutaneous coronary intervention and cardiac catheterization (ACC/AHA, 2007a).

Heparin, an anticoagulant given by the intravenous (IV) or subcutaneous (SC) route, is used in conjunction with antiplatelets (aspirin, clopidogrel, or both) in unstable angina to prevent thrombus formation. The use of low-molecular-weight heparin instead of unfractionated heparin is fairly common

because it provides a more stable pharmacodynamic response and is easier to use. Low-molecular-weight heparin has been shown to be as effective as traditional, unfractionated heparin and appears to be most beneficial to patients who are at the highest risk for complications from unstable angina. Heparin is discussed in Chapter 32. Bivalirudin (Angiomax), an anticoagulant, is used in patients with unstable angina who are undergoing percutaneous transluminal coronary angioplasty. This specific and reversible direct thrombin inhibitor is also discussed in Chapter 32. Warfarin, an oral anticoagulant, may be added to aspirin and/or clopidogrel therapy for chronic angina if needed, however, it increases the risk of bleeding and requires close monitoring of the patient and their clotting times (ACC/AHA, 2007b).

Lipid-lowering agents called statins are used in conjunction with drugs to treat both chronic and unstable angina to slow the progression of coronary heart disease if the low density lipid-type cholesterol (LDL-C) levels are 100 mg/dL or greater (ACC/AHA, 2007b). Decreasing circulating fats in the blood decreases the rate at which fatty deposits are deposited on the walls of the vessels. These fatty deposits narrow the vessel and block the blood flow, causing angina. Such blockages are especially problematic in the coronary arteries. Intensive statin therapy has been shown to decrease the risk of hospitalization for heart failure after ACS by 27% (Scirica, Morrow, Cannon, et al., PROVE IT-TIMI 22 Investigators, 2006). Lipid-lowering agents are discussed in Chapter 26.

An ACE inhibitor is used in patients with chronic angina if they also have: left ventricular ejection fraction of 40% or less, diabetes, hypertension, or chronic kidney disease unless contraindicated (ACC/AHA, 2007b). ACE inhibitors are discussed in detail in Chapter 26.

Angiotensin receptor blockers (ARBs) are recommended for patients with chronic angina who also have: indications for an ACE inhibitor but are intolerant of them, hypertension, heart failure, or have had an MI with left ventricular ejection fraction of 40% or less. ARBs may also be considered to be used in combination with ACE inhibitors in chronic angina (ACC/AHA, 2007b). ARBs are discussed in detail in Chapter 26.

Aldosterone blockers are also recommended for use in patients with chronic angina who are post MI without significant renal dysfunction or hyperkalemia and already are receiving therapeutic doses of an ACE inhibitor and/or a beta blocker, have left ventricular ejection fraction of 40% or less, have diabetes, or have heart failure (ACC/AHA, 2007b).

The most current clinical guidelines for chronic angina also recommend that these patients receive an annual flu vaccine (ACC/AHA, 2007b).

If the pain of unstable acute angina is not controlled by nitrates or anti-ischemic therapy, morphine, a narcotic, may be used. Morphine is discussed in Chapter 23.

NITRATES

Nitrates include nitroglycerin (Nitrostat), which is the prototype; isosorbide; and amyl nitrate (see Table 30.1).

Nursing Management of the Patient Receiving P Nitroglycerin

Core Drug Knowledge

Pharmacotherapeutics

Therapeutic uses of nitroglycerin vary by the route of administration. Given sublingually or by transmucosal or translingual spray or aerosol, nitroglycerin is used to treat acute angina. It also is used through topical, transdermal, translingual spray or aerosol, and oral sustained-release methods to prevent chronic recurrent angina. When given intravenously, nitroglycerin is used to treat to treat angina unresponsive to sublingual nitrates or beta blockers, to treat CHF associated with acute MI; to treat hypertension secondary to surgical procedures; and to create controlled hypotension during anesthesia. An unlabeled use for intravenous nitroglycerin includes reducing cardiac workload in patients with acute MI and CHF; although this is an unlabeled use, it is widely accepted in clinical practice.

Pharmacokinetics

Nitroglycerin is absorbed rapidly sublingually; it also is absorbed through the skin. Metabolism occurs in the liver, and the drug has an extensive first-pass effect when given orally. It is excreted in the urine. Absorption of sublingual products depends on salivary secretion; dry mouth decreases absorption. The drug is absorbed directly into the vascular system through this route; it is not swallowed and absorbed through the gastrointestinal (GI) tract. Thus, it bypasses the first-pass effect. Absorption of transdermal products is through the skin and into the vascular system. Ointments and transdermal systems provide a gradual release of drug into the circulatory system. The drug reaches its target organs before it is inactivated by the liver. Transdermal absorption will be increased with physical exercise, with elevated external temperatures (e.g., saunas), and if the drug is applied to broken skin.

Pharmacodynamics

Nitroglycerin relaxes vascular smooth muscle and dilates both arterial and venous vessels. Dilation of veins is more predominant than dilation of arteries, resulting in peripheral pooling of blood and decreased preload. Blood pressure will decrease as a result of venous dilation. Reflex tachycardia may follow the drop in blood pressure. Arteriolar dilation reduces systemic vascular resistance and arterial pressure, thus reducing afterload. Myocardial oxygen consumption is decreased. Nitroglycerin redistributes blood flow in the heart, improving circulation to ischemic areas.

Tolerance to the vascular and antianginal effects may develop. Tolerance is minimized by starting with as small a dose as possible and removing the nitroglycerin (paste or transdermal patches) from the patient for 10 to 12 hours a day. The sublingual and translingual spray forms of the drug are the least likely to produce tolerance. The transmucosal form also appears to produce minimal tolerance.

Contraindications and Precautions

Nitroglycerin is contraindicated with the use of phosphodiesterase inhibitors (drugs to treat erectile dysfunction) such as sildenafil or vardenafil because of a significant increase in the hypotensive effect. Nitroglycerin is contraindicated in hypersensitivity or idiosyncratic reactions to nitrates or to adhesives (transdermal patches only), severe anemia, orthostatic hypotension, when there is or is a risk for increased intracranial pressure, as it will further increase the pressure (such as in head trauma or cerebral hemorrhage; sublingual route), pericardial tamponade (intravenous route), constrictive pericarditis (intravenous route), restrictive cardiomyopathy (intravenous); and symptomatic hypotension.

Caution must be used when using nitroglycerin in patients with: hypotension secondary to volume depletion that is uncorrected, as increases in intraocular pressure can occur; hypertrophic cardiomyopathy; cerebral hemorrhage or head trauma; gastric hypermotility (sustained-release dosage form); hyperthyroidism; concurrent use of alcohol, CNS depressants, antihypertensives, or other drugs which cause hypotension (additive hypotension); or patients undergoing MRI procedures (transdermal patches), as the metal contained in patches can overheat. Caution also is advised when administering IV nitroglycerin to patients with hepatic disease and severe renal disease. Nitroglycerin is in pregnancy category C, and it is not known whether nitrates are excreted in breast milk; therefore, cautious use is advised.

Adverse Effects

The most common adverse effect of nitroglycerin is headache, which may be persistent and severe. Cardiovascular effects may include hypotension, postural hypotension, tachycardia, palpitations, and syncope. Other effects on the central nervous system (CNS) include dizziness, vertigo, anxiety, and weakness. These adverse effects are related to the vasodilation and cardiovascular effects that occur with nitroglycerin use. Dermatitis can occur from topical application. Local burning under the tongue can occur with sublingual administration. Alcohol intoxication can develop in patients receiving high doses of IV nitroglycerin because many of the IV products contain alcohol as a diluent.

Overdosage results in hypotension, tachycardia, flushing, perspiring skin turning cold and cyanotic, headache, vertigo, palpitations, visual disturbances, diaphoresis, dizziness, syncope, nausea, vomiting, and anorexia. Other signs and symptoms of overdose include initial hyperpnea, dyspnea and slow breathing, heart block, and increased intracranial pressure exhibited by cerebral symptoms of confusion, moderate fever, and paralysis. These signs and symptoms are related to excessive cardiovascular action.

Drug Interactions

A few drugs interact with nitroglycerin (Table 30.2), most notably the phosphodiesterase inhibitors such as sildenafil, which is noted above as a contraindication for nitroglycerin

TABLE 30.2	Agents That Interact with [P] Nitroglycerin	
Interactants	**Effect and Significance**	**Nursing Management**
acetylcysteine	Enhanced hypotension and nitroglycerin-induced headache when both are concurrently administered intravenously	Monitor blood pressure carefully if both therapies are indicated. Warn patient about risk of headache.
alteplase, recombinant	Possibly less coronary artery reperfusion, longer time to reperfusion, and more coronary artery reocclusion	Concomitant use of nitroglycerin and alteplase should be avoided if possible. If coadministration is necessary, the lowest effective dose of nitroglycerin should be used. Be aware that alteplase efficacy may be decreased and the risk of reocclusion may be increased.
alcohol, CNS depressants, antihypertensives	Severe hypotension and cardiovascular collapse	Ensure patient does not consume alcohol. Educate patient about risks of interaction. Monitor blood pressure if coadministration is necessary.
aspirin	Increase in nitroglycerin concentrations and additive platelet function depression	Use this interaction therapeutically to benefit patients with acute myocardial infarction. In patients taking analgesic doses of aspirin, monitor for an exaggerated response to nitroglycerin, as evidenced by headache and syncope. Teach patients to use another analgesic.
dihydroergotamine	Induction of dihydroergotamine toxicity (peripheral ischemia, paresthesias, nausea, vomiting) related to decreased metabolism; induction of angina	Monitor patient for signs of ergotism or loss of antianginal efficacy of nitroglycerin. Dose reductions of the ergot preparation may be needed. Ergonovine, ergotamine, or methylergonovine may be less susceptible to major fluctuations in metabolism and could be considered as substitutionary ergot preparations.
heparin	Possibly decreased pharmacologic effects of heparin	Monitor for therapeutic effect of heparin.
pancuronium	Increase in pancuronium duration of action	Concurrent administration of nitroglycerin and pancuronium is not recommended. If concurrent use cannot be avoided, carefully titrate the dose of the neuromuscular blocking agent and monitor for increased or prolonged respiratory depression or paralysis (apnea).
sildenafil, tadalafil, vardenafil	Potentiation of vasodilation from nitrates, resulting in significant hypotension	Educate patients not to use these drugs for erectile dysfunction

use. Nitroglycerin may interfere with the Zlatkis-Zak color reaction, causing a false report of decreased serum cholesterol levels.

Assessment of Relevant Core Patient Variables

Health Status

Ascertain whether the patient has acute angina or chronic recurrent angina. Assess the patient's pulse rate and blood pressure. Determine whether the patient has any of the following conditions, which are contraindications to nitroglycerin use: severe anemia, constrictive pericarditis, increased intracranial pressure, pericardial tamponade, restrictive cardiomyopathy, or symptomatic hypotension. If hepatic or severe renal disease exists, caution must be used with IV administration. Assess for use of the following drugs, as these will have additive hypotensive effects with nitroglycerin: erectile dysfunction drugs such as sildenafil, other CNS depressants, anti-hypertensives, or other drugs that can cause hypotension.

Life Span and Gender

Older adults may have a more pronounced venous dilation from nitroglycerin than younger adults and may experience more hypotension from the drug. Nitroglycerin is in pregnancy category C, so determine whether the patient

CRITICAL THINKING SCENARIO

NITROGLYCERIN

Peter Riley, age 4 years, is staying at his grandparents' house for the weekend. He finds his grandfather's nitroglycerin ointment in the bathroom. He squeezes some out and spreads it over his entire left arm. When his grandparents realize what he has done, they call the Advice Nurse hotline for their HMO.

1. If you were the Advice Nurse, what would you tell the grandparents to do?

2. What is the major risk to Peter?

is pregnant. Assess whether the patient is breast-feeding, because cautious use is advised in that case. Safety and efficacy in children have not been established. Note the age and sex of the patient (Box 30.1). Assess men for use of erectile dysfunction drugs.

Lifestyle, Diet, and Habits

If the patient has chronic stable angina, it is important to determine how much or what type of activity precipitates an anginal attack, or if angina occurs at rest, which may indicate unstable angina. In patients who smoke cigarettes, smoking constricts the blood vessels and may cause angina. Patients whose diet is high in cholesterol or saturated fats risk developing fatty deposits within the vessels, which contribute to narrowing the vessels. Monitor for use of alcohol, as this may increase the hypotensive effect.

Environment

Be aware of the environment in which the drug will be administered. Nitroglycerin can be administered in any environment, with the exception of IV nitroglycerin, which is administered in the hospital with continuous monitoring for blood pressure and heart rate. Sublingual tablets are likely to lose effectiveness if exposed to light, excessive heat, or moisture. Assess how patients store their medication at home.

Nursing Diagnoses and Outcomes

- Acute Pain, Chest, related to cardiac disease
  Desired outcome: *Acute chest pain will be resolved with the use of drug therapy without injury to the heart occurring.*
- Decreased Cardiac Output related to therapeutic effects of drug

Desired outcome: *Patient's blood pressure will decrease to therapeutic levels but will not decrease to the level of hypotension.*

- Risk for Injury, related to orthostatic hypotension and dizziness secondary to adverse effects of drug therapy
  Desired outcome: *Patient will not sustain injury because of orthostatic hypotension and dizziness.*
- Acute Pain, Headache, related to adverse effects of drug therapy
  Desired outcome: *Patient's headache, if it occurs, will be managed successfully by analgesics so that patient will adhere to drug therapy.*

Planning and Intervention

Maximizing Therapeutic Effects

SUBLINGUAL TABLETS

Place one tablet under the patient's tongue, where it should be allowed to dissolve. It is important to administer a tablet every 5 minutes, up to three in 15 minutes if necessary, to achieve full therapeutic effect. Have the patient sit or lie down to allow for rest and decrease the oxygen needs of the heart.

It is a good idea to keep tablets in the original dark bottle and keep the lid on when not in use to prevent deterioration and loss of efficacy. Avoid exposure of tablets to high temperatures.

TOPICAL OINTMENT AND TRANSDERMAL PATCHES

Apply to areas that do not have excessive hair, to promote absorption. Apply to the chest, upper arm, or upper thigh to promote absorption and increase onset of systemic action. Do not apply to distal parts of extremities (i.e., near the hands or feet).

BOX 30.1 FOCUS ON RESEARCH

Symptoms Across the Continuum of Acute Coronary Syndromes: Differences Between Women and Men

DeVon, H. A., Ryan, C. J., Ochs, A. L., & Shapiro, M. (2008). *Am J Crit Care,* 17(1):14–24.

The Study

This study set out to "detect differences between women and men in the type, severity, location, and quality of symptoms across the three clinical diagnostic categories of acute coronary syndromes (unstable angina, myocardial infarction without ST-segment elevation, and myocardial infarction with ST-segment elevation). "The authors controlled the following variables: age, diabetes, functional status, anxiety, and depression. The patients were from two urban teaching hospitals in the Midwest; a convenience sample of 112 women and 144 men admitted through the emergency department and hospitalized for acute coronary syndromes were enrolled in the study. These patients were interviewed using a structured interview tool. The authors assessed forty-eight symptom descriptors. Demographic characteristics, health history, functional status, anxiety, and depression levels also were measured. Regardless of their final exact diagnosis, women in the study

were more likely to experience indigestion, palpitations, nausea, numbness in the hands, and unusual fatigue. Both sexes experienced chest pain as a symptoms, but more than twice as many women as men (21% versus 10%) did not have chest pain. In this particular study, the differences between the sexes was not significant.

Nursing Implications

Although this study did not show any significant differences among men and women in terms of their symptoms of angina or MI, the sample size and selection most likely account for this, as larger epidemiological studies have found significant differences. The study does emphasize that patients may present with symptoms other than substernal chest pain when they are experiencing unstable angina or an MI. Many of these symptoms are somewhat vague and nonspecific. It is important to assess for these other symptoms and to recognize that taken together, they may help confirm the diagnosis of acute coronary syndrome (ACS) as opposed to representing other disease entities or pathological problems. Failure to recognize these symptoms as ACS can lead to delayed diagnosis, treatment, and potentially death for the patient if they are not diagnosed in a time effective manner.

TRANSLINGUAL SPRAY

Spray nitroglycerin onto or under the tongue to promote absorption. Do not allow the patient to inhale the drug. If used to treat acute angina, spray one or two metered doses. The dose may be repeated but not more than three times in 15 minutes. If used prophylactically, administer one metered dose 5 to 10 minutes before onset of activity that may precipitate angina.

INTRAVENOUS

Proper reconstitution and administration technique will increase the dose delivered. Between 40% and 80% of the IV nitroglycerin dose migrates into many plastics. Therefore, dilute the drug only into glass parenteral solution bottles, and administer using IV tubing not made from polyvinyl chloride (PVC), which is provided by the drug manufacturer. Use an IV pump to control the infusion rate.

Minimizing Adverse Effects
ALL ROUTES

Assess the patient's pulse and blood pressure before administering drug therapy. It also is important to monitor for orthostatic hypotension and to assist the patient to a standing position gradually when arising. Treat any headache that develops with aspirin or acetaminophen until tolerance to this adverse effect occurs. When withdrawing nitroglycerin as a treatment for angina, it is important to reduce the dosage gradually to prevent withdrawal reactions.

SUBLINGUAL

Do not give more than three tablets—one every 5 minutes—to relieve acute angina. If three tablets do not alleviate angina, the patient is considered to be having an acute MI, and it is urgent to obtain emergency help immediately.

TRANSDERMAL

This route is not appropriate for acute angina. Do not apply the drug to broken or irritated skin. It is important to remove the patch for 10 to 12 hours every 24 hours to prevent nitrate tolerance from developing. If anginal symptoms develop at night, the use of a beta blocker or calcium channel blocker should be considered. Patients who normally have angina only during daytime hours are not at substantial risk for developing nighttime angina with a nightly nitrate-free period.

Do not discharge a cardioversion or defibrillation paddle through a transdermal system. Arcing may develop, which may concentrate local current, damaging the paddles and burning the patient. Remove the patches before the patient receives an MRI, as the metal on the patch may allow the patient to be burned.

INTRAVENOUS

Monitor the patient's blood pressure and heart rate while IV therapy continues. It is important to assess for alcohol intoxication if giving high doses for a prolonged period. Use an IV pump to regulate the infusion rate.

Providing Patient and Family Education

Nurses may be asked to teach community groups about emergency care for someone with chest pain. In this circumstance the person offering emergency assistance will not know the patient's medical history. Early recognition of a heart attack and seeking emergency medical assistance for these patients helps to save lives (Box 30.2).

ALL ROUTES
- Explain the purpose and adverse effects of nitroglycerin.
- Instruct patients to sit or lie down when experiencing angina.
- Explain that postural hypotension may occur (especially if standing still after a dose). If feelings of dizziness, weakness, or fainting occur, patients should lie down or place the head in a low position (if sitting) and take deep breaths.

SUBLINGUAL TABLETS
- Teach patients to place a sublingual tablet under the tongue at the first sign of an anginal attack, and not to wait for the pain to become severe.
- Explain that if angina is not relieved, up to two more tablets may be taken; one 5 minutes after the first tablet and the other 5 minutes after the second tablet. Instruct the patient to go the nearest emergency department if angina is not relieved after the above measures are taken.
- Teach patients to keep the sublingual tablets in their original bottle and to keep the cap on the bottle. It also is important to explain the importance of not storing the bottle in the sun.

TRANSLINGUAL SPRAY
- Instruct patients on proper administration—spraying it onto or under the tongue, not inhaling it.

BOX 30.2 COMMUNITY BASED CONCERNS

Chest Pain or Heart Attack?

Many community groups request health education topics for their members. Nurses are often the health care professionals who respond to these requests. If called on to discuss public response to chest pain, be sure to include the following points when teaching families and the public how to respond appropriately when someone is experiencing an angina attack:

- Instruct them to have the person rest (sit or lie down).
- If the person is known to take nitroglycerin tablets, give one and have the person place it under the tongue.
- Repeat in 5 minutes and again in another 5 minutes if chest pain does not go away.

If after three tablets of nitroglycerin the pain does not go away, the person should be considered to be having a heart attack. Call the emergency medical number, and get the person to the nearest hospital.

OR

If the person with chest pain does not take nitroglycerin, have him or her sit or lie down. If the pain does not go away within 5 minutes, assume that the person is having a heart attack. Call the emergency medical number and get the person to the nearest hospital.

• Explain that the drug may be used prophylactically or to treat the onset of angina.

TRANSMUCOSAL TABLETS

• Instruct patients on the proper placement of the tablet—under the upper lip, between the lip and gum above the incisor, or in the pouch between the cheek and gum. It is important to explain that it will dissolve slowly over a 3- to 5-hour period.

• Emphasize the importance of not chewing or swallowing the tablet.

• Explain that the rate of dissolution may be increased by touching the tablet with the tongue or by drinking hot fluids.

SUSTAINED-RELEASE TABLETS

• Instruct patients to swallow these tablets, not to chew them or place them sublingually, because doing so alters onset of the drug effects.

OINTMENTS

• Explain that ointments do not provide immediate relief of acute angina pain and should be used only prophylactically.

• Instruct patients to use an applicator or dose-measuring papers, not the hands, to measure and apply the prescribed amount of nitroglycerin ointment.

• Instruct patients not to rub the drug into the skin.

• Teach patients to choose a different area on the skin when applying a new dose. Tell patients to use a tissue to remove any old ointment left on the skin before applying a new dose.

• Instruct patients to wipe off any ointment that gets on the outside of the tube to prevent it from getting on the hands, and to recap the tube securely.

TRANSDERMAL PATCHES

• Teach patients to apply the patch to as hairless a skin area as possible. Typically the chest or upper arm is used; avoid placing the patch in the distal portion of the extremities.

• Instruct patients to remove the patch for 10 to 12 hours as prescribed.

• Explain the importance of avoiding saunas and other environments that increase the external temperature.

• If the adhesive becomes loose during the "on" period, instruct patients to place additional tape over the patch to guarantee contact with the skin.

• A discarded patch still contains active nitroglycerin, which can be a hazard for children and pets. Therefore, it is important to advise patients to flush used patches down the toilet.

Ongoing Assessment and Evaluation

Monitor the patient's blood pressure and heart rate throughout nitroglycerin therapy. If given intravenously, this monitoring should be continuous. Assess for relief of angina or control of chronic angina. Therapy is effective when angina is controlled or prevented without the development of hypotension or damage to the heart.

MEMORY CHIP

P Nitroglycerin

• Used in treating angina; IV route is used to decrease blood pressure (BP)
• Usually given sublingually or topically, sometimes IV in acute care setting
• Relaxes smooth muscles and dilates vascular beds
• Most common adverse effect: headache followed by hypotension
• Most serious adverse effect: can be hypotension
• Maximizing therapeutic effects: Keep tablets out of sunlight (keep in original dark bottle), moisture (keep cap sealed tightly when drug not in use), and excessive heat; give one tablet every 5 minutes, up to 3 in 15 minutes; and have patient rest or lie down during anginal attacks.
• Minimizing adverse effects: Take BP before and during therapy; to prevent orthostatic hypotension, keep the patient lying down during therapy.
• Most important patient education: If three sublingual tablets do not alleviate pain, seek immediate emergency medical treatment; use prophylactic doses before activities that may precipitate angina; and remove patches or ointment for 10 or 12 hours out of every 24 to prevent tolerance.
• **Patient safety alert: avoid using drugs to treat erectile dysfunction (e.g., sildenafil) as severe hypotension can occur.**

Drugs Closely Related to P Nitroglycerin

Isosorbide (Isordil) is a nitrate, like nitroglycerin, and is used for treating and preventing angina. It is not used to treat hypertension. Isosorbide is given sublingually or orally. Sublingual isosorbide has a slower onset and a longer duration of action compared with sublingual nitroglycerin. Because sublingual isosorbide does not relieve chest pain as rapidly as nitroglycerin, isosorbide is limited to treating acute angina in patients intolerant of or unresponsive to sublingual nitroglycerin. Oral preparations include tablets, sustained-release tablets, and chewable tablets. Oral sustained-relief routes of isosorbide also have a slower onset and longer duration than comparable forms of nitroglycerin. Although nitroglycerin may be used occasionally with adequate monitoring during the early phases of an acute MI, isosorbide should never be used, because of its greater sustained effects.

Amyl nitrate is another nitrate that can be used to treat angina, however it is seldom used for this now, as nitroglycerin sublingual is the standard treatment. It is available only as a capsule that is crushed, releasing vapors that are inhaled. To administer the drug, wave the crushed capsule under the patient's nose for two to six inhalations. Therapeutic effects occur within 30 seconds and last for 3 to 5 minutes. Unlike nitroglycerin, amyl nitrate has no effect on the coronary arteries, but it systemically decreases afterload by causing peripheral vasodilation. It is also the initial treatment for cyanide poisoning and is administered prior to an intravenous infusion of sodium nitrite. Amyl nitrate is a highly flammable substance; therefore, it must not be exposed to heat or flame. Amyl nitrate is otherwise similar to nitroglycerin.

Drug Significantly Different From
P Nitroglycerin

Ranolazine (Ranexa), a new antianginal drug, is used in the treatment of chronic angina. Ranolazine has been found to be effective in reducing angina in a broad group of patients with angina (Wilson, Scirica, Braunwald, et al., 2009). Because it can cause prolongation of the QT interval on an ECG (a potentially dangerous alteration), it should be used only in patients whose angina has not been controlled using standard therapy. The effect on the QT interval is dose dependent. Ranolazine should be used only in combination with other antianginal therapy (either nitrates, beta blockers (metoprolol or atenolol), or amlodipine, a calcium channel blocker. It does not achieve its effects by lowering the heart rate or the blood pressure. It should be added on when other therapy has not controlled angina effectively (Rodriguez-Ospina L, Montano-Soto, L, 2008).

Management of Chronic Stable Angina Pectoris

Exactly how ranolazine works is unknown. Ranolazine is not a nitrate but is a piperazine derivative with chemical structure similar to several groups of drugs such as antidepressants, antipsychotics, and antihistamines. At therapeutic levels, ranolazine allows more activation of the sodium current, but precisely how this relates to anginal symptoms is not clear. Ranolazine also prolongs the ventricular action potential. It has been hypothesized that ranolazine can change cardiac muscle metabolism from using fatty acids to using carbohydrates. The antianginal and anti-ischemic effects of the drug are more pronounced in men than in women. When combined with amlodipine, ranolazine has been found to decrease the frequency of angina and the need for nitroglycerin use significantly. A large clinical trial (Metabolic Efficiency with Ranolazine for Less Ischemia in Non-ST elevation Acute Coronary Syndromes or MERLIN-TIMI 36 Trial), found that when ranolazine was added to standard therapy of aspirin, statins,, and beta blockers it minimized the worsening of angina and the need for more intense antinational medication, and it increased exercise duration at 8 months. Ranolazine did not decrease mortality from cardiovascular or events or IM, however (Wilson, Scirica, Braunwald, 2009).

Ranolazine is taken orally twice a day. Food has no effect on absorption. It is extensively metabolized in the gut and the liver, mostly by P-450 3A and to a lesser extent by P-450 2D6. Steady state is considered to be reached in 3 days of twice-daily dosing. The drug and metabolites are primarily eliminated renally; about 25% of elimination occurs through the GI tract.

Cardiovascular changes from ranolazine are normally minimal. The mean changes in pulse rate are less than 2 beats per minute. The systolic blood pressure increases less than 3 mm Hg, and the diastolic blood pressure normally increases only a few points in most patients. However, for patients with severe renal dysfunction, systolic blood pressure may rise 10 to 15 mm Hg. Mild to moderate hepatic dysfunction increases circulating ranolazine levels significantly and creates wider QT intervals than those seen in patients with normal liver function. The QT-widening effect in liver impairment can be 3 times as much as that with normal renal function.

Because of the pharmacokinetic and pharmacodynamic effects of ranolazine, it has the following contraindications: pre-existing QT prolongation; use of drugs that prolong the QT interval (e.g., Class Ia or Class III antiarrhythmics, erythromycin, and some antipsychotics [thioridazine, ziprasidone]); hepatic impairment (mild, moderate, or severe); and current use of drugs that are potent or moderately potent CYP 3A inhibitors (e.g., ketoconazole, HIV protease inhibitors, macrolide antibiotics, diltiazem, verapamil, or grapefruit juice, which all increase serum levels of ranolazine). Ranolazine is a pregnancy category C drug. Whether it is excreted in breast milk is not known. The drug has not been tested in children.

Ranolazine has several drug interactions. Many of the drug interactions are related to changes in the P-450 system. Drugs that inhibit the 3A pathway, which is responsible for metabolism of ranolazine, will increase the circulating level of ranolazine. Because ranolazine inhibits the 2D6 pathway, drugs that are metabolized by this route will have higher circulating levels. Many drugs are metabolized by one of these pathways, so the nurse should always consult a source listing drug interactions with ranolazine prior to administering it. Two drug interactions of special note occur with coadministration of ranolazine with digoxin or simvastatin. Ranolazine greatly increases the circulating levels of each of these drugs, which may produce serious adverse effects.

The most common adverse effects from ranolazine are dizziness, headache, constipation, and nausea. Small, reversible elevations in serum creatinine and blood urea nitrogen have been observed, but they are not associated with renal toxicity. The most serious adverse effect is prolongation of the QT interval. Patients receiving other drugs that prolong the QT interval are likely to develop a form of ventricular tachycardia called torsades de pointes.

To minimize adverse effects of ranolazine, it is necessary to confirm that the patient has previously received other therapy for angina prior to starting ranolazine; the patient should currently be receiving nitrates, beta blockers, or amlodipine when ranolazine is started. The dose should not exceed the maximum recommended amount of 1,000 mg twice a day. The patient should be assessed for evidence of any liver disease. Baseline and follow-up ECGs are necessary to evaluate the effects on the QT interval. Coadministration of drugs that prolong the QT interval or that are inhibitors of P3A isoenzyme should be avoided. Patients also receiving either digoxin or simvastatin may need a decreased dose of those drugs, depending on their serum levels. Blood pressure of patients with renal dysfunction should be monitored while they are taking ranolazine. Patients should be taught to avoid grapefruit juice or grapefruit in their diets. They may take the drug either with or without food as long as it is swallowed whole and not crushed, broken, or chewed.

CHAPTER SUMMARY

- Nitroglycerin is used to treat angina and to prevent angina. When given intravenously, it also is used to reduce hypertension.
- Nitroglycerin relaxes vascular smooth muscle and dilates both arterial and venous beds. Dilation of veins is more predominant than dilation of arteries, resulting in peripheral pooling of blood and decreased preload.
- Blood pressure decreases as a result of venous dilation. Reflex tachycardia may follow the drop in blood pressure. Thus, the patient's blood pressure is assessed before each dose and during drug therapy with nitroglycerin, and the pulse should be assessed during therapy.
- Arteriolar dilation reduces systemic vascular resistance and arterial pressure, thus reducing afterload. Reduced afterload decreases the work the heart must perform to eject blood from the left ventricle and thereby decreases the oxygen needs of the heart.
- The most common adverse effect of nitroglycerin is headache.
- When nitroglycerin is given intravenously because of elevated blood pressure, the patient must be continually monitored in an intensive care setting. For safety, the drug should be administered by pump.

QUESTIONS FOR STUDY AND REVIEW

1. If the patient is taking nitroglycerin through a transdermal patch to prevent recurrent angina, why should he or she wear the patch only 12 to 14 hours a day?
2. How often should a tablet of sublingual nitroglycerin be administered to treat an episode of angina? How many tablets can be administered?
3. Why should you take the patient's blood pressure before administering a dose of nitroglycerin ointment topically?
4. When measuring the dose of nitroglycerin ointment, you get some on your hands. Later, you experience a throbbing headache. What is the explanation for this headache?
5. How does nitroglycerin decrease anginal pain?

NEED MORE HELP?

Chapter 30 of the Study Guide to Accompany *Drug Therapy in Nursing*, 4th Edition, contains NCLEX-style questions and other learning activities to reinforce your understanding of the concepts presented in this chapter. For additional information or to purchase the study guide, visit thePoint.

REFERENCES

American College of Cardiology/American Heart Association (2007a). ACC/AHA 2007 Guidelines for the Management of Patients With Unstable Angina/Non–ST-Elevation Myocardial Infarction

A Report of the American College of Cardiology/American Heart Association Task Force on Practice Guidelines (Writing Committee to Revise the 2002 Guidelines for the Management of Patients With Unstable Angina/Non–ST-Elevation Myocardial Infarction) *Developed in Collaboration with the American College of Emergency Physicians, the Society for Cardiovascular Angiography and Interventions, and the Society of Thoracic Surgeons Endorsed by the American Association of Cardiovascular and Pulmonary Rehabilitation and the Society for Academic Emergency Medicine.*

Journal of the American College of Cardiology, 2007; 50:1–157. Retrieved from: http://content.onlinejacc.org/cgi/content/full/50/7/e1

American College of Cardiology/American Heart Association. (2007b). 2007 chronic angina focused update of the ACC/AHA 2002 Guidelines for the management of patients with chronic stable angina: A report of the American College of Cardiology/American Heart Association Task Force on Practice Guidelines Writing Group to develop the focused update of the 2002 Guidelines for the management of patients with chronic stable angina. Retrieved from *http://circ.ahajournals.org/cgi/reprint/CIRCULATIONAHA.107.187930.*

American Heart Association. Heart attack and angina statistics. Retrieved from http://www.americanheart.org/presenter.jhtml?identifier=4591. Accessed on September 20, 2009.

Antman, E. M., Tanasijevic, M. J., Thompson, B., et al. (1996). Cardiac-specific troponin I levels to predict the risk of mortality in patients with acute coronary syndromes. *New England Journal of Medicine*, 335:1342–1349.

Cannon, C. P., & Turpie, A. G. G. (2003). Unstable angina and non-ST-elevation myocardial infarction: Initial antithrombotic therapy and early invasive strategy. *Circulation*, 107(21): 2640–2645.

Canto, J. G., Shlipak, M. G., Rogers, W. J., et al. (2000). Prevalence, clinical characteristics, and mortality among patients with myocardial infarction presenting without chest pain *Journal of the American Medical Association*, 283:3223–3229.

Gabriel, H. M., & Oliveira, E. I. (2006). Role of abciximab in the treatment of coronary artery disease. *Expert Opinion on Biological Therapy*, 6(9):935–942.

James, S. K., Lindback, J., Tilly, J., et al. (2006). Troponin-T and N-terminal pro-B–type natriuretic peptide predict mortality benefit from coronary revascularization in acute coronary syndromes: A GUSTO-IV substudy. *Journal of the American College of Cardiology*, 48(6):1146–1154.

Januzzi, J. L., Jr., Newby, L. K., Murphy, S. A., et al. (2006). Predicting a late positive serum troponin in initially troponin-negative patients with non-ST elevation acute coronary syndrome: Clinical predictors and validated risk score results from the TIMI IIIB and GUSTO IIA studies. *American Heart Journal*, 151(2):360–366.

Lenderink, T., Boersma, E., Heeschen, C., et al., CAPTURE Investigators. (2003). Elevated troponin T and C-reactive protein predict impaired outcome for 4 years in patients with refractory unstable angina, and troponin T predicts benefit of treatment with abciximab in combination with PTCA. *European Heart Journal*, 24(1):77–85.

National Heart Lung and Blood Institute. Incidence and Prevalence: 2006 Chart Book on Cardiovascular and Lung Diseases. Retrieved from: http://www.nhlbi.nih.gov/resources/docs/06a_ip_chtbk.pdf.

Ohman, E. M., Armstrong, P. W., Christenson, R. H., et al. GUSTO IIA Investigators. (1996). Cardiac troponin T levels for risk stratification in acute myocardial ischemia. *New England Journal of Medicine*, 335:1333–1341.

Rodríguez-Ospina, L., & Montano-Soto, L. (2008). Management of chronic stable angina pectoris. *Boletín de la Asociación Médica de Puerto Rico*, 100(4):39-47.

Rosenson, R. S., & Koenig, W. (2003). Utility of inflammatory markers in the management of coronary artery disease. *American Journal of Cardiology*, 92(1A):10i–18i.

Sabatine, M. S., Morrow, D. A., Giugliano, R. P., et al. (2004). Implications of upstream glycoprotein IIb/IIIa inhibition and coronary artery stenting in the invasive management of unstable angina/non-ST-elevation myocardial infarction: A comparison of the Thrombolysis in Myocardial Infarction (TIMI) IIIB trial and the Treat angina with Aggrastat and determine Cost of Therapy with Invasive or Conservative Strategy (TACTICS)–TIMI 18 trial. *Circulation*, 109(7):874–880.

Scirica, B. M., Morrow, D. A., Cannon, C. P., et al., PROVE IT-TIMI 22 Investigators. (2006). Intensive statin therapy and the risk of hospitalization for heart failure after an acute coronary syndrome in the PROVE IT-TIMI 22 study. *Journal of the American College of Cardiologists*, 47(11):2326–2331.

See, R., & de Lemos, J. A. (2006). Current status of risk stratification methods in acute coronary syndromes. *Current Cardiology Reports*, 8(4):282–288.

Tadros, G. M., McConnell, T. R., Wood, G. C., et al. (2003). Clinical predictors of 30 day cardiac events in patients with acute coronary syndrome at a community hospital. *Southern Medical Journal*, 96(11):1113–1120.

Tanaka, H., Tsurumi, Y., & Kasanuki, H. (2006). Prognostic value of C-reactive protein and troponin T level in patients with unstable angina pectoris. *Journal of Cardiology*, 47(4): 173–179.

Vaglio, J., Safley, D. M., Rahman, M., et al. (2005). Relation of anemia at discharge to survival after acute coronary syndromes. *American Journal of Cardiology*, 96:496–499. Also available through Agency for Healthcare Research and Quality (AHRQ) online at *http://www.ahrq. gov/research/dec05/1205RA13.htm*.

Wilson, S. R., Scirica, B. M., Braunwald, E., et al. (2009). Efficacy of ranolazine in patients with chronic angina observations from the randomized, double- blinded, placebo-controlled MERLIN-TIMI (Metabolic Efficiency with Ranolazine for Less Ischemia inNon-ST Segment Acute Coronary Syndromes)36 Trial. *Journal of the American College of Cardiology*, 53(17):1510–1516.

Wiviott, S. D., de Lemos, J. A., & Morrow, D. A. (2004). Pathophysiology, prognostic significant and clinical utility of B-type natriuretic peptide in acute coronary syndromes. *Clinica Chimica Acta, International Journal of Clinical Chemistry*, 346:119–128.

31

Drugs Affecting Cardiac Rhythm

Learning Objectives

At the completion of this chapter the student will:

1. Identify core drug knowledge about drugs that affect cardiac rhythm.

2. Identify core patient variables relevant to drugs that affect cardiac rhythm.

3. Relate the interaction of core drug knowledge to core patient variables for drugs that affect cardiac rhythm.

4. Differentiate Class I, II, III, and IV antiarrhythmic drugs.

5. Describe the varied therapeutic effects of beta blockers and calcium channel blockers.

6. Generate a nursing plan of care from the interactions between core drug knowledge and core patient variables for drugs that affect cardiac function.

7. Describe nursing interventions to maximize therapeutic and minimize adverse effects for drugs that affect cardiac rhythm.

8. Determine key points for patient and family education for drugs that affect cardiac rhythm.

9. Differentiate the three main sources of data used in assessment of core drug variables.

Key Terms		
action potential	dysrhythmia	repolarization
arrhythmia	ectopic foci	resting membrane potential
atrial fibrillation	electrocardiogram	transmembrane potential
atrial flutter	proarrhythmia	ventricular fibrillation
automaticity	re-entry phenomenon	ventricular tachycardia
depolarization	refractory period	

Drugs Affecting Cardiac Rhythm

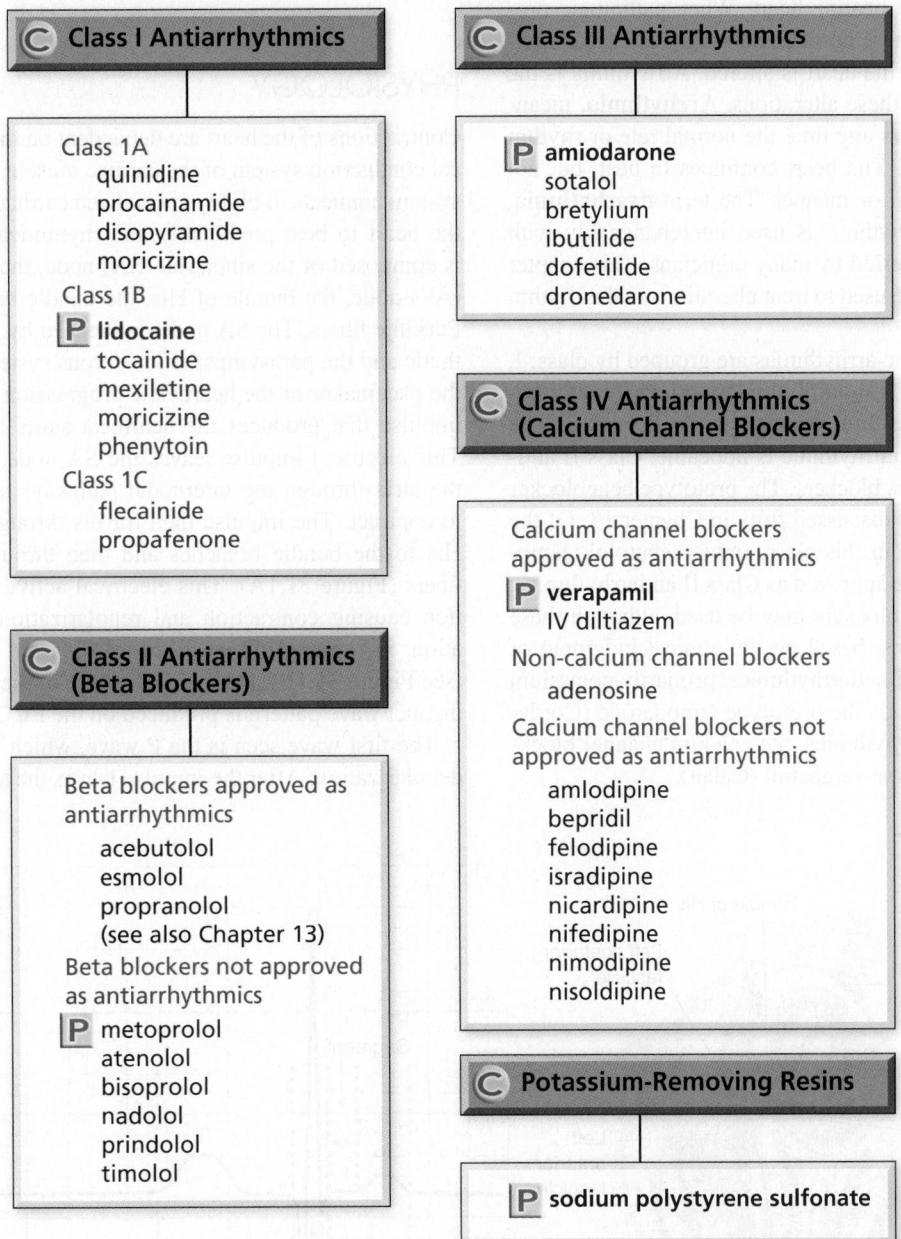

Class I Antiarrhythmics

Class 1A
- quinidine
- procainamide
- disopyramide
- moricizine

Class 1B
- lidocaine
- tocainide
- mexiletine
- moricizine
- phenytoin

Class 1C
- flecainide
- propafenone

Class II Antiarrhythmics (Beta Blockers)

Beta blockers approved as antiarrhythmics
- acebutolol
- esmolol
- propranolol
- (see also Chapter 13)

Beta blockers not approved as antiarrhythmics
- metoprolol
- atenolol
- bisoprolol
- nadolol
- prindolol
- timolol

Class III Antiarrhythmics

- amiodarone
- sotalol
- bretylium
- ibutilide
- dofetilide
- dronedarone

Class IV Antiarrhythmics (Calcium Channel Blockers)

Calcium channel blockers approved as antiarrhythmics
- verapamil
- IV diltiazem

Non-calcium channel blockers
- adenosine

Calcium channel blockers not approved as antiarrhythmics
- amlodipine
- bepridil
- felodipine
- isradipine
- nicardipine
- nifedipine
- nimodipine
- nisoldipine

Potassium-Removing Resins

- sodium polystyrene sulfonate

The symbol **C** indicates the drug class.
Drugs in **bold type** marked with the symbol **P** are prototypes.
Drugs in blue type are closely related to the prototype.
Drugs in red type are significantly different from the prototype.
Drugs in black type with no symbol are also used in drug therapy; no prototype.

The heart is the muscle responsible for pumping blood through the circulatory system. The contraction of the heart depends on changes in electrical stimulation in cardiac muscle cells. These changes in electrical activity occur at regular, set intervals. These set interval patterns establish a normal rhythm for the beating heart. When pathologic processes interfere with these normal changes in electrical stimulation, the rhythm of the heart is altered. Arrhythmia is the term used to describe these alterations. **Arrhythmia,** meaning "no rhythm," occurs any time the normal rate or rhythm of the heart is altered. The heart continues to beat, but not in the expected pattern or manner. The term **dysrhythmia,** meaning "abnormal rhythm," is used interchangeably with arrhythmia and is preferred by many clinicians. This chapter identifies drugs that are used to treat alterations in the rhythm of the heart.

Drugs to treat cardiac arrhythmias are grouped by class: I, II, III, and IV. Class 1 antiarrhythmics, primarily sodium-channel blockers, have three subclasses, A, B, and C. The prototype Class IB antiarrhythmic is lidocaine. Class II antiarrhythmics are the beta blockers. The prototype beta blocker is metoprolol, and it is discussed fully in Chapter 13. Of the other numerous drugs in this class, only acebutolol, esmolol, and propranolol are approved as Class II antiarrhythmics. Any of the other beta blockers may be used, although these are off-label indications, based on the clinical judgment of the physician. Class III antiarrhythmics, primarily potassium channel blockers, include the prototype amiodarone (Cordarone). Class IV antiarrhythmics, the calcium channel blockers, include the prototype verapamil (Calan).

Because hyperkalemia is an electrolyte imbalance that may cause potentially lethal arrhythmias, drugs to prevent arrhythmias are the potassium-removing resins. The prototype potassium-removing resin is sodium polystyrene sulfonate (Kayexalate).

PHYSIOLOGY

Contractions of the heart are dependent on the unique electrical conduction system of the cardiac muscle. The conduction system connects to highly specialized cardiac cells that allow the heart to beat predictably and rhythmically. The system is composed of the sinoatrial (SA) node, the atrioventricular (AV) node, the bundle of His, the bundle branches, and the Purkinje fibers. The SA node, influenced by both the sympathetic and the parasympathetic nervous systems, is known as the pacemaker of the heart. The progression of the electrical impulse that produces the heartbeat starts in the SA node. This electrical impulse leaves the SA node, travels through the atria through the internodal pathways and causes them to contract. The impulse then travels through the bundle of His to the bundle branches and then through the Purkinje fibers (Figure 31.1A). This electrical activity of depolarization causing contraction and repolarization causing relaxation, is captured on an electrocardiogram (ECG or EKG) (see Figure 31.1B). During each phase of the cardiac cycle, a distinct wave pattern is produced on the ECG.

The first wave seen is the P wave, which represents atrial depolarization. After the impulse leaves the atria, it is slowed

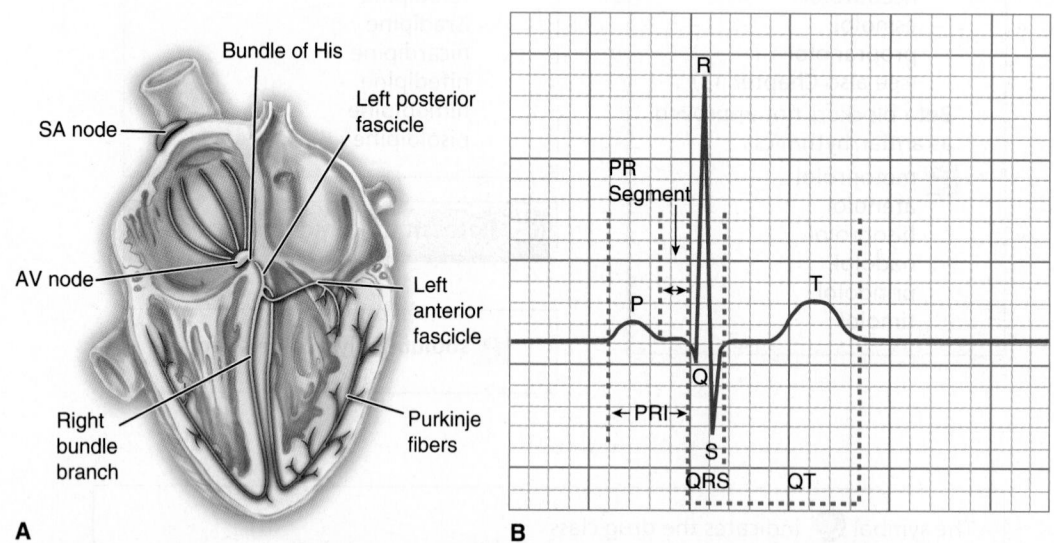

• FIGURE 31.1 Cardiac conduction. **(A)** The heart's electrical circuitry has a profound effect on efficient blood flow to the tissues. An electrical impulse from the sinoatrial (SA) node travels over the internodal pathways to produce atrial contraction. The impulse slows slightly as it nears the ventricles at the atrioventricular (AV) node (the AV junction). After passing through the bundle of His, the impulse descends along the left and right bundle branches to the Purkinje fibers, stimulating ventricular contraction and proceeding on to the SA node to continue the cycle. The efficiency of the conduction system has a major influence on cardiac rhythm and output reflected by blood flow. **(B)** This is the pattern of one cardiac cycle on an EKG. Note the components of the complex including the waves and intervals. P wave, PR interval, PR segment; Q,R and S waves, QRS complex; ST segment, QT interval.

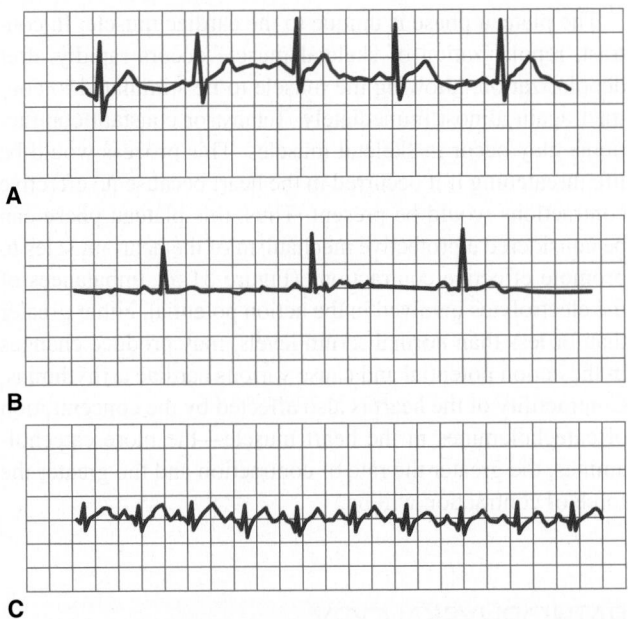

• FIGURE 31.2 **(A)** Normal sinus rhythm, ECG. **(B)** Bradycardia, slow heart rate. **(C)** Tachycardia, fast heart rate.

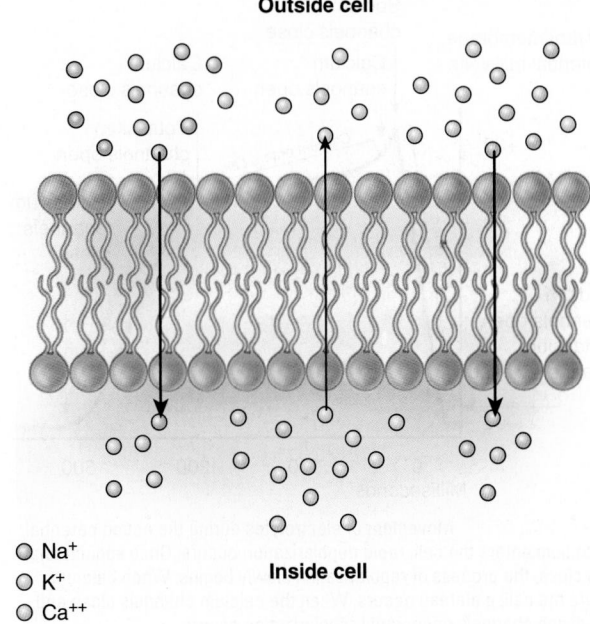

• FIGURE 31.3 Intracellular and extracellular ions. Potassium is the predominant intracellular ion. It will move to the outside of the cell, following its concentration gradient. Sodium and calcium are predominantly extracellular ions; they will move into the cell.

at the AV node to allow the ventricles to fill and to ensure that the atria and the ventricles do not contract simultaneously. On the ECG, this slowing is translated into a period of inactivity called the PR segment: a straight line between the end of the P wave and the start of the first deflection of the next wave. All of the electrical activity in the heart that takes place before the impulse reaches the ventricles is seen in the PR interval, which includes the P wave and the PR segment. The ventricular depolarization is shown by a large complex of three waves: The Q, the R, and the S, called the QRS complex. After the ventricles depolarize, they begin the repolarization phase, which results in another wave on the ECG called the T wave. The atria also repolarize, but their repolarization usually occurs at the same time as ventricular depolarization; thus, the atrial repolarization wave is usually hidden in the QRS complex.

Figure 31.2A shows a normal-rate ECG. Compare this normal rate to the slow heart rate (bradycardia: a resting heart rate less than 60 beats per minute [bpm]) shown in Figure 31.2B and to the fast heart rate (tachycardia: a resting heart rate greater than 100 bpm) shown in Figure 31.2C.

To best comprehend this unique conduction system, it is important to understand how the movement of potassium, sodium, and calcium ions bring about electrical changes in the cardiac cells to stimulate contraction. Potassium is predominantly an intracellular (within the cell) ion, and sodium and calcium are predominantly extracellular (outside the cell) ions (Figure 31.3). Calcium is also stored in sarcoplasmic reticulum within the cell, but it is not active as long as it is stored.

These ions (potassium, sodium, and calcium) all flow following the normal concentration gradient (moving from areas of high concentration to areas of low concentration). Because

of the different concentrations of intracellular and extracellular ions, an electrical gradient exists across the membrane of the cell. This electrical gradient is called the **transmembrane potential.** All changes that occur in the transmembrane potential during an entire cycle of contraction and relaxation are, as a unit, called the **action potential.** At rest, the electrical charge of the transmembrane potential, also known as the **resting membrane potential,** is −90 millivolts (mV). This means that there is a 90-mV difference between the electrical charge inside and outside of the cell, and that the charge is negative inside the cell. As sodium moves into the cell, **depolarization** occurs. At this point, the transmembrane potential changes from negative to positive. Depolarization occurs rapidly and is called phase 0 of the action potential. During this rapid depolarization, the sodium channels open quickly for only a brief period. While these "fast channels" are open, sodium rushes into the cell. The influx of sodium ions into the cell increases the transmembrane potential to about +30 (meaning that the charge is now positive inside the cell relative to outside the cell). As soon as this positive charge is achieved, the voltage-regulated sodium channels close, and the cell begins to return to a negative state. This movement of the transmembrane potential away from a positive value and toward the negative resting potential is called **repolarization.** The initial downward movement toward zero is phase 1 of the action potential. As the charge reaches 0 mV, a plateau occurs. This plateau is what differentiates the action potential of cardiac muscle from the action potential of skeletal muscle. In this plateau phase, called phase 2, the calcium channels open slowly. These "slow channels" allow calcium ions to enter the cell. The positively charged calcium channels

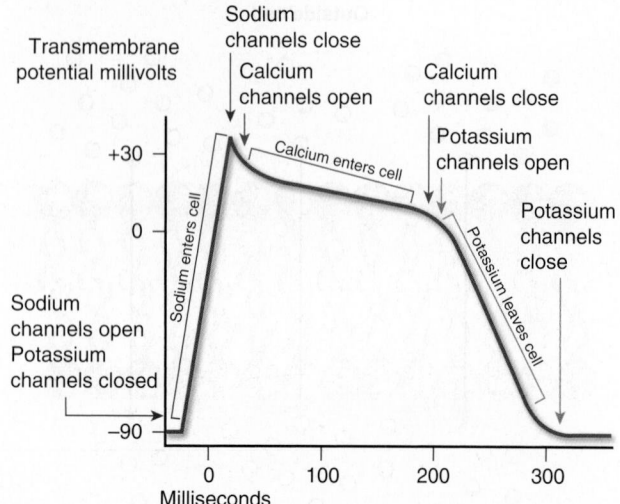

- FIGURE 31.4 Movement of electrolytes during the action potential. As sodium enters the cell, rapid depolarization occurs. Once sodium channels close, the process of repolarization slowly begins. When calcium enters the cell, a plateau occurs. When the calcium channels close and potassium channels open, rapid repolarization occurs.

close, potassium channels open, and potassium moves out of the cell. The cell then begins a rapid acceleration of repolarization: phase 3 of the action potential. When full polarization is achieved once more, the cell is in phase 4 of the action potential; sodium and potassium have gradually returned to their original locations (sodium outside of the cell, and potassium inside the cell). The cell remains polarized until stimulated again to depolarize. In other words, the cycle will start over (Figure 31.4).

After the cell depolarizes, and until it restores its normal electrical charge, it cannot be stimulated to fire again. This interval is termed the **refractory period.** Initially after depolarization, the cell cannot be stimulated to fire, no matter how great the stimulus. This state is the absolute refractory period. As repolarization continues, the cell eventually responds, even though it is not at the resting state. However, the intensity of the stimulus needed to depolarize the cell is greater than when the cell is in the resting state. This ability to respond, but only to a larger than normal stimulus, is termed the relative refractory period.

In addition to its role in the propagation of the action potential, calcium is also required for the mechanical contraction of the heart. In contracting cells of the heart, calcium links excitation (from polarization) to contraction. The contraction of cardiac and vascular smooth-muscle tissues is dependent on the movement of extracellular calcium into these cells. However, the influx of calcium is only approximately 20% of the calcium needed to initiate a contraction. The calcium that enters the cell stimulates the release of calcium that is stored inside the sarcoplasmic reticulum. This process is called calcium-induced calcium release. The process occurs during the plateau phase of the action potential. This release of additional calcium is what actually induces a contraction.

The plateau phase is unique to the cardiac muscle. In contrast, repolarization of skeletal muscle occurs rapidly after depolarization, allowing the muscle to be stimulated to contract again almost immediately. Tetany, or constant contractions, may occur in skeletal muscles. This process would be life threatening if it occurred in the heart because no effective contractions would be present. Thus, this plateau phase can be considered a protective mechanism of the heart muscles to promote effective contractions (Figure 31.5). Imbalances of the electrolytes involved in the action potential, either greater than or less than normal serum levels, may produce changes in the action potential and cause various cardiac arrhythmias. Contractility of the heart is also affected by the concentration of catecholamines in the heart muscle—the more catecholamines, the greater the rate of contraction and the greater the force of contraction will be.

PATHOPHYSIOLOGY

Arrhythmias, also called dysrhythmias, are a disturbance in the electrical activity of the heart. Some arrhythmias are insignificant and do not create any problems for the patient. Others disrupt the function of the heart, increase the oxygen demand of the heart, and interfere with cardiac output. Some are considered life threatening or lethal.

Changes in the ionic currents through ion channels of the myocardial cell membrane are the main cause of cardiac arrhythmia. The ions are sodium, potassium, and calcium. These ionic changes allow arrhythmias to develop in one of three ways: through a disorder with impulse formation, through a disorder of the impulse conduction system, or through a combination of both. When a disorder of impulse formation is present, the rate of SA nodal discharges is altered, allowing changes in the **automaticity** (ability to generate an impulse spontaneously) of the heart. Decreased automaticity results in sinus bradycardia; increased automaticity results in sinus tachycardia. These changes may be the result of drug toxicity, such as from digoxin, or of excessive sympathetic activity. Eliminating the contributing factor controls the arrhythmia. A different problem with automaticity occurs when the SA nodal rate decreases excessively and other excitable heart tissue reaches the threshold potential earlier than the SA node, thus generating an impulse. These abnormal sites of impulse formation are **ectopic foci.** These ectopic pacemakers may result from hypokalemia, myocardial ischemia, emotional stress, or hypoxia. Ectopic foci may arise in atrial, nodal, Purkinje, or ventricular muscle.

Disorders of impulse conduction may result from an alteration in either the rate or the pathway of impulse conduction. When conduction of the impulses through the AV node is delayed, heart block occurs.

Re-entry phenomenon is a more common source of alterations of impulse formation. Electrical impulses normally travel along a Purkinje fiber and divide at the small branch points in the fiber. When they meet each other in the connecting

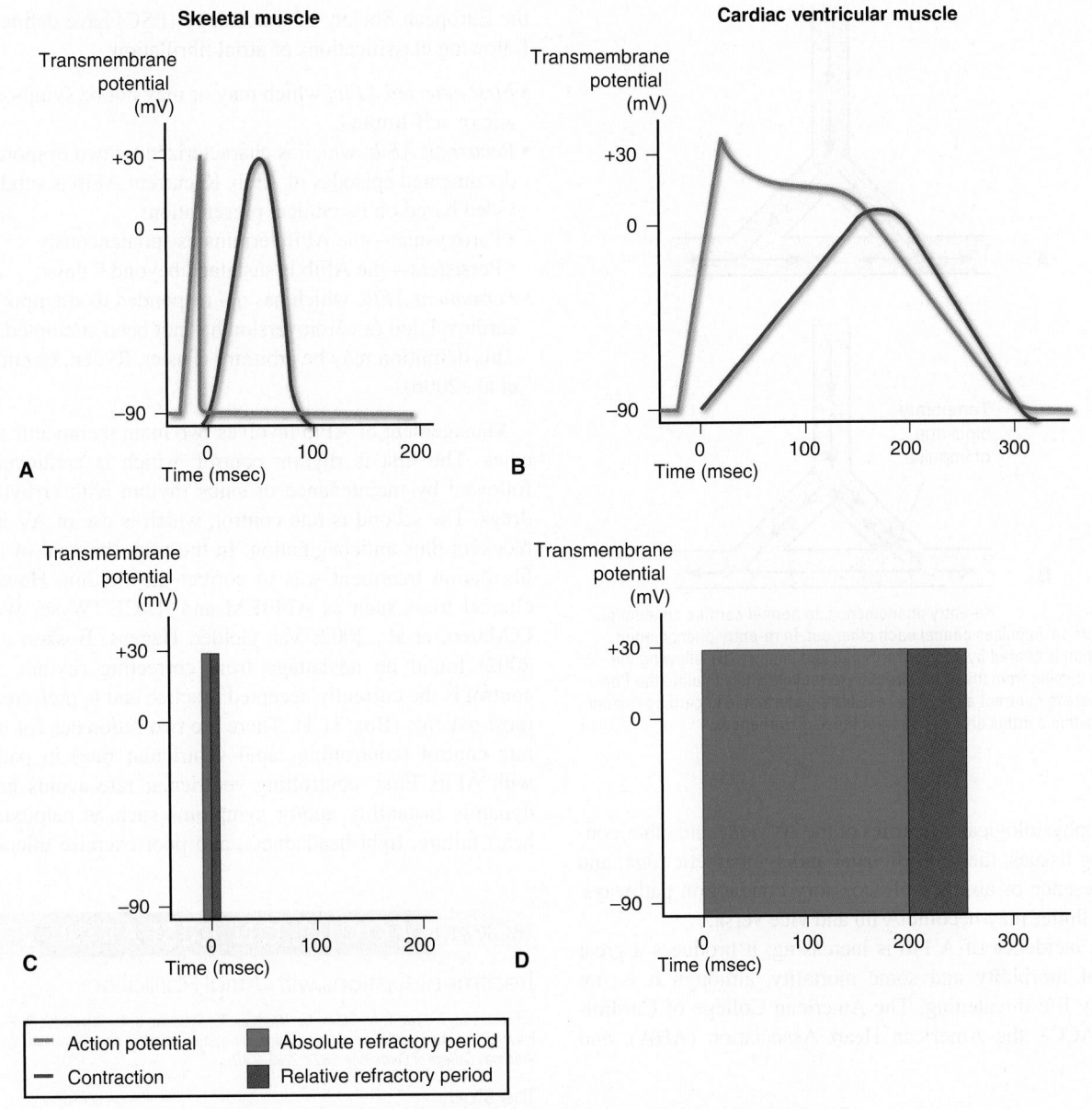

Skeletal muscle

Cardiac ventricular muscle

- Action potential
- Contraction
- Absolute refractory period
- Relative refractory period

• FIGURE 31.5 Comparisons of action potential, contraction, and refractory periods in skeletal and cardiac muscle.

branch, they normally extinguish each other. However, where there is a temporary block in one of the branches because of an alteration in nerve impulse conduction, the impulse cannot continue to travel in its normal forward path, canceling itself out in the common branch. Instead, the impulse is carried through the unopposed side and re-enters the branch from the opposite direction. Re-entry, or the **re-entry phenomenon**, causes repetitive cardiac stimulation, firing, and arrhythmias (Figure 31.6).

Arrhythmias can occur in the atria or in the ventricles. **Atrial flutter** (Figure 31.7A) is an arrhythmia originating in the atria: rapid atrial beating (approximately 240 to 320 bpm) but a slower, regular or irregular, ventricular beating (120 to 160 bpm; usually about 150 bpm). The slower ventricular rate results because atrial flutter commonly occurs with a 2:1 AV block, meaning that the ventricle is protected

from excessive stimulation; only half of the impulses pass through the AV node. The ECG pattern shows a sawtooth pattern for atrial activation with a normal QRS complex. **Atrial fibrillation** (AF or Afib) (see Figure 31.7B) is the most commonly seen arrhythmia in clinical practice. This arrhythmia is caused by rapid, irregular discharges from multiple atrial ectopic foci. The result is quivering of the atria without the occurrence of a true diastole or atrial contraction. Impulses are transmitted irregularly through the AV node, producing an irregular ventricular response, which is often rapid. Atrial fibrillation is a supraventricular tachyarrhythmia characterized by uncoordinated atrial activation, resulting in a loss of effective atrial contractions. The ECG pattern shows an absence of a normal P wave, which is replaced by rapid oscillating waves of various amplitudes, shapes, and timing. The exact response of the ventricles depends on several factors: the

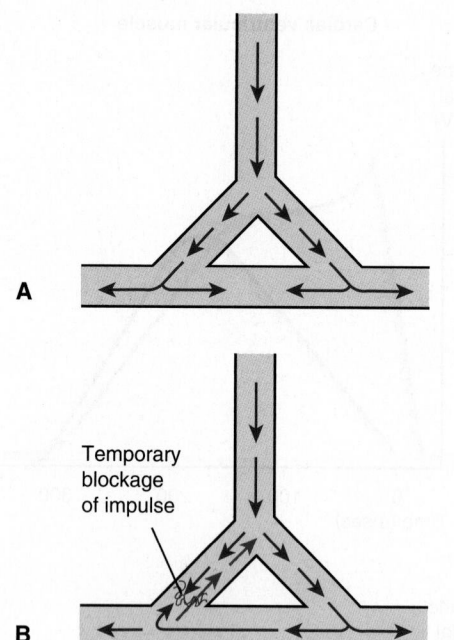

- FIGURE 31.6 Re-entry phenomenon. In normal cardiac conduction (**A**), electrical impulses cancel each other out. In re-entry phenomenon, conduction is altered by a temporarily blocked impulse (**B**), allowing the impulse coming from the other direction to recycle and stimulate the Purkinje fibers to contract again. The result is a disturbance in cardiac rhythm. Antiarrhythmic drugs are used to treat these disturbances.

electrophysiological properties of the AV node and other conducting tissues, the level of vagal and sympathetic tone, and the presence or absence of accessory conduction pathways. Atrial flutter may become A fib and vice versa.

The incidence of A Fib is increasing; it produces a great deal of morbidity and some mortality, although it is not directly life threatening. The American College of Cardiology (ACC), the American Heart Association (AHA), and

the European Society of Cardiology (ESC) have defined the following classifications of atrial fibrillation:

- *First detected AFib*, which may or may not be symptomatic or self-limited.
- *Recurrent AFib*, which is characterized by two or more documented episodes of AFib. Recurrent AFib is subdivided based on its clinical presentation:
  - Paroxysmal—the AFib terminates spontaneously
  - Persistent—the AFib is sustained beyond 7 days
- *Permanent AFib*, which has not responded to attempts at cardioversion or cardioversion has not been attempted. This definition may be arbitrary (Fuster, Ryden, Cannom, et al., 2006).

Management of AFib involves two main therapeutic strategies. The first is rhythm control, which is cardioversion followed by maintenance of sinus rhythm with arrhythmic drugs. The second is rate control, which is use of AV nodal blockers plus anticoagulation. In the past, the goal of atrial fibrillation treatment was to correct the rhythm. However, clinical trials such as AFFIRM and RACE (Wyse, Waldo, DiMarco, et al., 2002; Van Gelder, Hagens, Bosker, et al., 2002) found no advantage from correcting rhythm. Rate control is the currently accepted practice and is preferred for most patients (Box 31.1). There are two rationales for using rate control (controlling rapid ventricular rate) in patients with AFib. First, controlling ventricular rate avoids hemodynamic instability and/or symptoms such as palpitations, heart failure, light-headedness, and poor exercise tolerance.

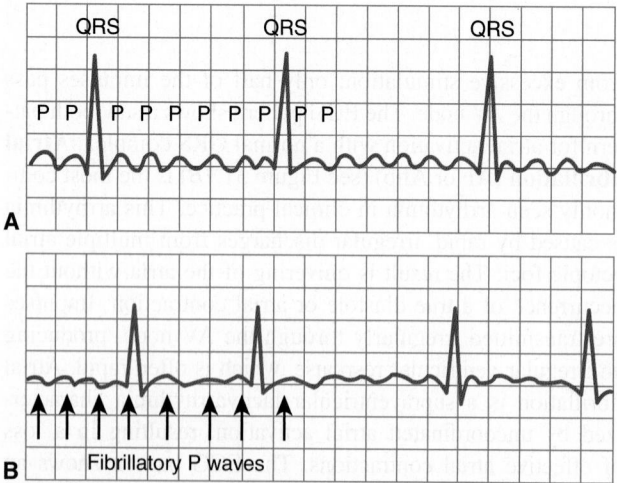

- FIGURE 31.7 (**A**) Atrial flutter. Note rapid flutter waves with occasional QRS complexes. (**B**) Atrial fibrillation. Note small, irregular waves. QRS complexes can be at an irregular rate but appear normal.

BOX 31.1 FOCUS ON RESEARCH

Treatment Options with Atrial Fibrillation

Schneider, M. P., Hua, T. A., Böhm, M., Wachtell, K., Kjeldsen, S. E., Schmieder, R. E. (2010). Prevention of atrial fibrillation by renin-angiotensin system inhibition a meta-analysis. *Journal of American College of Cardiology*, 55(21):2299–2307.

The Study

This meta-analysis reviewed 23 randomized controlled studies focusing on the treatment of atrial fibrillation (AF), both primary and secondary prevention, with renin-angiotensin system (RAS) inhibition. A total of 87,048 patients were included in the review. Both angiotensin converting enzyme and receptor blocker drugs were considered.

Results were variable based partly on the heterogeneity between the studies but it was concluded that RAS inhibition does have a role in the treatment of atrial fibrillation. More controlled studies are necessary.

Nursing Implications

This study is important because successful treatment of atrial fibrillation is hard to accomplish. A clear option has not been identified. Treatment with antiarrhymic drugs has limitations. At present, treatment options with antiarrhythmics lean more toward controlling rate rather than converting to sinus rhythm. This analysis demonstrated the possibility of preventing the occurrence or reoccurrence of AF with RAS inhibition. These studies will be ongoing. The nurse must be aware of new findings that will affect practice. Also, as with any drug therapy, patient education is a must. The patient must understand the dosage, side effects, and when to contact the prescriber.

Second, controlling ventricular rate has the long-term benefit of preventing a tachycardia-induced cardiomyopathy. Treatment of patients with AF should always include anticoagulant therapy, stroke risk assessment, and close follow-up if anticoagulation is discontinued.

Ventricular tachycardia is rapid ventricular beating (greater than 100 bpm; usually 150 to 200 bpm) arising from ventricular ectopic foci. The ECG from ventricular tachycardia consists of wide bizarre QRS complexes that can be regular or of varying shape and amplitude. **Ventricular fibrillation** is quivering of the ventricle without a systolic beat. If not terminated rapidly (2 to 3 minutes) with defibrillation, brain damage occurs because the brain is not receiving oxygen. The ECG from ventricular fibrillation shows rapid, oscillating waves of various amplitudes, shapes, and timing; it is varied and chaotic, with no discernible complexes.

Ventricular tachycardia and ventricular fibrillation are serious and potentially life-threatening arrhythmias. They may occur after an acute myocardial infarction (MI). These arrhythmias must be corrected quickly or the patient may die due to inadequate ventricular filling leading to a greatly reduced or nonexistent cardiac output. Once the patient has been converted by defibrillation to a normal rhythm, there may be a tendency to revert to ventricular tachycardia or ventricular fibrillation later. Patients who are deemed most at risk for reverting may be placed on long-term drug therapy, receive an implantable cardioverter defibrillator (ICD), or both.

DRUGS AND OTHER THERAPIES TO TREAT ARRHYTHMIAS

Drug therapy previously was the mainstay for treating arrhythmias; however, the latest research studies show it has become possible to prevent the recurrence of some arrhythmias with the use of ICDs. ICDs have an established and definitive role in preventing sudden cardiac death; technologic innovations and refinements in therapeutic capabilities of these devices have widened the spectrum of patients who can benefit from ICD. This therapy can improve myocardial function with physiologic AV sequential pacing, treat life-threatening ventricular tachyarrhythmias with electrical therapies, and prevent bradycardia with support pacing. Concomitant use of drug therapy with ICDs is often the rule for chronic AFib.

Other arrhythmias can be treated by catheter ablation. Catheter ablation is being used to treat supraventricular arrhythmias and is a highly successful and often curative intervention. The ablative procedure is performed in an electrophysiology laboratory with electrode catheters positioned in the area of the AV node to apply radiofrequency energy to the slow conducting pathway. The slow pathway is ablated, and the patient's conduction then uses the fast pathway, as it should with normal rhythm.

Antiarrhythmics are agents used to prevent, suppress, or treat a disturbance in cardiac rhythm. The primary outcomes are to decrease automaticity, decrease speed of conduction, and decrease re-entry. Clinical trials are providing new

information on the effectiveness of different drugs in treating various arrhythmias. Selection of an antiarrhythmic drug is based on outcomes from these clinical trials, such as the AFFIRM study, not solely on the electrophysiologic changes related to the drug class. One problem with all antiarrhythmics is that, because of their ability to modify the rhythm of the heart, they can cause a new arrhythmia or exacerbate the arrhythmia that they are treating. This adverse effect is termed **proarrhythmia.** Such effects range from an increase in frequency of premature ventricular contractions (PVCs) to the development of more severe ventricular tachycardia, ventricular fibrillation, or torsades de pointes. The latter is a rapid, unstable form of tachycardia in which the QRS complexes appear to twist around the axis line. It is usually associated with a prolonged Q-T interval (Figure 31.8), which may lead to death.

When antiarrhythmic drugs were developed, a system of classification was sought in an attempt to organize the complex information in a conceptually meaningful fashion. The classification system developed was fairly comprehensive and was grouped by the drugs' actions (not by the drugs, per se). Class I antiarrhythmic drugs block sodium channels. Several subtypes of sodium channels have been discovered, which depend on the kinetics of their sodium-channel properties (i.e., very fast, very slow, and intermediate). Class IA antiarrhythmic agents are intermediate. Class IB antiarrhythmic agents are very fast. Class IC antiarrhythmic agents are very slow; and Class IA antiarrhythmic agents are also known to suppress sodium-channel activity in all cardiac tissues, whereas Class IB antiarrhythmic agents suppress sodium-channel action only in diseased or depolarized tissue.

Class II antiarrhythmic drugs block adrenergic receptors (beta blockers), producing antisympathetic effects that slow the heart rate, lengthen the time needed for conduction, and increase the force of contraction. The effect seen with Class II antiarrhythmic drugs is depression of phase 4 of depolarization. Beta blockers are the most effective drugs that provide rate control for AF (Olshansky, Rosenfeld, Warner, et al., 2004). Class III antiarrhythmic drugs, or potassium channel blockers, lengthen the duration of the action potential, which prolongs phase 3 of repolarization. Class IV antiarrhythmic drugs block calcium channels, which depresses phase 4 of depolarization and lengthens phases 1 and 2 of repolarization

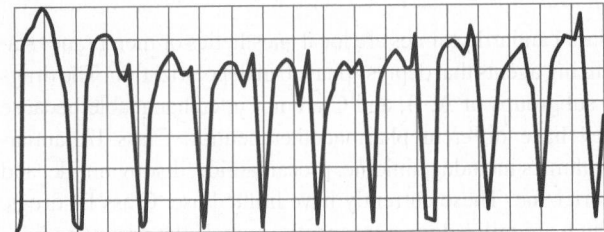

• FIGURE 31.8 Torsade de pointes. A rapid, unstable form of tachycardia where the amplitude and morphology of the QRS complexes are randomly varied. They appear to twist around the isoelectic line thus the name torsades. It is usually associated with a prolonged QT interval.

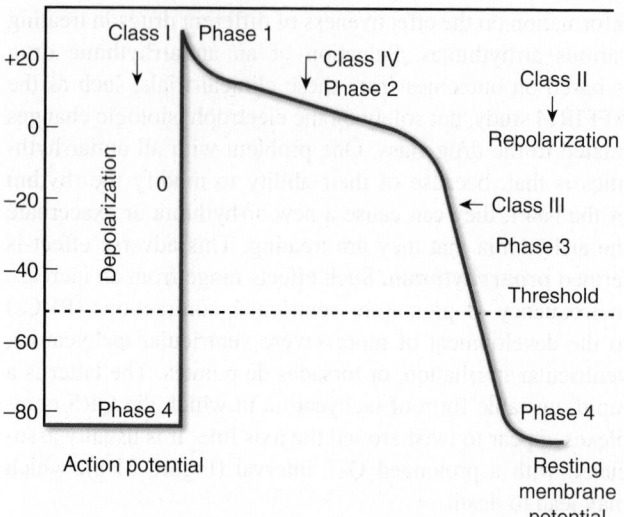

• FIGURE 31.9 Action potential and antiarrhythmic drugs. The change in the charge of the myocardial cell that occurs when sodium (Na+) and calcium (Ca++) flow into the cell and potassium (K+) flows out is called the action potential. Different antiarrhythmic drugs act at different phases of polarization and repolarization. Class I drugs (lidocaine) act during depolarization, class II drugs (propranolol) act during the resting period of repolarization, class III drugs (amiodarone) act during rapid repolarization, and class IV drugs (verapamil) act during early repolarization.

(Figure 31.9). Class IV antiarrhythmic drugs are effective in the control of rhythm in AF as well as in serious ventricular arrhythmias.

Although this classification system is widely used, it has substantial limitations. Some drugs have characteristics of more than one class; other drugs (such as digoxin and adenosine) used in specific types of arrhythmias do not fit in any of the classes. Despite these limitations, the antiarrhythmics discussed in this chapter are presented in the traditional groupings of Class I, II, III, and IV.

The major goals of antiarrhythmic therapy are to alleviate symptoms (e.g., palpitations, light-headedness, shortness of breath), improve quality of life, and prolong survival in patients with cardiac arrhythmias. The relief of symptoms in most patients can be achieved either by slowing the rate or by preventing recurrence. However, relief of the arrhythmia is not always associated with decreases in mortality.

Ⓒ CLASS I ANTIARRHYTHMIC DRUGS

Class I antiarrhythmics are local anesthetics or membrane-stabilizing agents that depress phase 0 in depolarization. The drugs in subgroups of A, B, and C are not interchangeable because they have different pharmacotherapeutics. Class IA antiarrhythmics include quinidine, procainamide, disopyramide, and moricizine. These currently have limited use. Class IB drugs, which are utilized most frequently, include the prototype lidocaine, tocainide, mexiletine, moricizine, and phenytoin. Class IC drugs include flecainide and propafenone. Table 31.1 presents a summary of selected Class IA antiarrhythmic drugs.

Nursing Management of the Patient Receiving Ⓟ Lidocaine

Core Drug Knowledge

Pharmacotherapeutics

Lidocaine (Xylocaine) may be used with all acute ventricular arrhythmias because these may be life threatening. In other strengths and routes, lidocaine also is used as a local and topical anesthetic.

Pharmacokinetics

Lidocaine is usually administered intravenously because it is ineffective orally. Under certain circumstances, it may be administered intramuscularly. Single intramuscular doses are justified in the following exceptional circumstances: lack of availability of ECG equipment to verify diagnosis (but the potential benefits must outweigh the possible risk) and when the facilities for IV administration are not readily available. When given intramuscularly, higher and more rapid serum levels are achieved by injection into the deltoid muscle over the gluteus or vastus lateralis. However, lidocaine given intramuscularly may increase creatine phosphokinase (CPK) levels. CPK is an enzyme used as a diagnostic test for acute MI. Lidocaine is about 50% protein bound. Lidocaine is metabolized extensively in the liver into at least two active metabolites. These metabolites have both antiarrhythmic and convulsant (inducing convulsions) effects. Metabolism of this drug is impaired substantially by any condition that impairs liver function. Although renal elimination processes only about 10% of the dose given, it is highly involved in the excretion of the metabolites. Accumulation of one of the metabolites (known as GX) because of renal disease or impaired renal function contributes to lidocaine toxicity.

Lidocaine has a biphasic half-life. The half-life involved with the distribution phase is less than 10 minutes. This brevity accounts for the short duration of action when an IV bolus is given. Because of the drug's very short half-life, repeated boluses may be required to quickly achieve therapeutic level when a continuous IV infusion is needed to maintain the therapeutic effects (see Table 31.1 for dosing information). The elimination half-life is 1.5 to 2 hours. It may be 3 hours or more if the lidocaine infusion has lasted longer than 24 hours.

Pharmacodynamics

Lidocaine, used to treat arrhythmias, in therapeutic levels, weakens phase 4 diastolic depolarization, decreases the automaticity, and decreases or causes no change in the excitability and membrane responsiveness. Additionally, it decreases the action potential duration and the effective refractory period of Purkinje fibers and ventricular muscle. However, the ratio of the effective refractory period to the action potential duration is increased. The effective refractory period of the AV node may increase, decrease, or remain unchanged; the atrial effective refractory period remains unchanged. Lidocaine raises the ventricular

TABLE 31.1	Summary of Selected Ⓒ Class I Antiarrhythmics		
Drug (Trade) Name	**Selected Indications**	**Route and Dosage Range**	**Pharmacokinetics**
quinidine (Quinaglute Dura-Tabs) Class 1A	Premature atrial and ventricular contractions Paroxysmal supraventricular tachycardias Atrial flutter	*Adult:* PO, 200–300 mg three or four times daily *Child:* PO, 30 mg/kg/24 h or 900 mg/m^2/24 h in five divided doses *Adult:* F 400–600 mg every 2 or 3 h until the paroxysm is terminated; administer after digitalization; dosage individualized *Child:* PO, 30 mg/kg/24 h or 900 mg/m^2/24 h in five divided doses *Adult:* After digitalization, dosage is individualized	*Onset:* PO, 1–3 h; IM; 30–90 min; IV, rapid *Duration:* 6–8 h $t_{1/2}$: 6–7 h
procainamide (Procan SR) Class 1A	Ventricular arrhythmias	*Adult:* PO, initially 50 mg/kg/d in divided doses every 3 h; PO, maintenance, 50 mg/kg/d in divided doses q6h; IV, loading (initial), 1 mL/min of 20 mg/mL solution or 100 mg every 5 min direct IV, up to 1 g total; maintenance, 1–3 mL/min of 2 mg/mL solution *Child:* PO, 15–50 mg/kg/d divided every 3–6 h; max of 4 g/d; IV, initial 3–6 mg/kg/dose over 5 min; maintenance, 20–80 μg/kg/min continuous infusion; maximum, 100 mg/dose or 2 g/d	*Onset:* PO, 30 min; IM, 10–30 min; IV, immediate *Duration:* 3–4 h $t_{1/2}$: 2.5–4.7 h
Ⓟ lidocaine (Xylocaine HCl IV for cardiac arrhythmias) Class 1B	Ventricular arrhythmias	*Adult:* Initial IV bolus 50–100 mg at rate of 25–50 mg/min; one-third to one-half the initial dose may be given after 5 min; do not exceed 200–300 mg in 1 h. Continuous infusion, 20–50 mg/kg/min *Child:* AHA recommends bolus of 1 mg/kg IV, followed by 30 μg/kg/min w/caution	*Onset:* IM, 5–10 min; IV, immediate *Duration:* IM; 2 h; IV, 10–20 min $t_{1/2}$: 10 min, then 1.5–3 h
flecainide (Tambocor) Class 1C	PSVT and PAF Sustained ventricular tachycardia	*Adult:* Starting dose of 50 mg every 12 h; increase in 50-mg increments twice a day every fourth day until efficacy is achieved. Max dose is 300 mg/d. *Child:* Not recommended *Adult:* 100 mg every 12 h; increase in 50-mg increments twice a day every fourth day until efficacy is achieved. Max dose is 400 mg/d. *Child:* Not recommended.	*Onset:* 30–60 min *Duration:* 24 h $t_{1/2}$: 20 h

PSVT, paroxysmal supraventricular tachycardia; PAF, paroxysmal atrial flutter.

fibrillation threshold, which is why it is effective in treating ventricular fibrillation.

Clinical electrophysiologic studies have demonstrated no change in sinus node recovery time, sinoatrial conduction time, and His-Purkinje fiber conduction time. AV node conduction time is unchanged or may be shortened. Lidocaine does increase the electrical stimulation threshold of the ventricle during diastole. This increase enables a longer diastole because the ventricle requires a longer time before it can be receptive to depolarization and contract again. This effect is helpful in treating ventricular arrhythmias. In therapeutic doses (serum levels of 1.5 to 6 mcg/mL), lidocaine has no effect on the contractility of the heart, blood pressure, or the absolute refractory period.

Contraindications and Precautions

Lidocaine is a pregnancy category B drug. However, caution should be used because no adequate and well-controlled studies have been done in pregnant women. Although safety and efficacy in children have not been established from clinical studies, the American Heart Association's Standards and Guidelines recommend using lidocaine when needed in children (see Table 31.1). Caution should be used, and lower doses are recommended, for patients who have CHF, reduced cardiac output, digitalis toxicity accompanied by AV block, hypovolemia, and shock; in all forms of heart block; and when used in older adults.

Adverse Effects

Adverse effects of lidocaine are seen particularly in the CV system and CNS. CV effects are related to serum levels, with the most severe cardiac depression coinciding with toxic levels of lidocaine. The most common CV effects are cardiac arrhythmias and hypotension. Other effects include bradycardia and CV collapse, which may lead to cardiac arrest. CNS adverse effects also are related to blood concentrations of lidocaine. The most common CNS effects are dizziness, light-headedness, fatigue, and drowsiness. These common, mild effects are seen with low blood levels of lidocaine and resolve rapidly. As blood levels of lidocaine rise, nervousness, confusion, mood changes, hallucinations, euphoria, tinnitus, blurred or double vision, and a sensation of heat, cold, or numbness may occur. In common health care jargon, these CNS effects are referred to as the "lidocaine crazies." With excessively high serum levels of lidocaine (greater than 6 mcg/mL), toxicity is present, and the patient develops seizures and loses consciousness.

It is very important to continually monitor the ECG of the patient receiving IV lidocaine. Emergency resuscitative equipment and drug therapy should be on hand in case the patient develops serious adverse effects. As soon as the patient is clinically stable, she or he should be switched to another antiarrhythmic that can be given orally.

Drug Interactions

Lidocaine interacts with many classes of drugs such as beta blockers, antimicrobials, protease inhibitors and other antiarrhythmics Typical effects are additive cardiac effects or decreasing metabolism with puts patients at risk for toxicity. Table 31.2 lists drugs that have a probable interaction with lidocaine.

Assessment of Relevant Core Patient Variables

Health Status

Before emergent use, the health care team must determine whether the patient has a type of ventricular arrhythmia that is an indication for therapy. It also is important to determine whether the patient has a sensitivity to lidocaine which would be a contraindication to therapy. Before initiating continuous therapy, it must be determined whether the patient is on any drugs which will interact with lidocaine.

Also, because lidocaine is largely metabolized in the liver and excreted through the kidneys, renal and liver status should be established. The patient with renal or hepatic disease may be at greater risk for toxicity. The patient with cardiac insufficiency will also be at risk for toxicity due to a decrease in hepatic blood flow. Conversely, the patient without heart disease and thus adequate cardiac output will have increased clearance of lidocaine, increasing the chance of recurrence of the arrhythmias.

Life Span and Gender

As stated earlier, lidocaine has not been linked to adverse effects in either pregnancy or breast-feeding but limited studies have been done. Caution is suggested. Dosage in children should be adjusted by weight.

Environment

Lidocaine should be given in a hospital or emergency setting where continuous ECG monitoring is possible.

Nursing Diagnoses and Outcomes

• Decreased Cardiac Output related to cardiac changes secondary to adverse effects of drug therapy

TABLE 31.2	Agents That Interact with P Lidocaine	
Interactants	**Effect and Significance**	**Nursing Management**
Amiodarone	May decrease metabolism	Monitor levels
Phenytoin	May increase metabolism; potential for increased cardiac effects	Avoid concomitant use
Propofol	Unknown mechanism, decreases dose necessary for desired effect of propofol	May need to decrease propofol dose
Arbutamine	Increased risk of life threatening arrhythmias due to additive cardiac effects	Avoid concomitant use
cimetidine	Rapid Increas in serum levels and risk of lidocaine toxicity	Monitor serum levels of lidocaine Assess for signs of adverse effects. Consider alternate GI prophylaxis
beta blockers ((propanolol, nadolol, penbutolol, metoprolol)	decrease in metabolism.	Monitor levels and adjust dosage as necessary.
Protease inhibitors (amprenavir, atazanavir, lopinavir)	Inhibition of P-450 3A metabolism of lidocaine.	Avoid concomitant use.
succinylcholine	Snergistic effect; may causeprolonged neuromuscular blockade	Monitor drug levels, and attempt to stagger doses.
St John's Wart	Unknown mechanism; prolonged anesthesia recovery time	Discontinue St John's wort at least 5 d prior to anesthesia
Dalfopristin/Quinupristin	Inhibition of P-450 3A metabolism of lidocaine.	Monitor for lidocaine toxicity; adjust dose as necessary

Desired outcome: The patient will not develop deleterious cardiac changes that alter cardiac output.

- Risk for Injury, such as hepatic toxicity, related to adverse effects of drug therapy

Desired outcome: The patient will not incur hepatic toxicity while on drug therapy.

- Change in level of consciousness related to CNS changes secondary to adverse effects of drug therapy

Desired outcome: The patient will not experience dangerous CNS changes while on therapy

Planning and Intervention

Maximizing Therapeutic Effects

To maximize the therapeutic effects of lidocaine, after an initial (or several) IV push dose of 50 to 100 mg, a continuous drip of 1 to 4 mg/min may be started.

Minimizing Adverse Effects

It is necessary to connect the patient to a cardiac monitor and monitor rhythm continuously

Notify the prescriber immediately if any of the following events occurs:

Prolongation of PR or QRS interval

- Sinus node dysfunstion
- Aggravation of the arrhythmia
- CNS depression or irritability
- Liver and kidney function tests. Reveal elevated values.

Providing Patient and Family Education

- Explain the purpose of the drug and the potential adverse effects.
- Explain the rationale for ECG monitoring and frequent blood testing, which is that these are methods used to detect early onset of adverse effects.

Ongoing Assessment and Evaluation

Monitor the patient's ECG and pulse throughout therapy. Check lidocaine blood levels to ensure that they are therapeutic, not toxic. Periodically, monitor liver enzymes, renal function, and complete blood counts. Drug therapy is considered effective if the ventricular arrhythmia is controlled without the patient developing serious adverse effect.

Drugs Closely Related to P Lidocaine

Other Class 1B antiarrhythics include tocainide, mexiletine, and phenytoin.

Tocainide (Tonocard) is used to treat life-threatening ventricular arrhythmias. As a Class IB antiarrhythmic, it is similar to lidocaine, producing dose-dependent decreases in sodium and potassium conduction and thereby decreasing the excitability of the cardiac cells. Most patients who respond to lidocaine respond to tocainide, and failure to respond to lidocaine usually indicates that the patient will not respond to tocainide, either. The electrophysiologic effects of tocainide are similar to those seen with lidocaine. Tocainide does not

prolong the QRS duration or QT intervals. Tocainide slightly depresses the left ventricular function and left ventricular end-diastolic pressure. Usually, this effect produces no changes in the cardiac output. It does slightly, but significantly, increase aortic and pulmonary arterial pressures. This effect is most likely related to increases in vascular resistance. Tocainide has been used safely in patients with acute MI, post-MI, and various degrees of CHF.

Tocainide is given orally because it does not have the high metabolism of lidocaine. Bioavailability of tocainide is nearly 100%; peak serum levels are reached in 0.5 to 2 hours after oral dosing. Protein binding is very low, at 10% to 20%. It is inactivated by conjugation in the liver. About 40% of the drug is excreted in the urine unchanged. Half-life is increased in severe renal dysfunction.

It is important to use tocainide cautiously in patients with known heart failure or minimal cardiac reserve, or when beginning or continuing antiarrhythmic therapy in the presence of signs of increasing depression of cardiac conductivity. Like all antiarrhythmics, tocainide can be proarrhythmic. The most common adverse effects are dizziness, vertigo, nausea, paresthesia, and tremor. These reactions are generally mild, transient, and dose related; they are reversible by reducing the dose, by taking the drug with food, or by discontinuing the therapy. The most serious adverse effect, although not common (less than 1% of patients), is the occurrence of blood dyscrasias (e.g., agranulocytosis, depressed bone marrow function, leukopenia, neutropenia, aplastic or hypoplastic anemia, and thrombocytopenia). Tocainide carries a Black Box warning about these potential blood dyscrasias. These effects, which usually occur during the first 12 weeks of therapy, can be fatal in about one fourth of patients who experience them. Monitor blood work weekly during this period for signs of any of these effects. If any of these disorders is diagnosed, discontinue the tocainide immediately. Blood work should return to normal within 1 month.

Fatalities also have occurred with patients who develop severe pulmonary disorders (such as pulmonary fibrosis, interstitial pneumonitis, fibrosing alveolitis, pulmonary edema, and pneumonia). Tocainide also carries a Black Box warning about the pulmonary fibrosis. Instruct patients to report immediately any pulmonary symptoms, such as shortness of breath on exertion, cough, or wheezing. Discontinue tocainide if any of these disorders develop.

Other potential adverse effects of tocainide include:

- CV: ventricular fibrillation, extension of acute MI, cardiogenic shock, angina, AV block, hypertension, increased QRS duration, pericarditis, prolonged QT interval, right bundle branch block, syncope, vasovagal episodes, cardiomegaly, sinus arrest, vasculitis, and orthostatic hypotension
- CNS: coma, convulsions/seizures, depression, psychosis, agitation, decreased mental acuity, dysarthria, impaired memory, increased stuttering, slurred speech, insomnia, sleep disturbances, local anesthesia, dream abnormalities, myasthenia gravis, and malaise
- Dermatologic: Stevens-Johnson syndrome, exfoliative dermatitis, erythema multiforme, urticaria, alopecia, pruritus, and pallor or flushed face
- GI: abdominal pain, constipation, stomatitis, dysphagia, dyspepsia, thirst, and dry mouth
- Hepatic: hepatitis and jaundice
- Respiratory: respiratory arrest and pulmonary edema or embolism

Mexiletine

Mexiletine (Mexitil) is another Class IB drug. It also is used in life-threatening ventricular arrhythmias and, like all antiarrhythmics, may produce arrhythmias. It is administered only orally. It has pharmacologic and electrophysiologic properties similar to those of lidocaine.

Phenytoin

Although treatment of arrhythmias is not a labeled use of phenytoin (Dilantin), an antiepileptic, it is used commonly in treating digitalis-induced arrhythmias. Like other Class IB drugs, it depresses phase 0 slightly and may shorten the action potential. A full discussion of phenytoin and its use in treating seizures can be found in Chapter 21.

Drugs Significantly Different From ⓟ Lidocaine

Class IA Antiarrhythmics

The Class IA drugs are similar to lidocaine (Class IB) and Class IC drugs because they depress phase 0 (although not as much) of the action potential. Also similar, these drugs may cause arrhythmias in addition to treating them. Unlike lidocaine, they prolong the effective refractory period, increasing

conduction time. Also unlike lidocaine their use in treating life-threatening ventricular arrhythmias has not been shown to improve survival, (see Table 31.1). The most important of these drugs are discussed below.

Quinidine

Quinidine is used primarily to treat atrial arrhythmias, including premature atrial, AV junctional, and paroxysmal atrial (supraventricular) tachycardia, paroxysmal AV junctional rhythm, atrial flutter, and paroxysmal and chronic AFib, but has decreased in use during the past decade for maintaining sinus rhythm and is being replaced by amiodarone (Fang, Stafford, Ruskin, et al., 2004). This Class IA antiarrhythmic can be used as maintenance therapy after electrical conversion of atrial fibrillation or flutter, but again, it is being replaced by amiodarone. Other uses include treating premature ventricular contractions (PVCs) and paroxysmal ventricular tachycardia not associated with complete heart block. Quinidine is also used in treating life-threatening ventricular arrhythmias; however, it is not used commonly for this purpose, because although it may correct the arrhythmia, it has not been shown to improve survival. Quinidine is available as two different salts: quinidine sulfate and quinidine gluconate. A noncardiac use of quinidine (quinidine gluconate only) is in treating life-threatening *Plasmodium falciparum*.

Quinidine is rapidly absorbed from the gastrointestinal (GI) tract. Normally given orally, quinidine gluconate may be given parenterally when oral therapy is not possible or when more rapid therapeutic effects are required, such as for cardioversion (see Table 31.1). Quinidine sulfate is given only orally. The concentration of quinidine varies among the different quinidine salts. Quinidine gluconate contains 62% active quinidine, whereas quinidine polygalacturonate contains 80% active quinidine, and quinidine sulfate contains 83% active quinidine. Quinidine distributes to all body tissues except the brain. It is fairly highly protein bound at 80% to 90% and is metabolized by the liver and excreted unchanged by the kidneys. The influence of renal dysfunction on the disposition of quinidine is controversial; volume of distribution and renal clearance may be reduced. Acid urine promotes elimination of quinidine. In patients with cirrhosis, quinidine may have a prolonged half-life and an increased volume of distribution. In chronic heart failure (CHF), total clearance and volume of distribution are decreased. In elderly patients, elimination half-life may be increased.

Quinidine depresses myocardial excitability, conduction velocity, and contractility. The effective refractory period is prolonged, increasing conduction time. Re-entry phenomenon is therefore prevented. Quinidine also exerts an indirect anticholinergic effect; it decreases vagal tone and may promote conduction in the AV junction.

Quinidine is contraindicated in the presence of hypersensitivity or a history of idiosyncratic reaction to quinidine or other cinchona derivatives. Hypersensitivity and idiosyncratic reaction are manifested by thrombocytopenia, skin eruption, or fever. The drug carries the Black Box warning that when it is used to prevent or defer recurrence of atrial flutter or fibrillation, it is associated with increased mortality, which appears to be greater than the risk of mortality from other antiarrhythmics. Therefore, quinidine is contraindicated in the following cardiovascular (CV) conditions:

- Digitalis intoxication manifested by arrhythmias or AV conduction disorders
- Complete heart block
- Left bundle branch block or other severe intraventricular conduction defects exhibiting marked QRS widening or bizarre ECG complexes
- Complete AV block with an AV nodal or idioventricular pacemaker
- Aberrant ectopic impulses and abnormal rhythms due to escape mechanisms
- Drug-induced torsades de pointes (ventricular tachycardia associated with QT prolongation)
- Long QT syndrome

Also, quinidine is contraindicated in myasthenia gravis

Extreme caution should be used when giving quinidine to patients with incomplete AV block because complete block may develop. Care also must be taken when administering quinidine to patients with:

- Digitalis toxicity, because unpredictable arrhythmias may result.
- Partial bundle branch block, severe CHF, and hypotension, because quinidine will further depress myocardial contractility and arterial pressure.
- Patients with renal, hepatic, or cardiac insufficiency, because toxicity is more likely to occur.

Quinidine crosses the placenta and achieves fetal serum levels similar to maternal levels. It is in pregnancy category C, indicating that safety has not been established. Quinidine also is excreted in breast milk. Milk-to-serum ratios have been found to be 0.71. Although safe use during breast-feeding has not been established clearly, the American Academy of Pediatrics considers the drug compatible with breast-feeding. Safety and efficacy in children have not been established.

The most common adverse effects involve the GI system and include nausea, vomiting, abdominal pain, diarrhea, and anorexia. These may occur after a fever. Arrhythmias also occur commonly, but most are not life threatening. Other common cardiovascular effects include hypotension and syncope. Another common adverse effect is a syndrome of cinchonism, related to the tree bark source of quinidine, usually associated with chronic toxicity but also described after a brief exposure to a moderate dose in sensitive patients. The symptoms of cinchonism include tinnitus, high-frequency hearing loss, deafness, headache, nausea, dizziness, vertigo, lightheadedness, and disturbed vision. Additionally, some dermatologic adverse effects (dermatitis, photosensitivity, rash) are fairly common.

The most serious adverse effect, although not common, is cardiotoxicity, which is manifested by increased PR and QT intervals, 50% widening of the QRS complex, ventricular tachyarrhythmias (including ventricular tachycardia, fibrillation, and torsades de pointes), frequent ventricular ectopic beats, or tachycardia. If signs of cardiotoxicity are present, quinidine should be discontinued at once, and the ECG of the patient should be monitored closely.

Other CV adverse effects include cardiac asystole, arterial embolism, ventricular extrasystole occurring at the rate of one or more for every six normal beats, complete AV block, ventricular flutter, and serious hypotension. Although large oral doses cause peripheral vasodilation that decreases blood pressure, the most serious hypotension is more likely to occur when quinidine is given intravenously.

Hepatic toxicity can occur, including granulomatous hepatitis. This reaction is believed to be the result of quinidine hypersensitivity. Fever occurs, and liver enzymes are elevated. Other hypersensitivity reactions, which are rare but may occur, are angioedema, acute asthma, vascular collapse, respiratory arrest, and purpura vasculitis.

Quinidine overdosage may be associated with depressed mental function even if the patient is hemodynamically stable. In addition, CNS symptoms (e.g., lethargy, confusion, coma, respiratory depression or arrest, seizures, headache, paresthesia, and vertigo) may occur after the onset of CV toxicity. GI effects include vomiting, abdominal pain, diarrhea, and nausea. The CV effects are tachyarrhythmias, depressed automaticity and conduction, hypotension, syncope, and heart failure.

Some of the adverse effects of quinidine may be similar to reasons the drug is prescribed. For this reason, it is important to monitor blood levels to determine whether the drug is in therapeutic range or is elevated excessively.

Drugs Closely Related to P Quinidine

The other Class IA antiarrhythmics are procainamide (Procan SR), disopyramide (Norpace). Like the prototype quinidine, they carry Black Box warnings that they may increase mortality, especially in patients with non–life-threatening ventricular arrhythmias and in post-MI patients. Procainamide has an additional Black Box warning; it may cause blood dyscrasia and development of a positive antinuclear antibody titer, with or without the development of lupus erythematosus–like syndrome. These three drugs have characteristics that make them similar to quinidine. However, unlike quinidine, these other Class IA drugs are labeled only for use in life-threatening ventricular arrhythmias; procainamide can also be used for AFib (off-label use).

Class IC Antiarrhythmics

Class IC drugs are flecainide (Tambocor) , propafenone (Rythmol), and moricizine (see Table 31.1). These drugs depress phase 0 considerably. In addition, they have a slight effect on repolarization and decrease conduction substantially. They are given orally. These drugs are labeled for use in atrial fibrillation and flutter but because of their strong proarrhythmic effects, their use is limited to patients with life-threatening arrhythmias.

One last note on Class 1 Antiarrhythmics:It is important to examine the relationship of Class I antiarrhythmics to mortality. In patients without structural heart disease, the use of Class I drugs rarely causes proarrhythmia serious enough to be life threatening. However, in studies of patients with ventricular tachycardia and ventricular fibrillation, no controlled study has produced decisive evidence demonstrating that Class I antiarrhythmics have the potential for prolonging survival of patients at high risk for dying suddenly. In fact, data from meta-analysis of several studies show that most, if not all, Class I antiarrhythmics are inclined to increase mortality. Thus, drugs that prolong the action potential only (Class I) are not the answer for decreasing mortality in patients with arrhythmias and structural heart disease. Class I agents are still widely used to decrease the number of shocks that patients with implantable cardioversion defibrillators receive. The efficacy for this use is unknown.

© CLASS II ANTIARRHYTHMIC DRUGS

Antiarrhythmic Class II drugs (beta blockers) depress phase 4 depolarization. Beta blockers slow heart rate by suppressing the SA node, slow the speed of conduction through the AV node, and decrease the force of contraction. They effectively reduce mortality in patients who have had a recent MI, those with symptomatic heart failure, and those with congenital long-QT syndrome. The prototype Class II drug metaprolol is discussed fully in Chapter 13. However, only acebutolol, esmolol, and propranolol are labeled as antiarrhythmics. Researchers have found that beta blockers are the most effective drugs for controlling the ventricular rate in AFib (Olshansky, Rosenfeld, Warner, et al., 2004). It is important to keep in mind that only some of the beta blockers are approved for use as antiarrhythmics. A brief discussion of their use as antiarrhythmics follows. Other uses of beta blockers relevant to CV function are found in Chapters 28, 29, and 30.

Propranolol

Propranolol (Inderal) is used for treating cardiac arrhythmias, specifically ventricular arrhythmias post-MI, tachyarrhythmias secondary to digoxin toxicity, and SVT (atrial fibrillation or flutter). Like other beta blockers, propranolol is used in AFib because it effectively slows ventricular rate and protects the heart from excessive ventricular contractions. It may be used either intravenously for acute control or orally for long-term chronic AFib. Propranolol, like other beta blockers, is especially helpful in controlling exercise-induced increases in ventricular rate, exercise-induced angina, acute MI, or heart failure, because it provides treatment for all these problems. The drug is also used to treat hypertension (Fuster, Ryden, Cannom, et al., 2006).

Propranolol blocks the beta-adrenergic receptor sites, which means it is a beta blocker. This blockage of the receptor sites occurs as the drug competes with beta-adrenergic

agonists for available beta receptor sites. Propranolol blocks both the beta-1 sites, which are located chiefly in the cardiac muscle, and beta-2 receptors, which are located chiefly in the bronchial and vascular musculature. Propranolol also has a membrane-stabilizing effect, like that of anesthetics, which depresses the cardiac action potential, causing the antiarrhythmic response.

Several mechanisms have been proposed to explain how propranolol achieves its various effects on the CV system. First, propranolol competitively blocks catecholamines at non-CNS adrenergic neuron sites, especially in the heart, thereby leading to decreased cardiac output. Second, propranolol has a central effect, resulting in reduced sympathetic outflow to the periphery. Third, because stimulation of beta receptors is responsible for the release of renin from the kidneys, beta blockade with propranolol prevents the release of renin. Total peripheral resistance initially increases slightly because of these mechanisms. However, it readjusts to the pretreatment level or lower with chronic use. Because the decrease in cardiac output is greater than the increase in peripheral resistance, blood pressure is lowered.

Propranolol is contraindicated in sinus bradycardia, greater than first-degree heart block, cardiogenic shock, CHF (unless secondary to a tachyarrhythmia treatable with beta blockers), overt cardiac failure, diabetes, bronchial asthma or bronchospasm, severe chronic obstructive pulmonary disease, and hypersensitivity to beta blockers.

Propranolol carries a black box warning regarding discontinuation of therapy. If discontinued abruptly, angina and myocardial infarction may be exacerbated. Dosages should be gradually decreased. Important patient teaching should include a warning about abruptly stopping therapy.

Acebutolol and Esmolol

Acebutolol (Monitan) differs from propranolol in that it is selective in beta-1 receptors and has little effect on beta-2 receptors. It is approved for use in hypertension and to treat ventricular arrhythmias. In terms of use in arrhythmias it has similar actions to propranolol. It is only administered orally.

Esmolol (Brevibloc) is approved for use in intraoperative and postoperative hypertension, as well as for supraventricular arrhythmia. Off-label uses include treatment of acute MI and as preinduction for rapid sequence intubation. Esmolol is administered only intravenously. It is relatively selective for beta-1 receptors, although it also can inhibit beta-2 receptors at high doses. It has a very short half-life of 9 minutes. Actions in treating arrhythmias are similar to those of propranolol.

© CLASS III ANTIARRHYTHMIC DRUGS

Class III antiarrhythmics produce a prolongation of phase 3 (repolarization). Action potential duration and refractory periods are prolonged, leading to reduction in membrane

TABLE 31.3	Summary of Selected ⓒ Class III Antiarrhythmics		
Drug (Trade) Name	**Selected Indications**	**Route and Dosage Range**	**Pharmacokinetics**
Ⓟ amiodarone (Cordarone)	Ventricular fibrillation	*Adult:* PO, 800–1,600 mg/d in divided doses for 1–3 wk; reduce to 600–800 mg/d in divided doses for 1 mo *Child:* Not established	*Onset:* 2–3 q *Duration:* 6–8 h $t_{1/2}$: 2.5–10 d, then 40–55 d
sotalol (Betapace; *Canadian:* Sotacor)	Ventricular arrhythmias	*Adult:* PO, 80 mg bid; adjust gradually q2–3d; may require 240–320 mg/d	*Onset:* Varies *Duration and* $t_{1/2}$: 12 h *Duration:* IV, 24 h $t_{1/2}$: 6.9–8.1 h
ibutilide (Corvert)	Atrial fibrillation Atrial flutter	*Adult: (= 60 kg):* IV, 1 mg infused over 10 min (<60 kg): 0.01 mg/kg infused over 10 min; may repeat 1×	*Onset:* Within 10 min *Duration:* Variable $t_{1/2}$: 2–12 h

excitability of all myocardial tissue. The drugs in this class include the prototype amiodarone (Cordarone, Pacerone), sotalol, bretylium, ibutilide, dofetilide and dronedarone. Table 31.3 presents a summary of selected drugs in this class.

Nursing Management of the Patient Receiving Ⓟ Amiodarone

Core Drug Knowledge

Pharmacotherapeutics

Because of severe and potentially lethal adverse effects, amiodarone is approved for use only in life-threatening arrhythmias. Orally, amiodarone is used in treating only the following documented life-threatening ventricular arrhythmias that do not respond to documented adequate doses of other antiarrhythmics or when alternative agents are not tolerated:

- Recurrent ventricular fibrillation
- Recurrent, hemodynamically unstable ventricular tachycardia

If the patient is nonresponsive to other therapy, intravenous amiodarone is used in the initiation of treatment and as prophylaxis for frequently recurring ventricular fibrillation and hemodynamically unstable ventricular tachycardia. IV amiodarone also can be used in patients who meet the requirements for oral amiodarone but who cannot take oral medication.

Amiodarone is often used in patients with an ICD to reduce the frequency of arrhythmias and decrease the need for future shocks; it appears to be more effective for this purpose when combined with a beta blocker (UpToDate, 2007). Amiodarone is also used as preventive therapy in patients who have survived sudden cardiac death who are not candidates for an ICD.

Although amiodarone is not specifically approved for treating AFib, it has been found to be effective in patients with paroxysmal or persistent AFib (VerNooy & Mounsey, 2004). For chronic maintenance therapy of AFib, research has established that amiodarone is the antiarrhythmic

with the highest efficacy (VerNooy & Mounsey, 2004). The drug is used to control rhythm in AFib. One study showed amiodarone was more effective at 1 year than either sotalol or Class I agents for maintaining sinus rhythm without cardioversion (AFFIRM First Antiarrhythmic Drug Substudy Investigators, 2003). Another small study showed that it was effective in maintaining normal sinus rhythm in patients with chronic AFib, even if the AFib was of long enough duration to have induced electrical atrial remodeling (Komatsu, Tachibana, Sato, et al., 2007). Despite these findings that demonstrate effectiveness, many authorities consider using amiodarone for AFib controversial, because it has many significant adverse effects (Fuster, Ryden, Cannom, et al., 2006; UpToDate, 2007).

Pharmacokinetics

With oral administration, amiodarone is absorbed slowly, and the absorption is highly variable. The bioavailability of a single dose of the drug (oral or IV) is about 50% of the dose given, although it can range from 35% to 65%. Some researchers suggest that the incomplete bioavailability is caused by incomplete absorption related to amiodarone's high lipid solubility. Incomplete bioavailability has ramifications for dosing when the patient is being switched from oral to IV (or vice versa). The patient may require a smaller IV dose than the oral dose.

Amiodarone is widely distributed throughout the body, with much variability. It is extensively distributed in some sites, such as adipose tissue and highly perfused organs (e.g., liver, lung, and spleen). Variability in distribution contributes to variability in response to drug therapy, which is exhibited by the patient. The drug is highly protein bound (96%). This high protein binding also complicates the distribution of amiodarone. Individual variability in protein levels may cause some of the variability of drug action. Free drug levels are difficult to measure in extensive protein binding. Because of its high lipid solubility, amiodarone and its metabolite are thought to concentrate in cell membranes, especially of the liver, heart, and fat cells.

Research supports the idea that the slow distribution of amiodarone into tissue sites is an important component of the drug's unusual pharmacokinetic and pharmacodynamic activities.

Metabolism occurs in the liver, apparently by cytochrome P-450 3A4, forming an active metabolite, diethanolamine (DEA), which accumulates in most tissues to an even greater extent than the parent. DEA has pharmacologic properties similar to amiodarone; DEA is highly protein bound, although its distribution is concentrated in the heart.

The actual route of amiodarone elimination is not well understood. Amiodarone has a biphasic elimination with an initial one-half reduction of plasma levels after 2.5 to 107 days. A much slower terminal plasma elimination has a mean half-life of 53 days for amiodarone and 61 days for DEA. Thus, it takes almost a year for the drug to reach steady state with chronic oral administration. Because of this, a loading regimen of the drug is needed to achieve an initial pharmacologic effect. With prolonged administration, serum concentrations of amiodarone and DEA are similar. The main route of excretion is hepatic, into the bile. Some enterohepatic recirculation may occur.

Pharmacodynamics

Although amiodarone produces electrophysiologic changes characteristic of all four antiarrhythmic classes, it predominantly has Class III effects. Amiodarone has two major properties: prolongation of the refractory period, and noncompetitive alpha- and beta-adrenergic inhibition. It also modulates thyroid function (one molecule of amiodarone contains two iodine atoms, and amiodarone shares some structural similarities with thyroid hormones), phospholipid metabolism, and production of certain cytokines (extracellular factors that are important in controlling the inflammatory response).

Like Class I antiarrhythmic drugs, amiodarone blocks the fast sodium channel. It may do this when the channel is in the inactivated state. Unlike Class I antiarrhythmic drugs, amiodarone also blocks potassium channels. These activities contribute to the slowing of conduction and increased refractory period. Amiodarone blocks multiple potassium channels, including inward and outward currents. Like Class II antiarrhythmic drugs, amiodarone has a noncompetitive antisympathetic action. Like Class IV antiarrhythmic drugs, it has a negative chronotropic effect (slowing heart rate) from blocking the slow calcium channel. All these actions (blocking sodium, potassium, and calcium channels, and inhibition of sympathetic action) have an effect on slowing conduction (negative dromotropic effect) at the SA node and on slowing conduction and increasing the refractory period at the AV node. Amiodarone does have some vasodilating effects, which decrease the oxygen needs of the heart.

The effect on sodium channels appears to be limited to acute dosing (by IV) and is not present in chronic dosing. The effect on calcium and potassium channels may be both acute and chronic. However, unlike oral dosing, IV dosing has little or no effect on the length of the sinus cycle, the refractoriness of the right atrium or right ventricle, repolarization, intraventricular conduction, and infranodal (below or beneath the nodes) conduction. These differences suggest that the initial acute effects of amiodarone IV are focused predominantly on the AV node (because of sodium channel blockade).

Several electrophysiologic effects occur with the administration of amiodarone. An increased cardiac refractory period occurs, usually without influencing the resting membrane potential. Sinus rate decreases by 15% to 20%. The PR and QT intervals increase by about 10%. U waves appear, and T waves are altered. These changes do not usually require discontinuation of amiodarone, although marked sinus bradycardia or sinus arrest and heart block can occur. QT prolongation can be associated with worsening of the arrhythmia, but this event is rare.

After IV dosing, amiodarone relaxes the vascular smooth muscle, reduces peripheral vascular resistance (decreasing afterload), and slightly increases the cardiac index (ratio of cardiac output per minute to the body surface area). With oral dosing, amiodarone produces no appreciable change in left ventricular ejection fraction. After acute IV dosing, amiodarone may have a mild negative inotropic effect on left ventricular ejection fraction, decreasing the force of contractility. Oral dosing, however, produces no meaningful change in left ventricular ejection fraction.

Because of its ability to lengthen repolarization and refractoriness in atria and ventricles, while also blocking adrenergic stimulation, amiodarone is a potentially valuable drug in treating AFib. One reason that amiodarone's use in AFib is attractive to researchers is its ability to increase the duration of the action potential in atrial and ventricular tissues following chronic drug administration, while producing lesser effects in Purkinje fibers and M cells (special cardiac cells). Additionally, its effect on repolarization is not influenced by heart rate. Despite producing marked slowing of the heart rate and substantial increases in the QT interval, the drug only seldom produces torsades de pointes (see Adverse Effects). Amiodarone is known to be effective in maintaining normal sinus rhythm, which is now considered crucial in treating atrial fibrillation. Low doses of amiodarone have been found to maintain sinus rhythm in patients with paroxysmal or chronic AFib who were previously nonresponsive to other drug therapies. Furthermore, amiodarone has been found to effectively treat and prevent AFib in patients who have CHF. Few other drugs have this benefit, yet almost 40% of patients with CHF develop atrial fibrillation.

Contraindications and Precautions

Contraindications for giving the drug orally include severe sinus-node dysfunction producing marked sinus bradycardia, second- and third-degree AV block, and a history of episodes of bradycardia that have caused syncope (unless the drug is used with a pacemaker). Contraindications for giving the drug intravenously are similar and include marked sinus bradycardia, second- and third-degree AV block (unless the patient has a functioning pacemaker), and cardiogenic shock. Additionally, if patients have a known hypersensitivity response to the drug, it should be avoided. Amiodarone carries a Black Box warning regarding the difficulty of using the drug safely because of its long half-life, P-450 effects, variability in effects, and frequent drug interactions.

Amiodarone inhibits peripheral conversion of thyroxine (T_4) to triiodothyronine (T_3), prompting increased T_4 levels, increased levels of inactive reverse T_3, and decreased levels of T_3. It also is a potential source of large amounts of inorganic iodine. Because it releases inorganic iodine, and perhaps for other unknown reasons, amiodarone can cause hypothyroidism or hyperthyroidism. Because of the slow elimination of amiodarone and its metabolite, high plasma iodide levels, altered thyroid function, and abnormal thyroid function tests may persist for several weeks or months after the drug is discontinued.

Amiodarone is in pregnancy category D. It can cause congenital goiter/hypothyroidism or hyperthyroidism. Amiodarone is excreted into breast milk. In animal studies, nursing offspring are less viable and have reduced body weight gains.

Adverse Effects

Amiodarone has several adverse effects that are potentially fatal. Pulmonary toxicity is the most important of these serious adverse effects. The frequency of pulmonary toxicity with amiodarone is between 2% and 17%. About 10% of the patients who develop pulmonary toxicity die. The syndrome, seen frequently with oral dosing, is cough, progressive dyspnea, and test findings (e.g., radiographic, gallium scan, or pulmonary function tests) consistent with pulmonary toxicity. Phospholipidosis (foamy cells, foamy macrophages) is present in most cases of amiodarone-induced pulmonary toxicity. However, this finding is not a specific marker for amiodarone toxicity; these changes are also present in about 50% of patients taking the drug.

Any new changes in the respiratory system warrant reexamining the patient to determine whether pulmonary toxicity is present. Amiodarone is prescribed to patients with life-threatening arrhythmias. Therefore, the drug must be discontinued cautiously if pulmonary toxicity is suspected, because more patients die from sudden cardiac death (the most common cause of death in these patients) than from pulmonary toxicity. Before discontinuing amiodarone because of suspected pulmonary toxicity, other causes of respiratory impairment (e.g., infection) should be ruled out.

Another potentially fatal adverse effect of amiodarone is exacerbation of the arrhythmia it is treating. It also may make the arrhythmia more difficult to reverse. This event occurs in about 2% to 5% of patients treated. The risk for exacerbation is increased if more than one type of arrhythmia is present. Exacerbation can include new ventricular fibrillation, incessant ventricular tachycardia, increased resistance to cardioversion, and polymorphic (more than one form) ventricular tachycardia associated with QT prolongation (torsades de pointes). Amiodarone also has caused symptomatic bradycardia, heart block, and sinus arrest with suppression of escape foci (ectopic foci picking up as pacemaker when SA is not functioning to maintain a heartbeat) in 2% to 4% of patients. Drug-related bradycardia does not appear to be dose related.

A final potentially lethal adverse effect is liver disease. However, this effect is very rare. Some liver injury, evidenced only by elevated liver enzyme levels, is common with amiodarone, but such injury is normally mild and not serious.

Amiodarone carries a Black Box warning related to the three serious adverse effects just described: pulmonary toxicity, fatal arrhythmia, and hepatotoxicity.

Optic neuritis or optic neuropathy, although not a fatal adverse effect, can be potentially serious because visual impairment can occur and may result in permanent blindness. However, this adverse effect is rare.

Other adverse effects include common CNS effects (e.g., malaise, dizziness, paresthesia, tremor, headache, and insomnia). These can occur in 20% to 40% of patients. The effects are not serious, rarely require discontinuing the drug, and often are alleviated with dosage reduction or dividing the dose. GI complaints (e.g., nausea, vomiting, constipation, anorexia, and abdominal pain) also are common; about 25% of patients have these complaints. The drug rarely needs to be discontinued because of these effects. The GI effects are seen mostly with high doses and usually are alleviated with dose reduction or divided doses.

Photosensitivity is a problem for about 10% of patients taking amiodarone. With long-term treatment, a blue-gray discoloration of the exposed skin may be seen. The risk, which may be increased in patients with fair complexions or excessive sun exposure, may be related to cumulative dose and the duration of therapy. It reverses slowly after the drug is discontinued, although sometimes it is irreversible. Hypothyroidism or hyperthyroidism may occur, as may edema, coagulation abnormalities, flushing, epididymitis, vasculitis, pseudotumor cerebri, thrombocytopenia, and angioedema.

When amiodarone is given intravenously, hypotension is its most frequent adverse effect, although it is not normally serious. Clinically significant hypotension occurs in the first few hours of drug administration and appears to be related to the rate of infusion, not the drug concentration. Blood pressure should return to normal if the rate is slowed down.

Drug Interactions

Amiodarone increases the plasma concentration of digoxin. This effect is believed to be caused by amiodarone's inhibition of P-glycoprotein. P-glycoprotein pumps drugs entering the enterocyte back into the intestinal lumen. It also is active on the tubular side of the renal epithelium and the biliary side of hepatocytes and serves to promote drug excretion at these sites. By inhibiting P-glycoprotein excretion, the elimination of digoxin is decreased, increasing blood levels of this drug.

Amiodarone also decreases the clearance of many other drugs, including flecainide and warfarin. Most likely, multiple mechanisms underlie these effects. Amiodarone's impairment of flecainide elimination appears to be mostly renal. Its impairment of warfarin clearance is most likely related to amiodarone being an inhibitor of CYP2C9 (another major isoenzyme of metabolism); warfarin relies solely on CYP2C9 for metabolism. Research

on amiodarone's effects on metabolism and elimination of other drugs is continuing. Table 31.4 provides additional information on drug interactions. Amiodarone also interferes with laboratory tests. It alters thyroid function tests because of its effects on T_3 and T_4 and also may alter liver function tests (alanine aminotransferase and aspartate aminotransferase).

Assessment of Relevant Core Patient Variables
Health Status
Determine the patient's cardiac status using an ECG. This verifies whether the patient has an arrhythmia that is responsive to amiodarone and ensures that none of the pathologic conditions that contraindicate amiodarone's use is present.

TABLE 31.4 Agents That Interact with P Amiodarone

Interactants	Effect and Significance	Nursing Management
anticoagulants	Potentiation of anticoagulant response; prothrombin may be increased	Dose decrease usually needed; monitor prothrombin
beta blockers	May increase risk of bradycardia and hypotension from additive effect	Monitor pulse and blood pressure
calcium channel blockers	Increased risk of atrioventricular block or hypotension	Monitor for electrocardiographic (ECG) changes; monitor blood pressure
cyclosporine	Increased plasma levels of cyclosporine, resulting in elevated creatinine	Reduce dose; monitor creatinine levels
dextromethorphan	Impairs metabolism of dextromethorphan	Assess for adverse effects
digoxin	Increased digoxin serum levels	Monitor digoxin levels; decrease dose of digoxin; consider stopping digoxin
disopyramide	Increases QT prolongation; may cause arrhythmias	Monitor for ECG changes
fentanyl	Increases effect of fentanyl and may cause hypotension and bradycardia	Monitor blood pressure and pulse
flecainide	Increases the effect of flecainide	Decrease the dose of flecainide; therapeutic levels will be maintained
hydantoins	Impairs metabolism of hydantoins; elevated serum levels of hydantoins may occur; amiodarone level also may be decreased	Monitor blood levels; assess for adverse effects
lidocaine	Increased levels of lidocaine	Monitor blood pressure (rare complications)
methotrexate	Impairs metabolism of methotrexate	Assess for adverse effects
procainamide	Increased procainamide serum levels may occur	Monitor for adverse effects
quinidine	Increased quinidine levels; potential for fatal arrhythmias	Assess ECG for changes
theophylline	Increased theophylline levels with toxicity	Monitor levels; assess for adverse effects
cholestyramine	Increased enterohepatic elimination of amiodarone; reduced serum levels and half-life may occur	Monitor for therapeutic effects
cimetidine	Increased serum levels of amiodarone may occur	Assess for adverse effects
ritonavir	Large increases in amiodarone blood levels may occur, increasing the risk of adverse effects	Assess for adverse effects; monitor ECG

Also, obtain baseline results of thyroid function tests and liver function tests. It is important to assess respiratory status through chest x-ray, pulmonary function studies (including diffusion capacity), and auscultation of breath sounds before treatment.

Life Span and Gender
Determine the patient's age because safety and efficacy have not been established in children. The benzyl alcohol that is contained in some of these products as a preservative has been associated with a fatal "gasping syndrome" in premature infants. In older adults, amiodarone has a lower clearance rate and an increased half-life. It also is important to determine whether the patient is pregnant because amiodarone is a pregnancy category D drug. The drug should be used only if the potential benefits outweigh the substantial risks to the fetus. If the patient is breastfeeding, she should be advised to discontinue nursing while on amiodarone.

Environment
Be aware of the setting in which amiodarone is administered. IV amiodarone is given in an intensive care unit, where the patient can receive continuous cardiac monitoring. Oral doses can be given in any environment, except when giving a loading dose; during this time, the patient needs to be hospitalized. While the patient is taking oral doses, assess the patient's exposure to sunlight because photosensitivity can occur.

Culture and Inherited Traits
Variations in response to amiodarone may be genetically related. However, little is yet known about this genetic variation.

Nursing Diagnoses and Outcomes
- Decreased Cardiac Output related to cardiac arrhythmia.
  Desired outcome: *Cardiac rhythm will return to normal, allowing for normal cardiac output.*
- Risk for Injury related to adverse effects of drug therapy
  Desired outcome: *The patient will not suffer permanent injury or death as a result of drug therapy.*

Planning and Intervention
Maximizing Therapeutic Effects
To maximize the therapeutic effect of amiodarone, administer the prescribed loading doses. When giving amiodarone intravenously, mix the drug in glass bottles or polyolefin bags of 5% dextrose in water (D_5W). Although some of the amiodarone dose is lost during administration because it is absorbed by polyvinyl chloride (PVC) tubing, this tubing should be used because the clinical trials that established dosage used this particular type of tubing, and recommended doses account for this loss. Surface properties of solutions of amiodarone are altered so that drop size may be reduced. This size reduction can account for an underdosage of up to 30%. Use a volumetric infusion pump to prevent underdosage.

Minimizing Adverse Effects
ORAL AND INTRAVENOUS DOSES
It is important to correct electrolyte disturbances before beginning therapy. Hypokalemia and hypomagnesemia can exaggerate the degree of QT prolongation and increase the potential for torsades de pointes. Assess for proarrhythmic changes. Use pulse oximetry or arterial blood gases to assess for changes in respiratory function, including breath sounds, dyspnea, and oxygen delivery to the tissues. If changes occur, it is important to repeat the chest x-ray physical examination, gallium scan, and pulmonary function tests to rule out pulmonary toxicity.

Assess for symptoms of visual impairment. Regular eye examinations are recommended throughout therapy. Ophthalmic examination should be sought immediately if impairment occurs. It also is important to assess T_3 and T_4 levels to determine thyroid function. Assess for signs of hyperthyroidism or hypothyroidism. Liver function studies also should be monitored.

ORAL DOSES
Monitor the patient closely during the loading phase until the risk for recurrent ventricular tachycardia or fibrillation has abated. It is important to attempt to discontinue prior antiarrhythmic drugs gradually. Reduce the dose of these other drugs by 30% to 50% several days after initiating amiodarone, when arrhythmias should be suppressed.

In patients whose arrhythmias are not well controlled on amiodarone alone, introduce other agents, using half of the usual recommended dosage. It is a good idea to divide the dose or give amiodarone with food to minimize or prevent nausea, vomiting, and other GI effects.

INTRAVENOUS DOSES
Adjust the starting dose to suppress life-threatening arrhythmias based on individual response to therapy. Monitor the patient continuously during therapy, using a cardiac monitor. It is important to monitor blood pressure carefully because hypotension is most likely to occur in the early period, and to reduce the infusion rate if hypotension occurs.

Avoid administering amiodarone with aminophylline, cefamandole, cefazolin, mezlocillin, heparin, and sodium bicarbonate because these agents are incompatible with amiodarone and form precipitates. If possible, administer amiodarone using a central venous catheter to prevent phlebitis.

Use an in-line filter. It is important to use IV therapy until the ventricular arrhythmia is stabilized. Transfer the patient to oral therapy either during or after IV treatment, and adjust the IV dose to a new, lower oral dose. If the patient is treated with IV infusion for less than 1 week, give an oral dose of 800 to 1,600 mg/d initially. If the patient is treated with IV for 1 to 3 weeks, give an oral dose of 600 to 800 mg/d initially. If the patient is treated with IV for longer than 3 weeks, give an oral dose of 400 mg/d initially. When adequate arrhythmia control is achieved, decrease to

600 to 800 mg/d (orally) in one to two doses for 1 month; the maintenance dose is 400 mg/d.

Providing Patient and Family Education
- Explain the purpose of the drug and possible adverse effects of the drug.
- Emphasize the importance of returning for follow-up blood work and ECGs.
- Teach patients to use appropriate protection when out in the sun and to limit sun exposure.
- Instruct the patient to notify the physician for new onset of cough, shortness of breath, and changes in visual acuity.

Ongoing Assessment and Evaluation

The patient's ECG should be monitored intermittently throughout therapy and after the initial stabilization and loading dose period for new arrhythmias or worsening of the current arrhythmia being treated. Make recurrent assessments of respiratory function, visual acuity, thyroid function, and liver function. Amiodarone therapy is considered effective if the arrhythmia is corrected and the patient does not develop serious adverse effects.

Drugs Closely Related to 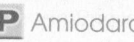 Amiodarone
Sotalol

Like amiodarone, sotalol (Betapace) prolongs repolarization (phase 3). These Class III effects are seen in doses greater than 160 mg/d. Additionally, like amiodarone, sotalol decreases automaticity at the SA node and ectopic pacemakers. It also decreases conduction velocity at the AV node, although unlike amiodarone, it does not decrease it at the atrium, bundle of His, or Purkinje fibers. ECG changes are similar except that sotalol does not lengthen the QT interval. Although sotalol and amiodarone both have antiadrenergic

CRITICAL THINKING SCENARIO

AMIODARONE THERAPY

Mr. Bowen is 74 years old. He was brought to the hospital emergency department by ambulance. He was diagnosed with myocardial infarction and was in ventricular fibrillation. He is successfully defibrillated and converted to sinus rhythm. He is started on amiodarone by IV infusion. When he is transferred to the intensive care unit, his blood pressure drops to 88/50 mm Hg. The intensive care unit nurse examines Mr. Bowen's laboratory results; the only unexpected finding is that he has a low serum albumin level.

1. What possible causes may account for Mr. Bowen's hypotension?
2. What action should you take to manage the hypotension?
3. If you are unable to correct the hypotension, what might you do next?

MEMORY CHIP
P Amiodarone

- Class III antiarrhythmic used to treat life-threatening ventricular arrhythmias and prevent their recurrence
- Produces prolonged phase of repolarization (phase 3)
- Has properties of Classes I, II, and IV
- Has extremely long half-life and great variability in pharmacodynamics and pharmacokinetics
- Major contraindications: severe sinus bradycardia and second- or third-degree atrioventricular heart block
- Most common adverse effects: central nervous system effects (e.g., malaise, dizziness, paresthesia, tremor, headache, and insomnia); GI effects (e.g., nausea and vomiting); photosensitivity; and hypotension (IV use)
- Most serious adverse effects: pulmonary toxicity and cardiac arrhythmias
- **Life span alert: Drug is in pregnancy category D; use only if benefit outweighs risk.**
- Maximizing therapeutic effects: Use a loading dose.
- Minimizing adverse effects: Correct pre-existing electrolyte imbalances before giving the drug; adjust IV dose to control ventricular arrhythmia; monitor blood pressure (IV dosing); monitor electrocardiogram for changes; and assess for respiratory changes.
- Most important patient education: Take with food to minimize GI distress and notify the physician if cough or shortness of breath develops.

effects, they work by different mechanisms. Sotalol is actually a beta blocker, blocking both beta-1 and beta-2 sites. However, it is not considered a Class II antiarrhythmic like the other beta blockers, because it also has Class IC and Class III effects.

Sotalol is used in treating life-threatening ventricular arrhythmias. It is also approved for treating atrial arrhythmias. Sotalol has been shown to maintain sinus rhythm in about 50% of patients with AFib after cardioversion to their normal rhythm. When sotalol is used in patients with an implanted cardioverter-defibrillator, patients are less likely to require a shock (Bollmann, Husser, & Cannom, 2005). Like all other antiarrhythmics, sotalol may induce arrhythmias as well as treat them. Torsades de pointes, although possible, is not likely to occur if the dose is controlled, if the patient has normal renal function, and if the patient does not have severe CHF. Sotalol is administered only orally, so it is started after the patient has been on IV antiarrhythmics for ventricular arrhythmias. The other antiarrhythmic should have been withdrawn for at least two to three half-lives before starting sotalol.

Sotalol should be initiated in a facility that can provide cardiac resuscitation, continuous ECG monitoring, and creatinine clearance values. Patients should be cared for by health care providers who are familiar with managing serious ventricular arrhythmias. Patients should continue to be monitored for a minimum of 3 days on the maintenance dose and should not be discharged within 12 hours of electrical or pharmacologic conversion to normal sinus rhythm.

Ibutilide

Ibutilide (Corvert) is a new drug in the category termed the "pure" Class III antiarrhythmics. It is not as multifaceted as amiodarone. The goal of developing these new Class III drugs was to find a drug as effective as amiodarone but without its adverse effects.

Ibutilide was the first of the pure Class III drugs approved for use in the United States. It is approved only for IV use to convert atrial flutter and fibrillation to normal sinus rhythm. It is about twice as effective in converting atrial flutter as AFib. Ibutilide increases the atrial effective refractory period and prolongs the QT interval. This effect on the QT interval is dose dependent. Ibutilide also causes some blockade of potassium channels. As a result, duration of the action potential in the ventricles is also prolonged somewhat. For these reasons, ibutilide should be used with caution in patients with bradycardia, CHF or low ejection fraction, hypokalemia or hypomagnesemia, recent MI, or significantly prolonged QT intervals prior to treatment, or in those who are taking other Class I or III antiarrhythmics (within 4 hours of ibutilide transfusion) or other drugs that prolong QT intervals. Patients who have had AF for more than 3 days must be anticoagulated for at least 2 weeks prior to starting ibutilide.

Ibutilide is metabolized extensively in the liver; its high first-pass effect is the reason it must be given intravenously. Unlike amiodarone, ibutilide has a short half-life of 4 to 8 hours; its metabolites have a similar half-life. Ibutilide distributes rapidly to a large volume, and its electrophysiologic effects decrease quickly after IV administration. Proarrhythmia effects are therefore greatest within the first hour of administration. Ibutilide use is associated with an estimated 8% risk for torsades de pointes. When it occurs, it often is transient. However, if ibutilide is given concurrently with beta blockers or calcium channel blockers, torsades de pointes is more likely to occur.

Dofetilide

Dofetilide (Tikosyn) is another new "pure" Class III drug, like ibutilide. It can be given IV or PO. Similarly, it has more limited effects than amiodarone. Dofetilide is used to convert patients in atrial fibrillation to normal sinus rhythm and maintain them in sinus rhythm. The drug delays repolarization by lengthening the effective refractory period in the atria, ventricles, and Purkinje fibers by blocking some of the potassium channels. It has no effect on sodium or calcium channels and thus little effect on conduction velocity, force of contraction, and systemic hemodynamics. Dofetilide also has no effect on alpha or beta receptors. It is not approved for managing ventricular arrhythmias, and its efficacy for these arrhythmias is under investigation (Khan, 2004). It increases repolarization and refractoriness in both atrial and ventricular tissue, although the predominant effect is on the atrial tissue. It is administered orally and is well absorbed with a bioavailability of more than 90%. Most of the drug is excreted unchanged in the urine, and the rest is metabolized in the liver

via the CYP 3A4 pathway. Systemic half-life is 10 hours. Because dofetilide is mostly excreted unchanged, it is important to monitor for kidney function, as decreasing function will make the patient more at risk of adverse effects.

Dofetilide has a reverse use-dependent effect, and at slow rates it has the tendency to increase the QT interval. Dofetilide is not likely to cause torsades de pointes. It carries the Black Box warning, relative to its risk of inducing arrhythmias, that a patient beginning dofetilide should be placed for a minimum of 3 days in a facility that can provide calculations of creatinine clearance, continuous ECG monitoring, and cardiac resuscitation. Dofetilide is available only to hospitals and prescribers who have received appropriate dofetilide dosing and treatment initiation education. Unlike other antiarrhythmics, dofetilide does not increase mortality in patients with a recent MI or CHF (Roukoz & Saliba, 2007). Common adverse effects include chest pain, dizziness, headache, dyspnea, respiratory tract infection, and GI problems. It is a pregnancy class C drug.

Dronedarone

Dronedarone is another new Class III antiarrhythmic. It was recently approved by the FDA for use in treating atrial fibrillation or flutter. It can be given PO. It is a synthetic analog of amiodarone, missing the iodine component. Similar to amiodarone, it has sodium, potassium, and calcium channel blocking properties as well as being a adrenergic receptor antagonist. Differences from amiodarone include: a shorter half life, quicker achievement of therapeutic drug levels, and fewer adverse effects primarily due to the missing iodine component (Cheng, 2010).

Dronedarone carries a Black Box warning related to its use in patients with class IV heart failure or class II or III decompensating heart failure. A study has shown a doubling of mortality when used in those patients. In addition to being contraindicated in those heart failure patients, it is also contraindicated in patients with bradycardia of less than 50, severe hepatitis, second or third degree block without a pacemaker, patients on other QT prolonging drugs, and patients who are pregnant or nursing.

Dronedarone is metabolized in the liver. Care must be taken to monitor liver function. In addition to nausea, vomiting, diarrhea, an increased serum creatinine, other adverse effects include a prolonged QT interval or heart failure. Patients should be taught to take this drug with meals and to avoid any form of grapefruit.

Bretylium

Bretylium (bretylium tosylate), a Class III antiarrhythmic also has adrenergic blocking properties. It was used for the treatment of life-threatening ventricular arrhythmias. It is no longer recommended by the AHA due to the frequent occurrence of adverse effects and the accessibility of other more effective alternatives such as amiodarone (AHA guidelines). There were also issues with the drug's availability. In 1999 the drug was not available due to limited quantities of the raw materials necessary for manufacture. There is a recent effort to evaluate the current ACLS guidelines specifically looking at the use of bretylium during resuscitation. Bretylium's ability to produce chemical defibrillation by prolonging the QT interval and blocking re-entery pathways is being examined. By raising the threshold for ventricular fibrillation, it may be considered a safer, more effective alternative to excessive doses of epinephrine and electrical defibrillation (Bacaner, Dembo, 2009).

© CLASS IV ANTIARRHYTHMIC DRUGS

Class IV antiarrhythmics depress phase 4 depolarization and lengthen phases 1 and 2 of repolarization (see Figure 31.6). This class is the calcium channel blockers, but only two have been approved specifically as antiarrhythmics: verapamil (Calan) and diltiazem (Cardizem). Table 31.5 presents a summary of selected Class IV antiarrhythmics and other calcium channel blockers. The prototype Class IV antiarrhythmic calcium channel blocker is verapamil.

Calcium channel blockers prescribed for other purposes include amlodipine (Norvasc), bepridil (Vascor), felodipine (Plendil), isradipine (Dyna Circ), nimodipine (Nimotop), nisoldipine (Sular), nicardipine (Cardene), and nifedipine (Procardia, Adalat). Other uses of calcium channel blockers are described in Chapters 28 and 30.

Nursing Management of the Patient Receiving ℗ Verapamil

Core Drug Knowledge

Pharmacotherapeutics

Verapamil is used as an antiarrhythmic. Verapamil, used alone or in conjunction with digoxin, controls ventricular rate in chronic atrial flutter or fibrillation. However, calcium channel blockers are not as effective as beta blockers for this purpose (Olshansky, Rosenfeld, Warner, et al., 2004). It also can be used prophylactically for repetitive paroxysmal SVT. IV verapamil also is used to treat supraventricular tachyarrhythmias, while the oral form may be used to sustain normal rhythm. The antiarrhythmic effects seem similar in adults and children.

Verapamil also is used in treating angina (including Prinzmetal angina) and hypertension. An unlabeled use is preventing migraine headache.

Pharmacokinetics

Well absorbed after oral administration, verapamil undergoes a substantial first-pass effect, resulting in considerably less bioavailability. Verapamil is excreted by the kidneys. It crosses the placenta and appears in breast milk. When sustained-release verapamil is administered with food, it takes longer to reach maximum plasma levels. However, bioavailability is not affected appreciably; hence, verapamil may be administered without regard to meals.

TABLE 31.5 Summary of Selected © Class IV Antiarrhythmics and Selected Other Calcium Channel Blocker

Drugs (Trade) Name	Selected Indications	Route and Dosage Range	Pharmacokinetics
℗ verapamil (Calan, Isoptin)	Angina pectoris Supraventricular tachyarrhythmias	*Adult:* PO, 80–120 mg tid, increase q1–2d as needed *Adult:* IV, 5–10 mg over 2 min; may repeat dose of 10 mg 30 min after first dose. Give dose over 3 min for elderly. *Child:* IV, >1 y, 0.1–0.2 mg/kg over 2 min; 1–15 y, 0.1–0.3 mg/kg over 2 min; do not exceed 5 mg; repeat after 30 min, if necessary.	*Onset:* PO, 30 min; IV, rapid *Duration:* PO, 3–7 h; IV, 2 h $t_{1/2}$: 3–7 h
	Hypertension	*Adult:* PO, 240 mg qd; sustained-release form in morning; 80 mg tid. May need to individualize dose by titration.	
diltiazem (Cardizem, Tiazac)	Angina pectoris Essential hypertension Atrial fibrillation or flutter (IV only)	*Adult:* PO, 30 mg qid before meals and hs, increase gradually at 1–2 d intervals to 180–360 mg in three to four divided doses; SR, cardizem CD, 180–240 mg/d PO for hypertension; 120–180 mg/d PO for angina IV, 0.25 mg/kg over 2 min; second bolus of 0.35 mg/kg given over 2 min IV infusion: 5–15 mg/h for up to 24 h *Child:* Safety and efficacy not established	*Onset:* PO and SR, 30–60 min; IV, immediate *Duration:* Unknown $t_{1/2}$: $3_{1/2}$–6 h; SR, 5–7 h
Non-Antiarrhythmic Calcium Channel Blockers			
amlodipine (Norvasc)	Angina pectoris Essential hypertension	*Adult:* PO, 5 mg qd, may increase over 10–14 d to a max dose of 10 mg/d *Child:* Safety and efficacy not established	*Onset:* PO, unknown *Duration:* Unknown $t_{1/2}$: 30–50 h
nicardipine (Cardene)	Stable angina	*Adult:* PO, 20 mg tid; range, 20–40 mg tid; allow 3 d before increasing dosage *Child:* Safety and efficacy not established	*Onset:* 20 min *Duration:* Unknown $t_{1/2}$: 2–4 h
	Hypertension	*Adult:* PO, 20 mg tid; range 20–40 mg tid. Adjust dosage based on BP response; allow 3 d before increasing *Child:* Safety and efficacy not established	

Pharmacodynamics

Verapamil acts by inhibiting the movement of calcium ions across the cardiac and arterial muscle cell membrane. It works preferentially in "slow response" myocardial tissue, such as the SA and AV nodes. Calcium currents through these tissues generate the slowly propagating action potentials. Verapamil slows phase 4 depolarization. Blocking calcium movement results in slowing conduction through the AV node (conduction velocity), prolonging the effective refractory phase (automaticity), depressing myocardial contractility, and producing dilation of both coronary arteries and peripheral arterioles. Verapamil interrupts re-entry at the AV node and thus can restore normal sinus rhythm in paroxysmal SVT. When calcium channel blockers such as verapamil cause peripheral vasodilation, they can induce reflex activation of the sympathetic nervous system, causing reflex tachycardia. This prevents a drop in cardiac output. Other outcomes of verapamil therapy are decreased oxygen demand, decreased cardiac effort, and increased oxygen to the myocardium.

Contraindications and Precautions

Verapamil is contraindicated in sick sinus syndrome or second- or third-degree heart block (except with a functioning pacemaker), hypotension (systolic pressure less than 90 mm Hg), cardiogenic shock, and severe CHF. Precaution should be used in severe left ventricular dysfunction (ejection fraction less than 30%). Verapamil may cause a greater hypotensive effect in elderly patients than in younger ones; thus, it should be administered cautiously to older patients. Caution should also be used in patients with cirrhosis of the liver (the half-life is greatly increased) and with renal disease. Caution should be used if the patient has Duchenne muscular dystrophy because verapamil may decrease neuromuscular transmission. IV verapamil can induce respiratory muscle failure in these patients.

Verapamil is in pregnancy category C.

Adverse Effects

The most common adverse effect of verapamil is constipation. Other common adverse effects include dizziness, headache, nausea, hypotension, and peripheral edema. Verapamil may produce potentially lethal ventricular arrhythmias and, rarely, MI.

Drug Interactions

Several drugs interact with verapamil (see Table 31.6). Ranolazine and dofetilide are both contraindicated

TABLE 31.6	Agents That Interact with P Verapami	
Interactants	**Effect and Significance**	**Nursing Management**
barbiturates	Clearance of verapamil possibly increased and bioavailability decreased	Monitor pulse, blood pressure, and respiration carefully. Monitor patient responses and blood levels.
calcium salts	Antagonism of effects of verapamil with calcium	Administer 2 h apart.
hydantoins	Serum verapamil levels possibly decreased	Monitor for therapeutic effect.
quinidine	Hypotension bradycardia, ventricular tachycardia, atrioventricular (AV) block, and pulmonary edema possible	Use concomitantly only when no other alternatives exist.
rifampin	Possible loss of clinical effectiveness of oral verapamil	Use of IV verapamil may circumvent the interaction.
vitamin D	Therapeutic efficacy of verapamil possibly reduced	Stagger dosage and monitor vital signs.
beta blockers	Coadministration, potential increased adverse effects due to depressant effects on myocardial contractility of AV conduction	Concurrent use normally avoided.
cardiac glycosides (digoxin)	Possible increased digoxin levels	Monitor for adverse effects of cardiac glycoside.
dofetilide	Coadministration of dofetilide and verapamil results in a significant increase in peak plasma levels of dofetilide, thus increasing the risk of serious ventricular arrhythmias associated with QT interval prolongation, including torsades de pointes.	Concurrent administration is contraindicated.
ranolazine	Verapamil inhibits the metabolism of ranolazine by the cytochrome P450-3A enzymes, increasing serum levels of ranolazine, which then increases the risk of QT prolongation.	Coadministration is contraindicated.

when taken in combination with verapamil, because coadministration increases the risk of QT prolongation. Verapamil may elevate serum transaminases, with and without concomitant elevations in alkaline phosphatase and bilirubin. Usually, the elevations are transient, although several cases of hepatocellular injury have occurred.

Verapamil forms a crystalline precipitate if administered into an infusion line containing 0.45% sodium chloride solution with sodium bicarbonate. A milky white precipitate forms when it is given as an IV push into the same line being used for nafcillin infusion.

Assessment of Relevant Core Patient Variables
Health Status
Determine whether the patient has chronic atrial flutter or fibrillation, which is causing elevated ventricular rate, or chronic repetitive paroxysmal SVTs, both of which pose a need for therapy. Also, determine whether the patient has any of the following conditions, because they are contraindications to treatment with verapamil: sick sinus syndrome or second- or third-degree heart block (except with a functioning pacemaker), hypotension (with systolic pressure less than 90 mm Hg), severe left ventricular dysfunction, cardiogenic shock, or severe CHF. It also is important to determine whether the patient has renal or liver impairment or Duchenne muscular dystrophy, because verapamil must be used with caution in these patients.

Life Span and Gender
Determine whether the patient is pregnant, because verapamil is in pregnancy category C and must be used cautiously during pregnancy. Also, note the patient's age before administering verapamil: the safety and efficacy of oral verapamil have not been established in children, but experience has shown that treatment results in children are similar to those for adults. IV verapamil is contraindicated in neonates and infants, but only when given to treat SVT, because of a high risk for electromechanical dissociation. In children older than 5 years and in adolescents, IV verapamil may be administered with the same restrictions as in adults (a wide QRS complex tachycardia or substantial hemodynamic compromise). Verapamil may have greater hypotensive effects on older adults.

Lifestyle, Diet, and Habits
Assess whether patients drink alcohol, as caution is required if there is cirrhosis of the liver. Assess for intake of grapefruit and grapefruit juice because these foods affect the verapamil level. Assess diet for normal intake of fiber.

Environment
Know the setting in which verapamil may be administered. IV verapamil is administered only in the hospital, where the patient is monitored constantly using ECG and blood pressure measurements. Oral verapamil can be administered in any setting.

Nursing Diagnoses and Outcomes
• Risk for Constipation related to adverse effects of the drug
Desired outcome: The patient will prevent or minimize constipation by increasing fluid intake and adding fruit and fiber to the diet.
• Decreased Cardiac Output related to decreased rate and force of contraction and return to normal rhythm related to therapeutic effects of drug
Desired outcome: The patient's decreased cardiac output will reduce symptoms of cardiac alterations without developing adverse cardiac effects from drug therapy.

Planning and Intervention
Maximizing Therapeutic Effects
Verify that the IV line is patent before IV administration. Digoxin may be given with verapamil to achieve the additive effect of slowing at the AV node.

Minimizing Adverse Effects
When administering verapamil by an IV route, do not dilute it with a sodium lactate injection in PVC bags, which may not be stable. It is important to administer IV slowly (bolus, 5 to 10 mg over 2 minutes; infusion, 5 mg/h) and to use an IV pump to regulate the drip rate.

Do not administer IV verapamil simultaneously with (or within a few hours of) IV beta blockers, because both drugs suppress contractility and AV conduction. Monitor the patient's ECG and blood pressure constantly during IV therapy. Throughout oral therapy too, monitor for ECG changes and hypotension. Encourage patients on oral verapamil therapy to increase fluid intake and include fresh fruit and fiber in their diets to help prevent constipation.

Providing Patient and Family Education
• Explain the purpose of the drug and its adverse effects.
• Stress the importance of adequate fluid intake and dietary fruit and fiber to help prevent constipation.
• Teach patients how to take the pulse daily while on oral verapamil, instructing them to notify the prescriber if irregular beating (arrhythmia) occurs.
• Teach patients how to take their own blood pressure, urging them to monitor their blood pressure on a regular basis. If the blood pressure falls below 90/60 mm Hg or any other parameter set by the prescriber, instruct patients to contact a member of the health care team.
• Emphasize the importance of scheduling follow-up visits and blood studies.

Ongoing Assessment and Evaluation
Monitor the patient's ECG and blood pressure throughout therapy with verapamil. It is important to monitor liver function periodically to detect elevated serum drug levels. Therapy is effective when normal rhythm is re-established without onset of new arrhythmias, hypotension, or other clinically important adverse effects.

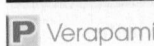

MEMORY CHIP

P Verapamil

- Class IV antiarrhythmic and a calcium channel blocker; may be given intravenously, orally, or sublingually
- Inhibits movement of calcium ions across the cardiac and arterial muscle cell membrane
- Slows conduction, depresses automaticity, depresses myocardial contractility, and dilates coronary arteries and peripheral arterioles
- Antiarrhythmic uses: controls ventricular rate in chronic atrial flutter or fibrillation; used prophylactically with digoxin for repetitive paroxysmal supraventricular tachycardia; used to treat supraventricular tachyarrhythmias (IV administration)
- Also used in angina and hypertension
- Major contraindications: significantly depressed cardiac function, including second- or third-degree heart block, severe hypotension, severe left ventricular dysfunction, severe chronic heart failure, or cardiogenic shock
- Most common adverse effect: constipation
- Most serious adverse effect: ventricular arrhythmias
- **Life span alert: IV routes are contraindicated in neonates and infants, and older adults are more sensitive to hypotensive effects.**
- Maximizing therapeutic effects: Shield drug solution from light; give with digoxin for additive effect of slowing at the atrioventricular node.
- Minimizing adverse effects: Monitor electrocardiogram and blood pressure constantly while on IV, and monitor periodically throughout oral therapy.
- Most important patient education: techniques to prevent constipation

Drug Closely Related to P Verapamil

Diltiazem is another calcium channel blocker like verapamil. It is indicated for rate control in atrial fibrillation, flutter, or paroxysmal supraventricular tachycardia. It is also used to treat stable chronic angina. It has similar actions and averse effects as verapimil. Unlike verapamil, it is not approved for use in children.

Drug Significantly Different From P Verapamil

Adenosine, unlike verapamil, is not a calcium channel blocker. Adenosine is not related chemically to verapamil or any other antiarrhythmic. It is an endogenous nucleoside occurring in all cells of the body. Adenosine, like verapamil, decreases automaticity, decreases conduction velocity at the AV node, and increases the refractory period at the AV node. It may produce first-, second-, or third-degree heart block of short duration. Unlike verapamil, it increases heart rate. It is used in the conversion of paroxysmal SVT to normal sinus rhythm and is given only as a rapid IV bolus. The IV boluses should be administered directly into the vein, or in an IV as proximally to the vein as possible, and followed by a rapid saline flush. The bolus may be repeated if necessary.

Adenosine is removed from the circulatory system very rapidly. It is taken up by erythrocytes and vascular endothelial cells. Its half-life is estimated to be less than 10 seconds. Adenosine is metabolized primarily to inosine and adenosine monophosphate. Conversion to normal sinus rhythm frequently occurs within 1 minute after dosing.

Adenosine is contraindicated in second- or third-degree AV block, sick sinus syndrome (unless a previously inserted pacemaker is functional), atrial flutter, AFib, and ventricular tachycardia, because the drug does not convert these arrhythmias.

The most common adverse effects of adenosine are facial flushing and shortness of breath and dyspnea. Other adverse effects that may occur include:

- CV: sweating, palpitations, chest pain, hypotension (rare), prolonged systole, ventricular fibrillation, ventricular tachycardia, and transient increase in blood pressure
- CNS: headache, light-headedness, dizziness, tingling in arms, numbness, apprehension, blurred vision, burning sensation, heaviness in arms, and pain in neck or back
- GI: nausea, metallic taste, tightness in throat, pressure in groin (rare)
- Respiratory: chest pressure, hyperventilation, and head pressure (rare)

C POTASSIUM-REMOVING RESINS TO PREVENT ARRHYTHMIAS

Because hyperkalemia may lead to cardiac arrhythmias, potassium-removing resins are drugs used to prevent arrhythmias from occurring. These resins bind with potassium and allow it to be excreted. The prototype and sole drug in this class is sodium polystyrene sulfonate (Kayexalate).

Nursing Management of the Patient Receiving P Sodium Polystyrene Sulfonate
Core Drug Knowledge
Pharmacotherapeutics

Sodium polystyrene sulfonate is a potassium-removing resin used in treating hyperkalemia. Because of its slow onset of action, it may not be appropriate to use if the potassium levels are severely elevated (see Pharmacokinetics below). It can be given orally or as an enema. Table 31.7 presents a summary of information about this drug.

Pharmacokinetics

The exchange of potassium ions after administration of sodium polystyrene sulfonate occurs in the large intestine. The drug is not absorbed systemically and is excreted through the GI tract. The onset of action after oral administration is 2 to 12 hours; after rectal administration, onset of action takes more time, although exact numbers are unknown.

TABLE 31.7	C Potassium-Removing Resin			
Drug (Trade) Name	**Selected Indications**	**Route and Dosage Range**	**Pharmacokinetics**	
sodium polystyrene sulfonate (Kayexalate)	Treatment of hyperkalemia	*Adult:* PO, 15 g 1–4×/d *Child:* PO, 1 g/kg q6h *Adult:* Enema, 30–50 g q6h	*Onset:* PO, 2–12 h Enema, >12 h *Duration:* Unknown $t_{1/2}$: Unknown	

Pharmacodynamics

As sodium polystyrene sulfonate moves through the intestine or is maintained in the intestine, it releases sodium ions that are replaced with potassium ions. The efficiency of this process is limited and unpredictable. The ion exchange capacity is approximately 1 mEq potassium per 1 g of drug. Small amounts of calcium and magnesium also can be lost during the exchange process. Effective lowering of serum potassium may take several hours or days.

Contraindications and Precautions

Caution must be used when giving this drug to anyone who cannot tolerate a small increase in sodium intake, such as patients with severe CHF, hypertension, or marked edema. Because therapeutic effects are slow, this should not be the only drug used to treat patients with severe hyperkalemia, in whom the hyperkalemia poses a medical emergency.

Adverse Effects

Hypokalemia may result from therapy and is the most serious adverse effect. Other electrolyte imbalances that may result include hypocalcemia and hypernatremia. Common adverse GI-related effects include gastric irritation, anorexia, nausea, vomiting, and constipation. The constipation occasionally may be severe and cause fecal impaction. Diarrhea occurs occasionally.

Drug Interactions

When administered with nonabsorbable cation-donating antacids and laxatives, such as magnesium hydroxide and aluminum carbonate, systemic alkalosis can occur.

Assessment of Relevant Core Patient Variables

Health Status

Monitor the patient's serum potassium level, and if it is severely elevated, the patient's total physiologic condition and ECG should be reviewed. Also, determine whether the patient has been receiving potassium supplements or replacements in IV fluids.

Life Span and Gender

Note the patient's age before administering sodium polystyrene sulfonate. Large doses of sodium polystyrene sulfonate can cause fecal impaction in elderly patients.

Lifestyle, Diet, and Habits

It is important to investigate the patient's dietary history and preferences, particularly if the patient normally consumes a potassium-rich diet.

Environment

Be aware that sodium polystyrene sulfonate is administered in the hospital.

Nursing Diagnoses and Outcomes

- Risk for Constipation related to adverse effects of drug therapy
  Desired outcome: *Constipation will be prevented by administering sorbitol, orally or rectally, if warranted.*
- Potential complication: hypokalemia.
  Desired outcome: *The patient's potassium level will be lowered only to the normal range.*

Planning and Intervention

Maximizing Therapeutic Effects

Clear the GI tract with a cleansing enema before administering the drug by enema. For adults, insert a soft, large (28-French) rubber tube about 20 cm into the rectum. Mix the resin in an aqueous vehicle, such as 100 mL sorbitol or 20% dextrose, to make a suspension; infuse the drug by gravity. During infusion, it is important to stir the fluid to keep the particles in suspension.

After the fluid has run into the patient, flush the tube with 50 to 100 mL of fluid to make a total of 150 to 200 mL of fluid as infused. It is important to clamp the tube and leave it in place for at least 30 to 60 minutes, preferably several hours (keeping the solution in the colon allows the resin to work; the longer the resin is in the colon, the more ion exchange can occur).

If back-leakage develops, elevate the patient's hips on pillows or have the patient assume a knee-chest position temporarily. These positions help keep the solution in the sigmoid colon.

Irrigate the colon using a Y-tube connection with approximately 2 L of a nonsodium flushing solution at body temperature to remove the resin. The Y-tube allows the returns to drain as the colon is being irrigated.

When the drug is administered orally, create a suspension of the powdered formula with water or syrup for greater palatability.

MEMORY CHIP

P Sodium Polystyrene Sulfonate

- Used to lower serum potassium levels
- Given orally or as enema
- Major contraindication: extremely high potassium levels
- Most common adverse effects: related to GI system
- Most serious adverse effect: hypokalemia
- Maximizing therapeutic effects: Give a cleansing enema first (if drug is given as enema), and leave resin in place at least 30 minutes after administering as enema.
- Minimizing adverse effects: Monitor serum electrolytes and electrocardiogram.

Minimizing Adverse Effects

If the potassium serum level is severely elevated, use other methods to reduce potassium. Sodium polystyrene sulfonate alone may be insufficient to correct an imbalance before a medical emergency occurs. Other methods include the use of IV calcium to antagonize the effect of hyperkalemia on the heart; IV sodium bicarbonate, glucose and insulin together to cause an intracellular shift of potassium (without causing hypoglycemia); the definitive treatment for severe hyperkalemia is dialysis.

Monitor serum electrolytes for changes in potassium and other electrolytes. It also is important to monitor the ECG for changes indicative of hypokalemia (lengthened QT interval; widening, flattening, or inversion of the T wave; prominent U waves; or arrhythmias).

Monitor the pulse rate for arrhythmias and irregularities. It is a good idea to administer sorbitol, orally or rectally, to prevent constipation if warranted.

Providing Patient and Family Education

- Explain the therapeutic and possible adverse effects of the drug.
- It is important to emphasize the importance of repeated blood work to monitor blood electrolyte concentrations.

Ongoing Assessment and Evaluation

Monitor serum electrolytes throughout therapy. Assess for signs of hypokalemia and monitor the patient's pulse and ECG periodically throughout sodium polystyrene sulfonate therapy. Therapy is considered effective in patients whose serum potassium levels return to normal and who do not develop cardiac arrhythmias from hyperkalemia, hypokalemia, or other electrolyte imbalances.

CHAPTER SUMMARY

- Antiarrhythmics restore normal rhythm and rate by varied mechanisms.
- All drugs given to treat an arrhythmia also may cause an arrhythmia.
- Class I drugs block the influx of sodium in the myocardial membrane. They are local anesthetics or membrane stabilizing agents that depress phase 0 of the action potential.

- Quinidine, a Class I antiarrhythmic, is used for treating atrial fibrillation and flutter. Quinidine depresses myocardial excitability, conduction velocity, and contractility. The effective refractory period is prolonged, increasing conduction time. Re-entry phenomenon is therefore prevented. Quinidine also exerts an indirect anticholinergic effect; it decreases vagal tone and may promote conduction in the AV junction.
- Potassium enhances the effect of quinidine, and hypokalemia reduces the effectiveness.
- Class IB antiarrhythmics depress phase 0 of the action potential, but not as much as Class IA drugs. They also suppress automaticity. Like quinidine, these drugs may also cause arrhythmias, in addition to treating them. Unlike quinidine, they are used primarily with ventricular arrhythmias, and they may shorten the action potential duration. Lidocaine is a Class IB drug; it may be used with all acute ventricular arrhythmias that occur in association with cardiac surgery or acute MI.
- Class IC antiarrhythmics also depress phase 0 but markedly so. In addition, they have a slight effect on repolarization and decrease conduction substantially. They have been found to increase mortality significantly when used in patients who have had an MI.
- All Class I antiarrhythmics have the potential to increase mortality; none have been proved to decrease mortality.
- Class II antiarrhythmics block the beta-1 and beta-2 adrenergic receptors and stabilize the cardiac cell membranes. They depress phase 4 depolarization.
- Propranolol, a beta blocker and Class II antiarrhythmic, is used to treat supraventricular, ventricular, and tachyarrhythmias secondary to digoxin toxicity or arising from excessive catecholamine action during anesthesia.
- Propranolol slows the sinus heart rate, depresses AV conduction, decreases cardiac output, reduces systolic and diastolic blood pressure at rest and on exercise, and reduces supine and standing blood pressure.
- Class II antiarrhythmics are the only antiarrhythmics that have been shown to decrease mortality.
- Class III drugs slow heart action by prolonging the action potential or myocardial repolarization (prolonged phase 3).
- Amiodarone, a Class III antiarrhythmic, is used to treat life-threatening ventricular arrhythmias. It also has actions from other classifications. These diverse actions of amiodarone are why the drug is being considered as potentially appropriate for treating atrial fibrillation as well.
- Amiodarone has unusual pharmacokinetic and pharmacodynamic properties. These unique effects include incomplete bioavailability, distribution to multiple tissue sites, extreme lipid solubility, biotransformation to an active metabolite, and extremely slow elimination of amiodarone and its metabolite. These effects may be attributable to genetic variations, although this possibility is not yet confirmed. Because of these unique effects, the effect on patients is variable.

- Adverse effects of amiodarone can be serious and potentially fatal. The patient needs to be monitored closely while on amiodarone therapy.
- Class IV drugs alter the action potential, decrease AV conduction, and prolong repolarization by inhibiting the influx of calcium in cardiac muscle cells. A few calcium channel blocker drugs are in this class.
- Verapamil, a calcium channel blocker and Class IV antiarrhythmic, controls ventricular rate in chronic atrial flutter or fibrillation (used in conjunction with digoxin). It is also used prophylactically for repetitive paroxysmal SVT. IV verapamil is used to treat SVT.
- Verapamil also is used in treating angina (including Prinzmetal angina) and hypertension.
- Sodium polystyrene sulfonate is a potassium-removing resin used in treating hyperkalemia. Because hyperkalemia may lead to cardiac arrhythmias, this drug prevents arrhythmias from occurring.
- Sodium polystyrene sulfonate is given orally or as an enema.
- Although sodium polystyrene sulfonate is in the GI tract, sodium ions are exchanged for potassium ions, which are then excreted in the stool. Onset is slow and unpredictable. Therefore, if the serum potassium level is quite elevated, other mechanisms of lowering the potassium level should be used.

QUESTIONS FOR STUDY AND REVIEW

1. Why are ventricular arrhythmias considered potentially life-threatening?
2. What is meant by proarrhythmia?
3. Why do all antiarrhythmics have proarrhythmic qualities?
4. Describe the phase of the action potential affected by Class I, Class II, Class III, and Class IV antiarrhythmics.
5. Amiodarone, a Class III drug, is used to treat which type of arrhythmias?
6. What changes in the ECG do you commonly see with amiodarone?
7. Why is a loading dose (or doses) necessary to administer when using the Class III drug amiodarone?
8. What suggestions can you give to a patient taking verapamil, a Class IV antiarrhythmic, to prevent constipation?

NEED MORE HELP?

Chapter 31 of the Study Guide to Accompany *Drug Therapy in Nursing*, 4th Edition, contains NCLEX-style questions and other learning activities to reinforce your understanding of the concepts presented in this chapter. For additional information or to purchase the study guide, visit thePoint.

REFERENCES

AFFIRM First Antiarrhythmic Drug Substudy Investigators. (2003). Maintenance of sinus rhythm in patients with atrial fibrillation: An AFFIRM substudy of the first antiarrhythmic drug. *Journal of the American College of Cardiology,* 42(1):20–29.

American Heart Association. Guidelines 2000 for cardiopulmonary resuscitation and emerging cardiovascular care. Part 6: advanced cardiovascular life support. *Circulation,* 8/2000:102, 112–165.

Bacaner, M., & Dembo, D. (2009). Arrhythmia and acute coronary syndrome suppression and cardiac resuscitation management with bretylium. *American Journal of Therapeutics,* 16(6): 534–542.

Blomstrom-Lundqvist, C., Scheinman, M. M., Aliot, E. M., et al., for the European Society of Cardiology Committee, NASPE-Heart Rhythm Society. (2003). ACC/AHA/ESC guidelines for the management of patients with supraventricular arrhythmias: Executive summary. A report of the American College of Cardiology/American Heart Association Task Force on Practice Guidelines and the European Society of Cardiology Committee for Practice Guidelines (writing committee to develop guidelines for the management of patients with supraventricular arrhythmias), developed in collaboration with NASPE-Heart Rhythm Society. *Journal of the American College of Cardiology,* 42(8):1493–1531.

Bollmann, A., Husser, D., & Cannom, D. S. (2005). Antiarrhythmic drugs in patients with implantable cardioverter-defibrillators. *American Journal of Cardiovascular Drugs,* 5(6):371–378.

Cheng, J. (2010). New and emerging antiarrhythmic and anticoagulant agents for atrial fibrillation. *American Journal of Health System Pharmacy,* 67(9):526–534.

Eisenberg, M. J., Brox, A., & Bestawros, A. N. (2004). Calcium channel blockers: An update. *American Journal of Medicine,* 116(1):35–43.

Fang, M. C., Stafford, R. S., Ruskin, J. N., et al. (2004). National trends in antiarrhythmic and antithrombotic medication use in atrial fibrillation. *Archives of Internal Medicine,* 164(1): 55–60.

Fuster, V., Ryden, L. E., Cannom, D. S., et al., American College of Cardiology/American Heart Association/European Society of Cardiology Board. (2006). ACC/AHA/ESC 2006 guidelines for the management of patients with atrial fibrillation: A report of the American College of Cardiology/American Heart Association Task Force on Practice Guidelines and the European Society of Cardiology Committee for Practice Guidelines (writing committee to revise the 2001 guidelines for the management of patients with atrial fibrillation), developed in collaboration with the European Heart Rhythm Association and the Heart Rhythm Society. *Journal of the American College of Cardiology,* 48(4):e149–e246.

Khan, M. H. (2004). Oral class III antiarrhythmics: What is new? *Current Opinion in Cardiology,* 19(1):47–51.

Komatsu, T., Tachibana, H., Sato, Y., et al. (2007). Efficacy of amiodarone for preventing the recurrence of symptomatic paroxysmal and persistent atrial fibrillation after cardioversion. *Circulation Journal: Official Journal of the Japanese Circulation Society,* 71(1):46–51.

Olshansky, B., Rosenfeld, L. E., Warner, A. L., et al. (2004). The Atrial Fibrillation Follow-up Investigation of Rhythm Management (AFFIRM) study: Approaches to control rate in atrial fibrillation. *Journal of the American College of Cardiology,* 43(7):1201–1208.

Prasun, M. A., & Kocheril, A. G. (2003). Treating atrial fibrillation: Rhythm control or rate control. *Journal of Cardiovascular Nursing,* 18(5):369–373.

Roukoz, H., & Saliba, W. (2007). Dofetilide: A new class III antiarrhythmic agent. *Expert Review of Cardiovascular Therapy,* 5(1):9–19.

Schneider, M. P., Hua, T. A., Böhm, M., Wachtell, K., Kjeldsen, S. E., Schmieder, R. E. Prevention of Atrial Fibrillation By Renin-Angiotensin System Inhibition A Meta-Analysis. (2010). *Journal of American College of Cardiology,* 55(21):2299–2307.

UpToDate. (2007). Control of ventricular rate in atrial fibrillation: Pharmacologic therapy. Retrieved from *www.uptodate.com.*

Van Gelder, I. C., Hagens, V. E., Bosker, H. A., et al. (2002). A comparison of rate control and rhythm control in patients with recurrent persistent atrial fibrillation. *New England Journal of Medicine,* 347(23):1834–1840.

VerNooy, R. A., & Mounsey, J. P. (2004). Antiarrhythmic drug therapy of atrial fibrillation. *Cardiology Clinics,* 22(1):21–34.

Wyse, D. G., Waldo, A. L., DiMarco, J. P., et al., Atrial Fibrillation Follow-up Investigation of Rhythm Management (AFFIRM) Investigators. (2002). A comparison of rate control and rhythm control in patients with atrial fibrillation. *New England Journal of Medicine,* 347(23):1825–1833.

Drugs Affecting Coagulation

Learning Objectives

At the completion of this chapter the student will:

1. Identify core drug knowledge about drugs affecting coagulation.
2. Differentiate between the anticoagulants heparin and warfarin.
3. Understand the differences between anticoagulants and thrombolytics.
4. Differentiate antiplatelet drugs from hemorrheologic drugs.
5. Differentiate clotting factors from hemostatic agents.
6. Identify core patient variables relevant to drugs affecting coagulation.
7. Relate the interaction of core drug knowledge to core patient variables for drugs affecting coagulation.
8. Generate a nursing plan of care from the interactions between core drug knowledge and core patient variables for drugs affecting coagulation.
9. Describe nursing interventions to maximize therapeutic and minimize adverse effects for drugs affecting coagulation.
10. Determine key points for patient and family education for drugs affecting coagulation.

Key Terms			
anticoagulants	fibrin	plasmin
clotting cascade	fibrinolysis	platelets
clotting factors	hemophilia	thrombin
coagulation	hemostasis	thromboembolus
embolus	International Normalized Ratio (INR)	thrombus

Drugs Affecting Coagulation

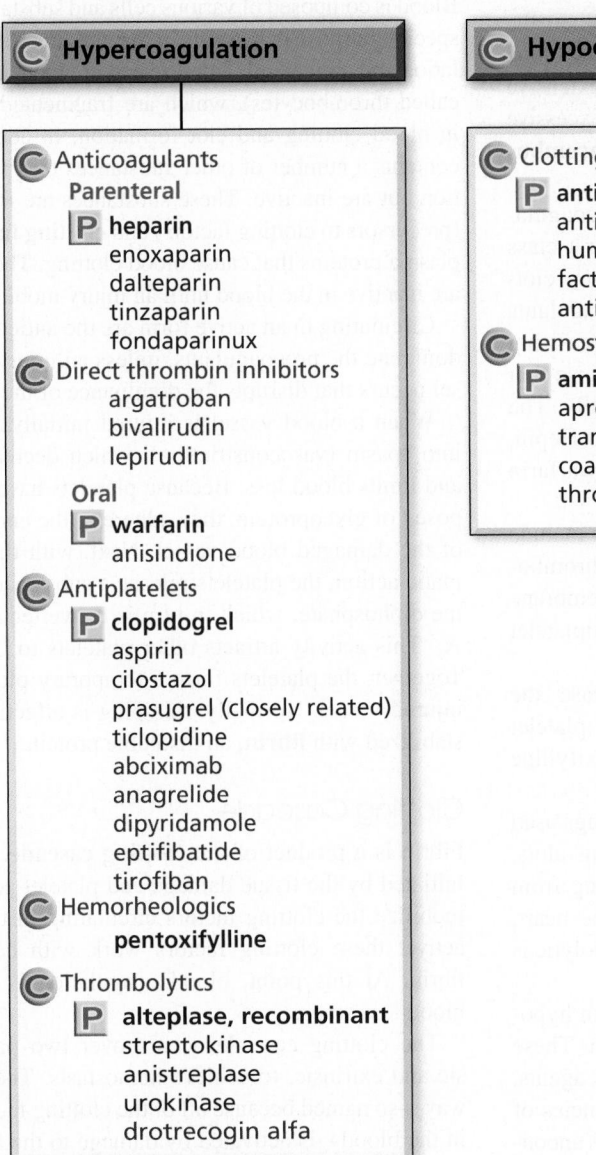

Hypercoagulation

Hypocoagulation

Anticoagulants
Parenteral
- **heparin**
- enoxaparin
- dalteparin
- tinzaparin
- fondaparinux

Direct thrombin inhibitors
- argatroban
- bivalirudin
- lepirudin

Oral
- **warfarin**
- anisindione

Antiplatelets
- **clopidogrel**
- aspirin
- cilostazol
- prasugrel (closely related)
- ticlopidine
- abciximab
- anagrelide
- dipyridamole
- eptifibatide
- tirofiban

Hemorheologics
pentoxifylline

Thrombolytics
- **alteplase, recombinant**
- streptokinase
- anistreplase
- urokinase
- drotrecogin alfa

Clotting factors
- **antihemophilic factor**
- anti-inhibitor coagulant complex
- human factor IX complex
- factor IX, recombinant
- anti-inhibitor coagulant factor

Hemostatics
- **aminocaproic acid**
- aprotinin
- tranexamic acid
- coagulation factor VIIa
- thrombin

The symbol **C** indicates the drug class.
Drugs in **bold type** marked with the symbol **P** are prototypes.
Drugs in blue type are closely related to the prototype.
Drugs in red type are significantly different from the prototype.
Drugs in black type with no symbol are also used in drug therapy; no prototype.

This chapter examines drugs used to treat **coagulation** (blood aggregation, or clotting) disorders. Disturbances in the coagulation balance cause abnormalities in the body's ability to transport blood through the vessels to the cells or to form blood clots. Pathophysiologic effects may result from an excess of or a deficit in coagulation factors. When the body begins bleeding, a series of events occurs to slow blood flow, stop blood loss at the injury site, and prevent extensive blood loss. This process is known as **hemostasis.** Excessive coagulation, or hypercoagulation, will result in a **thrombus** (blood clot).

Several drug classes that are used to treat hypercoagulation disorders are discussed in this chapter. The first class is **anticoagulants** (substances that keep blood from clotting). Existing naturally and in drug form, anticoagulants prevent thrombus formation and the extension of existing thrombi. There are two types of anticoagulants—those that are given parenterally and those that are given orally. The prototype parenteral anticoagulant is heparin (Lipo-Hepin, Hep-Lock). The prototype oral anticoagulant is warfarin (Coumadin).

Other drug classes used to treat hypercoagulability include the antiplatelet agents, the hemorheologics, and the thrombolytics. Antiplatelet agents interfere with platelet membrane function and platelet aggregation. The prototype antiplatelet is clopidogrel (Plavix).

Hemorheologics reduce blood viscosity, increase the flexibility of red blood cells (RBCs), and decrease platelet aggregation. The prototype hemorheologic is pentoxifylline (Trental).

Thrombolytics, unlike anticoagulants and other drugs used to treat hypercoagulation, actually dissolve existing clots. They are used to treat medical emergencies resulting from thrombus formations' blocking of blood flow to the heart, lung, or deep veins of the legs. The prototype thrombolytic is alteplase, recombinant (Activase).

This chapter also describes drug classes used when hypocoagulation, or subnormal coagulation, is a problem. These drug classes include clotting factors and hemostatic agents. Clotting factors are replacements for genetic deficiencies of normal clotting factors, which lead to **hemophilia** (uncontrollable bleeding). The prototype drug is antihemophilic factor (AHF, factor VIII). Hemostatics inhibit **fibrinolysis,** the process of breaking down a formed clot. They are either systemic or topical. The prototype systemic hemostatic drug is aminocaproic acid (Amicar). Topical hemostatics are used to control minor bleeding, usually after surgery. The various agents work differently. No prototype is identifiable for topical hemostatics.

PHYSIOLOGY OF COAGULATION

Normal circulation requires blood to circulate freely through large and small blood vessels. However, blood must also be able to form clots to prevent excessive blood loss from injuries. To perform both of these functions requires the body's ability to balance coagulation and anticoagulation.

Blood Components and Balanced Blood Flow

Blood is composed of various cells and substances, each with a specific purpose that assists in maintaining a balance of coagulation and anticoagulation. Present in blood are **platelets** (also called thrombocytes), which are fragmented cells that assist in blood clotting and clot formation. In addition, the blood contains a number of other substances that promote coagulation but are inactive. These substances are the procoagulants (precursors to clotting factors) and **clotting factors,** which are plasma proteins that cause blood clotting. The clotting factors are inactive in the blood until an injury mobilizes them.

Circulating in an active form are the anticoagulants, which dominate the procoagulants, unless an injury to a blood vessel occurs that disrupts the dominance of the anticoagulants.

When a blood vessel is injured initially, the vessel goes into spasm (vasoconstriction), which decreases blood flow and limits blood loss. Because platelets have a surface composed of glycoprotein, they adhere to the endothelial surface of the damaged blood vessel. Next, with the help of enzymatic action, the platelets release a substance called adenosine diphosphate, which in turn is converted to thromboxane A_2. This activity attracts other platelets to the damage site. Together, the platelets form a temporary plug that seals the injured vessel. Normally, this plug is effective because it is stabilized with **fibrin,** an insoluble protein.

Clotting Cascade

Fibrin is a product of the **clotting cascade.** The cascade is initiated by the tissue damage and platelet activation, which mobilize the clotting factors circulating in the blood. Once active, these clotting factors work with calcium to form fibrin. At this point, blood coagulation is completed and blood loss stops.

The clotting cascade occurs over two pathways, intrinsic and extrinsic, to achieve hemostasis. The intrinsic pathway—so named because all of the clotting factors are present in the blood—is activated by damage to the blood vessel. In the extrinsic pathway, the clotting factors are activated by the damaged tissue. One or both pathways may be activated in response to injury. Figure 32.1 depicts the intrinsic and extrinsic pathways in the clotting cascade.

Intrinsic Pathway

Activity in the intrinsic pathway begins with an enzyme reaction that modifies factor XII from its inactive to active form. In turn, factor XII helps modify factor XI so that it can activate factor IX. Factor IX acts on factor VIII, and factor VIII activates factor X. Activated factor X affects factor V and promotes the conversion of prothrombin (factor II) to **thrombin.** Thrombin in turn converts factor I (fibrinogen) to fibrin. Thrombin also activates factor XIII, a fibrin-stabilizing factor. The fibrin threads that are produced trap the clotting

P H Y S I O L O G Y

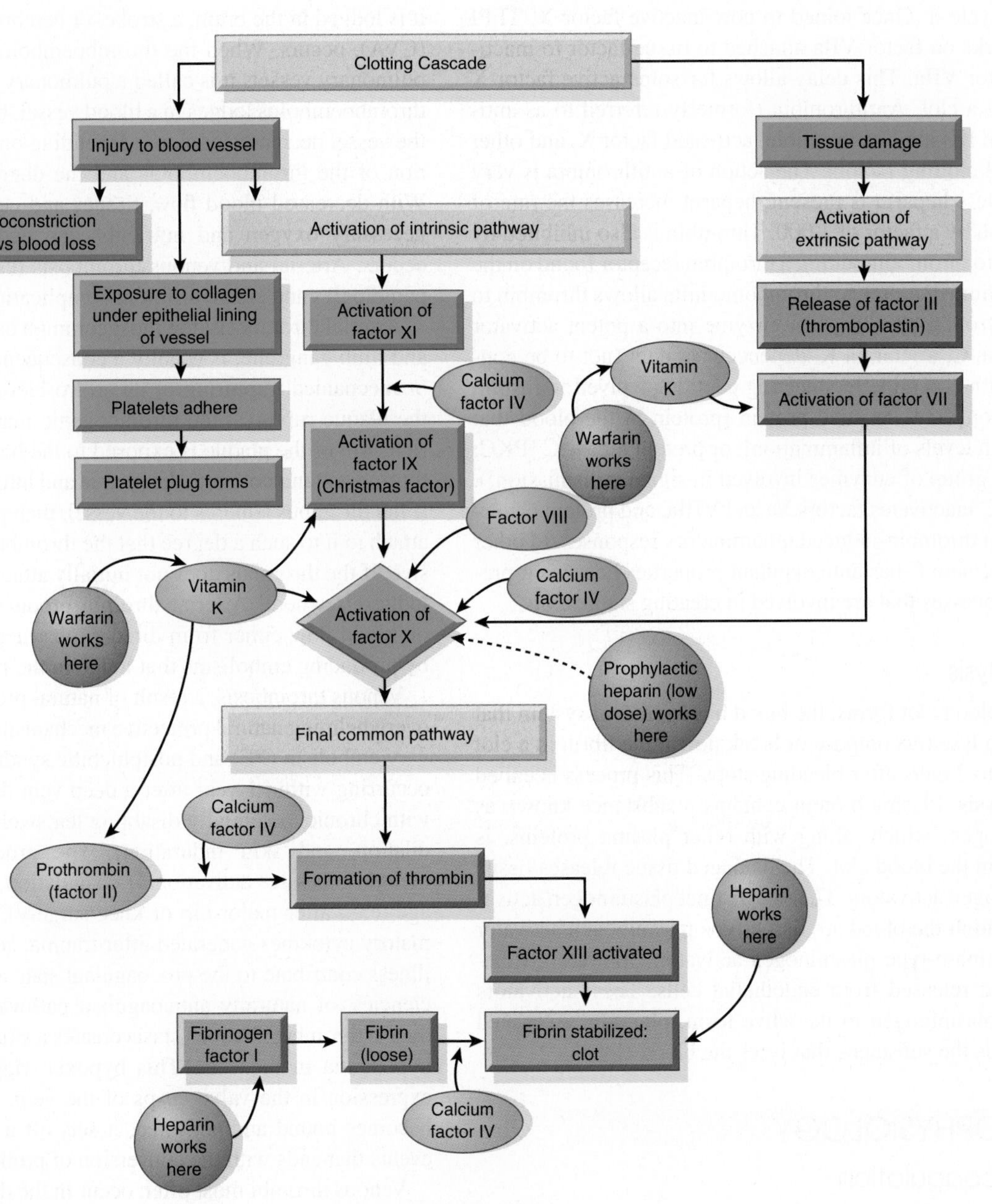

• FIGURE 32.1 Events in the clotting cascade.

factors that remain in the injured area, preventing the extension of the blood clot beyond the injury. The cascade thus ends in the formation of a stable blood clot.

Extrinsic Pathway

Activity in the extrinsic pathway begins with the activation of factor III, followed by the activation of factor VII. Tissue factor is a cellular receptor for this activated factor, or factor VIIa. The initiation of a clot in arteries or veins is triggered by tissue factor; factor VIIa has little or no enzymatic activity until it is bound to tissue factor. Factor VIIa then activates

factor X. The remaining steps in the extrinsic pathway follow those of the intrinsic pathway and are referred to as the final common pathway. The prevention of clot extension, which occurs at the end of the clotting cascade, is assisted by the release of heparin. Heparin, a naturally occurring anticoagulant normally found in small amounts in the blood, is released from mast cells at the time of the initial injury.

Coagulation Inhibitors

The key inhibitors of coagulation are tissue factor pathway inhibitor (TFPI), antithrombin, and the protein C pathway.

TFPI inhibits the complex made from tissue factor and clotting factor VIIa. TFPI first joins with activated factor X to inactivate it. Once joined to now-inactive factor X, TFPI then works on factor VIIa attached to tissue factor to inactivate factor VIIa. This delay allows for some active factor X to create a clot. Antithrombin (formerly referred to as antithrombin III) inhibits thrombin, activated factor X, and other activated clotting factors. The action of antithrombin is very slow unless heparin is present; heparin increases the rate of inhibition by a factor of 1,000. Thrombin is also inhibited by binding to thrombomodulin, a thrombin receptor found on the endothelium. Binding to thrombomodulin allows thrombin to change from a procoagulant enzyme into a potent activator of protein C, a vitamin K–dependent protein (not to be confused with c-peptide [connecting peptide involved in insulin production] or C-reactive protein [protein in the blood that rises with levels of inflammation], or protein kinase C [PKC: one of a group of enzymes involved in signal transmission]). Protein C inactivates factors Va and VIIIa, and protein C may also limit thrombin-induced inflammatory responses. In other words, protein C has anticoagulant properties because it prevents processes that are involved in creating stable clots.

Hemolysis

After a blood clot forms, the blood has a removal system that begins to lyse (decompose or break down) the fibrin in a clot about 1 to 2 days after bleeding stops. This process is called **fibrinolysis.** Plasma protein contains a substance known as plasminogen, which, along with other plasma proteins, is trapped in the blood clot. The damaged tissue releases tissue plasminogen activators. The two distinct plasminogen activators found in the blood are tissue-type plasminogen activator and urokinase-type plasminogen activator. Both are synthesized and released from endothelial cells. These activators change plasminogen to its active form, **plasmin.** Activated plasmin is the substance that lyses the blood clot.

PATHOPHYSIOLOGY

Hypercoagulation

When blood flow is impeded and slowed in an area, coagulation occurs, leading to formation of a thrombus. Any excessive action from the coagulating factors may also produce a thrombus that obstructs blood flow. A thrombus can form anywhere in the cardiovascular system. The components of a thrombus vary, depending on whether the thrombus is arterial (formed under high flow conditions) or venous (formed from stasis). Arterial thrombi consist mostly of platelet aggregates held together with thin fibrin strands, whereas venous thrombi are mostly red cells, a large amount of fibrin, and only a few platelets. An **embolism (embolus)** is any undissolved matter carried in a blood or lymph vessel to another location where it lodges and occludes the vessel. When a portion of a thrombus breaks off, the fragment may travel through the bloodstream and lodge in a vessel (**thromboembolus**), again

occluding blood flow. When the thromboembolus is lodged in a coronary vessel, a myocardial infarction (MI) occurs. When it is lodged in the brain, a stroke, or cerebrovascular accident (CVA), occurs. When the thromboembolus is lodged in the pulmonary vessels it is called a pulmonary **embolus.** When a thromboembolus lodges in a blood vessel, blood flow through the vessel decreases or stops, depending on the size and position of the thromboembolus and the degree of obstruction. With decreased blood flow, tissues and cells do not receive necessary oxygen and nutrients, and necrosis (cell death) occurs. Arterial and venous thrombosis result from different pathologies and create different complications for the patient.

Arterial thrombosis, the most common cause of MI, stroke, and limb gangrene, is usually a consequence of spontaneous or mechanical rupturing of an arthrosclerotic plaque. When the plaque ruptures, the thrombogenic material in the lipid-rich core of the plaque is exposed to the blood. The resulting thrombi extend both into the plaque and into the vessel lumen. If the thrombus adheres to the vessel, then platelets and fibrin attach to it to such a degree that the thrombus becomes occlusive. If the thrombus does not initially attach, it may float and lodge elsewhere. Arterial thrombi produce negative effects on blood flow either from directly obstructing blood flow or by producing embolisms that lodge in the microcirculation.

Venous thrombosis, a result of natural procoagulant stimuli overwhelming natural protective mechanisms, leads to pulmonary embolism (PE) and postphlebitic syndrome (a syndrome occurring within 1 year after a deep vein thrombosis [DVT], with chronic, potentially disabling leg swelling, pain, venous dilation, and skin induration). The procoagulant stimuli include excessive activation of coagulation, vessel wall damage (e.g., after major hip or knee surgery), or stasis. Inflammatory cytokines generated after trauma, surgery, or medical illness contribute to the procoagulant state and inherited deficiencies, of naturally anticoagulant pathways may also produce a thrombus. Venous stasis creates a situation of localized hypoxemia in the vein. This hypoxia triggers tissue factor expression in the valve cusps of the vein. Once factor VIIa becomes bound and activated, it sets off a series of clotting events that ends with the conversion of prothrombin to fibrin.

Venous thrombi most often occur in the deep vessels of the lower limbs (referred to as deep vein thrombosis, or DVT) and produce serious effects from inflaming the vessel wall, from direct obstruction of blood flow, or through pulmonary embolism. DVT may be secondary to surgery or trauma (as previously stated), as well as malignancy, hereditary thrombotic disorders, stroke, spinal cord injury, or unexplained causes. Trauma to the vein can result from central venous catheters; this can cause DVT of an upper extremity.

A relationship between cancer and thrombosis has been identified. The exact mechanism of the relationship between cancer and thrombosis is not known. It is known that cancer patients have an increased risk of developing thrombosis (this is possibly related to chemotherapy). The opposite is also true, in that patients who present with thromboembolism of unknown causes have a higher risk for developing cancer. It has been hypothesized that early presymptomatic cancer may be present in these people and may be producing hypercoagulability. It is also possible that because the patient hospitalized with a blood clot has many tests performed to determine the cause of the clot that the cancer is found serendipitously during this screening. At this time, no extensive screening is recommended to detect cancer in patients with thrombosis. Routine accepted tests for cancer screening (such as Pap smears, mammography, and prostate screening) may be done at the time of hospitalization if they have not been done recently.

Acute coronary syndromes are also related to thrombus. Acute coronary syndromes include unstable angina, non–ST-elevation MI, and ST-elevation MI. All of these conditions have an underlying pathology of unstable coronary plaque on a coronary vessel, with an overlying intracoronary thrombus. Thrombus formation can also be a problem in atrial fibrillation. In this condition, the blood is not moving, which may lead to coagulation of the blood into clots.

Some conditions of hypercoagulability result from increased platelet activity. Constriction of, or fatty deposits in, a blood vessel narrows its lumen, leading to decreased or slowed blood flow through the vessel. The decreased flow causes stasis, which results in blood coagulation. Platelet activity is responsible for the formation of the blood clot. This is a particular problem for patients with chronic, obstructive vascular disease because blood clots further impair or entirely block an already diminished blood flow, thereby posing a risk for tissue death from lack of oxygen and nutrients.

In peripheral vascular disease, the blood vessels in the extremities, particularly the legs, are narrowed. This narrowing prevents the flow of oxygenated blood to the tissues. Lack of oxygenation causes pain, especially with use of the extremity. This condition is known as intermittent claudication. Rest relieves the pain because it decreases the oxygen needed by the tissue. With the impaired circulation, venous stasis occurs, which in turn leads to platelet aggregation and thrombus formation. This thrombus further impairs circulation through the vessel to the tissue.

Hypocoagulation

When clotting factors are deficient, blood clotting does not occur in a timely manner. A minor injury or trauma can cause prolonged bleeding, or hemorrhage, either internally or externally. Bleeding may occur into a joint, such as the elbow or knee, and cause serious damage.

Inherited deficiencies of specific clotting factors produce three major hemophilic conditions: hemophilia A (classic hemophilia), hemophilia B (Christmas disease), and von Willebrand disease. Hemophilia A results from lack of factor VIII. Hemophilia B results from lack of factor IX. Hemophilias A and B are transmitted on recessive, sex-linked genes. The genes are carried by women and transmitted to male children. von Willebrand disease results from deficiency of factor VIII, factor VIII antigen, and von Willebrand factor. It is transmitted by an autosomal dominant gene and inherited by both sexes.

Decreased synthesis of clotting factors is characteristic of diseases that affect the liver, such as cirrhosis and hepatitis, because most clotting factors are produced in the liver. A second cause of decreased synthesis is an absence of vitamin K, which is necessary for the formation of four of the clotting factors: II (prothrombin), VII, IX, and X.

Fibrinolysis normally occurs in balance with blood coagulation. A clot forms to prevent extensive blood loss. When the vessel heals, the clot is broken down (fibrinolysis) by activating plasminogen so that it becomes plasmin. Plasmin breaks down fibrin, fibrinogen, and other plasma proteins. When fibrinolysis is not in balance with the other phases of coagulation (i.e., an excess of plasmin exists), excessive bleeding occurs because the body cannot form a stable clot in response to injury.

DRUG THERAPY FOR HYPERCOAGULATION

In general, disorders of hypercoagulability result from either an increase in platelets or an increase in the activity of the clotting system, or combinations of both. Treatment is aimed at interfering with the clotting cascade. The desired goals of drug therapy are to lengthen the time necessary for blood to clot, to alter platelet aggregation preventing clotting, or both. Anticoagulant drug therapy is used to prevent new clots from forming, to avoid extension of the thrombus, or to deter a thromboembolus. Antiplatelet therapy decreases the ability of platelets to stick together. Therapy to block platelet function is used primarily for arterial thrombi, because these clots consist of platelet aggregates held together by small amounts of fibrin; however, treatment often also includes some anticoagulant drugs to prevent deposits of fibrin. Anticoagulant therapy is the preferred choice for treatment or prevention of venous thrombi, which are mostly composed of fibrin.

When an existing clot may be fatal to the patient because of blocked blood flow to vital organs, thrombolytic agents are used to break it up. When the clot or obstruction blocks a coronary artery, the heart is affected; damage to the heart from an MI can be permanent or fatal. When the clot blocks the pulmonary artery, the blood supply to the lungs is altered; this alteration in turn decreases the oxygenation of blood to be circulated. This is a life-threatening condition. If the clot is in the brain, ischemia of the tissue results in brain cell death with loss of brain function and permanent neurologic deficits or disabilities in the patient. If the injury is severe or an extensive portion of the brain is affected, death can result. Because brain cells are highly dependent on sufficient oxygen for survival, rapid treatment to break apart a thrombus and relieve hypoxia is crucial. When the thrombus is large and blocks the great veins in the legs, circulation is impaired in the limb. If the circulatory impairment is severe enough, the patient may risk losing the limb as a result of tissue death. This event also is considered a medical emergency. Thrombolytic agents are indicated in these emergency situations to prevent severe damage to the body or death.

TABLE 32.1	Summary of Selected Drugs for Hypercoagulability		
Drug (Trade) Name	**Selected Indications**	**Route and Dosage Range**	**Pharmacokinetics**
P heparin	Anticoagulation	*Adult:* IV, 5,000 U bolus (or 35–70 U/kg) followed by 20,000–40,000 U/24 h or 15–25 U/kg/h *Child:* IV, 50 U/kg bolus, followed by 100 U/kg/4 h or 20,000 U/m2/24 h	*Onset:* Immediate *Duration:* 2–6 h $t_{1/2}$: 30–180 min *Onset:* 20–60 min *Duration:* 8–12 h
	Prophylaxis	*Adult:* SC, 5,000 U q8–12h	
enoxaparin (Lovenox)	Prophylaxis	*Adult:* SC, 30 mg, bid or 40 mg/d	*Onset:* 20–60 min *Duration:* 12 h $t_{1/2}$: 4.5 h
P warfarin (Coumadin)	Prophylaxis and treatment	*Adult:* PO, 5–10 mg/d for 2–4 d, then adjust according to results of PT or INR values	*Onset:* 24 h *Duration:* 2–5 d $t_{1/2}$: 1–2.5 d
P clopidogrel (Plavix)	Reduction of atherosclerotic events	*Adult:* PO, 75 mg/d	*Onset:* Rapid *Duration:* Unknown $t_{1/2}$: 8 h
aspirin (Bayer)	Prophylaxis for MI Decrease risk of TIA in men	*Adult:* PO, 300–325 mg/d *Adult:* PO, 1,300 mg/d divided into two to four doses	*Onset:* 5–30 min *Duration:* Varies $t_{1/2}$: 15–20 min
P pentoxifylline (Trental)	Intermittent claudication	*Adult:* PO, 400 mg tid	*Onset:* Rapid *Duration:* Unknown $t_{1/2}$: 0.4–0.8 h
P alteplase, recombinant (Activase)	Acute MI	*Adult* (>67 kg): 100 mg total: 15 mg bolus, 50 mg infusion over 30 min, then 35 mg infusion over 60 min	*Onset:* Rapid *Duration:* Unknown $t_{1/2}$: Unknown
	Acute ischemic stroke	*Adult:* IV, 0.9 mg/kg (max 90 mg) 10% given as bolus over 1 min, 90% infused over 60 min	
	Pulmonary embolism (PE)	*Adult:* IV, 100 mg infusion over 2 h	

When the patient has a less urgent need for therapy, has a high risk of developing arterial thrombi, or requires additional treatment after the use of thrombolytic drugs, antiplatelet drugs are used. Antiplatelets decrease clumping or aggregating of platelets. Platelet aggregation is also affected by hemorheologic drugs. In addition, the hemorheologics increase the flexibility of RBCs and decrease the blood viscosity.

Table 32.1 presents a summary of selected drugs used to treat hypercoagulability.

ⓒ ANTICOAGULANT DRUGS

Heparin, a naturally occurring anticoagulant, is produced by mast cells located in connective tissue throughout the body. The blood cells known as basophils produce a small amount as well. The areas that produce the largest amount of heparin are the lungs and, to a lesser degree, the liver. This fact reflects a natural protective mechanism of the body because these two areas receive the smallest emboli.

All anticoagulants interfere with the clotting cascade and prolong blood clotting time. They vary by their route and their method of action. There are two types of anticoagulants: those that can be administered only parenterally and those that can be administered only orally. The parenteral anticoagulants work by preventing the conversion of fibrinogen to fibrin. The oral anticoagulants work by preventing the synthesis of factors dependent on vitamin K for synthesis: factors II (prothrombin), VII, VIII, IX, and X. Two different laboratory tests, one for drugs administered orally and one for those administered parenterally, are therefore used to measure the therapeutic effects of these anticoagulants.

The prototype parenteral anticoagulant is heparin, which is unfractionated (containing both low-molecular and high-molecular weights). Most heparin is available as generic heparin sodium; lower concentrations may be labeled heparin lock flush.

Nursing Management of the Patient Receiving **P** Heparin

Core Drug Knowledge

Pharmacotherapeutics

Heparin is the prototype parenteral anticoagulant. It interferes with the final steps of the clotting cascade. It is used to prevent the extension of a blood clot, particularly in patients with DVT or PE. It is also used prophylactically in patients with short-term increased risk of thrombus formation, such as in the postoperative period after a total hip replacement. When used for treating disseminated intravascular coagulation (DIC), heparin prevents further clotting in the microcirculation, leaving the procoagulants available to work at other sites in the body. In addition, heparin is also used to maintain the patency of venous access devices. It has several off-label uses: in the treatment of acute coronary syndrome or acute MI and with peritoneal dialysis

The heparin dosage is tailored to the patient and the severity of the condition. Continuous intravenous (IV) infusion of heparin is used to achieve full anticoagulation. In adults, a heparin IV drip is usually started by giving an IV bolus of the drug, followed by continuous infusion. Standardized heparin administration protocols are frequently used to prevent medication error and to improve achieving full therapeutic response. These protocols may be based on a standard therapy of units per hour or patient weight. The weight-based nomograms have been found to achieve a therapeutic range more rapidly than methods of estimating the appropriate dose using clinical experience alone or any dose-based protocol. Other methods to achieve the full anticoagulating effects from heparin include intermittent IV boluses or subcutaneous injections of heparin, although these methods are not frequently used today. In adults, subcutaneous administration of heparin may also prevent thromboembolic events. Recently, the potency of U.S. heparin solutions was decreased 10% to match international standards. This decrease should not significantly alter the dose needed for most patients to receive the therapeutic effect; dosing recommendations on the label have not been modified. The FDA does not recommend that practitioners routinely adjust the dose initially prescribed for all patients based on this change in potency. Dosing as always is individually titrated to achieve the therapeutic effect as measured by blood tests (FDA, 2009).

The duration of anticoagulation therapy for venous thromboembolism is based on the patient's risk of thrombosis if anticoagulation is stopped, as well as the patient's risk of bleeding if drug therapy is continued. Risk of recurrent thrombosis is considered low if it was precipitated by a reversible factor, such as surgery (because the surgery and the postoperative period are past, so that risk is no longer present). Risk of recurrence is high if the thromboembolism occurred with no apparent risk factors, or if the patient has persistent risk factors (e.g., cancer). Patients at low risk of recurrence should receive anticoagulation therapy for 3 months. Those at higher risk should receive anticoagulation therapy for 6 months to indefinitely, depending on the patient's variables. Initially, treatment involves heparin for at least 5 days but then continues with the oral anticoagulant warfarin.

Pharmacokinetics

Heparin is not absorbed from the gastrointestinal (GI) tract because it is destroyed by gastric acid; hence, it must be administered parenterally. When administered intravenously, heparin has an immediate onset of action. When administered subcutaneously, its onset of action is 20 to 60 minutes. After administration, the drug is widely distributed in the body, although it does not cross the placenta, and it is not found in breast milk. Heparin metabolism occurs in the liver, where it is inactivated. It is eliminated from the body in the urine.

Pharmacodynamics

Heparin, along with antithrombin, rapidly promotes the inactivation of factor X, which, in turn, prevents the conversion of prothrombin to thrombin. Heparin also has an effect on fibrin, limiting the formation of a stable clot. In blood tests measuring activated partial thromboplastin time (aPTT or APTT), heparin prolongs the clotting time. Low-dose heparin therapy, which is prophylactic dosing, deactivates factor X but has minimal effect on already produced thrombin; thus, it does not normally alter aPTT levels. However, full anticoagulation effects can occur in some individuals. Heparin has no effect on blood clots that have already formed. Therapeutic doses of heparin release TFPI that was bound to the endothelial wall surface. It is not certain whether released TFPI contributes to the anticoagulant properties of heparin (Weitz, Hirsh, & Samama, 2008). A less important action of heparin is that it binds directly to platelets.

Contraindications and Precautions

Heparin is contraindicated in patients who are hypersensitive to beef or pork because some heparin products are derived from the intestinal mucosa of pigs and others from beef lung. Heparin is also contraindicated in patients with thrombocytopenia, bleeding disorders, and active bleeding other than DIC.

This drug should be used with caution in patients with the potential for hemorrhage (e.g., immediately after surgery, with peptic ulcer disease and liver disease).

Adverse Effects

The most common adverse effect of heparin is bleeding. Although heparin-induced thrombocytopenia (HIT) occurs rarely, it is potentially life threatening. Treatment for HIT is discussed under the section Minimizing Adverse Effects below. Other adverse effects of heparin, although uncommon, include hepatitis, rashes, urticaria, hypersensitivity, and fever. In addition, treatment with heparin for more than 6 months may lead to the development of osteoporosis; this is related to bone demineralization.

If a patient receives an overdose of heparin or shows signs of bleeding, then protamine sulfate, the antagonist for heparin, may be administered. Protamine sulfate, a strong base, reacts with heparin, a strong acid, to form a stable salt, thereby neutralizing the anticoagulant effects of heparin. The protamine sulfate dose is based on the heparin dose: 1 mg of protamine sulfate per 100 units of heparin, or 0.5 mg of protamine sulfate per 100 units of heparin if the heparin was administered more than 30 minutes before the protamine sulfate. No more than 100 mg of protamine sulfate should be given within a 2-hour period, because this drug can cause anticoagulation in its own right. Administering protamine sulfate too rapidly may result in hypotension, bradycardia, dyspnea, and anaphylaxis. Hypersensitivity reactions may occur in some patients because of the fish base of protamine sulfate. Symptoms include flushing and feelings of warmth.

If the patient is not actively bleeding after heparin overdosage, the patient is usually monitored closely, and the protamine sulfate is not administered because heparin has a short half-life. The patient will recover from the overdosage without the added risk of complications from the protamine sulfate.

Drug Interactions

Several different drugs affect the action of heparin. Table 32.2 identifies these drugs and the significance of the reactions.

Assessment of Relevant Core Patient Variables

Health Status

Before administering the first dose of heparin, review the patient's record for evidence of allergy or a pre-existing prolonged bleeding time that would contraindicate administering heparin. A baseline aPTT and platelet count should be obtained. Assess the patient's renal function, because if the creatinine clearance is less than 25 mL/min, heparin is preferred over low-molecular-weight heparins for treatment of venous thrombosis.

Life Span and Gender

Be aware that heparin is safe for pregnant women, although it places other patients at risk for injury, particularly those who are confused, cognitively impaired, unable to modify behavior to prevent injuries, or incapable of complying with requests to modify behavior.

Lifestyle, Diet, and Habits

Because heparin prolongs both internal and external bleeding, slight injuries may potentially cause serious adverse effects. Ask patients about their activity level. Patients who normally engage in active behaviors in which bumping or body injuries frequently occur are more at risk for injury when receiving subcutaneous heparin therapy at home. Assess hospitalized patients for falls; consider such factors as a recent history of falls, impaired mobility, and other known risk factors.

Environment

Be aware of the environment in which the drug will be administered. Heparin is normally administered in an acute care setting.

Nursing Diagnoses and Outcomes

• Risk for Injury, Hemorrhage, related to heparin therapy
Desired outcome: Hemorrhage will not occur.
• Risk for Injury, Heparin-induced thrombocytopenia, related to heparin therapy
Desired outcome: Heparin-induced thrombocytopenia will not occur.

Planning and Intervention

Maximizing Therapeutic Effects

Monitor laboratory values (e.g., the aPTT) to confirm that a therapeutic lengthening of the clotting time has been achieved. The therapeutic lengthening of the clotting time is generally measured as one and one half to two times the control aPTT. Because control times vary from laboratory to laboratory, depending on the test equipment used, the difference between the two times is used to measure effectiveness. To determine the therapeutic range, multiply the control by 1.5 and then by 2; the therapeutic range is between these two products. For example, if the aPTT control time is 30 seconds, a therapeutic level for the patient would be 45 to 60 seconds (30 × 1.5 = 45; 30 × 2 = 60). If the laboratory uses a

TABLE 32.2	Agents That Interact with P Heparin	
Interactants	**Effect and Significance**	**Nursing Management**
cephalosporins	Additive effect with heparin is possible, which increases risk of bleeding.	Monitor for signs of bleeding. Monitor activated partial thromboplastin time carefully. Use drug cautiously when it is required.
nitroglycerin	Information is conflicting, but effect of heparin may be increased, increasing risk of bleeding.	Same as above.
penicillins	Parenteral administration can alter platelet aggregation and coagulation test findings. They may have additive effect with heparin to increase the risk of bleeding.	Same as above.
salicylate	Antiplatelet effect increases risk of bleeding.	Concurrent use is normally avoided.

standard range for aPTT rather than a control (where the range can vary), then the heparin dose should be 1.5 to two times the upper limit of the normal aPTT range. It is important that patients reach the minimum of 1.5 times the control or upper normal range within the first 24 hours of therapy. Failure to promptly achieve this therapeutic level in patients with a clot increases the risk of developing additional clots.

Heparin levels should be allowed to reach steady state before measuring aPTT, usually 6 to 8 hours after the infusion starts. If the aPTT is less than one and one half to two times the control, contact the prescriber to seek new drug therapy orders. If the aPTT is below the desired therapeutic range, the dosage needs to be increased. Repeated testing is needed after each dosage change has reached steady state (6–8 hours after the dosage change). In institutions with established protocols for adjusting heparin infusion rates to meet therapeutic levels, the rate may be changed by a registered nurse. If aPTT values deviate from the protocol limits, the prescriber must be notified.

Do not interrupt IV heparin therapy, because this lowers the blood levels of heparin and affects the therapeutic response. If occlusion or infiltration necessitates changing the IV site, insert the new IV line as soon as possible to minimize the disruption of the infusion.

Doses of SC heparin should not be missed; they should be administered at the regularly prescribed times to maintain blood levels.

Minimizing Adverse Effects
Before initiating therapy, review such laboratory values as aPTT, hematocrit, and platelet count. These tests provide baseline information regarding clotting abilities and identify patients with conditions that contraindicate heparin therapy. However, these tests are not usually performed for prophylactic heparin use.

If the aPTT during treatment exceeds the desired range, the dosage should be decreased. Contact the prescriber to seek new drug therapy orders, or act on the standard protocol (if one is used).

Use an IV controller or pump for continuous IV drip heparin to promote a steady rate of delivery and prevent rapid overdosage, which may occur when IV flow rates are regulated by gravity. Use of a pump is a standard safety precaution. When selecting a vial of heparin, either to mix in a bag of fluid for infusion for SC use or to flush a venous catheter, confirm that the appropriate concentration of the heparin has been selected. Heparin comes in a wide variety of concentrations, from 10 units per mL to 10,000 units per mL. Selection of the wrong concentration is a medication error that can lead to serious adverse effects, especially hemorrhage.

Do not interrupt administration of IV heparin to give another drug. Doing so increases the risk of thrombus formation because therapeutic levels may not be maintained. Do not administer other drugs through the same tubing as heparin because heparin is incompatible with many other drugs and fluids. Instead, use an additional peripheral IV line or a multilumen central venous catheter.

To minimize the risk of heparin-induced thrombocytopenia (HIT), the American College of Chest Physicians recommends that the platelet count be monitored every day for 14 days or until the heparin is discontinued (whichever comes first). When the heparin is administered to prevent a clot, the platelet count should be monitored every 2 to 3 days from day 4 to 14, or until it is stopped (whichever comes first). Patients who have received heparin therapy in the past 100 days and are starting treatment again with heparin are at risk for accelerated thrombocytopenia, so a baseline platelet count should be obtained and then repeated within 24 hours. If patients are receiving heparin just as a flush for a venous catheter, they do not require platelet count monitoring (Hirsh, Albers, & Schunemann, 2008). HIT should be suspected if the patient is receiving heparin or has received heparin within the last 2 weeks and there is a 50% or more drop in the platelet count. Nurses should work jointly with the physician in monitoring the platelet count and bring changes in the platelet count to the physician's attention.

If the patient is determined to have HIT, the treatment includes discontinuing heparin, allowing the platelet count to return to normal, and treating any thrombosis with a nonheparin anticoagulant (such as danaparoid, lepirudin, argatroban, fondaparinux, or bivalirudin, which are discussed below in the section Drugs Significantly Different From Heparin) over further use of unfractionated heparin or low molecular weight heparin..

Monitor patients for bleeding from the gums, nose, vagina, or wounds. Examine urine and stools to detect blood as well. Inspect the skin for ecchymoses or hematomas that indicate bleeding into the tissues. If the patient develops active bleeding from an orifice or a wound, notify the prescriber immediately. Protamine sulfate is administered if significant active bleeding occurs.

Place pressure on IV sites when removing the line until bleeding stops. Use a 25-gauge or finer needle for SC administration (Box 32.1). Do not aspirate or massage the area after SC administration. Avoid intramuscular (IM) injections to prevent bleeding into the muscle.

To protect the patient from injury or falls, use standard fall precaution measures. Raise or pad the top side rails, particularly if the patient is confused, disoriented, restless, or unable to comprehend or follow activity restrictions during therapy.

Providing Patient and Family Education
• Before heparin therapy begins, inform patients why the drug is needed and what it is expected to accomplish. Heparin should be described as an anticoagulant, not a blood thinner. Although this is a common description, it is not correct.

Box 32.1 | **RESEARCH-BASED SUBCUTANEOUS ADMINISTRATION TECHNIQUES FOR HEPARIN**

Traditionally, the abdomen, 2 inches from the umbilicus, was the preferred site for injection because it was believed that this site carried less risk for developing hematoma. The limited research done to date has shown, however, that site selection of the arm or thigh, as opposed to the abdomen, does not increase bruising or alter aPTT (Fahs & Kinney, 1991). Research further indicates that technique affects hematoma formation. As early as 1988, Wooldridge found that changing the needle after drawing the drug into the syringe, having an air bubble in the syringe to follow the dose and lock the drug into the subcutaneous space, injecting at a 90-degree angle, and avoiding aspiration and massage after injection helped to prevent hematoma formation. The use of a 3-cc syringe rather than a 1-mL syringe has been found to cause smaller bruises when administering heparin (Hadley, Chang, & Rogers, 1996).

  MEMORY CHIP

P Heparin

- Anticoagulant that prevents formation or extensions of blood clots
- Has no effect on existing blood clots
- Parenteral administration (IV or SC)
- Major contraindications: thrombocytopenia, bleeding disorders, and active bleeding other than DIC
- Most common adverse effect: bleeding (antidote for heparin overdose is protamine sulfate)
- Most serious adverse effect: thrombocytopenia
- **Life span alert: Heparin is the anticoagulant that can be used during pregnancy.**
- **Patient safety alert: Check concentration of heparin carefully. Use of the wrong concentration for the route of administration is a common medication error with serious/potentially life-threatening ramifications.**
- Maximizing therapeutic effects: Monitor APTT for therapeutic range; adjust dose until therapeutic range achieved.
- Minimizing adverse effects: Use IV pump; assess for signs of bleeding.
- Most important patient education: Instruct patients to report any blood in urine or stools or bleeding from gums, nose, vagina, or wounds.

- Explain that frequent blood samples will need to be analyzed to measure patients' clotting time and determine whether they are receiving a safe amount of heparin.
- Instruct patients to report any blood in urine or stools and any bleeding from the gums, nose, vagina, or wounds.
- Educate patients to use a soft toothbrush and an electric razor during therapy to prevent bleeding and to follow activity restrictions to prevent bruising and internal bleeding from injuries.

Ongoing Assessment and Evaluation

Throughout therapy, monitor for signs of bleeding and review aPTT values to maintain heparin levels in the therapeutic range. Monitor platelet counts at appropriate intervals. Drug therapy is considered effective when a thrombus or extension of an existing thrombus is avoided and adverse effects are prevented or minimized.

Drugs Closely Related to **P** Heparin

Low-molecular-weight heparin is derived from standard heparin through either chemical or enzymatic depolymerization (breakdown of polymers into monomers, their basic building block). Whereas standard heparin has a molecular weight of 5,000 to 30,000 daltons, low-molecular-weight heparin ranges from 1,000 to 10,000 daltons, resulting in properties that are distinct from those of traditional heparin. Low-molecular-weight heparin binds to protein (although less strongly than traditional heparin), has enhanced bioavailability, interacts less with platelets, and yields a very predictable dose response, eliminating the need to monitor the aPTT. Low-molecular-weight heparin, like standard heparin, binds to antithrombin; however, low-molecular-weight heparin also inhibits thrombin to a lesser degree (and actual factor X to a greater degree) than standard heparin.

Low-molecular-weight heparins also have prolonged half-lives compared with unfractionated heparin (standard heparin

that has not been depolymerized). This characteristic, in combination with the increased bioavailability, allows once-daily SC dosing. Such dosing enables treatment for stabilized patients in their own homes, while they are followed as outpatients.

Low-molecular-weight heparins cause less bleeding when given in therapeutic doses, compared with unfractionated heparin, as well as less heparin-induced thrombocytopenia and osteoporosis. Traditional heparin is recommended when patients have severe renal insufficiency, as evidenced by a creatinine clearance less than 30 mL/min; if low-molecular-weight heparin is used, the dose should be decreased by 50% (Hirsh, Albers, & Schünemann, 2008). Obese patients are recommended to be dosed with LMWH based on body weight (Hirsh, Albers, & Schünemann, 2008).

Low-molecular-weight heparins are now used successfully for several therapeutic purposes. In multiple clinical trials and in meta-analyses of trials, these heparins have been found to be at least as safe and effective as unfractionated heparin in treatment of pulmonary embolism, as prophylaxis for venous thromboembolism, and in treatment of DVT; in many cases these drugs have replaced traditional heparin (Weitz, Hirsh & Samama, 2008; van Dongen, van den Belt, Prins, et al., 2004). They are also as effective as heparin in preventing thromboembolism prior to long-term anticoagulation after a mechanical heart valve replacement and in patients with a mechanical valve who have a contraindication to oral anticoagulation. In addition, a 14-day course of therapy of low-molecular-weight heparin may be used in patients who are at high risk for stent thrombosis. Patients who have major orthopedic surgery, particularly hip surgery, remain at risk for clinically important venous thrombosis for at least 4 weeks after the surgery; this risk is significantly reduced if they continue to receive a low-molecular-weight heparin, fondaparinux, or warfarin during this period (Hirsh, Albers & Schünemann, 2008). Low-molecular-weight heparins are currently being studied for their use in preventing thromboembolism in patients with cancer (Box 32.2).

All low-molecular-weight heparins have a Black Box warning regarding the use of epidural/spinal anesthesia or spinal puncture. Patients who either have received or will receive a low-molecular-weight heparin are at increased risk for the development of an epidural or spinal hematoma, which can result in long-term permanent paralysis. The risk of these events is increased by the use of indwelling epidural catheters for administration of analgesia or by the concomitant use of drugs affecting hemostasis, such as nonsteroidal anti-inflammatory drugs (NSAIDs), platelet inhibitors, or other anticoagulants. The risk also appears to be increased by traumatic or repeated epidural or spinal puncture. Other anticoagulants should be used for patients in these situations.

Commercially available low-molecular-weight heparins differ in their method of production, molecular weight, and degree of sulfation. They also differ somewhat in terms of pharmacokinetics. These differences may or may not have any clinical significance. Three low-molecular-weight heparins are used in the United States: enoxaparin, dalteparin, and tinzaparin. Another drug, fondaparinux, has a slightly different composition and is not in the same class but will be considered with these drugs.

Enoxaparin

Enoxaparin (Lovenox), which is considered safer than and equally effective as heparin, has an effect on activated factor X and has limited effect on thrombin. Thus, its effect on aPTT is decreased. Enoxaparin also affects clotting factor C and antithrombin. Most enoxaparin is absorbed after SC administration and is widely distributed. Enoxaparin has been found to be superior to unfractionated heparin in reducing death, MI, and emergency revascularization in patients with Q-wave MI. Enoxaparin and other LMWHs are considered the preferred treatment for deep venous thrombosis over traditional non-fractionated heparin. Enoxaparin is also approved to be used to prevent ischemia that may result from non-Q-wave myocardial infarction or unstable angina.

Enoxaparin appears to have greater efficacy but similar safety as unfractionated heparin when used to treat ST-segment-elevation myocardial infarction. Low-molecular- weight heparins, like enoxaparin, appear to be safe and effective for treating acute coronary syndrome when combined with platelet glycoprotein IIB/IIIa inhibitors (Ferguson, Antman, Bates, et al., 2003). When given to patients with a creatinine clearance of 30 mL/min or less, enoxaparin results in elevated levels of antiactivated factor X, and patients have an increased risk of bleeding. Dosage adjustments may be warranted (Lim, Dentali, Eikelboom, et al., 2006). Enoxaparin is a pregnancy category B drug.

Patients who are to receive enoxaparin by SC injection after discharge should be taught how to administer the drug to themselves (Box 32.3). It is important that they understand the reason for therapy, the necessity of taking the drug on time, and the importance of following a regular dosage schedule and having follow-up blood analyses done as recommended. They should also be advised about scheduling and keeping appointments with the prescriber.

Other important teaching points focus on safety (e.g., clearing pathways, removing loose scatter rugs, wearing nonskid

---

BOX 32.2 FOCUS ON RESEARCH

Low-Molecular-Weight Heparins and Cancer Patients

Hull, R. D., Pineo, G. F., Brant, R. F., et al. (2006). Long-term low-molecular-weight heparin versus usual care in proximal vein thrombosis patients with cancer. *The American Journal of Medicine*, 119(12):1062–1072.

Deitcher, S. R., Kessler, C. M., Merli, G., et al. (2006). Secondary prevention of venous thromboembolic events in patients with active cancer: Enoxaparin alone versus initial enoxaparin followed by warfarin for a 180-day period. *Clinical and Applied Thrombosis/ Hemostasis: Official Journal of the International Academy of Clinical and Applied Thrombosis/Hemostasis*, 12(4):389–396.

The Study

Although patients with cancer are known to be at increased risk of thromboembolism, anticoagulant trials have not frequently included these patients. Recently, two small trials examined patients with cancer and thromboembolism and evaluated their response to low-molecular-weight heparin. Patients with cancer frequently experience myelosuppression secondary to chemotherapy. With decreased platelets, they are at increased risk of bleeding, although they are also at increased risk of clotting. Warfarin may additionally increase the risk of bleeding.

The first study examined the effectiveness of a low-molecular-weight heparin, tinzaparin, compared with warfarin. Patients received one of these drugs for 3 months. Tinzaparin was found to be more effective than warfarin in preventing recurrent venous thromboembolism in patients with cancer and proximal venous thrombosis.

The second study compared the incidence of bleeding from a low-molecular-weight heparin, enoxaparin, with warfarin. Patients were treated for 6 months. No significant differences in the incidence of major or minor bleeding were found between the two groups.

Nursing Implications

Patients with cancer and a thromboembolism have needs that are unique from those of other patients with clots. Because these patients have an increased risk of both clotting and bleeding, the use of anticoagulant therapy can be challenging. These two small studies show that low-molecular-weight heparins are more effective and cause no more bleeding effects than traditional warfarin. Because the low-molecular-weight heparins are administered subcutaneously, this may be an advantage for patients with cancer who have nausea, vomiting, or difficulty swallowing due to myositis. Nurses should discuss with the other members of the health care team the possibility of using low-molecular-weight heparins in appropriate patients.

BOX 32.3 COMMUNITY BASED CONCERNS

Enoxaparin at Home

Patients receiving subcutaneous injections of enoxaparin at home are typically responsible for self-administering the medication. These patients need information on the following topics:

- Locating appropriate injection sites and rotating injection sites
- Performing subcutaneous injections using appropriate technique
- Disposing of used syringes and needles in an impervious container, such as a plastic milk jug or a coffee can. The lid should be taped shut before placing the container in the regular home trash.
- Recapping needles: Patients may recap their own used needle. If a family member is administering the medication, the needle and syringe should be placed in the container uncapped. The product may come in a self re-capping syringe to prevent accidental needle stick injuries.

footwear, obtaining adequate lighting, and using handrails on stairways in bathtubs). Additional teaching and management concerns are similar to those for heparin therapy.

Dalteparin

Dalteparin (Fragmin), another low-molecular-weight heparin, is used to prevent DVT. It is also used in treating unstable angina and non–Q-wave MI for preventing ischemic complication in patients on concurrent aspirin therapy. A unique feature of dalteparin is that the multiple-dose vial contains benzyl alcohol as a preservative; benzyl alcohol has been associated with "fatal gasping" syndrome in premature infants. Because of this possibility, dalteparin should not be used in infants or in pregnant women (because it crosses the placenta). Other characteristics of dalteparin are similar to those of enoxaparin.

Tinzaparin

Tinzaparin (Innohep) is very similar to enoxaparin. Its major difference is that it is approved for use only in treating DVT in conjunction with warfarin. It is administered subcutaneously for 6 days, at least, until the patient is adequately anticoagulated with warfarin (the patient should have an International Normalized Ratio [INR] of 2 for at least 2 days).

Fondaparinux

Like heparin, fondaparinux (Arixtra) is an anticoagulant. However, fondaparinux works differently. A synthetic polysaccharide that inhibits antithrombin, it is thus a direct inhibitor of activated factor X. Neutralization of activated factor X disrupts the blood coagulation cascade, inhibiting thrombin formation and thrombus development. However, fondaparinux has no direct effect against thrombin. It is administered subcutaneously.

Like heparin, fondaparinux is used to prevent postoperative DVT from hip, knee, or abdominal surgery. It is also used to treat DVT and PE in conjunction with warfarin. Research indicates that fondaparinux may be more effective than enoxaparin in preventing DVT, especially in high-risk orthopedic

patients (Weitz, Hirsh, & Samama, 2008). Although it may have a place in the treatment of acute coronary syndrome, more research is required to confirm this.

Like the low-molecular-weight heparins, fondaparinux carries a Black Box warning about a serious interaction that can occur if given before or after spinal or epidural anesthesia. A disadvantage of fondaparinux is that it cannot be reversed by protamine sulfate.

Like heparin, fondaparinux can cause bleeding, but unlike heparin it does not cause HIT with thrombosis. It can also cause anemia.

Drugs Significantly Different From Heparin

A new group of drugs are the direct thrombin inhibitors. This group includes argatroban, bivalirudin, and lepirudin. The direct thrombin inhibitors bind to the active thrombin site and inhibit both free and clot-bound thrombin. Thus, unlike heparin, they inactivate fibrin-bound as well as circulating thrombin (Weitz, Hirsh, & Samama, 2008). Because direct thrombin inhibitors do not bind to plasma proteins, they produce a more predictable anticoagulant response.

Argatroban and lepirudin (Refludan) are direct thrombin inhibitors that are both labeled for use in heparin-induced thrombocytopenia-thrombotic disorder. Argatroban may be used for both treatment and prophylaxis, whereas lepirudin may be used for prophylaxis only. Off-label uses for argatroban include stroke and MI, and off-label uses for lepirudin include prevention of MI. Argatroban has a slightly shorter half-life. Both these drugs are administered intravenously.

Both argatroban and lepirudin can cause serious bleeding (including hematuria, intracranial bleeding, GI bleeding, and hemoptysis), cardiovascular (CV) effects, pneumonia, and sepsis. Precise CV adverse effects differ; argatroban causes angina, cardiac arrest, hypotension, and ventricular arrhythmias, whereas lepirudin causes heart failure. The overall adverse effect profile of these two drugs differs. Argatroban can commonly cause the following adverse effects: GI (abdominal pain, diarrhea, nausea, and vomiting), neurologic (headache, pain), renal (urinary tract infections), respiratory (cough), as well as fever and infectious diseases. Lepirudin can commonly cause adverse effects such as anemia, fever, and cutaneous hypersensitivity. In addition, lepirudin also produces abnormal liver function tests, renal failure, and extrinsic allergic respiratory disease. Both argatroban and lepirudin are pregnancy category B drugs, and their effect in children is unknown.

Bivalirudin (Angiomax) is also a direct thrombin inhibitor. Unlike the other drugs, it is labeled only for use during percutaneous coronary intervention (PCI) in conjuncture with a glycoprotein IIb/IIIa inhibitor and during percutaneous transluminal coronary angioplasty for unstable angina. Its systemic half-life is short: 25 minutes. It is administered intravenously. The most frequent adverse effects of bivalirudin are back pain, headache, and hypotension. Serious adverse effects include bleeding and hemorrhage that requires transfusion. Like argatroban and lepirudin, bivalirudin is a pregnancy category B drug.

Nursing Management of the Patient Receiving P Warfarin

Core Drug Knowledge

Pharmacotherapeutics

Warfarin (Coumadin) is an oral anticoagulant. It is administered after heparin therapy for 3 to 6 months to complete treating a thrombus or embolism. Warfarin is also used prophylactically for patients with a long-term risk for thrombus formation (e.g., when the mitral valve has been replaced or when hypercoagulability is a chronic concern related to venous stasis). It is also used prophylactically in patients with atrial fibrillation who are at high risk for a cardioembolic stroke; about one third of patients with atrial fibrillation are at such risk. Women with atrial fibrillation especially seem to benefit from preventative treatment (Hart, Halperin, Pearce, et al., 2003).

The American College of Chest Physicians' clinical guidelines suggest that the starting dose should be 5 to 10 mg initially for the first 1 to 2 days, and then adjusted based on the clinical response achieved based on changes to the International Normalized Ratio (INR) (Hirsh, Albers, & Schünemann, 2008). INR has been developed to measure therapeutic levels of warfarin. The INR is determined by a mathematical equation and reflects the patient's prothrombin time (PT) compared with the standardized PT value. The INR has essentially replaced the more traditional PT in which the patient's PT is measured against a control PT. In the traditional PT test, the control times vary with laboratory test methods and equipment, so the effectiveness of the drug therapy is determined by completing a math equation; the patient should take longer to clot than the control. The use of the INR is simpler, as the lab results are standardized; all computation is reflected in the reported lab value. The INR is reported as a number; INRs of 1 indicate that the patient and the control are identical. For treatment or prophylaxis of a thrombus or embolus, the INR should be equal to 2 to 3; the patient's PT should be 1.4 to 1.6 times the control time. For prophylaxis in patients with mechanical heart valves, the PT should be 1.5 to 1.7 times the control, or the INR should be 2.5 to 3.5. While INR is considered the new standard, some institutions still utilize the traditional PT lab value to assess warfarin's effectiveness; others may still report both INR and PT.

After absorption, warfarin is bound to albumin in the plasma. The drug action peaks in 1 to 9 hours; however, the anticoagulant effects do not begin for 24 hours. Maximum effect occurs 3 to 4 days after dosing starts, which is the time required for the drug to reach a steady state in the blood. The time factor is related to previously activated factors that are still circulating in the blood. Each time the dose changes, another 3 to 4 days are needed for the drug to reach its full effect. The effects of warfarin persist for 4 to 5 days after discontinuation (see Table 32.1). The drug crosses the placenta but is not present in breast milk. It is metabolized in the liver and excreted in the bile.

Patients receiving heparin therapy begin taking warfarin before they discontinue heparin. This overlap allows the warfarin to reach a therapeutic level before heparin is discontinued. The practice is safe because the two drugs affect different clotting factors.

Pharmacodynamics

Warfarin works by competitively blocking vitamin K at its sites of action. Thus, it prevents the activation of factors II (prothrombin), VII, IX, and X. It has no effect on factors that have already been activated. Because of this action, the full therapeutic response to a warfarin dose cannot be measured until after 3 days of therapy. In practice however, even though the drug is not at steady state, most of the clinical effects can be seen after 2 days of treatment, so INR can be measured after 2 to 3 days of treatment (Hirsh, Albers, & Schünemann, 2008). For this reason, warfarin therapy is started while patients are still receiving heparin therapy for blood clots. The heparin can be discontinued once the INR is between 2 and 3 for 2 days in a row.

Contraindications and Precautions

Warfarin is contraindicated for patients with active bleeding, open wounds or ulcerations of the GI tract, or bleeding disorders, such as hemophilia or thrombocytopenia. It is not recommended for use in patients with subacute endocarditis, pericarditis, or pericardial effusions. Warfarin is also contraindicated for patients who are undergoing surgery in which hemorrhage is possible (spinal, eye, GI, cranial, and arterial bypass grafting). Usually, the drug is discontinued 7 days before elective surgery.

Cautious use is recommended in patients with renal and hepatic impairment. Warfarin use is primarily determined by comparing the risks of the drug with the benefits to the patient.

Adverse Effects

The most frequent adverse effects of warfarin are bleeding and hemorrhage. Nausea, vomiting, diarrhea, and abdominal cramps can occur as well. Tissue necrosis is a rare adverse effect. A fetal warfarin syndrome has been identified when warfarin is given to pregnant women. (See discussion under Life Span and Gender.)

Drug Interactions

Several drug–drug and drug–food interactions must be considered when a patient begins warfarin therapy (Table 32.3). Many of these drug interactions may be related to effects on the P-450 system. Many herbal preparations also interact with warfarin (Table 32.4). Because drug and herbal interactions are numerous, a complete assessment of all other drug therapies should be conducted when starting a patient on warfarin. Dose adjustments for warfarin may be indicated, depending on other required drug therapy for comorbidities.

TABLE 32.3 Agents That Interact with P Warfarin

Interactants	Effect and Significance	Nursing Management
acetaminophen, androgens, beta blockers, clofibrate, corticosteroids, cyclophosphamide, dextrothyroxine, disulfiram, erythromycin, fluconazole, gemfibrozil, glucagon, hydantoins, influenza virus vaccine, isoniazid, ketoconazole, miconazole, moricizine, propoxyphene, quinolones, sulfon-amides, tamoxifen, thioamines, thyroid hormones, urokinase	They may increase the effect of warfarin by unknown or complicated mechanism, increasing risk of bleeding.	Monitor for bleeding carefully. Monitor PT or INR carefully. Anticipate dose adjustments of warfarin if these drugs are started after titrating the dose of warfarin.
amiodarone, chloramphenicol, cimetidine, ifosfamide, lovastatin, metronidazole, omeprazole, phenylbutazones, propafenone, quinidine, quinine, sulfamethoxazole-trimethoprim (SMZ-TMP), sulfinpyrazone	The effect of warfarin may be increased by inhibiting its metabolism, increasing the risk of bleeding.	Same as above.
chloral hydrate, loop diuretics, nalidixic acid	The effect of warfarin may be increased because of displacement from binding sites, increasing the risk of bleeding.	Same as above.
aminoglycosides, mineral oil, tetracyclines, vitamin E	The effect of warfarin may be increased because of interference with vitamin K, increasing the risk of bleeding.	Same as above.
cephalosporins, diflunisal, NSAIDs, penicillins, salicylate	The effect of warfarin may be increased because of effects on platelets and GI irritation (from NSAIDs), increasing the risk of bleeding.	Avoid administering NSAIDs and salicylates if possible. Other considerations are the same as above.
ascorbic acid, dicloxacillin, ethanol, ethchlorvynol, griseofulvin, nafcillin, sucralfate, trazodone	The effect of warfarin may be decreased by an unknown action.	Be aware that dose of warfarin may need to be adjusted to be in therapeutic range. Monitor PT or INR to assess drug effectiveness.
aminoglutethimide, barbiturates, etretinate, carbamazepine, glutethimide, rifampin	The effect of warfarin may be decreased by induction of the anticoagulant's hepatic microsomal enzymes.	Avoid variation in vitamin K–rich food after titrating warfarin dose. Vitamin K is considered an antidote to warfarin. Otherwise nursing considerations are the same as above.
cholestyramine, contraceptives, oral estrogens, thiazide diuretics, thiopurines, spironolactone, vitamin K	The effect of warfarin may be decreased by various mechanisms.	Same as above.

Assessment of Relevant Core Patient Variables

Health Status

Because deficiencies of vitamin K increase the bleeding risk in patients receiving warfarin, assess the availability of vitamin K. Patients with vitamin K deficiency experience decreased synthesis of normal clotting factors and are at greater risk for hemorrhage if they receive warfarin. Besides the body's production of vitamin K in the GI tract, one source of vitamin K is food. Vitamin K is a fat-soluble vitamin and depends on the absorption of fat for its own absorption. Bile is necessary for fats to be digested and absorbed. A patient with decreased available bile (e.g., from obstructed bile ducts) absorbs less vitamin K. Patients with poor dietary intake of vitamin K are also deficient in the vitamin. Vitamin K deficiency may also occur in adults whose normal GI flora has been affected by long-term antibiotic therapy or whose dietary intake consists of parenteral nutrition without vitamin K supplements.

Life Span and Gender

Consider the patient's age before therapy begins. Because vitamin K is continually produced in the GI tract, deficiencies are rare in healthy adults. However, newborns may have a vitamin K deficiency because intestinal flora is not active at birth. In addition, bleeding complications with anticoagulant drugs appear to occur more frequently in older adults (those older than 75 years) than in younger adults. Older adults also have an increased sensitivity to the effects of warfarin, in both the early induction phase and the maintenance phase of drug therapy.

It is important to determine the stage of the reproductive cycle for women. Warfarin should not be used during pregnancy and is in pregnancy category X because it is associated with a described syndrome of fetal defects.

Lifestyle, Diet, and Habits

Obtain information about the patient's dietary habits. Because vitamin K competes with warfarin, high vitamin

TABLE 32.4 Interactions of Herbs and Warfarin*

Effect	Herbs
Increase the effects of warfarin	Boldo, bromelains, dan shen, dong quai (*Angelica sinensis*), garlic, ginkgo (*Ginkgo biloba*), *Lycium barbarum* L
Decrease the effects of warfarin	Coenzyme Q$_{10}$, green tea, ginseng (*Panax*), St. John's wort
Additive bleeding effects with warfarin	Herbs with potential anticoagulant effects: Alfalfa, dong quai (*Angelica sinensis*), aniseed, arnica, asafoetida, bladder wrack (*Fucus*), bogbean, boldo, buchu, capsicum, cassia, celery, chamomile (German and Roman), dandelion, fenugreek, horse chestnut, horseradish, licorice, meadowsweet, nettle, parsley, passion flower, pau d'arco, prickly ash (Northern), quassia, red clover, sweet clover, sweet woodruff, tonka beans, wild carrot, wild lettuce Herbs that contain salicylate or have antiplatelet properties: Agrimony, aloe gel, aspen, black cohosh, black haw, bogbean, cassia, clove, dandelion, feverfew, garlic, German sarsaparilla, ginger, ginkgo (*Ginkgo biloba*), ginseng (*Panax*), licorice, meadowsweet, onion, policosanol, poplar, senega, tamarind, willow, wintergreen Herbs with fibrinolytic properties: Bromelains, capsicum, garlic, ginseng (*Panax*), inositol nicotinate, onion
May decrease the effectiveness of warfarin	Herbs with coagulant properties: Agrimony, goldenseal, mistletoe, yarrow

*Other herbal interactions are possible.

K levels decrease the effectiveness of warfarin. Diets rich in vitamin K, therefore, should be avoided. If the diet was normally rich in vitamin K when the warfarin dosage was adjusted, restricting these foods is not as important. However, if the patient's diet does not normally include vitamin K–rich foods, these foods should be avoided. Consider lifestyle behaviors that place the patient taking heparin at increased risk for falls and injuries for the patient taking warfarin, as well. Many herbal medications interact with warfarin: assess for their use.

Environment
Be aware that warfarin therapy may be started in the hospital, but most treatment is self-administered by the patient at home. Explore with the patient potential risks in the home environment.

Culture and Inherited Traits
Because warfarin is metabolized via the P-450 system, inherited variations of this system may alter drug response. Variations in this system are believed to be responsible for the difficulty in finding a dose for some patients that is therapeutic but does not cause adverse effects. At this time, there is no way to determine which patients have inherited traits that will cause these problems.

Nursing Diagnosis and Outcome
• Risk for Injury, Bleeding, related to adverse effects of warfarin
  Desired outcome: *The patient will not experience bleeding.*

Planning and Intervention
Maximizing Therapeutic Effects
Warfarin dosage should be individualized until PT or the INR is in therapeutic range. An initial loading dose is given to attain a rapid therapeutic level. This dose is then followed by a maintenance dose. Doses are usually given in the evening, at 6:00 PM. This timing allows for early morning blood draws for PT or INR by hospital laboratory personnel.

Minimizing Adverse Effects
Assess the patient's response to warfarin therapy using either the ratio of the patient's PT compared with the control PT, or the INR. Notify the prescriber if the patient's clotting time is greater than the therapeutic level. (See Box 32.4 for guidelines of suggested responses to various INR levels.) Usually, drug dosage is decreased if clotting time exceeds this level. Skipping one dose may be all that is required to lower the PT or INR to the therapeutic level. In case of warfarin overdose where bleeding is present, the antidote, vitamin K (phytonadione), is administered intravenously.

Falls may cause internal bleeding. Assess all patients for fall risk. Ensure that the patient's home is also assessed for factors that may lead to falls. Encourage the use of proper lighting and handrails on stairways, which may help prevent falls.

Providing Patient and Family Education
• Teach patients the signs of bleeding and methods to prevent bleeding (which are the same as for heparin).
• Instruct patients to take the drug at the same time each day because this dosing schedule helps prevent a drop in warfarin blood levels. After the drug level is stabilized and daily PT is not needed, patients may switch to morning dosing. Doing so may increase absorption and improve adherence to drug therapy. Advise patients to return for follow-up blood work.
• Teach patients that skipping a dose of warfarin could alter therapeutic levels. If patients forget a dose, they should take it as soon as they remember. However, they should not double up on the next dose to prevent bleeding.
• Instruct patients that taking aspirin, large doses of acetaminophen, or other over-the-counter drugs with these ingredients can affect warfarin's action.

Box 32.4 CLINICAL GUIDELINE RECOMMENDATIONS FOR NON-THERAPEUTIC INR LEVELS

INR level	Significant Bleeding	Recommendation	Resume warfarin
>3 but <5	no	Omit a dose; monitor more frequently;	When INR has returned to therapeutic range with adjusted dose
≥5 but <9	no	Omit one or two doses; monitor more frequently; OR skip a dose and administer oral vitamin K (1–2.5 mg) if patient at increased risk of bleeding (may give ≤ 5 mg vitamin K if patient requires urgent surgery)	When INR has returned to therapeutic range with adjusted dose
>9	no	Hold warfarin; administer oral vitamin K (2.5–5 mg); monitor INR more frequently; administer additional vitamin K as needed	When INR has returned to therapeutic range with adjusted dose
Any elevation	yes	Hold warfarin therapy; give vitamin K 10 mg by slow IV infusion; supplemented with fresh frozen plasma, prothrombin complex concentrate, or recombinant factor VIIa, depending on the urgency of the situation. Repeat vitamin K administration every 12 h for persistent INR elevation	When INR has returned to therapeutic range with adjusted dose
Any elevation	yes, life threatening	Holding warfarin therapy and administering fresh frozen plasma, prothrombin complex concentrate, or recombinant factor VIIa supplemented with vitamin K, 10 mg by slow IV infusion, repeated, if necessary, depending on the INR	If indicated, when INR has returned to therapeutic range with adjusted dose

Based on American College of Chest Physicians Evidence-Based Clinical Practice Guidelines (8th Edition) CHEST June 2008 vol. 133 no. 6 suppl 71S-109S.

• Warn women to avoid becoming pregnant while taking this drug.
• Dietary teaching should focus on the need to avoid increased intake of foods rich in vitamin K, primarily green vegetables.
• Emphasize the importance of informing other health care providers (e.g., dentist, podiatrist) that they are taking

warfarin. Patients should also be instructed to wear or carry medical identification stating that they are receiving warfarin.

Ongoing Assessment and Evaluation

To determine the therapeutic effects of warfarin, the patient's PT or INR is monitored. Therapy is effective when a thrombus is prevented and bleeding does not occur.

CRITICAL THINKING SCENARIO

SOLVING PROBLEMS RELATED TO ANTICOAGULANT THERAPY

Melanie Graves is diagnosed with a left leg deep vein thrombosis (DVT). She is started on heparin 1,000 U/h by intravenous infusion. After 3 days, she will start taking warfarin in addition to the heparin.

1. Explain the rationale for starting warfarin while the patient is receiving heparin. Three days have passed. The first dose of warfarin (5 mg) is given at 6 PM. The following morning, blood is drawn to evaluate the PT. The control is 30 seconds, Ms. Graves' PT is 30 seconds, and the INR is 1.

2. Discuss the information about the dosage of the warfarin that can be obtained from this initial blood work. Explain how you arrived at this conclusion.

3. Ms. Graves complains that she doesn't like having her blood drawn so frequently. She says she cannot wait to go home so that she does not have to have any more blood work. What elements will you develop in the initial teaching plan for her?

MEMORY CHIP

P Warfarin

• Anticoagulant used to complete treatment with heparin after clot formation; is used prophylactically in patients at high risk of thrombus formation
• Administered orally
• May be given with heparin until therapeutic level of warfarin is obtained
• Major contraindications: active bleeding, ulcerations of the GI tract, or bleeding disorders
• Most common adverse effect: bleeding (vitamin K is the antidote for warfarin toxicity)
• Most serious adverse effect: fetal warfarin syndrome
• **Life span alert: Warfarin is not for use in pregnancy because it causes fetal defects.**
• Maximizing therapeutic effects: Monitor PT for therapeutic range; adjust dosage until therapeutic range is attained.
• Minimizing adverse effects: Monitor for signs of bleeding.
• Most important patient education: Teach patients to monitor for bleeding, to modify behavior to avoid injuries, and to avoid greatly increased vitamin K intake.

Drug Significantly Different From P Warfarin

Anisindione

Anisindione (Miradon) is an oral anticoagulant like warfarin, but it does not work in the same manner. An indanedione, anisindione is a synthetic anticoagulant drug that acts by reducing the prothrombin activity of the blood. Like warfarin, it can be used to treat or prevent PE and venous thrombosis and can be used in atrial fibrillation where there is thrombosis. It is also indicated as adjunct treatment in coronary occlusion. In contrast to warfarin, anisindione commonly has adverse effects, including dermatologic (alopecia, dermatitis, urticaria) and GI (nausea, mouth ulcers, vomiting) conditions. Fever may also occur. Many of the serious adverse effects of anisindione are similar to warfarin: cholesterol embolus syndrome, skin necrosis, hemorrhage, and hepatitis. Like warfarin, anisindione is in pregnancy category X and is contraindicated in pregnant women because of the risk of teratogenic effects. Anisindione should be reserved for patients who cannot tolerate warfarin.

C ANTIPLATELET DRUGS

Drugs that prevent platelet aggregation are called antiplatelet drugs. They are used when overactive platelets pose long-term risks for hypercoagulability. Platelet aggregation is important in hemostasis and is also involved in thrombus formation, particularly in the arterial circulation.

Antiplatelet drugs reduce platelet aggregation and are used to prevent further thromboembolic events in patients who have suffered MI, ischemic stroke or transient ischemic attack (TIAs), or unstable angina, and for primary prevention of a thromboembolic event in patients at risk. Some are also used for the prevention of reocclusion or restenosis following angioplasty and bypass procedures.

Antiplatelet drugs differ in their modes of action and adverse effects. Aspirin is the most widely used and studied; it acts by irreversibly inhibiting platelet cyclo-oxygenase (COX) and thus preventing synthesis of thromboxane A_2. Although aspirin may be the most frequently prescribed antiplatelet drug, it is also used frequently for other clinical reasons. The prototype NSAID is discussed in Chapter 24.

Heparin and the direct-acting thrombin inhibitors, as previously mentioned, have antiplatelet and anticoagulant effects. Glycoprotein IIb/IIIa-receptor antagonists, such as abciximab, eptifibatide, and tirofiban, interfere with the final step in platelet aggregation and are used in unstable angina and as adjuncts in reperfusion and revascularization procedures.

Drugs that interfere with adenosine metabolism have an antiplatelet effect, and those used include the thienopyridines clopidogrel and ticlopidine, which interfere with adenosine diphosphate–mediated platelet activation, and the adenosine reuptake inhibitor dipyridamole. Ticlopidine was previously identified as the prototype antiplatelet drug, but clopidogrel (Plavix) has replaced it because it is associated with fewer adverse effects and is now more widely used.

Nursing Management of the Patient Receiving P Clopidogrel

Core Drug Knowledge

Pharmacotherapeutics

Clopidogrel is used to reduce the occurrence of atherosclerotic events (MI, stroke, and vascular death) in patients who have atherosclerosis and have had a recent MI or stroke, or who risk having one of these events because they have acute coronary syndrome or peripheral arterial disease. Its use in peripheral arterial disease is unique from aspirin

It is also used in patients undergoing PCI where there is a coronary stent implanted or coronary artery bypass graft (CABG). Use of clopidogrel for 1 year after stent implantation significantly reduces the risk of major vascular events. Clopidogrel is administered orally; in some circumstances, a loading dose is used prior to starting the maintenance dose.

Pharmacokinetics

Clopidogrel is rapidly absorbed by the GI tract. At least 50% is absorbed. The bioavailability is not changed from food. The drug is metabolized in the liver via CYP2C19 to an active form and then eliminated by the kidneys and GI tract. The drug and metabolite are both highly protein bound. Steady state occurs between 3 and 7 days with daily dosing. Platelet aggregation and bleeding time gradually return to baseline levels, generally within 5 days after drug therapy is stopped. For more information, see Table 32.1.

Pharmacodynamics

Clopidogrel inhibits the binding of adenosine diphosphate (ADP) to its platelet receptor and the subsequent ADP-mediated activation of the glycoprotein IIb/IIIa complex and thus inhibits platelet aggregation. It thus prolongs the bleeding time. Clopidogrel must be metabolized to an active metabolite to produce this effect, although the active metabolite has not been isolated. Clopidogrel irreversibly modifies the platelet ADP receptor so that platelets exposed to the drug are affected for the remainder of their life span. The inhibition of platelet aggregation is dose dependent, and effects can be seen within 2 hours after a single oral dose of clopidogrel. By the time the drug is at steady state, the average inhibition of platelet aggregation is between 40% and 60% of normal. Clinical studies have identified a wide variation in response to a dose of clopidogrel, with the assumption that some patients are "nonresponders" to clopidogrel therapy. However, because clopidogrel relies on metabolism to its active metabolite to achieve therapeutic effect, it is probable that the decrease in clopidogrel's effectiveness is not due to an inherited trait but rather to a drug interaction from drugs that inhibit either the CYP3A4 or CYP2C19 pathway. Thus, it decreases conversion to an active, antiplatelet form (Lee et al., 2009).

When clopidogrel was added to aspirin therapy in the treatment of acute coronary syndromes with ST-segment elevation, a significant additive effect was found, reducing the number of deaths, reinfarctions, and strokes without producing significant excess risk of adverse effects. This was seen in all patients, including those who had received fibrinolytic therapy or who were older than 70 years of age (Chen, Jiang, Chen, et al., 2005). Although clopidogrel does not seem to improve early reperfusion when given before fibrinolysis therapy, it does improve late coronary patency and clinical outcomes by preventing reocclusion of open arteries (Scirica, Sabatine, Morrow, et al., 2006).

Contraindications and Precautions

Clopidogrel's black box warning states that poor metabolizers of the drug via CYP2C19 will form less active therapeutic levels. Genotype testing is necessary to determine an appropriate dose. Clopidogrel is contraindicated in patients with hypersensitivity and in those with active bleeding disorders such as peptic ulcers or intracranial hemorrhage. Caution should be used when administering clopidogrel to patients with severe hepatic dysfunction because knowledge regarding the effects on such patients is limited. Caution should be used if the patient is at risk for increased bleeding from trauma, surgery, or other pathologic conditions. Long-term use of a combination of aspirin and clopidogrel in patients with recent TIA or stroke is not recommended, as it has not been found to be more effective than treatment solely with clopidogrel; the combination has been shown to increase major bleeding. To achieve its full therapeutic effect, the length of therapy needs to be adequate; patients who receive clopidogrel post-stent (PCI) are at risk for stent thrombosis, MI, or death if the therapy is prematurely discontinued.

Assigned to pregnancy risk category B, clopidogrel should be used only if absolutely necessary during pregnancy. The drug is not recommended for use in breast-feeding mothers; it is not known whether the drug is excreted in breast milk.

Adverse Effects

Adverse reactions to clopidogrel are similar to those with aspirin. The most common adverse effect is GI distress, which can include abdominal pain, indigestion, diarrhea, nausea. The serious GI problems of bleeding and ulcers occur less frequently with clopidogrel than with aspirin. Clopidogrel is similar in chemical structure to ticlopidine, which is associated with a small (0.8%) risk of severe neutropenia. Clopidogrel appears to have a much smaller risk of producing severe neutropenia, and its incidence of neutropenia may be no greater than that found in the general population. However, the possibility of neutropenia should be considered if the patient develops a fever or other sign of infection while taking the drug.

Drug Interactions

Because clopidogrel is metabolized to an active metabolite by CYP2C19 concurrent use of any drug that inhibits the activity of isoenzyme CYP2C19 can reduce the plasma concentration of activated clopidogrel. Two proton pump inhibitors (PPIs, used in the prevention of excessive gastric acid) are known to decrease the therapeutic effectiveness of clopidogrel via this mechanism. These drugs are omeprazole and pantoprazole. If patients on clopidogrel require restrictions on their gastric acidity they should receive other drug classes than PPIs.

Because clopidogrel increases bleeding risk, especially from GI ulcers, caution should be used if clopidogrel is coadministered with other drugs that can cause GI ulcers and bleeding, such as aspirin or NSAIDs, because additive effects are likely. Coadministraton with warfarin will also increase the risk of bleeding from clopidogrel. While at high concentrations in laboratory studies, clopidogrel inhibits the hepatic isoenzyme P-450 2C9 and warfarin is a substrate of CYP2C9 (meaning it is metabolized by the isoenzyme) substantial impairment of warfarin's metabolism has not been noted when co-administered with clopidogrel in normal doses. So the increased risk of bleeding that occurs from giving the two drugs concurrently does not appear to be related to this pathway. The potential for an adverse reaction exists with warfarin and other drugs that are CYP2C9 substrates, however.

Additionally, clopidogrel may interact with numerous herbs. Patients taking herbal remedies or multiple prescription drugs should be monitored closely for either toxic or subtherapeutic effects of clopidogrel. Agents that interact with clopidogrel are listed in Table 32.5.

Assessment of Relevant Core Patient Variables

Health Status

Review the patient's history and physical examination findings for any contraindications to the use of this drug. The patient should have a baseline complete blood count (CBC) with differential to determine platelet functioning. Liver function studies should also be done. A baseline cardiovascular assessment is indicated when starting therapy. Neurologic status should also be assessed when clopidogrel is given to prevent stroke.

Life Span and Gender

Determine the patient's age before therapy begins. Caution must be used in children younger than 18 years because safety has not been established. The exact effects of clopidogrel on pregnancy and lactation are not known, and caution must be used. In older adults, no differences in platelet aggregation and bleeding time have been noted; thus, no dosage adjustment is needed.

Lifestyle, Diet, and Habits

Assess for lifestyle behaviors that would place the patient at increased risk for bleeding while taking this drug. Because patients take clopidogrel to decrease the risk of atherosclerotic events (such as MI and stroke), assess whether the patient is following a heart-healthy diet that is low in fat and cholesterol. Assess for use of herbs that may interact with clopidogrel.

Environment

Be aware of the environment in which the drug will be administered. Clopidogrel may be administered in the hospital. However, most of the time, it is self-administered by

TABLE 32.5	Agents That Interact with P Clopidogrel	
Interactants	**Effect and Significance**	**Nursing Management**
anticoagulants; thrombolytics; antiplatelets	Additive anticoagulation effects may increase risk of bleeding.	Concurrent use requires additional monitoring for complications. Observe for external and internal bleeding. Monitor PT, aPTT, platelet counts. Use full precautions to prevent internal injuries and bleeding.
NSAIDs	Decreased platelet function and decreased coagulation can occur, making bleeding, especially GI bleeding, more likely.	Avoid coadministration if possible. Use caution if coadministration is necessary. Monitor closely for GI bleeding.
Proton pump inhibitors (omeprazole, pantoprazole)	Prevents metabolism of clopidogrel to active form via CYP2C19. This significantly decreases therapeutic effect, and increases risk for developing life threatening clots.	Avoid this combination. Use H_2 antagonists or antacids instead of PPIs.
herbs and vitamins: angelica; anise; arnica; astragalus; bilberry; black currant; bladderwrack; bogbean; boldo; borage; capsaicin; cat's claw, celery; clove oil; curcumin; dandelion; evening primrose; feverfew; garlic; ginger; ginkgo; guggul; hawthorn; kava; licorice; meadowsweet; motherwort; skullcap; tan-shen; vitamin A	Increased risk of bleeding	Minimize or avoid coadministration. If coadministered, monitor for signs of bleeding.
drugs metabolized by CYP2C9 (warfarin; fluvastatin; phenytoin; tamoxifen; tolbutamide; torsemide)	Clopidogrel inhibits CYP2C9 in large dose. Less CYP2C9 means less metabolism of drugs via this pathway. Increased risk of adverse effects in these drugs is possible.	Administer together with caution. Monitor for adverse effects of CYP2C9-metabolized drug.
ibritumomab	Severe and prolonged thrombocytopenia that can be an adverse effect from ibritumomab may make patients more likely to bleed if they are taking drugs that interfere with platelet function.	Monitor for thrombocytopenia more frequently when using ibritumomab and antiplatelet agents concomitantly.

the patient at home. Discuss with the patient potential risks in the home environment. Falls and activities that are likely to produce internal or external bleeding should be avoided while taking clopidogrel.

Nursing Diagnoses and Outcomes
- Risk for Injury: Increased Risk for Bleeding related to decreased platelet aggregation from drug therapy
  Desired outcome: The patient will suffer no injury related to bleeding while on clopidogrel.
- Risk for Nausea related to adverse effects of clopidogrel.
  Desired outcome: Nausea and GI distress will not be extreme enough to warrant stopping clopidogrel therapy.

Planning and Intervention
Maximizing Therapeutic Effects
Ensure that clopidogrel is administered routinely to achieve its maximum therapeutic effects. Do not co-administer with omeprazole or pantoprazole.

Minimizing Adverse Effects
Have patients take clopidogrel with food to decrease GI problems if they occur. Make sure that the home environment

is assessed for safety hazards that may contribute to falls or other accidents. Remember that severe neutropenia is a potential risk, and evaluate the patient's white blood cell count (WBC) if the patient develops signs of infection.

Providing Patient and Family Education
- Inform patients and families about laboratory tests that are needed on a regular basis and the reasons for their frequency.
- Emphasize to patients and families the importance of informing all health care providers (e.g., dentists and other physicians) of the drug regimen. If surgery is needed, and the antiplatelet effect is not desired, drug therapy should be discontinued 7 days before the procedure to prevent excessive bleeding.
- Instruct patients and families to apply pressure on wounds until bleeding stops.
- Emphasize to patients that behaviors that may lead to injury should be avoided (e.g., roller-blading, ice skating, motorcycle riding, use of nonmotorized scooters, walking on icy patches).
- Instruct patients and families to make the home environment more "fall proof" by removing scatter rugs, placing handrails on stairs, and fastening any loose carpet edges.

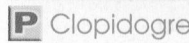

 Clopidogrel

- Used to prevent atherosclerotic events in patients who have had myocardial infarction or stroke, or who are at risk for having these events
- Prevents platelet aggregation and prolongs bleeding time
- Major contraindication: active bleeding disorders
- Most common adverse effect: GI distress
- Most serious adverse effect: bleeding
- Maximizing therapeutic effects: Administer regularly.
- Minimizing adverse effects: Take with food to decrease GI distress; assess for risk for falls and injuries.
- Most important patient education: Avoid activities that increase risk for falls or injury, remove scatter rugs or other hazards that may contribute to falls in the home; apply pressure to any bleeding cut.
- **Black box warning: This drug relies on metabolism via CYP2C19 to become active. Loss of therapeutic effect in poor metabolizers. Genetic test required to determine therapeutic dose. Consider alternative therapy in poor metabolizers.**

Ongoing Assessment and Evaluation

Periodic measurement of bleeding time and platelet function is needed throughout clopidogrel therapy. Neutrophil counts should be assessed if the patient develops signs of infection, to rule out severe neutropenia. Therapy is evaluated as effective when the outcomes are achieved and atherosclerotic events have been prevented.

Drugs Closely Related to Clopidogrel

Prasugrel

Like clopidogrel, prasugrel is an antiplatelet. Its labeled indications are more limited than clopidogrel. It is approved to prevent clots (including stent thrombosis) in patients with acute coronary syndrome who are to be managed with percutaneous coronary intervention. Prasugrel's onset of antiplatelet effect is achieved more quickly than clopidogrel. Prasugrel causes more bleeding than clopidogrel. Prasugrel carries several Black Box warnings. These include:

1) Can cause significant, sometimes fatal, bleeding in patients with active pathologic bleeding or a propensity to bleed, a history of transient ischemic attack or stroke, a body weight of less than 60 kg, or concomitant use of medications that increase the risk of bleeding (e.g., warfarin, heparin, fibrinolytics, chronic use of NSAIDs). Do not use in patients with active pathologic bleeding or a history of transient ischemic attack or stroke.
2) Do not use in patients 75 years of age and older because of the increased risk of fatal and intracranial bleeding with the exception of high-risk situations (patients with diabetes or a history of prior myocardial infarction) where its effect appears to be greater.

3) Do not start prasugrel in patients likely to undergo urgent coronary artery bypass graft surgery (CABG). When possible, discontinue prasugrel at least 7 days prior to any surgery.
4) Suspect bleeding in any patient who is hypotensive and has recently undergone coronary angiography, percutaneous coronary intervention (PCI), CABG, or other surgical procedures in the setting of prasugrel. (FDA label for EFFIENT, 2009).

Patients should be taught to watch for bleeding such as nose bleeds, coughing up blood, black tarry stools from gastrointestinal hemorrhage, and bruising.

Aspirin

Aspirin, a drug used for its antiplatelet properties, has a mechanism of action that differs from that of clopidogrel in that it irreversibly inhibits platelet cyclo-oxygenase (COX) and the subsequent synthesis of thromboxane A_2 for the life of the platelet. Thromboxane A_2 is a vasoconstrictor that facilitates platelet aggregation. Inhibiting its synthesis, therefore, inhibits platelet aggregation. The antiplatelet effects of aspirin, which result from its effect on COX-1 sites, can be achieved with low doses of aspirin, between 50 and 100 mg daily. Aspirin can also act on COX-2 to create anti-inflammatory effects, but a much larger dose and more frequent administration of doses are required (Tourmousoglou, Rokkas, 2008).

As an antiplatelet drug, it is recommended that aspirin be given within 24 to 48 hours of the onset of a stroke. Use of aspirin concurrently or within 24 hours of the use of thrombolytic agents, such as alteplase, is not recommended. Long-term aspirin therapy provides a significant reduction in the risk of MI, stroke, or vascular death in patients who have an intermediate to high risk of vascular complications. These risk factors include chronic stable angina, prior MI, unstable angina, TIA or minor stroke, as well as other high-risk conditions (Grant, Brotman, Jaffer, 2009). Aspirin is also used to decrease the incidence of coronary heart disease in adults who are at increased risk for heart disease.

Patients who should be considered for cardiac preventive therapy with aspirin include men older than 40 years, postmenopausal women, and younger adults with risk factors for coronary heart disease (hypertension, diabetes, smoking, elevated lipid levels, obesity, family history). Aspirin is used prophylactically against thromboembolic complications in cardiovascular disease, including MI and TIA. Aspirin in low doses is recommended after MI to prevent future infarcts and in patients with atrial fibrillation to prevent stroke; however, it is not as effective as warfarin for this purpose (Grant, Brotman, Jaffer, 2009). Aspirin prevents noncardioembolic strokes primarily. In patients with diabetes, low-dose aspirin is a primary prevention therapy if the patient has cardiovascular risk factors (family history of coronary vascular disease, cigarette smoking, hypertension, obesity, albuminuria, elevated lipid levels, and age older than 40 years). Aspirin is a secondary prevention strategy in patients with diabetes with large vessel disease; indications include history of MI, vascular bypass surgery, stroke or

TIAs, peripheral vascular disease, claudication, angina, or any combination of these factors. The American Diabetes Association recommends an aspirin dosage of 75 to 162 mg/d in patients with diabetes (American Diabetes Association, 2004).

A major adverse effect of aspirin is its ability to cause bleeding, especially GI bleeding; GI ulceration is also problematic. GI ulceration caused by overexposure to aspirin or other NSAIDS is a result of systemic inhibition of COX, which is an enzyme in prostaglandin formation that helps produce a protective mucous lining of the stomach and duodenum. Because of this systemic effect, GI complications are related to the use of aspirin no matter what form it is in (UpToDate, 2009b).

These adverse effects may limit the use of aspirin in some patients. Although the antiplatelet effect of aspirin is not dose related, the GI adverse effects are dose related, so administering as low a dose as possible helps minimize the risk of these adverse effects. Aspirin may pose a risk of neutropenia, but compared with clopidogrel, aspirin poses a much smaller risk of this complication.

For more information on aspirin, see Chapter 24.

Cilostazol

Cilostazol (Pletal) is a platelet aggregation inhibitor with vasodilating activity. It is used to treat the symptoms of intermittent claudication, which occur in about one third of patients who have peripheral arterial disease. The drug improves pain-free walking distance. Off-label uses include secondary prevention of repeat CVAs and during percutaneous coronary intervention. In addition to its antiplatelet effects, cilostazol also decreases triglycerides and increases high-density lipoprotein cholesterol. Cilostazol is contraindicated for use in patients with heart failure, hemostatic disorders, or active bleeding. Precaution is necessary in severe renal impairment. Cilostazol is extensively metabolized in the liver by the CYP3A4 and, to a lesser extent, CYP2C9 isoenzymes; thus, potential drug–drug interactions are similar to those of clopidogrel.

Cilostazol is a pregnancy category C drug. Breast-feeding should be ceased during cilostazol therapy, to avoid potential harm to the infant.

Ticlopidine

Ticlopidine works very similarly to clopidogrel with one major exception. Ticlopidine, unlike clopidogrel, can cause life-threatening hematologic adverse reactions, including neutropenia/agranulocytosis, thrombotic thrombocytopenic purpura (TTP) and aplastic anemia. Because of these serious adverse effects, ticlopidine is not frequently used to prevent platelet aggregation.

Drugs Significantly Different From
P Clopidogrel

Dipyridamole

Unlike clopidogrel, dipyridamole is primarily a coronary vasodilator that increases functional levels of adenosine, which produces vasodilation and inhibits platelet aggregation.

Dipyridamole also inhibits the enzyme phosphodiesterase, which increases cyclic adenosine monophosphate (cAMP) and decreases platelet activation. Data from the literature are conflicting as to whether dipyridamole actually has an antiplatelet effect. Dipyridamole dilates coronary arteries, increasing flow in narrowed vessels. It does not usually produce much systemic vasodilation. A mild positive inotropic effect has also been documented.

Dipyridamole is used with anticoagulants and other antiplatelets in patients after surgery, such as prosthetic heart valve placement and vascular grafting procedures, to prevent thrombus formation. It is used diagnostically during thallium myocardial perfusion imaging. A combination of aspirin and dipyridamole (Aggrenox) appears to increase the antiplatelet effect of aspirin and is approved for use in preventing recurrent thromboembolic stroke.

Dipyridamole is moderately absorbed after oral administration. Its distribution is widespread; it crosses the placenta and enters breast milk. It is metabolized in the liver and excreted by the GI tract. It should be used cautiously in patients with hypotension because some vasodilation occurs.

The most frequent adverse effects of dipyridamole are headache, dizziness, and nausea. After IV administration, MI, arrhythmias, and bronchospasm may occur, although they are uncommon.

Dipyridamole has additive effects on platelet aggregation when given with aspirin. Bleeding risk is increased when dipyridamole is used concurrently with anticoagulants, thrombolytics, NSAIDs, or sulfinpyrazone. Ingesting alcohol increases the risk for hypotension. Theophylline may negate the effects of dipyridamole during diagnostic thallium imaging.

Glycoprotein IIb/IIIa Inhibitors

Tirofiban (Aggrastat), eptifibatide (Integrilin), and abciximab (ReoPro) are all antagonists of the platelet glycoprotein IIb/IIIa receptor, the major platelet surface receptor involved in platelet aggregation. This receptor is found only on platelets and their progenitors. Glycoprotein IIb/IIIa inhibitors block the final common pathway leading to platelet aggregation. Activation of the glycoprotein IIb/IIIa receptors leads to the binding of fibrinogen and von Willebrand factor to platelets and thus to platelet aggregation. American College of Cardiology/American Heart Association guidelines recommend glycoprotein IIb/IIIa inhibitors as an integral component to prevent thromboembolic-induced myocardial ischemia in non-ST-elevation acute coronary syndromes and the ischemic complications of percutaneous coronary intervention.

Both tirofiban and eptifibatide reversibly prevent fibrinogen and von Willebrand factor from binding to the glycoprotein IIb/IIIa receptor, thereby inhibiting platelet aggregation. Eptifibatide has been found to achieve the highest level of consistent platelet inhibition compared with abciximab and tirofiban (Jennings, 2005). Eptifibatide, when combined with the low-molecular-weight heparin enoxaparin, has been found to be safe and effective in the treatment of acute coronary syndrome (unstable angina or non–Q-wave MI)

(Diez, Medina, Cheong, et al., 2009). Both tirofiban and eptifibatide are administered by IV infusion. One difference between these two drugs is their rate of ability to bind with protein in the blood. Tirofiban is moderately protein bound (65%), whereas eptifibatide has low protein binding (25%).

Contraindications for tirofiban and eptifibatide are the same and include active internal bleeding or a history of bleeding within the last 30 days; a history of thrombocytopenia following a prior exposure to tirofiban; history of stroke within 30 days or any history of hemorrhagic stroke; a major surgical procedure or severe physical trauma within the last 30 days; severe hypertension; concomitant use of another parenteral glycoprotein IIb/IIIa inhibitor; any history of intracranial hemorrhage, intracranial neoplasm, arteriovenous malformation, or aneurysm; history, symptoms, or findings suggestive of aortic dissection or acute pericarditis; platelet counts less than 1,000,000/mm³; a serum creatinine level of 2 mg/dL or higher; or dependency on renal dialysis.

The most frequent adverse effect for both tirofiban and eptifibatide is bleeding, which can be a minor or major event. Nonbleeding adverse effects for tirofiban (when coadministered with heparin) include nausea, fever, and headache. The only nonbleeding adverse effect of eptifibatide is hypotension, which may be serious. Tirofiban may cause bradycardia.

Abciximab is different from the other glycoprotein IIb/IIIa inhibitors in that it is a chimeric human-murine monoclonal antibody Fab (fragment antigen binding) fragment. It inhibits platelet aggregation by specifically binding to the glycoprotein GPIIb/IIIa receptor. Abciximab is used as an adjunct to percutaneous transluminal coronary angioplasty or atherectomy, to prevent acute cardiac ischemic complications in patients at high risk for abrupt closure of the treated coronary vessel. Off-label uses include treatment of myocardial infarction. It is used with aspirin and heparin. Low-dose, weight-adjusted heparin regimens are recommended to minimize the risk of bleeding. Like tirofiban and eptifibatide, bleeding is the major adverse effect of abciximab. Unlike tirofiban and eptifibatide, abciximab is a pregnancy category C drug.

Anagrelide

Anagrelide (Agrylin) is a platelet-reducing agent that is significantly different from clopidogrel. It is used in treating essential thrombocytosis, secondary to myeloproliferative disorders, to decrease the elevated platelet count and the risk of thrombosis and to reduce the associated symptoms of the disorder. Anagrelide hydrochloride, a phosphodiesterase III inhibitor, inhibits cAMP and reduces blood platelet production. WBCs and other coagulation factors are not affected. RBC counts may be altered, but these alterations are not clinically important. The most common adverse effects of anagrelide are headache, diarrhea, edema, palpitations, and abdominal pain. Serious potential adverse effects, none of which are common, include chronic heart failure, MI, cardiomyopathy, cardiomegaly, complete heart block, atrial fibrillation, CVA, pericarditis, pulmonary infiltrates, pulmonary fibrosis, pulmonary hypertension, pancreatitis, gastric or duodenal ulcers, and seizures.

C HEMORHEOLOGIC DRUGS

The hemorheologic drugs differ from the antiplatelet drugs in that they act on RBCs to reduce blood viscosity and increase the flexibility of RBCs. This effect helps prevent thrombus formation and allows the RBCs to enter the microcirculation, thereby increasing oxygenation at the cellular level. These effects are helpful in treating peripheral vascular disease. The prototype hemorheologic drug is pentoxifylline (Trental).

Nursing Management of the Patient Receiving P Pentoxifylline

Core Drug Knowledge

Pharmacotherapeutics

Pentoxifylline is used to manage the symptoms of intermittent claudication from peripheral vascular disease. Using this drug improves the patient's ability to walk for longer distances without pain. It has also been used to treat acute and chronic cerebral vascular disease because it improves the psychopathologic symptoms. Unlabeled uses include treating diabetic angiopathies, neuropathies, TIAs, chronic leg ulcers, Raynaud disease, and disorders of the circulation of the eye (see Table 32.1). Although an off-label use, the American College of Chest Physicians recommends that pentoxifylline, 400 mg po tid, be part of the treatment for venous leg ulcers (Hirsh, Albers, & Schünemann, 2008).

Pharmacokinetics

Pentoxifylline is absorbed readily from the GI tract. It undergoes first-pass effect in the liver with about 50% of the drug remaining. It is widely distributed. Onset of therapeutic effects takes 2 to 4 weeks. However, full therapeutic effects are not evident until 4 to 8 weeks after therapy starts. The drug is metabolized by RBCs and the liver and is excreted in urine.

Pharmacodynamics

Pentoxifylline increases the flexibility of RBCs by increasing cAMP levels. In turn, this effect decreases platelet aggregation and promotes vasodilation. Blood fibrinogen concentration is lowered. In addition, the drug increases cellular adenosine triphosphate levels, which stabilizes the cell membrane and reduces the RBC aggregation, thus lowering blood viscosity.

Contraindications and Precautions

Because pentoxifylline is derived from the methylxanthines (caffeine and theophylline), it is contraindicated in patients who have an intolerance to it or to the methylxanthines. Patients with impaired renal function may require a reduced dose to prevent toxicity. Caution is also necessary when administering pentoxifylline to patients with coronary artery or cardiovascular disease, such as angina, arrhythmias, or severe hypotension. Pentoxifylline should be used with care in pregnant or nursing women. The drug is in pregnancy risk category C and is excreted in breast milk. Caution should also be used for children younger than 18 years, because safety in this age group has not been established.

Adverse Effects

Pentoxifylline's adverse effects occur primarily in the central nervous, CV, and GI systems. The effects on these systems may result from this drug's similarity to caffeine and theophylline.

Headache, dizziness, tremor, dyspepsia, nausea, and vomiting are all common adverse effects. Other adverse effects can occur occasionally. These effects include agitation, nervousness, insomnia, angina, chest pain, arrhythmia, tachycardia, edema, hypotension, abdominal discomfort, bloating, belching, flatus, diarrhea, blurred vision, epistaxis, bad taste, rash, urticaria, pruritus, and brittle fingernails.

Drug Interactions

Pentoxifylline may interact with a few drugs, which are listed in Table 32.6.

Assessment of Relevant Core Patient Variables

Health Status

Determine whether the patient is hypersensitive to the drug or to methylxanthines before beginning therapy. Assess the patient's baseline walking tolerance, circulation, and pulses in the affected extremities. Ask the patient to describe any pain experienced with activity and the effect of rest on the pain.

Life Span and Gender

Determine whether the patient is pregnant or breast-feeding.

Lifestyle, Diet, and Habits

Find out whether the patient smokes tobacco. Usual patterns of exercise and activity should be compared with desired level of exercise and activity.

Environment

Be aware that pentoxifylline is generally self-administered in the home, although it may also be administered in the hospital. Discuss potential risks in the home environment with the patient.

Nursing Diagnosis and Outcome

- Risk for Injury related to adverse pentoxifylline effects (dizziness, drowsiness, blurred vision)
  Desired outcome: The patient will remain injury free while on pentoxifylline.

Planning and Intervention

Maximizing Therapeutic Effects

Pentoxifylline must be taken for several weeks before the full therapeutic effects are evident. Therefore, confirm that a patient discharged on this medication has a prescription for continued use.

Minimizing Adverse Effects

Give pentoxifylline with food to minimize GI upset.

Providing Patient and Family Education

- Inform patients that pentoxifylline does not have an immediate effect and that they should not stop taking the drug before the therapeutic effects are achieved.
- Instruct patients to avoid driving or operating machinery until it is known whether dizziness or blurred vision will occur from the drug. If these problems continue after the initial phase of drug therapy, the prescriber should be contacted in case the dosage needs to be decreased.
- Advise patients not to smoke because smoking constricts the blood vessels.
- Instruct patients to keep all follow-up visits with the prescriber.

Ongoing Assessment and Evaluation

Peripheral circulation should be reassessed periodically to measure improvement. Throughout pentoxifylline therapy, the patient's exercise tolerance should be assessed, with improvement being noted over time if therapy is effective. For patients also taking antihypertensive drugs, monitor blood pressure throughout therapy.

TABLE 32.6   Agents That Interact with P Pentoxifylline

Interactants	Effect and Significance	Nursing Management
cimetidine	Cimetidine decreases hepatic metabolism of pentoxifylline, which can lead to adverse effects from pentoxifylline.	Monitor for pentoxifylline toxicity (e.g., flushing, hypotension, or seizures) and adjust the dose accordingly. Suggest switching to another H₂-antagonist (e.g., ranitidine or famotidine), which has less potential to alter metabolism of pentoxifylline.
dicumarol	Hypoprothrombinemic effect of dicumarol may be increased, increasing the risk of bleeding.	Monitor PT and INR frequently; lower dose of pentoxifylline if necessary.
insulin glulisine; inhaled human insulin	The blood glucose–lowering effect of insulin may be increased, and hypoglycemia may result.	Monitor blood glucose levels closely if adding or subtracting pentoxifylline from insulin therapy.
theophylline	Overdoses of pentoxifylline can interfere with theophylline assay levels and falsely elevate the levels of theophylline when EMIT assay test is used.	Alternate assay tests can be used if large doses of pentoxifylline are indicated.

MEMORY CHIP

P Pentoxifylline

- Hemorheologic agent that reduces blood viscosity and increases flexibility of red blood cells
- Used to manage symptoms of intermittent claudication
- Needs to be taken for several weeks before full therapeutic effect is seen
- Major contraindication: sensitivity to methylxanthines
- Most common adverse effects: headache, dizziness, tremor, dyspepsia, nausea, and vomiting
- Most serious adverse effect: tachycardia

C THROMBOLYTIC DRUGS

Thrombolytic drugs assist in breaking down formed blood clots. These drugs are used for patients who are diagnosed with an evolving, acute MI; a PE; or acute ischemic stroke. They may also be given to unclog central venous catheters. These drugs may be given systemically or directly at the site of the blood clot. Although these drugs are given during emergency situations and can save lives, their adverse effects can be life threatening. Therefore, these drugs should be administered by clinicians who are familiar with them and skilled in using them. Patients receiving these drugs need to be monitored carefully for adverse effects. The prototype of the thrombolytic drugs, also known as the tissue plasminogen activators(tPA), is alteplase, recombinant (Activase; Cathflo Activase). Drugs closely related to alteplase, recombinant, are reteplase, recombinant; tenecteplase (TNKase); streptokinase; and urokinase. A significantly different drug is drotrecogin alfa (activated).

Nursing Management of the Patient Receiving P Alteplase, Recombinant

Core Drug Knowledge

Pharmacotherapeutics

Alteplase, recombinant (Activase) is indicated in a number of thromboembolic conditions considered medical emergencies (e.g., acute evolving MI from an acute coronary artery thrombus). Therapy for this condition is most effective when it is initiated as soon as possible after the onset of symptoms (within 3 hours after the onset of symptoms is preferred; Hirsh, Albers, & Schünemann, 2008). Alteplase, recombinant is also indicated for acute ischemic stroke; it is the only drug therapy approved for treating ischemic stroke. Treatment has shown to be safe and effective if initiated within 3 hours after the onset of stroke and after intracranial bleeding (hemorrhagic stroke) has been ruled out by a computed tomography (CT) scan (Hacke, 2008; Matthews, 2009). Box 32.5 describes management of patients who are receiving alteplase, recombinant, for ischemic stroke. Patients should be at least 18 years of age and have a clinical diagnosis of ischemic stroke with clinically meaningful neurologic deficit.

Box 32.5 MANAGEMENT OF PATIENTS RECEIVING ALTEPLASE, RECOMBINANT, FOR TREATMENT OF ISCHEMIC STROKE

- Infuse 0.9 mg/kg (maximum, 90 mg) over 60 minutes with 10% of the dose given as a bolus over 1 minute.
- Admit the patient to an intensive care unit or stroke unit for monitoring.
- Perform neurologic assessment every 15 minutes during infusion, every 30 minutes for the next 6 hours, and then every hour until 24 hours from treatment.
- Delay placing nasogastric tubes, indwelling bladder catheters, or intra-arterial pressure catheters.
- If the patient develops severe headache, acute hypertension, nausea, or vomiting, discontinue infusion (if still being administered), and obtain computed tomography scan of brain immediately.
- Monitor blood pressure every 15 minutes for the first 2 hours, every 30 minutes for the next 6 hours, and then every hour until 24 hours after treatment.
- Increase frequency of blood pressure monitoring if systolic is equal to or greater than 180 mm Hg or diastolic is equal to or greater than 105 mm Hg. Administer antihypertensive drug therapy to maintain blood pressure below these levels.
- If diastolic is 105 to 140 mm Hg or systolic is 180 mm Hg or greater, give IV labetalol, 10 mg over 1 to 2 minutes. Repeat or double the dose every 10 to 20 minutes to a maximum dose of 300 mg. Or, give initial bolus of labetalol followed by continuous IV infusion of 2 to 8 mg/min. If this approach does not control blood pressure and diastolic is 121 to 140 mm Hg or systolic is greater than 230 mm Hg, consider starting nitroprusside infusion.
- If diastolic is greater than 140 mm Hg, start nitroprusside infusion at 0.5 mg/kg/min.

From Adams, H. P., Adams, R. J., Brott, T., et al. (2003). Guidelines for the early management of patients with ischemic stroke: a scientific statement from the Stroke Council of the American Stroke Association. *Stroke*, 34(4):1056–1083. Available: *http://stroke.ahajournals.org/cgi/content/full/ 34/4/1056.*

Alteplase, recombinant is also indicated to treat massive pulmonary embolism. However, this use of alteplase, as well as other thrombolytics, is somewhat controversial. Although thrombolytics accelerate clot lysis and are associated with short-term physiologic benefits, current research does not clearly show that thrombolytics decrease mortality better than heparin (UpToDate, 2009a; Wan, Quinlan, Agnelli, et al., 2004; Dong, Jirong, Liu, et al., 2009). Persistent hypotension due to PE is the most accepted indication for the use of thrombolytics. Because thrombolytics have potential serious adverse effects, it has been recommended that their use be limited to confirmed PE or DVT. For these uses, alteplase, recombinant is administered by IV infusion.

A form of alteplase is designed and approved for clearing clots that have formed in central venous catheters (Cathflo Activase); this is a labeled use for the drug in patients 2 years or older. Unlabeled uses for alteplase, recombinant include managing peripheral arterial thromboemboli and treatment of massive proximal lower extremity or iliofemoral

DVT associated with severe symptomatic swelling or limb-threatening ischemia (see Table 32.1).

Pharmacokinetics

Alteplase is infused intravenously so that distribution begins immediately. Steady state is higher if accelerated infusion of alteplase is used. Alteplase is rapidly cleared from the plasma, primarily by the liver. About 80% of the drug is cleared within 10 minutes after the infusion has completed.

Pharmacodynamics

Alteplase, recombinant is a tissue plasminogen activator (tPA) synthesized by recombinant DNA technology. It acts in the same way as endogenous tPA. Alteplase, recombinant is actually an enzyme that, when fibrin is present, converts plasminogen to plasmin. It has limited effect if fibrin is not present. When administered, alteplase, recombinant binds to the fibrin in a clot and converts the trapped plasminogen to plasmin. Fibrinolysis, or breakdown of the clot, then occurs.

Contraindications and Precautions

Alteplase, recombinant should be used only in clinical settings in which hematologic function and clinical response can be adequately monitored. It should be administered by a clinician with experience and knowledge in treating the thromboembolic disorders.

Contraindications to the use of alteplase are numerous and include hypersensitivity to alteplase; active internal bleeding; evidence of intracranial bleeding (ischemic stroke) on pretreatment evaluation; history of intracranial bleeding; suspicion of subarachnoid hemorrhage; recent (within the past 2 months) stroke; recent intracranial or intraspinal surgery or severe head trauma (within 3 months); intracranial neoplasm; seizure at onset of stroke; conditions (including other prescribed drug therapy) that make the patient likely to bleed; severe uncontrolled hypertension (systolic blood pressure ≥180 mm Hg or diastolic blood pressure ≥110 mm Hg); platelet count less than 100,000/mm³ (ischemic stroke); and administration of heparin 48 hours preceding the onset of stroke and an elevated active partial thromboplastin time (aPTT) at presentation (ischemic stroke).

Risks of alteplase, recombinant when used to treat acute ischemic stroke may be increased if the patient has severe neurologic deficits or major early infarct signs visible in the CT scan (e.g., substantial edema, mass effect of midline shift). Several studies have looked at the risk for intracerebral hemorrhage following thrombolytic therapy for actue ischemic stroke, as it is associated with a high rate of morbidity and mortality. Risk factors include: hyperglycemia, history of diabetes, stroke severity, advanced age, increased time to treatment, high blood pressure, low platelets, early CT changes, large baseline diffusion lesion volume, a history of congestive heart failure and low plasminogen activator

inhibitor levels (Lansberg, Albers, & Wijman, 2007; Derex & Nighoghossian, 2008).Certain conditions may increase the risk of bleeding from alteplase, recombinant. If any of the following are present, the benefits must be weighed against this increased risk:

- Recent (≤10 days) major surgery (e.g., CABG, obstetrical delivery, organ biopsy, previous puncture of noncompressible vessels such as internal jugular)
- Cerebrovascular disease
- Recent (≤10 days) GI or genitourinary (GU) bleeding
- Recent (≤10 days) trauma
- Hypertension (systolic blood pressure ≥180 mm Hg; diastolic blood pressure ≥110 mm Hg)
- Likelihood of left heart thrombus (e.g., mitral stenosis with atrial fibrillation)
- Acute pericarditis
- Subacute bacterial endocarditis
- Hemostatic defects, including secondary to severe hepatic or renal disease
- Serious liver dysfunction
- Pregnancy
- Diabetic hemorrhagic retinopathy or other ophthalmic hemorrhaging
- Septic thrombophlebitis or occluded arteriovenous cannula at seriously infected site
- Older adult (greater than 75 years)
- Currently receiving oral anticoagulants
- Any other condition in which bleeding would pose a major hazard or would be very difficult to manage because of its location

Adverse Effects

Bleeding is the most frequently occurring adverse effect. It can be internal, involving GI, GU, or respiratory tracts or the retroperitoneal or intracranial areas. On the other hand, it can be surface or superficial bleeding at puncture sites (e.g., IV sites or arterial punctures) or surgical incisions. Predictors of major hemorrhage after alteplase administration for acute PE include receiving a catecholamine to increase blood pressure, cancer, diabetes, and elevated INR before fibrinolysis (Fiumara, Kucher, Fanikos, et al., 2006). Nausea, vomiting, hypotension, and fever can occur with alteplase use; however, these are common sequelae after an MI and therefore may not be related to drug therapy. Other possible adverse effects, although not common, include occasional, mild hypersensitivity reactions; urticaria; fat embolism (which can occur with any thrombolytic); cerebral edema with fatal brain herniation (if administered when ≥3 hours have elapsed since onset of ischemic stroke); and CV complications (bradycardia, cardiogenic shock, arrhythmias, pulmonary edema, heart failure, cardiac arrest, recurrent ischemic reinfarction, myocardial rupture, mitral regurgitation, pericardial effusion, pericarditis, cardiac tamponade, venous thrombosis and embolism, and electromechanical dissociation).

Drug Interactions

For a complete list of the drugs that interact with alteplase, recombinant, see Table 32.7. Anticoagulant therapy with heparin should be discontinued before starting to infuse alteplase. When the alteplase infusion is complete, heparin can be resumed when the aPTT is less than twice the upper limit of normal. Heparin, or other anticoagulants, and alteplase together may increase the risk of bleeding; however, heparin is used to help prevent additional clots. Many herbs may also increase the risk of bleeding. Drugs that alter platelet function (e.g., aspirin, dipyridamole, and abciximab) may potentially increase the risk of bleeding if administered prior to or after alteplase therapy.

Antiplatelet therapy, such as aspirin, is often indicated post-thrombus, especially post-MI, and is given after alteplase infusion; however, large doses may increase the risk of bleeding. Aminocaproic acid and other antifibrinolytic agents decrease the effects of alteplase, because they have the opposite effect on blood clotting. The use of nitroglycerin should be avoided during alteplase therapy because it may decrease antithrombotic effects.

Assessment of Relevant Core Patient Variables

Health Status

Assess the patient for conditions that contraindicate or are precautions for administering alteplase. If the patient has an acute ischemic stroke, confirm that the onset was less than 3 hours ago, because this is the recommended time frame for starting alteplase therapy. Laboratory values, such as hematocrit, hemoglobin level, platelet count, PT, and aPTT, can provide baseline clotting information. Assess the patient's skin for old puncture sites or incisions from which bleeding may likely occur during alteplase therapy. Determine whether the patient is receiving or will be receiving other drug therapy that increases the risk for bleeding from alteplase treatment. If the patient has a pulmonary embolism, assess whether the patient has received a catecholamine to increase blood pressure, has cancer or diabetes, or has an elevated baseline INR. If any of these are present, the patient is more likely to suffer severe hemorrhage from alteplase therapy.

Life Span and Gender

Determine the patient's age and whether pregnancy is an issue. If the patient is currently pregnant or has delivered a child within 10 days, the risk of bleeding with alteplase is increased. Alteplase is a pregnancy category C drug. Assess whether the woman is breast-feeding, because it is not known whether alteplase is secreted in breast milk. Safety and efficacy in children have not been established. Although increasing age (greater than 76 years) decreases the benefits received from alteplase therapy, treatment is still effective in reducing death rates from these cardiovascular events. Older adults have an increased risk of intracranial bleeding when they are treated for acute ischemic stroke, but treatment is still beneficial and should be provided. Accelerated infusion of alteplase (within 90 minutes) slightly increases the risk of stroke in older adults.

Environment

Be aware of the environment in which the drug will be administered. Alteplase must be administered in an acute care setting because the patient needs close monitoring.

TABLE 32.7	Agents That Interact with P Alteplase		
Interactants	**Effect and Significance**	**Nursing Management**
Drugs: anticoagulants; antithrombin; antiplatelets; other thrombolytics	May increase the risk of bleeding.	Use with caution if both must be used. Assess for signs of bleeding.
Herbs: angelica; anise; arnica; asafetida; astragalus; bilberry; black currant; bladderwrack; bogbean; boldo; borage; bromelains; buchu; capsaicin; cat's claw; celery; certoparin; chaparral; cilostazol; clove oil; curcumin; dandelion; dong quai; evening primrose; fenugreek; feverfew; garlic; ginger; ginkgo; guggul; kava; licorice; meadowsweet; motherwort; red clover; skullcap; tan-shen	May increase the risk of bleeding. Risk is considered theoretical.	Use with caution if both must be used. Assess for signs of bleeding.
nitroglycerin	By increasing hepatic blood flow, nitroglycerin infusions may increase the clearance of alteplase, resulting in decreased alteplase plasma concentrations. Reduced alteplase plasma concentrations may be associated with reocclusion of the coronary arteries, less coronary artery reperfusion, and longer time to reperfusion.	Concomitant use of nitroglycerin and alteplase should be avoided if possible. If coadministration is necessary, the lowest effective dose of nitroglycerin should be used. Be aware that alteplase efficacy may be decreased and the risk of reocclusion may be increased.

Nursing Diagnosis and Outcome

• Risk for Injury related to drug-induced bleeding from alteplase

Desired outcome: *The patient will not suffer injury from alteplase.*

Planning and Intervention

Maximizing Therapeutic Effects

Reconstitute alteplase, recombinant in sterile water for injection without preservatives. Do not use bacteriostatic water. The reconstituted solution is colorless to pale yellow and transparent. Dilute the 50-mg vial using a large-bore (e.g., 18-gauge) needle. Direct the sterile water without preservatives at the dry drug. The 100-mg vial does not have a vacuum, unlike the 50-mg vial. Use the transfer device provided to reconstitute the alteplase. Mix the drug and diluent by gentle swirling; avoid shaking or excessive agitation. Once reconstituted, it may be administered intravenously, or it may be further diluted in either 0.9% normal saline or 5% dextrose for IV infusion. The drug may be infused either by accelerated infusion, over 90 minutes (current recommended method), or by a 3-hour infusion. Make yourself familiar with the protocol of the institution regarding which method is to be used or ensure that the order specifies the preferred administration technique. With both methods, more of the dose is administered in the first part of the infusion. Check the manufacturer's instructions for exact information about drug administration.

Minimizing Adverse Effects

Throughout the time the drug is administered, closely and continually monitor vital signs and observe for signs of active bleeding. Frank bleeding may occur at access sites, such as old IM injection or arterial puncture sites; or from orifices such as the vagina or rectum. Internal bleeding may be signaled by abdominal pain with coffee grounds–like emesis; black, tarry stools; joint pain; and changes in level of consciousness.

Closely assess for possible bleeding throughout therapy. If it is necessary to perform an arterial puncture during therapy, the site chosen should be one in which external pressure can be applied, such as the femoral artery. A pressure dressing should be applied to the site and checked carefully for evidence of bleeding. Venipuncture, if it must be done, should be done carefully to prevent bleeding. IM injections and unnecessary handling of patients should be avoided to prevent internal injury while they are receiving alteplase. If bleeding occurs and is not controllable with pressure, stop the infusion and notify the prescriber.

Multiple IV lines are usually indicated to enable administration of the alteplase and other drugs and to provide a route for obtaining blood samples during therapy. Start these lines before initiating alteplase therapy.

The patient should be connected to a cardiac monitor, both during the treatment and afterward, if alteplase is given as treatment for an MI. Arrhythmias may occur, especially after the clot has dissolved and the heart has

been reperfused. Antiarrhythmic therapy should be on hand when starting alteplase therapy. Notify the prescriber if substantial arrhythmias occur.

When therapy is given to treat a PE, monitor respiratory status carefully. Note respiratory rate, dyspnea, pulse oximetry, and arterial blood gas findings in addition to all the assessments described previously.

When alteplase is given to treat acute ischemic stroke, monitor the blood pressure closely during therapy. Avoid starting alteplase if 3 hours or more have elapsed from the onset of the stroke, because the benefits of treatment during this time frame are not known, and this timing increases the risk of cerebral edema with fatal brain herniation and may increase the risk of cerebral hemorrhage.

Providing Patient and Family Education

• Emphasize to patients and families the need for frequent assessment, pressure dressings, and activity limitations.
• Instruct patients to notify their nurse if they experience signs of adverse reactions.

Ongoing Assessment and Evaluation

Vital signs, evidence of bleeding, and laboratory test results should be assessed throughout therapy with alteplase, recombinant as described previously. Therapy is judged effective if the patient sustains no injury or adverse effects of the drug, the clot dissolves, and circulation is restored.

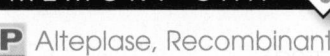

MEMORY CHIP

P Alteplase, Recombinant

• Used to break up blood clots posing acute medical emergencies such as acute myocardial infarctions, acute ischemic strokes, and pulmonary embolus
• Works by binding to the fibrin in a clot and converting the trapped plasminogen to plasmin. Fibrinolysis then occurs.
• Major contraindications: current internal bleeding, especially intracranial; recent surgeries or medical events in which patient bled or which put patient at increased risk for bleeding now; seizure at onset of stroke; or severe uncontrolled hypertension
• Most common adverse effect: bleeding
• Most serious adverse effect: bleeding
• **Life span alert: Current pregnancy or delivery of a child within the last 10 days increases risk for bleeding; older adults are more likely to have intracranial bleeding.**
• Maximizing therapeutic effects: Avoid vigorous shaking or agitation when reconstituting; administer IV over 90 minutes to 3 hours.
• Minimizing adverse effects: Monitor for bleeding; avoid venipuncture and arterial puncture if possible, use pressure dressings when needed; handle patient gently; when treating ischemic stroke, give within 3 hours of onset of symptoms.
• Most important patient education: need for frequent assessment and limitations on activity

Drugs Closely Related to Alteplase, Recombinant

Thrombolytic Enzymes: Streptokinase, Urokinase, and Anistreplase

Streptokinase (Streptase) is used in treating acute evolving MI, pulmonary embolism DVT, arterial thrombosis, or embolism, and to open occluded arteriovenous cannulas. Unlike alteplase, which works by attaching to the fibrin in a thrombus and converting the trapped plasminogen to plasmin, streptokinase works indirectly to activate plasminogen. Streptokinase acts with plasminogen to produce an "activator complex" that converts plasminogen to plasmin. Because fibrin is not necessary for streptokinase to activate plasminogen, streptokinase can produce more systemic bleeding than alteplase, recombinant. Allergic reactions are more common in streptokinase than with alteplase because it is not produced from DNA recombinant technology. Fever and chills are the common allergic reactions. Hypotension is also more common in streptokinase and may be severe. Because adverse effects are more common with streptokinase, its use has become more limited, and alteplase, recombinant is the drug most frequently used.

Urokinase (Abbokinase) is used in treating pulmonary embolism, lysis of coronary artery thrombi, and re-establishing patency of occluded IV catheters. Anistreplase (Eminase) is used in treating acute MI. It has a longer half-life than streptokinase or urokinase but otherwise possesses similar characteristics.

Drug Significantly Different From Alteplase, Recombinant

Drotrecogin Alfa (Activated)

Drotrecogin alfa, activated (Xigris) is an anticoagulant and profibrinolytic drug. Unlike alteplase, recombinant, drotrecogin alfa is used to reduce mortality in adults with severe sepsis who are at high risk for death. Very specific criteria must be met for the patient to be a candidate for use of this drug, because it is appropriate only if the patient is likely to die from the sepsis.

Drotrecogin alfa rapidly increases protein C and antithrombin levels, and it normalizes levels of plasminogen. Remember that protein C inactivates factors V and VII and may also limit thrombin-induced inflammatory responses. In other words, protein C prevents processes that are involved in creating stable clots. As an agent that increases the level of active protein C, drotrecogin alfa also has anti-inflammatory effects. As with alteplase, recombinant, bleeding is the most common adverse effect of drotrecogin alfa. The drug may prolong aPTT but has minimal effect on PT; the PT should be used to monitor the status of the coagulopathy. Drotrecogin alfa may cause serious hemorrhage. It should be discontinued 2 hours before procedures with an inherent risk of bleeding.

DRUG THERAPY FOR HYPOCOAGULATION

In addition to preventing blood coagulation, drug therapy may also be used to promote coagulation. Drug classes used to treat hypocoagulation, or subnormal coagulation, are clotting factors and hemostatic agents.

Table 32.8 presents a summary of information about drugs used to treat hypocoagulation.

C CLOTTING FACTORS

Deficiencies of normal blood clotting factors are associated with prolonged bleeding and clot formation times. These deficiencies result from an inherited absence of the factor (hemophilia) or from a decreased synthesis of the factor or factors. Replacement of these factors with clotting factors is the treatment of choice. The prototype clotting factor is antihemophilic factor (AHF). Other drugs in the class include

TABLE 32.8 Summary of Selected Drugs for Hypocoagulation			
Drug (Trade) Name	**Selected Indications**	**Route and Dosage Range**	**Pharmacokinetics**
P antihemophilic factor (Alphanate, Bioclate, Helixate, Hemofil M, Humate-P, Koate-HP, Kogenate, Monoclate-P, Profilate HP, Recombinate)	Temporarily replaces clotting factors missing because of hemophilia Prevents or corrects bleeding episodes Prophylaxis Mild to severe hemorrhage	*Adult:* administered so that factor VIII level assay is 20%–40% of normal or up to 80%–100% of normal after trauma or major surgery*	*Onset:* Immediate *Duration:* Unknown $t_{1/2}$: 12 h
anti-inhibitor coagulant complex (Autoplex T, FEIBA VH)	Controls bleeding in patients with factor VIII inhibitors Joint hemorrhage	*Adult:* IV, 50–100 U/kg at 12-h intervals (FEIBA VH) 25–100 U/kg, may repeat in 6 h (Autoplex I)	*Onset:* Immediate *Duration:* Unknown $t_{1/2}$: Unknown
P aminocaproic acid (Amicar)	Controls fibrinolysis and stops bleeding	*Adult:* PO or IV, 4–5 g over the first hour followed by 1–1.25 g/h for 8 h	*Onset:* PO, rapid; IV immediate *Duration:* IV, 2–3 h $t_{1/2}$: IV, 3 h

*Dosing is highly individualized to achieve desired results. See manufacturer's instructions.

anti-inhibitor coagulant complex and factor IX complex. AHF is from pooled human blood sources. It is screened for hepatitis antibodies and heated to prevent the transmission of hepatitis. Blood donors are screened for human immunodeficiency virus (HIV) as well, and positive sources are screened again. The chance of disease transmission, therefore, still exists but is quite small.

Nursing Management of the Patient Receiving P Antihemophilic Factor

Core Drug Knowledge

Pharmacotherapeutics

In patients with a demonstrated deficiency of clotting factor VIII, hemophilia A, AHF is used to prevent and control excessive bleeding. The drug effect is short term because the factor is used up in the clotting process (see Table 32.8).

Pharmacokinetics

Administered intravenously, AHF is totally absorbed. It is rapidly removed from the plasma because it is used in the clotting process. Its half-life is from 4 to 24 hours, with a 12-hour average half-life (see Table 32.8).

Pharmacodynamics

Factor VIII is an essential component of blood clotting. It is required for the conversion of prothrombin to thrombin. Patients with factor VIII deficiencies have markedly prolonged bleeding and clotting times.

Contraindications and Precautions

A contraindication to AHF is a hypersensitivity to mouse protein (limited to products that contain monoclonal antibodies). Considered a pregnancy risk category C drug, AHF should be used in pregnancy only if necessary. The pooled blood product may contain minute amounts of blood type A or B. If the patient receives a large quantity of the preparation, a risk of hemolysis from blood type incompatibility exists. In patients who have not previously received multiple infusions of blood or plasma products, signs or symptoms of some viral infections, especially hepatitis C, are likely to develop. These patients, particularly those with mild hemophilia, should receive single-donor products. AHF also carries risk of HIV transmission, although current viral-depleting processes and donor-screening practices have reduced the potential for transmission considerably.

Adverse Effects

Several adverse effects may result from AHF, although none is common. Allergic reactions include anaphylaxis, urticaria, nausea, and chills. Other adverse effects include tachycardia, hypotension, headache, drowsiness, lethargy, vision disturbances, loss of consciousness, vomiting, hepatitis, intravascular hemolysis, back pain, chest constriction, and wheezing.

Drug Interactions

No important interactions are associated with AHF.

Assessment of Relevant Core Patient Variables

Health Status

Important lab values to assess before administration of antihemophilic factor include factor VIII level assays, CBC, direct Coombs test, urinalysis, aPTT, thromboplastin generation test, and prothrombin generation test. These results provide data regarding current clotting times and serve as baseline information to determine whether therapeutic reactions are occurring during therapy. In the physical examination, be alert for signs of active bleeding and extent of the bleeding.

Life Span and Gender

Because the safety of AHF during pregnancy has not been established, determine whether the patient is pregnant.

Lifestyle, Diet, and Habits

During assessment, investigate any patient behaviors likely to result in injury, such as participation in contact sports.

Environment

Be aware that AHF is generally self-administered at home by the patient or family.

Culture and Inherited Traits

Patients with religious views that forbid receiving blood products may be opposed to receiving AHF. Discuss with the patient beliefs that may have an impact on drug therapy.

Nursing Diagnosis and Outcome

• Risk for Injury, Hemorrhage, related to deficiency of clotting factor VIII

  Desired outcome: The patient will receive enough factor VIII to prevent injury.

Planning and Intervention

Maximizing Therapeutic Effects

Refrigeration is required for AHF until it is used. Before reconstitution, warm the concentrate and the diluent provided by the manufacturer to room temperature. Add the diluent to the concentrate in the vial, and rotate the vial carefully until the contents dissolve. To help prevent gel formation, the vial should not be shaken. If a gel forms during reconstitution of AHF, notify the pharmacy or blood bank and withhold the AHF. Use only plastic syringes for drawing up the reconstituted drug, because the AHF solution can stick to glass surfaces.

Monitor coagulation studies during therapy to assess the effectiveness of AHF.

Minimizing Adverse Effects

After dilution, administer AHF within 3 hours to prevent bacterial growth. Use only the IV route. Apply pressure to all venipuncture sites for at least 5 minutes. Avoid IM injections to prevent bleeding into the muscle. Other measures include monitoring intake and output ratios and inspecting urine for color. If there is a discrepancy in ratios or if urine becomes red or orange, a sign of hemolytic reaction, notify the prescriber.

Monitor for decreased hematocrit and increased Coombs test, both of which are indications of hemolytic anemia, and assess for allergic reaction. If present, stop the infusion and notify the prescriber.

Providing Patient and Family Education

- Instruct patients and families to observe for bleeding from gums, skin, urine, stools, or emesis.
- Caution patients to avoid products containing aspirin or ibuprofen because they may further impair clotting.
- Discuss strategies to prevent bleeding, such as using a soft toothbrush, avoiding IM and SC injections, and avoiding behaviors and activities that are likely to cause injury.
- Advise patients to wear medical identification that identifies their disease.
- Emphasize that improved screening factors have decreased the risk of transmission of hepatitis or HIV substantially, although a slight risk of disease transmission remains.

Ongoing Assessment and Evaluation

Blood studies are monitored as previously described when AHF is administered. Therapy is effective when prolonged bleeding is prevented or stopped.

Drugs Closely Related to P Antihemophilic Factor

Anti-inhibitor coagulant complex (Autoplex T; FEIBA-VH Immuno) treats blood coagulation disorders associated with inhibitors of factors VIII, XI, or XII; the drug is used to treat and prevent hemorrhage. It is also used in hemophilia A or B for spontaneous bleeding or to cover surgical interventions. The exact mechanism of action of anti-inhibitor

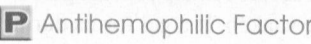

MEMORY CHIP

P Antihemophilic Factor

- Provides factor VIII for those with hemophilia; made from pooled human sources
- Temporarily meets needs for clotting factor to prevent or stop bleeding
- Dosage is individualized to needs of patient
- No common adverse effects
- Most serious adverse effects: slight risk of hemolytic anemia and transmission of hepatitis or HIV
- Minimizing adverse effects: monitor hematocrit and Coombs test result (hemolytic anemia)
- Most important patient education: Teach patients to avoid injury to prevent bleeding, and to carry or wear identification of the disease.

coagulant complex is unknown, although it may be related to one or more of the active clotting factors and their ability to bypass the factor VIII inhibitor. Anti-inhibitor coagulant complex is not used to treat bleeding that results from deficiencies of coagulation factors, in DIC, in fibrinolysis, or if there are normal coagulation mechanisms present; the drug is made from human plasma and may therefore contain infectious agents.

Human factor IX complex is used to treat hemophilia B (Christmas disease), although it is not a substitute for fresh-frozen plasma used in mild factor IX deficiency. The complex contains factors II (prothrombin), VII, IX, and X. Factors II (prothrombin), VII, and X are required for converting prothrombin to thrombin, and factor IX is necessary for prothrombin production. The complex prevents or controls bleeding in hemophilia B, controls bleeding episodes in patients with factor VIII inhibitors, and reverses oral anticoagulant-induced hemorrhage. Human factor IX complex (Konyne 80, Profilnine SD, Proplex T, and AlphaNine SD) has one variant: mononine. Mononine contains factor IX, but after reconstitution, it has undetectable levels of factors II (prothrombin), VII, and X. It also contains histidine, mannitol, and mouse protein. Factor IX is also available in a recombinant form called BeneFix. A Chinese hamster ovary cell line has been genetically engineered to secrete recombinant factor IX into a culture medium that contains no proteins derived from human or animal sources, thus producing this form of the drug.

Factor IX, human contains only factor IX. Human factor IX complex and factor IX are administered intravenously. Dosage depends on the condition of the patient and the manufacturer's instructions, which vary according to the manufacturer. For additional information, refer to Table 32.8.

Anti-Inhibitor Coagulant Factor

Made from pooled human plasma, anti-inhibitor coagulant factor is a concentrate of activated and precursor clotting factors. It differs from AHF in that it is useful in treating patients with hemophilia who have significant levels of factor VIII inhibitors. It therefore allows clotting to occur in patients with hemophilia who are not responsive to AHF (see Table 32.8).

© HEMOSTATIC DRUGS

Hemostatics stop blood loss by enhancing blood coagulation. There are two types of hemostatic agents: systemic and topical. Systemic agents interfere with the breakdown of clots. Topical agents are used to control small amounts of bleeding or oozing, usually following surgery. The prototype systemic hemostatic drug is aminocaproic acid (Amicar). Tranexamic acid is also a hemostatic drug. Additional topical hemostatic drugs are presented in Table 32.9.

TABLE 32.9 Topical Hemostatic Agents

Hemostatic Agent and Action	Indication	Dosage	Contraindications and Adverse Effects	Nursing Management
Topical thrombin (Thrombinar, Thrombogen, Thrombostat). When applied directly on the wound, thrombin converts fibrinogen to fibrin.	Used in oozing wounds after dental surgery, plastic surgery, neurosurgery, epistaxis, and graft procedures. Also used with absorbable gelatin sponges for hemostasis during surgery	The amount of bleeding determines the strength of solution, 100 to 2,000 U/mL.	This is included in pregnancy risk category C. The drug may cause a hypersensitivity reaction. If the drug enters the bloodstream, intravascular coagulation occurs and may result in death. Reported adverse effects include febrile episodes and allergic reaction when used to treat epistaxis.	Clean blood from affected area with gauze pads. Apply solution soon after it is reconstituted (within 3 h of reconstitution if it has to be refrigerated). Monitor the application site frequently to detect any recurrence of blood loss.
Microfibrillar collagen hemostat (Avitene Hemostat, Hemotene, Hemoped). Attracts platelets when applied to a bleeding area. Platelet aggregation fills the space with a fibrin clot.	Adjunct in controlling bleeding when traditional methods are not effective or useful	The dose is impregnated into a web or sponge form. The amount used depends on the amount of bleeding.	The drug should not be resterilized after use; its use in infected wounds is not recommended. Its effect during pregnancy is not known. Excess drug should be removed after use to prevent complications. Adverse effects include increase in infection, formation of adhesions, and hypersensitivity.	Avoid handling the substance with wet gloves or instruments, because it will adhere to a wet surface. After application to the wound, apply pressure using a dry gauze sponge. Discard any unused material; this agent may not be resterilized.
Absorbable gelatin sponge (Gelfoam). Product absorbs and holds many times its weight in whole blood. Wound may be closed over sponge, which will dissolve slowly.	Used in dental and oral surgery, neurosurgery, and prostatectomy to control bleeding	It is supplied in several different sizes to match size of the wound and the amount of bleeding.	The preparation should not be resterilized using heat, because heat may alter the product's effectiveness. The sponge should not be used on incisions. It has no indication for use in postpartum bleeding. It should be used sparingly in areas where expansion may be detrimental to surrounding structures. Adverse effects include potential for infection or abscess formation.	Assess wound frequently for bleeding. Apply during surgery as recommended by the surgeon—either dry or saturated in saline solution. Squeeze sponge to remove any air bubbles when the sponge is to be moistened on application. After application, apply pressure with a gauze pad for 10–15 s.
Absorbable gelatin film (Gel- film, Gelfilm Ophthalmic). Cellophane-like material that becomes rubbery when wet and may be implanted into body tissue; will be slowly absorbed.	Used in neurosurgery, thoracic surgery, and ocular surgery	This is supplied in a standard size and cut to fit the area	Using this film in contaminated wounds is contraindicated.	Soak the film in a sterile saline solution until pliable. The surgeon will cut the film to the desired size.
Oxidized cellulose (Oxycel, Surgicel). Exact mechanism of action is unknown but provides hemostasis when applied directly on bleeding area. It does not affect normal blood clotting, but in con-tact with blood, this product forms an artificial clot.	Used to control bleeding when sutures or clipping are not possible. Primarily for bleeding from capillaries, venioles, or arterioles. Used for oral and dental surgery	This is supplied impregnated into pads, pledgets, and strips. Number used depends on amount of bleeding and size of wound.	This product is contraindicated for use as wound packing. Product should not be used in fractures or spinal surgery because it may interfere with bone regrowth or cause cyst formation. It is not recommended for use in bleeding from large arteries or with serous oozing. This drug product should not be used if it has been autoclaved because this method of sterilization causes it to break down. The product may be left in the wound, but its removal once hemostasis is achieved is recommended. If used during a laminectomy, it must be removed. Adverse effects include nasal burning, encapsulation of fluid, antibody reactions.	Use a surgical clamp to remove substance from its container. Do not wet the product; instead, apply it dry. Monitor wounds of patients using oxidized cellulose for signs of bleeding.

Nursing Management of the Patient Receiving Aminocaproic Acid

Core Drug Knowledge

Pharmacotherapeutics

Aminocaproic acid treats severe, life-threatening hemorrhage from systemic hyperfibrinolysis or urinary fibrinolysis. Systemic hyperfibrinolysis has occurred with heart surgery, abruptio placentae, cirrhosis of the liver, and neoplastic disorders. Urinary hyperfibrinolysis is associated with severe trauma, shock, prostatectomy, nephrectomy, and renal cancers.

Unapproved uses of aminocaproic acid include: preventing recurrent subarachnoid hemorrhage, to control bleeding in thrombocytopenia or oral bleeding, as well as the prevetion of perioperative bleeding associated with cardiac surgery. Aminocaproic acid is also used to treat overdoses of fibrinolytic drugs, such as streptokinase.

Pharmacokinetics

Aminocaproic acid is administered orally or by IV infusion. After oral administration, the drug is quickly absorbed; through both routes, it is widely distributed. Most of the drug is excreted unchanged in the urine.

Pharmacodynamics

Aminocaproic acid prevents fibrinolysis in two ways. First, it blocks the action of plasminogen activators, thus interfering with the formation of active plasmin. Second, it interferes with the binding of active plasmin to fibrin, thus preventing breakdown of fibrin. The result is stabilization of the blood clot and control of bleeding.

Contraindications and Precautions

Aminocaproic acid should be used only in life-threatening situations and then only when overactivity of the fibrinolytic system is verified by laboratory testing. The drug is not to be used in patients with active intravascular clotting, such as DIC.

Rapid I.V. injection (IVP) of undiluted solution is not recommended due to possible hypotension, bradycardia, and arrhythmia.

This drug is used with caution in patients with uremia or hepatic disease. Cautious use is recommended in patients with upper renal tract bleeding and in those with cardiac, liver, or renal disease. Cautious use is also recommended in pregnancy or lactation because safety has not been established.

Adverse Effects

The most common adverse effect of aminocaproic acid is GI distress (anorexia, nausea). Life-threatening or serious adverse effects are rare; these include convulsions, rhabdomyolysis (acute, sometimes fatal disease with destruction of the skeletal muscle), and renal failure. Other adverse effects that may occur include headache, dizziness, seizures, malaise, thrombophlebitis, hypotension (after IV administration), arrhythmias, tinnitus, nasal congestion, vomiting, abdominal cramps, diarrhea, and diuresis. Symptoms of overdosage include nausea, diarrhea, delirium, hepatic necrosis, and thromboembolism.

Drug Interactions

An increase in clotting factors leading to hypercoagulation may occur if aminocaproic acid is administered concurrently with oral contraceptives or estrogen (Table 32.10).

Assessment of Relevant Core Patient Variables

Health Status

Initially, identify contraindications to the drug by determining clotting factor levels and platelet counts to assess the severity of the patient's condition.

Life Span and Gender

During assessment, evaluate the patient's possible pregnancy or breast-feeding status. If the patient is a child, measure his or her weight so that a correct dosage can be calculated.

Environment

Be aware of the environment in which the drug will be administered. Aminocaproic acid is administered in an acute care setting, such as a hospital.

Nursing Diagnosis and Outcome

- Risk for Altered Cardiovascular Perfusion related to volume loss secondary to uncontrolled bleeding or thrombophlebitis secondary to adverse effects of aminocaproic acid

  Desired outcome: *Adequate perfusion will be maintained as evidenced by presence of pulses, normal skin color and warmth, and capillary refill.*

Planning and Intervention

Minimizing Adverse Effects

Monitor vital signs at start of therapy and throughout therapy at intervals appropriate to the patient's condition. Every

TABLE 32.10	Agents That Interact with P Aminocaproic Acid	
Interactants	**Effect and Significance**	**Nursing Management**
oral contraceptives	Increase in clotting factors may lead to hypercoagulant state and may possibly increase risk of thrombus formation.	Monitor for signs of thrombus.
estrogens	Same as above.	Same as above.

15 to 30 minutes, assess the patient for bleeding, particularly at incision and old injection sites.

To administer aminocaproic acid, use an IV infusion pump to regulate the flow rate. Assess the IV site and line for patency. Verify that the line is secured to prevent thrombophlebitis. Do not mix aminocaproic acid with other drugs.

Connect the patient to a cardiac monitor to detect arrhythmias, and observe for signs of thromboembolic complications, such as chest pain, dyspnea, changes in skin color and temperature, pain in an extremity, or changes in peripheral pulses. Notify the prescriber if these changes occur.

Additional ways to guard against adverse drug effects include monitoring intake and output and monitoring neurologic status in patients with subarachnoid hemorrhage. Notify the prescriber of major discrepancies or changes.

To combat nausea, encourage patients to eat small, frequent meals.

Providing Patient and Family Education

- Teach patients and families about the role of aminocaproic acid in controlling bleeding. They also must understand the importance of reporting any bleeding or symptoms of thromboembolism immediately.
- Instruct patients to change positions slowly to prevent orthostatic hypotension.

Ongoing Assessment and Evaluation

Monitor the patient throughout treatment and recovery for signs and symptoms of bleeding or embolism or any other untoward event. Drug therapy is effective if bleeding is controlled.

Drugs Closely Related to Aminocaproic Acid

Tranexamic acid (Cyklokapron) is another systemic hemostatic agent. It competitively inhibits activation of plasminogen. It is used to reduce or prevent hemorrhage during and after tooth extraction in patients with hemophilia. After oral administration, between 30% and 50% of the drug is absorbed. The drug remains in serum for 7 to 8 hours and is excreted from the body in the urine.

Tranexamic acid is contraindicated for patients with subarachnoid hemorrhage. It should be used cautiously in patients with acquired defective color vision because altered color vision is an early sign of visual toxicity. Caution should be used in pregnant or lactating women and in patients with renal insufficiency.

Aprotinin, also a systemic hemostatic agent, is indicated to reduce perioperative blood loss and the need for blood transfusion in patients undergoing cardiopulmonary bypass in the course of CABG surgery. It has also been studied for use in other types of surgery. The exact mechanism by which it reduces bleeding is unclear.

Coagulation factor VIIa (NovoSeven) is used to prevent or treat bleeding related to factor VII deficiency. Factor VIIa is a vitamin K–dependent glycoprotein that is structurally similar to human plasma-derived factor VIIa. Administered intravenously, it promotes hemostasis by complexing with tissue factor and activating coagulation factors IX and X. Activated factor X, when it forms a complex with other factors, converts prothrombin to thrombin and fibrinogen to fibrin to form a hemostatic plug.

Thrombin (Thrombin-JMI; Thrombogen), unlike aminocaproic acid, is applied topically to control hemorrhage. Thrombin is a protein substance of bovine origin that immediately clots the fibrinogen of the blood without the aid of a physiological agent.

CHAPTER SUMMARY

- Anticoagulants do not break down existing clots; they prevent clots from forming.
- The parenteral anticoagulant heparin and the oral anticoagulant warfarin are used in treating thrombus or thromboembolic disorders to prevent extension of the clot or formation of an embolism. They are also used in high-risk patients to prevent formation of an initial clot. Patients may be taking both drugs at the same time during dose regulation of warfarin.
- Low-molecular-weight heparins are administered subcutaneously daily. They have been found to be effective for the same conditions as infusions of heparin. They require less monitoring of blood clotting times, because they have a very predictable effect. Patients can be taught to self-administer the SC injection at home.
- Education for patients taking anticoagulant therapy should include safety measures to prevent bleeding, instructions to be alert for signs of bleeding, and directions for what to do if bleeding occurs.
- Antiplatelet drugs prevent platelet aggregation and thereby prevent thrombus formation. They are used prophylactically to prevent CVAs (also called strokes) and MIs (also

---

MEMORY CHIP

Aminocaproic Acid

- Used to treat life-threatening bleeding from systemic hyperfibrinolysis or urinary fibrinolysis
- Prevents breakdown of the stable clot and controls bleeding
- Major contraindications: Use only in life-threatening situations and only when the overactivity of the fibrinolytic system is verified by laboratory testing; DIC.
- Most common adverse effect: GI distress
- Most serious adverse effects: renal failure (rare), rhabdomyolysis (rare), thromboembolism, and arrhythmias
- Minimizing adverse effects: Use IV pump, assess for bleeding or signs of thromboembolism, and place patient on cardiac monitor to detect arrhythmias.
- Most important patient education: Teach patients to report symptoms of thromboembolism

called heart attacks). They are used as part of treatment for ischemic strokes, after thrombolytic therapy.

- Hemorheologic agents promote the flexibility of the RBCs and decrease blood viscosity to prevent thrombus formation.
- Thrombolytic drugs break down existing clots. They are used in acute medical emergencies, such as evolving MI, pulmonary embolism, and acute ischemic stroke. Although they can save lives, these drugs carry a risk for inducing hemorrhage. The patient must be closely monitored during this drug therapy.
- Clotting factors are administered when the patient has a deficiency of clotting factors resulting from heredity or disease. These drugs allow natural clotting to occur and prevent massive blood loss.
- Hemostatics are drugs used to promote blood coagulation. Hemostatics come in systemic and topical forms. Systemic hemostatics also interfere with the breaking down of clots.

QUESTIONS FOR STUDY AND REVIEW

1. Describe how heparin and warfarin differ in their effects on the clotting cycle.
2. What interventions would promote safety while the patient is receiving heparin by continuous IV infusion?
3. Describe which laboratory values need to be monitored if the patient is receiving heparin and warfarin. What criteria do you use to determine whether these drugs are in a therapeutic range?
4. Why is it important to assess the usual vitamin K intake for a patient who will be receiving warfarin, but not for the patient who will be receiving heparin?
5. What assessment should be performed if the patient is receiving the antiplatelet drug clopidogrel and the antilipid drug fluvastatin?
6. What is the difference between an anticoagulant and a thrombolytic drug?
7. What drug therapy would be used for a patient who has hemophilia and who requires an inguinal hernia repair?

NEED MORE HELP?

Chapter 32 of the Study Guide to Accompany *Drug Therapy in Nursing*, 4th Edition, contains NCLEX-style questions and other learning activities to reinforce your understanding of the concepts presented in this chapter. For additional information or to purchase the study guide, visit thePoint.

REFERENCES

American Heart Association/American Stroke Association Council on Stroke. (2006). AHA/ASA guidelines for prevention of stroke in patients with ischemic stroke or transient ischemic attack. Retrieved from *http://stroke.ahajournals.org/cgi/content/full/37/2/577.*

American Diabetes Association. (2004). Clinical practice guidelines: Aspirin therapy in diabetes. Retrieved from *http://care.diabetesjournals.org/cgi/content/full/27/suppl_1/s72#SEC5.*

Buller, H. R., Agnelli, G., Hull, R. D., et al. (2004). Antithrombotic therapy for venous thromboembolic disease: The seventh ACCP conference on antithrombotic and thrombolytic therapy. *Chest*, 126(3 Suppl.):401S–428S.

Chen, Z. M., Jiang, L. X., Chen, Y. P., et al.; The COMMIT Collaborative Group Members. (2005). Addition of clopidogrel to aspirin in 45,852 patients with acute myocardial infarction: Randomized placebo-controlled trial. COMMIT (Clopidogrel and Metoprolol in Myocardial Infarction Trial) collaborative group. *Lancet*, 366:1607–1621.

Derex, L., & Nighoghossian, N. (2008). Intracerebral haemorrhage after thromboysis for acute ischaemic stroke: An update. *Journal of Neurology, Neurosurgery and Psychiatry* 79(10):1093–1099.

Diez, J. G., Medina, H. M., Cheong, B. Y., O'Meallie, L., & Ferguson, J. J. (2009). Safety of enoxaparin versus unfractionated heparin during percutaneous coronary intervention. *Texas Heart Institute Journal / from the Texas Heart Institute of St.Luke's Episcopal Hospital, Texas Children's Hospital,* 36(2):98–103.

Dong, B., Hao, Q., Yue, J., Wu, T., & Liu, G. (2009). Thrombolytic therapy for pulmonary embolism. *Cochrane Database Systematic Review,* (3):CD004437.

Fahs, P. S. S., & Kinney, M. R. (1991). The abdomen, thigh, and arm as sites for subcutaneous sodium heparin injections. *Nursing Research,* 40(4):204–207.

FDA. Label for prasugrel. (2009). Retrieved from : http://www.accessdata.fda.gov/scripts/cder/drugsatfda/index.cfm?fuseaction=Search.Label_ApprovalHistory. Accessed November 1, 2009

Fiumara, K., Kucher, N., Fanikos, J., et al. (2006). Predictors of major hemorrhage following fibrinolysis for acute pulmonary embolism. *American Journal of Cardiology,* 97(1):127–129.

Grant, P. J., Brotman, D. J., & Jaffer, A. K. (2009). Perioperative anticoagulant management. *The Medical Clinics of North America,* 93(5):1105–1121.

Hacke, W., Kaste, M., Bluhmki, E., et al. (2008). Thrombolysis with alteplase 3 to 4.5 hours after acute ischemic stroke. *New England Journal of Medicine,* 359:1317.

Hadley, S. A., Change, M., & Rogers, K. (1996). Effect of syringe size on bruising following subcutaneous heparin injection. *American Journal of Critical Care,* 5(4):271–276.

Hart, R. G., Halperin, J. L., Pearce, L. A., et al.; Stroke Prevention in Atrial Fibrillation Investigators. (2003). Lessons from the stroke prevention in atrial fibrillation trials. *Annals of Internal Medicine,* 138(10):832–838.

Hirsh, J., Albers, G.W., & Schünemann, H. J. (2008). Executive Summary. American College of Chest Physicians Evidence-Based Clinical Practice Guidelines (8th Edition), *CHEST* ; 133(6 suppl);71S–109S. Retrieved from: http://chestjournal.chestpubs.org/content/133/6_suppl/71S.full#sec-22. Accessed on November 1, 2009.

Jennings, L. K. (2005). Current strategies with eptifibatide and other antiplatelet agents in percutaneous coronary intervention and acute coronary syndromes. *Expert Opinion on Drug Metabolism and Toxicology,* 1(4):727–737.

Lansberg, M., Albers, G., & Wijman, C. (2007). Symptomatic intracerebral hemorrhage following thrombolytic therapy for actue ischemic stroke: a review of the risk factors. *Cerebrovascular Diseases,* 24(1):1–10.

Lee, J. M., Park, S., Shin, D. J., Choi, D., Shim, C. Y., Ko, Y. G., et al. (2009). Relation of genetic polymorphisms in the cytochrome P450 gene with clopidogrel resistance after drug-eluting stent implantation in Koreans. *The American Journal of Cardiology,* 104(1):46–51.

Lim, W., Dentali, F., Eikelboom, J. W., et al. (2006). Meta-analysis: Low molecular weight heparin and bleeding in patients with severe renal insufficiency. *Annals of Internal Medicine,* 144(9):673–684.

Matthews, M., Sharma, J., Snyder, K., Nataragjan, S., Siddiqui, A., Hopkins, L., Levy, E. L. (2009). Safety, effectiveness and practicality of endovascular therapy within the first 3 hours of acute ischemic stroke onset. *Neurosurgery,* 65(5):860–865.

Scirica, B. M., Sabatine, M. S., Morrow, D. A., et al. The TIMI Study Group. (2006). The role of clopidogrel in early and sustained arterial patency after fibrinolysis for ST-segment elevation myocardial infarction: The ECG CLARITY-TIMI 28 Study. *Journal of the American College of Cardiology,* 48(1):37–42.

Tourmousoglou, C. E., & Rokkas, C. K. (2008). Clopidogrel and aspirin in cardiovascular medicine: Responders or not–current best available evidence. *Cardiovascular & Hematological Agents in Medicinal Chemistry,* 6(4):312–322.

UpToDate. (2009). Therapeutic uses of heparin and low molecular weight heparin. Retrieved from http://www.uptodate.com.

UpToDate. (2009a). Fibrinolytic (thrombolytic) therapy in pulmonary embolism and deep vein thrombosis. Retrieved from http://www.uptodate.com

UpToDate. (2009b). NSAIDs (including aspirin): Pathogenesis of gastroduodenal toxicity. Retrieved from http://www.uptodate.com

van Dongen, C. J., van den Belt, A. G., Prins, M. H., et al. (2004). Fixed dose subcutaneous low molecular weight heparins versus adjusted dose unfractionated heparin for venous thromboembolism. *Cochrane Database of Systematic Reviews,* (4):CD001100.

Wan, S., Quinlan, D. J., Agnelli, G., et al. (2004). Thrombolysis compared with heparin for the initial treatment of pulmonary embolism: A meta-analysis of the randomized controlled trials. *Circulation,* 110(6):744–749. (No updated version)

Wardlaw, J. M., Zoppo, G., Yamaguchi, T., et al. (2003). Thrombolysis for acute ischemic stroke. *Cochrane Database System Review,* (3):CD000213.

Warkentin, T. E., & Greinacher, A. (2004). Heparin-induced thrombocytopenia: Recognition, treatment, and prevention: The Seventh ACCP Conference on Antithrombotic and Thrombolytic Therapy. *Chest,* 126:321S.

Weitz, J. I., Hirsh, J., & Samama, M. M. (2008). New antithrombotic drugs: American College of Chest Physicians Evidence-Based Clinical Practice Guidelines (8th Edition). *Chest,* 133(6 Suppl):234S–256S.

Wooldridge, J. B., & Jackson, J. G. (1988). Evaluation of bruises and areas of induration after two techniques of subcutaneous heparin injection. *Heart and Lung,* 17(5):476–82.

33

Drugs Affecting Hematopoiesis

Learning Objectives

At the completion of this chapter the student will:

1. Identify core drug knowledge about drugs that affect hematopoiesis.
2. Identify core patient variables relevant to drugs that affect hematopoiesis.
3. Relate the interaction of core drug knowledge to core patient variables for drugs that affect hematopoiesis.
4. Generate a nursing plan of care from the interactions between core drug knowledge and core patient variables for drugs that affect hematopoiesis.
5. Describe nursing interventions to maximize therapeutic and minimize adverse effects for drugs that affect hematopoiesis.
6. Determine key points for patient and family education for drugs that affect hematopoiesis.

Key Terms

anemia	hematopoiesis	neutrophils
aplastic	leukocytes	phagocytosis
erythrocytes	lymphocytes	platelets
erythropoiesis	macrophages	thrombocytopenia
erythropoietin	monocytes	thrombopoietin
granulocytes	neutropenia	

Drugs Affecting Hematopoiesis

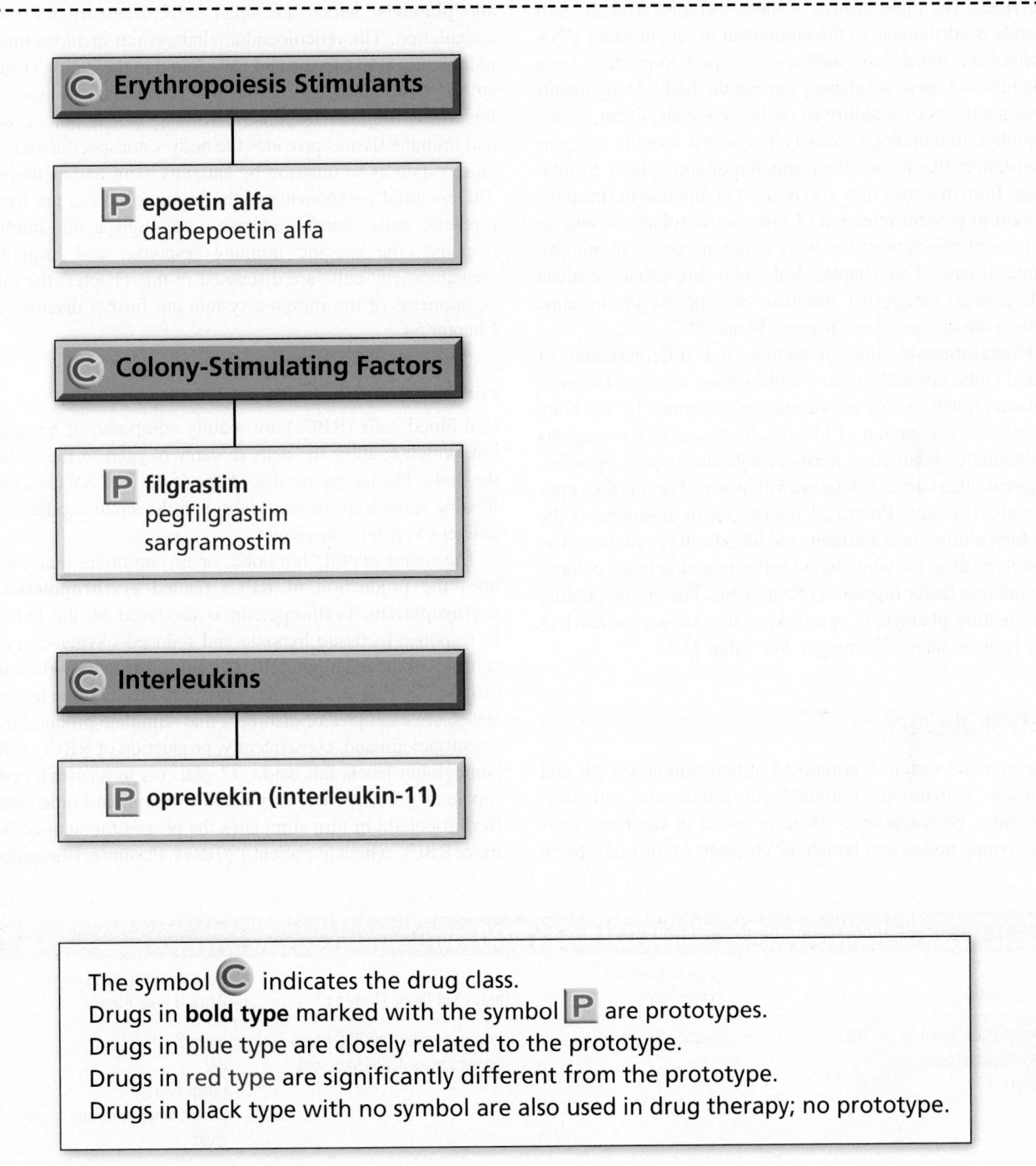

Erythropoiesis Stimulants

epoetin alfa
darbepoetin alfa

Colony-Stimulating Factors

filgrastim
pegfilgrastim
sargramostim

Interleukins

oprelvekin (interleukin-11)

The symbol C indicates the drug class.
Drugs in **bold type** marked with the symbol P are prototypes.
Drugs in blue type are closely related to the prototype.
Drugs in red type are significantly different from the prototype.
Drugs in black type with no symbol are also used in drug therapy; no prototype.

Biologic modulators, or biologic modifiers, are a group of biopharmaceuticals that are naturally occurring proteins used to alter the body's hematologic or immunologic responses. These substances are sometimes called biologic therapies. The rapid growth of these therapies over the past decade is attributable to the refinement of recombinant DNA technology, which has enabled researchers to produce large quantities of these substances outside the body. Many agents enhance the body's ability to create new cells. Other agents stimulate immunologic activity to combat specific antigens (substances that induce the formation of antibodies). Similar drugs from this class may also be used to suppress the immune system to prevent rejection of foreign transplanted tissue or to prevent rejection of the body's own tissue, as in autoimmune disease. This chapter deals with drugs that stimulate cell growth. Drugs that stimulate or suppress the immune system are discussed in Chapters 54 and 55.

Hematopoiesis, the production and differentiation of blood cells, normally occurs within bone marrow. Hematopoietic growth factors are substances generated by the body to enhance production of blood cells. Some of these agents are actually classified as hormone substances (e.g., epoetin), whereas others are cytokine growth factors. For this text, epoetin alfa (Epogen, Procrit), a hematopoietic hormone, is the prototype drug for stimulating red blood cell production. The prototype drug for white blood cell production is the colony-stimulating factor filgrastim (Neupogen). The prototype drug for creating platelets is oprelvekin (also known as interleukin-1; brand name, Neumega). See Table 33.1.

PHYSIOLOGY

The immune system is composed of hematopoietic cells and multiple hematologic-immunologic production and storage sites. Hematopoietic tissue is found in the bone marrow, lymph nodes, and lymphatic channels of the body. Stem cells located in the red bone marrow, found in the long bones and vertebral skeleton, produce the three types of functional hematopoietic cells: **erythrocytes** (also called red blood cells [RBCs]), **leukocytes** (also called white blood cells [WBCs]), and **platelets,** which are small cells necessary for blood coagulation. The reticuloendothelial system includes immunologically active tissue and cells found in the lymph system, spleen, liver, lungs, gastrointestinal (GI) tract, and brain. An integrated immune response involving hematopoietic cells and immune tissues provides the body's nonspecific and specific responses to invasion by antigens identified as nonself. The essential components of the immune system are hematopoietic cells, barrier defenses, the nonspecific immune response, the specific immune response, and immunity. Hematopoietic cells are discussed in this chapter; the other components of the immune system are further discussed in Chapter 54.

Hematopoietic Cells

Red blood cells (RBCs) are mainly composed of hemoglobin, which enables the cells to carry oxygen to the cells in the body. The biconcave disc shape of the RBCs makes them flexible enough to maneuver through the small capillaries to deliver oxygen to the tissues.

The major peptide hormone, or glycoprotein, that stimulates the production of RBCs (called **erythropoiesis**) is **erythropoietin.** Erythropoietin is produced by the kidneys in response to tissue hypoxia and reduced oxygen-carrying capacity of the red blood cells. Chronic obstructive pulmonary disease (COPD) and anemia, which produce chronic hypoxic states, are examples of disorders that stimulate production of erythropoietin and, consequently, production of RBCs. When hemoglobin levels fall below 12 g/dL (as in anemia), erythropoietin production is stimulated to maintain homeostasis. Erythropoietin in turn stimulates the progenitor stem cells to make RBCs, which live about 120 days. Plasma erythropoietin

TABLE 33.1	Understanding Drug Therapy That Affects Blood Cells			
Cell Picture	Cell Type	Drug to Increase Production	Impact of Drug Therapy	Patients may Require this Drug if they have:
<leave blank space for red blood cell figure to come>	RBC	Epoetin alfa	elevates or maintains RBC levels- improves oxygenation to tissues	Anemia HIV kidney disease Cancer, or receiving anti cancer drugs
<leave blank space for white blood cell figure to come>	WBC	Filgrastim	increase neutrophil count- fight infection, decrease risk of infection	Cancer Need fo astem cell harvest Or receiving anti cancer drugs
<leave blank space for platelet blood cell figure to come>	Platelets	Oprelvekin	Increase platelet production, prevent bleeding, allows for clot formation	cancer or patients receiving anti cancer drugs

P H Y S I O L O G Y

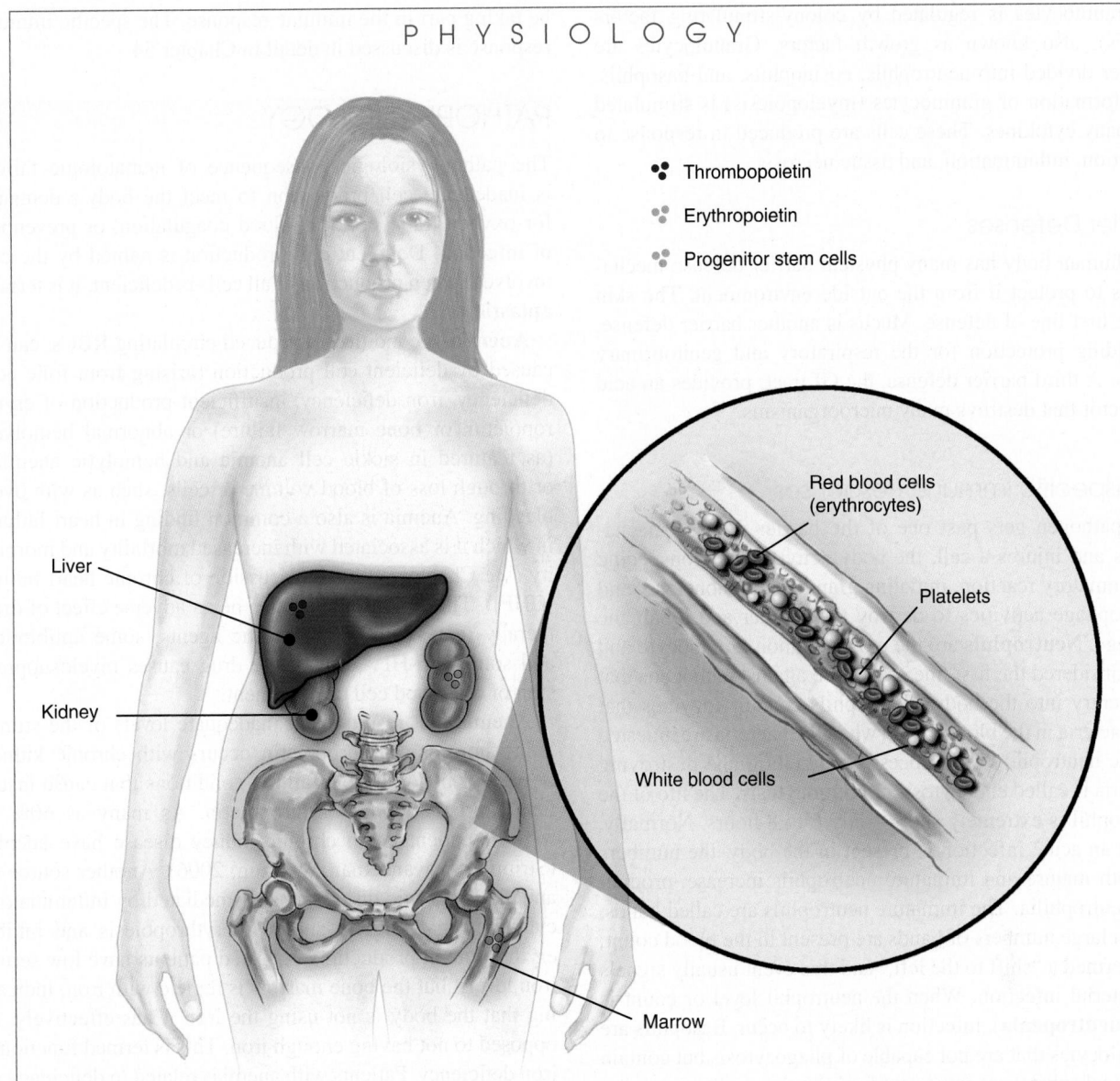

- **FIGURE 33.1** The kidney releases erythropoietin, which stimulates the progenitor cells in the bone marrow to produce red blood cells (erythrocytes). The liver produces thrombopoietin, which, along with interleukin-6, stimulates the production of platelets in the bone marrow. Colony-stimulating factors work on the developing white blood cells (leukocytes), allowing them to differentiate into granulocytes, monocytes, and lymphocytes. Granulocytes are further specialized as either neutrophils, eosinophils, or basophils.

levels vary from 0.01 U/mL to 0.03 U/mL and increase 100- to 1,000-fold during hypoxia or anemia. When hemoglobin levels are elevated, erythropoietin production is halted, ending the stimulation to produce new RBCs.

Iron, the primary ion reversibly bound to oxygen in the heme molecule, is necessary to support erythropoiesis. It is held stable in the ferrous form by the other atoms that are in heme. When iron deficiency exists, the final step in heme synthesis is interrupted.

Platelets are the formed element involved in blood coagulation. Platelets are small cells that arise from the bone marrow precursor cells, called megakaryocytes. Platelet production,

although stimulated by many cytokines, is mostly dependent on the action of interleukin-6 and a peptide called **thrombopoietin.** Thrombopoietin is produced in the liver. A low platelet count stimulates the production of thrombopoietin. Platelets are important in normal blood clotting. (For more information on blood clotting, see Chapter 32.)

Leukocytes (white blood cells, or WBCs) are key components of all immune system responses. During maturation in the bone marrow, WBCs differentiate into three main cell types—**granulocytes, monocytes,** and **lymphocytes**—that respond to cell injury or foreign invaders (Figure 33.1). Granulocytes are the most common type of WBC. Production of granulocytes is regulated by colony-stimulating factors (CSFs), also known as growth factors. Granulocytes are further divided into neutrophils, eosinophils, and basophils. The formation of granulocytes (myelopoiesis) is stimulated by many cytokines. These cells are produced in response to infection, inflammation, and tissue necrosis.

Barrier Defenses

The human body has many physical barrier defense mechanisms to protect it from the outside environment. The skin is the first line of defense. Mucus is another barrier defense, providing protection for the respiratory and genitourinary tracts. A third barrier defense, the GI tract, provides an acid protector that destroys many microorganisms.

Nonspecific Immune Responses

If a pathogen gets past one of the barrier defense mechanisms and injures a cell, the body activates the nonspecific inflammatory reaction, initiating granulocyte, monocyte, and macrophage activities to destroy the invader and repair the damage. **Neutrophils** are the most common granulocyte and are considered the first line of defense against pathogens that gain entry into the body. Neutrophils contain enzymes that kill bacteria in the bloodstream when the bacteria are ingested by the neutrophil. This process of engulfing and destroying bacteria is called endocytosis or **phagocytosis.** The life of the neutrophil is extremely short—only 6 to 8 hours. Normally, when an acute infection is present in the body, the numbers of both mature and immature neutrophils increase, producing neutrophilia. The immature neutrophils are called bands. When large numbers of bands are present in the blood count, it is termed a "shift to the left," and this event usually signals a bacterial infection. When the neutrophil level or count is low (**neutropenia**), infection is likely to occur. Basophils are granulocytes that are not capable of phagocytosis but contain chemical substances important for initiating and maintaining an immune response. These substances include histamine, heparin, and chemicals used in the inflammatory response. Monocytes differentiate into immunologically active cells called **macrophages.** Macrophages can be circulating phagocytes or can be fixed in specific tissues.

Specific Immune Responses

If an invader gets past the barrier and nonspecific immune systems and enters the tissues or bloodstream, a specific immune response involving lymphocytes is initiated.

Bone marrow stem cells develop into two types of lymphocytes: T lymphocytes, or T cells, and B lymphocytes, or B cells. These T and B lymphocytes may also differentiate into specialized cells such as natural killer cells and lymphokine-activated killer cells, which have been identified as the cells that aggressively attack and destroy neoplastic cells. Because research in the area of lymphocyte identification is relatively new and ongoing, other not-yet-identified lymphocytes may be taking part in the immune response. The specific immune response is discussed in detail in Chapter 54.

PATHOPHYSIOLOGY

The pathophysiologic consequence of hematologic failure is inadequate cell production to meet the body's demands for oxygen transportation, blood coagulation, or prevention of infection. Deficient cell production is named by the cell involved; when production of all cells is deficient, it is termed **aplastic.**

Anemia, a condition of reduced circulating RBCs, can be caused by deficient cell production (arising from folic acid deficiency, iron deficiency, insufficient production of erythropoietin, or bone marrow failure) or abnormal hemolysis (as featured in sickle cell anemia and hemolytic anemia), or through loss of blood volume or cells, such as with overt bleeding. Anemia is also a common finding in heart failure, in which it is associated with increased mortality and morbidity (see Chapter 29 for a discussion of chronic heart failure [CHF]). The condition may also be an adverse effect of drug therapy (e.g., with antineoplastic agents, some antibiotics, and some anti-HIV drugs); the drug causes myelosuppression of red blood cell development.

Anemia that results from inadequate levels of the stimulating hormone erythropoietin occurs with chronic kidney disease or bone marrow failure, conditions that cause insufficient production of erythropoietin. As many as 60% to 80% of patients with chronic kidney disease have anemia (Strippoli, Navaneethan, & Craig, 2006). Another source of anemia is chronic disease; this is mediated by inflammatory cytokines that directly suppress erythropoiesis and inhibit erythropoietin production. Affected patients have low serum iron levels, but the bone marrow is replete with iron, indicating that the body is not using the iron it has effectively, as opposed to not having enough iron. This is termed functional iron deficiency. Patients with anemias related to deficiency of erythropoietin have RBCs that are normal in size and color. Those with anemias related to iron deficiency or aluminum overload have smaller RBCs than normal, whereas those with anemias related to vitamin B_{12} or folate deficiency have larger than normal RBCs.

Anemias related to decreased erythropoietin levels can be treated with exogenous erythropoietin (epoetin alfa). In chronic kidney disease, hemoglobin levels that are below 10 g/dL induce the heart to work harder to meet the tissue's needs for oxygen. This phenomenon eventually leads to left ventricular hypertrophy and left ventricular dilation, creating greater morbidity with severely altered quality of life, as well as greater cardiac mortality. Early normalization of the hemoglobin level can prevent development of left ventricular dilation and improve quality of life. Children with chronic kidney disease and anemia have impaired cognitive function, growth retardation, reduced quality of life, and an increased risk of developing left ventricular hypertrophy (National Kidney Foundation, 2006).

To effectively manage early anemia in chronic kidney disease, it should be assumed that an erythropoietin deficiency exists and any iron deficiency that may be contributing to the problem should be ruled out. Assessment and evaluation of the anemia in a patient with chronic renal disease should occur when the hemoglobin (Hb) is less than 13.5 g/dL in men and postmenopausal women, or when it is less than 12 g/dL in women. Anemia for children is defined as less than the 5th percentile of normal Hb when adjusted for age and sex. Therapy with replacement erythropoietin should begin if the evaluation determines that the patient has normal serum iron levels. The target goal for both sexes and all ages is greater than 11 g/dL; this level has been found to increase quality of life without great risk of adverse effects (National Kidney Foundation, 2006). Functional iron deficiency (normal ferritin levels but low transferrin saturation) is a common occurrence in patients who have started epoetin alfa therapy, even if they originally had normal iron levels. This deficiency occurs because stimulation of erythropoiesis increases the demand for iron, and eventually not enough iron is available.

If anemia is related to cancer and its treatment, an Hb of less than 11 g/dL requires erythropoietic therapy, and the optimum maximum treatment goal is 12 g/dL (National Comprehensive Cancer Network, 2009). A relationship between anemia and fatigue, common among patients with cancer, is believed to exist. Cancer-related fatigue is a multifactorial and common problem that decreases quality of life. Treatment of anemia to the desired treatment goal has been shown to improve quality of life in patients with cancer (National Comprehensive Cancer Network, 2009). Raising the hemoglobin level greater than 12 g/dL increases the risk for adverse effects (see below).

Abnormalities in WBC counts are fairly common, although abnormalities of WBC function are rare. Decreased numbers of neutrophils, called neutropenia, are related to two basic causes: decreased marrow activity and decreased neutrophil survival. When neutropenia is related to decreased marrow activity, it may be related to drug therapy (e.g., with antineoplastics, some antibiotics, gold, certain diuretics, antithyroid agents, antihistamines, and antipsychotics). Other causes include radiation exposure, megaloblastic anemia (anemia in which large nucleated abnormal RBCs are present in the blood), cyclic neutropenia (a benign disease), Kostmann (infantile) neutropenia, aplastic anemia (anemia from complete suppression, or loss of function, of the bone marrow), myelodysplastic syndrome, and marrow replacement by tumor.

Because neutrophils are the first line of defense for infection, neutropenia increases the risk of infection. Chemotherapy-induced neutropenia is a major dose-limiting toxicity of systemic cancer chemotherapy; it increases the risk of morbidity, mortality, and the overall cost of treating patients with cancer. Febrile neutropenia may occur, and it often requires hospitalization for evaluation and treatment with antibiotics. Patients with chemotherapy-induced neutropenia are more likely to die from an infection than from cancer.

A low platelet count is termed **thrombocytopenia.** Thrombocytopenia can result from decreased production, shortened survival, or loss of platelets. Decreased production is caused by aplastic anemia (which may be drug induced), marrow infiltration, deficiencies of vitamin B_{12} and folate, radiation, and hereditary factors. Decreased survival of platelets is related to immune-mediated factors (idiopathic, systemic lupus erythematosus, drug induced, neonatal from maternal immunoglobulin G [IgG]); hypersplenism; disseminated intravascular coagulation; thrombotic thrombocytopenic purpura; hemolytic uremic syndrome; and prosthetic valves.

Hematopoietic growth factors are exogenous replacements of endogenous growth factors. They are used when the internal mechanism for producing sufficient blood cells does not meet the body's needs. Drugs that affect hematopoiesis include erythropoiesis stimulants, colony-stimulating factors, and interleukins. Table 33.2 provides a summary of selected hematopoietic agents.

Ⓒ ERYTHROPOIESIS STIMULANTS

The prototype drug used to create RBCs is epoetin alfa (Epogen, Procrit), a 165–amino acid glycoprotein manufactured by recombinant DNA technology. It is recombinant human erythropoietin. The product contains the same amino acid sequence as natural erythropoietin. The human erythropoietin gene is introduced into mammalian cells, which then produce erythropoietin that has the same biologic effects as endogenous erythropoietin.

Nursing Management of the Patient Receiving Ⓟ Epoetin Alfa

Core Drug Knowledge

Pharmacotherapeutics

Epoetin alfa, also referred to as erythropoietin or EPO, is used to treat anemia associated with chronic kidney disease, to elevate or maintain the RBC level (assessed through Hb determinations) and to decrease the need for transfusion (see Table 33.2). Epoetin alfa is also used to treat anemia related to zidovudine therapy in HIV-positive patients. It is used when the endogenous erythropoietin levels are 500 mU/ mL or less and the dose of zidovudine is 4,200 mg/wk or less. Although clinical reviews have found some evidence that supports the use of epoetin alfa to reduce transfusion requirements, increase hemoglobin levels, and improve the quality of life in HIV-infected patients with anemia, the review authors felt this evidence was weak. These authors stated: "There is a need for randomized trials of high methodological quality to evaluate the effect of interventions on anemia in persons infected with human immunodeficiency virus" (Martí-Carvajal & Solà, 2009). It has historically been used to treat chemotherapy-induced anemia in patients with cancer and it may reduce the need for blood transfusions. Improving Hb levels in patients with cancer appears to also decrease the fatigue that often accompanies cancer.

TABLE 33.2 Summary of Selected Hematopoietic Agents

Drug (Trade) Name	Selected Indications	Route and Dosage Range	Pharmacokinetics
C Erythropoiesis Stimulants			
P epoetin alfa or erythropoietin or EPO (Epogen, Procrit)	Anemia from chronic renal disease (CRD)	CRD: 50–100 U/kg 3×/wk IV or SC injection to maintain Hct of 30%–36%	*Onset:* IV, immediate; SC, within 5–24 h
	Anemia related to zidovudine therapy in HIV-associated illness	HIV: 100 U/kg 3×/wk for 8 wk IV or SC injection	*Duration:* IV, = 24 h; SC levels fall slowly after 24 h
	Anemia related to chemotherapy in cancer patients	Cancer: 150 U/kg 3×/wk SC injection (weekly injections under investigation)	$t_{1/2}$: 4–13 h
C Colony-Stimulating Factors			
P filgrastim or granulocyte-colony stimulating factor (G-CSF) (Neupogen)	Neutropenia due to chemotherapy, after bone-marrow transplantation (BMT), or severe chronic neutropenia	Chemotherapy: 5 mcg/kg/d SC injection, or infusion, or IV BMT: 10 mcg/kg/d IV or SC infusion Chronic: congenital 6 mcg/kg bid SC injection Idiopathic or cyclic: 5 mcg/kg once/d SC injection	*Onset:* IV, immediate *Duration:* Unknown $t_{1/2}$: 3.5 h
	Prior to peripheral blood progenitor cell (PBPC) collection	PBPC collection: 10 mcg/kg/d SC (injection or infusion) starting at least 4 d prior to procedure	
C Interleukins			
P oprelvekin or interleukin-11 (IL-11) (Neumega)	Thrombocytopenia from chemotherapy	*Adult:* 50 mcg/kg/d SC injection *Child:* Safety and efficacy not established	*Onset:* Unknown *Duration:* Unknown $t_{1/2}$: 6.9 h

However, two recent meta-analyses concluded that erythropoietin treatment shortens survival in cancer patients. It appears that all cancer patients are equally at risk, no matter what cancer treatment they receive or what type of cancer they have (Bohlius, Schmidlin, Brillant, 2009; Lambin, Ramaekers, van Mastrigt, et al., 2009). Finally, epoetin alfa is used in patients with anemia who will be undergoing elective, noncardiac, or nonvascular surgery, and in patients who are at high risk for substantial blood loss during surgery, to reduce their need for postoperative blood transfusions.

Off-label uses of epoetin alfa include treatment of anemia in a variety of other conditions, including critical illness, CHF, anemia due to radiation, anemia during puerperium, hepatitis C (in patients being treated with a combination of ribavirin and interferon alfa or ribavirin and peginterferon alfa), multiple myeloma, myelodysplastic syndrome, myelofibrosis, prematurity, and pre-donation for autologous blood transfusion.

Dosage and frequency of administration of epoetin alfa vary by its intended purpose. Multiple effective regimens have been studied and seem effective, including two or

three times per week, weekly, and biweekly. Most protocols recommend that epoetin alfa be administered subcutaneously, but it may also be given intravenously.

Pharmacokinetics

Epoetin alfa can be administered either intravenously or subcutaneously. When epoetin alfa is given intravenously, its circulating half-life is 4 to 13 hours. For chronic renal failure patients, it lasts approximately 20% longer than in healthy adults. Therapeutic levels are maintained for 24 hours or longer. After subcutaneous (SC) administration, peak levels are achieved within 5 to 24 hours and decline slowly afterward. Elimination is through the kidneys. Half-life is not affected by dialysis (see Table 33.2).

Pharmacodynamics

Epoetin alfa has the same effects on the body as endogenous erythropoietin. It stimulates production of RBCs. In patients with chronic kidney disease, the first evidence that epoetin alfa is producing a positive response is an increase in the reticulocyte (immature RBC) count within 10 days. Next seen, within 2 to 6 weeks, is an increase in the RBC count and Hb level. Once the target Hb level has been reached, it can be maintained by using epoetin alfa. The rate of hemoglobin increase varies among patients and is dose dependent; however, doses over 300 units/kg three times weekly (or 60,000 units once weekly) are unlikely to produce any additional biologic response. Other factors affecting rate and extent of response include the availability of iron stores, baseline hemoglobin, and concurrent illnesses. A recent study showed that erythropoietin (in addition to oral iron) given to patients with CHF and anemia yielded not only a significant increase in their hemoglobin levels but also the following improvements related to their heart failure: an improvement in New York Heart Association functional class; increased exercise endurance (including tolerating longer periods of exercise and an ability to walk greater distances); a significant improvement in oxygen use during exercise; a fall in plasma B–type natriuretic peptide levels; improved renal function (as evidenced by a significant decrease in serum creatinine and an increase in estimated creatinine clearance); and decreased need for hospitalization. Patients who received only the oral iron preparation did not experience these benefits (Palazzuoli, Silverberg, Iovine, et al., 2006). Another small study showed that patients with chronic kidney disease but not receiving dialysis who received epoetin alfa had a significant increase in their high-density lipid cholesterol; this may represent an important cardiovascular benefit of epoetin alfa (Siamopoulos, Gouva, Katopodis, et al., 2006).

Responsiveness of HIV-positive patients to epoetin alfa is based on endogenous erythropoietin levels. Those with levels above 500 mU/mL do not appear to respond to therapy. An increased Hb and a decreased need for transfusion are evidence of a response.

Epoetin alfa is no longer recommended for the treatment of anemia caused by cancer associated with solid tumors or hematologic malignancies other than myelodysplastic syndromes (National Comprehensive Cancer Network, 2009). The use of epoetin alpha in patients receiving myelosuppressive chemotherapy depends on symptoms of anemia and hemoglobin levels. For example, epoetin alfa is an option in someone with symptoms of anemia and a hemoglobin level of less than 11g/dL. In patients with no symptoms of anemia, it should only be considered as an option if hemoglobin levels are less than 10 g/dL and if the patient is at risk of development of symptomatic anemia requiring transfusion. Furthermore, the use of epoetin alfa for cancer-related anemia should be limited to the period during chemotherapy and a short period following (usually 6 weeks). The use of epoetin alfa in cancer-associated anemia must be monitored very closely because recent evidence indicates that there is decreased survival of cancer patients who receive epoetin alfa.

Research has shown that premature infants who are given epoetin alfa to prevent or treat anemia require fewer transfusions than those who did not receive the drug (Ohlsson & Aher, 2006; Haiden, Schwindt, Cardona, et al., 2006).

Contraindications and Precautions

Use of epoetin alfa should be avoided in uncontrolled hypertension and in cases of hypersensitivity to mammalian cell–derived products or human albumin; anaphylaxis can occur. Although epoetin alfa therapy does not appear to have direct vasopressor effects, blood pressure may rise during therapy, especially during the early phase of treatment, when the Hb is rising. An elevation in blood pressure is especially problematic for patients with chronic kidney disease, who typically have hypertension already.

Increasing the Hb to greater than 12 g/dL (in an attempt to raise it to normal levels) appears to increase the risk of cardiovascular complications, including death, myocardial infarction, hospitalization for CHF, or stroke; thus, treatment goals for Hb should be below this level. Hypertensive encephalopathy has also been reported with the use of epoetin alfa, and a reduction or interruption of the dose may be required.

In patients with chronic kidney disease who require correction for severe anemia, epoetin alfa therapy should not be used as a replacement for transfusion. Patients with chronic kidney disease who are taking epoetin alfa may suffer thrombotic events, such as myocardial infarction, transient ischemic attacks, and cerebrovascular accident, or clotting of the artificial kidney during dialysis. Patients receiving hemodialysis may need increased anticoagulation with heparin to prevent their artificial kidneys from clotting. The risk of thrombotic events is greatly increased in patients with ischemic heart disease or CHF when the prescriber is trying to increase the Hb to normal levels with epoetin alfa therapy.

In patients with cancer, epoetin alfa should only be used when anemia is due to concomitant myelosuppressive chemotherapy and should be discontinued when the chemotherapy course is completed. The use of epoetin alfa during cancer may shorten survival and/or increase the risk of tumor progression or recurrence. Patients with cancer are also at risk for serious cardiovascular and thrombovascular events and should use the lowest dose needed to avoid red blood cell transfusions.

Increasing the Hb level too quickly, with a rise of greater than 1 g/dL in any 2-week period, increases the risk of neurologic and cardiovascular events, including seizure, death, myocardial infarction, stroke, CHF, exacerbation of hypertension, and hemodialysis graft occlusion in all patient populations.

Several other patient variables require cautious use of epoetin alfa. Patients with porphyria may experience exacerbations. Patients with underlying hematologic disease (i.e., sickle cell anemia, myelodysplastic syndrome, hemolytic anemia) may have problems with epoetin alfa; the safety and efficacy of the drug in such patients have not been determined. Patients taking epoetin alfa who require surgery may require iron supplementation. Use of epoetin alfa during the peri-surgery period should be monitored due to increased risk of DVT and DVT prophylaxis may be considered. Epoetin alfa is a pregnancy class C drug. Premature infants are at increased risk of neurologic and sometimes-fatal complications, due to benzyl alcohol contained in the multidose-preserved formulation. Resumption of menses in some postmenopausal female patients has occurred; unplanned pregnancy may result. Also, because small amounts of human albumin are found in epoetin alfa, theoretically the drug may transmit viral illnesses or Creutzfeldt-Jakob disease; however, no known cases have been documented. Lastly, patients with several conditions may fail to respond or maintain a response to epoetin alfa. These include possible iron deficiency, underlying infection, inflammatory, or malignant processes, occult blood loss, underlying hematologic diseases, vitamin deficiencies, hemolysis, aluminum intoxication, osteitis fibrosa cystic, and pure red cell aplasia.

In contrast, there does not seem to be any association between epoetin alfa therapy in HIV-positive patients and exacerbation of hypertension, seizures, or thrombotic events. However, therapy should not be started until blood pressure is controlled. Epoetin alfa should not be used to treat anemia caused by iron or folate deficiencies, hemolysis, or GI bleeding in HIV-positive patients with cancer.

Adverse Effects

Adverse effects occurring during epoetin alfa therapy appear to reflect the patients' underlying disease process or their postoperative state. Although fever, headache, cough, rash, nausea, diarrhea, vomiting, and edema were all noted in the original clinical trials of epoetin alfa prior to Food and Drug Administration approval, these were also found in those patients who did not receive epoetin alfa. It is difficult to determine, then, exactly what the adverse effects of epoetin alfa are. Exacerbation of hypertension may occur in patients with chronic kidney disease who are on dialysis (see Contraindications and Precautions). Seizures have been reported less often; they occur most commonly in patients with renal disease who have lower Hb targets (less than 12 g/dL) (Strippoli, Navaneethan, & Craig, 2006). Porphyria (excretion of nitrogen-containing compounds in the urine) may be exacerbated in patients with chronic kidney disease, although this effect is rare.

Although it is difficult to determine adverse effects of epoetin alfa per se, there is mounting evidence that raising the hemoglobin level to 13.5 g/dL in patients with chronic kidney disease increases the risk of serious adverse effects such as hypertension, hospitalization for CHF, myocardial infarction, and stroke (Singh, Szczech, Tang, et al., 2006). Whether it increases the risk of death is inconclusive in the literature at this time (Strippoli, Navaneethan, & Craig, 2006). Patients with cancer receiving epoetin alfa have a significant increased risk of thromboembolic events (Bohlius, Wilson, Seidenfeld, et al., 2006).

Premature infants less than 8 days of age who received epoetin alfa experienced an increased risk of retinopathy of prematurity (Ohlsson & Aher, 2006).

Drug Interactions
No drug interactions are known to occur with epoetin alfa.

Assessment of Relevant Core Patient Variables
Health Status
Determine whether the patient has pre-existing uncontrolled hypertension, which is a contraindication for the use of epoetin alfa. Verify that the anemia is not caused by iron or folate deficiency, hemolysis, or GI bleeding, because these anemias should be treated differently. Determine whether the patient has pre-existing vascular disease, because it may increase the patient's risk for developing thrombotic adverse effects. Before and during therapy, assess the patient's iron status, including transferrin saturation (serum iron divided by iron-binding capacity) and serum ferritin (the iron-phosphorous-protein complex that is the form in which iron is stored in the tissues). Transferrin saturation should be at least 20%, and ferritin should be at least 100 ng/mL (200 ng/mL if the patient is receiving dialysis). Iron is needed to support erythropoiesis. Absolute or functional iron deficiency may develop during therapy. Functional iron deficiency, in which the ferritin level is normal but the transferrin saturation is low, is believed to be caused by the body's inability to mobilize iron stores rapidly enough to support increased erythropoiesis.

Life Span and Gender
Determine whether the patient is pregnant, because epoetin alfa is a pregnancy category C drug. Adverse effects have occurred in rats given epoetin alfa in doses five times the comparable human dose; however, no adequate studies have been performed in humans. Use caution if administering epoetin alfa to a woman who is breast-feeding, because it is not known whether the drug is excreted in breast milk. Because menstruation may resume in some female patients who take epoetin alfa, discuss birth control strategies.

Safety and efficacy in children are not established. If giving epoetin alfa for unlabeled purposes to premature infants, use the form without the benzyl alcohol (the preservative), because benzyl alcohol has been associated with a fatal "gasping syndrome" in premature infants. Administration of epoetin alfa to premature infants before 8 days of age is not recommended because of the increased risk of retinopathy of prematurity.

Ask the patient's age, which may affect the adverse effects from the drug. Carefully assess the older adult with cancer who is receiving epoetin alfa for adverse effects related to anemia, because these patients are more sensitive to the anemia that results from chemotherapy. Older adults are also likely to experience adverse effects from other, concurrent drug therapy. Some drugs bind to RBCs, and without adequate RBCs, epoetin alfa has no binding sites. In this case, levels of the drug rise, increasing the incidence of adverse effects).

Lifestyle, Diet, and Habits

Verify that patients with chronic kidney disease are continuing the dietary restrictions necessary in this disease. As the hemoglobin rises and patients begin to feel better, they may feel that they no longer need a restrictive diet. Determine whether patients are at risk for iron deficiency; if so, encourage them to consume foods high in iron.

Environment

Be aware of the setting in which epoetin alfa will be administered. The drug is administered in many ambulatory settings as well as in the hospital or dialysis center. For patients who receive home dialysis or intermittent ambulatory treatment (antiretroviral therapy, chemotherapy, or radiation therapy), therapy can be self-administered at home. Assess the patient factors in the home environment that may affect adherence to drug therapy. Be careful to review the reimbursement policies of the patient's health care insurance, because injectable medications are often not reimbursed as a home therapy.

Culture and Inherited Traits

No cultural barriers exist to the use of epoetin alfa. If your assessment reveals that the patient has a religious affiliation (such as the Jehovah Witnesses) in which blood transfusions are forbidden, epoetin alfa may still be administered. Epoetin alfa is not considered a blood component by religious affiliations that object to transfusions and hence offers an excellent alternative to RBC transfusion for those individuals.

Nursing Diagnoses and Outcomes

- Impaired Tissue Oxygenation related to anemia
  Desired outcome: Tissues will be oxygenated satisfactorily, and hemoglobin will reach desired level with epoetin alfa therapy.
- Risk for Injury related to adverse effects of epoetin alfa
  Desired outcome: Adverse effects will be prevented or minimized to prevent injury.

Planning and Intervention

Maximizing Therapeutic Effects

To maintain the biologic activity of epoetin alfa, do not shake the drug after reconstituting it. Vigorous shaking may denature the glycoprotein, making it biologically inactive. Do not further dilute the drug. Direct intravenous (IV) administration can be performed at the end of dialysis.

Allow time for the Hb level to rise before seeking an order to adjust the dose. An increase in Hb should not exceed 1 g/dL in 2 weeks. The accepted range for target Hb for all patients is 10 to 12 g/dL. When epoetin alfa is given, the time required to elicit a clinically meaningful change is 2 to 6 weeks. After dosage adjustment, measure Hb in patients with chronic kidney disease twice weekly for 2 to 6 weeks, and measure Hb in zidovudine-treated patients with HIV and patients with cancer once weekly until stabilized.

Iron stores (including transferrin saturation and ferritin) should be assessed prior to initiating therapy and periodically during therapy. Supplemental iron should be administered during therapy with epoetin alfa. Although oral iron preparations are most common, parenteral iron preparations are helpful in treating functional iron deficiency and may be more effective. Because allergic responses are possible from IV iron, it is often recommended that patients receive pretreatment with diphenhydramine and acetaminophen to minimize adverse effects.

If response to epoetin alfa is delayed or diminished, assess for other reasons that may cause a low Hb (e.g., functional iron deficiency; underlying infectious, inflammatory, or malignant processes; occult blood loss; underlying hematologic diseases; folic acid or vitamin B_{12} deficiencies; hemolysis; aluminum intoxication; or osteitis fibrosa cystica [overactivity of the parathyroid gland that results in disturbances of calcium and phosphorus metabolism]). Patients who fail to respond to epoetin alfa should be evaluated for these problems.

Minimizing Adverse Effects

Cancer patients should discuss with the physician if they are more at risk from taking epoetin alfa or from blood transfusions, as epoetin alfa appears to increase the rate of mortality from cancer, but blood transfusion also carries some risk to the patient (Bohlius, Schmidlin, Brillant, 2009).

Remember that the single-dose 1-mL vials have no preservative. To prevent contamination, use only one dose per vial, do not re-enter the vial, and discard any unused portion. In contrast, the multidose 2-mL vial has preservative in it. Store it at 2°C to 8°C after initial entry and between doses. Discard the vial 21 days after initial entry to prevent use of a possibly contaminated product. Never use the multidose preparation with preservatives in premature infants; use only the single-use, preservative-free preparations. The preservative has been found to cause potentially lethal adverse effects in premature infants. Although dilution is not generally recommended for adults, it may be done with bacteriostatic normal saline in a 1 to 1 ratio to help relieve injection site discomfort. Always monitor the patient closely after the first dose; anaphylactic reactions have occurred.

Monitor the blood pressure of all patients receiving epoetin alfa throughout therapy to assess for hypertension.

Monitor the Hb level to prevent adverse effects. Dosage adjustments to achieve the desired Hb level are not uncommon. These adjustments, or titrations, may be stated in the original drug order or in a unit or hospital protocol. If neither guideline exists, contact the prescriber for further orders. The nurse is responsible for verifying that the dose being administered is safe, based on the patient's current physiologic status, and does not promote serious adverse effects. Withhold a dose if hemoglobin exceeds 13 g/dL; reinitiate with 25% dose reduction when hemoglobin is less than 12 g/dL; an alternative to this would be to immediately decrease the dose instead of withholding the drug for a period of time. This method may help prevent the hemoglobin level from falling too greatly. If a very rapid hemoglobin response (increase of more than 1 g/dL in any 2-week period) occurs, the dose should be reduced by 25%. Consult with the prescriber for changes in the prescribed dose.

Assess for the presence of premonitory neurologic symptoms, particularly during the first 90 days of therapy. Assess renal function and fluid and electrolyte balance in patients with chronic renal failure.

Providing Patient and Family Education

- Teach patients and families the purpose of the drug and the need for follow-up blood work to check the Hb.
- Instruct patients to maintain adequate iron intake, which may aid in the effectiveness of epoetin alfa. Foods high in iron include green leafy vegetables, beans, and organ meats. High-iron-content foods or supplements are best absorbed if taken with ascorbic acid, such as that found in citrus drinks.
- If patients are to take an iron supplement, teach them that it is best taken without food or phosphate binders, and that the best time to take it is at bedtime.
- Explain to patients with chronic kidney disease the importance of continuing with diet restrictions and dialysis (if used) while receiving epoetin alfa.
- For patients who will be self-administering epoetin alfa at home, teach proper SC injection technique and safe disposal of used needles and syringes.
- Instruct patients to avoid activities requiring coordination until the drug effects are realized, as epoetin alfa may cause dizziness.
- Teach patients to stop using epoetin alfa when the chemotherapy course is complete.

Ongoing Assessment and Evaluation

Monitor patients' blood pressure and hemoglobin throughout epoetin alfa therapy. Check the hemoglobin twice weekly until the target hemoglobin has been achieved and the dose has been established. Monitor iron levels throughout therapy to verify that enough iron is available to support erythropoiesis. Therapy is effective when the Hb rises to a desired treatment level, the need for transfusions is reduced, and the patient does not have major adverse effects.

CRITICAL THINKING SCENARIO

EPOETIN ALFA AND IRON DEFICIENCY

Ada Greene, 65 years of age, has chronic kidney disease. Her blood work shows that her hemoglobin is 9 g/dL. An anemia evaluation shows that her serum iron levels are normal, and she is started on epoetin alfa. After 3 weeks of epoetin alfa therapy, her hemoglobin count is 10.5 g/dL, and her serum iron levels show normal ferritin levels but low transferrin saturation. She is diagnosed as having functional iron deficiency.

1. What would account for these changes in her iron levels?

2. What treatment would you expect to be ordered for Ms. Greene?

Drug Closely Related to Epoetin Alfa

Darbepoetin alfa (Aranesp) is in the same class as epoetin alfa. Darbepoetin alfa has a slightly different chemical structure (it contains five N-linked oligosaccharide chains, as compared to three) and a much longer half-life. Approved for use in treating anemia from chronic kidney disease or from chemotherapy, darbepoetin alfa should be avoided in cancer patients with anemia that is not secondary to drug therapy, because it is not effective in reducing the need for blood transfusions and it increases the mortality rate in these patients (FDA MedWatch, 2007). It appears to have a reduced efficacy in renal dialysis. In one study (Papatheofanis, Smith, Mody et al., 2007), short-term measurements of effectiveness (4 to 12 weeks) showed that darbepoetin alfa was not as effective as epoetin alfa; however, by 24 weeks of therapy, target Hb levels had been reached equally in patients receiving therapy with either drug. Darbepoetin alfa was 33% more expensive than epoetin alfa.

MEMORY CHIP

Epoetin Alfa

- Recombinant human erythropoietin works exactly as endogenous erythropoietin; it stimulates the production of RBCs (erythropoiesis)
- Used to treat anemia in chronic kidney disease, HIV infection (when zidovudine is used), and cancer (when chemotherapy is used), and in preoperative anemic patients (when high blood loss and transfusion are anticipated)
- **Black box warning: Renal failure patients experienced greater risks for death and serious cardiovascular events if hemoglobin level raised too high; treatment goal should be 10 to 12 g/dL only.**
- **Black box warning: Cancer patients may shorten overall survival and/or increased the risk of tumor progression or recurrence; use the lowest ESA dose needed to avoid red blood cell transfusion.**
- **Black box warning: For pre-operative use, administer anticoagulants to prevent DVT.**
- Major contraindication: uncontrolled hypertension
- Difficult to determine true adverse effects, because those reported are also present in disease process or post procedure
- Most common adverse effects: hypertension (in chronic kidney disease (CKD)); fever (all other uses); nausea and vomiting (surgical patients)
- Most serious adverse effects: thrombotic effects (in CKD, and preoperative patients)
- **Patient safety alert: Attempting to raise the Hb level to typical normal levels increases the risk of cardiovascular complication; raising the Hb level too quickly can result in seizures, doses should be individualized and the lowest effective dose should be used.**
- Maximizing therapeutic effects: Consult with prescriber about dose adjustment and verify iron availability; monitor hemoglobin levels in CKD patients; do not shake vial.
- Minimizing adverse effects: Monitor hemoglobin; do not use high target levels for hemoglobin.
- Most important patient education: Advise patients of the need for follow-up blood work and the importance of dietary iron.

© COLONY-STIMULATING FACTORS

Colony-stimulating factors are glycoproteins that assist in the production of blood cells by binding to specific cell-surface receptors and stimulating proliferation, differentiation commitment, and some end-cell functional activation. Filgrastim (Neupogen), a granulocyte colony-stimulating factor (G-CSF), is the prototype drug for stimulating WBC production.

Nursing Management of the Patient Receiving P Filgrastim

Core Drug Knowledge

Pharmacotherapeutics

Filgrastim is licensed for use in both adults and children with cancer to increase their neutrophil count. For patients with cancer who have nonmyeloid malignancies (cancers that are not related to blood cell components) and are receiving myelosuppressive chemotherapy (which suppresses the production of blood cells in the bone marrow), it is used to decrease the incidence of infection, as manifested by febrile neutropenia (Box 33.1). Primary administration of filgrastim or other CSFs as prophylaxis should be reserved for patients expected to experience febrile neutropenia at an incidence equal to or greater than 20% (National Comprehensive Cancer Network, Myeloid Growth Factors, 2009). Filgrastim is used for patients with cancer who receive chemotherapy following bone marrow transplantation to reduce the duration of neutropenia and neutropenia-related clinical sequelae (e.g., febrile neutropenia). In addition, it is used in patients with cancer before leukapheresis (removal of WBCs from blood, which are saved and then later transfused back into the patient). Other uses for filgrastim include severe, chronic neutropenia that is congenital, cyclic, or idiopathic in origin. The goal is to reduce the incidence and duration of sequelae of neutropenia (e.g., fever, infections, and oropharyngeal ulcers).

Off-label uses of filgrastim include treating neutropenia in patients with AIDS, prevention of febrile neutropenia in myeloid malignancies following a bone marrow transplantation, myelodysplastic syndrome, aplastic anemia, hairy cell leukemia, and drug-induced neutropenia.

Filgrastim is administered as a single daily SC injection bolus, by short IV infusion (15 to 30 minutes), or by continuous SC or IV infusion.

Pharmacokinetics

Filgrastim begins to work as soon as it can bind with its receptor sites. Absorption and excretion occur through the kidneys; the elimination half-life is about 3.5 hours (Quirion, 2009).

Pharmacodynamics

Filgrastim is produced by *Escherichia coli* bacteria that have had the human G-CSF gene inserted. G-CSF regulates the production of neutrophils within the bone marrow. Recombinant DNA G-CSF (filgrastim) acts the way that endogenous G-CSF does.

Filgrastim stimulates and mobilizes the cells that are the progenitor cells for neutrophils into the peripheral circulation. When this additional volume of progenitor cells is infused back into the patient by leukophoresis, the neutrophil count rises more rapidly. It also affects some end-cell functional activation, including phagocytic activity, cellular metabolism, and antibody-dependent killing.

Contraindications and Precautions

The only contraindication to administration of this agent is hypersensitivity to *E. coli*–derived proteins, filgrastim, or any of the product components. Caution should be used when a patient has a myeloid malignancy or requires concomitant cytotoxic (destructive to cells) chemotherapy or

BOX 33.1 FOCUS ON RESEARCH

Determining Cost-effective Treatment in Breast Cancer

Lyman, G., Lalla, A., Barron, R., & Dubois, R. (2009). Cost-effectiveness of pegfilgrastim versus filgrastim primary prophylaxis in women with early-stage breast cancer receiving chemotherapy in the United States. *Clinical Therapeutics*, 31(5):1092–1104.

The Study

Filgrastim has been used in women with early stage breast cancer to prevent febrile neutropenia. The newer drug pegfilgrastim has advantages related to the dosing schedule, but is more expensive. This study sought to assess the incremental cost effectiveness of pegfilgrastim versus filgrastim as a prophylaxis for febrile neutropenia in women with early stage breast cancer who have received myelosuppressive chemotherapy. The model included the cost of the treatment, other direct medical costs, the costs related to reduced risk for febrile neutropenia, and potential survival benefits associated with reduced risk for febrile neutropenia. The study found that despite an initial higher cost of treatment with pegfilgrastim, it is ultimately more cost effective than either an 11-day or a 6-day treatment with filgrastim. The factors most significant factors in the analysis were: cost of the medication and its administration, base line, and relative risk for febrile neutropenia and febrile neutropenia case fatality rate.

Nursing Implication

Despite the higher cost for the medication with pegfilgrastim, which can be as much as $7,000 per dose (Quirion, 2009), treatment with pegfilgrastim has been found to be over all more cost effective than filgrastim (which is comparatively inexpensive at approximately $150 to 350 per dose). Pegfilgrastim has the additional advantage of being given as a single dose rather than 6 or 11 days of injections needed for treatment with filgrastim. This is much more comfortable and more supportive of patient adherence. Nurses are often consulted by patients regarding both the financial cost and personal impact of treatment options. This study demonstrates that sometimes the most cost-effective regimen is not with the drug that is least expensive. Understanding the true cost of drug therapy allows the nurse to more accurately address patients' concerns over the potential financial burden from drug therapy.

radiotherapy, because the rapidly dividing myeloid cells may be sensitive to these substances.

Filgrastim should not be used from 24 hours before to 24 hours after chemotherapy with cytotoxic substances, because extremely elevated WBC counts have occurred as a result. Although no specific adverse effects have been noted with this use, the WBC count should be monitored closely during therapy. Be careful not to discontinue treatment with filgrastim prematurely. Although a transient increase in neutrophil count occurs 1 to 2 days after starting therapy, this increase should not be mistaken for the full therapeutic effect of drug therapy. This drug should be administered throughout the time when the marrow-suppressing therapy's full nadir (lowest level) of neutrophils should have occurred before therapy is discontinued.

Caution is also recommended if the patient has adult respiratory distress syndrome (specifically, neutropenic patients with sepsis), sickle cell disease, or severe sickle cell crisis. Filgrastim is a pregnancy category C drug and should be used with caution.

Adverse Effects

Determining the adverse effects of filgrastim in patients receiving chemotherapy is difficult because all of the effects recorded during clinical trials with the drug can also be consequences of the malignancy or the cytotoxic chemotherapy. In other words, adverse effects may mimic the disease being treated or the effects of other treatments for the disease. Medullary bone pain (pain within the marrow) is the only consistently observed adverse effect that can be attributed to drug therapy; it is mild to moderate in severity and is reported in 56% of patients taking filgrastim (Quirion, 2009).

In patients receiving intensive chemotherapy or total-body irradiation followed by bone marrow transplantation, few unique adverse effects have been attributable to the G-CSF therapy.

In patients in whom filgrastim is used during collection of peripheral blood progenitor cells, adverse effects have included decreased platelet count (although it usually remains in the normal range), anemia, mild to moderate musculoskeletal symptoms, medullary bone pain, headache, and increases in alkaline phosphatase levels. Patients with severe chronic neutropenia have also experienced mild to moderate bone pain.

Drug Interactions

Drug interactions with filgrastim have not yet been fully evaluated. Drugs such as lithium carbonate that can potentiate the release of neutrophils should be used with caution because a synergistic effect may result; consequently, CBC levels should be taken more than twice per week during treatment. Because cytotoxic treatment may attack the proliferating cells effected by filgrastim, it should not be used concurrently with chemotherapy or during radiation treatment (Amgen Inc., 2007).

Assessment of Relevant Core Patient Variables
Health Status
Determine whether the patient has nonmyeloid cancer, has neutropenic fevers or severe chronic neutropenia, has had a bone marrow transplantation, or is a candidate for peripheral blood progenitor cell collection, because these states are indications for the use of filgrastim.

Life Span and Gender
Determine whether the patient is pregnant or breast-feeding; caution is warranted in these patients because filgrastim is a pregnancy category C drug. Whether the drug is excreted in breast milk is unknown. Ask the patient's age. Filgrastim has been used in pediatric patients aged 4 months to 17 years, and no long-term risks have been identified. However, safety and efficacy in neonatal autoimmune neutropenia have not been established, and long-term effects of this agent have not been evaluated in neonates. Older adults with cancer are especially sensitive to adverse effects from neutropenia; the more severe and the longer the duration of the neutropenia, the more likely the older adult will develop a fatal infection. Neutropenia can also require that a lower dose of chemotherapy be given to older adults, thus making them less likely to receive the full therapeutic effect from chemotherapy. Prophylactic administration of filgrastim or pegfilgrastim (see below) to prevent febrile neutropenia is as effective for older adults as for younger adults in reducing the severity and duration of neutropenia. Administering filgrastim during the first cycle of chemotherapy may be especially valuable for older adults.

Environment
Determine the environment in which filgrastim is to be administered. IV infusions of filgrastim are administered in either a hospital or outpatient setting. SC injections may be administered in the hospital, in an outpatient center, or by the patient at home. Assess whether the patient will be able to return for daily injections or whether he or she has the ability to self-administer the drug. The drug should be kept refrigerated between 2°C and 8°C but not allowed to freeze. Assess whether there is a refrigerator at home if the patient is to self-administer the drug. The drug may be allowed to come to room temperature before administration and is stable at room temperature for up to 24 hours.

Nursing Diagnoses and Outcomes
• Risk for Altered Body Temperature related to neutropenia
Desired outcome: Febrile neutropenia will be avoided while receiving filgrastim.
• Risk for Caregiver Role Strain related to need to bring patient daily to clinic for treatment with filgrastim
Desired outcome: Caregiver role strain will not develop.
• Risk for Infection related to neutropenia
Desired outcome: The patient will not develop an infection while receiving filgrastim.

- Risk for Pain, Medullary Bone, related to adverse effect of filgrastim

  Desired outcome: Bone pain will not develop or will not be unmanageable if it develops while the patient is taking filgrastim.

- Management of Individual, Effective Therapeutic Regimen, as evidenced by using correct technique daily to administer filgrastim subcutaneously and returning for all follow-up appointments

  Desired outcome: Patient will be adept at self-administering filgrastim before discharge home and will be able to demonstrate technique when he or she returns for first follow-up appointment.

Planning and Intervention

Maximizing Therapeutic Effects

To achieve the maximum therapeutic effect from the filgrastim, take the following actions:

- Keep it refrigerated. Allow the drug to reach room temperature before administering it.
- If giving the drug intravenously, dilute it in 5% dextrose solution with albumin added, to prevent absorption by plastic materials.
- Do not dilute the drug in saline, because it may precipitate.
- Avoid shaking the drug, which can damage the protein.
- Administer filgrastim with the first cycle of chemotherapy for those at high risk for febrile neutropenia, including older adults.
- Administer filgrastim within 24 hours of the completion of chemotherapy.

Minimizing Adverse Effects

To prevent adverse effects, be careful not to decrease the dose prematurely (before the expected neutrophil nadir, or lowest point, is expected). Additionally, discard any vial that has been at room temperature for more than 24 hours, use only one dose per vial, and never re-enter a used vial. Because filgrastim is preservative free, these actions guard against bacterial growth. If the absolute neutrophil count remains above 1,000/mm³ for 3 consecutive days, discontinue filgrastim to prevent excessively high neutrophil counts. Patients should be monitored with biweekly CBCs during treatment because the increased blood viscosity caused by overproduction of white blood cells can lead to acute respiratory distress or sickle-cell crisis (Quirion, 2009).

Providing Patient and Family Education

Patients with neutropenia are at increased risk for contracting an infection. When providing patient education, instruct the patient and those in contact with the patient to wash their hands frequently, avoid crowds, and avoid people with illnesses (Box 33.2).

Ongoing Assessment and Evaluation

Monitor the patient's temperature closely (at least daily) throughout therapy for fever indicating infection. Monitor

Keeping Neutropenic Patients Infection Free

Patients who are neutropenic are at increased risk if they contract an infection, because they cannot defend themselves against the infecting organism. The infection may become severe or even life threatening. This is true for even "common" infections, which most people can overcome fairly easily on their own. Patients who are immunocompromised by either disease or drug therapy should be taught how to minimize their risk of becoming sick with an infection, as follows:

- Wash hands frequently. Family members and others in the household should also wash their hands frequently.
- Avoid people with acute illnesses.
- Avoid going out in crowds, especially during cold and flu season. This precaution would include such places as malls, movie theaters, and worship services.
- Handle food safely. Cook meats to an appropriately high temperature to kill bacteria. Clean thoroughly all surfaces that have come into contact with raw food products. Refrigerate leftover food as soon as possible.

---

the WBC count throughout filgrastim therapy, two to three times per week. The WBC count should rise and return to a normal level but should not become unduly elevated. If patients must use drugs that potentiate neutrophil release, monitoring the WBC is especially important, because a synergistic effect may occur. Once the absolute neutrophil count remains above 1,000/mm³ for 3 consecutive days, discontinue filgrastim. The other components of a complete blood count (CBC) should also be monitored to detect any adverse effects from filgrastim. Filgrastim therapy is effective when infection is avoided (or is minimal if it occurs) and the WBC count rises to a normal level.

Drugs Closely Related to 🅿 Filgrastim

Pegfilgrastim

Pegfilgrastim (Neulasta) is produced by recombinant DNA technology. Like filgrastim, pegfilgrastim is used in myelosuppressive chemotherapy to decrease the incidence of infection manifested as febrile neutropenia in patients who have nonmyeloid cancer and are receiving chemotherapy that suppresses the WBC count. However, unlike the prototype, it should not be used for peripheral blood progenitor cell mobilization. Pegfilgrastim is filgrastim that has been chemically altered by attaching a polyethylene glycol molecule to the filgrastim molecule. Although this change in molecular size does not alter the way the drug acts to increase the WBC count, it does have substantial effects on the pharmacokinetics and thus on the dosing of the drug. Pegfilgrastim, unlike filgrastim, has poor renal excretion. Its sole mechanism of elimination is related to binding on receptors of neutrophils (Quirion, 2009). When mature neutrophil counts remain low (as a result of myelosuppression from chemotherapy), unbound, circulating levels of pegfilgrastim remain high, stimulating more neutrophil development. Once the mature

MEMORY CHIP

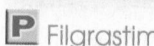 Filgrastim

- Used in patients with cancer to increase their neutrophil counts and to support stem cell harvest
- A DNA recombinant granulocyte colony-stimulating factor (G-CSF) that stimulates white blood cell development just as endogenous G-CSF does
- Administered by IV infusion or daily SC injections
- Most common adverse effect: medullary bone pain; nausea and vomiting
- Most serious adverse effects: none
- **Life span alert: Older adults are more at risk from complications with neutropenia; prophylactic use of G-CSF is usually appropriate.**
- **Patient safety alert: Patients have a high risk of infection until neutropenia is corrected.**
- Maximizing therapeutic effects: Do not dilute in saline use D5W; avoid shaking; do not use 24 hours pre- or post-chemotherapy; administer with the first cycle of chemotherapy in those at high risk for febrile neutropenia, including older adults.
- Minimizing adverse effects: Do not decrease the dose before the expected neutrophil nadir; keep refrigerated and use aseptic technique to minimize risk of bacterial growth.
- Most important patient education: how to decrease risk of infection

---

neutrophil cell count has increased sufficiently, receptors are present to enable binding and elimination of the pegfilgrastim. The elimination half-life of pegfilgrastim is much longer than for filgrastim: 15 to 80 hours instead of 3.5 hours. The advantage of this pharmacokinetic difference is that pegfilgrastim has to be given only once per chemotherapy cycle, instead of daily. Although the current labeling of pegfilgrastim states not to administer the drug between 14 days prior to and 24 hours after the administration of chemotherapy, one study showed that pegfilgrastim could be safely given simultaneously with chemotherapy in weekly chemotherapy schedules (Lokich, 2005). This difference may increase patients' adherence to therapy because they do not need to return daily for injections as they do with filgrastim. Patients may also prefer this therapy because they receive fewer injections.

Effectiveness, contraindications, precautions, drug interactions, and adverse effects of pegfilgrastim are similar to those of filgrastim. Pegfilgrastim, which is administered subcutaneously, comes in prefilled syringes that should be protected from light. Although it is kept refrigerated, it should be allowed to come to room temperature before administration. Like filgrastim, it should not be shaken. Because the solution is preservative free, only one injection should be administered per syringe; any remaining medication should be discarded. Pegfilgrastim should not be administered to patients weighing less than 45 kg (Quirion, 2009).

As with filgrastim, the patient's CBC with differential must be monitored after pegfilgrastim therapy. However, because patients are not seen as frequently when they receive

pegfilgrastim as when they receive filgrastim, it is especially important that they are taught the signs of infection and know when to contact the clinic or the prescriber.

Sargramostim

Sargramostim (Leukine), a granulocyte-macrophage colony-stimulating factor (GM-CSF), is produced by recombinant DNA technology in a yeast expression system. This 127-amino-acid glycoprotein has an amino acid sequence that differs from the natural human GM-CSF by substitution of leucine at position 23; the carbohydrate portion may also be different than in the native protein. Unlike G-CSF (filgrastim), which induces production only of granulocytes, specifically neutrophils, GM-CSF induces partially committed progenitor cells to divide and differentiate into the granulocyte and the macrophage pathways. Sargramostim increases the cytotoxicity of monocytes toward certain neoplastic cell lines and activates neutrophils to inhibit the growth of pathogens or tumor cells.

Sargramostim is used to treat patients with non-Hodgkin lymphoma, acute lymphoblastic leukemia, and Hodgkin disease who are undergoing autologous bone marrow transplantation (transplantation of their own bone marrow that was previously collected). It accelerates myeloid recovery in these patients. Sargramostim is also used in bone marrow transplant failure or when engraftment delays occur. It can be used after the induction of chemotherapy in older adults with acute myelogenous leukemia to shorten their neutrophil recovery time and reduce severe, life-threatening infections. Sargramostim can also be used to mobilize the hematopoietic progenitor cells into the peripheral circulation, where they can be collected by leukapheresis. The additional progenitor cells are later returned after chemotherapy, enabling more rapid engraftment and decreasing the need for supportive care. The drug is administered after collection and transplantation of peripheral blood progenitors, to rapidly increase monocyte production. Sargramostim is also used after allogenic (from a matched donor) bone marrow transplantation to accelerate the myeloid recovery.

Unlabeled uses of sargramostim include increasing WBC counts in patients with myelodysplastic syndromes and in patients with AIDS who are receiving zidovudine; limiting the duration of leukopenia secondary to myelosuppressive chemotherapy and decreasing myelosuppression in preleukemic patients; correcting neutropenia in aplastic anemia; and decreasing transplantation-associated organ system damage, particularly liver and kidney disease (neutropenia correlates with organ system injury). Sargramostim is administered by IV infusion for most applications. It may be given subcutaneously when used after peripheral blood progenitor cell transplantation.

Contraindications to sargramostim use include presence of excess leukemic myeloid blasts in the bone marrow or peripheral blood, known hypersensitivity to the drug, simultaneous administration of chemotherapy or radiotherapy, or administration of sargramostim 24 hours preceding or following chemotherapy or radiotherapy. Like filgrastim, sargramostim is a pregnancy category C drug. Whether it is excreted into breast milk is unknown. It does not appear to produce any greater toxicity in children than in adults.

Although most of the adverse effects that occur with sargramostim can also be attributed to the disease process or the chemotherapy used to treat it, it is necessary to be alert for unique events that may occur with sargramostim. Bone pain can occur, as with filgrastim. Sargramostim should be administered in the evening to minimize this problem; administration of acetaminophen 20 to 30 minutes before injection is also helpful. Site reactions are possible. Special attention to injection technique, as recommended by Buchsel and colleagues (2002), minimizes site pain. These steps include:

- Allowing enough time for the drug to come to room temperature before administration
- Choosing a short (⅝-inch), fine-gauge (25–27) needle
- Icing the injection site before and after injection
- Avoiding pinching the skin if possible
- Injecting no more than 2 mL into any injection site
- Injecting the medication slowly into the SC space, avoiding IM injections
- Not rubbing after injection
- Rotating injection sites among the upper arms, abdomen, and thighs

Occasional transient supraventricular arrhythmias may occur during administration of sargramostim, especially if the patient has a history of cardiac arrhythmias. These arrhythmias are reversible when the drug is discontinued. Trapping of granulocytes in the pulmonary circulation has occurred following sargramostim infusion, sometimes producing dyspnea. The recommended treatment for patients who become dyspneic is to reduce the rate of infusion by half. In patients with pre-existing pleural and pericardial effusions, sargramostim may aggravate fluid retention. This condition is usually reversible with dose interruption or reduction, although occasionally a diuretic is needed.

A first-dose effect has occurred rarely following the first dose of sargramostim. In this syndrome, respiratory distress, hypoxia, flushing, hypotension, syncope, or tachycardia occurs. The patient should be monitored for these problems for the first 20 minutes after the first injection, and the first dose should be administered in a clinical setting where the patient can be observed. The syndrome should be treated by stopping the infusion and treating the patient according to symptoms. Oxygen, methylprednisone, and diphenhydramine may be indicated. When symptoms have resolved, the infusion is resumed at half the rate. These effects do not usually happen again with future doses.

Excessively high WBC counts have sometimes rapidly occurred with sargramostim therapy (absolute neutrophil count [ANC] above 20,000 cells/mm³ or platelet count above 500,000/mm³). If this effect occurs, the dose should be reduced or temporarily stopped.

In some patients with pre-existing renal or hepatic dysfunction, sargramostim has induced elevation of serum creatinine or bilirubin and hepatic enzymes.

© INTERLEUKINS

Unlike other interleukins, oprelvekin (Neumega)—also known as interleukin-11—primarily alters hematopoietic activity and stimulates the production of platelets. Other interleukins are presented in Chapter 54. Interleukin-11, the sole drug in this class, is by necessity also the prototype.

Nursing Management of the Patient Receiving Ⓟ Oprelvekin

Core Drug Knowledge

Pharmacotherapeutics

Oprelvekin is used to prevent severe thrombocytopenia and to reduce the need for platelet transfusions following myelosuppressive chemotherapy in adult patients with non-myeloid malignancies who are at high risk for severe thrombocytopenia. It is administered as an SC dose once daily.

Pharmacokinetics

The peak serum level of oprelvekin is reached 3.2 hours after it is given subcutaneously. Although the drug is thought to be metabolized, the exact mechanism is not known. It is eliminated by the kidney.

Pharmacodynamics

Oprelvekin is produced in *E. coli* by recombinant DNA technology. The resultant polypeptide is 177 amino acids long and differs from the 178-amino-acid length of endogenous interleukin-11 by a missing amino-terminal proline residue. Bone-forming and bone-resorbing cells are potential targets of interleukin-11. Its primary hematopoietic activity is to directly stimulate the production of megakaryocyte progenitor cells and thrombopoietin. This action stimulates production of platelets that are structurally and functionally the same as those platelets produced by endogenous interleukin-11. Platelet counts begin to rise 5 to 9 days after starting drug therapy with oprelvekin. When treatment with oprelvekin is stopped, platelet levels continue to rise for about 7 days; they fall toward baseline in about 14 days.

Contraindications and Precautions

Oprelvekin is contraindicated only if the patient has hypersensitivity to the drug or any of its components. Caution should be used if oprelvekin is used in patients with pre-existing cardiomyopathy or CHF, because fluid retention is a common effect of therapy. Use caution if the patient has a history of atrial arrhythmia, which may increase the risk of developing an atrial arrhythmia from oprelvekin use. Do not use this drug with or immediately following cytotoxic chemotherapy. Oprelvekin is a pregnancy category C drug and has caused increased rates of fetal death in animal studies.

Adverse Effects

Nausea and vomiting are the most common adverse effects from oprelvekin, occurring in about 77% of patients. Fluid retention with weight gain is the next most common adverse effect, occurring in 59% of patients; this is a potentially very serious adverse effect. This condition may be evidenced by peripheral edema, dyspnea on exertion, an increase in pleural effusion (if effusion was present before therapy), pulmonary edema, and decreases of about 10% to 15% in hemoglobin concentration, hematocrit, and RBCs (dilutional anemia caused by an increase in plasma volume). The cardiovascular adverse effects of oprelvekin may also be related to fluid retention (tachycardia, vasodilation, palpitations, syncope, and atrial fibrillation and flutter). Other fairly common adverse effects include headache, fatigue, dizziness, rash, bone pain, and febrile neutropenia. Transient, mild blurred vision, conjunctival fluid, and papilledema have been reported. Papilledema, conjunctival fluid, and tachycardia are more common when oprelvekin is administered to children; the drug is not approved for use in children Anaphylaxis is possible, although not common.

Drug Interactions

There are no known drug interactions with oprelvekin.

Assessment of Relevant Core Patient Variables

Health Status

Assess for CHF, pleural or pericardial effusion, or susceptibility to developing CHF, because fluid retention is possible from oprelvekin. Also assess for a history of atrial fibrillation or flutter, other cardiac disorders, or cardiac medications, because these factors may increase the risk of atrial arrhythmia during drug therapy. Determine that at least 6 hours have elapsed after the completion of chemotherapy before starting oprelvekin. The patient should not have received myeloablative therapy (therapy in which myelocytes are destroyed), because this therapy is not an indication for oprelvekin use.

Life Span and Gender

Determine whether the patient is pregnant, because oprelvekin is a pregnancy category C drug. Ask the patient's age and whether she is breast-feeding. Whether oprelvekin crosses into breast milk is unknown, and the safety and efficacy for children under 12 years of age also are not known. Older adults may be more likely to develop atrial arrhythmias while taking oprelvekin.

Lifestyle, Diet, and Habits

Assess for poor potassium intake, as hypokalemia may increase the risk of atrial arrhythmias.

Environment

Find out whether refrigeration is available for storing oprelvekin. Oprelvekin must be kept refrigerated because neither it nor its diluent contains preservatives. The drug is also sensitive to light and must be stored accordingly.

Nursing Diagnoses and Outcomes

- Risk for Injury related to bleeding secondary to low platelet counts
  Desired outcome: *Injury will not occur while treating low platelet counts with oprelvekin.*
- Risk for Fluid Volume Excess related to adverse effects of oprelvekin
  Desired outcome: *Retention of fluid will not occur or will be controllable while on oprelvekin therapy.*
- Risk for Infection related to lack of medical asepsis in storage, preparation, and administration of subcutaneous oprelvekin
  Desired outcome: *The patient will remain free of infection.*
- Risk for Caregiver Role Strain related to the need to bring patient daily to clinic for treatment with oprelvekin
  Desired outcome: *Caregiver role strain will not occur.*

Planning and Intervention

Maximizing Therapeutic Effects

Store the powdered drug and the diluent in the refrigerator but do not freeze it. Keep the drug out of direct light. Reconstitute oprelvekin with the sterile water for injection (without preservative) that is provided with the medication. When injecting the sterile water into the vial, direct the spray of fluid toward the glass wall. To prevent excessive agitation, do not aim it directly into the powdered drug. Do not shake or excessively agitate the vial, which can denature the protein. To fully reconstitute the powder, gently swirl the vial.

Administration of oprelvekin should begin 6 to 24 hours after chemotherapy is completed. Continue until the post-nadir platelet count is greater than or equal to 50,000 cells/mm³. Clinical trials showed the need to dose for 10 to 21 days; the effect of giving oprelvekin for more than 21 days is not known. Discontinue oprelvekin treatment at least 2 days before starting the next round of chemotherapy.

Minimizing Adverse Effects

Because neither oprelvekin nor the sterile water used to dilute it contains preservatives, take care to maintain aseptic technique when reconstituting and drawing up the medication. Do not re-enter or reuse the single-dose vial. Be certain to use the reconstituted drug within 3 hours of reconstitution.

Monitor fluid intake and output carefully. Diuretics may be indicated if the patient is experiencing fluid retention from oprelvekin therapy.

Providing Patient and Family Education

If the patient will self-administer at home, teach the patient how to administer the drug safely and correctly into the subcutaneous tissue. Patient education should emphasize the importance of telling the physician or nurse when fluid retention occurs and should also emphasize the need to avoid activities that may cause bleeding until platelet counts are in the normal range.

MEMORY CHIP

P Oprelvekin (Interleukin-11)

- Used to prevent severe thrombocytopenia in cancer patients
- A recombinant DNA polypeptide that stimulates production of platelets in the same way that endogenous interleukin-11 does
- Administered daily by SC injection
- Major contraindication: Do not use with or immediately following cytotoxic chemotherapy.
- Most common adverse effects: nausea and vomiting, fluid retention, febrile neutropenia
- Most serious adverse effects: CHF or pulmonary edema from fluid retention; atrial arrhythmias
- **Life span alert: Older adults may be more likely to develop atrial arrhythmias.**
- Maximizing therapeutic effects: Do not shake or excessively agitate the vial; begin administration 6 to 24 hours after the completion of chemotherapy; continue until the postnadir platelet count is greater than or equal to 50,000 cells/mm³; discontinue 2 days prior to next chemotherapy.
- Minimizing adverse effects: Monitor fluid intake and output; maintain aseptic technique.
- Most important patient education: Contact prescriber if fluid retention occurs; avoid activities that increase risk for bleeding.

Ongoing Assessment and Evaluation

Monitor the patient's platelet count throughout oprelvekin therapy. Continue with therapy until the post-nadir platelet count is greater than or equal to 50,000 cells/mm³. Also, monitor the other components of the CBC to detect any adverse effects. Until the platelet count is adequate, monitor the patient for bleeding. Therapy with oprelvekin is effective if the platelet count rises to normal and severe bleeding is prevented.

CHAPTER SUMMARY

- The immune system is a complex system of cells and chemical mediators that prevents foreign pathogens or cells from invading the body.
- The mature blood cells differ in structure and function, but all develop from a common progenitor cell, or stem cell, from within the bone marrow.
- Blood cell components may be altered because of pathophysiology or drug therapy to treat a disease process.
- Drugs that stimulate the immune system to produce blood cells are hematopoietic growth factors. Drugs that stimulate production of RBCs are erythropoietics, those that produce WBCs are colony-stimulating factors, and those that increase platelets include a special interleukin. These drugs perform the same function as their endogenous counterparts.
- Recombinant human erythropoietin, also known as epoetin alfa, is used to treat anemias that result from decreased production of RBCs (erythropoiesis). Tissue oxygenation cannot occur optimally with anemia. Anemia is common

in chronic kidney disease, in CHF, and after some types of drug therapy.

- Iron is also needed to form RBCs. Epoetin alfa therapy that is not effective or has a diminished effect is likely attributable to iron deficiency, which may be absolute or functional. Most patients who receive epoetin alfa therapy need iron supplementation at some time for RBCs to be produced.
- The colony-stimulating factors are the granulocyte colony-stimulating factors (G-CSF) and the granulocyte-macrophage colony-stimulating factors (GM-CSF). They stimulate WBC production. Neutropenia and other suppression of the WBC count frequently occur after chemotherapy and use of some other types of drugs. Low WBC counts, especially low neutrophil counts, place the patient at increased risk for contracting an infection.
- Unlike other interleukins, interleukin-11 (oprelvekin) has hematopoietic properties and stimulates the production of platelets. Without an adequate number of platelets, proper blood clotting cannot take place. The patient is at risk for excessive bleeding (internal or external).
- Drugs that promote production of blood cells should not be given at the same time as chemotherapy because the rapidly producing cells are likely to be killed by the drug therapy.

QUESTIONS FOR STUDY AND REVIEW

1. What are the principal polypeptides and glycoproteins involved in hematopoiesis?
2. Why are people with chronic kidney disease anemic?
3. What is the major risk to people who are neutropenic after chemotherapy?
4. How are platelets produced?
5. Why do patients with CHF require close monitoring of their intake and output of fluids when they are started on oprelvekin?
6. Your patient has CHF and chronic kidney disease and is receiving epoetin alfa. Why should the target range for hemoglobin be set lower than what is usually considered "normal"?

NEED MORE HELP?

Chapter 33 of the Study Guide to Accompany *Drug Therapy in Nursing*, 4th Edition, contains NCLEX-style questions and other learning activities to reinforce your understanding of the concepts presented in this chapter. For additional information or to purchase the study guide, visit **the Point**.

REFERENCES

Aapro, M., Coiffier, B., Dunst, J., et al. (2006). Effect of treatment with epoetin beta on short-term tumour progression and survival in anemic patients with cancer: a meta-analysis. *British Journal of Cancer*, 95(11):1467–1473.

Amgen Inc. (2007). *Neupogen® (filgrastim)* [Prescribing information]. Retrieved October 28, 2009, from http://www.neupogen.com/pdf/Neupogen_PI.pdf

Bohlius, J., Schmidlin, K., Brillant, C., Schwarzer, G., Trelle, S., Seidenfeld, J., et al.(2009). Erythropoietin or Darbepoetin for patients with cancer—meta-analysis based on individual patient data. *Cochrane Database of Systematic Reviews,* (3):CD007303.

Buchsel, P. C., Forgey, A., Grape F. B., et al. (2002). Granulocyte macrophage colony-stimulating factor: current practice and novel approaches. *Clinical Journal of Oncology Nursing,* 2002;6(4):198–205.

Food and Drug Administration MedWatch. (January 26, 2007). 2007 Safety Alert: Aranesp (darbepoetin alfa). Accessed October 31, 2009, from *http://www.fda.gov/Safety/MedWatch/SafetyInformation/SafetyAlertsforHumanMedicalProducts/ucm150816.htm*

Haiden, N., Schwindt, J., Cardona, F., et al. (2006). Effects of a combined therapy of erythropoietin, iron, folate, and vitamin B_{12} on the transfusion requirements of extremely low birth weight infants. *Pediatrics,* 118(5):2004–2013.

Lokich, J. (2005). Same-day pegfilgrastim and chemotherapy. *Cancer Investigation,* 23(7):573–576.

Lambin, P., Ramaekers, B. L. T., van Mastrigt, G. A. P. G., et al. (2009). Erythropoietin as an adjuvant treatment with (chemo) radiation therapy for head and neck cancer. *Cochrane Database of Systematic Reviews,* (3):CD006158.

Martí-Carvajal, A. J., & Solà, I. (2007). Treatment for anemia in people with AIDS. *Cochrane Database of Systematic Reviews,* (1):CD004776.

Mircescu, G., Garneata, L., Ciocalteu, A., et al. (2006). Once-every-2-weeks and once-weekly epoetin beta regimens: Equivalency in hemodialyzed patients. *American Journal of Kidney Disease,* 48(3):445–455.

National Comprehensive Cancer Network. (2009). NCCN clinical practice guidelines in oncology: Cancer- and treatment-related anemia. Retrieved from *http://www.nccn.org/professionals/physician_gls/PDF/anemia.pdf*

National Comprehensive Cancer Network. (2009). NCCN clinical practice guidelines in oncology: Myeloid growth factors. Retrieved from *http://www.nccn.org/professionals/physician_gls/PDF/myeloid_growth.pdf*

National Kidney Foundation. (2006). Clinical practice guidelines and clinical practice recommendations for anemia in chronic kidney disease. Retrieved from *http://www.kidney. org/professionals/KDOQI/guidelines_anemia/guide1.htm.*

Ohlsson, A., & Aher, S. M. (2006). Early erythropoietin for preventing red blood cell transfusion in preterm and/or low birth weight infants. *Cochrane Database of Systematic Reviews,* (3):CD004863.

Palazzuoli, A., Silverberg, D., Iovine, F., et al. (2006). Erythropoietin improves anemia exercise tolerance and renal function and reduces B-type natriuretic peptide and hospitalization in patients with heart failure and anemia. *American Heart Journal,* 152(6):1096.e9–e15.

Papatheofanis, F. J., Smith, C., Mody, S. H., et al. (2007). Dosing patterns, hematologic outcomes, and costs of erythropoietic agents in anemic predialysis chronic kidney disease patients from an observational study. *American Journal of Therapeutics,* 14(4):322–327.

Quirion, E. (2009). Filgrastim and pegfilgrastim use in patients with neutropenia. *Clinical Journal of Oncology Nursing,* 13(3):324–328. http://search.ebscohost.com

Siamopoulos, K. C., Gouva, C., Katopodis, K. P., et al. (2006). Long-term treatment with EPO increases serum levels of high-density lipoprotein in patients with CKD. *American Journal of Kidney Disease,* 48(2):242–249.

Singh, A. K., Szczech, L., Tang, K. L., et al.; CHOIR Investigators. (2006). Correction of anemia with epoetin alfa in chronic kidney disease. *New England Journal of Medicine,* 355(20):2085–2098.

Straus, D. J., Testa, M. A., Sarokhan, B. J., et al. (2006). Quality-of-life and health benefits of early treatment of mild anemia: A randomized trail of epoetin alfa in patients receiving chemotherapy for hematologic malignancies. *Cancer,* 107(8):1909–1917.

Strippoli, G. F., Navaneethan, S. D., & Craig, J. C. (2006). Haemoglobin and haematocrit targets for the anaemia of chronic kidney disease. *Cochrane Database of Systematic Reviews,* (4):CD003967. current

UNIT 8

Respiratory System Drugs

Drugs Affecting the Upper Respiratory System

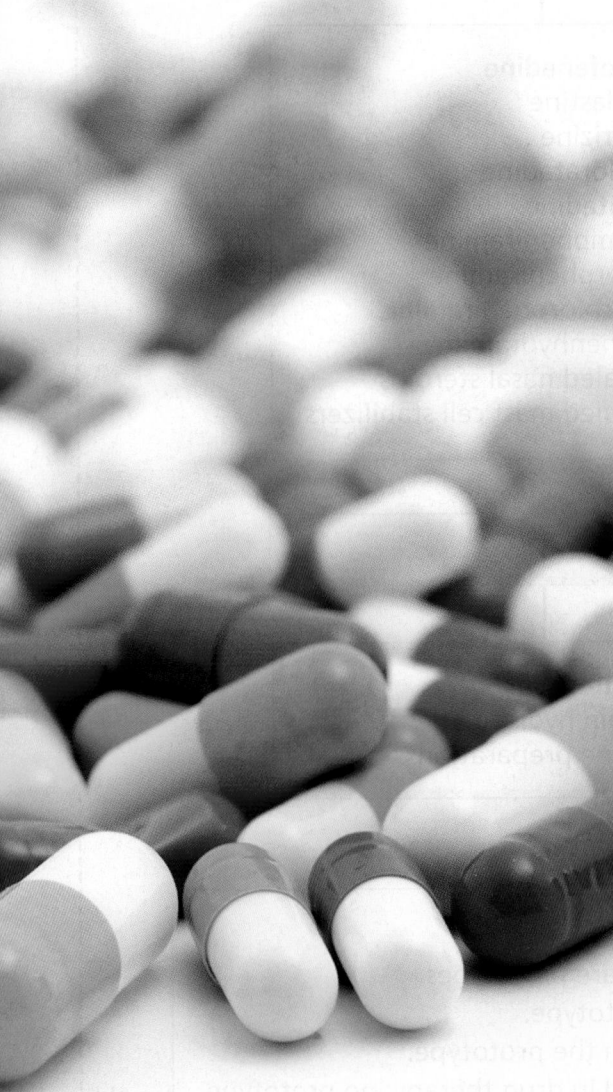

Learning Objectives

At the completion of this chapter the student will:

1. Describe the anatomy and physiology of the upper respiratory system.

2. Identify core drug knowledge pertaining to drugs that affect the upper respiratory system.

3. Identify core patient variables pertaining to drugs that affect the upper respiratory system.

4. Relate the interaction of core drug knowledge to core patient variables for drugs that affect the upper respiratory system.

5. Generate a nursing plan of care from the interactions between core drug knowledge and core patient variables for drugs that affect the upper respiratory system.

6. Describe nursing interventions to maximize therapeutic effects and minimize adverse effects for drugs that affect the upper respiratory system.

7. Determine key points for patient and family education for drugs that affect the upper respiratory system.

Key Terms

angioedema	expectorants	pharyngitis
antihistamines	enantiomer	rebound congestion
antitussives	histamine	rhinitis
common cold	influenza	sinusitis
decongestants	laryngitis	urticaria

Drugs Affecting the Upper Respiratory System

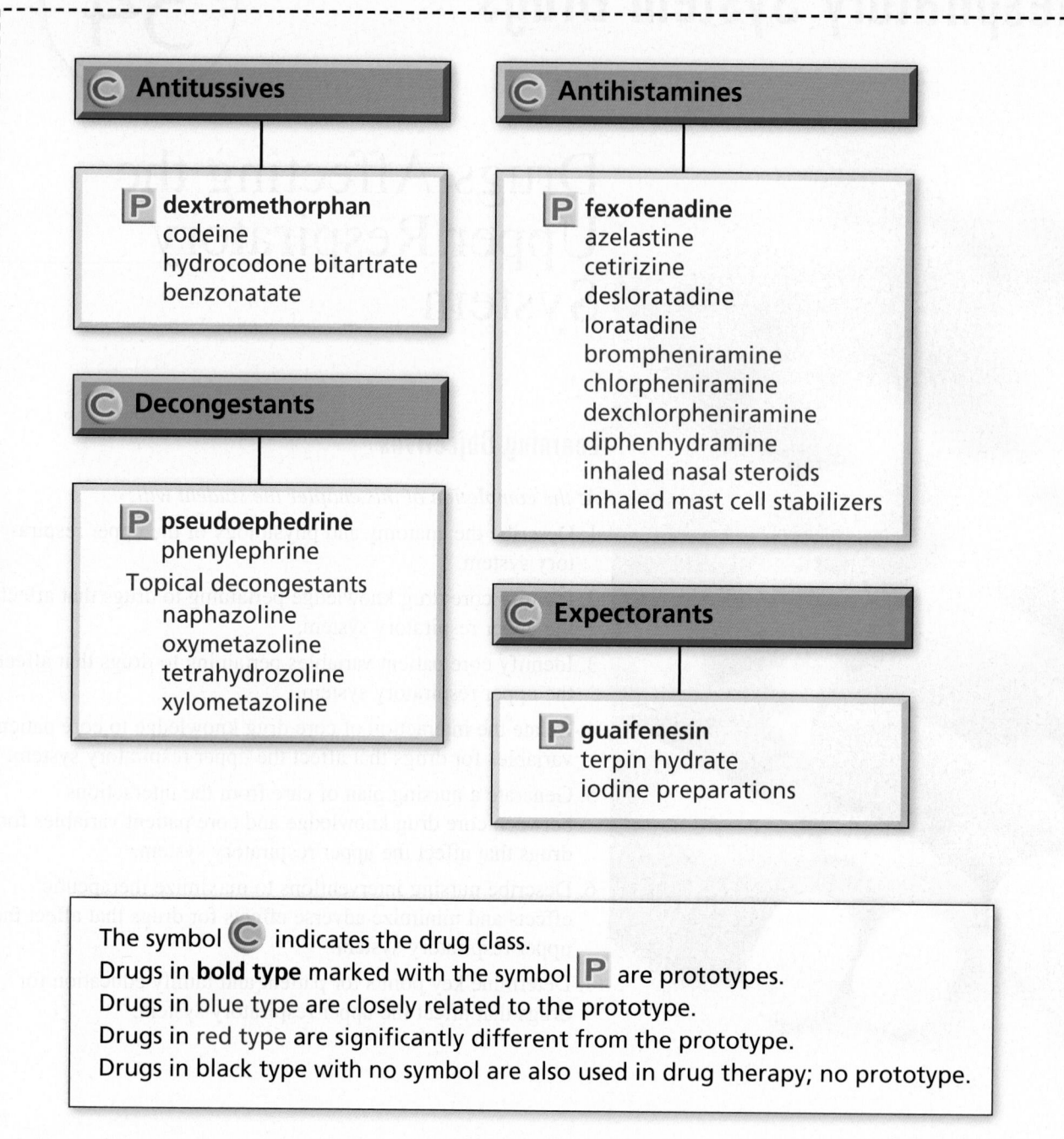

C Antitussives

P dextromethorphan
codeine
hydrocodone bitartrate
benzonatate

C Decongestants

P pseudoephedrine
phenylephrine
Topical decongestants
naphazoline
oxymetazoline
tetrahydrozoline
xylometazoline

C Antihistamines

P fexofenadine
azelastine
cetirizine
desloratadine
loratadine
brompheniramine
chlorpheniramine
dexchlorpheniramine
diphenhydramine
inhaled nasal steroids
inhaled mast cell stabilizers

C Expectorants

P guaifenesin
terpin hydrate
iodine preparations

The symbol C indicates the drug class.
Drugs in **bold type** marked with the symbol P are prototypes.
Drugs in blue type are closely related to the prototype.
Drugs in red type are significantly different from the prototype.
Drugs in black type with no symbol are also used in drug therapy; no prototype.

This chapter discusses drugs that affect the upper respiratory system. The upper respiratory system is essential for bringing oxygen into the body and body tissues. The classes of drugs that affect the upper respiratory system work to keep the airways open. The following drug classes are discussed in this chapter:

- **Antitussives**—drugs that block the cough reflex
- **Decongestants**—drugs that decrease the blood flow to an area and thus decrease overproduction of secretions
- **Antihistamines**—drugs that block the release or action of **histamine,** a chemical released during inflammation, which increases secretions and narrows airways
- **Expectorants**—drugs that increase productive cough to clear the airways

PHYSIOLOGY

The respiratory system is composed of the upper and lower respiratory systems. The upper respiratory system, or conducting airway, is composed of the nose, mouth, pharynx, larynx, trachea, and the bronchial tree (Figure 34.1). Air moves from the nasal cavity through the pharynx and into the larynx. The larynx contains the vocal chords and the epiglottis, the latter of which closes during swallowing to protect the lower respiratory tract from any foreign particles. From the larynx, air proceeds to the trachea, the main conducting airway into the lungs.

Air Filtration

Air usually moves into the nasal cavity through the nose. Nasal hairs catch and filter foreign substances, and the air is warmed and humidified as it passes by blood vessels close to the surface of the epithelial lining in the nasal passage. This epithelial lining contains goblet cells that produce mucus, which traps dust, microorganisms, pollen, and other foreign substances. These actions help purify the air and increase the efficiency of gas diffusion when the air reaches the lower respiratory tract.

The cells of the epithelial lining also contain cilia, microscopic hair-like projections of the cell membrane. The cilia are in constant motion, moving the mucus and any trapped substances toward the throat, where they are swallowed and destroyed. Three pairs of sinuses (air-filled passages through the skull) open into the nasal passage. The epithelial lining of the nose is continuous with the lining of the sinuses, and the mucus produced in the sinuses drains into the nasal cavity. The mucus drains into the throat, is swallowed, and proceeds to the gastrointestinal (GI) tract, where foreign materials are destroyed by the stomach acids.

Other Air-Purifying Mechanisms

The walls of the nasal cavity are sensitive to irritation. When receptors in these walls are stimulated, a central nervous system (CNS) reflex is initiated, and a sneeze results. The sneeze causes air to push through the nasal cavity under tremendous pressure, cleaning out any foreign irritant and opening the passages for more efficient flow of air. Throughout the airways, many macrophage scavengers are free to move throughout the epithelium and destroy invaders. Mast cells are present in abundance and release histamine, serotonin, adenosine triphosphate, and other chemicals to ensure a rapid and intense inflammatory reaction to any cell injury.

PATHOPHYSIOLOGY

The most common conditions that affect the upper respiratory system can be classified as inflammatory responses. For example, the rhinovirus and adenovirus are two types of common cold viruses that invade the tissues of the upper respiratory tract, initiating the release of histamine and prostaglandins and causing an inflammatory response.

Common Cold

The **common cold** is a viral infection that starts in the upper respiratory tract, sometimes spreads to the lower structures, and may contribute to secondary infections in the eyes or middle ears. The main differences between the common cold and other respiratory infections are the absence of fever and the relative mildness of the symptoms. Cold symptoms vary from person to person. Manifestations may include sneezing, headaches, fatigue, chills, sore throat, inflammation of the nose (**rhinitis**), and nasal discharge. Usually, there is no fever. The secretions are generally watery and clear. Pathologic changes occurring in the mucous membrane that lines the nose, the nasal sinuses, the nasopharynx, and other upper respiratory passages may include tissue swelling, congestion of blood, and oozing of fluids.

Allergic or Seasonal Rhinitis

A condition similar to the common cold that afflicts many people is called allergic or seasonal rhinitis. This inflammation

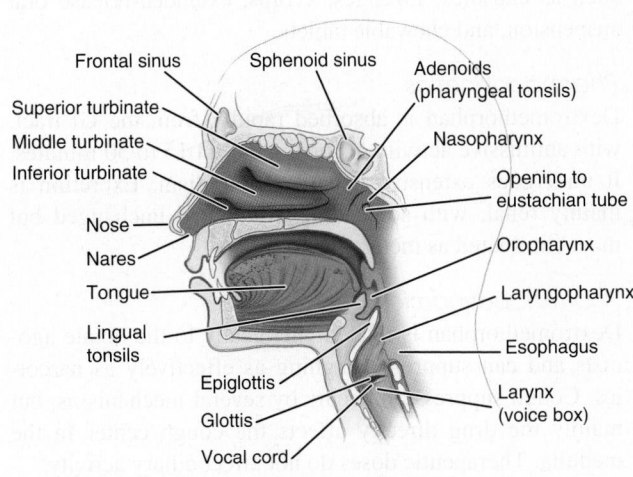

- FIGURE 34.1 Structures of the upper airway.

of the nasal cavity also is commonly called hay fever. It occurs when the upper airways respond to a specific allergen (e.g., pollen, mold, or dust) with a vigorous inflammatory response, resulting in nasal congestion, sneezing, stuffiness, and watery eyes. Other areas of the upper respiratory tract can become irritated or infected, resulting in inflammation.

Sinusitis

Sinusitis occurs when the epithelial lining of the sinus cavities becomes inflamed. It can be caused by bacteria or viruses. The resultant swelling often causes severe pain because the bony cavity cannot stretch and the swollen tissue pushes against the bone and blocks the sinus passages. The danger of a sinus infection is that if it is untreated, the causative microorganisms can move up the sinus passages and into brain tissue.

Pharyngitis

Pharyngitis is an inflammation or infection of the pharynx (throat) caused by bacteria or viruses. The symptoms of pharyngitis caused by bacteria are generally redness and swelling of the throat, a pustulant fluid on the tonsils or discharged from the mouth, extreme soreness of the throat that is felt during swallowing, swelling of lymph nodes, and a slight fever. Viral pharyngitis infections produce raised whitish to yellow lesions in the pharynx that are surrounded by reddened tissue. They also cause fever, headache, and sore throat that last for 4 to 14 days. Lymphatic tissue in the pharynx also may become involved.

Laryngitis

Laryngitis is an inflammation of the larynx or voice box, caused by chemical or mechanical irritation, viral infections, or bacterial infections. Simple laryngitis usually is associated with the common cold or similar infections. Usually, the mucous membrane lining the larynx is the primary site of infection; it becomes swollen and filled with blood, secretes a thick mucous substance, and contains many inflammatory cells.

When the epiglottis, which closes the larynx during swallowing, becomes swollen and infected by influenza viruses, the larynx can become obstructed, and suffocation may result. Excessive smoking, alcoholism, or overuse of the vocal cords may cause chronic laryngitis. The mucous membrane becomes dry and covered with polyps, small lumps of tissue that project from the surface. In addition, the wall of the larynx may thicken and become inflamed. Additional causes of laryngitis include diphtheria, tuberculosis, and syphilis—serious infections that require aggressive treatment.

Influenza

Influenza is an infection caused by any of several strains of myxoviruses, categorized as types A, B, and C. Influenza is transmitted from person to person through the respiratory tract by inhalation of infected droplets ejected by coughing and sneezing. As the virus particles gain entrance to the body, they selectively attack and destroy the ciliated epithelial cells that line the upper respiratory tract, bronchial tubes, and trachea. The onset of symptoms is abrupt, with sudden and distinct chills, fatigue, and high temperature. A diffuse headache and severe muscular aches throughout the body are experienced and often are accompanied by irritation or a sense of rawness in the throat. Symptoms associated with other respiratory tract infections, such as coughing and nasal discharge, also may occur.

C ANTITUSSIVE DRUGS

Antitussives are drugs that suppress the cough reflex. Many disorders of the upper and lower respiratory tracts, including the common cold, sinusitis, pharyngitis, and pneumonia, are accompanied by an uncomfortable, nonproductive cough. Coughing normally is a protective mechanism that forces foreign irritants out of the respiratory system, opening it for more efficient flow of air. However, persistent coughing can be exhausting, cause muscle strain, and further irritate the respiratory tract. A cough that occurs without an active disease process or that persists after treatment may be a symptom of another disease process and should be investigated before any drug is given to alleviate it. Antitussive drugs include dextromethorphan, codeine, and hydrocodone bitartrate. Dextromethorphan (Robitussin, PediaCare, Vicks 44, Benylin Pediatric) is selected as the prototype antitussive. Table 34.1 presents a summary of antitussive drugs.

Nursing Management of the Patient Receiving ☐P Dextromethorphan

Core Drug Knowledge

Pharmacotherapeutics

Dextromethorphan is used in treating nonproductive cough. It is available widely in a variety of nonprescription forms, such as capsules, lozenges, syrups, extended-release oral suspension, and chewable tablets.

Pharmacokinetics

Dextromethorphan is absorbed rapidly from the GI tract, with antitussive activity occurring within 15 to 30 minutes. It undergoes extensive hepatic metabolism. Excretion is mainly renal, with some drug eliminated unchanged but most eliminated as metabolites.

Pharmacodynamics

Dextromethorphan is related chemically to the opiate agonists and can suppress coughing as effectively as narcotics. Cough suppression occurs by several mechanisms, but mainly the drug directly affects the cough center in the medulla. Therapeutic doses do not affect ciliary activity.

TABLE 34.1 Summary of Selected © Antitussives

Drug (Trade) Name	Selected Indications	Route and Dosage Range	Pharmacokinetics
P dextromethorphan (Benylin, Delsym, Robitussin Maximum Strength Cough, Robitussin Cough Calmers, Sucrets Cough Control Formula, Vicks 44 Cough)	Cough suppression	*Adult and adolescent:* PO, regular-release formulation: 10–20 mg PO every 4 h; or 30 mg every 6–8 h; Max: 120 mg/d *Child 6–11 y:* PO, 5–10 mg every 4 h; or 15 mg every 6–8 h; Max: 60 mg/d *Child 2–5 y:* 2.5–5 mg every 4 h; or 7.5 mg every 6–8 h; Max: 30 mg/d *Child <2 y:* Safe and effective usage is not established. Extended-release formulation: *Adult and adolescent:* 10 mL every 12 h; Max: 20 mL/d *Child 6–11 y:* 5 mL every 12 h; Max: 10 mL/d *Child 2–5 y:* 2.5 mL every 12 h; Max: 5 mL/d *Child <2 y:* Safe and effective usage is not established.	*Onset:* 15–30 min *Duration:* 5–6 h $t_{1/2}$: 11 h
benzonatate (Tessalon Perles)	Cough suppression	*Adult and child >10 y:* PO, 100 mg 3∞/d or every 4 h; Max: 600 mg/day *Child <10 y:* Safe and effective usage is not established.	*Onset:* 15–20 min *Duration:* 3–8 h $t_{1/2}$: Unknown
codeine	Cough suppression	*Adult:* PO, 10–20 mg every 4–6 h; Max: 120 mg/24 h *Elderly:* May require reduced doses *Child 6–12 y:* 5–10 mg every 4–6 h; Max: 60 mg/d *Child 2–5 y:* 2.5–5 mg every 4–6 h; Max: 30 mg/d *Child and infant <2 y:* Safe dosage has not been established.	*Onset:* 15–20 min *Duration:* 4–6 h $t_{1/2}$: 1.5–4 h
hydrocodone bitartrate (Hycodan, Hydromet, Hydropane, Mycodone, Tussigon)	Cough suppression	*Adult:* PO, 5–10 mg every 4–6 h; Max single dose: 15 mg *Adolescent >12 y:* PO, 0.6 mg/kg/d in 3–4 divided doses; Max single dose: 10 mg *Child 2–11 y:* 0.6 mg/kg/d in 3–4 divided doses; Max single dose: 5 mg	*Onset:* 10–20 min *Duration:* 3–6 h $t_{1/2}$: 3–8 h

Contraindications and Precautions

Dextromethorphan is contraindicated for treating chronic coughs resulting from emphysema and asthma. Because of its extensive hepatic metabolism, dextromethorphan is used with caution in patients with hepatic impairment. It also is used with caution during pregnancy. Although teratogenic effects have not been demonstrated, dextromethorphan is in pregnancy category C.

Adverse Effects

Although adverse effects are generally rare, dextromethorphan toxicity can occur and is characterized by nausea and vomiting, drowsiness, dizziness, irritability, and restlessness. In excessive doses, dextromethorphan poisoning may occur and induce symptoms similar to those associated with phencyclidine (Box 34.1).

Drug Interactions

Dextromethorphan may potentiate sedation when used with other CNS depressants. It may interact with monoamine oxidase inhibitors (MAOIs), resulting in serotonin syndrome, a dangerous condition that consists of nausea, hypotension, excitation, hyperpyrexia, and possible coma. It also may interact with fluoxetine, quinidine, and sibutramine. Table 34.2 lists drugs that interact with dextromethorphan.

Box 34.1 DEXTROMETHORPHAN POISONING

In excessive amounts, dextromethorphan (DMX) may induce euphoric, stimulant, and dissociative effects in children and adolescents. Neurobehavioral effects begin in as little as 30 minutes and can last up to 6 hours. In 2008, 5 teenage deaths were attributed to DMX poisoning.

	Dose	Effect
First Plateau	100–200 mg 1.5 mg/kg	Mild stimulation
Second Plateau	200–400 mg 2.5–7.5 mg/kg	Euphoria and hallucinations
Third Plateau	300–600 mg 7.5–15 mg/kg	Dissociate state
Fourth Plateau	>600 mg >15 mg/kg	Complete dissociation with unresponsiveness

TABLE 34.2 Agents That Interact with P Dextromethorphan		
Interactants	Effect and Significance	Nursing Management
juice: grapefruit, orange	Grapefruit and orange juice inhibit metabolism and intestinal efflux of dextromethorphan, resulting in increased risk of pharmacologic and adverse effects that last for several days.	Avoid administration of dextromethorphan with grapefruit or orange juice. Monitor for adverse effects.
monoamine oxidase inhibitors	Dextromethorphan can block neuronal uptake of serotonin and may produce serotonin syndrome.	Maintain interval of at least 2 wk between administration of these drugs.
Sibutramine	Coadministration of these agents may have additive serotonergic effects.	Avoid coadministration if possible. Monitor for CNS irritability, motor weakness, shivering, myoclonus, and altered consciousness. Ensure safety.

Assessment of Relevant Core Patient Variables

Health Status

Before administering dextromethorphan, review the patient's record to determine whether dextromethorphan may be administered safely. This drug is contraindicated for patients with emphysema or asthma. If coughing is suppressed in these patients, they may retain secretions that exacerbate their disease. It is also necessary to review the patient's record for drugs that may interact with dextromethorphan, especially antidepressants. Also, evaluate the patient for a history of hepatic insufficiency, because dextromethorphan is processed by the liver. Finally, perform a baseline evaluation of the head, eyes, ears, nose, and throat in addition to a complete lung assessment.

Life Span and Gender

Determine whether the patient is pregnant. Dextromethorphan, a pregnancy category C drug, should be used with caution during pregnancy. Dextromethorphan is not indicated for use in children younger than 2 years old. With adolescent patients, assess the potential for abuse. Dextromethorphan abuse is a growing problem in high schools.

Lifestyle, Diet, and Habits

Investigate the patient's need to drive or operate potentially dangerous equipment and advise the patient to refrain from these activities until the sedative effects of dextromethorphan use are known. It is important to assess the patient's typical intake of alcohol. Caution the patient about the potentially additive effects of dextromethorphan when used with alcohol, because both are CNS depressants. Assess the frequency of grapefruit or orange juice ingestion, because these juices can substantially increase the concentration of dextromethorphan.

Environment

Dextromethorphan is used commonly in over-the-counter (OTC) cough and cold preparations, and prescribed dextromethorphan is just as commonly self-administered by patients at home. Therefore, caution patients to read labels of all drugs they are taking to avoid a possible overdose.

Nursing Diagnoses and Outcomes

- Risk for Injury related to sensory-perceptual alteration from drug-induced drowsiness and sedation
  Desired outcome: The patient will remain free from injury related to sedation and drowsiness.
- Risk for Ineffective Airway Clearance related to suppression of cough reflex
  Desired outcome: The patient will maintain his or her baseline respiratory function.

Planning and Intervention

Maximizing Therapeutic Effects

In acute or long-term care settings, administer dextromethorphan at evenly spaced intervals to maintain blood levels of the drug at steady state. Provide environmental controls, including appropriate lighting, reduced noise, and comfortable temperature, to ease sensory-perceptual alteration and aid relaxation.

Minimizing Adverse Effects

During therapy, ensure that safety precautions are used, such as side rails and ambulation assistance. Assess respiratory status and movement of air periodically during drug use. Refrain from administering dextromethorphan with grapefruit or orange juice.

Providing Patient and Family Education

- Explain to patients and their families that taking dextromethorphan will help quiet a cough.
- Emphasize that sedation, drowsiness, and impaired orientation can occur. Because it can be sedating, tell patients to take dextromethorphan only as directed and not to drive or perform other tasks that require alertness. Some patients may require assistance walking if they react strongly to dextromethorphan.
- Explain to patients that they should not take dextromethorphan if they have ever had a reaction to it, are pregnant or breast-feeding, or have a history of liver problems.

- Caution patients who are taking certain antidepressants or drugs for obesity about the potential for serious drug–drug interactions.
- Alert patients not to take any OTC drugs or consume alcohol while taking dextromethorphan because doing so could increase sedation.
- Caution patients to keep dextromethorphan out of the reach of children.
- Tell patients to report immediately any chest tightness, difficulty breathing, noisy breathing, or shortness of breath. These symptoms may indicate that the drug is not working, or that a patient is having a reaction to the drug.
- Caution parents about the potential for abuse of dextromethorphan.

Ongoing Assessment and Evaluation

Monitor the effect of dextromethorphan on the patient's motor control, sedation, and respiratory status. By the end of therapy, the patient should remain free of injury related to sedation and have cough relief.

Drugs Closely Related to P Dextromethorphan

Codeine

Codeine is a controlled substance used in treating cough. Like dextromethorphan, it works directly on the medullary center to suppress the cough reflex. Codeine is more sedating than dextromethorphan and also may induce respiratory depression. It is contraindicated for patients who must cough to maintain a patent airway (e.g., postoperative patients). Codeine is used with caution in patients who are pregnant or breast-feeding and in patients with head injuries. It also is used cautiously in patients with chronic cough (e.g., that caused by emphysema or asthma) or in patients with a history of drug addiction. Adverse effects include sedation, dry mouth, nausea, vomiting, and constipation. Codeine also is discussed in Chapter 23.

MEMORY CHIP

P Dextromethorphan

- Used to manage nonproductive cough
- Major contraindication: cough resulting from emphysema or asthma
- Most common adverse effects: nausea, vomiting, and irritability
- Most serious adverse effects: drowsiness and dizziness
- Maximizing therapeutic effects: Administer at evenly spaced intervals throughout the day.
- Minimizing adverse effects: Institute precautions to ensure safety during potential drowsiness or dizziness.
- Most important patient education: Advise the patient to seek medical attention if cough does not resolve.

Hydrocodone Bitartrate

Hydrocodone bitartrate (Hycodan), also a controlled substance, is a derivative of codeine and acts directly on the cough reflex center in the medulla. It is combined with homatropine methylbromide. Hydrocodone is more sedating than codeine and has the same properties, contraindications, and adverse effects.

Drug Significantly Different From P Dextromethorphan

Benzonatate

Benzonatate (Tessalon, Tessalon Perles) is an oral nonnarcotic antitussive agent that is rarely used because it is not as effective as other antitussives. Benzonatate works by anesthetizing the stretch receptors in the respiratory tract, lung tissue, and pleura, interfering with their activity, and thereby reducing the cough reflex. At normal doses, it does not affect the respiratory center.

Benzonatate is used to coat the oropharynx to depress the gag reflex before intubation or endoscopy. The "Perles" are also topically applied to discrete areas of the body, such as a defined lesion or abnormality, before magnetic resonance imaging, because they show up as "markers" for more accurate mapping and measurement. Of course, neither of these uses is approved by the Food and Drug Administration.

C DECONGESTANT DRUGS

Decongestants are drugs taken to decrease nasal congestion related to the common cold, sinusitis, and allergic rhinitis, a condition that is caused by an inflammatory response in the upper respiratory tract. Nasal decongestants work by constricting the nasal arterioles, thereby decreasing the swelling of the nasal membrane. These drugs can be administered orally or topically. When decongestants are taken orally, they are absorbed in the body, thus increasing the chance of adverse effects. When used topically, the drug has the same therapeutic effects; however, the potential for adverse effects is diminished.

Many of the decongestants have abuse potential. Several OTC decongestant drugs have been used to make methamphetamine. In 2006, the Combat Methamphetamine Abuse Act (Box 34.2) was signed into law. This act regulates the sale of pseudoephedrine, ephedrine, and phenylpropanolamine. Although ephedrine and phenylpropanolamine have been removed from the market, pseudoephedrine is still the active ingredient in a number of OTC cough and cold medications.

Pseudoephedrine, which is discussed as the prototype decongestant, is most frequently known by the trade name Sudafed. In accordance with the Combat Methamphetamine Abuse Act, Sudafed and any combination drugs that contain pseudoephedrine have been removed from the shelves of drug stores, *but they have not been taken off the market*

Box 34.2 COMBAT METHAMPHETAMINE ACT

The Combat Methamphetamine Act stipulates that merchants who sell pseudoephedrine must:

- Keep a retrievable record of all purchases, identifying the name and address of each party, for two years.
- Require verification of proof of identity of all purchasers.
- Use protection and disclosure methods in the collection of personal information.
- Report to the Attorney General any suspicious payments or disappearances of the regulated products.
- Sell the nonliquid dose form of regulated product only in unit-dose blister packs.
- Sell regulated products behind the counter or in a locked cabinet in such a way as to restrict access.
- Have daily sales of regulated products not exceed 3.6 g, without regard to the number of transactions.
- Have monthly sales not exceed 9 g of pseudoephedrine base in regulated products.
- With mail order purchases, have monthly sales that do not exceed 7.5 g

(Table 34.3). Consumers must purchase drugs containing pseudoephedrine from a pharmacy, despite the fact the drugs do not require a prescription. The amount of pseudoephedrine that may be purchased is regulated by this act, so the medication is kept behind the pharmacy counter. Sudafed PE is the drug on the shelves of drug stores, supermarkets, and other consumer stores. It is not regulated because it does not contain pseudoephedrine. Table 34.4 presents a summary of decongestant drugs.

TABLE 34.3 Over-The-Counter Drugs Available From the Pharmacy

Active Ingredient(s)	Trade Name	Dosage
Pseudoephedrine	Sudafed	pseudoephedrine, 30 mg
pseudoephedrine ER, naproxen	Aleve Cold and Sinus	pseudoephedrine ER, 120 mg naproxen, 220 mg
pseudoephedrine, loratadine	Claritin-D 12-hour	pseudoephedrine, 120 mg loratadine, 5 mg
	Claritin-D 24-h	pseudoephedrine, 240 mg loratadine, 10 mg
pseudoephedrine, chlorpheniramine, Acetaminophen	Coricidin-D	pseudoephedrine, 30 mg chlorpheniramine, 2 mg acetaminophen, 325 mg
pseudoephedrine,	Drixoral	pseudoephedrine, 60 mg dexbrompheniramine, dexbrompheniramine, 3 mg acetaminophen acetaminophen, 500 mg
pseudoephedrine, guaifenesin	Mucinex-D	pseudoephedrine, 30 mg guaifenesin, 600 mg

Nursing Management of the Patient Receiving P Pseudoephedrine

Core Drug Knowledge

Pharmacotherapeutics

Pseudoephedrine can reduce the volume of nasal mucus and is recommended for the temporary relief of nasal congestion related to the common cold, allergic rhinitis, and sinusitis. It also is used to relieve the pressure of otitis media by promoting drainage of the eustachian tubes.

Pharmacokinetics

Pseudoephedrine is an oral drug readily absorbed from the GI tract, with onset of activity occurring within 30 minutes. Duration of action ranges from 4 to 6 hours, in regular formulations, to 8 to 12 hours in extended-release preparations Pseudoephedrine is metabolized by the liver and excreted in the urine. This drug also crosses the placenta and is secreted in breast milk.

Pharmacodynamics

Pseudoephedrine mimics the actions of the sympathetic nervous system and achieves its nasal decongestant effects by causing vasoconstriction in the nasal mucous membranes. This shrinkage decreases membrane size and promotes sinus drainage and improved airflow. Stimulation of other sympathetic receptors while the patient is taking pseudoephedrine can result in cardiovascular stimulation, constriction of renal arterioles, and anxiety.

Contraindications and Precautions

Pseudoephedrine is a pregnancy category C drug and should be used with caution during pregnancy or lactation because of its possible effects on the fetus and neonate. This drug should not be used by patients with severe hypertension and coronary artery disease for a prolonged period because it produces sympathomimetic effects such as increased heart rate and blood pressure. Special caution should be used in patients with diabetes, thyrotoxicosis, coronary artery disease, benign prostatic hypertrophy, and increased intraocular pressure because of the risk for sympathomimetic adverse effects, which could aggravate these conditions.

Adverse Effects

Adverse effects related to pseudoephedrine use are related primarily to its sympathomimetic effects on the CNS and cardiovascular systems. They occur almost immediately and include feelings of tension, anxiety, restlessness, tremor, insomnia, and weakness. Severe CNS reactions have included hallucinations, delusions, and convulsions. Adverse cardiovascular effects include palpitations, tachycardia, hypertension, and arrhythmias. Allergic reactions that have been reported with pseudoephedrine use include skin rashes and urticaria. Extreme dryness of the mucous membranes, resulting in pain and irritation, has been reported in some cases.

When sympathomimetic adverse effects occur, patients with diabetes, thyrotoxicosis, coronary artery disease,

TABLE 34.4 Summary of Selected Ⓒ Decongestants

Drug (Trade) Name	Selected Indications	Route and Dosage Range	Pharmacokinetics
Oral Decongestants			
Ⓟ pseudoephedrine (Sudafed, PediaCare, Triaminic, Contac)	Nasal decongestion	*Adult and child >12 y:* PO, 60 mg q4–6 h *Child >6 y:* PO, 30 mg q4–6 h *Child <6 y:* PO, 15 mg q4–6 h Sustained release: *Adult and child >12 y:* PO, 120 mg q12 h *Child <12 y:* not recommended Controlled release: *Adult and Child >12 y:* PO, 240 mg q24 h *Child <12 y:* not recommended	*Onset:* 30 min *Duration:* 4–6 h $t_{1/2}$: 7 h
phenylephrine (Sudafed PE, Neo-Synephrine, Neofrin; *Canadian:* Dionephrine)	Nasal decongestion	*Adult and Child >12 y:* PO, 10–20 mg q4 h *Child >6 y:* PO, 10 mg q4 h	*Onset:* 5–10 min *Duration:* 3–4 h $t_{1/2}$: Unknown
Topical Decongestants			
naphazoline (Albalon, Nafazair, Naphcon-A, Opcon-A, Vasocon-A, Visine-A)	Nasal decongestion	Intranasal dosage (0.05% nasal spray): *Adult:* 1–2 sprays in each nostril q4–6 h as needed Intranasal dosage (0.05% nasal drops): *Adult:* 1–2 drops in each nostril q3 h as needed *Child:* not recommended	Minimal systemic absorption
oxymetazoline (Afrin 12 Hour Nasal, Dristan 12 Hr Nasal, Visine, Ocu-Clear plus many others)	Nasal decongestion	Nasal dosage: *Adult and Child >6 y:* 1–2 drops or sprays of 0.05% solution in each nostril 2∞/d or as required, but no more frequently than q6 h *Child <6 y:* not recommended	Minimal systemic absorption
phenylephrine (Neo-Synephrine)	Nasal decongestion	*Adult and Child >12 y:* 2–3 drops or 2–3 sprays of 0.25%–1% solution in each nostril q4 h as needed *Child 6–12 y:* 2–3 drops of 0.25% solution in each nostril q4 h as needed *Child <6 y:* not recommended	Minimal systemic absorption
tetrahydrozoline (Tyzine)	Nasal decongestion Occular erythema (Visine)	*Adult and Child ε 2 y:* 3–4 sprays of 0.1% nasal solution in each nostril q3 h *Child <6 y:* not recommended *Adult and Child >12 y:* 2–4 drops of 0.1% solution q3 h *Child <6 y:* 2–3 drops of 0.05% solution in each nostril q3 h	Minimal systemic absorption
xylometazoline (Otrivin)	Nasal decongestion	*Adult and Child >12 y:* 1–3 sprays of 0.1% solution in each nostril q8–10 h *Child 2–12 y:* 1 spray of 0.05% solution in each nostril q8–10 h *Adult and Child >12 y:* 2–3 drops of 0.1% solution in each nostril q8–10 h *Child 2–12 y:* 2–3 drops of 0.05% solution in each nostril q8–10 h	Minimal systemic absorption

hypertension, benign prostatic hypertrophy, or increased intraocular pressure should discontinue using pseudoephedrine. Patients without concurrent disease may continue taking the drug, unless the adverse effects create a safety problem.

Drug Interactions
Increased hypertension may occur if pseudoephedrine is taken concurrently with MAOIs, guanethidine, methyldopa, or furazolidone. Instruct the patient to avoid such combinations. The duration of pseudoephedrine's effect may increase if it is taken with any urinary alkalinizer (e.g., potassium citrate, sodium citrate, sodium lactate, tromethamine, sodium acetate, and sodium bicarbonate) because the drug cannot be excreted into alkaline urine. An increased dose of pseudoephedrine may be necessary when giving it with urinary acidifiers, such as ammonium chloride, potassium phosphate, or sodium acid phosphate. Table 34.5 lists drugs that interact with pseudoephedrine.

TABLE 34.5	Agents That Interact with P Pseudoephedrine	
Interactants	**Effect and Significance**	**Nursing Management**
furazolidone	May increase the pressor sensitivity to mixed and indirect-acting sympathomimetics, such as pseudoephedrine, resulting in hypertension	Avoid coadministration. If used concurrently, monitor for hypertension. If hypertensive crisis results, consider the use of phentolamine.
Guanethidine	Depletes norepinephrine stores, resulting in hypertension	Use an alternative antihypertensive therapy.
monoamine oxidase inhibitors	Increase the amount of norepinephrine available for release by pseudoephedrine, resulting in severe headache, hypertension, and hyperpyrexia; hypertensive crisis possible	Avoid coadministration. If these are used together and hypertension develops, administer phentolamine.
methyldopa	Coadministration of methyldopa and pseudoephedrine may result in an increased pressor response, resulting in hypertension	Monitor the blood pressure during coadministration. Discontinue pseudoephedrine if hypertension occurs.
urinary acidifiers	Tubular reabsorption of pseudoephedrine possibly decreased due to a decreased urinary pH by urinary acidifiers	Monitor possible need for an increased dose of pseudoephedrine to achieve desired results. Acidification of the urine may be useful in the treatment of sympathomimetic intoxication.
urinary alkalinizers	Tubular reabsorption of pseudoephedrine possibly increased due to an increased urinary pH by urinary alkalinizers	Decrease the dose of pseudoephedrine during coadministration of a urinary alkalinizer.

Assessment of Relevant Core Patient Variables

Health Status

Review the patient's health history and perform a physical examination to determine any contraindications to the use of this drug. Contraindications include hypersensitivity to the drug, thyrotoxicosis, diabetes, hypertension, benign prostatic hypertrophy, cardiovascular disorders, pregnancy, and lactation.

Assess the patient's baseline orientation, affect, respiratory rate and sounds, blood pressure, and pulse.

Life Span and Gender

Be aware of the patient's age before administering pseudoephedrine. Pseudoephedrine must be given cautiously to elderly patients because they may experience more serious adverse effects than other patients. Avoid sustained-release preparations and use short-duration preparations in the elderly. Assess female patients for pregnancy. Pseudoephedrine is in pregnancy category C; pregnant women should avoid it unless the benefits outweigh the risks.

Lifestyle, Diet, and Habits

Assess the use of OTC medications. Pseudoephedrine is used in combination with many other agents, including antihistamines. Teach the patient to read ingredient labels carefully.

Environment

Pseudoephedrine is generally taken in the outpatient setting. Because it is an OTC medication and patients have easy access to the drug, caution them about overuse of pseudoephedrine and other decongestants. Frequent, long-term, or excessive use of decongestants induces rebound congestion. **Rebound congestion** occurs when the nasal passages become congested as the drug effect wears off and the body compensates by vasodilating the same nasal arterioles that the drug constricted. When rebound occurs, patients tend to use more of the drug to decrease the congestion, and a vicious cycle of congestion–drug use–congestion develops.

Nursing Diagnoses and Outcomes

• Risk for Injury caused by visual sensory-perceptual alterations (hallucinations) related to drug-induced CNS effects
  Desired outcome: The patient will be protected from injury related to drug use and will demonstrate safety procedures to use if these effects occur.
• Ineffective Tissue Perfusion: Cerebral or Cardiopulmonary, related to sympathomimetic effects
  Desired outcome: The patient will be monitored and dosage adjusted to minimize potential perfusion deficits or CNS effects.

Planning and Intervention

Maximizing Therapeutic Effects

In conjunction with pseudoephedrine therapy, encourage patients to use a humidifier, drink plenty of fluids, and avoid smoke-filled rooms, because dry air, dry mucous membranes, and airborne irritants may render the drug less effective.

Minimizing Adverse Effects

Provide the patient with appropriate safety measures, such as side rails, adequate lighting, and assistance with movement to avoid injury if CNS effects are experienced.

Providing Patient and Family Education

- Explain to patients that the purpose of pseudoephedrine is to promote breathing and relieve congestion.
- Tell patients not to take pseudoephedrine if they have ever had a reaction to it, have high blood pressure, or are breast-feeding. In addition, instruct patients to take the drug exactly as prescribed. Higher doses may cause nervousness, dizziness, chest pain, or sleeplessness.
- Tell patients not to take pseudoephedrine for more than 4 days. They should contact their health care providers to schedule an appointment if respiratory symptoms do not subside after 4 days.
- Caution patients to avoid using other OTC drugs, many of which also contain pseudoephedrine, because a serious overdose could occur.
- To avoid rebound congestion, teach patients strategies for decreasing the discomfort of nasal congestion and explain why excessive drug use should be avoided.
- Outline safety measures that may be necessary if CNS effects occur, such as getting assistance with ambulation, using adequate lighting, and avoiding driving or other tasks that require alertness.
- Urge patients to report excessive dizziness, weakness, palpitations, and sleeplessness, and to keep pseudoephedrine out of the reach of children.

Ongoing Assessment and Evaluation

Monitor patients receiving pseudoephedrine for rebound congestion, sedation, dizziness, weakness, tremor, urinary retention, and cardiovascular effects. By the end of therapy, the patient should be free from nasal congestion and free from potential CNS or cardiovascular adverse effects.

Drugs Closely Related to
P Pseudoephedrine

Phenylephrine

Phenylephrine (Sudafed PE, Neo-Synephrine) is a powerful alpha-adrenergic stimulant that decreases nasal congestion. It is available in oral, spray, and drop formulations. Special caution must be taken to avoid use in abraded nasal membranes,

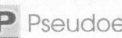

CRITICAL THINKING SCENARIO

PROLONGED USE OF NASAL DECONGESTANTS

Noah Rightman, age 16 years, comes to the clinic for a recheck of his allergic rhinitis. He uses a nasal decongestant daily. Lately, he has needed to use his nasal decongestant "10 times a day," and asks, "What's wrong with this drug? I want something stronger." Understanding the sympathetic nervous system, how would you respond to Noah?

MEMORY CHIP

P Pseudoephedrine

- Used to relieve nasal congestion
- Major contraindications: severe hypertension, severe cardiac disorders
- Most common adverse effects: tachycardia, palpitations, and nervousness
- Most serious adverse effects: dysrhythmias, hypertension, and coronary vasospasm
- Maximizing therapeutic effects: Use humidifier and increase fluid intake.
- Minimizing adverse effects: Adhere to safety precautions.
- Most important patient education: Take pseudoephedrine exactly as prescribed to avoid rebound congestion.

because systemic absorption of this drug can result in severe cardiac, CNS, and urinary effects. As with other decongestants, continuous use may induce rebound congestion.

Topical Decongestant Drugs

Topical decongestants include naphazoline (Naphcon and others), oxymetazoline (Afrin), phenylephrine (Neo-Synephrine), tetrahydrozoline (Tyzine), and xylometazoline (Otrivin). They stimulate alpha-adrenergic receptors in the nasal passages, causing constriction in the nasal arterioles. As a result, the nasal membrane is reduced in size, swelling is limited, and the size of the nostril is increased, allowing for more efficient airflow. Although topical decongestants have the same potential adverse effects as pseudoephedrine, the risks are diminished because their action is localized rather than systemic. In very young children, the vascularity of the nasal membranes, developing nasal passages, and eustachian tubes increases the risk for systemic absorption and adverse effects.

Use of topical decongestants for longer than 5 continuous days can lead to rebound congestion. Patients should be instructed to stop using the drug if rebound congestion occurs.

C ANTIHISTAMINES

Antihistamines are used to relieve symptoms of allergies. These drugs, which block the action of histamine as it is released during the inflammatory response to an antigen, are very effective for allergic rhinitis. Their action restores normal airflow through the upper respiratory system. Because of their OTC availability, these drugs are often misused to treat colds and influenza. Drugs within the antihistamine class can be separated into first-generation and second-generation agents. First-generation antihistamines are also referred to as sedating antihistamines. Second-generation antihistamines are known as nonsedating antihistamines, although a better term might be less-sedating antihistamines. Fexofenadine (Allegra), a second-generation drug, is the prototype antihistamine. Table 48.6 presents a summary of antihistamine drugs.

(text continues on page 705)

TABLE 34.6 **Summary of Selected ⓒ Antihistamines**

Drug (Trade) Name	Selected Indications	Route and Dosage Range	Pharmacokinetics
Second-Generation Antihistamines			
Ⓟ fexofenadine (Allegra)	Allergy relief	*Adult and Child >12 y:* PO, 60 mg 2×/d or 180 mg daily	*Onset:* 1–2 h
		Child 6–11 y: PO, 30 mg 2×/d	*Duration:* 12 h
	Chronic idiopathic urticaria	*Child 2–11 y:* Oral suspension, 30 mg (5 mL) 2×/d	$t_{1/2}$: 14 h
		Child 2–11 y: 30 mg (5 mL) 2×/d	
		Child 6 mo to <2 y: 15 mg (2.5 mL) 2∞/d	
cetirizine (Zyrtec, Zyrtec-D)	Allergy relief	*Adult and Child >6 y:* PO, tablets, chewable tablets, or oral syrup, 5–10 mg daily	*Onset:* 30 min
		Child 2–5 y: 2.5 mg (1/2 tsp or 2.5 mL of oral syrup) daily or 5-mg chewable tablet daily	*Duration:* 24 h
		Child 1–2 y: PO, 2.5 mg (1/2 tsp or 2.5 mL) q12 h	$t_{1/2}$: 8–11 h
		Child 6–11 mo: PO, 2.5 mg (1/2 tsp or 2.5 mL) daily	
desloratadine (Clarinex)	Allergy relief	*Adult and Child >12 y:* PO, 5 mg daily	*Onset:* 1 h
			Duration: 24 h
			$t_{1/2}$: 27 h
Levocetirizine (Xyzal)	Allergy relief	*Adult and Child > 12y PO:*	*Onset:* unk
		5 mg daily	*Duration:* 24 h
		Child 6–11 y PO:	$t_{1/2}$: 7-8 h
		2.5 mg daily	
		Child: 2-6 y PO:	
		1.25 mg daily	
loratadine (Alavert, Claritin)	Allergy relief	*Adult and Child >6 y:* PO, 10 mg daily	*Onset:* 1–3 h
		Child 2–5 y: PO, 5 mg (5 mL oral syrup) daily	*Duration:* 24 h
		Child <2 y: Safe and effective use has not been established.	$t_{1/2}$: 8.4 h
Inhaled Antihistamine			
azelastine (Astelin)	Allergy relief	*Adult and Child >12 y:* 2 sprays in each nostril 2∞ daily	Minimal systemic absorption
		Child 5–11 y: 1 spray in each nostril 2∞ daily	
First Generation Antihistamines			
brompheniramine (Veltane)	Allergy relief	*Adult and Child >12 y:* PO, 4 mg q4–6h	*Onset:* 1 h
		Child 6–11 y: 2–4 mg q6–8h	*Duration:* 9–24 h
		Child <6 y: 0.125 mg/kg q6h	$t_{1/2}$: 12–34 h
	Anaphylaxis	*Adult and Child >12 y:* IV, IM, SQ, 5–20 mg q6h	
		Child <12 y: IV, IM, SQ, 0.5 mg/kg/d	
Clemastine (Tavist Allergy)	Allergy relief	*Adult and Child >12 PO:*	*Onset:* 15–30 min
		1.34 mg 2×/day	*Duration:* 12 h
		Child 6–12 y PO:	$t_{1/2}$: 3–4 h
		0.67 mg as syrup 2×/d	
	Urticaria	*Adult and Child >12y PO:*	
		2.68 mg 1–3×/d	
		Child 6-12 y PO:	
		1.34 mg as syrup 2×/d	
chlorpheniramine (Chlor-Trimeton)	Allergy relief	*Adult and Child >12 y:* 4 mg PO q4–6h; max, 24/mg/d	*Onset:* 15–30 min
		Extended-release: 8–12 mg q8–12h	*Duration:* 4–12 h
		Child 6–11 y: 2 mg PO q4–6 h; max, 12/mg/d	$t_{1/2}$: 20–24 h
		Child 2–5 y: 1 mg PO q4–6 h; max, 4/mg/d	
		Adult: SC, IM, IV, 5–40 mg single dose; max, 40 mg/d	
		Child: SC (only), 87.5 mcg/kg q6 h	

TABLE 34.6 Summary of Selected ⊖ Antihistamines (continued)

Drug (Trade) Name	Selected Indications	Route and Dosage Range	Pharmacokinetics
dexchlorpheniramine (Polaramine)	Allergy relief	*Adult:* PO, 2 mg q4–6 h or 4–6 mg timed release at bedtime or q8–10 h *Child 2–5 y:* PO, 0.5 mg q4–6 h (do not use timed release) *Child 6–11 y:* PO, 1 mg q4–6 h or 4 mg timed release at bedtime	*Onset:* 15–30 min *Duration:* Unknown $t_{1/2}$: 12–15 h
diphenhydramine (Benadryl)	Allergy relief	*Adult:* PO, 25–50 mg qid; IV/IM, 10–50 mg; max, 400 mg *Child:* PO, 5 mg/kg/d; max, 300 mg daily; IV/IM, same	*Onset:* 15–30 min *Duration:* 4–8 h $t_{1/2}$: 2.5–7 h
Combination Drugs			
acrivastine and pseudo-ephedrine (Semprex-D)	Allergy and congestion relief	*Adult and Child >12 y:* PO, 1 capsule (acrivastine 8 mg and pseudoephedrine 60 mg) q4–6 h	See individual components
brompheniramine, dex-tromethorphan, pseudo-ephedrine (Bromfed-DM, Myphetane DX)	Allergy and congestion relief	*Adult and Child >12 y:* PO, 10 mL q4 h *Child 6–12 y:* PO, 5 mL q4 h *Child 2–6 y:* PO, 2.5 mL q4 h	See individual components
brompheniramine, pseudoephedrine (Bromfed-PE, Efidac 24)	Allergy and congestion relief	*Adult and Child >12 y:* PO, 1–2 capsules q12 h *Child 6–12 y:* PO, 1 capsule q12 h	See individual components
chlorpheniramine and pseudoephedrine (Allerest Maximum Strength)	Allergy and congestion relief	*Adult and Child >12 y:* PO, 1 tablet q4–6 h *Child 6–12 y:* PO, 1/2 tablet q4–6 h	See individual components
chlorpheniramine pseu-doephedrine, ibuprofen (Advil Allergy Sinus)	Allergy and congestion relief	*Adult:* PO, 2 mg chlorpheniramine, 60 mg pseudoephedrine, 200 mg ibuprofen; 1 tablet q4–6 h	See individual components
loratadine and pseudoephedrine (Claritin-D, Claritin-D 12-hour)	Allergy and congestion relief	12-h extended-release tablets: *Adult and Child >12 y:* PO, 1 tablet q12 h 24-h extended-release tablet: *Adult and child >12 y:* PO, 1 tablet q24 h *Child <12 y:* Safe and effective use has not been established.	See individual components
fexofenadine and pseu-doephedrine (Allegra-D)	Allergy and congestion relief	*Adult and Adolescent:* PO, 1 tablet 2×/d *Child:* Safe and effective use has not been established.	See individual components
triprolidine pseudoephedrine (Actifed Cold and Allergy)	Allergy and congestion relief	*Adult:* PO, 2.5 mg triprolidine, 60 mg pseudoephedrine q4–6 h	Minimal systemic absorption
Ophthalmic Antihistamine/Mast Cell Stabilizers			
alcaftadine (Lastacaft)	Allergic Conjunctivitis	*Adult and child >2y:* *Instill 1 drop daily*	Minimal systemic absorption
azelastine (Optivar)	Allergic Conjunctivitis	*Adult and child >3y:* Instill 1 drop 2×/d	Minimal systemic absorption
bepotastine (Bepreve)	Allergic Conjunctivitis	*Adult and Child >2y:* Instill 1 drop 2×/d	Minimal systemic absorption
epinastine (Elestat)	Allergic Conjunctivitis	*Adult and Child >3y:* Instill 1 drop every 8–12 h	Minimal systemic absorption
ketotifen (Zaditor, Alaway)	Allergic Conjunctivitis	*Adult and Child >3y:* Instill 1 drop every 8–12 h	Minimal systemic absorption
olopatadine (Pataday, Patanol)	Allergic Conjunctivitis	*Adult and Child >3y:* 0.2% 1 drop daily 0.1% 1 drop 2×/d	Minimal systemic absorption

(Continued)

TABLE 34.6 Summary of Selected © Antihistamines *(continued)*

Drug (Trade) Name	Selected Indications	Route and Dosage Range	Pharmacokinetics
Inhaled Nasal Steroids			
beclomethasone (Beconase, Vancenase)	Allergy and congestion relief	**Metered-dose inhalers (42 mcg/spray)** *Adult and Child >12 y:* 1 spray in each nostril 2–4×/d *Child 6–12 y:* 1 spray in each nostril 3×/d **AQ pump nasal sprays (42 mcg/spray)** *Adult and Child >6 y:* 1–2 sprays in each nostril 2×/d **AQ double-strength pump nasal spray (84 mcg/spray)** *Adult and Child >6 y:* 1–2 sprays in each nostril once daily in the morning *Children <6 y:* not recommended	beclomethsone (Beconase, Vancenase)
budesonide (Rhinocort)	Allergy and congestion relief	**Metered-dose inhaler (32 mcg/spray)** *Adult and Child >6 y:* 2 sprays in each nostril in the morning and in the evening, or 4 sprays in each nostril in the morning **AQ pump nasal sprays (32 mcg/spray)** *Adult and Adolescent:* 1 spray in each nostril once daily in the morning; max, 256 mcg/d *Child >6 y:* 1 spray in each nostril once daily in the morning; max, 128 mcg/d	budesonide (Rhinocort)
ciclesonide (Omnaris)	Allergic rhinitis	**AQ pump nasal spray (50 mcg/spray)** *Adult and Child >12 y:* 2 sprays in each nostril daily	ciclesonide (Onmaris)
flunisolide (Nasalide)	Allergy and congestion relief	**AQ pump nasal sprays (25 mcg/spray)** *Adult and Child >14 y:* 2 sprays in each nostril 2×/d; max, 200 mcg in each nostril per day *Child 6–14 y:* 1 spray in each nostril 3×/d, or 2 sprays in each nostril 2×/d; max, 100 mcg in each nostril per day *Child <6 y:* Safe and effective use has not been established.	flunisolide (Nasalide)
fluticasone (Flonase)	Allergy and congestion relief	**AQ pump nasal sprays (50 mcg/spray)** *Adult >18 y:* 2 sprays in each nostril once daily or 1 spray in each nostril 2×/d; max, 200 mcg/d *Child 4–17 y:* 1 spray in each nostril 1×/d *Child <4 y:* Safe and effective dosage has not been established.	fluticasone (Flonase)
mometasone (Nasonex)	Allergy and congestion relief	**AQ pump nasal sprays (50 mcg/spray)** *Adult and Child >11 y:* 2 sprays in each nostril once daily (total daily dose of 200 mcg) *Child 2–11 y:* 1 spray in each nostril once daily (total daily dose of 100 mcg) *Child <2 y:* Safe and effective use has not been established.	mometasone (Nasonex)
triamcinolone (Nasacort)	Allergy and congestion relief	**Metered-dose inhaler (55 mcg/pump)** *Adult and Adolescent >12 y:* 2 sprays in each nostril once daily Max: 440 mcg/d *Child 6–11 y:* 2 sprays in each nostril 1×/d; max, 220 mcg/d **AQ pump nasal sprays (55 mcg/spray)** *Adult and Child >12 y:* 2 sprays in each nostril once daily (total dose of 220 mcg) *Child 6–11 y:* 1–2 sprays in each nostril once daily	triamcinolone (Nasacort)
Inhaled Mast Cell Stabilizers			
cromolyn sodium (NasalCrom)	Allergy and congestion relief	**Metered-dose inhaler (5.2 mg/spray)** *Adult and Child >2 y:* 1 spray in each nostril 3–4×/d	Minimal Systemic Absorption
cromolyn sodium (Opticrom, Crolom)	Allergic conjunctivitis	*Adult and Child >4y:* 1–2 drops 4–6×/d	Minimal Systemic Absorption
lodoxamide (Alomide)	Vernal keratitis, conjunctivitis, and keratoconjunctivitis	*Adult and Child >2y:* 1–2 drops 4×/d for up to 3 months	Minimal Systemic Absorption
nedocromil (Alocril)	Allergic conjunctivitis	*Adult and Child >3y:* 1–2 drops 2×/d	Minimal Systemic Absorption

Nursing Management of the Patient Receiving P Fexofenadine

Core Drug Knowledge

Pharmacotherapeutics

Fexofenadine is used to relieve symptoms associated with seasonal and perennial allergic rhinitis, allergic conjunctivitis, uncomplicated urticaria, and angioedema. It is most effective if used before the onset of symptoms.

Pharmacokinetics

Fexofenadine is taken orally and is absorbed rapidly. The peak drug effect is seen within 2 to 6 hours Fexofenadine is only slightly (5%) metabolized in the liver and is excreted in the feces (80%) and urine (11%).

Pharmacodynamics

Fexofenadine selectively blocks the effects of histamine at H_1-receptor sites, decreasing the allergic response. Fexofenadine also has anticholinergic and antipruritic effects. However, fexofenadine, a second-generation antihistamine, has less of an anticholinergic effect than the first-generation antihistamines because it binds to lung receptors substantially more than it binds to cerebellar receptors, resulting in a reduced sedative potential.

Contraindications and Precautions

Fexofenadine should not be used in a patient with hypersensitivity to fexofenadine or terfenadine or any of their components or in children younger than 2 years of age. This drug is in pregnancy category C; because it crosses the placenta and enters breast milk, it should be avoided or used with caution by pregnant and lactating women. Fexofenadine also should be used with caution in patients with renal impairment, because the drug's half-life is prolonged in these patients. In addition, peak plasma levels in patients with renal impairment are increased.

Adverse Effects

The most common adverse reactions associated with fexofenadine include viral infection (e.g., colds and flu), nausea and vomiting, dysmenorrhea, drowsiness, dyspepsia, and fatigue. Fexofenadine is a metabolite of terfenadine, which has been associated with QT-interval prolongation and ventricular tachycardias and is no longer manufactured. Fexofenadine has not induced QT-interval prolongation, but patients should still be monitored for this adverse effect.

Drug Interactions

Only a few drug interactions are associated with fexofenadine. They are presented in Table 34.7.

Assessment of Relevant Core Patient Variables

Health Status

Assess the patient's history for allergy to any antihistamine and for pregnancy, lactation, or renal impairment. Before beginning therapy, assess the patient's respiratory system, orientation and affect, and skin condition. If long-term therapy is anticipated, renal function should be assessed as well.

Life Span and Gender

Note the age of the patient before administering fexofenadine. Use special precautions in elderly patients, who are more likely than others to experience dizziness, sedation, and syncope. Determine whether the patient is pregnant, because fexofenadine should not be used during pregnancy.

Lifestyle, Diet, and Habits

Evaluate how often the patient drinks apple, grapefruit, or orange juice because these juices decrease the absorption of fexofenadine. Teach the patient to avoid these juices for 1 hour before and 2 hours after taking fexofenadine.

Caution patients taking fexofenadine to assess the level of sedation caused by the drug before driving a vehicle or performing tasks that require concentration.

Environment

Fexofenadine usually is administered at home and in the community setting. Caution patients taking fexofenadine to read the labels of nonprescription products to be sure that they are not taking another product that also contains an antihistamine, which could potentiate the effects of both drugs.

Nursing Diagnosis and Outcome

- Risk for Injury caused by drowsiness and fatigue related to drug-induced CNS effects
  Desired outcome: *Safety precautions will prevent injury related to drug-induced CNS effects.*

TABLE 34.7	Agents That Interact with P Fexofenadine	
Interactants	**Effect and Significance**	**Nursing Management**
Juices Apple Grapefruit Orange	Apple, grapefruit, and orange juice decrease the absorption of fexofenadine.	Monitor for continued allergy symptoms. May require increased dose of fexofenadine.
Rifampin	Rifampin reduces the absorption of fexofenadine.	Monitor for continued allergy symptoms.

Planning and Intervention

Maximizing Therapeutic Effects

Institute measures to prevent dangers associated with thickening of respiratory secretions. Examples of appropriate measures include use of a humidifier, forcing fluids as appropriate, and encouraging the patient to avoid dry or smoke-filled areas.

Minimizing Adverse Effects

Refrain from giving the patient apple, grapefruit, or orange juice with fexofenadine, because these juices decrease its absorption.

Provide safety measures, such as side rails, and assistance with ambulation if CNS effects occur.

Providing Patient and Family Education

- Explain that fexofenadine is formulated to relieve allergy symptoms.
- Caution patients not to take fexofenadine if they have ever had a reaction to it, are pregnant, or are breast-feeding.
- Caution patients to take the drug as prescribed. If they miss a dose, they should take it as soon as they remember, unless it is almost time for the next dose; two doses should not be taken at the same time.
- Tell patients to avoid the use of other OTC drugs, many of which contain similar antihistamines that could cause serious adverse effects if taken concurrently with fexofenadine.
- Inform patients to avoid alcohol while taking fexofenadine and not to drive or perform tasks that require alertness until the drug's effect has been determined.
- Tell patients to take fexofenadine with food if GI upset occurs and to suck on sugarless lozenges if dry mouth is a problem.
- Teach patients to take fexofenadine with a glass of water. Explain why apple, grapefruit, and orange juices should not be taken at the same time as fexofenadine.
- Warn patients to report difficulty breathing, tremors, hallucinations, and palpitations; teach patients and their families about safety measures that may be needed if these CNS effects occur. Caution patients to keep fexofenadine out of the reach of children.
- Encourage patients to use a humidifier, drink fluids, and avoid overly dry spaces and smoke-filled areas to help decrease the problems associated with the drying effects of antihistamines.

Ongoing Assessment and Evaluation

After several days taking fexofenadine, the patient should experience little discomfort associated with the drug's adverse effects. The patient should be free of injury related to the CNS effects of fexofenadine. The patient should not experience respiratory difficulty related to the anticholinergic effects of the drug.

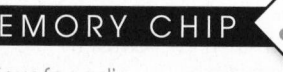

MEMORY CHIP

P Fexofenadine

- Used for allergic disorders
- Major contraindication: use in children younger than 12 years old
- Most common adverse effects: flu-like symptoms, nausea and vomiting, dysmenorrhea, and drowsiness
- Most serious adverse effect: potential for QT-interval prolongation
- Maximizing therapeutic effects: Use a humidifier and increase fluid intake.
- Minimizing adverse effects: Adhere to safety precautions.
- Most important patient education: Use for symptoms related to allergic disorders; do **not** use for symptoms related to common viral illness, such as colds and flu.

Drugs Closely Related to P Fexofenadine

Azelastine

Azelastine (Astelin) is a second-generation H_1-receptor antagonist that is administered as a nasal spray. It is approved to treat the symptoms of seasonal allergic rhinitis and vasomotor rhinitis such as rhinorrhea, nasal congestion, sneezing, nasal pruritus, and postnasal drip. It acts by locally antagonizing the effects of histamine at the H_1-receptor sites but does not bind to or inactivate histamine. Adverse effects include drowsiness, dizziness, epistaxis, nasal burning, sneezing, dry mouth, and a bitter taste. A pregnancy category C drug, it is approved for use in children older than 5 years.

Cetirizine

Cetirizine (Zyrtec) is the active metabolite of hydroxyzine; it differs from the parent compound by having greater affinity for the H_1 receptor. Cetirizine is effective in treating chronic idiopathic urticaria, perennial allergic rhinitis, and seasonal allergic rhinitis. It causes more sedation than other second-generation antihistamines such as desloratadine, loratadine, and fexofenadine but much less sedation than first-generation antihistamines. Cetirizine is approved for use in children as young as 6 months of age.

Cetirizine is classified as a pregnancy category B drug. It is excreted in human breast milk; because the concentration of drug in breast milk has not been quantified, the manufacturer recommends against using cetirizine during breast-feeding.

Desloratadine

Desloratadine (Clarinex) is the **enantiomer** (mirror image) of loratadine. It is a potent, long-acting antihistamine. Because it penetrates poorly into the CNS and has low affinity for CNS H_1 receptors, it does not cause intense drowsiness. It is available as regular or rapidly disintegrating tablets. It is approved for use in children older than 12 years.

Desloratadine is a pregnancy category C drug. It enters breast milk and reaches a concentration equal to that in maternal serum. Potential adverse effects in the infant include irritability, disturbed sleeping patterns, drowsiness, hyperexcitability, and excessive crying.

Levocetirizine (Xyzal)

Levocetirizine (Xyzal) is the enantiomer of cetirizine. It is used in the management of idiopathic urticaria, chronic uncomplicated skin manifestations, and both perennial and seasonal allergic rhinitis. It is approved for children as young as 6 months of age. Levocetirizine is contraindicated for patients receiving hemodialysis and those with renal impairment. It is a pregnancy category B drug.

Loratadine

Loratadine (Claritin), like fexofenadine, is a second-generation antihistamine. It has fewer CNS effects than other H_1 receptor blockers and can be administered once a day. It is not indicated for children younger than 2 years of age. Loratadine should be given cautiously to patients with pre-existing hepatic dysfunction. To minimize the risk of hepatotoxicity, these patients should take loratadine on an every-other-day regimen. Loratadine is most effective when taken on an empty stomach.

Loratadine is a pregnancy category C drug. Like desloratadine, it enters breast milk in a concentration equal to that in maternal serum.

Drugs Significantly Different From P Fexofenadine

Brompheniramine, Chlorpheniramine, and Dexchlorpheniramine

Brompheniramine (Veltane), chlorpheniramine (Chlor-Trimeton), clemastine (Tavist Allergy), and dexchlorpheniramine (Polaramine) are antihistamines which also may be used in conjunction with decongestants. They are nonselective H_1 blockers (first-generation antihistamines) and thus have sedative effects. These drugs are given to treat allergies such as hay fever, allergic conjunctivitis, **urticaria** (hives), and **angioedema** (allergic swelling). They reduce sneezing, runny nose, and itching eyes in hay fever. In addition, they have a mild anticholinergic action that suppresses mucus secretion. Their advantage is that they are relatively inexpensive. The major detriment is that they must be taken every 4 to 6 hours.

Brompheniramine causes less sedation than other first-generation antihistamine agents. A pregnancy category C drug, it is contraindicated during the first trimester of pregnancy and should be avoided during the following trimesters. If brompheniramine must be used during pregnancy, extended-release products should be avoided to limit fetal exposure. Chlorpheniramine is a pregnancy category B drug, although it also should be avoided during pregnancy. Clemastine is another less sedating first generation antihistamine. It is frequently used for pruritus. Clemastine is a pregnancy category B drug. Dexchlorpheniramine is the predominant active isomer of chlorpheniramine and is approximately twice as active. It has the same indications and precautions as brompheniramine and chlorpheniramine. Like chlorpheniramine, it is a pregnancy category B drug.

Diphenhydramine

Diphenhydramine (Benadryl) is a first-generation antihistamine known as an ethanolamine. Ethanolamine antihistamines have substantial antimuscarinic activity and produce marked sedation in most patients. In general, GI effects are minimal. In addition to treating allergic symptoms, diphenhydramine is effective in relieving nausea, vomiting, and vertigo associated with motion sickness. Because of its sedating effects, it is frequently used to induce sleep. It also is used commonly to treat drug-induced extrapyramidal symptoms and mild cases of Parkinson disease.

Diphendydramine is a pregnancy category B drug. Although the use of H_1 antagonists is discouraged during pregnancy, diphenhydramine is the parenteral antihistamine of choice for managing acute or severe allergic reactions in pregnant patients. First-generation H_1 antagonists are not used during breast-feeding because they may inhibit lactation. In addition, they may induce paradoxical CNS stimulation in neonates or seizures in premature infants.

Ophthalmic Antihistamines and Mast Cell Stabilizers

The drugs in this class include alcaftadine (Lastacaft), azelastine (Optivar), bepotastine (Bepreve), epinastine (Elestat), ketotifen (Alaway, Zaditor), and olopatadine (Patanol, Pataday). As antihistamines, they reversibly block H-1 receptors in the conjunctiva and eyelid. As mast cell stabilizers, they inhibit the first step of the allergic cascade by inhibiting mast cell degranulation. The combination of these effects is more efficacious than utilizing antihistamines or mast cell stabilizers as a single topical agent. Common adverse effects include eye irritation, nasopharyngitis, bitter taste, and headache. Emedastine (Emadine) is an H-1 antihistamine. It does not have mast cell stabilizing effects.

Inhaled Nasal Steroids

Inhaled nasal steroidal preparations are used to treat seasonal or perennial allergic rhinitis. Drugs in this class include beclomethasone (Beconase), budesonide (Rhinocort), ciclesonide (Omnaris), flunisolide (Nasalide), fluticasone (Flonase), mometasone (Nasonex), and triamcinolone (Nasacort). Studies have shown that they are superior to oral antihistamines for alleviating nasal, eye, and global allergy symptoms.

Two types of inhaled nasal steroids are available: aqueous sprays that spray a liquid from a bottle through a nozzle fixed at the top of the unit, and metered-dose nasal inhalers that deliver the drug from a pressurized canister through a nozzle on the side near the bottom of the unit. Aqueous sprays are less irritating than those delivered by metered-dose inhaler.

Common adverse effects of inhaled nasal steroids include a burning or itching sensation and a drying effect on the nasal mucosa. By delivering steroids directly to the nasal passage, inhaled nasal steroids maximize the beneficial therapeutic effects of corticosteroids while minimizing their potential systemic adverse effects, although systemic adverse effects may still occur during long-term or high-dose therapy.

Despite these drugs' reduced risk for systemic adverse effects, children receiving inhaled nasal steroids should be evaluated routinely for possible growth retardation, although the risk is extremely small.

Inhaled Mast Cell Stabilizer

Cromolyn sodium (NasalCrom Nasal Spray) is available OTC. Cromolyn sodium provides a protective layer that shields mast cells lining the nasal passage and prevents them from breaking down and releasing histamines. Common adverse effects include irritation inside of the nose, flushing, and an increase in sneezing. Cromolyn sodium has been approved for adults and children older than 2 years. For best results, cromolyn sodium should be taken for 1 full week before coming in contact with allergens and should then be taken three to four times daily.

Ophthalmic Mast Cell Stabilizers

Cromolyn sodium (Opticrom), lodoxamide (Alomide), nedocromil (Alocril), and pemirolast (Alamast) are mast cell stabilizers for allergic conjunctivitis. They are not used for acute symptoms because their onset of action is 5 to 14 days. These drugs are generally used for patients who experience only mild to moderate symptoms. They require more frequent dosing than the combination antihistamine/mast cell stabilizer formulation.

© EXPECTORANT DRUGS

Expectorants are drugs that liquefy lower respiratory tract secretions. This effect decreases the viscosity of the secretions (which makes it easier for the patient to cough them up) and improves airflow. Expectorants are available in many OTC preparations, making them widely available to the patient without advice from a health care provider. Guaifenesin (Robitussin) is the prototype expectorant drug. Table 48.8 presents a summary of selected expectorant drugs.

Nursing Management of the Patient Receiving P Guaifenesin
Core Drug Knowledge
Pharmacotherapeutics
Guaifenesin is used to relieve the symptoms of respiratory conditions characterized by a dry, nonproductive cough. These disorders include the common cold, acute bronchitis, and influenza. Guaifenesin is often found in combination with antihistamines and decongestants (see Table 34.8).

Pharmacokinetics
Guaifenesin is taken orally and is absorbed readily from the GI tract, with an onset of action of 30 minutes. The duration of action is 4 to 6 hours.

Pharmacodynamics
Guaifenesin enhances the output of respiratory tract fluids by reducing the adhesiveness and surface tension of the fluids, thus allowing easier movement of the less viscous secretions. Thinned secretions result in a more productive cough. With a more productive cough, the frequency of coughing should decrease.

Contraindications and Precautions
The only known contraindication to guaifenesin is a known allergy to the drug. The most important consideration in the use of this drug is discovering the cause of the underlying cough. Prolonged use of the OTC preparation could result in masking important symptoms of a serious underlying disorder. The drug should not be used for more than a week; if the cough persists, encourage the patient to visit the prescriber.
Guaifenesin is a pregnancy category C drug.

Adverse Effects
The most common adverse effects of guaifenesin use are GI symptoms, including nausea, vomiting, and anorexia.

TABLE 34.8 Summary of Selected © Expectorants

Drug (Trade) Name	Selected Indications	Route and Dosage Range	Pharmacokinetics
P guaifenesin (Robitussin, Scot-Tussin, Mytussin, Fenesin, and many more)	Relief of conditions characterized by dry, nonproductive cough. Presence of mucus in the respiratory tract	*Adult:* PO, 100–400 mg q4 h, not to exceed 2.4 g/d. *Child >12 y:* PO, adult dosage. 6–12 y: PO, 100–200 mg q4 h, not to exceed 1.2 g/d. 2–6 y: PO, 50–100 mg q4 h, not to exceed 600 mg/d	*Onset:* 30 min. *Duration:* 4–6 h. $t_{1/2}$: Unknown
terpin hydrate (various)	Symptomatic relief of dry, nonproductive cough	*Adult:* PO, 85–170 mg tid–qid. *Child:* Do not give unless prescribed. 10–12 y: 85 mg tid–qid. 5–9 y: 40 mg tid–qid. 1–4 y: 20 mg tid–qid	*Onset:* 30–60 min. *Duration:* Unknown. $t_{1/2}$: Unknown
iodine preparations (SSKI, potassium iodide)	Symptomatic treatment of COPD diseases in which tenacious mucus complicates the problem	*Adult:* PO, 300–1,000 mg after meals bid–tid. *Child:* PO, 150–500 mg after meals bid–tid	*Onset:* 30 min. *Duration:* Unknown. $t_{1/2}$: Unknown

Some patients experience headache or dizziness, and an occasional person will develop a mild rash.

Drug Interactions

Guaifenesin has no important drug–drug interactions. However, it may interfere with colorimetric tests and give false results with urinary catecholamine determinations.

Assessment of Relevant Core Patient Variables

Health Status

Assess the patient for any past hypersensitivity to guaifenesin; history of persistent cough for more than 1 week; cough caused by smoking, asthma, or emphysema; or a very productive cough. In addition, perform a physical assessment, which should include an examination of the patient's skin condition (as a baseline if a rash develops), temperature (to monitor for underlying problems), respiratory status, and adventitious breath sounds.

Life Span and Gender

Determine whether the patient is pregnant. Guaifenesin is a pregnancy category C drug and should be used very cautiously by pregnant patients.

Lifestyle, Diet, and Habits

It is important to assess the patient's smoking habits and typical alcohol intake. Smokers do not benefit from the action of guaifenesin because the etiology of their cough is irritation. When using guaifenesin, the patient should take care not to drink alcohol or use other drugs containing alcohol. Although guaifenesin and alcohol do not interact, both cause drowsiness; therefore, they should not be taken together.

Nursing Diagnoses and Outcomes

- Imbalanced Nutrition: Less than Body Requirements, related to GI symptoms of nausea and vomiting
  Desired outcome: The patient will maintain baseline weight and nutritional status.
- Ineffective Airway Clearance related to increased viscosity of secretions
  Desired outcome: The patient will demonstrate effective coughing technique and make use of several methods to increase airway clearance.

Planning and Intervention

Maximizing Therapeutic Effects

Teach the patient about good pulmonary hygiene, which includes coughing, deep breathing, drinking plenty of fluids, and using a humidifier. Show the patient how to perform effective coughing technique. Family members may assist with percussion and postural drainage as appropriate.

Minimizing Adverse Effects

Suggest that the patient eat small, frequent meals to alleviate GI upset. Additionally, give the drug with meals if symptoms become intolerable.

Providing Patient and Family Education

- Explain to patients that guaifenesin will help make it easier to cough up secretions from the lungs.
- Warn patients not to take guaifenesin if they have ever had a reaction to it, if their cough is caused by smoking, or if their cough is chronic (unless use of the drug is approved by their provider).
- Tell patients not to use guaifenesin for longer than 1 week, and that if the cough persists after that time, or if fever or rash develops, they should consult with their prescriber.
- Caution patients taking guaifenesin not to take any other drugs without their provider's approval and not to drink alcohol while taking this drug.
- Tell patients that if a dose is missed, it should be taken as soon as remembered unless it is time for the next dose. Two doses should never be taken at the same time.
- Teach patients ways to augment guaifenesin therapy, such as drinking a glass of water with each dose. Lots of water helps the body thin the secretions in the lungs and helps guaifenesin work more efficiently. Other ways to augment drug therapy include use of a humidifier, deep breathing, chest percussion, and positional drainage if needed. In addition, teach patients good coughing technique and encourage patients to use the technique regularly.

Ongoing Assessment and Evaluation

Monitor the patient's reaction to guaifenesin carefully; fever, rash, or persistent cough may indicate a more serious underlying medical problem, and appropriate follow-up should be arranged. The patient should tolerate drug adverse effects through use of small, frequent meals and proper timing of dosage. Within 1 week, the patient should exhibit an increasingly productive cough and good movement of respiratory secretions, as demonstrated by productive cough and clearing breath sounds.

Drugs Closely Related to Guaifenesin

Terpin Hydrate

Terpin hydrate stimulates the glands of the respiratory tract to increase the amount of fluid secreted. Actions

---

MEMORY CHIP

P Guaifenesin

- Used to manage dry cough
- Major contraindication: hypersensitivity
- Most common adverse effects: nausea, vomiting, and anorexia
- Maximizing therapeutic effects: good pulmonary hygiene
- Minimizing adverse effects: small, frequent meals to decrease GI distress
- Most important patient education: Seek medical attention if cough does not resolve.

and management related to this drug are very similar to those for guaifenesin. However, terpin hydrate contains about 42% alcohol, which crosses the placenta and may result in congenital abnormalities. The alcohol in terpin hydrate also is excreted in breast milk and can be harmful to infants.

Iodine Preparations

These drugs have been used for many years to stimulate an increase in the fluid produced by the lungs. They are used in treating chronic obstructive pulmonary disease and as adjunctive treatment in respiratory tract conditions, such as cystic fibrosis and chronic sinusitis, and after surgery to prevent atelectasis. These drugs tend to have a bitter flavor, which limits their popularity. They must be used with caution in many conditions because of the effect of iodine on the thyroid gland. Iodine preparations are assigned to pregnancy category X because of potential damage to the fetal thyroid.

CHAPTER SUMMARY

- The upper respiratory system is composed of upper or conducting airways, including the nares, nasal sinus, pharynx, larynx, and trachea.
- Disorders of the upper respiratory system include inflammation and irritation of the upper airways.
- Antitussives, such as dextromethorphan, are drugs used to suppress the cough reflex when dry, nonproductive coughing is tiring and irritating to the respiratory system.
- Decongestants, such as pseudoephedrine, are drugs used to decrease the swelling and blood flow to the mucosa of the respiratory tract. Oral decongestants have greater potential than topical decongestants, which are applied directly to the mucosa, to cause systemic adverse effects. However, the topical decongestants are more likely to cause rebound congestion if used longer than 5 consecutive days.
- Antihistamines are classified as first- or second-generation drugs. First-generation antihistamines are more sedating than second- generation drugs.
- Antihistamines, such as fexofenadine, are used to block the action of histamine as it is released in response to an inflammatory reaction. These drugs block the swelling and congestion that follow histamine release.
- Antihistamines may be taken orally or by nasal or topical administration.
- Topical antihistamines with both antihistamine and mast cell stabilizing effects are most effective for allergic conjunctivitis.
- Inhaled nasal steroids are also used to manage allergic rhinitis and vasomotor rhinitis.
- Expectorants, such as guaifenesin, are drugs used to increase the viscosity and volume of the respiratory tract secretions, which helps patients to clear the lower respiratory tract of tenacious secretions.

QUESTIONS FOR STUDY AND REVIEW

1. What is the difference between dextromethorphan and narcotic antitussive agents?
2. Why are antihistamines inappropriate for treating the common viral cold?
3. What property of fexofenadine makes it an excellent antihistamine?
4. What are the advantages of inhaled antihistamine or steroid drugs over oral formulations?
5. How does guaifenesin assist in controlling cough?

NEED MORE HELP?

Chapter 34 of the Study Guide to Accompany *Drug Therapy in Nursing*, 4th Edition, contains NCLEX-style questions and other learning activities to reinforce your understanding of the concepts presented in this chapter. For additional information or to purchase the study guide, visit thePoint.

REFERENCES

Bepotastine (Bepreve) – An Ophthalmic H1-Antihistamine. *The Medical Letter*, 2010;52:11.

Drug Enforcement Administration. (2008). Title 21 CFR, Part 1300–1399. Retrieved from http://www.deadiversion.usdoj.gov/21cfr/cfr/index.html.

Drugs for allergic disorders. *Treatment Guidelines Medical Letter*, 2010; 90:9.

Facts and Comparisons. (2010). *Drug facts and comparisons*. Philadelphia, PA: Lippincott Williams & Wilkins.

Friedman, N. D., & Sexton, D. J. (2009). The common cold in adults: Treatment and prevention, *Up To Date*. Retrieved from www.uptodate.com July 24, 2010.

Karch, A. M. (2010). *Nursing Drug Guide*, Philadelphia, PA: Lippincott Williams& Wilkins.

Koda-Kimbal, M. A., Young, L. Y., Kradian, W. A., et al. (2008). *Applied Therapeutics: The Clinical Use of Drugs (9th Ed)*, Philadelphia, PA: Lippincott Williams& Wilkins.

Leonardi, A., & Quintieri, L. (2010). Olopatadine: a drug for allergic conjunctivitis targeting the mast cell, *Expert Opinion on Pharmacotherapy*, 11(6):969–981.

Logan, B.K., Goldfogel, G., Hamilton, R., Kuhlman, J. (2009). Five deaths resulting from abuse of dextromethorphan sold over the internet, *Journal of Analytical Toxicology*, 33(2): 99–103.

Meltze, E. O., Munafo, D. A., Chung, W., et al. (2010). Intranasal mometasone furoate therapy for allergic rhinitis symptoms and rhinitis-disturbed sleep, *Annals of Allergy, Asthma, and Immunology*, 105(1):65–74.

Micromedex Healthcare Series. Retrieved from *http://thomsonhc.com*.

Reza-Dana, M. (2009). Allergic Conjunctivitis, *Up To Date*, Retrieved from www.uptodate.com on July 24, 2010.

Rosenbaum, C., & Boyer, E.W. (2009). Dextromethorphan poisoning: Epidemiology, pharmacology and clinical features, *Up To Date*. Retrieved from www.uptodate.com July 24, 2010.

Tatro, D. S. (2011). *Drug Interaction Facts: The Authority on Drug Interactions*. Philadelphia, PA: Lippincott Williams & Wilkins.

Weinberger, S. E., & Silvestri, R. C. (2009). Treatment of subacute and chronic cough in adults, Up-To-Date. Retrieved from www.uptodate.com July 24, 2010.

Drugs Affecting the Lower Respiratory System

Learning Objectives

At the completion of this chapter the student will:

1. Describe the anatomy and physiology of the lower respiratory system.
2. Identify core drug knowledge pertaining to drugs that affect the lower respiratory system.
3. Identify core patient variables pertaining to drugs that affect the lower respiratory system.
4. Relate the interaction of core drug knowledge to core patient variables for drugs that affect the lower respiratory system.
5. Generate a nursing plan of care from the interactions between core drug knowledge and core patient variables for drugs that affect the lower respiratory system.
6. Describe nursing interventions to maximize therapeutic and minimize adverse effects for drugs that affect the lower respiratory system.
7. Determine key points for patient and family education for drugs that affect the lower respiratory system.
8. Compare and contrast drugs used for maintenance treatment of lower respiratory disorders with those used to manage acute exacerbations of lower respiratory disorders.

Key Terms

bronchodilators
bronchospasm
chemoreceptors
chronic airway limitation (CAL)

chronic obstructive pulmonary disease (COPD)
mucolytics
perfusion

respiration
status asthmaticus
ventilation

Drugs Affecting the Lower Respiratory System

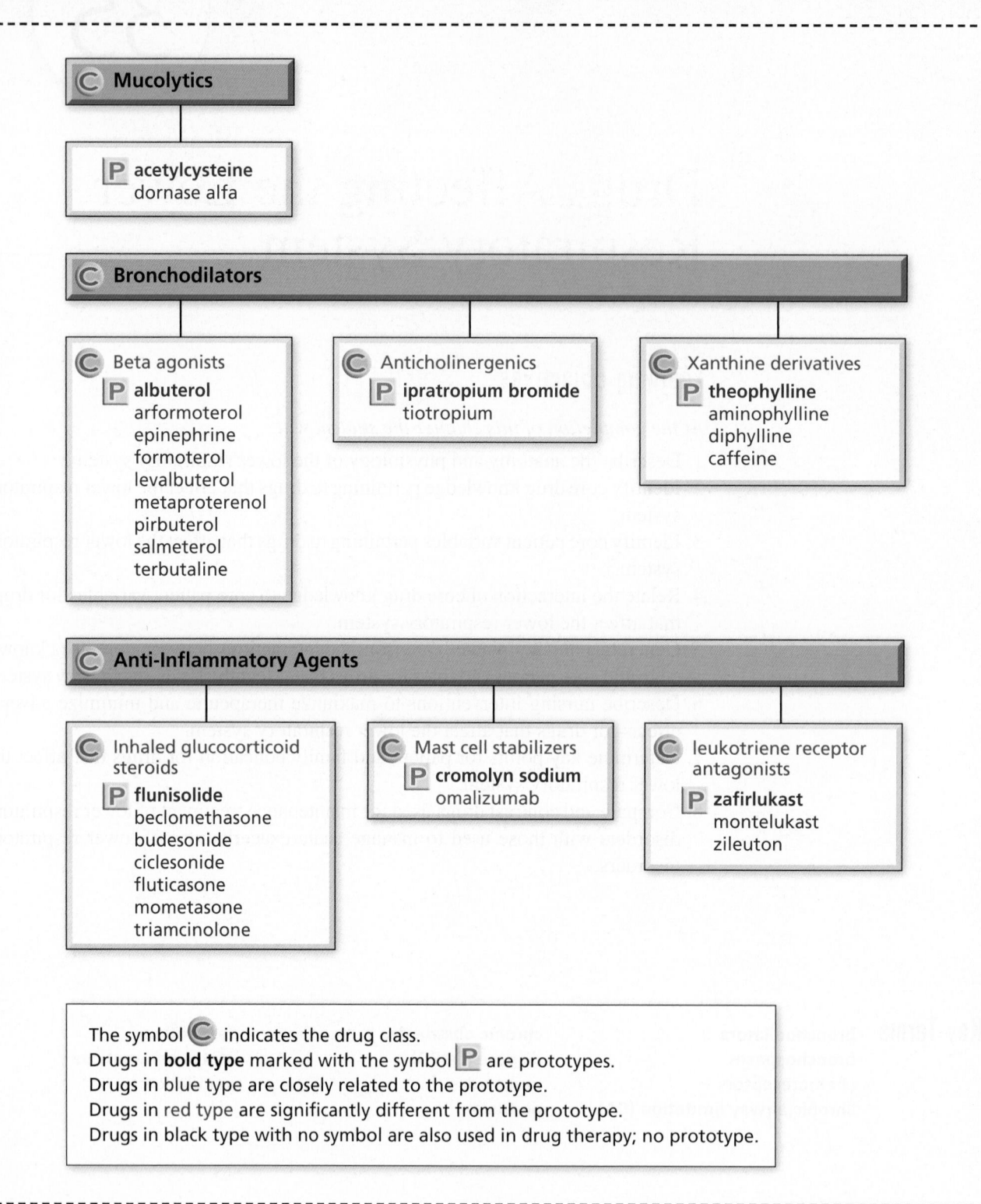

Mucolytics

P **acetylcysteine**
dornase alfa

Bronchodilators

Beta agonists
P **albuterol**
arformoterol
epinephrine
formoterol
levalbuterol
metaproterenol
pirbuterol
salmeterol
terbutaline

Anticholinergenics
P **ipratropium bromide**
tiotropium

Xanthine derivatives
P **theophylline**
aminophylline
diphylline
caffeine

Anti-Inflammatory Agents

Inhaled glucocorticoid steroids
P **flunisolide**
beclomethasone
budesonide
ciclesonide
fluticasone
mometasone
triamcinolone

Mast cell stabilizers
P **cromolyn sodium**
omalizumab

leukotriene receptor antagonists
P **zafirlukast**
montelukast
zileuton

The symbol C indicates the drug class.
Drugs in **bold type** marked with the symbol P are prototypes.
Drugs in blue type are closely related to the prototype.
Drugs in red type are significantly different from the prototype.
Drugs in black type with no symbol are also used in drug therapy; no prototype.

This chapter discusses drugs that affect the lower respiratory system. The lower respiratory system is affected by many serious conditions, which all, to some extent, affect the ability to move air in and out of the lungs. Examples of these conditions include pneumonia, bronchitis, chronic obstructive pulmonary diseases, and cystic fibrosis.

Drugs used to manage lower respiratory system disorders include mucolytics such as acetylcysteine; bronchodilators, which include several subclasses, such as sympathomimetics (respiratory beta agonists), anticholinergics, and xanthines; and anti-inflammatory drugs, which also have several subclasses, including glucocorticoids, mast cell stabilizers, monoclonal antibodies, and leukotriene receptor antagonists.

PHYSIOLOGY

The lower respiratory tract is virtually sterile because of the various defense mechanisms in the upper respiratory system. The lower respiratory system, or the bronchial tree, begins at the trachea, which is surrounded by cartilaginous C-shaped rings that reinforce it and maintain its patency. The trachea bifurcates into two bronchi at a segment called the carina. The right main stem bronchus is wider, shorter, and more vertical. It divides into the upper, middle, and lower lobar bronchi, which then divide into 10 segmental (tertiary) bronchi. The left main stem bronchus is narrower, longer, and more horizontal. It divides into two lobar bronchi, which then divide into 8 to 10 segmental bronchi. Segmental bronchi supply the bronchopulmonary segments, which are the functional units of the lung. Within each bronchopulmonary segment, the segmental bronchi branch 6 to 18 times, producing 50 to 70 respiratory bronchioles that oxygenate the alveolar sacs composed of alveoli (Figure 35.1).

Protective Mechanisms

The bronchial tubes have three layers: cartilage, muscle, and epithelial cells. The cartilage keeps the tube open and becomes progressively less abundant as the bronchi divide and get smaller. The muscles also help to keep the bronchi open, and they too become smaller and less abundant, with only a few muscle fibers remaining in the terminal bronchi and alveoli.

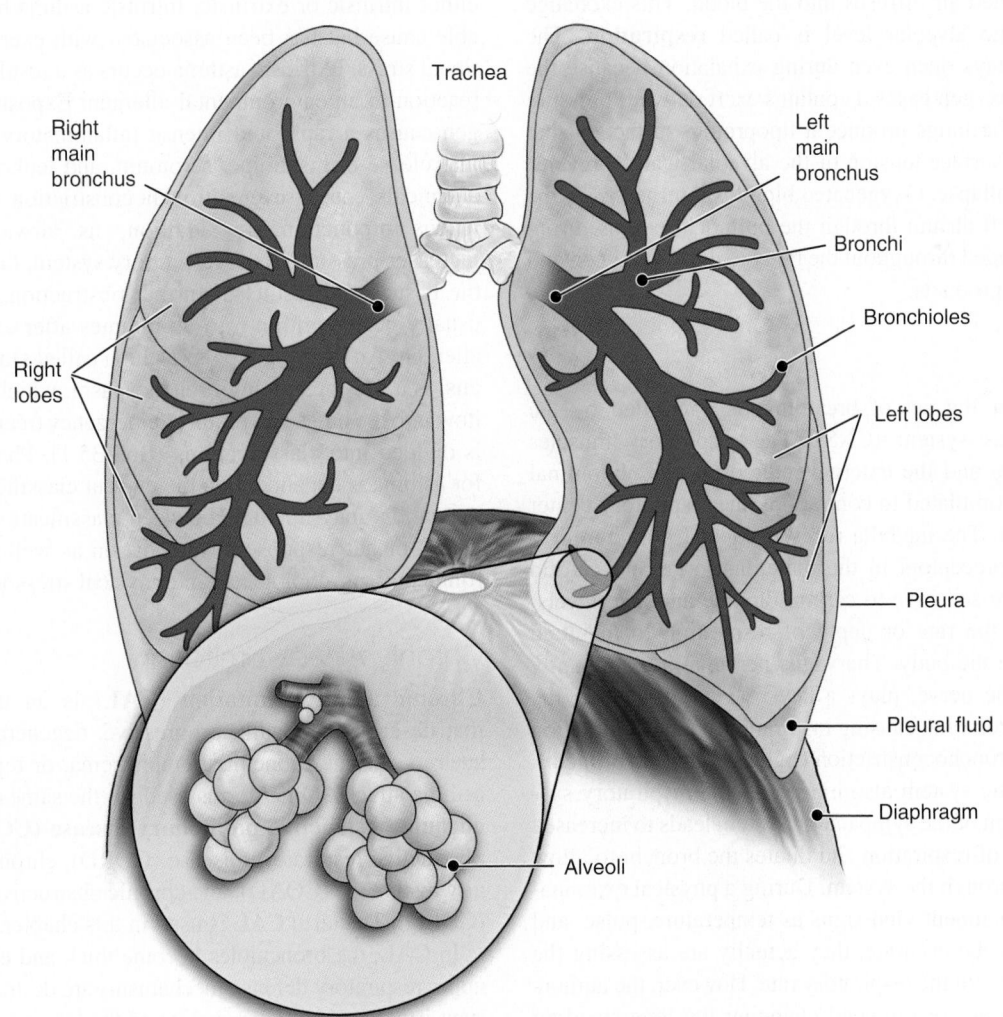

• FIGURE 35.1 Lower respiratory system.

All the tubes in the lower airway contain goblet cells, which secrete mucus to entrap any particles that may have escaped the upper airway protective mechanisms. In addition, during the passage through the bronchi, microorganisms and other foreign bodies are removed from the air by tiny hair-like structures called cilia, which project from the cells that line the bronchial wall. With a wave-like motion, these cilia sweep the foreign material and mucus upward toward the trachea and larynx. The walls of the trachea and the conducting bronchi are very sensitive to irritation. Foreign material and mucus stimulate nerve endings in the bronchial wall and initiate the cough reflex. Coughing completes the expulsion of the foreign material and mucus from the bronchial tree.

Gas Exchange, Perfusion, and Respiration

Lung tissue receives its blood supply from the bronchial artery, which branches directly off the thoracic aorta. The alveoli receive unoxygenated blood from the right ventricle by way of the pulmonary artery. Blood delivery to the alveoli is referred to as **perfusion.** In the alveoli, gas exchange occurs; carbon dioxide is removed from the blood, while oxygen from inhaled air diffuses into the blood. This exchange of gases at the alveolar level is called **respiration.** The alveolar sac stays open even during exhalation because the nitrogen and oxygen gases it contains exert outward pressure and because the lungs produce a lipoprotein surfactant that decreases the surface tension of the alveolar walls, preventing alveolar collapse. Oxygenated blood is returned from the lungs to the left atrium through the pulmonary veins. From there, it is pumped throughout the body to deliver oxygen and pick up waste products.

Ventilation

Ventilation, or the act of breathing, is controlled by the central nervous system (CNS). The inspiratory muscles (the diaphragm and the external intercostal and abdominal muscles) are stimulated to contract by the respiratory center in the medulla. The medulla receives input from **chemoreceptors** (neuroreceptors in the medulla, aorta, and carotid arteries that are sensitive to carbon dioxide and acid levels) and increases the rate or depth of respiration to maintain homeostasis in the body. The vagus nerve, a predominantly parasympathetic nerve, plays a key role in stimulating the diaphragm to contract, causing inspiration. Vagal stimulation also leads to bronchoconstriction (tightening of the bronchi). The sympathetic system also innervates the respiratory system. Stimulation of the sympathetic system leads to increased rate and depth of respiration and dilates the bronchi to allow freer airflow through the system. During a physical examination, nurses document vital signs as temperature, pulse, and respirations. To be accurate, they actually are assessing the ventilatory rate, not the respiratory rate. However, the authors of this text do not recommend changing the long-standing method of charting vital signs.

PATHOPHYSIOLOGY

Acute Bronchitis

Acute bronchitis is caused most frequently by viruses. Therefore, it may be a sequela to the common cold, influenza, whooping cough, and measles. Bacteria such as streptococci and staphylococci also may cause acute bronchitis. Furthermore, bronchitis can be precipitated by a variety of physical and chemical agents, such as fumes of strong acids, ammonia, or organic solvents. Symptoms of acute bronchitis include fever, a productive cough, and purulent mucus. Inflammation often narrows or obstructs a person's airway, making bronchitis a potentially serious condition. Treatment includes bronchodilators and expectorants, plus antibiotic therapy if there is a bacterial infection. The course of the disease is commonly short: 2 to 4 days. However, untreated acute bronchitis may develop into chronic bronchitis.

Asthma

Asthma is a disorder characterized by recurrent episodes of **bronchospasm,** bronchial muscle spasm that leads to narrowed or obstructed airways. Asthma has been classified as either intrinsic or extrinsic. Intrinsic asthma has no identifiable cause but has been associated with exercise and emotional stress. Extrinsic asthma occurs as a result of an allergic reaction to an environmental allergen. Exposure to the antigen causes a rapid and intense inflammatory reaction with the release of histamine, serotonin, and leukotrienes. These chemicals cause severe bronchoconstriction and increased mucus production. In addition, as airway obstruction increases pressure in the respiratory system, fluid moves into the tissues and results in further obstruction. This reaction usually occurs within 5 to 30 minutes after exposure to the allergen. An extreme type of asthma called **status asthmaticus,** is a life-threatening bronchospasm, which occludes airflow into the lungs and requires emergency treatment. Asthma is divided into classifications (Box 35.1). Pharmacotherapy for asthma is dependent on the current classification because the patient may fluctuate between classifications, depending on his or her response to medication as well as daily environmental, psychological, and physical stressors (Box 35.2).

Chronic Airway Limitation

Chronic airway limitation (CAL) is an umbrella term that describes gradually progressive, degenerative diseases, such as chronic bronchitis, emphysema, or repeated, severe asthma attacks. Other terms used for the same conditions are **chronic obstructive pulmonary disease (COPD),** chronic obstructive respiratory disease (CORD), chronic obstructive airway disease (COAD), and chronic obstructive lung disease (COLD). The term CAL is used in this chapter.

In CAL, the bronchioles become thick and edematous, the upper respiratory defense mechanisms are destroyed, and constant irritation and inflammation of the lower respiratory tract are present. With time, the fragile alveoli enlarge and collapse

Box 35.1 CLASSIFICATION OF ASTHMA SEVERITY

Components of Severity		Classification of Asthma Severity ≥12 years of age			
		Intermittent	Persistent		
			Mild	Moderate	Severe
Impairment Normal FEV₁/FVC: 8–19 yr 85% 20–39 yr 80% 40–59 yr 75% 60–80 yr 70%	Symptoms	≤2 days/week	>2 days/week but not daily	Daily	Throughout the day
	Nighttime awakenings	≤2x/month	3–4x/month	>1x/week but not nightly	Often 7x/week
	Short-acting beta₂-agonist use for symptom control (not prevention of EIB)	≤2 days/week	>2 days/week but not daily, and not more than 1x on any day	Daily	Several times per day
	Interference with normal activity	None	Minor limitation	Some limitation	Extremely limited
	Lung function	• Normal FEV₁ between exacerbations • FEV₁ >80% predicted • FEV₁/FVC normal	• FEV₁ >80% predicted • FEV₁/FVC normal	• FEV₁ >60% but <80% predicted • FEV₁/FVC reduced 5%	• FEV₁ <60% predicted • FEV₁/FVC reduced >5%

Adapted from Expert Panel Report-3: Guidelines for the Diagnosis and Management of Asthma

Box 35.2 STEPWISE APPROACH TO ASTHMA THERAPY

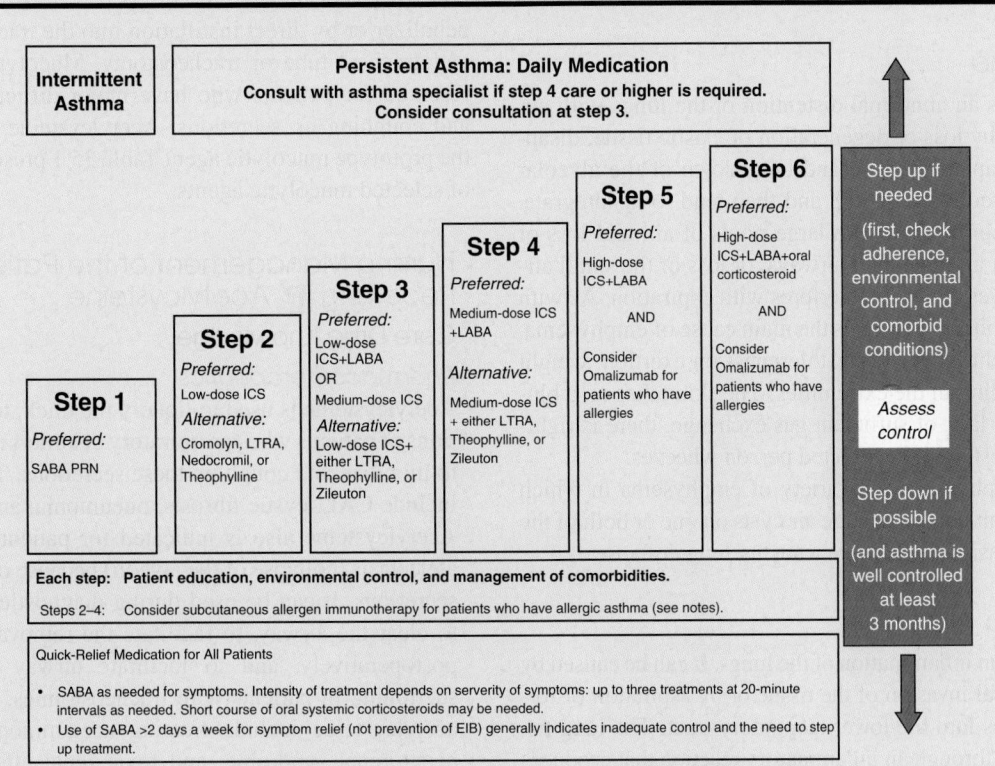

STEPWISE APPROACH FOR MANAGING ASTHMA IN YOUTHS ≥12 YEARS OF AGE AND ADULTS

Key: Alphabetical order is used when more than one treatment option is listed within either preferred or alternative therapy. EIB, excercise-induced bronchospasm; ICS, inhaled corticosteroid; LABA, long-acting inhaled beta₂-agonist; LTRA, leukotriene receptor antagonist; SABA, inhaled short-acting beta₂-agonist

or fuse. Air is trapped in the lungs as the elastic fibers are lost, and increasing amounts of energy are required to try to move the air through the narrowed bronchial tubes. The lungs overinflate and the efficiency of gas exchange is lost. The person suffering from CAL complains of dyspnea and shortness of breath. A barrel chest develops as the lungs overinflate. The person is fatigued from the poor oxygenation of the blood and from the increased expenditure of energy required for breathing.

Chronic Bronchitis

Chronic bronchitis is long-standing, largely irreversible inflammation of the bronchial tree. The continuous inflammatory injury to the lining of the bronchial tree has destroyed many of the cells, the cilia are absent, and the defense mechanism against invading foreign material is lost. The bronchial tubes are narrow, rigid, and distorted. Viscous mucous materials are hypersecreted, resulting in a chronic, deep, productive cough. The cough is difficult to suppress and in fact should not be, because the abundant secretions must be eliminated to avoid the danger of severe superimposed infection.

Excessive and prolonged tobacco smoking can cause chronic bronchitis and is certainly one of its most aggravating factors. Infections of the sinus cavities also provide a reservoir of microorganisms that can continually reinfect the lungs. Damaged bronchi are ideal sites for harboring infections and for accumulation of excess fluids and secreted mucus. Episodes of acute bronchitis and pneumonia are frequent because the respiratory tract is more susceptible to invasion by pathogenic microorganisms.

Emphysema

Emphysema is an abnormal distention of the lungs with air, characterized by loss or degeneration of elastic tissue, disappearance of capillary walls, and breakdown of the alveolar walls. The alveoli first stretch and then tend to disintegrate. The lungs become filled with large pools of air, and loss of elastic support around small airways, or loss of the small airways themselves, severely interferes with expiration. As with chronic bronchitis, smoking is the main cause of emphysema. Symptoms include severe breathlessness on exertion, weight loss, and swelling in the extremities. The skin takes on a bluish color from lack of sufficient gas exchange, there is tightness in the chest, and the affected person wheezes.

Bullous emphysema is a variety of emphysema in which the distended alveoli form large air cysts on one or both of the lungs and occasionally rupture, causing lung collapse.

Pneumonia

Pneumonia is an inflammation of the lungs. It can be caused by bacterial or viral invasion of the tissue or by aspiration of foreign substances into the lower respiratory tract. The lung tissue progresses through an inflammatory reaction that produces symptoms of difficulty breathing, fever, productive cough, shortness of breath, and sometimes chest pain. Pneumonia is more frequently seen when a person's immune system is compromised or when the person has an upper respiratory disorder that causes the normal protective mechanisms to be inefficient. Its etiology can be challenging to pinpoint.

Cystic Fibrosis

Cystic fibrosis is a hereditary disease that affects the functioning of the body's exocrine glands: the mucus-secreting and sweat glands. In persons with this disease, a protein is produced that lacks the amino acid phenylalanine. This flawed protein distorts the movement of salt and water across the membranes that line the lungs and gut, resulting in dehydration of the mucus that normally coats these surfaces. Thus, the normal mucous secretions in the respiratory and digestive systems become abnormally thick, sticky, and concentrated. The thick, sticky mucus accumulates in the lungs, plugging the bronchi and making breathing difficult. This condition results in chronic respiratory infections, often bacterial. Chronic cough, recurrent pneumonia, and progressive loss of lung function are the major manifestations of this disease. The goals of treatment are to keep the secretions fluid and moving and to maintain airway patency as much as possible. Because the disease increases tenacious mucous secretions, acetylcysteine, a mucolytic drug, is the drug of choice.

C MUCOLYTIC DRUGS

Mucolytics break down mucus and help the high-risk respiratory patient cough up thick, tenacious secretions to improve breathing and airflow. The drugs can be administered by a nebulizer or by direct instillation into the trachea through an endotracheal tube or tracheostomy. Mucolytics usually are reserved for patients who have major difficulty mobilizing and coughing up secretions. Acetylcysteine (Mucomyst) is the prototype mucolytic agent Table 35.1 presents a summary of selected mucolytic agents.

Nursing Management of the Patient Receiving P Acetylcysteine

Core Drug Knowledge

Pharmacotherapeutics

Acetylcysteine is used to liquefy the thick, tenacious secretions of patients whose respiratory disorders make it difficult to mobilize and cough up these secretions. These disorders include CAL, cystic fibrosis, pneumonia, and tuberculosis. Acetylcysteine also is indicated for patients who develop atelectasis (collapse of the alveoli) because of thick mucous secretions. It can be used during diagnostic bronchoscopy to clear the airway, to facilitate the removal of secretions postoperatively, and to facilitate airway clearance and suctioning in patients with tracheostomies. Other uses for acetylcysteine include treating acetaminophen overdose, hepatorenal syndrome, and toxic renal effects caused by cisplatin therapy. It is also used to prevent contrast-induced renal complications in high-risk patients receiving contrast agents for diagnostic imaging tests.

TABLE 35.1	Summary of Selected Ⓒ Mucolytics		
Drug (Trade) Name	Selected Indications	Route and Dosage Range	Pharmacokinetics
Ⓟ acetylcysteine (Mucomyst)	Mucolytic adjuvant therapy for abnormal or viscous mucous secretions in acute and chronic bronchopulmonary disease Diagnostic bronchial studies Acetaminophen antidote Contrast-induced nephropathy prophylaxis	Nebulization with face mask, mouthpiece, tracheostomy; 1–10 mL of 20% solution or 2–20 mL of 10% solution q2–6 h Nebulization with tent, croupette: up to 300 mL per treatment Instillation: Direct or by tracheostomy, 1–2 mL of a 10%–20% solution q1–4 h Diagnostic bronchogram: Before the procedure, give two to three administrations of 1–2 mL of a 20% solution or 2–4 mL of a 10% solution by nebulization or intratracheal instillation Acetaminophen antidote: PO, 140 mg/kg loading dose followed by 17 maintenance doses of 70 mg/kg starting 4 h after the loading dose Prevention of contrast-induced nephropathy: PO 600 mg 2×/d	Onset: Instillation and inhalation, 1 min Duration: 2–3 h $t_{1/2}$: 6–25 h
dornase alfa (Pulmozyme)	Management of respiratory symptoms associated with cystic fibrosis	Adult: Inhaled, 2.5 mg qid through nebulizer Child >5 y: Inhaled, adult dosage	Onset: Slow Duration: 1 wk $t_{1/2}$: Unknown

Pharmacokinetics

Acetylcysteine is delivered directly to the respiratory system by nebulizer (inhalation) or direct instillation. Onset of effect occurs within 1 minute, with a peak effect occurring within 5 to 10 minutes. The drug is metabolized in the liver and is excreted in the urine.

Pharmacodynamics

Acetylcysteine affects the mucoproteins in the respiratory secretions. It splits disulfide bonds that are responsible for holding the mucous material together. The result is a decrease in the tenacity and viscosity of the secretions. This drug also protects liver cells from being damaged during episodes of acetaminophen toxicity. For best results, acetylcysteine is given within 8 to 10 hours after ingestion of acetaminophen. It has this effect because it normalizes hepatic glutathione levels and binds with a reactive hepatotoxic metabolite of acetaminophen. In its role in preventing contrast-induced nephropathy, acetylcysteine acts as an antioxidant and vasodilator. Antioxidants prevent oxygen free radicals from bonding with other unbound radicals and thus reduce cell damage.

Contraindications and Precautions

Acetylcysteine is contraindicated in patients who are hypersensitive to the drug. It should be used with caution in patients with a history of respiratory compromise. For example, acetylcysteine should be used with caution in any condition that compromises the patient's ability to cough, because the increased volume of secretions can compromise the airway if it is not cleared. It should also be used with caution in patients who have asthma because bronchospasm can occur.

Intravenous (IV) acetylcysteine is used with caution in patients with serious hepatic disease because these patients may have higher serum concentrations of acetylcysteine than other patients do. Oral acetylcysteine may induce vomiting; thus, it should be given cautiously to patients with esophageal varices or peptic ulcer disease because vomiting can result in acute bleeding.

Acetylcysteine is a pregnancy category B drug.

Adverse Effects

Inhaled acetylcysteine may induce bronchospasm, bronchoconstriction, chest tightness, a burning feeling in the upper airway, and rhinorrhea. Some patients report stomatitis as well. Less common adverse effects are fever, chills, drowsiness, and clammy skin.

IV acetylcysteine may induce anaphylactoid reactions such as angioedema, chest tightness, rash, hypotension, and tachycardia. Both IV and oral acetylcysteine may cause nausea and vomiting.

Drug Interactions

No important drug interactions have been reported for acetylcysteine.

Assessment of Relevant Core Patient Variables

Health Status

Before initiating therapy, perform a physical examination to establish baselines. This examination should include temperature, skin evaluation, respiratory evaluation (including adventitious sounds and ability to cough), and an abdominal assessment for potential hepatomegaly.

Life Span and Gender

Determine whether the patient is pregnant or breast-feeding, because acetylcysteine should be avoided during pregnancy and lactation unless the benefit to the mother outweighs the potential risk to the fetus or child.

Environment

Inhaled acetylcysteine usually is administered under the supervision of a respiratory therapist or specially trained nurse, although some patients or caregivers trained to administer it may give it at home.

Patients receiving acetylcysteine for contrast-induced nephrotoxicity or acetaminophen overdose must be closely monitored; thus, acetylcysteine given for these purposes is administered in the acute care hospital.

Nursing Diagnoses and Outcomes

- Ineffective Airway Clearance related to drug effect or bronchospasm
  Desired outcome: *The patient's airway will be maintained without increased difficulty breathing.*
- Disturbed Sensory Perception, Olfactory, related to odor of drug and route of administration
  Desired outcome: *The patient will remain comfortable and able to tolerate drug therapy.*
- Imbalanced Nutrition: Less than Body Requirements, related to nausea and vomiting.
  Desired outcome: *The patient will maintain nutritional balance throughout therapy.*
- Risk for Injury related to anaphylactoid reaction
  Desired outcome: *Potential anaphylactoid reactions will be recognized and treated appropriately.*

Planning and Intervention

Maximizing Therapeutic Effects

Administer an inhaled beta agonist before administering acetylcysteine, to dilate the bronchial tree and enable the drug to permeate the entire tree. Read the instructions for using the inhalation mask before administering inhaled acetylcysteine. Monitor the nebulizer for any buildup of the drug in the mask from evaporation. Dilute oral acetylcysteine with any kind of diet soda to mask the taste.

Minimizing Adverse Effects

Inform the patient that nebulization may produce an initially disagreeable odor, but that this odor is transient. Remove residual drug from the patient's face after administration by face mask; the drug may irritate the face and will make it feel sticky and uncomfortable. Establish a routine for pulmonary hygiene to eliminate secretions as efficiently as possible; keep suction equipment available.

Carefully monitor the patient receiving IV acetylcysteine for signs of anaphylactoid reaction. If the patient's face becomes flushed, slow the administration of acetylcysteine and administer diphenhydramine as ordered.

Providing Patient and Family Education

- Explain the rationale for receiving acetylcysteine.
- Instruct patients to report all adverse effects, including difficulty breathing, severe nausea, and dizziness.
- Explain to patients that inhaled acetylcysteine will help to get rid of mucus in the lungs.
- Inform patients that they must not take this drug without the assistance of a respiratory therapist or other health care provider unless they have been taught how to prepare the drug and how to use the nebulizer for administration.
- Warn patients not to take any other drugs without their provider's approval and not to drink alcohol while taking this drug.
- Teach patients and their family members all aspects of pulmonary hygiene, including drainage, cupping, coughing, and deep-breathing exercises. Encourage other methods of keeping secretions loose: drinking plenty of fluids, using a humidifier, and avoiding dry or smoke-filled areas.
- Inform patients that nebulization may produce a disagreeable odor, but that this odor is transient. In addition, explain the need to wipe the face with water to remove residual drug after administration by face mask because the drug may irritate the face and make it feel uncomfortable. These patient education tips help increase adherence to drug therapy.

Ongoing Assessment and Evaluation

For the patient receiving acetylcysteine for acetaminophen overdose, monitor for anaphylactoid reactions and schedule serial liver function tests. For the patient receiving acetylcysteine to prevent contrast-induced nephrotoxicity, monitor kidney function tests, urinalysis, and intake and output of food and fluids. For the patient receiving acetylcysteine for its mucolytic effects, assess the patient for proper techniques of pulmonary hygiene and respiratory status.

Determinants of successful therapy depend on the pharmacotherapeutic use of acetylcysteine. In managing acetaminophen overdose, the patient recovers without permanent hepatic dysfunction. The patient receiving acetylcysteine before contrast imaging maintains his/her baseline renal function. The patient receiving acetylcysteine for its respiratory effects tolerates the procedure without breathing difficulty, maintains his/her respiratory status, and continues with drug therapy. There is evidence, by history and breath sounds, that secretions are loosening and the patient is having success coughing and moving secretions.

Drug Closely Related to P Acetylcysteine

Dornase alfa (Pulmozyme) is a mucolytic agent prepared by techniques that use recombinant deoxyribonucleic acid

P Acetylcysteine

- Used to liquefy thick, tenacious secretions
- Major contraindication: hypersensitivity
- Most common adverse effects: nausea, vomiting, and rhinorrhea
- Most serious adverse effects: bronchospasm and bronchoconstriction
- Maximizing therapeutic effects: Refrigerate the solution and use it within 96 hours.
- Minimizing adverse effects: Keep suction equipment close by.
- Most important patient education: correct use of special equipment

(DNA). The mucus of people with cystic fibrosis contains excess DNA. The drug selectively breaks down respiratory tract mucus by separating this extracellular DNA from proteins. This drug is used as adjunctive therapy to relieve the buildup of secretions in cystic fibrosis. It does not replace any other therapy for cystic fibrosis, but it does help keep the airways open and functioning longer. Caution must be used in anyone with a history of hypersensitivity to hamster protein because the drug is manufactured using Chinese hamster ovary cells. It is not yet approved for use in children younger than 5 years old. Adverse effects can include hoarseness and sore throat related to nebulizer use, skin rash, and conjunctivitis.

© BRONCHODILATORS

Bronchodilators are drugs used to facilitate respiration by dilating the airways. Sympathomimetics (beta-2 adrenergic agonists), such as albuterol; anticholinergics, such as ipratropium bromide; and xanthine derivatives, such as theophylline, are bronchodilators commonly used to treat respiratory diseases. Bronchodilators may be administered orally, parenterally, or by inhalation. Inhalation is the most frequent method using metered-dose inhalers (MDIs) or dry-powder inhalers (DPIs). Table 35.2 presents a summary of selected bronchodilators.

• © BETA AGONISTS (SYMPATHOMIMETICS)

As discussed in Chapter 13, sympathomimetics are drugs that mimic the effects of the sympathetic nervous system. As a quick review, the body has two subtypes of beta receptors: beta-1 and beta-2. Drugs that stimulate these receptors may be nonspecific or selective to either beta-1 or beta-2 receptors. Beta-2 receptors are more predominant in the lungs, whereas beta-1 receptors are more predominant in the heart. One of the actions of beta stimulation in the sympathetic nervous system is dilation of the bronchi and increased rate and depth of respiration. For respiratory disorders, the drugs of choice would be those that are beta-2 selective. Albuterol (Proventil, Ventolin) is the prototypical beta-agonist agent

Nursing Management of the Patient Receiving **P** Albuterol

Core Drug Knowledge

Pharmacotherapeutics

Albuterol is used as a bronchodilator in managing CAL and asthma

Pharmacokinetics

Albuterol may be administered orally in tablet or liquid form and by inhalation. Oral inhalation is by MDI, or nebulizer (Box 35.3). Following oral inhalation, bronchodilation occurs in 5 to 15 minutes, after which albuterol is absorbed over several hours from the respiratory tract. The kidneys excrete 80% to 100% of a dose within 72 hours, whereas 10% may be eliminated in feces.

When albuterol is administered orally in tablet or liquid form, bronchodilation occurs within 30 minutes. The kidneys excrete 75% of a dose within 72 hours as metabolites, and 4% may be found in feces.

Pharmacodynamics

Albuterol is a moderately selective beta-2 agonist. It selectively stimulates receptors of smooth muscle in the lungs, the uterus, and the vasculature that supplies skeletal muscle. The main result of albuterol binding to beta-2 receptors in the lungs is relaxation of bronchial smooth muscles. This relaxation of bronchial smooth muscle relieves bronchospasm, reduces airway resistance, facilitates mucus drainage, and increases vital capacity. Figure 35.2 shows where albuterol and other asthma medications exert their effects.

Contraindications and Precautions

The only absolute contraindication to albuterol is hypersensitivity to the drug or any components of the delivery system, such as fluorocarbons.

Precautions of albuterol use include hypertension, cardiac disease, cardiac arrhythmias, ischemic heart disease, hyperthyroidism, diabetes mellitus, and seizures. Selectivity is relative; therefore, potential beta-1 stimulation may exacerbate these conditions.

Albuterol, a pregnancy category C drug; should be used cautiously in pregnancy because beta-2 agonists may interfere with uterine contractility. This effect occurs more frequently when albuterol is administered orally than when it is inhaled.

Adverse Effects

Adverse effects to albuterol are related to its sympathomimetic action and occur more frequently when the drug is administered orally than when it is inhaled. The most common adverse effects of inhaled albuterol include throat irritation, palpitations, sinus tachycardia, anxiety, tremor, and increased blood pressure. Rarely, serious adverse effects such as bronchospasm, urticaria, or angioedema may occur.

Frequent adverse effects of oral albuterol include tachycardia or palpitations, anxiety, tremors, headache, insomnia,

TABLE 35.2 Summary of Selected Ⓒ Bronchodilators

Drug (Trade) Name	Selected Indications	Route and Dosage Range	Pharmacokinetics
Ⓒ Beta Agonists			
albuterol, inhaled (AccuNeb, Proventil HFA, Ventolin HFA, Ventolin Nebules, ProAir HFA) 90 mcg/spray MDI; 2.5/3 mL, 5/mL NEB	Asthma, bronchospasm	**Adult acute asthma exacerbation:** MDI: 4–8 inhalations every 20 min up to 4 h, then every 1–4 h as needed Nebulized solution: 2.5–5 mg every 20 min for 3 doses, then 2.5–10 mg every 1–4 h as needed, or 10–15 mg/h by continuous nebulization **Adult bronchospasm:** MDI: 2 inhalations every 4–6 h or 1 inhalation every 4 h as needed 0.083% nebulized solution: 2.5 mg (3 mL) by inhalation over 5 to 15 min, 3–4 times daily as needed 0.5% nebulized solution: 2.5 mg (0.5 mL diluted in 2.5 mL NS) by inhalation over 5 to 15 min, 3–4 times daily as needed **Adult maintenance PO:** Syrup and tablets, 2 or 4 mg 3–4×/d; MAX 32 mg/d in divided doses Extended-release tablets, 4 or 8 mg every 12 hr; MAX 32 mg/d in divided doses **Adult exercise-induced asthma prophylaxis:** MDI, 2 inhalations 15–30 min prior to exercise **Child acute asthma exacerbation:** MDI: 4–8 inhalations every 20 min for 3 doses, then every 1–4 h as needed; add mask for children <4 y of age Nebulized solution: 0.15 mg/kg (minimum dose 2.5 mg) every 20 min for 3 doses then 0.15–0.3 mg/kg up to 10 mg every 1–4 h as needed, or 0.5 mg/kg/h by continuous nebulization **Child bronchospasm > 4 y MDI:** 2 inhalations every 4–6 h or 1 inhalation every 4 h as needed **Child bronchospasm >12 y nebulizer:** 0.083% nebulized solution: 2.5 mg by inhalation over 5–15 min 3–4 times daily as needed **Child bronchospasm >2 y nebulizer:** (Ventolin Nebules(R)), 2.5 mg by inhalation over 5–15 min 3–4 times daily as needed; (Ventolin(R)), 0.1–0.15 mg/kg/dose (dilute in NS to total volume of 3 mL) by inhalation; MAX dose 2.5 mg 3–4 times daily as needed; AccuNeb(TM) nebulized solution 1.25 mg or 0.63 mg by inhalation over 5–15 min, 3 or 4 times daily, as needed **Child >12 maintenance PO:** Syrup and tablets, 2 or 4 mg 3–4×/d; MAX 32 mg/d in divided doses Extended-release tablets, 4 or 8 mg every 12 h; max 32 mg/d in divided doses **Child >6–12 maintenance PO:** Syrup and tablets: 2 mg 3–4×/d; MAX 24 mg per day in divided doses Extended-release tablets, 4 mg every 12 h; max 24 mg/d in divided doses **Child >2–6 maintenance PO:** Syrup: 0.1 mg/kg 3×/d; MAX starting dosage 2 mg 3 times daily; MAX 12 mg/d in divided doses **Child 4y exercise-induced asthma prophylaxis:** MDI, 2 inhalations 15–30 min prior to exercise	*Onset:* 5 min *Duration:* 3–8 h $t_{1/2}$: 2–4 h
Arformoterol (Brovana) 15 mcg/2mL NEB	Chronic Bronchitis Emphysema	*Adult:* INH, 15mcg 2x/d	*Onset:* SC, 7–20 min; *Duration:* unknown *T1/2:* 26 h

TABLE 35.2	Summary of Selected Ⓒ Bronchodilators *(continued)*		
Drug (Trade) Name	**Selected Indications**	**Route and Dosage Range**	**Pharmacokinetics**
epinephrine (S2, MicroNefrin) 2.25% NEB	Acute bronchospasm	*Adult:* NEB, 0.5 mL up to q3 h *Child >4 y:* 0.5 mL q3–4 h *Child <4y:* 0.05 mL/kg q2–4 h Max: 0.5 mL q3 h	*Onset:* SC, 5–10 min; IM, 5–10 min; inhalation, 1–5 min *Duration:* SC, 20–30 min; IM, 20–30 min; inhalation, 1–3 h $t_{1/2}$: SC, 5–6 h; IM, 5–6 h; inhalation, 5–6 h
formoterol (Foradil) 12 mcg/powder cap INH; formoterol fumarate (Perforomist) inhalation solution	Asthma, prophylaxis COPD	*Adult and child >5 y:* INH, 12 mcg (contents of one capsule) q12 h in Aerolizer Max: 24 mcg/d *Child <5 y:* Safety not established	*Onset:* 1–3 h *Duration:* Unknown $t_{1/2}$: 10 h
	Asthma, exercise induced	*Adult and child >12 y:* 12 mcg formoterol (contents of one capsule) via Aerolizer at least 15 min before exercise	
levalbuterol (Xopenex, Xopenex HFA) MDI 45 mcg/spray; 0.31/3 mL, 0.63/3 mL, 1.25/3 mL NEB	Bronchospasm	*Adult:* NEB, 0.63–1.25 mg q6–8 h MDI: 1–2 inhalations q4–6 h *Child >11 y:* NEB, 0.63 mg 3×/d Max: 1.25 mg 3×/d *Child 6–11 y:* NEB, 0.31 mg 3×/d Max: 0.63 mg 3×/d	*Onset:* Rapid *Duration:* 5–6 h $t_{1/2}$: 3.3–4 h
pirbuterol (Maxair) 0.2 mg/spray	Bronchospasm	*Adult and child >12 y:* INH, 1–2 puffs q4–6 h Max: 12 puffs/d	*Onset:* Rapid *Duration:* 6 h $t_{1/2}$: 2–3 h
salmeterol (Serevent Diskus)	Asthma, COPD Asthma, exercise induced	*Adult and child >4 y:* DPI, 50 mcg q12 h *Adult and child >4 y:* DPI, 50 mcg ∞1, 30–60 min before exercise Max: 50 mcg q12 h	*Onset:* 5–20 min *Duration:* 12 h $t_{1/2}$: 3–4 h
terbutaline	Asthma	*Adult and child >15 y:* PO, 5 mg 3×/d Max: 15 mg/d *Adult and child >15 y:* SC, 0.5 mg q4 h *Child 12–15 y:* PO, 2.5–5 mg 3×/d Max: 7.5 mg/d *Child 12–15 y:* SC, 0.5 mg q4 h *Child 6–12 y:* PO, 0.05 mg/kg 3×/d Max: 0.15 mg/kg/dose or 5 mg/d *Child 6–12 y:* SC, 0.005–0.01 mg/kg q15–30 min ×2 Max: 0.4 mg/d	*Onset:* PO, 30 min; SC, 30 min; inhalation, 5–30 min *Duration:* PO, 4–8 h; SC, 1.5–4 h; inhalation, 3–4 h $t_{1/2}$: PO, 3–4 h; SC, 3–4 h; inhalation, 3–4 h
Combination Inhalers			
albuterol/ipratropium (Combivent Duo-Neb) 120/21 mcg/spray MDI; 3/0.5/3 mL NEB	COPD	*Adult:* INH, 1–2 puffs 4×/d Max: 12 puffs/d *Adult:* NEB, 3 mL 4×/d Max: 6 doses/d *Child:* Safety not established	See individual drugs
budesonide/formoterol (Symbicort) budesonide 80 mcg/ formoterol 4.5 mcg;	Asthma maintenance	*Adult and Child >5 y:* 2 puffs 2×/d	See individual drugs
fluticasone/salmeterol (Advair HFA) 45/21, 115/21, 230/21 mcg/spray MDI	Asthma maintenance	*Adult and child >12 y:* INH, 2 inhalations 2×/d (45/21, 115/21, or 230/21)	See individual drugs
fluticasone/salmeterol (Advair Diskus) 100/50, 250/50, 500/50 mcg/spray DPI	Asthma maintenance	*Adult and child >12 y:* INH, 1 inhalation 2x/d (100/50, 250/50, or 500/50) *Child 4–11 y:* INH, 1 inhalation 2x/d (100/50 mcg)	See individual drugs
Mometasone/formoterol (Dulera) 100mcg/5mcg 200mcg/5mcg	Asthma maintenance	*Adult and Child >12y:* INH 2 inhalations 2×/d	

Box 35.3 TYPES OF INHALATION DEVICES

Metered-dose inhaler (MDI)

- A small, hand-held device that delivers a set amount of drug with each activation
- Requires coordination to inhale medication correctly
- Optimally, approximately 10% of drug reaches the lung
- Important to wait at least 1 minute between puffs
- May be used with a "spacer" to increase amount of drug delivered to the lungs

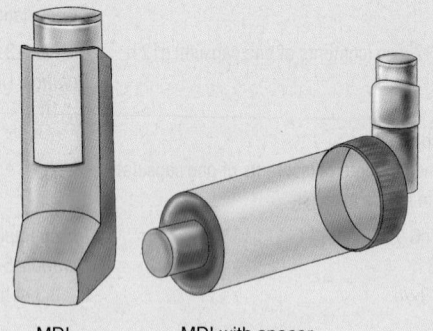

MDI   MDI with spacer

Dry-powder inhaler (DPI)

- A small, hand-held device that delivers a dry, micronized powder with each inhalation
- Does not require coordination
- Optimally, approximately 20% of drug reaches the lung
- Important to wait at least 1 minute between inhalations

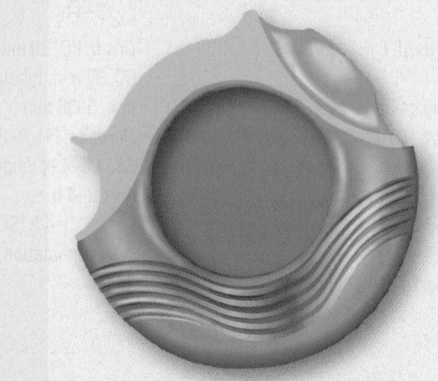

Dry-powder inhaler

Nebulizer

- A small machine that delivers misted droplets of drug into the lungs
- Delivered through a mouthpiece or mask
- Takes longer time to deliver medication to the lungs than MDIs or DPIs
- More effective for some patients than MDIs or DPIs

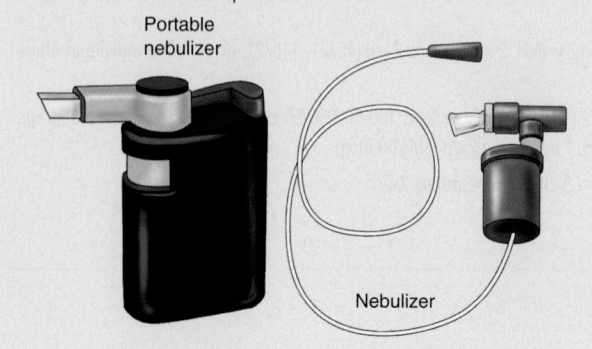

Portable nebulizer

Nebulizer

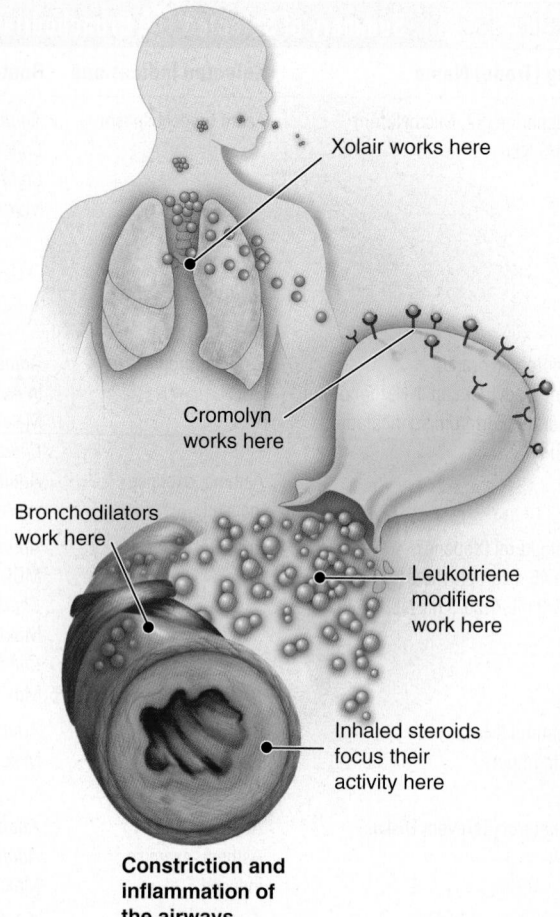

Xolair works here

Cromolyn works here

Bronchodilators work here

Leukotriene modifiers work here

Inhaled steroids focus their activity here

Constriction and inflammation of the airways

• FIGURE 35.2 Sites of action of drugs used in controlling asthma.

muscle cramps, and gastrointestinal (GI) symptoms such as dyspepsia, nausea, and vomiting.

Overuse of albuterol may induce rebound bronchoconstriction, regardless of the method of administration.

Drug Interactions

Albuterol may interact with other sympathomimetic agents, beta-adrenergic blocking agents, digoxin, antidepressants such as monoamine oxidase inhibitors (MAOIs) or tricyclic antidepressants, and potassium-losing diuretics. Table 35.3 presents these potential drug–drug interactions.

Assessment of Relevant Core Patient Variables

Health Status

Evaluate the patient for potential medical conditions or other drug therapy that contraindicates using albuterol or requires close patient monitoring. Any positive findings should be communicated to the health care provider.

Perform a baseline physical examination, concentrating on the cardiac and respiratory systems. Document the baseline findings for later comparison to evaluate efficacy of treatment or potential adverse effects.

TABLE 35.3 Agents That Interact with ℗ Albuterol

Interactants	Effect and Significance	Nursing Management
sympathomimetics	Additive effects may occur when albuterol is administered in combination with other sympathomimetic drugs. This increases risk of cardiovascular adverse effects.	Monitor vital signs frequently. Monitor neurologic status.
beta-adrenergic blocking agents	Albuterol has exact opposite effect on body as beta-adrenergic blocking agents. Additionally, beta blockers may induce bronchospasm.	Monitor for bronchospasm.
digoxin	Albuterol may decrease serum digoxin levels.	Monitor for therapeutic effects of digoxin. Monitor serum digoxin levels. Discuss adjustment of digoxin dose with health care provider.
diuretics	Beta agonist may worsen ECG changes or hypokalemia that may be induced by loop or thiazide diuretics.	Monitor potassium levels. Monitor for signs of hypokalemia. Monitor for ECG changes.
MAOI or tricyclic antidepressants	MAOI and tricyclic antidepressants potentiate albuterol's effect on peripheral vasculature. This may result in severe hypotension.	Monitor blood pressure. Ensure safety.

Life Span and Gender

Evaluate the pregnancy status of female patients. Albuterol is classified as a pregnancy class C drug because it can interfere with uterine contractility as a result of its beta-adrenergic– mediated relaxant effects on smooth muscle.

Determine the age of a pediatric patient before administering albuterol. Oral albuterol tablets and extended-release tablets are not recommended for children younger than 6 years of age, and liquid albuterol is not recommended for children younger than 2 years of age.

Lifestyle, Diet, and Habits

Assess the patient's intake of caffeine, including coffee, tea, soda, cocoa, candy, and chocolate. Caffeine has sympathomimetic effects that may increase the risk for adverse effects. Also, assess for use of over-the-counter (OTC) medications such as pain relievers, appetite suppressants, and cold medicines because they frequently contain caffeine.

Environment

Albuterol is most frequently used in the home environment. It is also the drug of choice for patients in the emergency department experiencing an acute asthma attack.

Nursing Diagnoses and Outcomes

- Anxiety related to sympathomimetic effects of albuterol administration
  Desired outcome: The patient will engage in interventions that decrease anxiety.
- Ineffective Tissue Perfusion: Cardiopulmonary, related to rebound bronchoconstriction caused by overuse of albuterol
  Desired outcome: The patient will use albuterol as prescribed by the health care provider and contact that person if symptoms do not abate.

Planning and Intervention

Maximizing Therapeutic Effects

To obtain the correct dose of albuterol, prime the device by releasing 2 test sprays when using a new MDI or if the MDI has not been used in more than 3 days. Because albuterol is most commonly administered by inhalation, it is important to supervise the patient's ability to use the MDI or nebulizer appropriately (Box 35.4).

Minimizing Adverse Effects

Patients who self-administer albuterol may use their MDIs more frequently than recommended. This practice can result in rebound bronchoconstriction, which may motivate the patient to increase MDI use, stimulating the cycle of rebound congestion. Explain the need to adhere to the recommended frequency of administration. The patient should be encouraged to contact the health care provider to obtain adjunctive medications if symptoms persist, rather than increase the frequency of albuterol use.

Providing Patient and Family Education

- Teach patients that inhaled albuterol is called a "rescue drug" and should be the *first drug* to use when symptoms of an acute attack occur.
- Teach patients how to use an MDI. Include the correct procedure for administering medication, methods of keeping the equipment clean, and how to assess when to change the canister (Box 35.5).
- Explain the importance of using the drug as prescribed and encourage patients to communicate with the health care provider if the symptoms do not abate with the recommended therapy.
- Explain the importance of limiting caffeine intake.
- Explain the importance of refraining from use of OTC drugs without the health care provider's knowledge.

BOX 35.4 COMMUNITY BASED CONCERNS

How to Use an Inhaler

When a patient is first diagnosed with asthma and prescribed inhalation therapy, he or she may need to learn how to use the inhaler that will deliver drug therapy. The nurse may be the health care provider who supplies instructions such as these:

Metered-Dose Inhaler (MDI)

1. When using a new inhaler, or one that has not been used in several days, point the inhaler away from you and prime the inhaler 1–2 times.
2. Hold the device upright and shake it.
3. Tilt the head back slightly.
4. Exhale and open mouth.
5. Position the inhaler in one of three ways:
   - Held 1 to 2 inches from the mouth (this is preferred)
   - Using a spacer
   - With the inhaler between the lips
6. Start to inhale slowly and press down on the inhaler to release the medication.
7. Breathe in for 3 to 5 seconds.

8. Hold your breath for 10 seconds to allow the drug to reach deep into the lungs.
9. Repeat for the ordered number of puffs, allowing 1 minute between each puff.

Spacers are recommended for children, older adults, and anyone who has difficulty using a nebulizer alone. Spacers are indicated when using inhaled steroids.

Dry-Powder Inhaler (DPI)

1. Prepare the medication for inhalation.
2. Place the mouthpiece to the lips.
3. Inhale quickly.
4. Hold your breath for 10 seconds to allow the drug to reach deep into the lungs.
5. Capsules for inhalation (such as those used in the Foradil Aerolizer or Spiriva HandiHaler) must not be swallowed.
6. Do not place your device in water.

When the patient is prescribed more than one type of inhaler, instruct the patient to use the bronchodilator first to open air passages, and then use other prescribed medications.

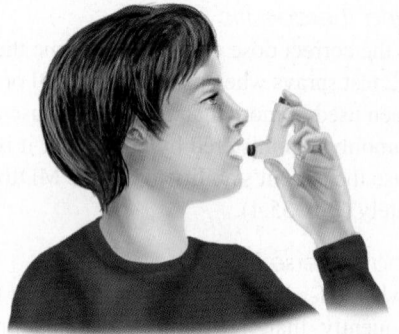
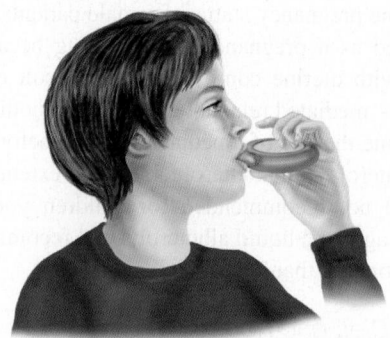

Ongoing Assessment and Evaluation

Evaluate for the symptoms of asthma or CAL in patients using albuterol. Evaluate for CNS symptoms, such as anxiety, tremors, insomnia, or CNS disturbances. Determine the frequency of use and refer the patient to the health care provider if albuterol is needed more frequently than prescribed.

BOX 35.5 COMMUNITY BASED CONCERNS

How to Care for Your Inhaler

- Keep the inhaler clean.
- Once a week, remove the medication canister from the plastic casing and wash the casing in warm, soapy water. When the casing is dry, replace the medication canister and place the cap on the mouthpiece. Ensure that the hole is clear.
- Check the expiration date.
- Keep a log of doses used to know when medication should be replaced.

Drugs Closely Related to [P] Albuterol

Several other beta-agonist agents are used as bronchodilators. The pharmacodynamics and pharmacokinetics of all of these drugs are very similar; slight variations or different vehicles make them the drugs of choice for different patients. A patient may need to try several of these before finding the one that works most effectively. In addition, combination inhalers, with beta agonists combined with either anticholinergic drugs or inhaled steroids, are available.

Short-Acting Beta-2 Agonists

Epinephrine

Epinephrine is the active ingredient in OTC inhalers such as Primatene Mist. It is a nonselective adrenergic agonist; therefore, it stimulates alpha-1, alpha-2, beta-1, and beta-2. For that reason, it is prone to induce multiple adverse reactions, especially tachycardia, hypertension, chest palpitations, and anxiety.

MEMORY CHIP

P Albuterol

- Used for acute and chronic management of CAL and asthma
- Major contraindication: hypersensitivity
- Most common adverse effects: throat irritation, palpitations, tachycardia, anxiety, tremors, and increased blood pressure
- Most serious adverse effects: bronchospasm, urticaria, and angioedema
- Maximizing therapeutic effects: Ensure correct use of inhalation device.
- Minimizing adverse effects: Do not use more than prescribed.
- Most important patient education: This rescue drug should be used first for all acute symptoms of shortness of breath or wheezing.

Levalbuterol

Levalbuterol (Xopenex) is the R-isomer of albuterol and has approximately twofold greater binding affinity than racemic albuterol and approximately 100-fold greater binding affinity than the S-isomer of albuterol. It is available as a solution for nebulization and as an MDI.

Pirbuterol

Pirbuterol (Maxair) is structurally very similar to albuterol. It is used to interrupt an acute asthmatic event or to prevent bronchospasm associated with asthma, exercise-induced bronchospasm, bronchitis, emphysema, and bronchiectasis.

Terbutaline

Terbutaline (Brethine) is shorter acting than albuterol or salmeterol. Its main pharmacotherapeutic use is the prevention of bronchospasm, but it is also used clinically to abort premature labor.

Long-Acting Beta-2 Agonists

Arformoterol

Arformoterol tartrate (Brovana) is a long-acting beta-2 agonist bronchodilator for nebulization. It is the isomer of formoterol specifically developed for maintenance of chronic obstructive disorders such as chronic bronchitis and emphysema. Arformoterol is used cautiously in patients being treated with MAOIs, tricyclic antidepressants, or other drugs known to prolong the QTC interval because these agents may potentiate the action of adrenergic agonists on the cardiovascular system. It should not be used in conjunction with other long-acting beta-2 agonists, or with any other medications that contain long-acting beta-2 agonists.

The most common adverse effects of arformoterol are back and chest pain, diarrhea, and sinusitis. A Black Box warning states that long-acting beta-2–adrenergic agonists such as arformoterol may increase the risk of asthma-related death. Data from a large placebo-controlled U.S. study comparing the safety of another long-acting beta-2–adrenergic agonist (salmeterol) or placebo added to usual asthma therapy showed an increase in asthma-related deaths of patients receiving salmeterol.

Instruct the patient who is making the transition from short-acting beta-2 agonists to stop routine use when starting arformoterol. Should acute symptoms occur, use a short-acting beta-2 agonist.

Formoterol

Formoterol (Foradil) is a highly selective long-acting beta-2 agonist administered as a DPI. The drug does not work fast enough to be used for an acute asthma attack. It is used primarily to prevent exercise- induced asthma, although it approved for use in patients with asthma, bronchospasm, and CAL. Formoterol has the same Black Box warning as arformoterol. Formoterol fumate (Performist) is an inhalation solution, approved for long-term maintenance, for emphysema and chronic bronchitis.

Salmeterol

Salmeterol (Serevent Diskus) is another highly selective long-acting beta-2 agonist with the same indications as formoterol. Like formoterol, it has a slow onset, which makes it useful for the prevention of attacks but not for an acute attack. Salmeterol also carries a Black Box warning because the Salmeterol Multicenter Asthma Research Trial (SMART) showed an increase in asthma-related deaths in patients receiving salmeterol (13 deaths among 13,176 patients treated for 28 weeks on salmeterol, versus 3 deaths among 13,179 patients on placebo).

• C RESPIRATORY ANTICHOLINERGIC AGENTS

Inhaled anticholinergic drugs are considered first-line treatment for patients with CAL whose symptoms have become persistent. Anticholinergic agents diminish the effect of acetylcholine, the terminal neurotransmitter in the parasympathetic nervous system. In the respiratory system, use of inhaled anticholinergic drugs stops the bronchoconstriction that is caused by stimulation of the parasympathetic nervous system. Ipratropium bromide (Atrovent) is the prototype respiratory anticholinergic agent (Table 35.4).

Nursing Management of the Patient Receiving P Ipratropium Bromide

Core Drug Knowledge

Pharmacotherapeutics

Ipratropium bromide is used for maintenance treatment of bronchospasm associated with asthma, bronchitis, or pulmonary emphysema.

Pharmacokinetics

Ipratropium bromide is administered by oral inhalation (MDI or nebulizer) or intranasal spray. Following oral inhalation, onset of action occurs between 15 and 30 minutes; action peaks in 1 to 2 hours and lasts 4 to 5 hours. Ipratropium bromide is not readily absorbed into the systemic circulation after inhalation either from the surface of the lung or from the

TABLE 35.4 Summary of Selected ⊖ Anticholinergic Agents

Ⓟ ipratropium (Atrovent HFA) MDI; 17 mcg/spray	Bronchospasm maintenance Asthma and COPD	*Adult:* HFA, 2 puffs 4×/d *Adult:* NEB, 0.25 mg every 6 h Max: 12 puffs/d	*Onset:* 15 min *Duration:* 3–4 h $t_{1/2}$: 2–3 h
tiotropium (Spiriva) 18 mcg/inhalation DPI	Bronchospasm maintenance	*Adult:* DPI, 1 inhalation every day *Child:* Safety not established	*Onset:* 5 min *Duration:* 24 h $t_{1/2}$: 5–6 d

GI tract. Approximately 50% of the absorbed drug is excreted unchanged in the urine. After intranasal dosing, less than 20% of an ipratropium dose is absorbed from the nasal mucosa into the systemic circulation. The metabolism of intranasal ipratropium bromide is the same as that of the inhaled drug.

Pharmacodynamics

Ipratropium antagonizes the action of acetylcholine by blocking muscarinic cholinergic receptors. Blockade of these cholinergic receptors decreases the formation of cyclic guanosine monophosphate, resulting in decreased contractility of smooth muscle and thereby reducing bronchospasm.

Contraindications and Precautions

Ipratropium aerosol inhalation is contraindicated in patients with sensitivity to ipratropium and atropine or any of its derivatives.

Because of its anticholinergic effects, ipratropium should be used with caution in patients with bladder obstruction, prostatic hypertrophy, or closed-angle glaucoma. Ipratropium may precipitate urinary retention in patients with pre-existing bladder obstruction or prostatic hypertrophy. It may increase intraocular pressure and aqueous outflow resistance in patients with closed-angle glaucoma, especially if the medication gets into the eyes.

Ipratropium is a pregnancy category B drug.

Adverse Effects

Ipratropium aerosols can produce a paradoxic acute bronchospasm that can be life threatening in some patients. This rare problem, when it occurs, is usually seen with the first inhalation from a newly opened MDI. Like a new albuterol MDI, a new ipratropium MDI should be primed with 2 sprays before use. Another serious, but rare, adverse effect is an anaphylactoid reaction. Symptoms include urticaria; angioedema of the tongue, lips, and face; maculopapular rash; bronchospasm; laryngospasm; pruritus; and oropharyngeal edema. This reaction may occur when a patient has an unknown allergy to soybeans, legumes, or soya lecithin.

More commonly, ipratropium may induce cough, hoarseness, throat irritation, or dysgeusia. The classic anticholinergic adverse effects—dry mouth, constipation, urinary retention, and blurred vision—may also occur, but

not as frequently or intensely as with systemic anticholinergic drugs.

Nasal administration of ipratropium may induce epistaxis, headache, rhinitis, nasal congestion, rhinorrhea, and general nasal irritation.

Temporary ocular irritation, ocular pain, mydriasis, cycloplegia, blurred vision, conjunctivitis, or visual impairment may result from spraying ipratropium products inadvertently into the eyes.

Drug Interactions

No serious drug–drug interactions are associated with ipratropium. Ipratropium inhalation solution forms a precipitate with cromolyn sodium inhalation solution if they are mixed together in a nebulizer. Theoretically, potential exists for ipratropium to have additive anticholinergic effects when administered with other antimuscarinics.

Assessment of Relevant Core Patient Variables

Health Status

Assess the patient for potential medical conditions or other drug therapy that contraindicates using ipratropium or requires close patient monitoring. Perform a baseline respiratory examination and document the findings. This baseline assessment will be used to evaluate the efficacy of treatment.

Life Span and Gender

Evaluate the pregnancy status of the patient, as needed. Ipratropium is classified as a pregnancy category B drug. However, human studies have not been performed. Therefore, ipratropium should be used during pregnancy only when the benefits to the mother outweigh the possible risk to the fetus. Minimal amounts of inhaled ipratropium reach breast milk; therefore, the potential risk to the breast-feeding infant is negligible. Safety and effectiveness of ipratropium have not been established in infants or in children younger than 5 years.

Lifestyle, Diet, and Habits

Determine whether the patient smokes. Smoking causes vasoconstriction, the opposite of the action of ipratropium.

Environment

Ipratropium is most frequently self-administered in the home environment. It is used on a daily basis, regardless of the presence or absence of symptoms. Although beta-agonist drugs, such as albuterol, are the drugs of choice for acute symptoms, ipratropium may still be delivered during exacerbations of asthma.

Nursing Diagnoses and Outcomes

- Risk for Injury (bronchospasm) related to use of new canister of ipratropium
  Desired outcome: *The patient will "test-spray" a new canister three times before inhaling the medication.*
- Risk for Injury (anaphylactoid reactions) related to allergies to soybeans, legumes, or soya lecithin.
  Desired outcome: *The patient will review past allergic responses to assess whether any of the causative foods may have been responsible.*

Planning and Intervention

Maximizing Therapeutic Effects

Explain the importance of taking ipratropium daily, despite the absence of symptoms. Watch the patient demonstrate the correct use of the MDI.

Minimizing Adverse Effects

Explain the importance of using the MDI as prescribed to avoid systemic absorption that leads to an increased risk of adverse effects.

Providing Patient and Family Education

- Advise patients that ipratropium is used prophylactically to reduce the frequency and severity of future asthma attacks. It will not abort an asthma attack in progress.
- Advise patients to avoid using ipratropium if they have a history of allergy to soybeans, legumes, or soya lecithin.
- Remind patients that ipratropium must be taken daily, despite the absence of symptoms of asthma.
- Remind patients that overuse of ipratropium may induce adverse effects or increase their intensity.
- Teach patients to use an MDI. Include the correct procedure for administering the medication, keeping the equipment clean, and assessing when to change the canister.

Ongoing Assessment and Evaluation

Assess the patient's need for beta-agonist drugs in addition to ipratropium. If the patient continues to need beta agonists more than twice a week, refer the patient to the health care provider for additional assessment.

Drug Closely Related to Ipratropium Bromide

Tiotropium

Tiotropium (Spiriva), administered as a DPI, is structurally close to ipratropium but pharmacodynamically different. It is selective for muscarinic receptors 1 to 3; however, it

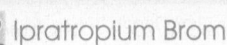

MEMORY CHIP

P Ipratropium Bromide

- Used for maintenance therapy of CAL or asthma
- Major contraindications: hypersensitivity to fluorocarbons or legumes, such as soybeans or peanuts
- Most common adverse effects: cough, hoarseness, throat irritation, dysgeusia, and anticholinergic effects
- Most serious adverse effects: bronchospasm and anaphylaxis
- Maximizing therapeutic effects: Administer the medication daily, despite the absence of symptoms.
- Minimizing adverse effects: Use only as directed to decrease potential systemic absorption.
- Most important patient education: This drug will not abort an acute asthma attack.

dissociates from them much slower than ipratropium does. This slow dissociation gives tiotropium a long duration of action and enables once-daily dosing. Another advantage is that tiotropium is minimally absorbed, which decreases the risk for systemic adverse effects.

Tiotropium should be used with caution in the elderly because they may experience anticholinergic effects such as blurred vision, constipation, urinary retention, and dry mouth despite the drug's minimal systemic absorption. It should also be used with caution in pregnant women. Tiotropium is a pregnancy category C drug; whether it crosses into breast milk is unknown.

As with ipratropium, there is potential for additive anticholinergic effects when tiotropium is administered with other antimuscarinics.

C XANTHINE DERIVATIVES

The xanthine derivatives, including theophylline, aminophylline, dyphylline, and caffeine, come from a variety of naturally occurring sources. They are excellent bronchodilators but do not work as rapidly as beta-adrenergic agonist drugs. Theophylline (Elixophyllin, Theo24, Uniphyl) is the prototype xanthine derivative bronchodilator (Table 35.5).

Nursing Management of the Patient Receiving P Theophylline

Core Drug Knowledge

Pharmacotherapeutics

Theophylline is indicated for the symptomatic relief or prevention of bronchial asthma and reversal of bronchospasm associated with CAL. An off-label use is treatment of apnea and bradycardia in premature infants.

Pharmacokinetics

Theophylline is given orally or intravenously. When given orally, it is well absorbed, with peak effects in 2 hours; it lasts from 4 to 8 hours. The drug is metabolized in the liver and excreted in the urine.

TABLE 35.5 **Summary of Selected C Xanthine Derivatives**

P theophylline (Elixophyllin, Theo24, Uniphyl) 100, 200, 300, 400 ER	Acute asthma/CAL/COPD	*Adult child and infant loading dose:* IV, 5.7 mg/kg of lean body weight *Adult and child 16 to 60 y, nonsmokers IV (after loading dose):* 0.4 mg/kg/h *Adult >60 IV:* 0.3 mg/kg/h *Child IV (after loading dose):* Neonates up to 24 days, 1 mg/kg every 12 h Neonates over 24 days, 1.5 mg/kg IV every 12 h Infants 6 to 52 wk, mg/kg/h = (0.008) × (age in wk) + 0.21 IV 1–9 y, initial 0.8 mg/kg/h 9–12 y, 0.7 mg/kg/h 12–16 y, smokers, 0.7 mg/kg/h 12–16 y, nonsmokers, 0.5 mg/kg/h	*Onset:* PO, varies; peak: 2 h *Duration:* 2–3 d $t_{1/2}$: 3–5 h for nonsmoker; 4–5 h for smoker
	Maintenance	*Adult and Child >45 kg PO:* 300 mg in divided doses every 6–8 h; after 3 days increase to 400 mg/d in divided doses every 6–8 h; after 3 more days increase to 600 mg/d in divided doses every 6–8 h; Note: ER formulation are administered every 12 h; Theo-24 and Uniphyl is given 1×/d.	
aminophylline	Acute asthma/CAL/COPD	*Adult child and infant loading dose:* IV, 5.7 mg/kg of lean body weight *Adult and child 16 to 60 y, nonsmokers IV (after loading dose):* 0.5 mg/kg/h *Adult >60 IV:* 0.38 mg/kg/h *Child IV (after loading dose):* Neonates up to 24 d, 1.25 mg/kg every 12 h Neonates over 24 d, 1.9 mg/kg IV every 12 h Infants 6 to 52 wk, (0.008) × (age in wk) + 0.21 IV 1–9 y, initial 1 mg/kg/h 9–12 y, 0.88 mg/kg/h 12–16 y, smokers, 0.88 mg/kg/h 12–16 y, nonsmokers, 0.625 mg/kg/h	*Onset:* PO, 15–60 min; IV, rapid *Duration:* 6–8 h $t_{1/2}$: Variable
	Maintenance	*Adult and child >16 y:* PO, 300 mg in divided doses every 6–8 h; after 3 d increase to 400 mg/d in divided doses every 6–8 h; after 3 more days increase to 600 mg/d in divided doses every 6–8 h; *Child 1–15 y:* PO, 12–14 mg/kg in divided doses every 4–6 h; after 3 days increase to 16 mg/kg in divided doses every 4–6 h; after 3 more days increase to 20 mg/kg in divided doses every 4–6 h.	
dyphylline (Lufyllin)		*Adult:* PO, 15/mg/kg qid; IM, 250–500 mg q6h *Child:* Safety not established	*Onset:* Unknown *Duration:* Unknown $t_{1/2}$: Unknown

Pharmacodynamics

Theophylline has a direct effect on the smooth muscles of the respiratory tract, both those in the bronchi and those in the blood vessels. Although the exact mechanism of action is not fully understood, it is believed that bronchodilation is caused by inhibiting phosphodiesterase (PDEs III and IV). Nonbronchodilation occurs through other molecular mechanisms. Theophylline also increases the force of contraction of diaphragmatic muscles to draw more air into the lungs.

Contraindications and Precautions

Theophylline is contraindicated in patients with hypersensitivity to any xanthines, in those with status asthmaticus, or in those with a peptic ulcer. Many diseases and disorders decrease the clearance of theophylline, including acute pulmonary edema, chronic heart failure, cor pulmonale, hypothyroidism, sepsis with multiorgan failure, and shock, resulting in an increased risk of toxicity. Theophylline should be used with caution with any patient with cardiovascular problems such as an arrhythmia or hypertension because of the drug's stimulatory effects. In addition, care also should be taken when theophylline is used in patients with renal or hepatic disease, because the drug is metabolized in the liver and excreted through the kidneys.

Theophylline is a pregnancy category C drug. It should be used with caution in pregnancy because it crosses the placenta and may enter breast milk.

Adverse Effects

Adverse effects related to theophylline use are related directly to serum levels of the drug. At serum levels less than 20 mcg/ mL, adverse effects are uncommon. At serum levels of 20 to 25 mcg/mL, the most common adverse effects are GI symptoms of nausea, vomiting, and diarrhea and CNS effects of headache, insomnia, and irritability. At serum levels exceeding 30 mcg/mL, adverse effects such as hyperglycemia, hypotension, arrhythmias, seizures, brain damage, and even death may occur. Even at therapeutic doses, theophylline may cause CNS effects, such as irritability (especially in children), restlessness, and muscle twitching. It also may cause GI effects, such as loss of appetite, hematemesis, and gastroesophageal reflux. Potential cardiovascular effects include palpitations, tachycardia, and circulatory failure. In the respiratory system, theophylline may cause tachypnea. Possible genitourinary effects include urinary retention in men with prostate enlargement and diuresis. Generalized effects, such as fever, flushing, rash, and elevated liver enzymes, also have occurred.

Drug Interactions

Theophylline may have a substantial interaction with a multitude of drugs (Table 35.6). These drugs decrease the clearance of theophylline, resulting in an increased risk of adverse effects and toxicity. Theophylline may also induce the metabolism of other drugs, resulting in decreased efficacy of those drugs. Many of these interactions require a dose adjustment of theophylline or the interactant drug. Potential dosage adjustments should be discussed with the health care provider.

Assessment of Relevant Core Patient Variables

Health Status

When taking the patient history before starting theophylline therapy, screen the patient for any hypersensitivity to xanthines and for peptic ulcer, active gastritis, coronary artery disease, hypothyroidism, renal or hepatic disorders, pregnancy, and lactation.

Patients with cardiac disease should be monitored closely during theophylline therapy because the drug may cause cardiovascular effects, such as palpitations, tachycardia, and elevated blood pressure.

Perform a baseline physical examination, including skin color, texture, and lesions; reflexes, orientation, and affect; and heart rate. Assess the respiratory system for breathing rate, adventitious sounds, and the patient's forced expiratory volume in 1 second (FEV_1). For patients on long-term therapy, obtain baseline thyroid, liver, and kidney function test results.

Life Span and Gender

Assess the patient for pregnancy and lactation because theophylline is contraindicated during pregnancy; newborns of mothers who used theophylline exhibit tachycardia, jitteriness, and withdrawal apnea. Assess older men carefully for possible enlargement of the prostate gland, because special precautions should be taken when administering theophylline to these patients: they should be monitored closely for any prostate changes.

Lifestyle, Diet, and Habits

Determine whether the patient smokes. Smoking cigarettes may decrease serum theophylline levels. In fact, some patients who smoke require an increase in theophylline dosage of up to 50%. Monitor patients who smoke for any change in smoking habits. It also is important to assess the diet of patients taking theophylline. Theophylline elimination is increased by a low-carbohydrate, high-protein diet and by charcoal-broiled beef. Theophylline elimination is decreased by a high-carbohydrate, low-protein diet. The effects of theophylline can be increased by foods containing xanthines, particularly caffeine. Caffeine is found in many beverages, such as coffee, tea, and cola, and in chocolate. OTC drug preparations also frequently contain caffeine.

Environment

Oral theophylline may be administered in any environment. IV theophylline is administered in an acute care setting.

Nursing Diagnoses and Outcomes

- Disturbed Sensory Perception: Kinesthetic, related to CNS effects of irritability, insomnia, and dizziness
  Desired outcome: The patient will be protected from injury caused by CNS effects, such as dizziness and loss of balance.
- Ineffective Tissue Perfusion: Cardiopulmonary, related to cardiac effects of drug
  Desired outcome: Adverse effects will be limited by proper administration and monitoring of drug serum levels.
- Risk for Injury related to headache, GI effects, and CNS effects
  Desired outcome: The patient will develop strategies to be able to tolerate the drug and remain injury free during drug therapy.

Planning and Intervention

Maximizing Therapeutic Effects

If serum levels of theophylline have not been stabilized, screen the patient's diet, other drugs taken (including OTC

TABLE 35.6 Agents That Interact with P Theophylline

Interactants	Effect and Significance	Nursing Management
Acyclovir cimetadine diltiazem disulfiram fluvoxamine fluoroquinolone hormonal contraceptives mexiletine ticlopidine zileuton	Coadministration decreases clearance of theophylline, resulting in increased risk of adverse effects and toxicity.	Monitor for headache, insomnia, irritability, nausea, vomiting, arrhythmias, and seizures. Monitor theophylline levels.
activated charcoal	Can reduce absorption of theophylline and remove it from systemic circulation, resulting in subtherapeutic levels of theophylline	Monitor for efficacy of theophylline.
adenosine	Mechanism of action unclear; theophylline may decrease effectiveness of adenosine.	Monitor heart rate. Monitor blood pressure.
barbiturates	May induce cytochrome P-450, stimulating theophylline metabolism and increasing clearance, resulting in subtherapeutic levels of theophylline	Monitor for efficacy of theophylline.
benzodiazepines	Possible antagonistic action by competitive binding to intracerebral adenosine receptors, resulting in decreased sedative effects of benzodiazepines	Monitor sedation level. Monitor for anxiety.
beta blockers	May reduce N-demethylation of theophylline, resulting in decreased effect of one or both agents	Monitor efficacy of both drugs.
halothane	Catecholamine-induced arrhythmias possible when halothane is administered after theophylline	Document theophylline use clearly on front of chart for patients scheduled for surgery.
hydantoins	Phenytoin and theophylline metabolism increased, resulting in subtherapeutic levels of both drugs	Monitor plasma levels of both drugs.
isoniazid	Isoniazid may induce and inhibit hepatic enzymes responsible for theophylline metabolism.	Monitor for both decreased efficacy and increased adverse effects of theophylline.
ketamine	Mechanism is unknown. Coadministration may increase risk of seizures.	Monitor for seizure activity. Ensure safety.
ketoconazole	Ketoconazole may decrease absorption of theophylline.	Monitor for theophylline efficacy.
macrolide antibiotics	Inhibit metabolism of theophylline; theophylline reduces bioavailability and increases renal clearance of oral erythromycin, resulting in theophylline toxicity and macrolide ineffectivity.	Monitor drug levels of both drugs.
non-depolarizing muscle relaxants	Antagonistic activity between theophylline and nondepolarizing muscle relaxants—nontherapeutic effects of muscle relaxants	Document theophylline use clearly on front of chart for patients scheduled for surgery.
rifampin	Appears to induce hepatic metabolism of theophylline, resulting in subtherapeutic levels	Monitor theophylline efficacy.
thyroid hormones and preparations	Direct correlation between plasma thyroid hormones/preparations and theophylline clearance; hypothyroid or hyperthyroid patients, alteration in theophylline clearance	Monitor theophylline levels closely. Achieving euthyroid state is critical in controlling theophylline clearance.

COMMUNITY BASED CONCERNS

Using a Peak Flow Meter

Patients receiving inhaled bronchodilators at home can monitor the effectiveness of drug therapy and lung function by using a peak flow meter to monitor peak expiratory flow rates (PEFR). These devices are inexpensive and may be available from the health care provider or by prescription from the pharmacist.

Peak flow values are a way to quantify and evaluate lung function. Daily monitoring helps detect trends and subtle changes in lung function, sometimes even before the patient experiences symptoms. Daily monitoring also permits early and prompt intervention before the patient experiences a setback and needs to seek emergency care.

The peak flow meter consists of a mouthpiece connected to a sealed measuring device. The patient inhales as deeply as possible and then places the mouthpiece in the mouth, making a tight seal. Next, the patient blows out as hard and as fast as possible. The exhaled air propels an indicator up a scale to a number. This number, signifying liters of air per minute, represents the peak flow rate. After consulting with the provider, the patient can determine his or her normal PEFR. The patient can then keep a record of the readings and report any changes in PEFR to the health care provider.

---

drugs), smoking habits, and adherence to prescribed regimen. In the hospital setting, administer theophylline at a rate of 20 mg/minute. If patients have frequent exacerbations of CAL, determine the patient's ability to use a peak flow meter in the home environment to assess the need for additional bronchodilation (Box 35.6).

Minimizing Adverse Effects

Monitor serum theophylline levels carefully and discuss dosage adjustment with the health care provider to keep serum levels at 10 to 20 mcg/mL, which is the optimal therapeutic level. Never infuse theophylline rapidly; rapid infusion may cause hypotension, arrhythmias, syncope, or even death.

Administer immediate-release preparations with a meal to decrease GI distress. Administer sustained-release preparations on an empty stomach, 1 hour before or 2 hours after meals. To prevent injuries, be prepared to institute safety precautions if CNS effects occur. Additionally, provide environmental control—including adjusting lighting, heat, and noise—if irritability, restlessness, or insomnia occurs.

Providing Patient and Family Education

• Explain that theophylline will help make breathing easier.
• Caution patients not to take theophylline if they are allergic to it, if they have reactions to caffeine, or if they are breast-feeding.
• Make sure that patients report to their health care providers the names of all drugs they are currently taking.
• Explain the importance of taking theophylline exactly as prescribed and instruct patients to make a list of things that can interfere with their drug concentrations (e.g., diet, OTC drugs, and smoking). Make sure that patients

and their families are aware of precautions they should take and know when to contact the health care provider if they change their diets, use OTC drugs, or change their smoking habits.

• Teach patients never to chew or crush time-release capsules; they should be swallowed whole. In addition, time-release capsules should always be taken on an empty stomach, 1 hour before or 2 hours after meals. If patients are using a solution, it should be shaken well before use. Encourage patients to take immediate-release and liquid preparations of the drug with food if GI upset occurs.
• Caution patients not to change the drug dosage without consulting the health care provider and to schedule regular checkups or blood tests so that progress can be evaluated.
• Instruct patients to take the drug around the clock; if a dose is missed, it should be taken as soon as it is remembered unless it is almost time for the next dose. However, two doses should never be taken at the same time.
• Instruct patients to avoid consuming large quantities of caffeine-containing foods (e.g., chocolates) or beverages (e.g., coffee, cola, and tea) while taking theophylline and to contact their health care provider if they change their consumption substantially. In addition, alert patients to check the ingredients of any OTC drug for caffeine before using it.
• Advise patients to ingest small, frequent meals if GI distress occurs.

CRITICAL THINKING SCENARIO

THINKING ABOUT THEOPHYLLINE AND OTHER ASTHMA THERAPIES

Martin Kell is a 12-year-old boy with a history of allergic asthma. Skin testing has revealed allergies to trees, molds, and dust. His mother, Mrs. Kell, is bringing him to the clinic for sensitization treatment. She reports that Martin has had a stuffy nose, dry cough, and occasional wheezing. On examination, scattered wheezes are noted throughout the lung fields. The physician orders the following:

Theophylline, 200 mg bid
Albuterol inhaler, 2 puffs bid
Beclomethasone inhaler, 2 puffs bid

You review all of the medications with Martin's mother, who exclaims, "All these medicines! How is he ever going to be able to take them all?"

1. Prioritize concerns to be discussed with Mrs. Kell.
2. Explain the rationale for using both inhalers.
3. Construct written instructions about using the inhalers to give to Mrs. Kell.
4. Consider what adaptations may be necessary with Martin to help ensure therapeutic adherence and effective drug therapy.
5. Propose some assessments that you can plan to make during the next visit to evaluate the effectiveness of therapy.

- Advise a quiet environment or exercise to decrease agitation or insomnia from theophylline therapy.
- Caution against using oral theophylline for an acute asthma attack because its onset is not quick enough to subdue an acute attack. IV theophylline may be used for an acute attack.
- Urge patients to report such adverse effects as headaches, insomnia, restlessness, muscle twitching, nausea, vomiting, severe GI pain, palpitation, and convulsions.

Ongoing Assessment and Evaluation

Monitor the patient taking theophylline for potential CNS and cardiovascular adverse effects. The patient's serum theophylline level should be maintained between 10 and 20 mcg/mL for optimal therapeutic effects and minimal adverse effects. After 1 to 2 weeks on theophylline, the patient should report no more than minimal discomfort from adverse effects and continue to adhere to the therapy prescribed.

Drugs Closely Related to [P] Theophylline

Aminophylline

Aminophylline, a theophylline salt, is pharmacologically identical to theophylline. It is more soluble than theophylline; thus, it is preferred when IV administration is needed. It is important to administer IV aminophylline at a rate not to exceed 25 mg/min. Aminophylline also can be administered as a rectal suppository (Truphylline).

Dyphylline

Dyphylline (Lufyllin) is structurally similar to theophylline. Dyphylline works by direct stimulation of the bronchial smooth muscles but is not converted into theophylline to achieve its action. It is approximately one tenth as potent as theophylline, and therefore it induces fewer adverse effects.

Caffeine

Caffeine is a naturally occurring xanthine derivative used as a CNS and respiratory stimulant, or as a mild diuretic. Caffeine often is combined with analgesics or with ergot alkaloids to

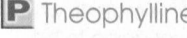 MEMORY CHIP

[P] Theophylline

- Used for symptomatic relief of bronchoconstriction and bronchospasm
- Major contraindications: status asthmaticus and peptic ulcer
- Most common adverse effects: nausea, vomiting, headache, and insomnia
- Most serious adverse effects: seizures and arrhythmias
- Maximizing therapeutic effects: Evaluate patient care variables if serum concentration not stable.
- Minimizing adverse effects: Monitor serum theophylline levels periodically.
- Most important patient education: Take the drug exactly as prescribed to avoid adverse effects.

treat migraine and other types of headache. Caffeine also is sold without a prescription in products marketed to treat drowsiness, or in products used for mild water-weight gain.

Caffeine is administered both orally and parenterally as a respiratory stimulant in neonates with apnea of prematurity. It reduces the frequency of apneic episodes by 30% to 50% within 24 hours of administration. Caffeine is an excellent drug for neonates because of its once-daily administration, reliable oral absorption, and wide therapeutic margin.

[C] ANTI-INFLAMMATORY AGENTS

In addition to bronchodilators, anti-inflammatory agents are used to manage respiratory disorders, especially asthma. These agents include glucocorticoid steroids, mast cell stabilizers, and leukotriene receptor antagonists.

• [C] INHALED GLUCOCORTICOID STEROIDS

Glucocorticoid steroids are the most effective anti- inflammatory drugs available for managing respiratory disorders. They can be given orally, parenterally, or by inhalation. Oral and parenteral agents (discussed in Chapter 48) are the most potent and are reserved for an exacerbation of CAL or asthma that occurs despite the use of inhaled steroids. Inhaled corticosteroid (ICS) agents have become the first-line treatment for persistent asthma. Although there may be regional preferences, the prototype ICS in this chapter is flunisolide (AeroBid). Table 35.7 provides a summary of selected inhaled glucocorticosteroids.

Nursing Management of the Patient Receiving [P] Flunisolide

Core Drug Knowledge

Pharmacotherapeutics

Inhaled flunisolide is used to prevent bronchospasm associated with asthma, CAL, and other respiratory disorders. A maintenance drug, it is not helpful during an acute attack. Intranasal flunisolide is used to treat allergic rhinitis.

Pharmacokinetics

As with the anticholinergic ipratropium bromide, flunisolide obtains its peak effect only after 1 to 2 weeks of regular use. Despite flunisolide being an inhaled drug, systemic absorption does occur. During inhalation, especially when a spacer is not used, flunisolide is deposited in the mouth and pharynx, where some of the drug is swallowed. Also, ICS deposited in the lungs is not inactivated; therefore, any portion of the inhaled drug not used by the lungs eventually becomes systemically absorbed.

Pharmacodynamics

Inhaled glucocorticoid steroids such as flunisolide have several actions. They inhibit the production of leukotrienes and prostaglandins through interference with arachidonic acid metabolism, reduce migration and activity of the

TABLE 35.7 Summary of Selected ⊖ Inhaled Steroids

Drug (Trade) Name	Selected Indications	Route and Dosage Range	Pharmacokinetics
ℙ flunisolide (AeroBid), 250 mcg/ spray; (AeroSpan), 80 mcg/spray	Asthma prophylaxis	*Adult and child >15 y:* INH, 2 puffs 2×/d Max: 8 puffs/d *Child 6–15 y:* INH, 2 puffs 2×/d Max: 4 puffs/d	Not systemically absorbed
beclomethasone HFA (QVAR), 40, 80 mcg/puff INH	Asthma prophylaxis	*Adult and child >12 y:* INH, 40–160 mcg 2×/d Max: 320 mcg 2×/d *Child 4–11 y:* INH, 40–80 mcg 2×/d Max: 160 mcg/d	Not systemically absorbed
budesonide DPI (Pulmicort Flexhaler), 90, 180 mcg/actuation INH	Asthma prophylaxis	*Adult:* INH, 180–360 mcg/ 2×/d *Child >6y:* INH 180–360 mcg 2×/d Max: 720 mcg/d Max: 1 mg/d	Not systemically absorbed
budesonide (Pulmicort Respules), 0.25, 0.5 mg/2 mL INH solution	Asthma prophylaxis	*Adult: Not recommended* *Child 1–8 y:* INH via nebulizer, 0.25–0.5 mg 1–4×/d; max: 0.5 mg/d	Onset: PO, 30 min Inhalation: Immediate Duration: 8–12 h $t_{1/2}$: PO, 2–3.6 h; inhalation, 2.8 h
ciclesonide (Alvesco) 80, 160 mcg/puff	Asthma prophylaxis	*Adult and Child >12 y:* INH 80–160 mcg 2×/d	Not systemically absorbed
fluticasone (Flovent HFA), 44, 110, 220 mcg/spray	Asthma prophylaxis	*Adult:* INH, 88–440 mcg 2×/d; max: 880 mcg 2×/d *Child:* INH, 88 mcg 2×/d; max 176 mcg	Not systemically absorbed
fluticasone (Flovent Diskus), 50 mcg DPI	Asthma prophylaxis	*Adult and child >12 y:* INH, 100–500 mcg 2×/d; max 1000 mcg *Child 4–11 y:* INH, 50–100 mcg 2×/d; max: 100 mcg 2×/d	Not systemically absorbed
mometasone (Asmanex Twisthaler) 110, 200 mcg/activation	Asthma prophylaxis	*Adult and child >12 y:* INH, 220–440 mcg 1–2×/d *Child 4–11y:* INH 110 mcg/d	Not systemically absorbed

inflammatory cells, increase the number of beta receptors, enhance the responsiveness of beta receptors in airway smooth muscle, and decrease the production of mucus.

Contraindications and Precautions

Flunisolide is contraindicated for use in patients with an active systemic fungal infection. It should be used with caution in patients with active infection of the respiratory tract; untreated systemic fungal, bacterial, parasitic or viral infections; or ocular herpes simplex because it depresses the immune response, an effect that could result in serious illness.

Flunisolide, a pregnancy category C drug, should be used during pregnancy only if the benefits outweigh the risks to the fetus, because animal studies have shown teratogenic and fetotoxic effects.

Adverse Effects

Adverse effects are limited with flunisolide because of the route of administration. Sore throat, hoarseness, coughing, dry mouth, and pharyngeal and laryngeal fungal infections are the most common adverse effects. Dysphonia and oro-pharyngeal *Candida albicans* infection are common adverse effects associated with daily use of ICS. In children, long-term use of ICS may delay growth patterns. Suppression of the hypothalamic-pituitary-adrenal (HPA) axis is possible, but this effect is very rare.

Drug Interactions

Because of the route of administration, no important drug–drug interactions occur with flunisolide.

Assessment of Relevant Core Patient Variables

Health Status

Assess for signs of an active lung infection because flunisolide may exacerbate the infection. Contact the prescriber if you suspect that the patient has a systemic fungal infection. Assess for recent oral corticoid steroid use. Patients making the transition from oral corticoid steroids to ICS have an increased risk of adrenal insufficiency if they experience trauma, surgery, or infections, particularly gastroenteritis.

To accurately assess for delayed growth patterns during flunisolide therapy, obtain baseline height and weight of children.

Life Span and Gender

Flunisolide is approved for use in children older than 6 years. Schedule periodic clinic visits for children to monitor for possible adverse effects on growth patterns. Assess whether women of childbearing age are pregnant. Flunisolide is a pregnancy category C drug and should be used during pregnancy only if the benefits outweigh the risks to the fetus. It is not known whether flunisolide enters breast milk.

Lifestyle, Diet and Habits

Caution the patient to avoid cigarette smoking because smoking will decrease the efficacy of flunisolide.

Environment

Flunisolide is used primarily in the home care setting. Evaluate the patient's inhalation technique during each outpatient visit to ensure proper drug administration at home.

Nursing Diagnoses and Outcomes

- Impaired Verbal Communication related to dysphonia and cough
  Desired outcome: *The patient will report symptoms to the health care provider.*
- Risk for Infection related to immunosuppression
  Desired outcome: *The patient will remain free of infection throughout therapy.*

Planning and Intervention

Maximizing Therapeutic Effects

Instruct the patient to take flunisolide every day, regardless of how well she or he feels. As a maintenance drug, flunisolide must be taken twice daily in order to affect its maximal response. Using a beta-2 agonist before flunisolide dilates the bronchial tree and allows the drug to be dispersed throughout the lungs. The use of a spacer may also help increase the intrapulmonary delivery of the drug if the patient's inhalation technique is poor.

Minimizing Adverse Effects

Spacers may help alleviate dysphonia by filtering larger aerosol particles that ordinarily deposit in the oropharynx and extrathoracic airways (this precaution also reduces the risk of oropharyngeal candidiasis). Spacers also help decrease systemic absorption because less flunisolide is swallowed. Rinsing the mouth after use decreases the potential for thrush as well as decreases the amount of drug swallowed, thus reducing the potential for systemic effects. With children, be especially vigilant for signs of HPA axis suppression, even in children with normal growth patterns, because growth is not a reliable predictor of HPA axis suppression. Monitor patients making the transition from oral corticosteroid to ICS frequently. Monitor for signs of

adrenal insufficiency, especially if the patient is experiencing additional stressors such as infection.

Providing Patient and Family Education

Patient education is important for inhaled steroid therapy. Include the following topics in patient education:

- Good oral hygiene
- Proper use of MDI
- Signs and symptoms of oropharyngeal candidiasis (e.g., mouth ulcers, white spots on oral mucous membranes, and painful swallowing)
- Importance of rinsing the mouth after each administration to decrease the potential for fungal infections of the mouth
- Importance of daily use, regardless of the absence of symptoms, and of using a short-acting sympathomimetic inhaler for acute symptoms
- Symptoms of HPA suppression. Advise the patient to resume taking oral steroids if symptoms of HPA suppression occur.

Ongoing Assessment and Evaluation

Assess for a decreased incidence of acute asthma attacks. Evaluate the correct use of the MDI or DPI at each visit. Although the risk for developing HPA suppression is very low with inhaled flunisolide, monitor for this possibility at each visit. In children, document growth patterns at each visit.

Drugs Closely Related to Flunisolide

Beclomethasone

Beclomethasone (Qvar) is used to treat steroid-dependent asthma, prevent allergic or nonallergic rhinitis, and prevent recurrent nasal polyps after removal. It is available for both nasal and oral inhalation for use in patients older than 5 years. It is a pregnancy category C drug.

Budesonide

Budesonide is available as intranasal inhalation (Rhinocort), oral inhalation (Pulmicort DPI, Pulmicort Respules), or orally (Entocort EC). It is also available as a combination MDI

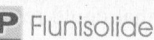

MEMORY CHIP

P Flunisolide

- Used for maintenance treatment of CAL and asthma
- Major contraindication: active respiratory infection
- Most common adverse effects: dry mouth, dysphonia
- Most serious adverse effects: oral candidiasis, systemic absorption
- Maximizing therapeutic effects: Administer the drug daily, despite the absence of symptoms.
- Minimizing adverse effects: Use a spacer device.
- Most important patient education: This drug will not abort an acute attack.

with the long-acting beta-2 agonist formoterol (Symbicort). Budesonide is used to manage symptoms associated with allergic rhinitis, asthma, ulcerative colitis, or Crohn disease. Given as an oral inhaled drug, it is approved for use in children older than 6 years of age. Given by nebulizer, it may be given to children 1 to 8 years of age. Budesonide is a pregnancy category C drug.

Ciclesonide

Ciclesonide (Alvesco) is the same steroid used in the nasal spray Omnaris. It has a smaller particle size that, theoretically, should be able to disperse into smaller airways. As a prodrug, it is activated in the lungs. This decreases the potential for oral or esophageal candidiasis. Ciclesonide is indicated for adults and children over the age of 12. It is a pregnancy category C drug.

Fluticasone

Fluticasone is also used in managing rhinitis, asthma, and CAL. It is available for nasal inhalation (Flonase), for oral inhalation (Flovent HFA, Flovent Diskus), and in combination with salmeterol (Advair Diskus). High-dose fluticasone is associated with suppression of the HPA axis. It is approved for use in children older than 4 years of age. It is a pregnancy category C drug.

Mometasone

Mometasone DPI (Asmanex Twisthaler) is the same steroid as the nasal spray Nasonex. It is approved for the management of asthma, but not bronchospasm. Studies have demonstrated better compliance with mometasone due to its once-daily administration. Better compliance may decrease the frequency of exacerbations and the need for short-acting beta agonist rescue drugs. Instruct the patient to discard when the counter reaches "00" or 45 days after it was removed from its foil package.

Triamcinolone

Triamcinolone (Azmacort) was the first ICS on the market. It is used to manage rhinitis, asthma, and CAL. It is available for nasal inhalation (Nasacort) and oral inhalation (Azmacort). It is approved for use in children older than 6 years. Like other ICS drugs, it is a pregnancy category C drug.

• Ⓒ Mast Cell Stabilizers

Vasoactive substances such as histamine, serotonin, bradykinin, and leukotrienes are located within the mast cell. When the mast cell ruptures, these substances cause an inflammatory response, such as bronchial constriction, which accounts for the symptoms of an acute asthma attack. The prototype mast cell stabilizer is cromolyn sodium (Table 35.8).

Nursing Management of the Patient Receiving Ⓟ Cromolyn Sodium

Core Drug Knowledge

Pharmacotherapeutics

Cromolyn sodium is used as a prophylactic agent in treating mild to moderate asthma (Intal) and acute bronchospasm induced by exercise, environmental pollutants, and known antigens. The drug also is used as a nasal inhaler

TABLE 35.8	Summary of Selected Ⓒ Mast Cell Stabilizers			
Ⓟ cromolyn sodium (Intal)	Asthma prophylaxis	Oral inhalation (800 mcg/spray): *Adult and child >5 y:* 2 puffs qid until stabilized, then 2 puffs bid Exercise-induced asthma: 2 puffs 10–60 min before exercise *Child 2–4 y:* 20 mg Spinhaler qid until stabilized, then bid	*Onset:* 15 min *Duration:* Unknown $t_{1/2}$: 80–90 min
(NasalCrom)	Allergic rhinitis	Nasal inhalation (40 mg/mL): *Adult and child >6 y:* 1 spray each nostril, 3–4/d	
(Crolom)	Allergic conjunctivitis	Ophthalmic (4% drops): *Adult and child >4 y:* 1–2 drops each eye, 4–6/d	
nedocromil ophthalmic (Alocril)	Allergic conjunctivitis	Ophthalmic (2%) drops) Adult and child > 3 y: 1–2 drops each eye 2×/d	
omalizumab (Xolair)	Allergic asthma	*Adult and child >12 y:* SC, 150–375 mg q2–4 wk	*Onset:* Slow *Duration:* Unknown $t_{1/2}$: 26 d

(NasalCrom) to treat seasonal allergic rhinitis, as an ophthalmic solution (Crolom) to treat allergic conjunctivitis, and orally (Gastrocrom) to treat systemic mastocytosis (a rare disease characterized by an abnormal increase in mast cells in various body organs and tissues) and ulcerative colitis. Off-label uses include refractory forms of chronic urticaria/ angioedema, treatment of food allergies, and mucosal and serosal eosinophilic gastroenteritis.

Pharmacokinetics

Cromolyn sodium may be administered orally for a systemic effect to treat mastocytosis. There is no systemic absorption when used by either intranasal or ophthalmic administration. Approximately 10% of inhaled cromolyn reaches the lungs, but this percentage may be decreased by the degree of bronchoconstriction present. About 98% of the drug is eliminated unchanged in feces. Minimal amounts of the drug cross the placenta or enter the breast milk. Improvement of symptoms requires several weeks of therapy.

Pharmacodynamics

Cromolyn sodium is an anti-inflammatory agent that works at the surface of the mast cell to inhibit mast cell rupture and degranulation after contact with an antigen. This action, in turn, prevents the release of histamine and SRS-A, mediators of type I allergic reactions. Cromolyn also may reduce the release of inflammatory leukotrienes. Although its exact mechanism of action is unclear, it is thought to produce these effects by inhibiting calcium influx.

Contraindications and Precautions

Cromolyn sodium is absolutely contraindicated in patients with a demonstrated hypersensitivity because anaphylaxis can occur. Cromolyn sodium is not a bronchodilator. Therefore, it is contraindicated for treating acute bronchospasm or status asthmaticus. The aerosol preparation of cromolyn sodium is contraindicated in patients with coronary artery disease or cardiac dysrhythmias because the aerosol contains fluorocarbon as a propellant, and fluorocarbons irritate cardiac cells.

Precautions include patients with lactose intolerance because oral preparations contain lactose. Patients who wear soft contact lenses should use ophthalmic cromolyn sodium cautiously because it contains benzalkonium chloride, which can cause ocular irritation.

Cromolyn sodium is a pregnancy category B drug.

Adverse Effects

In general, cromolyn is well tolerated. When it is administered by oral inhalation, the most common adverse effects are bronchospasm, throat irritation, and cough. Because preparations for oral inhalation can contain lactose, patients with lactose intolerance may experience nausea and vomiting, bloating, abdominal cramps, and flatulence.

Intranasal cromolyn spray can produce sneezing and nasal irritation, but these are generally transient effects following application. Ocular cromolyn ophthalmic drops may produce ocular irritation, especially in patients with soft contact lenses. The most frequent adverse effects from cromolyn powder for oral solution are headache and diarrhea.

Drug Interactions

No clinically important drug interactions are known with cromolyn sodium.

Assessment of Relevant Core Patient Variables

Health Status

Evaluate for previous adverse effects to cromolyn sodium before administration. Perform a baseline physical assessment, including the head, eyes, ears, nose, throat, and lung sounds.

Life Span and Gender

Cromolyn sodium can be administered to both adults and children. Note whether the patient is pregnant or lactating. Cromolyn sodium is classified as a pregnancy category B drug because only a minimal amount of the drug crosses the placenta or enters the breast milk.

Lifestyle, Diet, and Habits

Monitor patients with lactose intolerance for adverse effects to oral cromolyn sodium. Advise patients who experience exercise-induced bronchospasm to take cromolyn sodium 15 to 20 minutes before exercise.

Environment

Cromolyn sodium can be administered in any setting. If it will be administered at home, remind the patient to administer it before engaging in an activity that causes bronchospasm.

Nursing Diagnoses and Outcomes

- Imbalanced Nutrition: Less than Body Requirements, related to nausea and vomiting, bloating, abdominal cramps, and flatulence
  Desired outcome: The patient will maintain body weight throughout therapy.
- Ineffective Breathing Pattern related to bronchospasm and cough
  Desired outcome: The patient will have a patent airway throughout therapy.

Planning and Intervention

Maximizing Therapeutic Effects

Cromolyn sodium is available in a variety of administration vehicles, such as a nebulizer, an MDI, or an oral tablet. Evaluate the patient's ability to correctly use these devices (see Box 35.4). Cromolyn sodium is used for long-term management of respiratory disorders. Except in the case of exercise-induced asthma, the patient should take the medication daily, even when symptoms are absent.

Minimizing Adverse Effects

Caution patients who have a known intolerance to lactose or who experience symptoms of lactose intolerance (nausea and vomiting, bloating, abdominal cramps, and flatulence) while taking oral cromolyn sodium. Changing to a different route of administration may be necessary to avoid losing weight from GI effects.

Providing Patient and Family Education

- Stress that cromolyn sodium should not be taken by anyone who has a hypersensitivity to this drug.
- Emphasize that cromolyn sodium is not useful for managing acute symptoms and that it is used for prophylaxis only. Patients should use a sympathomimetic drug for acute symptoms of respiratory distress.
- Demonstrate the correct use of administration devices and then have patients demonstrate it while you watch.
- Be sure that patients understand that cromolyn sodium must be taken daily, whether or not symptoms are present, except for exercise-induced asthma.
- Instruct patients to use cromolyn sodium 15 to 20 minutes before engaging in any activity, such as exercise, that is known to induce bronchospasm in that patient.
- Teach patients how to use a peak flow meter to monitor his or her personal respiratory status.

Ongoing Assessment and Evaluation

Evaluate the effectiveness of cromolyn sodium, demonstrated by a decrease in the frequency and severity of symptoms. For example, the patient should remain free from symptoms such as itchy and watery eyes, nasal congestion, or respiratory distress. Monitor for potential adverse effects in patients with lactose intolerance and in those who wear soft contact lenses, as previously mentioned.

MEMORY CHIP

Cromolyn Sodium

- Used for prophylaxis of allergic symptoms, including asthma
- Major contraindications: hypersensitivity and acute symptoms
- Most common adverse effects: dry throat, cough, and wheezing
- Most serious adverse effects: bronchospasm and anaphylaxis
- Maximizing therapeutic effects: Teach use of delivery systems.
- Minimizing adverse effects: Use only as directed.
- Most important patient education: Take the medication daily, despite the absence of symptoms; the drug is to be used only for prophylaxis and not as a "rescue" drug.

Drug Significantly Different From
P Cromolyn Sodium

Omalizumab (Xolair) is the first monoclonal antibody directed against immunoglobulin E (IgE) and the first biologic therapy developed to treat asthma. It is used to manage asthma in patients with moderate to severe persistent asthma and a positive skin test for perennial allergens that inhaled corticosteroids do not control. Omalizumab is also being studied for use in other IgE-related conditions, including allergic rhinitis, peanut allergy, latex sensitivity, atopic dermatitis, chronic urticaria, and allergic bronchopulmonary aspergillosis. Omalizumab is a subcutaneous injection. Reconstituting this medication correctly is important, and you must be sure to wait 20 minutes to ensure that the powder dissolves.

Omalizumab binds to mast cells, preventing mast cell rupture and degranulation. In addition to binding mast cells, it binds to receptors on monocytes, eosinophils, dendritic cells, epithelial cells, and platelets, thereby interfering with release of inflammatory mediators and cytokines.

The only contraindication to the use of omalizumab is hypersensitivity to hamster protein because it is derived from this source. Omalizumab is used cautiously in patients with pre-existing neoplasm because it has induced several types of malignancy.

Omalizumab may induce anaphylaxis in susceptible patients. Anaphylaxis can occur at any time, even with the first dose. It occurs most frequently within the first 2 hours after administration; however, delayed reactions of up to 24 hours have been reported. More common adverse effects include injection-site reaction, viral infections (including upper respiratory tract infections), sinusitis, headache, and pharyngitis.

Monitor the patient for a minimum of 2 hours after administering the injection. Teach the patient the signs and symptoms of anaphylaxis and the importance of obtaining immediate medical care, such as calling 911 for assistance should any symptoms occur. Omalizumab is a pregnancy category B drug; whether it enters breast milk is not known. It is not approved for use in children younger than 12 years of age.

C LEUKOTRIENE RECEPTOR ANTAGONISTS

Leukotrienes are inflammatory mediators that are powerful bronchoconstrictors and vasodilators. Within the past decade, leukotrienes have been identified as important mediators in the pathology and symptomatology of asthma, both acute and chronic. Even patients with mild asthma show airway inflammation, including infiltration of the mucosa and epithelium with activated T cells, mast cells, and eosinophils. T cells and mast cells release the cytokines leukotriene, histamine, bradykinin, and serotonin, which increase microvascular permeability, disrupt the epithelium, and stimulate neural reflexes and mucus-secreting glands. The result is airway hyperreactivity, bronchoconstriction, and hypersecretion, manifested by wheezing, coughing, and dyspnea. Leukotriene receptor antagonists include zafirlukast, montelukast, and zileuton. Zafirlukast (Accolate) is the prototype leukotriene receptor antagonist (Table 35.9).

TABLE 35.9　Summary of Selected Ⓒ Leukotriene Receptor Antagonists

Ⓟ zafirlukast (Accolate) 10, 20 mg	Asthma maintenance	*Adult and child >12:* PO, 20 mg bid *Child 5–11 y:* PO, 10 mg bid	*Onset:* Rapid *Duration:* 12–24 h $t_{1/2}$: 10 h
montelukast (Singulair) 4, 5 mg chewable; 10 mg; 4-mg granule packet	Asthma maintenance	*Adult and child >15 y:* PO, 10 mg in the evening *Child 6–14 y:* PO, 5 mg in the evening *Child 2–5 y:* 4 mg in the evening *Child 12–24 mo:* 4-mg granule	*Onset:* Rapid *Duration:* 12–24 h $t_{1/2}$: 5.5 h
zileuton (Zyflo CR) 600 mg	Asthma maintenance	*Adult and child >12 y:* 1,200 mg bid *Child <12 y:* Not recommended	*Onset:* Rapid *Duration:* Unknown $t_{1/2}$: 2.5 h

Nursing Management of the Patient Receiving Ⓟ Zafirlukast

Core Drug Knowledge

Pharmacotherapeutics

Zafirlukast is used as prophylaxis or for treating chronic asthma. It is not indicated for symptoms of an acute attack. Off-label uses of zafirlukast are chronic idiopathic urticaria and dermatographism.

Pharmacokinetics

Zafirlukast is administered orally. It is distributed to tissues to some degree, but it distributes across the blood–brain barrier only minimally. In treating asthma, the peak action is noted as early as day 1 of therapy but more commonly takes up to 2 weeks. For that reason, it is not useful for managing an acute asthma attack.

Food reduces the bioavailability of zafirlukast by approximately 40%; therefore, this drug should be taken either 1 hour before or 2 hours after meals. Zafirlukast is metabolized extensively through the P-450 (CYP3A4 and CYP2C9) system. Elimination is primarily in feces, with approximately 10% excreted in urine.

Pharmacodynamics

Several kinds of leukotrienes have been identified. Zafirlukast blocks receptors for the leukotrienes bound to the amino acid cysteine. The cysteinyl leukotrienes are potent bronchoconstrictors, approximately 100 to 1,000 times more potent than histamine. By blocking their receptors, which mediate bronchoconstriction, vascular permeability, and mucous secretion, zafirlukast substantially improves the wheezing, coughing, and dyspneic symptoms of asthma.

Contraindications and Precautions

Zafirlukast is contraindicated in any patient with a known hypersensitivity to zafirlukast or to povidone, lactose, titanium dioxide, or cellulose derivatives, which are all inactive ingredients in the tablet. The drug is a pregnancy category B drug and is contraindicated for use in women who breastfeed because it is not approved for use in children younger than 6 years. Finally, zafirlukast is contraindicated for use against acute symptoms of wheezing, shortness of breath, or bronchospasm.

Zafirlukast should be given cautiously to patients with hepatic disease or those older than 65 years of age because clearance of the drug is decreased in these patients. It also is used cautiously in patients taking warfarin because both drugs use the same P-450 metabolism pathway.

Adverse Effects

The most common adverse effects of zafirlukast are headache, gastritis, pharyngitis, and rhinitis. Other reported adverse effects include dizziness, nausea and vomiting, diarrhea, abdominal pain, arthralgia, myalgia, fever, and back pain.

Serious adverse effects include asymptomatic elevated hepatic enzymes, symptomatic hepatitis with hyperbilirubinemia or jaundice, and, rarely, hepatic failure.

In patients taking zafirlukast at the same time that systemic steroids are being withdrawn, Churg-Strauss syndrome (CSS), a form of vasculitis with migratory lung infiltrates and eosinophilia, may occur. In patients in whom this event has occurred, it has been unclear whether CSS is caused by the use of zafirlukast or is already present but masked by the use of glucocorticosteroids.

Drug Interactions

Zafirlukast interacts with theophyllines, warfarin, and macrolides such as erythromycin and clarithromycin.. Table 35.10 presents these potential drug–drug interactions. Food decreases the bioavailability of zafirlukast by approximately 40%.

Assessment of Relevant Core Patient Variables

Health Status

Assess the patient for potential medical conditions, such as hepatic insufficiency or drug therapy, that contraindicate using zafirlukast or require close patient monitoring. Assessing the patient for use of theophylline, aspirin, warfarin, or other drugs that use the P-450 metabolism pathway

TABLE 35.10	Agents That Interact with P Zafirlukast	
Interactants	Effect and Significance	Nursing Management
erythromycin and clarithromycin	In asthmatic patients, erythromycin decreases bioavailability of zafirlukast by approximately 40%.	Monitor for efficacy of antibiotic therapy.
theophylline	Zafirlukast may increase serum concentration of theophylline resulting in an increased risk for pharmacologic and toxic effects. Zafirlukast levels may decrease.	Monitor serum theophylline levels. Monitor for signs and symptoms of theophylline toxicity. Monitor for efficacy of zafirlukast therapy.
warfarin	Zafirlukast increases elimination half-life of S-warfarin by ~36% and prolongs prothrombin time by 35%.	Prothrombin times and international normalized ratios should be carefully monitored in patients on warfarin therapy. Anticoagulant dosage should be adjusted as indicated.

is especially important. Assess for hypersensitivity to povidone, lactose, titanium dioxide, and cellulose derivatives, all of which are ingredients in zafirlukast tablets. Finally, evaluate the plan of care to see whether the patient is being withdrawn from glucocorticoid steroid therapy. Communicate any positive findings to the health care provider. Perform a baseline respiratory assessment and document the findings. The baseline data will be used to evaluate the efficacy of zafirlukast therapy.

Life Span and Gender

Evaluate the pregnancy status of the patient, as needed. Zafirlukast is a pregnancy category B drug, but human studies have not been performed. Zafirlukast should be administered during pregnancy only when the benefits to the mother outweigh the risk to the fetus. The drug enters breast milk. Therefore, it should not be administered to women who breast-feed because it is not approved for use in children younger than 5 years.

Note the age of the patient taking zafirlukast. Arrange for frequent follow-up appointments for patients older than 65 years of age. Elderly patients may experience decreased clearance of zafirlukast, which increases the risk of adverse effects and toxicity.

Lifestyle, Diet, and Habits

Assess the patient's understanding that zafirlukast must be taken on an empty stomach. Remind the patient that food decreases the bioavailability of zafirlukast.

Environment

Zafirlukast generally is administered in the home environment.

Nursing Diagnoses and Outcomes

- Risk for Injury (poisoning) related to interaction between drugs metabolized by the P-450 enzyme system
  Desired outcome: The patient will adhere to dosage adjustment of medications, undergo serial laboratory testing, and report adverse effects immediately to the health care provider.

- Diarrhea related to drug therapy
  Desired outcome: The patient will remain well hydrated throughout therapy.
- Acute Pain related to drug therapy
  Desired outcome: The patient will take nonnarcotic analgesics if headache occurs.

Planning and Intervention
Maximizing Therapeutic Effects

Ensure that the patient takes zafirlukast twice daily despite the absence of symptoms. Remind the patient to take zafirlukast 1 hour before or 2 hours after a meal to increase the bioavailability of the drug.

Minimizing Adverse Effects

Ensure that the patient takes the medication only as prescribed. Assess for potential need to change CAL or asthma therapy when zafirlukast is added, especially if the patient is taking systemic glucocorticoid steroid medications. Carefully review the patient's medications to establish whether he or she is taking other medications that use the P-450 metabolism pathway.

Providing Patient and Family Education

- Explain that zafirlukast is used in maintenance therapy for CAL and asthma and should not be used if acute shortness of breath or wheezing occurs.
- Advise patients to report symptoms such as abdominal pain, jaundice, nausea, vomiting, or dark urine immediately, because these symptoms may indicate hepatic injury.
- Encourage patients to take nonnarcotic analgesics if headache occurs and to drink plenty of fluids if they experience diarrhea while taking zafirlukast. Patients also should report these adverse effects to the health care provider.
- Caution patients not to stop or decrease systemic glucocorticoid steroid therapy without speaking with the health care provider first.
- Emphasize the importance of contacting the primary health care provider if any new medications are prescribed by any other member of the health care team.

Ongoing Assessment and Evaluation

Assess whether the patient needs beta-agonist drugs in addition to zafirlukast. If the patient continues to need beta-agonist drugs more than twice weekly, refer the patient to the health care provider for additional assessment.

Assess the patient for symptoms that may reflect hepatic injury. If the patient takes other medications that are metabolized by the P-450 enzyme system, evaluate the patient for potential adverse effects or toxicities of these drugs.

Drugs Closely Related to P Zafirlukast

Montelukast

Montelukast (Singulair) is similar to zafirlukast in its mechanism of action. It has the advantage of once-daily dosing, and it is also approved for use in children 2 years of age and older. Unlike zafirlukast, montelukast does not inhibit specific hepatic cytochrome isozymes. Therefore, it is not expected to affect the hepatic clearance of drugs metabolized by these enzymes.

Zileuton

Zileuton (Zyflo) inhibits the first enzyme in the lipoxygenase pathway, thus preventing the formation of potent leukotrienes. Although this mechanism of action may be beneficial in other disorders, such as rheumatoid arthritis and ulcerative colitis, at this time, zileuton is approved only for managing asthma.

In animal studies, zileuton produced developmental defects. Therefore, it is assigned to pregnancy category C. During pregnancy, zileuton should be used only if the potential benefit to the mother outweighs the potential risks to the fetus. It is not known whether zileuton is excreted in human milk, and therefore, it should be avoided by women who breast-feed.

Most adverse effects attributed to zileuton therapy have been mild and self-limited. Adverse effects include flu-like syndrome, headache, dizziness, dyspepsia, drowsiness, abdominal pain, and insomnia. In rare cases, hepatotoxicity and neutropenia have occurred.

MEMORY CHIP

P Zafirlukast

- Used for maintenance treatment of CAL and asthma
- Major contraindications: hypersensitivity to povidone, lactose, titanium dioxide, and cellulose; breast-feeding
- Most common adverse effects: headache, gastritis, pharyngitis, and rhinitis
- Most serious adverse effects: hepatic failure and Churg-Strauss syndrome
- Maximizing therapeutic effects: Administer the drug daily, despite the absence of symptoms.
- Minimizing adverse effects: Take the drug only as prescribed.
- Most important patient education: This drug will not abort an acute attack.

Administer the extended release formula within 1 hour after morning and evening meals. Document the patient's baseline liver function tests prior to initiation of treatment. Instruct the patient to return for repeat liver function tests monthly for 3 months, then every 3 months thereafter.

CHAPTER SUMMARY

- Mucolytics, such as acetylcysteine, are drugs designed to break up the mucus produced in the respiratory tract, leading to thinner secretions that are more easily moved.
- Acetylcysteine is also used to manage acetaminophen overdose and in patients having contrast imaging to reduce the risk for contrast-induced nephrotoxicity.
- Drugs used to manage CAL (COPD) are generally grouped into two categories: bronchodilators and anti-inflammatory agents.
- Bronchodilators are composed of several different subclasses, such as sympathomimetics, anticholinergics, and xanthine derivatives.
- Short-acting beta-agonist drugs are the only types of inhaled drug that help during acute episodes of asthma or exacerbations of CAL. They are known as "rescue drugs."
- Inhaled anticholinergics are used for maintenance treatment for asthma and CAL and are not used for acute symptoms.
- Xanthine derivatives are most frequently used as maintenance drugs; however, they may be given intravenously during an acute exacerbation of CAL or asthma.
- Anti-inflammatory drugs are composed of several different subclasses, including inhaled glucocorticoids, such as beclomethasone, mast cell stabilizers, and leukotriene receptor antagonists.
- Anti-inflammatory drugs are used as maintenance therapy, not for an acute exacerbation of CAL or asthma.
- The glucocorticoids are the most effective anti-inflammatory drugs available for managing respiratory disorders.
- The mast cell stabilizer cromolyn sodium works by stabilizing mast cells and preventing rupture when these cells are exposed to an antigen. This action stops the release of histamine, serotonin, bradykinin, and leukotriene, all of which induce bronchoconstriction.
- The leukotriene receptor antagonist zafirlukast works by inhibiting the bronchoconstrictive properties of leukotrienes.

QUESTIONS FOR STUDY AND REVIEW

1. In managing lower respiratory tract disorders, which main classes of drugs are used?
2. Compare and contrast the pharmacodynamics of the different types of bronchodilators.
3. In a patient with acute respiratory distress, which of the bronchodilators would be most effective?
4. Which of the anti-inflammatory agents is the most effective?

5. What is the difference between glucocorticoid steroids given orally and by inhalation?

6. Compare and contrast the pharmacodynamics of the different types of antiinflammatory agents.

7. If a patient is taking inhaled steroids, an anticholinergic inhaler, and a beta-adrenergic agonist inhaler, which inhaler would you tell the patient to use first?

NEED MORE HELP?

Chapter 35 of the Study Guide to Accompany *Drug Therapy in Nursing*, 4th Edition, contains NCLEX-style questions and other learning activities to reinforce your understanding of the concepts presented in this chapter. For additional information or to purchase the study guide, visit thePoint.

REFERENCES

Facts and Comparisons. (2010). *Drug facts and comparisons*. Philadelphia, PA: Lippincott Williams & Wilkins.

Fanta, C. H, Fletcher, S. W. (2010). An Overview of Asthma Management, *Up To Date*. Retrieved from www.uptodate.com on July 25, 2010.

Fanta, C. H. (2010). Treatment of acute exacerbations of asthma in adults, *Up To Date*. Retrieved from www.uptodate.com on July 25, 2010.

Ferguson, G. T., Make, B. (2010). Management of stable chronic obstructive pulmonary disease, *Up To Date*. Retrieved from www.uptodate.com on July 25, 2010.

Friedman, H. S., Urdaneta, E., McLaughlin, J. M., & Navaratnam, P. (2010). Mometasone furoate versus beclomethasone dipropionate: effectiveness in patients with mild asthma, *The American Journal of Managed Care*, 16(7):e151–e156.

Karch, A. M. (2010). *Nursing Drug Guide*, Philadelphia, PA: Lippincott Williams& Wilkins.

Koda-Kimbal, M. A., Young, L. Y., Kradian, W. A., et al. (2008). *Applied Therapeutics: The Clinical Use of Drugs* (9th Ed), Philadelphia, PA: Lippincott Williams& Wilkins.

Mautone, A., & Brown, J. R. (2010). Contrast-induced nephropathy in patients undergoing elective and urgent procedures, *Journal of Interventional Cardiology*, 23(1):78–85.

Morjaria, J. B., & Polosa, R. (2009). Off-label use of omalizumab in non-asthma conditions: new opportunities, *Expert Review of Respiratory Medicine*, 3(3):299–308.

Micromedex Healthcare Series. Retrieved from *http://thomsonhc.com*.

National Heart, Lung, and Blood Institute. (2007). Expert Panel Report-3: Guidelines for the Diagnosis and Management of Asthma. Retrieved from http://www.nhlbi.nih.gov/guidelines/asthma/asthgdln.pdf on July 24, 2010.

Rudnick, M. R., & Tumlin, J. A. (2010). Prevention of contrast-induced nephropathy, *Up To Date*. Retrieved from www.uptodate.com on July 25, 2010.

Tatro, D. S. (2011). *Drug Interaction Facts: The Authority on Drug Interactions*. Philadelphia, PA: Lippincott Williams & Wilkins.

UNIT 9

Gastrointestinal Tract Drugs

36

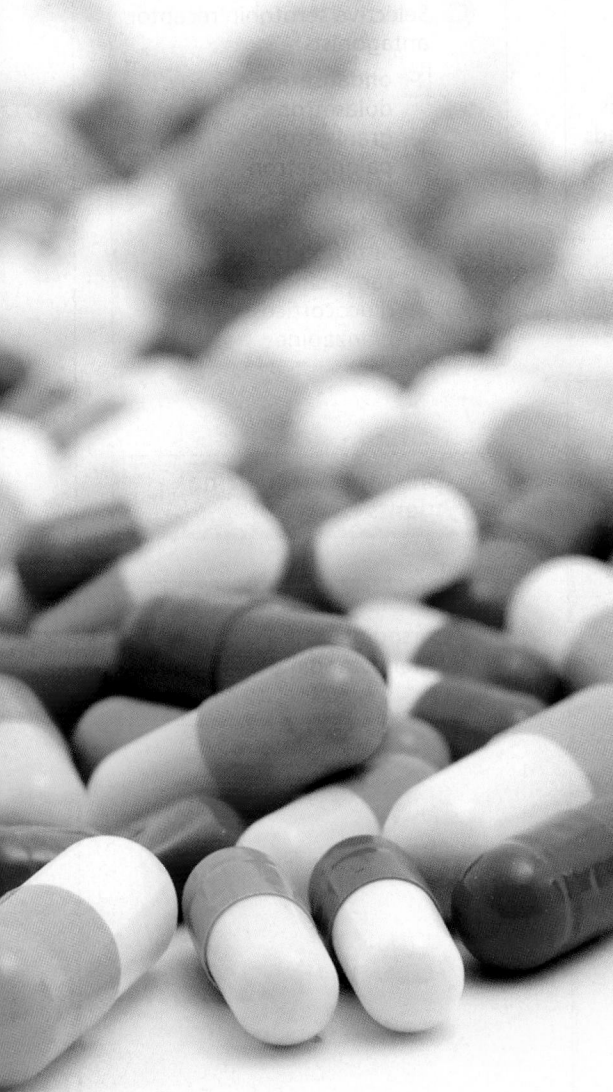

Drugs Affecting the Upper Gastrointestinal Tract

Learning Objectives

At the completion of this chapter the student will:

1. Identify core drug knowledge about drugs that affect the upper gastrointestinal (GI) tract.

2. Differentiate the drugs and drug classes used to treat peptic ulcer disease.

3. Differentiate histamine-1 (H_1) receptor antagonists from histamine-2 (H_2) receptor antagonists.

4. Identify core patient variables related to drugs that affect the upper GI tract.

5. Relate the interaction of core drug knowledge to core patient variables for drugs that affect the upper GI tract.

6. Generate a nursing plan of care from the interactions between core drug knowledge and the core patient variable for drugs that affect the upper GI tract.

7. Describe nursing interventions to maximize therapeutic effects and minimize adverse effects for drugs that affect the upper GI tract.

8. Determine key points for patient and family education for drugs that affect the upper GI tract.

Key Terms

antiemetics
chemoreceptor trigger zone
digestive enzymes
duodenum
dysphagia
emetics
gastroesophageal reflux disease

heartburn
Helicobacter pylori
hematemesis
melena
peptic ulcer
peristalsis
prokinetic agent

reflux
regurgitation
stress ulcer
vomit center
waterbrash

Drugs Affecting the Upper Gastrointestinal Tract

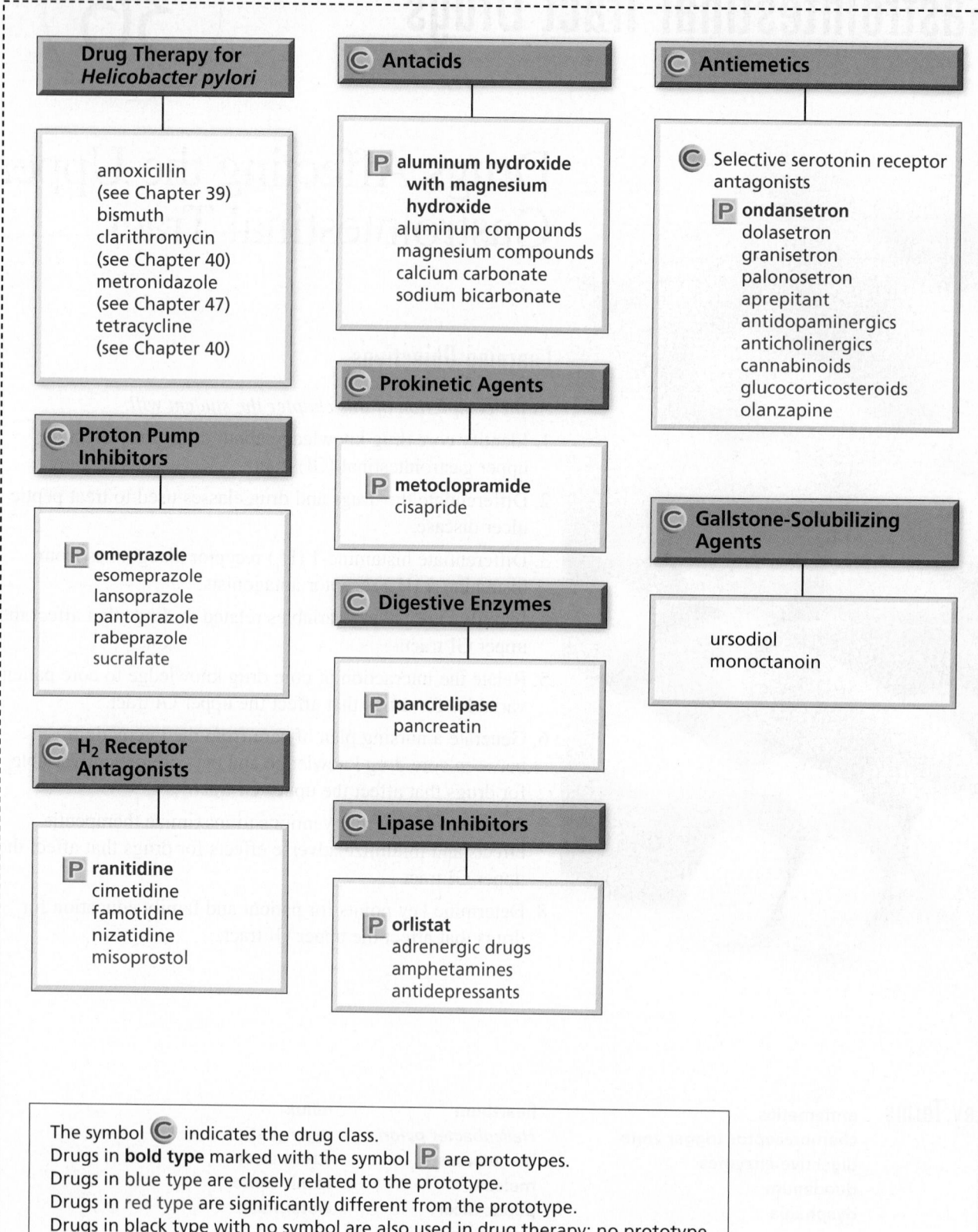

Drug Therapy for Helicobacter pylori

amoxicillin
(see Chapter 39)
bismuth
clarithromycin
(see Chapter 40)
metronidazole
(see Chapter 47)
tetracycline
(see Chapter 40)

C Proton Pump Inhibitors

P omeprazole
esomeprazole
lansoprazole
pantoprazole
rabeprazole
sucralfate

C H₂ Receptor Antagonists

P ranitidine
cimetidine
famotidine
nizatidine
misoprostol

C Antacids

P aluminum hydroxide with magnesium hydroxide
aluminum compounds
magnesium compounds
calcium carbonate
sodium bicarbonate

C Prokinetic Agents

P metoclopramide
cisapride

C Digestive Enzymes

P pancrelipase
pancreatin

C Lipase Inhibitors

P orlistat
adrenergic drugs
amphetamines
antidepressants

C Antiemetics

C Selective serotonin receptor antagonists
P ondansetron
dolasetron
granisetron
palonosetron
aprepitant
antidopaminergics
anticholinergics
cannabinoids
glucocorticosteroids
olanzapine

C Gallstone-Solubilizing Agents

ursodiol
monoctanoin

The symbol C indicates the drug class.
Drugs in **bold type** marked with the symbol P are prototypes.
Drugs in blue type are closely related to the prototype.
Drugs in red type are significantly different from the prototype.
Drugs in black type with no symbol are also used in drug therapy; no prototype.

Numerous prescription drugs and over-the-counter (OTC) preparations are used to treat or prevent disorders of the upper gastrointestinal (GI) tract, such as gastroesophageal reflux disease, hiatal hernia, peptic ulcer disease, digestive problems, nausea, and vomiting. These problems may be caused by innate physiologic problems, such as poor organ functioning or excessive acid production, or they may be secondary to therapeutic treatment, such as surgery or other drug therapy.

Many of these drugs have a local effect in the GI tract and can interfere with the absorption of other drugs that are administered orally. Other GI drugs act systemically and can produce interactions with other drugs. Because many of the drugs used to treat these disorders are available OTC, the potential for self-diagnosis and self-medication is great. Patients might not consider OTC drugs to be part of their drug therapy and therefore might not mention using these agents unless questioned directly. Therefore, it is important for the nurse to specifically ask about these preparations.

This chapter discusses the most common drug classes used to treat disorders of the upper GI tract, including:

- Drugs to treat *Helicobacter pylori* infection
- Proton pump inhibitors (PPIs)
- Histamine-2 receptor antagonists (H_2RAs)
- Antacids
- Prokinetic agents
- Digestive enzymes
- Lipase inhibitors
- Antiemetics
- Gallstone-solubilizing agents. These drugs are mentioned briefly in this chapter, but a prototype is not presented.

PHYSIOLOGY

The upper GI tract consists of the mouth, oropharynx, esophagus, stomach, and duodenum (small intestine). The **duodenum,** which is responsible for most digestive functions, is composed of four layers—the mucosa, submucosa, muscularis externa, and serosa. The mucosa is a mucous membrane covering the entire inner surface of the GI tract. In the duodenum, where some of the glands necessary for digestion and absorption are located, the mucosa forms folds and projections that increase the surface area of the intestine. The submucosa is composed of loose connective tissue containing blood, lymphatic vessels, and nerves. The blood vessels provide nutrients and oxygen to the tissues and remove the products of digestion. The muscularis externa is composed of two layers of smooth muscle. One layer encircles and constricts the tract; the other layer consists of longitudinal muscle fibers that contract to decrease the length of the tract. The serosa, which covers the outside of the GI tract, contains secretory cells that keep the outer surface of the tract moist and lubricated.

Digestion begins in the mouth, where food is chewed into fine particles, and salivary glands secrete substances that begin breaking down the food. The salivary glands consist of two types of secretory cells—serous and mucous. The serous cells contain amylase, an enzyme that splits the starch and glycogen contained in carbohydrates into disaccharides. This process is the first step of digestion. The mucous cells secrete mucus, which binds the food and facilitates swallowing. The tongue mixes food with the salivary gland secretions and moves the food toward the pharynx for swallowing.

Swallowing is a complex reflex that requires coordination of several muscle groups. After the bolus of food is moved toward the pharynx by the tongue, stimulated sensory nerves in the pharyngeal area trigger the swallowing reflex. Swallowing begins when the soft palate rises, preventing food from entering the nasal cavity. The epiglottis moves down over the trachea, preventing food from entering the lungs. Next, muscles in the lower pharynx relax, enabling food to move into the esophagus. **Peristalsis,** a rhythmic movement of contraction and expansion of the smooth muscle, propels the food toward the stomach.

The esophagus, a long, hollow tube that connects the mouth to the stomach, passes through the diaphragm and joins the stomach in the abdomen. The lower esophageal sphincter (LES) contains circular muscle fibers that contract to prevent regurgitation of gastric contents into the esophagus. Peristalsis causes these muscles to relax and allows food to enter the esophagus.

The stomach, which is situated between the esophagus and the duodenum, is a temporary storage and mixing site for food undergoing digestion. Three types of cells—mucous, chief, and parietal—secrete fluids commonly referred to as gastric juice. Chief cells in the stomach release pepsinogen, which is activated to form the digestive enzyme pepsin by hydrochloric acid (secreted from parietal cells). Pepsin begins the process of protein digestion. The mucus secreted by mucous cells in the stomach protects against pepsin and hydrochloric acid, which can help form or aggravate peptic ulcers (Figure 36.1).

Gastric secretions are regulated primarily by the parasympathetic nervous system. The sight, smell, or thought of food stimulate parasympathetic nerve impulses that trigger the release of the hormone gastrin, which stimulates production of gastric juice (chyme). The movement of food mixed with chyme into the duodenum inhibits further secretion of gastric juice. Fat-rich, acidic chyme entering the duodenum triggers the release of cholecystokinin, a hormone produced in the intestinal wall that decreases gastric motility.

The acid in chyme also triggers release of secretin, another hormone. Secretin and cholecystokinin stimulate the release of pancreatic juice that contains bicarbonate, which buffers the effects of gastric acid, and **digestive enzymes.** The digestive enzymes, which break down chyme into nutrients the body can absorb, are secreted by the pancreas in inactive forms and changed to their active forms in the duodenum. The duodenum also produces some digestive enzymes.

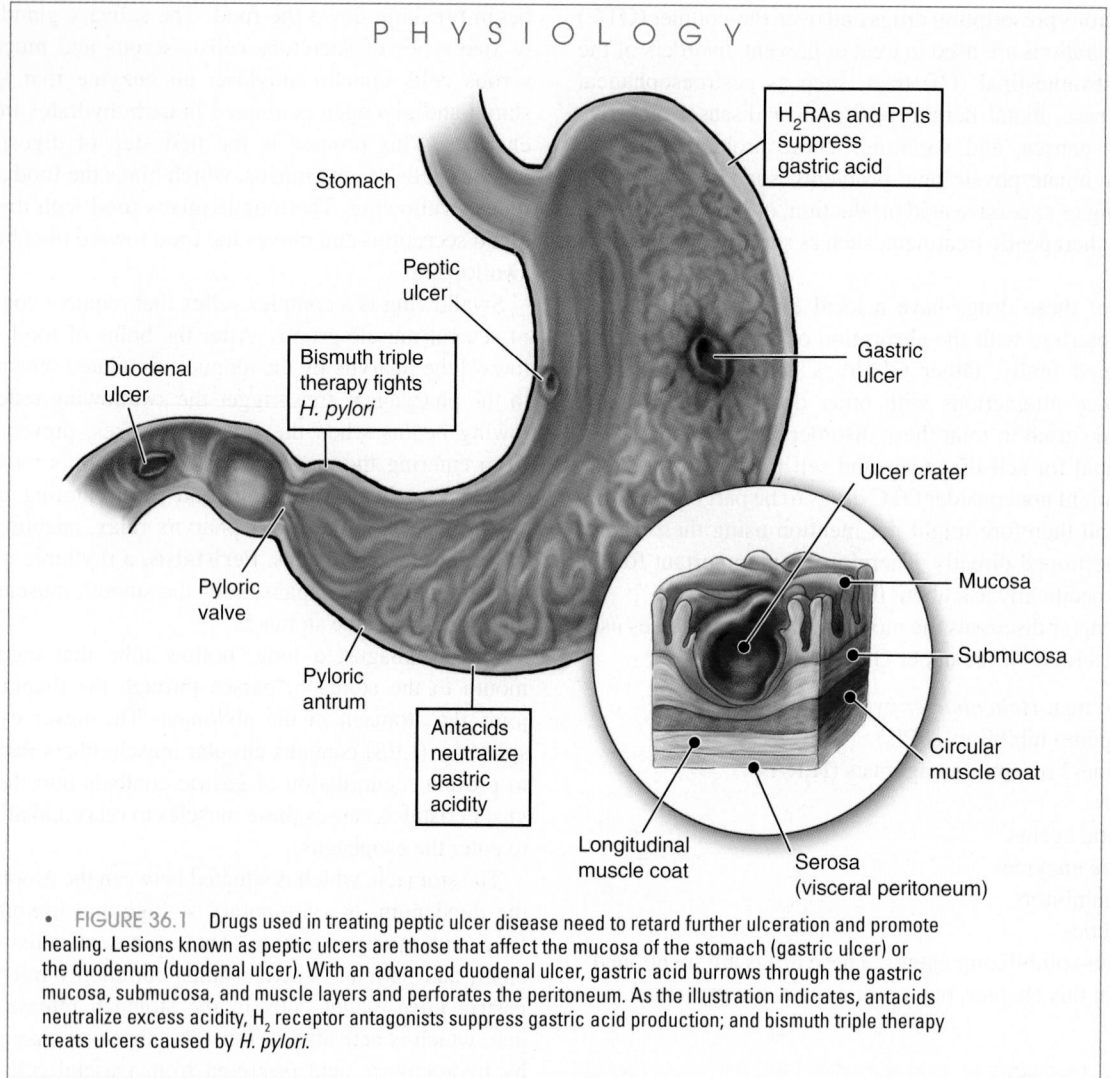

PHYSIOLOGY

Stomach

H₂RAs and PPIs suppress gastric acid

Peptic ulcer

Gastric ulcer

Duodenal ulcer

Bismuth triple therapy fights *H. pylori*

Ulcer crater

Mucosa

Submucosa

Pyloric valve

Pyloric antrum

Antacids neutralize gastric acidity

Circular muscle coat

Longitudinal muscle coat

Serosa (visceral peritoneum)

- FIGURE 36.1 Drugs used in treating peptic ulcer disease need to retard further ulceration and promote healing. Lesions known as peptic ulcers are those that affect the mucosa of the stomach (gastric ulcer) or the duodenum (duodenal ulcer). With an advanced duodenal ulcer, gastric acid burrows through the gastric mucosa, submucosa, and muscle layers and perforates the peritoneum. As the illustration indicates, antacids neutralize excess acidity, H₂ receptor antagonists suppress gastric acid production; and bismuth triple therapy treats ulcers caused by *H. pylori*.

The pancreatic enzymes include amylase (which splits starch and glycogen into disaccharides), lipase (which hydrolyzes fats to fatty acids), and trypsin, chymotrypsin, and carboxypeptidase (which split proteins into amino acids).

Vomiting of GI contents is controlled by the **vomit center** (VC) in the medulla of the brain. The GI tract contains sensory receptors that send nerve impulses to the brain in response to abdominal distention or irritation. Inflammation, spasms, and ischemia can also irritate nerve endings and activate the VC. These impulses are transmitted to the VC, which returns impulses that trigger abdominal contractions and reverse peristalsis, thereby inducing vomiting. The VC can also be directly stimulated through the cortical pathway by unpleasant olfactory and visual stimuli, pain, emotional factors, increased intracranial pressure, migraine headaches, or vestibular (inner ear) disturbances.

Additionally, the VC can be stimulated when the **chemoreceptor trigger zone** (CTZ) is stimulated. Located near the VC, the CTZ is stimulated by drugs, chemicals, toxins, radiation, hormonal changes, some disease states,

and altered metabolic states. It also is stimulated by vestibular mechanisms. When the CTZ is stimulated, it acts on the VC to maintain a state of excitability to other incoming vestibular impulses.

PATHOPHYSIOLOGY

Gastroesophageal Reflux Disease

The esophagus normally is not exposed to much gastric acid because the LES prevents **reflux** (upward movement of gastric juices into the esophagus). This condition is known as **gastroesophageal reflux disease** (GERD) or acid reflux disease. In patients with GERD, the LES opens either more frequently or at the wrong time, allowing stomach acid to back up into the esophagus. When gastric acids reflux into the esophagus over a long period of time, a portion of the esophagus can become "raw." This change in the esophagus, which is called erosive esophagitis, can lead to serious medical problems such as scarring, bleeding, and ulcers. Chronic GERD may result in a disorder called Barrett's esophagus, which is characterized by an abnormal lining of the esophagus; affected patients have an increased risk of cancer of the esophagus.

Although GERD frequently occurs alone, it may also result from a hiatal hernia, a condition in which the cardiac portion of the stomach moves up through an opening in a weakened diaphragm. The movement of the stomach through the diaphragm decreases the pressure of the LES, so that the acid easily moves into the esophagus.

Four major symptoms are characteristic of GERD: heartburn, regurgitation, dysphagia, and waterbrash. **Heartburn,** the most common symptom, is a burning sensation that rises from the stomach up the chest toward the neck. It can be quite painful. **Regurgitation** occurs when stomach acid washes through the esophagus into the mouth, causing a bitter or sour taste. **Dysphagia** is difficulty swallowing. **Waterbrash** is the sudden appearance of a slightly sour or salty fluid in the mouth that occurs when the salivary glands are stimulated by acid reflux.

There are four treatment options for GERD, depending on the severity of the symptoms: antacids, promotility agents, antisecretory agents, or mucosal protective agents may be used. Each of these drug classes has a different mechanism by which it decreases either the amount of acid in the stomach or inhibits damage to the GI tract.

Helicobacter pylori Infection

Helicobacter pylori (*H. pylori*) infection, the most common chronic bacterial infection worldwide, is found in more than half of the human population. The natural history of *H. pylori* infection and its transmission is still unknown. Current theories of transmission include the fecal–oral, oral–oral, and gastric–oral routes.

H. pylori is a gram-negative, spiral bacterium that weakens the protective mucous lining of the stomach and duodenum, allowing gastric acid to reach the sensitive lining of the GI tract. Both the bacterium and gastric acid irritate this sensitive lining, resulting in ulceration. *H. pylori* is not destroyed by gastric acid because it secretes enzymes that neutralize the acid. Infection with the bacterium is the major cause of gastritis and the gastritis-associated diseases: gastric ulcer, duodenal ulcer, gastric cancer, and primary gastric B-cell lymphoma (MALToma). *H. pylori* has been identified in 90% to 95% of patients with duodenal ulcers, 50% to 80% of patients with gastric ulcers, and almost 100% of patients with chronic active gastritis. Chronic *H. pylori* infection, particularly when acquired in early childhood, increases the risk of gastric cancer. *H. pylori* is not a causative factor in the development of GERD.

Diagnosis of *H. pylori* infection is determined by a blood test, stool test, urea breath test, or biopsy of an endoscopically obtained sample. It is possible to identify antibodies attached to the *H. pylori* bacteria in blood or the antigen in a stool sample. If the result of either test is positive, the patient is currently infected or has had an infection within the past 3 years. The only way to establish the definitive existence of a current infection is by a urea breath test, which

indirectly detects the presence of *H. pylori*–associated urease by measuring CO_2 in the patient's breath. The patient ingests urea labeled with a naturally occurring, nonradioactive carbon isotope. *H. pylori*–associated urease degrades the urea, producing ammonia and CO_2. The resultant CO_2 is absorbed in the blood, exhaled, and measured. An increased amount of labeled CO_2 indicates the presence of *H. pylori*–associated urease. To produce an accurate breath test, the patient must not have taken bismuth or antibiotics for 1 month, PPIs for 1 week, or H_2RAs for 24 hours, and should fast for 1 hour prior to the test.

Eliminating *H. pylori* from the GI tract improves healing and decreases the recurrence of ulcers. Once the infection has been eradicated, reinfection rates are less than 0.5% per year; ulcer recurrence rates also decline dramatically. The cure rate from the various treatment options ranges from about 70% to 90% or higher. Eradication therapy is the standard of care for patients with active or inactive peptic ulcers, including patients who use nonsteroidal anti-inflammatory drugs (NSAIDs).

The current treatment protocol of choice is called sequential therapy and has replaced legacy triple therapy, due primarily to increasing macrolide resistance (Graham, Fischbach, 2010). Classic quadruple therapy (bismuth, a PPI, 1,500 mg of metronidazole, and 1,500 mg of tetracycline) is highly effective and is frequently the regimen of choice. A newer sequential therapy (PPI plus amoxicillin followed by a PPI plus clarithromycin plus metronidazole) has been proposed and is expected to replace legacy therapy (Table 36.1).

Prophylactic and therapeutic vaccines have been developed against *H. pylori* in animals. Research toward developing vaccines against *H. pylori* for use in humans is now under way (Agarwal and Agarwal, 2009).

Peptic Ulcer Disease

Peptic ulcer disease (PUD) is a general term that refers to ulcer formation in the esophagus (esophageal ulcer), stomach (gastric ulcer), or duodenum (duodenal ulcer). Approximately 75% of ulcers, especially duodenal ulcers, are caused by the bacteria *H. pylori;* however, most infected persons do not develop PUD. Other causes of ulcer formation include drugs such as aspirin, NSAIDs, and glucocorticosteroids. Although many practitioners believe that stress may also be a factor in the development of ulcers, there is some controversy about this matter.

Pain is the most common symptom of an ulcer. The pain lasts from a few minutes to hours, may be worse when the stomach is empty, and may flare at night. It may be temporarily relieved when eating foods that buffer the stomach acid or by taking acid-reducing drugs. Severe symptoms that occur less frequently include **hematemesis** (vomiting of blood), **melena** (dark tarry stools), chest pain, unexplained weight loss, and nausea or vomiting.

Timing of the pain in relation to meals may differentiate between gastric and duodenal ulcers. Pain occurs with or just after meals with gastric ulcers because food increases

TABLE 36.1 — Therapies for *Helicobacter pylori* Infection Approved by the Food and Drug Administration

Regimen	Side Effect Rating	Cure Rate	Duration of Treatment
Two-Drug Regimen			
amoxicillin + PPI	Low-medium	66%–77%	14 d
clarithromycin + PPI	Low-medium	70%–74%	14–28 d
Three-Drug Regimen (Legacy Therapy)			
*clarithromycin + metronidazole + PPI	Medium	85%–95%	10–14 d
*amoxicillin + clarithromycin + PPI	Low-medium	85%–95%	10–14 d
amoxicillin + metronidazole + PPI	Medium	80%–90%	10–14 d
Four-Drug Regimen			
Bismuth + metronidazole + tetracycline + H₂RA	Medium-high	80%–90%	7–14 d
Bismuth + metronidazole + amoxicillin + H₂RA	Medium-high	70%–90%	7–14 d
†Bismuth + metronidazole + tetracycline + PPI	Medium-high	80%–90%	7–14 d
Bismuth + metronidazole + clarithromycin +	Medium-high	80%–90%	7–14 d
Sequential Therapy			
PPI + amoxicillin followed by PPI + clarithromycin PPI		90%–94%	14 d
Combination Drugs			
Helidac + H₂RA	Medium-high	Up to 82%	14 d
Prevpac	Low-medium	81%–92%	14 d

*First-line treatment; †second-line treatment; PPI, proton pump inhibitor; H₂RA, histamine-2 receptor antagonist.

the release of gastric acid. Pain occurs before a meal with duodenal ulcers because acid that is stimulated by hunger passes into the duodenum.

A **stress ulcer** is an ulcer that is caused by acute or chronic stress, especially in burn patients. Stress ulcers occur frequently in critically ill patients. Complications of stress ulcers include bleeding that requires transfusion and bleeding associated with hemodynamic instability. Stress ulcers may have significant impact on morbidity and mortality rates in an intensive care setting.

The gold standard for diagnosing an ulcer is an esophago-gastroduodenoscopy (EGD), which is also known as a gastroscopy. An EGD is a minimally invasive test that allows direct visualization of the upper part of the GI tract to the duodenum. In addition, during the EGD the health care provider may obtain tissue for biopsy to rule out gastric carcinoma because it has several symptoms that are similar to PUD.

Treatment for PUD depends on the etiology of the ulcer. Patients with *H. pylori* infection require multiple-drug therapy (see *H. pylori* section). Treatment protocols for patients without *H. pylori* include PPIs, H₂RAs, antacids, or mucosal protective agents.

The most serious complication of PUD is a perforated ulcer. This complication requires immediate surgical repair.

Pancreatitis

The pancreas contributes pancreatic juice and vital digestive enzymes to digestion. Production of these enzymes is reduced or no longer occurs in patients who have chronic pancreatitis or in those who have undergone a pancreatic resection or removal. In pancreatitis, digestive enzymes that normally are maintained in the pancreas in their inactive form become activated, destroying parts of the gland. With time, destruction of the pancreas decreases the amount of enzymes produced because the cells that produce the enzymes have been lost. Chronic pancreatitis generally occurs following repeated attacks of acute pancreatitis, but it may also be triggered by only one acute attack, especially if the pancreatic ducts are damaged.

Symptoms of chronic pancreatitis include abdominal pain that may become worse when eating or drinking, spread to the back, or become constant and disabling. Other symptoms include nausea, vomiting, weight loss, and fatty stools. Weight loss occurs because the body does not secrete enough pancreatic enzymes to break down food, so nutrients are not absorbed. Poor digestion leads to excretion of fat, protein, and sugar into the stool. If the insulin-producing cells of the pancreas (islet cells) have been damaged, diabetes may also develop at this stage.

Treatment for chronic pancreatitis includes replacement of digestive enzymes with pancrelipase.

Obesity

The incidence of overweight and obesity is increasing at an alarming rate, both in the United States and worldwide. Obesity and overweight reflect the extent to which a patient's body mass index (BMI) exceeds the normal range. The BMI is calculated as weight in kilograms divided by the square of height in meters. Normal BMI is 18.5 to 24.9 kg/m². The term overweight is used if the patient's BMI is 25 to 29.9 kg/m², whereas the term obesity is used if the BMI exceeds 29.9 kg/m². Overweight and obesity are the result of a mismatch between energy consumed in calories and energy expended in activities. The lifestyle in industrialized countries is increasingly sedentary. The energy expenditure of the average American worker at the beginning of the 21st century is estimated to be about half of that of the American worker at the start of the 20th century. Additionally, a high-fat diet, common in these countries, also contributes to obesity. High blood pressure, type 2 diabetes, coronary heart disease, elevated blood cholesterol, gallbladder disease, and osteoarthritis are associated with overweight and obesity. High blood pressure is the most common overweight- and obesity-related health condition, and its incidence increases as weight increases. Type 2 diabetes, gallbladder disease, and osteoarthritis also are more prevalent as weight increases. The risk of coronary heart disease, somewhat higher than normal in overweight patients, is substantially elevated if the patient is obese. Elevated blood cholesterol levels are found at all levels of overweight and obesity. Preventing and treating obesity are important to control these lifelong morbidities and the mortality that accompanies them.

Nausea and Vomiting

Disorders of the upper GI tract are often accompanied by nausea and vomiting. Increased activity of neurotransmitters—for example, dopamine in the CTZ and acetylcholine in the VC—appears to play an important role in inducing vomiting. Serotonin also has a role in vomiting, and special serotonin receptors are located in the CTZ. The CTZ is stimulated through peripheral and central pathways. Peripheral stimulation happens when chemotherapy causes damage to the GI mucosa, activating afferent input through the vagus nerve. Serotonin is the neurotransmitter for peripheral stimulation. The neurotransmitter substance P, found in the gut and the central nervous system, is capable of mediating emesis and is responsible for central pathway stimulation. Substance P exerts its antiemetic effect by binding to the tachykinin neurokinin (NK1) receptor, found throughout the central and peripheral systems and in the gut. The release of serotonin from the small intestine during chemotherapy stimulates these receptors and therefore stimulates vomiting. Because different substances are involved in the process of nausea and vomiting, several different classes of drugs may be used for management.

PROTON PUMP INHIBITORS

The secretion of gastric acid can be suppressed by inhibiting the H⁺/K⁺ adenosine triphosphatase (ATPase) enzyme system at the secretory surface of the gastric parietal cell. Because this enzyme system is the "acid pump," also known as the "proton pump," within the gastric mucosa, drugs that inhibit this system are known as PPIs. These drugs block the final step of gastric acid production. Their effect is dose related; they inhibit both basal and stimulated acid secretion.

The prototype PPI is omeprazole (Prilosec). Table 36.2 presents a summary of proton pump inhibitors.

Nursing Management of the Patient Receiving P Omeprazole
Core Drug Knowledge
Pharmacotherapeutics

Omeprazole is used for symptomatic treatment of heartburn and other symptoms of GERD. It also is used to treat duodenal ulcers associated with *H. pylori* infection. It is sometimes used for short-term treatment (4 to 8 weeks) of active duodenal and gastric ulcer when *H. pylori* is not present and is also used as short-term treatment for erosive esophagitis, diagnosed by endoscopy, to maintain healing. It can be used long term in chronic hypersecretory conditions, such as Zollinger-Ellison syndrome, multiple endocrine adenomas, and systemic mastocytosis. Off-label uses are treatment of GERD-related laryngitis, and adjunctive treatment to enhance the efficacy of pancreatin in treating steatorrhea (large quantities of fat in stool) in cystic fibrosis.

Pharmacokinetics

Omeprazole, like other PPIs, is unstable in an acid environment and therefore is enteric-coated to protect the drug until it passes through the stomach. It is well absorbed when it reaches the small intestine. An immediate-release formulation of omeprazole (Zegerid) works by adding sodium bicarbonate to protect omeprazole from gastric acid degradation.

Omeprazole is metabolized extensively by the cytochrome P-450 system in the liver, and several metabolites are formed. These metabolites have minimal antisecretory function. The antisecretory effect of omeprazole is long lasting and is not related closely to elimination half-life: its half-life in plasma is less than 2 hours, whereas the antisecretory effect lasts longer than 24 hours. This extended effect is attributed to prolonged binding of the drug to the parietal H⁺/K⁺ ATPase enzyme. When the drug is discontinued, normal secretory activity returns within 3 to 5 days. Little of the drug is excreted unchanged. The metabolites are excreted mostly in the urine, although about one fourth of them are eliminated in the feces.

Pharmacodynamics

Omeprazole suppresses the last phase of gastric acid production by suppressing the H⁺/K⁺ ATPase enzyme system. Intragastric pH is therefore elevated, and as a result, blood flow in the antrum, pylorus, and duodenal bulb is

TABLE 36.2 **Summary of Selected ⓒ Proton Pump Inhibitors**

Drug (Trade) Name	Selected Indications	Route and Dosage Range	Pharmacokinetics
Ⓟ omeprazole (Prilosec)		*Adult:* PO,	*Onset:* Within 1 h
	Active duodenal ulcer	20–40 mg/d × 4–8 wk	*Duration:* Unknown
	Gastric ulcer	40 mg/d × 4–8 wk	t$_{1/2}$: 30–60 min
	GERD	20 mg/d × 4–8 wk	
	Erosive esophagitis	20–40 mg/d × 4–8 wk	
	Hypersecretory conditions	60 mg once daily (max, 120 mg/d)	
	Helicobacter pylori	20 mg bid (in combination with other therapy) × 10–14 d	
esomeprazole (Nexium)	Erosive esophagitis, GERD	PO, 20–40 mg/d × 4–8 wk	*Onset:* 1–2 h
	H. pylori	IV, 20–40 mg/d up to 10 d	*Duration:* 17 h
	Hypersecretory conditions	PO, 40 mg/d × 10 d	t$_{1/2}$: 1–1.5 h
	Gastric ulcer prophylaxis	PO, 40 mg 2×/d (max, 240 mg/d)	
		PO, 20–40 mg/d	
lansoprazole (Prevacid)	Active duodenal ulcer	PO, 15 mg/d × 4 wk	*Onset:* Unknown
	Erosive esophagitis, GERD	PO, 15–30 mg/d × 8 wk	*Duration:* 24 h
	Hypersecretory conditions	60 mg/d	t$_{1/2}$: 1.5 h
	H. pylori	30 mg/d × 2 wk (in combination with other drug therapy)	
pantoprazole (Protonix)	Erosive esophagitis, GERD	PO, 40 mg 1–2×/d × 8 wk	*Onset:* PO, unknown; IV, 15–30 min
		IV, 40 mg/d × 7–10 d	*Duration:* 24 h
	Hypersecretory conditions	40–120 mg 2×/d	t$_{1/2}$: 1–1.5 h
		IV, 80 mg q8–12 h × 6 d	
	Upper GI bleed	IV, 80-mg bolus ×1, then 8 mg/h × 72 h	
rabeprazole (Aciphex)	GERD	PO, 20 mg/d × 4–8 wk	*Onset:* 1 h
	Erosive esophagitis	20 mg 1–2×/d × 8 wk	*Duration:* >24 h
	Duodenal ulcer	PO, 20 mg/d up to 4 wk	t$_{1/2}$: 1.5 h
	Hypersecretory conditions	60 mg 1–2×/d	
	H. pylori	PO, 20 mg 2×/d × 7 d	

decreased. Omeprazole increases serum pepsinogen levels and decreases pepsin activity. The increases in gastric pH are associated with increased numbers of nitrate-reducing bacteria and elevated nitrate concentrations in gastric juice in patients with gastric ulcers. Serum gastrin levels increase as acid secretion is inhibited. Continued treatment does not provoke serum gastrin levels to rise continually; however; they reach a certain degree of elevation and remain there. Omeprazole also has an antimicrobial affect against *H. pylori*. It inhibits *H. pylori* urease, which is necessary for gastric colonization.

Contraindications and Precautions

Omeprazole is contraindicated for patients who are hypersensitive to the drug or any of its components. It is given cautiously as empiric therapy because it may decrease the symptoms of gastric cancer, thus delaying treatment. Long-term PPI administration in rats has demonstrated an increased rate of gastric cancer. This finding has not been replicated in humans. PPIs do cause hypergastrinemia, which in turn causes diffuse, linear, or micronodular

hyperplasia and atrophic gastritis. These changes occur most frequently in patients with *H. pylori* infection and markedly increased gastrin levels. Gastric hyperplasia and atrophic gastritis in combination with *H. pylori* infection increase the risk of gastric cancer, but there are no studies that show a direct correlation between PPI administration and gastric cancer (Ito, et al., 2009).

Omeprazole is a pregnancy category C drug.

Adverse Effects

Omeprazole is generally well tolerated. The most common adverse effects are headache and diarrhea. However, during clinical trials, these effects also were found in patients receiving placebo. Other adverse effects reported in clinical trials include central nervous system (CNS) effects of dizziness and asthenia; GI effects of constipation, abdominal pain, nausea, and vomiting; and miscellaneous effects of upper respiratory infection, cough, rash, and back pain. Pneumonia is another potential adverse effect associated with all PPIs, including omeprazole, because bacterial colonization of the stomach and respiratory tract increases when gastric acidity is reduced. As people age, gastric pH rises, and omeprazole therapy raises the pH even further. Elevated gastric pH inhibits the dissolution and absorption of calcium, theoretically resulting in an increased risk of fractures. Several recent studies have been unable to validate this concern (Thompson et al., 2010; Gray et al., 2010; Targownik et al., 2010).

Rare adverse effects are numerous and diverse. They include confusion, drowsiness, blurred vision, tachycardia, diaphoresis, flushing, dry mouth, severe generalized skin reactions, blood dyscrasias, elevated liver enzyme levels, and overt hepatic disease. Study findings regarding an increased risk of *Clostridium difficile* diarrhea (Ananthakrishnan, Issa, and Binion, 2010) in patients taking proton pump inhibitors are conflicting.

Overdosage with omeprazole has been reported rarely, and no serious outcomes have been reported from overdosage. In patients who received 16 to 45 times the usual dose, symptoms were transient and included confusion, drowsiness, blurred vision, tachycardia, nausea, diaphoresis, flushing, headache, and dry mouth.

Drug Interactions

Omeprazole can interact with other drugs that also are metabolized through the cytochrome P-450 pathway. Such interactions can produce elevated levels of these other drugs because their metabolism is decreased. Because omeprazole causes prolonged and substantial decreases in gastric acidity, drugs that depend on an acid environment for absorption may not be absorbed optimally. Table 36.3 lists drugs that interact with omeprazole.

Assessment of Relevant Core Patient Variables

Health Status

Determine that the patient has a clinical indication for the use of omeprazole. Hepatic and renal diseases do not require a decreased dosage. For patients on long-term therapy, coordinate testing for *H. pylori* infection.

Life Span and Gender

Note the patient's age. Omeprazole's efficacy and safety in children have not been established. Although bioavailability of the drug may be increased in older adults, no dosage adjustment is needed. Coordinate bone density testing for elderly patients on long-term omeprazole therapy. Omeprazole decreases the dissolution and absorption of calcium, which may increase the risk of hip fracture. Men are more likely to have PPI-associated hip fractures than women.

Assess female patients for pregnancy or breast-feeding. Omeprazole is a pregnancy category C drug; no adequate or well-controlled studies of the drug have been done in pregnant women. Omeprazole should be used during pregnancy only if the potential benefit to the mother justifies the potential risk to the fetus. It is not known whether omeprazole is secreted in breast milk. Animal studies showed decreased weight gain from nursing when the mother received large doses (35 to 365 times the human dose) of omeprazole. Therefore, use in breast-feeding is not recommended.

Lifestyle, Diet, and Habits

Assess the patient's diet and smoking habits. Highly acidic foods, such as tomato juice, and highly spiced foods may worsen the symptoms of GERD or PUD until the ulcer heals. Omeprazole should be taken 30 minutes before eating a meal. Smoking also may aggravate the symptoms of PUD.

Environment

Omeprazole may be given in any environment. Advise elderly patients to clear the home of factors that increase the risk of falling such as loose rugs or highly waxed floors because of the association between PPI administration and hip fractures.

Culture and Inherited Traits

Assess the patient's culture and genetic background before administering omeprazole. The drug has a longer duration of action of omeprazole in Asians than in whites. In addition, Asians can experience elevated serum levels (up to fourfold higher) than whites and thus may need a decreased dose.

Nursing Diagnoses and Outcomes

• Altered Comfort related to symptoms of GERD, peptic ulcer disease, or chronically elevated acid production
  Desired outcome: *Drug therapy will relieve the symptoms from the GI disorder.*
• Imbalanced Nutrition: Less than Body Requirements, related to symptoms of GERD, peptic ulcer disease, or chronically elevated acid production
  Desired outcome: *Drug therapy will allow adequate dietary intake.*
• Collaborative Problem: *H. pylori* infection
  Desired outcome: *Treatment regimen to eradicate **H. pylori** will be effective, with minimal adverse effects.*

Planning and Intervention

Maximizing Therapeutic Effects

Optimal efficacy requires that omeprazole is taken daily, not just when the patient is symptomatic. Make sure that omeprazole is administered for the recommended time, based on the clinical indication for therapy, usually between 2 and 8 weeks. For chronic pathologic hypersecretory conditions, administer daily for as long as needed. Some patients are known to have received omeprazole for 5 years or longer.

Be sure the patient does not crush or chew the capsule. For patients who cannot swallow the capsule, open it and sprinkle the granules in 1 tablespoon of applesauce, and advise patients to swallow the applesauce without chewing the granules.

TABLE 36.3 **Agents That Interact with P Omeprazole**

Interactants	Effect and Significance	Nursing Management
azole antifungal agents	Bioavailability of azole antifungal agents may be decreased because of elevated gastric pH induced by omeprazole.	Monitor for antifungal treatment failure.
benzodiazepines	Omeprazole may reduce clearance, prolong $t_{1/2}$, and increase serum levels of certain benzodiazepines.	Ensure safety. Monitor for sedation. Discuss dosage adjustment of benzodiazepine with health care provider.
calcium citrate	Omeprazole may decrease pH-dependent calcium absorption.	Ensure safety, especially of elderly patients. Discuss increasing dose of calcium with health care provider.
cilostazol	Omeprazole inhibits metabolism of cilostazol, resulting in increased therapeutic and pharmacologic activity.	Monitor PT and INR. Monitor for bleeding or bruising. Discuss possible dosage adjustment of cilostazol with health care provider.
clarithromycin	Increases plasma levels of both clarithromycin and omeprazole; this may be beneficial because the two are given as cotherapy to treat *Helicobacter pylori*.	Administer as ordered. Assess for possible adverse effects.
cyclosporine	Omeprazole alters metabolism of cyclosporine, resulting in alterations of serum concentration (may be increased or decreased).	Verify order with health care provider. Monitor renal status. Discuss dosage adjustment of cyclosporine with health care provider as needed.
digoxin	Omeprazole may increase absorption of digoxin.	Monitor digoxin levels. Monitor heart rate. Monitor for anorexia, nausea, or vomiting.
herbal drugs ginkgo biloba St. John's wort	Ginkgo biloba induces metabolism of omeprazole, resulting in decreased serum concentration of omeprazole.	Monitor for efficacy of PPI therapy.
methotrexate	Omeprazole decreases renal clearance of methotrexate.	Monitor CBC. Monitor renal and hepatic function. Monitor for signs of methotrexate toxicity.
phenytoin	Reduced plasma clearance of phenytoin and increased half-life, most likely caused by inhibition of its metabolism.	Monitor phenytoin levels. Monitor for ataxia, difficulty thinking, difficulty speaking.
protease inhibitors (PIs)	Omeprazole may decrease dissolution of certain PIs, resulting in decreased absorption and lower serum concentrations.	Monitor viral load. Monitor T-cell count. Monitor for opportunistic infections.
salicylates	Enteric-coated salicylates may dissolve more rapidly in increased pH environment caused by omeprazole.	Monitor for gastric adverse effects. Advise patients to avoid enteric-coated preparations.
selective serotonin reuptake inhibitors (SSRIs)	Omeprazole may inhibit metabolism of SSRIs, resulting in an increased serum concentration.	Monitor for increased SSRI adverse effects.
sulfonylureas	Omeprazole inhibits metabolism of sulfonylurea drugs, resulting in increased serum concentration of sulfonylureas.	Monitor blood glucose. Monitor for signs of hypoglycemia. Discuss dosage adjustment of sulfonylurea drug with health care provider.
Sucralfate	Delayed absorption and reduced bioavailability of omeprazole (by about 17%) when the two are given at same time; this decreases desired therapeutic effect.	Give omeprazole ≥30 min before sucralfate.

TABLE 36.3	Agents That Interact with P Omeprazole *(continued)*	
Interactants	Effect and Significance	Nursing Management
tacrolimus	Omeprazole inhibits metabolism of tacrolimus, resulting in increased therapeutic and pharmacologic activity.	Monitor for CNS effects such as seizures, headache, insomnia, and tremors. Discuss possible dosage adjustment of tacrolimus with health care provider.
theophylline	Omeprazole induces hypochlorhydria that increases peristalsis in the small intestine and antiperistalsis in the proximal colon. This allows increased absorption of sustained-release theophylline formulations.	Monitor for signs of theophylline toxicity.
Warfarin	Omeprazole inhibits metabolism of warfarin, increasing its therapeutic and pharmacologic activity.	Monitor PT and INR. Monitor for bleeding or bruising. Discuss possible dosage adjustment of warfarin with health care provider.

Minimizing Adverse Effects

Daily dosages larger than 80 mg should be given in divided doses. Because the drug is enteric coated, it cannot be crushed before use. Monitor the patient for the development of diarrhea and notify the health care provider should it occur. Suggest calcium citrate supplementation for elderly patients on long-term therapy.

Providing Patient and Family Education

• Teach patients to take omeprazole 1 hour before meals and to continue therapy for the duration prescribed.
• Emphasize that the drug should not be crushed or chewed, because doing so alters absorption and effectiveness.
• Explain the importance of taking the drug daily to ensure an adequate therapeutic response.
• Encourage calcium citrate supplementation for patients on long-term therapy to decrease the potential for PPI-induced hip fracture.
• Discuss potential adverse effects and interventions
• Avoid driving if dizziness occurs.
• Ensure adequate nutrition if nausea, vomiting, or diarrhea occurs. Contact the health care provider if these symptoms are persistent.
• Do not self-medicate for symptoms of an upper respiratory infection because this is a drug effect, not an infection. Contact the health care provider if the symptoms are intolerable.
• Explain that antacids can be used while taking omeprazole if symptoms require additional management.
• Advise patients to contact the health care provider immediately if they experience persistent diarrhea.

Ongoing Assessment and Evaluation

Omeprazole therapy is considered effective when the symptoms of GERD, PUD, or hypersecretory conditions are controlled or the duodenal ulcer is healed.

Drugs Closely Related to P Omeprazole

Four additional PPIs are available in the United States: esomeprazole, lansoprazole, pantoprazole, and rabeprazole. The major difference between these PPIs and omeprazole is that they are all available in both oral and intravenous (IV) forms and none is marketed as a generic drug. Indications, precautions, and adverse effects are similar to omeprazole, including the risk of pneumonia and GI cancer. Most health care providers believe all of the PPIs to be similarly effective.

Esomeprazole

Esomeprazole (Nexium) is the S-isomer of omeprazole. It is metabolized more slowly than omeprazole; therefore, it suppresses gastric acid for a longer period. This finding has not been proven to be clinically significant.

Lansoprazole

Lansoprazole (Prevacid) is very similar to omeprazole. It is available as an orally disintegrating tablet, delayed-release tablet, and enteric-coated granules that form a suspension.

Rabeprazole

Rabeprazole (Aciphex) has a shorter duration of action than omeprazole. However, it also has antibacterial activity that works in conjunction with other antibiotics to eradicate *H. pylori*. Rabeprazole interacts with digoxin and increases its serum concentration. It is necessary to monitor for signs of digoxin toxicity when these drugs are given together.

Pantoprazole

Pantoprazole (Protonix) is also very similar to omeprazole. It is used frequently because it is the least expensive of all the PPIs.

MEMORY CHIP

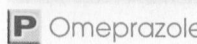

P Omeprazole

- Used to treat peptic ulcers resulting from *H. pylori*, GERD, erosive esophagitis, and chronic hypersecretory conditions (e.g., Zollinger-Ellison syndrome)
- May interact with other drugs metabolized by CYP 450
- Most common adverse effects: headache and diarrhea
- **Life span alert: use not recommended during breast-feeding**
- Most important patient education: Take omeprazole before meals; do not crush or chew drug.

Drug Significantly Different From P Omeprazole

Sucralfate (Carafate), like omeprazole, is used to treat duodenal ulcers (Table 36.4). Off-label uses of sucralfate include accelerating the healing of gastric ulcers and long-term management of gastric ulcers. Other off-label uses include treating reflux ulcers, reflux and peptic esophagitis, and NSAID-induced GI symptoms (including those caused by aspirin), and preventing stress ulcers and GI bleeding in critically ill patients. Sucralfate suspension also has been used to treat oral and esophageal ulcers caused by radiation, chemotherapy, and sclerotherapy.

Unlike omeprazole, sucralfate is not a PPI and does not prevent the secretion of gastric acid. Sucralfate is an aluminum salt of sulfated sucrose, a polysaccharide with antipeptic activity. In the acidic medium of gastric fluid, the aluminum ion splits off, leaving a highly polar anion. An essentially nonabsorbent paste forms and adheres to the ulcer lesion, protecting the lesion from acid, pepsin, and bile salts. This protection allows the ulcer to heal. The drug also has minimal antacid effects, but these effects do not contribute to ulcer healing.

Sucralfate should be used cautiously during pregnancy (pregnancy category B) and breast-feeding because it is not known whether the drug is secreted in breast milk. Safety and efficacy in children have not been established. In dialysis patients and others with chronic renal failure, sucralfate given concurrently with aluminum antacids increases the risk of aluminum toxicity because small amounts of aluminum, given off by sucralfate, are absorbed from the GI tract. This toxicity is not a potential problem for patients with normal renal function.

Adverse effects from sucralfate are usually mild. The drug rarely had to be discontinued during clinical trials. The most common adverse effect was constipation, which occurred in only 2% of patients. Sucralfate may decrease the effectiveness of anticoagulants, digoxin, hydantoins, ketoconazole, quinidine, and the quinolones.

Patients should be taught to take sucralfate at least 1 hour before meals and at bedtime to maximize the therapeutic effect. Sucralfate may block the absorption of other drugs; therefore, it should be taken 1 hour before or after other drugs are administered. Antacids should be taken 30 minutes before or after sucralfate.

C HISTAMINE-2 RECEPTOR ANTAGONISTS

Various terms are used to describe the H_2 receptor antagonists, including H_2RAs, H_2 receptor blockers, H_2 antagonists, H_2 blockers, and histamine blockers. H_2RAs block the effect of histamine at H_2 receptors, particularly those in the parietal cells of the stomach. Antihistamines that block histamine-1 (H_1) receptors, the most frequent site of action for antihistamines, do not affect H_2 receptor sites, and H_2RAs do not block H_1 sites; they also are not anticholinergic.

By blocking histamine at the parietal cells, these drugs inhibit gastric acid secretion in all phases, and other secretions caused by histamine, muscarinic agonists, and gastrin are also inhibited. H_2RAs also inhibit the fasting secretions that occur during the night, as well as secretions stimulated by food, insulin, caffeine, pentagastrin, and betazole. These drugs also reduce the volume of, and the hydrogen ion concentration in, gastric secretions.

Although cimetidine was the first drug in this class, it is not used frequently because of its numerous drug interactions that are not found with other H_2RA drugs. The prototype H_2RA is ranitidine (Zantac). Table 36.5 presents a summary of H_2RAs.

Nursing Management of the Patient Receiving P Ranitidine

Core Drug Knowledge

Pharmacotherapeutics

Ranitidine is used to treat patients with active duodenal or benign gastric ulcers and (at reduced dosage) in maintenance therapy after acute ulcers have healed. It is also used to treat pathologic hypersecretory conditions, such as

TABLE 36.4	Summary of Miscellaneous Drugs Used to Treat Ulcers		
Drug (Trade) Name	**Selected Indications**	**Route and Dosage Range**	**Pharmacokinetics**
misoprostol (Cytotec)	Prevention of NSAID-induced gastric ulcers	PO, 200 mcg qid with food; if not well tolerated, may use 100 mcg/dose	*Onset*: Rapid *Duration*: 3 h $t_{1/2}$: 20–40 min
sucralfate (Carafate)	Duodenal ulcer	PO, 1 g qid 1 h before meals and at bedtime for 4–8 wk	*Onset*: 30 min *Duration*: 5 h $t_{1/2}$: 6–20 h

TABLE 36.5 Summary of Selected ⒸHistamine-2 Receptor Antagonists

Drug (Trade) Name	Selected Indications	Route and Dosage Range	Pharmacokinetics
Ⓟ ranitidine (Zantac, EFFERdose, Zantac 75 [OTC]; Zantac 150 [OTC];	Duodenal and gastric ulcers	PO, 150 mg bid, or 300 mg at bedtime (for duodenal) as short-term use for active ulcers; maintenance dose, 150 mg at bedtime Parenteral (any use): IM, 50 mg (2 mL premixed) q6–8h; IV push, 50 mg (2 mL) diluted with 0.09% NaCl solution (normal saline) to make 20 mL, over 5 min or more; intermittent IV, 50 mg diluted in 100 mL dextrose 5% in water (D_5W) or other compatible solution, run over 15–20 min, q6–8h, not to exceed 400 mg/d	*Onset:* PO, varies; IM, rapid; IV, immediate *Duration:* 8–12 h $t_{1/2}$: 2–3 h
	GERD	PO, 150 mg bid	
	Pathologic hypersecretory conditions (i.e., Zollinger-Ellison syndrome)	PO, 150 mg bid (max, 6 g/d); continuous IV infusion (dilute in compatible solution to no more than 2.5 mg/mL), run at 1 mg/kg/h; after 4 h may be adjusted upward in 0.5-mg/kg/h increments up to 2.5 mg/kg/h	
	Erosive esophagitis	PO, 150 mg qid; maintenance, 150 mg bid	
cimetidine (Tagamet [DSC], Tagamet HB 200 [OTC])	Duodenal and gastric ulcers	PO, 800 mg at bedtime, or 300 mg qid with meals and at bedtime for 4–6 wk (duodenal) or 8 wk (gastric); IV or IM, 300 mg q6–8 h, not to exceed 2,400 mg/d	*Onset:* PO, varies; IV, rapid *Duration:* 4–13 h (depending on dose and regimen) $t_{1/2}$: 2 h
	Prevention of upper GI bleeding	IV, infusion at 50 mg/h	
	Erosive GERD	PO, 1,600 mg/d divided into 2 or 4 doses for 12 wk; IV or IM, dosing and regimen not established	
	Pathologic hypersecretory conditions	PO, 300 mg qid with meals and at bedtime, not to exceed 240 mg/d, given as long as clinically needed	
	Heartburn/acid indigestion	PO, OTC, 200 mg twice daily; continuous IV infusion, 300 mg q6–8 h	
famotidine (Pepcid, Pepcid AC, Pepcid RPD, Fluxid)	Same as ranitidine, for ulcers and related conditions	PO (acute duodenal ulcer), 40 mg/d at bedtime or 20 mg bid for 6–8 wk; maintenance, 20 mg/d at bedtime or (for acute benign gastric ulcer) 40 mg/d at bedtime; IV (patient NPO), 20 mg q12 h (dilute 2 mL, or 20 mg, in 5 or 10 mL normal saline or other compatible solution, and inject over at least 2 min); intermittent IV, 20 mg (dilute in 100 mL D5W or other compatible solution; infuse over 15–30 min)	*Onset:* PO, ≤1 h; IV, rapid *Duration:* 10–12 h $t_{1/2}$: 2.5–3.5 h
	Hypersecretory conditions	PO (individualize), 20 mg q6 h to start, up to 160 mg q6 h; continue as long as needed	
	GERD	PO, 20 mg bid up to 6 wk	
	Esophagitis due to GERD	PO, 20 or 40 mg bid up to 12 wk	
	Heartburn, acid indigestion	PO, OTC, 10 mg (1 tablet); prevention, 1 h before eating a meal expected to cause GI distress; up to 2 tablets in 24 h	
nizatidine (Axid, Axid AR [OTC])	Duodenal ulcer, benign active gastric ulcer	PO (for active ulcer), 300 mg once daily at bed-time or 150 mg bid (less for patients with renal insufficiency); maintenance, 150 mg once daily at bedtime	*Onset:* Varies *Duration:* 3–10 h $t_{1/2}$: 1–2 h
	GERD	*Adult:* PO, 150 mg bid	

Zollinger-Ellison syndrome. It is used to treat GERD and endoscopically diagnosed erosive esophagitis and as maintenance therapy to promote healing of erosive esophagitis.

Pharmacokinetics
Ranitidine is a competitive, reversible inhibitor of the action of histamine at the H_2 receptors, including receptors on the

gastric cells. The drug is 50% absorbed after oral administration. It is metabolized by the liver to N-oxide, S-oxide, and desmethyl ranitidine.

The drug's principal route of excretion is in the urine, with approximately 30% of the orally administered dose collected in the urine as unchanged drug in 24 hours. The elimination half-life is 2.5 to 3 hours.

Pharmacodynamics

Ranitidine inhibits both daytime and nocturnal basal gastric acid secretions as well as gastric acid secretion stimulated by food, betazole, and pentagastrin. Ranitidine does not affect pepsin secretion. It has little or no effect on fasting or postprandial serum gastrin secretion. It has no effect on prolactin levels, gonadotropins, thyroid-stimulating hormone, growth hormone, cortisol, aldosterone, androgen or estrogen levels, or sperm count.

Contraindications and Precautions

Ranitidine is contraindicated in patients who are hypersensitive to the drug. It is a pregnancy category B drug; no adequate, well-controlled studies of this drug have been performed in pregnant women. It also is not recommended for use by nursing mothers because it has been found in breast milk. The safety and effectiveness of ranitidine have been established in patients 1 month to 16 years of age.

Ranitidine should be used cautiously in patients with hepatic or renal impairment because the drug is metabolized by the liver and excreted by the kidneys. Patients with gastric ulcers should be monitored closely when using ranitidine because the drug can mask symptoms of GI cancer temporarily. Such patients should be evaluated thoroughly to rule out cancer. Ranitidine is also used cautiously in elderly patients, in patients with chronic obstructive pulmonary disease, and in those who are immunocompromised because of an increased risk of community-acquired pneumonia. In geriatric populations, as compared with younger subjects, no overall differences in safety or effectiveness have been observed. However, greater sensitivity of some older individuals to the drug cannot be ruled out.

Adverse Effects

Ranitidine generally is well tolerated. Headache, sometimes severe, seems to be related to drug administration. Blood count changes (leukopenia, granulocytopenia, and thrombocytopenia) have occurred. These effects are usually reversible. Rash has been reported. GI effects include constipation, diarrhea, nausea and vomiting, and abdominal discomfort or pain; pancreatitis has also been reported, but rarely. Hepatocellular, cholestatic, or mixed hepatitis, with or without jaundice, occurs occasionally. CNS, cardiovascular, musculoskeletal, integumentary, and other effects such as hypersensitivity are rare.

IV ranitidine may cause increased liver function enzymes when given for a prolonged period. Rapid IV infusion may induce bradyarrhythmias. Low-weight neonates who receive IV ranitidine have an increased risk of necrotizing enterocolitis.

Drug Interactions

Ranitidine has a favorable drug interaction profile because it does not inhibit the cytochrome P-450 system. Table 36.6 presents drug interactions with ranitidine.

Assessment of Relevant Core Patient Variables

Health Status

Before administering ranitidine, assess the patient for epigastric, abdominal, and esophageal pain, commonly described as heartburn or a burning sensation that occurs after eating. Also, explore complaints of dyspepsia; nausea and vomiting; dark, tarry stools; hepatic dysfunction; and

TABLE 36.6 Agents That Interact with Ⓟ Ranitidine

Interactants	Effect and Significance	Nursing Management
alcohol	Ranitidine may increase absorption and decrease gastric first-pass metabolism of alcohol by inhibiting gastric alcohol dehydrogenase activity.	Advise patients to avoid alcohol.
azole antifungal agents	Ranitidine increases gastric pH, which results in decreased dissolution and absorption of itraconazole and ketoconazole.	Monitor for azole antifungal efficacy.
cephalosporins	Ranitidine increases gastric pH, which results in decreased absorption of cephalosporins.	Monitor for cephalosporin efficacy.
Diltiazem	Ranitidine may increase the bioavailability of diltiazem.	Monitor for diltiazem toxicity.
phenytoin	Ranitidine inhibits metabolism of phenytoin, resulting in an increased serum concentration.	Monitor phenytoin levels. Monitor for ataxia, difficulty thinking, difficulty speaking.
Procainamide	Ranitidine may alter bioavailability and renal clearance of procainamide.	Monitor for procainamide toxicity.
Sulfonylureas	Ranitidine inhibits metabolism of sulfonylureas, resulting in an increased serum concentration.	Monitor glucose. Monitor for signs of hypoglycemia.

renal impairment. If the patient has a nasogastric tube in place, inspect for frank or occult bleeding.

The drug history should include the prescription and OTC drugs the patient is taking currently because many drugs, including aspirin, other NSAIDs, and corticosteroids, can cause gastric irritation. Additional drug history involves determining whether the patient is taking any OTC H$_2$RA drugs and asking how long and why the patient has been using these drugs.

Ensure that a baseline complete blood count as well as liver and renal functions tests are obtained when long-term therapy is anticipated or patients have a history of hematopoietic, renal, or liver dysfunction.

Life Span and Gender

Assess whether the patient is pregnant or breast-feeding because pregnant and breast-feeding patients should take ranitidine only if necessary. Ranitidine is a pregnancy category B drug. Determine the patient's age. Elderly patients should be assessed carefully for decreased renal and hepatic function. Monitor low-birth-weight neonates carefully for signs of necrotizing enterocolitis.

Lifestyle, Diet, and Habits

Assess the patient's diet and smoking habits. Caffeine, alcohol, and certain foods may aggravate gastric symptoms from GERD, PUD, and hypersecretory conditions. Assess for meals that frequently include spices, onion, citrus, tomato, and pepper. Evaluate the use of peppermint, chocolate, or carbonated beverages. Decreasing the intake of these foods may decrease the severity of GERD symptoms. Smoking reverses the drug-induced inhibition of nocturnal gastric acid production and hinders ulcer healing. Cigarette smoking also is related closely to ulcer recurrence.

Question the patient about napping and sleep patterns. Lying down within 3 hours of eating increases the risk of acid reflux.

Environment

Ranitidine can be administered in any setting. The oral form is self-administered easily. Administration through the IV route is done most commonly in an inpatient setting.

Culture and Inherited Traits

Cultural influences on dietary patterns must be considered if the patient normally eats a diet consisting of highly spiced foods, such as jalapeño peppers, Thai curries, or Szechwan cuisine.

Nursing Diagnoses and Outcomes

- Chronic Pain related to alteration in the gastric mucosa, ulceration, or irritation
  Desired outcome: The patient will report decreased pain while receiving drug therapy.
- Acute Pain related to adverse drug effects, such as headache

Desired outcome: The patient will not experience adverse effects while taking ranitidine.
- Risk for Injury related to drug-induced somnolence, dizziness, confusion, or hallucinations
  Desired outcome: The patient will not suffer injury from adverse effects of drug therapy.
- Diarrhea related to adverse effects of drug therapy
  Desired outcome: The patient will remain well hydrated and elimination patterns will remain within normal parameters.

Planning and Intervention

Maximizing Therapeutic Effects

If both ranitidine and antacids are prescribed, give them at least 2 hours apart to prevent decreased absorption of ranitidine. If administration is intramuscular, inject undiluted ranitidine into a large muscle.

Minimizing Adverse Effects

Monitor serum trough levels in patients with renal or hepatic impairment because CNS effects are more likely to occur when serum levels are elevated above the therapeutic level. Drug therapy may have to be discontinued if serious adverse effects occur.

Administer IV ranitidine slowly to prevent hypotension and cardiac arrhythmias. It is important to administer single IV push doses, diluted in 20 mL of normal saline or other compatible solution, over at least 2 minutes. Intermittent IV infusions of 300 mg in at least 50 mL of D$_5$W or other compatible solution should be administered over at least 15 minutes or 20 minutes. Give a continuous IV infusion at a rate of 37.5 mg/h.

Providing Patient and Family Education

- Instruct patients to take the drug exactly as directed for the entire course of therapy, even if symptoms disappear (it usually takes 4 to 6 weeks for an ulcer to heal but less time for the symptoms to subside).
- Caution patients not to take a double dose if a dose is missed.
- Counsel patients on smoking cessation. OTC or prescription smoking cessation aids may be recommended, if appropriate.
- Explain that alcohol, caffeine, spicy foods, products containing aspirin or ibuprofen, and smoking all contribute to gastric irritation and slow healing of the ulcer.
- Discuss potential adverse effects and interventions.
  - Avoid driving if dizziness occurs.
  - Ensure adequate nutrition if nausea, vomiting, or diarrhea occurs. Contact the health care provider if these symptoms are persistent.
  - Adjust lights or temperature, and avoid noise if headache occurs. Contact the health care provider if the symptoms are intolerable.
- Caution patients not to substitute OTC ranitidine for prescribed ranitidine because these products have different potencies (Box 36.1).

BOX 36.1 COMMUNITY BASED CONCERNS

Using Over-the-Counter (OTC) Gastrointestinal Drugs Responsibly

Various antacids, such as Maalox and Mylanta, and histamine-2 receptor antagonists (H₂RAs) such as cimetidine (Tagamet HB), ranitidine (Zantac HB), famotidine (Pepcid AC), and nizatidine (Axid AR), are available OTC. Nurses who provide home care or who treat patients on an outpatient basis need to be aware that many patients self-medicate with these preparations. They may use them alone, as an adjunct to prescribed therapy, or in place of their prescribed drug. The following guidelines may help nurses help such patients use these drugs responsibly:

- Assess specifically for OTC antacid and H₂RA use. The patient may not think of OTC products as "real drugs" and so fail to identify them during the drug history.
- Advise the patient taking a prescribed H₂RA to take only that drug and not to substitute any OTC preparation for it. Explain that the dosages and drug formulations may be different.
- Caution the patient not to take any OTC H₂RA in addition to the prescribed drug. In such cases, "more is not better."
- If a particular antacid has been prescribed for a patient, warn the patient not to switch brands or type of antacid without consulting the prescriber. Some forms of antacids are contraindicated in certain medical conditions (e.g., chronic heart failure, renal failure, and hypertension).
- Urge the patient to consult his or her own health care provider before taking antacids in conjunction with an H₂RA.

- Teach patients to stagger ranitidine and antacid dosing schedules to allow at least 2 hours between doses.
- Advise patients to contact the health care provider immediately if they experience:
  - Sharp, sudden or persistent stomach pain
  - Bloody or black stools
  - Bloody vomit or vomit that looks like coffee grounds
  - Sore throat, fever, unusual bruising, confusion, hallucinations, severe headache, or severe muscle or joint pain.

Ongoing Assessment and Evaluation

During long-term ranitidine therapy, the patient's blood count should be monitored to detect changes from baseline. Drug therapy is effective when epigastric pain decreases, peptic ulcers heal, hypersecretion of gastric acid declines, or GI bleeding is prevented without adverse effects.

Drugs Closely Related to Ranitidine

Cimetidine

Cimetidine (Tagamet) was the first H₂RA on the market. It is available as a prescription and OTC drug. Unlike ranitidine, cimetidine is a potent inhibitor of P-450 drugs. For this reason, cimetidine use is decreasing, and ranitidine, famotidine, and nizatidine have become the drugs of first choice.

Cimetidine has the same indications as ranitidine. It has two additional indications: acute upper GI hemorrhage and systemic mast cell disease (mastocytosis). Mastocytosis is

 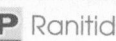
P Ranitidine

- Blocks histamine competitively at histamine-2 (H₂) receptors in the gastric parietal cells; these receptors are not affected by H₁ antagonists.
- Inhibits all phases of gastric acid secretion
- Used for gastroesophageal reflux disease, duodenal ulcer, gastric ulcer, pathologic hypersecretory conditions; to prevent upper GI bleeding; and for heartburn and acid indigestion (OTC strength only)
- Interacts with numerous other drugs, many by decreasing their hepatic metabolism
- Most serious adverse effects (all rare): neutropenia, agranulocytosis, thrombocytopenia, autoimmune hemolytic or aplastic anemia
- Maximizing therapeutic effects: Give ranitidine at least 2 hours apart from antacids.
- Most important patient education: Do not substitute OTC drug for prescription drug nor add OTC drug to prescribed drug therapy.

a rare disorder characterized by abnormal accumulations of mast cells in skin, bone marrow, and internal organs such as the liver, spleen, and lymph nodes.

Famotidine

Famotidine (Pepcid), another frequently used H₂RA, is also available as a prescription and OTC drug. It has the same indications as ranitidine with two additions: esophagitis and common indigestion. The most common adverse effect of famotidine is dizziness. Patients with moderate to severe renal dysfunction may experience increased CNS effects and longer elimination half-life than other patients.

Nizatidine

Nizatidine (Axid), another H₂RA, is also available OTC and has the same indications as ranitidine. Nizatidine is used with caution in patients who are immunocompromised because of an increased risk of strongyloidosis (tapeworm infection). The most common adverse effects are abdominal pain, headache, and GI symptoms.

Drug Significantly Different From P Ranitidine

Misoprostol (Cytotec), unlike ranitidine, is not an H₂ antagonist. It is a synthetic form of prostaglandin E and is used to prevent NSAID-induced gastric ulcers in high-risk patients, such as older adults, patients with other debilitating diseases, and patients with a history of gastric ulcers (see Table 36.4). An off-label use is treating duodenal ulcers. Misoprostol may be useful in treating duodenal ulcers refractory to treatment with H₂ receptor antagonists. Although misoprostol does not prevent duodenal ulcers, it is effective in decreasing the incidence of gastric ulcers associated with the use of NSAIDs.

NSAIDs inhibit prostaglandin synthesis, causing diminished bicarbonate and mucus secretion in the gastric mucosa. Misoprostol binds at the prostaglandin receptors and can increase bicarbonate and mucus secretion, thereby protecting the stomach lining. This action results in decreased peptic ulcer formation in patients taking NSAIDs. Misoprostol decreases pepsin concentration moderately during basal conditions but not during histamine stimulation. It has no significant effect on gastrin levels, either before or after meals. Misoprostol does decrease normal daytime and nocturnal gastric acid secretion. It also decreases the gastric acid that is produced in response to stimuli, including meals, histamine, pentagastrin, and coffee. Activity of the drug begins within 30 minutes of administration and lasts for 3 hours or more.

Misoprostol is classified as a pregnancy category X drug because it has abortifacient properties. The drug causes uterine contractions and miscarriage. Women of childbearing potential must receive written and oral warnings about the hazards of misoprostol, be able to adhere to effective contraceptive measures, and have had a negative serum pregnancy test result in the 2 weeks before beginning therapy. Therapy should be started on the second or third day of the next normal menstrual cycle. It is not known whether the drug enters breast milk; thus, its use by nursing mothers is not recommended. Efficacy and safe use in children have not been established. Additionally, elderly patients may not be able to tolerate the usual dose. Cautious use is recommended for patients with renal failure. However, a dosage reduction is not normally necessary.

The most common adverse effect of misoprostol therapy is diarrhea; the next most common is abdominal pain. Other adverse effects are nausea and vomiting, dyspepsia, flatulence, constipation, and headache. Possible gynecologic problems include spotting, cramps, and menstrual disorders.

When antacids are administered with misoprostol, the availability of misoprostol is reduced, but this effect does not appear to be important clinically. Although food decreases plasma concentrations of misoprostol, the specific receptors for misoprostol in the GI tract are still activated, and a therapeutic response is evident. The effect of misoprostol is topical, rather than systemic. Patients should take misoprostol with food. If diarrhea is a problem, it can be diminished if the drug is taken after the meal.

ⓒ ANTACIDS

Antacids are drugs that increase the gastric pH, thereby neutralizing gastric acidity. These preparations are used for various upper GI disorders, including symptoms of GERD (heartburn, indigestion, and upset stomach), esophagitis, hiatal hernia, gastritis, and PUD. Antacids are composed of inorganic salts of aluminum, magnesium, calcium, or sodium used alone or in various combinations. Antacids include aluminum hydroxide with magnesium hydroxide, aluminum, magnesium, calcium, and sodium bicarbonate. The prototype antacid is aluminum hydroxide with magnesium hydroxide (Maalox, Mylanta). Table 36.7 presents a summary of antacid drugs.

Nursing Management of the Patient Receiving ⓟ Aluminum Hydroxide with Magnesium Hydroxide
Core Drug Knowledge
Pharmacotherapeutics
The combination drug aluminum hydroxide with magnesium hydroxide is used in conditions of hypersensitivity to relieve the symptoms of upset stomach, heartburn, gastric reflux, and sour stomach associated with GERD, and the discomfort from peptic ulcers. Off-label uses include treatment and maintenance therapy for duodenal ulcer.

Pharmacokinetics
A single oral dose of an aluminum and magnesium–based antacid typically results in minimal absorption from the GI tract. Patients taking this type of drug for a prolonged period may absorb between 5% and 20% of the magnesium and very little of the aluminum. The small amounts of magnesium and aluminum that are absorbed are distributed widely throughout the body. Small amounts of the drugs are found in breast milk. Aluminum hydroxide with magnesium hydroxide is eliminated in the feces.

The onset of action is rapid. Duration of action varies according to when the drug was taken in relation to meals. If it is taken on an empty stomach, the duration is 20 to 60 minutes; if it is taken following a meal, the duration is 3 hours.

Pharmacodynamics
Antacids do not coat the lining of the stomach, despite what is commonly believed. Aluminum hydroxide with magnesium hydroxide raises the gastric pH in the stomach and duodenal bulb above 4, which inhibits pepsin's proteolytic activity and increases the tone of the lower esophageal sphincter. Antacids, in general, may have a local astringent effect. The aluminum in this drug, and in other aluminum antacids, inhibits gastric emptying by inhibiting contraction of the smooth muscle of the stomach. The aluminum in the drug binds with phosphate in the GI tract and can lower phosphate levels effectively.

Antacids have different acid-neutralizing capacities (ANCs). The ANC is expressed in mEq/mL. The definition is the milliequivalent (mEq) of HCl required to keep the antacid suspension at a pH of 3.5 for 10 minutes, in vitro (in the laboratory). To be an antacid, a substance must neutralize 5 mEq/dose or more. Antacids with high ANCs are usually more effective in vivo (in the patient). Of the various forms of antacids available, suspensions have the greatest neutralizing capacity.

Contraindications and Precautions
Aluminum hydroxide with magnesium hydroxide may cause hypophosphatemia, especially if dietary intake of phosphorus is inadequate. Patients with renal insufficiency should use magnesium-containing antacids with caution because a small amount of magnesium is absorbed systemically, and hypermagnesemia is possible, especially if the

TABLE 36.7 Summary of Selected Ⓒ Antacids

Drug (Trade) Name	Selected Indications	Route and Dosage Range*	Pharmacokinetics
Ⓟ aluminum hydroxide with magnesium hydroxide (Maalox)	Hyperacidity; prevention of stress ulcer bleeding; treatment and maintenance of duodenal and gastric ulcers; initially for GERD	PO, 15–30 mL up to 4×/d	Onset: Immediate Duration: 20–40 min on empty stomach; 3 h if 1 h after meals $t_{1/2}$: Not systemically absorbed
magnesium hydroxide (Milk of Magnesia, MOM)	Hyperacidity; bleeding; treatment and maintenance of duodenal and gastric ulcers; initially for GERD	PO, liquid, 5–15 mL up to 4×/d; liquid concentrate, 2.5–7.5 mL up to 4×/d; tablets, 622–1,244 mg up to 4×/d	Onset: Immediate Duration: 20–40 min on empty stomach; 3 h if 1 h after meals $t_{1/2}$: Not systemically absorbed
aluminum hydroxide (Amphojel, LternaGEL)	Hyperacidity; prevention of stress ulcer bleeding; treatment and maintenance of duodenal and gastric ulcers; initially for GERD; reduction of phosphate absorption in hyperphosphatemia in chronic renal failure	PO, suspension, 5–30 mL as needed after meals and at bedtime; tablets/capsules, 500–1,500 mg 3–6×/d, between meals and at bedtime	Onset: Immediate Duration: 20–40 min on empty stomach; 3 h if 1 h after meals $t_{1/2}$: Not systemically absorbed
calcium carbonate (Tums, Caltrate 600, Nephro-Calci)	Hyperacidity (occasional use); calcium replacement	PO, tablets, 0.5–1.5 g as needed	Onset: Immediate Duration: 20–40 min on empty stomach; 3 h if 1 h after meals $t_{1/2}$: Unknown
magnesium oxide (Mag-Ox, Mag-Caps, MagGel)	Hyperacidity; magnesium replacement	PO, capsules, 140 mg tid–qid; tablets, 400–800 mg/d	Onset: Immediate Duration: 20–40 min on empty stomach; 3 h if 1 h after meals $t_{1/2}$: Not systemically absorbed
magaldrate/simethicone (Riopan Plus)	Hyperacidity; treatment and maintenance of duodenal and gastric ulcers; initially for GERD	PO, suspension liquid, 5–10 mL between meals and at bedtime	Onset: Immediate Duration: 20–40 min on empty stomach; 3 h if 1 h after meals $t_{1/2}$: Not systemically absorbed
sodium bicarbonate (Bell/ans)	Hyperacidity (occasional use)	PO, tablets, 0.3–2 g up to qid	Onset: Immediate Duration: 20–40 min on empty stomach; 3 h if 1 h after meals $t_{1/2}$: Unknown
sodium citrate and citric acid (Bicitra, Oracit)	Hyperacidity (occasional use)	Adult: PO, liquid, 10–30 mL diluted in water, up to 4×/d Child: PO, liquid, 5–15 mL diluted in water, up to 4×/d	Onset: Immediate Duration: 20–40 min on empty stomach; 3 h if 1 h after meals $t_{1/2}$: Unknown

patient takes more than 50 mEq daily. Aluminum hydroxide with magnesium hydroxide is a pregnancy category B drug; pregnant or breast-feeding patients should consult the prescriber before taking this medication.

Aluminum hydroxide with magnesium hydroxide should be used cautiously in patients who have recently experienced massive upper GI bleeding.

Adverse Effects

Antacids that contain aluminum alone can cause constipation, whereas antacids that contain magnesium alone can cause diarrhea. Aluminum and magnesium are combined to balance the constipating effects of aluminum with the diarrheal effects of magnesium. Other possible adverse effects

include hypermagnesemia (in patients with renal failure) and hypophosphatemia. Less common adverse effects are accumulation of aluminum in serum, bone, and the CNS (with large doses); osteomalacia; and encephalopathy. Acid rebound may occur, although this effect may not be important clinically because the buffers in the antacid may neutralize any elevation in acidity.

Drug Interactions

Magnesium and aluminum affect the action of many orally administered drugs (Table 36.8). This interaction may stem from decreased acidity of gastric juices, which affects absorption; absorption or binding by the magnesium and aluminum to the surface of drugs, which decreases their

TABLE 36.8	Agents That Interact with Ⓒ Antacids	
Interactants	**Effect and Significance**	**Nursing Management**
allopurinol	Decreased effect with aluminum salts	Monitor for drug effectiveness. Separate administration of drugs by 2 h. Discuss possible dosage adjustment with health care provider.
Amphetamines	Increased effect with sodium bicarbonate	Same as above
benzodiazepines	Increased effect with aluminum salts; decreased effect with magnesium salts, sodium bicarbonate, and magnesium/aluminum combinations	Same as above
Captopril	Decreased effect with magnesium/aluminum combinations	Same as above
Chloroquine	Decreased effect with aluminum and magnesium salts	Same as above
corticosteroids	Decreased effect with aluminum, magnesium, and magnesium/aluminum combinations	Same as above
Dicumarol	Increased effect with magnesium salts	Same as above
Diflunisal	Decreased effect with aluminum salts	Same as above
Digoxin	Decreased effect with aluminum and magnesium salts	Same as above
Ethambutol	Decreased effect with aluminum salts	Same as above
Flecainide	Increased absorption with sodium bicarbonate	Same as above
fluoroquinolones	Decreased effect with calcium salts and magnesium/aluminum combinations	Same as above
H₂RAs	Decreased effect with aluminum salts, magnesium salts, and magnesium/aluminum combinations	Same as above
hydantoins	Decreased effect with calcium salts, magnesium salts, and magnesium/aluminum combinations	Same as above
iron salts	Decreased effect with all antacids	Same as above
Isoniazid	Decreased effect with aluminum salts	Same as above
ketoconazole	Decreased effect with sodium bicarbonate and magnesium/aluminum combinations	Same as above
Levodopa	Increased effect with magnesium/aluminum combinations	Same as above
Lithium	Decreased effect with sodium bicarbonate	Same as above
Methenamine	Decreased effect with sodium bicarbonate	Same as above
Methotrexate	Decreased effect with sodium bicarbonate	Same as above
Nitrofurantoin	Decreased effect with magnesium salts	Same as above
penicillamine	Decreased effect with aluminum salts and magnesium salts	Same as above
phenothiazines	Decreased effect with aluminum salts, magnesium salts, and magnesium/aluminum combinations	Same as above
quinidine	Increased effect with calcium salts, magnesium salts, sodium bicarbonate, and magnesium/aluminum combinations	Same as above
salicylates	Decreased effect with calcium salts, sodium bicarbonate, and magnesium/aluminum combinations	Same as above

(Continued)

TABLE 36.8 **Agents That Interact with ⓒ Antacids** *(continued)*

Interactants	Effect and Significance	Nursing Management
sodium polystyrene sulfonate	Concurrent use, possible metabolic alkalosis in patients with renal impairment	Same as above
Sulfonylureas	Increased effect with magnesium salts and magnesium/aluminum combinations; decreased effect with sodium bicarbonate	Same as above
Sympathomimetics	Increased effect with sodium bicarbonate	Same as above
Tetracycline	Decreased effect with all antacids	Same as above
thyroid hormones	Decreased effect with aluminum salts	Same as above
ticlopidine	Decreased effect with aluminum salts, magnesium salts, and magnesium/aluminum combinations	Same as above
valproic acid	Increased effect with magnesium/aluminum combinations	Same as above

bioavailability; or increased urine alkalinity, which changes the rate of drug elimination (slowing the excretion of basic drugs and speeding the elimination of acidic drugs).

Assessment of Relevant Core Patient Variables

Health Status

Determine whether the patient has symptoms that warrant the use of aluminum hydroxide with magnesium hydroxide. Assess for GI bleeding; coffee grounds–like emesis indicates GI bleeding, as do dark, tarry stools if the patient is not taking iron supplements. Assess for a history of recent upper GI bleeding. Patients who have had massive upper GI bleeding should use caution when taking products that contain aluminum. Also assess for renal insufficiency. Patients with a history of renal insufficiency should not receive aluminum hydroxide with magnesium hydroxide. Although antacids that are solely aluminum based are used to decrease elevated phosphate levels found in renal failure, aluminum in combination with magnesium hydroxide should be avoided because these patients do not excrete magnesium at the normal rate. The additional magnesium that can be absorbed from this product and all magnesium-containing antacids may be sufficient to cause hypermagnesemia in the patient with renal failure. Also, determine the patient's serum phosphate level because aluminum binds with phosphate.

Ask the patient about use of OTC drugs because the patient may not consider these agents important to mention during the drug history. Assess which type of drugs the patient uses and determine why they are being used, to detect possible drug interactions.

Lifestyle, Diet, and Habits

Evaluate the patient's normal dietary, alcohol, and smoking habits. Caffeine, alcohol, spicy food, and smoking may contribute to the severity of symptoms experienced.

Environment

Aluminum hydroxide with magnesium hydroxide is easily self-administered. It may be used in any care setting, including the home (see Box 36.1).

Nursing Diagnoses and Outcomes

- Chronic Pain related to alteration in the gastric mucosa, ulceration, or irritation
  Desired outcome: *The patient will report that pain has decreased while on drug therapy.*
- Potential Complication: Electrolyte Imbalance related to hypophosphatemia, hypermagnesemia, or hyperalbuminemia secondary to drug therapy
  Desired outcome: *The patient's electrolyte levels will remain within normal limits.*
- Diarrhea or Constipation secondary to drug therapy
  Desired outcome: *The patient's elimination patterns will remain within normal parameters.*

Planning and Intervention

Maximizing Therapeutic Effects

Liquid preparations are usually preferred, because of their rapid action. Shake suspensions well before use to disperse the drug evenly. If tablets are used, they must be chewed thoroughly before swallowing and followed with a glass of water. Tablets should be administered 1 to 3 hours after meals and at bedtime for the best therapeutic effects.

Minimizing Adverse Effects

Administer or teach the patient to administer aluminum hydroxide and magnesium hydroxide 2 hours after other drugs to prevent drug interactions. Assess for use of antacids and other OTC preparations during drug history; patients might not consider these to be drugs and might fail to mention them unless asked.

Monitor for signs of acid rebound, such as increased GI pain and complaints of acid reflux. Monitor serum phosphorus and magnesium levels in patients receiving high doses of aluminum hydroxide and magnesium hydroxide (the maximum dosage for more than 2 weeks) or in patients on long-term therapy or with renal impairment. Monitor for signs of aluminum deposits in serum, bone, and CNS and for dialysis encephalopathy and osteomalacia syndromes when high doses are given to patients with renal failure.

Providing Patient and Family Education

- Teach patients to take the antacid 2 hours after other drugs and 1 hour after meals and at bedtime.
- Caution patients not to take the maximum dose for longer than 2 weeks unless directed by the prescriber.
- Instruct patients not to substitute this drug for prescription drugs to treat PUD.
- Urge patients to contact the prescriber if diarrhea or constipation occurs, if abdominal pain does not diminish, or if black, tarry stools, or coffee grounds–like emesis is seen.
- Teach patients to shake liquid forms well and measure the proper dose; they should not just drink some undetermined amount.
- Instruct patients to chew the tablet form thoroughly and then drink water.

Ongoing Assessment and Evaluation

Therapy using aluminum hydroxide with magnesium hydroxide is considered effective if the patient's pain is decreased or eliminated, electrolytes remain at normal levels, elimination patterns remain normal, and GI symptoms are controlled.

MEMORY CHIP

 Aluminum Hydroxide with Magnesium Hydroxide

- Treats hyperacidity and its symptoms in GERD and peptic ulcers; prevents stress ulcer bleeding
- Interacts with many other drugs by increasing the pH (i.e., increasing alkalinity), which alters absorption, adsorption, or binding with drugs; or by increasing urinary pH (i.e., affecting drug elimination rate)
- Major contraindication: Avoid use in chronic renal failure (multiple doses).
- Most common adverse effects: constipation (aluminum antacids) and diarrhea (magnesium antacids); combination usually negates the adverse effect of each, although either may occur
- Most serious adverse effect: potential electrolyte imbalance
- Minimizing adverse effects: Administer 2 hours after other drugs to prevent drug interactions.
- Most important patient education: Do not substitute this drug for prescription drugs to treat peptic ulcer disease.

Drugs Closely Related to P Aluminum Hydroxide with Magnesium Hydroxide

All antacid preparations are related closely and are used in various combinations to produce the desired results. In addition to the prototype aluminum hydroxide with magnesium hydroxide, aluminum preparations and magnesium preparations may be used individually. Additionally, sodium bicarbonate and calcium carbonate are used as antacids, either alone or in combination with other antacids. Various combinations of aluminum salts, magnesium salts, calcium carbonate, and sodium bicarbonate are useful. The aluminum salts used in antacids include aluminum carbonate, aluminum hydroxide, aluminum phosphate, and dihydroxy-aluminum aminoacetate. The magnesium salts include magnesium carbonate, magnesium hydroxide, magnesium oxide, and magnesium trisilicate. The calcium salt *calcium carbonate* is often given with simethicone (an antiflatulent), magnesium carbonate, magnesium hydroxide, or aluminum hydroxide. However, it can be used alone.

The pharmacotherapeutics of the antacids vary. Unlike aluminum or magnesium preparations, neither calcium carbonate nor sodium bicarbonate is recommended for long-term use, such as in treating PUD. Aluminum hydroxide is used to treat hyperphosphatemia associated with chronic renal failure. Aluminum carbonate can be used to treat, control, or manage hyperphosphatemia. It can also be used with low-phosphate diets to prevent phosphate-based renal calculi (kidney stones) from developing. Calcium carbonate is used in treating hypocalcemia. Magnesium sulfate is used to treat hypomagnesemia.

The pharmacokinetics of the antacids varies slightly because sodium bicarbonate and calcium carbonate undergo much more systemic absorption than the aluminum or magnesium preparations.

The main variation in pharmacodynamics is in the ANC of the antacids.

Sodium bicarbonate and calcium carbonate have the greatest ANC. Suspension forms of antacids have greater ANC than tablets. Box 36.2 lists selected antacids according to their acid-neutralizing ability.

Box 36.2 ACID-NEUTRALIZING CAPACITY OF ANTACIDS

The antacids listed below appear in descending order of their acid-neutralizing capacity (e.g., sodium bicarbonate most effective). Aluminum phosphate has the lowest acid-neutralizing effect.

- sodium bicarbonate
- calcium carbonate
- magnesium hydroxide
- magnesium and aluminum hydroxide mixtures
- magaldrate
- magnesium trisilate
- aluminum hydroxide
- aluminum phosphate

Sodium bicarbonate and calcium carbonate can cause metabolic alkalosis and acid rebound because of their systemic absorption, especially with large doses and frequent use. When given together in large doses, they may cause milk alkali syndrome. Milk alkali syndrome can be acute (with symptoms of weakness, headache, nausea, and irritability) or chronic (with alkalosis, hypercalcemia, and possible renal impairment).

The major core patient variable that must be considered for the different forms of antacids is health status. It is necessary to bear in mind the following points:

• Aluminum hydroxide may be used therapeutically in patients with renal failure.
• Multiple doses of magnesium oxide are avoided in renal failure because of the risk of magnesium toxicity.
• Sodium bicarbonate should not be given to people on low-sodium diets or those who have underlying pathologies that make sodium restrictions necessary, such as hypertension, chronic heart failure, or renal failure because of its high sodium content.
• Neither sodium bicarbonate nor calcium carbonate is recommended for PUD.

ⓒ PROKINETIC AGENTS

The **prokinetic agents** increase the effect of acetylcholine on the GI system. Acetylcholine is responsible for normal GI function. Prokinetic agents increase peristalsis and gastric emptying. The prototype prokinetic agent is metoclopramide (Reglan). Table 36.9 presents an overview of metoclopromide.

Nursing Management of the Patient Receiving Ⓟ Metoclopramide

Core Drug Knowledge

Pharmacotherapeutics

Metoclopramide is used to relieve symptoms of diabetic gastroparesis, also known as diabetic gastric stasis. Symptoms of this disorder include nausea, vomiting, heartburn, persistent fullness after meals, and anorexia. Metoclopramide also is used short-term to treat GERD in patients who do not respond to usual therapy. It is used parenterally to prevent nausea and vomiting associated with postoperative states, opioid administration, and cancer chemotherapy or radiation therapy. It may be administered as a single dose before small bowel intubation, especially in instances in which the tube does not pass through the pylorus easily. It may be used to promote the transit of barium through the GI tract after a diagnostic procedure if the delayed passage of barium interferes with further radiographic diagnostic procedures in the stomach and small intestine.

Off-label uses of metoclopramide include improving lactation (it can increase milk production by elevating serum prolactin levels); minimizing nausea and vomiting in a variety of conditions, including during pregnancy and labor; treating gastric ulcers and anorexia nervosa; improving response to ergotamine, analgesics, and sedatives used in migraine headache; treating postoperative gastric bezoars (boluses of food that have hardened and remain in the stomach); treating diabetic atonic bladder; and treating esophageal variceal bleeding.

Pharmacokinetics

Metoclopramide is given orally and is absorbed readily from the GI tract. The drug is distributed widely throughout the body; it crosses the blood–brain barrier and placenta and is found in breast milk. The drug is not highly protein bound (30%).

A small amount of the drug is metabolized by the liver, and most is excreted in the urine. Patients with renal insufficiency may require a dosage reduction.

Pharmacodynamics

Metoclopramide's mechanism of action is unclear. However, it appears to sensitize tissues to the effect of acetylcholine. It has the cholinergic-like effect on the upper GI tract of stimulating motility but does not stimulate gastric, pancreatic, or gallbladder secretions. Metoclopramide increases peristalsis of the duodenum and jejunum, thus shortening the transit time through the stomach and small intestine. It also increases the tone of the lower esophageal sphincter, increases gastric contractions, and relaxes the pyloric sphincter.

TABLE 36.9   Overview of Metoclopromide

Drug (Trade) Name	Selected Indications	Route and Dosage Range	Pharmacokinetics
Ⓟ metoclopramide (Reglan, Octamide, Metozolv ODT)	Diabetic gastroparesis, GERD, prevention of postoperative nausea and vomiting, prevention of chemotherapy-induced vomiting	*Adult:* PO, 10 mg 30 min before each meal and at bedtime for 2–8 wk; IM, 10–20 mg near end of surgery; IV, infuse over at least 15 min, 30 min before chemotherapy, repeat every 2 h for two doses, then every 3 h for three doses; for highly emetogenic drugs, such as cisplatin and dacarbazine, give 2 mg/kg for first two doses; for less emetogenic drugs, give 1 mg/kg Metozolv ODT is an orally disintegrating tablet that usually dissolves within 1 minute.	*Onset:* PO, 30–60 min; IM, 10–15 min; IV, 1–3 min *Duration:* PO, IM, IV, 1–2 h $t_{1/2}$: PO, IM, IV, 5–6 h

Dopamine and serotonin produce nausea and vomiting by stimulating the medullary CTZ. Metoclopramide blocks these receptors, inducing an antiemetic effect directly on the CTZ. It is believed to lessen the sensitivity of visceral nerves to stimuli that induce nausea and vomiting.

Contraindications and Precautions

Metoclopramide is contraindicated when stimulation of GI motility may be dangerous, as in GI hemorrhage, perforation, or mechanical obstruction. Other contraindications include hypersensitivity to the drug; pheochromocytoma (the drug may cause a hypertensive crisis that probably results from a release of catecholamines from the tumor); history of seizure disorders (seizure activity may increase with this drug); and concomitant use of drugs that produce extrapyramidal effects (because these effects may increase).

Depression, from mild to severe, including suicidal ideation, has occurred in patients with and without a history of depression. Use caution in giving metoclopramide to patients with a history of depression; it should be given only if the benefits of the drug outweigh the potential risks from depression. Metoclopramide should be given very cautiously, if at all, to patients with Parkinson disease because they may experience an exacerbation of symptoms. Use caution if giving this drug to patients with hypertension. Theoretically, metoclopramide may increase the pressure on a suture line following a gut anastomosis or closure. Although this effect has not been reported in the literature, use some caution when giving this drug to postoperative patients. Elevated prolactin levels will persist during chronic administration of metoclopramide. One third of human breast cancers are prolactin dependent in vitro. Therefore, use caution if the patient has previously detected breast cancer. Studies have not, however, shown a definite link between elevated prolactin levels and breast cancer in animals or in humans.

Metoclopramide is a pregnancy category B drug.

Adverse Effects

Approximately 20% to 30% of patients receiving metoclopramide experience adverse effects of the drug. The adverse effects are usually mild, transient, and reversible after discontinuing the drug. Incidence correlates with dose and duration of therapy. Effects on the CNS are common and include restlessness, drowsiness, fatigue, insomnia, headache, dizziness, confusion, anxiety, dystonia, mental depression (even in patients who had never experienced clinical depression before) with suicidal ideation and suicide, convulsive seizures, and hallucinations. Extrapyramidal symptoms, Parkinson-like reactions, tardive dyskinesia, and akathisia also may occur. Extrapyramidal symptoms are manifested primarily as acute dystonic reactions. They occur more commonly in children and young adults during the first 24 to 48 hours of treatment. They occur even more frequently when metoclopramide is used in high doses to control vomiting caused by chemotherapy. Tardive dyskinesia, potentially irreversible, occurs most often in the elderly, particularly older women and is identified as a black box warning. Additional adverse effects are nausea, diarrhea, and transient hypertension.

Drug Interactions

Metoclopramide interacts with several drugs because it increases gastric motility, thereby altering absorption. The most important drug interactions are with levodopa, anticholinergics, and narcotics. Levodopa and metoclopramide have opposite effects on dopamine receptors. Metoclopramide's effects on GI motility are antagonized by anticholinergics and narcotics. Table 36.10 presents agents that interact with metoclopramide.

Assessment of Relevant Core Patient Variables

Health Status

Before beginning therapy with metoclopramide, assess the patient indications for metoclopramide use, such as diabetic gastroparesis, GERD, cancer that requires chemotherapy or radiation therapy, postoperative status, or opioid administration. Also, assess for depression, Parkinson disease, seizures, or hypertension because these conditions are precautions to its use. In addition, assess the patient's drug history; it should not include current use of levodopa, anticholinergics, or narcotics. Any renal or hepatic impairment should be noted because the dosage may need to be adjusted.

Life Span and Gender

Determine whether the patient is pregnant. Metoclopramide is classified as a pregnancy category B drug. Several case reports show no adverse effects on the fetus with the use of metoclopramide; however, no adequate and well-controlled studies exist. Although metoclopramide is excreted into breast milk, the levels are well below the maximum therapeutic infant dose. Therefore, there appears to be no contraindication to breast-feeding if the mother receives no more than 45 mg/d of metoclopramide. Note the patient's age and gender because older adults, especially older women, are more likely than others to develop the adverse effect of tardive dyskinesia.

Environment

Oral metoclopramide can be given in any setting and can be self-administered. IV administration of metoclopramide is performed in an acute care setting or an outpatient center.

Nursing Diagnoses and Outcomes

• Risk for Self-Directed Violence secondary to adverse effects of drug therapy

   Desired outcome: The patient will do no self-harm related to depression from drug therapy.

TABLE 36.10 Agents That Interact with P Metoclopramide

Interactants	Effect and Significance	Nursing Management
alcohol	Increases the rate of absorption, raising blood levels more quickly	Advise patient to avoid alcohol while on drug therapy.
Anticholinergics	Antagonize effects of metoclopramide on GI motility	Monitor for therapeutic effects.
cyclosporine	Faster gastric emptying, which may allow for increased absorption, possibly increasing immunosuppression and adverse effects from cyclosporine	Monitor CBC. Monitor for other adverse effects, such as tremor, hypertension, and renal dysfunction.
digoxin	Absorption, plasma levels, and therapeutic response may be decreased; capsule, elixir, and tablets with a high dissolution rate least affected	Monitor digoxin level. Monitor efficacy of digoxin therapy. Discuss dosage adjustment of digoxin with health care provider.
levodopa	Has opposite effect on dopamine receptors; bioavailability of levodopa may be increased; may decrease effect of metoclopramide on gastric emptying and lower esophageal pressure	Monitor for therapeutic and adverse effects of both. Administration of metoclopramide to patients with Parkinson disease is relatively contraindicated.
mefloquine	Increased gastric emptying could increase rate of mefloquine absorption in small intestine.	Monitor for GI, CNS, and cardiovascular adverse effects of mefloquine.
selective serotonin reuptake inhibitors	Increased risk of serotonin syndrome. Mechanism unknown.	Monitor for irritability, increased muscle tone, shivering, myoclonus, and altered consciousness.
succinylcholine	Metoclopramide inhibits plasma cholinesterase, may increase neuromuscular blocking effects of succinylcholine.	Monitor respiratory function.
Tacrolimus	Increased gastric emptying could increase rate of tacrolimus absorption in small intestine.	Monitor for signs of tacrolimus toxicity.

- Powerlessness related to extrapyramidal effects, Parkinson-like symptoms, or tardive dyskinesia secondary to adverse effect of drug therapy
  Desired outcome: The patient will make decisions regarding own care, treatment, and future (when possible) while on drug therapy.
- Risk for Injury related to drowsiness, fatigue, insomnia, confusion, and hallucination secondary to adverse effects of drug therapy
  Desired outcome: The patient will not suffer injury while on drug therapy.

Planning and Intervention
Maximizing Therapeutic Effects
Give oral doses 30 minutes before each meal to allow for onset of action and give an intramuscular injection near the end of surgery to prevent postoperative nausea and vomiting. Administer IV metoclopramide over at least 15 minutes, 30 minutes before the start of chemotherapy, to prevent chemotherapy-induced vomiting. Repeat every 2 hours for two doses, then every 3 hours for three doses. Do not administer metoclopramide concurrently with anticholinergic drugs.

Minimizing Adverse Effects
Monitor for evidence of depression and report positive findings to the prescriber. Institute interventions to protect the patient if he or she expresses suicidal ideas. If extrapyramidal symptoms (e.g., involuntary movements of the limbs, facial grimacing, and rhythmic protrusion of the tongue) occur, especially during the first 48 hours of therapy, withhold the metoclopramide dose, notify the health care provider, and seek orders for diphenhydramine (Benadryl), 50 mg intramuscularly, or benztropine (Cogentin), 1 to 2 mg intramuscularly. Either of these drugs usually reverses the symptoms.

Withhold the dose and notify the prescriber if Parkinson-like symptoms (e.g., bradykinesia, tremor, cog-wheel motions, and mask-like faces) occur, particularly in the first 6 months of therapy. Effects usually subside gradually within 2 to 3 months after drug discontinuation. Contact the prescriber regarding discontinuing the drug if signs of tardive dyskinesia (involuntary movements of the face, tongue, mouth, or jaw and sometimes involuntary movements of trunk or extremities) occur because tardive dyskinesia may be irreversible.

Providing Patient and Family Education

- Tell patients to take metoclopramide 30 minutes before meals.
- Caution patients to prevent injury by avoiding activities that require mental alertness, coordination, or physical dexterity (e.g., operating motor vehicles or other heavy machinery) until the effects of the drug are known.
- Caution patients to avoid alcoholic beverages, sedatives, and other CNS depressants during metoclopramide therapy because these substances may cause additive sedation.
- Explain to patients how to recognize any involuntary movements of the eyes, face, or limbs, such as tremors or cogwheel motion of the arms; depression; or serious diarrhea, and report these to the prescriber at once. In such cases, the patient should not take any more of the drug without discussing these signs and symptoms with the prescriber.

Ongoing Assessment and Evaluation

With careful monitoring and follow-up assessments, nursing care and metoclopramide therapy can be considered successful if the patient's GI complaints diminish and the patient does not experience depression or other adverse effects, such as nausea or Parkinson-like symptoms.

Drug Significantly Different From P Metoclopramide

Cisapride

Cisapride (Propulsid) is a prokinetic agent that was removed from the U.S. market because of its potential to induce fatal cardiac arrhythmias. It is now available through a limited access program—to be used only as a last resort—to treat refractory GERD, gastroparesis, severe chronic constipation, and pseudo-GI obstruction. Cisapride promotes the release of acetylcholine from neurons of the myenteric plexus, resulting in increased tone and motility of GI smooth muscle. It is contraindicated for patients with a risk of cardiac arrhythmias. This includes those with heart failure, ischemic heart disease, prolonged QT interval, sinus node dysfunction, second- or third-degree atrioventricular block, and a history of ventricular arrhythmias or torsades de pointes. Cisapride interacts with many drugs that increase the risk of cardiac arrhythmias. Certain drugs that inhibit CYP3A4, loop and thiazide diuretics, and class 1 and 2 antidysrhythmic drugs are contraindicated for use with cisapride.

C DIGESTIVE ENZYMES

Digestive enzymes are responsible for breaking down food into forms that can be absorbed easily in the GI tract. The digestive process normally begins in the mouth with digestive enzymes in salivary secretions and then continues in the stomach with the action of gastric acid and pepsin. It is completed in the duodenum with the release of the pancreatic enzymes that change protein, carbohydrate, and fat into absorbable forms.

Replacement of many of these enzymes is not necessary or truly useful, because rarely does a deficiency of endogenous enzymes actually cause GI problems. Many of the drug preparations of digestive enzymes are combinations of various enzymes, frequently paired with anticholinergics, barbiturates, or antacids. In those few situations in which an endogenous deficit does exist, it is nearly impossible to correct the deficit adequately with these combinations. In addition, combination therapy increases the risk of adverse effects from the other drug entities in the compound.

Pancreatic enzymes comprise one group of digestive enzymes that is an exception. Replacement of these enzymes is indicated. The prototype pancreatic digestive enzyme is pancrelipase (Pancrease MT, Viokase, Creon, Lipram, Pancrecarb, Panocaps). Table 36.11 presents a summary of selected digestive enzymes.

Nursing Management of the Patient Receiving P Pancrelipase

Core Drug Knowledge

Pharmacotherapeutics

Pancrelipase is enzymatic replacement therapy for patients with deficient exocrine pancreatic secretions; cystic fibrosis; chronic pancreatitis; ductal obstructions caused by cancer of the pancreas or common bile duct; pancreatic insufficiency; or steatorrhea from malabsorption syndrome; and after pancreatectomy, gastrectomy, or post-GI surgery, such as Billroth II gastroenterostomy. Pancrelipase also can be used as a presumptive test to evaluate pancreatic function. Pancrelipase is administered orally.

MEMORY CHIP

P Metoclopramide

- Used as a GI stimulant in diabetic gastric stasis, and GERD; as an antiemetic postsurgery and with chemotherapy for cancer
- Major contraindication: when stimulation of GI motility might be dangerous
- Most common adverse effects: CNS complaints
- Most serious adverse effects: tardive dyskinesia and severe depression
- **Life span alert: Older women are more likely to experience tardive dyskinesia as an adverse effect.**
- Maximizing therapeutic effects: Give metoclopramide 30 min before meals or chemotherapy.
- Minimizing adverse effects: Monitor for depression, Parkinson-like symptoms, extrapyramidal effects, and tardive dyskinesia; hold further drug administration and contact the prescriber if noted.
- Most important patient education: Teach patient to recognize signs of serious adverse effects; to call prescriber at once when noted.
- **Black box warning: May cause tardive dyskinesia in the elderly, especially in women.**

TABLE 36.11 Summary of Selected C Digestive Enzymes

Drug (Trade) Name	Selected Indications	Route and Dosage Range	Pharmacokinetics
P pancrelipase (Pancrease, Ku-Zyme, Viokase, Ilozyme, Zymase, Ultrase)	Deficient exocrine pancreatic secretions Pancreatic insufficiency, steatorrhea from malabsorption syndrome and post-gastrectomy, or post-GI surgery, Billroth II gastroenterostomy	Adjust dosage until steatorrhea minimizes and good nutritional status is maintained *Adult:* PO, 4,000 to 50,000 U with each meal and with snacks; severe deficiencies, increase to 64,000–88,000 U with each meal or increase hourly if tolerated *Child <6 mo:* PO, dose not established; *6–12 mo,* 2,000 U with each meal; *1–6 y,* 4,000–8,000 U with each meal and 4,000 U with each snack; *7–12 y,* 4,000–12,000 U with each meal and snack	Unknown
	Postpancreatectomy, ductal obstructions caused by cancer of the pancreas or common bile duct Cystic fibrosis	*Adult:* PO, 8,000–16,000 U at 2-h intervals, or as prescribed Use powder form: 0.7 g with meals	
pancreatin (Dizymes, Entozyme, Donnazyme, Hi-Vegi-Lip, Creon)	Same as above	*Adult:* PO, 1 or 2 tablets with meals and snacks; adjust according to individual meals *Child:* Dosage not established	Unknown

Pharmacokinetics

Absorption, distribution, metabolism, and excretion of this drug are unknown. The onset, peak, and duration are also unknown. Because pancrelipase is affected by gastric acid, the drug is enteric coated. However, this formulation may decrease absorption in the duodenum. The site of metabolism and route of elimination from the body are unknown.

Pharmacodynamics

Pancrelipase contains the enzymes lipase, protease, and amylase, which are responsible for the final phase of digestion. During this phase, fats are hydrolyzed to fatty acids, proteins to proteoses and derived substances, and starches to sugars and dextrins so that they can be absorbed in the small intestine. Pancreatic enzymes normally exert their effects in the duodenum and in the first part of the jejunum.

Contraindications and Precautions

Pancrelipase is contraindicated in patients who are hypersensitive to pork protein or enzymes, because the drug is derived from pork. It should not be used by patients with acute pancreatitis or acute exacerbations of chronic pancreatitis. Pancrelipase is a pregnancy category C drug and should be used only if necessary. It is not known whether it crosses into breast milk; therefore, it should be administered with caution to nursing mothers.

Caution must be used not to spill the powder on one's hands because it may irritate the skin. Inhaling the powder irritates the nasal mucosa and the respiratory tract, triggering an asthma attack in those susceptible.

Adverse Effects

Caution must be used with large doses because they may cause nausea, abdominal cramps, and diarrhea. Hyperuricosuria and hyperuricemia have occurred with extremely high doses. Less often, allergic reactions have occurred.

Drug Interactions

The antacids calcium carbonate and magnesium hydroxide can interfere with the beneficial effects of pancrelipase. Serum iron response to oral iron supplements may be decreased by concurrent dosing of pancrelipase. Table 36.12 lists agents that interact with pancrelipase.

TABLE 36.12 Agents That Interact with C Pancrelipase

Interactants	Effect and Significance	Nursing Management
calcium carbonate, magnesium hydroxide	May negate effect of enzymes	Administer 2 h apart. Monitor for therapeutic effect.
Iron	Serum levels may not increase as expected with oral supplements	Monitor blood iron levels. Seek order to adjust dose if iron levels are significantly affected.

Assessment of Relevant Core Patient Variables

Health Status

Assess the patient's health history for chronic pancreatitis, cystic fibrosis, ductal obstructions from cancer, pancreatic insufficiency, pancreatectomy, gastrectomy, or other GI surgery. Results of laboratory studies to review include serum amylase and lipase levels to determine pancreatic functioning and findings of steatorrhea. Foul-smelling, frothy stools are a sign of steatorrhea. Assess the patient's nutritional status because deficiency of pancreatic enzymes prevents the absorption of fats, proteins, and starches and may leave the patient malnourished. Also, determine whether the patient is allergic to pork, because pancrelipase is derived from pork.

Life Span and Gender

Determine whether the patient is pregnant or breast-feeding. Because pancrelipase is in pregnancy category C, it should be given only if clearly necessary. Caution should be used when administering pancrelipase to a breast-feeding woman. The drug can be given to children, but the dosage for children younger than 6 months old has not been established.

Environment

Pancrelipase can be administered in any setting, including the home.

Culture and Inherited Traits

Consider the religious affiliation of patients taking pancrelipase. Some religious groups, such as Muslims and Orthodox Jews, forbid the consumption of pork products in any form, and pancrelipase is pork based. Therefore, these patients may not accept this drug therapy.

Nursing Diagnoses and Outcomes

- Imbalanced Nutrition: Less than Body Requirements, related to impaired digestion secondary to insufficient pancreatic enzymes
  Desired outcome: *The patient's nutrient absorption will be adequate to meet body needs while on drug therapy.*
- Risk for Pain, acute abdominal, secondary to adverse effects of drug therapy
  Desired outcome: *The patient will not develop pain as an adverse effect of drug therapy.*

Planning and Intervention

Maximizing Therapeutic Effects

Brands of pancrelipase should not be changed without consulting the prescriber because the various brands do not have equal bioavailability. Administer antacids or H_2 receptor antagonists, if prescribed, to maintain the patient's gastric pH within an alkaline range. An alkaline pH prevents pancrelipase tablets from dissolving in the stomach and becoming inactivated.

Minimizing Adverse Effects

Be sure to administer or make sure the patient is administering pancrelipase exactly as prescribed to prevent excessive dosing.

Providing Patient and Family Education

- Explain to patients and families the need to learn about the role of the digestive enzyme in digesting and absorbing food. Insufficient amounts of enzyme result in weight loss and steatorrhea (foul-smelling and frothy stools). Although it is not usually possible to dose pancrelipase to eradicate steatorrhea completely, pancrelipase should greatly decrease steatorrhea.
- Tell patients to take the drug every time they eat, either before or with meals and snacks.
- Caution patients not to crush or chew pancrelipase because doing so will destroy the enzyme by exposing it to gastric acid.
- Urge patients to notify the prescriber of any abdominal pain, diarrhea, nausea, or return of steatorrhea.
- If the form of pancrelipase is a capsule that is to be opened and mixed with food, caution patients to avoid getting the powder on the hands or sniffing the powder contained in the capsules. Asthma attacks can occur in susceptible patients who inhale pancrelipase powder.

Ongoing Assessment and Evaluation

Assess patients taking pancrelipase for decreased steatorrhea, weight gain, and improved nutritional status. Drug therapy is considered successful if digestion and nutritional status improve without the occurrence of adverse effects.

Drug Closely Related to Ⓟ Pancrelipase

Pancreatin (Dygase, Hi-Vegi-Lip, Ku-Zyme, Kutrase, Lapase) is a digestive enzyme that has the same action and indication for use as pancrelipase. This agent is not as concentrated as pancrelipase and therefore may not control steatorrhea as well. Pancreatin may be from beef or pork sources.

DRUGS FOR WEIGHT MANAGEMENT

Lipase inhibitors and anorexiants are Food and Drug Administration (FDA)–approved drug classes for the management of obesity. Other drug classes used for weight

---

MEMORY CHIP

Ⓟ Pancrelipase

- Used as enzyme replacement therapy for patients deficient in this pancreatic enzyme
- Most common adverse effects: nausea, abdominal cramps, and diarrhea at large doses
- Most important patient education: Do not crush or chew tablets; take before or with meals; avoid breathing powder and skin contact.

TABLE 36.13 Summary of Selected Drugs for Weight Management

Drug (Trade) Name	Indication	Dosage Range	Pharmacokinetics
P orlistat (Xenical)	Obesity	*Adult:* PO, 120 mg tid with meals that contain fat	*Onset:* Immediate *Duration:* Unknown $t_{1/2}$: Not absorbed
benzphentermine (Didrex)	Obesity	*Adult and child* >12 y: PO, 25–50 mg daily; maximum, 50 mg 3×/d	*Onset:* Unknown *Duration:* Unknown $t_{1/2}$: Unknown
diethylpropion (Tenuate)	Obesity	*Adult and child* >16 y: PO, Immediate release: 25 mg 3×/d Controlled release: 75 mg/d	*Onset:* Rapid *Duration:* Immediate release, 4 h; controlled release, 12 h $t_{1/2}$: 4–8 h
phendimetrazine (Bontril)	Obesity	*Adult and child* >12 y: PO, Immediate release: 35 mg 2–3×/d Sustained release: 105 mg/d	*Onset:* Immediate release, rapid; controlled release, 1–2 h *Duration:* Unknown $t_{1/2}$: 2–4 h
phentermine (Adipex-P)	Obesity	*Adult and child* >16 y: PO, 37.5 mg/d; may be divided	*Onset:* 1–2 wk *Duration:* 12 wk $t_{1/2}$: 20 h

management include amphetamines and some antidepressant drugs, but they are not approved for this use (Table 36.13).

C LIPASE INHIBITORS

Lipase inhibitors are used specifically for long-term weight reduction in patients with an initial BMI of 30 kg/m^2 or more, or a BMI of 27 kg/m^2 or more in those who have other cardiovascular risk factors (e.g., hypertension, diabetes, or dyslipidemia). The prototype lipase inhibitor is orlistat (Xenical).

Nursing Management of the Patient Receiving P Orlistat

Core Drug Knowledge

Pharmacotherapeutics

Orlistat with the trade name Xenical is a prescription drug used to manage obesity by promoting weight loss and weight maintenance. Orlistat with the trade name Alli is also available as an OTC drug. It is used in conjunction with a weight-loss diet and exercise program as well to reduce the risk of regaining weight after weight loss.

Pharmacokinetics

Very little orlistat is absorbed into the systemic circulation after oral administration; most of its effect is from its local action in the GI tract. In laboratory studies, orlistat was more than 99% protein bound. Metabolism appears to occur predominantly within the GI wall. Two metabolites are formed, but they do not seem to be pharmacologically important. Fecal excretion is the main route of elimination.

Pharmacodynamics

Orlistat is a reversible lipase inhibitor. By inhibiting the action of lipase, it decreases the absorption of dietary fats. Its therapeutic effect occurs in the lumen of the stomach and small intestine, where it prevents the formation of active gastric and pancreatic lipases. The inactivated enzymes are unable to hydrolyze dietary fat, in the form of triglycerides, into absorbable free fatty acids and monoglycerides. Undigested triglycerides are not absorbed, and therefore fewer calories are absorbed. This reduced caloric intake enables weight loss. At the recommended therapeutic dose of 120 mg three times a day, orlistat inhibits dietary fat absorption by about 30%.

Contraindications and Precautions

Orlistat is contraindicated if the patient has chronic malabsorption syndrome or cholestasis. It also is contraindicated if the patient is hypersensitive to the drug or any of its elements. Organic causes of obesity, such as hypothyroidism, should be ruled out before prescribing orlistat.

Some patients may develop increased levels of urinary oxalate following treatment. Caution should be used if the patient has a history of hyperoxaluria or calcium oxalate nephrolithiasis. The weight loss brought about by orlistat use may improve metabolic control in diabetic patients. They may require a reduced dose of oral hypoglycemic medication or insulin. Orlistat is a pregnancy category B drug.

Adverse Effects

The adverse effects of orlistat are extensions of its treatment effects. GI symptoms, the most common adverse effects, are related to the pharmacodynamics of the drug. These adverse effects are generally mild and transient, although for some patients, they may last for 6 months or longer and be severe enough to warrant discontinuing the drug. These GI symptoms are oily spotting, flatus with discharge of stool, fecal urgency, fatty or oily stool, oily evacuation, increased defecation, and fecal incontinence.

Other adverse effects that can occur, but are not common, include:

- CNS: anxiety, depression, dizziness, and headache
- Dermatologic: dry skin and rash
- GI: abdominal pain, gingival disorder, infectious diarrhea, nausea, rectal pain or discomfort, tooth disorders, and vomiting
- Musculoskeletal: arthritis, back pain, joint disorders, myalgia, tendonitis, and pain in the lower extremities
- Reproductive, female: menstrual irregularity and vaginitis
- Respiratory: ear, nose, and throat symptoms, influenza, lower respiratory tract infection, and upper respiratory tract infection
- Miscellaneous: fatigue, otitis, pedal edema, sleep disorder, and urinary tract infection

No adverse effects related to overdose are known to have occurred. If necessary, stop the drug and observe the patient for 24 hours. The systemic effects attributable to lipase inhibition should be rapidly reversible.

Drug Interactions

Because orlistat impairs fat absorption, the absorption of fat-soluble vitamins (A, D, E, beta-carotene) decreases. A few other known drug interactions are listed in Table 36.14.

Assessment of Relevant Core Patient Variables

Health Status

Verify that the patient does not have a physiologic cause for obesity before starting orlistat. Assess for a history of hepatic dysfunction. Assess for thyroid disease, diabetes mellitus, and anticoagulant therapy. Patients with these conditions require direct supervision by a health care provider when taking orlistat (Xenical) rather than the OTC formulation (Alli).

Life Span and Gender

Assess the pregnancy status of female patients. Orlistat is a pregnancy category B drug, which poses a risk to the fetus. Suggest use of barrier contraceptives while taking orlistat. It is not known whether orlistat is excreted in breast milk; therefore, its use is not recommended during breast-feeding. Determine the patient's age because safety and efficacy have not been established in children.

Lifestyle, Diet, and Habits

Take a dietary history to determine how many calories in the patient's diet, and what percentage of the calories, come from fat. The patient should eat a nutritionally balanced, reduced-calorie diet; no more than 30% of the patient's caloric intake should come from fat while he or she receives orlistat. Assess the patient's exercise pattern. Weight loss is accomplished best when a diet and exercise plan are used together.

Environment

Orlistat is normally self-administered in the patient's home.

Nursing Diagnoses and Outcomes

- Imbalanced Nutrition: More than Body Requirements
  Desired outcome: *The patient will lose weight during drug therapy.*
- Risk for Imbalanced Nutrition: Less than Body Requirements, related to impaired absorption of fat-soluble vitamins during drug therapy

TABLE 36.14	Agents That Interact with P Orlistat	
Interactants	**Effect and Significance**	**Nursing Management**
Amiodarone	Orlistat may decrease absorption of amiodarone.	Monitor for arrhythmias.
cyclosporine	Exact clinical effect is unknown. Changes in cyclosporine absorption have been reported with variations in dietary intake.	Monitor immunosuppressive effects of cyclosporine.
fat-soluble vitamins	Decreased absorption rate of fat-soluble vitamins; 30% decrease in beta-carotene and about 60% reduction in vitamin E absorption have been shown. Decreases in other vitamin levels not known exactly; vitamin deficiency may result.	Teach patient to take multivitamin that includes fat-soluble vitamins to prevent deficiencies.
Warfarin	Possible decrease in vitamin K absorption. No known effect on pharmacokinetics or pharmacodynamics of warfarin currently.	Monitor PT/INR. Monitor for bruising or bleeding.

Desired outcome: *The patient will not have serious vitamin deficiencies while taking drug therapy.*

- Risk for Bowel Incontinence related to adverse effects of drug therapy
Desired outcome: *Bowel incontinence will not occur or will be minimal and transient.*
- Risk for Diarrhea related to adverse effects of drug therapy
Desired outcome: *Diarrhea will not occur or will be minimal and transient.*

Planning and Intervention

Maximizing Therapeutic Effects

Ensure that the patient takes orlistat with all meals that contain fat and that he or she limits dietary fat to 30% of calories. Omit the dose of orlistat if the meal does not contain fat. The patient should also be encouraged to participate in exercise while on drug therapy.

Minimizing Adverse Effects

Advise the patient to take a multivitamin that contains fat-soluble vitamins to prevent imbalances from drug therapy. Separate the administration of orlistat and multivitamins by 2 hours.

GI symptoms are more pronounced when the fat content of a meal is high. Emphasize the need to alter fat ingestion.

Providing Patient and Family Education

- Teach patients to limit dietary fat. Calories from fat should be no more than 30% of daily calories. This percentage promotes weight loss and prevents and minimizes GI adverse effects.
- Instruct patients to divide daily fat intake equally between meals and to take the drug with each meal containing fat (during or up to 1 hour after eating). Patients should skip a dose if the meal has no fat or if the meal is missed.
- Encourage patients to take a vitamin supplement that includes fat-soluble vitamins. Remind patients to separate these drugs by at least 2 hours.
- Discuss possible adverse effects and potential interventions:
  - Suck sugarless lozenges and perform frequent mouth care for dry mouth
  - Decrease the amount of fat in meals for continued loose stools

Ongoing Assessment and Evaluation

Orlistat therapy is considered effective if weight loss occurs without major GI adverse effects or vitamin deficiency arising.

Drugs Significantly Different From 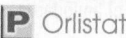 Orlistat
Adrenergic Drugs

The adrenergic drugs benzphetamine (Didrex), diethylpropion (Tenuate, Dospan), phentermine (Adipex-P, Ionamin),

ADVERSE EFFECTS FROM ORLISTAT

Ms. Benson has been taking orlistat, a lipase inhibitor, to promote weight loss for 1 month. She returns to the clinic for follow-up. You, the nurse, ask her how she is tolerating the medication. She tells you that initially she only had some problems with "needing to go to the bathroom a couple of times a day." However, she says that in the last few days she has been bothered by "real oily poop." She tells you that she has to run to the bathroom "like mad, 'cause I can't hold it. Sometimes I can't get there fast enough and spot my panties with that stuff."

What questions should you ask Ms. Benson to assess her problem thoroughly?

and phendimetrazine (Bontril) are used for weight control. They decrease the appetite by stimulating the CNS. They also effects similar to those of amphetamines, such as tachycardia, hypertension, nervousness, and anxiety. Although they are safer than amphetamines, they still have an abuse potential; thus, they are scheduled drugs. They are not useful for long-term management of obesity because tolerance develops in 6 to 12 weeks. They are contraindicated during pregnancy because of an increased risk of cleft palate and congenital heart defects.

Amphetamines

Amphetamines work by decreasing the appetite. Although they are effective, the risk of abuse outweighs the benefit of weight loss. Some health care providers do prescribe these drugs; however, they are not approved for use in weight management.

Antidepressant Drugs

Bupropion (Wellbutrin), fluoxetine (Prozac), venlafaxine (Effexor), and sertraline (Zoloft) are antidepressant drugs. None are approved for weight loss. Bupropion blocks reuptake of norepinephrine and dopamine, while fluoxetine, venlafaxine, and sertraline block the reuptake of serotonin. All of these drugs are discussed in Chapter 16.

MEMORY CHIP

P Orlistat

- Used to promote weight loss in obesity; prevents absorption of dietary fat
- Major contraindication: chronic malabsorption syndrome or cholestasis
- Most common adverse effects: GI (oily spotting, flatus with stool, and fecal urgency)
- Most important patient education: Take with all meals containing fat; limit dietary fat to 30% of calories; take a multivitamin with fat-soluble vitamins.

C ANTIEMETICS

Nausea and vomiting related to oncologic therapy are frequently difficult to manage. The American Society of Clinical Oncology (ASCO) categorizes their antiemetic guidelines according to type of emesis: acute, delayed, anticipatory, special emetic problems, and radiation emesis. The special emetic problems category includes emesis in pediatric oncology, high-dose chemotherapy, and nausea and vomiting despite prophylaxis, also referred to as refractory or breakthrough emesis.

Antiemetics, which suppress stimulation of the CTZ and the VC, are used to treat nausea and vomiting. Antiemetic drugs are primarily from three main drug classifications—selective serotonin receptor antagonists, antidopaminergic drugs, and anticholinergic drugs. Other classes of drugs that may be used include glucocorticoids, cannabinoids, and benzodiazepines (Table 36.15).

• C SELECTIVE SEROTONIN RECEPTOR ANTAGONISTS

The selective serotonin receptor antagonists, also known as the 5-HT$_3$ receptor antagonists, prevent the stimulation of type 3 serotonin receptors in the CTZ. The prototype selective serotonin receptor antagonist is ondansetron (Zofran).

Nursing Management of the Patient Receiving P Ondansetron
Core Drug Knowledge
Pharmacotherapeutics
Ondansetron is used to prevent nausea and vomiting associated with cancer chemotherapy and radiotherapy, and in postoperative states when expectation is high that nausea or vomiting will occur or when nausea and vomiting must be avoided (Box 36.3).

Off-label uses of ondansetron include treating nausea and vomiting associated with acetaminophen poisoning; hyperemesis gravidarum; and treatment of early-onset alcoholism. Alcoholism that occurs relatively early in life is associated with serotonergic abnormality and antisocial behaviors. Ondansetron appears to be effective treatment for these patients, presumably by relieving an underlying abnormality in serotonin stimulation.

Pharmacokinetics
Ondansetron is metabolized by the liver. It is moderately protein bound (about 75%). It crosses the placenta, may enter breast milk, and is excreted in the urine.

Pharmacodynamics
Serotonin receptors of the 5-HT$_3$ type are located peripherally on the vagal nerve terminal and centrally in the CTZ. During chemotherapy, special mucosal cells in the small intestine release serotonin, which stimulates these receptors.

Ondansetron blocks these receptor sites, thus preventing nausea and vomiting.

Contraindications and Precautions
Ondansetron is contraindicated in patients with hypersensitivity to the drug or its components. Ondansetron is a pregnancy category B drug.

Adverse Effects
The most common adverse effects of ondansetron are headache, constipation, and malaise. Potentially serious adverse effects are arrhythmias, hypotension, and extrapyramidal effects (e.g., Parkinson-like symptoms). Other adverse effects that can occur include:

- Cardiovascular: hypertension
- CNS: anxiety, dizziness, drowsiness, and chills or shivering
- GI: abdominal pain, diarrhea, and xerostomia
- Miscellaneous: wound problems, musculoskeletal pain, cold sensation, fever, gynecologic disorders, hypoxia, injection-site reaction, paresthesia, pruritus, urinary retention, weakness, increases in aspartate transaminase and alanine aminotransferase, and pain.

Drug Interactions
Because ondansetron is metabolized by the cytochrome P-450 enzymes, drug interactions may occur with other drugs that are metabolized by these enzymes or those that inhibit P-450 metabolism. However, no dosage adjustment has been recommended based on available data regarding this finding. Table 36.16 presents drugs that interact with ondansetron.

Assessment of Relevant Core Patient Variables
Health Status
Verify that the patient has clinical indications for receiving ondansetron and is not known to have a hypersensitivity to it. Assess baseline skin color and texture and urinary output. Perform an abdominal examination.

Life Span and Gender
Assess whether the patient is pregnant. Ondansetron is a pregnancy category B drug. Therefore, it should be used only if the potential benefit to the mother justifies potential risks to the fetus. Determine the patient's age. Ondansetron is used to prevent nausea and vomiting associated with cancer chemotherapy in children. However, dosage information for children 3 years of age or younger is limited. Dosage adjustment is not needed in older adults.

Environment
Ondansetron normally is administered in an acute care setting. Oral ondansetron is frequently self-administered in the home environment.

TABLE 36.15 **Summary of Selected ⒸAntiemetics**

Drug (Trade) Name	Selected Indications	Route and Dosage Range	Pharmacokinetics
Ⓒ 5-HT3 Receptor Antagonists			
Ⓟ ondansetron	Prevention and treatment of chemotherapy-induced nausea and vomiting; prevention and treatment of postoperative nausea and vomiting; prevention of radiation-induced nausea and vomiting	*Adult:* PO, 8 mg 30 min before chemotherapy; repeat 8 h later, then q12 h for 1–2 d; increase to 8 mg 3×/d for radiotherapy *Adult:* IV, 0.15 mg/kg infused over 15 min, beginning 30 min before chemotherapy; repeat 4 and 8 h later	*Onset:* PO, 30–60 min; IV, immediate *Duration:* Unknown $t_{1/2}$: 3.5–6 h
dolasetron (Anzemet)	Prevention of chemotherapy-induced nausea and vomiting; prevention and treatment of postoperative nausea and vomiting	*Adult:* PO, 100 mg 1 h before chemotherapy or 2 h before surgery *Child* 2–16 y: PO, 1.8 mg/kg 1 h before chemotherapy; 1.2 mg/kg 2 h before surgery *Adult:* IV, 1.8 mg/kg 30 min before chemotherapy; 12.5 mg 15 min prior to stopping anesthesia *Child:* IV, 1.8 mg/kg 30 min before chemotherapy; 0.35 mg/kg 15 min before stopping anesthesia	*Onset:* PO, rapid; IV, immediate *Duration:* Unknown $t_{1/2}$: 3.5–5 h
granisetron (Kytril)	Prevention and treatment of chemotherapy-induced nausea and vomiting; prevention and treatment of postoperative nausea and vomiting; prevention and treatment of radiation-induced nausea and vomiting	*Adult and child* >2 y: PO, 1 mg 2×/d or 2 mg/d. Start 1 h before chemotherapy and give second dose 12 h later. IV, 10 mcg/kg over 5 min, starting within 30 min of chemotherapy	*Onset:* PO, moderate; IV, rapid *Duration:* 24 h $t_{1/2}$: 3–14 h
palonosetron (Aloxi)	Prevention of acute and delayed nausea and vomiting associated with chemotherapy	*Adult:* IV, 0.25 mg over 30 s, 30 min before start of chemotherapy. Do not repeat use for 7 d.	*Onset:* IV, immediate *Duration:* Unknown $t_{1/2}$: 40 h
Ⓒ Substance P/NK1 Receptor Antagonist			
aprepritant (Emend)	Prevention of chemotherapy-induced nausea and vomiting; prevention and treatment of postoperative nausea and vomiting	*Adult:* PO, 125 mg 1 h before chemo on day 1, then 80 mg on day 2–3; *Postop:* 40 mg within 3 h of anesthesia induction.	*Onset:* unknown *Duration:* unknown $t_{1/2}$: 9–14 h
Ⓒ Anticholinergic Drugs			
dimenhydrinate	Nausea and vomiting, vertigo, motion sickness	*Adult:* PO/IM/IV, 50–100 mg q4–6 h	*Onset:* 15–30 min *Duration:* 3–6 h $t_{1/2}$: Unknown
diphenhydramine (Benadryl)	Nausea and vomiting, motion sickness	*Adult:* PO/IM/IV, 10–50 mg q4–6 h	*Onset:* 15–30 min *Duration:* 4–8 h $t_{1/2}$: 2.5–7 h
hydroxyzine (Vistaril)	Nausea and vomiting	*Adult:* PO/IM, 25–100 mg q6 h *Child* >6 y: PO, 50–100 mg/d in divided doses *Child* <6 y: PO, 50 mg/d in divided doses	*Onset:* 15–30 min *Duration:* 4–6 h $t_{1/2}$: 3 h
meclizine (Antivert)	Nausea and vomiting, vertigo Motion sickness	*Adult:* PO, 25–100 mg daily in divided doses *Adult:* PO, 25–50 mg 1 h before travel; may repeat q24 h	*Onset:* 1 h *Duration:* 12–24 h $t_{1/2}$: 6 h
scopolamine (Transderm Scop)	Nausea and vomiting, motion sickness	*Adult:* Transdermal patch, 0.5 mg q72 h *Child:* Not recommended	*Onset:* 4–5 h *Duration:* 72 h $t_{1/2}$: 8 h
Ⓒ Antidopaminergic Drugs			
chlorpromazine (Thorazine)	Nausea and vomiting	*Adult and child* >12 y: rectal suppository, 0.5 mg/lb q6–8 h *Child* >6 mo: rectal suppository, 1 mg/kg q6–8 h	*Onset:* 1 h *Duration:* 3–4 h $t_{1/2}$: 20–24 h

TABLE 36.15 Summary of Selected ⒸAntiemetics *(continued)*

Drug (Trade) Name	Selected Indications	Route and Dosage Range	Pharmacokinetics
droperidol (Inapsine)	Nausea and vomiting	*Adult*: IM/IV, 2.5–5 mg q4–6 h *Child* 2–12 y: IM/IV, 0.1 mg/kg	*Onset*: 3–10 min *Duration*: 2–12 h $t_{1/2}$: 2 h
haloperidol (Haldol)	Nausea and vomiting	*Adult*: PO/IM/IV, 1–5 mg q12 h *Child*: Not recommended	*Onset*: 1 h *Duration*: Unknown $t_{1/2}$: 21–24 h
prochlorperazine (Compazine)	Nausea and vomiting	*Adult*: PO/IM/IV/rectal, 5–10 mg 3–4×/d *Child* >2 y: PO/rectal suppository 20–29 lb: 2.5 mg 1–2×/d 30–39 lb: 2.5 mg 2–3×/d 40–85 lb: 2.5 mg 3×/d or 5 mg 2×/d	*Onset*: 30–40 min *Duration*: 3–4 h $t_{1/2}$: 6.8–9 h
promethazine (Phenergan)	Nausea and vomiting, vertigo, motion sickness	*Adult*: PO/IM/IV/rectal, 12.5–25 mg q4–6 h *Child* >2 y: PO/rectal, 1.1 mg/kg q4–6 h	*Onset*: PO/IM, 20 min; IV, 3–5 min *Duration*: 12 h $t_{1/2}$: 7–15 h
thiethylperazine (Torecan)	Nausea and vomiting	*Adult and child* >12 y: PO, 10 mg 3×/d *Child* <12 y: Not recommended	*Onset*: 30 min *Duration*: 4 h $t_{1/2}$: Unknown
Ⓒ **Cannabinoids**			
dronabinol (Marinol)	Nausea and vomiting not responsive to other antiemetics	*Adult*: PO, 5–7.5 mg/m² q24 h *Child*: PO, 5 mg/m² 1–3 h before chemotherapy, 5 mg/m² q2–4 h after chemotherapy for a total of 4–6 doses/d	*Onset*: 30–60 min *Duration*: 4–6 h $t_{1/2}$: 25–36 h
nabilone (Cesamet)	Nausea and vomiting not responsive to other antiemetics	*Adult*: PO, 1–2 mg 1–3 h before chemotherapy; may be administered 2–3× during course of therapy, up to 48 h after last dose of chemotherapy	*Onset*: 60–90 min *Duration*: 8–12 h $t_{1/2}$: 2 h

Nursing Diagnoses and Outcomes

- Imbalanced Nutrition: Less than Body Requirements, related to severe nausea and vomiting
  Desired outcome: *Nutritional needs will be met, and ondansetron therapy will prevent severe nausea and vomiting.*

- Risk for Altered Comfort related to severe nausea and vomiting
  Desired outcome: *Comfort will be maintained, and ondansetron therapy will prevent severe nausea and vomiting.*

BOX 36.3 FOCUS ON RESEARCH

Control of Stress-Related Gastrointestinal Bleeding in the Critical Care Setting

Lin, P. C., Chang, C. H., Hsu, P. I., Tseng, P. L., & Huang, Y. B. (2010). The efficacy and safety of proton pump inhibitors vs histamine-2 receptor antagonists for stress ulcer bleeding prophylaxis among critical care patients: A meta analysis. *Critical Care Medicine*, 38(4):1197–1205.

The Study

A meta-analysis was conducted to compare the efficacy and safety of proton pump inhibitors and histamine-2 receptor antagonists in the management of stress related bleeding in critical care patients. A search for randomized, controlled studies that compared these two therapies was completed and resulted in the identification of seven randomized, controlled trials with a total of 936 patients. Results demonstrated no significant difference in stress bleeding prophylaxis, pneumonia, or mortality between the two treatment options. Recommendations included more well-designed and powered randomized, clinical trials to be conducted.

Nursing Implications

Stress-related gastrointestinal disease and bleeding are associated with increased mortality and morbidity. While gastrointestinal prophylaxis is routine care in most critical care units, there is a need to better manage these patients. According to Lin et al. (2010), there is a 48.5% mortality rate in patients with stress-related gastrointestinal bleeding as compared to 9.1% in those without bleeding.

TABLE 36.16 Drugs that Interact with P Ondansetron

Interactants	Effect and Significance	Nursing Management
cisplatin	Ondansetron may decrease cisplatin levels, resulting in subtherapeutic effect.	Monitor for efficacy of cisplatin therapy. Discuss possible dosage adjustment with health care provider.
cyclophosphamide	Ondansetron may decrease cyclophosphamide levels, resulting in subtherapeutic effect.	Monitor for efficacy of cyclophosphamide therapy. Discuss possible dosage adjustment with health care provider.
Rifamycins	Rifamycins may decrease serum ondansetron levels.	Monitor for continued nausea or vomiting. Discuss alternative antiemetic therapy with health care provider.

- Potential Complication: Altered Cardiac Output related to adverse effects of ondansetron
  Desired outcome: Cardiac output will not be affected adversely by possible hypotension and arrhythmias from ondansetron.

Planning and Intervention

Maximizing Therapeutic Effects

Administer ondansetron 30 minutes before the start of chemotherapy. Infusions should be given over 15 minutes. Additional doses are used after chemotherapy. When used for postoperative nausea and vomiting, ondansetron should be given immediately before induction into anesthesia. If ondansetron is used with radiation therapy, the dose should be given orally, 1 to 2 hours before treatment. Oral disintegrating tablets should be removed from the pack by peeling back the foil, not by pushing the drug tablet through the foil. Place ondansetron on the patient's tongue and have the patient swallow it. The drug does not have to be administered with a fluid.

Minimizing Adverse Effects

For IV administration, dilute ondansetron in 50 mL of 5% dextrose or 0.9% sodium chloride. Do not mix with alkaline solutions. Administer slowly over 15 minutes. Undiluted ondansetron may be given by IV push over 2 to 5 minutes.

Providing Patient and Family Education

- Explain the purpose of the drug.
- Advise patients to take ondansetron every 8 hours for 1 to 2 days after chemotherapy or radiation therapy to maximize prevention of nausea and vomiting.
- Teach patients to change positions slowly to avoid weakness or dizziness.
- Advise patients to refrain from driving or performing tasks that require alertness until the effects of ondansetron are assessed.
- Teach patients to report any tremor, gait problems, or other Parkinson-like symptoms.

Ongoing Assessment and Evaluation

Ondansetron therapy is considered effective if nausea and vomiting are controlled and adverse effects are controlled or do not occur.

Drugs Closely Related to P Ondansetron
Dolasetron

Dolasetron (Anzemet) is available as an oral and parenteral drug. It is approved for treatment of acute nausea and vomiting associated with emetogenic chemotherapy and prevention and treatment of postoperative nausea and vomiting. Off-label uses include the treatment and prevention of radiation therapy–induced nausea and vomiting. The drug is also used cautiously in patients with atrioventricular block or in those who are at risk for developing prolongation of cardiac conduction intervals.

Granisetron

Granisetron (Kytril) is very similar to ondansetron with the same indications, precautions, and adverse effects. The most common adverse effect is headache.

Palonosetron

Palonosetron (Aloxi), the newest drug in this class, is available only for parenteral administration. It has the same indications as ondansetron. In comparison with other selective serotonin receptor antagonists, palonosetron has a prolonged half-life, which makes it an excellent drug for delayed emesis from chemotherapy.

Drugs Significantly Different From P Ondansetron
Aprepitant

A new drug, aprepitant (Emend), is a substance P/NK1 receptor antagonist that has been approved for preventing delayed

MEMORY CHIP
P Ondansetron

- Used to prevent nausea and vomiting associated with cancer chemotherapy, radiation, and certain postoperative states
- Most common adverse effects: headache, constipation, and malaise
- Most serious adverse effects: arrhythmias, hypotension, and extrapyramidal effects
- Maximizing therapeutic effects: Administer 30 minutes before treatment.
- Most important patient education: Notify the nurse if any adverse effects occur

emesis from chemotherapy. It has little or no affinity for serotonin (5-HT), dopamine, and corticosteroid receptors, the targets of other antiemetics. Aprepitant is highly protein bound at 95%. The drug is extensively metabolized by the P-450 system, primarily by CYP3A4. Aprepitant is also a moderate inhibitor of CYP3A4. Minor metabolism occurs through CYP1A2 and CYP2C19. Metabolism is the route of elimination; aprepitant is not renally excreted. The half-life is 9 to 13 hours. No clinically statistical pharmacokinetic differences in aprepitant use exist among men and women, older and younger adults, and Hispanics, blacks, and whites. No dosage adjustments are indicated for any of these groups. Aprepitant has not been studied in children younger than 18 years.

Studies show that, given orally once a day for 3 days (the day of therapy, and then 2 days afterward) 1 hour before administration of chemotherapy, this drug decreased delayed emesis by 30% over placebo. Aprepitant is used in combination with ondansetron and dexamethasone as a standardized regimen. It is not used alone. The aprepitant regimen prevents acute and delayed nausea and vomiting associated with highly emetogenic drugs, including high doses of cisplatin. Aprepitant is not effective in treating current conditions of nausea.

Aprepitant is generally well tolerated and in clinical trials had an adverse effect pattern similar to that of placebo. The most common adverse effects were tiredness, hiccups, constipation, diarrhea, and loss of appetite.

A major difference between aprepitant and ondansetron is the potential for drug interactions. Aprepitant must be used with extreme caution in patients who also receive other drugs that are primarily metabolized through CYP3A4, and elevations of their plasma levels are likely to occur. It should not be used at all concurrently with pimozide, cisapride, terfenadine, or astemizole, because inhibition of CYP3A4 in these drugs and the elevated plasma concentrations of these drugs can potentially cause serious or life-threatening reactions. Several chemotherapy drugs are metabolized by CYP3A4, including docetaxel, paclitaxel, etoposide, vinblastine, vincristine, irinotecan, ifosfamide, and imatinib. During clinical trials, aprepitant was commonly coadministered with etoposide, vinorelbine, or paclitaxel. These drugs did not require dosage adjustments. Use of the other chemotherapeutic CYP3A4 substrates has not been studied, and they may require downward dosage adjustments if coadministered with the aprepitant regimen. Aprepitant also interacts substantially with warfarin, which may result in a clinically significant decrease in the International Normalized Ratio (INR), leading to a risk of clotting. Patients need to have their INR monitored for 14 days, especially between days 7 and 10, following initiation of the 3-day aprepitant regimen. The efficacy of oral contraceptives may also be reduced by aprepitant. A backup method of contraception should be used.

Antidopaminergic Drugs

The antidopaminergic drugs (also referred to as phenothiazines) block the action of dopamine, a neurotransmitter found in both the GI tract and the CTZ. Used for nausea and vomiting, they also have sedative properties. Drugs in this class include chlorpromazine (Thorazine), prochlorperazine (Compazine), promethazine (Phenergan), and thiethylperazine (Torecan). In addition to nausea and vomiting, chlorpromazine is used for intractable hiccups. Other drugs that affect dopamine receptors, but are not phenothiazines, include the butyrophenones droperidol (Inapsine) and haloperidol (Haldol), and the dopamine-2 antagonist metoclopramide (Reglan).

These drugs have limited use in children with prolonged vomiting because of their possible adverse effects. Drowsiness should be anticipated, and patient safety should be a priority. Patients should be advised not to drive or perform activities requiring mental alertness until the effects of the drug are known. Patients should be taught to avoid alcohol and other CNS depressants because of possible additive effects. Additional information regarding the phenothiazines and butyrophenones is found in Chapter 17.

Anticholinergic Drugs

The anticholinergic antiemetics block the action of acetylcholine in the VC. They prevent motion sickness by reducing the sensitivity of the labyrinthine apparatus, thus inhibiting vestibular input to the CNS. This process decreases stimulation of the CTZ and the VC. The anticholinergics are used to treat nausea, vomiting, and motion sickness, and some of these agents, such as meclizine (Antivert) and dimenhydrinate, are used to treat vertigo. Other drugs in this class that are used as antiemetics include scopolamine (Transderm-Scop), diphenhydramine (Benadryl), hydroxyzine (Vistaril), and trimethobenzamide (Tigan).

Anticholinergic drugs are used with caution in patients with glaucoma, obstructive diseases of the GI or GU tract, and elderly men with possible prostatic hypertrophy. Like antidopaminergic drugs, anticholinergic drugs may cause significant sedation. It is necessary to caution patients about possible additive effects with alcohol and other CNS depressants. Patients should be taught to wash their hands after handling scopolamine transdermal patches, because temporary dilation of the pupil and blurred vision are possible if the drug comes in contact with the eyes.

Cannabinoids

Dronabinol (Marinol) and nabilone (Cesamet) are used for nausea and vomiting associated with cancer chemotherapy that does not respond to other antiemetic drugs. Also used for its psychoactive activity in marijuana, dronabinol is also known as tetrahydrocannabinol (THC). Its use is also approved by the FDA for the treatment of anorexia in patients who are HIV antibody positive. As an antiemetic, the exact mechanism of action of dronabinol is unknown, but it is thought to work by inhibiting the vomiting control mechanism in the medulla oblongata. Dronabinol is a schedule III drug because of its abuse potential. It may induce CNS effects such as ataxia, confusion, problems with coordination,

TABLE 36.17 **Summary of Selected © Gallstone-Solubilizing Agents**

Drug (Trade) Name	Selected Indications	Contraindications and Precautions	Adverse Effects	Route and Dosage Range
ursodiol (Actigall)	Dissolution of radiolucent, noncalcified, smaller than 20-mm gallstones in patients who are not candidates for surgery due to age, disease states, or idiosyncratic reactions to anesthesia	Will not dissolve calcified, radiopaque, or radiolucent bile pigment stones in patients with compelling needs for cholecystectomy	Nausea, vomiting, dyspepsia	*Adult:* PO, 8–20 mg/kg/d in two to three doses, for 1 y or more (if partial or full dissolution does not occur in 1 y, likelihood of success is reduced)
monoctanoin (Moctanin)	Dissolution of radiolucent gallstones retained in biliary tract after cholecystectomy when other means have failed or cannot be used	Impaired hepatic function, significant biliary tract infection, recent history of duodenal ulcer or duodenitis, portosystemic shunting, acute pancreatitis, or any life-threatening problem that would be complicated by biliary tract infusion	Abdominal pain, nausea, vomiting, diarrhea, anorexia, indigestion, fever	*Adult* (direct infusion into biliary tract only after a catheter has been placed endoscopically as close to the stones as possible): Dilute 120-mL vial with 13 mL of sterile water; perfuse stone 3–5 mL/h for 2–10 d

dizziness, somnolence, and vertigo. Psychiatric adverse effects such as delusion of persecution, depersonalization, depression, disturbance in thinking, and euphoria may occur. Potential cardiovascular adverse effects include hypertension or hypotension, palpitations, tachyarrhythmia, and vasodilatation. Because of these potential effects, dronabinol is used cautiously in patients with a history of substance abuse, psychiatric disorders, and cardiovascular disorders.

Nabilone is a schedule II drug. Precautions are similar to those for dronabinol. In addition, nabilone is used cautiously in patients with hepatic dysfunction. It has a high incidence of adverse effects such as asthenia, ataxia, drowsiness, dizziness, dry mouth, headache, poor concentration, somnolence, vertigo, and hypotension. Orthostatic hypotension, euphoria, dysphoria, depression, visual hallucinations, and psychosis can occur, especially in older patients.

Patients should be taught to take these drugs exactly as prescribed. Because of the potential adverse effects, a responsible adult should be with the patient while taking these drugs. Patients taking cannabinoids should be advised not to drive or perform activities that require concentration. Patients should refrain from alcohol or other CNS depressants. It is important to reporting symptoms such as bizarre thoughts, uncontrollable behavior or thought processes, fainting, dizziness, or irregular heartbeat to the health care provider immediately. In the acute care setting, it is necessary to ensure the safety of the patient.

Glucocorticoid Steroids

Dexamethasone (Decadron) and methylprednisolone (Depo-Medrol) are used for cancer-induced nausea and vomiting, although this is not a FDA-approved indication. The ASCO recommends the use of glucocorticoids for every type of cancer-induced emesis. The drugs are administered intravenously just prior to chemotherapy. Adverse effects are rare due to the short duration of treatment.

Olanzapine

Olanzapine (Zyprexa) is actually a drug for schizophrenia and bipolar mania. Olanzapine blocks multiple neurotransmitters, including D_1, D_2, and D_4 receptors; the serotonin receptors $5\text{-}HT_{2a}$, $5\text{-}HT_{2c}$, and $5\text{-}HT_3$; alpha-1 adrenergic receptors; acetylcholine; and histamine-1 receptors. Because many of these receptors have a role in nausea and vomiting, olanzapine may be effective for its management. It is hypothesized that olanzapine decreases nausea and vomiting because of its antagonism of D_2 receptors and its blockade of $5\text{-}HT_3$ receptors. Olanzapine is also discussed in Chapter 17.

© GALLSTONE-SOLUBILIZING AGENTS

Gallstone-solubilizing agents, including ursodiol (Actigall) and monoctanoin (Moctanin), work to dissolve gallstones. They are used only under specific circumstances and are summarized in Table 36.17.

CHAPTER SUMMARY

• Drug therapy for the upper GI tract is related to problems from bacterial infection, acid production, digestion, and nausea and vomiting.
• Dietary factors can influence symptoms experienced from the disease process; can contribute to the effectiveness of the therapy; and can contribute to adverse effects from therapy. Current dietary habits should be explored, and additional dietary teaching provided as indicated, with all patients requiring drug therapy for upper GI problems.
• *Helicobacter pylori* causes a bacterial infection that is a causative factor in peptic ulcers and gastric cancer. When

H. pylori is eradicated, an ulcer rarely reoccurs. Treatment involves various drug choices but optimally includes the combination of antibiotics (usually two) and a proton pump inhibitor. A bismuth salicylate may be added as well. H$_2$ receptor antagonists sometimes are used instead of a proton pump inhibitor.

- PPIs, such as omeprazole, decrease gastric acid production. They are used to manage the symptoms of GERD and peptic ulcers and to treat hypersecretory conditions.
- H$_2$RAs, such as ranitidine, block histamine at parietal cells, thus reducing the hydrogen ion concentration and the volume of gastric acid. Common uses of H$_2$RAs include treating PUD, GERD, and hypersecretory conditions and preventing stress ulcers. OTC H$_2$RAs are used for heartburn and indigestion.
- Antacids are basic salts that increase the gastric pH, thereby neutralizing gastric acidity. These preparations are used for upper GI disorders such as gastroesophageal reflux esophagitis, hiatal hernia, gastritis, and PUD. Antacids do not cure these conditions but help manage the symptoms and discomfort associated with them. All antacids are closely related and are used in various combinations to produce the desired effects and to minimize adverse effects.
- Two antacids are absorbed systemically: sodium bicarbonate and calcium carbonate. In large doses, they can cause metabolic alkalosis. Sodium bicarbonate contains large quantities of sodium. It should not be given to patients who have pathologies that require salt restriction.
- Magnesium antacids should not be given to patients with chronic renal failure because these drugs increase the risk of developing magnesium toxicity in such patients. Aluminum carbonate is used in patients with chronic renal failure because it binds with phosphorus, reducing serum phosphate levels.
- Sucralfate, although an aluminum salt, is not an antacid. When it dissolves in the stomach, it forms a sticky paste that adheres to ulcerated areas, preventing gastric acids from touching the ulcer and allowing healing to occur.
- The GI stimulants, such as metoclopramide, are used in diabetic gastroparesis and with symptomatic gastroesophageal reflux. They increase GI motility, apparently by sensitizing the tissues to acetylcholine. Metoclopramide, because of its dopamine antagonist characteristics, also is used as an antiemetic postoperatively and during chemotherapy.
- Digestive enzymes are a replacement for the body's intrinsic enzymes when the body does not produce enough to meet the needs for digestion. The enzymes that are replaced most frequently and with the greatest therapeutic effects are the pancreatic enzymes. They should be taken with meals and with snacks.
- Orlistat, a lipase inhibitor, prevents the absorption of dietary fat. It is used in obesity to promote and maintain weight loss.
- Antiemetics prevent nausea and vomiting; they prevent stimulation of the CTZ and the VC by interfering with neurotransmitter receptors. They are primarily selective serotonin receptor antagonists, antidopaminergics, or anticholinergics.
- Selective serotonin receptor antagonists, such as ondansetron, are used to prevent the nausea and vomiting associated with cancer chemotherapy and radiation therapy, and after some types of surgery.

QUESTIONS FOR STUDY AND REVIEW

1. If a patient is treated for active peptic ulcer disease solely with an antisecretory drug, such as the proton pump inhibitor (PPI) omeprazole or an H$_2$ receptor antagonist (H$_2$RA) such as ranitidine, is it likely that the ulcer will recur?
2. Your patient is receiving the PPI omeprazole for GERD. Explain how dietary factors may interact with the therapeutic action of omeprazole.
3. Why is it important to assess the pharmacokinetics of other drugs that a patient is receiving when you plan to start the patient on omeprazole therapy?
4. How do H$_1$ receptor antagonists (H$_1$RAs) differ from H$_2$ receptor antagonists (H$_2$RAs)?
5. What is the advantage of combining aluminum hydroxide with magnesium hydroxide as an antacid?
6. Why are aluminum antacids given to patients with chronic renal failure?
7. What are the main adverse effects of orlistat, a lipase inhibitor used in treating obesity?
8. Why is ondansetron especially helpful in preventing nausea and vomiting caused by cancer chemotherapy?

NEED MORE HELP?

Chapter 36 of the Study Guide to Accompany *Drug Therapy in Nursing*, 4th Edition, contains NCLEX-style questions and other learning activities to reinforce your understanding of the concepts presented in this chapter. For additional information or to purchase the study guide, visit the**Point**.

REFERENCES

Agarwal, K., & Agarwal, S. (2008). *Helicobacter pylori Vaccine: From past to future. Mayo Clinic Proceedings,* 83(2):169–175.

Ananthakrishnan, A. N., Issa, M., & Binion, D. G. (2010). *Clostridium Difficile* and inflammatory bowel disease. *Medical Clinics of North America,* 94(1):135–153. Camilleri, M. (2007). Clinical practice: Diabetic gastroparesis. *New England Journal of Medicine,* 356(8):820–829.

Chua, D., Lo, A., & Jung, J. (2010). Evidence for interaction between clopidogrel and proton pump inhibitors. *American Journal of Health-System Pharmacy,* (67):604–606.

Facts and Comparisons. (2010). *Drug facts and comparisons.* Philadelphia, PA: Lippincott Williams & Wilkins.

Gatta, L., Vakil, N., Leandro, G., et al. (2009). Sequential therapy or triple therapy for Helicobacter pylori infection: systematic review and meta-analysis of randomized controlled trials in adults and children. *Am J Gastroenterol,* 104(12):3069–3079.

Gray, S. L., LaCroix, A. Z., Larson, J., et al. (2010). Proton pump inhibitor use, hip fracture, and change in bone mineral density

Gray, S. L., LaCroix, A. Z., Larson, J., et al. (2010). Proton pump inhibitor use, hip fracture, and change in bone mineral density in postmenopausal women: results from the Women's Health Initiative, *Archives of Internal Medicine,* 170(9):765–771.

Graham, D., & Fischback, L. (2010). Heicobacter pylori treatment in the era increasing antibiotic resistance. *Gut,* 59(8):1143–1153.

Habib, A. S., Reuveni, J., Taguchi, A., et al. (2007). A comparison of ondansetron with promethazine for treating postoperative nausea and vomiting in patients who received prophylaxis with ondansetron: a retrospective database analysis. *Anesthesia and Analgesia,* 104(3):548–551.

Ito, M., Takata, S., Tatsugami, M., Wada, W., Imagawa, S., et al. (2009). Clinical prevention of gastric cancer by *Helicobacter pylori* eradication therapy: a systemic review. *Journal of Gastroenterology,* 44:365–371.

Last, E. J., & Sheehan, A. H. (2009). Review of recent evidence: Potential interaction between clopidogrel and proton pump inhibitors. *American Journal Health-System Pharmacy,* 66:2117–2122.

Lin, P. C., Chang, C. H., Hsu, P. I., Tseng, P. L., & Huang, Y. B. (2010). The efficacy and safety of proton pump inhibitors vs histamine-2 receptor antagonists for stress ulcer bleeding prophylaxis among critical care patients: A meta analysis. *Critical Care Medicine,* 38(4):1197–1205.

Micromedex Healthcare Series. Retrieved from *http://thomsonhc.com.*

Naeim, A., Dy, S. M., Lorenz, K. D., Sanati, H., Walling, A., & Asch, S. M. (2008). Evidence-based recommendations for cancer nausea and vomiting. *Journal of Clinical Oncology,* 28(23):3903–3910.

Navari, R. M. (2009). Pharmacological management of chemotherapy-induced nausea and vomiting. *Drugs,* 69(5):515–533.

Roila, F., Herrstedt, J., Aapro, M., et al. (2010). Guideline update for MASCC and ESMO in the prevention of chemotherapy- and radiotherapy-induced nausea and vomiting: results of the Perugia consensus conference, *Annals of Oncology,* 21(Suppl 5):v232–v243.

Rupinow, M. F. T., Chang, A. H., Shacter, R. D., Owens, D. K., & Parsonnet, J. (2009). Cost effectiveness of a potential pro-phylactic *Helicobacter pylori* vaccine in the Unites States. *The Journal of Infectious Diseases,* 200:1311–1317.

Targownik, L.E., Lix, L.M., Leung, S., et al. (2010). Proton-pump inhibitor use is not associated with osteoporosis or accelerated bone mineral density loss, *Gastroenterology,* 138(3):896–904.

Thomson, A. B., Sauve, M. D., Kassam, N., et al. (2010). Safety of the long-term use of proton pump inhibitors, *World Journal of Gastroenterology,* 16(19):2323–2330.

Vilaichone, R. K., Mahachai, V., & Graham, D. Y. (2006). *Helicobacter pylori* diagnosis and management. *Gastroenterology Clinics of North America,* 35(2):229–247.

White, P. F., Tang, J., Song, D., et al. (2007). Transdermal sco-polamine: An alternative to ondansetron and droperidol for the prevention of postoperative and postdischarge emetic symp-toms. *Anesthesia and Analgesia,* 104(1):92–96.

Yang, L. P. H., & Scott, L. J. (2009). Palonosetron: In the prevention of nausea and vomiting. *Drugs,* 69(16): 2257–2258.

37

Drugs Affecting the Lower Gastrointestinal Tract

Learning Objectives

At the completion of this chapter the student will:

1. Identify core drug knowledge about drugs that affect the lower gastrointestinal (GI) tract.

2. Identify core patient variables related to drugs that affect the lower GI tract.

3. Relate the interaction of core drug knowledge to core patient variables for drugs that affect the lower GI tract.

4. Generate a nursing plan of care from the interactions between core drug knowledge and core patient variables for drugs that affect the lower GI tract.

5. Describe nursing interventions to maximize therapeutic effects and minimize adverse effects for drugs that affect the lower GI tract.

6. Determine key points for patient and family education for drugs that affect the lower GI tract.

Key Terms

constipation
Crohn disease
diarrhea

fecal impaction
flatus
inflammatory bowel disease (IBD)

irritable bowel syndrome (IBS)
peristalsis
ulcerative colitis

Drugs Affecting the Lower Gastrointestinal Tract

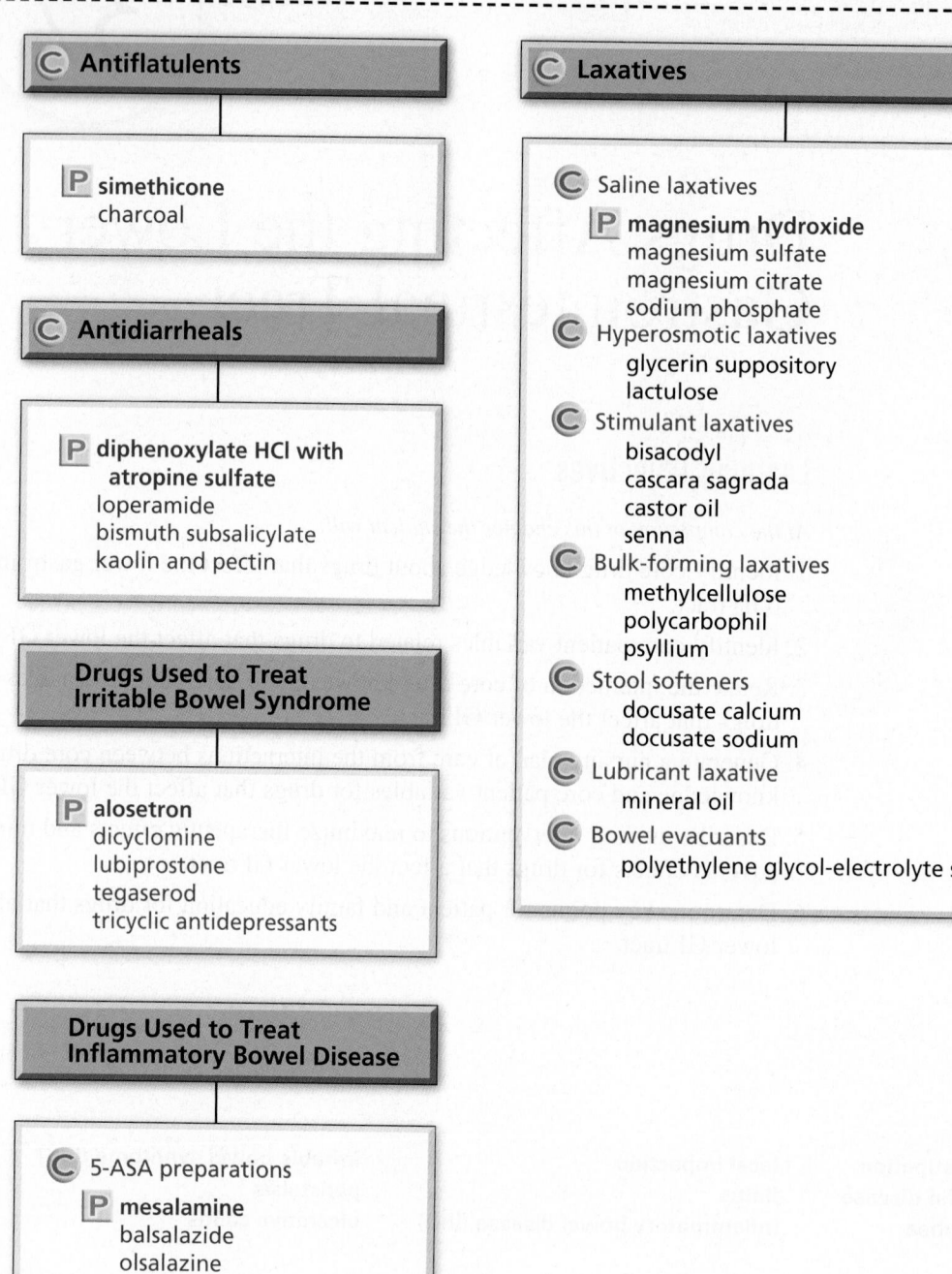

© Antiflatulents

P **simethicone**
charcoal

© Antidiarrheals

P **diphenoxylate HCl with atropine sulfate**
loperamide
bismuth subsalicylate
kaolin and pectin

Drugs Used to Treat Irritable Bowel Syndrome

P **alosetron**
dicyclomine
lubiprostone
tegaserod
tricyclic antidepressants

Drugs Used to Treat Inflammatory Bowel Disease

© 5-ASA preparations

P **mesalamine**
balsalazide
olsalazine
sulfasalazine
infliximab

© Laxatives

© Saline laxatives

P **magnesium hydroxide**
magnesium sulfate
magnesium citrate
sodium phosphate
© Hyperosmotic laxatives
glycerin suppository
lactulose
© Stimulant laxatives
bisacodyl
cascara sagrada
castor oil
senna
© Bulk-forming laxatives
methylcellulose
polycarbophil
psyllium
© Stool softeners
docusate calcium
docusate sodium
© Lubricant laxative
mineral oil
© Bowel evacuants
polyethylene glycol-electrolyte solution

The symbol **©** indicates the drug class.
Drugs in **bold type** marked with the symbol **P** are prototypes.
Drugs in blue type are closely related to the prototype.
Drugs in red type are significantly different from the prototype.
Drugs in black type with no symbol are also used in drug therapy; no prototype.

This chapter discusses drugs used to treat the most common alterations of the lower gastrointestinal (GI) tract, including flatus (gas), diarrhea, constipation, irritable bowel syndrome, and irritable bowel disease. All are digestive disorders. Their occurrence may be mild and episodic or severe, debilitating, and chronic. Patients may self-treat these problems with over-the-counter (OTC) medications, or they may seek medical attention. These problems may be related to other drug therapy, diet, emotions, or changes in activity. The drug classes used to treat flatus, diarrhea, and constipation are called antiflatulents, antidiarrheals, and laxatives, respectively. In addition, drugs used to treat irritable bowel syndrome and inflammatory bowel disease (including ulcerative colitis and Crohn disease) are presented.

Some drugs begin acting in the lower GI tract. However, their therapeutic uses are for alterations of other systems. These drugs include potassium-removing resins, such as sodium polystyrene sulfonate (Kayexalate), and a lipid-lowering agent, such as cholestyramine (Questran). These drugs are discussed in Chapters 26 and 31, respectively.

PHYSIOLOGY

The large intestine is approximately 5 feet long (1.5 m) and 2.5 inches (6.5 cm) in diameter. The longitudinal muscle fibers on the outer surface of the large intestine are in three layers and do not cover the entire colon uniformly. This arrangement of the muscle exerts a tension on the wall of the intestine, drawing it up and giving it a puckered appearance.

The large intestine is composed of the cecum, colon, rectum, and anal canal. The cecum, located on the right side of the abdomen, is a small pouch-like structure. The appendix is a blind tube of lymphoid tissue attached to the cecum. The colon has four sections—ascending, transverse, descending, and sigmoid. The area immediately after the sigmoid colon is the rectum, which is followed by the anal canal. The anal canal has two sphincters—the internal and the external.

The contents from the small intestine enter the cecum through the ileocecal valve. **Peristalsis,** wave-like muscular contractions and squeezing of the intestines, moves the contents through the small and large intestines. The movement of fecal material into the rectum triggers defecation. The distended rectum activates the defecation reflex, relaxing both the internal and external anal sphincters. As peristaltic action increases, the diaphragm lowers, and the abdominal muscles contract, forcing the feces out of the body through the anus. Defecation is controlled in the healthy person by maintaining a contracted external anal sphincter. The normally brown color of fecal material is caused by the breakdown of bilirubin. The normal content of fecal matter includes dead bacteria, fat, inorganic matter, protein, dried digestive juices, and indigestible components of food.

Large amounts of mucus are secreted by goblet cells in the epithelial layer of the large intestine. This mucus protects the epithelial surface from abrasive fecal material and aids in holding the fecal material together. Certain bacteria normally present in the large intestine produce some needed vitamins, including vitamin K, vitamin B_{12}, riboflavin, and thiamine. The bacteria produce gases that contribute to the formation of flatus.

During the movement of stomach contents through the large intestine, water and some electrolytes are reabsorbed. Absorption of fluid and electrolytes occurs primarily in the proximal colon. The longer the contents remain in the large intestine, the greater the amount of water that is reabsorbed (Figure 37.1).

PATHOPHYSIOLOGY

Flatus

Flatus is a normal by-product of digestion. Flatus becomes problematic, causing discomfort or pain from excessive production (caused by ingesting gas-producing foods) or from an inability to pass the gas through the large intestine (a disruption of peristalsis, such as occurs temporarily after surgery).

Diarrhea

Diarrhea is the frequent passage of loose or liquid stools. It is a symptom rather than a disease. Causes include decreased fluid absorption, increased fluid secretion, or motility disturbances. Decreased fluid absorption may result from malabsorption syndrome, lactulose intolerance, osmotic diarrhea, or mucosal injury due to celiac disease, Crohn disease, radiation injury, ulcerative colitis, or ischemic bowel disease. Increased fluid secretion most frequently results from infectious bacterial endotoxins such as *Vibrio cholerae, Escherichia coli, Shigella, Salmonella, Staphylococcus,* and *Clostridium difficile,* as well as viral agents such as rotavirus and parasites such as *Giardia lamblia.* Other causes of increased fluid secretion include gastrin secretion from Zollinger-Ellison syndrome, calcitonin secretion from carcinoma of the thyroid, and polypeptide secretion from adenoma of the pancreas. The motility disturbance that most frequently causes diarrhea is irritable bowel syndrome. Patients with a previous gastrectomy may experience "dumping syndrome" that leads to increased motility and diarrhea.

Diarrhea may be acute or chronic. Acute diarrhea is usually self-limiting or responds to treatment within 48 hours. It is generally associated with bacterial or viral infections. Symptoms include explosive diarrhea, tenesmus (spasmodic contraction of the anal sphincter with pain and persistent desire to defecate), and abdominal cramping. Anal skin irritation frequently occurs because of the frequency of liquid stool. In contrast, chronic diarrhea lasts more than 4 weeks. It is associated with chronic disease states. Chronic diarrhea can be life-threatening due to electrolyte imbalance, acid-base imbalance, or dehydration. Malabsorption and malnutrition are other complications. Children and the

PHYSIOLOGY

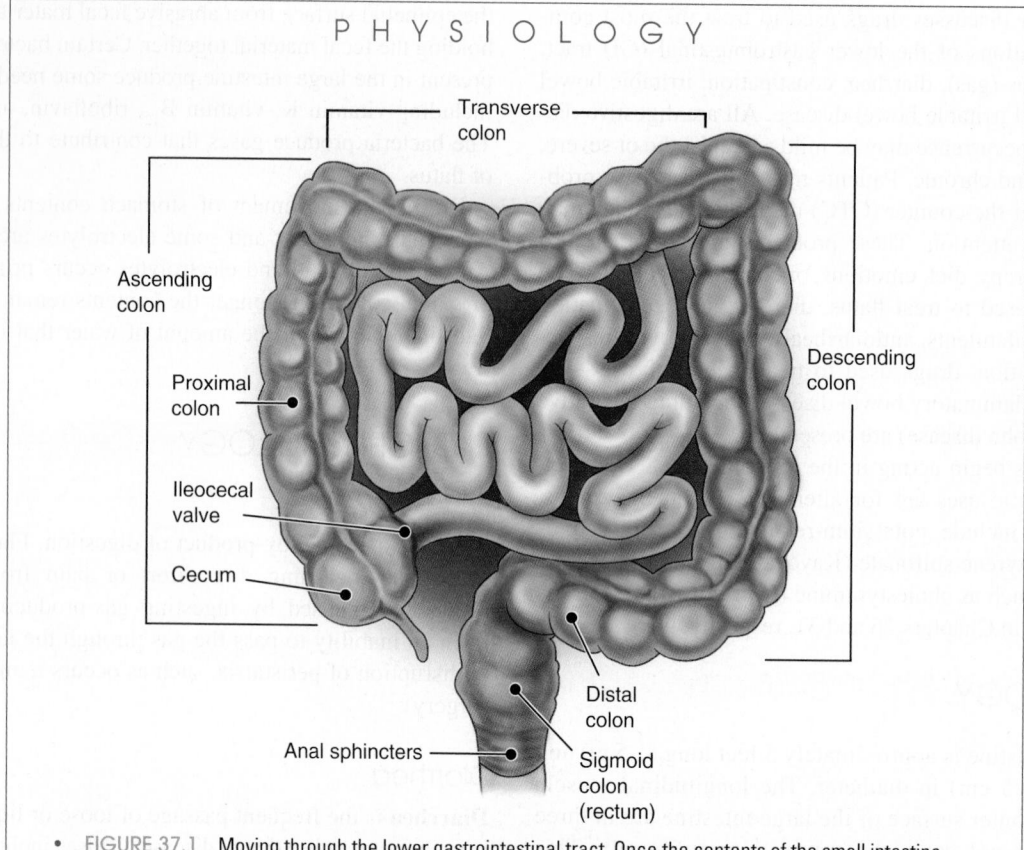

Transverse
colon

Ascending
colon

Descending
colon

Proximal
colon

Ileocecal
valve

Cecum

Distal
colon

Anal sphincters

Sigmoid
colon
(rectum)

• FIGURE 37.1 Moving through the lower gastrointestinal tract. Once the contents of the small intestine enter the cecum through the ileocecal valve, they are transported through the large intestine by peristalsis (wave-like propulsion of gastric contents). The three segments of the large intestine are termed the ascending colon, the transverse colon, and the descending colon. When the contents leave the distal colon and enter the sigmoid colon (rectum), the distended rectum activates the defecation reflex, which causes the internal and external anal sphincters to relax. As peristaltic activity increases, the diaphragm lowers and the abdominal muscles contract, forcing the feces out of the body through the anus. Certain bacteria normally present in the intestine produce gases that are commonly known as flatus. Absorption of fluid and electrolytes occurs primarily in the proximal colon, although some absorption occurs throughout the length of the large intestine. The longer the contents remain in the large intestine, the more water is absorbed.

elderly are most vulnerable. Treatment of the underlying disease usually eliminates the diarrhea. However, when diarrhea becomes chronic, antidiarrheal drug therapy may be needed for an extended period.

Constipation and Fecal Impaction

Constipation is infrequent or incomplete passage of hard stools resulting from a decrease in peristaltic activity and slow movement of fecal material through the colon. This slow movement through the colon allows more water to be absorbed from the feces, resulting in hard, dry stools. The hard, dry fecal material is more difficult to pass and can cause painful defecation. Other symptoms associated with constipation include abdominal distention or bloating, increased flatulence, increased rectal pressure, straining, and tenesmus. Box 37.1 presents possible causes of constipation.

Normal bowel frequency varies substantially among individuals. "Normal" may range from a bowel movement 3 times a day to one every 3 days. For this reason, an individual's

definition may not reflect the actual slowed movement through the colon and the resultant dry, hard stools.

Prolonged constipation may lead to **fecal impaction,** in which the patient is unable to pass the hardened mass of feces. Fecal impaction may be resistant to pharmacotherapy, and digital stool removal may be required.

Irritable Bowel Syndrome

Irritable bowel syndrome (IBS) is a common disorder of the intestines characterized by altered bowel habits and abnormal sensations (discomfort or pain) in the absence of specific organic pathology. In the United States, IBS is the most common GI diagnosis made by gastroenterologists, affecting 10% to 20% of the general population.

IBS is a complex syndrome with a varying clinical presentation. For some people, the primary problem is diarrhea; for some, it is constipation; and for others, it is alternating diarrhea and constipation. No definitive test exists for IBS; thus, a clear diagnosis is difficult. A consensus panel of gastroenterologists has developed a set of conditions for the diagnosis

Box 37.1 CAUSES OF CONSTIPATION

Colonic Disorders

- IBS
- Diverticular disease
- Inflammatory strictures
- Luminal obstruction
- Rectocele

Metabolic/Endocrine Systemic Disorders

- Hypothyroidism
- Diabetes mellitus
- Hypokalemia
- Pheochromocytoma
- Pregnancy

Neurologic Disorders

- Multiple sclerosis
- Parkinson disease
- Spinal cord lesions
- Cerebrovascular accident
- Autonomic neuropathy

Drug Induced

- Laxative abuse
- Opioids
- Anticholinergics
- Antihypertensives
- Antidepressants
- Antacids (calcium and aluminum)
- Calcium and iron supplements

Box 37.2 ROME III CRITERIA USED IN THE DIAGNOSIS OF IRRITABLE BOWEL SYNDROME

The patient must have recurrent abdominal pain or discomfort at least 3 d/mo during the previous 3 months that is associated with two or more of the following:

- Improvement with defecation
- Onset associated with a change in frequency of stool
- Onset associated with a change in form (appearance) of stool

Supporting symptoms include the following:

- Altered stool frequency
- Altered stool form
- Altered stool passage (straining and/or urgency)
- Mucorrhea
- Abdominal bloating or subjective distention

of IBS known as the Rome III Criteria (Box 37.2). There are four subtypes of IBS: IBS-D (diarrhea predominant), IBS-C (constipation predominant), IBS-A (alternating diarrhea and constipation), and IBS-M (mixed diarrhea and constipation).

IBS is called a functional disorder because no evidence of disease is seen when the colon is examined. It does not lead to any serious, organic diseases, and it does not cause cancer of the bowel. IBS has not been linked to inflammatory bowel diseases such as Crohn disease or ulcerative colitis. However, IBS is a chronic disorder that can be very painful, limiting the ability of a person to fully participate in life, diminishing quality of life, and incurring substantial cost.

The symptoms of IBS are painful diarrhea or constipation, or diarrhea that alternates with constipation. Other symptoms are crampy abdominal pain, bloating, gas pain, excessive flatulence, increased belching, mucus in the stool, small stools ("rabbit-like pellets"), or flat "ribbon" stools. Bleeding, fever, weight loss, and persistent severe pain are not symptoms of IBS and may indicate other problems. IBS symptoms negatively affect general health, vitality, social functioning, bodily pain, diet, sexual function, and sleep, and they also contribute to time lost from work.

For individuals with IBS, the symptoms of spastic contractions may be triggered by stress because the bowel is controlled partly by the nervous system. However, IBS is not related to a personality disorder; it is a disorder of digestion. Stress management or use of stress-reduction techniques may help relieve some of the symptoms or make them less severe. Diet also can trigger flares of IBS. An increase in peristalsis is normal after eating. For people with IBS, strong contractions of the colon may come sooner after eating than usual, accompanied by cramps and diarrhea. Because fat is a strong stimulus for colonic contractions, eating a high-fat meal induces contractions in some people that may be stronger or more violent than usual. Large meals also can cause cramping and diarrhea in people with IBS. Lack of fiber may potentiate constipation in IBS. Finally, women with IBS experience more symptoms when they have their menstrual period, which is hypothesized to be related to female sex hormones increasing the susceptibility of the colon to spasm.

The exact cause of IBS is not known. The theory of IBS pathogenesis includes altered GI motility and visceral hyperalgesia. In IBS, the bowel is hypersensitive and overreacts to mild stimulation. The normal distention of the bowel that can occur with food intake, gas, or a high-fiber diet can be enough to trigger IBS. Thus, patients with IBS exhibit pain and discomfort at lower volumes of gastric distention than occur in patients who do not have IBS. Some researchers also believe that psychopathology may contribute to IBS. Whether psychopathology induces the development of IBS or IBS induces the development of psychopathology is unclear.

It is not unusual for the symptoms of one subtype of IBS to change to those of another; therefore, treatment of IBS focuses on the symptoms the patient is currently experiencing. Although antidiarrheals, antispasmodics, and laxatives are commonly used, some patients require drugs that either stimulate or block serotonin (5-HT$_3$) receptors. Serotonin is a primary neurotransmitter affecting the enteric tract, and it plays a role in visceral sensation and the normal functioning of the tract, including secretion and motility. Abnormalities in motility and visceral sensation correspond to the pathology of many of the symptoms of IBS. Although seven serotonin receptor sites have been identified, 5-HT$_3$ and 5 HT$_4$ receptors are the most important sites in IBS.

Lifestyle modification may also be used in the treatment of patients with IBS. However, research has not shown that stress reduction or dietary modification is helpful or effective in all patients with IBS. Even in patients who experience a positive effect, these lifestyle modifications may not replace the need for drug therapy.

Inflammatory Bowel Disease

Inflammatory bowel disease (IBD) is a general term that includes both ulcerative colitis and Crohn disease. **Ulcerative colitis** is an inflammatory disease of the large intestine in which ulcers form in the mucosa of the colon or rectum. Diarrhea, blood, and pus may result. **Crohn disease** is an inflammation extending into the deeper layers of the intestinal wall. It is most often found in the ileum and the cecum. However, Crohn disease can develop anywhere along the intestines. It may cause ulcers along the entire colon, form a string of ulcers in one part of the colon, or cause multiple scattered clusters of ulcers in the colon. The main symptom of IBD is diarrhea, which may, especially in ulcerative colitis, contain blood. Constipation also may develop during active flare-ups. Cramps and intestinal pain may occur. Fever, fatigue, loss of appetite, and weight loss also may occur.

Approximately 1 to 2 million Americans have IBD (the wide variation is because of the difficulty of diagnosing IBD and because people may have long remissions and not be identified as having IBD). Men and women seem to be affected equally. IBD most often is diagnosed between 15 and 40 years of age. Jewish Americans of European descent have a risk for IBD that is five times that of the general population. IBD is more common among city dwellers than country dwellers and is more prevalent in developed countries.

Although the exact cause is not known, genetic factors have been implicated. Up to 25% of people with IBD have family members with the disease. Genetic abnormalities linked to the two disorders may share locations on chromosomes 1, 3, 4, 7, 12, and 16. Some researchers believe that the disease develops in people who have a genetic susceptibility that allows an agent, such as a virus or bacterium, to trigger an abnormal immune response. When an organism injures the lining of the intestine in a normal, healthy person, the immune system reduces the inflammation and injury by producing suppressor T cells. In people with

IBD, however, when an organism injures the lining of the intestine, the immune system produces helper T cells. Helper T cells produce a protein called a cytokine. Cytokines cause intestinal inflammation and damage, which attract even more helper T cells to the area. Because IBD is more prevalent in industrialized countries, environmental factors, such as diet, are believed to also play a role in producing IBD. No clear insight into this phenomenon is yet available from research.

Post-operative Ileus

Post-operative ileus is a temporary decrease in gastrointestinal motility observed in patients after undergoing gastrointestinal, as well as other procedures requiring general anesthesia (Bream-Rouwnehorst and Cantrell, 2009). Opiate receptors are located in the gastrointestinal tract and play a role in gastrointestinal motility, secretion, and transportation of electrolytes. Secondary to surgical manipulation or trauma, inhibitory sympathetic neural reflexes are triggered in the gut, resulting in decreased gastrointestinal mobility. Post-operative ileus is most often associated with bowel manipulation or surgical trauma, and usually resolves within 24 to 72 hours.

C ANTIFLATULENTS

Antiflatulents decrease gas production, coalesce gas bubbles, and facilitate the passage of gas through belching and expelling flatus. Antiflatulents include simethicone and charcoal. The prototype antiflatulent is simethicone (Mylicon) Table 37.1. It is available alone or combined with antacids and digestants (see Chapter 36).

Nursing Management of the Patient Receiving P Simethicone
Core Drug Knowledge
Pharmacotherapeutics
Antiflatulents are drugs used to relieve the discomfort of excess gas in the GI tract caused by swallowing air, postoperative gas distention, peptic ulcer, spastic or irritable colon, or diverticulitis. These drugs relieve pain and discomfort by promoting belching and the passing of flatus.

Pharmacokinetics
Simethicone is inert and is not absorbed from the GI tract. Because the drug is inactive, it is excreted unchanged in feces and does not interfere with absorption of water

TABLE 37.1	Summary of Selected C Antiflatulent Drugs		
Drug (Trade) Name	Selected Indications	Route and Dosage Range	Pharmacokinetics
P simethicone (Mylanta Gas, Gas Relief, Gas-X, Major-Con, Phazyme, Flatulex, Mylicon)	Relief of symptoms and pressure from excess gas in intestinal tract	*Adult:* PO, 125-mg capsules qid with meals; 40–125-mg tablets qid with meals; 40–80-mg drops qid up to 500 mg/d *Child <2 y:* PO, 20 mg qid up to 240 mg/d *Child 2–12 y:* 40 mg qid	*Onset:* Not absorbed systemically *Duration:* None t$_{1/2}$: None

or nutrients or the secretion of mucus in the GI tract. Simethicone is not distributed systemically in the body and is excreted unchanged in the feces. It begins to act immediately in the GI tract and has a duration of approximately 3 hours. Its peak and half-life are unknown.

Pharmacodynamics

Simethicone has a defoaming action that alters the surface tension of gas bubbles. As the surface tension is changed, gas bubbles unite, forming larger gas bubbles that are eliminated more easily by belching or expulsion as flatus. It also is combined with antacids to decrease flatulence, but it has no antacid properties. An off-label use is treating the symptoms of infant colic.

Contraindications and Precautions

Simethicone has no contraindications or precautions.

Adverse Effects

No substantial adverse reactions have been reported with the use of simethicone.

Drug Interactions

No drug interactions with simethicone are known.

Assessment of Relevant Core Patient Variables

Health Status

Before administering simethicone, assess for abdominal pain, distention, and bowel sounds.

Lifestyle, Diet, and Habits

Assess the patient's dietary choices for gas-producing foods such as cucumbers, cabbage, onions, beans, and radishes.

Environment

Simethicone is easily self-administered and can be given in any setting. Some preparations are available OTC.

Nursing Diagnosis and Outcome

• Acute Pain related to the presence of flatus
  Desired outcome: *Within 2 to 3 hours of using simethicone, the patient will experience a decrease in abdominal pain and distention.*

Planning and Intervention

Maximizing Therapeutic Effects

Simethicone should be given after meals and at bedtime to increase its effectiveness. Have the patient chew tablets thoroughly or allow them to dissolve in the mouth to promote dispersion. The suspension form of the drug must be shaken to ensure that the active ingredients are well dispersed.

To ensure accuracy of dosing liquid forms of the drug, use or teach the patient to use a calibrated dropper. When administering to infants, simethicone should be mixed

with 30 mL of a suitable liquid, preferably formula or cool water.

Providing Patient and Family Education

• Teach patients to take simethicone after each meal and at bedtime, to chew tablets thoroughly before swallowing, and to shake the liquid suspension form well before measuring a dose.
• Tell patients to expect to pass gas and have increased belching after taking this drug.
• Caution patients not to increase the dosage unless instructed to do so by the prescriber.
• Instruct patients to avoid gas-producing foods. A high-fiber diet increases peristalsis, and a low-fat diet decreases production of carbon dioxide gas.

Ongoing Assessment and Evaluation

Assess abdominal pain and distention periodically throughout simethicone therapy to monitor the effectiveness of the drug. It is effective if abdominal distention is decreased and the patient reports feeling more comfortable. If effectiveness is not observed, the dose may need to be increased. Verify that the patient does not have any increase in abdominal pain, nausea, vomiting, or fever because these findings are not symptoms of excessive flatus and may indicate that the patient requires medical attention.

Drug Closely Related to P Simethicone

Charcoal is an absorbing, detoxifying, and soothing agent. The drug relieves gas and cramping by absorbing toxins and gas on the surfaces of its carbon particles. Like simethicone, it is useful for the relief of gas, diarrhea, and GI distress associated with indigestion and cramping.

Unlike simethicone, charcoal is used as an antidote in poisonings from drug overdose because it reduces absorption of certain drugs and chemicals and can actually remove them from the systemic circulation. Charcoal also is used for preventing nonspecific pruritus associated with kidney dialysis. It should not be given to children younger than 3 years of age. Charcoal can be combined with simethicone to treat gas pains; the charcoal decreases the amount of gas produced, and the simethicone promotes elimination of gas.

MEMORY CHIP

P Simethicone

• Relieves the pain of excess gas in the GI tract; antifoaming action changes surface tension of gas bubbles, causing them to coalesce and pass more easily
• Most important patient education: Chew tablets to promote effectiveness; take after meals and at bedtime.

C ANTIDIARRHEALS

Antidiarrheals slow intestinal motility, allowing time for fluid reabsorption and better stool formation. The most effective antidiarrheal drugs include opiate derivatives, the opiates themselves, and loperamide, a drug related to the antipsychotic drug haloperidol. These drugs act systemically to reduce intestinal motility and slow peristalsis. Several locally acting drugs are available OTC and are effective in mild cases of diarrhea The prototype antidiarrheal drug is diphenoxylate HCl with atropine sulfate (Lomotil, Lonox) (Table 37.2).

Nursing Management of the Patient Receiving P Diphenoxylate HCl with Atropine Sulfate

Core Drug Knowledge

Pharmacotherapeutics

Diphenoxylate HCl with atropine sulfate is used as an adjunct in treating diarrhea.

Pharmacokinetics

Diphenoxylate HCl with atropine sulfate is absorbed readily in the GI tract. When the tablet form is used instead of the solution, bioavailability is decreased by approximately 10%. Diphenoxylate HCl with atropine sulfate is found in breast milk; however, the distribution is unknown. The drug is metabolized in the liver to difenoxin, which is an active metabolite that produces the desired therapeutic effects. It leaves the liver as bile and is excreted in feces. A tiny amount is excreted unchanged in the urine.

Pharmacodynamics

Diphenoxylate HCl with atropine sulfate is a synthetic narcotic similar in structure to meperidine, and it is classified as a schedule V drug. The dosage used in treating diarrhea is not high enough to provide pain relief. The drug acts on the smooth muscle of the intestine to slow intestinal motility and prolong intestinal transit time, allowing for the reabsorption of fluid. This preparation is very effective in treating diarrhea. A small amount of atropine sulfate is combined with diphenoxylate to discourage deliberate abuse. When excessive dosages are taken, the adverse reactions of atropine sulfate, which include dry mouth and tachycardia, are particularly unpleasant.

Contraindications and Precautions

Hypersensitivity to diphenoxylate HCl with atropine sulfate or to atropine sulfate alone is a contraindication. Use is contraindicated for diarrhea caused by GI organisms that penetrate the gastric mucosa (e.g., *Shigella*, *Salmonella*, and some toxic strains of *E. coli*) because the drug slows peristalsis and may aggravate and prolong the diarrhea. The drug is contraindicated in patients with pseudomembranous colitis that occurs with broad-spectrum antibiotic therapy because it may worsen and prolong diarrhea. It also is contraindicated in patients

TABLE 37.2	Summary of Selected C Antidiarrheal Drugs			
P diphenoxylate HCl with atropine sulfate (Lomotil, Lonox, Logen, Lomanate)	Acute diarrhea	*Adult:* PO, 5 mg qid *Child 2–12 y:* 0.3–0.4 mg/kg/d in 4 doses		*Onset:* Unknown *Duration:* Unknown $t_{1/2}$: 12–14 h
bismuth subsalicylate (Pepto-Bismol, Bismatrol, Kao-Tin, Kaopectate)	Indigestion, nausea, diarrhea (including traveler's diarrhea), abdominal cramps	*Adult:* PO, 2 tablets or 30 mL every 30 min to 1 h as needed, up to 8 doses in 24 h *Child 9–12 y:* PO, 1 tablet or 15 mL *Child 6–9 y:* ⅔ tablet or 10 mL *Child 3–6 y:* ⅓ tablet or 5 mL, same dosing schedule as for adults		bismuth subsalicylate (Pepto-Bismol, Bismatrol, Pink Bismuth, Kaopectate)
loperamide (Imodium, Kaopectate II Caplets, Pepto Diarrhea Control)	Acute and chronic diarrhea	*Adult (acute):* PO, 4 mg initially, then 2 mg after each loose stool, not to exceed 16 mg/d; *Adult (chronic):* 4 mg initially, then 2 mg after each loose stool until diarrhea controlled *Child (acute):* PO, first day, 13–20 kg weight, 1 mg tid; 20–30 kg, 2 mg bid; >30 kg, 2 mg tid; after first day, 1 mg/10 kg after loose stools (not to exceed first-day recommended doses) *Child (chronic):* not established		loperamide (Imodium, Kaopectate II Caplets, Pepto Diarrhea Control)
	OTC: traveler's diarrhea (acute diarrhea)	*Adult:* PO, 4 mg initially, then 2 mg after each loose stool, no more than 8 mg/d for no more than 2 d *Child 9–11 y:* PO, 2 mg initially, then 1 mg after each loose stool up to 6 mg/d for no more than 2 d *Child 6–8 y:* 1 mg initially and after each loose stool up to 4 mg/d for up to 2 d		

with obstructive jaundice caused by hepatic impairment. Diphenoxylate HCl with atropine sulfate is contraindicated in children younger than 2 years of age. The drug is a pregnancy category C drug.

Caution is used when administering diphenoxylate HCl with atropine sulfate to patients with advanced hepatic and renal disease because of the risk of hepatic coma, to those with ulcerative colitis because of the risk of inducing toxic megacolon, and to those with severe dehydration because it may cause variability of drug response that may predispose to delayed diphenoxylate intoxication. Caution should be used in lactating women and in children because adverse effects from the atropine sulfate are more likely to occur in these patients. Children with Down syndrome are at special risk of atropine sulfate toxicity when taking diphenoxylate, even if it is taken in recommended doses. Although diphenoxylate HCl with atropine sulfate does not produce morphine-like effects or addiction in recommended dosages, at high doses, addiction can occur.

Adverse Effects

The most common adverse effects of diphenoxylate HCl with atropine sulfate are drowsiness and dizziness related to the drug's chemical similarity to meperidine, an opioid. Dry mouth and other anticholinergic effects (e.g., flushing, tachycardia, hyperthermia, and urinary retention) from the atropine in the drug are not common in adults receiving normal, therapeutic doses of diphenoxylate HCl, although the risk of these effects is greater in children. Diphenoxylate HCl with atropine sulfate also may have the following adverse effects:

- GI: nausea, vomiting, abdominal discomfort, paralytic ileus, toxic megacolon, and pancreatitis
- Central nervous system (CNS): sedation, headache, malaise, lethargy, restlessness, euphoria, depression, and numbness of extremities
- Allergic: pruritus, swelling of gums, angioneurotic edema, urticaria, and anaphylaxis

Drug Interactions

When diphenoxylate HCl with atropine sulfate is given to patients taking monoamine oxidase inhibitors (MAOIs), the combination of the two drugs could precipitate a hypertensive crisis because diphenoxylate is similar chemically to meperidine. The antidiarrheal drug may potentiate the depressive effects of alcohol, barbiturates, and tranquilizers. Table 37.3 lists drugs that interact with diphenoxylate HCl with atropine sulfate.

Assessment of Relevant Core Patient Variables

Health Status

Before administering diphenoxylate HCl with atropine sulfate, assess the patient for abdominal pain and distention to have a baseline for monitoring therapy. Auscultate bowel sounds. Patients with diarrhea usually have frequent, high-pitched bowel sounds. Assess the condition of mucous membranes and the skin for signs of dehydration. It is necessary to assess and document pertinent information about stools; this includes frequency, color, consistency, and odor. Examine laboratory reports of stool specimens and do not administer diphenoxylate HCl with atropine sulfate if stool cultures are positive for *E. coli, Salmonella, Shigella,* or *C. difficile.* Determine whether the patient has a diagnosis of hepatic impairment, obstructive jaundice, pseudomembranous colitis, or ulcerative colitis. While taking a drug history, determine whether the patient is receiving MAOIs. Report any positive findings to the health care provider. If the patient is a child, observe for Down syndrome.

Life Span and Gender

Determine whether the patient is pregnant or breast-feeding because diphenoxylate HCl with atropine sulfate is a pregnancy category C drug. If the patient is a child, verify that he or she is older than 2 years of age. In children aged 2 to 12 years, liquid diphenoxylate is recommended. Monitor children and elderly patients closely because they have an increased risk of atropine toxicity.

Lifestyle, Diet, and Habits

Determine whether the patient has a history of substance abuse because it may make the patient more likely to use diphenoxylate HCl with atropine sulfate inappropriately. Assess the patient's use of alcohol. Encourage the patient to refrain from alcohol while taking diphenoxylate.

TABLE 37.3	Agents That Interact with ⓟ Diphenoxylate HCl with Atropine Sulfate	
Interactants	**Effect and Significance**	**Nursing Management**
monoamine oxidase inhibitors	Chemical structure of diphenoxylate similar to meperidine—hypertensive crisis possible	Administer together cautiously. Monitor blood pressure.
barbiturates, tranquilizers, and alcohol	Depressant effect on central nervous system may be potentiated, leading to respiratory depression or sedation	Monitor for sedation. Monitor vital signs. Ensure safety.

Environment

Although diphenoxylate HCl with atropine sulfate requires a prescription, oral doses are easily self-administered and can be given in any setting.

Culture and Inherited Traits

Cultural and social variations exist regarding how regular bowel movements and diarrhea are defined. Determine the patient's perception of normal elimination and diarrhea.

Nursing Diagnoses and Outcomes

• Diarrhea related to the causative factor (if identified)
  Desired outcome: *Diarrhea will be controlled through use of diphenoxylate HCl with atropine sulfate.*
• Risk for Injury related to drowsiness and dizziness secondary to drug therapy
  Desired outcome: *The patient will not sustain injury from drug therapy.*

Planning and Intervention

Maximizing Therapeutic Effects

To maximize the therapeutic effect, administer diphenoxylate HCl with atropine sulfate as ordered, four times daily, to obtain therapeutic results. Use the dropper provided when administering liquid preparations to ensure the correct dose.

Minimizing Adverse Effects

Decrease the dosage of diphenoxylate HCl with atropine sulfate when the number of stools decreases. The recommended dosage should not be exceeded. If the patient's condition does not improve with the maximum daily dose for 10 days, diarrhea symptoms are unlikely to be controlled with further use of the drug. In such cases, assess for adverse effects. Assess for toxic megacolon (abdominal distention and pain are possible indications). Because the massive dilation and atony of the colon from toxic megacolon can result in serious complications, signs of abdominal distention should be reported immediately.

Assess for and report signs of atropine sulfate toxicity (e.g., dry mouth, flushing, hypothermia, tachycardia, and urinary retention) because this condition requires immediate treatment. Children must be assessed very carefully because they are especially susceptible to atropine sulfate toxicity.

Providing Patient and Family Education

• Teach patients not to exceed the prescribed dosage and to lower the dosage as instructed as soon as symptoms of diarrhea are controlled. Furthermore, if a dose is missed, instruct the patient not to take two doses.
• Instruct patients to notify the prescriber if diarrhea persists for more than 2 days.
• Encourage patients to avoid alcohol and other CNS depressants and not to drive or perform tasks that require mental alertness until the effects of diphenoxylate HCl with atropine sulfate on the individual are known.

CRITICAL THINKING SCENARIO

DIPHENOXYLATE IN ANTIDIARRHEAL THERAPY

Mr. Rothberg is 46 years old. He enters the emergency clinic with complaints of acute diarrhea for the last 36 hours. He also complains of abdominal pain and cramping. "Every time I eat," he says, "I have to run to the bathroom. I can't seem to keep anything in."

1. What questions would you ask when assessing Mr. Rothberg's condition?
2. After assessment is completed, Mr. Rothberg is diagnosed as having diarrhea secondary to an acute viral illness of the GI tract. He is given a prescription for diphenoxylate HCl with atropine sulfate. What additional core patient variables need to be assessed to provide patient education geared to Mr. Rothberg's personal learning needs?

• Caution patients to maintain adequate fluid intake during periods of diarrhea to prevent dehydration and electrolyte imbalance.
• Caution patients to store diphenoxylate HCl with atropine sulfate out of the reach of children.
• For liquid forms of diphenoxylate HCl with atropine sulfate, tell patients not to use a household teaspoon to measure doses but rather a specially marked dropper or measuring spoon.
• If dry mouth occurs, recommend that patients suck on hard candy or sip water.

Ongoing Assessment and Evaluation

In patients who take diphenoxylate HCl with atropine sulfate, it is important to assess skin turgor and mucous membranes for loss of moisture because these signs indicate dehydration. Monitoring electrolyte laboratory reports for electrolyte imbalance that may occur with the loss of fluid through diarrhea is also a priority. Weakness, muscular cramping, or dizziness should be reported because they are subjective symptoms of electrolyte imbalance. Any change in amount, color, consistency, or odor of stools should be noted. Drug therapy is considered effective when diarrhea is controlled without any adverse effects.

Drug Closely Related to Diphenoxylate HCl with Atropine Sulfate

Loperamide

Loperamide (Imodium) is also chemically similar to meperidine. However, it is not a scheduled drug. It comes in prescription and OTC strengths. Unlike diphenoxylate, loperamide may be used for chronic as well as acute diarrhea. Loperamide is contraindicated for diarrhea related to infections and pseudomembranous colitis. It is used cautiously in patients with hepatic impairment because of the risk of encephalopathy. The contraindications and adverse reactions related to atropine sulfate are not applicable because loperamide does not contain the anticholinergic drug atropine sulfate. For this

MEMORY CHIP

P Diphenoxylate HCI with Atropine Sulfate

- Used to treat diarrhea not responsive to symptomatic and supportive treatment
- This drug is related chemically to meperidine, an opioid, but lacks any analgesic effect. Atropine is added to discourage abuse.
- Major contraindications: diarrhea associated with organisms that penetrate intestinal mucosa; pseudo-membranous enterocolitis
- Most common adverse effects: drowsiness, dizziness, and dry mouth
- Most serious adverse effects: atropine overdose and toxic megacolon
- **Life span alert: Children are more likely to have adverse effects from atropine, especially if they have Down syndrome; variable response in children; avoid use if patient is less than 2 years old.**
- Minimizing adverse effects: Decrease the dose when diarrhea becomes less frequent; monitor for signs of atropine overdose (in children) and toxic megacolon.
- Most important patient education: Do not exceed the prescribed dose.

reason, it may also be better tolerated than diphenoxylate HCl with atropine sulfate. If no clinical improvement occurs, loperamide is generally discontinued after 48 hours.

Drugs Significantly Different From **P** Diphenoxylate HCI with Atropine Sulfate

Bismuth Subsalicylate

Bismuth subsalicylate (Pepto-Bismol, Bismatrol, Pink Bismuth, Kaopectate), a locally acting antidiarrheal, is available without a prescription and is used widely as an antidiarrheal agent. The salicylate component of this drug seems to have an antisecretory effect, whereas the bismuth component has a direct antimicrobial effect against bacteria and viral pathogens in the GI tract. Bismuth subsalicylate is used to treat diarrhea, indigestion, heartburn, nausea, and abdominal cramps. Off-label uses include treating chronic infantile diarrhea and the symptoms of Norwalk virus–induced gastroenteritis, as well as preventing traveler's diarrhea. Bismuth subsalicylate is not given to children or adolescents with viral diseases because of the possibility that the salicylate component may cause Reye syndrome.

Kaolin and Pectin

Kaolin and pectin (Kapectolin) are locally acting antidiarrheals frequently used in combination. These drugs are used widely to treat mild diarrhea, even though clinical studies have not firmly established their effectiveness. These drugs act as absorbents; that is, toxins, bacteria, and other irritants in the GI tract bind to them. Commercial products usually contain two or more adsorbents. For example, Kaopectate is a combination of kaolin and pectin. The adsorptive action

is not selective and therefore can interfere with normal GI absorption, particularly absorption of other drugs.

C LAXATIVES

Drugs used to treat constipation are referred to as laxatives. Laxatives are drugs that act directly on the intestine to promote peristalsis and evacuation of the bowel. Laxatives are classified as saline, hyperosmotic, stimulant (irritant), and bulk-forming. Table 37.4 presents a summary of laxative drugs. Stool softeners (surfactants) and emollients (lubricants) are also used to promote easy passage of stool, but they are not technically laxatives.

C SALINE LAXATIVES

Saline laxatives attract or retain water in the intestinal lumen, resulting in an increased intraluminal pressure that stimulates peristalsis. The increased amount of water also softens fecal material for easier evacuation. The prototype saline laxative is magnesium hydroxide (Milk of Magnesia).

Nursing Management of the Patient Receiving **P** Magnesium Hydroxide

Core Drug Knowledge

Pharmacotherapeutics

Magnesium hydroxide is used for acute or chronic constipation, preoperatively to prepare the bowel for surgery, and to clear the lower bowel tract before or after radiologic and other diagnostic studies. Magnesium hydroxide also is used as an antacid (see Chapter 36).

Pharmacokinetics

Magnesium hydroxide has a local effect in the lower GI tract and is absorbed poorly. Approximately 15% to 30% of the magnesium in magnesium hydroxide is absorbed in the small intestine. Onset of action is 30 minutes to 3 hours after administration. Low-dose administration produces effects in 6 to 12 hours, whereas high-dose administration produces effects in 2 to 6 hours. Excretion occurs in the kidneys and the GI tract.

Pharmacodynamics

Magnesium hydroxide is a salt. It works in the small and large intestines by attracting and retaining water in the intestinal lumen, thereby increasing pressure within the intestine. The retention of fluid in the intestine results in stimulation of the stretch receptors and an increase in peristalsis, which promotes evacuation of the bowel.

Contraindications and Precautions

Magnesium hydroxide should not be used if the patient has abdominal pain or any symptoms that indicate an acute abdomen (nausea, vomiting, or diarrhea). Magnesium salts must be used with caution in patients with renal failure because retention of magnesium could result in magnesium

TABLE 37.4 Summary of Selected Ⓒ Laxatives

Drug (Trade) Name	Selected Indications	Route and Dosage Range	Pharmacokinetics
Ⓒ Saline Laxatives			
Ⓟ magnesium hydroxide (Milk of Magnesia, Dulcolax)	Constipation, preparation for diagnostic tests of lower GI tract, post-GI diagnostic tests	*Adult:* PO, 30–60 mL/d; 15–30 mL/d if concentrated *Child 2–5 y:* PO, 5–15 mL/d *Child 6–11:* PO, 15–30 mL	*Onset:* 0.5–3 h *Duration:* Unknown $t_{1/2}$: None
magnesium sulfate (Epsom salts)	Same as above	*Adult:* PO, 10–15 g in glass of water *Child:* PO, 5–10 g in glass of water	*Onset:* 0.5–3 h *Duration:* Unknown $t_{1/2}$: None
magnesium citrate (Citrate of Magnesia, Citroma;	Same as above	*Adult:* PO, 240 mL *Child:* PO, 120 mL	*Onset:* 0.5–3 h *Duration:* Unknown $t_{1/2}$: None
sodium phosphate (Fleet, Phospho-Soda, sodium phosphates, OsmoPrep;	Same as above	*Adult:* PO, 20–45 mL mixed in half glass of cool water *Child (5–11 y):* PO, 5–20 mL mixed in half glass of cool water	*Onset:* 0.5–3 h *Duration:* Unknown $t_{1/2}$: None
Ⓒ Hyperosmotic Laxatives			
glycerin (Sani-Supp, Fleet Babylax)	Constipation	*Adult and child:* Rectal, 1 suppository, retain 15 min (sized for adults and children)	*Onset:* 0.25–1 h *Duration:* Unknown $t_{1/2}$: None
lactulose (Cholac, Constilac, Constulose, Enulose, Generiac, Kristalose)	Constipation Prevention and treatment of portal-systemic encephalopathy, including hepatic precoma and coma	*Adult:* PO, 15–30 mL/d up to 60 mL/d if needed *Child (infant):* PO, 2.5–10 mL in divided doses; older children and adolescents, 40–90 mL *Adult:* PO, 30–45 mL tid or qid; adjust dose every day or two to produce two or three soft but formed stools; may give hourly doses to induce rapid effect initially *Adult:* rectal, 300 mL in 700 mL water or normal saline solution, retain for 30–60 min; repeat every 4–6 h until patient is awake enough to take oral form	*Onset:* 24–48 h *Duration:* Unknown $t_{1/2}$: None
Ⓒ Stimulant/Irritant Laxatives			
bisacodyl (Bisac-Evac, Bisacodyl Uniserts, Bisco-Lax, Bisalax, Bisco-Lax, Carter's Little Pills, Correctol, Dacodyl, Dulcolax, Durolax, Feen-a-Mint, Modane, Theralax)	Constipation	*Adult and child >12 y:* PO, 5–15 mg/d, up to 30 mg/d before diagnostic study *Adult and child >12 y:* PR, 10 mg/d *Child 2–11 y:* PO/PR, 5–10 mg/d *Child 6 mo–2 y:* PR, 5 mg/d	*Onset:* PO, 6–10 h; PR, 0.25–1 h *Duration:* Unknown $t_{1/2}$: Unknown
cascara sagrada (Cascara Sagrada Fluid Extract Aromatic)	Constipation	*Adult:* PO, 325-mg tablet at bedtime or 5 mL *Child <12 y:* No recommended dosage	*Onset:* 6–8 h *Duration:* Unknown $t_{1/2}$: None
castor oil (Fleet flavored Castor Oil, Purge, Emulsoil)	Constipation Bowel prep	*Adult:* PO, 15–60 mL *Child 2–12 y:* PO, 5–15 mL	*Onset:* 2–6 h *Duration:* Unknown $t_{1/2}$: None
senna (Senokot, Senexon, Ex-Lax, Senna-Gen, SenokotXTRA, Black Draught, Gentlax, Dr. Caldwell Senna Laxative, Fletcher's Castoria)	Same as above	*Adult:* PO, 1 or 2 tablets, 1–2×/d *Child 6–12 y:* PO, 1 tablet once or twice/d	*Onset:* 6–10 h *Duration:* Unknown $t_{1/2}$: None

TABLE 37.4 **Summary of Selected C Laxatives** *(continued)*

Drug (Trade) Name	Selected Indications	Route and Dosage Range	Pharmacokinetics
C Bulk-Forming Laxatives			
polycarbophil (FiberCon, Equalactin, Mitrolan, Fiber-Lax, Fiberall)	Constipation or diarrhea associated with conditions such as irritable bowel syndrome and diverticulitis; acute nonspecific diarrhea	*Adult:* PO, 1 g/d to qid; not to exceed 4 g/d; severe diarrhea, repeat every 30 min; not to exceed maximum dose *Child 6–12 y:* PO, 500 mg no more than qid; not to exceed 2 g/d	*Onset:* 12–72 h *Duration:* Unknown $t_{1/2}$: None
psyllium (Fiberall, Hydrocil Instant, Konsyl, Metamucil, natural vegetable powder, Reguloid, Serutan, Syllact, Konsyl-D, Modane Bulk, V-Lax)	Constipation, promotion of regularity	*Adult:* PO, 1 rounded tsp in 8 oz water 1–3×/d	*Onset:* 12–72 h *Duration:* Unknown $t_{1/2}$: None
Methylcellulose (Citrucel)	Constipation	*Adult:* PO, 1 heaping tbsp 1–3×/d *Child:* Not recommended	*Onset:* 12–72 h *Duration:* Unknown $t_{1/2}$: None
C Stool Softeners/Surfactants			
docusate sodium (Colace, Disonate, DOK, DOS Softgel, D-S-S, Modane Soft, Pro-Sof, Regular SS, Dioeze, Surfak Liquigels, DC Softgels, Pro-Cal-Sof, Sulfalax Calcium, Diolose, Diocto-K, Kasof)	Softens stool to prevent constipation and straining in defecation	*Adult:* PO, 50–300 mg/d *Child 6–12 y:* PO, 40–150 mg/d 2–4×/d *Child 3–6 y:* PO, 20–60 mg/d 2–4×/d *Child <3 y:* PO, 10–40 mg/d 2–4×/d	*Onset:* 12–72 h *Duration:* Unknown $t_{1/2}$: None
C Emollient Laxatives			
mineral oil (Fleet Mineral Oil Enema, Kondremul, Liqui-Doss)	Constipation	*Adult:* PO, 15–45 mL/d *Child 6–12 y:* PO, 5–15 mL/d	*Onset:* 6–8 h *Duration:* Unknown $t_{1/2}$: None
C Bowel Evacuants			
polyethylene glycol-electrolyte solution (PEG-ES) (Colyte, GoLYTELY, NuLYTELY, TriLyte, MoviPrep;	Bowel prep	*Adult:* PO, 240 mL every 10 min until 4 L consumed or effluent is clear; may be given through nasogastric tube, 20–30 mL/min	*Onset:* 1–2 h *Duration:* About 4 h $t_{1/2}$: None
C Peripherally Selective Mu (μ) Opioid Receptor Antagonist			
alvimopan (Entereg)	Postoperative ileus	*Adult:* PO, 12 mg 30min-5 h prior to surgery, then 12 mg 2×/d for up to 15 doses	*Onset:* unknown *Duration:* unknown $t_{1/2}$: 10–17 h
methylnaltrexone (Relistor)	Opioid-Induced Constipation	*Adult:* SC <38 kg: 0.15 mg/kg every other day 38–61 kg: 8 mg every other day 62–114 kg: 12 mg every other day >114 kg: 0.15 mg/kg every other day	*Onset:* unknown *Duration:* unknown $t_{1/2}$: 8 h

TABLE 37.5 Agents That Interact with P Magnesium Hydroxide

Interactants	Effect and Significance	Nursing Management
Chloroquine	Magnesium may decrease absorption of chloroquine.	Separate administration of these drugs by 2 h.*
dicumarol	Magnesium may increase anticoagulant activity of dicumarol.	Monitor PT/INR. Monitor for bruising or bleeding.
digoxin	Magnesium may physically absorb digoxin in GI tract.	Monitor serum digoxin levels. Monitor for efficacy of digoxin therapy.
Fluoroquinolones	Magnesium may decrease absorption of fluoroquinolones.	Monitor for efficacy of fluoroquinolone therapy.
Ketoconazole	Magnesium may reduce tablet dissolution of ketoconazole.	Monitor for efficacy of ketoconazole therapy.
levodopa	Magnesium decreases gastric emptying times, allowing for more rapid and complete intestinal levodopa absorption.	Monitor for levodopa toxicity.
nifedipine	Neuromuscular blockade and hypotension have occurred with coadministration of nifedipine and magnesium.	Monitor blood pressure. Ensure safety.
Nitrofurantoin	Magnesium may absorb nitrofurantoin, decreasing its bioavailability.	Monitor for efficacy of nitrofurantoin.
penicillamine	Poor GI absorption of penicillamine may be result of chelation or adsorption with magnesium.	Administer penicillamine on an empty stomach.
Quinidine	Inhibition of excretion of quinidine, possibly leading to increased effect.	Monitor for arrhythmias.
salicylates	Magnesium-induced increase in urinary pH reduces renal reabsorption of salicylates, increasing their clearance.	Monitor for efficacy of salicylate therapy.
Tetracyclines	Binds to surface of tetracycline, preventing absorption, decreasing effect.	Monitor for efficacy of tetracycline therapy.
Ticlopidine	Decreases effect of ticlopidine	Monitor for bruising or bleeding.

*Whenever possible, magnesium hydroxide administration should be separated by 2 hours from that of any other drug in this table.

toxicity. Safe use in children younger than 2 years of age has not been established. Large doses in pregnancy may lead to serious fluid and electrolyte imbalances.

Adverse Effects
Adverse effects can occur with large doses. Overactive bowel (marked by cramps, diarrhea, or nausea) is the primary adverse effect. Fluid and electrolyte imbalance can occur with large doses given frequently.

Drug Interactions
Magnesium hydroxide may decrease or increase the effects of many drugs. Table 37.5 lists agents that interact with magnesium hydroxide.

Assessment of Relevant Core Patient Variables

Health Status
Determine whether the patient receiving magnesium salts has a history of renal insufficiency. Before drug administration, listen for bowel sounds, palpate for abdominal distention, and ask questions about the patient's usual pattern of bowel function. Be sure to determine whether the patient is receiving drug therapy that may interact with magnesium hydroxide.

Life Span and Gender
Determine the patient's age before administering magnesium hydroxide. The patient must be at least 2 years of age to receive magnesium hydroxide. Older adults may have weakened abdominal muscles and decreased peristalsis related to aging. They also may engage in less regular activity and eat fewer foods containing roughage. All of these factors may contribute to constipation.

Lifestyle, Diet, and Habits
Determine whether the patient's normal fluid intake is adequate (at least between 1,000 and 1,500 mL daily); whether the normal diet includes an adequate amount of fruits, vegetables, and roughage; and whether the patient engages in any regular physical activity. Assess whether the patient must frequently ignore the urge to defecate because of lifestyle patterns. These variables can contribute to constipation. In addition, it is important to determine whether the patient uses laxatives regularly because chronic use of laxatives may lead to dependency on the laxative to expel a bowel movement.

Environment

Magnesium hydroxide is sold OTC, and patients frequently self-medicate for constipation. The drug also is used in acute care settings before rectal and colonic examinations, diagnostic tests, or operations. Patients in an inpatient facility frequently are less active than when they are at home, which can contribute to constipation. Thus, magnesium hydroxide also may be used in a hospital setting to prevent constipation.

Culture and Inherited Traits

Cultural and social variations exist regarding how frequently bowel movements should occur for the individual to be considered regular or constipated. Ascertain what the patient means by normal elimination and constipation.

Nursing Diagnosis and Outcome

- Constipation related to dietary factors, fluid restrictions, decreased peristalsis, lack of activity, changes in activity, postoperative state, GI disease or malfunction, or adverse effects from other drug therapy.
  Desired outcome: *The patient will have a bowel movement after taking magnesium hydroxide.*

Planning and Intervention

Maximizing Therapeutic Effects

After taking magnesium hydroxide, the patient should follow with a full glass of water to prevent dehydration and to promote a more rapid effect.

Minimizing Adverse Effects

To prevent fluid and electrolyte imbalance, use of magnesium hydroxide should be limited to short-term treatment of constipation. Administer magnesium hydroxide with caution, if at all, in patients with renal disease. At least 2 hours should pass between administration of magnesium hydroxide and drugs that are known to interact with it.

Providing Patient and Family Education

- Teach patients that magnesium hydroxide should be used for short-term use only and that long-term use may cause electrolyte imbalance and dependency on laxatives (Box 37.3).
- Caution patients not to take magnesium hydroxide within 2 hours of drugs that may interact with it.

Ongoing Assessment and Evaluation

Assess color, consistency, and amount of stool produced to monitor effectiveness of magnesium hydroxide.

Drugs Closely Related to P Magnesium Hydroxide

Other Saline Laxatives

Magnesium sulfate (Epsom salts), magnesium citrate (Citrate of Magnesia), and sodium phosphate (Phospho-Soda) are all saline laxatives similar to magnesium hydroxide. Like

---

BOX 37.3 COMMUNITY BASED CONCERNS

Educating Patients in the Community About Laxative Use

Individual misuse of OTC and prescription laxatives is encountered commonly by nurses practicing in the community. Nurses have a vital educational role to play in this area by providing teaching programs for individuals or groups. These programs may focus on general principles of elimination and bowel health so that patients learn to use laxatives responsibly and to avoid laxative abuse. A general teaching program may include the following features:

- Assessing elimination patterns. Teach patients how to assess their own usual habits and daily elimination routines to identify what is a "normal bowel movement" pattern for them.
- Defining normality. Show patients how to analyze their assessment findings and recognize patterns that are normal for the individual. Emphasize that what is normal for one person may not be normal for another.
- Eating to promote regularity. Identify dietary measures that promote peristalsis and regular bowel movement. Emphasize adequate fluid intake of 1,000 to 2,000 mL/d and fiber-rich foods, such as whole-grain breads, cereals, and vegetables, and fluids, such as pulpy fruit juices.
- Exercising to promote regularity. Assist patients to incorporate regular exercise into their daily activities. Explain how exercise promotes peristalsis and regular bowel movements.
- Dealing with altered elimination patterns. Teach patients to observe for changes in the normal pattern, form, and color of stools. Help them decide when occasional use of laxatives, preferably bulk or stimulant types, may be appropriate and when medical attention may be advisable. Also point out the potential for dependence on laxatives and the disadvantages of dependence.

---

magnesium hydroxide, both magnesium sulfate and magnesium citrate are contraindicated for patients with renal dysfunction. Sodium phosphate is contraindicated for patients with disorders that are exacerbated by an increased fluid volume such as chronic heart failure, hypertension, or significant edema. Pharmacologic indications, adverse effects, and patient management are similar to those of magnesium hydroxide.

C Hyperosmotic Laxatives

The hyperosmotics act similarly to the saline laxative magnesium hydroxide. Drugs in this laxative subclass include lactulose (Cephulac, Cholac, Chronulac, Constilac, Constulose, Duphalac, Enulose) and glycerin suppository (Sani-Supp, Colace, Fleet Babylax).

Like the saline laxative magnesium hydroxide, lactulose pulls water into the colon. Unlike magnesium hydroxide, lactulose is a synthetic disaccharide of lactose. In the colon, lactulose is metabolized by bacteria into acids and carbon dioxide. These products increase the oncotic pressure in the colon and draw water into the stool. The acids formed also draw ammonia into the stool for evacuation. Because of this action, lactulose is used to decrease blood ammonia levels in hepatic coma and hepatic encephalopathy in addition to its use for constipation. Lactulose also can be given by enema.

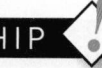

MEMORY CHIP

P Magnesium Hydroxide

- Laxative for short-term use. Works by pulling water into the bowel by distending it and promoting peristalsis.
- Major contraindications: signs of an acute abdomen and renal failure
- Most common adverse effect: overactive GI activity
- Most serious adverse effect: fluid and electrolyte imbalance (large, frequent doses only)
- Maximizing therapeutic effects: Follow administration with a glass of water.
- Most important patient education: Magnesium hydroxide is not for long-term use.

Glycerin suppositories are inserted into the rectum. They pull moisture into the bowel and provide local irritation to stimulate a bowel movement. Glycerin suppositories are considered a very gentle laxative.

Drugs Significantly Different From
P Magnesium Hydroxide

Stimulant (Irritant) Laxatives

Stimulant laxatives include bisacodyl (Bisac-Evac, Bisacodyl Uniserts, Bisacolax, Bisalax, Bisco-Lax, Carter's Little Pills, Correctol, Dacodyl, Dulcolax, Durolax, Feen-a-Mint, Modane, Theralax), cascara sagrada (Cascara Aromatic, Aromatic Cascara Fluid Extract), senna (Senokot, Senexon, Ex-Lax, Cenalax, Senna-Gen, Black Draught, Gentlax, Dr. Caldwell Senna Laxative, Fletcher's Castoria), and castor oil (Purge, Emulsoil, and Neoloid). Therapeutic uses are similar to those for magnesium hydroxide. These laxatives have a direct stimulatory effect on the intestinal mucosa or nerve plexus and increase peristalsis. They also alter water and electrolyte secretion. They all work in the colon, with the exception of castor oil, which works in the small intestine. Stimulant laxatives are the most frequently abused type of laxative. Chronic use may induce loss of normal bowel function and laxative dependency. They are contraindicated for use in patients with fecal impaction or obstipation (severe obstruction of fecal flow through the bowels).

Bulk-Forming Laxatives

Bulk-forming (fiber) laxatives are considered the safest and most physiologic of the laxatives. They include polycarbophil (FiberCon, Equalactin, Mitrolan, Fiber-Norm, and Konsyl Fiber), psyllium (Fiberall, Genfiber, Metamucil, Hydrocil Instant, Konsyl, Natural Fiber Laxative, Reguloid, Serutan, Syllact, Modane Bulk, and Perdiem Fiber Therapy), and methylcellulose (Citrucel). Bulk-forming laxatives pass through the body undigested. The fibers attract water to the large and small intestine, and they absorb the water and swell to form a soft, bulky stool. The bulky mass stimulates the intestinal muscles and increases peristalsis. Their

onset of action, normally 12 to 24 hours but rarely up to 72 hours, is more prolonged than that of the saline laxative magnesium hydroxide. Some of these preparations contain sodium and therefore must be used cautiously in patients for whom excess sodium can cause problems (e.g., patients with chronic heart failure or hypertension). Psyllium also appears to be useful in reducing cholesterol levels as an adjunct therapy to dietary control, although this use is off-label. In addition to its laxative use, polycarbophil can be used for diarrhea because it absorbs free fecal water and produces formed stools. Patients should be cautioned to increase fluid intake while taking bulk-forming laxatives. They will not work without increased fluid intake and can complicate constipation.

Stool Softeners

Docusate is a stool softener (surfactant). It has detergent activity and facilitates the addition of fat and water into the stool to soften it. It does not stimulate peristalsis. It is used prophylactically to prevent constipation in patients who are at risk for developing it, such as elderly patients after orthopedic surgery or patients for whom straining at stool is contraindicated (e.g., after myocardial infarction, eye surgery, or anorectal surgery).

Docusate is available in two formulations, either as docusate sodium (Colace, D-S-S, Modane Soft, Regulax SS, Diocto, Ex-lax Stool Softener, Non Habit Forming Stool Softener, Stool Softener, Genasoft, Phillips Liqui-Gels, Docu, and Silace) or as docusate calcium (Surfak, DC Softgels).

Emollient (Lubricant) Laxatives

Mineral oil (Fleet Mineral Oil Enema, Kondremul, Liqui-Doss) is an emollient (lubricant) laxative. It is also used as an enema in fecal impaction. Mineral oil lubricates the intestine and retards colonic absorption of water. The stool is thus softened because it contains more water. Because of its coating action, mineral oil may decrease absorption of fat-soluble vitamins. This is especially important for patients receiving warfarin because the patient is at risk of bleeding when decreased vitamin K stores affect the clotting mechanism.

Bowel Evacuants

Polyethylene Glycol-Electrolyte Solution (PEG-ES) is used not to treat constipation, but rather for bowel cleansing in preparation for GI examinations. PEG-ES is a combination of a nonabsorbable osmotic agent (polyethylene glycol) and an electrolyte solution containing potassium chloride, sodium chloride, sodium sulfate, and sodium bicarbonate. This combination results in practically no net absorption or excretion of ions or water, thus allowing for bowel evacuation while maintaining fluid and electrolyte balance. PEG-ES is used cautiously in patients with ulcerative colitis. Common adverse effects include anal irritation, bloating, epigastric fullness, nausea, stomach cramps, and vomiting.

Management of Opioid Induced Constipation

Chamberlain, B. H., Cross, K., Winston, J. L., Thomas, J., Wang, W., et al. (2009). Methylnaltrexone treatment of opioid-induced constipation in patients with advanced illness. *Journal of Pain and Symptom Management,* 38(5):683–690.

The Study
Opioid-induced constipation is a frequent complication for patients in the advanced stages of terminal diseases. Researchers conducted a double blind study comparing the effects of methylnaltrexone with placebo in 27 nursing homes. The study included 134 patients, with advanced disease defined as a terminal condition or end stage cancer, who had been on opioids for at least two weeks. Methylnaltrexone was found to induce a bowel movement within four hours of administration, with no effect on pain control. Because this drug has limited effect on the central nervous system, it is an acceptable option for those patients who develop severe constipation secondary to opioid administration.

Nursing Implications
This study provides evidence for management of constipation for patients in the late stages of terminal disease, where palliation and comfort are priorities. The results of this study found that methylnaltrexone was effective in inducing a bowel movement without affecting pain control. This treatment also decreased other uncomfortable procedures often associated with opioid induced constipation, including enemas.

© Peripherally Selective Mu (μ) Opioid Receptor Antagonist

Post-operative ileus and opiate induced bowel dysfunction (OBID) are treated with peripherally selective μ opioid receptor antagonists, such as alvimopan (Entereg) or methylnaltrexone (Relistor). These drugs act by blocking the μ opioid receptors, resulting in improved gastrointestinal motility. Alvimopan should only be administered in a hospital, and be limited to 15 doses. A major advantage of alvimopan is its ability to selectively block opioid receptors in the gastrointestinal system, with little to no effect in the central nervous system (CNS) secondary to its low systemic absorption and limited ability to cross the blood–brain barrier and enter the CNS. The health care provider should be made aware if any of the following side effects occur secondary to the administration of alvimopan: gas, constipation, heartburn, difficulty urinating, or back pain.

Methylnaltrexone (Relistor) was approved by the FDA in 2008 to treat opioid related constipation and ileus, and has been used with patients undergoing palliative therapy (Kyle, 2009). Intended for subcutaneous injection, the dose is based on the weight of the patient. This drug is to be used in combination with more conventional treatments for constipation, including laxatives. Methylnaltrexone must be discontinued when the opiates for pain control are discontinued. Common side effects of this drug include abdominal pain, flatus, nausea, dizziness, and diarrhea. The administration of methylnaltrexone longer than 4 months has not been extensively evaluated (Box 37.4).

DRUGS USED TO TREAT IRRITABLE BOWEL SYNDROME

Serotonin receptors in the bowel play a role in bowel motility and visceral sensations perceived from the bowel. Drugs that work at these receptors can alter symptoms of IBS such as diarrhea, constipation, and abdominal pain. Blockade of serotonin receptor subtype 3 (5-HT$_3$) decreases the diarrhea associated with IBS. The prototype drug for this group is alosetron (Lotronex). Table 37.6 presents a summary of drugs used to treat IBS.

Nursing Management of the Patient Receiving P Alosetron

Core Drug Knowledge
Pharmacotherapeutics
Alosetron is the only drug approved in the United States for the treatment of women with IBS-D. It is administered orally. Its use is restricted to those with severe symptoms that have not responded to other therapies. It is not used

---

TABLE 37.6	Summary of Selected Drugs to Treat Irritable Bowel Syndrome		
Drug (Trade) Name	**Selected Indication**	**Route and Dosage Range**	**Pharmacokinetics**
P alosetron (Lotronex)	IBS-D	PO, 1 mg daily; may increase to 1 mg bid after 4 wk if needed	*Onset:* Rapid *Duration:* Unknown t$_{1/2}$: Elimination, 1.5 h; pharmacodynamic, 6–10 h
dicyclomine (Bentyl)	IBS	*Adult and Child > 12 y:* 20 mg 4×/d *Child 2–12 y:* PO, 10 mg 3×/d *Child 6 mo–2 y:* PO, 5–10 mg 3×/d	*Onset:* 1–2 h *Duration:* 4 h t$_{1/2}$: 9–10 h
lubiprostone (Amitiza)	IBS-C, chronic idiopathic constipation	*Adult:* PO, 24 mcg 2∞/d with food *Child:* Not recommended	*Onset:* Rapid *Duration:* Unknown t$_{1/2}$: 0.9–1.4 h

in patients who have any degree of constipation from IBS. IBS-D is considered severe if it includes diarrhea and one or more of the following: frequent and severe abdominal pain or discomfort, frequent bowel urgency or fecal incontinence, or disability or restriction of daily activities caused by IBS. Less than 5% of IBS cases are considered severe.

Pharmacokinetics

Alosetron is rapidly absorbed. The oral availability of alosetron is about 60%. Absorption is decreased by about 25% when it is taken with food, but the drug can be taken with or without food. The presence of food delays the peak by about 15 minutes. Men achieve a 30% to 50% lower serum concentration than women who receive the same dose. Alosetron is moderately protein bound at 82%. Although the elimination half-life is 1.5 hours, the pharmacodynamic half-life is much longer at 6 to 10 hours. Alosetron is extensively metabolized by the P-450 isoenzymes (predominantly CYP2C9, and to a lesser extent, CYP3A4 and CYP1A2). Most of the drug is excreted as metabolites by the kidneys, and the rest is lost in the stool.

Pharmacodynamics

Alosetron blocks the 5-HT$_3$ receptor. It alters visceral sensation, decreasing abdominal discomfort and pain. It also lengthens the transit time in the bowel and decreases chloride and water secretion, which help control diarrhea in IBS.

Contraindications and Precautions

Alosetron should not be administered to anyone with IBS-C. Alosetron is also contraindicated for anyone with a history of chronic or severe constipation or with a history of sequelae from constipation; a history of intestinal obstruction, stricture, toxic megacolon, GI perforation, or adhesions; a history of ischemic colitis, impaired intestinal circulation, thrombophlebitis, or hypercoagulable state; a history of or current Crohn disease or ulcerative colitis; or a history of or active diverticulitis. Alosetron is also contraindicated in patients who are unable to understand or comply with the Patient–Physician Agreement or who have a known hypersensitivity to any component of the product.

Alosetron is a pregnancy category B drug. Whether it is excreted into breast milk is unknown; therefore, it must be used with caution. Because alosetron is extensively metabolized in the liver, patients with poor liver function are likely to have increased circulating levels of alosetron. No studies have been done on this phenomenon, but caution is warranted because these patients may be at increased risk for adverse effects.

Adverse Effects

The major adverse effect of alosetron is constipation, occurring in 22% to 39% of patients who received the drug during clinical trials. Most of the time, constipation is mild to moderate and stops either spontaneously or after an interruption in drug therapy. Constipation can be severe in some

patients, possibly even necessitating hospitalization or surgery for removal of part or all of the colon (colectomy). Serious complications of constipation include obstruction, perforation, impaction, and toxic megacolon. These patients are also at risk for ischemic colitis, which is a serious complication and potentially fatal, although rare. The signs of ischemic colitis include rectal bleeding, bloody diarrhea, and new or worsening abdominal pain. Alosetron was first approved and originally available in February 2000 but was taken off the market in November 2000 because of reports of eight possible cases of ischemic colitis. Owing to a large and rather unexpected public outcry over the withdrawal of the drug, the Food and Drug Administration (FDA) reviewed additional material and eventually reapproved the drug in June 2002. Use of the drug is now severely restricted because of these potential adverse effects. To prescribe the drug, physicians must have completed an educational training session, use special stickers on prescriptions, fully inform the patient about the potential risks, and obtain a signed consent form from the patient. The incidence of complications from alosetron is somewhat controversial because a large research study conducted after the drug was first put on the market did not find that alosetron users were at greater risk for bowel surgery or hospitalization caused by constipation than those patients not taking alosetron.

Drug Interactions

No important drug interactions with alosetron have been identified. Alosetron does not appear to inhibit the hepatic metabolism of drugs metabolized by the major P-450 enzymes.

Assessment of Relevant Core Patient Variables

Health Status

Assess whether the patient has IBS-D. Patients should not have IBS-C or any bowel problems that are considered contraindications for therapy. Assess whether the patient has liver disease or poor liver function, which may place the patient at increased risk for adverse effects. Assess whether the patient is generally debilitated or taking other medications that may slow GI motility. These factors may also increase the risk of adverse effects from alosetron.

Life Span and Gender

Assess the patient's age. The effectiveness of alosetron has not been established in pediatric patients. Older adults may be at increased risk for constipation. Alosetron is a pregnancy category B drug. Because it is not known whether the drug is excreted in breast milk, if the patient is breastfeeding, the infant should be cautiously monitored for signs of complications. The safety and effectiveness of alosetron cannot be determined in men, because few men were included in the clinical trials for the drug. Women are more likely than men to experience a positive effect from alosetron.

Nursing Diagnosis and Outcome

- Risk for Altered Elimination, Constipation, related to potential adverse effect of alosetron
  Desired outcome: *The patient will not develop serious constipation while on alosetron.*

Planning and Intervention

Maximizing Therapeutic Effects

No specific actions are recommended to maximize the therapeutic effects of alosetron.

Minimizing Adverse Effects

Confirm that the patient has received the Medication Guide from the prescriber before starting therapy and has read it and understands it. Answer any questions the patient may have regarding drug therapy and its potential adverse effects or contact the prescriber to answer patient questions. Confirm that the medical record contains the signed Patient–Physician Agreement and that the patient has a copy of this agreement. If the patient develops any constipation or signs of ischemic colitis, alosetron therapy should be discontinued at once. Although treatment can be resumed under medical direction for patients with constipation, it should not be resumed if the patient develops ischemic colitis.

Providing Patient and Family Education

- Help educate patients about the potential adverse effects of alosetron. If needed, repeat or clarify information that the prescribing physician was required to provide. Provide answers to any additional patient questions.
- Because the contents of the Medication Guide may change, emphasize to patients that they need to read the entire Medication Guide each time they get a prescription for alosetron.
- Instruct patients to report any constipation or signs of ischemic colitis (rectal bleeding, bloody diarrhea, or new or worsening abdominal pain) immediately.
- To help prevent or minimize constipation, encourage patients to drink sufficient fluids daily.

Ongoing Evaluation and Assessment

Assess the patient throughout alosetron therapy for constipation. Drug therapy is considered effective if the symptoms of IBS are decreased and the patient does not develop serious complications.

Drugs Significantly Different From Alosetron
Dicyclomine

Dicyclomine (Bentyl) is an antispasmodic that is commonly prescribed for IBS. It works by blocking the action of acetylcholine at parasympathetic sites in secretory glands, smooth muscle, and the CNS. Dicyclomine is contraindicated for patients with obstructive uropathy, myasthenia gravis, glaucoma, GI tract obstruction, paralytic ileus, and toxic megacolon. It is given cautiously to patients with hepatic or renal insufficiency,

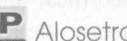

MEMORY CHIP

Alosetron

- Used to treat women with severe IBS, diarrhea type
- Works by blocking a specific serotonin receptor (5-HT4) to decrease bowel motility, bowel secretions, and abdominal pain and discomfort
- Major contraindication: constipation
- Most common adverse effect: constipation
- Most serious adverse effects: ischemic colitis, severe constipation
- **Life span alert: effectiveness in men not yet known**
- Minimizing adverse effects: Discontinue drug if patient develops constipation or signs of ischemic colitis; do not resume drug therapy if patient develops ischemic colitis.
- Most important patient education: Read Medication Guide every time a prescription is filled; contact prescriber at once if constipation or signs of ischemic colitis develop.
- **Black box warning: Risk for serious GI adverse effects; only indicated for women with severe diarrhea-predominant IBS without adequate response to conventional therapies; prescribers must enroll in Prometheus Prescribing Program**

cardiovascular disease, hyperthyroidism, or hypertension. Dicyclomine may cause sedation, constipation, urinary retention, tachycardia, blurred vision, dry mouth, or dizziness. Children 3 months of age and younger have been reported to experience respiratory distress, seizures, syncope, asphyxia, pulse rate fluctuation, muscular hypotonia, and coma within minutes of ingesting dicyclomine. These effects appear to be a result of local irritation or aspiration rather than the drug itself. However, because of these possible problems, dicyclomine should not be used in infants younger than 3 months of age.

Laxatives and Antidiarrheals

Laxatives, bulk agents, and antidiarrheals are sometimes also prescribed for symptoms of IBS and have already been discussed in this chapter.

Selective Chloride Channel Activator

Lubiprostone (Amitiza) is used in the treatment of chronic idiopathic constipation. It works by activating chloride channels on the apical part of the small bowel epithelium that results in a secretion of chloride ions. Sodium and water passively diffuse into the lumen to maintain isotonicity. The drug is contraindicated for use in patients with a history of mechanical GI obstruction or in those with a suspected obstruction. Common adverse effects include headache, abdominal distention, abdominal cramps, diarrhea, and flatulence. Lubiprostone is a pregnancy category C drug and is not recommended for use in children.

Tricyclic Antidepressants

Imipramine (Tofranil) and amitriptyline (Elavil) are tricyclic antidepressants used to manage IBS. They provide visceral analgesia by increasing the pain threshold in the GI system, thus reducing abdominal pain, mucorrhea, and stool frequency. The dose used for IBS is subtherapeutic for depression. Imipramine is contraindicated for patients with narrow-angle glaucoma, those in the acute recovery phase following myocardial infarction, and those who started taking MAOIs less than 2 weeks previously. Amitriptyline is also contraindicated for patients taking MAOIs as well as patients with a history of seizures, cardiac arrhythmias, glaucoma, and urinary retention. Both drugs may impair mental or physical abilities required for concentration and performance of hazardous tasks. They may also cause sedation, confusion, constipation, tachycardia, orthostasis, blurred vision, and dry mouth. Tricyclic antidepressants are fully discussed in Chapter 19.

DRUGS USED TO TREAT INFLAMMATORY BOWEL DISEASE

Drug therapy cannot cure IBD, but it is effective in reducing inflammation and symptoms of the disease in up to 80% of patients. The drug groups used to treat IBD include the 5-aminosalicylic acid (5-ASA) preparations, corticosteroids, and drugs that suppress the immune system (Table 37.7). Some antibiotics are also used in mild to moderate disease. Corticosteroids are discussed in Chapter 48, and drugs that suppress the immune system are discussed in Chapter 54. One drug that suppresses the immune system and has a role in treating IBD is infliximab.

• © 5-ASA Preparations

Aminosalicylates (5-ASA) are the anti-inflammatory drugs most commonly prescribed for IBD. A recent review of

the literature suggests that this group of drugs offers some protection against the development of colon cancer in patients with IBD. This finding is a positive one, because the sites of chronic inflammation with IBD are associated with an increased risk of developing cancer. The prototype 5-ASA preparation is mesalamine (Asacol, Pentasa, Lialda)

Nursing Management of the Patient Receiving P Mesalamine
Core Drug Knowledge
Pharmacotherapeutics
Mesalamine is approved for use for patients with ulcerative colitis and proctosigmoiditis. It is used off-label for the management of Crohn disease.

Pharmacokinetics
Mesalamine is available in tablet, capsule, extended release capsule, suppository, and rectal suspension formulations. Oral bioavailability is 20% to 30%; rectal bioavailability is 10% to 35%. Both formulas are metabolized in the liver. Oral drugs are also metabolized in the intestinal mucosal wall and rectal formulas in the colonic epithelium. Mesalamine is excreted in feces.

Pharmacodynamics
The action of mesalamine is unknown. Mucosal production of arachidonic acid metabolites is increased in patients with IBD through both the cyclooxygenase and lipoxygenase pathways. Mesalamine is thought to inhibit these pathways, thereby decreasing the production of prostaglandins, leukotrienes, and hydroxyeicosatetraenoic acids.

Contraindications and Precautions
Mesalamine is contraindicated for patients with a hypersensitivity to salicylates or with active peptic ulcer disease. It is

TABLE 37.7 Summary of Selected Drugs to Treat Inflammatory Bowel Disease

Drug (Trade) Name	Selected Indication	Route and Dosage Range	Pharmacokinetics
P mesalamine (Asacol, Pentasa, Rowasa, Lialda)	Ulcerative colitis	*Oral tablet:* 800 mg tid for 6 wk *Oral capsule:* 1 g qid up to 8 wk *Extended release capsule (Apriso):* 1.5 g daily *Oral tablet (Lialda):* 2.4 g once daily *Suppository:* 500 mg bid for 3–6 wk *Enema:* 4 g rectally at bedtime for 3–6 wk	*Onset:* Oral, unknown; rectal, 3–21 d *Duration:* Unknown $t_{1/2}$: Oral, 2–15 h; rectal: 5–10 h
balsalazide (Colazal)	Ulcerative colitis	*Adult:* PO, 2.25 g tid for 8–12 wk	*Onset:* Within 1 h *Duration:* Unknown $t_{1/2}$: Unknown
sulfasalazine (Azulfidine, Azulfidine Entabs) Certolizumab (Cimzia)	Ulcerative colitis Rheumatoid arthritis Crohn's Disease Rheumatoid arthritis	*Ulcerative colitis:* PO, 1 g tid–qid *Rheumatoid arthritis:* 500 mg to 2 g/d in 2–4 divided doses *Crohn's disease:* SQ, 400 mg initially and then at wk 2, 4 and then every 4 wk as maintenance *Rheumatoid Arthritis:* 400 mg initially and then at wk 2, 4 and then 200 mg every other weeks.	*Onset:* Unknown *Duration:* Unknown $t_{1/2}$: 5.7–10 h *Onset* *Duration*

TABLE 37.8	Agents That Interact with P Mesalamine		
Interactants	**Effect and Significance**		**Nursing Management**
thiopurines	Mesalamine may inhibit thiopurine-metabolizing enzyme, thiopurine methyltransferase.		Monitor for leukopenia.
Warfarin	Anticoagulant effect of warfarin may be decreased; mechanism is unknown.		Monitor PT/INR.

used cautiously in patients with renal and hepatic impairment and in women who are pregnant or breast-feeding. Mesalamine is a pregnancy category B drug.

Adverse Effects

Common adverse effects of mesalamine include diarrhea, abdominal pain, cramps, flatulence, nausea, and headache. Serious, but rare, adverse effects include blood dyscrasias, exacerbation of colitis, pericarditis, renal impairment, and hepatotoxicity.

Drug Interactions

Mesalamine interacts with thiopurines such as azathioprine and mercaptopurine. It also interferes with salicylates (Table 37.8).

Assessment of Relevant Core Patient Variables

Health Status

Assess for hypersensitivity to salicylates or sulfites prior to administration. Mesalamine contains potassium metabisulfite, so a hypersensitivity reaction may occur in patients with sulfite hypersensitivity. Evaluate reflexes, affect, urinary output, and thyroid and renal function tests. Evaluate hair pattern; hair loss may occur but is generally mild and transient. Communicate positive findings to the health care provider.

Life Span and Gender

Mesalamine is a pregnancy category B drug. It is contraindicated for women who are pregnant or breast-feeding. It is not approved for use in children.

Nursing Diagnoses and Outcomes

• Risk for Altered Elimination, Constipation, related to potential adverse effect of mesalamine
  Desired outcome: *The patient will not develop serious constipation while on mesalamine.*
• Acute pain related to drug induced adverse GI effects.
  Desired outcome: *The patient will take acetaminophen for pain as needed.*

Planning and Intervention

Maximizing Therapeutic Effects

To administer mesalamine as an enema or suppository, assist the patient into a side-lying position on his or her left side (to facilitate migration of the drug into the sigmoid colon) or a knee–chest position, whichever is most comfortable. Prior to administering the enema, shake the bottle thoroughly. Handle the suppository as little as possible, because it melts at body temperature. Explain the importance of retaining the enema for 8 hours and the suppository for 3 hours.

Minimizing Adverse Effects

Administer the oral medication at even intervals throughout the day. Be sure the patient does not crush or chew the capsules or tablets.

Providing Patient and Family Education

• Educate patients about the potential adverse effects of mesalamine.
• Instruct patients to stop taking the drug if fever or rash occurs.
• Instruct patients how to administer an enema if ordered. Be sure they understand that the goal is to retain the enema for 8 hours.
• Instruct patients to limit handling of the suppository to avoid melting.
• Instruct patients to swallow capsules and tablets whole; emphasize the patient should not to crush or chew oral forms of mesalamine.
• To help prevent or minimize constipation, encourage patients to drink sufficient fluids daily.

Ongoing Evaluation and Assessment

Assess the patient throughout mesalamine therapy for relief of pain. Drug therapy is considered effective if the symptoms of IBD are decreased and the patient does not develop serious complications.

Drugs Closely Related to P Mesalamine

Balsalazide

Balsalazide (Colazal), the newest IBD drug, is delivered intact into the colon, where it is cleaved to release mesalamine. More free and active mesalamine is delivered by balsalazide than by the other preparations. Balsalazide is used in the treatment of mildly to moderately active ulcerative colitis. It should not be used in patients with sensitivity to aspirin. The most common adverse effect is headache, followed by abdominal pain, nausea, and diarrhea. Balsalazide is a safe and effective first-line drug for treating ulcerative colitis.

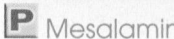

MEMORY CHIP

P Mesalamine

- Used to treat IBD
- Works by decreasing the production of prostaglandins, leukotrienes, and hydroxyeicosatetraenoic acids.
- Major contraindication: hypersensitivity to salicylates and sulfites
- Most common adverse effects: GI effects and headache
- Most serious adverse effects: blood dyscrasias, exacerbation of colitis, pericarditis, renal impairment, and hepatotoxicity
- Minimizing adverse effects: Ensure the oral formulation is swallowed whole.
- Most important patient education: Contact the health care provider if fever or rash occurs.

Olsalazine

Olsalazine (Dipentum) is used to maintain remission of ulcerative colitis when the patient is intolerant to sulfasalazine. It is a sodium salt of a salicylate compound that is bioconverted to mesalamine in the colon by bacteria. The very slow absorption rate from the colon results in very high local concentrations in the colon. Olsalazine produces diarrhea in approximately 17% of patients taking the drug, a finding that may be difficult to distinguish from the diarrhea caused by IBD.

Sulfasalazine

Sulfasalazine (Azulfidine) is used to treat ulcerative colitis; it also is used to treat rheumatoid arthritis. It is a combination of mesalamine (5-ASA) and sulfapyridine, a sulfa antibiotic that prevents mesalamine from being absorbed until it reaches the colon. In the colon, the intestinal bacteria break sulfasalazine into the two main components. The sulfapyridine plays no active role in the treatment of IBD, and all of the therapeutic effects come from the mesalamine. Because of its sulfa component, sulfasalazine should not be used in people allergic to sulfa. The sulfa component accounts for most of the adverse and allergic reactions in up to 33% of the people who take the drug. These common adverse effects are heartburn, headache, loss of appetite, nausea, vomiting, and temporarily lower sperm count in men. Sulfasalazine also may turn the urine bright orange-yellow. Rare but serious adverse effects include a lupus-like disorder, pancreatitis, liver damage, and potentially life-threatening blood disorders (including aplastic anemia, leukopenia, and neutropenia).

Drug Significantly Different From
P Mesalamine

Infliximab

Infliximab (Remicade) is an immune response modulator used to treat moderate to severe Crohn disease or ulcerative colitis, as well as ankylosing spondylitis. In combination with methotrexate, it is used for severe active rheumatoid arthritis and psoriatic arthritis. It reduces the signs and symptoms of IBD, induces and maintains clinical remission in patients with moderate to severe IBD, and reduces the number of draining enterocutaneous fistulas associated with Crohn disease. Infliximab is a monoclonal antibody produced using recombinant technology. It neutralizes the biological activity of tumor necrosis factor-alpha by inhibiting its binding to receptor sites. This effect reduces the infiltration of inflammatory cells and tumor necrosis factor-alpha production in inflamed areas of the intestine. Infliximab is administered as an infusion. Its most common adverse effect, which requires discontinuing the therapy, is an infusion-related reaction (characterized by dyspnea, flushing, headache, and rash). Potentially serious infections are possible with infliximab, and GI complaints (nausea, diarrhea, abdominal pain, vomiting, painful digestion) are fairly common. Monoclonal antibodies are discussed further in Chapter 55.

Certolizumab

Certolizumab (Cimzia) is a TNF (tumor necrosis factor) blocker that is used in the treatment of Crohn disease. It is also used in the treatment of rheumatoid arthritis. Administered as a subcutaneous injection, the usual dose is is 400 mg (initially administered as two separate injections), at weeks 2 and 4. If the patient responds to the medication, the recommended maintenance dose is 400 mg every 4 weeks. Patients taking Cimzia are at increased risk of developing significant infections that may require hospitalizations. The risk of serious infection is exacerbated if the patient is also taking immunosuppressants or corticosteroids.

CHAPTER SUMMARY

- Drugs used to treat digestive disorders of the lower GI tract include antiflatulents, antidiarrheals, laxatives, and drugs used to treat IBS and IBD.
- Antiflatulents are drugs that decrease gas production and cause gas bubbles to coalesce, facilitating the passage of gas through belching and expelling flatus. These drugs are used to provide relief from postoperative gastric distention, dyspepsia, peptic ulcer, spastic colon, and diverticulosis. Simethicone is the prototype antiflatulent.
- Charcoal is another antiflatulent. Unlike simethicone, it interferes with the absorption of many drugs and is therefore useful in the treatment of poisoning and drug overdose.
- Diarrhea occurs when GI motility is too rapid, which prevents water from being reabsorbed from the stool. Infections of the GI tract may cause some diarrhea. Changes in diet and emotional stress also may contribute to diarrhea.
- Antidiarrheals are used to slow motility of the GI tract. OTC antidiarrheals are used widely, although specific data on their efficacy are lacking. The prototype antidiarrheal is diphenoxylate HCl with atropine sulfate. This drug is structurally similar to meperidine. A small amount of

atropine sulfate is combined with diphenoxylate to discourage deliberate abuse. It acts systemically to reduce intestinal motility and slow peristalsis.

- Constipation occurs when excessive water is reabsorbed from the stool while it is in the colon, drying and preventing passage of the stool. Lacking or deficient peristalsis, dietary factors, and changes in activity also may contribute to constipation. Laxatives are used to treat constipation. Types of laxatives include saline laxatives, hyperosmotics, stimulants and irritants, stool softeners, and lubricants.

- Laxatives are contraindicated in patients who have undiagnosed severe abdominal pain, who are nauseated and vomiting, or who have a bowel obstruction.

- Magnesium hydroxide, the prototype saline laxative, works by attracting water into the colon, increasing intracolonic pressure, and increasing peristalsis. It should not be used if the patient has renal failure because the additional magnesium is not excreted renally and may cause hypermagnesemia.

- Lactulose, a hyperosmotic laxative, also attracts water into the colon. A unique feature of this laxative is that it additionally produces acid in the colon, which attracts ammonia from the blood. Lactulose is therefore also used therapeutically to decrease serum ammonia levels in patients with hepatic coma.

- Peripherally selective Mu (μ) opioid receptor antagonists are not used for routine constipation. They are reserved for prophylaxis of postoperative ileus or opioid-induced constipation.

- Serotonin stimulates receptors in the bowel, producing bowel motility, bowel secretions, and visceral sensations. Drug therapy to treat IBS is directed at these serotonin (5-HT) receptors. Alosetron is a 5-HT$_3$ blocker that is used to treat severe IBS-D.

- Other medications that treat any one of the symptoms of IBS may not be as effective as the drugs that affect 5-HT.

- The inflammation seen in IBD is treated with 5-ASA preparations (e.g., mesalamine), corticosteroids, and immunosuppressant agents (e.g., infliximab).

QUESTIONS FOR STUDY AND REVIEW

1. What instructions should be given to the patient taking simethicone tablets?
2. Why is atropine sulfate added to diphenoxylate HCl?
3. What class of laxative would be used prophylactically for a patient recovering from a cataract extraction? Why?
4. Should a patient with severe constipation and renal failure receive magnesium hydroxide?
5. What nonlaxative effect of lactulose is desired for patients with severe hepatic disease?
6. Why is the sale of alosetron limited to women with severe IBS-D?
7. Why are drugs that affect serotonin receptors used to treat IBD?

NEED MORE HELP?

Chapter 37 of the Study Guide to Accompany *Drug Therapy in Nursing*, 4th Edition, contains NCLEX-style questions and other learning activities to reinforce your understanding of the concepts presented in this chapter. For additional information or to purchase the study guide, visit thePoint.

REFERENCES

Belavic, J. M. (2009). Methylnaltrexone for opioid-induced constipation. *The Nurse Practitioner,* 34(3):6–7.

Belling, R., McLaren, S., & Woods, L. (2009). Specialist nursing interventions for inflammatory bowel disease. *Cochran Database of Systemic Reviews,* (4).

Bream-Rouwenhorst, H. R., & Cantrell, M. A. (2009). Alvimopan for postoperative ileus. *American Journal of Health-SystemPharmacy,* 66:1267–1276.

Cannom, R. R., Kaiser, A. M., Ault, G. T., Beart, R. W. Jr, & Etzioni, D. A. (2009). Inflammatory bowel disease in the United States from 1998 to 2005: has infliximab affected surgical rates? *The American Surgeon,* 75(10):976–980.

Carter, N. J., & Scott, L. J. (2009). Lubiprostone: In constipation predominant irritable bowel syndrome. *Drugs,* 69(9):1229–1237.

Chey, W. D., Howden, C. W., Tack, J., Ligozio, G., & Earnest, D. I. (2010). Long-term tegaserod treatment for dysmotility-like functional dyspepsia: results of two identical 1-year cohort studies. *Digestive Diseases and Science,* 55(3):684–697.

Crowell, M. D., Harris, L. A., DiBaise, J. K., & Olden, K. W. (2007). Activation of type-2 chloride channels: A novel therapeutic target for the treatment of chronic constipation. *Current Opinion in Investigational Drugs,* 8(1):66–70.

Devlin, S. M., & Panaccione, R. (2010). Evolving inflammatory bowel disease treatment paradigms: Top-down versus step-up. *Medical Clinics of North America,* 94(1):1–18. Facts and Comparisons. (2010). *Drug facts and comparisons.* Philadelphia, PA: Lippincott Williams & Wilkins.

Fried, M., Johanson, J. F., & Gwee, K. A. (2007). Efficacy of tegaserod in chronic constipation in men. *American Journal of Gastroenterology,* 102(2):362–370.

Gershon, M. D., & Tack, J. (2007). The serotonin signaling system: From basic understanding to drug development for functional GI disorders. *Gastroenterology,* 132(1): 397–414.

Kamm, M. A., Sandborn, W. J., & Gassull, M. (2007). Once-daily, high-concentration MMX mesalamine in active ulcerative colitis. *Gastroenterology,* 132(1):66–75.

Katzung, B. G., Masters, S. B., & Trevor, A. J. (2009). *Basic and Clinical Pharmacology,* (11th ed.). New York, NY: McGraw-Hill.

Kraft, M. D. (2009). Alvimopan for post-operative ileus: One piece of the puzzle. *American Journal of Health-System Pharmacy,* 66(14):1309–1310.

Kyle, G. (2009). Methylnaltrexone: a subcutaneous treatment for opioid-induced constipation in palliative care patients. *International Journal of Palliative Nursing,* 15(11): 533–540.

Lai, E. J., Calderwood, A. H., Doros, G., Fix, O. K., & Jacobsen, B. C. (2009). The Boston bowel preparation scale: a valid and reliable instrument for colonoscopy. *Gastrointestinal Endoscopy,* 69(3 Pt 2):620–625. Micromedex Healthcare Series. Retrieved from *http://thomsonhc.com.*

Nielsen, O. H., & Munck, L. K. (2007). Drug insight: Aminosalicylates for the treatment of IBD. *Nature Clinical Practice Gastroenterology and Hepatology,* 4(3):160–170.

37Porth, C. M. (2008). *Pathophysiology: Concepts of Altered Health States* (8th ed.). Philadelphia, PA: Lippincott Williams & Wilkins.

Rao, S. S. C. (2009). Constipation: Evaluation and treatment of colonic and anorectal motility disorders. *Gastrointestinal Endoscopy Clinics of North America,* 19(1):117–139.

Rivkin, A., & Chagan, L. (2006). Lubiprostone: Chloride channel activator for chronic constipation. *Clinical Therapeutics,* 28(12):2008–2021.

Sandborn, W. J. (2009). The future of inflammatory bowel syndrome. *Reviews in Gastroenterological Disorders,* 9(3):E69–E77.

Shan, Y. (2009). Irritable bowel syndrome treatment and management. *Primary Health Care,* 19(8):28–34.

Spinz, G., Amato, A., Imperiali, G., Lenoci, N., Mandelli, G., Paggi, S., Ragaelli, F., Terreni, N., & Terruzzi, V. (2009).

Drugs and Aging, 26(6):469–474. Tatro, D. S. (2011). *Drug Interaction Facts: The Authority on Drug Interactions.* Philadelphia, PA: Lippincott Williams & Wilkins.

Toglia, M. R. (2009). Pathophysiology of anal incontinence, constipation, and defecatory dysfunction. *Obstetrics and Gynecology Clinics of North America,* 36(3):659–671.

Trentacosti, A. M., He, R., Burke, L. B., Griebel, D., & Kennedy, D. L. (2010). Evolution of clinical trials for irritable bowel syndrome: Issues in end points and study design. *American Journal of Gastroenterology,* 105(4):731–737.

Wald, M. D. (2010). Treatment of Irritable Bowel Syndrome, Up To Date. Retrieved from http://www.uptodate.com on July 26, 2010.

Wood, J. D. (2010). Enteric nervous system: Sensory physiology and constipation. *Current Opinion in Gastroenterology,* 26(2):102–108.

UNIT 10
Antimicrobial Drugs

38

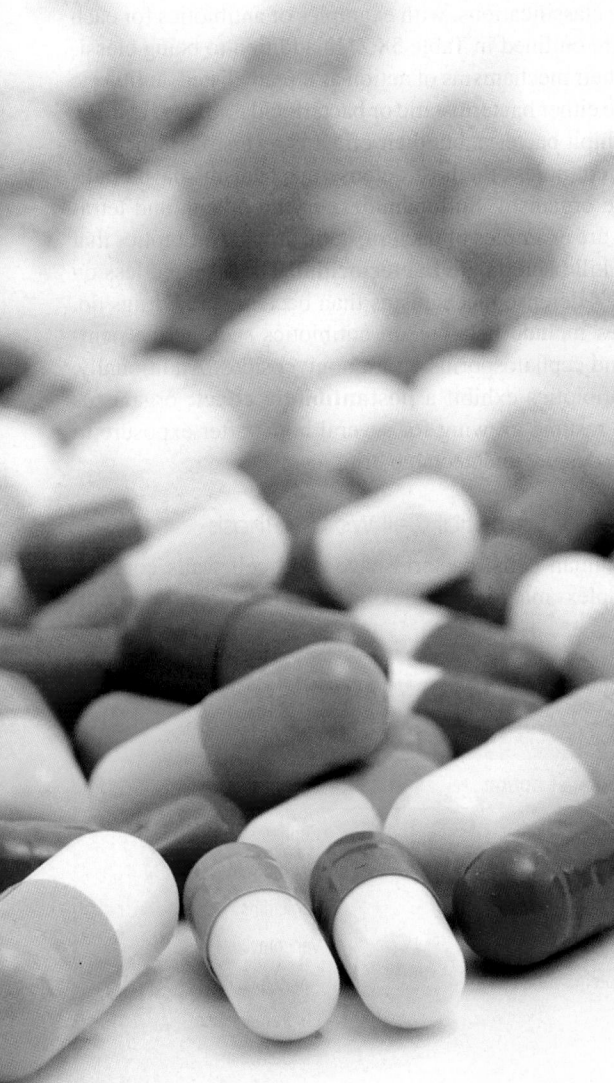

Principles of Antimicrobial Therapy

Learning Objectives

At the completion of this chapter the student will:

1. Describe the classifications of antimicrobial drugs.
2. Describe the principle of selective toxicity and how it applies to antimicrobial therapy.
3. Explain the emergence of drug-resistant microbes.
4. Identify and discuss the four most common drug-resistant pathogens.
5. Distinguish between drug of choice and alternative drugs used to manage infections.
6. Discuss the procedures used to identify pathogens.
7. Relate the principle of drug susceptibility to antimicrobial therapy.
8. Identify patient care variables that influence the choice of antimicrobial agents.
9. Describe appropriate laboratory tests to monitor antimicrobial therapy.

Key Terms

anthelminthic
antibacterial
antifungal
anti-infectives
antimicrobials
antiprotozoal
antiviral

bacteriocidal
bacteriostatic
culture
empiric therapy
Gram stain
microbe
nosocomial

pathogen
postantibiotic effect
selective toxicity
sensitivity
spectrum
superinfection

rugs used to manage infections are called **antimicrobials, anti-infectives,** or **antibiotics.** The first effective antimicrobial drug was penicillin. Since its introduction, morbidity and mortality from infections have steadily declined. However, as we grow in our knowledge of how specific types of microbes work and how to eradicate them, microbes also continue to develop ways to mutate or to secrete enzymes that make current antimicrobials ineffective. This chapter focuses on the basics of antimicrobial therapy, including classification of antimicrobial drugs, selective toxicity, antimicrobial resistance, general considerations of antimicrobial therapy, and monitoring of antimicrobial therapy.

CLASSIFICATION OF ANTIMICROBIAL DRUGS

Two popular ways to classify antimicrobial drugs are by susceptible organism and by mechanism of action.

Classification by Susceptible Organism

A **microbe** is a unicellular or small multicellular organism. Microbes that are capable of producing disease are called **pathogens.** Types of microbes include bacteria, viruses, protozoa, some algae and fungi, and some worms (helminths). Drugs used to treat infection can be classified according to the type of microbe they affect. The major classifications include **antibacterial** drugs, **antiviral** drugs, **antiretroviral** drugs, **antifungal** drugs, **antiparasitic** drugs, **antiprotozoal** drugs, and **anthelminthic** drugs. Antibacterial drugs are subdivided into narrow-spectrum, broad-spectrum, or antimycobacterial drugs. As the name implies, a narrow-spectrum drug is effective against a few types of bacteria, whereas a broad-spectrum drug is effective against many types of bacteria. The antiviral classification also has a subdivision: antiretroviral agents. Table 38.1 outlines these classifications.

TABLE 38.1	Classification of Antimicrobial Drugs by Susceptible Organism
Susceptible Organisms	**Antimicrobial Classification**
Bacteria	Antibacterial drugs
• Mycobacterium	
Viruses	Antiviral drugs
Retroviruses	Antiretroviral drugs
Fungi	Antifungal drugs
Parasites	Antiparasitic drugs
Protozoa	Antiprotozoal drugs
Helminths (worms)	Anthelminthic drugs

Classification by Mechanism of Action

Antimicrobial drugs work in a variety of ways:

- Inhibition of bacterial cell wall synthesis
- Inhibition of protein synthesis
- Inhibition of nucleic acid synthesis
- Inhibition of metabolic pathways (antimetabolites)
- Disruption of cell wall permeability
- Inhibition of viral enzymes

These classifications, with examples of antibiotics for each group, are outlined in Table 38.2. In addition to being classified by their mechanisms of action as already listed, antibiotic drugs are either bacteriostatic or bacteriocidal. **Bacteriostatic** drugs inhibit bacteria, but their effect is reversible if the drug is removed, unless the host defense mechanisms have eradicated the organism. Sulfonamides, erythromycin, and tetracyclines are examples of bacteriostatic drugs. Antibiotics that actually kill bacteria are **bacteriocidal.** They depend less on the body's defense mechanisms than bacteriostatic drugs do. Examples include beta-lactam antibiotics such as the penicillins and cephalosporins or aminoglycosides. Additionally, some antibiotics exhibit a **postantibiotic effect:** organisms may not resume growing for several hours after exposure to the drug, despite undetectable drug levels.

Inhibition of Bacterial Cell Wall Synthesis

Unlike human cells, bacteria have rigid cell walls containing complex macromolecules, which are formed through

TABLE 38.2	Classification of Antimicrobial Drugs by Mechanism of Action
Mechanism of Action	**Antimicrobials**
Inhibit cell wall synthesis	Cephalosporins
	Daptomycin
	Penicillins
	Vancomycin
Inhibit protein synthesis	Aminoglycosides
	Chloramphenicol
	Clindamycin
	Erythromycin
	Tetracyclines
Inhibit nucleic acid synthesis	Fluoroquinolones
	Rifampin
Disrupt cell membrane permeability	Polymyxins
	Polyene antimicrobials
	Imidazole antifungal agents
Work as an antimetabolite	Sulfonamides
	Trimethoprim
Inhibit viral enzymes	Acyclovir
	Saquinavir

biosynthetic pathways. The osmotic pressure within the cell is very high and relies on the integrity of the cell wall to resist the absorption of water. Without the rigid cell wall, the bacteria would absorb water, swell, and then lyse. Several antimicrobial drugs weaken the cell wall, allowing the cell to absorb water, a process that causes bacterial death. Penicillins and cephalosporins bind to specific proteins located within the bacterial cytoplasmic membrane, the portion of the cell wall that borders the cytoplasm. Binding to these proteins causes inhibition of transpeptidase, an enzyme needed for the final step of cell wall synthesis. The result is decreased cell wall synthesis. These antibiotics also activate autolytic enzymes that are destructive to the cell wall. Another antibiotic, vancomycin, interferes with bacterial cell wall synthesis by inhibiting the synthesis of precursors of murein or by preventing the formation of linear peptidoglycan chains. These chains are polysaccharides and polypeptides that are cross-linked to form the bacterial cell wall.

Inhibition of Protein Synthesis

Both human and bacterial cells require ribosomes to synthesize protein for use by the cell (see Chapter 40). However, human cell ribosomes are structurally different than bacterial cell ribosomes. Because of this difference, many of the commonly used antimicrobial drugs are able to disrupt bacterial protein synthesis without affecting protein synthesis in human cells.

Tetracyclines, aminoglycosides, erythromycin, clindamycin, and chloramphenicol all inhibit protein synthesis; however, they do so by binding or inhibiting different subunits of the process of protein binding.

Inhibition of Nucleic Acid Synthesis

Many bacteria use enzymes for replication that do not exist in human cells. For instance, fluoroquinolones inhibit deoxyribonucleic acid (DNA) gyrase, an enzyme needed for bacterial DNA replication. Although human cells contain an enzyme that functions in the same manner, the human enzyme is not affected by fluoroquinolones.

Inhibition of Metabolic Pathways (Antimetabolites)

Nucleic acid synthesis is dependent on folic acid (folate), which acts as a coenzyme in many biosynthetic reactions. Humans obtain folate in the diet, but many microorganisms must synthesize folate. Sulfonamides inhibit bacterial folate synthesis by acting as an antimetabolite of the precursor to folate, para-aminobenzoic acid (PABA). Similarly, trimethoprim is an antimetabolite of folic acid that selectively inhibits dihydrofolate reductases of bacteria and protozoa.

Disruption of Cell Wall Permeability

Drugs that disrupt the integrity of the bacterial cell wall cause the cell to leak components that are vital to its survival. The polymyxins disrupt the membranes of the bacterial cell wall by inserting themselves into the lipid bilayer and forming artificial pores. The polyene antimicrobials bind to membrane components that are present only in microbial cells. The imidazole antifungal agents act as selective inhibitors of enzymes involved in the synthesis of sterols that are essential components of fungal membranes.

Inhibition of Viral Enzymes

The replication of viruses requires multiple enzymatic activities. Nucleoside analogues, such as acyclovir, and protease inhibitors, such as saquinavir, interrupt important enzymes required for viral replication.

SELECTIVE TOXICITY

An important principle of antimicrobial therapy is **selective toxicity,** which is the ability to suppress or kill an infecting microbe without injury to the host. Selective toxicity is achievable because the drug accumulates in a microbe at a higher level than in human cells; the drug has a specific action on cellular structures or biochemical processes that are unique to the microbe; or an action of a drug on biochemical processes is more harmful to the microbe than to host cells. For example, differences in the chemical compositions of the cell walls of microbes and human cells permit the selective toxicity of polymyxins, polyene antimicrobials, and imidazole antifungal agents. Tetracycline and chloramphenicol do not have absolute selective toxicity: they are able to inhibit protein synthesis in some human cells as well. Understanding selective toxicity has made antimicrobial drugs safe and effective for managing infection in humans.

ANTIMICROBIAL RESISTANCE

Antimicrobial resistance refers to the resistance of the microbe, not the patient, to the drug. Because of antimicrobial resistance, pharmaceutical companies are constantly looking for new ways to eradicate microbes despite the large number of antimicrobial agents available. Antimicrobial resistance is a major problem, especially in developed countries where antimicrobial agents are used daily. In the United States, the Centers for Disease Control and Prevention (CDC) issued a "Campaign to Prevent Antimicrobial Resistance in Healthcare Settings" in 2002 (Box 38.1). The campaign focuses on hospitals because they are most likely to harbor resistant bacteria, and it is most useful to prescribers such as physicians, nurse practitioners, and physician assistants. However, certain sections are clearly within the domain of the nurse. For instance, use of aseptic technique for all procedures, obtaining culture specimens appropriately, timely communication of culture and sensitivity results, adherence to isolation procedures, clear documentation of improvement or worsening of symptoms of infection, and most important, washing hands between contact with patients, are all among the CDC's campaign objectives.

Box 38.1 TWELVE STEPS FOR PREVENTION OF ANTIMICROBIAL RESISTANCE IN HOSPITALIZED ADULTS

Prevent Infection

Step 1. Vaccinate
- Give influenza/pneumococcal vaccine to at-risk patients before discharge
- Get influenza vaccine annually

Step 2. Get the Catheters Out
- Use catheters only when essential
- Use the correct catheter
- Use proper insertion and catheter-care protocols
- Remove catheters when they are no longer essential

Diagnose and Treat Infection Effectively

Step 3. Target the Pathogen
- Culture the patient
- Target empiric therapy to likely pathogens and local antibiogram
- Target definitive therapy to known pathogens and antimicrobial susceptibility test results

Step 4. Access the Experts
- Consult infectious diseases experts for patients with serious infections

Use Antimicrobials Wisely

Step 5. Practice Antimicrobial Control
- Engage in local antimicrobial control efforts.

Step 6. Use Local Data
- Know your antibiogram.
- Know your patient population.

Step 7. Treat Infection, Not Contamination
- Use proper antisepsis for blood and other cultures.

- Culture the blood, not the skin or catheter hub.
- Use proper methods to obtain and process all culture specimens.

Step 8. Treat Infection, Not Colonization
- Treat pneumonia, not the tracheal aspirate.
- Treat bacteremia, not the catheter tip or hub.
- Treat urinary tract infection, not the indwelling catheter.

Step 9. Know When to Say "No" to Vanco
- Treat infection, not contaminants or colonization.
- Fever in a patient with an intravenous catheter is not a routine indication for vancomycin.

Step 10. Stop Antimicrobial Treatment:
- When infection is cured
- When cultures are negative and infection is unlikely
- When infection is not diagnosed

Prevent Transmission

Step 11. Isolate the Pathogen
- Use standard infection control precautions.
- Contain infectious body fluids. (Follow airborne, droplet, and contact precautions.)
- When in doubt, consult infection control experts.

Step 12. Break the Chain of Contagion
- Stay home when you are sick.
- Keep your hands clean.
- Set an example.

Fact sheet from the CDC's Campaign to Prevent Antimicrobial Resistance in Healthcare Settings. Retrieved from http://www.cdc.gov/drugresistance/healthcare/tools. htm#factsheets.

Contributing Factors

Antimicrobial resistance may occur for several reasons: production of drug-inactivating enzymes, changes in receptor structure, changes in drug permeation and transport, development of alternative metabolic pathways, emergence of drug-resistant microbes, or factors that facilitate the development of resistance.

Production of Drug-Inactivating Enzymes

This common mechanism causes resistance to many beta-lactam antibiotics. The microbe synthesizes hydrolytic beta-lactamases, enzymes that are specific for certain penicillin and cephalosporin structures called beta-lactams. The beta-lactam structure must remain intact for the antibiotic to be effective; thus, when these enzymes affect the beta-lactam structure, the antibiotic becomes ineffective. To date, more than 100 beta-lactamases have been identified. Pathogens such as *Staphylococcus aureus*, *Haemophilus* species, and *Escherichia coli* have specificity to affect penicillins but not cephalosporins. *Pseudomonas aeruginosa* and *Enterobacter* species have a broader spectrum and may affect cephalosporins as well as penicillins.

Changes in Receptor Structure

Bacteria contain molecules that act as targets, or receptors, for antimicrobial drugs. These molecules may undergo

changes in their structures. These structural changes make the microbe less susceptible to the toxic action of antibiotics. For example, alteration in penicillin-binding proteins (PBPs) decreases the affinity for binding beta-lactam antibiotics.

Changes in Drug Permeation and Transport

The antimicrobial action of many drugs depends on their ability to penetrate the cell membranes of an organism and reach effective intracellular concentrations. The organism's defense starts in the efficiency of its cell wall. If an antibiotic reaches the interior structures of the cell rapidly, the cell is unable to overcome the activity of the drug. However, if the antibiotic has difficulty passing through the cell wall, the bacteria are able to hydrolyze the antibiotic as it slowly enters the cell. Another bacterial defense mechanism is the production of an efflux pump, which effectively extrudes certain drugs, such as tetracycline, from the cell.

Development of Alternative Metabolic Pathways

Some bacteria are affected by antibiotics, such as sulfonamides, that act as antimetabolites by interrupting their metabolic pathway for replication. In the case of sulfonamides, the antibiotic inhibits dihydropteroate synthase, the enzyme necessary to metabolize folic acid. Resistant bacteria may produce levels of PABA, the precursor to folic acid, that are high enough to overcome the inhibition of dihydropteroate synthase. Additionally, certain bacteria are able to use pre-formed folic acid from their environment, thus bypassing the inhibitory actions of the sulfonamides.

Emergence of Drug-Resistant Microbes

All antimicrobials have the ability to promote the emergence of drug-resistant microbes. However, resistance is more likely to occur in organisms exposed to broad-spectrum drugs. Although the use of antimicrobials promotes the potential for drug resistance to occur, they do not directly cause the resistance. Drug-resistant microbes develop in two ways: by spontaneous mutation and by conjugation. Spontaneous mutation is exactly what the name infers: a change in the genetic composition of the microbe that may just be a random occurrence, or the microbe may have mutated by acquiring DNA from an external source. The resistance developed is drug specific. Conjugation is a form of sexual reproduction in which two individual microbes join in temporary union to transfer genetic material. Conjugation may occur between two microbes of the same species or between different species.

Factors That Facilitate the Development of Resistance

Several factors facilitate the development of resistance. Drug concentrations in tissues that are too low to kill resistant organisms contribute to the development of resistance. The minimum inhibitory concentration (MIC) of a drug must be present to stop or slow the replication of the microbe. When a tissue does not reach MIC, the microbe can become resistant to the antimicrobial. Inadequate tissue concentrations may occur because of an improper dose of drug or improper length of time between doses. Insufficient duration of therapy may allow resistant organisms to repopulate and re-establish an infection. Patients frequently stop taking antibiotics when they feel better "to save some in case the infection comes again." Treatment must be continued beyond clinical improvement, especially if there is any problem with host defenses.

Prophylactic use of antibiotics may also contribute to the development of resistant organisms. Prophylactic use of antimicrobial drugs means that the drug is given to prevent an infection rather than to treat an infection. This practice increases the risk of the development of resistant microbes; therefore, antimicrobial prophylaxis should be reserved for appropriate indications. Such indications include:

- Exposure to sexually transmitted diseases
- Recurrent urinary tract infections
- Neutropenia
- Surgery, especially within the gastrointestinal tract
- Bacterial endocarditis

COMMON ANTIBIOTIC-RESISTANT MICROBIAL INFECTIONS

Although any microbe may become drug resistant, four important microbes are most prevalent: methicillin-resistant *Staphylococcus aureus* (MRSA), penicillin-resistant *Streptococcus pneumoniae,* vancomycin-resistant *Enterococcus* (VRE), and multiple drug–resistant *Mycobacterium tuberculosis* (MDR-TB). Microbes that cause antimicrobial-resistant nosocomial infections may also develop.

Methicillin-Resistant *Staphylococcus Aureus* (MRSA)

The abbreviation MRSA is commonly used for this infection; however, the abbreviation is somewhat misleading. In actuality, the pathogen is widely resistant to all of the anti-staphylococcic penicillins, not just methicillin. In MRSA, PBPs are altered, reducing the ability of penicillins to inhibit cell wall synthesis, except at very high drug concentrations that may not be achievable because of poor tissue penetration and toxicity concerns. Many strains of MRSA are also resistant to aminoglycosides, tetracyclines, erythromycin, and clindamycin.

Closely related to MRSA is methicillin-resistant *Staphylococcus epidermidis* (MRSE). MRSE frequently colonizes the nasal passages of health care workers, resulting in the spread of nosocomial infections, especially in critical care units.

Vancomycin is the drug of choice to manage infections caused by MRSA and MRSE. Because vancomycin is also used for many other drug-resistant microbes, vancomycin resistance is emerging. New drugs with different mechanisms of action, such as linezolid (Zyvox), dalfopristin-quinupristin (Synercid), and daptomycin (Cubicin), have been developed to treat vancomycin-resistant microbes. Older drugs such as sulfamethoxazole/trimethoprim (Septra/Bactrim) and rifampin also have been found to be effective in the treatment of MRSA.

Penicillin-Resistant *Streptococcus Pneumoniae*

In the past, penicillins have successfully treated pneumococcal infections such as otitis media in children, community-acquired pneumonia, and meningitis. Because they are used so frequently, particularly in children and the elderly, strains of penicillin-resistant streptococci are emerging. To decrease penicillin resistance among *Streptococcus pneumoniae,* the CDC suggested that clinicians stop using penicillins and cephalosporins as prophylaxis for otitis media and that patients over the age of 65 years or those under the age of 2 years, who have an increased risk for pneumococcal infections, be immunized.

Vancomycin-Resistant *Enterococcus* (VRE)

Infection due to *Enterococcus* is generally treated with a combination of antibiotics: an aminoglycoside with a penicillin or an aminoglycoside with a cephalosporin. The penicillin or cephalosporin damages the bacterial cell wall and allows the aminoglycoside to penetrate the cell. Strains of *Enterococcus* have developed resistance to penicillin, gentamicin, and vancomycin, however. Potential alternative drugs for VRE include teicoplanin (Targocid), minocycline (Minocin), ciprofloxacin (Cipro), quinupristin-dalfopristin (Synercid), and daptomycin (Cubicin).

Multiple Drug–Resistant *Mycobacterium Tuberculosis* (MDR-TB)

Multiple drug–resistant TB is increasingly common. Although some of the bacilli are inherently resistant, others develop resistance over the long course of TB treatment, which can last up to 2 years. The cause of MDR-TB is inadequate drug therapy, a category that includes a duration of therapy that is too short; a dose that is too low; or, more commonly, patient adherence that is only intermittent. To decrease the incidence of MDR-TB, multiple-drug therapy is implemented at the onset of treatment, followed by a decrease in the number of drugs, but no less than four drugs are given at any time.

Nosocomial Infections

A **nosocomial** infection is an infection that originates or occurs in a hospital or hospital-like setting. Such infections occur because the hospital setting has a high prevalence of pathogens, a high prevalence of compromised hosts, and an efficient mechanism of transmission from patient to patient. According to the World Health Organization, an estimated 2 million patients per year in the United States acquire a nosocomial infection, resulting in 247 deaths per day. Nosocomial infections with antibiotic-resistant bacteria such as MRSA, which are difficult to treat, are transmitted primarily by the contaminated hands of health care providers. Handwashing with soap and water or with waterless, alcohol-based hand antiseptics after leaving the bedside of each patient and before touching the next patient results in an immediate and profound reduction in the spread of resistant bacteria.

GENERAL CONSIDERATIONS FOR SELECTING ANTIMICROBIAL THERAPY

The most important factor in managing infections is to "match the drug with the bug." Each pathogen has a "drug of choice" and "alternative drugs." Several factors must be considered when choosing the drug of choice or an alternative:

1. Identification of the pathogen
2. Drug susceptibility
3. Drug spectrum
4. Drug dose
5. Time to affect the pathogen
6. Site of infection
7. Patient assessment

Identification of the Pathogen

To eradicate an infection, drugs must be specific to the type of pathogen involved. An antiviral agent will not eradicate bacteria, nor will an antibacterial agent eradicate fungi. In fact, an antibiotic may not affect the bacteria causing a particular infection. Thus, effective treatment requires identification of the specific pathogen.

The first step in the identification of the pathogen is viewing a Gram-stained preparation under a microscope. A **Gram stain** is a simple test done with a dye and a glass slide. A sample of the pathogen is obtained from body fluids, sputum, blood, or exudates. Visualization under the microscope shows the shape of the pathogen, which aids in identifying it (Figure 38.1). The Gram stain indicates whether the pathogen is gram-positive or gram-negative type. Gram-positive bacteria absorb Gram stain and are often aerobic. Aerobic bacteria need a fresh and continuous supply of oxygen to reproduce. Gram-negative bacteria do not absorb Gram stain and tend to be anaerobic. Anaerobic bacteria are much more difficult to eradicate than aerobic bacteria because anaerobes can reproduce in an environment that is oxygen-free. Some drugs affect only gram-positive microbes; some affect only gram-negative microbes; and some affect both, but not to the same extent. In some cases, the pathogen must be grown in a culture medium for identification.

Drug Susceptibility

To choose the right drug for the infection, a drug susceptibility test is optimal. However, it is not always required. The site of infection is frequently a clue to the causative agent. For instance, *E. coli* causes most urinary tract infections. The health care practitioner therefore initially chooses a drug that can eradicate *E. coli*. Prescribing antibiotic treatment before the pathogen has been definitively identified is called **empiric therapy.** When multiple microbes may be the causative agent, empiric therapy may be started, but a culture specimen of the infected area should be taken before treatment with antimicrobial agents is started because antimicrobial use may make identification of the microbe difficult. The culture is then used to determine drug susceptibility.

The most common test to identify drug susceptibility is called a culture and sensitivity. A sample of the exudate,

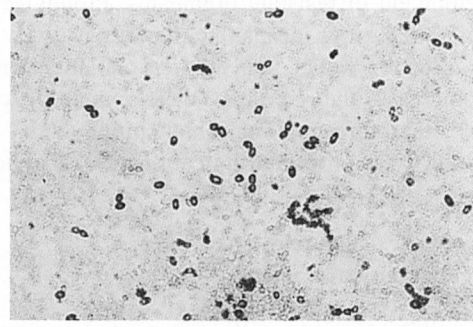

• FIGURE 38.1   Gram-stained slide. This slide contains a type of gram-positive bacilli.

CRITICAL THINKING SCENARIO

WORKING WITH CULTURE AND SENSITIVITY REPORTS

Your patient has been receiving IV ciprofloxacin (Cipro) for a pulmonary infection, and you are about to hang a new infusion. The culture and sensitivity report has just arrived and shows an "R" next to ciprofloxacin. What should you do?

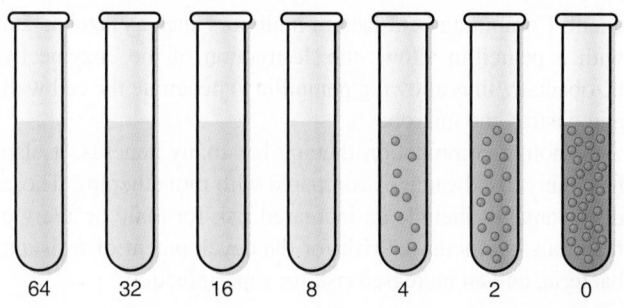

64   32   16   8   4   2   0

mcg/mL Antibiotic

• **FIGURE 38.3** Broth dilution procedure. Bacteria are inoculated into a liquid medium containing graduated concentrations of the test antimicrobial. A clear test tube indicates that the concentration of the antimicrobial is sufficient to eradicate the microbe.

body fluids, or serum is sent to the laboratory. The **culture** determines the identity of the microbe, and the **sensitivity** determines which antimicrobial agent will be therapeutic. Check the sensitivity test result of a patient receiving empiric therapy and notify the prescriber immediately if the current antibiotic is rated as "resistant." Sensitivity testing can be done by a disk diffusion test or broth dilution procedure.

Disk Diffusion Test

This is the most commonly performed test to determine drug susceptibility. In the disk diffusion method, disks containing a standardized amount of an antimicrobial agent are placed on an agar plate inoculated with the infecting organism. The plate is placed in an incubator, and the bacterial lawn is allowed to grow. A growth inhibition zone will appear around each antibiotic that affects the microbe (Figure 38.2). The diameter of the visible growth inhibition zone correlates with the MIC, which is the lowest concentration of an antibiotic that prevents visible growth of a microbe. Organisms are rated as sensitive (S) to a particular antibiotic if they are affected by it and resistant (R) if they are not.

Broth Dilution Procedure

In the broth dilution procedure, the bacteria are inoculated into a liquid medium containing graduated concentrations of

the test antimicrobial. This method directly determines the MIC (Figure 38.3). The broth dilution procedure also determines the minimum bactericidal concentration (MBC), that is, the lowest concentration that will kill more than 99.9% of the original inoculum of the microbe. The broth dilution procedure is particularly helpful in managing difficult infections because it demonstrates both MIC and MBC.

Drug Spectrum

Choosing a drug with the narrowest possible **spectrum** is important. The range of microbes against which a drug is active is its spectrum. Narrow-spectrum drugs affect only a few microorganisms, whereas broad-spectrum drugs affect many microorganisms. The benefit of a narrow-spectrum antimicrobial agent is that it limits the potential for adverse effects, such as superinfection. A **superinfection** is one that occurs during the course of treatment for a primary infection. For example, an antibiotic suppresses all susceptible microbes, including the body's natural flora, which may keep other microbes in check. In the absence of these bacteria, non-susceptible microbes can proliferate because they no longer have other microbes secreting toxins in their proximity and because they no longer need to compete for available nutrients. Two consequences may occur: secondary infections and the development of drug-resistant microbes.

An alternative to the use of broad-spectrum antimicrobials is combination therapy. Combination therapy is used frequently for an initial severe infection in which the pathogen is unknown. Once the pathogen is known, the appropriate drug can be administered. Another use for combination therapy is to treat an infection that is caused by more than one pathogen. This kind of infection is known as a mixed infection. Combination therapy is also used to prevent resistant microbes from developing. For instance, drug resistance occurs frequently during TB treatment as a result of its duration. When multiple drugs are given at the same time, the pathogen is less likely to be able to become resistant to all of the drugs employed. Another benefit of combination therapy is enhanced antibacterial action. For instance, some bacteria are capable of secreting enzymes that inhibit the action of the antibacterial

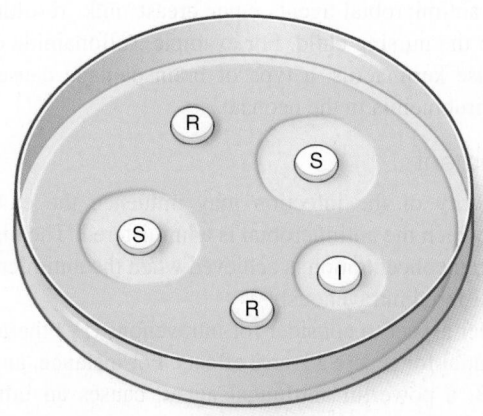

S = sensitive   I = intermediate   R = resistant

• **FIGURE 38.2** Disk diffusion test. In the disk diffusion test, samples of antibiotics are placed on a plate of the infecting organism. The organism is "sensitive" (S) to the antibiotic if there is a bacteria-free zone around the antibiotic, "resistant" (R) if the bacteria remain around the antibiotic, and "intermediate" (I) if there is a zone of inhibition but not sufficient to eradicate the organism.

agent. Combining beta-lactam inhibitors such as tazobactam with a penicillin allows the destruction of the enzyme by tazobactam, thus allowing penicillin to penetrate the cell wall and destroy the microbe.

Although combination therapy has many benefits, it also has many disadvantages compared with monotherapy. These disadvantages include an increased risk for toxic or allergic reactions, an increased risk for the development of resistant bacteria, and an increased risk for superinfection.

Drug Dose

Choosing the antimicrobial agent with the lowest effective dose is important. The dose of the antimicrobial agent is adjusted to affect the MIC at the site of infection. Pediatric doses are calculated as mg/kg/d.

Duration

Choosing the antimicrobial agent that takes the shortest time to affect the pathogen is equally important. The drug must remain at the site of infection at drug concentrations equal to or greater than MIC. The duration of treatment depends on the type of pathogen, the site of infection, and the presence or absence of host defenses. The duration of antimicrobial treatment is generally 7 to 10 days, but it may be extended to 30 days or more for infections such as prostatitis.

It is important to instruct the patient to take antimicrobial medication until all the medication is gone. Stopping therapy early may result in reinfection with the same pathogen, which will have become more drug resistant as a result of inadequate treatment.

Site of Infection

To be effective, a drug must be able to reach the site of infection at a concentration equal to or greater than the MIC. Achieving this concentration is a particular problem when the infection is in the meninges, because many drugs do not cross the blood–brain barrier. Another difficult site is within an abscess because abscesses are poorly vascularized, and the presence of pus impedes drug concentrations. Specific types of infections, such as endocarditis, are difficult to treat because the vegetative growths are hard to penetrate.

Infections that occur in foreign objects such as pacemakers or prosthetic joints are also difficult to treat. When a foreign object enters the body, the immune system attempts to destroy the object by phagocytosis. While the phagocytes are busy attacking the foreign object, they are less able to attack bacteria that are multiplying at the site. Frequently, the infected foreign object must be removed to eradicate the bacterial infection.

Patient Assessment

Nurses need to evaluate the individual patient before starting antimicrobial drugs. Important core patient variables include health status, life span, gender, environment, and culture.

Health Status

The type of antimicrobial agent chosen must reflect the immune status of the patient. Remember that most antimicrobial agents cannot eradicate infection without the assistance of the immune response. Immunocompetent patients may receive either bacteriocidal or bacteriostatic drugs because their immune systems can function with adequate response from phagocytic cells such as macrophages and neutrophils. Immunocompromised patients should receive drugs that are quickly bacteriocidal because such patients' immune responses are limited.

The patient must also be assessed for previous allergic responses to a particular drug class. When the patient states she or he has an allergy to a certain drug, find out what symptoms occurred when they took the drug. Many patients think that nausea, diarrhea, or headaches reflect an "allergy" to a certain drug. True allergic symptoms reflect an antigen–antibody reaction and are characterized by symptoms such as rash, itching, hives, periorbital swelling, and shortness of breath.

Life Span and Gender

Infants and the elderly are the populations most vulnerable to drug toxicity. In the infant, the liver and kidneys are still immature and may have difficulty metabolizing or excreting the drug, which results in accumulation. The same process in the elderly is related to the age of their liver and kidneys, which may no longer be functioning at an optimal level.

Prescribers may request lower doses of antimicrobial agents for these two populations to minimize the risk for toxicity.

During pregnancy, antimicrobial drugs may cross the placenta and cause damage to the developing fetus. For instance, tetracycline binds to developing teeth, producing a gray mottled discoloration.

Most antimicrobial agents enter breast milk, resulting in injury to the nursing child. For example, sulfonamide drugs may cause kernicterus, a type of brain damage caused by hyperbilirubinemia in the neonate.

Environment

The severity of the infection may influence the environment in which the antimicrobial is administered. The highest serum drug concentration is achieved when the antimicrobial is administered intravenously.

Another aspect to consider for intravenous (IV) therapy is the potential for severe adverse effects. For instance, amphotericin B, a powerful antifungal agent, causes an infusion reaction when administered. For that reason, most patients receiving amphotericin B are admitted to a facility that employs licensed nurses to administer the drug.

Culture and Inherited Traits

Certain genetic factors may influence antimicrobial therapy. For example, some groups, especially African Americans, have a predisposition to glucose-6-phosphate deficiency (G6PD). This deficiency causes red blood cells to be destroyed, resulting in hemolytic anemia, which is potentially lethal. Patients with this deficiency should not receive antimicrobials such as sulfonamides, which may induce red blood cell lysis.

MONITORING ANTIMICROBIAL THERAPY

Successful antimicrobial therapy eradicates the infection. Some antimicrobial agents have the ability to induce toxic adverse effects. Serum drug levels should be monitored for drugs that have a high potential for severe adverse effects. In addition, serum peak and trough levels may be measured, although in some hospitals, only trough levels are taken. Blood for a peak level is generally drawn 1 hour after IV or intramuscular (IM) administration. Trough levels are drawn just prior to the next dose of medication, once steady state has been reached. Individual drugs may need to have the peak level drawn at a different time, so it is prudent to verify the appropriate timing of the peak level with the laboratory performing the test. The goal is to keep the serum drug level within the therapeutic margin.

For patients receiving long-term or high-dose antimicrobial therapy, other laboratory testing may be indicated. For instance, if an antimicrobial is known to cause anemia, the patient should be monitored using serial complete blood counts (CBCs).

The very young and the very old should also be monitored closely. Immaturity or advanced maturity may affect liver and kidney functioning. Appropriate testing includes hepatic and renal function tests.

The bottom line for patient monitoring is that it must be individualized according to the type of pathogen, site of infection, potential for adverse effects during therapy, and the patient care variables associated with each patient.

CHAPTER SUMMARY

- Bacteriocidal drugs kill bacteria, whereas bacteriostatic drugs inhibit bacterial growth but rely on the immune system to eradicate the pathogen.
- Antimicrobial therapy is effective because of the principle of selective toxicity: the ability of the drug to harm the pathogen without injuring the host.
- Drug resistance is an ever-present danger to effectively managing infection.
- Prophylactic use of antimicrobial drugs must be limited to appropriate indications to decrease the potential development of drug-resistant microbes.
- There are four major drug-resistant pathogens in the United States: methicillin-resistant *Staphylococcus aureus* (MRSA), penicillin-resistant *Streptococcus pneumoniae*, vancomycin-resistant *Enterococcus* (VRE), and multiple drug–resistant *Mycobacterium tuberculosis* (MDR-TB).

- Nosocomial infections are difficult to treat because hospital settings have a high prevalence of pathogens, a high prevalence of compromised hosts, and an efficient mechanism of transmission from patient to patient.
- Handwashing before contact with each patient is the most effective way of limiting the patient's risk of a nosocomial infection.
- The most important principle in managing infection is to use the right drug for the right bug.
- A culture determines which pathogen is present, whereas a sensitivity test determines the susceptibility of the pathogen to a particular antibiotic.
- The antimicrobial agent used should be the one with the narrowest spectrum, at the lowest dose, that needs to be taken for the shortest time to affect the pathogen.
- Narrow-spectrum drugs affect only a few microorganisms, whereas broad-spectrum drugs affect many microorganisms.
- The minimum inhibitory concentration (MIC) is the minimum concentration of an antibiotic that completely suppresses bacterial growth.
- The minimum bactericidal concentration (MBC) is the concentration of an antibiotic that kills 99.9% of the initial inoculum in a broth dilution.
- Treatment with the drug of choice to eradicate a particular pathogen may have to be changed to an alternative drug because of specific core patient variables such as health status, life span, gender, environment, and culture and inherited traits.
- The most important element of patient education is to advise the patient to complete the entire course of therapy, taking the prescribed dose at the prescribed intervals.

QUESTIONS FOR STUDY AND REVIEW

1. What is the most important principle of antimicrobial therapy?
2. How are antimicrobials classified?
3. How do most antimicrobials work?
4. What is the principle of selective toxicity?
5. How does a superinfection occur?
6. In the United States, what microbes have developed substantial resistance to antimicrobials?
7. How can nurses assist in the CDC's "Campaign to Prevent Antimicrobial Resistance in Healthcare Settings"?
8. What is the best method to limit the patient's risk for acquiring a nosocomial infection?

NEED MORE HELP?

Chapter 38 of the Study Guide to Accompany *Drug Therapy in Nursing*, 4th Edition, contains additional NCLEX-style questions and other learning activities to reinforce your understanding of the concepts presented in this chapter. For additional information or to purchase the study guide, visit thePoint.

REFERENCES

Centers for Disease Control and Prevention. (2006). *Campaign to prevent antimicrobial resistance in healthcare settings*. Retrieved June 6, 2009 from *http://www.cdc.gov/drugresistance/healthcare/ha/HASlideSet.pdf*

Facts and Comparisons. (2009). *Drug facts and comparisons*. Philadelphia, PA: Lippincott Williams & Wilkins.

Gould, D. (2009). Infection Control: Hand Hygiene, *British Journal of Healthcare Assistants,* 3(3):110–113.

Kilpatrick, C. (2009). Save lives: clean your hands. A global call for action at the point of care, *American Journal of Infection Control*, 37(4):261–262.

Koda-Kimbal, M. A., Young, L. Y., Kradian, W. A., et al. (2008). *Applied Therapeutics: The Clinical Use of Drugs*, Philadelphia, PA: Lippincott Williams & Wilkins.

Kuban, C. J. (2008). Antimicrobial stewardship programs: role in optimizing infectious disease outcomes, *Disease Management and Health Outcomes*, 16(6):403–410.

Mulvey M. R., & Simor A. E. (2009). Antimicrobial resistance in hospitals: how concerned should we be? *Canadian Medical Association Journal*, 180(4):408–415.

Rybak, M., Lomaestro, B., Rotschafer, J. C., et al. (2009). Therapeutic monitoring of vancomycin in adult patients: a consensus review of the American Society of Health-System Pharmacists, the Infectious Diseases Society of America, and the Society of Infectious Diseases Pharmacists, *American Journal of Health System Pharmacy*, 66(1):82–98.

Tatro, D. S. (2010). *Drug interaction facts*. Philadelphia, PA: Lippincott Williams & Wilkins.

Weston, Debbie. (2008). *Infection Prevention and Control: Theory and Practice for Healthcare Professionals*, United Kingdom: John Wiley and Sons.

World Health Organization. (2009). WHO Global Strategy for the Containment of Antibiotic Resistance. Retrieved June 6, 2009 from http://www.who.int/drugresistance/WHO_Global_Strategy_English.pdf

Antibiotics Affecting the Bacterial Cell Wall

Learning Objectives

At the completion of this chapter the student will:

1. Identify the antibiotic drug classes that affect the bacterial cell wall and name at least one drug in each class.

2. Describe the primary therapeutic uses for each antibiotic drug class that affects the bacterial cell wall.

3. Identify core drug knowledge pertaining to antibiotics that affect the bacterial cell wall.

4. Identify core patient variables pertaining to antibiotics that affect the bacterial cell wall.

5. Relate the interaction of core drug knowledge to core patient variables for antibiotics that affect the bacterial cell wall.

6. Generate a nursing plan of care from the interactions between core drug knowledge and core patient variables for antibiotics that affect the bacterial cell wall.

7. Describe nursing interventions to maximize therapeutic and minimize adverse effects for antibiotics that affect the bacterial cell wall.

8. Determine key points for patient and family education for antibiotics that affect the bacterial cell wall.

Key Terms bacterial cell envelope   beta-lactamases   penicillinases
beta-lactam   cephalosporinases   penicillin-binding proteins (PBPs)

Antibiotic Affecting the Bacterial Cell Wall

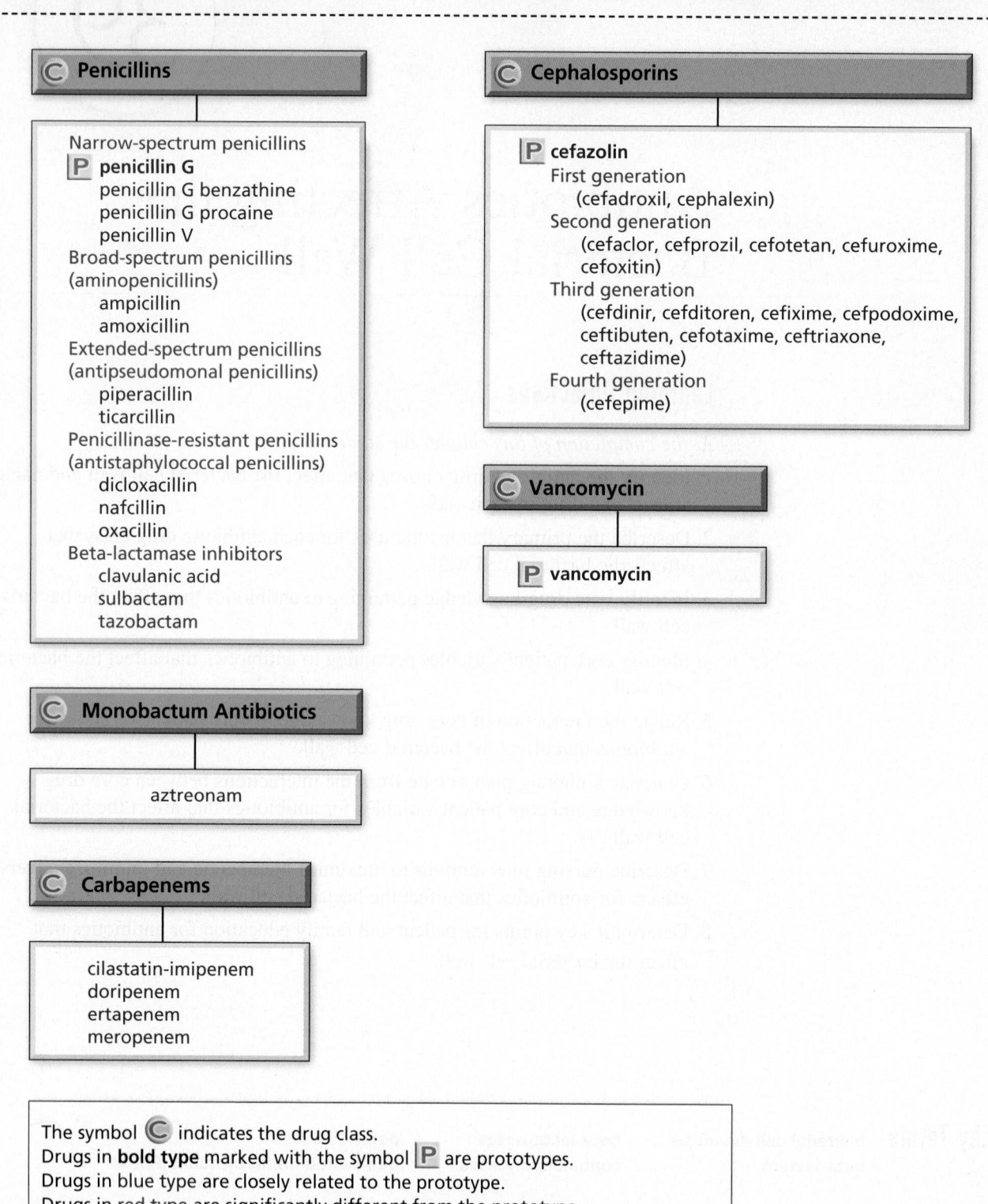

C Penicillins

Narrow-spectrum penicillins
P penicillin G
penicillin G benzathine
penicillin G procaine
penicillin V
Broad-spectrum penicillins
(aminopenicillins)
ampicillin
amoxicillin
Extended-spectrum penicillins
(antipseudomonal penicillins)
piperacillin
ticarcillin
Penicillinase-resistant penicillins
(antistaphylococcal penicillins)
dicloxacillin
nafcillin
oxacillin
Beta-lactamase inhibitors
clavulanic acid
sulbactam
tazobactam

C Cephalosporins

P cefazolin
First generation
(cefadroxil, cephalexin)
Second generation
(cefaclor, cefprozil, cefotetan, cefuroxime,
cefoxitin)
Third generation
(cefdinir, cefditoren, cefixime, cefpodoxime,
ceftibuten, cefotaxime, ceftriaxone,
ceftazidime)
Fourth generation
(cefepime)

C Vancomycin

P vancomycin

C Monobactum Antibiotics

aztreonam

C Carbapenems

cilastatin-imipenem
doripenem
ertapenem
meropenem

The symbol **C** indicates the drug class.
Drugs in **bold type** marked with the symbol **P** are prototypes.
Drugs in blue type are closely related to the prototype.
Drugs in red type are significantly different from the prototype.
Drugs in black type with no symbol are also used in drug therapy; no prototype.

Drugs affecting the bacterial cell wall include the antibiotics known as the penicillins, monobactams, carbapenems, cephalosporins, and vancomycin. Penicillin G is the prototype drug for the penicillin drug class; drugs significantly different from penicillin are the beta-lactamase inhibitors and bacitracin. Other prototype drugs discussed in this chapter include aztreonam for the monobactam drug class; imipenem for the carbapenem drug class; cefazolin for the cephalosporin drug class; and vancomycin, which is the only drug in its class.

In addition to explaining how these drugs work, this chapter discusses nursing management related to evaluating the patient's condition, monitoring the patient's response, and teaching the patient and family about antibiotic therapy.

PHYSIOLOGY

Bacteria are surrounded by a rigid cell wall that is responsible for maintaining the integrity of the internal cellular environment. The interior of the cell has a high osmotic pressure. If the bacterial cell wall is not intact, the internal osmotic pressure draws fluid into the cell until it bursts.

Even when the cell wall is breached by an antibiotic, bacterial death may not occur because of bacterial resistance. Bacterial resistance occurs for one of two reasons: the drug is unable to reach binding sites within the cell, or the bacteria produce an enzyme that inactivates the drug.

Bacterial Cell Envelope

Drugs that affect the bacterial cell wall must be able to penetrate the cell wall to bind to molecular targets on the cytoplasmic membrane within the cell. Gram-positive bacteria have a **cell envelope** with only two layers: a thick cell wall and a

cytoplasmic membrane. Despite the thickness of the cell wall, many drugs are capable of penetrating this wall and attaching to the targets on the cytoplasmic membrane. Gram-negative bacteria have a cell envelope with an additional outer membrane, and the cell wall is much thinner. Although the cell wall can be penetrated easily, the outer membrane cannot. Only drugs that can pass through the very small pores of the outer membrane can reach the target sites on the cytoplasmic membrane (Figure 39.1).

Bacterial Enzymes

Beta-lactamases are enzymes that disrupt the beta-lactam ring. This mechanism inactivates **beta-lactam** drugs, such as penicillins and cephalosporins, because their antibiotic activity is derived from characteristics of the beta-lactam ring. Enzymes that affect penicillins are called **penicillinases**, whereas enzymes that affect cephalosporins are called **cephalosporinases.**

PATHOPHYSIOLOGY

Bacteria may cause infections in any body organ, structure, or fluid. In addition to the original bacterial infection, the loss of certain "good" bacteria may result in a superinfection, such as that caused by *Candida* species.

Ⓒ PENICILLINS

Penicillins were the first antibiotics introduced for clinical use. They are also called beta-lactam antibiotics because their chemical structure contains a beta-lactam ring that is essential for antibacterial activity. All penicillins contain this essential beta-lactam ring; however, adding a side chain to

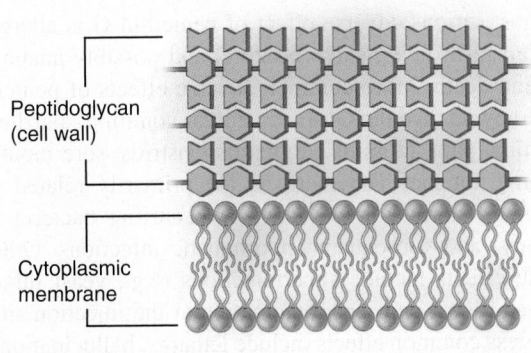

Gram-positive cell envelope

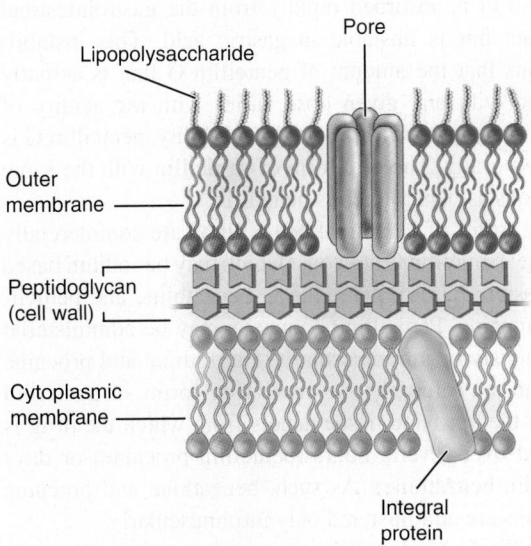

Gram-negative cell envelope

• FIGURE 39.1 Although the gram-positive cell wall is much thicker than the gram-negative cell wall, antibiotics can attach to targets on the cytoplasmic membrane. In the gram-negative cell, the wall is thinner, but the cell also contains an outer membrane that makes it difficult for antibiotics to permeate the cell.

specific types of penicillins influences their pharmacokinetic properties, binding capabilities, penicillinase resistance, and resistance to stomach acids. Penicillins are most effective against cells undergoing active growth and division. Penicillins are classified as narrow-spectrum penicillins, aminopenicillins (broad-spectrum penicillins), extended-spectrum penicillins, and penicillinase-resistant penicillins. Table 39.1 presents a summary of selected penicillins. Penicillin G aqueous, a narrow-spectrum penicillin, is the prototype for the penicillin class.

Nursing Management of the Patient Receiving P Penicillin G

Core Drug Knowledge

Pharmacotherapeutics

Penicillin G is indicated for use in infections caused by susceptible gram-positive bacteria, anaerobes, and spirochetes, including streptococci, non–penicillinase-producing staphylococci, and *Treponema pallidum*. Clinically, these bacteria cause infections such as pneumonia, pharyngitis, tonsillitis, endocarditis, and scarlet fever. Other clinical uses include therapy for tetanus, anthrax, meningitis, syphilis, diphtheria, rat-bite fever, and fusospirochetal infections.

Penicillin G may also be used as prophylaxis in special patient populations to prevent bacterial endocarditis prior to procedures likely to produce temporary bacteremia. These patients include those with prosthetic heart valves, mitral valve prolapse, most congenital heart diseases, and acquired valvular heart disease. It may also be used as prophylaxis in patients with recurrent rheumatic fever or rheumatic heart disease.

Pharmacokinetics

Penicillin G is absorbed rapidly from the gastrointestinal (GI) tract but is unstable in gastric acid. This instability means that the amount of penicillin G that is actually absorbed with any given dose varies with the acidity of stomach contents. Because of this instability, penicillin G is not given orally. The oral form of penicillin with the same indications as penicillin G is penicillin V.

Three forms of parenteral penicillin G are commercially available: penicillin G aqueous (which may be sodium based or potassium based), penicillin G benzathine, and penicillin G procaine. Penicillin G aqueous may be administered intravenously or intramuscularly. Benzathine and procaine penicillin are referred to as repository forms of penicillin because they provide tissue depots from which the drug is absorbed over several hours (penicillin procaine) or days (penicillin benzathine). As such, benzathine and procaine penicillins are administered only intramuscularly.

Penicillin G binds to plasma proteins and circulates in the blood to be released at various tissue sites. The average peak drug effect is 4 hours after administration. Penicillin G crosses the placenta and is secreted in breast milk. It does not penetrate the blood–brain barrier very well except in the presence of meningeal inflammation, a fact that makes it somewhat useful in treating meningitis.

Penicillin G is rapidly cleared unchanged from the plasma by the kidneys (by glomerular filtration and renal tubular secretion). Because this rapid clearance of the drug makes it somewhat difficult to maintain therapeutic levels, around-the-clock administration is needed for therapy to be truly effective.

Pharmacodynamics

Penicillin G inhibits the third and final stage of bacterial cell wall synthesis by binding to specific **penicillin-binding proteins** (PBPs) located inside the bacterial cell wall. After binding with specific PBPs, penicillin inhibits transpeptidase, an enzyme that is responsible for developing cross-bridges within the cell wall. These cross-bridges give the cell wall its strength. Additionally, penicillin affects autolytic enzymes (autolysins) that promote active cell wall destruction. The relationship between PBPs and autolysins is unclear; possibly, penicillin interferes with an autolysin inhibitor. As the cell wall weakens, the internal osmotic pressure of the bacteria changes, allowing the cell to swell, then burst. The body's immune system completes the process of fighting the infection and cleans up debris from ruptured bacteria.

Penicillin has selective toxicity to bacteria because human cells do not use the biochemical process that the bacteria use to form a cell wall and are thus protected from destruction.

Contraindications and Precautions

Penicillin G is contraindicated in the presence of known allergies to penicillin, cephalosporins, or imipenem. Penicillin sensitivity tests are available if the patient's history of allergy is unclear and penicillin is the drug of choice. Caution should be exercised in the presence of renal disease, pregnancy, and lactation.

Adverse Effects

The most serious adverse effect of penicillin G is allergic reaction: rash, fever, and wheezing, and possibly anaphylaxis and death. More common adverse effects of penicillin therapy involve the GI tract: nausea, vomiting, diarrhea, abdominal pain, glossitis, stomatitis, gastritis, sore mouth, and furry tongue. These effects are primarily related to the loss of normal flora (naturally occurring bacteria in the body) and subsequent opportunistic infections. Other adverse effects include superinfections (e.g., yeast infections) and local pain or inflammation at the injection site. Other, less common effects include lethargy, hallucinations, anemia, thrombocytopenia, nephritis, and sodium overload (especially with the sodium salt of penicillin G).

Drug Interactions

The effectiveness of penicillin G is decreased when it is taken concurrently with tetracyclines. Parenteral aminoglycosides (amikacin, gentamicin, kanamycin, neomycin,

TABLE 39.1	Summary of Selected ⓒ Penicillins and Other Beta-Lactam Antibiotics		
Drug (Trade) Name	**Selected Indications**	**Route and Dosage Range**	**Pharmacokinetics**
ⓒ Penicillins			
ⓟ penicillin G (Pfizerpen)	Pneumococcal infections Streptococcal infections (Group A) Bacterial endocarditis Diphtheria Neurosyphilis Congenital syphilis	Penicillin G is administered IV as penicillin G aqueous and IM as penicillin G procaine or benzathine. Dosages highly individualized. *Adult:* IM, 300,000–8 million units daily in divided doses; IV, 6–20 million units daily by continuous or intermittent infusion (q2–4 h) *Child:* IM/IV, 25,000–250,000 U/kg/d in divided doses	*Onset:* IM, rapid; IV, rapid *Duration:* Varies $t_{1/2}$: 30–60 min
penicillin G benzathine (Bicillin-CR, Bicillin LA Permapen)	Streptococcal infections Early syphilis Syphilis of >1-y duration	*Adult:* IM, 1.2 million U q4wk *Adult:* IV, 2.4 million U in one single dose *Adult:* Parenteral, 2.4 million U once weekly for 3 wk *Child:* >27 kg, parenteral, 900,000–1.2 million U in one dose; < 27 kg, 300–600,000 U in one dose	*Onset:* IM, slow *Duration:* 1–4 wk $t_{1/2}$: 30–60 min
penicillin G procaine	Pneumococcal infections Staphylococcal infections	*Adult and child:* IM, 600,000–1.2 million U/d in one or two doses for 10 d–2 wk	*Onset:* IM, slow *Duration:* 15–20 h $t_{1/2}$: 30–60 min
penicillin V (Pen-Vee K, Veetids)	Fusospirochetal infections Streptococcal infections	*Adult:* PO, 250–500 mg q6–8 h *Adult:* PO, 125–250 mg q6–8 h for 10 d *Child:* PO, 25–50 mg/kg/d q6–8h	*Onset:* Rapid *Duration:* Varies $t_{1/2}$: 30–60 min
ⓒ Aminopenicillins			
ampicillin (Omnipen)	Septicemia Bacterial meningitis Respiratory/soft-tissue infections	*Adult:* IV, 150–200 mg/kg/d for 3 d, then IM q3–4 h *Child:* Same as adult *Adult:* IV, 150–200 mg/kg/d by continuous infusion and then IM injections q3–4 h *Child:* Same as adult *Adult:* PO, ≥40 kg; IV or IM, 250–500 mg q6 h; <40 kg, IV or IM, 25–50 mg/kg at 6–8 h intervals; <20 kg, PO, 50 mg/kg/d in equal doses q6–8 h	*Onset:* PO, 30 min; IM, 15 min; IV, immediate *Duration:* 6–8 h $t_{1/2}$: 1–2 h
amoxicillin (Amoxil)	URI, GU infections Lower respiratory tract infections	*Adult:* PO, 250–500 mg q8h *Child:* Same as adult *Adult:* PO, 500 mg q8h *Child:* Same as adult	*Onset:* Varies *Duration:* 6–8 h $t_{1/2}$: 1–1.4 h
ⓒ Extended-Spectrum Penicillins			
piperacillin (Pipracil)	Lower respiratory tract infections Skin and skin structure infections Bone and joint infections Intra-abdominal infections Gynecologic infections Bacteremia Septicemia	*Adult:* IV, 3–4 g infusion over 20–30 min q4h *Child:* Although safety and efficacy in children have not been fully established, pediatric patients have received 76–100 mg/kg/d IV or IM in divided doses q4h	*Onset:* IV, rapid *Duration:* 4–6 h $t_{1/2}$: 0.7–1.3 h
ⓒ Penicillinase-Resistant Penicillins			
dicloxacillin (Dynapen)	Infections due to penicillinase-producing staphylococci	*Adult and child >40 kg:* PO, 125 mg q6h; up to 250 mg q6h in severe infections *Child <40 kg:* PO, 12.5–25 mg/kg/d in equally divided doses q6h; up to 25 mg/kg/d in equally divided doses q6h in severe infections	*Onset:* Varies *Duration:* 6–8 h $t_{1/2}$: 30–90 min

(Continued)

TABLE 39.1 Summary of Selected ⓒ Penicillins and Other Beta-Lactam Antibiotics *(continued)*

Drug (Trade) Name	Selected Indications	Route and Dosage Range	Pharmacokinetics
nafcillin (Nallpen)	Infections due to penicillinase-producing staphylococci Infections caused by group A beta-hemolytic streptococci, *Streptococcus viridans*	*Adult:* IV, 0.5–2 g q4 h *Child:* IV, 50–100 mg/kg/d in equally divided doses q6 h; for severe infections, 100–200 mg/kg/d *Adult:* IM, 500 mg q4–6 h *Child:* IM, 50–100 mg/kg/d in equally divided doses q6 h; for severe infections, 100–200 mg/kg/d *Adult:* PO, 0.25–1 g q4–6 h *Child:* PO, 50–100 mg/kg/d in divided doses q6 h	*Onset:* PO, varies; IM, rapid; IV, immediate *Duration:* PO and IV, 4 h; IM, 4–6 h $t_{1/2}$: 1 h
oxacillin (Bactocill)	Infections due to penicillinase-producing staphylococci Infections caused by streptococci	*Adult and child >40 kg:* IM/IV, 0.25–2 g q4–6 h; maximum daily dose, 23 g *Child <40 kg:* IM/IV, 50–100 mg/kg/d in equally divided doses q4–6 h *Adult and child ≥40 kg:* PO, 0.5–1 g q4–6 h *Child <40 kg:* PO, 50–100 mg/kg/d in equally divided doses q4–6 h	*Onset:* PO, varies; IM/IV, rapid *Duration:* PO/IM, 4–6 h; IV, length of infusion $t_{1/2}$: 0.5–1 h

ⓒ Monobactams

Drug (Trade) Name	Selected Indications	Route and Dosage Range	Pharmacokinetics
aztreonam (Azactam)	Moderately severe systemic infection with *Pseudomonas aeruginosa* Urethritis Endocervicitis Proctitis Gonococcal infections	*Adult:* IV, 0.5–2 g q6–12 h *Infant and child ≥1 mo:* IV, 30 mg/kg q6–8 h; for patients with cystic fibrosis, 50 mg/kg q6–8 h *Infant and child ≥1 mo:* IV, 50 mg/kg q4–6 h *Adult:* IM, 1 g as a single dose	*Onset:* IM, varies; IV, rapid *Duration:* 6–8 h $t_{1/2}$: 1.5–2 h

ⓒ Carbapenems

Drug (Trade) Name	Selected Indications	Route and Dosage Range	Pharmacokinetics
cilastatin-imipenem (Primaxin)	Intra-abdominal infections Gynecologic infections Lower respiratory tract infections Skin and skin structure infections Bone and joint infections Bacteremia or septicemia Endocarditis Febrile neutropenia	*Adult:* IV, 250–500 mg q 6 h to a maximum of 4 g/d *Adult:* IM, 500–750 mg q 12 h, depending on severity of infection *Child >3 mo:* IV, 15–25 mg/kg q6 h to a maximum dose of 2 g/d	*Onset:* IM, rapid; IV, immediate *Duration:* 6–12 h $t_{1/2}$: 90–120 min
doripenem (Doribax)	Complicated abdominal or urinary tract infections Pyelonephritis	*Adult IV:* 500 mg every 8 h	*Onset:* rapid *Duration:* length of infusion *T1/2:* 1 hour
ertapenem (Invanz)	Community-acquired pneumonia Skin and skin structure infections Complicated GI infections Complicated intra-abdominal infections Acute pelvic infections	*Adult:* IM/IV, 1 g/d *Child:* Safety in children not established	*Onset:* IM, 10 min; IV, rapid *Duration:* Unknown $t_{1/2}$: 4 h
meropenem (Merrem)	Intra-abdominal infections Bacterial meningitis	*Adult and child >50 kg:* IV, 1–2 g q8 h *Child <50 kg:* IV, 20–40 mg/kg q8 h	*Onset:* Immediate *Duration:* 10–12 h $t_{1/2}$: 1 h

TABLE 39.1 Summary of Selected ⓒ Penicillins and Other Beta-Lactam Antibiotics *(continued)*

Drug (Trade) Name	Selected Indications	Route and Dosage Range	Pharmacokinetics
ⓒ **Combination Drugs**			
ampicillin/sulbactam (Unasyn)	Skin and skin structure infections Soft-tissue infections Otitis media Sinusitis Respiratory tract infections GU infections Septicemia	*Adult and child >40 kg:* IV/IM, 1.5–3 g q6–8 h *Child >1 y:* IV, 75 mg/kg q6 h	*Onset:* IM, rapid; IV, immediate *Duration:* 6–8 h $t_{1/2}$: 1–1.5 h
amoxicillin/clavulanic acid (Augmentin)	Otitis media Respiratory tract infections Skin and skin structure infections Urinary tract infections Community-acquired pneumonia SARS	*Adult:* PO, 250–500 q8 h *Child <40 kg:* PO, 20–40 mg/kg in divided doses q8 h	*Onset:* 30 min *Duration:* 8 h $t_{1/2}$: 1–1.5 h
ticarcillin/clavulanic acid (Timentin)	Skin and skin structure infections Bone and joint infections Septicemia Respiratory tract infections Intra-abdominal infections Gynecologic infections Urinary tract infections	*Adult and child >40 kg:* IV, 3 g q4 h or 4 g q6 h *Child <40 kg:* IV, 33.3–50 mg/kg q4 h or 50–75 mg/kg q6 h *Neonate >2 kg:* IV, 75 mg/kg q8 h *Neonate <2 kg:* IV, 75 mg/kg q12 h	*Onset:* IM/IV, rapid *Duration:* 4–6 h $t_{1/2}$: 1 h
piperacillin/tazobactam (Zosyn)	Intra-abdominal infections Skin and skin structure infections Gynecologic infections Respiratory tract infections	*Adult:* IV, 3–4 g q6–8 h	*Onset:* IM/IV, rapid *Duration:* 4–6 h $t_{1/2}$: 0.7–1.5 h

paromomycin, streptomycin, tobramycin) are inactivated when these drugs are administered with penicillin G. Table 39.2 lists agents that interact with penicillin G.

Oral probenecid, a drug used in the treatment of gout, is sometimes given with intravenous (IV) penicillin G because it slows the excretion of the drug by competing with the penicillin molecule for excretion sites in the renal tubule. The result is that penicillin levels stay high for a longer time, achieving a greater effect.

Assessment of Relevant Core Patient Variables

Health Status

Take a careful health history to assess for any known reactions to antibiotics. Examine the skin for any rash or lesions to provide a baseline to avoid misdiagnosis of an allergic reaction. Assess the respiratory status of the patient as a baseline for possible wheezing associated with an allergic reaction.

For patients with a questionable history of allergic reaction to penicillin, perform a skin test to determine current allergic status. Because the skin test itself may cause an anaphylactic response in susceptible patients, it should be performed only in a setting staffed and equipped to respond to a potential emergency. In rare situations, it may be necessary to give penicillin to a penicillin-allergic patient. In these rare cases, penicillin is administered according to a desensitization schedule. Desensitization does not always stop an allergic response; therefore, it must be performed in an acute care setting. Epinephrine and respiratory support must be immediately available for either skin testing or desensitization.

For elderly patients or patients with kidney disease, evaluate kidney function (including blood urea nitrogen [BUN] and creatinine clearance) to determine baseline functioning. Patients with severe decreased kidney function may need a reduced dose of penicillin G. For long-term therapy, also

TABLE 39.2	Agents That Interact with P Penicillin G	
Interactants	**Effect and Significance**	**Nursing Management**
aminoglycosides	GI absorption of penicillins may be impaired by aminoglycosides. Penicillins may inactivate certain aminoglycosides.	Avoid combination therapy if possible. Administer at least 2 h apart. Tailor dose of penicillin as needed. Monitor peak and trough levels of aminoglycoside.
anticoagulants	Large IV doses of penicillin may prolong bleeding time.	Monitor for signs of bleeding. Monitor PT/INR
food	GI absorption of penicillins are impaired by the presence of food.	Administer at least 1 h before or 2 h after meals.
oral contraceptives	Penicillins may suppress intestinal flora, which provide an enzyme essential for enterohepatic recirculation for certain oral contraceptives. This may result in a decreased contraceptive plasma level.	Advise patients taking oral contraceptives to use an additional method of birth control while taking penicillins.
methotrexate	Coadministration may increase serum methotrexate levels, resulting in toxicity.	Avoid if possible. Monitor signs and symptoms of methotrexate toxicity.
tetracyclines	The bacteriostatic action of tetracyclines may impair the bactericidal activity of penicillins.	Avoid combination therapy.

perform baseline liver function tests (LFTs). In addition, assess for previously prescribed drugs that may interact with penicillin to cause undesired effects.

When penicillin G is used for gram-negative infections, always perform culture and sensitivity tests to be sure that the causative bacteria are sensitive to penicillin G.

Life Span and Gender

Document the method of birth control used by a woman of childbearing age because antibiotics, such as penicillin G, can counteract the effects of an oral contraceptive. Assess women of childbearing age for pregnancy and lactation. Give pregnant and lactating women penicillin G with caution because superinfections may occur in the fetus or infant, or the infant may develop diarrhea. If the patient is elderly, he or she may need a reduced dose because of decreased kidney function.

Lifestyle, Diet, and Habits

Instruct patients self-administering penicillin G to administer the drug around the clock to ensure that drug levels stay within a therapeutic range. Assess the patient's daily schedule to ensure that the patient who is self-administering penicillin G can complete the therapy as prescribed.

Environment

Be aware of the environment in which the drug will be administered. Whether administered at home or in an acute care setting, penicillin G solution should be mixed and stored in a refrigerator between 2° and 8°C (36° and 46°F) for up to 7 days. It should never be frozen. Commercially prepared infusion solutions may be kept at room temperature for 24 hours. Oral penicillin does not have specific environmental requirements.

Nursing Diagnoses and Outcomes

- Risk for Injury related to drug-related allergic reactions
  Desired outcome: The patient will recognize symptoms of allergy and contact the prescriber immediately to minimize ill effects.
- Imbalanced Nutrition: Less than Body Requirements related to drug-induced GI effects, such as diarrhea, GI upset, altered taste sensation, or superinfection
  Desired outcome: The patient will maintain consistent body weight and consult prescriber about persistent adverse effects that affect nutritional status.
- Diarrhea related to drug therapy
  Desired outcome: The patient will avoid dehydration, maintain fluid intake, and contact prescriber about persistent diarrhea.
- Risk for Infection related to overgrowth of nonsusceptible organisms.
  Desired outcome: The patient will report signs of superinfection to the prescriber.

Planning and Intervention

Maximizing Therapeutic Effects

Review culture and sensitivity reports to make sure that penicillin G is appropriate for the patient, especially for gram-negative infections. Administer penicillin G as prescribed, spaced evenly around the clock to increase effectiveness. For oral preparations, administer the dose on an empty stomach. Optimally, drug therapy should continue for at least 7 to 10 days, but it may continue for 2 weeks.

In acute care settings, retrieve the antibiotic from the refrigerator approximately 15 minutes before administration, and evaluate the IV site for signs of phlebitis before and after administration.

Administer intramuscular (IM) penicillin deep into the muscle mass. Aspirate the syringe to avoid accidental injection into the vasculature. Assess landmarks for IM administration to avoid injection into a nerve.

Minimizing Adverse Effects

Provide small, frequent meals; mouth care; and ice chips for the patient to suck on if stomatitis and sore mouth are problems. Monitor the patient to ensure that adequate fluids are given to replace fluid lost with an adverse effect such as diarrhea. Monitoring fluid intake and output is especially important. Notify the prescriber if a substantial change develops in the intake-to-output ratio, because such a change may be the first indication of kidney dysfunction.

When administering penicillin parenterally (IM or IV), monitor the patient for a minimum of 30 minutes. Epinephrine and respiratory support should be immediately available whenever parenteral penicillin is administered.

Read the penicillin label carefully prior to administration. Penicillin G benzathine and penicillin G procaine must be given intramuscularly. Inadvertent administration into the vasculature has been associated with cardiopulmonary arrest and death.

Providing Patient and Family Education

• Teach patients that penicillin is one drug within a class of drugs. Advise patients who have ever had any type of allergic reaction to penicillin never to take any other drug with a name that ends with "cillin."

• Explain to patients with penicillin allergy the importance of wearing some form of identification (e.g., MedicAlert necklace or bracelet) to alert health care personnel of the allergy in an emergency.

• Stress the importance of completing the full course of antibiotics, explaining the purpose of the drug and stating that it may not work for other types of infection.

• Emphasize the need to take penicillin G exactly as prescribed at evenly spaced intervals around the clock. Instruct the patient that oral drugs should be taken on an empty stomach 1 hour before or 2 hours after a meal.

• Instruct patients to take missed doses as soon as remembered but not at the time that the next dose is scheduled.

• If patients must mix the solution, instruct them to do so just before administration. When premixed solutions are used, they should be kept in the refrigerator and retrieved approximately 15 minutes before administration.

• Advise patients to contact the prescriber if no improvement occurs within 3 days.

• Because any patient may develop sensitivity to penicillin G at any time, discuss the signs and symptoms of allergic reaction and instruct patients to stop the drug and call the prescriber if a rash, welts, itching, or shortness of breath develops.

• Review common adverse effects and home interventions that may relieve discomfort. Patients who experience abdominal cramps or GI distress may try eating small,

Taking Antibiotics Safely

Every year, families in the community face colds, sore throats, flu, and other types of infections. Should all of these conditions be treated with antibiotics? Even as a new member of the health care team, you can answer questions concerning antibiotic safety with ease. Be sure to emphasize these key points:

• Illnesses with very similar symptoms may be caused by entirely different types of microbes.
• Illnesses caused by microbes other than bacteria are generally not affected by antibiotics.
• Overuse, including inappropriate use of antibiotics, leads to bacterial resistance (super-strains of microbes that are very difficult to kill).
• Antibiotics take time to work, so it will take a couple of days to feel better.
• Take the medication exactly as prescribed—don't take fewer pills per day to make the prescription last longer.
• Never take medication from a previous illness—if its expiration date has passed, it might not work.
• Never take medication prescribed for another person, even if your symptoms are similar to theirs.
• All medications can cause adverse effects, especially nausea or diarrhea, but these effects are not signs of allergy.
• Signs of allergy include reddened skin, rash, itching, hives, swelling of one or more body parts, shortness of breath, wheezing, or chest palpitations. If you have these symptoms, do not take any more of the drug! Call the person who prescribed the medication immediately.

frequent meals. To relieve a sore mouth or throat, sucking on ice chips may help. If diarrhea occurs, teach patients to increase fluid intake and to contact the prescriber if symptoms do not resolve in 24 hours.

• Teach patients about other adverse effects, such as a change in tongue color, fatigue, easy bruising, and vaginal discharge. Instruct patients to report these signs and symptoms of superinfection to the prescriber immediately.

• Advise women of childbearing age to use a backup method of birth control for the duration of therapy.

• Explain the importance of sterile technique if family members administer IV therapy at home (Box 39.1).

Ongoing Assessment and Evaluation

Monitor for signs of allergic reaction and for resolution of the presenting symptoms of infection (e.g., fever, lethargy, or hot and reddened or inflamed skin). Failure of these symptoms to resolve may indicate a treatment failure. Monitor for signs of superinfection and notify the prescriber immediately to arrange for treatment. For patient comfort, provide warm compresses and gentle massage to painful or swollen injection sites and observe for signs of phlebitis or abscess formation.

Monitor patients receiving parenteral sodium penicillin G for potential fluid overload. Monitoring is especially important in patients with cardiac disease or hypertension. Monitor patients receiving potassium penicillin G for signs

MEMORY CHIP

P Penicillin G

- Used for infections caused by gram-positive bacteria, anaerobes, and spirochetes. Also used as prophylaxis to prevent bacterial endocarditis.
- Major contraindications: hypersensitivity to penicillin, cephalosporins, or imipenem
- Most common adverse effects: nausea, vomiting, diarrhea
- Most serious adverse effect: hypersensitivity
- **Life span alert: Elderly patients may need reduced dosage because of decreased kidney function.**
- Maximizing therapeutic effects: Oral preparations should be given on an empty stomach. When using for gram-negative infections, be sure culture and sensitivity tests are done before administration.
- Minimizing adverse effects: Monitor intake and output because it may be the first sign of kidney dysfunction. Blood levels may become toxic if the kidneys cannot excrete penicillin.
- Most important patient education: Take the medication exactly as prescribed until the entire prescription is completed, despite the absence of symptoms. Monitor for signs and symptoms of allergic response and stop the medication if any occur.
- **Black box warning: Penicillin G has three formulations— penicillin G aqueous, penicillin G procaine, and penicillin G benzathine. Only penicillin G aqueous may be given intravenously.**

---

of hyperkalemia that may result in cardiac arrhythmias. Arrange for periodic electrolyte studies for patients receiving either preparation.

When treatment ends, the initial infection should be resolved. The patient should be adequately nourished and hydrated, and any adverse drug effects should be resolved.

Drugs Closely Related to P Penicillin G

Other Narrow-Spectrum Penicillins

Penicillin G benzathine is the benzathine salt of penicillin G. It has low solubility and provides an IM reservoir for low levels of penicillin over a long time. It can be detected in serum for up to 12 weeks after injection. It is used primarily for treating syphilis and preventing rheumatic fever.

Penicillin G procaine is the procaine salt of penicillin G. Because it is given by IM injection only, its use has been limited by the advent of IV antibiotics and newer broad-spectrum IM antibiotics. This drug must be stored in the refrigerator. Because it is viscous, it must warm at room temperature for approximately 15 minutes before being injected. Patients may react to procaine with confusion or agitation. This response is sometimes mistaken for a penicillin allergy.

Both penicillin G procaine and penicillin G benzathine have a Black Box warning that these two forms of penicillin G must be administered by the IM route. IV administration is associated with cardiorespiratory arrest and death.

Penicillin V (Pen-Vee-K, V-cillin-K) is the acid-stable oral form of penicillin G. It is indicated for the same infections

CRITICAL THINKING SCENARIO

IMPLEMENTING PENICILLIN V THERAPY

You have a patient who has been taking penicillin V for 2 days to "cure" an infection. You find out that this antibiotic was left over from an upper respiratory infection for which it had been prescribed 2 years earlier. The patient states that he stopped the drug when he felt better and kept it around just in case he got sick again. Describe how you would explain the dangers of taking antibiotics in this manner in a way that makes sense to the patient and leads to his adherence to antibiotic therapy in the future.

---

as penicillin G and for prophylaxis during dental and upper respiratory procedures for patients who are immunocompromised or who are prone to bacterial endocarditis.

The contraindications, precautions, drug interactions, and adverse effects associated with penicillin V are the same as those associated with penicillin G. Penicillin V should be given only on an empty stomach, 1 hour before or 2 to 3 hours after meals, with a full glass of water. Advise the patient to continue the drug for the full course of the drug therapy, usually 7 to 10 days. Advise the patient neither to save the drug for self-medication at a later date nor to share the drug with any other person.

Broad-Spectrum Penicillins (Aminopenicillins)

Ampicillin and amoxicillin are aminopenicillins. The aminopenicillins have a slightly altered side chain that makes them effective against many gram-negative microorganisms, including *Haemophilus influenzae*, *Escherichia coli*, *Salmonella* and *Shigella* species, and indole-positive *Proteus mirabilis*. Aminopenicillins are ineffective against most infections caused by *Staphylococcus aureus* because they are easily inactivated by penicillinase produced by this species.

The benefits of these drugs include their higher oral absorption, higher serum levels, and longer half-lives. Ampicillin is the only drug that may be is available for both oral and intravenous administration.

Because these drugs are available for oral use and are effective against some of the most serious pediatric infections, they are frequently used to treat otitis media, upper respiratory infections, tonsillitis, skin infections, and pneumonia in children. Aminopenicillins should be used only for infections that are not sensitive to penicillin G or penicillin V because they have a broader spectrum of activity and therefore pose a greater opportunity for resistant strains to develop and adverse effects to occur.

Teach parents or other caregivers to follow storage and administration instructions exactly, to discard leftover drug and not save it for later use, to report frequently occurring rash or diarrhea, and to watch for signs of superinfections.

Extended-Spectrum Penicillins (Antipseudomonal Penicillins)

Piperacillin and ticarcillin are the extended-spectrum penicillins. They have an even broader spectrum than the aminopenicillins. The extended-spectrum penicillins are effective against all of the organisms susceptible to the aminopenicillins, plus *Pseudomonas aeruginosa, Enterobacter* species, *Bacteroides fragilis,* many *Klebsiella* species, *Proteus vulgaris, Proteus morganii,* and *Proteus rettgeri.* Like the aminopenicillins, extended-spectrum penicillins are easily inactivated by penicillinase produced by *S. aureus.* They are available for oral or parenteral administration.

When given to combat *Pseudomonas,* extended-spectrum penicillins are frequently given concurrently with aminoglycoside antibiotics. When administered appropriately, this combination is highly effective. Remember to administer these two antibiotics at least 2 hours apart to avoid an antagonist drug–drug interaction.

The extended-spectrum penicillins should be reserved for use in serious infections by susceptible organisms. Again, caution patients to take oral preparations on an empty stomach, to complete the full course, and to monitor for side effects.

Penicillinase-Resistant Penicillins (Antistaphylococcal Penicillins)

With the use of penicillins over the years, increasing numbers of bacterial species are developing the enzyme penicillinase to counteract the effects of penicillin. The penicillinase-resistant drugs (dicloxacillin, nafcillin, and oxacillin) were developed to remain effective against bacteria that produce penicillinase and thus are resistant to penicillin. Although the penicillinase-resistant antibiotics are highly effective against strains of staphylococci, they are inactive against many other bacteria that secrete penicillinase, especially gram-negative bacteria. Culture and sensitivity tests are mandatory when using a penicillinase-resistant drug. The drugs in this group include dicloxacillin, which is an oral preparation, and nafcillin and oxacillin, which are IV preparations.

Certain strains of staphylococci are resistant to the drugs in this class. A patient infected with these strains of staphylococci may have an infection known as methicillin-resistant *Staphylococcus aureus* (MRSA). Resistance to methicillin implies resistance to any drug in this class. Methicillin (which is no longer available in the United States) is used infrequently because it can cause interstitial nephritis, whereas nafcillin and oxacillin are equally effective and do not have this adverse effect. The oral use of these drugs is now recommended for treating all gram-positive infections, because staphylococci are almost entirely penicillin resistant. Again, urge the patient to complete the full course of drug therapy, to take oral drugs on an empty stomach, and not to self-medicate with this drug at another time.

Drugs Significantly Different From P Penicillin G

Beta-Lactamase Inhibitors

Resistance to beta-lactams, such as penicillin, may occur because of the bacteria's ability to produce beta-lactamase. Clavulanic acid, sulbactam, and tazobactam are beta-lactamase inhibitors. On their own, they exhibit only weak antibacterial effects, and they are combined with other penicillin antibiotics to act as competitive "suicide" inhibitors of

bacterial beta-lactamases. They accomplish this feat by binding to the enzyme's active site, thus allowing the penicillin to reach its target site. Clavulanic acid, sulbactam, and tazobactam do not alter the actions of the beta-lactam antibiotics. They simply prevent penicillins from being destroyed. Box 39.2 identifies the most common combination drugs that contain beta-lactamase inhibitors.

Bacitracin

Bacitracin is an oral, parenteral, and topical polypeptide antibiotic. It acts principally against gram-positive bacteria. Thus, it is combined frequently with drugs such as neomycin and polymyxins, which are active against gram-negative bacteria. The most common use of bacitracin is as a topical agent to prevent superficial skin and eye infections following minor injuries. It is available as a cream or ointment as well as ophthalmic drops or ointment.

Oral bacitracin is designated as an orphan drug to treat pseudomembranous colitis caused by *Clostridium difficile.* IM bacitracin is used rarely because of the risk for serious nephrotoxicity. However, IM bacitracin may be used to treat infants with pneumonia or empyema. Oral or parenteral bacitracin is used only in clinical situations in which less toxic drugs have not been effective.

To avoid systemic absorption of topical bacitracin, do not apply it to serious burns, deep wounds, or animal bites, over large areas of the body, or into a perforated tympanic membrane. Although topical bacitracin has few adverse effects, rare cases of anaphylaxis have been reported. Ophthalmic bacitracin may cause blurred vision that resolves spontaneously.

MONOBACTAM ANTIBIOTICS

Aztreonam (Azactam) is a monobactam with a mechanism of activity similar to that of penicillin: it inhibits bacterial cell wall synthesis. It is used to manage infections caused by gram-negative aerobic bacteria. It has no activity against gram-positive bacteria or anaerobes. The structure of aztreonam differs substantially from the structures of other beta-lactam antibiotics; this drug may be given safely to penicillin-allergic patients because there is little cross-sensitivity.

Aztreonam is administered intravenously or intramuscularly and is eliminated by renal tubular secretion. It is also available as an inhaled drug (Cayston) for cystic fibrosis patients with *Pseudomonas aeruginosa.* Half-life is prolonged in patients with renal failure. It is widely distributed throughout the body, including the central nervous system (CNS).

Hypersensitivity is the only contraindication to aztreonam therapy. Common adverse effects include vertigo and headache. Serious, but rare, adverse effects include GI distress with possible superinfection, hepatotoxicity, seizures, and blood dyscrasias, including neutropenia.

Important drug–drug interactions include synergistic effects when aztreonam is given with aminoglycosides and other beta-lactam antibiotics. Antagonistic effects may occur when it is given with cefoxitin or imipenem. Toxic aztreonam levels may occur when probenecid is given at the same time.

When giving aztreonam intravenously, check frequently for signs of thrombophlebitis at the IV insertion site. For long-term therapy, monitor laboratory studies, such as complete blood count (CBC), LFTs, prothrombin time (PT), partial thromboplastin time (PTT), and platelet count.

C CARBAPENEMS

Like monobactams, carbapenems are chemically different from penicillins but retain the beta-lactam ring structure. They are very broad-spectrum antibiotics with activity against gram-positive cocci, gram-negative cocci, and bacilli, and they are the most effective beta-lactam antibiotics for use against anaerobes. Imipenem, meropenem, and ertapenem, and doripenem are the carbapenems approved for use in the United States.

Cilastatin-Imipenem

Imipenem is rapidly inactivated by renal dehydropeptidase 1. Therefore, imipenem is always administered with cilastatin, a drug that inhibits this enzyme. Cilastatin-imipenem (Primaxin) given IV or IM has a high affinity for bacterial PBPs and thus penetrates the cell wall efficiently. It also has a high resistance to bacterial enzymes, making it a very effective antibiotic.

Cilastatin-imipenem is structurally similar to penicillin and cephalosporins. For that reason, patients with a severe hypersensitivity to either of these agents should not be given cilastatin-imipenem. Cilastatin-imipenem is given cautiously to patients with head trauma, brain lesions, and pre-existing seizure disorders because these patients have a high risk for cilastatin-imipenem–induced seizures. Because cilastatin-imipenem is substantially excreted by the kidneys, patients with renal insufficiency, including the elderly, need a reduced dose. Cilastatin-imipenem is a Food and Drug Administration (FDA) pregnancy category C drug; however, whether it is excreted in human milk is unknown. Drug–drug interactions include cyclosporine, ganciclovir, or theophylline; the CNS effects of these drugs may be additive. Serious adverse effects include seizures, pseudomembranous colitis, and blood dyscrasias. More common adverse effects include GI distress, superinfections such as candidiasis, injection-site reactions, phlebitis, and elevations of LFT, BUN, and creatinine.

Doripenem

Doripenem (Doribax) is the newest carbapenem drug to be approved in the United States. It is FDA approved for the management of complicated abdominal or urinary tract infections and pyelonephritis. Like the other carbapenems, hypersensitivity is the only contraindication. Doripenem should not be given cautiously with probenecid or valproic acid. When administered with probenecid, doripenem levels are increased resulting in an increased risk for adverse effects. Like meropenem, doripenem may decrease serum valproic acid levels. Doripenem is a pregnancy category B; whether it is excreted into breast milk is unknown. Like ertapenem, it is not approved for use in children. Common adverse effects include phlebitis, rash, GI distress, and headache. Serious adverse effects are similar to those of cilastatin-imipenem.

Ertapenem

Ertapenem (Invanz) is administered either intramuscularly or intravenously. Its spectrum of activity is less than that of cilastatin-imipenem or meropenem. Most important, ertapenem has little or no activity against *P. aeruginosa* or *Acinetobacter* species. Ertapenem is indicated to manage moderate to severe complicated intra-abdominal infections, skin and skin structure infections, pyelonephritis, acute pelvic infections, and community-acquired pneumonia. Like meropenem, ertapenem is administered as a single agent. It is also excreted primarily by the kidneys, and reduced doses are required for patients with renal compromise. It belongs to FDA pregnancy category B and is secreted in breast milk. Ertapenem is not indicated for use in children. Contraindications and precautions are similar to those for cilastatin-imipenem and meropenem. Probenecid decreases the renal clearance of ertapenem. Adverse effects are similar to those of other carbapenems, and although seizures may occur, they are less likely to occur with ertapenem.

Meropenem

Meropenem (Merrem) is an IV antibiotic that is similar to cilastatin-imipenem. It is used to manage abdominal infections, such as appendicitis and peritonitis, and bacterial meningitis. It is also useful in managing nosocomial infections that are resistant to other antibiotics. Meropenem is not degraded by renal dipeptidases and can therefore be given as a single agent. As with cilastatin-imipenem, hypersensitivity is the only contraindication. Precautions to meropenem use are the same as for cilastatin-imipenem. Meropenem is excreted substantially unchanged; thus, a reduced dose is necessary for patients with renal insufficiency. It belongs to FDA pregnancy category B; whether it is excreted into breast milk is unknown. Meropenem may interact with valproic acid; thus, patients receiving valproic acid should be monitored to ensure that their treatment is effective. Adverse effects are similar to those of cilastatin-imipenem; however, seizures are less likely to occur.

C CEPHALOSPORINS

The cephalosporins were first introduced in the 1960s. They are similar to the penicillins in structure and in activity and are also considered beta-lactam antibiotics. Four generations of cephalosporins have been introduced, each group with its own spectrum of activity. Selecting an antibiotic from this class depends on the sensitivity of the involved organism, the preferred route of administration, and sometimes the cost of therapy. The major differences between the generations include their activity against gram-negative bacteria, their resistance to beta-lactamases, and their ability to distribute into cerebrospinal fluid. The first-generation cephalosporins have the least activity against gram-negative bacteria, and the fourth-generation cephalosporins have the most. The first-generation cephalosporins have little resistance to beta-lactamases; resistance increases in second and third generations, with the fourth generation having the most resistance. First- and second-generation cephalosporins have poor distribution into cerebrospinal fluid, and third- and fourth-generation cephalosporins have good distribution. Cefazolin (Ancef, Kefzol), a first-generation agent, is the prototypical cephalosporin. See Table 39.3 for a summary of selected cephalosporins.

Nursing Management of the Patient Receiving [P] Cefazolin

Core Drug Knowledge

Pharmacotherapeutics
Cefazolin can be used to treat many kinds of infections: skin, bone, heart, blood, respiratory tract, GI tract, sinus, ear, and urinary tract. Cefazolin is also used for perioperative prophylaxis in surgeries involving the GI or genitourinary tracts, bone, and skin.

Pharmacokinetics
Cefazolin is rapidly absorbed after IM injection. Peak effect occurs within 1.5 to 2 hours. It is also administered by the IV route, with immediate onset and peak effect in 5 minutes. Only two of the first-generation cephalosporins are available exclusively for oral use: cefadroxil and cephalexin.

Cefazolin is widely distributed to body fluids and tissues, including bone. It does not cross the blood–brain barrier, but it does cross the placenta and enters breast milk. It is excreted unchanged in the urine.

Pharmacodynamics
Cefazolin, like penicillin G, has no direct effect on the body. Cefazolin produces its bactericidal effects by binding with PBPs, which disrupts bacterial cell wall synthesis. Like penicillin, it also activates autolysins, which results in additional damage to the cell wall, allowing the cell to swell and then burst from the osmotic pressure within the cell. Like penicillins, it is most effective against cells undergoing active growth and division.

Contraindications and Precautions
Cefazolin is contraindicated in anyone with a known allergy to cephalosporins. Caution must be used in patients with renal failure and in pregnant or lactating patients. Because of the structural similarities between cephalosporins and penicillins, patients who are allergic to one type of drug may experience cross-sensitivity to the other. Cephalosporin

hypersensitivity occurs in 5% to 10% of patients with penicillin allergy. Patients with a history of severe allergic reactions to penicillins should not receive cephalosporins because of the increased risk for cross-sensitivity reactions in these patients.

Adverse Effects
Hypersensitivity reactions occur frequently with cephalosporin drugs. Severe immediate reactions are rare. Hypersensitivity presents most frequently as a maculopapular rash that develops several days after the onset of therapy.

Other common adverse effects of cefazolin involve the GI tract. Nausea, vomiting, diarrhea, anorexia, abdominal pain, and flatulence are common side effects. Pseudomembranous colitis, a potentially dangerous disorder, has also been reported with cefazolin. The drug should be discontinued immediately at any sign of violent, bloody diarrhea and abdominal pain.

CNS symptoms include headache, dizziness, lethargy, and paresthesias. Nephrotoxicity is also associated with the use of cefazolin, most particularly with patients who have predisposing renal insufficiency. Superinfections are also common with cephalosporin use. As with the penicillins, this adverse effect is related to the normal flora having been destroyed. Thrombophlebitis and an abscess at the injection site are potential adverse effects of administering cephalosporins intravenously.

Serum sickness–like reactions, such as erythema multiforme or skin rashes accompanied by polyarthritis, arthralgia, and fever, may occur following a second course of therapy. Symptoms resolve after the patient stops taking the drug.

Drug Interactions
Risk for nephrotoxicity is greater when cefazolin is given concurrently with aminoglycoside antibiotics. Patients receiving oral anticoagulants may experience increased bleeding when also given cefazolin. Like penicillin, cefazolin may have prolonged effects when given concurrently with probenecid. Table 39.4 presents agents that interact with cefazolin. A disulfiram-like reaction may occur in patients taking cephalosporins with a chemical structure similar to that of disulfiram (see Chapter 9). Symptoms of a disulfiram-like reaction include flushing, shortness of breath, nausea and vomiting, chest pains, palpitations, dizziness and faintness, confusion, sweating, blurred vision, and possibly respiratory depression, seizures, and unconsciousness.

Effects on Test Results
False-positive results may occur in tests of urine glucose using Benedict solution, Fehling solution, and Clinitest tablets. Blood glucose monitoring is therefore recommended in patients with diabetes who are receiving cefazolin. False-positive results have also been noted in direct Coombs tests and measurements of urinary 17-ketosteroids. These tests should be avoided in patients receiving any cephalosporins.

TABLE 39.3 Summary of Selected Ⓒ Cephalosporins

Drug (Trade) Name	Selected Indications	Route and Dosage Range	Pharmacokinetics
Ⓒ First-Generation Cephalosporins			
Ⓟ cefazolin (Kefzol, Ancef)	Respiratory tract infections Skin, joint, biliary, genital infections Endocarditis Surgical prophylaxis Septicemia	*Adult:* IM/IV Life-threatening infections, 1–2 g q6 h Moderate infections, 250 mg–1 g q8 h *Child:* IM/IV Life-threatening infections, 100 mg/kg in 3–4 divided doses Moderate infections, 25–50 mg/kg in 3–4 equal doses	*Onset:* IM, 30 min; IV, 10 min *Duration:* 6–12 h $t_{1/2}$: 90–120 min
cefadroxil (Duricef)	Respiratory tract infections Skin infections Otitis media Tonsillitis/pharyngitis UTI Endocarditis prophylaxis	*Adult:* PO, 1–2 g every day or q12 h in divided doses Loading dose of 1 g initially *Adult:* 2 g 1 h before procedure *Child:* PO, 30 mg/d divided, twice daily, up to a maximum of 2 g/d; 50 mg/kg 1 h before procedure	*Onset:* Rapid *Duration:* 12–24 h $t_{1/2}$: 1 1/2–2 h
cephalexin (Keflex, Biocef)	Respiratory tract infections Skin, bone infections Otitis media UTI	*Adult:* PO Severe infections, 500 mg–1 g q6 h Moderate infections, 250–500 mg q6 h *Child:* PO Severe infections, 50–100 mg/kg in 4 equal doses Moderate infections, 25–50 mg/kg day in 4 equal doses	*Onset:* 15–30 min *Duration:* 6–12 h $t_{1/2}$: 50–80 min
Ⓒ Second-Generation Cephalosporins			
cefaclor (Raniclor)	Respiratory tract infections UTI Skin, bone, joint infections Gynecologic infections Septicemia Otitis media	*Adult:* PO, 250–500 mg q8 h *Child:* PO, 20–40 mg/kg/d in divided doses q8 h	*Onset:* 15 min *Duration:* 6–12 h $t_{1/2}$: 30–60 min
cefprozil (Cefzil)	Respiratory tract infections UTI Skin infections Otitis media	*Adult:* PO, 250–500 mg 1–2 ×/d *Child:* PO, 7.5–15 mg/kg q12 h	*Onset:* Varies *Duration:* 12–24 h $t_{1/2}$: 1–1 1/2 h
cefotetan	Respiratory tract infections Skin and bone infections Gynecological infections Intra-abdominal infections Urinary Tract Infections Surgical prophylaxis	*Adults IM/IV: 1–2 g every 12 h* *500 mg every 12 h* *1–2 g 30–60 min before surgery*	*Onset:* rapid *Duration:* unknown $t_{1/2}$: 3–4.5 h
cefuroxime (Ceftin, Zinacef)	Severe respiratory tract infections Skin infections Otitis media Surgical prophylaxis	*Adult:* PO, 250–500 mg PO q12 h *Adult:* IM/IV, 750 mg q8 h *Child:* PO, 125 mg PO q12 h *Child and infant ≥3 mo:* IM/IV, 50–100 mg/ kg/d in equally divided doses q6–8 h *Neonate:* IM/IV, 20–100 mg/kg/d in equally divided doses q12 h	*Onset:* PO, varies; IM, 20 min; IV, rapid *Duration:* 18–24 h $t_{1/2}$: 1–2 h
cefoxitin	Lower respiratory tract infections Skin and bone infections Gynecologic infections Gonococcal infections Septicemia Peritonitis	*Adult:* IM/IV, 1–2 g q6–8 h *Child >3 mo:* IM/IV, 80–160 mg/kg/d in divided doses q4–6 h	*Onset:* IM, 5–10 min; IV, immediate *Duration:* 6–8 h $t_{1/2}$: 40–60 min
Ⓒ Third-Generation Cephalosporins			
cefdinir (Omnicef)	Pneumonia CAL exacerbations Otitis media Maxillary sinusitis Pharyngitis/tonsillitis Skin infections	*Adult:* PO, 600 mg/d *Child:* PO, 14 mg/kg/d *Infants ≥6 mo:* PO, 14 mg/kg/d Note: All may be divided into 2 doses given q12 h	*Onset:* 2 h *Duration:* 8–10 h $t_{1/2}$: 1.7 h

TABLE 39.3 **Summary of Selected ⓒ Cephalosporins** *(continued)*

Drug (Trade) Name	Selected Indications	Route and Dosage Range	Pharmacokinetics
cefditoren (Spectracef)	Bronchitis, chronic Acute bacterial infection Community-acquired pneumonia Infection of skin and/or subcutaneous tissue Pharyngitis Tonsillitis	*Adult:* PO, 400 mg 2×/d for 10 d 400 mg 2×/d for 14 d 200 mg 2×/d for 10 d	*Onset:* Rapid *Duration:* 8–10 h $t_{1/2}$: 1.6–2 h
cefixime (Suprax)	Acute exacerbation of COPD Acute bronchitis Acute otitis media Pharyngitis Tonsillitis Uncomplicated UTI Gonococcal infections	*Oral Suspension Only* *Adult:* PO, 400 mg daily (may be divided) *Adult:* 400 mg one time only *Child 60 mo–12 y:* PO, 8 mg/kg/d (may be divided) *Child >12 y or 50 kg:* same as for an adult	*Onset:* Unknown *Duration:* Unknown $t_{1/2}$: 3–4 h
cefpodoxime (Vantin)	Respiratory tract infections UTI Skin infections Otitis media STDs	*Adult:* PO, 200–400 mg q12 h *Child:* PO, 5 mg/kg q12 h	*Onset:* Varies *Duration:* 12 h $t_{1/2}$: 2–3 h
ceftibuten (Cedax)	Respiratory tract infections Otitis media	*Adult:* PO, 400 mg every day *Child >6 mo:* 9 mg/kg to a maximum of 400 mg/d	*Onset:* Rapid *Duration:* 24 h $t_{1/2}$: 1–1.5 h
cefotaxime (Claforan)	Serious lower respiratory tract infections UTI Skin and bone infections Gonococcal infections Bacteremia Septicemia Meningitis	*Patient ≥50 kg:* IM/IV, 1 g q12 h Moderate to severe infections: 1–2 g q8 h Severe infections: 2 g q6–8 h Life-threatening infections: 2 g q4 h; maximum dosage is 12 g/d *Child and infant 1 mo–12 y, <50 kg:* 75–100 mg/ kg/d given in 3–4 divided doses Severe infections: 150–225 mg/kg/d given in 3–4 equally divided doses *Neonate 1–4 wk:* IM/IV, 50 mg/kg every 6 or 8 h *Neonate >7 d, ≤ 2 kg:* 50 mg/kg IV or IM every 8 h (or every 12 h in neonates weighing >2 kg)	*Onset:* IM, 30 min; IV, 5–10 min *Duration:* 4–12 h $t_{1/2}$: 1 h
ceftriaxone (Rocephin)	Serious lower respiratory tract infections UTI Skin, bone, joint infections Gonococcal infections Intra-abdominal infections	*Adult:* IM/IV, 1–2 g q12–24 h; maximum dosage is 4 g/d *Child and infant ≥1 mo:* IM/IV, 50–75 mg/kg/d divided, every 12–24 h; maximum dose is 2 g/d *Neonate ≤ 7 d, <2000 g:* IM/IV, 50 mg/kg/d q24 h *Neonate ≤7 d:* IM/IV, 50 mg/kg/d q24 h *Neonate >7 d, >2000 g:* IM/IV, 50–75 mg/kg/d q24 h	*Onset:* IM, 30 min; IV, immediate *Duration:* 12–24 h $t_{1/2}$: 5–8 h
ceftazidime (Fortaz, Tazicef)	Serious respiratory tract infections UTI Skin, bone, joint infections Gynecologic infections Intra-abdominal infections Septicemia Meningitis	*Adult:* IM/IV, 1–2 g q8 h; maximum dose is 6 g/d *Child and infant ≥1 mo:* IV, 30–50 mg/kg q8h; maximum dose is 6 g/d *Neonate 0–4 wk:* IV, 30 mg/kg q12 h	*Onset:* IM, 30 min; IV, immediate *Duration:* 6–12 h $t_{1/2}$: 1/2–1 h

ⓒ Fourth-Generation Cephalosporins

Drug (Trade) Name	Selected Indications	Route and Dosage Range	Pharmacokinetics
cefepime (Maxipime)	Lower respiratory tract infections UTI Skin and bone infections Gonococcal infections Septicemia Peritonitis	*Adult and adolescent >16 y:* IV, 2 g IV q8 h *Infant and child ≤40 kg:* IV, 50 mg/kg/dose q8 h	*Onset:* IM, 30 min; IV, immediate *Duration:* 10–12 h $t_{1/2}$: 2–2.3 h

TABLE 39.4 Agents That Interact with P Cefazolin

Interactants	Effect and Significance	Nursing Management
alcohol	Combination may cause disulfiram-like reaction.	Advise patient to refrain from alcohol for 72 h.
aminoglycosides	Increased risk of nephrotoxicity, although the mechanism of action is unknown.	Monitor peak and trough levels of aminoglycoside. Monitor BUN and creatinine levels closely. Contact provider to discuss decreasing dose or discontinuing drug if signs of kidney dysfunction occur.
oral anticoagulants	Some cephalosporins may have a warfarin-like activity and antiplatelet effects. This results in an augmentation of the action of oral anticoagulants and an increased risk of bleeding.	Advise patients of the signs and symptoms of overanticoagulation. Monitor oral anticoagulant levels. Discuss reducing oral anticoagulant dose with the provider.

Assessment of Relevant Core Patient Variables

Health Status

Follow the same guidelines used for evaluating the health status of a patient receiving penicillin.

Life Span and Gender

Document the age of the patient and, if appropriate, assess for pregnancy and lactation. In elderly patients who have any degree of renal insufficiency, cefazolin should be used cautiously, and the dosage should be adjusted. Adjusted dosage recommendations are based on creatinine clearance levels. Cefazolin is not recommended for infants younger than 1 month because of their immature renal and hepatic functioning.

Lifestyle, Diet, and Habits

Assess the patient's lifestyle and dietary practices to ensure that the drug can be taken consistently, completely, and on an empty stomach, if possible. Assess for the patient's use of alcoholic beverages. Although not all cephalosporins cause a disulfiram-like reaction, it is preferable to refrain from drinking alcohol while on cephalosporin therapy.

Environment

Be aware of the environment in which the drug will be administered. After dilution, cefazolin can be kept at room temperature for 24 hours or in a refrigerator between 2°C and 8°C (36°C and 46°F) for 96 hours (4 days). In acute care settings, retrieve the antibiotic from the refrigerator and let it warm at room temperature for about 15 minutes before administering it. The IV site should be evaluated for signs of phlebitis before and after drug administration. Premixed solutions should be kept in the refrigerator and retrieved approximately 15 minutes before administration as well.

Nursing Diagnoses and Outcomes

- Diarrhea related to drug effects

  Desired outcome: The patient will avoid dehydration, maintain fluid intake, and contact the prescriber if diarrhea persists.

- Imbalanced Nutrition: More or Less than Body Requirements, related to GI effects, alteration in taste, superinfections

  Desired outcome: The patient will maintain body weight and contact the prescriber if persistent adverse effects alter nutritional status.

- Risk for Infection related to overgrowth of nonsusceptible organisms

  Desired outcome: The patient will report signs of superinfection to the prescriber.

Planning and Intervention

Maximizing Therapeutic Effects

Review culture and sensitivity tests to evaluate the efficacy of treatment. Oral suspensions of cephalosporins should be kept in the refrigerator. Be sure that the patient receives injections of cefazolin as prescribed around the clock for increased effectiveness. Monitor the site of infection and presenting signs and symptoms throughout the course of drug therapy. Failure of the signs and symptoms of infection to resolve may indicate the need to repeat culture and sensitivity testing. For optimal effect, drug therapy should continue for at least 2 days after all signs and symptoms resolve.

Minimizing Adverse Effects

Cefazolin may be taken with food or fluids to decrease GI distress. Provide small, frequent meals; mouth care; and ice chips to suck on if stomatitis and sore mouth are problems. Monitor the patient's hydration status and ensure that adequate fluids are given to replace fluid lost with diarrhea. Evaluate the patient for CNS effects and use safety precautions, such as elevating side rails.

Administer IM cefazolin deep into a large muscle. Forewarn the patient that the injection may be uncomfortable. The patient receiving IM cefazolin should be monitored for an abscess at the injection site. IV administration may be as an IV push or IV piggyback. Administer IV cefazolin exactly as prescribed by the prescriber. In addition, monitor the patient receiving IV cefazolin for the possibility of thrombophlebitis.

Monitor the patient receiving combination therapy with aminoglycoside antibiotics (serum BUN and creatinine

MEMORY CHIP

P Cefazolin

- Used for infections caused by gram-positive bacteria, anaerobes, and spirochetes. Also used as prophylaxis in patients having GI or GU surgery.
- Major contraindication: hypersensitivity to cephalosporins or penicillin
- Most common adverse effects: nausea, vomiting, diarrhea
- Most serious adverse effect: hypersensitivity
- **Life span alert: Cefazolin should be used cautiously and the dosage adjusted in elderly patients who have any degree of renal insufficiency.**
- Maximizing therapeutic effects: When using for gram-negative infections, be sure culture and sensitivity tests are done before administration.
- Minimizing adverse effects: Inject IM preparations into a large muscle mass. Be sure IV preparations are administered according to the health care prescriber's orders, either IV push or IV piggyback.
- Most important patient education: Take the medication exactly as prescribed until the entire prescription is completed, despite the absence of symptoms. Monitor for signs and symptoms of allergic response and stop the medication if any occur.
- **Patient safety alert: The generic names of the cephalosporins are very similar. Triple-check the order before administering the medication.**

---

levels) frequently for nephrotoxicity. Give the patient receiving oral anticoagulants in addition to cefazolin instructions about monitoring for signs of blood loss, for example, bleeding gums and easily bruised skin. Dosage of the oral anticoagulant may have to be reduced.

Providing Patient and Family Education

- Because cefazolin and the other cephalosporins are similar to penicillins, follow the same guidelines for providing patient and family education to a patient receiving penicillin.
- In addition, inform patients about possible interactions between cephalosporins and alcohol, urging the patient to refrain from drinking alcohol for 72 hours after drug therapy stops.
- Educate patients on hidden sources of alcohol, such as over-the-counter cough and cold preparations.

Ongoing Assessment and Evaluation

Monitor the patient for any signs of superinfection and notify the prescriber immediately to arrange for treatment if superinfection does occur. Monitor also for signs of allergic or serum sickness-like reactions (fever, hives, swollen glands, neutropenia, arthralgia, and edema). Implement comfort measures as needed and monitor for signs of phlebitis, abscess formation, and other complications. When treatment ends, the initial infection should be resolved. The patient should be adequately nourished and hydrated, and any adverse drug effects should be resolved.

Drugs Closely Related to **P** Cefazolin

First-Generation Cephalosporins

Cefadroxil and cephalexin are oral first- generation cephalosporins. Both of these drugs cover basically the same spectrum of pathogens. They are most active against gram-positive bacteria, especially staphylococci and nonenterococcal streptococci. They have minor activity against gram-negative bacteria. Most first-generation cephalosporins are destroyed by beta-lactamases and have minimal ability to concentrate in the cerebrospinal fluid (CSF). Oral forms are not affected by food and are best taken with food to decrease the GI upset that accompanies their use.

Second-Generation Cephalosporins

Second-generation cephalosporins include cefaclor and cefprozil which are available for oral administration; cefuroxime, which is available in oral, IM, or IV preparations; and cefotetan, cefoxitin, and cefuroxime, which are available for IM or IV administration. These drugs are less sensitive to destruction by beta-lactamases than first-generation drugs but still cannot achieve effective concentrations in the CSF.

The second-generation cephalosporins have broader coverage against gram-negative bacteria than first-generation cephalosporins because they are better able to penetrate the gram-negative cell envelope and have an increased affinity for the PBPs of gram-negative bacteria. They are used in the same way as first-generation cephalosporins as well as uncomplicated gonorrhea.

Third-Generation Cephalosporins

Third-generation cephalosporins include the oral drugs cefdinir, cefditoren, cefixime, cefpodoxime, and ceftibuten and the IM and/or IV drugs cefotaxime, ceftriaxone, and ceftazidime. These drugs are highly resistant to destruction by beta-lactamases and are highly effective against gram-negative aerobes. Ceftazidime is especially effective for bacterial strains resistant to aminoglycosides and is also effective against *P. aeruginosa*. This generation of cephalosporins is used for severe infections or in immunocompromised patients. The exception is ceftriaxone, which is the drug of choice for gonorrhea. With the exception of cefixime, third-generation cephalosporins can penetrate the blood–brain barrier to treat CNS infections.

Cefditoren contains a milk protein. Thus, it is contraindicated for patients with a milk-protein allergy, although it may be given to patients who are lactose intolerant. Cefditoren is excreted with carnitine, an amino acid responsible for transport of fatty acids into mitochondria, and should be given cautiously to patients with carnitine deficiency. This may occur during periods of growth or pregnancy, when the body needs more carnitine than it naturally produces. Carnitine deficiency may also occur in patients with vitamin C deficiency because vitamin C is necessary for synthesis of carnitine.

Fourth-Generation Cephalosporins

Cefepime is the first fourth-generation cephalosporin. It is active against both gram-positive and gram-negative organisms. It has a greater spectrum than third-generation drugs, is more active against organisms such as *P. aeruginosa* or Enterobacteriaceae that have developed resistance to third-generation drugs, and has good penetration into the CSF. Like third-generation cephalosporins, cefepime is highly resistant to destruction by beta-lactamases.

Ⓒ VANCOMYCIN

Vancomycin (Vancocin) is a complex and unusual tricyclic glycopeptide antibiotic. It is the only drug in its class. The use of vancomycin is limited by its ability to produce toxic effects. Because of its toxicity, vancomycin is used only when other antibiotics fail to resolve an infection. It has been touted as able to eradicate most gram-positive pathogens; however, the emergence of vancomycin-resistant enterococci (VRE) has become problematic. Table 39.5 presents an overview of vancomycin.

Nursing Management of the Patient Receiving Ⓟ Vancomycin

Core Drug Knowledge

Pharmacotherapeutics

Vancomycin is used in treating bacterial septicemia, endocarditis, bone and joint infections, and pseudomembranous colitis caused by *C. difficile*. Vancomycin is exceptionally effective for treating gram-positive infections in penicillin-allergic patients. It is also used for penicillin- and methicillin-resistant staphylococcal infections.

Vancomycin is used with aminoglycosides to combat *Streptococcus faecalis* and methicillin-resistant organisms. However, this synergism also increases possible toxicity.

Gram-negative bacteria and mycobacteria are resistant to vancomycin. Vancomycin is not used in treating meningitis because of poor penetration into CSF.

Pharmacokinetics

Oral bioavailability of vancomycin is extremely low; therefore, it is generally administered intravenously. Oral administration is used in treating some GI infections, such as pseudomembranous colitis, but only after a trial of another antimicrobial—metronidazole. Some patients, especially those with renal impairment, have developed detectable vancomycin serum levels following oral administration.

After IV administration, plasma concentrations reach a peak approximately 1 hour after infusion. In patients with normal renal function, vancomycin has a serum half-life of 4 to 6 hours, but in elderly patients or those with renal impairment, half-life can be as long as 146 hours.

Vancomycin is distributed widely into most body tissues and fluids, including pericardial, pleural, ascitic, and synovial fluids, and the meninges if they are inflamed. It is not known whether any metabolism takes place. Excretion is mainly by glomerular filtration; only small amounts are excreted in the feces. With oral administration, excretion is mainly fecal.

Pharmacodynamics

Vancomycin is bactericidal because it inhibits cell wall synthesis by altering the cell's permeability. Vancomycin also inhibits the synthesis of ribonucleic acid (RNA). Because of this dual mechanism of action, resistance to vancomycin has been limited to strains of group D streptococci. The body is not directly affected.

Contraindications and Precautions

Vancomycin is contraindicated for patients with hypersensitivity to it and for pregnant patients. Although it is excreted into breast milk, vancomycin is not contraindicated for breast-feeding women. However, breast-feeding neonates

TABLE 39.5 Overview of Vancomycin

Drug (Trade) Name	Selected Indications	Route and Dosage Range	Pharmacokinetics
Vancomycin (Vancocin)	MRSA	*Adult IV:* 2 g/d IV divided every 6–12 h *Child IV:* 10 mg/kg IV every 6 h *Neonate IV:* 15 mg/kg IV, followed by 10 mg/kg IV every 12 h for neonates in the first week of life, and every 8 h thereafter up to the age of 1 mo	*Onset Oral:* varies *Onset IV:* rapid *Duration:* unknown $t_{1/2}$: 6–6 h
	Bacterial meningitis	*Adult IV:* 30–45 mg/kg/d divided every 8–12 h 2 g/d IV divided every 6–12 h administered over at least 60 min *Child IV > 28 d:* 60 mg/kg/d divided every 6 h *Neonate IV 8–28 d:* 8–28 d, 30–45 *Neonate 0–7 d:* 20–30 mg/kg/d divided every 8–12 h;	
	Infective endocarditis	*Adult IV:* 2 g/d IV divided every 6–12 h *Child IV:* 10–15 mg/kg IV every 6 h	
	Antibiotic induced pseudomembranous enterocolitis	*Adult Oral:* 500 mg to 2 g daily divided every 6–8 h *Child Oral:* 40 mg/kg/d divided every 6–8 h	

and infants should be monitored for vancomycin serum concentration to avoid potential toxicities. Use it with caution in patients with renal disease, such as renal failure or renal impairment, and in patients receiving other drugs with the potential for nephrotoxicity, such as aminoglycosides.

Oral vancomycin should be used with caution in patients with inflammatory bowel disease because this disorder increases absorption of oral vancomycin, thereby increasing the risk for toxicity.

Adverse Effects

The most serious toxicities caused by vancomycin are ototoxicity and nephrotoxicity. Ototoxicity can take the form of cochlear toxicity (tinnitus, hearing loss) or vestibular toxicity (ataxia, vertigo, nausea and vomiting, nystagmus).

Nephrotoxicity can also occur with vancomycin, although its incidence has decreased since the newer formulations have less impurities. Nephrotoxicity and elevated serum concentrations are more likely to occur in patients receiving other nephrotoxic drugs, such as aminoglycosides. Cases of interstitial nephritis, a hypersensitivity reaction, have been reported.

Vancomycin can cause histamine release, resulting in anaphylactoid reactions. Symptoms include fever, chills, sinus tachycardia, and pruritus. Paresthesias, flushing, rash, or redness in the face, neck, upper body, arms, or back are also symptoms of histamine release. In some cases, hypotension occurs. Because of the presenting symptoms, this histamine-release reaction is often called the "red man" or "red neck" syndrome. Other adverse reactions include phlebitis or other injection-site reactions, leukopenia, and thrombocytopenia.

Drug Interactions

Orally administered vancomycin should be avoided in patients receiving antihyperlipidemic drugs (HMG-CoA reductase inhibitors, statins). Vancomycin should be used with caution in combination with other drugs that have potential nephrotoxic or ototoxic effects and in patients receiving nondepolarizing muscle relaxants. Table 39.6 presents drugs that interact with vancomycin.

Assessment of Relevant Core Patient Variables

Health Status

Assess the patient for contraindications or precautions to the use of vancomycin, including other drugs with potential nephrotoxicity and ototoxicity. Lower doses of vancomycin are recommended for patients with renal dysfunction or for patients receiving other ototoxic or nephrotoxic drugs. Assess gross hearing in patients with pre-existing hearing impairment. Periodic audiograms may be necessary during therapy. For patients with expected long-term therapy, perform a baseline CBC and hepatic and renal function tests. Consult with the prescriber about any laboratory abnormalities before vancomycin therapy begins.

Life Span and Gender

Ask women of childbearing age about their contraceptive methods and assess for pregnancy and lactation. Vancomycin should not be given to pregnant women and should be given cautiously to breast-feeding women. Note whether patients are elderly, because such patients are at higher risk for toxicity and drug accumulation because of their age-related decreases in renal function.

Environment

Be aware of the environment in which the drug will be administered. Generally, vancomycin is administered in an inpatient setting because of its potentially serious toxicities and the need to closely monitor vancomycin serum concentrations.

Nursing Diagnoses and Outcomes

- Risk for Injury related to drug-induced histamine-release reactions
  Desired outcome: The patient will experience no preventable reaction related to vancomycin.
- Disturbed Sensory Perception (auditory) related to drug-induced ototoxicity
  Desired outcome: The patient will report any unusual auditory sensations and have periodic audiograms to detect early ototoxicity.
- Excess Fluid Volume related to nephrotoxicity from drug therapy
  Desired outcome: The patient will remain normovolemic throughout therapy.
- Risk for Infection related to overgrowth of nonsusceptible organisms
  Desired outcome: The patient will report signs of superinfection to the prescriber.

Planning and Intervention

Maximizing Therapeutic Effects

Ensure that the patient receives the full course of vancomycin as prescribed, divided around the clock to increase effectiveness. Coordinate administering drugs to decrease potential drug–drug interactions. In addition, culture and sensitivity results should be monitored to be sure that vancomycin is the drug of choice for this patient.

Minimizing Adverse Effects

Administer vancomycin over at least 60 minutes. This rate diminishes effects such as flushing, tachycardia, hypotension, or rashes that occur when administration is too fast. Slowing the IV rate also decreases the potential for phlebitis. Assess the IV site frequently for signs of phlebitis.

Ototoxicity after IV administration is believed to be associated with serum concentration ranges above 60 to 80 mcg/mL, which may occur when doses are too large or infused too rapidly. Administering IV vancomycin too rapidly may also lead to red man syndrome. In addition, take care to avoid extravasation because vancomycin is extremely irritating to tissues.

TABLE 39.6	Agents That Interact with Vancomycin	
Interactants	**Effect and Significance**	**Nursing Management**
methotrexate	Coadministration may increase methotrexate serum concentration.	Monitor CBC. Monitor for myelosuppression.

Nephrotoxic drugs
  aminoglycosides
  amphotericin B
  bacitracin
  cisplatin
  cyclosporine
  polymyxin B
	Parenteral vancomycin with other nephrotoxic drugs can lead to additive risks for nephrotoxicity.	Monitor renal function closely.
		Consider lower doses of vancomycin.

Nondepolarizing muscle relaxants	Vancomycin may affect presynaptic and postsynaptic myoneural function and act synergistically with nondepolarizing muscle relaxants.	Avoid this combination when possible. When given, monitor neuromuscular function closely, and be prepared to initiate mechanical ventilation.

Ototoxic drugs
  aminoglycosides
  salicylates
  ethacrynic acid
  furosemide
  paromomycin
  succinylcholine
	Parenteral vancomycin with other ototoxic drugs can lead to additive risks for ototoxicity.
	
	Vancomycin may potentiate the neuromuscular blocking effects of succinylcholine.
		Monitor sensory/hearing functions closely. Consider lower doses of vancomycin. Monitor for neuromuscular paralysis and respiratory collapse.

Peak and trough levels are terms associated with serum concentration measurements. Obtain the peak serum level 1 hour after completion of the infusion and the trough serum level 30 minutes before beginning the next infusion. Some hospitals obtain only a trough level unless the patient is at high risk for nephrotoxicity.

MEMORY CHIP

P Vancomycin

- Used for serious gram-positive infections, especially *Clostridium difficile* and methicillin-resistant *Staphylococcus aureus*.
- Major contraindications: hypersensitivity and pregnancy
- Most common adverse effects: histamine release resulting in "red-man" syndrome
- Most serious adverse effects: ototoxicity and nephrotoxicity
- **Life span alert: Elderly patients may need vancomycin concentration monitoring because of a higher risk of toxicity and drug accumulation secondary to age-related decreases in renal function.**
- Maximizing therapeutic effects: Obtain culture and sensitivity report before administration.
- Minimizing adverse effects: Administer over 60 minutes.
- Most important patient education: Need for periodic CBC when taking for prolonged period or high doses. Need to advise the health care team for changes in hearing.

Providing Patient and Family Education
- Advise the patient of the importance of completing therapy.
- Explain the potential adverse effects and need for periodic blood monitoring.
- Advise the patient to report symptoms such as tinnitus, hearing loss, vertigo, or nausea and vomiting.
- Teach the patient the importance of accurate fluid intake and output measurements.

Ongoing Assessment and Evaluation

Elderly patients may need vancomycin concentration monitoring because age-related decreases in renal function put them at risk for toxicity and drug accumulation.

Monitor for signs of ototoxicity. Factors that may increase the risk for developing ototoxicity include excessive dose, serum concentrations above 60 mcg/mL, prolonged exposure to the drug, multiple ototoxic drugs, dehydration, excessive noise, and bacteremia. Assess for symptoms, such as ataxia and nystagmus, which may indicate ototoxicity. Monitor fluid intake and output to assess for potential nephrotoxicity.

For patients receiving long-term or high-dose therapy, coordinate periodic audiometric testing and serial CBCs, LFTs, and kidney function tests. As with other potent antibiotics, monitor for signs of superinfection. When treatment ends, the initial infection should be resolved. The patient should be adequately nourished and hydrated, and any adverse drug effects should be resolved.

CHAPTER SUMMARY

- Penicillins are classified as narrow-spectrum, penicillinase-resistant, aminopenicillins (broad-spectrum), and extended-spectrum (antipseudomonal) penicillins. They are also known as beta-lactam antibiotics.
- Penicillins may be inactivated by beta-lactamase, an enzyme produced by the bacteria. Penicillinase-resistant penicillins or penicillin–beta-lactamase combination drugs decrease the effects of penicillinase.
- Penicillins are most effective against gram-positive bacteria because they have difficulty penetrating the gram-negative cell envelope.
- Penicillins are the safest antibiotics available, except in patients with a hypersensitivity to penicillin.
- Penicillins can be administered orally, intramuscularly, or intravenously.
- Patients with a possible history of penicillin allergy should receive skin testing before administration.
- Patients with hypersensitivity to any penicillin should be considered allergic to all penicillins.
- Monobactam and carbapenem antibiotics are also beta-lactam antibiotics. Imipenem has the broadest spectrum of activity of all antibiotics.
- Cephalosporins are the antibiotics most widely used today.
- Cephalosporin antibiotics are structurally similar to penicillins. Between 5% and 10% of patients with hypersensitivity to penicillin will also react to cephalosporins.
- Cephalosporin antibiotics are grouped according to "generations."
- As cephalosporin generations progress, the drugs have increased activity against gram-negative bacteria and anaerobes, increased resistance to destruction by beta lactamases, and increased ability to reach the CSF.
- Most of the cephalosporins are administered parenterally.
- Vancomycin is very effective against most gram-positive infections; however, its use is limited by its potential to cause severe adverse effects.
- Vancomycin is the drug of choice for pseudomembranous colitis caused by *Clostridium difficile,* infections caused by methicillin- resistant *Staphylococcus aureus,* and serious infections in patients who are allergic to penicillin.
- Patients with an antibiotic allergy should wear a MedicAlert necklace or bracelet.

QUESTIONS FOR STUDY AND REVIEW

1. How do penicillins work?
2. Why are most penicillins ineffective against gram-negative bacteria?
3. On what basis are the penicillins classified into four groups?
4. Why are clavulanic acid, tazobactam, and sulbactam added to some penicillin preparations?
5. Compare and contrast the carbapenem antibiotics.
6. What is the difference between the generations of cephalosporins?
7. What classes of antibiotics are called beta-lactam antibiotics? Why?
8. Why is vancomycin reserved for serious infections?

NEED MORE HELP?

Chapter 39 of the Study Guide to Accompany *Drug Therapy in Nursing,* 4th edition, contains additional NCLEX-style questions and other learning activities to reinforce your understanding of the concepts presented in this chapter. For additional information or to purchase the study guide, visit thePoint.

REFERENCES

Aschenbrenner, D. (2008). Complicated intraabdominal infection and UTI. *American Journal of Nursing,* 108(3):36–36.
Baldwin, C., Lyseng-Williamson, K., & Keam, S. (2008). Meropenem: a review of its use in the treatment of serious bacterial infections. *Drugs,* 68(6):803–838.
Calderwood, S. B. (2009). Overview of the beta-lactam antibiotics, *Up To Date.* Retrieved from *http://uptodate.com.*
Calderwood, S. B. (2009). Combination beta-lactamase inhibitors, carbapenems, and monobactams, *Up To Date.* Retrieved from *http://uptodate.com.*
Calderwood, S. B. (2009). Cephalosporins, *Up To Date.* Retrieved from *http://uptodate.com.*
Cronin, H., & Mowad, C. (2009). Anaphylactic reaction to bacitracin ointment, *Cutaneous Medicine for the Practitioner,* 83(3):127–129.
Facts and Comparisons. (2010). *Drug facts and comparisons.* Philadelphia, PA: Lippincott Williams & Wilkins.
Forouzesh, A., Moise, P. A., Sakoulas, G. (2009). Vancomycin ototoxicity: a reevaluation in an era of increasing doses, *Antimicrobial Agents and Chemotherapy,* 53(2):483–486.
Koda-Kimbal, M. A, Young, L. Y., Kradian, W. A., et al. (2008). *Applied Therapeutics: The Clinical Use of Drugs.* Philadelphia, PA: Lippincott, Williams, and Wilkins.
Livermore, D. M. (2009). Doripenem: antimicrobial profile and clinical potential, *Diagnostic Microbiology and Infectious Disease,* 63(4):455–458.
Micromedex Healthcare Series. Retrieved from *http://thomsonhc.com.*
Rosen, T., Vandergriff, T., & Harting, M. (2009). Antibiotic use in sexually transmissible diseases. *Dermatologic Clinics,* 27(1):49–61.
Rybak, M., Lomaestro, B., Rotschafer, J. C., et al. (2009), Therapeutic monitoring of vancomycin in adult patients: a consensus review of the American Society of Health-System Pharmacists, the Infectious Diseases Society of America, and the Society of Infectious Diseases Pharmacists, *American Journal of Health System Pharmacy,* 66(1):82–98.
Shahid, M., Sobia, F., Singh, A., et al. (2009). Beta-lactams and Beta-lactamase-inhibitors in current- or potential-clinical practice: A comprehensive update. *Critical Reviews in Microbiology,* 35(2):81–108.
Tatro, D. S. (2010). *Drug interaction facts.* Philadelphia, PA: Lippincott Williams & Wilkins.
Vancomycin dosing and monitoring. (2009). *Medical Letter on Drugs & Therapeutics,* 51(1309):25.
Vergidis, P. I., & Falagas, M. E. (2008). New antibiotic agents for bloodstream infections. *International Journal of Antimicrobial Agents,* 32(Suppl 1):S60–S65.

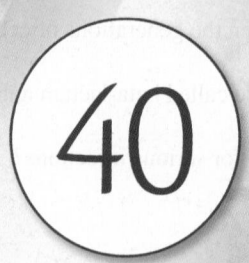

Antibiotics Affecting Protein Synthesis

Learning Objectives

At the completion of this chapter the student will:

1. Identify core drug knowledge pertaining to drugs affecting protein synthesis.

2. Identify core patient variables pertaining to drugs affecting protein synthesis.

3. Relate the interaction of core drug knowledge to core patient variables for drugs affecting protein synthesis.

4. Generate a nursing plan of care from the interactions between core drug knowledge and core patient variables for drugs affecting protein synthesis.

5. Describe nursing interventions to maximize therapeutic and minimize adverse effects for drugs affecting protein synthesis.

6. Determine key points for patient and family education for drugs affecting protein synthesis.

Key Terms

azotemia	ototoxicity	xeroderma
cylindruria	peak and trough	xerophthalmia
hyposthenuria	proteinuria	
nephrotoxicity	pyuria	

Antibiotics Affecting Protein Synthesis

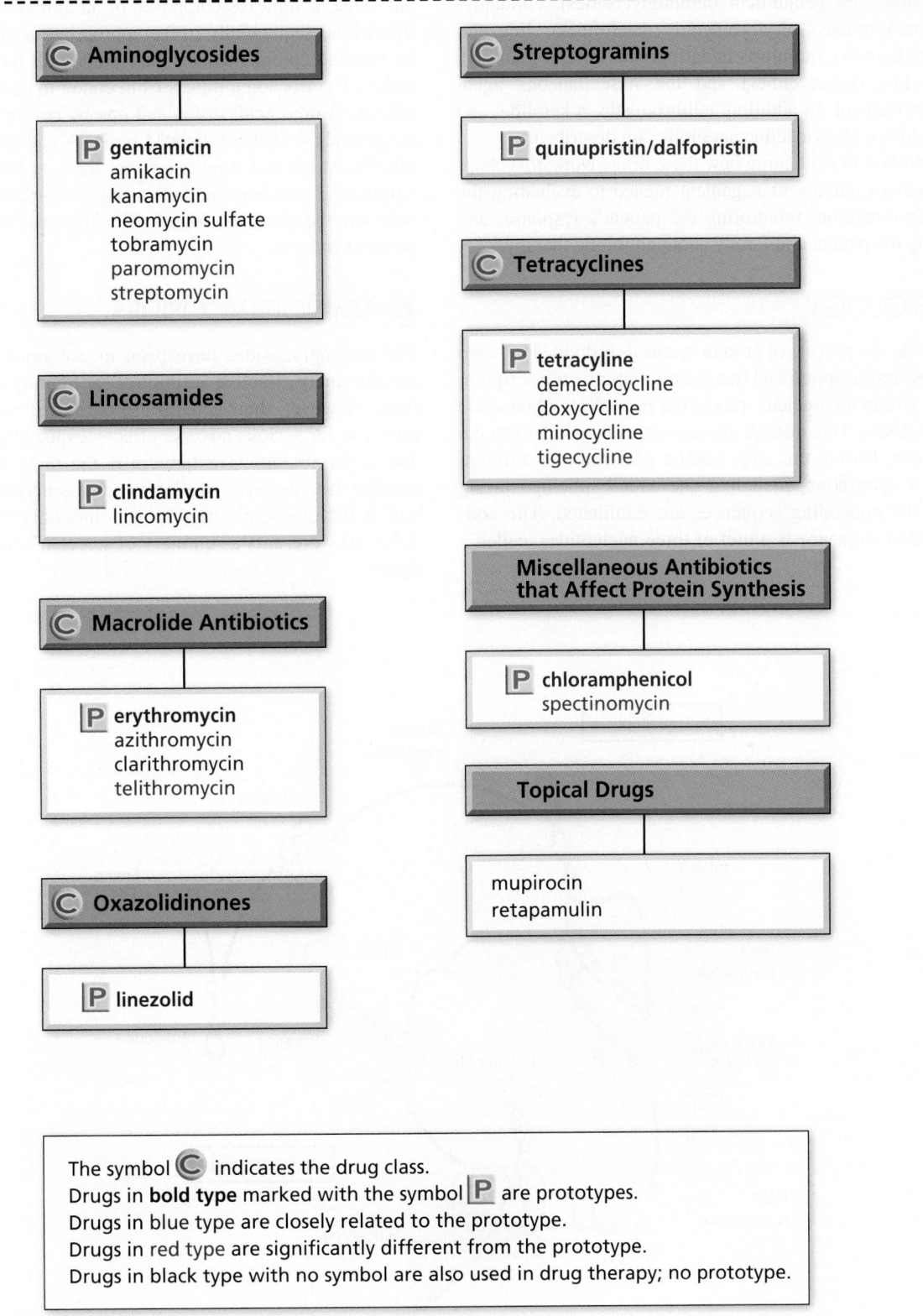

C Aminoglycosides

P gentamicin
amikacin
kanamycin
neomycin sulfate
tobramycin
paromomycin
streptomycin

C Lincosamides

P clindamycin
lincomycin

C Macrolide Antibiotics

P erythromycin
azithromycin
clarithromycin
telithromycin

C Oxazolidinones

P linezolid

C Streptogramins

P quinupristin/dalfopristin

C Tetracyclines

P tetracyline
demeclocycline
doxycycline
minocycline
tigecycline

Miscellaneous Antibiotics that Affect Protein Synthesis

P chloramphenicol
spectinomycin

Topical Drugs

mupirocin
retapamulin

The symbol C indicates the drug class.
Drugs in **bold type** marked with the symbol P are prototypes.
Drugs in blue type are closely related to the prototype.
Drugs in red type are significantly different from the prototype.
Drugs in black type with no symbol are also used in drug therapy; no prototype.

Drugs affecting protein synthesis include aminoglycoside agents, ketolide agents, lincosamide agents, macrolide agents, oxazolidinones, streptogramins, tetracyclines, and miscellaneous antibiotics. The prototype drugs discussed in this chapter are gentamicin (aminoglycosides), clindamycin (lincosamides), erythromycin (macrolides), linezolid (oxazolidinones), quinupristin/dalfopristin (streptogramins), tetracycline (tetracyclines) and the miscellaneous agent chloramphenicol. In addition, telithromycin, a ketolide, and tigecycline, a glycylcycline antibiotic, are described.

In addition to explaining how these drugs work, this chapter discusses nursing management related to evaluating the patient's condition, monitoring the patient's response, and teaching the patient and family about antibiotic therapy.

PHYSIOLOGY

In all cells, the process of protein synthesis is divided into two sections: transcription and translation. Initially, transcription occurs within the nucleus, producing messenger ribonucleic acid (mRNA). This mRNA migrates from the nucleus to the cytoplasm. During this step, mRNA goes through different types of maturation, including one called splicing, during which the noncoding sequences are eliminated. The coding mRNA sequence is a unit of three nucleotides, called a codon.

Translation occurs in the cytoplasm. The ribosome binds to the mRNA at the start codon (AUG) that is recognized only by initiator tRNA (transfer ribonucleic acid). The ribosome proceeds to the elongation phase of protein synthesis. During this stage, complexes composed of an amino acid linked to tRNA bind sequentially to the appropriate codon in mRNA by forming complementary base pairs with the tRNA anticodon. The ribosome moves from codon to codon along the mRNA. Amino acids are added one by one, translated into polypeptide sequences dictated by DNA and represented by mRNA. At the end, a release factor binds to the stop codon, terminating translation and releasing the completed polypeptide from the ribosome. Figure 40.1 illustrates the process of protein synthesis.

Ⓒ AMINOGLYCOSIDES

The aminoglycosides have been in use since 1944. They are extremely effective antibiotics for treating severe infections. However, their general use is limited because of the potential for serious adverse effects, especially ototoxicity and nephrotoxicity. Gentamicin is the most widely used, possibly because of its availability as a generic formulation, and is the prototype drug for the aminoglycoside family. Table 40.1 presents a summary of selected aminoglycoside agents.

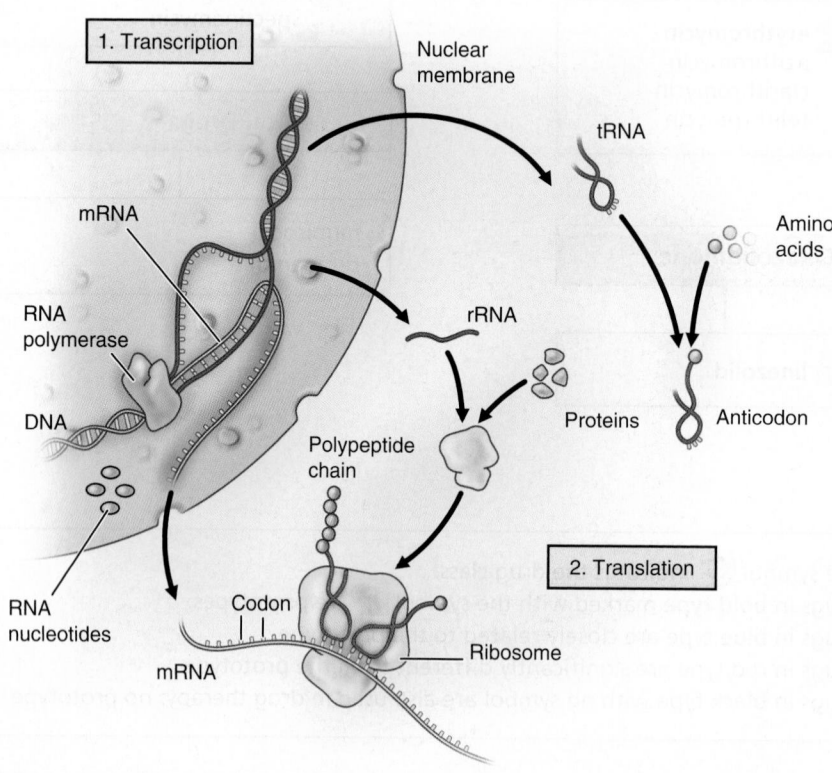

• FIGURE 40.1   Protein synthesis.

TABLE 40.1	Summary of Selected Ⓒ Aminoglycoside Antibiotics		
Drug (Trade) Name	**Selected Indications**	**Route and Dosage Range**	**Pharmacokinetics**
Ⓟ gentamicin (Garamycin;	Gram-negative infections Staphylococcal infections	*Adult:* IM/IV, 3–5 mg/kg/d in divided doses *Child:* 6–7.5 mg/kg in divided doses *Infants and neonates:* 7.5 mg/kg in divided doses q8 h	*Onset:* Rapid *Duration:* 6–8 h $t_{1/2}$: 2–3 h
	Localized eye infections	*Adult and Child:* 1 drop every 1–4 h	
amikacin (Amikin)	Gram-negative infections Staphylococcal infections	*Adult:* IM/IV, 15 mg/kg/d *Child:* Same as adults *Neonate:* IM/IV, 10 mg/kg initially then 7.5 mg/kg q12 h	*Onset:* IM, varies; IV, immediate *Duration:* 6–8 h $t_{1/2}$: 2–3 h
kanamycin (Kantrex)	*Escherichia coli* and other infectious agents Suppression of intestinal flora	*Adult:* IM, 15 mg/kg/d; IV, dilute 500 mg vial with 100–200 mL sterile diluent per day PO, 1 g every hour for 4 h then 1 g q6h for 36–72 h	*Onset:* IM/IV, rapid *Duration:* 8–12 h $t_{1/2}$: 2–3 h
neomycin (Mycifradin Sulfate)	Preoperative suppression of intestinal bacteria Hepatic coma	*Adult:* 1 g at 19, 18 and 9 h before surgery *Adult:* 4–12 g/d	*Onset:* PO, varies *Duration:* 6–8 h $t_{1/2}$: 3 h
paromomycin (Humatin)	Intestinal amebiasis Hepatic coma	*Adult and child:* 25–35 mg/kg/d in three divided doses *Adult:* 4 g/d in divided doses	*Onset:* Poorly absorbed *Duration:* Excreted $t_{1/2}$: Unchanged in feces
streptomycin	Non-tubercular Infections	*Adult:* IM, 1–2 g/d in divided doses *Child:* IM, 20–40 mg/kg/d q12 h	*Onset:* Rapid *Duration:* 8–12 h $t_{1/2}$: 2.5 h
	TB in conjunction with other drug therapy, prophylaxis of TB	*Adult:* IM, 15 mg/kg with a maximum of 1 g/d; reduce to 25–30 mg/kg or maximum of 1.5 g two to three times a week *Child:* IM, 20–40 mg/kg/d in divided doses q6–12 h to a maximum of 1 g/d; reduce to 25–30 mg/kg two to three times a week	
tobramycin (Nebcin)	Gram-negative infections especially Pseudomonas staphylococcal infections, burns Soft tissue wounds	*Adult and child:* 3–5 mg/kg every 12 h *Neonate <1 w:* IM/IV: up to 4 mg/kg every 12 h	*Onset:* Rapid *Duration:* 8–12 h $t_{1/2}$: 2–3 h

Nursing Management of the Patient Receiving Ⓟ Gentamicin

Core Drug Knowledge

Pharmacotherapeutics

Clinically, gentamicin is useful in serious infections that include urinary tract infections (UTIs), such as pyelonephritis; gynecologic infections; peritonitis; endocarditis; pneumonia; bacteremia and sepsis; respiratory infections, including those associated with cystic fibrosis; osteomyelitis; and foot and other soft-tissue infections associated with diabetes.

Gentamicin is effective in managing infections caused by gram-negative bacilli. Susceptible organisms include *Pseudomonas aeruginosa*, *Proteus mirabilis*, *Escherichia coli*; *Klebsiella*, *Enterobacter*, *Serratia*, and *Citrobacter* species; and staphylococci. Gentamicin must be transported across the cell membrane in order to enter the cell and disrupt protein synthesis. This process requires oxygen; therefore, gentamicin and other aminoglycosides are ineffective against anaerobes. Gentamicin is not considered useful in treating meningitis unless it is administered intrathecally.

Gentamicin is also indicated for topical treatment of eye or skin infections caused by susceptible organisms. It is used as a liposome injection for treating disseminated *Mycobacterium avium-intracellulare* (MAC) infection, and it has an orphan drug indication as drug-impregnated polymethylmethacrylate (PMAA) beads on surgical wire for treating chronic osteomyelitis. Gentamicin liquid has been used successfully in bone cement for the management of musculoskeletal infections.

Pharmacokinetics

Parenteral gentamicin is widely distributed through the body in extracellular fluids; however, it does not penetrate appreciably into the central nervous system (CNS). It crosses the placenta and is secreted in breast milk. Gentamicin concentrates in the kidney, reaching levels 50 times higher than those in serum. It also concentrates in the endolymph and perilymph of the inner ear. High concentrations of gentamicin in these fluids are associated with its major adverse effects—**nephrotoxicity** and **ototoxicity.** Parenteral gentamicin is excreted unchanged in urine, whereas oral gentamicin is excreted unchanged in feces.

Because it is poorly absorbed when taken orally, gentamicin is usually reserved for parenteral use. It may be given orally to effect a decrease in gastrointestinal (GI) tract flora before colorectal surgical or other invasive procedures. It may also be used topically for infections of the skin, eyes, and ears.

Pharmacodynamics

Gentamicin, like all antibiotics, has no direct effect on the cells of the body. It exerts its effect by entering the bacterial cell and binding to the 30S ribosomal subunit (see Chapter 38). This event leads to a misreading of the information used within the cell to form proteins. The cell then produces amino acids that do not link correctly. The result is a change in metabolic function that in turn prevents bacterial reproduction and weakens the cell wall, leading to cell wall rupture and death. Many strains of bacteria are resistant to the aminoglycosides and do not allow them to enter the cell. Because of this, aminoglycosides are often given with synergistic antibiotics to increase their effectiveness or to alter the cell wall so that the aminoglycoside can enter.

Contraindications and Precautions

Gentamicin is contraindicated during pregnancy and lactation. It is also contraindicated in patients with known allergy to any aminoglycoside. It is used cautiously in patients with renal or hepatic disease, dehydration, pre-existing hearing loss, and myasthenia gravis, as well as in patients receiving other nephrotoxic or ototoxic drugs.

Adverse Effects

Many serious side effects are associated with gentamicin, limiting its usefulness. The most well-known adverse effects are neurotoxicity, nephrotoxicity, ototoxicity, and neuromuscular blockade, which are all Black Box warnings. Ototoxicity occurs most frequently when serum trough levels are elevated, in infants or elderly patients, or with prolonged or high-dose therapy. Gentamicin may induce both cochlear and vestibular damage to the inner ear. Cochlear damage, a high-frequency hearing loss, may be preceded by high-pitched tinnitus. Nephrotoxicity occurs most frequently in infants or the elderly or with prolonged or high-dose therapy. Acute tubular necrosis is the most common gentamicin-induced nephrotoxicity. Neuromuscular blockade may result in profound respiratory depression. It occurs most frequently in patients with myasthenia gravis and in patients receiving general anesthetics or nondepolarizing skeletal muscle relaxants.

In the CNS, gentamicin therapy may induce confusion, depression, disorientation, numbness, tingling, and weakness. Leukemoid reactions and depressed bone marrow function are potential adverse effects in the hematologic

system. GI symptoms include nausea, vomiting, diarrhea, weight loss, stomatitis, and hepatic toxicity. Gentamicin may induce palpitations, hypotension, and hypertension in the cardiovascular system. Hypersensitivity reactions include purpura, rash, urticaria, and exfoliative dermatitis. Other adverse effects such as superinfections, fever, apnea, and joint pain may also occur.

Drug Interactions

Gentamicin may interact with other drugs that are known to be ototoxic, nephrotoxic, or neurotoxic such as acyclovir, amphotericin B, cephalothin, cisplatin, cyclosporine, loop diuretics (especially ethacrynic acid), nonsteroidal anti-inflammatory drugs (NSAIDs), and vancomycin. Additionally, gentamicin may interact with general anesthetics, indomethacin, nondepolarizing skeletal muscle relaxants, extended penicillins, and cephalosporins. Table 40.2 lists drugs that interact with gentamicin.

Assessment of Relevant Core Patient Variables

Health Status

In assessing the health status of the patient taking gentamicin, elicit a thorough health history, particularly the renal history. Because gentamicin is excreted unchanged by glomerular filtration, patients with renal dysfunction or dehydration are at risk for nephrotoxicity. Evaluate patients for a history of hearing impairment and eighth cranial nerve impairment because these patients have an elevated risk for ototoxicity.

Investigate any patient with a history of myasthenia gravis or one who may have received neuromuscular blocking agents during surgical procedures. Gentamicin may cause severe neuromuscular weakness, lasting hours to days, because of its potential curare-like effect, and it may aggravate muscle weakness in these patients.

Perform a baseline gross hearing test before administering gentamicin. Evaluate laboratory test results that indicate the renal and hepatic function of the patient.

Life Span and Gender

Evaluate women for potential pregnancy. Although gentamicin is not absolutely contraindicated during pregnancy, it has been found to be ototoxic to the fetus. Evaluate neonates (younger than 1 month) and patients older than 65 years frequently because these patients have immature or decreased renal function, which increases their risk of ototoxicity and nephrotoxicity.

Lifestyle, Diet, and Habits

Assess the nutritional status of the patient. Patients whose oral intake is restricted and patients who eat poorly are at increased risk for hypomagnesemia during gentamicin therapy. Dehydrated patients have an increased risk of nephrotoxicity.

TABLE 40.2	Agents That Interact with P Gentamicin	
Interactant	Effect and Significance	Nursing Management
Cephalosporins	Synergistic bacterial activity, however it may also increase risk for nephrotoxicity.	Synergistic bacterial interaction is beneficial Assess peak and trough level of aminoglycoside drug Monitor BUN and creatinine levels Monitor input and output
Extended penicillins	Extended penicillins may inactivate gentamicin.	Avoid combination when possible. Administer these drugs at least 2 h apart.
Loop diuretics, especially ethacrynic acid	Synergistic ototoxicity may cause hearing loss of varying degrees, with possibly permanent hearing loss. Patients with renal insufficiency have highest risk for ototoxicity.	Perform baseline and daily hearing function test Inform patient to immediately report ringing or roaring in the ears, or muffled sounds Advise family members to be alert for evidence of hearing loss.
General anesthetics	Gentamicin may induce a synergistic interaction resulting in an increased risk for prolonged respiratory depression and gentamicin toxicity.	Monitor for respiratory depression Have ventilatory support available Monitor BUN and creatinine levels
NSAIDS	NSAIDS may reduce glomerular filtration rate (GFR) allowing gentamicin to accumulate thus increasing the risk for toxicity	Assess peak and trough level of aminoglycoside drug Monitor BUN and creatinine levels Monitor input and output Inform patient to immediately report ringing or roaring in the ears, or muffled sounds Advise family members to be alert for evidence of hearing loss.
Nondepolarizing muscle relaxants	The actions of nondepolarizing muscle relaxants may be enhanced resulting in protracted respiratory depression.	Mark patient's chart and arrange for extended monitoring and support following anesthesia. Monitor respirations and other vital signs following anesthesia.
Ototoxic, nephrotoxic, and neurotoxic drugs	Risk for ototoxicity, nephrotoxicity, or neurotoxic effects are increased when these drugs are coadministered with gentamicin.	Avoid these combinations if possible. Assess peak and trough level of aminoglycoside drug Monitor BUN and creatinine levels Monitor input and output Inform patient to immediately report ringing or roaring in the ears, or muffled sounds Advise family members to be alert for evidence of hearing loss. Reduce dose of one or both drugs as ordered.
succinylcholine	Gentamicin may increase neuromuscular effects of succinylcholine.	Monitor for respiratory depression. Have bag-mask-valve apparatus and ventilation equipment available.

Environment

Be aware of the environment in which gentamicin will be administered and, if appropriate, assess the home or living environment for potential risk factors. Parenteral gentamicin is usually administered in the acute hospital setting; however, it may also be given in the home environment by a home health care nurse. Oral or topical gentamicin may be given in any environment.

In the hospital setting, store gentamicin in the refrigerator and be sure that it does not freeze. Before administration, gentamicin solution should be inspected for discoloration or particulates. After administration, any unused solution should be discarded.

Nursing Diagnoses and Outcomes

- Risk for Injury related to potential drug-related allergic reactions or neuromuscular blockade or suppression of bone marrow function
  Desired outcome: The patient will remain free of injury and will contact the prescriber if unusual adverse effects occur.
- Diarrhea related to drug effects
  Desired outcome: The patient will avoid dehydration, maintain fluid intake, and contact the prescriber if diarrhea persists.
- Imbalanced Nutrition: Less than Body Requirements, related to drug-induced GI effects or superinfection

Desired outcome: The patient will maintain body weight and report to the health care provider any persistent adverse effects that affect nutritional status.
- Risk for Injury related to CNS effects
Desired outcome: The patient will remain free of injury and contact the provider if confusion, disorientation, or depression occurs.
- Disturbed Sensory Perception related to potential ototoxicity
Desired outcome: The patient will report sensory or perceptual changes to the prescriber.
- Excess Fluid Volume related to potential nephrotoxicity
Desired outcome: The patient will report any weight gain exceeding 3 lb to the health care prescriber.

Planning and Intervention

Maximizing Therapeutic Effects

Make sure that patients receive the full course of gentamicin as prescribed at around-the-clock intervals; coordinate the administration of drugs to decrease potential drug interactions; and evaluate culture and sensitivity reports to make sure that gentamicin is the appropriate drug.

Because gentamicin may be inactivated by extended penicillins, such as carbenicillin or ticarcillin, administer these drugs at least 2 hours apart to ensure the efficacy of gentamicin.

Minimizing Adverse Effects

To reduce the occurrence of adverse effects, it is imperative to maintain blood levels of gentamicin within a therapeutic margin that is very narrow. To do this, **peak and trough** drug levels are monitored throughout therapy. Blood for peak levels is drawn 30 minutes after the completion of a 30-minute intravenous (IV) administration or immediately after a 60-minute IV administration and 45 to 60 minutes after intramuscular (IM) administration. Blood for trough levels is drawn just before the next dose. Some hospitals obtain only a trough level unless the patient has an increased risk for nephrotoxicity.

Monitor for signs of ototoxicity. Before administering each dose, assess the patient's balance and gross hearing.

Monitor for signs of nephrotoxicity. Assess the hydration status of the patient and be alert for dilute urine or proteinuria. Monitor the patient for gentamicin-induced diarrhea because diarrhea may also cause dehydration.

If CNS effects occur, safety measures should be instituted to protect the patient. Small, frequent meals can be arranged for patients with GI effects, and frequent mouth care and ice chips can be offered to relieve stomatitis and sore mouth.

If a patient receiving gentamicin requires surgery, the chart should indicate prominently that gentamicin has been given. Remember that gentamicin may interact with neuromuscular blocking agents commonly used during surgery, resulting in prolonged neuromuscular blockade. The patient requires extended monitoring and support after surgery to detect problems and intervene if they occur.

Monitor laboratory tests such as renal and hepatic function tests, peak and trough levels of gentamicin, and the fluid intake and output status of the patient.

Providing Patient and Family Education

- Teach patients that gentamicin is one drug within a class of drugs. Ask if they have ever had a drug reaction to any drug with "micin" in its name.
- Advise female patients that they should not take this drug if they are pregnant or breast-feeding.
- Advise patients to take oral gentamicin on an empty stomach, 1 hour before or 2 hours after any meal or other drugs. Instruct patients to take forgotten doses as soon as they remember, but not to double the dose, and to contact the prescriber if symptoms do not improve in 3 days.
- Teach patients how to identify, report, and manage signs and symptoms of allergic reaction and adverse effects.
- Teach patients signs of ototoxicity such as persistent headache, nausea, balance difficulties, dizziness, vertigo, tinnitus, or high-frequency hearing loss. Instruct patients to contact their prescriber immediately if any of these symptoms occur.
- Instruct patients to take aspirin for headache or muscle pain because aspirin decreases the potential for gentamicin-induced hearing loss.
- Teach patients signs of nephrotoxicity, such as frequent or diminished urinary excretion. Instruct the patient to contact the prescriber immediately if such signs occur.
- Teach patients how to recognize superinfection and to watch for CNS effects such as confusion, depression, numbness, tingling, or weakness. Explain the importance of contacting the prescriber if any of these symptoms occur.
- Help patients develop strategies for minimizing GI upset and oral soreness.
- Show patients how to use gentamicin eye or ear drops correctly, making sure to stress the importance of keeping the dropper portion of the bottle from touching the eye or ear to avoid contamination.

Ongoing Assessment and Evaluation

Coordinate the care of the patient to ensure that other potentially nephrotoxic or ototoxic drugs are not added to the treatment plan. Notify the primary prescriber if any such drugs are added. Monitor peak and trough levels of gentamicin. Although maintaining gentamicin serum concentrations within traditional ranges is believed to minimize the risk for nephrotoxicity, some patients may still develop ototoxicity or nephrotoxicity. Monitor for **azotemia** (excessive urea levels in the blood), decreased creatinine clearance, **hyposthenuria** (loss of the ability to concentrate urine), **pyuria** (increased white blood cell count), **proteinuria,** and **cylindruria** (cells or casts in the urine).

Evaluate for signs of ototoxicity. Cochlear damage may be subtle; therefore, coordinate referrals for audiologic testing for patients who receive repeated or prolonged courses of gentamicin therapy. Vestibular damage is characterized by a headache followed by vertigo, dizziness, or nausea. To avoid permanent ototoxic damage, the drug should be withdrawn at the first sign of tinnitus or persistent headache.

EXPLAINING THE DRUG SELECTION PROCESS

Georgia James, age 64 years, is admitted to your unit with a diagnosis of pneumonia. She has just completed her first dose of IV gentamicin when her granddaughter arrives. The granddaughter comes to the nurses' station and is very upset. She states in a very loud voice, "Why is my grandmother getting gentamicin? I saw on the Internet that there is a new type of drug for pneumonia called syner-something. Why isn't she getting the strongest kind of medication?" How would you handle this situation?

Evaluate patients for signs of neuromuscular blockade, such as muscle weakness, especially of the respiratory muscles. Observe the injection site regularly because IM injection of gentamicin can cause irritation.

When therapy ends, the presenting infection should be resolved. The patient should be adequately nourished and hydrated and free from adverse drug effects.

Drugs Closely Related to P Gentamicin

Drugs closely related to gentamicin include amikacin, kanamycin, neomycin sulfate, and tobramycin. Contraindications, adverse effects (including Black Box warnings), drug interactions, and patient management for all these drugs are the same as those of gentamicin.

Amikacin

Amikacin (Amikin) is a parenteral aminoglycoside with a broader spectrum of activity than gentamicin for gram-negative bacilli. It is also less likely to induce bacterial resistance.

Kanamycin

Kanamycin (Kantrex) is used orally to reduce ammonia-forming bacteria in hepatic coma and as an adjunctive therapy to decrease GI flora. Its use for systemic infections is limited by the number of bacteria that are resistant to it and the availability of gentamicin in its less expensive generic formulation.

Neomycin Sulfate

Neomycin sulfate (Neo-Fradin) has the highest risk of toxicity of all the aminoglycosides. Because it is so toxic, it is not administered parenterally. It is available orally to decrease GI flora as a preparation for bowel surgery and to treat hepatic encephalopathy. Because it is not absorbed from the GI tract, it frequently causes superinfection within the bowel. Neomycin is an ingredient combined with other topical prescription medications and alone as an over-the-counter (OTC) drug as a topical antibiotic.

Tobramycin

Tobramycin (Nebcin) is similar to gentamicin in its antibacterial spectrum; however, it is more active than gentamicin against *Pseudomonas* species. It is given parenterally for

P Gentamicin

- Used for serious gram-negative infections
- Major contraindications: hypersensitivity, pregnancy, and breast-feeding
- Most common adverse effects: nausea, vomiting, diarrhea, and weight loss
- Most serious adverse effects: see black box warnings
- Maximizing therapeutic effects: Administer at least 2 hours before or after extended infusions of penicillins.
- Minimizing adverse effects: Monitor peak and trough levels throughout therapy.
- Most important patient education: Teach the patient the signs and symptoms of both nephrotoxicity and ototoxicity and also the importance of contacting the health care provider immediately if any symptoms should occur.
- **Black box warning: neurotoxicity, nephrotoxicity, ototoxicity, and neuromuscular blockade**

systemic infections or topically to treat superficial ophthalmic infections. Tobramycin solution for inhalation (TSI) is currently the only approved inhaled antibiotic in the United States. Peak and trough levels should be closely monitored in patients with serious infections or in disease states known to substantially alter aminoglycoside pharmacokinetics, such as cystic fibrosis, burns, or major surgery.

Drugs Significantly Different From P Gentamicin

Paromomycin

Paromomycin (Humatin) is an aminoglycoside antibiotic that differs from gentamicin because of its amebicidal and anthelminthic activity. Paromomycin has poor oral bioavailability; thus, it is used to treat intestinal amebiasis and various intestinal parasites by its local activity. It is also useful in managing hepatic encephalopathy or coma because it inhibits bacteria in the gut that produce urease, an enzyme that breaks down urea into carbon dioxide and ammonia.

Paromomycin is contraindicated in patients with renal failure or intestinal obstruction. Adverse GI effects of paromomycin include anorexia, nausea, vomiting, gastric burning and pain, abdominal cramps, and diarrhea.

The only important drug–drug interaction with paromomycin occurs with succinylcholine. When they are given in combination, paromomycin may potentiate the neuromuscular effects of succinylcholine.

Coordinate follow-up appointments for the patient. Stool cultures should be done weekly for 6 weeks after therapy, then monthly for 2 years.

Streptomycin

Streptomycin is a parenteral aminoglycoside. It is used as part of combination therapy both for active tuberculosis and

TABLE 40.3	Summary of Selected ⓒ Lincosamide Antibiotics		
Drug (Trade) Name	Selected Indications	Route and Dosage Range	Pharmacokinetics
Ⓟ clindamycin (Cleocin)	Skin and skin structure infection Respiratory tract infections Septicemia Intra-abdominal infections Osteomyelitis Gynecologic infection Endocarditis prophylaxis	*Adult:* PO, 150–450 mg q6 h; IM/IV, 600 mg–2.7 g q6–12 h up to 4.8 g/d for life-threatening infections *Child:* PO, 10–30 mg/kg/d in three divided doses every 6–8 h; IM/IV, 20–40 mg/kg q6–8 h up to 40 mg/kg/d for severe infection *Adult PO/IM/IV;* 600 mg *Child:* 20 mg/kg	*Onset:* PO, varies; IM, 20–30 min; IV, immediate *Duration:* 8–12 h $t_{1/2}$: 2–3 h
lincomycin (Lincocin)	Serious infections from streptococci, pneumococci, and staphylococci	*Adult:* PO, 500 mg q8 h; IM, 600–200 mg/d; IV, 600–1,000 mg q8–12 h	*Onset:* IM, 20–30 min; IV, immediate *Duration:* IM, 0.5 h; IV, 14 h $t_{1/2}$: 5 h

for treating streptococcal or enterococcal endocarditis. As a single agent, it is used for mycobacterial infections, plague, tularemia, and brucellosis. Streptomycin may induce the same Black Box adverse effects as gentamicin.

LINCOSAMIDES

The lincosamides include clindamycin (Cleocin) and lincomycin (Lincocin). They are very toxic drugs; thus, their use must be monitored and limited to situations with infections by bacteria with known sensitivity. Although lincomycin was the first drug developed in this class, it is rarely used. Clindamycin is discussed as the prototype lincosamide. Table 40.3 presents a summary of lincosamide antibiotics.

Nursing Management of the Patient Receiving Ⓟ Clindamycin

Core Drug Knowledge

Pharmacotherapeutics

Clindamycin is active against a wide range of aerobic gram-positive cocci and several anaerobic gram-negative and gram-positive organisms. Clindamycin is used in the treatment of skin and skin structure infections, respiratory tract infections, septicemia, intra-abdominal infections, osteomyelitis, and as prophylaxis for endocarditis. Topical forms are used to treat acne vulgaris. A vaginal preparation is available for treating bacterial vaginosis.

Pharmacokinetics

The oral absorption of clindamycin varies greatly, depending on the presence of food in the stomach. Peak levels are achieved in about 1 to 2 hours. Given intramuscularly, clindamycin is rapidly absorbed within 20 to 30 minutes, with peak levels occurring at 1 to 3 hours. IV administration produces a peak effect within minutes. Topical clindamycin is only minimally absorbed.

Clindamycin crosses the placenta and enters breast milk and cerebrospinal fluid (CSF). It is readily carried to most body tissues. Metabolized in the liver, it is excreted through the bile and urine.

Pharmacodynamics

Clindamycin is either bacteriostatic or bactericidal, depending on its concentration at the site of action and on the specific susceptibility of the organism being treated. It enters the bacterial cell and binds to bacterial ribosomes, suppressing protein synthesis and leading to cell death in susceptible bacteria. It has no direct effect on the body.

Contraindications and Precautions

Clindamycin is contraindicated in pregnancy and lactation and in patients with a known allergy to lincosamides, history of asthma or other allergies, allergy to tartrazine (a component of several oral preparations of clindamycin), or hepatic or renal dysfunction. Caution should be exercised in patients with a history of antibiotic-associated colitis, regional enteritis, or ulcerative colitis.

Adverse Effects

The most serious adverse effect is pseudomembranous colitis (a Black Box warning), also known as *Clostridium difficile* colitis. Diarrhea, abdominal cramps, and abdominal tenderness may suggest antibiotic-associated colitis. Nausea and vomiting and abdominal pain following oral administration are the most common adverse effects of clindamycin.

Thrombocytopenia, neutropenia, and eosinophilia have been reported during clindamycin therapy. Sore throat or fever may indicate neutropenia.

Maculopapular rash, erythema, and pruritus can develop from systemic or topical use of clindamycin. Pathologic dryness of the skin (**xeroderma**), conjunctiva (**xerophthalmia**), or mucous membranes is the most common effect of topical application. Alcohol in some topical formulations may irritate the eyes, mucous membranes, or abraded skin if allowed to come into contact with them.

Hypersensitivity reactions range from skin rashes and urticaria to anaphylactoid reactions. After injection, pain, abscess, and phlebitis are relatively common.

Drug Interactions

Neuromuscular blockers, aluminum salts, and cyclosporine interact with clindamycin. Topical preparations containing

TABLE 40.4	Agents that Interact with P Clindamycin	
Interactants	Effect and Significance	Nursing Management
aluminum salts or kaolin	Marked decreased GI absorption of oral clindamycin	Administer absorbent antidiarrheal product 2 h before or 3–4 h after administering oral clindamycin.
cyclosporine	Cyclosporine concentrations may be reduced, decreasing its pharmacologic effects	Monitor cyclosporine concentrations when clindamycin is started, stopped, or changed.
non-depolarizing muscle relaxants	Clindamycin potentiates the action of non- depolarizing muscle relaxants, resulting in increased neuromuscular blockade, respiratory depression, and extended paralysis.	Mark patient's chart with warning of the drug combination. Arrange for extended monitoring and support of patient after surgery or procedure. Monitor respiration and other vital signs. Be prepared for ventilatory support as needed

benzoyl peroxide, tretinoin, salicylic acid, or other topical preparations for acne, when used with clindamycin preparations, can cause a cumulative irritant effect, leading to excessive drying and peeling of the skin. Table 40.4 lists agents that interact with clindamycin.

Assessment of Relevant Core Patient Variables

Health Status
Assess patients for allergy to lincosamides or predisposition to such allergy as shown by a previous reaction to tartrazine. Some clindamycin preparations contain tartrazine dye, which can precipitate bronchial asthma or other allergic reactions in sensitive patients.

Next, investigate any history of GI disease because clindamycin predisposes patients to the overgrowth of nonsusceptible organisms and hence may induce pseudomembranous colitis.

Any previous renal or hepatic disease must be explored because the half-life of clindamycin is prolonged in patients with hepatic dysfunction, and toxicity can occur. Hepatic and renal function should be tested at baseline, and the results should be evaluated before beginning therapy. For patients with severe renal or hepatic impairment, dose reduction should be considered.

Patients on long-term therapy should have a baseline complete blood count (CBC) because of clindamycin's potential to induce blood dyscrasias.

Life Span and Gender
Explore the benefits of treatment versus potential risks with the pregnant or lactating woman. In general, clindamycin is prescribed for pregnant or lactating women only if the benefits outweigh the potential risks.

Assess the growth and developmental level of the child or infant. Clindamycin should be used cautiously in children. Neonates younger than 1 month (and premature infants) have a prolonged plasma half-life for clindamycin, probably because of an immature hepatic system.

Lifestyle, Diet, and Habits
Assess the patient's lifestyle to determine the likelihood that the patient will take the drug around the clock.

Environment
Be aware of the environment in which clindamycin will be administered and, if appropriate, assess the home or living environment for potential risk factors. Parenteral solutions of clindamycin must be used within 24 hours of reconstitution. Oral or topical clindamycin may be administered in any environment.

Nursing Diagnoses and Outcomes
- Risk for Injury related to allergic reactions
  Desired outcome: The patient will stop drug therapy and immediately report symptoms of allergic reaction to the prescriber.
- Diarrhea related to drug effects
  Desired outcome: The patient will avoid dehydration and report persistent diarrhea to the provider.
- Imbalanced Nutrition: Less than Body Requirements, related to drug-related GI effects, alteration in taste, superinfections
  Desired outcome: The patient will maintain body weight and report persistent symptoms affecting nutritional status.
- Risk for Injury related to possible blood dyscrasias
  Desired outcome: The patient will remain injury free throughout drug therapy.

Planning and Intervention
Maximizing Therapeutic Effects
Make sure that the patient receives the full course of clindamycin as prescribed, at around-the-clock intervals for maximal effectiveness. Coordinate the administration of drugs to decrease potential undesired interactions. Culture and sensitivity reports may be reviewed periodically to confirm that clindamycin is the appropriate drug for the patient.

Minimizing Adverse Effects
Clindamycin should be administered on an empty stomach with a full glass of water. For patients with GI effects,

provide a small meal with administration. Provide frequent mouth care and ice chips to suck on if stomatitis and sore mouth are problems. It is also important to keep this drug out of the reach of children to avoid accidental overdose. Report diarrhea to the provider immediately.

Providing Patient and Family Education

- Ensure that patients understand that they should not take clindamycin or any other lincosamide antibiotic if they have ever had a reaction to a drug with a generic name that ends with "mycin" or "micin."
- Advise patients to contact the prescriber immediately if they experience diarrhea.
- Advise pregnant or breast-feeding patients to avoid clindamycin.
- Discuss general dosage and safe storage recommendations.
- Advise patients to take clindamycin on an empty stomach with a full glass of water. If GI distress occurs, take with food.
- Urge patients to contact their prescriber if clindamycin therapy does not improve symptoms in 3 days.
- Teach patients to recognize and report symptoms of allergic reaction and superinfection (sore throat, easy bruising or bleeding, and fatigue).
- Advise women of childbearing age who are taking birth control pills to use a backup method of contraception while taking clindamycin.
- Advise patients using clindamycin lotion that dry skin may occur. Instruct patients to drink plenty of fluids and to keep the skin moisturized.

Ongoing Assessment and Evaluation

Monitor the patient for the onset of diarrhea. If it occurs, the prescriber should be notified immediately because diarrhea may be the presenting sign of pseudomembranous colitis. Obtain an order for the stool to be evaluated for white blood cells (WBCs), blood, and mucus. Arrange for a proctoscopy to be performed.

During therapy, monitor for potential procedures that would require the use of neuromuscular blocking agents. If a procedure is scheduled, note prominently on the patient's chart the current use of clindamycin. After the procedure, the patient should be monitored and supported for an extended period once the neuromuscular blocker is discontinued.

Monitor for sore throat and fever, which may be signs of thrombocytopenia, neutropenia, or eosinophilia.

When treatment ends, the initial infection should be resolved. The patient should be adequately nourished and hydrated, and any adverse drug effects should be resolved.

Drug Closely Related to P Clindamycin

Lincomycin (Lincocin) is a parenteral lincosamide antibiotic. It is used for serious staphylococcal and streptococcal infections. Lincomycin is usually reserved for patients who

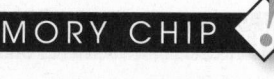

MEMORY CHIP

P Clindamycin

- Used for serious infections caused by gram-positive cocci and both gram-positive and gram-negative anaerobes.
- Major contraindications: hypersensitivity, pregnancy, breast-feeding, and renal or hepatic dysfunction
- Most common adverse effects: nausea, vomiting, abdominal pain, rash, and pruritus
- Most serious adverse effect: pseudomembranous colitis
- Maximizing therapeutic effects: Administer at evenly spaced intervals.
- Minimizing adverse effects: Give with food to minimize GI distress.
- Most important patient education: Teach the patient the signs and symptoms of superinfection, especially pseudomembranous colitis, and explain the importance of contacting the health care provider immediately if any symptoms occur.
- **Black box warning: Pseudomembranous colitis: May range from severe to mild to life threatening.**

cannot take penicillins or clindamycin. It is not a drug of choice because it has been associated with severe or fatal colitis. Like clindamycin, lincomycin is used with caution in patients with asthma, liver disease, GI disease, colitis, and tartrazine sensitivity. Adverse effects, drug interactions, and patient management are similar to those of clindamycin.

C MACROLIDE ANTIBIOTICS

The macrolide antibiotics have been in use since 1952. They are characterized by molecules made up of large-ring lactones. Macrolides are bacteriostatic or bactericidal in susceptible bacteria. They include erythromycin and troleandomycin. Synthetic derivatives of erythromycin, also classified as macrolide antibiotics, include azithromycin and clarithromycin. Erythromycin was the first macrolide discovered and is the prototype for this class. Table 40.5 presents a summary of macrolide antibiotics.

Nursing Management of the Patient Receiving P Erythromycin

Core Drug Knowledge

Pharmacotherapeutics

Erythromycin is commonly used in treating Legionnaire disease, *Mycoplasma pneumoniae* pneumonia, diphtheria, chlamydial infections, and chancroid, and as an alternative to beta-lactam antibiotics in patients who are allergic to penicillin. Erythromycin may have benefits in hypomotility conditions, such as diabetic gastroparesis, because it increases gastric motility and emptying.

Erythromycin is generally more effective against gram-positive organisms than against gram-negative organisms because of its ability to penetrate into gram-positive organisms.

TABLE 40.5	Summary of Selected Ⓒ Macrolide Antibiotics		
Drug (Trade) Name	**Selected Indications**	**Route and Dosage Range**	**Pharmacokinetics**
Ⓟ erythromycin (E-Mycin, Ilosone, EES, Erythrocin stearate)	Urethral, endocervical, or rectal infections Syphilis Legionnaire disease Rheumatic fever Bacterial endocarditis *Mycoplasma* infections Bronchitis Pharyngitis Skin infections	*Adult*: PO, 250–500 mg q6 h (maximum 4g) *Child*: PO, 30–50 mg q6–12 h (maximum 100 mg/kg in divided doses) (*Note*: EES dosage is slightly higher)	*Onset*: 1–2 h *Duration*: 6–8 h $t_{1/2}$: 3–5 h
azithromycin (Zithromax)	Lower respiratory tract infection Nongonococcal urethritis and cervicitis Skin infections Acute otitis media Pharyngitis/tonsillitis *Helicobacter pylori* infection *Mycobacterium avium* (prevention or treatment)	*Adult*: PO, 500 mg/d on first day, then 250 mg for days 2 through 5 *Child 6 mo–2 y*: PO, 10 mg/kg on d 1, then 5 mg/kg on days 2–5; >2 y, PO, 10 mg/kg as single dose (not to exceed 500 mg) first day; then 5 mg/kg (not to exceed 250 mg) once daily for 4 d *Adult*: PO, 500 mg q12 h *Adult*: PO, 250–500 mg q12 h for 7–14 d	*Onset*: Rapid *Duration*: 24 h $t_{1/2}$: 11–48 h
clarithromycin (Biaxin)	Respiratory infections Skin infections	*Adult*: PO 250–500 mg every 12 h for 7–14 d *Child*: PO 7.5 mg/kg 2×/d, to a maximum of 500 mg 2×/d	*Onset*: Rapid *Duration*: 8–12 h $t_{1/2}$: 3–7 h
telithromycin (Ketek)	Acute exacerbation of chronic bronchitis Acute bacterial sinusitis Community-acquired pneumonia Not approved for children	*Adult and Child >18 y*: PO 800 mg × 5 d *Adult and Child >18 y*: PO 800 mg qd 7–10 d	*Onset*: 1 h *Duration*: Unknown $t_{1/2}$: 10 h

Pharmacokinetics

Erythromycin base (E-Mycin, Ery-Tab) is easily inactivated by gastric acid; therefore, several formulations have been developed to overcome this problem. Erythromycin stearate (Erythrocin) is the most likely to yield to gastric acid destruction. Erythromycin estolate (Ilosone) is more acid stable, dissociates in the upper intestine, and releases an inactive ester that is absorbed and hydrolyzed in the blood to produce free erythromycin. Erythromycin ethylsuccinate (EES, EryPed) is first absorbed and then hydrolyzed in the blood to free erythromycin. The newest formulation of oral erythromycin is encapsulated pellets that are small enough to pass through the pyloric sphincter independent of gastric emptying and are absorbed as the base. None of the oral forms, however, allows complete absorption. The drug reaches peak levels 1 to 4 hours after administration. Erythromycin is also available for IV use as erythromycin lactobionate or erythromycin gluceptate. Administration of IV erythromycin is painful and is used only when high serum levels of erythromycin are required. When given intravenously, erythromycin peak effect occurs within 1 hour. Erythromycin is also available in an ophthalmic preparation.

Erythromycin crosses the placenta and is secreted in breast milk. It does not cross the blood–brain barrier. It is metabolized in the liver and excreted in the bile and urine. Table 40.5 has additional information.

Pharmacodynamics

Erythromycin has no direct effect on the body. The macrolides are bactericidal or bacteriostatic. They exert their effect by inhibiting RNA-dependent protein synthesis at the chain elongation step. This action can prevent the cell from dividing, or it can cause cell death, depending on the sensitivity of the bacteria and the concentration of the drug.

Contraindications and Precautions

Erythromycin is contraindicated in patients who are allergic to it. Caution should be used in any patient with hepatic insufficiency because the ability to break down erythromycin for excretion may be compromised. Caution should be exercised during pregnancy or lactation and in patients with impaired hearing, biliary function, GI disease, and cardiac arrhythmias. Ocular preparations are contraindicated in patients with viral, fungal, or mycobacterial infections of the eye.

Adverse Effects

Adverse effects suggesting allergic reaction to erythromycin include urticaria, maculopapular rash, erythema, and interstitial nephritis. Pruritus is a possible reaction to topical application of erythromycin.

The most common adverse effects related to erythromycin occur in the GI tract. They include nausea or vomiting, abdominal pain, and diarrhea. These effects are often dose related and may occur regardless of the route of administration.

Rare potential adverse effects include hepatotoxicity, pseudomembranous colitis, QT interval prolongation and ventricular tachycardia of the torsades de pointes type, tinnitus, and reversible hearing loss.

Drug Interactions

Erythromycin inhibits the metabolism of many drugs, resulting in an increased risk of adverse effects and toxicity. A potentially fatal interaction may occur with astemizole and terfenadine. Although these two drugs are not available in the United States, it is still prudent to ask the patient if he or she is taking these drugs, because they can be acquired from other sources. Table 40.6 presents the most important potential drug interactions.

Assessment of Relevant Core Patient Variables

Health Status

In assessing a patient's health status before administering erythromycin, explore any history of hypersensitivity to erythromycin or other macrolide antibiotics because of the risk for cross-sensitivity.

Assess for hepatic or biliary dysfunction. Moreover, monitor hepatic function in patients receiving prolonged treatment. Ilosone, the estolate salt of erythromycin, should not be used in patients with hepatic disease because of the potential for hepatotoxicity.

Review the patients' GI history, particularly because the normal flora of the colon may allow an overgrowth of *Clostridium* organisms. A toxin produced by *C. difficile* is a primary cause of antibiotic-associated colitis. Patients who develop diarrhea while taking or soon after taking erythromycin should be evaluated for potential antibiotic-associated pseudomembranous colitis.

Monitor the patient's hearing because high-dose therapy with erythromycin may cause a reversible loss of hearing, and patients with preexisting hearing impairment may be at especially great risk.

In addition, explore any possibility of cardiovascular disorder, specifically a history of torsades de pointes, because IV administration of erythromycin at a rate above 15 mg/min may place patients with such a history at risk for this arrhythmia.

Life Span and Gender

Evaluate women for pregnancy and lactation. Erythromycin should be used with caution in breast-feeding women because it is excreted in breast milk at about 50% of maternal plasma concentrations, which may induce diarrhea and superinfection in the infant. Consider the developmental level of the patient. Erythromycin lactobionate injection may contain benzyl alcohol as a preservative, which can cause toxicity in neonates. Infants less than 2 weeks of age are at risk for developing hypertrophic pyloric stenosis with erythromycin therapy.

Lifestyle, Diet, and Habits

Assess the patient's dietary habits for drug sensitivity when taking drugs on an empty stomach and the frequency of eating grapefruit or drinking grapefruit juice. Instruct the patient to avoid grapefruit or grapefruit juice because it increases the serum concentration of erythromycin and may cause adverse effects or toxicity. Food decreases the absorption of nonenteric-coated erythromycin. Advise the patient to take erythromycin at least 1 hour before or 2 hours after meals.

Environment

Be aware of the environment in which the drug will be administered. Oral or ophthalmic erythromycin may be given in any environment, whereas IV infusion should be given in a monitored setting.

Nursing Diagnoses and Outcomes

- Risk for Injury related to possible allergic reactions
  Desired outcome: *The patient will stop drug therapy and report any signs of allergic reaction immediately to the prescriber.*
- Diarrhea related to drug-induced GI upset
  Desired outcome: *The patient will avoid dehydration, maintain fluid intake, and contact the prescriber if diarrhea persists.*
- Risk for Infection related to potential for superinfection following drug therapy
  Desired outcome: *The patient will contact the provider if any signs of superinfection occur, such as sore throat or fever.*

Planning and Intervention

Maximizing Therapeutic Effects

Reconstitute erythromycin with sterile water only. Diluents containing preservatives or organic salts should not be used. Prepared infusion solutions that are stored at room temperature must be used within 8 hours. Prepared solutions that are refrigerated must be used within 24 hours.

Evaluate culture and sensitivity reports to verify that erythromycin is the drug of choice. Moreover, administer erythromycin as prescribed, at around-the-clock intervals to increase effectiveness. Because food interferes with drug absorption, administer erythromycin stearate at least 1 hour before or 2 hours after meals. Other formulations of erythromycin may be given without regard to meals. If GI irritation occurs, however, erythromycin stearate may be administered with food. Each dose should be administered with a full glass of water, not with fruit juice.

Minimizing Adverse Effects

Provide small, frequent meals; mouth care; and ice chips to suck on if stomatitis and sore mouth are problems. Additionally, monitor regularly to ensure adequate

TABLE 40.6 Agents That Interact with P Erythromycin

Interactants	Effect and Significance	Nursing Management
Antidysrhythmic Agents	Erythromycin increases drug effect, especially dysrhythmias	Monitor heart rate and rhythm.
Benzodiazepines	Decreases the metabolism of many benzodiazepines, resulting in an increased CNS depression and prolonged effect	Monitor for sedation. Ensure safety precautions for patients. Discuss reduction of dosage of benzodiazepine with the prescriber.
bromocriptine	Increased pharmacologic effect of bromocriptine resulting in an increased risk for toxicity.	Monitor for bromocriptine toxicity. Discuss bromocriptine dose adjustment with the prescriber.
Calcium channel blockers (CCBs)	Decrease the metabolism of certain CCBs, resulting in hypotension	Monitor vital signs. Ensure safety precautions for patients. Discuss changing to azithromycin with the prescriber.
carbamazepine	Decreases the metabolism of carbamazepine, resulting in an increased risk for carbamazepine toxicity	Monitor carbamazepine levels closely. Discuss reduction of dosage of carbamazepine with the prescriber.
colchicine	Decreases the metabolism of colchicine, resulting in an increased risk for colchicine toxicity	Monitor for adverse effects, especially diarrhea.
cyclosporine	Decreases the metabolism of cyclosporine, resulting in an increased risk for adverse effects and toxicity	Avoid combination if possible. Monitor cyclosporine levels carefully. Monitor for cyclosporine toxicity. Adjust cyclosporine as ordered.
digoxin	Increases the serum concentration of digoxin, resulting in toxicity	Monitor digoxin levels carefully. Monitor for signs of toxicity. Discuss adjustment of digoxin dose with the prescriber.
Ergot Alkaloids	Acute ergotism such as peripheral ischemia may occur	Monitor peripheral circulation and sensation. Contact prescriber immediately if symptoms occur.
felodipine	Erythromycin may inhibit the metabolism of felodipine resulting in adverse effects	Monitor for tachycardia, palpitations, flushing, and ankle edema. Contact the prescriber if any occur.
Fluoroquinolone antibiotics	Sparfloxacin and moxifloxacin may induce life-threatening cardiac arrhythmias	Contact prescriber prior to administering this combination.
HMG-CoA Reductase Inhibitors (Statins)	Increases serum concentration of statins increasing risk for severe myopathy or rhabdomyolysis.	Monitor for muscle pain, weakness, or tenderness Avoid combination if possible. Discuss with the prescriber.
methylprednisolone	Decreases the metabolism of methylprednisolone, resulting in an increased risk for adverse effects and toxicity	Monitor therapeutic effects of methylprednisolone. Monitor for adverse effects and toxicity. May be beneficial effect for patients with asthma.
pimozide	Decreases the metabolism of pimozide, resulting in QT interval prolongation	Avoid combination. Discuss with the prescriber.
Rifamycins	The antimicrobial effects of erythromycin may be decreased and the GI adverse effects of rifamycins may be increased.	Monitor for efficacy of erythromycin therapy Monitor for GI distress.
repaglinide	Erythromycin may inhibit the metabolism of repaglinide resulting in an increased risk for adverse effects	Monitor blood glucose frequently Monitor for signs of hypoglycemia such as hunger dizziness, shakiness, sweating, or confusion
sildenafil	Decreases the metabolism of sildenafil, resulting in an increased risk for adverse effects and toxicity	Advise patient to seek medical attention for prolonged erection.
tacrolimus	Erythromycin inhibits tacrolimus metabolism resulting in an increased risk for toxicity.	Monitor renal status carefully. Discuss alternate antibiotic therapy with the prescriber.

(Continued)

TABLE 40.6 Agents That Interact with ▣ Erythromycin *(continued)*

Interactants	Effect and Significance	Nursing Management
theophylline	Macrolides inhibit the metabolism of theophylline. Theophylline reduces the bioavailability and increases the renal clearance of erythromycin. These actions result in increased efficacy of theophylline and decreased efficacy of erythromycin.	Monitor theophylline levels closely. Monitor for theophylline toxic effects. Monitor for treatment failure of erythromycin.
vinblastine	Increased risk for severe vinblastine toxicity	Monitor for neutropenia, constipation, and myalgias. Contact the prescriber immediately if any occur.
warfarin	Decreases the metabolism of warfarin, resulting in an increased risk for warfarin toxicity	Monitor warfarin levels carefully. Monitor INR or PT frequently. Discuss adjustment of warfarin dose with the prescriber.

hydration, and provide fluids to replace those lost with diarrhea. Because erythromycin can be very irritating to veins, it is important to administer IV infusions over 30 to 60 minutes. If pain persists, reduce the rate of infusion. If pain persists, apply ice and notify the prescriber.

Providing Patient and Family Education
• Encourage patients to take the complete course of antibiotics.
• Explain safe drug handling and storage.
• Explain the importance of taking erythromycin around the clock to maintain a therapeutic drug level.
• Teach patients the potential adverse effects and the measures to alleviate discomfort if such events occur.
• Advise patients to take erythromycin on an empty stomach, unless GI distress is unbearable.
• Advise patients to contact the prescriber if there is no improvement in 3 days.

Ongoing Assessment and Evaluation

Monitor for signs of allergic reactions, resolution of presenting signs and symptoms of infection, signs of superinfection, and for patients receiving IV erythromycin, signs of phlebitis or abscess formation. When therapy ends, the patient should be free of the initial infection. The patient will be adequately nourished and hydrated, and adverse effects will be resolved.

Drugs Closely Related to ▣ Erythromycin

Azithromycin and clarithromycin are similar to erythromycin. All of these drugs are comparable to erythromycin in terms of their adverse effects, drug interactions, and patient management.

Azithromycin

Azithromycin (Zithromax) is available in oral, ophthalmic and IV formulations. Generally active against organisms that are also usually susceptible to erythromycin, it produces less GI intolerance than erythromycin. Azithromycin is the drug of choice in the management of chlamydial infection.

Azithromycin is unique in that it can reach exceptionally high levels in tissues, thus increasing its efficacy and duration of action. For this reason, it is administered only once a day. Absorption of azithromycin *capsules* is decreased in the presence of food, and capsules should be given on an empty stomach. The absorption of azithromycin *suspension* is increased in the presence of foods, so much so that the serum concentration may be too high. For that reason, the suspension should be taken on an empty stomach. Conversely, azithromycin *tablets* have an increased absorption when given with a meal with high-fat content and may be given with or without food.

Clarithromycin

Clarithromycin (Biaxin, ZMAX) is an oral macrolide antibiotic similar to erythromycin and azithromycin. Like azithromycin, clarithromycin penetrates tissues to a greater degree than erythromycin. Clarithromycin is generally active against organisms that are usually susceptible to erythromycin. Combined with omeprazole, clarithromycin is useful for *Helicobacter pylori*–associated peptic ulcer disease. Clarithromycin is contraindicated during pregnancy. It is unknown whether clarithromycin is excreted in breast milk. It is used cautiously in patients with either hepatic or renal insufficiency because it is partially renally excreted.

MEMORY CHIP

▣ Erythromycin

• Used for infections caused by gram-positive organisms. Less effective for gram-negative organisms.
• Major contraindication: hypersensitivity
• Most common adverse effect: GI distress
• Most serious adverse effects: hepatotoxicity, QT prolongation, pseudomembranous colitis, and ventricular tachycardia
• Maximizing therapeutic effects: Administer on an empty stomach, unless GI distress is pronounced.
• Minimizing adverse effects: Provide small, frequent meals.
• Most important patient education: Complete the entire course of medication, even when feeling better.

Drug Significantly Different From P Erythromycin

Telithromycin (Ketek) is the first drug in a new class of antibiotics called ketolides. A semisynthetic drug structurally similar to macrolides, telithromycin is approved to treat community-acquired pneumonia caused by *S. pneumoniae* (including multidrug-resistant isolates [MDRSP]), *H. influenzae, M. catarrhalis, Chlamydophila* (formerly *Chlamydia*) *pneumoniae,* and *Mycoplasma pneumoniae*. Its advantages include once-daily dosing and a short duration of administration (5 to 10 days).

Contraindications to telithromycin include patients with a history of myasthenia gravis, hepatitis or jaundice that occurred when taking other macrolide antibiotics, and patients with concomitant use of cisapride or pimozide. Telithromycin is given cautiously in cases of congenital prolongation of the QT interval, uncorrected hypokalemia and hypomagnesia, and clinically important bradycardia because these are considered prodysrhythmic conditions.

Telithromycin may induce several serious adverse effects. There is a black box warning regarding the use of telithromycin in patients with myasthenia gravis because of the potential to induce an exacerbation that may include life-threatening acute respiratory failure. Telithromycin may also cause liver dysfunction such as acute hepatic failure, severe liver injury, fulminant hepatitis, and hepatic necrosis. In addition, it may cause fainting spells and visual disturbances, both of which place the patient at risk for injury. Lastly, telithromycin may cause a prolonged QT interval or Torsades de pointes.

The common adverse effects for telithromycin are similar to that for erythromycin—mainly nausea, diarrhea, headache, and dizziness. In addition, telithromycin may cause. A potent CYP3A4 inhibitor, telithromycin has a long list of potential drug–drug interactions. Telithromycin is a pregnancy category C drug and is not recommended for patients under the age of 18 years.

C OXAZOLIDINONES

Oxazolidinones are the first new class of antibiotics developed specifically for treating methicillin-resistant *Staphylococcus aureus* (MRSA) infections. Linezolid (Zyvox) is the prototype for this new class of drugs (Table 40.7).

Nursing Management of the Patient Receiving P Linezolid

Core Drug Knowledge

Pharmacotherapeutics

Linezolid is approved for use in treating bacteremia associated with vancomycin-resistant *Enterococcus faecium* or *E. faecalis* (VRE); complicated skin infections; nosocomial or community-acquired pneumonia; bacteremia associated with nosocomial or community-acquired pneumonia; and infective endocarditis. It is also being used in the management of peritonitis in patients receiving peritoneal dialysis in certain circumstances.

Pharmacokinetics

Linezolid is available in both oral and parenteral formulations. Oral linezolid is 100% bioavailable, which means that the IV and oral forms are interchangeable without making dosage adjustments. Oral linezolid is rapidly absorbed from the GI tract and is widely distributed. Food delays absorption but does not decrease peak plasma concentrations. Linezolid is partly metabolized in the liver and is excreted in urine.

Pharmacodynamics

Linezolid attacks bacteria by blocking the early stages of the process bacteria use to make proteins, whereas other antibiotics act at later stages of protein synthesis. This unique mechanism of action suggests that bacteria may not be able to develop resistance as quickly and that cross-resistance between linezolid and other antibiotics is less likely to occur.

Contraindications and Precautions

The only contraindication for linezolid is hypersensitivity. Linezolid oral suspension should be used with caution in patients with phenylketonuria because the linezolid oral suspension is formulated with aspartame, which supplies roughly 20 mg of phenylalanine in each 5-mL suspension. Other linezolid products do not contain phenylalanine. Linezolid is given cautiously to patients with pre-existing blood dyscrasias because it may suppress bone marrow function. For the same reason, it should be given cautiously to patients receiving other drugs known to suppress bone marrow function. Because linezolid is a nonselective inhibitor of

TABLE 40.7	Overview of C Linezolid		
Drug (Trade) Name	**Selected Indications**	**Route and Dosage Range**	**Pharmacokinetics**
P linezolid (Zyvox)	Vancomycin-resistant *Enterococcus faecium* infection	*Adult IV/PO:* 600 mg every 12 h for 14–28 d Child < 11 y IV/PO: 10 mg/kg every 8 h	*Onset IV/PO:* rapid *Duration:* unknown
	Community-acquired pneumonia, complicated skin and skin-structure infections, diabetic foot ulcers	*Adult IV/PO: 600 mg every 12 h for a minimum of 8 wk*	$t_{1/2}$: 5 hours
	Infective endocarditis		
	Uncomplicated skin and skin-structure infections	*Adult PO:* 400–600 mg every 112 h for 10–14 d *Child 5–11 y PO:* 10 mg/kg every 12 h *Child <5 y PO:* 10 mg/kg every 8 h	

monoamine oxidase (MAO), it should be used with caution in patients with hypertension, untreated hyperthyroid disease, severe cardiac disease, cerebrovascular disease, or pheochromocytoma. These patients have an increased risk of poor sequelae because linezolid-induced MAO inhibition reduces the metabolism of pressor amines, which may increase blood pressure in these individuals. Linezolid is classified as an FDA pregnancy category C drug.

Adverse Effects

Linezolid is generally well tolerated. The most common adverse effects associated with linezolid therapy are rash, fever, diarrhea, headache, nausea, and vomiting, usually mild to moderate in intensity and limited in duration. Serious adverse effects include seizures, blood dyscrasias, myelosuppression, lactic acidosis, serotonin syndrome, elevated hepatic enzyme levels, and pseudomembranous colitis. Hypertension is another potentially serious adverse effect in people with existing hypertension, untreated hyperthyroid disease, severe cardiac disease, cerebrovascular disease, or pheochromocytoma. As with other antibiotics, superinfections may occur during linezolid treatment.

Drug Interactions

Because linezolid is a reversible, nonselective MAO inhibitor, most potential drug interactions are related to this action of the drug. Linezolid interactions include adrenergic and serotonergic agents. Table 40.8 presents potential drug interactions.

Dietary interactions with linezolid can be serious. Foods containing tyramine should be avoided.

Assessment of Relevant Core Patient Variables

Health Status

Elicit a complete history from the patient focusing on pre-existing medical conditions that require cautious use of linezolid. Evaluate the patient's current medications for drugs that may interact with linezolid. Communicate positive findings to the prescriber before administering linezolid.

Review the culture and sensitivity report to establish that linezolid is an appropriate therapy. For patients requiring therapy longer than 14 days, obtain a baseline CBC and liver function test values.

Life Span and Gender

Assess the patient for potential pregnancy or breast-feeding because linezolid is a pregnancy category C drug. Linezolid is not approved for use in children.

Lifestyle, Diet, and Habits

Ask the patient about dietary intake, focusing on foods that are rich in tyramine. Evaluate for potential alcohol abuse because alcohol consumption during therapy increases the risk for a hypertensive crisis.

Because linezolid may interact with many OTC medications, assess for self-medicating of coughs, colds, or allergies or to achieve weight loss.

Environment

Be aware of the environment in which linezolid will be administered. Parenteral linezolid should be administered in an acute hospital setting. Oral linezolid may be administered in any setting.

Nursing Diagnoses and Outcomes

- Deficient Fluid Volume related to nausea, vomiting, and diarrhea from linezolid therapy
  Desired outcome: *The patient will remain well hydrated throughout therapy.*
- Risk for Injury related to thrombocytopenia and pseudomembranous colitis
  Desired outcome: *The patient will remain free from injury and contact the health care provider immediately if any signs of bleeding or abdominal pain occur.*
- Risk for Injury related to hypertensive crisis
  Desired outcome: *The patient will remain normotensive by adhering to antihypertensive therapy and limiting foods or beverages with tyramine, caffeine, or alcohol.*

TABLE 40.8	Agents That Interact with ℗ Linezolid	
Interactants	**Effect and Significance**	**Nursing Management**
Rifamycins	Rifamycins may decrease the serum concentration of linezolid	Monitor for linezolid efficacy
SSRI	Linezolid is a reversible, non-selective MAOI and can potentially interact with serotonergic agents, precipitating the serotonin syndrome.	Monitor for symptoms of "serotonin syndrome" such as irritability, increased muscle tone, shivering, myoclonus, and altered consciousness. Contact the prescriber if any occur.
tyramine	Linezolid may inhibit tyramine metabolism resulting in a severe pressor response	Avoid administration of large quantities of foods or beverages with high tyramine content (greater than 100 mg tyramine per meal)

Planning and Intervention

Maximizing Therapeutic Effects

Administer linezolid at evenly spaced intervals throughout the day (Box 40.1).

Minimizing Adverse Effects

To avoid hypertensive crisis, monitor the patient's intake of food or beverages containing tyramine, caffeine, or alcohol. Serial blood pressure readings should be obtained throughout therapy.

Providing Patient and Family Education

- Explain the importance of taking linezolid exactly as prescribed for the entire course of treatment, even if the patient feels better.
- Explain the need for periodic laboratory tests if therapy is anticipated to last longer than 14 days.
- Explain dietary restrictions, focusing on food or beverages containing tyramine, caffeine, or alcohol.
- Explain the importance of not using OTC drugs that may interact with linezolid.

BOX 40.1 FOCUS ON RESEARCH

Nosocomial MRSA

Henderson, D. K. (2006). Managing methicillin-resistant staphylococci: A paradigm for preventing nosocomial transmission of resistant organisms. *American Journal of Infection Control, 34*(5 Suppl. 1), S46–S54; discussion S64–S73.

The Study

Multidrug-resistant bacteria, such as methicillin-resistant *Staphylococcus aureus* (MRSA), are endemic in health care settings in the United States and many other countries of the world. MRSA causes serious infections commonly seen in clinical settings. Nosocomial transmission of MRSA serves as a source of hospital outbreaks, and recent reports of vancomycin-resistant *S aureus* strains in the United States emphasize the need for better control of MRSA and other resistant bacteria within health care settings. Colonization with *S aureus* or MRSA is relatively common in both healthy and hospitalized people; it most often involves the anterior nares and is frequently asymptomatic. Colonization increases risk of infection. Patient-to-patient transmission of MRSA within health care settings primarily occurs via carriage on the hands of health care workers. The Society for Healthcare Epidemiology of America (SHEA) has developed guidelines for the prevention of transmission of MRSA and vancomycin-resistant enterococci within health care settings, and chief among the recommendations is an emphasis on adherence to hand hygiene guidelines.

Nursing Implications

Health care providers have been identified as a primary route of MRSA transmission. The SHEA guidelines mimic the Centers for Disease Control and Prevention (CDC) guidelines developed in 2003 to control the spread of MRSA. The CDC and SHEA guidelines include those listed below. In addition, the SHEA guidelines emphasize improved antibiotic stewardship, staff cohorting, maintenance of appropriate staffing ratios, reductions in length of hospital stays, contact isolation, active microbiologic surveillance, and better staff education.

Patient Considerations

- Place the patient with MRSA in a private room. When a private room is not available, the patient may be placed in a room with patients who have active infection with MRSA but no other infections (a practice called cohorting).
- Limit the movement and transport of the patient from the room for essential purposes only.
- Ensure that patient-care items, bedside equipment, and frequently touched surfaces receive daily cleaning.
- Dedicate the use of noncritical patient-care equipment and items, such as stethoscope, sphygmomanometer, bedside commode, or electronic rectal thermometer, to a single patient (or cohort) infected or colonized with MRSA and avoid sharing such items between patients.

Handwashing

- Wash hands after touching blood, body fluids, secretions, excretions, and contaminated items, whether or not gloves are worn.
- Wash hands immediately after gloves are removed, between patient contacts, and when otherwise indicated, to avoid transferring microorganisms to other patients or environments.
- Wash hands between tasks and procedures on the same patient to prevent cross-contamination of different body sites.

Gloving

- Wear gloves (clean nonsterile gloves are adequate) when touching blood, body fluids, secretions, excretions, and contaminated items.
- Put on clean gloves just before touching mucous membranes and nonintact skin.
- Remove gloves promptly after use, before touching noncontaminated items and environmental surfaces, and before going to another patient.
- Wash hands immediately after glove removal to avoid transferring microorganisms to other patients or environments.

Masking

- Wear a mask and eye protection or a face shield to protect mucous membranes of the eyes, nose, and mouth during procedures and patient-care activities that are likely to generate splashes or sprays of blood, body fluids, secretions, and excretions.

Gowning

- Wear a gown (a clean nonsterile gown is adequate) to protect skin and prevent soiling your clothes during procedures and patient-care activities that are likely to generate splashes or sprays of blood, body fluids, secretions, and excretions or otherwise soil clothing.

Appropriate Device Handling

- Handle used patient-care equipment soiled with blood, body fluids, secretions, and excretions in a manner that prevents exposure to skin and mucous membranes, contamination of clothing, and transfer of microorganisms to other patients and environments.
- Ensure that reusable equipment is not used to care for another patient until it has been appropriately cleaned and reprocessed and that single-use items are properly discarded.

Appropriate Handling of Laundry

- Handle, transport, and process used linen soiled with blood, body fluids, secretions, and excretions in a manner that prevents exposure to skin and mucous membranes, contamination of clothing, and transfer of microorganisms to other patients and environments.

TABLE 40.9	Overview of Quinupristin/Dalfopristi		
Drug (Trade) Name	**Selected Indications**	**Route and Dosage Range**	**Pharmacokinetics**
P quinupristin/dalfopristin (Synercid)	Life-threatening vancomycin-resistant *Enterococcus.faecium* bacteremia Infective endocarditis Complicated skin Infections	Adult IV; 7.5 mg/kg every 8 h 7.5 mg/kg every 8 h for a minimum of 8 wk 7.5 mg/kg every 12 h	*Onset:* immediate *Duration:* unknown $t_{\frac{1}{2}}$: 3 h quinupristin 1 h dalfopristin

- Explain that linezolid may interact with many types of prescription medications. Patients should contact their prescriber before taking any other medications, even those prescribed by another health care professional.
- Teach patients the signs and symptoms of thrombocytopenia and pseudomembranous colitis. Advise patients to contact their prescriber immediately if any symptoms occur.

Ongoing Assessment and Evaluation

Monitor for efficacy of treatment and the resolution of the presenting infection. Monitor for signs and symptoms of thrombocytopenia and pseudomembranous colitis and advise the prescriber if any occur. Monitor the patient's blood pressure and intake of foods or beverages containing tyramine, caffeine, or alcohol. Coordinate serial CBC and liver enzyme tests if therapy lasts more than 14 days.

When treatment ends, the initial infection should be resolved. The patient should be adequately nourished and hydrated, and any adverse drug effects should be resolved.

© STREPTOGRAMINS

Streptogramins are the newest class of antibiotics, specifically designed to eradicate "superbugs" resistant to other antibiotics. Quinupristin and dalfopristin are the only streptogramins

---

MEMORY CHIP ❗

P Linezolid

- Used for infections caused by vancomycin-resistant Enterococcus faecium or E. faecalis (VRE), methicillin-resistant Staphylococcus aureus (MRSA), and penicillin-susceptible Streptococcus pneumoniae.
- Major contraindication: hypersensitivity
- Most common adverse effects: nausea, vomiting, headache, and diarrhea.
- Most serious adverse effects: thrombocytopenia and pseudo-membranous colitis.
- Maximizing therapeutic effects: Administer at evenly spaced intervals.
- Minimizing adverse effects: Monitor the patient's intake of foods and beverages containing tyramine, caffeine, or alcohol.
- Most important patient education: Teach the patient dietary restrictions and the importance of not taking any medications, including OTC medications, without the health care provider's approval.

---

approved for use in the United States by the FDA; they are marketed as the combination drug quinupristin/ dalfopristin (Synercid) (Table 40.9).

Nursing Management of the Patient Receiving **P** Quinupristin/Dalfopristin

Core Drug Knowledge

Pharmacotherapeutics

Quinupristin/dalfopristin is indicated for the treatment of serious or life-threatening infections associated with VRE bacteremia, infective endocarditis, and for complicated skin and skin-structure infections. It is also used off label to treat MRSA and in the management of peritonitis in patients receiving peritoneal dialysis in certain circumstances.

Pharmacokinetics

Quinupristin/dalfopristin is administered by the IV route only. Both drugs are converted to several active major metabolites and are excreted primarily through bile.

Pharmacodynamics

Quinupristin/dalfopristin inhibits bacterial protein synthesis by irreversibly blocking ribosome functioning. When used as single agents, these drugs are bacteriostatic. When used in combination, quinupristin/dalfopristin has up to 16 times the activity of each agent alone and is bacteriocidal against most organisms.

Contraindications and Precautions

The only contraindication to use of quinupristin/dalfopristin is hypersensitivity. Because quinupristin/dalfopristin received accelerated FDA approval based on the drug's ability to clear VRE from the bloodstream, there is a black box warning that there are no clinical studies to confirm efficacy of the drug.

Adverse Effects

Serious adverse effects include pseudomembranous colitis, superinfection, and angioedema. Common adverse effects include injection site reaction, injection site pain, nausea, vomiting, diarrhea, thrombophlebitis, arthralgias and myalgias, rash, pruritus, and hyperbilirubinemia.

Drug Interactions

Quinupristin/dalfopristin is a potent inhibitor of CYP3A4, a cytochrome of P-450. Serum concentrations of drugs metabolized through this pathway may be increased. Table 40.10

TABLE 40.10	Agents That Interact with P Quinupristin/Dalfopristin	
Interactants	**Effect and Significance**	**Nursing Management**
P-450 3A4 drugs	Quinupristin/dalfopristin inhibits cytochrome P-450 3A4 and will decrease the elimination of drugs metabolized by this pathway. This results in an increased risk for toxicity and adverse effects.	Avoid these drugs if possible. Monitor for toxicity if coadministration is unavoidable.
Calcium Channel Blockers (CCBs)	Quinupristin/dalfopristin may decrease the metabolism of CCBs	Monitor BP—may increase if quinupristin/dalfopristin is initiated/dose increased, or decreased if quinupristin/dalfopristin is discontinued/dose decreased.
Cyclosporine	Quinupristin/dalfopristin may decrease the metabolism of cyclosporine	Monitor for signs of toxicity if quinupristin/dalfopristin is started; monitor for decreased efficacy of cyclosporine if quinupristin/dalfopristin is discontinued.

presents drugs metabolized through this pathway, which may therefore interact with quinupristin/dalfopristin.

Assessment of Relevant Core Patient Variables

Health Status

Elicit a complete medical history to evaluate for potential contraindications or precautions to the administration of quinupristin/dalfopristin. Be especially alert for a history of liver dysfunction. Evaluate the patient's current medications for drugs that are metabolized through the CYP3A4 enzyme system. Be sure to communicate any positive findings to the prescriber before administering this drug.

Coordinate baseline liver function and bilirubin tests on blood drawn before administration of quinupristin/ dalfopristin. Coordinate liver function and bilirubin tests twice weekly for the first week of therapy and once weekly thereafter.

Life Span and Gender

Evaluate the patient for pregnancy and lactation. Quinupristin/dalfopristin is an FDA pregnancy category B drug. It is unknown whether quinupristin/dalfopristin is secreted in breast milk. Consider the ratio of benefits to potential risks for the pediatric patient. Quinupristin/dalfopristin has not been approved for use in children; however, it has been administered to children in emergency situations.

Environment

Be aware of the environment in which the drug will be administered. Quinupristin/dalfopristin should be administered in an acute hospital setting. Review the policy of the parent institution and be sure that approval by the Infectious Disease Committee is documented if needed.

Nursing Diagnoses and Outcomes

• Pain related to IV administration
Desired outcome: The patient will inform you immediately should pain at the injection site occur.

• Diarrhea related to potential pseudomembranous colitis
Desired outcome: The patient will remain well hydrated throughout therapy and report any diarrhea immediately.
• Risk for Injury related to potential superinfection or hepatotoxicity
Desired outcome: The patient will remain free of injury throughout therapy.
• Risk for Impaired Skin Integrity related to rash or pruritus.
Desired outcome: The patient will report itching or rash immediately to minimize potential for infection.

Planning and Intervention

Maximizing Therapeutic Effects

Quinupristin/dalfopristin should not be administered with any other medications through a Y-site infusion unless compatibility with both the drug and diluent is established. Flush the line before and after administration with 5% dextrose and water (D_5W) to minimize venous irritation. *DO NOT FLUSH* the IV line with saline or heparin after administering quinupristin/dalfopristin because this procedure is not compatible with these solutions.

Minimizing Adverse Effects

Because injection site problems are very common with the administration of quinupristin/dalfopristin, administer these drugs in a peripherally inserted central catheter (PICC) or central line whenever possible. If administering them peripherally, dilute them in 250 mL of D_5W and infuse over 1 hour.

Providing Patient and Family Education

Because quinupristin/dalfopristin is used for serious life-threatening infections, the patient may not be able to comprehend patient teaching at the onset of therapy. When appropriate, teaching should include the following:
• Encourage patients to report any pain during infusion.
• Teach patients the potential adverse effects associated with quinupristin/dalfopristin such as arthralgias and myalgias, rash, and pruritus.

- Advise patients to report cough, congestion, rash, or feeling warm because these may indicate a superinfection.
- Advise patients to report any diarrhea immediately to avert pseudomembranous colitis, if possible.

Ongoing Assessment and Evaluation

During infusion, monitor the IV site for signs of infiltration, edema, or phlebitis. Question the patient regarding pain at the injection site. During therapy, monitor for signs and symptoms of hyperbilirubinemia. Monitor for diarrhea. Pseudomembranous colitis may develop from a toxin produced by *C. difficile*. Therefore, this diagnosis should be considered in any patient who complains of diarrhea after administration of quinupristin/dalfopristin.

At the end of therapy, the initial infection should be resolved. The patient will be adequately nourished and hydrated and will have normal liver function and bilirubin test results, and any adverse effects will be resolved.

Ⓒ TETRACYCLINES

The tetracyclines were developed as semisynthetic antibiotics based on the structure of a common soil mold. They are broad-spectrum antibiotics that affect both gram-positive and gram-negative bacteria. The first syllables of their name derive from the four-ring structure common to all of these drugs. Over the years, major resistance has developed to tetracyclines, and less toxic, more effective drugs have been discovered. Still, tetracyclines are effective against certain organisms for which they remain the drug of choice. Tetracyclines include tetracycline, demeclocycline, doxycycline, and minocycline. Table 40.11 provides a summary of tetracycline antibiotics. The prototype for the tetracycline class is tetracycline

---

MEMORY CHIP

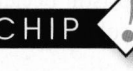 Quinupristin/Dalfopristin

- Used for vancomycin-resistant Enterococcus faecium bacteremia and for complicated skin and skin-structure infections due to *Staphylococcus aureus*
- Major contraindication: hypersensitivity
- Most common adverse effects: injection site pain, swelling, or phlebitis
- Most serious adverse effect: hepatotoxicity
- Maximizing therapeutic effects: Do not use saline or heparin to flush the solution because they are not compatible with this drug.
- Minimizing adverse effects: Administer through PICC or central line whenever possible.
- Most important patient education: Teach the patient about the potential for injection-site adverse effects and about the importance of notifying the nurse if injection site pain occurs.
- **Black box warning: FDA accelerated approval, no clinical studies to ensure efficacy**

Nursing Management of the Patient Receiving Ⓟ Tetracycline

Core Drug Knowledge

Pharmacotherapeutics

Oral tetracycline (Sumycin) is FDA approved for many types of infection, however, it has acquired substantial resistance patterns so it not used for all of its indications. It is used for infections caused by *Borrellia burgdorferi, Rickettsia* species, *Mycoplasma pneumoniae,* and *Chlamydia trachomatis*. It is also used to treat brucellosis, cholera, anthrax, Lyme disease, and *H. pylori* infection.

Pharmacokinetics

Tetracycline is administered orally because it is no longer available for parenteral administration. In the fasting state, tetracycline is about 75% to 77% absorbed. Absorption takes place mainly in the stomach and upper intestine. As the dosage is increased, the percentage absorbed decreases. Absorption is decreased in the presence of food, iron preparations, and antacids containing calcium, magnesium, and aluminum salts.

Tetracycline is widely distributed into body fluids, including CSF. Tetracycline tends to concentrate in bone, liver, tumors, spleen, and teeth. It crosses the placenta and is distributed in breast milk. Tetracycline is about 65% bound to plasma protein and does not appear to undergo hepatic metabolism; however, it undergoes enterohepatic circulation and is excreted in the feces by way of the bile. The primary excretion route is the kidney. About 60% of a dose is excreted unchanged from both routes. The serum half-life of tetracycline is between 6 and 12 hours in adults with normal renal function but is greatly increased in patients with severely impaired renal function.

Pharmacodynamics

The tetracyclines are bacteriostatic; they inhibit or retard the growth of bacteria but do not kill them. They retard bacterial growth by inhibiting protein synthesis in sensitive bacteria and by preventing cell division and replication. Like other antibiotics, their effect on the body is indirect.

Contraindications and Precautions

Tetracycline is contraindicated in patients with a known allergy to tetracyclines or to tartrazine (specific oral preparations contain tartrazine) and during pregnancy and lactation. Tetracycline should be used with caution in children younger than 8 years and in patients with hepatic and renal dysfunction.

Adverse Effects

The common adverse effects of tetracycline therapy involve the GI tract and the CNS; they include nausea, vomiting, diarrhea, abdominal or epigastric discomfort, headache, dizziness, and photosensitivity. Rare but serious adverse effects include anaphylaxis, angioedema, blood dyscrasias, damage to the teeth (in children < 8 years), and hepatotoxicity or nephrotoxicity. Like other broad-spectrum antibiotics,

TABLE 40.11 **Summary of Selected ⓒ Tetracycline Antibiotics**

Drug (Trade) Name	Selected Indications	Route and Dosage Range	Pharmacokinetics
P tetracycline (Sumycin; Bristacycline)	Brucellosis Syphilis Uncomplicated gonorrhea Gonococcal urethritis Uncomplicated chlamydial infections Severe acne	Adult PO: 500 mg 4x d 30–40 g in divided doses over 10–15 d 1.5 g initially followed by 500 mg every 6 h to a total of 9 g 1.5 g initially followed by 500 mg every 4–6 h for 4–6 d 500 mg 4x d for at least 7 d 125–500 mg/d	*Onset:* PO, varies *Duration:* Varies $t_{1/2}$: 6–12 h
demeclocycline (Declomycin)	Same as tetracycline	*Adult:* PO, 600 mg in four doses of 150 mg each *Child >8 y:* PO, 6–12 mg/kg in two to four doses	*Onset:* Varies *Duration:* 18–20 h $t_{1/2}$: 12–16 h
doxycycline (Vibramycin)	Same as above and for anti-diuretic hormone-secreting tumors, bacterial enteritis and Lyme disease	*Adult:* PO, 200 mg initially; maintenance, 100 mg/d; IV, 200 mg/d initially, then 100–200 mg depending on infection *Child 8 y:* PO, 4.4 mg/kg divided in two doses initially; maintenance, 2.2 mg/kg in one or two doses per day; IV, 4.4 mg/kg on first day in one or two infusions depending on infection	*Onset:* PO, varies; IV rapid *Duration:* 24–36 h $t_{1/2}$: 15–25 h
doxycycline (Oracea)	Rosacea	*Adult PO:* 40 mg daily	
minocycline (Minocin)	Same as tetracycline and Neisseria meningitidis	*Adult:* PO, 200 mg initially followed by 100 mg q12h; IV, 200 mg followed by 100 mg q12 h not to exceed 400 mg/d *Child >8 y:* PO, 4 mg/kg initially, followed with 2 mg/kg q12h; IV, 4 mg/kg followed by 2 mg/kg q12 h	*Onset:* PO, varies; IV, rapid *Duration:* 24–36 h $t_{1/2}$: 11–18 h
tigecycline (Tygacil)	Complicated skin and skin structure infections Complicated intra-abdominal nfections	*Adult and Child >18 y:* IV, 100 mg initially followed by 50 mg every 12 h	*Onset:* Immediate *Duration:* Unknown $t_{1/2}$: 42.4 h

tetracycline has a high potential to cause superinfections, such as candidiasis.

Drug Interactions

The effectiveness of penicillin G decreases if it is taken concurrently with tetracyclines. If this combination is used, the dosage of the penicillin will have to be increased. Oral contraceptives may be less effective if taken with tetracycline. Patients taking oral contraceptives should be advised to use an additional form of birth control while receiving tetracycline. Tetracycline forms an insoluble chelate with aluminum, bismuth, calcium, iron, magnesium, and zinc salts, which are frequently an ingredient in antacids. This chelate decreases absorption of either tetracycline or the salt. For more information on drug interactions, see Table 40.12.

Assessment of Relevant Core Patient Variables

Health Status

Follow the same guidelines for evaluating health status as those for a patient receiving penicillin. Assess for known allergies to any drug with a name ending in the suffix "cycline." Additionally, closely evaluate the renal and hepatic status of

patients prescribed tetracycline. Anuric patients should not receive tetracycline, and the dosage should be decreased in patients with renal insufficiency. If renal impairment exists, even usual doses may lead to excessive systemic accumulation of tetracycline, resulting in liver or kidney toxicity.

Life Span and Gender

Evaluate women for potential pregnancy because tetracycline is an FDA pregnancy category D drug. Because the tetracyclines bind to calcium in developing teeth and bones, women in the second and third trimesters of pregnancy should not take this drug. In infants born to mothers who take tetracyclines during pregnancy, mottled and discolored deciduous teeth may develop. To prevent damage to the developing permanent teeth, tetracycline should not be given to children younger than 8 years.

Lifestyle, Diet, and Habits

Because many OTC drugs contain mineral salts that may decrease the absorption of tetracycline, obtain an OTC drug history from the patient or an appropriate caregiver. Explore the dietary habits of the patient, because tetracycline is not absorbed effectively when taken with food or dairy products.

TABLE 40.12 Agents That Interact with P Tetracycline

Interactants	Effect and Significance	Nursing Management

Antacids
  aluminum salts
  bismuth salts
  calcium salts
  iron salts
  magnesium salts
  zinc salts
	Tetracycline forms an insoluble chelate with antacids, decreasing absorption and serum levels of either or both.	Avoid simultaneous administration.
		Separate administration by 3–4 h.

digoxin	In some patients, digoxin is metabolized by bacteria in the GI tract. Tetracycline may reverse the process by altering GI flora, allowing more digoxin to be absorbed and increasing digoxin levels.	Monitor digoxin levels. Monitor pulse rate. Monitor patient for signs of digoxin toxicity.
Food	Foods such as milk and dairy products contain calcium, which forms poorly absorbed chelates with tetracyclines.	Administer tetracycline at least 1 h before or 2 h after meals.
insulin	Tetracycline may increase extrapancreatic response to insulin, resulting in hypoglycemia.	Monitor blood glucose frequently. Monitor for signs of hypoglycemia such as hunger, dizziness, shakiness, sweating, or confusion.
lithium	Increased serum concentration of lithium resulting in increased risk for lithium toxicity.	Monitor for drowsiness, slurred speech, tremor, and thirst. Contact the prescriber immediately should symptoms occur.
methotrexate	Increased serum concentration of methotrexate resulting in increased risk for adverse effects and toxicity	Monitor CBC. Monitor for signs and symptoms of bone marrow suppression. Contact the prescriber immediately should symptoms occur.
methoxyflurane	Tetracycline may induce biotransformation and impairment of renal excretion of toxic metabolites of methoxyflurane, resulting in an increased risk of nephrotoxicity.	Avoid this combination.
Oral contraceptives	Tetracyclines may suppress intestinal flora, which provides an enzyme essential for enterohepatic recirculation for certain oral contraceptives. This may result in a decreased contraceptive plasma level.	Advise patients taking oral contraceptives to use an additional method of birth control while taking tetracyclines.
Penicillins	The bacteriostatic action of tetracyclines may impair the bactericidal activity of penicillins.	Avoid combination therapy.
Retinoids	Increased risk of pseudotumor cerebri (benign intracranial hypertension) due to additive or synergistic effect	Monitor for headache, nausea, vomiting, and visual disturbances. Notify the prescriber immediately should symptoms occur.
theophylline	There is an increased risk for adverse effects to theophyllines.	Monitor theophylline level. Monitor for theophylline toxicity.
Urinary alkalinizers	This combination may alter tubular reabsorption of tetracycline, resulting in a decreased absorption of tetracycline.	Separate administration of these drugs by 3–4 h. Monitor for efficacy of tetracycline therapy. Tetracycline dosage may need to be increased.
warfarin	Elimination of vitamin K–producing gut bacteria by tetracycline may increase the activity of warfarin.	Monitor PT and INR frequently. Monitor for bruising or bleeding.

Environment

Assess for the patient's potential to be outdoors while taking tetracycline. Because this drug causes photosensitivity, teach the patient to avoid direct sunlight, and if going outdoors is unavoidable, encourage the patient to wear appropriate cover-up clothing, hat, and sunglasses, plus a sunscreen that has a sun protection factor (SPF) of at least 30.

Nursing Diagnoses and Outcomes

• Risk for Injury related to potential superinfection or allergic drug reaction
Desired outcome: The patient will experience no new infection and no preventable allergic reaction related to tetracycline.
• Diarrhea related to drug-induced GI effects

Desired outcome: *The patient will report any incidence of diarrhea and follow the prescriber's recommendation.*
- Imbalanced Nutrition: Less than Body Requirements, related to adverse GI effects of nausea, vomiting, diarrhea, and altered taste
  Desired outcome: *The patient will maintain dietary intake to provide adequate nutrition.*
- Risk for Impaired Skin Integrity related to drug-induced photosensitivity
  Desired outcome: *The patient will dress appropriately and take adequate precautionary measures while outdoors to avoid sunburn.*

Planning and Intervention

Maximizing Therapeutic Effects

To judge the efficacy of ongoing treatment, evaluate results of initial culture and sensitivity tests performed on samples from the infection site. Make sure that the patient receives tetracycline as prescribed, divided around the clock to increase effectiveness. To maximize absorption, oral preparations should be administered on an empty stomach either 1 hour before or 2 hours after any meals or other drugs. In addition, remind the patient to avoid antacids within 3 hours of tetracycline administration. It is optimal to continue drug therapy for at least 7 to 10 days.

Minimizing Adverse Effects

Provide small, frequent meals; mouth care; and ice chips or sugarless candy to suck on if stomatitis and sore mouth are problems. Monitor the patient to ensure that adequate fluids are given to replace fluid lost with diarrhea. In addition, remind patients of the potential for photosensitivity and the need to wear protective clothing and a sunscreen with a minimum 15 SPF.

Caution patients about taking outdated tetracycline. The shelf life of tetracycline is limited, and ingestion of outdated tetracycline has been associated with the development of nausea, vomiting, and renal failure. These reactions are thought to be a result of the effects of degradation products.

Providing Patient and Family Education

- Explain that tetracycline is one drug in a class of drugs. It is important that patients understand that they should not take this drug if they have ever had a reaction to a drug with a name that ends with "cycline."
- Advise women of childbearing age that tetracycline should not be taken during pregnancy or breast-feeding.
- Explain that tetracycline is prescribed for a particular infection and should not be used to self-medicate or treat any other infection.
- Emphasize that tetracycline should not be given to any other person, especially a child, and that it must be kept out of the reach of children.
- Advise patients to complete the full course of drug therapy, even if they feel better, and to avoid taking any outdated tetracycline because it may cause liver damage.

- Advise patients to take tetracycline on an empty stomach, with water and not dairy products.
- Advise patients to take OTC medications, such as antacids, that contain mineral salts at least 3 hours after administration of tetracycline.
- Teach patients to take forgotten doses as soon as they remember, but not if it is almost time for the next dose.
- Instruct patients to call the prescriber if the symptoms do not improve in 3 days.
- Explain the potential adverse effects of tetracycline and the potential remedies for these discomforts. Measures to relieve GI upset include taking small, frequent meals if patients experience GI distress and increasing fluid intake for diarrhea. Patients with a sore mouth or throat should be advised to suck on ice chips or hard candy.
- Teach patients signs and symptoms of superinfection, such as discoloration of the tongue, fatigue, easy bruising, or vaginal discharge. Caution patients about the potential for photosensitivity and the importance of staying out of direct sunlight and wearing sunscreen.
- Advise women who use oral contraceptives to use a backup method of contraception while taking tetracycline.

Ongoing Assessment and Evaluation

Monitor the site of infection and compare it with presenting signs and symptoms throughout the course of drug therapy. Failure to resolve these signs and symptoms may indicate a treatment failure. Also, monitor the patient to ensure that the full course of therapy is completed.

Monitor renal status to detect and prevent hepatotoxicity and to observe for any signs of superinfection. Notify the provider immediately if they occur.

At the end of therapy, the patient should be free of the initial infection. The patient will have maintained adequate nutrition and hydration, and any adverse effects will be resolved.

MEMORY CHIP

P Tetracycline

- Used for Rickettsia, Mycoplasma pneumoniae, chlamydia, and acne
- Major contraindications: pregnancy, breast-feeding, and in children younger than 8 years of age
- Most common adverse effects: discoloration of teeth, nausea, vomiting, and photosensitivity
- Most serious adverse effect: azotemia
- Maximizing therapeutic effects: Administer at evenly spaced intervals on an empty stomach.
- Minimizing adverse effects: Give frequent small meals and increase mouth care when GI distress is present.
- Most important patient education: Teach the patient to complete the entire course of medication, despite feeling better. Teach the patient to keep medication out of the reach of children.

Drugs Closely Related to [P] Tetracycline

Demeclocycline, doxycycline, and minocycline are similar to tetracycline. Contraindications, other adverse effects, drug interactions, and patient management are comparable to those for tetracycline.

Demeclocycline

Demeclocycline (Declomycin) has the same FDA indications as tetracycline. In addition, it is used for treating Syndrome of Inappropriate Antidiuretic Hormone secretion (SIADH) and fluid imbalances. Demeclocycline inhibits ADH-induced water reabsorption in the kidneys, resulting in diuresis.

Demeclocycline has similar contraindications, precautions, drug interactions, and adverse effects as tetracycline. There is an increased risk of photosensitivity with demeclocycline. It is a pregnancy category D drug.

Doxycycline

Doxycycline (Vibramycin) is a new type of tetracycline. It has the same pharmacotherapeutics as tetracycline and is used frequently for nongonococcal urethritis or cervicitis, as well as prophylaxis against STDs after sexual aggression. Taken orally, it is better absorbed than tetracycline, even in the presence of food and dairy products. It is excreted mainly through feces, unlike the other tetracyclines. Because of its excretion pattern, doxycycline is useful in patients with compromised renal function. Its half-life is longer than that of tetracycline, allowing for twice-daily dosing.

A new formulation of doxycycline (Oracea) is specifically used to manage inflammatory lesions of rosacea, not infections generally treated with doxycycline. Oracea contains 30 mg of immediate-release doxycycline and 10 mg of delayed-release doxycycline that targets the underlying inflammatory pathophysiology of rosacea, without exerting antimicrobial effects.

Minocycline

Minocycline (Minocin, Dynacin, Solodyn) is another fairly new tetracycline. Like doxycycline, minocycline has a long half-life. In addition to sharing the utility of other tetracyclines, minocycline is also used to treat meningococcal carrier states of *Neisseria meningitidis*. Minocycline is also useful in decreasing the symptoms of rheumatoid arthritis.

Solodyn is an extended-release formulation of minocycline specifically used for acne.

Minocycline may cause vestibular toxicity with symptoms of dizziness, light-headedness, or vertigo. Patients should be cautioned to assess for these symptoms before driving a motor vehicle or performing hazardous tasks.

Drugs Significantly Different From [P] Tetracycline

Tigecycline (Tygacil) is the first drug in a new class of drugs called glycylcycline antibiotics. They are structurally similar to tetracyclines but are designed to circumvent key bacterial resistance mechanisms. Tigecycline is indicated for the management of complicated skin and skin structure infections, complicated intra-abdominal infections, and community-acquired pneumonia. Its spectrum of activity is broad and includes resistant organisms such as methicillin-resistant *Staphylococcus aureus* (MRSA), vancomycin-resistant enterococcus (VRE), extended-spectrum beta-lactamase (ESBL) producing bacteria, like *E. coli* and *Klebsiella pneumoniae*, and *Acinetobacter* species.

Because tigecycline is structurally similar to tetracycline, it may induce many of the same adverse effects. The most common adverse effects are nausea and vomiting. Tigecycline is contraindicated during pregnancy because it may cause fetal harm. It is given cautiously to patients with a known sensitivity to tetracyclines, patients less than 8 years of age, those with intestinal perforation, and in patients taking warfarin. The PT and international normalized ratio (INR) of patients taking warfarin should be monitored. To maintain the effectiveness of tigecycline, it should be used only to treat infections caused by susceptible bacteria.

[C] MISCELLANEOUS ANTIBIOTICS THAT AFFECT PROTEIN SYNTHESIS

Miscellaneous antibiotics include chloramphenicol and spectinomycin. Chloramphenicol is the prototypical miscellaneous antibiotic (Table 40.13). In 1947, chloramphenicol was isolated from *Streptomyces venezuelae* and used to treat large outbreaks of typhus. It is now available synthetically as chloramphenicolor chloramphenicol succinate.

TABLE 40.13	Overview of [C] Chloramphenicol		
Drug (Trade) Name	**Selected Indications**	**Route and Dosage Range**	**Pharmacokinetics**
[P] chloramphenicol	Serious infections caused by *Salmonella*, *Haemophilus influenzae*, rickettsiae, lymphogranuloma	*Adult IV:* 50–100 mg/kg/d in divided doses every 6 h *Child IV:* 50–75 mg/kg/d in divided doses every 6 h *Ophthalmic Adult and Child:* As prescribed	*Onset:* 20–30 min *Duration:* 48–72 h t ½: 1.5–4 h

Nursing Management of the Patient Receiving P Chloramphenicol

Core Drug Knowledge

Pharmacotherapeutics

Chloramphenicol is a true broad-spectrum antibiotic. It is active against a wide range of gram-positive and gram-negative bacteria, many anaerobic bacteria, *Bacteroides* species, and *Salmonella* species. However, it is inactive against fungi.

Chloramphenicol is relatively toxic and thus has a Black Box warning for use only in serious infections against which other antibiotics have been ineffective or in patients who cannot take safer drugs because of resistance or allergies. It is the drug of choice for treating meningitis caused by *Streptococcus pneumoniae, Neisseria meningitidis,* or *Haemophilus influenzae.* It is also used in treating brain abscesses, rickettsial infections, and acute typhoid fever.

Pharmacokinetics

Chloramphenicol base is administered orally; chloramphenicol succinate is administered intravenously. For chloramphenicol succinate to be active, it must be hydrolyzed to free chloramphenicol. Free chloramphenicol is rapidly absorbed from the GI tract. Peak action occurs within 1 to 3 hours. Peak concentrations rise with repeated administration. The goal is to keep plasma concentrations below 25 mcg/mL to decrease the risk for adverse hematologic effects. Plasma concentration levels of chloramphenicol are increased in patients with hepatic and renal dysfunction and in premature or newborn infants with immature systems.

Chloramphenicol is widely distributed throughout most body tissues and fluids, with highest concentrations in the liver and kidneys. Chloramphenicol can reach substantial CSF concentrations, especially in patients with inflamed meninges.

Following oral administration, between 5% and 15% of chloramphenicol is excreted unchanged in the urine by glomerular filtration, and the remainder is excreted by tubular secretion, mostly as inactive metabolites. Small amounts are excreted unchanged in the bile and feces.

Pharmacodynamics

Chloramphenicol is usually bacteriostatic but may be bactericidal in high concentrations or against more susceptible organisms, such as *H. influenzae* and *S. pneumoniae.* It works by inhibiting the protein synthesis of bacterial cells. Chloramphenicol also inhibits mitochondrial protein synthesis in both bacterial and human cells. In humans, the protein synthesis of rapidly proliferating cells, such as erythrocytes, may be affected. This effect may explain the mechanism of reversible depression of bone marrow function associated with chloramphenicol therapy.

Contraindications and Precautions

Chloramphenicol should not be given to patients who have had known toxic reactions to the drug because some fatal reactions have occurred. It should not be used systemically for minor infections because of the potential for serious toxicity. Chloramphenicol is also contraindicated in breast-feeding women because it can suppress bone marrow function in breast-feeding infants. The drug should be used with caution in patients with depressed bone marrow function and in those who have received cytotoxic drug therapy or radiation therapy. It can cause dose-related depression of bone marrow function and an idiosyncratic aplastic anemia.

Chloramphenicol should be given with extreme caution to pregnant women, infants, and children. Other patients at high risk during chloramphenicol therapy include patients with hepatic disease, renal impairment, glucose-6-phosphate dehydrogenase (G6PD) deficiency, and acute intermittent porphyria.

Adverse Effects

A serious and potentially life-threatening adverse effect of chloramphenicol is "gray baby" syndrome. It is most common in premature infants or newborns receiving chloramphenicol, whose hepatic systems have difficulty conjugating or excreting chloramphenicol. This syndrome is characterized by failure to feed, abdominal distention, possible vomiting, progressive blue-gray skin, and vasomotor collapse. The infant may also have irregular breathing.

Other serious and potentially life-threatening adverse effects of chloramphenicol are blood dyscrasias, which are a Black Box warning. These include aplastic anemia, hypoplastic anemia, thrombocytopenia, pancytopenia, and granulocytopenia. These adverse effects have all occurred following short-term or long-term therapy as a result of depressed bone marrow function.

Bone marrow toxicity may or may not be dose related. Irreversible depression of bone marrow function, a type of toxicity unrelated to dose, can result in aplastic anemia, which has a high mortality rate. This type of aplasia or hypoplasia can develop months after the drug has been discontinued or from a single dose. Reversible depression of bone marrow function usually is dose related and is characterized by anemia, reticulocytopenia, leukopenia, or thrombocytopenia.

Other adverse effects, which may be dose related, are optic neuritis, which can cause blindness, and peripheral neuritis. Patients with either of these effects should discontinue the drug immediately.

Other neurotoxic effects include headache, mild depression, confusion, and delirium, but these reactions are usually mild. Patients should be monitored for other signs of peripheral neuropathy.

GI effects are usually minimal during therapy with chloramphenicol but can include nausea, vomiting, diarrhea, dysgeusia, glossitis, stomatitis, pruritus ani, or enterocolitis. Adverse GI symptoms should be reported immediately because they can indicate more severe reactions, such as superinfection.

Maculopapular rash and urticaria can occur from either systemic administration or topical application of

TABLE 40.14 **Agents That Interact with P Chloramphenicol**

Interactants	Effect and Significance	Nursing Management
Barbiturates	Coadministration may decrease chloramphenicol serum levels and may decrease barbiturate clearance resulting in increased adverse effects or toxicity.	Monitor for chloramphenicol efficacy. Monitor for signs of barbiturate poisoning. Contact the prescriber if symptoms occur.
cyclosporine	Coadministration may increase cyclosporine serum concentration resulting in increased risk for adverse effects and toxicity	Monitor BUN and creatinine levels. Monitor intake and output.
Hydantoins	Chloramphenicol alters metabolism of hydantoins, resulting in an increased risk for hydantoin toxicity.	Monitor serum concentration of hydantoins. Adjust hydantoin dosage as needed.
Iron salts	Chloramphenicol decreases iron clearance and erythropoiesis due to bone marrow toxicity. This may result in iron overload and anemia.	Monitor CBC. Monitor serum iron levels. Discuss iron dosage adjustment with prescriber as needed.
Oral anticoagulants	Chloramphenicol may interfere with hepatic metabolism of the anti-coagulant and possibly the hypoprothrombinemic effect. This results in an increased risk of bleeding.	Monitor PT and INR closely. Monitor for signs of bleeding. Contact prescriber immediately if symptoms occur. Discuss adjustment of oral anticoagulant dose with the prescriber.
Oral hypoglycemic agents	Chloramphenicol may reduce hepatic clearance of oral hypoglyce-mics, resulting in clinical hypoglycemia.	Monitor blood glucose concentrations. Monitor for signs of hypoglycemia such as hunger dizziness, shakiness, sweating, or confusion.
penicillin	Synergistic effects may develop in the treatment of certain microorganisms, but antagonism may also occur.	Monitor for penicillin efficacy.
rifampin	Coadministration may decrease chloramphenicol serum concentration resulting in subtherapeutic effects	Monitor for chloramphenicol efficacy. Discuss chloramphenicol dose adjustment with the prescriber.
tacrolimus	Chloramphenicol inhibits the metabolism of tacrolimus resulting in an increased risk for adverse effects and toxicity	Monitor BUN and creatinine levels in renal transplant patients carefully. Monitor for fatigue, lethargy, headache, and tremors. Contact the prescriber immediately if symptoms occur.

chloramphenicol. Topical use can also cause pruritus and burning, vesicular dermatitis, or maculopapular rash. Adverse reactions require discontinuing the drug. Transient burning or itching of the eye can occur following ophthalmic application. Repeated or prolonged use of eye or topical preparations should be discouraged.

Drug Interactions

Chloramphenicol interacts with many different types of drugs. Table 40.14 describes potential interactions.

Assessment of Relevant Core Patient Variables

Health Status

Because therapeutic benefits generally do not outweigh the risks for chloramphenicol therapy, assess the culture and sensitivity findings to evaluate the efficacy of chloramphenicol.

Evaluate the patient for risk factors that would increase the potential for severe toxicities. Such factors include recent cytotoxic or radiation therapy, anemia, depressed bone marrow function, hepatic disease, renal impairment, acute intermittent porphyria, or G6PD deficiency. Patients with recent cytotoxic or radiation therapy are at risk for blood dyscrasias. Administering chloramphenicol increases the risk of these dyscrasias. Chloramphenicol therapy may also exacerbate acute intermittent porphyria or G6PD deficiency.

Evaluate the patient for the use of other drugs, such as oral hypoglycemics, oral anticoagulants, or antiepileptic agents, which may interact with chloramphenicol. Other drugs to consider are those with a high risk of hematologic toxicity, hepatic toxicity, or nephrotoxicity because blood, liver, or kidney problems increase the risk of adverse effects with chloramphenicol therapy.

Before initiating therapy, evaluate baseline laboratory test results, including CBC and hepatic and renal function. Communicate abnormal test findings to the prescriber immediately. Perform a baseline neurologic examination because chloramphenicol may induce adverse CNS effects.

Life Span and Gender

Evaluate women for pregnancy. Chloramphenicol is contra-indicated for pregnant women who are near term because it may depress bone marrow function or cause gray baby syndrome in the neonate. Determine whether the patient is breast-feeding. Chloramphenicol is contraindicated for use in nursing mothers. Because it is excreted into breast milk, chloramphenicol may depress bone marrow function in infants.

Assess the developmental status of infants. Premature infants and neonates may develop gray baby syndrome. This syndrome can affect children up to 2 years of age, but infants receiving chloramphenicol within the first 48 hours of life are at highest risk. Chloramphenicol should be discontinued at the first signs of gray baby syndrome because it can be fatal in a matter of a few hours.

Environment

Be aware of the environment in which the drug will be administered. Administration of chloramphenicol must occur in a setting where appropriate serum level and patient monitoring can be undertaken. Evaluate the patient frequently and contact the provider immediately for discontinuation of therapy at the first sign of adverse reactions.

Nursing Diagnoses and Outcomes

- Risk for Injury related to drug-induced adverse effects, such as blood dyscrasias, gray baby syndrome, and CNS effects, including optic or peripheral neuritis, headache, depression, confusion, or delirium
  Desired outcome: Regular and careful monitoring will protect the patient from permanent drug-related adverse effects.
- Risk for Impaired Skin Integrity, rash and pruritus, related to topical drug use
  Desired outcome: The nurse and patient will observe for and report signs of unusual skin reaction and contact the prescriber.

Planning and Intervention

Maximizing Therapeutic Effects

Oral chloramphenicol should be administered on an empty stomach 1 hour before or 2 hours after meals. However, for patients with GI distress, chloramphenicol may be administered with meals.

Minimizing Adverse Effects

Although adverse effects may occur when therapeutic concentrations are within normal limits, they are more likely to occur if they are high. Monitor plasma concentrations at least weekly or more often in patients with hepatic or renal impairment. Peak levels should be in the range of 10 to 20 mcg/mL, whereas trough levels should be 5 to 10 mcg/mL.

Avoid IM injections because they may cause bleeding, bruising, or hematomas as a result of thrombocytopenia resulting from chloramphenicol-induced depression of bone marrow function.

Providing Patient and Family Education

- Explain the importance of completing therapy.
- Point out the potential adverse effects and the need for periodic blood monitoring and daily assessment.
- Teach patients the importance of measuring fluid intake and output accurately.
- Advise patients to report any symptoms to the health care team immediately.

Ongoing Assessment and Evaluation

Serum concentrations and patients' responses to systemic chloramphenicol therapy are unpredictable. For patients receiving systemic therapy, coordinate serial monitoring of chloramphenicol plasma concentrations.

Assess patients receiving chloramphenicol therapy for signs of anemia and depressed bone marrow function; these signs include bleeding, easy bruising, and fatigue. Bone marrow function should be monitored with serial CBCs throughout therapy.

Monitor for signs of hepatic or renal insufficiency. For long-term or high-dose therapy or for patients with a history of hepatic or renal insufficiency, serial hepatic and renal function tests are important. In addition to increasing the risk for toxicities, impaired hepatic function has resulted in adult reactions similar to gray baby syndrome.

Other important assessments are GI and CNS effects. Although GI effects occur infrequently, they may indicate a more serious problem, such as superinfection. In the CNS, monitor for optic or peripheral neuritis, headache, depression, confusion, or delirium.

Because most adverse effects require that therapy be discontinued, assessing the patient frequently and communicating findings to the prescriber are the most important aspects of chloramphenicol therapy.

When treatment ends, the initial infection should be resolved. The patient should be adequately nourished and hydrated, and any adverse drug effects should be resolved.

Drug Significantly Different From P Chloramphenicol

Spectinomycin is related to the aminoglycosides but is somewhat different structurally. Spectinomycin is usually given as a one-time injection, followed by other antibiotic therapy, and is used to treat acute gonorrheal urethritis and prostatitis in men and acute gonorrheal cervicitis and proctitis in women. It is also a prophylactic treatment after known recent exposure to gonorrhea.

Spectinomycin is active against a number of other gram-negative bacteria, although it is inferior to other antibiotics commonly used to treat these organisms. It is contraindicated in patients with a known hypersensitivity to the drug. Soreness at the injection site is the most common adverse effect. Other serious adverse effects are limited because the drug is given only once.

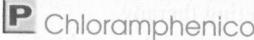

MEMORY CHIP

P Chloramphenicol

- Used for serious gram-positive or gram-negative infections, especially brain abscesses or meningitis
- Major contraindications: hypersensitivity and breastfeeding
- Most common adverse effects: headache, nausea, vomiting, and diarrhea
- Most serious adverse effects: blood dyscrasias, "gray-baby" syndrome
- Maximizing therapeutic effects: Administer oral preparations on an empty stomach.
- Minimizing adverse effects: Monitor peak and trough levels throughout therapy.
- Most important patient education: Teach the patient the signs and symptoms of bone marrow suppression and the importance of contacting the health care provider immediately if any symptoms occur.
- **Black box warning: Serious and fatal blood dyscrasias including aplastic anemia, hypoplastic anemia, thrombocytopenia, and granulocytopenia.**

TOPICAL DRUGS

Mupirocin (Bactroban) and retapamulin (Altabax) are topical antibiotics used to treat impetigo and other minor skin infections due to *Staph aureus* or *Strep pyogenes*. Mupirocin is also approved for nasal decolonization of methicillin-resistant *Staph aureus* (MRSA). Retapamulin is not approved for MRSA nor is it intended to be used inside the nose. Both mupirocin and retapamulin inhibit bacterial growth by disrupting protein synthesis; however, they bind at different sites. Mupirocin is applied three times per day for up to 12 days, and retapamulin is applied two times per day for 5 days. Mupirocin is available as a generic drug, making it less expensive than retapamulin. More severe skin infections require oral antibiotics.

CHAPTER SUMMARY

- Drugs that inhibit protein synthesis may be bacteriocidal or bacteriostatic.
- Gentamicin is the prototype for aminoglycoside agents.
- Gentamicin is used for serious infections caused by gram-negative bacilli.
- Gentamicin use is limited by its potential for adverse effects, especially neurotoxicity, nephrotoxicity, ototoxicity, and neuromuscular blockade which are all Black Box warnings.
- Gentamicin is generally given parenterally but may be given orally to exert a local effect on the GI tract because oral drugs are more poorly absorbed.
- Clindamycin, the lincosamide prototype, is used for infections caused by gram-positive cocci and many gram-negative or gram-positive anaerobes.

- Clindamycin is reserved for treating serious infections that have not responded to less toxic antibiotics.
- Clindamycin therapy is limited by its potential for adverse effects, especially pseudomembranous colitis which is a Black Box warning.
- Macrolides, such as erythromycin, are used to treat an array of infections caused by gram-positive organisms. They are less effective against gram-negative organisms.
- Erythromycin is used for patients with a hypersensitivity to penicillin.
- Erythromycin has a spectrum of activity similar to that of penicillins and cephalosporins.
- Oxazolidinones and streptogramins are the newest classes of antibiotics developed to manage "superbugs" that do not respond to vancomycin.
- The prototype oxazolidinone is linezolid.
- The unique mechanism of action of linezolid may reduce the emergence of resistance.
- Quinupristin/dalfopristin, the prototype streptogramin, is a combination drug that is 16 times more potent than each drug alone.
- The tetracyclines have been used for many types of infections in the past; therefore, resistance to these drugs is now a problem.
- Tetracyclines remain useful in treating infections caused by *Rickettsiae* species, *Mycoplasma pneumoniae*, and *Chlamydia* species. They are also used to treat acne.
- Tigecycline, a glycylcycline antibiotic, is structurally similar to tetracycline but is designed to circumvent key bacterial resistance mechanisms.
- Chloramphenicol is used for serious gram-positive or gram-negative infections that have not responded to less toxic antibiotics.
- Chloramphenicol passes the blood–brain barrier and is useful in treating brain abscesses or meningitis.
- Chloramphenicol therapy is limited by its potential for adverse effects, especially blood dyscrasias which is a Black Box warning.

QUESTIONS FOR STUDY AND REVIEW

1. List disadvantages of tetracycline therapy.
2. Why are aminoglycosides used only in serious infections?
3. What are the most serious adverse effects of chloramphenicol therapy?
4. After a patient receives erythromycin for 10 days for a severe skin infection, the patient develops a vaginal yeast infection. Explain why this infection occurred.
5. A patient who is taking clindamycin at home calls you to report violent, watery, and bloody diarrhea. Explain the probable cause for these symptoms. What advice would you give to this patient?
6. Describe the differences between quinupristin/dalfopristin and linezolid for managing VRE and MRSA.

NEED MORE HELP?

Chapter 40 of the Study Guide to Accompany *Drug Therapy in Nursing,* 4th Edition, contains additional NCLEX-style questions and other learning activities to reinforce your understanding of the concepts presented in this chapter. For additional information or to purchase the study guide, visit thePoint.

REFERENCES

Apicella, M. (2009). Treatment and prevention of meningococcal infection, *Up To Date*. Retrieved from *http://uptodate.com.*

Brown, S. (2008). Benefit-risk assessment of telithromycin in the treatment of community-acquired pneumonia. *Drug Safety,* 31(7):561–575.

Brooks, N. (2009). Prophylactic antibiotic treatment to prevent infective endocarditis: new guidance from the National Institute for Health and Clinical Excellence, *Heart,* 95(9):774–780.

Del Rosso, J. (2009). Oral antibiotic drug interactions of clinical significance to dermatologists. *Dermatologic Clinics,* 27(1):91–94.

Del Rosso, J., & Kim, G. (2009). Optimizing use of oral antibiotics in acne vulgaris. *Dermatologic Clinics,* 27(1):33–42.

Drew, R. H. (2009). Aminoglycosides, *Up To Date.* Retrieved from *http://www.uptodate.com.*

Facts and Comparisons. (2010). *Drug facts and comparisons.* Philadelphia, PA: Lippincott Williams & Wilkins.

Falagas, M., & Vardakas, K. (2008). Benefit-risk assessment of linezolid for serious gram-positive bacterial infections. *Drug Safety,* 31(9):753–768.

File, T. M. (2009). Antibiotic studies for the treatment of community-acquired pneumonia in adults, *Up To Date.* Retrieved from *http://uptodate.com.*

Fowler, V. G., & Sexton, D. J. (2009). Treatment of *S. aureus* bacteremia in adults, *Up To Date.* Retrieved from *http://uptodate.com.*

Furgeson, S. B., & Teitelbaum, I. (2009). New Treatment Options and Protocols for Peritoneal Dialysis-Related Peritonitis. *Contributions to Nephrology,* 163:169–176.

Geller, D. E. (2009). Aerosol Antibiotics in Cystic Fibrosis. *Respiratory Care,* 54(5):658–670.

Gentamicin (Systemic). (2008, December 3). Retrieved June 12, 2009, from CINAHL Plus with Full Text database.

Graziani, A. L. (2009). Azithromycin, clarithromycin, and telithromycin, *Up To Date.* Retrieved from *http://uptodate.com*

Hsieh, P. H., Huang, K. C., & Tai, C. L. (2009). Liquid gentamicin in bone cement spacers: in vivo antibiotic release and systemic safety in two-stage revision of infected hip arthroplasty, *The Journal of Trauma,* 66(3):804–808.

Koda-Kimbal, M. A, Young, L. Y., Kradian, W. A., et al. (2008). *Applied Therapeutics: The Clinical Use of Drugs,* Philadelphia, PA: Lippincott Williams & Wilkins.

Linezolid. (2008, December 3). Retrieved June 13, 2009, from CINAHL Plus with Full Text database.

MacGowan, A. P. (2008). Tigecycline pharmacokinetic/pharmacodynamic update. *The Journal of Antimicrobial Chemotherapy,* 62(suppl 1); i11–i16.

May, D. B. (2009). Tetracyclines, *Up To Date.* Retrieved from *http://uptodate.com.*

Micromedex Healthcare Series. Retrieved from *http://thomsonhc.com.*

Murray, B. E. (2009). Treatment of enterococcal infections, *Up To Date.* Retrieved from *http://www.uptodate.com*

Popovich, K. J., Hota, B. (2008). Treatment and prevention of community-associated methicillin-resistant Staphylococcus aureus skin and soft tissue infections, *Dermatologic Therapy,* 21(3):167–179.

Powell, J. P., & Wenzel, R. P. (2008). Antibiotic options for treating community-acquired MRSA. *Expert Review of Anti-Infective Therapy,* 6(3):299–307.

Rosen, T., Vandergriff, T., & Harting, M. (2009). Antibiotic use in sexually transmissible diseases. *Dermatologic Clinics,* 27(1):49–61.

Shneker, B., Baylin, P., & Nakhla, M. (2009). Linezolid inducing complex partial status epilepticus in a patient with epilepsy. *Neurology,* 72(4):378–379.

Sobel, J. D. (2009). Bacterial Vaginosis, *Up To Date.* Retrieved from *http://uptodate.com.*

Tatro, D. S. (2009). *Drug interaction facts.* Philadelphia, PA: Lippincott Williams & Wilkins.

Vergidis, P. I., & Falagas, M. E. (2008). New antibiotic agents for bloodstream infections. *International Journal of Antimicrobial Agents,* 32(Suppl 1):S60–S65.

Wang, J. L., & Hsueh, P. R. (2009). Therapeutic options for infections due to vancomycin-resistant enterococci. *Expert Opinion on Pharmacotherapy,* 10(5):785–796.

41

Drugs That Are Miscellaneous Antibiotics

Learning Objectives

At the completion of this chapter the student will:

1. Identify core drug knowledge pertaining to miscellaneous antibiotic agents.

2. Identify core patient variables pertaining to miscellaneous antibiotic agents.

3. Relate the interaction of core drug knowledge to core patient variables for miscellaneous antibiotic agents.

4. Generate a nursing plan of care from the interactions between core drug knowledge and core patient variables for miscellaneous antibiotic agents.

5. Describe nursing interventions to maximize therapeutic and minimize adverse effects for miscellaneous antibiotic agents.

6. Determine key points for patient and family education for miscellaneous antibiotic agents.

Key Terms   arthropathy   fluoroquinolones
                cyclic lipopeptides quinolones

Drugs That Are Miscellaneous Antibiotics

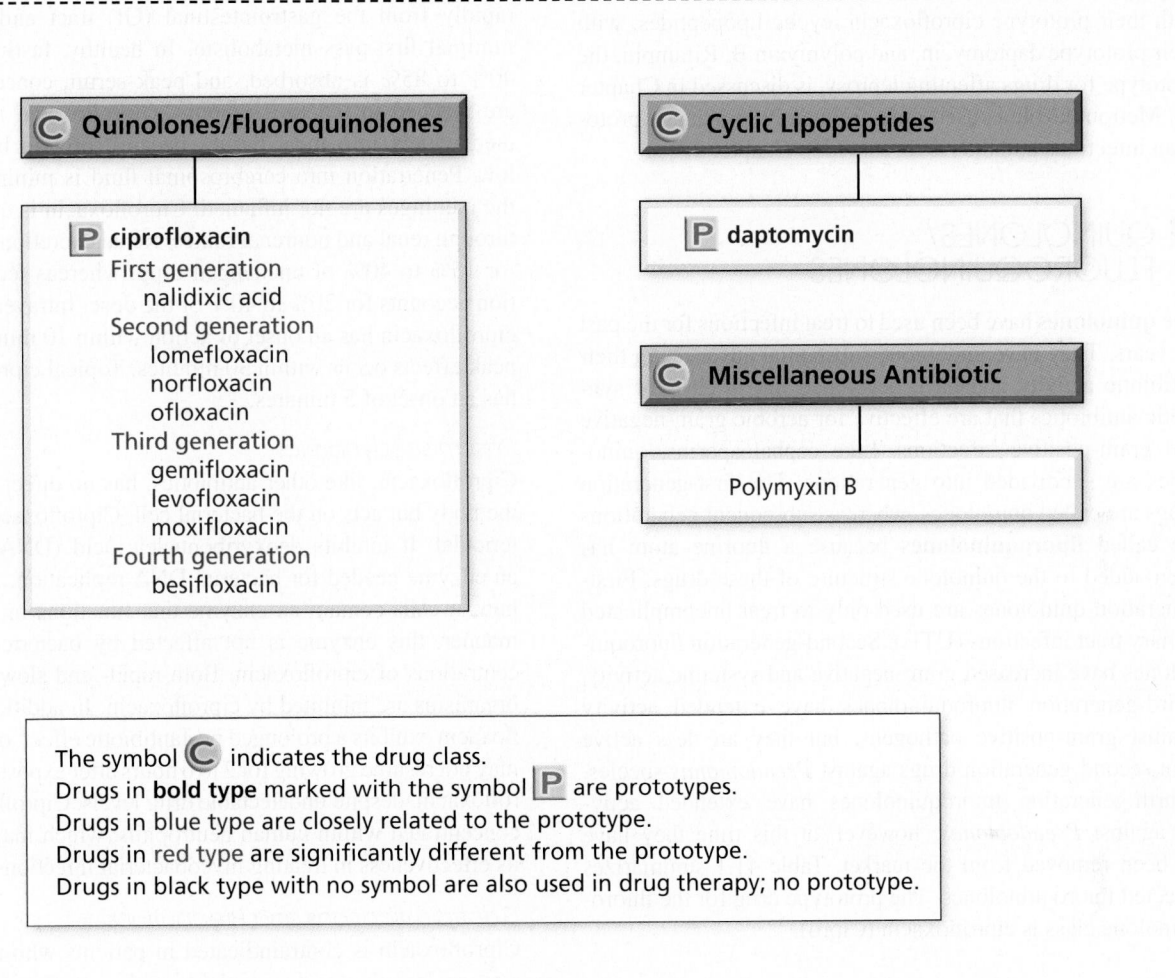

C Quinolones/Fluoroquinolones

P ciprofloxacin
First generation
nalidixic acid
Second generation
lomefloxacin
norfloxacin
ofloxacin
Third generation
gemifloxacin
levofloxacin
moxifloxacin
Fourth generation
besifloxacin

C Cyclic Lipopeptides

P daptomycin

C Miscellaneous Antibiotic

Polymyxin B

The symbol **C** indicates the drug class.
Drugs in **bold type** marked with the symbol **P** are prototypes.
Drugs in blue type are closely related to the prototype.
Drugs in red type are significantly different from the prototype.
Drugs in black type with no symbol are also used in drug therapy; no prototype.

Miscellaneous antibiotics are those that have a mechanism of action other than disrupting the cell wall or protein synthesis of bacteria. These drugs include the fluoroquinolones, cyclic lipopeptides, rifampin, metronidazole, and polymyxin B. This chapter discusses the fluoroquinolones, with their prototype ciprofloxacin; cyclic lipopeptides, with their prototype daptomycin; and polymyxin B. Rifampin, the prototype for drugs affecting leprosy, is discussed in Chapter 43. Metronidazole is used most frequently to manage protozoan infections and thus is discussed in Chapter 47.

QUINOLONES/ FLUOROQUINOLONES

The **quinolones** have been used to treat infections for the past 40 years. They have undergone substantial advances in their antibiotic activity and have developed into a class of synthetic antibiotics that are effective for aerobic gram-negative and gram-positive infections. Like cephalosporins, quinolones are subdivided into generations. The first-generation drugs are called quinolones, whereas subsequent generations are called **fluoroquinolones** because a fluorine atom has been added to the quinolone structure of these drugs. First-generation quinolones are used only to treat uncomplicated urinary tract infections (UTIs). Second-generation fluoroquinolones have increased gram-negative and systemic activity. Third-generation fluoroquinolones have extended activity against gram-positive pathogens, but they are less active than second-generation drugs against *Pseudomonas* species. Fourth-generation fluoroquinolones have extended activity against *Pseudomonas;* however, at this time they have all been removed from the market. Table 41.1 summarizes selected fluoroquinolones. The prototype drug for the fluoroquinolone class is ciprofloxacin (Cipro).

Nursing Management of the Patient Receiving [P] Ciprofloxacin
Core Drug Knowledge
Pharmacotherapeutics
Ciprofloxacin is most active against aerobic gram-negative organisms and group D streptococci.

Ciprofloxacin also has been used extensively to treat serious gram-negative infections; however, resistance has developed in strains of *Pseudomonas aeruginosa* and *Serratia marcescens*. Ciprofloxacin is generally active against aerobic gram-positive organisms, but resistance has been noted in *S. aureus* and *Pneumococcus* species. It is not active against anaerobic organisms.

Ciprofloxacin is useful in treating infections in the urinary tract (Box 41.1) and upper and lower respiratory tract; gonorrhea; infections in bone, skin, subcutaneous tissues, and joints; bacterial conjunctivitis; and otitis externa. Ciprofloxacin is also used in the treatment of and prophylaxis against anthrax and for the treatment of typhoid fever.

Pharmacokinetics
Ciprofloxacin is available in oral, parenteral, and topical formulations. Topical formulations include both otic and ophthalmic preparations. Oral preparations are absorbed rapidly from the gastrointestinal (GI) tract and undergo minimal first-pass metabolism. In healthy, fasting adults, 40% to 85% is absorbed, and peak serum concentrations are reached in 0.5 to 2.3 hours. Ciprofloxacin is distributed widely into most tissues because protein binding is low. Penetration into cerebrospinal fluid is minimal when the meninges are not inflamed. Ciprofloxacin is eliminated through renal and nonrenal routes. Renal excretion accounts for 15% to 40% of unchanged drug, whereas fecal excretion accounts for 20% to 40% of the dose. Intravenous (IV) ciprofloxacin has an onset of action within 10 minutes, and peak effects occur within 30 minutes. Topical ciprofloxacin has an onset of 5 minutes.

Pharmacodynamics
Ciprofloxacin, like other antibiotics, has no direct effect on the body but acts on the bacterial cell. Ciprofloxacin is bactericidal. It inhibits deoxyribonucleic acid (DNA) gyrase, an enzyme needed for bacterial DNA replication. Although human cells contain an enzyme that functions in the same manner, this enzyme is not affected by bactericidal concentrations of ciprofloxacin. Both rapid- and slow-growing organisms are inhibited by ciprofloxacin. In addition, ciprofloxacin exhibits a prolonged postantibiotic effect; organisms may not resume growing for 2 to 6 hours after exposure to ciprofloxacin, despite undetectable drug levels. Ciprofloxacin is concentrated within human neutrophils, which may explain its effectiveness in treating mycobacterial infections.

Contraindications and Precautions
Ciprofloxacin is contraindicated in patients who are pregnant or lactating and in patients with a known allergy to any fluoroquinolone. Oral and parenteral ciprofloxacin is contraindicated for children younger than 18 years, with the exception of complicated UTIs and the treatment of anthrax. Topical ciprofloxacin may be used in children without restriction.

Caution should be used in patients with GI disease (especially colitis), diabetes mellitus, renal dysfunction, hepatic dysfunction, and in patients who are dehydrated and those receiving warfarin. Because ciprofloxacin can stimulate the central nervous system (CNS), it should be used with caution in patients with CNS disorders (such as seizures) or cerebrovascular disease (e.g., cerebral arteriosclerosis).

Adverse Effects
Ciprofloxacin is generally well tolerated. The most clinically important adverse reaction is **arthropathy** (joint disease). This often irreversible adverse reaction tends to occur in children under 18 years of age and adults over the age of 60. There is a black box warning for ciprofloxacin related to an increased risk of tendinitis and tendon rupture. This risk

TABLE 41.1 Summary of Selected Miscellaneous Antimicrobials

Drug (Trade) Name	Selected Indications	Route and Dosage Range	Pharmacokinetics
Ⓒ Fluoroquinolones			
Ⓟ ciprofloxacin (Cipro)	Uncomplicated UTI	*Adult:* PO, 250 mg bid × 7–14 d; IV, 200 mg q12 h	*Onset:* PO, varies; IV, 10 min
	Respiratory, bone, joint infections	*Adult:* PO, 500 mg q12 h; IV, 400 mg q12 h	*Duration:* 4–5 h
	Severe skin infections	*Adult:* PO, 750 mg q12 h	$t_{1/2}$: 3.5–4 h
	Infectious diarrhea	*Adult:* PO, 500 mg bid 5–7 d	
		Child: Not recommended	
	Complicated UTI	*Adult:* PO, 500 mg bid 10–21 d; IV, 40 mg q12 h	
		Child: IV, 6–10 mg/kg twice daily	
		Child: PO, 10–20 mg/kg twice daily	
	Inhalation anthrax	*Adult:* IV, 400 mg every 12 h, then switch to PO, 500 mg twice daily, after susceptibility tests returned	
		Child: IV, 10 mg/kg every 12 h, then switch to 15 mg/kg twice daily after susceptibility tests returned	
First Generation			
nalidixic acid (NegGram)	UTI	*Adult and child >12 y:* PO, 1 g qid 1–2 wk; prolonged therapy, 2 g/d	*Onset:* varies
		Child 3 mo–12 y: PO, 55 mg/kg/d in four divided doses; prolonged therapy, 33 mg/k/d	*Duration:* unknown
			$t_{1/2}$: 1–2.5 h
Second Generation			
lomefloxacin (Maxaquin)	Lower respiratory tract infections, uncomplicated UTI	*Adult:* PO, 400 mg qd × 10 d	*Onset:* Varies
	Complicated UTI	*Adult:* PO, 400 mg qd × 14 d	*Duration:* 8–10 h
	Prophylaxis	*Adult:* PO, 400 mg 2–6 h prior to surgery	$t_{1/2}$: 8 h
		Child: Not recommended	
norfloxacin (Noroxin)	Uncomplicated UTI	*Adult:* PO, 400 mg q12h × 7–10 d	*Onset:* Varies
	Complicated UTI	*Adult:* PO, 400 mg q12h × 10–21 d	*Duration:* Unknown
	STD	*Adult:* 800 mg single dose	$t_{1/2}$: 3–4.5 h
	Prostatitis	*Adult:* PO, 400 mg q12h for 28 d	
		Child: Not recommended	
ofloxacin (Floxin)	Uncomplicated UTI	*Adult:* PO, 200 mg bid for 3 d	*Onset:* Varies
	Complicated UTI, lower respiratory tract infections, skin infections	*Adult:* PO, 200 mg bid for 10 d	*Duration:* 9 h
		Adult: PO, 300 mg bid for 6 wk	$t_{1/2}$: 5–10 h
		Adult: PO, 400 mg single dose	
	Prostatitis	*Adult:* PO, 300 mg bid for 7 d	
	Uncomplicated gonorrhea Cervicitis, urethritis	*Child:* Not recommended	
Third Generation			
gemifloxacin (Factive)	Pneumonia	*Adult:* PO, 320 mg qd	*Onset:* Rapid
	Chronic bronchitis	*Child:* Not recommended	*Duration:* 24 h
			$t_{1/2}$: 7 h
levofloxacin (Levaquin)	Pneumonia, skin infections	*Adult:* PO/IV, 500 mg qd for 7–14 d	*Onset:* Varies
	Sinusitis	*Adult:* PO/IV, 500 mg qd 10–14 d	*Duration:* 3–5 h
	Chronic bronchitis	*Adult:* PO/IV, 500 mg qd × 7 d	$t_{1/2}$: 4–7 h
	UTI, nephritis	*Adult:* PO/IV, 250 mg qd × 10 d	
		Child: Not recommended	
moxifloxacin (Avelox)	Pneumonia, sinusitis	*Adult:* PO, 400 mg qd × 10 d	*Onset:* Varies
	Chronic bronchitis	*Adult:* PO, 400 mg qd × 5 d	*Duration:* Unknown
		Child: Not recommended	$t_{1/2}$: 12–13.5 h

(Continued)

TABLE 41.1 Summary of Selected Miscellaneous Antimicrobials *(continued)*

Drug (Trade) Name	Selected Indications	Route and Dosage Range	Pharmacokinetics
C Cyclic Lipopeptide			
P daptomycin (Cubicin)	Serious infections, especially MRSA and VRE	*Adult*: IV, 4 mg/kg once a day for 7–14 d *Child*: Not recommended	*Onset*: Rapid *Duration*: Unknown $t_{1/2}$: 8 h
C Miscellaneous Antibiotic			
Polymyxin B	Bacterial corneal ulcer Bacterial infection of eye Infection due to Pseudomonas aeruginosa Meningitis	*Adult*: Topical, 1–3 drops every hour; increase interval as response indicates; Ointment, apply every 3–4 h for 7–10 d IV, 15,000 to 25,000 U/kg/d divided every 12 h; maximum 25,000 U/kg/d IM, 25,000 to 30,000 U/kg/d divided every 4 to 6 h *Child >1 y*: IM, 25,000 to 30,000 U/kg/d divided every 4–6 h *Adult*: Intrathecal, 50,000 U once daily for 3 to 4 d, then 50,000 U every other d	*Onset*: IV, rapid; IM, gradual *Duration*: Unknown $t_{1/2}$: 4.3–6 h

is further increased in older patients, usually over age 60; in kidney, heart, and lung transplant recipients; and with patients taking concomitant steroid therapy. Other potential serious adverse effects include pseudomembranous colitis, superinfection, hepatotoxicity, nephrotoxicity, myelosuppression, and peripheral neuropathy.

The most common adverse reactions are GI effects, including nausea and vomiting, diarrhea, and abdominal pain. For the most part, CNS reactions, such as headache and restlessness, occur in only 1% to 2% of patients. Other CNS effects that occur in fewer than 1% of patients include dizziness, vertigo, insomnia, nightmares, hallucinations, confusion, agitation, drowsiness, anxiety, malaise, depression, paresthesias, and increased intracranial pressure. In predisposed patients, seizures may occur.

Cardiovascular adverse effects, such as palpitations, atrial flutter, premature ventricular contractions, syncope, angina, myocardial infarction, cardiac arrest, and cerebral thrombosis, have been reported with ciprofloxacin, but they occur rarely.

Photosensitivity may occur with ciprofloxacin. However, this adverse effect occurs more frequently with other fluoroquinolones. Lastly, ciprofloxacin may induce dysglycemia (either hyperglycemia or hypoglycemia).

Adverse reactions to ophthalmic ciprofloxacin usually are associated with local effects, such as burning or discomfort. Other adverse effects of ophthalmic ciprofloxacin include lid margin crusting, crystals, scales, foreign body sensation, pruritus, conjunctival hyperemia, and a bad taste following administration.

BOX 41.1 FOCUS ON RESEARCH

Ciproflaxin Therapy for UTI

How Long is Long Enough?
Lutters, M., Vogt-Ferrier, N. B. (2008). Antibiotic duration for treating uncomplicated, symptomatic lower urinary tract infections in elderly women. *Cochrane Database of Systematic Reviews*, 16(3):CD001535.

The Study
The purpose of this study was to determine the optimal duration of antibiotic treatment for uncomplicated symptomatic lower UTI in elderly women. The authors researched all randomized controlled trials comparing different treatment durations of oral antibiotics for uncomplicated symptomatic lower UTIs in elderly women. Fifteen studies were evaluated. Three studies compared single dose with short-course treatment (3 to 6 days), six compared single dose with long-course treatment (7 to 14 days) and six compared short- with long-course treatment. There was a significant difference for persistent UTI between single dose and short-course treatment

and single versus long-course treatment. Short versus longer treatments showed no significant difference in efficacy. Rate of adverse drug reactions increased significantly with longer treatment durations in one study.

Conclusion
Short-course treatment (3 to 6 days) could be sufficient for treating uncomplicated UTIs in elderly women, although more studies on specific commonly prescribed antibiotics are needed.

Nursing Implications
UTIs are the most common infection for elderly women. Elderly women are more likely to forget to take medication when prolonged treatment is prescribed. They are also more likely to have difficulty affording prescriptions. Short-term therapy appears to be as efficacious as long-term therapy and will be a cost saving for the patient. Nurses should continue to keep abreast of the latest information to appropriately answer questions from their patients.

Drug Interactions

Ciprofloxacin has many potential drug–drug interactions. Most interactions are related to either inhibiting the metabolism of the interacting drug or decreasing the absorption of ciprofloxacin. Many of the precautions for use of ciprofloxacin stem from the potential drug–drug interactions. For example, patients receiving warfarin may obtain subtherapeutic levels for anticoagulation, those receiving sulfonylureas may have hypoglycemia, and those receiving cyclosporin are at risk for nephrotoxicity. Table 41.2 summarizes drug interactions with ciprofloxacin.

Assessment of Relevant Core Patient Variables

Health Status

Elicit a patient history to evaluate for pre-existing GI disease, renal or hepatic dysfunction, CNS disorder, pregnancy,

or lactation. Communicate any positive finding to the prescriber. Assess for any known reactions to antibiotics.

Physical examination should include an examination of the skin for any rash or lesions, to provide a baseline for comparison if an allergic reaction is suspected. For the same reason, assess respiratory status, checking breath sounds for wheezing. When ciprofloxacin is proposed for long-term use, additional assessments should be done. For patients with pre-existing renal or hepatic disease obtain baseline blood tests to document current functioning. Patients with pre-existing anemias should have a complete blood count (CBC). Patients with pre-existing cardiac disorders should have an electrocardiogram.

Life Span and Gender

Assess the patient for pregnancy and lactation. Because ciprofloxacin crosses the placenta and enters breast milk, pregnant

TABLE 41.2	Agents That Interact with P Ciprofloxacin	
Interactants	**Effect and Significance**	**Nursing Management**
Antacids	Concurrent administration of antacids and ciprofloxacin may decrease the absorption of ciprofloxacin.	Administer antacids 6 h before or 2 h after ciprofloxacin.
cyclosporine	Ciprofloxacin may decrease cyclosporine metabolism, resulting in increased risk for adverse effects and toxicity.	Monitor for nephrotoxicity. Contact the prescriber if symptoms occur.
didanosine	The magnesium and aluminum cations in the buffers of didanosine decrease GI absorption of ciprofloxacin.	Administer ciprofloxacin 2 h before or 6 h after didanosine.
Food	Food interferes with the absorption of ciprofloxacin.	Administer on an empty stomach. Lengthen interval between milk and ciprofloxacin as much as possible.
Hydantoins	The mechanism of action is unclear, but ciprofloxacin may reduce serum phenytoin concentrations. This may result in seizure activity.	Monitor serum phenytoin levels. Discuss adjustment of dose with the prescriber.
methadone	Ciprofloxacin may decrease methadone metabolism, resulting in increased risk for adverse effects and toxicity.	Monitor for CNS depression and hypotension. Ensure patient safety.
procainamide	Ciprofloxacin may decrease procainamide metabolism, resulting in increased risk for adverse effects and toxicity.	Monitor for QT interval prolongation. Contact prescriber immediately if symptoms occur.
Salts iron zinc	GI absorption of ciprofloxacin may be decreased by the formation of iron–ciprofloxacin complex.	Avoid coadministration.
sucralfate	GI absorption of ciprofloxacin may be decreased by sucralfate.	Administer sucralfate 6 h after ciprofloxacin.
Sulfonylureas	Severe and persistent hypoglycemia may occur.	Increase frequency of blood glucose monitoring. Monitor for signs of hypoglycemia.
Theophyllines	Ciprofloxacin inhibits the hepatic metabolism of theophyllines. This may result in theophylline toxicity.	Monitor for theophylline levels. Observe for signs of toxicity. Discuss adjustment of dose with the prescriber.
tizanidine	Ciprofloxacin may decrease tizanidine metabolism, resulting in increased risk for adverse effects and toxicity.	Monitor for dizziness and hypotension. Contact prescriber if symptoms occur.
warfarin	Ciprofloxacin may decrease warfarin metabolism, resulting in increased risk for adverse effects and toxicity.	Monitor PT and INR. Monitor for signs of bleeding. Contact prescriber immediately if symptoms occur. Discuss adjustment of dose with the prescriber.

or breast-feeding women should not take ciprofloxacin. As with other fluoroquinolones, the patient's age should be noted before administering ciprofloxacin. Fluoroquinolone antibiotics have caused arthropathies, such as cartilage deterioration, when administered to immature animals. Although similar consequences of therapy have not been demonstrated in humans, ciprofloxacin should not be used in patients younger than 18 years except for the treatment of complicated urinary tract infections or anthrax. However, ciprofloxacin ophthalmic solution is approved for use in children. Elderly patients should be monitored carefully for renal or hepatic dysfunction and receive reduced dosages of ciprofloxacin as needed. Older patients taking warfarin should be monitored closely. Studies have shown they have an increased risk for upper GI bleeding while on ciprofloxacin therapy.

Lifestyle, Diet, and Habits

It is important to assess the patient's typical food, caffeine, and over-the-counter drug use. Caution the patient that food or caffeine may interrupt the action of ciprofloxacin. Remind patients with frequent dyspepsia that antacids can decrease the absorption of ciprofloxacin and that some vitamins also can decrease the absorption of ciprofloxacin. The safest advice would be to take any vitamin therapy at least 2 hours before or after administration of ciprofloxacin.

Environment

Ciprofloxacin is administered in a variety of environments. In acute care settings, administer parenteral ciprofloxacin over 60 minutes through a large vein to minimize discomfort and reduce the risk of venous irritation.

In the home, the patient should take ciprofloxacin every 12 hours on an empty stomach. Advise patients using the ophthalmic or otic solutions not to contaminate the tip of the dispenser by contact with the eye, ear, fingertips, or other surface.

Nursing Diagnoses and Outcomes

- Diarrhea related to adverse drug effects
  Desired outcome: *The patient will avoid dehydration, maintain fluid intake, and contact the prescriber if diarrhea persists.*
- Imbalanced Nutrition: More or Less than Body Requirements, related to GI effects, alteration in taste, and superinfections
  Desired outcome: *The patient will maintain body weight and contact the prescriber if persistent adverse effects alter nutritional status.*
- Risk for Injury related to drug-induced dizziness, confusion, and other CNS effects
  Desired outcome: *The patient will remain free of injury and contact the prescriber about persistent CNS disturbances.*
- Risk for Impaired Tissue Integrity related to drug-induced photosensitivity
  Desired outcome: *The patient will take measures to protect his or her skin from prolonged sun exposure*

Planning and Intervention

Maximizing Therapeutic Effects

Ensure that the patient receives the full course of ciprofloxacin as prescribed, around the clock, to increase effectiveness. Coordinate the administration of drugs to decrease potential drug–drug interactions.

Review culture and sensitivity reports to confirm that the causative bacteria are sensitive to ciprofloxacin.

Minimizing Adverse Effects

Institute safety measures to protect the patient if CNS effects occur. For patients with adverse GI effects, provide small, frequent meals as tolerated.

Frequent mouth care and sucking on ice chips may relieve stomatitis and sore mouth.

Providing Patient and Family Education

- One of the most important features of patient and family education is teaching patients that ciprofloxacin is one drug in a class of drugs. Advise patients who have had any type of allergic reaction to a fluoroquinolone never to take any other drug with a name that ends with "oxacin."
- Advise patients who are pregnant or breast-feeding not to take ciprofloxacin.
- It is important to explain that ciprofloxacin is prescribed for a particular infection. Tell patients that ciprofloxacin should not be used to self-medicate or treat any other infection or any other person, especially not a child.
- Instruct patients to call the prescriber if their symptoms do not improve within 3 days.
- It is important to instruct patients to complete the full course of drug therapy, even when they feel better.
- Advise patients to take ciprofloxacin every 12 hours. A forgotten dose can be taken as soon as it is remembered, but not if it is almost time for the next dose.
- Teach patients symptoms of an allergic reaction to ciprofloxacin (i.e., rash, welts, itching, or shortness of breath) and instruct patients to stop taking the drug at once and notify the prescriber if these symptoms occur.
- Advise patients who experience GI upset to eat small, frequent meals and to increase their fluid intake, particularly if they have diarrhea. For patients with a sore mouth or throat, sucking on ice chips may provide relief.
- Caution patients about possible photosensitivity and encourage them to avoid sunlight or ultraviolet light, to wear appropriate clothing, and to apply a sunscreen with a sun protection factor of at least 15 if exposure is unavoidable.
- Advise patients of signs and symptoms of a superinfection, such as discoloration of the tongue, fatigue, easy bruising, or vaginal discharge. In addition, tell patients that ciprofloxacin may cause CNS disturbances or cardiovascular symptoms, and that patients should contact the prescriber immediately if these adverse reactions occur.
- Tell patients to report any tendon pain to the prescriber immediately because of the potential for tendon rupture as an adverse effect of ciprofloxacin therapy.

acid is not commonly used because fluoroquinolones are more efficacious.

Second-Generation Fluoroquinolones

Second-generation fluoroquinolones include lomefloxacin, norfloxacin, and ofloxacin. Contraindications, adverse effects, and drug interactions for lomefloxacin and norfloxacin are the same as those listed for ciprofloxacin.

Lomefloxacin (Maxaquin) is used to treat lower respiratory tract infections, such as bronchitis, and UTIs. It also may be given as a preoperative prophylaxis to patients undergoing transurethral procedures or transrectal prostate biopsy. Lomefloxacin is a once-a-day oral preparation. The drug may induce serious photosensitivity reactions and should be discontinued at the first sign of rash, redness, or burning sensation on the skin.

Norfloxacin (Noroxin) is used to treat UTIs, prostatitis, and urethral or endocervical gonorrhea. It is an oral agent very similar to ciprofloxacin, with the same antimicrobial spectrum.

Ofloxacin (Floxin), which is available in oral and topical formulations, is very similar to ciprofloxacin in antimicrobial spectrum, pharmacotherapeutics, and adverse effects. However, ofloxacin is considered to be less efficacious. Drug interactions also are similar to those of ciprofloxacin, except that ofloxacin does not affect theophylline levels.

Third-Generation Fluoroquinolones

The third-generation fluoroquinolones include gatifloxacin, gemifloxacin, levofloxacin, and moxifloxacin.

Gatifloxacin (Tequin) has been removed from the market because of its ability to induce serious cases of diabetes and other potentially fatal blood sugar abnormalities. It is still available for ophthalmologic application as the drug Zymar.

Gemifloxacin (Factive) is used to manage acute exacerbations of chronic bronchitis caused by susceptible organisms such as *Streptococcus pneumoniae*, *Haemophilus influenzae*, *Haemophilus parainfluenzae*, and *Moraxella catarrhalis*. It is also used to manage community-acquired pneumonia caused by these bacteria or by *Mycoplasma pneumoniae*, *Chlamydia pneumoniae*, or *Klebsiella pneumoniae*. It is a once-a-day oral drug that is well tolerated. Common adverse effects include rash, photosensitivity, and elevations in liver enzymes.

Levofloxacin (Levaquin) may be more active than other fluoroquinolones against pneumococci and certain "atypical" respiratory pathogens. It is indicated for acute maxillary sinusitis, acute bacterial exacerbation of chronic bronchitis, community-acquired pneumonia, uncomplicated skin and skin-structure infections, complicated UTIs, acute pyelonephritis, cystitis, and prostatitis; sexually transmitted diseases such as urethral and cervical gonorrhea, nongonococcal urethritis, and cervicitis; and mixed infections of the urethra and cervix. It is administered orally or parenterally. Oral preparations require once-a-day dosing.

Important precautions related to levofloxacin involve giving the drug to patients with CNS disorders that predispose them

CRITICAL THINKING SCENARIO

HOW DID THAT HAPPEN?

Keri H., age 25 years, comes to your clinic after a weekend of skiing in the mountains with a complaint of chest pain, cough, and shortness of breath. She is diagnosed with pneumonia and is started on ciprofloxacin, 400 mg bid. Four days after starting the medication, Keri calls the clinic and asks, "Can I come back and get seen again? My chest pain and cough are gone but I am limping and my left heel hurts. I guess I must have done something while I was skiing, but I don't remember hurting myself." How would you respond to Keri? Can you correlate this scenario with why ciprofloxacin is contraindicated during pregnancy?

- Inform women who use oral contraceptives to use a backup method of contraception during ciprofloxacin therapy because their birth control pills may be less effective while they are taking ciprofloxacin.

Ongoing Assessment and Evaluation

Antibiotic therapy can result in superinfection with nonsusceptible organisms. Due to the possibility for overgrowth of candidal organisms with ciprofloxacin therapy, monitor patients closely during treatment. In addition, patients who develop diarrhea while taking—or soon after taking—ciprofloxacin should be considered for differential diagnosis of antibiotic-associated pseudomembranous colitis.

Drugs Closely Related to
 P Ciprofloxacin

First-Generation Quinolone

Nalidixic acid (NegGram) is an oral quinolone agent that is indicated for use in UTIs because it concentrates in the urine and achieves only low concentrations in serum, making it ineffective for infections outside the urinary tract. Nalidixic

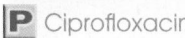 MEMORY CHIP

P Ciprofloxacin

- Used for infections caused by aerobic gram-negative organisms
- Major contraindications: hypersensitivity, children younger than 18 years, pregnancy, or breast-feeding
- Most common adverse effects: GI
- Most serious adverse effect: arthropathy (in children younger than 18 years)
- Maximizing therapeutic effects: Complete the full course of antibiotic therapy.
- Minimizing adverse effects: Provide small, frequent meals for GI distress.
- Most important patient education: Importance of completion of therapy and, for women, use of a backup method of contraception
- **Black box warning: increased risk of tendinitis and tendon rupture.**

to seizure activity and kidney failure. Severe renal impairment requires dosage reduction. Levofloxacin is associated with QT prolongation and can cause photosensitization, but incidence of these adverse effects is relatively low. Interaction studies have shown that levofloxacin, unlike other fluoroquinolones, causes few or no problems with drugs such as theophylline, warfarin, digoxin, and cyclosporine. However, levofloxacin is more likely than ciprofloxacin to cause dysglycemia.

Moxifloxacin (Avelox) is indicated for treating acute exacerbations of chronic bronchitis, acute sinusitis, and pneumonia. It is especially efficacious in eradicating pathogens that cause exacerbations of chronic bronchitis. An important consideration for moxifloxacin is that to date, because it is a new drug, no organisms have been shown to be resistant to it. Moxifloxacin is being investigated currently for use in managing tuberculosis. Moxifloxacin is administered orally once a day for 5 to 10 days.

Like levofloxacin, moxifloxacin is reportedly associated with substantial prolongation of the QT segment. It should be avoided in patients who have conditions or are taking medications known to prolong the QT interval and in patients with a predisposition to arrhythmias.

Fourth Generation

Fourth generation besifloxacin (Besivance), an opthalmic fluoroquinolone for bacterial conjunctivitis, may be considered a 4th generation fluoroquinolone, although it has similar characteristics to 2nd generation fluoroquinolones as well. Historically, opthalmic fluoroquinolones were first used systemically then became approved for opthalmologic uses. Besifloxacin is the first fluoroquinolone to be initially used in opthalmology.

C CYCLIC LIPOPEPTIDES

Daptomycin (Cubicin) is the only drug in a new class of antibiotics called **cyclic lipopeptides.** This class of antibiotics has a substantially different mechanism of action than other antibiotic drugs. Another benefit of daptomycin is its ability to retain potency against antibiotic-resistant gram-positive bacteria. Table 41.3 presents an overview of daptomycin.

Nursing Management of the Patient Receiving P Daptomycin
Core Drug Knowledge
Pharmacotherapeutics
Daptomycin is FDA approved for treatment of bacteremia due to *S. aureus* (including MRSA and right-sided

endocarditis) and complicated skin and skin structure infections caused by a wide variety of gram-positive bacteria. Daptomycin may also be used in the treatment of vancomycin-resistant enterococcal (VRE) bacteremia.

Pharmacokinetics
Daptomycin is a once-daily IV medication. It reaches maximum serum concentration within 1 hour. 78% of daptomycin is excreted as unchanged drug by the kidneys. For that reason, a patient with severe renal impairment should receive a lower dose of medication.

Pharmacodynamics
Daptomycin is a bacteriocidal antibiotic that has a unique mechanism of action. It works by binding to the bacterial membrane and interfering with the integrity of the cell wall. This disruption causes a rapid depolarization of the membrane potential that leads to inhibition of protein, DNA, and RNA synthesis and, eventually, bacterial cell death. Daptomycin also has a postantibiotic effect that lasts approximately 6 hours.

At this time, no mechanism of resistance to daptomycin has been identified, there are no known transferable elements (plasmids) that confer resistance, and cross-resistance has not been reported.

Contraindications and Precautions
The only contraindication to the use of daptomycin is hypersensitivity. Precautions include pre-existing GI disorders, myopathy, and peripheral neuropathy. It should be used cautiously in elderly people and in patients with pre-existing renal dysfunction. Whether daptomycin enters breast milk is unclear; therefore, it should be given cautiously to women who breast-feed.

Like other antibiotics, daptomycin may alter the normal flora of the GI tract. Patients with pre-existing GI disorders have a higher risk of developing pseudomembranous colitis. Daptomycin has also been associated with inducing muscle weakness and pain. For that reason, patients with pre-existing myopathy and peripheral neuropathy should be monitored closely during daptomycin therapy.

Adverse Effects
Daptomycin is generally well tolerated. The most common adverse effects are constipation, diarrhea, nausea and vomiting, and injection site reactions. In the CNS, daptomycin may induce headache, insomnia, or dizziness. Cardiovascular adverse effects include hypotension or hypertension and unspecified chest pain. Hematopoietic

TABLE 41.3	Overview of Daptomycin		
Drug (Trade) Name	Selected Indications	Route and Dosage Range	Pharmacokinetics
daptomycin (Cubicin)	Complicated skin and skin structure	*Adult:* IV, 4 mg/kg once a day for 7–14 d	*Onset:* Rapid
		Adult IV: 6 mg/kg once a day for 2–6 wk	*Duration:* Unknown
	Bacteremia	*Child:* Not recommended	$t_{1/2}$: 8 h

effects such as anemia, eosinophilia, leukocytosis, and thrombocytopenia may occur.

Metabolic and nutritional adverse reactions such as electrolyte disturbance, hyperglycemia, hypoglycemia, hypokalemia, hypomagnesemia, and increased serum bicarbonate have been reported. Elevations of creatine kinase (CK), hepatic enzymes, alkaline phosphatase, and INR may also occur.

In addition, daptomycin may induce problems with the musculoskeletal system, including arthralgia, back pain, limb pain, muscle cramps, muscle weakness, myalgia, and osteomyelitis. Cases of rhabdomyolysis also have been reported

Drug Interactions
Daptomycin may interact with other drugs that have the ability to cause myopathy, such as HMG-CoA reductase inhibitors. Another theoretical drug–drug interaction is warfarin because daptomycin may elevate INR.

Assessment of Relevant Core Patient Variables
Health Status
Assess the patient for contraindications or precautions to the use of daptomycin. Be especially vigilant for a history of renal insufficiency or current medications that may induce myopathy, such as HMG-CoA reductase inhibitors. Review the culture and sensitivity report to ensure that daptomycin is recommended for the invading organism. Review the CBC, renal function tests, liver function tests, comprehensive metabolic panel, and a baseline CK. Alterations in these laboratory values should be discussed with the prescriber before starting therapy.

Life Span and Gender
Daptomycin is in FDA pregnancy category B. Caution the patient to avoid breast-feeding while taking daptomycin, because it is unclear whether the drug enters breast milk. Dosing for the elderly should be adjusted if the patient has renal insufficiency. Daptomycin is not approved for use in children.

Environment
Daptomycin is used for serious infections that have not responded to other types of medications; thus, the patient will be admitted to an acute care hospital. In rare circumstances, daptomycin may be administered in the home environment by a home health nurse.

Nursing Diagnoses and Outcomes
• Acute Pain related to myopathy
Desired outcome: *The patient will contact the health care provider should pain or tingling in the extremities occur.*
• Imbalanced Nutrition: Less than Body Requirements, related to drug-induced GI effects, such as nausea, vomiting, diarrhea, or dyspepsia

Desired outcome: *The patient will maintain consistent body weight and consult prescriber about persistent adverse effects that affect nutritional status.*
• Diarrhea related to drug therapy
Desired outcome: *The patient will avoid dehydration, maintain fluid intake, and contact prescriber about persistent diarrhea.*
• Risk for Infection related to overgrowth of nonsusceptible organisms
Desired outcome: *The patient will report signs of superinfection to the prescriber.*
• Fatigue related to metabolic and hematopoietic alterations
Desired outcome: *The patient will immediately report signs of fatigue to the health care provider.*

Planning and Intervention
Maximizing Therapeutic Effects
Review the culture and sensitivity report to ensure that daptomycin is an appropriate drug. Before administration, visually inspect daptomycin for particulate matter and discoloration. Administer daptomycin with 0.9% sodium chloride or lactated Ringer's solution because daptomycin is not compatible with dextrose-containing solutions. Check your hospital's policy prior to administration. Daptomycin may be infused over 30 minutes without any other IV substances, additives, or other medications. Recent studies have shown that daptomycin also may be given IVP over 2 minutes without altering its pharmacokinetics or increasing its adverse effects. Before and after daptomycin infusion, flush the primary line with a compatible solution.

Minimizing Adverse Effects
Evaluate the IV site before administering daptomycin. Teach the patient the importance of reporting diarrhea, muscle pain or tingling, dark-colored urine, and fatigue immediately because these signs and symptoms signal potentially severe adverse effects.

Providing Patient and Family Education
• Explain the potential adverse effects and need for periodic blood monitoring.
• Teach patients the importance of reporting diarrhea, muscle pain or tingling, dark-colored urine, and fatigue to the prescriber immediately.
• Advise patients to stop taking HMG-CoA reductase inhibitors until advised to resume the medication by the prescriber.

Ongoing Assessment and Evaluation
Evaluate for resolution of the presenting infection. Question the patient frequently concerning the onset of musculoskeletal pain or tingling, and arrange for a weekly CK to be drawn. Notify the provider if the patient has symptoms of myopathy and the CK is five times the upper limit of normal. If the CK elevates to 10 times the normal limit, it is necessary to discontinue the drug even if the patient is asymptomatic.

MEMORY CHIP

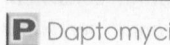

P Daptomycin

- Used for serious aerobic gram-positive complicated skin and skin structure infections caused by *Enterococcus faecalis, Staphylococcus aureus, methicillin-resistant S. aureus, Streptococcus agalactiae, Streptococcus dysgalactiae,* and *Streptococcus pyogenes.*
- Major contraindication: hypersensitivity
- Most common adverse effects: nausea, vomiting, diarrhea, dyspepsia
- Most serious adverse effect: myopathy
- **Life span alert: Elderly patients may need a reduced dose of daptomycin because of renal insufficiency.**
- Maximizing therapeutic effects: Obtain culture and sensitivity report before administration.
- Minimizing adverse effects: Administer over 30 minutes. Monitor weekly CK.
- Most important patient education: Notify prescriber if diarrhea, muscle pain, or tingling occurs.

By the end of daptomycin therapy, the initial infection should be resolved. Any adverse effects should be resolved or at least should be addressed. The patient should have normal laboratory values or be receiving appropriate electrolyte or hematopoietic replacement.

MISCELLANEOUS ANTIBIOTIC: POLYMYXIN B

Polymyxin B is an older antibiotic that is completely different from the fluoroquinolones and cyclic lipopeptides. Its spectrum of activity is limited to gram-negative bacteria, with the exception of *Proteus* and *Neisseria* species. Polymyxin B binds to phospholipids in the cell membranes of gram-negative bacteria. This binding increases the permeability of the cell membrane, which results in loss of metabolites essential to bacterial existence.

Polymyxin B is administered commonly as either a topical, ophthalmic, or otic drug. It rarely is used systemically, because of its potential for causing nephrotoxicity or neurotoxicity. It frequently is used in combination with other drugs such as trimethoprim B (Polytrim) or bacitracin and neomycin (Neosporin). It also is used in combination with neomycin alone as a urinary tract irrigant.

CHAPTER SUMMARY

- Quinolone antibiotics inhibit an enzyme needed for bacterial DNA replication.
- Quinolone antibiotics, like cephalosporin antibiotics, are categorized into generations.
- First-generation quinolones are used only to treat uncomplicated UTIs.
- The second, third, and fourth generations of quinolone drugs are called fluoroquinolone antibiotics.

- All fluoroquinolones have systemic activity.
- Third-generation fluoroquinolones have extended activity against gram-positive pathogens but are less active than second-generation drugs against *Pseudomonas* species.
- Ciprofloxacin is the prototype fluoroquinolone.
- Fluoroquinolones should not be used during pregnancy, while breast-feeding, or in children because of their potential to cause arthropathies in children.
- Daptomycin, a cyclic lipopeptide, is the only member of this new class of antibiotics.
- To decrease the possibility of antibiotic resistance development, daptomycin should be reserved for infections that do not respond to other antibiotics.
- Polymyxin B is another type of miscellaneous antibiotic.

QUESTIONS FOR STUDY AND REVIEW

1. Describe the spectrum of activity of the four generations of quinolone antibiotics.
2. How do fluoroquinolone drugs, such as ciprofloxacin, inhibit bacteria?
3. In addition to hypersensitivity, which other contraindications are associated with ciprofloxacin use?
4. Why is it important that patients take ciprofloxacin on an empty stomach?
5. What are the characteristics of daptomycin that are different from other antibiotics? Why is one of its characteristics so important?
6. Why is polymyxin B rarely used in its parenteral form?

NEED MORE HELP?

Chapter 41 of the Study Guide to Accompany *Drug Therapy in Nursing,* 4th Edition, contains NCLEX-style questions and other learning activities to reinforce your understanding of the concepts presented in this chapter. For additional information or to purchase the study guide, visit the**Point.**

REFERENCES

Aspinall, S. L., Good, C. B., Jiang, R., et al. (2009). Severe Dysglycemia with the Fluoroquinolones: A Class Effect? Jun 22.

Chakraborty, A., Roy, S., Loeffler, J., Chaves, R. L. (2009). Comparison of the pharmacokinetics, safety and tolerability of daptomycin in healthy adult volunteers following intravenous administration by 30 min infusion or 2 min injection. *Journal of Antimicrobial Chemotherapy,* 64(1):151–158.

Drugs for MRSA with Reduced Susceptibility to Vancomycin. (2009). *The Medical Letter on Drugs and Therapeutics,* 51(1309):25.

Facts and Comparisons. (2010). *Drug facts and comparisons.* Philadelphia, PA: Lippincott Williams & Wilkins.

File, T. M. (2009). Antibiotic studies for the treatment of community-acquired pneumonia in adults, *Up To Date.* Retrieved from *http://uptodate.com.*

Fischer, H. D, Juurlink, D. N., Mamdani, M. M., et al. (2010). Hemorrhage During Warfarin Therapy Associated With Cotrimoxazole and Other Urinary Tract Anti-infective Agents. *Arch Intern Med,* 170(7):617–621.

Fowler, V. G, Sexton, D. J. (2009). Treatment of *S. aureus* bacteremia in adults, *Up To Date.* Retrieved from *http://uptodate.com.*

Fowler, V. G, Sexton, D. J. (2009). Treatment of *S. aureus* bacteremia in adults, *Up To Date*. Retrieved from *http://uptodate. com*.

Fluoroquinolones and tendon injuries. *Obstetrics & Gynecology* [serial online]. May 2009;113(5):1162–1162. Retrieved from: CINAHL Plus with Full Text, Ipswich, MA. Accessed June 24, 2009.

Koda-Kimbal, M. A, Young, L. Y., Kradian, W. A., et al. (2008). *Applied Therapeutics: The Clinical Use of Drugs*. Philadelphia, PA: Lippincott Williams & Wilkins.

Lowy, F. D. (2009). In Up-To-Date, Treatment of invasive methicillin-resistant Staphylococcus aureus infections in adults. Retrieved June 8, 2011 from *uptodate.com*

Mave, V., Garcia-Diaz, J., Islam, T., & Hasbun,R. (2009). Vancomycin-resistant enterococcal bacteraemia: is daptomycin as effective as linezolid? *Journal of Antimicrobial Chemotherapy*, 64(1):175–180.

Mehlhorn, A. J., Brown, D. A. (2007). Safety concerns with fluoroquinolones. *The Annals of Pharmacotherapy*, 41(11):1859–1866.

Micromedex Healthcare Series. Retrieved from *http://thomsonhc. com*.

Odero, R. O., Cleveland, K. O., Gelfand, M. S. (2009). Rhabdomyolysis and acute renal failure associated with the co-administration of daptomycin and an HMG-CoA reductase inhibitor. *Journal of Antimicrobial Chemotherapy*, 63(6):1299–1300.

Raygada, J., & Levine, D. (2009). Managing CA-MRSA infections: current and emerging options. *Infections in Medicine*, 26(2):49.

Tatro, D. S. (2009). *Drug interaction facts*. Philadelphia, PA: Lippincott Williams & Wilkins.

Wang, J. L., & Hsueh, P. R. (2009). Therapeutic options for infections due to vancomycin-resistant enterococci. *Expert Opinion on Pharmacotherapy*, 10(5):785–796.

42

Drugs Treating Urinary Tract Infections

Learning Objectives

At the completion of this chapter the student will:

1. Describe the primary therapeutic uses for sulfonamides, urinary tract antiseptics, and urinary tract analgesics.

2. Identify core drug knowledge about drugs that are used for treating urinary tract infections.

3. Identify core patient variables relevant to drugs that are used for treating urinary tract infections.

4. Relate the interaction of core drug knowledge to core patient variables for drugs that are used for treating urinary tract infections.

5. Generate a nursing plan of care from the interactions between core drug knowledge and core patient variables for drugs that are used for treating urinary tract infections.

6. Describe nursing interventions to maximize therapeutic and minimize adverse effects for drugs that are used for treating urinary tract infections.

7. Determine key points for patient and family education for drugs that are used for treating urinary tract infections.

Key Terms

crystalluria	pyelonephritis	relapse
cystitis	recurrent infection	sulfonamides
prostatitis	reinfection	urethritis

Drugs Treating Urinary Tract Infections

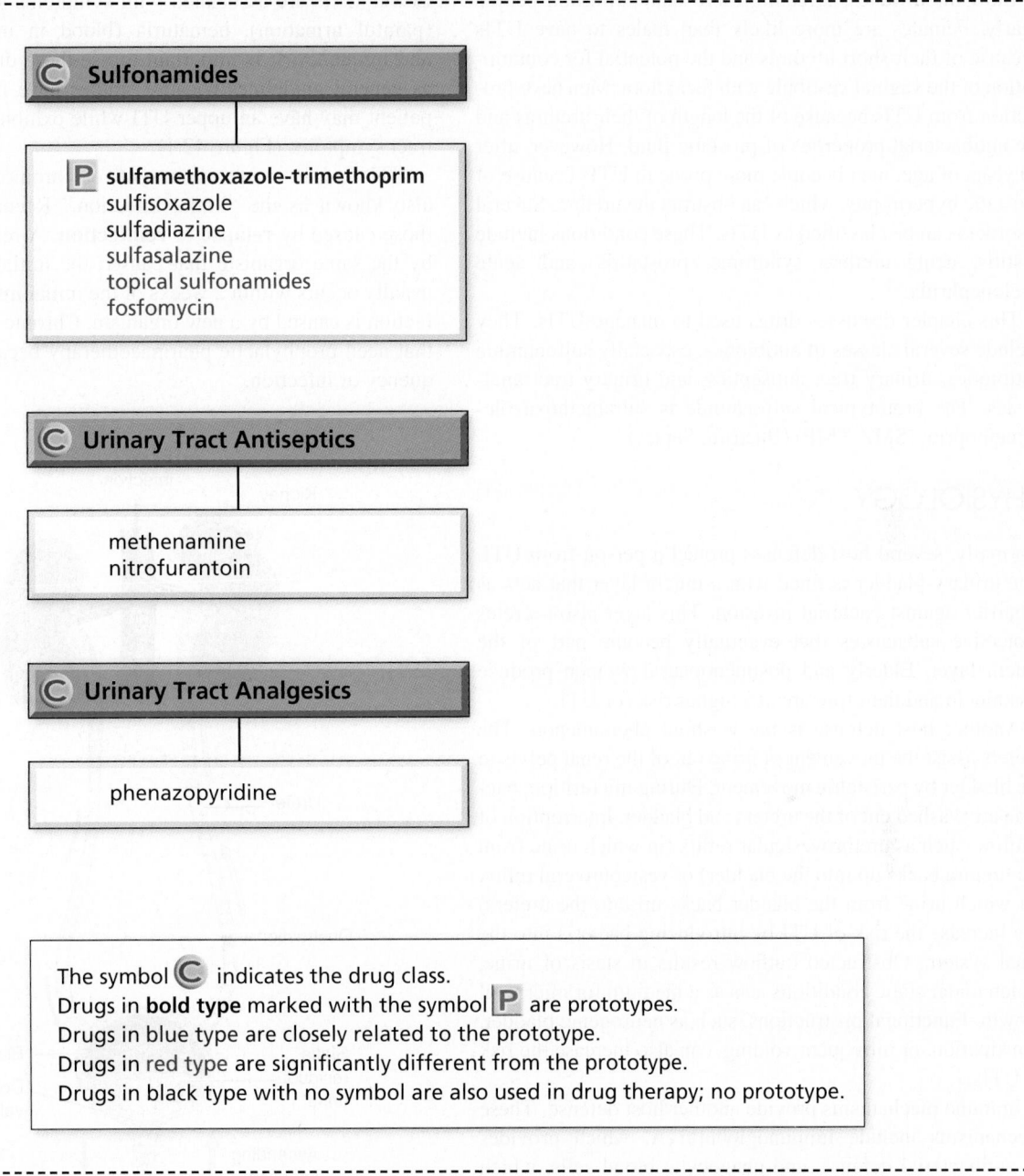

C Sulfonamides

P **sulfamethoxazole-trimethoprim**
sulfisoxazole
sulfadiazine
sulfasalazine
topical sulfonamides
fosfomycin

C Urinary Tract Antiseptics

methenamine
nitrofurantoin

C Urinary Tract Analgesics

phenazopyridine

The symbol **C** indicates the drug class.
Drugs in **bold type** marked with the symbol **P** are prototypes.
Drugs in blue type are closely related to the prototype.
Drugs in red type are significantly different from the prototype.
Drugs in black type with no symbol are also used in drug therapy; no prototype.

A urinary tract infection (UTI) is a clinical condition caused by microorganisms infecting structures within the urinary system. It is the most common cause of infection in the United States, affecting more than 7 million people yearly. Females are more likely than males to have UTIs because of their short urethras and the potential for contamination of the vaginal vestibule with fecal flora. Men have protection from UTIs because of the length of their urethras and the antibacterial properties of prostatic fluid. However, after 50 years of age, men become more prone to UTIs because of prostatic hypertrophy, which can obstruct the urethra. Several disorders can be classified as UTIs. These conditions include cystitis, acute urethral syndrome, prostatitis, and acute pyelonephritis.

This chapter discusses drugs used to manage UTIs. They include several classes of antibiotics, especially sulfonamide antibiotics, urinary tract antiseptics, and urinary tract analgesics. The prototypical sulfonamide is sulfamethoxazole-trimethoprim (SMZ-TMP) (Bactrim, Septra).

PHYSIOLOGY

Normally, several host defenses protect a person from UTI. The urinary bladder is lined with a mucin layer that acts as a barrier against bacterial invasion. This layer also secretes protective substances that eventually become part of the mucin layer. Elderly and postmenopausal women produce less mucin and therefore are at a higher risk for UTI.

Another host defense is the washout phenomenon. The ureters assist the movement of urine out of the renal pelvis to the bladder by peristaltic movement. During micturition, bacteria are washed out of the ureters and bladder. Interruption of outflow, such as urethrovesicular reflux (in which urine from the urethra backs up into the bladder) or vesicoureteral reflux (in which urine from the bladder backs up into the ureters) can increase the risk of UTI by introducing bacteria into the renal system. Obstructed outflow results in stasis of urine, which under static conditions acts as a medium for microbial growth. Functional obstructions, such as neurogenic bladder, constipation, or infrequent voiding, can also increase the risk of UTIs.

Immune mechanisms provide another host defense. These mechanisms include immunoglobulin A, which provides an antibacterial defense, and phagocytic blood cells, which remove bacteria from the urinary tract. Alterations in the immune system increase the risk of UTIs.

PATHOPHYSIOLOGY

Urinary tract infections are generally classified as complicated or uncomplicated. An uncomplicated UTI is a bacterial infection, whereas a complicated UTI, also caused by bacteria, is associated with some anatomical or structural abnormality. UTIs are also divided into upper and lower UTIs. Upper UTIs are commonly associated with symptoms such as fever, nausea and vomiting, and flank or back pain. Lower UTIs are associated with symptoms such as dysuria (painful urination), hematuria (blood in urine), urgency, and frequency. It is important to use these distinctions only as general guidelines because studies have indicated that a patient may have an upper UTI while exhibiting only lower tract symptoms (Figure 42.1).

UTIs can be acute, **recurrent,** or chronic. Acute UTI is also known as the "initial infection." Recurrent UTIs are those caused by **relapse** or **reinfection.** A relapse is caused by the same organism that caused the initial infection and usually occurs within 2 weeks of the initial infection. A reinfection is caused by a new organism. Chronic UTIs are those that need prophylactic pharmacotherapy because of the frequency of infection.

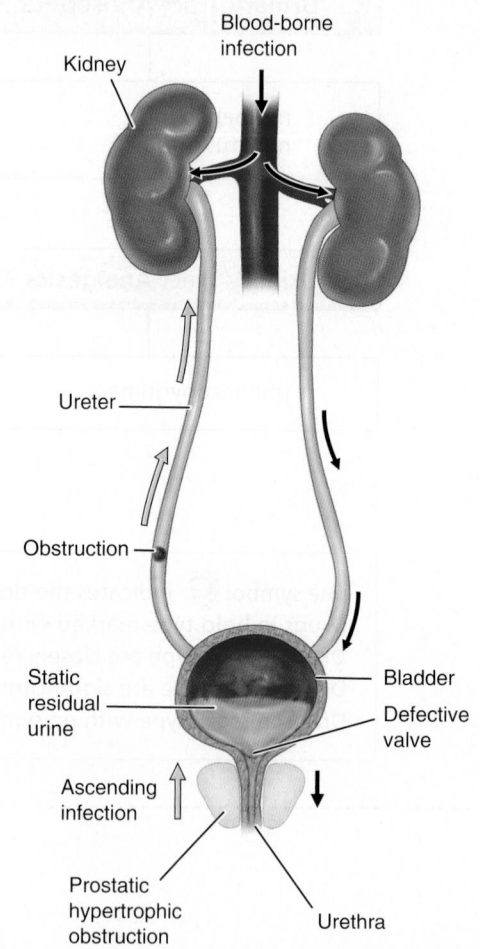

• FIGURE 42.1 Urinary tract infections (UTIs) result from various causes: blood-borne infections that cycle through the renal system; ascending infection from external or other sources; stagnant urine (urinary stasis) caused by immobility or obstructions, which allows microorganisms to colonize; defective valves that may allow infected urine to flow backward; and other problems.

Asymptomatic Bacteriuria

Asymptomatic bacteriuria is diagnosed when the patient has no symptoms but the urinalysis shows significant numbers of bacteria. The condition is usually harmless but can increase the risk for symptomatic UTI. Asymptomatic bacteriuria is common during pregnancy. It is important to identify in pregnant women because it increases the risk for pyelonephritis during the second and third trimesters. Additionally, untreated UTI is associated with an increased risk for miscarriage.

Cystitis

Cystitis is an infection of the lower urinary tract caused by introduction of a pathogen into the bladder. This infection results in redness, inflammation, irritation, and edema of the bladder mucosa, with multiple submucosal hemorrhages and sometimes pus. Symptoms may include urgency, frequency, incontinence, dysuria, hematuria, burning or a feeling of warmth on urination, bladder cramps or spasms, perineal itching, suprapubic discomfort, mild backache, or a low-grade fever. Nosocomial bladder infections, which are infections acquired in the hospital, are frequently caused by instrumentation and urinary catheterization. They are more difficult to treat because the bacteria that cause them are often resistant to drug treatment and patients are often in poor health. More commonly, bladder infections occur in the community. Factors that increase the risk of community-acquired UTIs include pregnancy, diaphragm with spermicide use, sexual intercourse, and delayed postcoital micturition. Complications include chronic cystitis, acute pyelonephritis, or urosepsis, especially in the elderly (Box 42.1).

Urethritis

Urethritis is a term that is generally associated with a syndrome of sexually transmitted infections (STIs) and is most commonly divided into nongonococcal urethritis (NGU) and gonococcal urethritis. NGU is characterized by redness, irritation, and edema of the urethral mucosa. Common pathogens causing NGU include *Chlamydia trachomatis*, *Ureaplasma urealyticum*, *Mycoplasma hominis*, *Mycoplasma genitalium*, or *Trichomonas vaginalis*. In women, urethritis may also be associated with irritation by chemicals in feminine deodorants, suppositories, bubble baths, and spermicidal gels. In postmenopausal women, NGU is commonly caused by tissue changes related to low estrogen levels. Gonococcal urethritis has symptoms similar to NGU with the addition of a discharge that may be yellow, green, brown, or tinged with blood, and production is unrelated to sexual activity. Many patients, including approximately 25% of those with NGU, are asymptomatic and present only after partner screening.

Complications of urethritis include chronic urethritis, cystitis, periurethral abscess, urethral stricture or fistula, pyelonephritis, and in men, prostatitis or epididymitis.

In cases of either type of urethritis, the nurse explains the importance of partner notification. If the partner is not simultaneously treated, the infection will recur in the patient.

Prostatitis

Prostatitis is usually associated with urethritis or cystitis. Organisms can infect the prostate gland through the bloodstream or by ascending from the urethra. Symptoms include fever, chills, dysuria, urethral discharge, and a boggy, tender prostate. Diagnosis may be made by massaging the prostate, which results in a urethral discharge of prostatic secretions full of white blood cells. Complications include chronic prostatitis, epididymitis, and pyelonephritis.

Acute Pyelonephritis

Acute pyelonephritis is an infection of the kidneys and renal pelvis. Infection can occur by way of the bloodstream or ascending organisms from the bladder. Approximately 80% of cases of pyelonephritis are caused by a uropathogenic strain of *Escherichia coli* that has specific fimbriae that attach to the epithelial cells of the kidney. When microorganisms invade the kidney, an inflammatory process is initiated, resulting in local edema. As the edema subsides with treatment, fibrosis and scar tissue develop. This scarring may lead to impaired tubular reabsorption and diminished renal function.

Predisposing factors are UTI, urinary tract instrumentation, catheterization, pregnancy, vesicoureteral reflux, and neurogenic bladder. Symptoms include acute onset of chills and fever, flank pain, hematuria, general malaise or fatigue, headache, and costovertebral angle tenderness. Complications of pyelonephritis include chronic pyelonephritis, scarring of the kidneys, and permanent kidney damage.

DIAGNOSIS OF UTI

Diagnosis of UTI is frequently based on the patient's subjective description of symptoms and a positive urine dipstick test. The dipstick test is recommended for nonpregnant women at low risk for recurrent infection and without symptoms suggesting other problems, such as vaginitis. The dipstick is placed in a fresh specimen of urine and examined for a positive reaction to nitrates, leukocytes, and blood. This test is difficult to read if the patient has been taking an over-the-counter urinary analgesic because it will discolor the urine bright orange.

A urinalysis (UA) is required for women who are pregnant or over the age of 55, men with urinary symptoms, and patients with recurrent symptoms. A successful UA requires a midstream or clean-catch urine specimen. When obtaining urine for a UA from a catheterized patient, the urine must be withdrawn from the proximal port on the catheter tubing and not from the urine collection bag.

When the specimen is obtained from a noncatheterized patient, the nurse instructs the patient to:

- Wash his/her hands thoroughly before starting the procedure
- Cleanse the penis or vulva and surrounding area three times, using a new sponge each time, with a front to back motion.
- Urinate into the toilet, then place the sterile container to capture the mid portion of the stream
- Complete urination into the toilet after the specimen is obtained
- Secure the container lid without touching the inside of the container

A urine culture and sensitivity test are usually performed on the clean-catch urine specimen to identify the organism for appropriate antimicrobial therapy (see Chapter 38).

C SULFONAMIDES

Sulfonamides have been the mainstay of treatment for UTIs for many years. Unfortunately, the incidence of sulfonamide-resistant bacteria has steadily increased. Sulfonamides have similar structures, functions, and therapeutic indications. These drugs are categorized as short acting, intermediate acting, topical, and long acting, although the long-acting sulfonamides are not available for use in the United States because of their ability to cause Stevens-Johnson syndrome. Sulfamethoxazole (SMZ) is an intermediate-acting sulfonamide that is only available in the United States in combination with the drug trimethoprim (TMP). The prototype sulfonamide, SMZ-TMP, is a combination of these two drugs. Table 42.1 provides a summary of sulfonamides and other selected drugs that are used to treat UTIs.

Nursing Management of the Patient Receiving P Sulfamethoxazole-Trimethoprim

Core Drug Knowledge

Pharmacotherapeutics

SMZ-TMP (Cotrimoxazole, Bactrim DS, Septra DS) has a broad range of therapeutic uses. It is indicated for uncomplicated UTIs and systemic infections caused by susceptible organisms. SMZ-TMP is frequently used for respiratory infections caused by *Haemophilus influenzae* or *Streptococcus pneumoniae*. It is an alternative treatment for *Legionella pneumophila* pneumonia. Gastrointestinal (GI) infections treated with SMZ-TMP include shigellosis and salmonella infection. SMZ-TMP concentrates in prostate and vaginal fluids and thus is an effective treatment for infections at these sites. SMZ-TMP is also effective treatment for sexually transmitted diseases, such as acute gonococcal urethritis and oropharyngeal gonorrhea. In some circumstances, SMZ-TMP may be used for skin and skin structure community-acquired MRSA.

For patients with HIV, SMZ-TMP is used for prophylaxis and treatment of *Pneumocystis jiroveci* pneumonia (formerly known as *P. carinii*) and toxoplasma encephalitis.

Pharmacokinetics

SMZ-TMP is completely absorbed following oral administration. It is metabolized in the liver to inactive by-products and excreted primarily in the urine. Peak plasma levels generally occur within 4 hours. After intravenous (IV) administration of SMZ-TMP, peak plasma levels occur in approximately 1 hour; the half-life is age dependent. SMZ-TMP is well distributed throughout the body, crosses the blood–brain barrier and the placenta, and is excreted in breast milk.

Pharmacodynamics

SMZ-TMP inhibits microorganisms by interfering with the synthesis of tetrahydrofolic acid (THF). Reduced availability of THF inhibits thymidine synthesis and subsequently DNA synthesis. SMZ, which is structurally similar to para-aminobenzoic acid (PABA), displaces PABA and blocks the synthesis of dihydrofolic acid, which is an interim step in the production of tetrahydrofolic acid. TMP binds to bacterial dihydrofolate reductase (in preference to human dihydrofolate reductase), also preventing the formation of THF. Although TMP and SMX are weak bactericidal agents when given alone, the combination is highly bactericidal. The presence of necrotic tissue, pus, or serum interferes with the action of SMZ-TMP because these materials contain PABA.

Contraindications and Precautions

SMZ-TMP is contraindicated in patients with hypersensitivity to sulfonamides, deficiency of glucose-6-phosphate dehydrogenase (G6PD) or other folate deficiency disorders, porphyria (porphobilinogen in urine), and urinary obstruction. Patients with G6PD deficiency may develop dose-related hemolytic anemia. SMZ-TMP is used cautiously in patients with hepatic or renal failure. Patients with hypersensitivity to thiazide diuretics or sulfonylureas may have cross-sensitivity to sulfonamides because of the related sulfa structures of these drugs.

Use in pregnant women at term, in children younger than 2 months (except for treating congenital toxoplasmosis), and in mothers nursing infants younger than 2 months is also contraindicated because sulfonamides may promote kernicterus (staining of certain areas of the brain by bilirubin) in the newborn by displacing bilirubin from plasma proteins.

Adverse Effects

SMZ-TMP is well tolerated in routine use. However, in patients with HIV, the adverse effect rate is 25% to 50%, with many of the reactions being severe. Although nausea, vomiting, and diarrhea occur most frequently with SMZ-TMP, there are three classic potential adverse reactions to this drug: hematologic effects (such as anemia), allergic reactions, and crystalluria.

Hematologic effects are related to the direct action of SMZ-TMP on bone marrow. SMZ-TMP can induce megaloblastic anemia in patients with folate deficiency. Other blood

TABLE 42.1	Summary of Selected Drugs to Treat Urinary Tract Infections		
Drug (Trade) Name	**Selected Indications**	**Route and Dosage Range**	**Pharmacokinetics**
Ⓒ Sulfonamides			
Ⓟ sulfamethoxazole-trimethoprim (SMZ-TMP; Bactrim) single strength (SS): 80 mg TMP/400 mg SMZ; double strength (DS): 160 mg TMP/800 mg SMZ; pediatric suspension: 40 mg TMP/200 mg SMZ per tsp (5 mL)	UTIs, otitis media, acute bronchitis, skin or soft tissue infections	*Adult:* 1 DS or 2 SS or 4 tsp suspension q 12 h for 10–14 d *Alternate:* 6 tablets at one time *Child >2 mo:* Up to 10 kg: 1 tsp; 11–20 kg: 2 tsp or 1 SS tab; 21–30 kg: 3 tsp or 1.5 SS tab; 31–40 kg: 4 tsp or 2 SS tab or 1 DS tab for 10–14 d	*Onset:* Varies *Duration:* 6–12 h $t_{1/2}$: 8–12 h
	Diarrhea or shigella	Same dose as above but stop after 5 days	
	PCP	*Adult and child:* 15–20 mg/kg TMP and 75–100 mg/kg SMZ in 24 h in divided doses every 6 h for 14–21 d *Adult:* 1 DS every day	
	PCP prophylaxis	*Child:* 150 mg/m²/d TMP with 750 mg/m²/d SMZ in equally divided doses 2 ×/d on 3 consecutive days per week	
sulfadiazine	Chancroid, trachoma, inclusion conjunctivitis, nocardiosis	*Adult:* PO, initially 2–4 g, followed by 2–4 g, divided into 3–6 doses, every 24 h *Child >2 mo:* PO, initially 1/2 the 24-h dose of 150 mg/kg or 4 g/m², divided into 4–6 doses, every 24 h, with a maximum of 6 g every 24 h.	*Onset:* Varies *Duration:* Unknown $t_{1/2}$: Unknown
Sulfisoxazole/erythromycin (Eryzole, Pediazole)	Otitis media	*Adult:* PO, 400 mg erythromycin/1,200 mg sulfisoxazole (10 mL) every 6 h *Child >2 mo:* PO, 50 mg/kg/d (erythromycin component) and 150 mg/kg/d (sulfisoxazole component) in 3 or 4 divided doses for 10 d	*Onset:* Varies *Duration:* Unknown $t_{1/2}$: 4.5–7.8 h
sulfasalazine (Azulfidine)	Ulcerative colitis	*Adult:* PO 3–4 g/d in evenly divided doses not exceeding 8-hour intervals; maintenance, 2 g/d in divided doses not exceeding 8-h intervals; *Child >6 y:* PO, 40–60 mg/kg/d divided in 3–6 doses; maintenance 30 mg/kg/d divided in 4 doses up to a maximum of 2 g/d	*Onset:* 1 h *Duration:* 6–12 h $t_{1/2}$: 5–10 h
	Rheumatoid arthritis	*Adult PO:* 0.5–1 g/d once daily or in divided doses twice daily; maintenance, 1 g twice daily up to a maximum of 3 g/d *Child >6 y:* PO, 30–50 mg/kg/d in 2 evenly divided doses up to a maximum of 2 g/d	
	Crohn's disease	*Adult:* PO, 3–6 g/d in divided doses	
fosfomycin (Monurol)	UTIs	*Adult:* PO, 3 g, one time only *Child <18 y:* not recommended	*Onset:* Rapid *Duration:* Unknown $t_{1/2}$: 5.7 h
Ⓒ Urinary Tract Antiseptics			
methenamine (Hiprex, Urex)	UTIs	*Adult:* PO, 1 g >qid *Child 6–12 y:* PO, 500 mg qid; <6 y: PO, 50 mg/kg in 3 divided doses	*Onset:* Rapid *Duration:* Unknown $t_{1/2}$: 3–6 h
nitrofurantoin (Furadantin, Macrodantin, Macrobid)	UTIs	*Adult:* 50–100 mg qid 10–14 d; suppressive history: 50–100 mg PO hs *Child >1 mo:* 5–7 mg/kg/d in 4 divided doses; suppressive history: 1 mg/kg/d	*Onset:* Rapid *Duration:* Unknown $t_{1/2}$: 20–60 min
Ⓒ Urinary Tract Analgesic			
phenazopyridine (Pyridium)	UTIs	*Adult:* PO, 200 mg tid after meals *Child 6–12 y:* 12 mg/kg/d in three divided doses	*Onset:* Rapid *Duration:* Unknown $t_{1/2}$: Unknown

dyscrasias, such as hemolytic anemia, agranulocytosis, leukopenia, thrombocytopenia, and aplastic anemia, may occur. Patients at high risk for folate deficiency are elderly adults, patients with long-term alcoholism, patients with malabsorption disorders, and patients with malnutrition.

Allergic reactions are common. SMZ-TMP is associated with several cutaneous reactions, including urticaria, maculopapular rashes, pruritus, contact dermatitis, and erythema nodosum. More severe reactions, such as Stevens-Johnson syndrome and exfoliative dermatitis, have been reported. Photosensitivity reactions may also occur and can continue for months after discontinuing the drug. Immunocompromised patients have a higher risk for photosensitive cutaneous eruptions. The mechanism for this increase in cutaneous eruptions is not clear.

Although the newer sulfonamides are much more soluble than older formulations, sulfonamides in general have poor solubility in water. If the urine volume and pH value drop, these drugs may crystallize in the renal tubules. This condition, called **crystalluria,** results in severe renal damage. To avoid crystalluria, patients should be instructed to maintain hydration by drinking at least 1.5 L of water every day.

Other potential adverse reactions may involve the central nervous system (CNS). Effects such as drowsiness, dizziness, and ataxia may occur. Additionally, depression and psychosis have been reported, although these effects are rare.

Drug Interactions

Certain sulfonamides are highly bound to serum proteins. When given in combination with other drugs that are also protein bound, sulfonamides may displace those drugs from their binding sites and enhance their action. This interaction occurs most frequently with drugs such as oral hypoglycemics, phenytoin, oral anticoagulants, and the antineoplastic drug methotrexate. The action of sulfonamides may be diminished when administered with local anesthetics, such as procaine, that are derived from PABA. Table 42.2 lists drugs that interact with SMZ-TMP.

Foods that can acidify the urine (such as cranberry juice) should be avoided. When the urine pH falls, the sulfonamides may precipitate and cause crystalluria.

Assessment of Relevant Core Patient Variables
Health Status

Carefully assess for potential hypersensitivity to sulfonamides and other contraindications for drug therapy. Cross-sensitivity may also occur with chemically related drugs, such as the thiazide or loop diuretics and the oral sulfonylureas. SMZ-TMP should not be administered to patients with hepatic or renal dysfunction, porphyria, blood dyscrasias, or G6PD deficiency. Closely monitor patients with folate deficiency or with increased risk for folate deficiency.

When therapy is anticipated to last more than 2 weeks, complete blood counts (CBCs) should be performed to establish a baseline value before starting therapy.

Life Span and Gender

Evaluate the patient's pregnancy or breast-feeding status. To avoid inducing kernicterus, do not administer SMZ-TMP and the other sulfonamides to pregnant or lactating women. Do not give these drugs to infants younger than 2 months. Monitor elderly patients taking warfarin closely. Studies have indicated they have an increased risk for upper GI bleeding when on SMZ-TMP therapy.

TABLE 42.2	Agents That Interact With P Sulfamethoxazole-Trimethoprim (SMZ-TMP)	
Interactants	**Effect and Significance**	**Nursing Management**
Anticoagulants	Sulfonamides inhibit the hepatic metabolism of oral anticoagulants, resulting in an increased risk for hemorrhage.	Monitor PT and INR closely. Monitor for signs of bleeding. Consult with prescriber about adjusting dose as needed.
cyclosporine	Although the mechanism is unknown, sulfonamides may increase the risk of nephrotoxicity associated with cyclosporine.	Monitor cyclosporine levels. Monitor serum creatinine frequently. Monitor I/O. Avoid coadministration if possible.
dofetilide	TMP inhibits the renal cation transport system responsible for dofetilide elimination.	Avoid coadministration if possible. Monitor for cardiac arrhythmias.
Hydantoins	Sulfonamides inhibit the hepatic metabolism of hydantoins, resulting in an increased risk for toxicity.	Monitor hydantoin levels. Monitor for speech, cognitive, or motor changes. Consult with prescriber about adjusting dose as needed.
methotrexate	Sulfonamides may displace methotrexate from protein binding sites and decrease renal clearance of drug. This results in an increased risk for methotrexate-induced bone marrow suppression.	Monitor closely for signs of hematologic toxicity. Monitor CBC. Consult with prescriber about adjusting dose as needed.
Oral Hypoglycemics	Trimethoprim may inhibit the metabolism of oral hypoglycemics, resulting in hypoglycemia.	Monitor blood glucose frequently. Monitor for signs of hypoglycemia.

Lifestyle, Diet, and Habits

Ask the patient about dietary intake of foods and fluids that acidify the urine, because many drugs are affected by urine's pH, and acidic urine increases the risk for crystalluria. Determine whether the patient has a condition that contraindicates an increased fluid intake, because increasing fluids decreases the potential for crystalluria. Assess the patient for alcohol use or abuse. Advise the patient to refrain from alcohol while taking SMZ-TMP, because it may cause a disulfiram-like reaction.

Environment

Evaluate the amount of time the patient spends outdoors because photosensitivity may occur. The patient should avoid direct sunlight; if going outdoors is unavoidable, encourage the patient to wear sunscreen with a minimum skin protective factor of 15 and appropriate clothing.

Nursing Diagnoses and Outcomes

- Pain related to altered comfort level (nausea, vomiting, diarrhea, dizziness, or headache) from adverse effects of SMZ-TMP

Desired outcome: The patient will develop strategies to cope with pain and take the drug as directed for the full course of therapy.

- Risk for Injury related to drug-induced hypersensitivity reactions, liver or kidney dysfunction, or blood dyscrasias

Desired outcome: By the end of therapy, the patient will be free from avoidable drug therapy–related injuries and infection.

- Risk for Impaired Tissue Integrity related to drug-induced photosensitivity

Desired outcome: The patient will take measures to protect his or her skin from prolonged sun exposure.

Planning and Intervention

Maximizing Therapeutic Effects

Administer SMZ-TMP 1 hour before or 2 hours after a meal with a full glass of water to enhance the absorption of the drug. Patients who experience adverse GI effects may take the drug with food.

Minimizing Adverse Effects

Administer SMZ-TMP with a full glass of water. Unless contraindicated, the patient's fluid intake should increase by 1.5 L/day. Increasing fluid intake decreases the potential for crystalluria and decreases the ability of bacteria to multiply because the urine is diluted. Encourage the patient to take precautions before exposure to the sun. When administering SMZ-TMP by the IV route, infuse the drug slowly, over 60 to 90 minutes. After completing the infusion, flush all lines to remove any residual SMZ-TMP.

Providing Patient and Family Education

- Teach patients the optimal way to take SMZ-TMP, advising them to take it 1 hour before or 2 hours after a meal. However, if the patients become nauseated, vomit, or cannot eat, the drug may be taken with meals to minimize discomfort.
- Teach interventions to decrease the risk for adverse effects. Patients should avoid foods that may acidify the urine and drink at least 1.5 L of water a day. They should also wear sunscreen and protective clothing when outside. These interventions decrease the risk of crystalluria and photosensitivity reactions, respectively.
- Explain the potential adverse effects of SMZ-TMP and advise patients to contact the prescriber immediately if a skin rash, fever, sore throat, blood in the urine, easy bruising, or nose bleeds develop.
- Advise patients to refrain from alcohol while taking SMZ-TMP.

Ongoing Assessment and Evaluation

Monitor patients for signs of hematologic dysfunction, such as sore throat, fever, bruising, or bleeding. Also, carefully monitor fluid intake and output of hospitalized patients. Optimally, patients should maintain an output of 1,500 mL daily. Monitor urine pH as well. Urine pH below 5.5 may potentiate crystalluria. Patients with acidic urine may need sodium bicarbonate to neutralize the urine. With prolonged therapy, monitor hematologic function and kidney function. Perform periodic urine testing to check for crystals. For patients receiving parenteral SMZ-TMP, monitor the IV site for signs of phlebitis.

Drug Closely Related to P Sulfamethoxazole-Trimethoprim

Of the short-acting sulfonamides, sulfisoxazole (Eryzole, Pediazole) is the most frequently used. Sulfisoxazole is highly water soluble, which minimizes the risk for crystalluria. It is also approved for management of otitis media.

Sulfadiazine, another oral short-acting sulfonamide, is a Food and Drug Administration (FDA)-indicated treatment and prophylaxis for AIDS and toxoplasmosis, as well as meningitis. A non-FDA indication for sulfadiazine is rheumatic fever. The drug is also used as adjunctive therapy in the management of malaria and toxoplasmosis encephalitis. Sulfadiazine is less soluble than sulfamethoxazole; thus, there is an increased risk of crystalluria.

CRITICAL THINKING SCENARIO

TEACHING STRATEGIES FOR SULFAMETHOXAZOLE-TRIMETHOPRIM (SMZ-TMP) THERAPY

Melissa Hawthorne, a 25-year-old graduate student, comes to the campus health clinic with a complaint of dysuria and urinary frequency and urgency. She is diagnosed with a UTI and given a prescription for SMZ-TMP.

1. Prepare some instructions related to drug therapy for Melissa, explaining the rationale for the instructions.

2. How would you vary the instructions if Melissa were 78 years of age or had a history of chronic heart failure?

MEMORY CHIP

Sulfamethoxazole-Trimethoprim (SMZ-TMP)

- Used for UTI, prophylaxis and treatment of *Pneumocystis jiroveci* pneumonia, and infection by *Legionella*, *Shigella*, or *Salmonella* species; *Haemophilus influenzae*; or *Streptococcus pneumoniae*
- Major contraindications: hypersensitivity, deficiencies in G6PD or other folates, porphyria, urinary obstruction, term pregnancy just ready to deliver, and age less than 2 months old
- Most common adverse effects: nausea, vomiting, diarrhea
- Most serious adverse effects: hematopoietic effects, crystalluria, Stevens-Johnson syndrome
- **Life span alert: to avoid inducing kernicterus, this drug should not be given to pregnant or breast-feeding women or to infants younger than 2 months old.**
- Maximizing therapeutic effects: Administer 1 hour before or 2 hours after a meal.
- Minimizing adverse effects: Increase fluids by 1.5 L/d to avoid crystalluria.
- Most important patient education: Teach the patient strategies to avoid disulfiram-like reactions, photosensitivity, and crystalluria.

Drugs Significantly Different From Ⓟ Sulfamethoxazole-Trimethoprim

Other Sulfonamides

Sulfasalazine

Sulfasalazine (Azulfidine), another short-acting sulfonamide, is given as an enteric-coated tablet for treating ulcerative colitis. Within the colon, sulfasalazine splits into its components aminosalicylic acid and sulfapyridine, which are the active antimicrobial metabolites. Its action begins in the bowel lumen instead of systemically. Its potential adverse effects and adverse reactions are similar to those of other sulfonamides.

Topical Sulfonamides

Mafenide (Sulfamylon) and silver sulfadiazine (Silvadene, SSD, Thermazene) are used topically to prevent bacterial or fungal infection in burn patients. Both drugs may be used in children who are at least 2 months of age. When applied, mafenide may cause pain or a burning feeling, whereas silver sulfadiazine does not. When topically applied, both drugs are absorbed in amounts that cause systemic effects.

It is important to use topical sulfonamides appropriately. Before applying them, cleanse the wound completely and remove dead or burned skin and other debris. Take care to remove all of the left-over medication when cleansing the wound. Wear sterile gloves to apply a thin layer (about 1/16 inch) to the wound. After application, leave the wound covered or uncovered, as ordered by the health care provider.

Drugs That Belong to Other Antibiotic Classes

Several other classes of antibiotics can also be used to manage UTIs.

Aminoglycoside drugs such as gentamicin, tobramycin, and amikacin are used for infections that originated in the urinary tract but have become systemic. This kind of infection is known as urosepsis. These drugs are all administered intravenously.

Cephalosporins may be given orally or parenterally. Oral drugs include cephalexin, cephradine, and cefadroxil. Ceftazidime and ceftriaxone may be given orally or parenterally. Although these drugs are effective, they offer no clear advantage over less expensive drugs.

The fluoroquinolones ciprofloxacin, norfloxacin, and ofloxacin are very effective for managing UTIs. Fluoroquinolones have a broad spectrum of activity that affects most microbes that cause UTIs. Many prescribers use these drugs as first-line agents, despite their expense, because of the increasing resistance to SMZ-TMP. Other prescribers use these drugs after treatment failure with SMZ-TMP.

The penicillin drugs ampicillin, amoxicillin, and amoxicillin-clavulanate may also be administered. Ampicillin may be given orally or parenterally. Other parenteral penicillin drugs include ticarcillin, mezlocillin, and piperacillin. Penicillins are useful against most microbes that cause UTI; however, some penicillin resistance has been reported among *Escherichia coli* isolates.

Tetracycline drugs are most useful in managing UTIs caused by *Chlamydia* species, but incidence of resistance is high among other causative microbes. Both tetracycline and doxycycline are effective against sensitive organisms.

BOX 42.1 FOCUS ON RESEARCH

UTI in Women

Juthani-Mehta, M., Quagliarello, V., Perrelli, E., et al. (2009). Clinical features to identify urinary tract infection in nursing home residents: a cohort study. *Journal of the American Geriatrics Society*, 57(6):963–970.

The Study

The objective of the study was to identify clinical features associated with bacteriuria plus pyuria in non-catheterized nursing home residents with clinically suspected urinary tract infection (UTI).

The researchers developed a prospective, observational cohort study utilizing 5 nursing homes in New Haven, Connecticut between the years 2005 to 2007. The study had 228 participants with 399 episodes of clinically suspected UTI with a urinalysis and urine culture performed; 36.8% of participants were found to have bacteriuria plus pyuria. The clinical features associated with bacteriuria plus pyuria were dysuria, change in character of urine, and change in mental status.

Conclusions

Dysuria, change in character of urine, and change in mental status were significantly associated with the combined outcome of bacteriuria plus pyuria. Absence of these clinical features identified residents at low risk of having bacteriuria plus pyuria, whereas presence of dysuria plus one or both of the other clinical features identified residents at high risk of having bacteriuria plus pyuria.

Nursing Implications

Elderly patients are more likely to be admitted to an acute care facility. They also have physical changes related to aging that increase the risk for UTI. The nurse should frequently assess elderly patients for dysuria, change in character of urine, and change in mental status because these symptoms are highly associated with UTI. Early identification of infection decreases the risk for complications of UTI such as urosepsis.

Fosfomycin

Fosfomycin (Monurol) is classified as a miscellaneous antibiotic. It works by inhibiting an enzyme, pyruvoyl transferase, which is critical in the synthesis of bacterial cell walls. Fosfomycin is active against most urinary tract pathogens and has a prolonged post-antibiotic effect of 3.4 to 4.7 hours. The drug is distributed to the kidneys, bladder wall, prostate, and seminal vesicles. Fosfomycin has been shown to cross the placenta; however, whether it enters breast milk is unknown. It is not metabolized, and excretion occurs through both urine and feces.

Fosfomycin is administered orally for acute UTI as a one-time dose, without regard to meals. Advise the patient to place the entire contents of a sachet containing the equivalent of 3 g of fosfomycin into 3 to 4 oz (1/2 cup) of water, then stir to dissolve it. It is best not to use hot water. The patient should take the medication immediately after dissolving the powder.

Fosfomycin is in FDA pregnancy category B. It is not recommended for children younger than 12 years.

The most frequent adverse effects with fosfomycin therapy are asthenia, diarrhea, dizziness, dyspepsia, headache, nausea and vomiting, rash, and vaginitis. Although rare, serious adverse effects such as angioedema, aplastic anemia, asthma exacerbation, cholestatic jaundice, hepatic necrosis, and toxic megacolon have been reported.

© URINARY TRACT ANTISEPTICS

Urinary tract antiseptics are drugs that work by local action because high serum levels are not achievable. Because of their local action, few systemic effects occur. No true prototype exists; thus, each drug is discussed separately here.

Methenamine

Methenamine (Hiprex, Urex) is indicated for suppressing or eliminating bacteriuria (bacteria in urine) associated with chronic cystitis and other chronic UTIs. It is effective against both gram-positive and gram-negative organisms. In fact, the only resistance to methenamine comes from organisms such as *Proteus vulgaris* and *Pseudomonas aeruginosa,* which raise urine pH.

In acidic urine, methenamine is hydrolyzed to ammonia and formaldehyde in the bladder. Because methenamine must be hydrolyzed into its components to be effective, it does not work for upper UTIs because the time through the upper urinary tract is insufficient for this action to occur. Additionally, patients with indwelling catheters have a constant outflow of urine, again negating the time needed for hydrolysis occur. Therefore, methenamine is not useful in patients with upper UTIs and indwelling catheters.

Methenamine is contraindicated in patients with hepatic dysfunction because ammonia is also a product of its hydrolysis. Patients with hepatic dysfunction cannot eliminate ammonia, and the high ammonia levels that result can adversely affect the CNS. Methenamine should not be given concurrently with sulfonamides because the combination forms an insoluble precipitate in acidic urine.

Adverse reactions are minimal. The most common are nausea, vomiting, and anorexia. Methenamine may also cause bladder irritation, dysuria, hematuria, and crystalluria when administered as long-term prophylaxis.

Nitrofurantoin

Nitrofurantoin (Furadantin, Macrodantin, Macrobid) is another synthetic urinary tract antiseptic. It works by interfering with several bacterial enzyme systems, which may explain the lack of bacterial resistance to it. Although nitrofurantoin has a broad spectrum of activity, it is not an effective systemic drug because it is rapidly excreted by the kidneys and thus does not achieve high blood levels. It is highly effective against gram-negative and gram-positive organisms in the urinary system because high concentrations are found in urine. Resistant microbes include *Enterobacter, Klebsiella, Proteus,* and *Pseudomonas* species.

Nitrofurantoin is available in two pill formulations: microcrystalline nitrofurantoin (Furadantin) and macrocrystalline nitrofurantoin (Macrodantin, Macrobid). Although both types of nitrofurantoin have equal therapeutic efficacy, macrocrystalline nitrofurantoin is absorbed more slowly and induces less GI distress.

Nitrofurantoin is contraindicated in patients with renal impairment, in infants younger than 1 month because of the possibility of hemolytic anemia, and in pregnant women at term. As previously mentioned, nitrofurantoin achieves high concentrations in urine but low concentrations in blood. In the presence of kidney dysfunction, its concentration in urine decreases and concentration in blood increases. This effect decreases the efficacy of treatment and increases the risk of toxic adverse effects. Nitrofurantoin should be used with caution in the elderly (because of their decreased renal function) and in patients with G6PD deficiency, anemia, vitamin B deficiency, diabetes mellitus, or electrolyte abnormalities. It is a pregnancy category B drug.

The most common adverse reactions are anorexia, nausea, and vomiting. Other adverse reactions include abdominal pain, diarrhea, parotitis, and pancreatitis. Hepatic reactions, including hepatitis, have occurred. Nitrofurantoin may induce an asthma attack in patients with a history of asthma. As with other urinary tract antiseptics, nitrofurantoin may cause hematopoietic effects, especially in patients with folate deficiency.

Nitrofurantoin has potentially serious adverse reactions. Peripheral neuropathy is one of the most serious toxic effects; however, it is reversible if detected early. Permanent damage may result if the drug is not discontinued. Peripheral neuropathy may be enhanced in debilitating diseases, such as diabetes mellitus, anemia, and vitamin B deficiency.

Nitrofurantoin is also associated with acute and chronic pulmonary reactions. Acute reactions are manifested by sudden onset of fever, cough, chills, myalgias, and dyspnea. As with other drugs, the effects are reversible if the drug is discontinued. Subacute pulmonary reactions develop over time with many of the same symptoms; however, diffuse interstitial pulmonary fibrosis may be irreversible. Subacute pulmonary reactions occur most frequently in patients on therapy longer than 6 months.

C URINARY TRACT ANALGESIC

Phenazopyridine (Pyridium) is used frequently for UTIs but does not itself have any antibacterial activity. It is excreted in the urine, where it exerts a topical analgesic effect. It is indicated for the symptomatic relief of pain, burning, frequency, and urgency caused by the irritation that infection produces in the urinary tract mucosa. The precise mechanism of action is not known. Phenazopyridine is contraindicated for patients with known hypersensitivity or renal insufficiency. Adverse reactions include headache, rash, pruritus, and GI disturbances. Phenazopyridine is an azo dye, which colors the patient's urine orange or red. It is important to inform the patient to expect this change in urine color.

Phenazopyridine is available as an over-the-counter (OTC) medication (AZO Urinary Pain Relief). It is important to teach patients that they must contact their provider for urinary pain even if the pain is relieved by the OTC product because an untreated UTI may become a more serious problem such as pyelonephritis. Chronic use of phenazopyridine may cause a cumulative toxicity, resulting in hemolytic anemia, thrombocytopenia, acute renal failure, hepatitis, and skin pigmentation.

CHAPTER SUMMARY

- A urinary tract infection (UTI) is caused by microorganisms infecting any structure within the urinary system.
- UTI is the most frequent type of infection in the United States.
- Sulfamethoxazole-trimethoprim (SMZ-TMP) is the prototype sulfonamide, which is the drug class most commonly used to treat UTI.
- Many other drug classes may be used to treat UTI. These include aminoglycosides, cephalosporins, fluoroquinolones, penicillins, tetracyclines, and fosfomycin.
- Urinary tract antiseptics work directly in the urinary tract and have minimal systemic activity. These drugs include methenamine, nitrofurantoin, nalidixic acid, and cinoxacin.
- Phenazopyridine has no antimicrobial effects. It is used as a urinary analgesic in combination with antimicrobial drugs.

QUESTIONS FOR STUDY AND REVIEW

1. In addition to UTI, which other diseases or disorders are treated with SMZ-TMP?
2. Why are sulfonamides ineffective against organisms that do not synthesize their own folate?
3. What is the difference between antibiotics used to manage UTI and urinary tract antiseptics?
4. What is the purpose of prescribing phenazopyridine (Pyridium) for a UTI, if it has no antibacterial activity?
5. What are the key points in the proper application of a topical sulfonamide cream?

NEED MORE HELP?

Chapter 42 of the Study Guide to Accompany *Drug Therapy in Nursing*, 4th Edition, contains NCLEX-style questions and other learning activities to reinforce your understanding of the concepts presented in this chapter. For additional information or to purchase the study guide, visit thePoint.

REFERENCES

Béraud, G., Pierre-François, S., Foltzer, A., et al. (2009). Cotrimoxazole for treatment of cerebral toxoplasmosis: an observational cohort study during 1994-2006. *American Journal of Tropical Medicine and Hygiene*, 80(4):583–587.

Caterino, J. M., Weed, S. G., Espinola, J. A, & Camargo, C. A. Jr. (2009). National trends in emergency department antibiotic prescribing for elders with urinary tract infection, 1996–2005. *Academic Emergency Medicine*, 16(6):500–507.

Facts and Comparisons. (2010). *Drug facts and comparisons*. Philadelphia, PA: Lippincott Williams & Wilkins.

Fischer, H. D, Juurlink, D. N., Mamdani, M. M., et al. (2010). Hemorrhage During Warfarin Therapy Associated With Cotrimoxazole and Other Urinary Tract Anti-infective Agents. *Arch Intern Med*, 170(7):617–621.

Hooten, T. M., Stamm, W. E. (2009). *Up To Date*. Acute cystitis in women. Retrieved from *http://uptodate.com*.

Kashanian, J., Hakimian, P., Blute, M. Jr. (2008). Nitrofurantoin: the return of an old friend in the wake of growing resistance. *BJU International*, 102(11):1634–1637.

Koda-Kimbal, M. A, Young, L. Y., Kradian, W. A., et al. (2008). *Applied Therapeutics: The Clinical Use of Drugs*, Philadelphia, PA: Lippincott Williams & Wilkins.

Kovacs, J. A., & Masur, H. (2009). Evolving health effects of Pneumocystis: one hundred years of progress in diagnosis and treatment. *Journal of the American Medical Association*, 301(24):2578–2585.

Magilner, D., Byerly, M. M., & Cline, D. M. (2008). The prevalence of community-acquired methicillin-resistant Staphylococcus aureus (CA-MRSA) in skin abscesses presenting to the pediatric emergency department. *North Carolina Medical Journal*, 69(5):351–354.

May, D. B. (2009). *Up To Date*. Trimethoprim-sulfamethoxazole: An overview. Retrieved from *http://uptodate.com*.

Micromedex Healthcare Series. Retrieved from *http://thomsonhc.com*.

Roberts, S. S., & Kazragis, R. J. (2009). Methicillin-resistant Staphylococcus aureus infections in U.S. service members deployed to Iraq. *Military Medicine*, 174(4):408–411.

Schito, G. C., Naber, K. G., & Botto, H. (2009). The ARESC study: an international survey on the antimicrobial resistance of pathogens involved in uncomplicated urinary tract infections, *International Journal of Antimicrobial Agents*, Jun 6.

Tatro, D. S. (2009). *Drug interaction facts*. Philadelphia, PA: Lippincott Williams & Wilkins.

Tietjen, P. A., & Bartlett, J. G. (2009). Prophylaxis against Pneumocystis carinii (P. jirovecii) in HIV-infected patients, *Up To Date*. Retrieved from *http://uptodate.com*.

Thi, L., Shaw, D., & Bird, J. (2009). Warfarin Potentiation: A Review of the "FAB-4" Significant Drug Interactions. *The Consultant Pharmacist*, 24(3):227–230.

Wanat, K. A., Anadkat, M. J., & Klekotka, P. A. (2009). Seasonal variation of Stevens-Johnson syndrome and toxic epidermal necrolysis associated with trimethoprim-sulfamethoxazole. *Journal of the American Academy of Dermatology*, 60(4): 589–594.

Drugs Treating Mycobacterial Infections

Learning Objectives

At the completion of this chapter the student will:

1. Identify core drug knowledge about drugs that are used for treating mycobacterial infections.

2. Identify core patient variables relevant to drugs that are used for treating mycobacterial infections.

3. Relate the interaction of core drug knowledge to core patient variables for drugs that are used for treating mycobacterial infections.

4. Generate a nursing plan of care from the interactions between core drug knowledge and core patient variables for drugs that are used for treating mycobacterial infections.

5. Describe nursing interventions to maximize therapeutic and minimize adverse effects for drugs that are used for treating mycobacterial infections.

6. Determine key points for patient and family education for drugs that are used for treating mycobacterial infections.

Key Terms

chemoprophylaxis
leprosy

Hansen disease
MDR TB

Mycobacteria
XDR TB

Drugs Treating Mycobacterial Infections

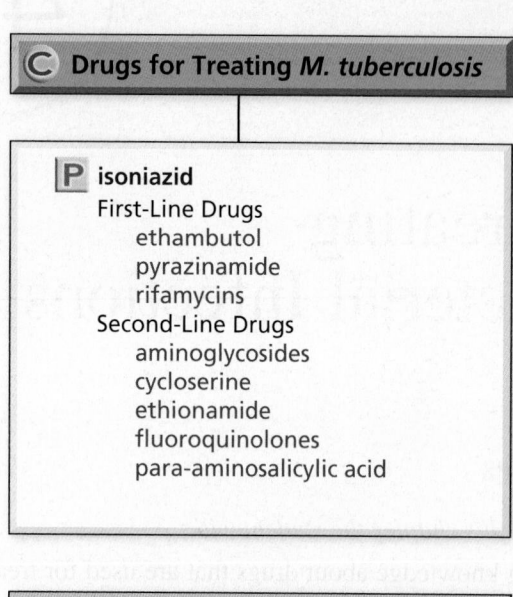

C Drugs for Treating *M. tuberculosis*

P isoniazid
First-Line Drugs
ethambutol
pyrazinamide
rifamycins
Second-Line Drugs
aminoglycosides
cycloserine
ethionamide
fluoroquinolones
para-aminosalicylic acid

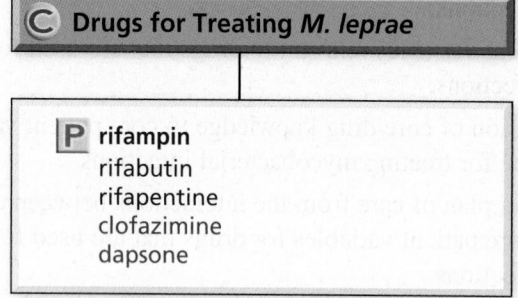

C Drugs for Treating *M. leprae*

P rifampin
rifabutin
rifapentine
clofazimine
dapsone

The symbol **C** indicates the drug class.
Drugs in **bold type** marked with the symbol **P** are prototypes.
Drugs in blue type are closely related to the prototype.
Drugs in red type are significantly different from the prototype.
Drugs in black type with no symbol are also used in drug therapy; no prototype.

This chapter discusses pharmacologic management of mycobacterial infections. **Mycobacteria** are slow-growing microbes that require prolonged treatment, generally with multiple medications. Many of the antimycobacterial drugs may be used for more than one type of infection. Table 43.1 presents a summary of antimycobacterial drugs.

Although many *Mycobacterium* species exist, this chapter focuses on three species: *M. tuberculosis*, *M. leprae*, and *M. avium*. The prototype drug for treating *M. tuberculosis* infection is isoniazid (INH), and the prototype for treating *M. leprae* infection is rifampin. The drugs of choice for *M. avium* are clarithromycin and azithromycin; both of these macrolide drugs are discussed in Chapter 40.

PATHOPHYSIOLOGY

Tuberculosis

Tuberculosis (TB) is a mycobacterial infection that is found most frequently in the lungs; however, it may invade any organ of the body. The two types of TB are *Mycobacterium tuberculosis hominis* (human) and *Mycobacterium tuberculosis bovis* (bovine). Human TB is an airborne disease spread by tiny, invisible particles called droplet nuclei. Bovine TB is spread through the gastrointestinal (GI) system after drinking milk from infected cows. In the United States, bovine TB is very rare because dairy herds are strictly monitored, and pasteurization of milk is widespread. Symptoms of active TB include night sweats, cough, low-grade fever, fatigue, weight loss, and anorexia.

TABLE 43.1	Summary of Selected Antimycobacterial Drugs		
Drug (Trade) Name	**Selected Indications**	**Route and Dosage Range**	**Pharmacokinetics**
P isoniazid (Nydrazid; Laniazid)	TB in conjunction with other drug therapy, prophylaxis of TB	*Adult:* PO, active TB, 5 mg/kg/d up to 300 mg in single dose; prophylaxis, 300 mg/d in single dose *Child:* PO, active TB, 10–20 mg/kg/d; prophylaxis, 10 mg/kg/d in single dose	*Onset:* Varies *Duration:* 24 h $t_{1/2}$: 1–4 h
clofazimine (Lamprene)	Leprosy	*Adult:* 50 mg qd self-administered and 300 mg q mo *Child:* 1 mg/kg/d	*Onset:* 1 h *Duration:* Unknown $t_{1/2}$: Terminal 8 d, tissue 70 d
cycloserine (Seromycin Pulvules)	Tuberculosis	*Adult:* PO, 250 mg every 12 h × 2 wk, then 250 mg every 6–8 h *Child:* PO, 10–20 mg/kg/d every 12 h	*Onset:* Rapid *Duration:* Unknown $t_{1/2}$: 10 h
dapsone (Avlosulfon)	Leprosy	*Adult:* PO, 100 mg qd *Child:* 1–2 mg/kg/d	*Onset:* 2 h *Duration:* Unknown $t_{1/2}$: 30 h
ethambutol (Myambutol; *Canadian:* Etibi)	TB in conjunction with other drug therapy, prophylaxis of TB	*Adult:* PO, mg/kg/d as single oral dose; retreatment, 25 mg/kg/d, reduced after 60 d to 15 mg/kg/d once daily *Child:* Not recommended for children younger than 13 y	*Onset:* Rapid *Duration:* 20–24 h $t_{1/2}$: 3.3 h
ethionamide (Trecator)	Tuberculosis	*Adult:* PO, 15–20 mg/kg/d in 2–3 divided doses *Child:* PO, 10–20 mg/kg/d in 2–3 divided doses	*Onset:* Rapid *Duration:* 9.5 h $t_{1/2}$: 2–3 h
para-aminosalicylic acid (PAS, Paser)	Tuberculosis Crohn's disease	*Adult:* PO, 4 g 3 × d *Child:* PO, 275–420 mg/kg/d in 4 divided doses *Adult:* PO, 500 mg 3 × d	*Onset:* Rapid *Duration:* Unknown $t_{1/2}$: 26.4 min
pyrazinamide	TB in conjunction with other drug therapy, prophylaxis of TB	*Adult:* PO, 15–30 mg/d once daily *Child:* Same	*Onset:* Rapid *Duration:* 9.5 h $t_{1/2}$: 9–10 h
rifabutin (Mycobutin)	TB, leprosy, MAC	*Adult:* 300 mg PO qd, may be given 150 mg bid to decrease GI distress *Child:* Not approved	*Onset:* 1 h *Duration:* Unknown $t_{1/2}$: 16–69 h
rifapentine (Priftin)	TB	*Adult and child >12 y:* 600 mg 2 × wk for 2 mo, then 1 × wk for 4 mo *Child:* Not recommended	*Onset:* 5–6 h *Duration:* Unknown $t_{1/2}$: 13 h

Human TB can become a devastating disease, although the bacteria themselves are not particularly virulent. The damage to the human host is a result of a hypersensitivity response evoked by the bacteria. Untreated TB may result in death, whereas inadequately treated TB may result in multidrug-resistant TB.

TB may be latent or active. Latent tuberculosis infection (LTBI) occurs when the patient has been infected with *M. tuberculosis*, but does not have active disease and is not infectious. Approximately 10% of patients with LTBI will develop active TB later in life. The diagnosis is made by administering a purified protein derivative (PPD) test, the screening test for TB. The PPD test involves a solution that is placed intradermally on the forearm of the patient. After 48 to 72 hours, the injection site is evaluated for induration. More than 10 mm of induration at the site of injection (or 5 mm of induration for an immunocompromised patient) is a positive reaction. Another method for diagnosing LTBI is Interferon Gamma Release Assays (IGRA) testing, sometimes referred to as ELISPOT. There are two available tests: the QuantiFERON-T Gold (QFT-G) and TB SPOT.TB. The IGRA test are more sensitive than the PPD and the results are obtainable in 24 hours. Another advantage of IGRA testing is that they are unlikely to produce false positives because of Bacillus Calmette-Guérin (BCG) vaccination, or because of the boosting effect from serial PPD testing that is done with heath care workers and other people at high risk of exposure. The BCG vaccine is not used in the United States because of its variable efficacy, however, it is used extensively in countries throughout the world (Box 43.1).

People with latent TB may benefit from chemoprophylaxis. Chemoprophylaxis greatly decreases the potential for LTBI to progress to active disease. The CDC has identified certain groups that have an increased risk for the development of active disease (Box 43.2)

Active TB results from activation of previously healed primary lesions. Activation may occur as the body's defenses decline as the patient ages or acquires other diseases that weaken the immune system. Active TB is diagnosed by chest radiography, sputum smear microscopy, and then sputum culture and drug susceptibility testing. Patients with active or reactivated TB require multidrug therapy (MDT) for 6 to 24 months. Therapy is based on the susceptibility of the infecting organism and the immunocompetence of the patient. Immunocompromised patients need a longer duration of therapy because their ability to fight infections is reduced.

Treatment of active TB is done by Direct Observed Treatment (DOTS), Short Course (Box 43.3); inadequate drug therapy due to patient nonadherence is the most common cause of multidrug-resistant TB. Multi-drug resistant tuberculosis (**MDR-TB**) is defined as TB that is resistant at least to isoniazid (INH) and rifampin, the two most powerful first-line anti-TB drugs. Extensively drug resistant TB (**XDR TB**) is defined TB that is resistant to

isoniazid and rifampin and to any fluoroquinolone and at least one of three injectable second-line drugs (amikacin, kanamycin, or capreomycin). These types of TB infection require extremely close supervision throughout treatment.

BOX 43.1 FOCUS ON RESEARCH

Vaccine on the Horizon?

Sander, C. R., Pathan, A. A., Beveridge, N. E., et al. (2009). Safety and immunogenicity of a new tuberculosis vaccine, MVA85A, in Mycobacterium tuberculosis-infected individuals, *American Journal of Respiratory and Critical Care Medicine*, 179(8):724–733.

The Study

The purpose of the study is to evaluate the safety and immunogenicity of a leading new TB vaccine, recombinant Modified Vaccinia Ankara expressing Antigen 85A (MVA85A) in individuals with latent TB infection (LTBI). The researchers completed a phase I clinical study with patients recruited from TB clinics in Oxford and London, England. Patients were assessed clinically and had blood samples drawn for immunological analysis over a 52-week period after vaccination with MVA85A. Thoracic computed tomography scans were performed at baseline and at 10 weeks after vaccination. The study determined that MVA85A is safe and highly immunogenic in individuals with LTBI. Further trials in TB-endemic areas are needed.

Nursing Implications

The United States does not currently utilize a vaccine for TB prophylaxis, but many countries throughout the world use the Bacillus Calmette-Guérin vaccine (BCG). BCG has a variable efficacy and does not provide life-long immunity. Because multi-drug resistant TB has become a global concern, the need for a more efficacious vaccine has become even more important. The nurse must consistently update his/her knowledge regarding infectious diseases such as TB and potential new treatment options for our patients.

Box 43.2 CDC RECOMMENDATIONS FOR TREATMENT OF LTBI

Chemoprophylaxis is considered for patients with a positive PPD greater than 10 mm if they are:

- Recent arrivals (less than 5 years) from high-prevalence countries
- Injectable drug users
- Residents and employees of high-risk settings (e.g., correctional institutions, nursing homes, homeless shelters, hospitals)
- Mycobacteriology laboratory personnel
- Persons with clinical conditions that make them high risk (e.g., diabetes, chronic malnutrition, ESRD, pre-existing lung disease)
- Children less than 4 years of age or children or adolescents exposed to adults in high-risk categories

Chemoprophylaxis is considered for patients with a positive PPD greater than 5 mm if they are:

- HIV infected persons
- Recent contacts of a TB case
- Patients with fibrotic lung changes consistent with old TB
- Patients with organ transplants
- Patients who are immunocompromised (e.g., prolonged corticosteroid therapy, taking TNF-Alpha antagonists)

THE FIVE ELEMENTS OF THE DOTS STRATEGY FOR THE TREATMENT OF TUBERCULOSIS

- Political commitment with increased and sustained financing
- Case detection through quality-assured bacteriology
- Standardized treatment, with supervision and patient support
- An effective drug supply and management system
- Monitoring and evaluation system, with impact measurement

Leprosy

Leprosy was first described in 1873 by G. A. Hansen; thus, its alternate name is **Hansen disease.** It is a chronic infectious disease caused by *M. leprae,* an acid-fast, rod-shaped bacillus. The disease affects mainly the skin, the peripheral nerves, the mucosa of the upper respiratory tract, and the eyes.

The two classifications of leprosy are paucibacillary leprosy (PB) and multibacillary leprosy (MB). They can be classified on the basis of skin-smear results or clinical manifestations. In the classification based on skin smears, patients who have negative smears at all sites are grouped as having PB, whereas those who have positive smears at any site are grouped as having MB. However, in practice, most prescribers use clinical criteria for classifying the disease and deciding the appropriate treatment regimen for individual patients because skin-smear services are not always available or dependable. The clinical system of classification uses the number of skin lesions and nerves involved as the basis for grouping leprosy. Patients with fewer than five lesions are diagnosed with PB leprosy, and patients with six or more lesions are diagnosed with MB leprosy.

The correct classification is important because the treatment regimens differ between the two types of leprosy. Like TB, leprosy must be treated with a multidrug regimen for 6 to 12 months. For MB leprosy, rifampin, clofazimine, and dapsone are used, and for PB leprosy, rifampin and dapsone are used. For patients with single-skin lesion PB leprosy, ofloxacin and minocycline are used in combination with rifampin.

Mycobacterium Avium Complex

Mycobacterium avium complex (MAC) is the term used to describe an opportunistic infection caused by two similar types of bacteria named *M. avium* and *M. avium-intracellulare.* Because these bacteria are so similar, they are referred to together as a "complex." However, *M. avium* is the predominant infective organism seen in most MAC infections in people with AIDS.

M. avium and *M. intracellulare* are very common. They are found in water, soil, dust, and food, and almost everyone has them in their body. A healthy immune system controls MAC, but immunocompromised people can develop a MAC infection. MAC can be localized or disseminated (sometimes called DMAC). It often occurs in the lungs, intestines, bone marrow, liver, and spleen. Symptoms of MAC include high fevers, chills, diarrhea, weight loss, stomachaches, fatigue, and anemia. When MAC disseminates, it can cause blood infections, hepatitis, pneumonia, and other serious problems.

MAC bacteria can mutate and develop resistance to pharmacotherapy. As with other mycobacterial infections, a combination of antibacterial drugs is used to manage MAC. Immunocompromised patients are started on MAC prophylaxis when their T-cell count drops below 50. Once an immunocompromised patient develops a MAC infection, treatment must continue for life to avoid recurrence. The drugs of choice for MAC prophylaxis and treatment are azithromycin and clarithromycin. These drugs are discussed in Chapter 40. Additional drugs that may be used against MAC include rifampin, rifabutin, and clofazimine, which are described in this chapter in the section on drugs for *M. leprae* infection.

C DRUGS FOR TREATING *MYCOBACTERIUM TUBERCULOSIS* INFECTION

Antitubercular drugs are divided into two major categories: first- and second-line drugs. First-line drugs are those that are effective for treatment and have manageable toxicities. First-line drugs include isoniazid, rifampin, rifapentine, rifabutin, ethambutol, and pyrazinamide. Because TB can easily become drug resistant, combination therapy with three to four drugs is common

Isoniazid is referred to as INH, an abbreviation related to its clinical structure. Isoniazid is included in all therapeutic regimens, except in those for INH-resistant TB. For that reason, INH is the prototype for antitubercular drugs. Table 43.1 presents a summary of drugs used to treat TB.

Nursing Management of the Patient Receiving P Isoniazid

Core Drug Knowledge

Pharmacotherapeutics

INH is an antibacterial drug used to treat or prevent TB and other susceptible mycobacterial infections. *Mycobacterium* organisms generally considered susceptible to INH therapy include *M. avium, M. bovis, M. intracellulare, M. kansasii, M. szulgai,* and *M. xenopi.*

Pharmacokinetics

INH is administered orally and intramuscularly. It is absorbed rapidly from the GI tract, with peak serum levels attained within 12 hours. It is distributed into all body tissues and fluids and crosses the blood–brain barrier to achieve therapeutic levels in the cerebrospinal fluid (CSF). It also crosses the placenta and is distributed into breast milk. INH is metabolized in the liver to inactive metabolites. About 75% of the drug and its metabolites are excreted in the urine, and the rest is excreted in the feces, saliva, and sputum.

Pharmacodynamics

INH is bactericidal or bacteriostatic, depending on the drug concentration within an infected site and the susceptibility of the organism. It works by disrupting the synthesis of the bacterial cell wall. Some patients have experienced adverse effects after ingesting tyramine-containing foods. This interaction suggests that INH may inhibit plasma monoamine oxidase, although this action has not been documented. INH has no direct effect on the body.

Contraindications and Precautions

INH is contraindicated in patients with acute hepatic disease and in patients with a history of INH-induced hepatic disease. INH should be used with caution in patients with chronic hepatic disease, alcoholism, or severe renal impairment because these conditions can prolong elimination of the drug, increasing the likelihood of adverse reactions.

INH should also be given with caution to patients with diabetes mellitus, malnutrition, or alcoholism because its effects (antagonism or increased excretion) on pyridoxine (vitamin B_6) can cause peripheral neuropathy in these patients. Pyridoxine generally is given concurrently with INH to decrease the risk for this adverse effect.

Data conflict about INH use during pregnancy; it is classified as a U.S. Food and Drug Administration (FDA) pregnancy category C drug. Because INH is given as part of a multidrug regimen to combat TB, studies have not been able to elicit the exact risk that INH poses to the fetus. INH appears to be safe for use during lactation.

Adverse Effects

The major adverse effect of INH therapy is hepatotoxicity, which is a Black Box warning. Hepatitis, elevated hepatic enzyme levels (aspartate transaminase, alanine transaminase), bilirubinemia, and jaundice may also occur.

Another frequent adverse effect is peripheral neuropathy. This effect may present with paresthesias in the hands and feet. As previously mentioned, malnourished patients and those with diabetes and alcoholism have a higher risk for this adverse effect. Encephalopathy, convulsions, memory impairment, toxic psychosis, and optic neuritis have been reported, but these events are rare.

INH may induce endocrine changes, such as pellagra, hyperglycemia, metabolic acidosis, and gynecomastia. Because it alters vitamin D metabolism, INH may cause hypocalcemia and hypophosphatemia.

Infrequently, INH may also cause adverse effects in the GI, hematologic, and integumentary systems. GI effects include diarrhea, abdominal pain, nausea, and vomiting.

Hematologic effects are agranulocytosis, hemolysis with anemia, sideroblastic anemia, aplastic anemia, pancytopenia, and thrombocytopenia. Integumentary effects include maculopapular rash, acneiform rash, or exfoliative dermatitis. Injection site reaction can be seen with intramuscular (IM) administration of INH. Rarely, INH may cause interstitial nephritis or central nervous system (CNS) toxicity, resulting in seizures.

Drug Interactions

Isoniazid interacts with a variety of drugs, including antiseizure drugs (carbamazepine and the hydantoins), alcohol, aluminum-based antacids, benzodiazepines, disulfiram, enflurane, ketoconazole, meperidine, warfarin, and rifampin. Table 43.2 lists drugs that interact with INH.

Because INH has some monoamine oxidase inhibitor activity, interactions may occur with tyramine-containing foods. INH may also interact with foods containing histamine.

Assessment of Relevant Core Patient Variables

Health Status

Prophylaxis with INH is given for 9 months, whereas treatment for active TB may last up to 24 months. Assess for pre-existing hepatic disease or disorders such as drug or alcohol abuse, which would predispose the patient to hepatic toxic effects. Coordinate baseline liver function tests (LFTs) and schedule serial LFTs throughout therapy. Some prescribers believe all patients should have these baseline tests, whereas others believe only those patients with an increased risk should be tested.

Evaluate the patient for other pre-existing disorders, such as diabetes mellitus or anemias,. Patients with diabetes should have a baseline A_{1C} evaluation because INH may cause hyperglycemia. This test indicates the general glucose control for the patient over the preceding 3 months. Patients with pre-existing anemias should have a baseline complete blood count (CBC) because they are at risk for hematologic disorders.

Life Span and Gender

INH is classified as FDA pregnancy category C. Therefore, evaluate the patient's pregnancy or breast-feeding status. Although no studies have demonstrated potential fetal risk, INH use in pregnant women should be restricted to active TB therapy. Pregnant women who need INH prophylaxis should begin therapy after delivery because the risk that TB will become active increases after childbirth. Assess infants of nursing mothers for signs of peripheral neuritis and hepatitis.

Determine the patient's age before therapy begins. Patients 35 years or older are three times more likely to develop drug-induced hepatitis than those younger than 35 years. INH prophylaxis for patients older than 35 years should be restricted to patients who are immunocompromised or whose PPD results indicate recent seroconversion. Monitor these patients closely with serial LFTs for signs of hepatotoxicity. There is also an increased risk for hepatitis in females, especially black and Hispanic women.

Lifestyle, Diet, and Habits

Ask the patient about diet and alcohol consumption. INH has some monoamine oxidase inhibitor (MAOI) activity

TABLE 43.2 Agents That Interact with P Isoniazid

Interactants	Effect and Significance	Nursing Management
alcohol	Isoniazid and alcohol may induce hepatotoxicity.	Advise the patient to limit ingestion of alcohol throughout therapy. Monitor for signs of hepatitis.
carbamazepine	Isoniazid is suspected to inhibit carbamazepine metabolism, resulting in carbamazepine toxicity. Carbamazepine may increase isoniazid degradation to hepatotoxic metabolites, resulting in an increased risk for hepatotoxicity.	Monitor carbamazepine serum concentrations. Monitor liver function test results.
chlorzoxazone	INH may inhibit the metabolism of chlorzoxazone, resulting in an increased risk for adverse effects.	Monitor for an ataxic gait. Monitor for dizziness or drowsiness Maintain a safe environment.
disulfiram	The combination of disulfiram and isoniazid may induce excess dopaminergic activity.	Monitor patient for acute behavioral and coordination changes. Refer to health care provider immediately if any occur.
enflurane	Fast acetylation of isoniazid produces high concentrations of hydrazine, facilitating defluoridation of enflurane. This may result in high-output renal failure.	Monitor renal function, especially in fast acetylators.
Hydantoins	Isoniazid inhibits the metabolism of hydantoins, resulting in increased serum hydantoin concentrations and increased risk for toxicity.	Monitor serum hydantoin levels frequently. Monitor for signs of hydantoin toxicity.
meperidine	These drugs in combination may induce hypotension or CNS depression. The mechanism of action is unknown.	Use combination cautiously. Monitor blood pressure. Monitor for CNS depression. Maintain a safe environment.
rifampin	Hepatotoxicity may occur more frequently when combined.	Monitor liver function test results.
warfarin	The anticoagulant activity is increased when given concurrently with isoniazid. This results in an increased risk for hemorrhage.	Monitor PT and INR frequently. Monitor for bruising or bleeding

and some providers believe patients should refrain from a tyramine-rich diet. Foods that contain tyramine include cheese and dairy products, beef or chicken liver, beer and ale, red wine, avocados, bananas, figs, raisins, caffeine, and chocolates. Other providers believe that INH is a very weak MAO inhibitor that rarely causes symptoms. Monitor the patient and advise the provider if flushing, sweating, diarrhea, elevated BP, or other unusual symptoms occur.

Patients should also refrain from foods containing histamine. Foods in this category include tuna, brine, or yeast extract. The patient may experience headache, palpitations, sweating, hypotension, flushing, diarrhea, or itching.

Daily consumption of alcohol increases the risk of INH-induced hepatitis and can increase the clearance of INH.

Environment

INH therapy is routinely conducted in the home. Because of its long duration (up to 24 months), adherence is an issue. With the patient, explore factors in the home environment that may affect adherence. Additionally, stress that he or she needs to have periodic follow-up examinations and laboratory testing to monitor for severe and potentially fatal adverse reactions.

Culture and Inherited Traits

INH is metabolized in the body by a process called acetylation. In some people, this process occurs more rapidly than it does in others. Fast acetylators are at higher risk for hepatic toxicity from INH therapy, whereas slow acetylators are at higher risk for high serum levels and more frequent adverse effects. Because the determination of fast acetylators or slow acetylators is genetically controlled, it is important to be aware of the patient's ethnic background. Eskimos, Asians, and about 50% of African Americans or European Americans from North America are fast acetylators. The remainder of African Americans and European Americans, Scandinavians, and people of Arab or Jewish heritage are slow acetylators.

Nursing Diagnoses and Outcomes

- Altered Protection related to drug-induced hepatitis
  Desired outcome: The patient will call the prescriber immediately if signs or symptoms of hepatitis occur.
- Risk for Infection related to drug-induced blood dyscrasias
  Desired outcome: The patient will monitor for signs of infection and contact the prescriber if any occur.
- Risk for Peripheral Neurovascular Dysfunction related to drug-induced neuropathy
  Desired outcome: The patient will take pyridoxine throughout INH therapy to decrease potential for peripheral neuropathy.
- Risk for Trauma related to adverse CNS effects
  Desired outcome: The patient will encounter no injury related to CNS effects brought on by using INH.
- Impaired Skin Integrity related to drug-induced acne
  Desired outcome: The patient will practice careful skin care to prevent breakdown from acne resulting from drug effects.

Planning and Intervention

Maximizing Therapeutic Effects

Administer INH to the patient with an empty stomach 1 hour before or 2 hours after meals to increase absorption. For patients with GI distress, INH may be given with meals. To avoid possible drug interactions, do not administer antacids less than 1 hour before or 2 hours after administering INH.

Minimizing Adverse Effects

The early identification of symptoms of potential adverse effects is the best way to minimize complications of INH therapy. Advise patients to report any of the prodromal symptoms of hepatitis, including anorexia, malaise, fatigue, jaundice, or nausea. Also advise patients to report burning or pain in the extremities, numbness or tingling, or symptoms of anemia. The drug should be discontinued if clinical symptoms of hepatitis occur.

Most prescribers discontinue the drug if LFT results indicate elevations ranging from three to five times higher than the upper limit of normal values.

Providing Patient and Family Education

- Advise patients to take the drug on an empty stomach every day and emphasize the importance of taking the drug as prescribed. Patients who stop and start INH therapy repeatedly are at risk for developing drug-resistant TB. Although it is important to take the drug as prescribed, it is more important not to double the dosage if a drug dose is forgotten.
- Explain diet and alcohol restrictions to limit the risk of adverse reactions. A written list of foods that contain tyramine or histamine is most helpful to patients.
- Teach patients the signs of hepatotoxicity such as anorexia, malaise, fatigue, jaundice, or nausea. Explain

the importance of notifying the prescriber if any of these symptoms occur.
- Teach patients the signs of peripheral neuropathy such as burning or pain in the extremities, numbness, or tingling. Advise them to contact the prescriber if any of these symptoms occur.
- Explain the importance of follow-up visits, including laboratory testing and eye examinations.

Ongoing Assessment and Evaluation

Ongoing assessment is extremely important in INH therapy. Monitor for signs of adverse effects, especially hepatitis. Question the patient about symptoms such as yellow skin or eyes, anorexia, nausea, vomiting, fatigue, malaise, or weakness. Also, ask about rash, itching, or darkened urine. It is also important to question the patient regarding symmetric numbness or tingling in the extremities. Optimally, results of the patient's serial blood tests will be available for evaluation during the visit.

INH should be discontinued if signs or symptoms of hepatic damage become evident. Discontinuing INH should be considered if LFT values exceed three to five times the upper limit of normal ranges.

At each visit, review diet and alcohol recommendations. Also, review the signs and symptoms of hepatitis and peripheral neuropathy and remind the patient to call the prescriber if any symptoms occur. It may be preferable to arrange for the next follow-up appointment rather than wait for the patient to call.

CRITICAL THINKING SCENARIO

EXPOSURE TO THE TUBERCULOSIS (TB) MYCOBACTERIUM

David Haversham, age 32 years, works as a correctional officer in the local jail. Following policy, David goes to the clinic for his yearly TB test. His test result last year was negative, and David does not recall having been exposed to TB. Two days later, you call David to tell him that his purified protein derivative (PPD) measured 12 mm and to arrange for him to have a chest x-ray (CXR). David calls the clinic today and learns that his CXR is normal and then asks, "So, what does all this mean?"

1. How would you answer David's question?
2. What therapy, if any, would you anticipate for this patient?
3. Would this therapy change if the patient were 40 years of age?
4. What questions would you ask the patient before initiating therapy?
5. Develop a patient teaching plan for the patient.
6. How would this scenario change if David were HIV-positive?

MEMORY CHIP

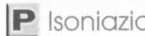 Isoniazid

- Used for prophylaxis and management of tuberculosis and for other susceptible mycobacterial infections
- Important contraindications: acute hepatic diseases
- Most common adverse effects: peripheral neuropathy, elevated liver enzyme levels
- Most serious adverse effects: hepatotoxicity, optic neuritis
- **Life span alert: patients over the age of 35 years have an increased risk for isoniazid-induced hepatic dysfunction**
- Maximizing therapeutic effects: Administer on an empty stomach, unless GI distress occurs.
- Minimizing adverse effects: Promptly identify signs and symptoms of potential adverse effects, especially hepatitis.
- Most important patient education: Teach patients about the role of adherence in avoiding drug resistance.
- **Black box warning: hepatotoxicity**

Drugs Significantly Different From 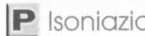 Isoniazid

First-Line Drugs

Ethambutol

Ethambutol (Myambutol) appears to be more effective and less toxic than other antitubercular drugs. It works by inhibiting the synthesis of certain metabolites, with subsequent impairment of cell metabolism leading to cell death. Ethambutol is effective against INH and rifampin-resistant bacilli.

Ethambutol is administered orally, partially metabolized in the liver, and excreted primarily in urine, with approximately 25% excreted unchanged in feces. A widely distributed drug, it reaches high concentrations in the kidneys, lungs, and saliva. It penetrates inflamed meninges to reach therapeutic levels in the CSF. Although ethambutol crosses the placenta and is distributed into breast milk, no adverse effects on the fetus or nursing infant have been reported. It is not recommended for use in children under the age of 13.

One of the main adverse effects of ethambutol is optic neuritis. Patients with pre-existing ocular disease should have a baseline ophthalmologic examination and be closely monitored for changes in visual acuity and color discrimination. The drug should not be used in children whose visual acuity cannot be adequately assessed. Other serious adverse effects include hepatotoxicity, peripheral neuropathy, and blood dyscrasias. Ethambutol may also cause hyperuricemia; therefore, patients with a history of gout should be closely monitored for exacerbations.

Pyrazinamide

Like ethambutol, pyrazinamide (PZA) appears to be more effective and less toxic than other antitubercular drugs. It is indicated only for use in treating *M. tuberculosis*. The exact mechanism of action of PZA is not known; however, it exhibits bacteriocidal action. Studies indicate that PZA is most effective in the induction phase of treatment.

PZA is administered orally, metabolized into active metabolites, and excreted in the urine, primarily by way of glomerular filtration. It is widely distributed and penetrates inflamed meninges. Whether PZA crosses the placenta is unknown, but the drug does enter breast milk.

PZA should be given cautiously to patients who are pregnant and those with alcoholism, gout, or hepatic disease. The most severe adverse effect is hepatotoxicity. In rare instances, liver atrophy and fatalities have occurred. Common adverse effects include arthralgias, GI disturbances, and photosensitivity. Nongouty arthritis may occur because PZA inhibits urate excretion, resulting in hyperuricemia. Rarely, hematopoietic effects, such as thrombocytopenia and sideroblastic anemia, may occur.

Patients receiving PZA should have baseline laboratory tests completed before initiating treatment and periodically throughout therapy. These tests include a CBC, liver and renal function tests, and uric acid level.

Rifamycins

The rifamycins rifampin, rifapentine, and rifabutin are also first-line drugs used to manage TB. Rifampin is the drug of choice for managing leprosy and thus will be discussed as the prototype for that disease.

Second-Line Drugs

Aminoglycoside Antibiotics

Amikacin (Amikin), capreomycin sulfate (Capastat), kanamycin (Kantrex), and streptomycin are aminoglycoside antibiotics that are effective against *M. tuberculosis*. They are all given by the parenteral route. As with other aminoglycoside antibiotics, adverse effects include damage to the eighth cranial nerve, resulting in hearing loss or balance disturbances and nephrotoxicity. For detailed information regarding aminoglycoside antibiotics, see Chapter 40.

Cycloserine

Cycloserine (Seromycin), a bacteriostatic drug, works by inhibiting cell wall synthesis. It is always given in conjunction with another antitubercular drug. Cycloserine is contraindicated in patients with epilepsy, depression, anxiety, psychosis, severe renal insufficiency, and alcohol abuse. Major adverse effects include seizures, confusion, dizziness, headache, and somnolence.

Ethionamide

Ethionamide (Trecator) is structurally similar to INH but less effective. It is always given in conjunction with another antitubercular drug. Ethionamide is used infrequently in the management of TB because of its severe affects on the GI system. In addition to the GI adverse effects, ethionamide may induce hepatotoxicity, orthostatic hypotension, hypoglycemia, and impotence. Because of its structural similarity to INH, INH-resistant TB also may be resistant to ethionamide.

Fluoroquinolones

The fluoroquinolones are used for multidrug-resistant TB, although they are not FDA approved for this indication. Moxifloxacin (Avelox) has the most *in vitro* activity against tuberculosis, followed by levofloxacin (Levaquin), ofloxacin (Floxin), and ciprofloxacin (Cipro). For detailed information regarding the fluoroquinolones, see Chapter 41.

Aminosalicylic Acid

Aminosalicylic acid (Paser), also known as para-aminosalicylic acid (PAS), is similar to sulfonamides. It works by inhibiting the synthesis of folic acid. Aminosalicylic acid is usually used for TB in children, in place of ethambutol. In addition, aminosalicylic acid is used for the maintenance of Crohn's disease. Aminosalicylic acid may induce GI adverse effects such as nausea, vomiting, and diarrhea. Rarely, hepatotoxicity may occur.

Check the packet for granules that appear swollen or have lost their tan color and have turned dark brown or purple. Do not use if these changes have occurred. To administer, sprinkle granules on applesauce or yogurt or suspend in tomato, orange, grapefruit, grape, cranberry, or apple juice or in punch that contains fruit juice.

ⓒ DRUGS FOR TREATING *MYCOBACTERIUM LEPRAE* INFECTION

MDT, the standard approach for other mycobacterial infections, is also recommended for treating leprosy. Rifampin is the drug of choice for both types of leprosy (see Pathophysiology), except in cases of rifampin resistance. For that reason, rifampin is the prototype drug for treating leprosy. Table 43.3 presents a summary of selected rifamycins.

Nursing Management of the Patient Receiving Ⓟ Rifampin

Core Drug Knowledge

Pharmacotherapeutics

Rifampin is one of the first-line drugs used in treating TB, although it should never be used as a single drug, because resistance develops rapidly. Its only other FDA-approved use is meningococcal infectious disease. Rifampin frequently is used as an off-label drug. It is a primary drug for leprosy, although it is always a part of MDT for this purpose. In addition, it is used in the treatment of other mycobacterial infections, MAC infection, staphylococcal infections (including MRSA), bacterial meningitis, osteomyelitis, infective endocarditis, and as prophylaxis against *Neisseria meningitidis* and *H. influenzae*.

Pharmacokinetics

Rifampin may be administered orally or parenterally. It is well absorbed from the GI tract, except in the presence of food, which decreases both the rate and extent of absorption. Rifampin is widely distributed into most body tissues and fluids including CSF, and concentrates intracellularly (up to five times that of extracellular concentrations), primarily in leukocytes. Rifampin is metabolized in the liver to an active metabolite and undergoes enterohepatic circulation with substantial reabsorption. It is excreted primarily through biliary elimination in feces.

Pharmacodynamics

Rifampin works by blocking initiation of RNA transcription by inhibiting bacterial DNA-dependent RNA polymerase. It is bactericidal or bacteriostatic, depending on the concentration reached within an infected site and the

TABLE 43.3	Summary of Selected Rifamycins		
Drug (Trade) Name	Selected Indications	Route and Dosage Range	Pharmacokinetics
Ⓟ rifampin (Rifadin)	TB in conjunction with other drug therapy, prophylaxis of TB	*Adult:* PO or IV, 600 mg in single daily dose until improvement occurs; direct observed treatment (DOTS) 10 mg/kg 2 × wk *Child:* 10–20 mg/k not to exceed 600 mg qd	*Onset:* PO, varies; IV, rapid *Duration:* 6 h $t_{1/2}$: 3–5.1 h
	Leprosy	*Adult:* PO or IV 600 mg 1 × mo for 6–24 mo *Child:* Not recommended	
	Mycobacterium avium complex (MAC)	*Adult:* 600 mg PO or IV in combination with other antimycobacterials *Child:* 10–20 mg/kg PO or IV in combination with other antimycobacterials	
rifabutin (Mycobutin)	TB, leprosy, MAC	*Adult:* 300 mg PO qd, may be given 150 mg bid to decrease GI distress *Child:* Not approved	*Onset:* 1 h *Duration:* Unknown $t_{1/2}$: 16–69 h
rifapentine (Priftin)	TB	*Adult and child >12 y:* 600 mg 2 × wk for 2 mo, then 1 × wk for 4 mo *Child:* Not recommended	*Onset:* 5–6 h *Duration:* Unknown $t_{1/2}$: 13 h

susceptibility of the organism. It does not bind to RNA polymerase in human cells; thus, RNA synthesis in the host is not affected.

Contraindications and Precautions

Rifampin should not be administered to patients with known rifamycin hypersensitivity, including rifabutin, because cross-sensitivity between agents is possible. Parenteral rifampin contains sulfite sodium formaldehyde sulfoxylate. Therefore, parenteral rifampin is contraindicated in patients with sulfite hypersensitivity because it has been associated with serious or potentially fatal anaphylactoid reactions, although the incidence of such reactions is low. Rifampin is also contraindicated for use in patients taking nonnucleoside reverse transcriptase inhibitors (NNRTIs).

Because of its potential adverse effects on the liver, rifampin is used cautiously in patients with a history of hepatic dysfunction and in patients known to have alcoholism. It is also used cautiously with patients taking other medications known to be hepatotoxic.

Adverse Effects

Rifampin may cause adverse effects similar to those of INH, especially hepatic injury. Additionally, rifampin can discolor bodily fluids, such as urine, saliva, tears, and sputum. Wearers of soft contact lenses should be cautioned that the lenses may be permanently discolored.

Although rifampin is generally well tolerated, it may cause GI disturbances such as nausea and vomiting, anorexia, flatulence, cramps, and diarrhea. Other common adverse effects include headache, drowsiness, fatigue, dizziness, and rash. Rarely, rifampin may induce pseudomembranous colitis or thrombocytopenia or other blood dyscrasias, and acute renal failure.

Drug Interactions

Rifampin is a potent inducer of the cytochrome P-450 hepatic enzyme system and its subsets. Induction may result in reduced plasma concentrations of other drugs metabolized by the P-450 enzyme system. When these drugs are given concurrently with rifampin, their dosage may need to be increased. In some cases, the drugs are contraindicated for concurrent use. Table 43.4 lists drugs that interact with rifampin.

Assessment of Relevant Core Patient Variables

Health Status

Assess for diseases or disorders that contraindicate the use of rifampin or require strict monitoring during therapy, especially those that increase the risk of hepatotoxicity. Assess for any medications that may interact with rifampin or other drugs known to be hepatotoxic. Communicate any positive findings to the prescriber before starting therapy.

Pay special attention to patients with a diagnosis of HIV infection or AIDS. Many drugs used to treat these disorders are contraindicated for use with rifampin. Additionally, patients with HIV infection or AIDS need TB therapy

for a longer duration than other patients do, increasing the problem of drug resistance.

Arrange for baseline laboratory tests before administering rifampin. These tests include a CBC and hepatic and renal studies.

Life Span and Gender

Rifampin is an FDA pregnancy category C drug; therefore, it is important to evaluate the patient's pregnancy status. The drug may be used in children younger than 1 month. Rifampin may increase the metabolism of oral contraceptives, placing the patient at risk for pregnancy. Advise women taking oral contraceptives to use another form of birth control while taking rifampin.

Lifestyle, Diet, and Habits

Assess for alcohol consumption and explain the increased risk for hepatotoxicity when alcohol consumption is combined with rifampin therapy. Because rifampin can discolor body fluids red-orange, suggest that soft contact lens wearers change to a different type of contacts or regular glasses throughout therapy. Dietary changes are not needed.

Environment

Rifampin can be given in any environment. Oral rifampin is most frequently used in the home environment; intravenous (IV) rifampin is most frequently administered in an acute care hospital. Be aware of the environment in which the drug will be administered and explore with the patient any factors in the home setting that may affect adherence to drug therapy.

Nursing Diagnoses and Outcomes

- Risk for Injury related to hepatic injury
  Desired outcome: *The patient will remain free of injury and contact the prescriber if signs such as yellow skin, itching, or fatigue occur.*
- Imbalanced Nutrition: Less than Body Requirements, related to potential nausea, vomiting, anorexia, and diarrhea
  Desired outcome: *The patient will have balanced nutrition throughout therapy.*
- Ineffective Protection related to blood dyscrasias
  Desired outcome: *The patient will remain without injury throughout therapy.*

Planning and Intervention

Maximizing Therapeutic Effects

Administer IV rifampin by slow infusion over 2 hours. Oral rifampin should be given 1 hour before or 2 hours after a meal to avoid decreasing absorption. Promote adherence to oral rifampin therapy by explaining the importance of taking the medication daily.

Minimizing Adverse Effects

Evaluate the patient for contraindications to its use and avoid administering rifampin to a patient with signs of

TABLE 43.4	Agents That Interact with Ⓟ Rifampin	
Interactants	**Effect and Significance**	**Nursing Management**
Drugs affected by induction: • anticoagulants • beta blockers • oral contraceptives • corticosteroids • cyclosporine • digitoxin • disopyramide • doxycycline • estrogens/progestins • haloperidol • HMG Co-A reductase inhibitors • hydantoins • nifedipine • ondansetron • oral antidiabetic agents • quinine derivatives • tacrolimus tamoxifen • theophyllines • tricyclic antidepressants • zolpidem	Increased hepatic microsomal enzyme metabolism (induction) by rifampin results in decreased action of interactant drugs.	Monitor for efficacy of interactant drugs. Discuss adjustment of interactant drug dosages with provider.
azole antifungal agents	Rifampin may induce the metabolism of azole antifungal drugs resulting in decreased action of azole antifungal drugs. Additionally, azole antifungal drugs interfere with the absorption of rifampin resulting in decreased serum rifampin levels.	Monitor for efficacy of azole antifungal drugs. Monitor for efficacy of rifampin. Consult with prescriber about adjusting drug dosages as needed.
benzodiazepines	The oxidative metabolism of benzodiazepines may be increased resulting in decreased pharmacologic effects.	Monitor for efficacy of benzodiazepine drugs. Consult with prescriber about adjusting benzodiazepine drug dosages as needed.
buspirone, verapamil	Rifampin induces first-pass metabolism of these drugs resulting in decreased plasma concentration.	Monitor for efficacy of interactants. Consult with prescriber about adjusting dosages of interactants as needed.
isoniazid	Rifampin may cause an alteration in the metabolism of isoniazid. Hepatotoxicity may occur at a rate higher than with either agent alone.	Monitor for signs of hepatotoxicity. Monitor liver function studies. Discontinue as needed.
macrolide antibiotics	The metabolism of rifampin may be inhibited while the metabolism of macrolide antibiotics may be increased, resulting in decreased antimicrobial effects and increased GI adverse effects.	Monitor for efficacy of macrolide antibiotics. Monitor for adverse GI effects of macrolide antibiotics. Consult with prescriber about using azithromycin or dirithromycin as alternative drugs because they do not undergo metabolism.
NNRTI	Rifampin may increase the metabolism of NNRTI drugs, resulting in a decreased efficacy of both drugs.	Monitor NNRTI drug levels. Discuss increasing rifampin dose with provider.
Opioids	Rifampin stimulates the metabolism of opioid analgesics, resulting in decreased efficacy.	Monitor the patient's clinical response to opioids. Monitor for signs of withdrawal. Discuss an alternative analgesic with the provider.
Protease inhibitors (PIs)	Rifampin may reduce PI plasma levels, decreasing their effect. PI drugs may increase rifampin levels, resulting in an increased risk for toxicity.	Discuss alternative drug therapy with the provider. If ordered, observe for efficacy of PI drugs and toxicity from rifampin.

hepatotoxicity. Assess patients taking other hepatotoxic drugs such as INH and PZA carefully, because the risk of hepatotoxicity is increased.

Providing Patient and Family Education

• Explain the potential effect of rifampin on the liver. Advise patients to contact the prescriber immediately if they experience anorexia, nausea, fatigue, malaise, jaundice, cola-colored urine, or pale stools. Also, explain that many drugs increase the risk for hepatic damage and that the patients should contact the prescriber before taking any new drugs, even those prescribed by another provider. In addition, explain that alcohol consumption may also increase the risk of hepatic damage.

• Advise patients with soft contact lenses to consult their ophthalmologist for an alternate form of contacts or glasses. Assure patients that the discoloration of body fluids is not harmful.

• Advise women using oral contraceptives to use another method of birth control while taking rifampin.

• Because adherence is always difficult when rifampin must be taken for a prolonged time, explain the importance of taking the medication consistently, even though patients will not feel different.

• Explain the importance of consistent follow-up visits to ensure that the microbes are eradicated and to monitor for adverse effects.

Ongoing Assessment and Evaluation

Ask patients whether they have experienced any symptoms suggestive of hepatic dysfunction. Periodic testing of hematopoietic, renal, and hepatic function should also be arranged.

By the end of therapy, the microbes should be eradicated, and the patient should be free from any adverse effects from rifampin therapy.

MEMORY CHIP

P Rifampin

• Used to manage acute TB and leprosy; also used to manage other mycobacterial infections
• Important contraindication: hypersensitivity
• Most common adverse effects: discoloration of body fluids, GI disturbances
• Most serious adverse effect: hepatotoxicity
• Maximizing therapeutic effects: Administer on an empty stomach.
• Minimizing adverse effects: Evaluate the patient for potential drug–drug interactions.
• Most important patient education: Teach patients the role of adherence in preventing resistance and the importance of contacting the prescriber if any signs of hepatic dysfunction occur.

Drugs Closely Related to P Rifampin

Two drugs, rifabutin and rifapentine, are similar to rifampin. Contraindications, precautions, adverse effects, and drug interactions for both of these drugs are the same as those for rifampin.

Rifabutin

Rifabutin (Mycobutin) is a derivative of rifamycin. It is used for prophylaxis or treatment of TB and MAC. *M. leprae* is also considered to be susceptible to rifabutin, but leprosy is not a labeled indication. Rifabutin appears to be a less potent hepatic enzyme inducer than rifampin, although similar drug–drug interactions may still occur. Rifabutin does not interfere with the metabolism of INH.

The most serious adverse effects of rifabutin are uveitis and blood dyscrasias. Like rifampin, rifabutin may cause discoloration of body fluids. Rifabutin is contraindicated for concurrent use with NNRTIs, hard-gel formulation saquinavir, or ritonavir. It can be given cautiously with other antiretroviral agents, but the dosage of those agents may need to be increased.

Rifapentine

Rifapentine (Priftin) is very similar to rifampin. Although many mycobacteria are considered susceptible to rifapentine, its only approved use is in managing TB. The major difference between rifapentine and rifampin is rifapentine's extended half-life, which allows for twice-a-week dosing.

Drugs Significantly Different From P Rifampin

Clofazimine

Clofazimine (Lamprene) is used as an antimycobacterial and anti-inflammatory agent, although access to this drug is restricted in the United States. It is bacteriocidal against *M. tuberculosis* and *M. leprae;* however, its action against *M. leprae* is very slow. It is bacteriostatic against *M. avium-intracellulare.* Clofazimine works by binding to mycobacterial DNA, thus inhibiting reproduction and growth. As an anti-inflammatory agent, it inhibits neutrophil motility and enhances the phagocytic activity of the polymorphonuclear cells and macrophages.

Clofazimine is insoluble in water and is incompletely absorbed from the GI tract. The extent of absorption varies with the person and with the form of the drug administered. Clofazimine concentrates and can crystallize in mesenteric lymph nodes, adipose tissue, adrenals, liver, lungs, gall-bladder, bile, and spleen. It crosses the placenta and enters breast milk. Clofazimine is excreted unchanged in feces.

The only contraindication to clofazimine therapy is hypersensitivity. Precautions include pre-existing GI disease and hepatic dysfunction. Common GI adverse effects to clofazimine include anorexia, diarrhea, nausea and vomiting, and colicky or burning abdominal pain. GI toxicity can include hepatitis (with elevated hepatic enzyme levels) or jaundice. Rare but serious adverse effects include splenic infarction, GI obstruction or ileus, and GI bleeding. Clofazimine can cause dark, black, or tarry stools that may be misinterpreted as GI hemorrhage.

In addition, clofazimine can cause long-lasting discoloration of the skin. In Caucasians, the skin may be bronze or dark tan. This effect may last months after clofazimine is discontinued. Like rifampin, clofazimine may discolor body fluids.

Dapsone

Dapsone (Avlosulfon) is a synthetic sulfone that is chemically similar to sulfonamides. It is used as an antimicrobial agent for leprosy, for *Pneumocystis carinii* pneumonia (PCP), and for the prophylaxis of malaria. It is also used as an immunosuppressive agent for systemic lupus erythematosus and as a dermatologic agent in a variety of integumentary disorders. In managing leprosy, dapsone is used in combination with other drugs such as rifampin and clofazimine. In the past, dapsone was the mainstay of therapy for leprosy. Now, resistance to dapsone monotherapy is common among *M. leprae.*

Dapsone works by inhibiting folic acid synthesis in susceptible organisms. Although the mechanism of dapsone in integumentary disorders is unknown, it has been suggested that it may act as an immunomodulator. Dapsone is orally administered and almost completely absorbed from the GI tract. It is widely distributed throughout the body, crosses the placenta, and enters into breast milk. Dapsone is metabolized in the liver. Approximately 20% of the drug is excreted unchanged in the urine, whereas 70% to 85% is excreted as metabolites. A small amount can be detected in the feces.

Hypersensitivity is the only contraindication to the use of dapsone. Caution is used in patients with sulfonamide hypersensitivity, but no direct cross-sensitivity occurs. Dapsone is also used with caution in cases of severe anemia, glucose-6-phosphate dehydrogenase (G6PD) deficiency, or methemoglobin reductase deficiency, because hemolytic anemia can occur.

Other serious effects that may be induced by dapsone include aplastic anemia, agranulocytosis, methemoglobinemia, acute tubular necrosis, and hepatotoxicity. More common adverse effects include fever, myalgias, headache, chills, fatigue, malaise, rash, and urticaria.

Probenecid may reduce renal excretion of dapsone, resulting in an increased risk of toxicity and adverse effects. Patients receiving other hemolytic agents, such as folic acid antagonists, should be closely monitored because concurrent use increases the potential for hematopoietic adverse effects.

Miscellaneous Drugs

Other drugs used to manage leprosy include ofloxacin, a fluoroquinolone antibiotic, and minocycline, a tetracycline antibiotic. These drug classes are discussed in Chapters 41 and 40, respectively.

CHAPTER SUMMARY

- The most common mycobacteria are *M. tuberculosis, M. leprae, M. avium,* and *M. intracellulare.*
- Isoniazid, or INH, the prototype for antitubercular drugs, is used for both prophylaxis and treatment of acute active tuberculosis (TB).
- Other first-line drugs for TB include rifampin, ethambutol, pyrazinamide, and streptomycin.
- Rifampin is the prototype drug for managing leprosy (Hansen disease).
- Other medications useful for leprosy include rifabutin, rifapentine, dapsone, clofazimine, ofloxacin, and minocycline.
- *M. avium* and *M. intracellulare* are the causative agents of *Mycobacterium avium* complex (MAC), a condition that frequently affects immunocompromised patients.
- Azithromycin and clarithromycin are the drugs of choice for MAC prophylaxis and treatment.
- Additional drugs used in managing MAC include rifampin, rifabutin, and clofazimine.

QUESTIONS FOR STUDY AND REVIEW

1. What type of patient has the highest risk for developing chemically induced hepatitis from isoniazid, or INH, therapy?
2. What is the difference between chemoprophylaxis and active tuberculosis (TB) therapy?
3. Why does multidrug-resistant TB occur?
4. What are the obstacles to successful drug therapy with rifampin?
5. Why is adherence an issue when treating mycobacterial infections?

NEED MORE HELP?

Chapter 43 of the Study Guide to Accompany *Drug Therapy in Nursing,* 4th Edition, contains NCLEX-style questions and other learning activities to reinforce your understanding of the concepts presented in this chapter. For additional information or to purchase the study guide, visit the**Point**.

REFERENCES

Al-Orainey, I. O. (2009). Diagnosis of latent tuberculosis: Can we do better? *Annals of Thoracic Medicine,* 4(1):5–9.

Bass, J. B. (2009). Treatment of tuberculosis in HIV-seronegative patients, *Up To Date.* Retrieved from *http://uptodate.com*

Could it really be leprosy? (2009). *Clinical Advisor for Nurse Practitioners,* Retrieved July 5, 2009, from CINAHL Plus with Full Text database.

CDC. (2007). Treatment of Latent TB Infection (LTBI), retrieved July 5, 2009 at www.cdc.gov/tb/publications/factsheets/treatment/treatment.html

Chan, E., & Iseman, M. (2008). Multidrug-resistant and extensively drug-resistant tuberculosis: a review, *Current Opinion in Infectious Diseases,* 21(6):587–595.

Drew, R. H. (2009). Rifampin and other rifamycins, *Up To Date.* Retrieved from *http://uptodate.com*

Donald, P., & van Helden, P. (2009). The global burden of tuberculosis–combating drug resistance in difficult times. *New England Journal of Medicine*, 360(23):2393–2395.

Facts and Comparisons. (2010). *Drug facts and comparisons*. Philadelphia, PA: Lippincott Williams & Wilkins.

Fiesinger, T. (2009). Latent tuberculosis. Retrieved July 5, 2009, from CINAHL Plus with Full Text database.

Hauck, F., Neese, B., Panchal, A., & El-Amin, W. (2009). Identification and management of latent tuberculosis infection. *American Family Physician*, 79(10):879–886.

Horsburgh, C. R. (2009). Treatment of latent tuberculosis infection in HIV-seronegative patients, *Up To Date*. Retrieved from *http://uptodate.com*

Koda-Kimbal, M. A, Young, L. Y., Kradian, W. A., et al. (2008). *Applied Therapeutics: The Clinical Use of Drugs*. Philadelphia, PA: Lippincott Williams & Wilkins.

LoBue, P. (2009). Extensively drug-resistant tuberculosis, *Current Opinion in Infectious Diseases*, 22(2):167–173.

Moadebi, S., Harder, C., Fitzgerald, M., et al. (2007). Fluoroquinolones for the treatment of pulmonary tuberculosis, *Drugs*, 67(14):2077–2099.

Micromedex Healthcare Series. Retrieved from *http://thomsonhc.com*

Mitnick, C. D., McGee, B., Peloquin, C. A. (2009). Tuberculosis pharmacotherapy: strategies to optimize patient care, Expert Opinion on Pharmacotherapy, 10(3):381–401.

Schluger, N. W. (2009). Diagnosis and treatment of drug-resistant tuberculosis, *Up To Date*. Retrieved from *http://uptodate.com*

Tatro, D. S. (2009). *Drug interaction facts*. Philadelphia, PA: Lippincott Williams & Wilkins.

44

Drugs Treating Fungal Infections

Learning Objectives

At the completion of this chapter the student will:

1. Identify core drug knowledge about drugs used to treat fungal infections.

2. Identify core patient variables relevant to drugs used to treat fungal infections.

3. Relate the interaction of core drug knowledge to core patient variables for drugs used to treat fungal infections.

4. Generate a nursing plan of care from the interactions between core drug knowledge and core patient variables for drugs used to treat fungal infections.

5. Describe nursing interventions to maximize therapeutic and minimize adverse effects for drugs used to treat fungal infections.

6. Determine key points for patient and family education for drugs used to treat fungal infections.

Key Terms

Candida	dermatophytes	tinea
cryptococcosis	dimorphic fungi	

Drugs Treating Fungal Infections

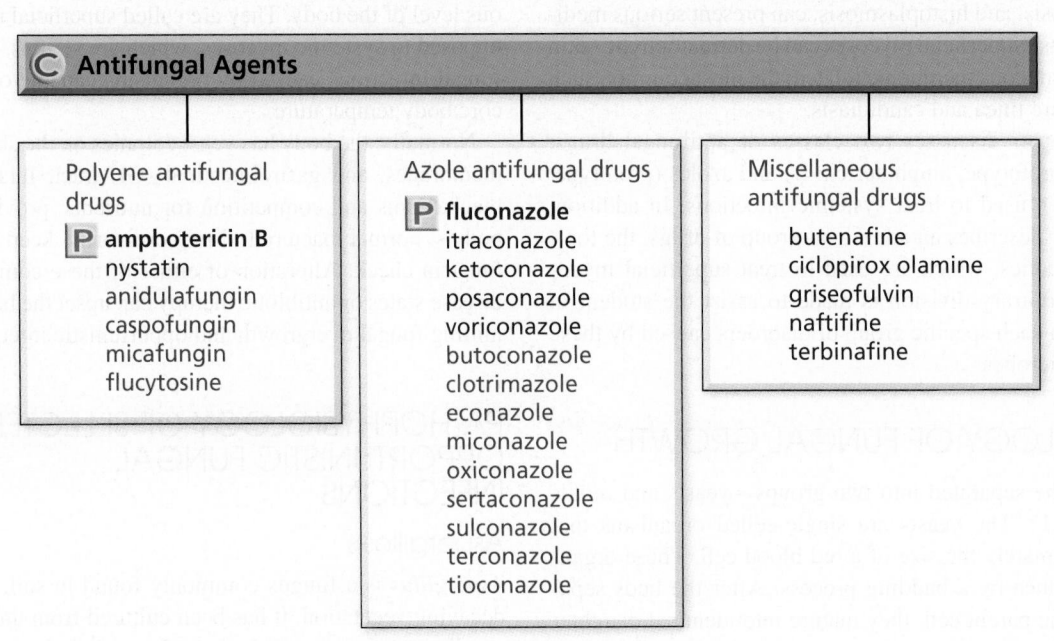

C Antifungal Agents

Polyene antifungal drugs
- **P** **amphotericin B**
- nystatin
- anidulafungin
- caspofungin
- micafungin
- flucytosine

Azole antifungal drugs
- **P** **fluconazole**
- itraconazole
- ketoconazole
- posaconazole
- voriconazole
- butoconazole
- clotrimazole
- econazole
- miconazole
- oxiconazole
- sertaconazole
- sulconazole
- terconazole
- tioconazole

Miscellaneous antifungal drugs
- butenafine
- ciclopirox olamine
- griseofulvin
- naftifine
- terbinafine

The symbol **C** indicates the drug class.
Drugs in **bold type** marked with the symbol **P** are prototypes.
Drugs in blue type are closely related to the prototype.
Drugs in red type are significantly different from the prototype.
Drugs in black type with no symbol are also used in drug therapy; no prototype.

Fungal infections can be life threatening in immunocompromised patients. Fungal infections can be divided into two categories: systemic infections and superficial mycoses. Systemic infections, such as aspergillosis, cryptococcosis, blastomycosis, and histoplasmosis, can present serious medical problems. Superficial mycoses can be dermatophytic (skin related) or mucous membrane related; the most common such infections are tinea and candidiasis.

This chapter discusses two classes of antifungal drugs: polyenes (prototype, amphotericin B) and azoles (prototype, fluconazole), used to treat systemic infections. In addition, this chapter describes an additional group of drugs, the topical antimycotics, which are used to treat superficial mycoses. This arbitrary division is made to assist the student in focusing on each specific group of disorders caused by these different microbes.

PHYSIOLOGY OF FUNGAL GROWTH

Fungi can be separated into two groups—yeasts and molds (Figure 44.1). The yeasts are single-celled organisms that are approximately the size of a red blood cell. These organisms reproduce by a budding process. After the buds separate from the parent cell, they mature into identical daughter cells. Molds produce long, hollow, branching filaments called hyphae. The term **dimorphic fungi** describes a limited number of fungi that are capable of growing as yeasts at one temperature and as molds at another. Reproduction for most fungi may be sexual or asexual.

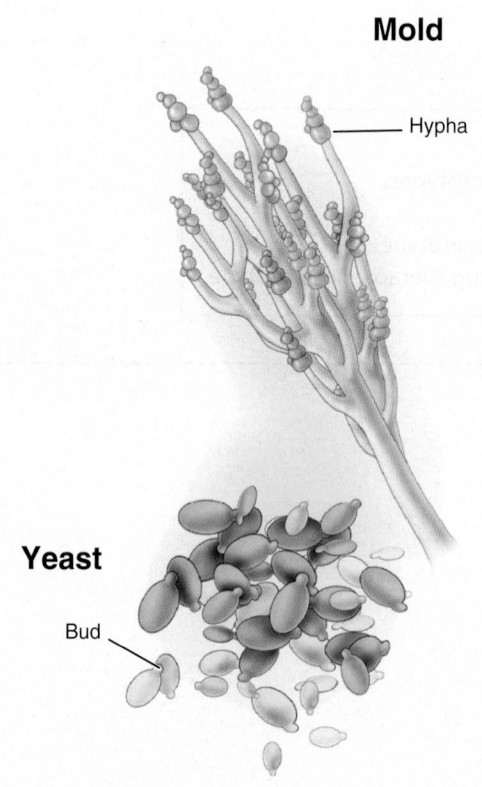

Mold

——— Hypha

Yeast

Bud

• FIGURE 44.1 Fungus family.

Fungi can produce disease in humans only if they can grow at the temperature of the infected body site. Fungi that cannot grow at core body temperature are called **dermatophytes.** Infections caused by these fungi are contained at the cutaneous level of the body. They are called superficial mycoses, as opposed to systemic mycoses, which are serious, deep-tissue fungal infections caused by organisms capable of growth at core body temperature.

Normally, the body has yeast colonies on the skin, mucous membranes, and gastrointestinal (GI) tract. Intact immune mechanisms and competition for nutrients, provided by the body's normal bacterial flora, ordinarily keep colonizing fungi in check. Alteration of either of these components by disease states or antibiotic therapy can upset the balance, permitting fungal overgrowth and opportunistic infections.

PATHOPHYSIOLOGY OF SELECTED OPPORTUNISTIC FUNGAL INFECTIONS

Aspergillosis

Aspergillus is a fungus commonly found in soil, water, and decaying vegetation. It has been cultured from unfiltered air, ventilation systems, contaminated dust dislodged during hospital renovation and construction, horizontal surfaces, food, and ornamental plants. It has been recognized increasingly as a cause of severe illness and mortality in highly immunocompromised patients, such as those undergoing chemotherapy, those with acquired immunodeficiency syndrome (AIDS), or those with bone marrow or vital organ transplants.

Infection with *Aspergillus* that is airborne may be acquired by inhaling the fungal spores. In severely immunocompromised patients, primary aspergillus pneumonia results from local lung tissue invasion. Colonization of the lower respiratory tract by *Aspergillus* in patients with pre-existing lung disease, such as chronic obstructive lung disease, cystic fibrosis, or inactive tuberculosis, can predispose patients to invasive pulmonary or disseminated infection. After pulmonary invasion, the fungus may disseminate through the bloodstream to involve multiple organs. The most reliable technique for diagnosis is a lung biopsy, although the fungus may be cultured from sputum or from specimens acquired by bronchoalveolar lavage.

Candidiasis

Candida is a yeast-like fungus that is almost always present as part of the normal population of organisms in the mouth, skin, intestinal tract, and vagina. The immune system and other organisms in the mucous membranes normally prevent it from growing in colonies. However, in immunocompromised patients, deterioration of the immune system can lead to candidal colonization; most outbreaks occur when the CD4+ T-cell count falls below 400 mm^3.

Human immunodeficiency virus (HIV)–infected infants and children are particularly prone to serious and extensive candidal infections. Other factors that can promote growth of *Candida* species in healthy individuals include use of broad-spectrum antibiotics (which alter the natural population of organisms in the mouth and vagina); use of topical and systemic corticosteroids; diabetes; ill-fitting dentures; drugs or conditions that alter saliva flow; radiation therapy; cancer; chemotherapy; nutritional deficiency in iron, folate, vitamin B_{12}, or zinc; oral contraceptives with a high estrogen content; pregnancy; poor oral or dental hygiene; smoking; stress; depression; and use of antihistamines.

Cryptococcosis

Cryptococcosis, which usually manifests as cryptococcal meningitis, is the most serious of the fungal infections in immunocompromised patients. Cryptococcosis rarely occurs when the CD4+ T-cell count is over 100 mm^3 and is most likely when the count drops below 50 mm^3. It is caused by a yeast-like organism, *Cryptococcus neoformans*. This fungus is widespread in the environment, especially in soil containing bird droppings. Exposure occurs when contaminated sources become airborne and are inhaled.

In people with intact immune systems, the fungus may form inactive fungal nodules in the lungs, which may be visible on x-ray films and can later produce active infection when the immune response decreases. As cryptococcosis progresses, from either the original infection or a later reactivation, it can take three forms (more than one of which may be present):

• Central nervous system (CNS) infection
• Pulmonary infection
• Disseminated infection

Meningitis, inflammation of the membranes surrounding the spinal cord or brain, is the most common manifestation of cryptococcal infection.

Mucormycosis

Mucormycosis, also known as zygomycosis, is a fungal infection of the sinuses, brain, or lungs caused by fungi such as *Mucor* or *Rhizopus*. These common fungi are found in soil and decaying vegetation. The spores are inhaled into the body through the mouth and nose. In the immunocompetent person, the spores are destroyed by phagocytosis. In the immunocompromised patient, the spores attach to the nasal or oral mucosa. The spores can then spread into the nasal cavity and maxillary sinuses. The spores can also invade the blood vessels, causing systemic spread, or a local inflammatory or thrombotic effect on the vessels.

Common syndromes associated with mucormycosis include rhinocerebral infection, pulmonary infection, or mucormycosis of the GI tract, skin, or kidneys. Symptoms associated with rhinocerebral infection include orbital and facial pain, headache, visual changes, acute sinusitis, fever, proptosis (protrusion of eye orbit), and erythema (redness) of skin overlying sinuses. Necrotic tissue may be seen on the nasal turbinates, septum, and palate. Symptoms of pulmonary involvement include cough, hemoptysis, and shortness of breath. Patients with GI involvement may have abdominal pain or vomiting.

Without treatment, mucormycosis has a mortality rate of 30% to 70%. Unlike other fungal diseases, mucormycosis requires surgical débridement of necrotic tissues in addition to pharmacotherapy to resolve the infection.

PATHOPHYSIOLOGY OF SELECTED NONOPPORTUNISTIC FUNGAL INFECTIONS

Blastomycosis

Blastomycosis is a chronic infection characterized by granulomatous and suppurative lesions. It is caused by inhaling the dimorphic fungus *Blastomyces dermatitidis*. Blastomycosis is endemic in eastern parts of the United States, but it also is seen throughout Canada and Central America.

Two basic forms of blastomycosis are recognized: pulmonary and chronic cutaneous. Most infections originate in the lungs and then disseminate to any organ, but usually to the skin and bones. In chronic cutaneous blastomycosis, the initial skin lesion presents as one or more subcutaneous nodules that eventually ulcerate. They are most common on exposed skin, such as that of the face, hands, wrist, and lower leg. Diagnosis is usually made by direct culture, agents that contain potassium hydroxide, special stains, and measurement of complement-fixing antibodies to various antigens.

Coccidioidomycosis

Coccidioidomycosis (valley fever) is primarily a disease of the lungs, which is common in the southwestern United States and northwestern Mexico. It is caused by the fungus *Coccidioides immitis,* which grows in soil. The fungal spores become airborne when the soil is disturbed by wind, construction, farming, and other activities. Within the lung, the spore changes into a larger, multicellular structure called a spherule. The spherule grows and bursts, releasing endospores, which develop into other spherules. Person-to-person transmission does not occur.

Most cases of coccidioidomycosis are mild. It is thought that more than 60% of infected people either have no symptoms or experience flu-like symptoms and never seek medical attention. Among patients who seek medical care, the most common symptoms are fatigue, cough, chest pain, fever, rash, headache, and joint aches. Some people develop erythema nodosum, which produces painful red bumps that gradually turn brown.

Disseminated disease occurs in less than 0.5% of patients. In patients with disseminated disease, spores may be found in lymph nodes and meningeal, spleen, liver, kidney, and adrenal tissues. Meningitis is the most common cause of death. Patients at risk for disseminated disease are immunocompromised and include patients who have undergone organ transplantation and those with lymphoma, HIV infection, adrenal corticosteroid therapy, or diabetes. Disseminated disease also occurs more frequently in men, in African Americans and Filipinos, and in pregnant women during the third trimester.

Dermatophytic Infections (Tinea, Ringworm)

Dermatophytic infections are commonly called **tinea** or ring-worm. It is not a worm infection as the name suggests; rather, it is a fungal infection caused by mold-like fungi called der-matophytes. Tinea lives on the dead tissues on the skin and any structures that grow from the skin (such as hair or nails).

Tinea can affect most skin sites, depending on the specific fungal type. The descriptive terms used in Figure 44.2 refer to the location of the infection and not to the specific type of fungus involved. A slightly different type of tinea infection is known as tinea versicolor. This chronic, noninflammatory infection is characterized only by patchy, hypopigmented dis-coloration of the skin (Figure 44.3).

The classic features of tinea are itching, redness on the skin, and a circular patchy lesion that spreads along its bor-ders and clears at the center. In time, it may appear as a ring or a series of rings around a clear center, hence its common name, ringworm. These particular characteristics may not always be seen in every infected person; lack of certain signs or symptoms or the presence of additional signs or symptoms depends on which site is infected and how advanced the dis-ease is. On the palms of the hands or soles of the feet, red-ness may be the only sign. Sometimes there are deep-seated blisters on the soles of the feet that, with time, dry and end up as brown crusts. There may be thick, white scales between the toes. Nails can turn thick and white and eventually crum-ble if untreated. On the scalp, there may be hair loss as the hairs break off at their shafts.

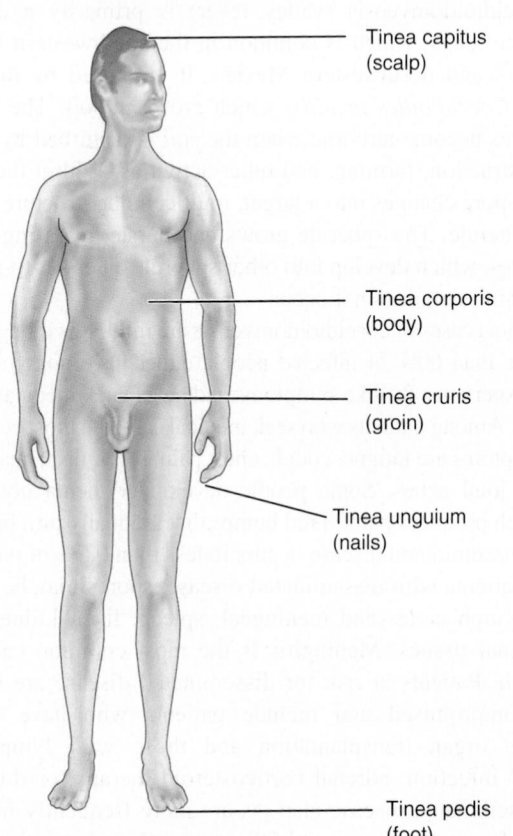

Tinea capitus
(scalp)

Tinea corporis
(body)

Tinea cruris
(groin)

Tinea unguium
(nails)

Tinea pedis
(foot)

• FIGURE 44.2   Types of tinea infections.

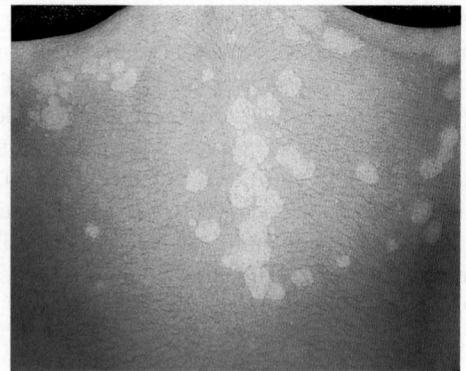

• FIGURE 44.3   Tinea versicolor.

Histoplasmosis

Histoplasmosis is a fungal infection that affects the lungs or other organs by dissemination. The disease is acquired by inhaling fungal spores. Outbreaks may occur in groups who have been exposed to bird or bat droppings or recently dis-turbed contaminated soil found in chicken coops or caves. Person-to-person spread of histoplasmosis does not occur. Although anyone can get histoplasmosis, it more often infects immunocompromised patients. Infection usually results in increased resistance to further infection, although the immu-nity is not complete. Symptoms vary from mild to severe, ranging from flu-like illness to serious lung infection.

There are four clinical forms of histoplasmosis. The most common is acute pulmonary histoplasmosis. Patients with this form of the infection experience a flu-like cough, chest pains, dyspnea, fever, weight loss, and hemoptysis. The symptoms may resolve spontaneously. In children, primary histoplas-mosis can lead to disseminated infection. Therefore, children who have HIV and histoplasmosis should receive suppres-sive therapy for life. The second form of histoplasmosis is chronic pulmonary histoplasmosis, which may develop after acute infection; this form resembles pulmonary tuberculosis. The third form is termed acute disseminated histoplasmosis. Patients with this form may develop hepatosplenomegaly, fever, and prostration. This type of histoplasmosis is usually fatal. The last form of histoplasmosis is termed chronic dis-seminated histoplasmosis, which may present a diagnostic problem because of the extremely varied presentation. Like the acute form, it also may be fatal.

ⓒ ANTIFUNGAL AGENTS

Antifungal drugs are generally grouped according to their pharmacotherapeutics into those used to manage systemic infections and those used to manage superficial infections, although some of the antifungal drugs may be used for both.

• POLYENE ANTIFUNGAL AGENTS

Polyene antimicrobials include amphotericin B and nystatin. These drugs have high affinity for fungal infections and are therefore useful for treating systemic fungal infections. Unfortunately, the polyene antifungal drugs also have the ability to induce severe adverse effects. Amphotericin B (Fungizone) is the prototype polyene antifungal drug. Table 44.1 presents a summary of selected antifungal agents.

Nursing Management of the Patient Receiving P Amphotericin B

Core Drug Knowledge

Pharmacotherapeutics

Amphotericin B is an antifungal agent used to treat progressive and potentially fatal systemic fungal or protozoal infections. It has a wide spectrum of activity against many fungi, including *Aspergillus*, *Blastomyces*, *Candida*, *Coccidioides*, *Cryptococcus*, and *Histoplasma*. Certain protozoan infections also are sensitive to amphotericin B, including *Leishmania*, and *Naegleria*.

Intravenous (IV) amphotericin B is available as its conventional formula (amphotericin B deoxycholate [Fungizone]) and three lipid- formulations: amphotericin B lipid complex (Abelcet), amphotericin B cholesteryl sulfate (Amphotec), and liposomal amphotericin B (AmBisome). All of the formulations are used for serious or life-threatening fungal infections. The lipid formulas induce less adverse effects than the conventional formula, especially nephrotoxicity.

TABLE 44.1	Summary of Selected C Antifungal Drugs		
Drug (Trade) Name	**Selected Indications**	**Route and Dosage Range**	**Pharmacokinetics**
P amphotericin B deoxycholate (Fungizone) amphotericin B lipid complex (Abelcet), amphotericin B cholesteryl sulfate (Amphotec), liposomal amphotericin B (AmBisome)	Progressive and potentially fatal systemic fungal or protozoal infections	Fungizone *Adult IV:* 0.1 – 1.5 mg/kg/d Abelcet *Adult IV:* 5 mg/kg/d Amphotec *Adult IV:* 3-4 mg/kg/d AmBisome *Adult IV:* 3-5 mg/kg/d	*Onset:* 20–30 min *Duration:* 20–24 h $t_{1/2}$: 24 h initially and then 15 d; Abelcet, 173.4 h
anidulafungin (Eraxis)	Candidemia or disseminated candidiasis Esophageal candidiasis	*Adult:* IV, 200 mg on first day, then 100 mg once daily	*Onset:* rapid *Duration:* 6 d $t_{1/2}$: 40–50 h
caspofungin (Cancidas)	Invasive aspergillosis Esophageal or oropharyngeal candidiasis	*Adult:* IV, 70 mg on first day then 50 mg/d *Adolescent and child:* Safety not established	*Onset:* Rapid *Duration:* Unknown $t_{1/2}$: Triphasic: alpha phase, short; beta phase, 9–11 h; terminal phase, 40–50 h
flucytosine (Ancobon)	Serious infections caused by susceptible strains of *Candida, Cryptococcus*	*Adult:* PO, 50–150 mg/kg/d q6h	*Onset:* Varies *Duration:* 10–12 h $t_{1/2}$: 2–5 h
micafungin (Mycamine)	Candidemia Esophageal candidiasis Prophylaxis of *Candida* infection in hematopoietic stem cell transplantation	*Adult:* IV, 100 mg daily *Adult:* IV, 150 mg daily *Adult:* IV, 50 mg daily *Adolescent and child:* Safety not established	*Onset:* Unknown *Duration:* Unknown $t_{1/2}$: 10–15 h
nystatin (Mycostatin)	Candidiasis—oropharyngeal, cutaneous, mucocutaneous, vulvovaginal, intestinal	*Adult:* PO, 500,000–1,000,000 U tid, continued for at least 48 h after clinical cure; PO suspension, 400,000–600,000 U qid (½ dose in each side of mouth; retain the drug as long as possible before swallowing); troche, dissolve 1–2 tablets in mouth 4–5× daily up to 14 daily; vaginal preparation, 1 tablet (100,000 U) intra-vaginally daily for 2 wk; topical, apply to affected area 2–3× daily until healing is complete *Child:* Oral suspension (infants), 200,000 U qid (100,000 in each side of mouth); oral suspension (premature and low-birth-weight infants), 100,000 U qid	Not generally absorbed systemically

Pharmacokinetics

Amphotericin B is no longer available in the United States as an oral preparation. Distribution of IV amphotericin B is limited; it crosses the placenta and may pass into breast milk. Lower concentrations are achieved in aqueous humor and pleural, pericardial, peritoneal, and synovial fluids. Because cerebrospinal fluid (CSF) concentrations are approximately 3% of those in serum, amphotericin B must be given intrathecally to achieve fungistatic concentrations within the CSF.

The metabolism of amphotericin B is unknown. It is presumed that the drug enters the tissues of the body and is released slowly over time. After therapy is discontinued, amphotericin B can be detected for up to 4 weeks in blood and 4 to 8 weeks in urine. The initial half-life is approximately 24 hours, followed by a second elimination phase with a half-life of about 15 days.

Pharmacodynamics

Amphotericin B works by binding to sterols in fungal cell membranes. This binding appears to form pores or channels and results in increased cell permeability, cell leakage, and death. Because human cells also contain sterols, damage to the host's cells also may occur. At low concentrations, amphotericin B is fungistatic; higher concentrations may induce fungicidal activity.

Contraindications and Precautions

Hypersensitivity is the only contraindication for all four of the formulations. Amphotericin B can cause anemia, hypokalemia, and hypomagnesemia. The drug should be administered cautiously to patients with any of these conditions because parenteral therapy with amphotericin B can cause substantial renal electrolyte loss. For patients with pre-existing renal impairment, the patient should be monitored for signs of nephrotoxicity. Amphotericin B is assigned to pregnancy category B and should be used with caution during pregnancy and lactation. Of course, for life-threatening infections, amphotericin B can be given despite the contraindications.

Adverse Effects

Amphotericin B has an extensive adverse effects profile. In fact, some clinicians refer to it as "amphoterrible." Nephrotoxicity occurs in 5% to 80% of patients receiving IV amphotericin B. Nephrotoxicity is manifested in many forms, including renal insufficiency, azotemia, hyposthenuria, renal tubular acidosis, and frank renal failure.

Administration of IV amphotericin B may induce infusion-related reactions, such as headache, chills, fever, rigors, hypotension, bronchospasm, and nausea and vomiting. Administration over more than 4 hours may decrease the severity of these symptoms. Infusion reactions are also less severe when a lipid-based formulation of amphotericin B is administered.

Electrolyte abnormalities, including hypokalemia, hypomagnesemia, hypochloremia, and hypocalcemia, also may occur with amphotericin B therapy. Patients with pre-existing cardiac problems may have exacerbations of their disorders when electrolyte abnormalities occur.

A normocytic, normochromic anemia occurs in most patients receiving amphotericin B. This reaction is believed to be caused by a suppressive effect on erythropoietin production and bone marrow. Transfusions are not usually necessary, and the anemia resolves when therapy is discontinued. Leukopenia and thrombocytopenia also may occur.

Less common adverse effects from amphotericin B consist of ventricular fibrillation, hypertension, cardiac arrest (primarily in situations when infusion is too rapid), hypersensitivity, peripheral neuropathy, and seizures.

Intrathecal amphotericin B can cause blurred vision and, in some cases, difficulty in urination. Polyneuropathy or paresthesias can occur in some patients, resulting in numbness, tingling, pain, or weakness.

Drug Interactions

Amphotericin B should not be coadministered with drugs known to be nephrotoxic or hemotoxic, such as antineoplastic agents, cyclosporine, tacrolimus, or aminoglycosides. It should not be used with drugs that may be affected by electrolyte imbalances, such as corticosteroids, digitalis glycosides, and thiazide diuretics. Other drugs that interact with amphotericin B include neuromuscular blocking agents, imidazoles, and flucytosine. Table 44.2 lists agents that interact with amphotericin B.

Assessment of Relevant Core Patient Variables

Health Status

Elicit a patient history to evaluate for pre-existing renal dysfunction, cardiac disease, electrolyte imbalance, or anemia. Also, assess for use of diuretics or for any concurrent drugs known to be nephrotoxic. Communicate any positive findings to the prescriber.

Perform a complete physical examination, especially assessing the renal system. For patients with pre-existing cardiac disease, a baseline electrocardiogram (ECG) should be performed. Baseline laboratory values should include complete blood count (CBC), complete metabolic profile, and renal function tests.

Life Span and Gender

Assess for pregnancy and lactation. Amphotericin B may be given during pregnancy. However, because of the potential adverse effects, it should be given only when absolutely needed. It should not be given to breast-feeding women because of its potential effects on the infant.

It is important to note the patient's age before administering amphotericin B. Safety of amphotericin B has not been demonstrated in children and older adults. Closely monitor patients when giving them this drug. Elderly patients are more likely to have decreased renal function, which may increase the risk of nephrotoxicity.

TABLE 44.2	Agents That Interact with Ⓟ Amphotericin B	
Interactants	**Effect and Significance**	**Nursing Management**
antineoplastic agents	Coadministration of antineoplastic agents and amphotericin B increases the risks for renal toxicity, bronchospasm, and hypotension.	Monitor for adverse effects. Monitor BUN and creatinine levels. Discuss adjustment of dosage with prescriber as needed.
corticosteroids	Concurrent use may cause potential hypokalemia.	Do not coadminister unless needed for control of adverse reactions.
cyclosporine	The nephrotoxic effects of cyclosporine are increased with the addition of amphotericin B. The mechanism of action is unknown.	Monitor BUN/creatinine. Monitor intake and output. Contact the provider immediately if signs of nephrotoxicity occur.
hemotoxic agents	Concurrent use increases the risk for anemia, neutropenia, and thrombocytopenia.	Monitor drug levels closely. Monitor CBC. Monitor for signs of blood dyscrasias. Discuss adjustment of dosage with prescriber as needed.
nephrotoxic agents	Concurrent use increases the risk for nephrotoxicity.	Monitor drug levels closely. Monitor BUN and creatinine levels. Monitor intake and output. Discuss adjustment of dosage with prescriber as needed.
zidovudine	Coadministration increases the risk of myelosuppression and nephrotoxicity.	Monitor BUN and creatinine levels. Monitor CBC. Discuss adjustment of dosage with prescriber as needed.

Lifestyle, Diet, and Habits

Assessing fluid intake in patients on amphotericin B therapy is important. Make sure that patients on amphotericin B therapy are kept well hydrated. This practice may minimize the potential for nephrotoxicity.

Environment

Amphotericin B should be administered in an acute care environment, although therapy with amphotericin B may last for months. Be familiar with administration of IV amphotericin B. Do not reconstitute the drug with a bacteriostatic agent in the solution because doing so may lead to precipitation.

Nursing Diagnoses and Outcomes

• Risk for Injury related to infusion reaction or to electrolyte imbalance imposed by drug therapy
Desired outcome: The patient will remain free from injury during drug administration or respond without injury to electrolyte replacement therapy.
• Ineffective Protection related to drug-induced leukopenia and thrombocytopenia
Desired outcome: The patient will remain free from opportunistic infections resulting from leukopenia and thrombocytopenia.
• Excess Fluid Volume related to renal dysfunction resulting from drug therapy

Desired outcome: The patient will have an appropriate ratio of fluid intake to output.
• Acute Pain related to infusion reaction
Desired outcome: The patient will have a decrease in pain after administration of analgesic drug, such as meperidine (Demerol).
• Ineffective Breathing Patterns due to drug-induced bronchospasm
Desired outcome: The patient will maintain adequate oxygenation.
• Ineffective Cardiopulmonary Tissue Perfusion related to cardiac arrest or arrhythmias resulting from drug therapy
Desired outcome: The patient will remain adequately perfused.
• Disturbed Sensory Perception: Visual, due to drug-related blurred vision
Desired outcome: The patient will regain adequate vision after therapy concludes.
• Risk for Injury related to drug effects of numbness, tingling, or weakness
Desired outcome: The patient will remain injury free throughout therapy.

Planning and Intervention

Maximizing Therapeutic Effects

Patients may desire to stop amphotericin B therapy if they have infusion reactions. Prepare the patient for the possibility of this reaction. Also, provide comfort measures, such as extra blankets, diversion therapy, or warm fluids, to offset the discomfort of this reaction. To reduce the potential for infusion reactions, flucytosine may be prescribed concurrently to decrease the dosage of amphotericin B. Because there is a positive drug–drug interaction between these two, the therapeutic effect remains constant.

Minimizing Adverse Effects

Administer test dose as ordered by provider. Be prepared for the possibility of an infusion reaction which may begin 15 minutes to 3 hours after the initiation of the infusion. Administer preordered drugs, such as diphenhydramine and acetaminophen, before starting therapy to minimize an infusion reaction. Be prepared to administer dantrolene or meperidine if rigors occur. In some cases, steroids may be required. Coordinate the administration of amphotericin B with possible blood transfusions. Infusion-related reactions can be more severe if administration occurs shortly after platelet or granulocyte transfusions.

Administer amphotericin B in a central line, if possible, and make sure that the IV administration set has an in-line filter. Place the solution on an infusion pump and deliver the drug over 2 to 4 hours. If using peripheral veins, rotate the infusion site to decrease the potential of phlebitis. Infuse at the appropriate rate for the specific type of amphotericin B being administered:

- Fungizone: over 6 hours
- Abelcet: 2.5 mg/kg/h
- Amphotec: 1 mg/kg/h over at least 2 hours
- AmBisome: over more than 2 hours

Monitor the patient carefully for signs of nephrotoxicity. In addition to accurately recording fluid input and output, monitor renal function tests and notify the prescriber immediately if the creatinine is higher than 3.5 mg/dL. Be sure the patient remains well hydrated. Administering 1 liter of saline on the day of infusion (sodium loading) decreases the potential for nephrotoxicity.

Coordinate the care of the patient when multiple prescribers are writing orders for the patient. To prevent orders for other nephrotoxic drugs, all prescribers must know that amphotericin B is being administered.

Providing Patient and Family Education
- Describe and explain the possibility of an infusion reaction and the importance of notifying staff immediately if symptoms occur.
- Explain possible adverse effects of amphotericin B and the need for serial blood tests. Because the adverse effects of amphotericin B can induce severe complications, it is important to explain the necessity of reporting any change from baseline that may occur.
- Another important area to discuss with patients and family is the importance of an accurate fluid intake and output record. It is necessary to enlist the assistance of patients and their families to document fluid intake and output as needed.

- Instruct patients to immediately report to the prescriber any symptoms of altered protection against infection, such as easy bruising, sore throat, or fatigue. In addition, tell patients to report CNS symptoms such as numbness, tingling, or weakness.

Ongoing Assessment and Evaluation
During the first dose of amphotericin B, take vital signs every 15 minutes. At this time, evaluate the patient for possible infusion reactions. Should a severe reaction occur, stop the infusion, call for another nurse to stay with the patient, and contact the prescriber immediately. Also, monitor the IV site during administration for signs of phlebitis, because amphotericin B is very irritating to tissues. Assess the infusion solution frequently and discontinue if a precipitate forms.

Throughout therapy, coordinate the collection of samples for laboratory tests, including a CBC, complete metabolic panel, and renal function tests. Renal function testing should be performed every 3 to 4 days. Weigh the patient daily and evaluate fluid intake and output every shift.

It is important to monitor patients with pre-existing cardiac disease for exacerbation of their symptoms. Fluid overload and electrolyte imbalances place these patients at high risk for a cardiac event.

Monitor for adverse effects that may place the patient at increased risk of injury. For patients with sensory-perceptual disturbances or numbness, tingling, and weakness, ensure that the patient understands the need for assistance to and from the bed. Keep the bed in the low position and the side rails up at all times.

MEMORY CHIP

P Amphotericin B

- Used for severe systemic fungal or protozoal infections
- Major contraindication: hypersensitivity
- Most common adverse effects: infusion reactions, electrolyte abnormalities, and anemia
- Most serious adverse effect: nephrotoxicity
- Maximizing therapeutic effects: Prepare the patient for the possibility of an infusion reaction so that the patient does not cease therapy.
- Minimizing adverse effects: Do not administer with other nephrotoxic drugs to minimize the potential for nephrotoxicity.
- Most important patient education: Discuss the potential for an infusion reaction and the need to monitor the hematopoietic and renal systems closely.
- **Black box warning: Amphotericin B deoxycholate should only be used for life-threatening systemic fungal infections.**
- **Patient safety alert: There are four formulations of amphotericin B. Use caution to administer the correct formula at the correct infusion rate.**

Use strict aseptic technique for patients receiving amphotericin B. Most patients have anemia related to the therapy, which increases the risk of infection.

By the end of therapy, the fungal infection should be resolved. In addition, all adverse effects should be identified and appropriate intervention should be started.

Drugs Closely Related to P Amphotericin B

Nystatin (Mycostatin) is an antifungal antibiotic that is nearly identical to amphotericin B in structure. It is available in topical, vaginal, and oral formulations. This agent is not used for systemic fungal infections, because it is poorly absorbed from the GI tract and has high potential for toxicity. Nystatin is used to treat oropharyngeal, cutaneous, mucocutaneous, and vulvovaginal candidiasis.

Adverse effects from nystatin are uncommon. Oral doses can cause mild and transient nausea and vomiting, diarrhea, and abdominal pain. Topical and vaginal forms may produce skin irritation, rash, or urticaria.

The oral suspension of nystatin is called a "swish and swallow" drug. Advise the patient to swish the solution throughout the mouth and then swallow or spit out the drug as directed by the prescriber. When nystatin troches are prescribed, advise the patient to allow them to dissolve completely in the mouth and not to chew or swallow the intact troche. The troche may take up to 30 minutes to dissolve.

Drugs Significantly Different From P Amphotericin B

Echinocandins

Echinocandins are a new class of drugs that have a different mechanism of action than amphotericin B. Echinocandins work by inhibiting the synthesis of a major fungal cell wall component, β-(1,3)-D-glucan, which is not present in human cell walls. Because of their unique mechanism of action, cross-resistance with other antifungal classes of drugs is unlikely.

Anidulafungin

Anidulafungin (Eraxis), an IV antifungal agent, is an echinocandin. It is indicated for candidemia, candida infection of the esophagus, and disseminated candidiasis such as intra-abdominal infection or peritonitis. Anidulafungin undergoes slow chemical degradation at physiologic temperature and pH and is excreted mostly in feces.

The only contraindication to anidulafungin use is hypersensitivity. It is given cautiously to patients with hepatic dysfunction or during pregnancy. Common adverse effects include hypokalemia, headache, nausea, and diarrhea. Less frequent but serious adverse effects include deep vein thrombosis, liver dysfunction, ECG changes, and seizures. Anidulafungin may also induce histamine-mediated symptoms such as rash, urticaria, flushing, pruritus, dyspnea, and hypotension. Limiting the rate of infusion to 1.1 mg/minute decreases

the frequency of these adverse effects. There are no significant drug–drug interactions with anidulafungin. It is a pregnancy category C and believed to be excreted in breast milk, so it should not be given to women who are breast-feeding. Anidulafungin has not been approved for use in children.

Caspofungin

Caspofungin (Cancidas) has the same indications as anidulafungin. In addition, it is given for invasive aspergillosis and empirically for febrile neutropenia.

Caspofungin has more precautions than anidulafungin. It is given cautiously to patients with liver impairment, myelosuppression, and renal insufficiency. Hypersensitivity reactions, including anaphylaxis, have occurred but are rare. Common adverse effects associated with the use of caspofungin include abdominal pain, diarrhea, elevated temperature, AST/ALT and alkaline phosphatase, and decreased potassium.

Several drug–drug interactions may occur with caspofungin. When it is given concurrently with P-450 inducers, serum caspofungin levels are substantially decreased. These drugs include carbamazepine, dexamethasone, efavirenz, phenytoin, fosphenytoin, nevirapine, and rifampin. When caspofungin is given concurrently with cyclosporine, caspofungin levels increase, thus increasing the risk of hepatotoxicity. When it is given concurrently with tacrolimus, serum tacrolimus levels are substantially decreased. Caspofungin has the same pregnancy and lactation precautions as anidulafungin and is not recommended for use in children.

Micafungin

Micafungin (Mycamine) is approved for use in the management of esophageal candidiasis, treatment of candidemia, acute disseminated candidiasis, and other candidal infections such as peritonitis and abscesses, and as prophylaxis for patients receiving a bone marrow transplant. It is given cautiously to patients with hepatic and renal dysfunction and in patients with prior hypersensitivity to the other echinocandins, anidulafungin and caspofungin. Common adverse effects include phlebitis at the infusion site, GI effects such as abdominal pain, diarrhea, nausea or vomiting, headache, fever, and abnormal liver function tests. Serious adverse effects include hemolytic anemia/hemoglobinuria, new onset or worsening hepatic failure, elevated BUN, serum creatinine, renal dysfunction, and/or acute renal failure. As with anidulafungin, a histamine-related reaction may occur. Rarely, life-threatening anaphylaxis has occurred.

Micafungin needs to be light-protected during infusion. To decrease the potential of a histamine reaction, the drug should be infused over 1 hour. Micafungin has the same pregnancy and lactation precautions as anidulafungin and caspofungin and is not recommended for use in children.

Flucytosine

Flucytosine (Ancobon) is an oral pyrimidine analog. It is approved for the treatment of meningitis or pulmonary infections caused by *Candida*. In addition, it is approved for septicemia, endocarditis, urinary tract infections, and pulmonary infections caused by cryptococcus. Frequently, flucytosine is given with amphotericin B to avoid resistance.

Flucytosine acts as an antimetabolite, interfering with pyrimidine metabolism and eventually disrupting both RNA and DNA synthesis. It is not metabolized; more than 90% is excreted by glomerular filtration as unchanged drug. Therefore, it is used cautiously in patients with pre-existing renal impairment. It also is used with caution in patients with pre-existing depression of bone marrow function, recent radiation therapy or cytotoxic drug therapy, dental disease, or a history of a hematologic disease, because these patients are most susceptible to flucytosine's myelosuppressive effects. In patients with hepatic disease, flucytosine can cause hepatitis or jaundice. There is a black box warning to avoid use as monotherapy because resistance develops rapidly.

Flucytosine can induce serious adverse effects. It carries a black box warning to closely monitor hematologic, renal, and hepatic status throughout therapy. All patients must be monitored weekly, especially those who are concurrently taking other drugs also known to cause these toxicities. Flucytosine is toxic to rapidly proliferating tissues, such as the bone marrow and the lining of the GI tract. Therefore, common hematologic adverse effects include anemia, leukopenia, and thrombocytopenia. GI adverse effects include abdominal pain, diarrhea, nausea, vomiting, and anorexia. Other adverse effects caused by flucytosine include hepatic dysfunction, photosensitivity, and CNS effects, such as dizziness, headache, and lightheadedness. Flucytosine is assigned to pregnancy category C and is contraindicated for use during pregnancy and breastfeeding. It is not approved for use in children.

• Azole Antifungal Drugs

The azole antifungal drugs can be classified into two subgroups: imidazoles and triazoles. These two groups differ slightly in their chemical structures but have similar clinical applications. Azole antifungal drugs can be used for both superficial mycoses and more serious systemic mycoses. Fluconazole (Diflucan) is the prototype azole antifungal drug. Table 44.3 presents a summary of azole antifungal agents and Table 44.4 lists topical azole agents.

Nursing Management of the Patient Receiving P Fluconazole
Core Drug Knowledge
Pharmacotherapeutics
Fluconazole is a triazole antifungal agent with a wide spectrum of activity. It is used for esophageal or oropharyngeal candidiasis, candida vaginitis, candiduria, disseminated candidiasis, and cryptococcal meningitis. It is also used prophylactically against fungal infections in patients receiving bone marrow transplants, in immunocompromised patients with a CD4+ T-cell count less than 200 mm³, and against coccidioidomycosis, cryptococcosis, and histoplasmosis in patients with CD4+ T-cell counts below 50 mm³.

Pharmacokinetics
Fluconazole is administered orally and intravenously. The pharmacokinetics of both oral and IV fluconazole are similar. GI absorption is rapid and almost complete. Oral bioavailability is more than 90% in fasting adults, and peak serum concentrations are attained within 1 to 2 hours after oral administration.

Fluconazole is distributed widely into body tissues and fluids. Saliva, sputum, nail, blister, and vaginal secretion concentrations are approximately equal to plasma concentrations. High concentrations also can be achieved in the cornea, aqueous humor, and vitreous body following IV administration. Fluconazole distributes well into the CSF and achieves CSF concentrations that are 60% to 80% of plasma concentrations, regardless of the degree of meningeal inflammation. Fluconazole crosses the placenta and enters breast milk. Elimination is mainly renal; about 60% to 80% of a dose is excreted in the urine unchanged and 11% as metabolites. Small amounts of fluconazole are excreted in the feces. Elimination of the drug can be impaired in elderly patients.

Pharmacodynamics
Fluconazole works directly by altering the fungal cell membrane. Fluconazole inhibits synthesis of ergosterol, a cytochrome P-450 enzyme that is an essential component of the fungal membrane. Inhibition of ergosterol synthesis results in increased cellular permeability, causing leakage of cellular contents. Other proposed antifungal effects of fluconazole include inhibition of endogenous respiration, interaction with membrane phospholipids, and inhibition of the transformation of yeasts to molds. It has no direct effects on the body.

Contraindications and Precautions
There are no absolute contraindications to fluconazole use. It should be used with caution during pregnancy and in patients with pre-existing hepatic and renal dysfunction.

Adverse Effects
Triazoles, such as fluconazole, are generally well tolerated. Gastrointestinal symptoms are most frequently reported, including nausea, abdominal pain, vomiting, and diarrhea. Mild elevations in levels of alanine transaminase, aspartate transaminase, alkaline phosphatase, and bilirubin may occur. These abnormalities usually return to pretreatment levels after therapy is completed. Rarely, hepatotoxicity has been reported.

Other symptoms that have occurred during fluconazole therapy include alopecia and exfoliative skin disorders, such as Stevens-Johnson syndrome. These conditions occur most frequently in HIV-infected patients and in patients with a concurrent malignancy who are taking multiple drugs. A direct causative relationship has not been determined. Rarely, fluconazole therapy may induce hypokalemia, eosinophilia, and thrombocytopenia.

TABLE 44.3	Summary of Selected Ⓒ Azole Antifungal Agents		
Drug (Trade) Name	**Selected Indications**	**Route and Dosage Range**	**Pharmacokinetics**
Ⓟ fluconazole (Diflucan)	oropharyngeal,	*Adult:* PO/IV, 200 mg on first day, followed by 100-200 mg/d for 7–14 d *Child:* PO/IV, 6 mg/kg on the day 1, followed by 3 mg/kg once daily	*Onset:* PO, slow; IV, immediate *Duration:* 2–4 days $t_{1/2}$: 30 hours
	Esophageal candidiasis	*Adult PO/IV:* 400 mg loading dose, then 200–400 mg daily for 14–21 d *Child PO/IV:* 6 mg/kg on the day 1, followed by 3 mg/kg once daily	
	Vaginal candidiasis	*Adult PO:* 150 mg one time only	
	Candidal urinary tract infections	*Adult PO:* 200 mg daily for 14 d	
	cryptococcal meningitis	*Adult:* PO/IV, 400 mg daily as consolidation dose; then 200 mg daily as maintenance dose *Child:* PO/IV, 12 mg/kg on first day, followed by 6 mg/kg once daily;	
	Histoplasmosis; blastomycosis; coccidioidomycosis	*Adult PO:* 400–800 mg daily	
	Candidemia/invasive candidiasis	*Adult PO/IV:* 800 mg loading dose followed by 400 mg daily *Child PO/IV:* 6–12 mg/kg/d	
itraconazole (Sporanox)	Oropharyngeal or esophageal candidiasis	*Adult solution:* 200 mg daily	*Onset:* rapid *Duration:* end of infusion $t_{1/2}$: 20–40 h
	Histoplasmosis/blastomycosis	*Adult PO/IV:* 200–400 mg daily	
	Coccidioidomycosis	*Adult PO/IV:* 400 to 600 mg in two divided doses	
	Allergic bronchopulmonary aspergillosis	*Adult PO/IV:* 200 mg twice daily	
	Onychomycosis	*Adult PO:* 200 mg daily (toenails) for 12 weeks 200 mg 2x day for 1 week (fingernails) *Child:* safety not established	
ketoconazole (Nizoral)	Systemic fungal infections	*Adult:* PO, 200 mg daily, up to 400 mg/d; treat from 3 wk to 6 mo, depending on infecting organism and site *Child:* PO, >2 y, 3.3–6.6 mg/kg/d as a single dose; <2 y, safety and efficacy not established	*Onset:* PO, varies; topical, slow, not appreciably systemically absorbed *Duration:* Unknown $t_{1/2}$: 8 h
	Dermatophytosis, tinea corporis, tinea cruris, tinea versicolor	*Adult:* Topical, apply daily to affected area; may be treated twice daily; continue treatment for at least 2 wk *Child:* Topical, >2 y, same as adult; <2 y, safety and efficacy not established	
posaconazole (Noxafil)	Prophylaxis for aspergillosis	*Adult:* PO, 200–300 mg 3×/d	*Onset:* 1–2 h *Duration:* Unknown $t_{1/2}$: 35 h
	Oropharyngeal candidiasis	*Adult PO:* 100 mg 2x first day, then 100 mg daily for 13 days	
voriconazole (Vfend)	Invasive aspergillosis	*Adult and child >12 y:* IV, 6 mg/kg every 12 h day 1 followed by 3–4 mg/kg 2×/d *Adult and child >12 y:* PO, 400 mg every 12 h day 1 followed by 200 mg 2×/d	*Onset:* 1 h *Duration:* 96 h $t_{1/2}$: 24 h
	Systemic candida infections	*Adult and child >12 y:* IV, 6 mg/kg q12h as an infusion leading dose on first day, followed by 3 mg/kg as an infusion q12h *Adult and child ≥12 y (≥40 kg):* PO, 200 mg 2×/d for 14 d and for at least 7 d following resolution of symptoms *Adult and child ≥12 y (<40 kg):* PO, 100 mg 2×/d for 14 d and for at least 7 d following resolution of symptoms *Child <12 y:* Safety and efficacy have not been established	

TABLE 44.4	Summary of Selected Topical ⓖ Azole Antifungal Agents		
Drug (Trade) Name	**Selected Indications**	**Route and Dosage Range**	**Pharmacokinetics**
butoconazole (Gynazole-1, Femstat-3)	Vaginal candidiasis	**Vaginal dosage (vaginal cream):** Apply 1 applicatorful of 2% cream at bedtime for 3 consecutive d (6 d if pregnant)	Not systemically absorbed
clotrimazole (Mycelex, Gyne-Lotrimin)	Tinea infections Candidal infections: skin and mouth	**Topical:** *Adult and child >2 y.* Apply to affected skin and surrounding areas twice daily, morning and evening **Oral (troche) dosage:** *Adult and child >3 y.* Dissolve a 10-mg troche slowly and completely in the mouth 5×/d for 14 d **Vaginal dosage (vaginal cream):** Apply 1 applicatorful of 1% cream once daily at bedtime for 7–14 d **Vaginal dosage (tablets):** 100-mg tablet at bedtime for 7 d; or one 200-mg tablet at bedtime for 3 d; or 500-mg tablet as a single dose at bedtime	Not systemically absorbed
econazole	Tinea infections Candidal infections: skin and mouth	**Topical dosage (1% cream or lotion):** *Adult, adolescent, and child.* Apply to the affected area(s) and the immediately surrounding area(s) 1–2×/d	Not systemically absorbed
miconazole (Oravig)	Oropharyngeal candidiasis	*Adults and children >16 y.* 50 mg buccal tablet against the upper gum above the incisor tooth once daily in the morning for 14 days	
oxiconazole (Oxistat)	Tinea infections	**Topical dosage (1% cream or lotion):** *Adult, adolescent, and child.* Apply to the affected area(s) and the immediately surrounding area(s) 1–2×/d	Not systemically absorbed
sertaconazole (Ertaczo)	Tinea infections	**Topical application (cream):** *Adult, adolescent, and child >12 y.* Apply a thin layer of the 2% cream to the cleansed, dry, infected area twice daily for 4 wk	Not systemically absorbed
sulconazole (Exelderm)	Tinea infections	**Topical dosage (cream and solution):** *Adult.* Apply 1% preparation topically to the cleansed, dry, affected area(s) once or twice daily, morning and evening, for 3 wk	Not systemically absorbed
terconazole (Terazol)	Vaginal candidiasis	**Intravaginal dosage (Terazol 7 cream):** *Adult and adolescent.* Insert 1 applicatorful intravaginally once daily at bedtime for 7 consecutive d **Intravaginal dosage (Terazol 3 cream):** *Adult and adolescent.* Insert 1 applicatorful once daily at bedtime for 3 consecutive d **Intravaginal dosage (Terazol 3 vaginal suppositories):** *Adult and adolescent.* Insert one 80-mg suppository intravaginally once daily at bedtime for 3 consecutive d	Not systemically absorbed
tioconazole (Vagistat-1)	Vaginal candidiasis	**Intravaginal dosage (cream):** *Adult and adolescent.* 1 applicatorful before bedtime as a single dose	Not systemically absorbed

Drug Interactions

Many drug–drug interactions are possible with fluconazole because it inhibits drugs metabolized by the CYP3A4 enzyme system. Several drugs no longer available in the United States—astemizole, cisapride, and terfenadine—can induce fatal arrhythmias when given concurrently with fluconazole. Table 44.5 lists drugs that interact with fluconazole.

TABLE 44.5	Agents That Interact with P Fluconazole	
Interactants	**Effect and Significance**	**Nursing Management**
antiarrhythmics agents	Fluconazole may decrease the metabolism of the antiarrhythmics such as dofetilide and quinidine.	Monitor antiarrhythmic drug levels. Monitor for arrhythmias.
antidiabetic agents	Fluconazole inhibits the metabolism of oral antidiabetic agents, resulting in an increased pharmacologic effect.	Monitor blood glucose. Monitor for edema.
antipsychotic agents	Fluconazole may decrease the metabolism of the antipsychotics such as haloperidol, quetiapine, and risperidone.	Monitor for CNS depression. Ensure a safe environment.
benzodiazepines	Metabolism of certain benzodiazepines and first-pass effect of benzodiazepines may be decreased.	Monitor for CNS depression. Ensure a safe environment. Discuss adjustment of benzodiazepine dosage with prescriber as needed.
calcium channel blockers	Fluconazole inhibits the metabolism of calcium channel blockers, resulting in an increased pharmacologic effect.	Monitor blood pressure carefully. Advise patient to change positions slowly. Monitor for constipation.
carbamazepine	Fluconazole inhibits the metabolism of carbamazepine.	Monitor carbamazepine levels. Monitor hepatic status.
Corticosteroids	Fluconazole inhibits the metabolism of corticosteroids.	Monitor for corticosteroids adverse effects and toxicity.
cyclosporine	Fluconazole may inhibit cyclosporine hepatic metabolism.	Monitor cyclosporine levels. Monitor serum BUN/creatinine levels. Monitor intake and output. Discuss adjustment of cyclosporine dosage with prescriber as needed.
Fentanyl	Fluconazole inhibits the metabolism of fentanyl.	Monitor for CNS depression. Monitor for respiratory depression.
HMG CoA reductase inhibitors	Fluconazole may decrease the metabolism of the statins.	Monitor for myalgias. Monitor for signs of rhabdomyolysis.
hydantoins	Fluconazole may decrease the metabolism of hydantoins, such as phenytoin.	Monitor hydantoin levels. Monitor patient for sign of toxicity. Monitor the patient's ability to walk, talk, and think. Discuss adjustment of hydantoin dosage with prescriber as needed.
oral contraceptives	Concurrent use with oral contraceptives containing ethinyl estradiol/levonorgestrel may decrease serum concentration of the oral contraceptives.	Advise women taking ethinyl estradiol or levonorgestrel BCP to use another method of contraception.
NSAIDS	Fluconazole inhibits the metabolism of NSAIDS.	Monitor for GI distress. Monitor for GI bleeding. Monitor for renal and hepatic insufficiency.
protease inhibitors	Fluconazole inhibits the metabolism of protease inhibitors.	Monitor protease inhibitor levels. Monitor blood glucose levels. Monitor CBC. Monitor for signs of pancreatitis.
proton pump inhibitors/ H$_2$ blockers/antacids	PPI/H$_2$ blockers decrease the absorption of fluconazole.	Monitor for efficacy. If not contraindicated, administer fluconazole with acidic beverage such as Coca-Cola or Pepsi.
rifamycins	Rifamycins may induce the metabolism of fluconazole. This may decrease plasma concentration of fluconazole and decrease antifungal activity.	Monitor for therapeutic efficacy of fluconazole. Discuss adjustment of fluconazole dosage with prescriber as needed.

(Continued)

TABLE 44.5	Agents That Interact with [P] Fluconazole *(continued)*	
Interactants	**Effect and Significance**	**Nursing Management**
risperidone	Fluconazole inhibits the metabolism of risperidone.	Monitor for risperidone toxicity. Monitor CBC.
tacrolimus	Fluconazole inhibits the metabolism of tacrolimus.	Monitor I/O carefully. Monitor renal function tests. Monitor tacrolimus levels.
tolterodine	Fluconazole inhibits the metabolism of tolterodine.	Monitor for urine retention. Monitor for excessive anticholinergic effects.
tricyclic antidepressants	Fluconazole may inhibit the metabolism of TCA drugs.	Monitor the patient's clinical response to tricyclic agents (TCAs). Monitor cardiac status. Discuss adjustment of TCA dosage with prescriber as needed.
warfarin	Fluconazole may decrease the metabolism of anticoagulants such as warfarin.	Monitor PT and INR at least every 2 d. Monitor patient for signs of bleeding. Discuss adjustment of anticoagulant dosage with prescriber as needed.

Assessment of Relevant Core Patient Variables

Health Status

Elicit a patient history to evaluate for pre-existing renal or hepatic dysfunction, pregnancy, or breast-feeding. It is important to communicate any positive findings to the prescriber. Also, assess for any known reactions to azole antifungal agents.

Perform a complete physical examination, documenting signs and symptoms of the fungal infection. For patients with pre-existing anemia, renal, or hepatic disease or patients expected to be on long-term therapy, obtain samples for baseline CBC, renal, and hepatic function tests to determine baseline organ function.

Life Span and Gender

Determine whether the patient is pregnant or breast-feeding. In animal studies, fluconazole has been teratogenic when used in higher doses. Similar teratogenic malformations have been reported in women taking more than 400 mg/d over an extended period of time. Although fluconazole is assigned to pregnancy category C, many providers believe it should be used during pregnancy only if the potential benefit to the mother outweighs the potential risk to the fetus. It achieves high concentrations in breast milk.

Note the patient's age before administering fluconazole. Although a dosage schedule has been established for children, the safety of fluconazole has not been demonstrated in children younger than 13 years. However, drug therapy has been successful, and complications have not occurred in neonates treated with IV fluconazole in emergency treatment situations. With these concerns in mind, closely monitor children throughout therapy. Elderly patients are more likely than others to have decreased renal and hepatic function, which may increase the risk for toxicities.

Lifestyle, Diet, and Habits

Assess whether fluconazole is causing gastric distress in the patient. Fluconazole absorption and bioavailability are not affected by food or changes in gastric pH. Encourage patients who experience GI distress to take the drug with food.

Ask questions to uncover information about alcohol ingestion and other substance use (such as drugs and tobacco). Fluconazole may elevate hepatic enzymes. Caution the patient to refrain from alcohol ingestion throughout therapy because it increases the risk of hepatotoxicity. As with other drugs used as prophylaxis against opportunistic diseases in immunocompromised patients, discuss potential substance abuse (other drugs, alcohol, tobacco) with the patient. Explain how a healthy lifestyle decreases the risk of opportunistic diseases.

Determine which type of over-the-counter (OTC) pain reliever the patient generally uses. Advise the patient to use aspirin instead of acetaminophen for relief of minor discomforts because acetaminophen has the potential to damage the liver or kidneys.

Environment

Fluconazole is administered orally and intravenously. The oral preparation is used in the home environment, often as long-term prophylaxis for fungal infections in immunocompromised patients. Be sure to explain the importance of follow-up visits to assess the efficacy of therapy and to evaluate the patient for possible adverse effects.

IV therapy is usually reserved for patients unable to tolerate or take fluconazole orally and is administered in the hospital setting. Before administration, visually inspect the solution for particulate matter and discoloration. Do not administer unless the solution is clear. Fluconazole should be administered with an infusion pump at a rate not to exceed 200 mg/h.

Nursing Diagnoses and Outcomes

- Acute Pain related to fluconazole-induced headache
  Desired outcome: The patient will self-administer aspirin to relieve headache.
- Ineffective Protection related to adverse effects of blood dyscrasias and Stevens-Johnson syndrome
  Desired outcome: The patient will report signs and symptoms of these adverse reactions immediately to the prescriber.
- Disturbed Body Image from drug-related alopecia
  Desired outcome: The patient will verbalize concerns of changes in body image to the prescriber and develop coping strategies.
- Imbalanced Nutrition: Less than Body Requirements, related to adverse effects of nausea, vomiting, and abdominal pain
  Desired outcome: The patient will remain within acceptable weight parameters throughout therapy.
- Risk for Injury related to elevated hepatic enzymes and hypokalemia resulting from drug therapy
  Desired outcome: The patient will remain injury free throughout therapy.

Planning and Intervention

Maximizing Therapeutic Effects
Administer fluconazole in evenly divided intervals throughout the day.

Minimizing Adverse Effects
Carefully screen patients for pre-existing disorders, which may increase the risk for adverse reactions. In the hospitalized patient, contact the prescriber if any drugs known to interact or increase the risk for adverse effects are added to the drug profile. Administer an antiemetic or antidiarrheal agent, if prescribed, for adverse GI effects.

Providing Patient and Family Education
- Advise patients that they should not take fluconazole if they have ever had a reaction to any drug whose name includes the ending "azole."
- Advise patients to notify the prescriber if they are pregnant or breast-feeding.
- Explain that fluconazole is prescribed for a particular infection and should not be used to self-medicate or treat any other infection.
- Unless such use is specified by a physician, caution that this drug should not be used in children younger than 13 years.
- Teach patients about the need to complete the full course of drug therapy, even if the infection resolves. Instruct patients to take forgotten doses as soon as they remember, but not if it is time for the next dose.

- Remind patients of the importance of remaining well hydrated while taking this drug.
- Explain potential adverse effects of fluconazole and potential remedies for these discomforts. Advise patients to contact the prescriber immediately if they experience unusual bruising or bleeding, skin rash (including inside the mouth), redness, blistering, peeling, or loosening of the skin. This advice is especially important for patients taking fluconazole as prophylaxis for opportunistic diseases.
- Discuss the possibility of hepatic injury. Advise patients to contact the prescriber if they experience dark urine, pale stool, jaundice, anorexia, nausea or vomiting, and persistent fatigue.
- Explain that fluconazole may decrease the effectiveness of oral contraceptives and suggest that patients use an alternative form of contraception while taking fluconazole.
- Advise patients taking sulfonylureas to monitor their blood glucose levels frequently and to notify the prescriber in the event of frequent episodes of hypoglycemia.
- Suggest that patients taking anticoagulants have blood tests performed frequently to detect altered prothrombin times. Patients should contact the prescriber if they experience easy bruising or bleeding.
- Advise patients of signs and symptoms of secondary bacterial infections that may occur with superficial mycoses. Recommend that patients contact the prescriber if the affected skin becomes red and hot or exudes pus.
- Assure patients with alopecia that the condition is temporary.

Ongoing Assessment and Evaluation

Monitor the effectiveness of therapy. When treating superficial mycoses, be sure to document new lesions and assess for possible secondary bacterial infections. In the hospital setting, monitor for hepatic or renal dysfunction. It is important to monitor fluid intake and output carefully; enlist the patient and family to document intake and output not observed by nurses.

Throughout therapy, arrange for serial blood testing to evaluate renal, hepatic, and hematopoietic function. For

CRITICAL THINKING SCENARIO

FLUCONAZOLE AND CHRONIC CANDIDIASIS

Janice Wind is a 40-year-old woman infected with HIV. She has been diagnosed with esophageal candidiasis, for which fluconazole therapy has been prescribed. This is her third episode of esophageal candidiasis for which she will receive prolonged therapy. Assume you are Ms. Wind's nurse.

1. Identify the assessments and evaluations you would find valuable before initiating therapy.

2. Propose or construct a patient-teaching plan. Which features would you include?

3. Develop some questions about the effects of therapy to explore with Ms. Wind when she returns to the clinic in 6 weeks for a follow-up evaluation.

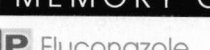

suspected electrolyte imbalance, reviewing complete metabolic panel test results is important.

Monitor the patient for GI distress, headache, dizziness, exfoliative skin disorders, and hepatic dysfunction. It is important to ensure the safety of the patient experiencing CNS effects by keeping the bed in the low position and the side rails up at all times. To avoid injury, be sure that the patient understands the need to ask for ambulatory assistance if he or she experiences dizziness. By the end of therapy, the patient should be without symptoms of fungal infection. In addition, adverse reactions should be controlled.

Drugs Closely Related to P Fluconazole

Itraconazole, posaconazole, and voriconazole are similar to fluconazole because they are also triazole antifungal agents. Ketoconazole is also closely related to fluconazole, but is an imidazole antifungal agent.

Itraconazole

Itraconazole (Sporanox) is an oral or IV triazole antifungal drug that is related closely to fluconazole. Itraconazole offers a broader spectrum of activity than fluconazole, including endemic fungi, *Sporothrix schenckii*, and *Aspergillus* species. The drug is used as an alternative to IV amphotericin B for the treatment of blastomycosis, histoplasmosis, paracoccidioidomycosis, and sporotrichosis. Absorption of oral itraconazole capsules may be increased when given concurrently with a meal, cola beverage, or cranberry juice because it requires an acidic gastric pH for solubilization. Conversely, drugs such as proton pump inhibitors, histamine-2 receptor blockers, and antacids interfere with its absorption. The oral solution of itraconazole is unaffected by gastric pH and administered on an empty stomach for optimal absorption. Adverse effects are the same as other triazole antifungal agents. In addition, itraconazole may have two serious adverse effects: an aldosterone-like effect, manifested by hypertension, hypokalemia, and peripheral edema and hepatotoxicity. Because of these potential adverse effects, itraconazole should be reserved for use in serious fungal infections,

especially in patients with pre-existing cardiac or hepatic disorders. Pregnancy and lactation precautions are the same as fluconazole.

Like fluconazole, itraconazole inhibits drugs metabolized by the CYP3A4 enzyme system but actually has more drug–drug interactions than fluconazole. Coadministration with dofetilide, oral midazolam, pimozide, quinidine, lovastatin, simvastatin, or triazolam is contraindicated. Serious cardiovascular events, including QT prolongation, torsades de pointes, ventricular tachycardia, cardiac arrest, and/or sudden death, have occurred in patients using pimozide or quinidine concomitantly with itraconazole. Patients taking itraconazole should be monitored for hepatotoxicity, neuropathy, and heart failure.

For patients with aspergillosis, histoplasmosis, or blastomycosis, arrange for periodic serum drug level monitoring.

Posaconazole

Posaconazole (Noxafil) is a new triazole antifungal agent approved for use as a prophylactic agent for fungal infections in stem cell transplant recipients and in patients who are neutropenic with either acute leukemia or myelodysplastic syndrome. It is also approved for oral but not systemic candidiasis. It is an oral solution that should be taken with a meal or nutritional supplement. Posaconazole has a chemical structure different than fluconazole and voriconazole; thus, it may inhibit mutated fungal strains resistant to these drugs. Liver and renal function tests should be coordinated at the start of and during the course of therapy. It is necessary to inform the prescriber immediately if serum potassium, magnesium, and calcium levels are elevated, because they must be corrected prior to initiation of therapy. The patient should shake the solution well prior to pouring it and should rinse the supplied spoon after each dose. Adverse effects are similar to other drugs in the triazole class.

Voriconazole

Voriconazole (Vfend) is another triazole antifungal agent that is structurally related to fluconazole. It is used for esophageal candidiasis, primary treatment of invasive aspergillosis, and salvage therapy for infections caused by *Scedosporium* species or *Fusarium* species in patients refractory to or intolerant of other antifungal therapy. Voriconazole can be administered by the oral or intravenous route. Give oral voriconazole on an empty stomach.

Voriconazole is given cautiously to patients with pre-existing hepatic or renal dysfunction, especially when using the intravenous formulation. It is also given cautiously to patients with pre-existing ocular disorders because of the potential for adverse effects to vision.

In addition to the usual adverse effects with triazole antifungal agents, voriconazole is associated with two distinct adverse reactions: transient vision changes and rash. Patients experience visual disturbances that involve enhanced brightness, blurred vision, photophobia, or color vision changes. Visual hallucinations may indicate voriconazole neurotoxicity. Neurotoxicity may also induce confusion, agitation, myoclonic movements, and auditory hallucinations A photosensitive rash may occur that is not prevented by use of sunscreens. Advise the patient to limit sun exposure throughout therapy. Rarely, severe rash such as Stevens-Johnson syndrome or toxic epidermal necrolysis have occurred. Patients with severe systemic illness have an increased risk for QT prolongation, torsade de pointes, cardiac arrest, and sudden death. Drug–drug interactions are similar to those with fluconazole. Voriconazole is a pregnancy category D drug. Teratogenicity, embryotoxicity, reduced fetal weight, and multiple skeletal abnormalities were noted in animal trials. It is not approved for use in children.

Ketoconazole

Ketoconazole (Nizoral) is available as an oral formulation and as a cream, gel, foam, and shampoo for topical use. Imidazole antifungal agents, such as ketoconazole, have largely been replaced by the triazoles because of superior pharmacokinetics, improved safety profiles, and higher efficacy for the treatment of systemic mycoses. It is effective against most systemic mycoses. In addition to its antifungal activity, ketoconazole possesses actions that may make it useful in other types of conditions. For example, ketoconazole has been used successfully for treating advanced prostate cancer. When used in high doses, ketoconazole can inhibit sterol synthesis in humans, including the synthesis of aldosterone, cortisol, and testosterone.

When ketoconazole is given orally, its bioavailability is affected by the pH of the stomach. Like itraconazole, absorption of oral ketoconazole may be increased when given concurrently with a meal, cola beverage, or cranberry juice because it requires an acidic gastric pH for solubilization. It should not be given concurrently with agents that increase gastric pH, such as food, antacids, histamine-2 blockers, and proton pump inhibitors. Adverse effects are similar to those with fluconazole. Like other azole antifungal agents, ketoconazole interacts with many drugs metabolized by the CYP3A4 enzyme system. Pregnancy and lactation precautions are the same as for fluconazole.

Drugs Significantly Different From P Fluconazole

Butoconazole

Butoconazole (Femstat-3, Gynezole-1) is a topical imidazole antifungal agent that is effective in treating vulvovaginal candidiasis. As other azole antifungals, it exerts its antifungal activity by altering cellular membranes, resulting in increased membrane permeability and growth inhibition.

The only contraindication to the use of butoconazole is hypersensitivity. Butoconazole should be used cautiously in patients with other azole hypersensitivities because cross-sensitivity may occur. Adverse effects associated with the use of butoconazole include vaginal irritation, burning, pruritus, stinging, vaginal pain or soreness, and vaginal discharge.

Women using butoconazole should be advised to refrain from sexual intercourse until 72 hours after therapy is completed because butoconazole contains mineral oil, which may weaken contraceptive devices, including condoms, diaphragms, and cervical caps. Butoconazole is available as an OTC medication. It is a pregnancy category C drug.

Clotrimazole

Clotrimazole (Mycelex, Gyne-Lotrimin) is another imidazole antifungal drug. It is not orally absorbed and is too toxic for IV administration. It is marketed in various forms, including vaginal suppositories and cream, topical lotion and cream, and oral solution and lozenges. It is active against a wide variety of fungi, yeast, and dermatophytes; certain gram-positive bacteria; and superficial fungal infections. These infections include dermatophytosis, vaginal and oral candidiasis, and tinea infections. The ability of clotrimazole's formulations to reach subcutaneous tissues is poor. Therefore, clotrimazole is not indicated for treating subcutaneous mycoses.

Clotrimazole is available as a prescription and an OTC medication. Contraindications are similar to those of butoconazole. Adverse effects include skin blistering, skin irritation, burning, pruritus, and stinging. It is a pregnancy category C drug.

Econazole

Econazole is a topical imidazole antifungal agent used primarily to treat cutaneous candidiasis and tinea infections, including tinea versicolor. Its spectrum of activity is similar to that of clotrimazole, miconazole, or tioconazole. Econazole is not approved for ophthalmic administration or vaginal administration. Contraindications and adverse effects are similar to those of butoconazole. It is a pregnancy category C drug and may be used in children older than 3 months of age.

Miconazole

Miconazole (Monistat, M-Zole, Monistat-derm, Vusion) is a topical imidazole-type antifungal agent. It is also available as a buccal tablet (Oravig). Miconazole is different than other azoles because it has two mechanisms of action. Like other azoles, it inhibits ergosterol synthesis, and it also inhibits peroxidases, which results in the accumulation of peroxide within the cell, resulting in cell death. It is most commonly used topically and intravaginally and is available as an OTC preparation. Prescriptions are required for Monistat-derm (a 2% cream) and Vusion, a topical ointment with zinc oxide and petrolatum for diaper rash caused by candidiasis.

Oxiconazole

Oxiconazole (Oxistat) is a topical imidazole antifungal agent used to manage tinea pedis, tinea corporis, and tinea cruris. It is available as both a cream and a lotion and is administered once daily. Oxiconazole is not approved for ophthalmic administration or vaginal administration. Contraindications and adverse effects are similar to those of butoconazole. It is a pregnancy category B drug and may be used in children.

Sertaconazole

Sertaconazole (Ertaczo) is an imidazole-type antifungal used for treating tinea pedis in immunocompetent patients. Sertaconazole is administered as a topical cream. Systemic absorption does not occur. Antifungal hypersensitivity is the only contraindication to it use. Skin irritation may occur when sertaconazole is used with other creams or lotions at the same site. Adverse effects include application site reaction, burning, and tenderness. It is a pregnancy category C drug and is generally considered safe to use while breast-feeding.

Sulconazole

Sulconazole (Exelderm) is a topical imidazole antifungal agent used in managing tinea pedis, tinea corporis, and tinea cruris. It has greater efficacy than clotrimazole and miconazole. Like oxiconazole, it is administered only once per day. It is not approved for ophthalmic or vaginal administration. Its contraindications and adverse effects are similar to those for oxiconazole. Topical sulconazole is classified as a pregnancy risk category C drug. It is not approved for use in children.

Terconazole

Terconazole (Terazol) is a triazole antifungal agent that is structurally related to imidazole antifungal drugs. It is available for intravaginal use only. Terconazole is as effective as clotrimazole or miconazole in managing vulvovaginal candidiasis. Contraindications and adverse effects are similar to those of butoconazole.

Tioconazole

Tioconazole (Vagistat-1) is an imidazole antifungal agent available for intravaginal use. It is the only topical antifungal agent approved in the United States as a single-dose treatment for vulvovaginal candidiasis. It is now available as an OTC medication. Contraindications and adverse effects are similar to those of butoconazole.

MISCELLANEOUS ANTIFUNGAL DRUGS

A summary of miscellaneous antifungal agents is presented in Table 44.6.

Butenafine

Butenafine (Mentax) is an allylamine topical antifungal drug indicated for treating tinea pedis, tinea corporis, and tinea cruris. It currently is under investigation for treatment of onychomycosis. Butenafine is similar to tolnaftate (discussed later in this chapter); however, it also is effective against Candida species, whereas tolnaftate is not. No important drug inter-actions or adverse effects have been identified at this time.

Ciclopirox Olamine

Ciclopirox olamine (Loprox) is a miscellaneous broad-spectrum antifungal drug used to treat infections caused by dermatophytes or Candida species. It is used primarily for tinea pedis, tinea cruris, tinea corporis, and tinea versicolor. It works by blocking transport of amino acids into the fungal cell, thus altering the cell membrane to allow leakage of intracellular material. Ciclopirox olamine also is manufactured as a nail lacquer (Penlac) for the topical treatment

TABLE 44.6 Summary of Miscellaneous Antifungal Agents

Drug (Trade) Name	Selected Indications	Route and Dosage Range	Pharmacokinetics
butenafine (Mentax)	Tinea pedis, tinea corporis, tinea cruris	*Adult*: Topical, apply to affected area once daily for 4 wk	Not generally absorbed systemically
ciclopirox olamine (Loprox)	Tinea pedis, tinea cruris, tinea corporis, tinea versicolor	*Adult*: Topical, apply to affected area as directed twice daily	Not generally absorbed systemically
griseofulvin (Grifulvin V, Gris-Peg)	Superficial dermatophyte infections (ringworm)—tinea corporis, tinea barbae, tinea capitis, tinea ungulum; tinea pedis and tinea cruris only when unresponsive to topical therapy	*Adult*: PO, 250–500 mg bid for 2 wk, up to 18 mo	*Onset*: 4 h *Duration*: 2 d $t_{1/2}$: 9–24 h
naftifine (Naftin)	Tinea pedis, tinea cruris, tinea corporis	*Adult*: Topical, massage into area bid; do not use longer than 4 wk	Not generally absorbed systemically
terbinafine (Lamisil)	Onychomycosis	*Adult*: PO, 250 mg/d; topical, apply to areabid up to 4 wk *Child*: ≤20 kg, PO, 62.5 mg/d *Child*: 20–40 kg, PO, 125 mg/d	*Onset*: 24 h *Duration*: 90 d $t_{1/2}$: 100 h

of mild to moderate onychomycosis of the fingernails and toenails without lunula involvement in immunocompetent patients.

Ciclopirox olamine is absorbed deeper into the dermal layers than other topical drugs. However, little is absorbed systemically. No important drug–drug interactions are known. Potential adverse effects include irritation, pruritus at the application site, redness, pain, burning, and worsening of clinical signs or symptoms.

Griseofulvin

Griseofulvin (Grifulvin-V, Gris-Peg) is a miscellaneous antifungal drug used in treating superficial dermatophytic infections, such as ringworm and tinea. It is available in a microsize or ultramicrosize formulation. These different formulations are meant to increase the bioavailability of, and to decrease the GI intolerance to, the drug.

Griseofulvin works by disrupting the mitotic spindle structure of the fungal cell, thereby stopping cell division. It also may cause defective DNA that is unable to replicate. It is very effective for superficial mycoses because it is deposited in keratin precursor cells, creating an unfavorable environment for fungal infection. Infected skin, cells, and hair are then replaced slowly by tissue that is not infected by the dermatophyte. Griseofulvin therapy lasts until the infected area has completely regrown. This therapy may take 6 to 12 months in treating tinea unguium.

Griseofulvin is contraindicated during pregnancy and breast-feeding. It should be given with caution to patients with hepatic dysfunction, porphyria, or systemic lupus erythematosus because the drug may exacerbate these conditions.

Griseofulvin has a moderate adverse effect profile. Common adverse effects include nausea, vomiting, flatulence, and epigastric distress. CNS effects may include headache, fatigue, dizziness, insomnia, confusion, psychotic symptoms, and paresthesias of the hands and feet. Integumentary adverse effects may include maculopapular rash, urticaria, and photosensitivity. In addition, hepatitis, elevated hepatic enzymes, granulocytopenia, and leukopenia have occurred after high-dose or long-term therapy.

Griseofulvin interacts with several drugs. Most importantly, it interacts with oral contraceptives by decreasing their effectiveness. Therefore, advise women taking birth control pills to use another method of contraception during griseofulvin therapy. Griseofulvin also may decrease the effectiveness of warfarin.

It is necessary to closely monitor prothrombin time if griseofulvin is either added to or discontinued from warfarin therapy. Barbiturates can decrease the antifungal activity of griseofulvin. Finally, griseofulvin may increase the adverse effects of alcohol when taken concurrently.

Naftifine

Naftifine (Naftin) is a topical allylamine antifungal drug. It is used primarily for tinea pedis, tinea cruris, and tinea corporis. Naftifine is believed to interfere with sterol biosynthesis, but by a different mechanism than azoles. No important drug interactions occur with naftifine. Adverse effects include burning, stinging, dryness, erythema, pruritus, local irritation, and rash.

Terbinafine

Terbinafine (Lamisil) is another allylamine antifungal drug administered either orally or topically. Its topical formulation is now available OTC. Terbinafine is pharmacologically similar to naftifine. Oral terbinafine is highly effective for treating onychomycosis because of its fungicidal activity and ability to concentrate within the nail. In fact, it has been found to be superior to griseofulvin and itraconazole for treating onychomycosis.

Oral terbinafine should be given with caution to patients with hepatic and renal insufficiency and during breast-feeding. The most common adverse effects are GI, followed by elevated hepatic enzyme levels, urticaria, pruritus, and occasionally a distorted sense of taste (dysgeusia). Rare but serious adverse effects include symptomatic idiosyncratic hepatobiliary dysfunction (including cholestatic hepatitis), serious skin reactions, severe neutropenia, and allergic reactions (including anaphylaxis). Some formulations of terbinafine are now available as OTC preparations.

CHAPTER SUMMARY

- Antifungal drugs can be arbitrarily divided into those used to manage systemic infections and those used to manage superficial infections.
- The two types of fungi are yeasts and molds.
- Systemic fungal diseases are categorized by those that are opportunistic and those that occur in every population.
- Amphotericin B is the prototype polyene antifungal and is the drug of choice for most systemic fungal infections.
- Amphotericin B induces severe adverse effects, including infusion reactions.
- Fluconazole is the prototype azole antifungal drug used for both systemic and superficial mycoses.
- Superficial fungal infections are treated with both oral and topical formulations of drugs.

QUESTIONS FOR STUDY AND REVIEW

1. List the potential adverse effects of amphotericin B.
2. What important adverse effects are associated with fluconazole therapy?
3. Which of the azole antifungal agents may be used in managing systemic fungal infections?
4. What follow-up should be performed for a patient taking griseofulvin?
5. Why are there so many adverse effects related to drug–drug interactions with azole drugs?

NEED MORE HELP?

Chapter 44 of the Study Guide to Accompany *Drug Therapy in Nursing,* 4th Edition, contains NCLEX-style questions and other learning activities to reinforce your understanding of the concepts presented in this chapter. For additional information or to purchase the study guide, visit **thePoint**.

REFERENCES

Ashley, E. D., Perfect, J. R. (2009). Pharmacology of azoles, *Up To Date*. Retrieved from *http://uptodate.com*

Chandwani, S., Wentworth, C., Burke, T., & Patterson, T. (2009). Utilization and dosage pattern of echinocandins for treatment of fungal infections in US hospital practice. *Current Medical Research and Opinion*, 25(2):385–393.

Cleary, J. D. (2009). Echinocandins: pharmacokinetic and therapeutic issues. *Current Medical Research and Opinion*, 25(7):1741–1750.

Cross, S., & Scott, L. (2008). Micafungin: a review of its use in adults for the treatment of invasive and oesophageal candidiasis, and as prophylaxis against Candida infections. *Drugs*, 68(15):2225–2255.

Davis, S., & Vazquez, J. (2008, June). Anidulafungin: an evidence-based review of its use in invasive fungal infections. *Core Evidence*, 2(4):241–249. Retrieved July 9, 2009, from CINAHL Plus with Full Text database.

Drew, R. H. (2009). Pharmacology of amphotericin B, *Up To Date*. Retrieved from *http://uptodate.com*

Facts and Comparisons. (2010). *Drug facts and comparisons*. Philadelphia, PA: Lippincott Williams & Wilkins.

Gafter-Gvili, A., Vidal, L., Goldberg, E., et al. (2008). Treatment of invasive candidal infections: systematic review and meta-analysis. *Mayo Clinic Proceedings*, 83(9):1011–1021.

Kaufman, C. A. (2009). Treatment of oropharyngeal and esophageal candidiasis, *Up To Date*. Retrieved from *http://uptodate.com*

Kaufman, C. A. (2009). Candidemia in adults, *Up To Date*. Retrieved from *http://uptodate.com*

Koda-Kimbal, M. A, Young, L. Y., Kradian, W. A., et al. (2008). *Applied Therapeutics: The Clinical Use of Drugs*. Philadelphia, PA: Lippincott Williams & Wilkins.

Micromedex Healthcare Series. Retrieved from *http://thomsonhc.com*

Moen, M. D., Lyseng-Williamson, K. A., Scott, L. J. (2009). Liposomal amphotericin B: a review of its use as empirical therapy in febrile neutropenia and in the treatment of invasive fungal infections. *Drugs*, 69(3):361–392.

Pappas, P. G., Kauffman, C. A., Andes, D. (2009). Clinical practice guidelines for the management of candidiasis: 2009 update by the Infectious Diseases Society of America. *Clinical Infectious Diseases*, 48(5):503–535.

Sugar, A. M. (2009). Treatment of invasive aspergillosis, *Up-To-Date*, Retrieved from www.uptodate.com

Tatro, D. S. (2009). *Drug interaction facts*. Philadelphia, PA: Lippincott Williams & Wilkins.

Walsh, T. J., Anaissie, E. J., Denning, D. W., et al. (2009). Treatment of aspergillosis: clinical practice guidelines of the Infectious Diseases Society of America. *Clinical Infectious Diseases*, 46(3):327–360.

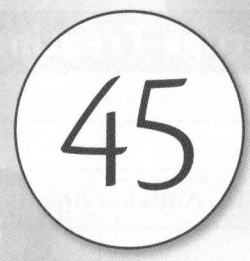

Drugs Treating Viral Infections

Learning Objectives

At the completion of this chapter the student will:

1. Identify core drug knowledge about drugs used to treat viral infections.

2. Identify core patient variables relevant to drugs used to treat viral infections.

3. Relate the interaction of core drug knowledge to core patient variables for drugs used to treat viral infections.

4. Generate a nursing plan of care from the interactions between core drug knowledge and core patient variables for drugs used to treat viral infections.

5. Describe nursing interventions to maximize therapeutic and minimize adverse effects for drugs used to treat viral infections.

6. Determine key points for patient and family education for drugs used to treat viral infections.

Key Terms cytomegalovirus   herpes zoster   respiratory syncytial virus
herpes simplex virus   phosphorylation

Drugs Treating Viral Infections

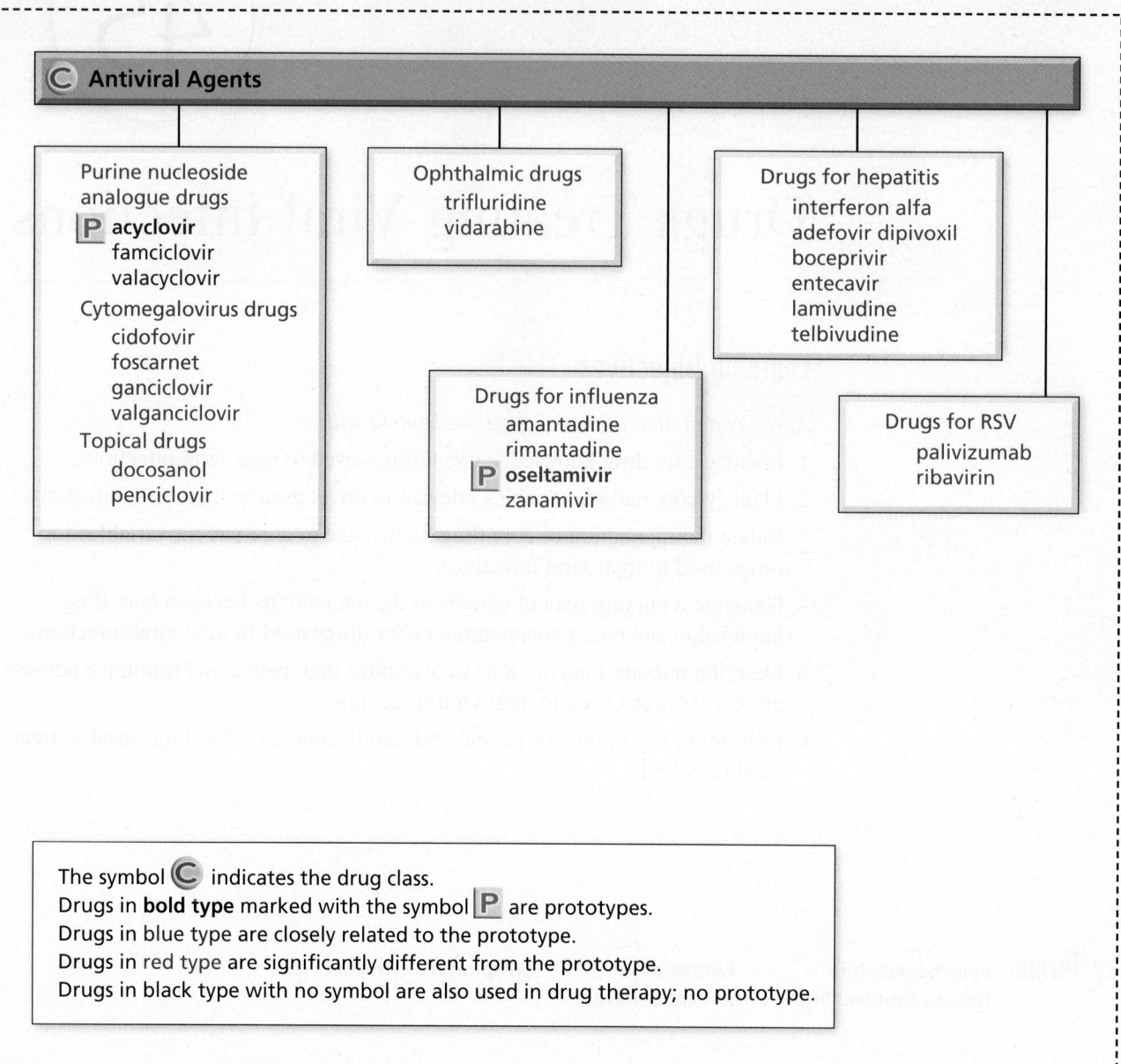

C Antiviral Agents

Purine nucleoside analogue drugs
P **acyclovir**
famciclovir
valacyclovir
Cytomegalovirus drugs
cidofovir
foscarnet
ganciclovir
valganciclovir
Topical drugs
docosanol
penciclovir

Ophthalmic drugs
trifluridine
vidarabine

Drugs for influenza
amantadine
rimantadine
P **oseltamivir**
zanamivir

Drugs for hepatitis
interferon alfa
adefovir dipivoxil
boceprivir
entecavir
lamivudine
telbivudine

Drugs for RSV
palivizumab
ribavirin

The symbol **C** indicates the drug class.
Drugs in **bold type** marked with the symbol **P** are prototypes.
Drugs in blue type are closely related to the prototype.
Drugs in red type are significantly different from the prototype.
Drugs in black type with no symbol are also used in drug therapy; no prototype.

Viral diseases affect people throughout the life span. In healthy people, these diseases may be considered an annoyance; in immunocompromised people, these diseases can be deadly. Viruses are responsible for many infectious disorders, ranging from the common cold to life-threatening meningitis. In contrast to the number of drugs that have been developed to treat bacterial disease, few antiviral drugs have been developed. Because viruses have no metabolic enzymes of their own, they can replicate only within a living host cell by using the metabolic processes of the host. Therefore, most drugs used to eliminate a virus may do substantial harm to the host. However, a few antiviral drugs have been developed that can target the invading virus yet leave the host intact. These drugs have a narrow spectrum of activity, and each drug has specific clinical applications.

This chapter discusses the purine nucleoside analogue drugs; the prototype is acyclovir. Drugs used to manage influenza are represented by oseltamivir, and drugs used in the management of hepatitis B and C are represented by interferon alfa.

PHYSIOLOGY OF VIRAL REPRODUCTION

The reproduction of viruses in humans requires five steps—adsorption, penetration, uncoating, replication, and transcription (the change of ribonucleic acid [RNA] to deoxy- ribonucleic acid [DNA]), all of which precede viral assembly and release. During the adsorption step, the virus attaches itself to receptor sites on the host cell surface. Once attached, the virus releases enzymes that enable the virus to penetrate the cell. After the virus enters the cell, the protein coat of the virus dissolves and releases viral genetic material. The virus then synthesizes new messenger RNA and, using host ribosomes, synthesizes viral proteins. The viral nucleic acids and proteins are assembled into mature viruses that are then released by budding off from infected cells or by lysis of the infected cell (Figure 45.1).

PATHOPHYSIOLOGY OF SELECTED VIRAL INFECTIONS

Cytomegalovirus

Cytomegalovirus (CMV) is a type of herpesvirus. CMV infection is extremely prevalent—approximately 80% of the population demonstrates evidence of infection. In most individuals, infection is asymptomatic. However, in some individuals, such as those with acquired immunodeficiency syndrome (AIDS) and bone marrow transplant recipients, CMV infection is associated with severe and usually fatal disease. CMV infection during pregnancy can be hazardous to the fetus, possibly leading to stillbirth, brain damage, and other birth defects or to neonatal illness.

Although CMV most frequently causes retinitis, it also can cause infection in the lungs, throat, brain, kidneys, gallbladder, liver, and colon. In immunocompromised patients, CMV prophylaxis is started when the CD4+ T-cell count measures less than 50 mm³.

Hepatitis

There are five types of hepatitis: hepatitis A (HAV), hepatitis B (HBV), hepatitis C (HCV), hepatitis D (HDV), and hepatitis E (HEV). In North America, the most prevalent types are HAV, HBC, and HCV. Symptoms of hepatitis include jaundice, fatigue, abdominal pain, nausea, and anorexia. Some patients may have dark urine or light-colored stool.

HAV infection is an acute viral syndrome spread by the oral–fecal route. It does not have the ability to become a chronic disease. Hepatitis A vaccine is the preferred method of prevention.

HBV infection is spread when blood or body fluid from an infected person enters the body of a person who is not immune. Infection may occur through having sex with an infected person, through needlesticks or sharps exposures, from an infected mother to the neonate during birth, or by sharing drugs or needles. HBV may present as a mild illness, lasting a few weeks (acute), to a serious long-term (chronic) illness that can lead to liver disease or liver cancer. Like hepatitis A, hepatitis B vaccine is the preferred method of prevention.

HCV is spread in the same manner as HBV. There are multiple genotypes and subtypes of HCV, a circumstance which makes treatment difficult. An estimated 4 to 5 million people in the United States have chronic HCV. HCV occurs most frequently in people who use intravenous (IV) illegal drugs. There is no preventive vaccine.

Herpes Simplex

Herpes simplex virus (HSV) has two types—type 1 (HSV-1) and type 2 (HSV-2). Both types cause similar infections. HSV-1 is associated generally with herpes labialis (cold sores or fever blisters), signs of which occur on or near the lips. HSV-2 may cause herpes labialis or herpes genitalis (genital lesions). Infection with either virus is characterized by the formation of painful vesicles, which rupture and form a crust when fluid from active lesions contacts parts of the body that have a break in the skin. In between outbreaks, the virus remains in a latent stage in sensory nerve ganglions. Recurrence may be triggered by other infections, sun exposure, or stress. Outbreaks are preceded by a burning or tingling sensation along the nerve and at the site of infection.

Herpes Zoster

Herpes zoster is an acute unilateral and segmental inflammation of the dorsal root ganglia caused by reactivation of the varicella-zoster virus (VZV), which also causes chickenpox. This infection usually occurs in adults and produces localized vesicular skin lesions, confined to a dermatome, and severe neuralgic pain in peripheral areas innervated by the nerves arising in the inflamed root ganglia.

PHYSIOLOGY

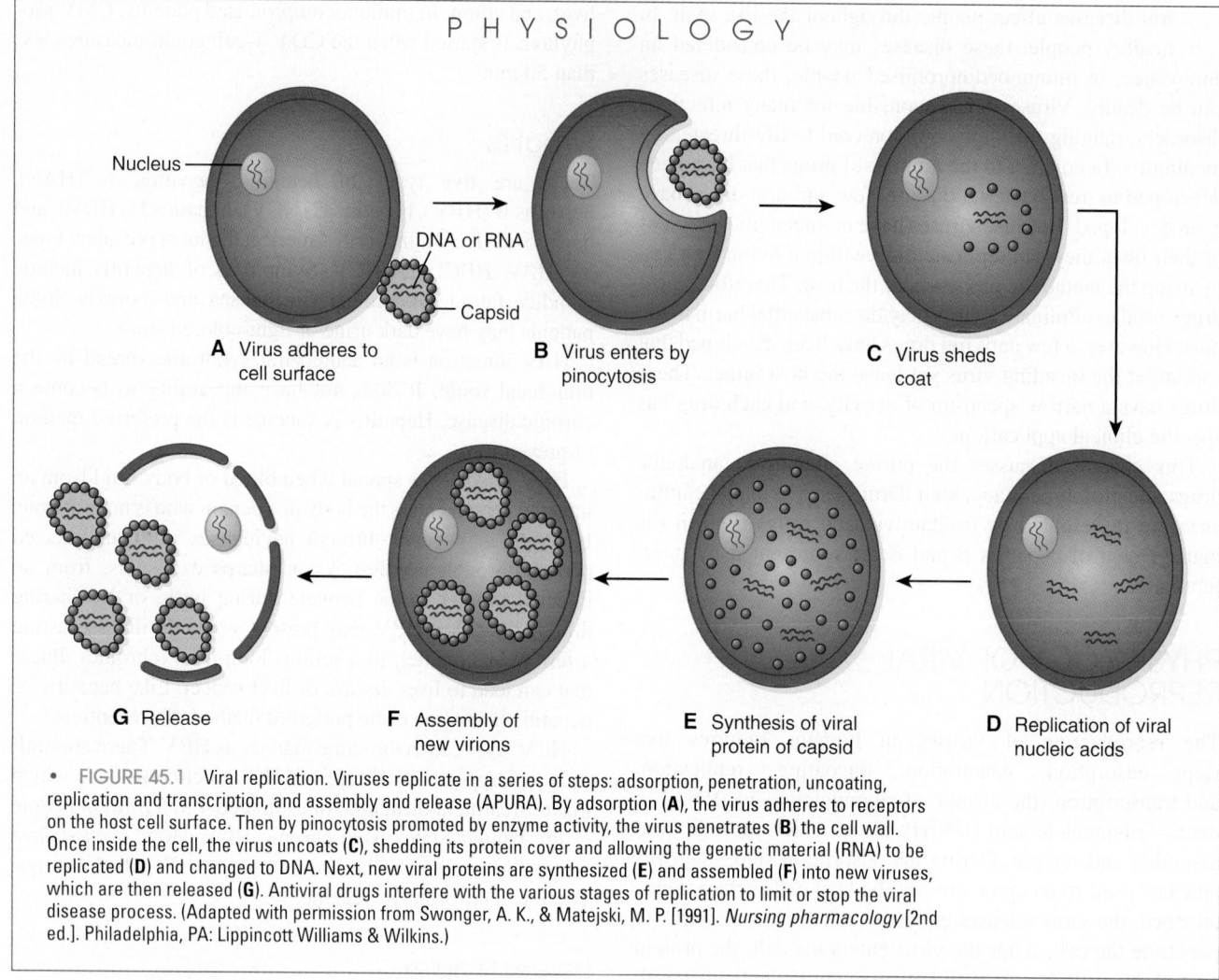

A Virus adheres to cell surface

B Virus enters by pinocytosis

C Virus sheds coat

D Replication of viral nucleic acids

E Synthesis of viral protein of capsid

F Assembly of new virions

G Release

• FIGURE 45.1 Viral replication. Viruses replicate in a series of steps: adsorption, penetration, uncoating, replication and transcription, and assembly and release (APURA). By adsorption (**A**), the virus adheres to receptors on the host cell surface. Then by pinocytosis promoted by enzyme activity, the virus penetrates (**B**) the cell wall. Once inside the cell, the virus uncoats (**C**), shedding its protein cover and allowing the genetic material (RNA) to be replicated (**D**) and changed to DNA. Next, new viral proteins are synthesized (**E**) and assembled (**F**) into new viruses, which are then released (**G**). Antiviral drugs interfere with the various stages of replication to limit or stop the viral disease process. (Adapted with permission from Swonger, A. K., & Matejski, M. P. [1991]. *Nursing pharmacology* [2nd ed.]. Philadelphia, PA: Lippincott Williams & Wilkins.)

Onset of herpes zoster is characterized by fever and malaise. Within 2 to 4 days, severe deep pain, pruritus, and paresthesia or hyperesthesia develop, usually on the trunk and occasionally on the arms and legs. The pain may be continuous or intermittent and usually lasts from 1 to 4 weeks. Up to 2 weeks after the first symptoms, small, red, nodular skin lesions erupt on the painful areas.

After the initial outbreak, the virus retreats back to the dorsal root ganglia, but outbreaks may recur. Postherpetic neuralgia is a common and potentially debilitating complication of herpes zoster that is difficult to manage, especially in elderly patients.

Influenza

Of the many types of influenza virus, influenza A and influenza B are the only types that can be affected by current antiviral agents. Influenza A and B have similar characteristics; however, infection with influenza A is more common and more severe. The virus attacks both the upper and lower respiratory tracts. It is transmitted directly by respiratory droplet or indirectly by contact with a contaminated object. Influenza virus is difficult to combat because it undergoes

constant antigenic changes, which limit vaccine development and the ability of individuals to develop long-term immunity.

Influenza has a sudden, acute onset with fever and chills, marked malaise, headache, general muscle aching, sore throat, unproductive cough, and nasal congestion. It may be self-limiting or may progress to pneumonia. Elderly patients, patients with chronic diseases, and immunocompromised patients should be immunized yearly.

Respiratory Syncytial Virus

Respiratory syncytial virus (RSV) is a major cause of respiratory illness in all age groups. In adults, infection with RSV tends to cause mild cold symptoms; in school-aged children, it can cause a cold and bronchial cough; and in infants and toddlers, it can cause bronchiolitis (inflammation of the smaller airways of the lungs) or pneumonia. Reinfection throughout life is common.

The highest rates of RSV illness occur in infants 2 to 6 months of age, with a peak at 2 to 3 months. RSV infection is often carried home by a school-aged child and passed to a younger one, especially an infant.

RSV infection is especially dangerous in infants younger than 1 year and in children with asthma, other lung disorders, or heart disease. It is a major cause of hospitalization among children during the winter months. The symptoms of bronchiolitis include a hacking cough and wheezing on exhalation. In addition, children typically have fever and a cloudy nasal drainage; infants often are irritable, and oral intake decreases, sometimes to the point of dehydration.

Ⓒ ANTIVIRAL AGENTS

• Purine Nucleoside Analogue Drugs

The largest group of antiviral drugs is the purine nucleoside analogue drugs, initially developed as antitumor drugs but used as antiviral drugs for more than 30 years. They have relatively selective toxicity to viruses because viral DNA polymerases are more sensitive than human polymerases to inhibition by these drugs. The prototype purine nucleoside analogue antiviral drug is acyclovir (Zovirax). Table 45.1 presents a summary of purine nucleoside analogue drugs

Nursing Management of the Patient Receiving Ⓟ Acyclovir
Core Drug Knowledge
Pharmacotherapeutics
Acyclovir is an oral, parenteral, and topical antiviral agent. Its antiviral spectrum is limited to the herpesviruses, including HSV, herpes zoster virus, Epstein-Barr virus, and CMV. Acyclovir is not active against human immunodeficiency virus (HIV). Acyclovir is used to treat herpes simplex (including encephalitis), herpes genitalis, recurrent herpes labialis, herpes zoster, and varicella.

Pharmacokinetics
After topical application, percutaneous absorption is minimal, and no drug is detected in the blood or urine. After oral administration, acyclovir is absorbed poorly from the gastrointestinal (GI) tract, with a bioavailability of approximately 20%. Peak serum concentrations occur in about 1.5 to 2 hours. Acyclovir distributes extensively, with the highest concentrations in the kidneys, liver, and intestines. Cerebrospinal fluid (CSF) concentrations are about 50% of plasma concentrations. Acyclovir crosses the placenta and enters breast milk. Acyclovir is metabolized minimally. Approximately 70% is eliminated by the kidneys unchanged. Half-life in patients with normal renal function is about 2.5 hours. In patients with impaired renal function, the half-life may extend to 20 hours.

Pharmacodynamics
To be active, acyclovir must undergo **phosphorylation,** a process by which a phosphate combines with an organic compound. In an infected cell, acyclovir is converted by the viral enzyme thymidine kinase. Fully active acyclovir triphosphate competes for a position in the DNA chain of the herpesvirus. Once incorporated, it terminates DNA synthesis. Uninfected cells show only minimal phosphorylation of acyclovir; thus, only a small amount of uptake into these cells occurs. Acyclovir is effective only against actively replicating viruses; it does not cure the latent herpesvirus. Acyclovir has only indirect effects on the body.

Contraindications and Precautions
Acyclovir should be used with caution in patients with ganciclovir or valganciclovir hypersensitivity because acyclovir has a similar chemical structure. It also should be given with caution to women who are pregnant or breast-feeding.

IV acyclovir should be used with caution in patients with renal disease and pre-existing neurologic disorders, especially seizures. Systemic acyclovir is excreted primarily by glomerular filtration and tubular secretion. Therefore, renal toxicity may occur in patients with renal disease. Patients with pre-existing neurologic disorders have an increased risk of developing tremors and myoclonus.

Adverse Effects
Acyclovir is well tolerated. Common adverse effects of acyclovir include light-headedness, anorexia, nausea, vomiting, abdominal pain, and headache. More serious adverse effects include confusion, tremors, hallucinations, seizures, or coma. IV acyclovir may be nephrotoxic. Acyclovir nephrotoxicity appears to result from crystallization of the drug in the nephron, which can lead to renal tubular obstruction.

Drug Interactions
Acyclovir may interact with valproic acid, hydantoins, theophyllines, and probenecid. The risk of nephrotoxicity increases when acyclovir is given concurrently with other drugs known to cause nephrotoxicity. Table 45.2 lists drugs that interact with acyclovir.

Assessment of Relevant Core Patient Variables
Health Status
Elicit a patient history to evaluate for pre-existing renal dysfunction, dehydration, pregnancy, or breast-feeding. Also, assess for concurrent use of any drugs known to be nephrotoxic. Communicate any positive finding to the prescriber. Physical examination should include a dermatologic inspection to verify that the patient has active lesions and does not have a secondary bacterial infection (acyclovir does not affect bacterial pathogens). Immunocompromised patients and patients with pre-existing renal dysfunction should have baseline renal function tests documented. For patients with pre-existing neurologic disorders, complete a baseline neurologic assessment.

Life Span and Gender
Determine whether the patient is pregnant or breast-feeding. Acyclovir is a pregnancy category B and should be used with caution during pregnancy. Breast milk concentrations

TABLE 45.1 Summary of Selected Purine Nucleoside Analogue Drugs

Drug (Trade) Name	Selected Indications	Route and Dosage Range	Pharmacokinetics
P acyclovir (Zovirax)	Herpes simplex Herpes genitalis Herpes zoster	*Adult:* IV, 5–10 mg/kg infused over 1 h, q8 h (15 mg/kg/d) for 7 d; PO (initial genital herpes), 200 mg q4h while awake (1,000 mg/d) for 10 d; PO (chronic suppressive therapy), 400 mg bid for up to 12 mo; topical, apply sufficient quantity to cover all lesions six times per day for 7 d; 1.25 cm (1/2 in) ribbon of ointment covers 2.5 cm^2 (4 in^2) surface area q3h *Child:* IV (>12 y), adult dosage; IV (<12 y), 250–500 mg/m^2 infused over 1 h, q8 h (750 mg/m^2/d); PO, safety not established	*Onset:* IV, immediate; PO, varies *Duration:* IV, 8 h; PO, unknown $t_{1/2}$: 2.5–5 h
cidofovir (Vistide)	CMV retinitis in AIDS patients	*Adult:* IV, 5 mg/kg IV infused over 1 h once/wk for 2 consecutive wk during induction (5 mg/kg once every 2 wk for maintenance); probenecid must be administered PO with each dose, 2 g PO 3 h before cidofovir and 1 g at 2 h and 8 h after infusion *Child:* Safety and efficacy not established for children younger than 12 y	*Onset:* Rapid *Duration:* 24 h $t_{1/2}$: 1 h
famciclovir (Famvir)	Acute herpes zoster	*Adult:* PO, 500 mg q8 h for 7 d *Child:* Safety and efficacy not established	*Onset:* Varies *Duration:* 24 h $t_{1/2}$: 2 h
ganciclovir (DHPG, Cytovene)	Recurrent genital herpes CMV infections (retinitis, colitis, esophagitis) in immunocompromised patients	*Adult:* PO, 125 mg bid for 5 d *Adult:* IV, 5 mg/kg given at a constant rate over 1 h, q12 h for 14–21 d (maintenance: 5 mg/kg given over 1 h once daily, 7 d/wk or 6 mg/kg/d 5 d/wk; PO, 1,000 mg tid with food or 500 mg six times daily q3 h with food while awake) *Child:* Safety and efficacy not established	*Onset:* IV, slow; PO, slow *Duration:* Unknown $t_{1/2}$: 2–4 h; PO, 4.8 h
	Prevention of CMV infection in transplant patients	*Adult:* IV, 5 mg/kg over 1 h q12 h for 7–14 d, then 5 mg/kg/d once daily for 7 d or 6 mg/kg/d once daily for 5 d	
penciclovir (Denavir)	Herpes labialis	*Adult:* Topical, apply thin layer to affected area q2h while awake. Therapy continues for 4 d	Not generally absorbed systemically
valacyclovir (Valtrex)	Initial or recurrent genital herpes Herpes zoster	*Adult:* PO, 500 mg bid for 5 d *Child:* Safety and efficacy not established *Adult:* PO, 1 g tid for 7 d, most effective if started within 48 h of onset of symptoms	*Onset:* Rapid *Duration:* 3 h $t_{1/2}$: 2.5–3.3 h
valganciclovir (Valcyte)	CMV retinitis Maintenance	*Adult:* PO, 900 mg 2 ×/d × 21 d 900 mg/d	*Onset:* Rapid *Duration:* 12–24 h $t_{1/2}$: 4.8 h
docosanol (Abreva)	HSV	*Adult and child:* Apply cream 5 times/d	*Onset:* Rapid *Duration:* Unknown $t_{1/2}$: Unknown
foscarnet (Foscavir)	CMV retinitis in patients with AIDS Acyclovir-resistant HSV infections in immunocompromised patients	*Adult:* IV induction, 60 mg/kg q8h for 2–3 wk; maintenance, 90–120 mg/kg *Adult:* IV, 40 mg/kg q8–12 h for 2–3 wk or until healed	*Onset:* Immediate *Duration:* Unknown $t_{1/2}$: 1.4–3 h

of acyclovir are greater than serum concentrations; therefore, it should be given cautiously to nursing mothers.

Note the patient's age before administering acyclovir. Although acyclovir is not contraindicated for use in elderly patients, these patients should be monitored closely for the onset of nephrotoxicity because renal function diminishes with age.

Lifestyle, Diet, and Habits

Advise patients with genital herpes that acyclovir is not a cure and that they are able to transmit the virus to another person, even when asymptomatic. To avoid transmitting the disease, patients should routinely use a condom. Instruct patients to refrain from sexual contact when genital lesions are active. Be aware of patients' economic status. Oral

TABLE 45.2 Agents That Interact with P Acyclovir

Interactants	Effect and Significance	Nursing Management
probenecid	Probenecid inhibits the renal tubular secretion of acyclovir, resulting in increased acyclovir serum concentration and potential for adverse effects of acyclovir.	Monitor I/O. Monitor BUN and creatinine levels. Discuss dosage adjustment with prescriber.
hydantoins	Serum phenytoin concentrations may be decreased, resulting in an increased risk for seizure activity.	Monitor the patient for seizure activity. Ensure patient safety. Discuss dosage adjustment with prescriber.
theophyllines	Acyclovir may inhibit the metabolism of theophyllines, resulting in an increased risk for adverse effects to theophylline.	Monitor theophylline levels closely. Monitor for adverse effects such as tachycardia, nausea, vomiting, diarrhea, seizures, restlessness, irritability, and headache. Discuss dosage adjustment with prescriber.
valproic acid	Serum valproic acid concentrations may be decreased, resulting in an increased risk for seizure activity.	Monitor the patient for seizure activity. Ensure patient safety. Discuss dosage adjustment with prescriber.

acyclovir is expensive. It is one of the drugs approved for reimbursement in many statewide AIDS programs. Patients may qualify for medical assistance from county, state, or federal funds or receive their drugs from local health departments. Refer patients with financial problems to the hospital or clinic's social service department.

Environment
Acyclovir is most frequently given in the outpatient community setting. Caution patients to take acyclovir only when active lesions are present to avoid inducing acyclovir-resistant virus. However, some immunocompromised patients with frequent or severe outbreaks may be placed on a prophylactic regimen. Acyclovir should be protected from light and moisture in the home environment.

Administer IV acyclovir in acute care settings to patients with a severe outbreak. Use reconstituted acyclovir within 12 hours. Administer the infusion over 60 minutes.

Nursing Diagnoses and Outcomes
- Disturbed Thought Processes related to drug-induced confusion, hallucinations, or seizures
  Desired outcome: The patient will be free of thought aberrations related to drug therapy.
- Acute Pain related to drug-induced headache
  Desired outcome: Drug-related pain will subside after administration of acetaminophen.
- Imbalanced Nutrition: Less than Body Requirements, related to acyclovir-related anorexia, nausea and vomiting, or abdominal pain
  Desired outcome: The patient will remain within an acceptable weight range.
- Excess Fluid Volume related to adverse effects of drug therapy, such as nephrotoxicity
  Desired outcome: The patient will have an adequate fluid intake and output profile.

Planning and Intervention
Maximizing Therapeutic Effects
Administer acyclovir tablets or capsules with a full glass of water, with or without food. Administering the drug at regular intervals is important.

Minimizing Adverse Effects
Oral acyclovir is well tolerated. However, for patients who report GI complaints, administer the drug with food. Advise the patient to drink at least eight 8-oz glasses of water a day.

To minimize potential nephrotoxicity, ensure that the patient is well hydrated. Administer IV acyclovir over 60 minutes. It is best to use an infusion pump to ensure that administration is timed correctly. Monitor the patient's urine output for 2 hours after the infusion and notify the prescriber if urine output is less than 500 mL/g of acyclovir administered.

Providing Patient and Family Education
- One of the most important points to stress with patients is that they should not take this drug if they have ever had a reaction to any drug with a name that ends in "vir."
- Advise patients to notify the prescriber if they are pregnant or breast-feeding.
- Explain that acyclovir is prescribed for a particular infection and should not be used to self-medicate or to treat any other infection.
- Emphasize that acyclovir does not prevent the transmission of infection to another person and does not cure the infection.
- Instruct patients to complete the full course of drug therapy, even if the lesions resolve. If patients are taking 200-mg tablets, advise them to take the drug five times a day. For patients who have difficulty taking pills, the drug may be taken in 400-mg doses three times a day. However, consult with the prescriber to be sure the alternate method is acceptable.

- It is important to advise patients to keep the drug away from light and moisture, and to instruct them to take forgotten doses as soon as they remember, but not if it is time for the next dose.
- Inform patients of the importance of remaining well hydrated while taking this drug.
- Teach patients to recognize the symptoms of an allergic reaction to acyclovir. Patients should stop taking the drug and contact their prescriber if a rash, welts, itching, or shortness of breath occurs.
- Explain the potential adverse effects of acyclovir and the potential remedies for these discomforts. If patients experience central nervous system (CNS) effects, such as confusion, tremors, hallucinations, or coma, or have signs of nephrotoxicity, such as weight gain or decreased urinary output, the prescriber should be contacted immediately.
- Because autoinoculation is possible with herpetic lesions, it is important to teach patients to wear a glove or finger cot when applying topical acyclovir. Explain the importance of washing the hands after each application, even when barriers are used. The drug should be applied to cover the lesions every 3 hours, six times a day for 7 days.
- Advise patients to contact the prescriber if the lesions turn red, become hot, or exude purulent material, all of which are indications of a secondary bacterial infection.
- Instruct patients to self-administer acetaminophen if headache occurs. For persistent pain, unrelieved by acetaminophen, patients should contact the prescriber.
- Instruct patients to consume frequent small meals if GI distress occurs. If weight loss persists, patients should contact the prescriber.

Ongoing Assessment and Evaluation

Monitor for the effectiveness of therapy, making sure to document new lesions and assess for possible secondary bacterial infections. Also, monitor for adverse effects, such as lethargy, tremors, headache, change in mental status, and GI complaints.

For immunocompromised and elderly patients, monitoring renal function to detect early nephrotoxicity is important. Patients on long-term therapy should have periodic renal function tests. Hospitalized patients receiving IV acyclovir also should be monitored closely for developing nephrotoxicity. Measure and monitor fluid intake and output to ensure adequate hydration. Also, monitor for the development of phlebitis when administering IV acyclovir. By the completion of therapy, herpetic lesions and any adverse effects should be resolved.

Drugs Closely Related to P Acyclovir

Famciclovir

Famciclovir (Famvir) is an alternative to acyclovir in treating acute herpes zoster and recurrent episodes of genital herpes. In patients with chronic HBV infection, famciclovir

ACYCLOVIR AND HERPES SIMPLEX VIRUS

Your patient Sara Thompson is HIV antibody positive and has a history of type 1 diabetes and steroid-dependent asthma. Current drugs include Combivir (150/300 mg bid), Kaletra (200/50 mg bid), Lantus (30 units daily), metformin (500 mg twice daily), and prednisone (20 mg daily). Ms. Thompson experienced severe headache, nausea, drowsiness, and confusion and was admitted to the hospital with a diagnosis of altered level of consciousness. After multiple laboratory tests, she is diagnosed with herpetic encephalitis, and the provider prescribes acyclovir (10 mg/kg every 8 hours).

1. What factors do you think contributed to this diagnosis?
2. What additional information do you need?
3. Would you administer this medication?
4. What body systems do you need to monitor closely in this patient?
5. What discharge instructions do you anticipate providing?

---

has decreased HBV, DNA, and aminotransferase activity. Famciclovir's spectrum of activity is similar to that of acyclovir, but its duration of action is longer. Recent studies have shown that 1-day famciclovir therapy is as efficacious as 3-day valacyclovir therapy when treating recurrent genital herpes. Despite famciclovir's advantages of better bioavailability and longer duration of action, acyclovir possesses a higher affinity for thymidine kinase, the enzyme that promotes metabolism.

The adverse effects and drug interactions of famciclovir are the same as those seen with acyclovir. Famciclovir is classified as an FDA pregnancy category B drug; however, it should be used in pregnancy only if the benefit clearly outweighs the potential risk.

Valacyclovir

Valacyclovir (Valtrex) was developed to improve acyclovir's oral bioavailability. Improved bioavailability means that less

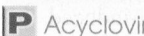 MEMORY CHIP

P Acyclovir

- Used for the management of herpes simplex virus, herpes zoster virus, Epstein-Barr virus, and cytomegalovirus
- Major contraindication: hypersensitivity or cross-sensitivity to ganciclovir
- Most common adverse effects: nausea, vomiting, anorexia, light-headedness, abdominal pain, and headache
- Most serious adverse effects: seizures and renal dysfunction
- Maximizing therapeutic effects: Administer the drug at regular intervals.
- Minimizing adverse effects: Ensure hydration to avoid nephrotoxicity.
- Most important patient education: Acyclovir treats the symptoms of the disease; it does not cure the disease or prevent its transmission to another person.

frequent dosing is required for valacyclovir than for acyclovir. Valacyclovir is the drug of choice in treating genital herpes, either as a first episode or as a recurrent episode. It also is the drug of choice in treating herpes zoster. Compared with acyclovir, it demonstrates earlier pain reduction or cessation of pain in treating herpes zoster.

The adverse effects and drug interactions of valacyclovir are similar to those of acyclovir. In immunocompromised patients, valacyclovir also may induce thrombotic thrombocytopenic purpura and hemolytic uremia syndrome. For that reason, it is not indicated for use in immunocompromised patients. It is used with caution in patients with renal dysfunction because accumulation of valacyclovir may induce acute renal failure or neuropsychiatric adverse effects, especially in the elderly. Post-marketing reports indicate the potential for psychosis with manic presentation in young, healthy patients without a psychiatric history. To prevent crystalluria, teach the patient to remain well hydrated to maintain a high urine volume and avoid dehydration. Valacyclovir is in FDA pregnancy category B.

Drugs Significantly Different From P Acyclovir
Drugs Used for Cytomegalovirus Infections
Cidofovir
Cidofovir (Vistide) is an IV drug indicated for treating CMV retinitis in patients with AIDS. Cidofovir gel has been effective for topical treatment of acyclovir-resistant mucocutaneous HSV infections in AIDS patients. Cidofovir may also be used in patients with ganciclovir resistance. Its major advantage is its long half-life, which allows for a once-weekly infusion.

Cidofovir use is limited by its serious potential toxic effects. Major adverse effects with cidofovir therapy include renal impairment, granulocytopenia, metabolic acidosis, uveitis, and ocular hypotony. To minimize possible nephrotoxicity, IV normal saline solution and oral probenecid must be used before and after each cidofovir dose. Renal function tests should be completed before each dose of cidofovir. Neutrophil counts also should be monitored throughout therapy. Cidofovir therapy is contraindicated in patients who are taking other nephrotoxic agents. Cidofovir is classified as an FDA pregnancy category C drug and should be used in pregnancy only if the benefit clearly outweighs the potential risk.

Foscarnet
Foscarnet (Foscavir) is an IV antiviral agent that is structurally unrelated to other antiviral agents. Foscarnet currently is indicated for treating CMV retinitis in patients with AIDS. It is also being investigated for treating CMV disease, herpes simplex, and varicella zoster infection in HIV-positive patients. Its mechanism of action is similar to that of acyclovir and ganciclovir, yet it does not require phosphorylation before becoming activated.

Foscarnet therapy should be given with caution to patients with anemia, dehydration, renal impairment, and electrolyte imbalances. Patients who have cardiac disease, are receiving other drugs that influence serum electrolytes, or have a pre-existing seizure disorder or other neurologic disease require close monitoring during treatment. Foscarnet is assigned to pregnancy category C and should therefore be used with caution during pregnancy.

Foscarnet has an extensive and serious adverse reaction profile. Anemia, granulocytopenia, or leukopenia develop in as many as 33% of patients on foscarnet therapy. Electrolyte imbalances, such as hypocalcemia, hypophosphatemia or hyperphosphatemia, hypomagnesemia, and hypokalemia also may occur. GI disturbances, such as anorexia, abdominal pain, nausea, and vomiting, occur in up to 30% of patients. Considerable renal impairment, resulting in azotemia or necrosis, develop in as many as 33% of patients. Patients with renal impairment also are at high risk for seizures. Other CNS effects include headache, peripheral neuropathy, and anxiety.

Foscarnet should be given with caution in combination with other drugs known to be nephrotoxic, such as acyclovir, aminoglycosides, amphotericin B, cisplatin, cyclosporine, gold compounds, lithium, nonsteroidal anti-inflammatory drugs, penicillamine, pentamidine, rifampin, and vancomycin. In combination with ciprofloxacin, foscarnet increases the risk of seizures, whereas the combination of foscarnet and zidovudine increases the risk of anemia.

Ganciclovir
Ganciclovir (Cytovene) is an antiviral agent used to treat CMV infections, especially retinitis, colitis, and esophagitis, in immunocompromised patients. It is the drug of choice to prevent CMV infection in immunocompromised patients, such as patients with HIV or transplant recipients. Its spectrum of activity also includes HSV-1 and HSV-2, herpesvirus type 6, Epstein-Barr virus, varicella zoster virus, and HBV.

Like acyclovir, ganciclovir works by terminating DNA synthesis. It is administered intravenously, orally, and by intravitreal implantation. After implantation, intravitreal ganciclovir is released at a steady rate over 5 to 8 months. After oral administration, ganciclovir is absorbed poorly from the GI tract. Bioavailability is increased when ganciclovir is administered with a high-fat meal. Following IV administration, distribution into body tissues and fluids, including the eyes, is extensive. Ganciclovir crosses the placenta and the blood–brain barrier.

Ganciclovir is not indicated for use in neonates and children and should not be taken during pregnancy and lactation. It must be used with caution in patients with depressed bone marrow function, dehydration, neutropenia, hematologic disease, thrombocytopenia, renal disease or impairment, or recent radiation therapy. Cross-sensitivity is also possible with acyclovir.

Ganciclovir can cause substantial hematologic toxicity. Granulocytopenia, neutropenia, and thrombocytopenia have all occurred during ganciclovir therapy. Like acyclovir, ganciclovir is potentially nephrotoxic. Slight-to-moderate increases in serum creatinine and azotemia have occurred. Elevated liver function test results also may occur during therapy with ganciclovir; such changes are generally reversible. Serial laboratory tests required during therapy include complete blood count (CBC), platelet counts, and renal and liver function tests.

Advise the prescriber immediately if the platelet count is less than 25,000 mm^3 or the neutrophil count is less than 500 mm^3.

Adverse effects, which occur most commonly with IV administration of ganciclovir, include diaphoresis, pruritus, pneumonia, chills, sepsis, and phlebitis. Adverse effects seen with intravitreal administration of ganciclovir may induce bacterial endophthalmitis, retinal detachment, vitreous hemorrhage, cataracts, corneal opacification, hyphema, floaters, ocular pain, posterior chamber inflammation, macular abnormalities, spikes of increased intraocular pressure, optic disc or nerve changes, and uveitis.

Ganciclovir is in FDA pregnancy category C. Based on animal studies, ganciclovir should be considered a potential teratogen in humans, with the potential to cause birth defects. It also suppresses spermatogenesis.

Valganciclovir

Valganciclovir (Valcyte) is an ester of ganciclovir. This oral drug is rapidly metabolized into its active form, ganciclovir. Pharmacotherapeutics for valganciclovir include treatment of active CMV retinitis in patients with AIDS, maintenance therapy for CMV retinitis, secondary prophylaxis in patients with inactive CMV retinitis, and prophylaxis against CMV infections in solid organ transplant patients. Oral valganciclovir has the same efficacy as IV ganciclovir for the management of active CMV retinitis. The drug is also approved for prophylaxis against CMV following heart, kidney, or kidney-pancreas transplantation.

Adverse effects and contraindications for valganciclovir are similar to those for ganciclovir. Serial laboratory tests required during therapy include CBC, renal function tests, and liver function tests.

Valganciclovir is classified in FDA pregnancy risk category C. In animal studies, ganciclovir was found to be mutagenic and teratogenic. Therefore, as a prodrug to ganciclovir, valganciclovir should be considered a potential teratogen in humans, with the potential to cause birth defects.

Topical Drugs

Docosanol

Docosanol (Abreva) is an over-the-counter (OTC) topical cream for recurrent oral-facial herpes simplex episodes. Docosanol works by inhibiting fusion between the plasma membrane and the HSV envelope, thereby preventing viral entry into cells and subsequent viral replication. Other antivirals, such as acyclovir, work by inhibiting viral DNA replication and carry a risk for mutating the virus. Because docosanol does not act directly on the virus, it is unlikely it will produce drug-resistant mutants of HSV. Docosanol has minimal adverse effects; headache is the most common. Successful therapy occurs when the drug is applied at the earliest sign of infection.

Penciclovir

Penciclovir (Denavir) is a topical antiviral agent used to treat herpes labialis. Penciclovir is the active metabolite of famciclovir. It works by inhibiting viral DNA. Penciclovir is applied every 2 waking hours.

Adverse effects associated with penciclovir use include headache, oral and pharyngeal edema, application site reactions, erythematous rash, pain, paresthesias, pruritus, skin discoloration, and urticaria.

Ophthalmic Drugs

Trifluridine

Trifluridine (Viroptic) is an ophthalmic solution used in primary keratoconjunctivitis and recurrent epithelial keratitis caused by HSV-1 and HSV-2. One drop of 1% solution should be instilled into the affected eye every 2 hours during waking hours, up to a maximum daily dose of nine drops. This therapeutic regimen should continue until the corneal ulcer has completely re-epithelialized. At this point, it is important to treat for an additional 7 days with one drop every 4 hours during waking hours, up to a maximum daily dosage of five drops.

No important interactions between trifluridine and other drugs have been reported. Adverse effects include mild transient burning or stinging on instillation, palpebral edema, epithelial keratopathy, irritation, keratitis sicca, hyperemia, and increased intraocular pressure.

Drugs Used for Influenza

While influenza is a debilitating virus, it generally subsides without pharmacotherapy. However, in certain populations, it can be a serious illness, possibly resulting in death. Oseltamivir (Tamiflu) is the prototype anti-influenza drug. Table 45.3 summarizes drugs used for influenza.

Oseltamivir

Pharmacotherapeutics

Oseltamivir phosphate (Tamiflu) is a neuraminidase inhibitor used to manage infection with influenza A or B virus. It is the drug of choice for H5N1 (avian or bird) influenza and the novel H1N1 (swine) influenza (Box 45.1). Since the H1N1 virus became pandemic in 2009, isolates of this virus have become oseltamivir-resistant in many countries. It is also used as prophylaxis against influenza A and B.

Pharmacokinetics

Oseltamivir phosphate is available as an oral capsule or as powder for reconstitution. It is a prodrug that is metabolized into oseltamivir carboxylate, which is the active drug. It is excreted 99% unchanged by the kidneys.

Pharmacodynamics

Influenza A and B viruses contain the viral enzyme neuraminidase on their surfaces, which facilitates the release of newly formed virus particles from infected cells. This mechanism enables infection of adjacent cells. Neuraminidase inhibitors, such as oseltamivir, appear to inhibit the release of viruses from infected cells, thus reducing spread to adjacent cells and limiting tissue damage and the duration of symptoms. The effectiveness of the drug depends on how early the treatment is initiated.

Contraindications and Precautions

Hypersensitivity is the only contraindication to the use of oseltamivir. Precautions include pregnancy, breastfeeding, asthma, CAL, and patients with renal insufficiency.

BOX 45.1   COMMUNITY BASED CONCERNS

Is it a bird, a plane, or a pig?

H5N1 influenza A virus (aka avian or bird flu) had been reported to be the next pandemic threat to the world. Who knew that a pig would take its place? A pandemic event requires three characteristics: it is a new strain of disease that most people do not have a natural immunity to resist, it has the ability to cause human illness, and it is transmissible from human to human.

On June 6, 2009 the World Health Organization (WHO) declared the novel H1N1 influenza A virus (aka swine flu) to be a pandemic event. As of July 27, 2009 there were 134,503 confirmed cases throughout the world with 816 deaths. The novel H1N1 virus was initially called the "swine flu" because laboratory testing showed that many of the genes were very similar to influenza viruses that normally occur in pigs in North America. However, further study has shown that this new virus is very different from the virus that occurs in North American pigs.

The novel H1N1 virus generally presents with symptoms of seasonal influenza: fever, cough, sore throat, malaise, nasal congestion, myalgias, chills, fatigue, and headache. Like seasonal influenza, H1N1 may also cause CNS symptoms including seizure activity. In addition, many patients also experienced vomiting and diarrhea which do not normally occur with seasonal influenza. The largest number of novel H1N1 flu confirmed cases have occurred in people between the ages of 5 and 24 years old. With seasonal influenza, over 90% of deaths and about 60% of hospitalization occur in people older than 65. At this time, there are few cases and no deaths reported in people older than 64 years old.

Not all patients with novel H1N1 virus require pharmacotherapy. Those with mild symptoms need acetaminophen, rest, and fluids. Patients who require hospitalization are treated with oseltamivir or zanamivir, optimally within 48 hours of the onset of symptoms. Pregnant women should receive pharmacotherapy. Influenza causes more severe disease and an increased rate of mortality during pregnancy. Use of acetaminophen is important when fever is present, because hyperthermia during the first trimester has been associated with birth defects and fever during labor is a risk factor for neonatal seizures, encephalopathy, cerebral palsy, and neonatal death. Both oseltamivir and zanamivir are pregnancy category C.

Nursing Implications

H1N1 influenza A is a potentially life-threatening illness, especially in the very young, immunocompromised patients, and those with chronic illness. The media has reported extensively on this pandemic event. Nurses have a special relationship with patients that allow the patient to express his/her fears and seek information from a person they trust. Continue to update yourself on the facts of the H1N1 influenza A virus. Rely on information from medical sources, rather than media sources. Advise your patients to take the same precautions as they would for any type of influenza: stay away from people known to be ill, especially children; wash hands frequently; use bacteriostatic hand gels; and get plenty of rest and fluids. Advise patients with a mild influenza-like illness to self-isolate at home for a minimum of 24 hours after the cessation of symptoms. Encourage patients with more severe symptoms to seek medical attention quickly.

Adverse Effects

The most common adverse effects of oseltamivir are nausea and vomiting, bronchitis, insomnia, and vertigo. In 2006, post-marketing reports indicated a risk for abnormal behavior with subsequent injury, especially in children. It is unclear if oseltamivir is the etiology because influenza itself may cause neurologic and behavioral symptoms such as hallucinations, delirium, and abnormal behavior.

Drug Interactions

There are no known significant drug-drug interactions.

Assessment of Relevant Core Patient Variables

Health Status

Assess the patient for influenza symptoms as the patient may not know the difference between influenza and the common cold (Box 45.2).

Life Span and Gender

For women, determine the potential for pregnancy and lactation. Oseltamivir is an FDA pregnancy category C drug. It is unclear whether it passes into breast milk. Weigh children to ensure an accurate dose of medication.

Lifestyle, Diet, and Habits

Assess for a history of fructose intolerance. Oseltamivir suspension contains 2 g of sorbitol per 75 mg dose. It may be taken with or without food.

Environment

Oseltamivir is most frequently given in the community environment. Occasionally, the patient may be severely ill and require hospitalization.

Nursing Diagnoses and Outcomes

• Disturbed Thought Processes related to drug-induced confusion, hallucinations, or seizures
  Desired outcome: The patient will be free of thought aberrations related to drug therapy
• Risk for Injury related to abnormal behaviors
  Desired outcome: The patient will remain free from injury
• Imbalanced Nutrition: Less than Body Requirements, related to anorexia, nausea and vomiting, or abdominal pain
  Desired outcome: The patient will remain within an acceptable weight range.

Planning and Intervention

Maximizing Therapeutic Effects

Question the patient regarding the duration of symptoms. Oseltamivir works best when begun within 48 hours of the onset of symptoms. To prepare the solution, add 23 mL of water to the bottle containing the powder and shake well for 15 seconds. Administer the solution directly in the mouth–do not mix with any liquid. Cleanse the dispenser under running water and allow to air dry. Store the unused solution in the refrigerator. Shake the solution prior to each dose. Store the oseltamivir capsules at room temperature.

Minimizing Adverse Effects

Nausea and vomiting can be reduced by administration with milk, a snack, or a meal.

TABLE 45.3 Summary of Selected Anti-Influenza Drugs

Drug (Trade) Name	Selected Indications	Route and Dosage Range	Pharmacokinetics
amantadine (Symmetrel; *Canadian*: Gen-Amantadine)	Influenza A	*Adults <65 y and adolescents:* PO, 200 mg/d daily and continue for 24–48 h after resolution of signs/symptoms *Elderly:* PO, 100 mg/d and continue for 24–48 h after resolution of signs/symptoms *Children:* PO, 10 y and >40 kg: 100 mg 2×/d; 10 y and <40 kg: 5 mg/kg/d PO in two divided doses, not to exceed 200 mg/d; <10 y: 5 mg/kg/d (up to 150 mg/d) in 2 divided doses	*Onset:* 2 h *Duration:* 12 h $t_{1/2}$: 15–24 h
rimantadine (Flumadine)	Influenza A	*Adults and adolescents >14 y:* PO, 100 mg 2×/d for 24–48 h after resolution of signs/symptoms *Elderly:* PO, 100 mg qd for 24–48 h after resolution of signs/symptoms *Children:* PO, 10–13 y and >40 kg: 200 mg qd; 10–13 y and <40 kg: 5 mg/kg/d or 200 mg qd, whichever is less; 1–9 y: 5 mg/kg/d or 150 mg qd, whichever is less	*Onset:* Slow *Duration:* Unknown $t_{1/2}$: 25.4 h
P Oseltamivir (Tamiflu)	Influenza A and B prophylaxis	*Adults and adolescents ≥13 y:* PO, 75 mg 2×/d for 5 d *Children 1–12y:* PO, 2×/d for 5 d >40 kg: 75 mg (6.2 mL) 24–40 kg: 60 mg (5 mL) 16–23 kg: 45 mg (3.8 mL) <15 kg: 30 mg (2.5 mL) 2×/d for 5 d *Infants <1 y:* Not indicated *Adult and Child:* PO Dose as above, once daily for 10 d	*Onset:* Rapid *Duration:* Unknown $t_{1/2}$: 6–10 h
zanamivir (Relenza)	Influenza A and B Influenza prophylaxis during outbreak or exposure	*Adults and children >7 y:* PO, 2 inhalations 2×/d for 5 d *Children <7 y:* Safety and efficacy have not been established *Adults and children >7 y:* PO, 2 inhalations (10 mg) daily *Children ≤7 y:* Safety and efficacy have not been established	*Onset:* 1 h *Duration:* 24 h $t_{1/2}$: 2.5–5.1 h

Providing Patient and Family Education

- Instruct the patient on the correct way to prepare, administer, and store the solution.
- Teach the patient the importance of using the dispenser that accompanies the product to assure an accurate dose of the solution.
- Encourage the patient to take the medication for the full course of therapy as prescribed (5 days for acute illness; 10 days for prophylaxis).
- Instruct families to monitor children closely throughout therapy and contact the provider immediately should any unusual behavior occur.
- Instruct the patient to contact the provider for severe nausea and diarrhea or worsening of symptoms.
- Teach the patient oseltamivir is not a substitute for yearly influenza vaccine.

Ongoing Assessment and Evaluation

Monitor for abnormal behavior; notify the provider immediately if it occurs. Monitor for elevated temperature, nausea, vomiting, and diarrhea. Assess for resolution of the symptoms.

Drugs Closely Related to Oseltamivir

Zanamivir

Zanamivir (Relenza) is the second neuraminidase inhibitor. Its mechanism of action is the same as that of oseltamivir.

Zanamivir is an orally inhaled agent that is approved for use in adults and in children older than 7 years of age. Like oseltamivir, the effectiveness of zanamivir is directly related to the promptness with which treatment is initiated.

Box 45.2 SYMPTOMS AT A GLANCE

Signs and Symptoms	Flu	Cold
Onset	Sudden	Gradual
Fever	Common, lasting 3–4 days	Rare
Cough	Dry, can become severe	Hacking, mild
Headache	Prominent	Rare
Muscle/joint aches, pain	Usual, often severe	Slight
Fatigue and weakness	Can last up to 2 weeks	Very mild
Extreme exhaustion	Early and prominent	Never
Chest discomfort	Common	Mild/Moderate
Stuffy nose	Sometimes	Common
Sneezing	Sometimes	Usually
Sore throat	Sometimes	Common

Roche patient information handout

Zanamivir is supplied on a Rotadisk containing four blisters of a powder mixture. The Rotadisk is loaded into a Diskhaler, the blister is punctured, and the patient inhales through the mouthpiece. The actual amount of drug delivered to the respiratory tract depends on the ability of the patient to inhale adequately. Approximately 10% of zanamivir is absorbed systemically. It is excreted renally as unchanged drug.

Adverse effects with zanamivir include headache, dizziness, nausea, diarrhea, and respiratory effects such as sinusitis, bronchitis, cough, nasal symptoms, and infections. Because zanamivir is administered by oral inhalation, it is more likely to cause local adverse effects, such as bronchospasm, than systemic reactions. For this reason, zanamivir is given cautiously to patients with underlying respiratory disorders, especially asthma. Instruct the patient to have a fast-acting inhaled bronchodilator, such as albuterol, available when administering zanamivir. It is an FDA pregnancy category B drug.

Like oseltamivir, zanamivir should not be substituted for yearly influenza vaccine in high-risk populations. The considerations for LAIV apply to zanamivir as well.

Drugs Significantly Different From Oseltamivir
Amantadine

Amantadine (Symmetrel) is a synthetic antiviral agent used for the prophylactic or symptomatic treatment of influenza A virus infection, especially in high-risk patients. It is not recommended for use in the United States because of substantial resistance. It also is used to relieve the symptoms of Parkinson disease. It is not effective for the novel H1N1virus.

As an antiviral, amantadine appears to block the uncoating of the virus particle and subsequent release of viral nucleic acid into the host cell. Amantadine also may interfere with penetration of the cell wall by adsorbed virus. In treating Parkinson disease, amantadine appears to potentiate CNS dopaminergic responses. It may release dopamine and norepinephrine from storage sites and inhibit the reuptake of dopamine and norepinephrine.

Amantadine is administered orally and is well absorbed from the GI tract. It crosses the blood–brain barrier and the placenta; distributes into tears, saliva, and nasal secretions; and is excreted into breast milk. About 90% of amantadine is excreted in the urine by way of glomerular filtration and tubular secretion.

Amantadine should be given with caution to patients with chronic heart failure, peripheral edema, seizure disorders, eczema, and history of psychosis. These conditions may be exacerbated by amantadine therapy. Patients with renal impairment, elderly patients, and pregnant women also should be given amantadine with caution because these conditions increase the risk of adverse effects. Abrupt withdrawal of amantadine should be avoided in patients with Parkinson disease because it may precipitate symptoms of increased rigidity, confusion, urinary retention, or bulbar palsy.

Amantadine has many potential adverse effects. In the GI system, amantadine may cause nausea and vomiting, diarrhea, constipation, anorexia, and xerostomia. CNS effects include dizziness, anxiety, impaired coordination, insomnia, and nervousness. Other CNS effects that occur less commonly are headache, irritability, nightmares, depression, ataxia, confusion, somnolence and drowsiness, agitation, fatigue, and hallucinations. Patients with a history of psychosis may experience an exacerbation of symptoms, including abnormal thinking, weakness, amnesia, slurred speech, and hyperkinesia. In rare cases, amantadine has been associated with more serious effects, including increased frequency of seizures, suicidal ideation, and neuroleptic malignant syndrome. Adverse cardiovascular effects include orthostatic hypotension and peripheral edema. Livedo reticularis, a persistent purplish network-patterned discoloration of the skin, is a common adverse reaction among patients taking amantadine for Parkinson disease. This reaction is believed to be caused by abnormal capillary permeability associated with peripheral vasoconstriction, which results in decreased skin temperature and peripheral blood flow. Amantadine also may cause adverse reactions in the eyes. Diffuse, white, subendothelial corneal opacification may occur. Other ophthalmic adverse reactions include corneal edema, light sensitivity, and optic nerve palsy.

Amantadine should not be used with CNS stimulants, alcohol (ethanol), opiate agonists, hydrochlorothiazide, or triamterene. Nervousness, irritability, insomnia, seizures, or cardiac arrhythmias may occur if amantadine is taken concurrently with CNS stimulants. Ethanol use with amantadine may increase CNS effects, such as dizziness, confusion, light-headedness, fainting, or orthostatic hypotension. Use of opiate agonists may increase the incidence of adverse effects. Hydrochlorothiazide or triamterene, used in conjunction with amantadine, can reduce renal clearance of amantadine, with subsequent increase in plasma amantadine concentrations and possible toxicity.

Rimantadine

Rimantadine (Flumadine) is an oral antiviral agent. It is indicated for prophylaxis and treatment of influenza A virus infection in adults and for prophylaxis only in children. Like amantadine, it is not recommended for use in the United States.

Rimantadine is related chemically and structurally to amantadine, but it does not produce the CNS effects seen with amantadine and does not have therapeutic value in treating Parkinson disease.

Rimantadine is contraindicated for use in infants and neonates. It should be used cautiously in elderly patients and in patients with hepatic or renal dysfunction because delayed metabolism or excretion of rimantadine may increase the risk for toxic effects.

Rimantadine has a much better adverse effects profile than amantadine. The most common adverse effects reported are nausea, vomiting, insomnia, dizziness, anorexia, xerostomia, abdominal pain, headache, asthenia, nervousness, and fatigue.

Clearance of rimantadine is reduced by concurrent administration of cimetidine. Decreased serum concentration may occur if rimantadine is coadministered with acetaminophen or aspirin.

Drugs Used for Hepatitis

Tables 45.4 and 45.5 summarize information about drugs used to treat hepatitis.

Interferons

The interferons are a family of glycoproteins that affect many types of viral illness. They are administered parenterally, either subcutaneously or intramuscularly. Although pharmacologically similar, each is used for specific viral illnesses. The three main classes of interferons are interferon alfa, interferon beta, and interferon gamma. Interferon alfa and interferon beta are used in the management of hepatitis, whereas interferon gamma is used for other types of viral illness. The interferons are presented in depth in Chapter 54.

TABLE 45.4	Summary of Selected Drugs for Hepatitis		
Drug (Trade) Name	Selected Indications	Route and Dosage Range	Pharmacokinetics
interferon alfa-2a (Roferon-A)	See Table 45.5.	Adult: IM/SC, 3 million international units 3×/wk for 12 mo	Onset: Rapid Duration: Unknown $t_{1/2}$: 3.7–8.5 h
interferon alfa-2b (Intron-A)	See Table 45.5.	Adult: IM/SC, 5 million international units/d or 10 million international units 3×/wk for 16 wk 3 million international units 3×/wk for up to 18–24 mo if a positive response	Onset: Rapid Duration: Unknown $t_{1/2}$: 2–3 h
peginterferon alfa-2a (Pegasys)	See Table 45.5.	Adult: SC, 180 mcg once weekly for 24 wk 180 mcg once weekly for 48 wk	Onset: Rapid Duration: Unknown $t_{1/2}$: 70–90 h
peginterferon alfa-2b (PEG-Intron)	See Table 45.5.	Adult: SC, 1 mcg/kg/wk	Onset: Rapid Duration: 42–72 h $t_{1/2}$: 4.6 h
interferon alfa-n3 (Alferon)	See Table 45.5.	Adult: IM/SC, 3–6 million international units 3×/wk	Onset: Unknown Duration: Unknown $t_{1/2}$: Unknown
interferon alfacon-1 (Infergen)	See Table 45.5.	Adult: SC, 9 mcg 3×/wk for 24 wk. At least 48 h should elapse between doses.	Onset: Rapid Duration: Unknown $t_{1/2}$: Unknown
interferon alfa-2b (SC) and ribavirin (PO) (Rebetron)	See Table 45.5.	Adults >75 kg: Ribavirin, PO, 600 mg 2×/d in combination with interferon alfa-2b, 3 million international units SC 3×/wk Adults, adolescents, and children >61 kg: Ribavirin, PO, 400 mg in the morning and 600 mg in the evening every day, in combination with interferon alfa-2b, 3 million international units SC 3×/wk Adults, adolescents, and children 50–61 kg: Ribavirin, PO, 400 mg 2×/d, in combination with interferon alfa-2b, 3 million international units/m² SC 3×/wk Adolescents and children 37–49 kg: Ribavirin, PO 200 mg in the morning and 400 mg in the evening every day, in combination with interferon alfa-2b, 3 million international units/m² SC 3×/wk Adolescents and children 25–36 kg: Ribavirin, PO 200 mg 2×/d, in combination with interferon alfa-2b, 3 million international units/m² SC 3×/wk	Onset: Rapid Duration: Unknown $t_{1/2}$: 3.7–8.5 h
adefovir (Hepsera)	See Table 45.5.	Adult: PO, 10 mg 1×/d	Onset: Unknown Duration: 24 h $t_{1/2}$: 7.5 h
boceprivir (Victrelis)	Hepatitis C	Adult PO: 800 mg 3× day	Onset: unknown Duration: unknown $t_{1/2}$: 12–15 h
entecavir (Baraclude)	Chronic hepatitis B	Adult: PO, 0.5–1 mg every day	Onset: Unknown Duration: Unknown $t_{1/2}$: 128–149 h
lamivudine (Epivir-HBV)	Chronic hepatitis B	Adult: PO 100 mg daily Child >2y: PO 3 mg/kg daily	Onset: Rapid Duration: 12 h $t_{1/2}$: 5–7 h

TABLE 45.5	Drugs for Managing Hepatitis	
	Hepatitis B	Hepatitis C
Name		
interferon alfa-2a (Roferon-A)		X
interferon alfa-2b (Intron-A)	X	X
peginterferon alfa-2a (Pegasys)	X	X
peginterferon alfa-2b (PEG-Intron)		X
interferon alfacon-1 (Infergen)		X
interferon alfa-2a and ribavirin (Rebetron)		X
adefovir (Hepsera)	X	
entecavir (Baraclude)	X	
lamivudine (Epivir HBV)	X	
tenofovir		
telbivudine	X	

Interferon Alfa

Interferon alfa is an immunomodulator. The name interferon alfa actually refers to several compounds that differ slightly in their amino acid sequence and duration of action. Conventional interferons include:

- Interferon alfa-2a (Roferon-A)
- Interferon alfa-2b (Intron-A)
- Interferon alfacon-1 (Infergen)
- Interferon alfa-n3 (Alferon)

Long-acting interferons include:

- Peginterferon alfa-2a (Pegasys)
- Peginterferon alfa-2b (PEG-Intron)

Interferon alfa is approved for treating hairy cell leukemia, AIDS-related Kaposi sarcoma, condylomata acuminatum, chronic HBV, and chronic HCV It also has been used investigationally for treating renal cell carcinoma, bladder carcinoma, chronic myelogenous leukemia, and lymphomas. Peginterferon combined with oral ribavirin is the treatment of choice for HCV. Ribavirin is discussed later in this chapter.

Other Drugs for Hepatitis

Lamivudine, adefovir, entecavir, tenofovir, and telbivudine are also used in the management of hepatitis B. They are nucleoside or nucleotide analogues (Table 45.4).

Adefovir Dipivoxil

Adefovir dipivoxil (Hepsera) is a nucleoside reverse transcriptase inhibitor (NRTI) used in managing chronic HBV infection. Although it was initially introduced as an antiretroviral drug, it led to a high incidence of nephrotoxicity at the dose needed to affect the HIV virus. Adefovir replaces a nucleotide in the HBV virus, resulting in DNA chain termination.

Common adverse effects of adefovir include GI complaints such as abdominal pain, diarrhea, dyspepsia, flatulence, and nausea, as well as headache or rash. Although the prevalence of nephrotoxicity is much lower with the current recommended

dosage of adefovir, it may still occur. The risk of nephrotoxicity is highest in patients with pre-existing renal impairment, and they require a reduction in dose. The drug should also be given cautiously to patients with liver dysfunction. Lactic acidosis and severe hepatomegaly with steatosis, including fatal cases, may occur with the use of nucleoside analogues alone or in combination with other antiretrovirals. Acute hepatitis may occur in patients who stop taking drugs, including adefovir, for HBV. Serial liver function tests should be performed for several months after ceasing therapy, to monitor for hepatitis.

Caution is necessary when adefovir is given to patients who are taking other drugs that increase the risk of renal or hepatic toxicity and lactic acidosis. Adefovir is an FDA pregnancy category C drug. It is not known whether adefovir passes into breast milk. It is not indicated for use in adolescents or children.

HIV testing should be offered to all patients prior to initiation of adefovir therapy. HIV drug resistance may occur in patients with chronic HBV infection and unrecognized or untreated HIV infection. The patient should be taught the signs of hepatic injury and advised to contact the prescriber immediately if any occur.

Boceprevir

Boceprevir (Victrelis) is a HCV protease inhibitor used in combination with peginterferon and ribavirin, to treat hepatitis C genotype 1. It is a direct acting antiviral drug against the hepatitis C virus. It is contraindicated during pregnancy because of its teratogentic effects. It is given cautiously to patients who also receive drugs that utilize the CYP3A4/5 pathway. Common adverse effects include fatigue, nausea, headache and dysgeusia. Serious adverse effects include birth defects and fetal death, anemia, and neutropenia. Both men and women receiving boceprivir must use 2 forms of birth control during therapy and avoid pregnancy for 6 months following completion of therapy. Women must have monthly pregnancy tests.

Entecavir

Entecavir (Baraclude) is an NRTI similar to adefovir. It is also approved for use in the management of chronic HBV infection. Entecavir works by competing with the substrate deoxyguanosine triphosphate, resulting in inhibition of all three activities of the HBV polymerase: base priming, reverse transcription of the negative strand from messenger RNA, and synthesis of HBV DNA. The drug is available as an oral solution or a tablet.

Common adverse effects of entecavir include nausea, dizziness, headache, and fatigue. Serious adverse effects are similar to those of adefovir. Dosage adjustments are required for patients with pre-existing renal impairment. As with adefovir, severe exacerbations of HBV may occur in patients who discontinue entecavir therapy. Entecavir is a pregnancy category C drug. Teratogenic effects have been seen in animal studies, but human studies have not been performed. Entecavir is not indicated for use in children under the age of 16 years.

Patient education for entecavir is the same as for adefovir. In addition, patients should be advised to take entecavir

2 hours before or after a meal. For patients taking the oral solution, the importance of using the measuring spoon that comes with the product and not diluting the solution with water or any other liquid should be explained.

Lamivudine

Lamivudine (Epivir-HBV) is another NRTI. Epivir-HBV tablets and oral solution contain a lower dose of the same active ingredient (lamivudine) as Epivir tablets and oral solution used to treat HIV infection. If treatment with Epivir-HBV is prescribed for chronic HBV for a patient with unrecognized or untreated HIV infection, rapid emergence of HIV resistance is likely because of the subtherapeutic dose and inappropriate monotherapy.

Common adverse effects of lamivudine include anorexia, nausea, vomiting, headache, and fatigue. Serious adverse effects are similar to those of adefovir and entecavir. The risk of lactic acidosis and severe hepatomegaly with steatosis is higher in women and obese patients who take lamivudine. Lamivudine is also an FDA pregnancy category C drug but may be given to children as young as 2 years.

Telbivudine

Telbivudine (Tyzeka) is another thymidine nucleoside analogue. It works by competitive inhibition of viral DNA polymerase (reverse transcriptase), resulting in DNA chain termination. Unlike the aforementioned NRTI drugs, telbivudine is not approved for the management of HIV infection. Its only approved use is the management of chronic hepatitis B. Telbivudine is used cautiously in patients who have pre-existing myopathy or are taking drugs that might cause myopathy, because of the potential increased risk for myopathy with the drug. Common adverse effects include headache, malaise, fatigue, upper respiratory infection, and abdominal pain. Telbivudine carries a Black Box warning regarding the potential for inducing lactic acidosis and severe hepatomegaly with steatosis and the potential for acute exacerbation of hepatitis B when discontinued. Telbivudine is a pregnancy category B drug. It is not approved for use in children.

Drugs Used for Respiratory Syncytial Virus

Most children with RSV bronchiolitis will not require hospitalization and can be treated successfully at home with albuterol, either as a nebulizer or MDI with spacer (see Chapter 35). For those who are more acutely ill and require hospitalization, one of the following drugs may be used.

Palivizumab

Palivizumab (Synagis) is a humanized monoclonal antibody to RSV prepared by using recombinant DNA technology. As a "humanized" monoclonal antibody, the drug tends to have little immunogenicity.

Palivizumab is administered to high risk children as an intramuscular (IM) injection that is given monthly during the RSV season, which is generally the beginning of fall to the end of spring. It may also be used for acute infection in hospitalized

children. In rare circumstances, palivizumab has induced hypersensitivity reactions, including anaphylaxis. Infants who experience any type of hypersensitivity reaction should not receive additional injections. Because palivizumab is given as an IM injection, it is given cautiously to infants with a history of thrombocytopenia or any coagulation disorder.

Common adverse effects include upper respiratory tract infection, otitis media, rhinitis, rash, cough, gastroenteritis, and wheezing. Rarely, infants may experience fever, diarrhea, or vomiting. Palivizumab does not have a risk of pulmonary edema because it is not given by infusion.

Palivizumab powder should be reconstituted with sterile water according to the dose of medication to be delivered. The vial is rolled between the hands but not shaken, and the solution is then allowed to sit for 20 minutes before the injection is administered.

Ribavirin

Ribavirin is a synthetic nucleoside antiviral drug. It is used as a primary agent to treat RSV infections. Intravenous ribavirin is available from the United States Centers for Disease Control and Prevention to treat hantavirus infection and Lassa fever. Oral ribavirin (Rebetol) is approved for treating chronic hepatitis C infection in combination with interferon alfa-2b (PEG-Intron) or interferon alfa-2b (Rebetron). The exact mechanism of antiviral activity of ribavirin is unclear; however, it is thought to increase the mutation rate of RNA viruses, leading to "error catastrophe."

Inhaled ribavirin (Virazole) should be administered using the SPAG-2 aerosol generator. Clinicians should make sure they are thoroughly familiar with the use of this device before administering ribavirin. Solutions placed in the SPAG-2 reservoir should be discarded every 24 hours and before adding newly reconstituted solutions. Reconstituted solutions may be stored at room temperature for 24 hours.

Ribavirin is one of the few antiviral drugs that is indicated for use in children. However, it is contraindicated for use in children who require ventilatory support, because it may precipitate in the respiratory equipment.

Ribavirin is teratogenic and embryotoxic in animals; therefore, it is contraindicated for use in adults because of its potential for producing testicular lesions and teratogenic effects. It is considered a pregnancy category X drug. Pregnant health care workers should not administer aerosolized ribavirin because it can disperse into the immediate bedside area. Additionally, ribavirin should not be given concurrently with zidovudine because it blocks the action of zidovudine.

CHAPTER SUMMARY

- Viral and fungal diseases range from annoying disorders to life-threatening infections.
- Antiviral drugs can be arbitrarily divided into purine nucleoside analogue drugs, ophthalmic antiviral drugs, topical antiviral drugs, drugs used for influenza, drugs used for hepatitis, and drugs for RSV.

- Few effective antiviral drugs exist because eradicating the virus also may severely damage the host.
- Acyclovir is the prototype purine nucleoside analogue drug used to treat viral infections.
- Oseltamivir is the prototype drug for influenza.
- Drugs used for influenza do not replace influenza vaccine.
- Drugs used for hepatitis include interferons nucleoside reverse transcriptase inhibitors and HCV protease inhibitors.
- Drugs used for RSV are divided into those that prevent RSV and those that treat RSV.

QUESTIONS FOR STUDY AND REVIEW

1. Why are there so few effective antiviral drugs?
2. How does acyclovir work to fight herpes infections?
3. Acyclovir should be given cautiously to patients with which types of diseases or disorders?
4. What type of antiviral agents are useful in managing hepatitis?
5. Why should all patients receiving nucleoside reverse transcriptase inhibitors for chronic HBV infection be offered HIV testing prior to treatment?
6. What are pharmacotherapeutic differences between amantadine (or rimantadine) and oseltamivir (or zanamivir)?
7. What special instructions should be given to immunosuppressed patients regarding oseltamivir and zanamivir?
8. Why is ribavirin not generally used in adults?
9. What are pharmacotherapeutic differences between ribavirin and palivizumab and RSV-IG?

NEED MORE HELP?

Chapter 45 of the Study Guide to Accompany *Drug Therapy in Nursing*, 4th Edition, contains NCLEX-style questions and other learning activities to reinforce your understanding of the concepts presented in this chapter. For additional information or to purchase the study guide, visit thePoint.

REFERENCES

Abudalu, M., Tyring, S., Koltun, W., et al. (2008). Single-day, patient-initiated famciclovir therapy versus 3-day valacyclovir regimen for recurrent genital herpes: a randomized, double-blind, comparative trial. *Clinical Infectious Diseases*, 47(5):651–658.

Antiviral drugs for influenza. (2008). *Medical Letter on Drugs & Therapeutics*, 50(1301–1302):98.

Aslam, S. P., Carroll, K. A., Naz, B., & Alao, A. O. (2009). Valacyclovir-induced psychosis and manic symptoms in an adolescent young woman with genital herpes simplex. *Psychosomatics*, 50(3):293–296.

Centers for Disease Control. (2009). Key Facts About Swine Influenza. Retrieved July 11, 2009 at http://www.cdc.gov/h1n1flu/key_facts.htm

Drew, W. (2008). Valacyclovir to reduce transmission of genital herpes simplex virus infection. *Journal of Infectious Diseases*, 198(8):1098–1100

Facts and Comparisons. (2010). *Drug facts and comparisons*. Philadelphia, PA: Lippincott Williams & Wilkins.

Fiore, A. E., Shay, D. K., Broder, K., et al. (2008). Prevention and Control of Influenza: Recommendations of the Advisory Committee on Immunization Practices. *MMWR*, 57(RR-7):1–60.

Hall, C. B. (2009). Antiviral drugs for the prevention and treatment of influenza in children, *Up To Date*. Retrieved from *http://uptodate.com*

Karch, A. M. (2010). *Nursing Drug Guide*. Philadelphia, PA: Lippincott Williams & Wilkins.

Koda-Kimbal, M. A., Young, L. Y., Kradian, W. A., et al. (2008). *Applied Therapeutics: The Clinical Use of Drugs*. Philadelphia, PA: Lippincott Williams & Wilkins.

Len, O., Gavaldà, J., Aguado, J. M., et al. (2008). Valganciclovir as treatment for cytomegalovirus disease in solid organ transplant recipients. *Clinical Infectious Diseases*, 46(1):20–27.

Merck. (2011). Boceprevir prescribing package insert. Retrieved from *http://www.victrelis.com/boceprevir/victrelis/hcp/index.jsp*

Micromedex Healthcare Series. Retrieved from *http://thomsonhc.com*

National Institute of Health. (2008). NIH Consensus Development Conference: Management of Hepatitis B.

Tappenden, P., Jackson, R., Cooper, K., et al. (2009). Amantadine, oseltamivir and zanamivir for the prophylaxis of influenza (including a review of existing guidance no. 67): a systematic review and economic evaluation. *Health Technology Assessment*, 13(11):1–268. Retrieved July 13, 2009, from CINAHL Plus with Full Text database.

Tatro, D. S. (2009). *Drug interaction facts*. Philadelphia, PA: Lippincott Williams & Wilkins.

Thorner, A. R. (2009). Treatment and prevention of swine H1N1 influenza, *Up To Date*. Retrieved from *http://uptodate.com*

Thorner, A. R. (2009). Epidemiology, clinical manifestations, and diagnosis of swine H1N1 influenza A, *Up To Date*. Retrieved from *http://uptodate.com*.

Update: drug susceptibility of swine-origin influenza A (H1N1) viruses, April 2009. MMWR: Morbidity & Mortality Weekly Report [serial online].58(16):433–435.

Weaver, B. S. (2009). Herpes zoster overview: natural history and incidence, *Journal Of the American Osteopathic Association*, 109(6 Suppl 2):S2–S6.

World Health Organization, Pandemic H1N1 2009. Retrieved July 11, 2009 at http://www.who.int/csr/don/2009_07_06/en/index.html

Zachary, A. C. (2009). Antiviral drugs for the prevention of influenza in adults, *Up To Date*. Retrieved from *http://uptodate.com*

Drugs Treating HIV Infection and AIDS

Learning Objectives

At the completion of this chapter the student will:

1. Describe the parameters that govern the choice of antiretroviral agents.

2. Identify core drug knowledge about drugs that are used in treating human immunodeficiency virus (HIV) infection and acquired immunodeficiency syndrome (AIDS).

3. Identify core patient variables relevant to drugs that are used in treating HIV infection and AIDS.

4. Relate the interaction of core drug knowledge to core patient variables for drugs that are used in treating HIV infection and AIDS.

5. Generate a nursing plan of care from the interactions between core drug knowledge and core patient variables for drugs that are used in treating HIV infection and AIDS.

6. Describe nursing interventions to maximize therapeutic effects and minimize adverse effects for drugs that are used in treating HIV infection and AIDS.

7. Determine key points for patient and family education for drugs that are used in treating HIV infection and AIDS.

Key Terms

CD4 cell count
Chemokine receptor antagonist (CCR5 Inhibitors)
enzyme immunoassay
enzyme-linked immunosorbent assay

fusion inhibitors
highly active antiretroviral therapy (HAART)
integrase inhibitors
HIV RNA count
nonnucleoside reverse transcriptase inhibitors (NNRTIs)
nucleoside reverse transcriptase inhibitors (NRTIs)

protease inhibitor (PI)
rapid HIV testing
resistance testing (genotype, phenotype)
salvage therapy
viral load
Western blot

Drugs Treating HIV Infection and AIDS

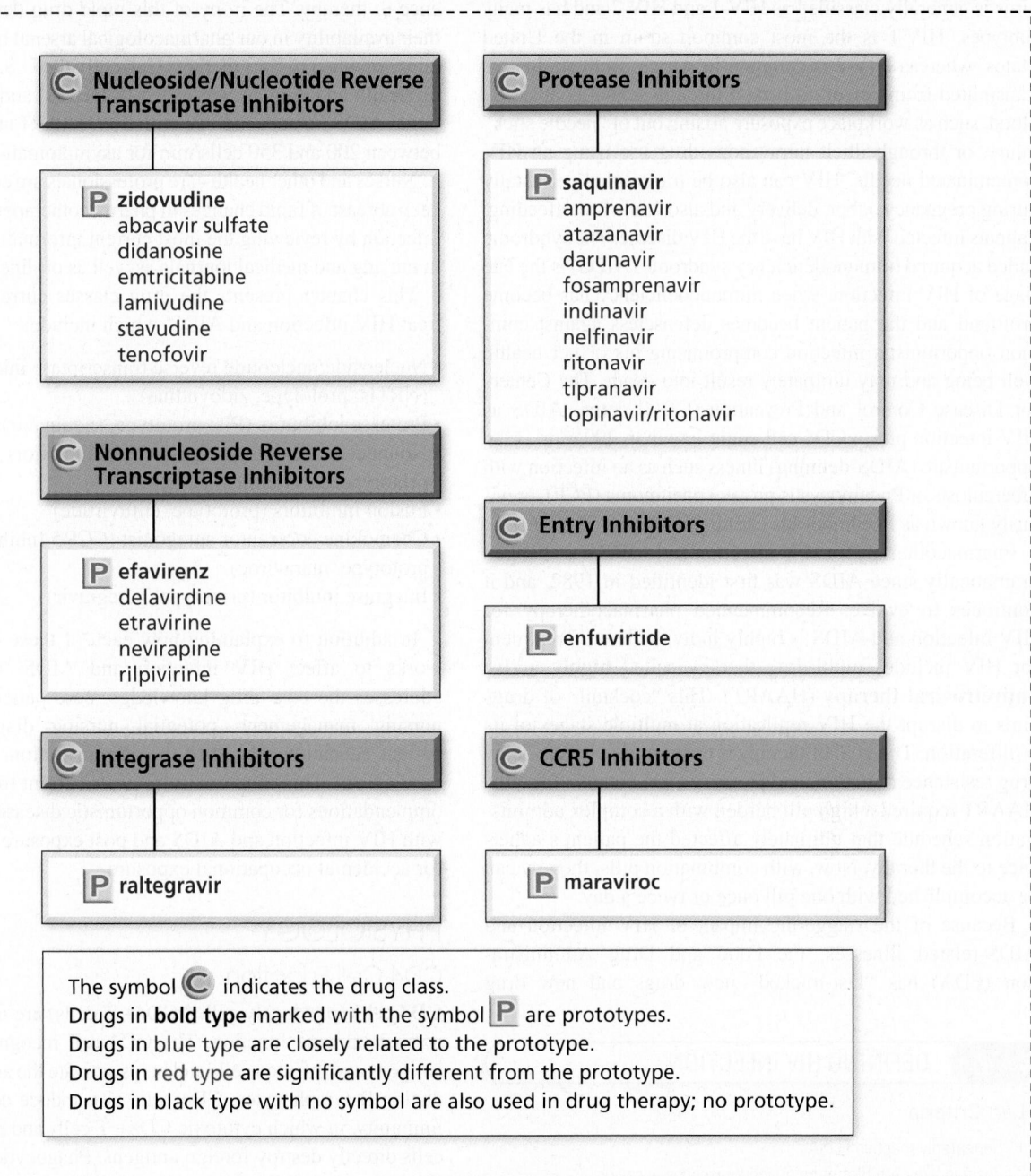

Nucleoside/Nucleotide Reverse Transcriptase Inhibitors

P zidovudine
- abacavir sulfate
- didanosine
- emtricitabine
- lamivudine
- stavudine
- tenofovir

Nonnucleoside Reverse Transcriptase Inhibitors

P efavirenz
- delavirdine
- etravirine
- nevirapine
- rilpivirine

Integrase Inhibitors

P raltegravir

Protease Inhibitors

P saquinavir
- amprenavir
- atazanavir
- darunavir
- fosamprenavir
- indinavir
- nelfinavir
- ritonavir
- tipranavir
- lopinavir/ritonavir

Entry Inhibitors

P enfuvirtide

CCR5 Inhibitors

P maraviroc

The symbol **C** indicates the drug class.
Drugs in **bold type** marked with the symbol **P** are prototypes.
Drugs in blue type are closely related to the prototype.
Drugs in red type are significantly different from the prototype.
Drugs in black type with no symbol are also used in drug therapy; no prototype.

Human immunodeficiency virus (HIV) is a virus that disables the human immune system and makes the infected person susceptible to common opportunistic infections. The virus is generally classified as HIV-1 and HIV-2 and has many subtypes. HIV-1 is the most common strain in the United States, whereas HIV-2 is common in Africa. Both strains are transmitted from person to person through sexual contact, by blood, such as workplace exposure arising out of "needle stick" injury, or through illicit intravenous drug use using an HIV contaminated needle. HIV can also be transmitted perinatally during pregnancy, labor, delivery and also while breastfeeding. Patients infected with HIV have the HIV disease. The syndrome called acquired immunodeficiency syndrome (AIDS) is the late stage of HIV infection, when immunodeficiency has become profound and the patient becomes defenseless against common opportunistic infection compromising his or her health, well being and may ultimately result into death. The Centers for Disease Control and Prevention (CDC) define AIDS as HIV infection plus a CD4 cell count less than 200/mm^3 or an opportunistic (AIDS-defining) illness such as an infection with tuberculosis or Pneumocystis jiroveci pneumonia (PCP), previously known as Pneumocystis carinii pneumonia (Box 46.1).

Pharmacotherapy for HIV infection and AIDS has changed dramatically since AIDS was first identified in 1982, and it continues to evolve. Recommended pharmacotherapy for HIV infection and AIDS is highly individualized. Treatment for HIV includes multi-drug therapy called **highly active antiretroviral therapy** (HAART). This "cocktail" of drugs aims to disrupt the HIV replication at multiple stages of its proliferation. The goal of therapy is to suppress virema, delay drug resistance mutation, and preserve CD4 counts.. Initially, HAART required a high pill burden with a complex administration schedule that ultimately affected the patient's adherence to the therapy. Now, with combination pills, therapy can be accomplished with one pill once or twice a day.

Because of the staggering impact of HIV infection and AIDS-related illnesses, the Food and Drug Administration (FDA) has "fast-tracked" new drugs and new drug

classes. Currently, there are 27 antiretroviral drugs, in 6 drug classes, with 6 fixed dose combination medications (2 or 3 antiretrovirals formulated in one pill) promoting easier adherence to therapy. The irony of this rapid drug development is their availability in our pharmacological arsenal but the uncertainty of when to start therapy. Currently the U.S. Department of Health and Human Services (US DHHS) and the International AIDS Society endorse initiation HAART at CD4 counts between 200 and 350 cells/mm for asymptomatic patients.

Nurses and other health care professionals are encouraged to keep abreast of rapid changes in pharmacotherapeutics for HIV infection by reviewing the most current information presented in nursing and medical journals as well as on-line resources.

This chapter presents the drug classes currently used to treat HIV infection and AIDS, which include:

- Nucleoside/nucleotide reverse transcriptase inhibitors (NRTIs; prototype, zidovudine)
- Protease inhibitors (PIs; prototype, saquinavir)
- Nonnucleoside reverse transcriptase inhibitors (NNRTIs; prototype, efavirenz)
- Fusion inhibitors (prototype, enfuvirtide)
- Chemokine coreceptor antagonist (CCR5 Inhibitor; prototype, maraviroc)
- Integrase inhibitor (prototype, raltegravir)

In addition to explaining how each of these drug classes works to affect HIV infection and AIDS, this chapter addresses the core drug knowledge, core patient variables, nursing management, potential nursing diagnoses, and patient education related to the administration of antiretroviral agents. This chapter also reviews current treatment recommendations for common opportunistic diseases associated with HIV infection and AIDS and post exposure prophylaxis for accidental occupational exposure.

PHYSIOLOGY

CD4 Cell Function

CD4 cells (previously called CD4+ T cells) are necessary for normal immune function. The CD4 cell recognizes foreign antigens and infected cells and helps activate the antibody-producing B lymphocytes. CD4 cells also induce cell-mediated immunity, in which cytotoxic CD8+ T cells and natural killer cells directly destroy foreign antigens. Phagocytic monocytes and macrophages also are influenced by CD4 cells. Figure 46.1 illustrates normal CD4 T-cell function. Chapter 54 presents a more thorough review of immune system physiology.

Human Immunodeficiency Virus

HIV is like all other viruses in structure. Its ribonucleic acid (RNA) is surrounded by core proteins, which are surrounded by a protein shell called a capsid. The capsid, in turn, is surrounded by a lipid bilayer envelope. The envelope contains glycoproteins that are used to attach to host cells. The two glycoprotein subunits, gp41 and gp120, are attached to each other and embedded in the lipid bilayer (Figure 46.2).

Box 46.1 DEFINING HIV INFECTION

Lab Criteria

1. Repeatedly reactive ELISA
2. Positive Western Blot or immunofluorescence assay or
3. Positive result or detectable quantity
   a. HIV nucleic acid detection test
   b. HIV p24 antigen test, including neutralization assay
   c. HIV isolation

Case Classification

	AIDS-Defining Illness	CD4+ Lymphocyte Count	CD4+ Lymphocyte % of total Lymphocytes
Stage 1	Absent	≥ 500 cells/mcL	≥29
Stage 2	Absent	200–499 cells/mcL	14–28
Stage 3	Positive	< 200 cells/mcL	< 14

RNA into deoxyribonucleic acid (DNA) to replicate. This process is completed by an enzyme called reverse transcriptase.

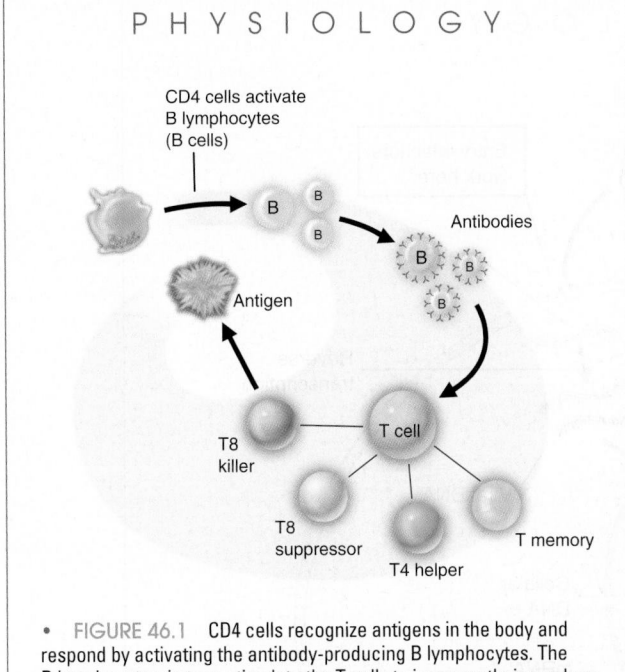

CD4 cells activate
B lymphocytes
(B cells)

Antibodies

Antigen

T8
killer

T cell

T8
suppressor

T4 helper

T memory

• FIGURE 46.1 CD4 cells recognize antigens in the body and respond by activating the antibody-producing B lymphocytes. The B lymphocytes, in turn, stimulate the T cells to increase their numbers in order to perform their various functions. T4 helper cells release lymphokines, which enhance macrophage and monocyte activity; T8 killer cells directly attack and destroy the antigen; T8 suppressor cells help to stop the immune response when appropriate; and T memory cells are stored for future use against returning antigens.

HIV is called a retrovirus. The difference between a virus and a retrovirus is in the genetic material. Like all viruses, HIV is an obligate parasite; it cannot replicate unless it is inside a living cell. Retroviruses have positive-sense single-stranded RNA and thus must transcribe their

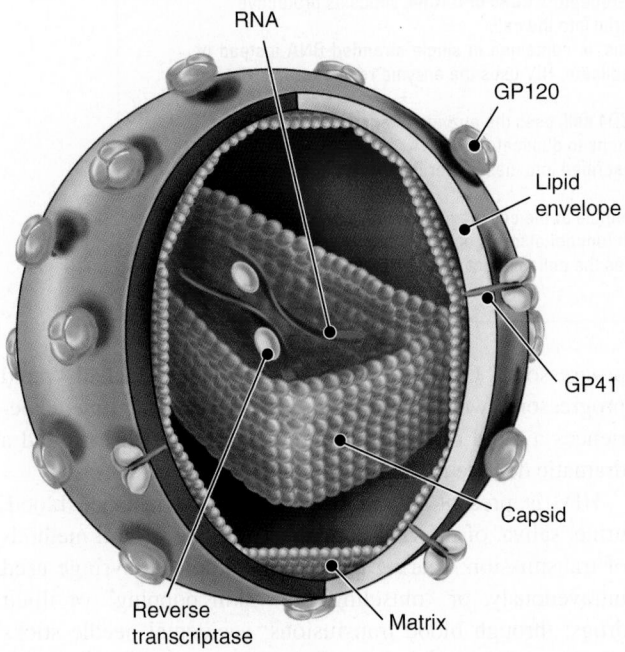

RNA

GP120

Lipid
envelope

GP41

Capsid

Reverse
transcriptase

Matrix

• FIGURE 46.2 Structure of HIV.

PATHOPHYSIOLOGY

HIV infection begins when gp120, a surface protein on the HIV viral envelope, binds to cells that have a CD4 protein receptor site. These cells include CD4 cells, monocytes, macrophages, and certain nerve cells. Once the virus is bound to the cell, the viral envelope and the plasma membrane fuse, and the genetic material from HIV enters the cell. In the cell, viral RNA is transcribed into a single strand of viral DNA with the assistance of reverse transcriptase, an enzyme made by HIV. This DNA strand replicates itself, becoming double-stranded viral DNA. At this point, viral DNA can enter the cell's nucleus and, using an enzyme called integrase, splice itself into the host cell's genome, thus becoming a permanent part of the cell's genetic structure.

This action results in two major problems. First, because all genetic material is replicated during cellular division, all daughter cells from the infected host cell also will be infected. Second, because the host cell's genome now contains viral DNA, the cell's genetic codes can direct the cell to make HIV. Production of new virus then occurs by translation and transcription of the code from the integrated DNA into viral RNA. Some of this RNA is messenger RNA that codes for HIV proteins. This complex process results in long strands of HIV RNA, which must be cut into viable lengths. Late in replication, when the newly formed virus separates from the host cell, these HIV proteins are cleaved into small proteins by the enzyme protease. Some of these proteins become part of the HIV core, and some become part of the viral protein shell. HIV protease thus is critical for viral infectivity and replication. It has been shown that HIV **provirus** (the virus before it exits the cell) manufactured without protease is non-infectious. Figure 46.3 represents HIV replication.

HIV has an affinity for CD4 cells. The virus destroys these important cells, responsible for normal immune function, which effectively strips the person of protection against common organisms.

Originally, researchers believed that after initial infection, HIV viral replication remained dormant until stimulated by an unknown event. Now we know that viral replication is never dormant as HIV replicates continuously from the time of infection although the *symptoms* of HIV disease may remain undetectable for many years. At the initial stage of infection, the **viral load** (the amount of virus in the body) is exceptionally high and quantifiable through a serological marker, the HIV RNA that measures the amount of virus in the blood. There are two reasons for this high initial viral load. First, because HIV is a new virus entering the host, the immune system is not yet sensitized to the foreign antigen, and the immune response is suboptimal. Second, because the immune system has not yet been affected by the virus, there are many CD4 cells to invade and infect.

PHYSIOLOGY

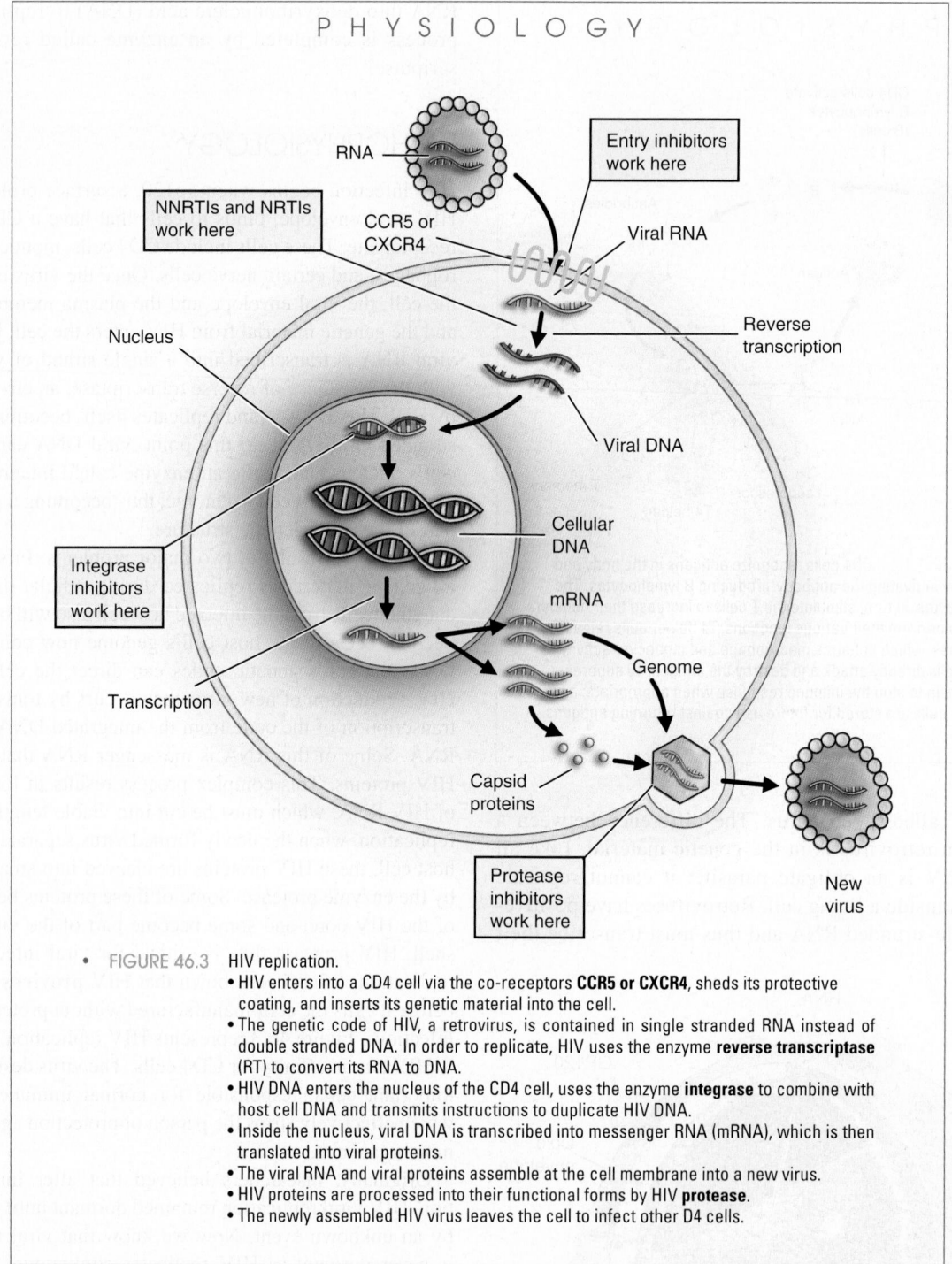

• FIGURE 46.3   HIV replication.
  • HIV enters into a CD4 cell via the co-receptors **CCR5 or CXCR4**, sheds its protective coating, and inserts its genetic material into the cell.
  • The genetic code of HIV, a retrovirus, is contained in single stranded RNA instead of double stranded DNA. In order to replicate, HIV uses the enzyme **reverse transcriptase** (RT) to convert its RNA to DNA.
  • HIV DNA enters the nucleus of the CD4 cell, uses the enzyme **integrase** to combine with host cell DNA and transmits instructions to duplicate HIV DNA.
  • Inside the nucleus, viral DNA is transcribed into messenger RNA (mRNA), which is then translated into viral proteins.
  • The viral RNA and viral proteins assemble at the cell membrane into a new virus.
  • HIV proteins are processed into their functional forms by HIV **protease**.
  • The newly assembled HIV virus leaves the cell to infect other D4 cells.

During this initial stage, the patient may experience an acute retroviral syndrome that includes fever, pharyngitis, rash, myalgia or arthralgia, diarrhea, and headache. Although these symptoms are common in HIV infection, they may be dismissed initially by the patient as "the flu." After the immune system responds to the viral invasion, the viral load decreases, and the patient may remain asymptomatic for many years. There are patients who harbor the virus but remain asymptomatic while maintaining a healthy number of CD4 over a long period of time. They are called "slow

progressors." On the other hand, there those called "rapid progressors" who, in a relatively short period of time, experiences a rapid downturn progression of their disease and a dramatic decline in their CD4 values.

HIV is present in the body fluids, for instance blood, urine, saliva, of infected patients. There are several methods of transmission: sharing of HIV contaminated syringe used intravenously, or "muscling," or "skin popping" of illicit drugs; through blood transfusions; accidental needle sticks injuries at the work place, and sexual contact with an infected sexual partner. HIV also can be transmitted though breast milk of an infected person; therefore, women with HIV are taught to avoid breast-feeding to limit the potential transmission of the virus to the infant. There is also mucotaneous exposure, such as a splash with a contaminated HIV body fluids, or penetration through an abraded skin, however this type of exposure rarely causes seroconversion.

HIV infection eventually induces symptoms in every body system. In addition to those already mentioned, common symptoms associated with HIV infection include lymphadenopathy, nausea and vomiting, hepatosplenomegaly, thrush (candidiasis of the oral tissues), and weight loss. Neurologic symptoms, such as meningoencephalitis or aseptic meningitis, peripheral neuropathy, radiculopathy, facial palsy, Guillain-Barré syndrome, brachial neuritis, cognitive impairment, or psychosis, affect up to 40% of patients.

DIAGNOSIS OF HIV INFECTION

Diagnosis of HIV infection is initially made by a screening test followed by a confirmatory assay. Screening tests are highly sensitive, whereas confirmatory assays are highly specific. The combination use of these two types of tests produces results that are highly accurate. In 2006, the CDC recommended universal, routine HIV screening for all adults in health care settings ages 13–64. This recommendation now makes HIV screening a routine test that no longer requires counseling or consent and effectively passed the responsibility of testing to the health care provider (Box 46.2). In addition, the CDC advises that pregnant women take the following steps:

• Include an HIV test in the routine panel of prenatal screening tests

Box 46.2 RECOMMENDATIONS FOR HIV SCREENING

• Routine, voluntary HIV screening for all persons 13–64 years of age in health care settings, not based on risk
• Repeat HIV screening of persons with known risk at least annually
• "Opt-out" HIV screening with the opportunity to ask questions and the option to decline
• Inclusion of consent for HIV testing with general consent for care (separate signed informed consent not necessary)
• No requirement for prevention counseling in conjunction with HIV screening in health care settings
• Availability of HIV testing in all health care settings, including inpatient services, emergency departments, urgent care clinics, sexually transmitted disease clinics, tuberculosis clinics, public health clinics, community clinics, substance abuse treatment centers, correctional health facilities, and primary care settings
• Communication of test results in same manner as other diagnostic/screening tests
• Provision of clinical HIV care or reliable referral to qualified providers

Adapted from Centers for Disease Control and Prevention. (2006). Revised recommendations for HIV testing of adults, adolescents, and pregnant women in healthcare settings. Retrieved from http://www.phppo.cdc.gov/hiv/topics/testing/resources/factsheets/pdf/healthcare.pdf.

• Consent to HIV testing in prenatal care
• May have an option to decline HIV testing
• Have a second HIV test in the third trimester (for women known to be at risk for HIV, in jurisdictions with elevated HIV incidence, or in health care facilities with high HIV prevalence).

Initially, the **enzyme immunoassay** (EIA) or **enzyme-linked immunosorbent assay** (ELISA) was the only test available. The EIA test poses some problems. It requires that the patient return to the provider to obtain the results of the test, and many patients have the test but never return to obtain the results. The EIA detects antibodies produced in response to infection and is based on the light absorbance of antigen–antibody complexes. If the patient tests positive with the EIA test, a confirmatory **Western Blot** (WB) assay test is administered. The Western Blot assay detects certain protein from the sample tissue and confirms an infection in the presence of HIV specific protein band in the tissue sample.

Now, several tests are approved by the FDA. In addition to EIA, the following tests are available:

• *Rapid HIV testing.* These screening tests produce a result within 30 minutes. Rapid testing is a valuable tool during an accidental workplace HIV exposure where a test can be conducted fairly quickly without compromising the time element crucial with post exposure prophylaxis. As with other screening tests, any positive result requires a confirmatory assay to ensure accuracy. There are several rapid HIV tests available:
  • OraQuick Advance Rapid HIV-1/2 may be used with whole blood (fingerstick or venipuncture), serum, or plasma. In addition, it may use oral fluid. Contrary to popular belief, it is not a saliva test but instead uses a small pad to draw fluids that are derived from blood from within the mouth and gums.
  • Reveal G-2 Rapid HIV-1 requires serum or plasma.
  • Uni-Gold Recombigen HIV test may be used with whole blood (fingerstick or venipuncture), serum, or plasma.
• *P24 antigen test.* This test is useful for patient with typical clinical features and negative or indeterminate HIV serologic test, that is the patient has negative HIV AB test. For these patients who are probably in the very early stage of infection, p24 is produced in high amount while the body is still in the process of producing the HIV antibody that normally will only be evident in 2–3 weeks after the infection.
• *Polymerase chain reaction (PCR).* This specialized blood test looks for HIV *genetic information* rather than HIV antibodies. This test can detect the virus, rather than the viral antibody, even in a person who has been only recently infected. This test is labor intensive and thus very expensive. DNA PCR test is crucial on new born babies who may have the maternal antibodies acquired perinatally, but not necessarily the disease, thus making the HIV antibody test inaccurate.

LABORATORY TESTS

Initial laboratory testing of patients with symptoms consistent with HIV include:

- HIV antibody testing
- Complete blood count (CBC)
- Complete metabolic panel
- Urinalysis
- Rapid plasma reagin (RPR) or Venereal Disease Research Laboratory (VDRL) testing for syphilis
- Tuberculosis (TB) skin test (unless contraindicated)
- Hepatitis A, B, and C serologies
- Fasting blood glucose and serum lipids
- *Toxoplasma gondii* immunoglobulin G (IgG)
- Papanicolaou smear and pregnancy test in women
- HIV RNA count
- CD4 cell count
- Chest X-ray for positive TST or pulmonary symptoms
- Gonorrhea, Chlamydia to identify high-risk sexual activities

The CD4 cell count and the plasma HIV RNA (viral load) assays are the essential parameters in the decision to initiate, monitor, and change antiretroviral therapies (Box 46.3).

CD4 Cell Count

CD4 cell counts are an indication of the current immunologic status of the patient. In the healthy patient, the CD4 cell count ranges from 800/mm^3 to 1,200/mm^3. In addition, the CD4 cell count is the most important consideration for initiating antiretroviral therapy and initiation and or discontinuation of chemoprophylaxis for opportunistic diseases. CD4 is the strongest predictor of disease progression and survival. As HIV infection progresses, the CD4 cell count generally decreases. The CD4 cell count is performed prior to

 Box 46.3 INDICATIONS FOR INITIATING ANTIRETROVIRAL THERAPY FOR THE PATIENT WITH CHRONIC HIV-1 INFECTION

Panel of Experts Recommendation:

- Antiretroviral therapy should be initiated on patients with AIDS defining illness or a CD4 of less than 350/mm3.
- Antiretroviral therapy should be initiated with the following patients regardless of CD4 count
  - Pregnant patients regardless of CD4
  - Patients with HIV associated nephropathy
  - Patients co-infected with HBV when treatment is indicated.
- Patients' scenario and co-morbidity conditions may be considered for initiation of antiretroviral for patients with CD4 greater than 350.
- The panel also recommends discussion of requirement for long term adherence and identification of barriers to adherence prior to initiation of therapy.

Adapted from the U.S. Department of Health and Human Services (2008) Guidelines for the Use of Antiretroviral Agents in HIV Infected Adolescent and Adults. Retrieved from: http://www.aidsinfo.nih.gov/Guidelines/GuidelineDetail.aspx?GuidelineID=7

initiation of HAART and then every 3 to 6 months thereafter to assess an optimal or sub-optimal response to therapy. When HAART is initiated, an increase in the CD4 cell count is ideally expected along with a stable clinical and virological response. Ideally, an accelerated improvement in the CD4 count is seen in the first months of therapy and levels off to a steady state as the treatment progress.

Viral Load (HIV RNA) Count

The **HIV RNA counts** are reported as copies per milliliter (mL). Viral load of HIV RNA indicates the risk for disease progression and the most important indicator of treatment response. Three tests are currently approved for use in the United States to measure viral load:

- HIV-1 reverse transcriptase PCR assay (Amplicor HIV-1 Monitor v1.5)
- Signal amplification nucleic acid probe assay (Versant HIV-1 RNA 3.0)
- Nucleic acid amplification test for HIV RNA (NucliSens HIV-1 QT)

These tests all measure the concentration of virions in blood plasma, although HIV replication occurs in other tissues as well. When the patient is receiving HAART, the virologic response in plasma corresponds with the decay of HIV-1 viral load in tissues; thus, there is currently no clinical indication for viral load testing of tissues other than blood plasma. Because these tests use different technologies, it is essential to know which type of test was used in order to interpret the results accurately.

The viral load is performed at the time of diagnosis and generally every 3 to 4 months thereafter in the asymptomatic HIV-positive patient not receiving HAART. The viral load is measured immediately before starting HAART and ideally again 2 to 8 weeks later. When the therapy proves effective, the viral load is monitored generally every 3 to 4 months to evaluate the continuing efficacy of therapy. Viral load is also measured in conjunction with any clinical event (i.e., opportunistic infection) or significant decrease of the CD4 cell count. The goal is to bring the viral load to undetectable levels (i.e., less than 50 copies/mL) within the shortest time possible and sustained it at the undetectable level overtime

When assessing the need to change antiretroviral therapy, viral load counts, CD4 cell counts and resistance testing should be evaluated at the same time. The goal of antiretroviral therapy is to increase the CD4 cell count overtime and a sustained decrease in the viral load burden for the longest time possible (Figure 46.4).

Resistance Assays

The biology of HIV infection is characterized by a high rate of replication and as a result, introduction of random mutation at each round of the replication process may occur. Drug-resistant HIV may occur due to ineffective drugs and or lack of adherence to medication regimen. The latest recommendation for resistance testing was developed in November 2008 (Box 46.4).

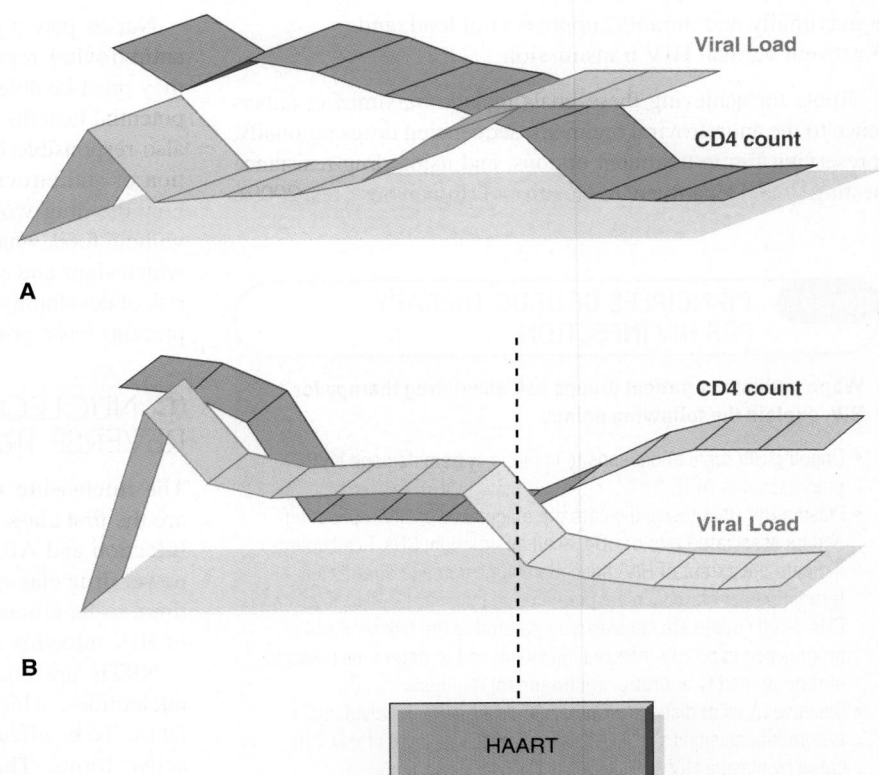

Viral Load

CD4 count

A

CD4 count

Viral Load

B

HAART

• FIGURE 46.4 **(A)** Natural progression of HIV infection. **(B)** Progression of HIV infection with highly active antiretroviral therapy (HAART). (Adapted with permission from slides designed by Dr. Gita Gupta.)

There are two types of resistance assays: genotypic and phenotypic. **Genotypic testing** evaluates the genetic makeup of a patient's virus and detects the presence of drug resistance mutations that exist in relevant genes. This information is then compared with data that document past trends in HIV treatment failure from a list of significant associated mutations maintained and updated by the International AIDS Society. If the genetic mutations in a patient's virus match genetic mutations that are presumed to be responsible for resistance to a certain drug, then his or her virus is presumed to be resistant to that drug. The test can be done rapidly and test result available in 1 to 2 weeks.

Phenotypic testing, on the other hand, is considered a direct way of measuring drug resistance. It places a sample of a patient's HIV in contact with antiretroviral drugs and observes how the virus reacts. Phenotypic testing is also considered quantitative because it can demonstrate how much of a drug is necessary to stop HIV from replicating. Phenotypic test is more expensive, takes 2 to 3 weeks to get the result, and interpretation is more complicated.

The end result of both types of genotypic and phenotypic testing is the identification of a drug or group of drugs that should not be used for a particular patient. Genotypic testing is more rapid and less costly than phenotypic testing; therefore, it is used more frequently.

Box 46.4 DRUG RESISTANCE TESTING

- HIV resistance testing is recommended for persons with HIV infection when they enter into care regardless of whether therapy will be initiated immediately. If therapy is deferred, repeat testing at the time of antiretroviral therapy initiation should be considered.
- A genotypic assay is generally preferred for antiretroviral-naïve persons.
- HIV drug resistance testing should be performed to assist in the selection of active drugs when changing antiretroviral regimens in cases of virologic failure and HIV RNA levels greater than 1,000 copies/mL. In persons with greater than 500 but less than 1,000 copies/mL, testing may be unsuccessful but should still be considered.
- Drugs resistance testing should also be performed when managing suboptimal viral load reduction.
- Drugs resistance testing in the setting virologic failure should be performed while the patient is taking his/her antiretroviral drugs, or immediately (within 4 weeks) of discontinuation of therapy.

Genotypic resistance testing is recommended for all pregnant women prior to initiation of therapy and for those entering pregnancy with detectable HIV RNA levels while on therapy.

PRINCIPLES OF DRUG THERAPY FOR HIV INFECTION

As researchers learn more about HIV and new drugs and drug classes are developed, the principles of drug therapy continues to evolve. The current goals of therapy include:

- reduce HIV-related morbidity and prolong survival
- improve quality of life
- restore and preserve immunologic function

- maximally and durably suppress viral load, and
- prevent vertical HIV transmission

Tools for achieving these goals include maximizing adherence to the antiretroviral regimens, sequencing drugs rationally, preserving future treatment options, and using drug-resistance testing (U.S. Department of Health and Human Services, 2009).

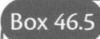

Box 46.5 PRINCIPLES OF DRUG THERAPY FOR HIV INFECTION

When patients or patient groups ask about drug therapy for HIV, explain the following points:

- Ongoing HIV replication leads to immune system damage and progression to AIDS.*
- Plasma HIV RNA levels indicate the magnitude of HIV replication and its associated rate of CD4 T-cell destruction; CD4 T-cell counts indicate the extent of HIV-induced immune damage already suffered. Regular periodic measurements of plasma HIV RNA levels and CD4 T-cell counts are necessary to determine the risk for disease progression in an HIV-infected individual and to determine when to initiate or modify antiretroviral treatment regimens.
- Because rates of disease progression differ among individuals, treatment decisions should be individualized by level of risk indicated by plasma HIV RNA levels and CD4 T-cell counts.
- Using potent combination antiretroviral therapy to suppress HIV replication below the limits of detection of sensitive plasma HIV RNA assays narrows the potential for selection of antiretroviral-resistant HIV variants, which is the major factor limiting the ability of antiretroviral drugs to inhibit virus replication and delay disease progression. Therefore, maximum achievable suppression of HIV replication should be the goal of therapy.
- The most effective means of accomplishing durable suppression of HIV replication is to simultaneously initiate combinations of effective anti-HIV drugs with which the patient has not been treated previously and that are not cross-resistant with antiretroviral agents with which the patient has been treated previously.
- Each antiretroviral drug used in combination-therapy regimens should always be used strictly according to optimal schedules and dosages.
- The available effective antiretroviral drugs are limited in number and mechanism of action, and cross-resistance between specific drugs has been documented. Therefore, any change in antiretroviral therapy increases future therapeutic constraints.
- Women should receive optimal antiretroviral therapy, regardless of pregnancy status.
- The same principles of antiretroviral therapy apply to both HIV-infected children and adults, although the treatment of HIV-positive children involves unique pharmacologic, virologic, and immunologic considerations.
- People with acute primary HIV infection should be treated with combination antiretroviral therapy to suppress virus replication to levels below the limit of detection of sensitive plasma HIV RNA assays.
- HIV-positive people, even those with viral loads below detectable limits, are infectious and should be counseled to avoid sexual and drug-use behaviors that are associated with transmission of HIV and other infectious pathogens.

*Long-term survival free from clinically important immune dysfunction has improved substantially since HAART was introduced.

Nurses play a pivotal role in maximizing adherence to the antiretroviral regimens. As patient advocates and educators, they must be able to discuss and inform the patient about the potential benefits and risks of HAART In addition, nurses are also responsible for educating patients about self-administration of antiretroviral therapy. It is important to teach patients how the drug works, when to take the drug, such as with or without food, what the potential adverse effects of the drug are, which signs and symptoms to report, and ways to decrease the risk of developing resistance to the HAART regimen. Box 46.5 presents basic principles of drug therapy for HIV infection.

© NUCLEOSIDE/NUCLEOTIDE REVERSE TRANSCRIPTASE INHIBITORS

The **nucleoside reverse transcriptase inhibitors (NRTIs)** are the first class of drugs approved by the FDA to treat HIV infection and AIDS. Although more potent newer drugs and newer drug classes have emerged, nucleoside analogues continue to be crucial drugs in the pharmacologic management of HIV infection and AIDS.

NRTIs are chemically similar to human nucleosides or nucleotides, which are considered the "building blocks" of DNA. To be effective, all of the NRTIs must convert to their active forms. These drugs inhibit reverse transcriptase, an enzyme critical to HIV replication (see Figure 46.3).

Zidovudine was first synthesized as an antineoplastic drug in the 1960s. In 1987, it was found to inhibit the in vitro infectivity of HIV-1 and that same year was approved as the first antiretroviral of its class. Zidovudine (AZT, ZDV, Retrovir) is the prototype NRTI. Table 46.1 presents a summary of drugs in this class.

Nursing Management of the Patient Receiving [P] Zidovudine

Core Drug Knowledge

Pharmacotherapeutics

Zidovudine is active against the Epstein-Barr virus and hepatitis B virus (HBV) and exerts some antibacterial activity against Enterobacteriaceae, but its main indication is for treating HIV infection in adults and children and preventing transmission of HIV to the fetus in pregnant, HIV-positive women. The parameters for starting antiretroviral therapy are controversial, complex, and constantly changing. However, the persisting theory is that symptomatic patients should begin therapy regardless of laboratory values. The recommendation for initiating treatment in asymptomatic patients is a CD4 cell count between 200–350 cell/mm, or those with HIV nephropathy, or patients with active HBV with the intent to treat the HBV.

Pharmacokinetics

Zidovudine, or AZT, is administered orally or parenterally. Following oral administration, zidovudine is absorbed rapidly from the gastrointestinal (GI) tract. The rate and extent of drug absorption may be decreased by fatty meals. The half-life of zidovudine is about 1 hour

TABLE 46.1   **Summary of Selected Ⓒ Nucleoside/Nucleotide Reverse Transcriptase Inhibitors**

Drug (Trade) Name	Route and Dosage Range	Pharmacokinetics	Special Considerations
ℙ zidovudine (AZT, ZDV, Retrovir)	*Adult and adolescent:* PO, 300 mg 2×/d PO 200 mg 3×/d *Adult and adolescent:* IV, 1 mg/kg 5–6×/d around the clock *Child and infant ≥90 d:* PO, 160 mg/m² q8h; maximum 200 mg Q8 hrs (syrup, capsules, or tablets) *Infant <90 d and neonate:* PO, 2 mg/kg q6h *Child and infant ≥90 d:* IV, 120 mg/m² q6h *Infant <90 d and neonate:* IV, 1.5 mg/kg q6h	*Onset:* Rapid *Duration:* 4 h $t_{1/2}$: 1.1 h	No food restrictions Assess for renal insufficiency. Advise provider if positive findings.
abacavir sulfate (ABC, Ziagen)	*Adult and adolescent >16 y:* PO, 300 mg 2×/d or 600 mg once daily *Infant and child 3 mo–16 y:* PO, 8 mg/kg 2×/d	*Onset:* 0.7 h *Duration:* Unknown $t_{1/2}$: 1.5 h	No food restrictions. Monitor closely for rash.
didanosine (ddI, Videx)	*Adult >60 kg:* PO, two 100-mg tablets 2×/d or two 200-mg tablets once daily or one 200-mg tablet 2×/d; 250 mg 2×/d (solution) *Adult and adolescent <60 kg:* PO, 125 mg 2×/d or one 250-mg tablet daily; 167 mg 2×/d (solution) *Child and infant ≥8 mo:* PO, 90–150 mg/m2 q12h *Neonates <2 wk:* PO, 50 mg/m2 PO q12h	*Onset:* Rapid *Duration:* 12 h $t_{1/2}$: 1.6 h	Administer on an empty stomach at least 30 min before or 2 h after a meal.
didanosine (ddI EC, Videx EC)	*Patients >60 kg:* 400 mg once daily *Patients <60 kg:* 250 mg once daily		Take on an empty stomach. Must be swallowed whole.
emtricitabine (FTC, Emtriva)	*Adult:* PO, 200 mg daily *Adolescent, child, and infant:* Safe and effective use has not been established.	*Onset:* Rapid *Duration:* 24 h $t_{1/2}$: 10 h	No food restrictions
lamivudine (3TC, Epivir)	*Adult and adolescent >16 y and >50 kg:* PO, 300 mg daily or 150 mg 2×/d *Adult and adolescent 12–16 y and <50 kg:* PO, 2 mg/kg 2×/d *Infant >3 mo and child:* PO, 4 mg/kg 2×/d	*Onset:* Rapid *Duration:* 12 h $t_{1/2}$: 3–6 h	No food restrictions
stavudine (d4T, Zerit, Zerit XR)	*Adult and adolescent >60 kg:* PO, 40 mg 2×/d *Adult and adolescent <60 kg:* PO, 30 mg 2×/d Extended-release capsules *Adult and adolescent >60 kg:* PO, 100 mg daily *Adult and adolescent < 60 kg:* PO, 75 mg daily Child: Safe and effective dosage has not been established	*Onset:* Rapid *Duration:* 12 h $t_{1/2}$: 1 h	No food restrictions
tenofovir disoproxil fumarate (PMPA, TDF, Viread)	*Adult:* PO, 300 mg daily *Adolescent, child, and infant:* Safe and effective dosage has not been established.	*Onset:* Rapid *Duration:* 24 h $t_{1/2}$: 17 h	No food restrictions Administer 1 h before or 2 h after Videx
Combination Drugs			
abacavir sulfate/lamivudine (ABC, 3TC, Epzicom)	*Adult:* PO, one tablet (600 mg ABC/300 mg 3TC) daily	See individual drugs	No food restrictions
tenofovir/emtricitabine (Truvada)	Adult: PO, 1 tablet (200 mg tenofovir/300 mg emtricitabine) daily *Adolescent, child, and infant:* Safe and effective dosage has not been established.	See individual drugs	No food restrictions
tenofovir/emtricitabine/efavirenz (Atripla)	*Adults:* PO, 1 tablet (600 mg efavirenz/200 mg emtricitabine/300 mg tenofovir) 1×/d *Adolescent, child, and infant:* Safe and effective dosage has not been established.	See individual drugs	Administer on empty stomach, preferably at bedtime
zidovudine/lamivudine (Combivir)	*Adult and child >12 y:* PO, 1 tablet (150 mg lamivudine/300 mg zidovudine) 2×/d	See individual drugs	No food restrictions
zidovudine/lamivudine/abacavir (Trizivir)	*Adult and adolescent >40 kg:* PO, 1 tablet 2×/d *Child:* Not intended for use in pediatric patients or adolescents weighing <40 kg	See individual drugs	No food restrictions

in patients with normal renal function and increases to 1.4 to 2.9 hours in patients with renal dysfunction. Hepatic dysfunction also causes a moderate prolongation of zidovudine half-life.

Zidovudine crosses the blood–brain barrier and the placenta. It is converted into zidovudine triphosphate, its active form, by intracellular conversion and its inactive metabolite by the liver. Both active drug and inactive metabolite are excreted by glomerular filtration and tubular secretion. It is now available in fixed dose combination in one pill, with lamivudine or abacavir.

Pharmacodynamics

Zidovudine inhibits the synthesis of DNA by reverse transcriptase (the viral enzyme that copies viral RNA into DNA). Zidovudine bears a structural resemblance to thymidine, a natural nucleoside. Reverse transcriptase fails to distinguish zidovudine from its natural counterpart, and the enzyme attempts to use the drug to synthesize viral DNA. When zidovudine is incorporated into a strand of DNA, the addition of further nucleotides is blocked, and the full-length viral DNA chain is prematurely terminated.

Contraindications and Precautions

Absolute contraindications to the use of zidovudine include hypersensitivity, breast-feeding, and existing lactic acidosis. Patients with pre-existing hepatic dysfunction, obesity, and prolonged nucleoside analogue therapy have a higher risk of developing lactic acidosis due to the association of NRTIs to liver mitochondrial toxicity. Zidovudine should be given with caution to patients with pre-existing depression of bone marrow function, folate deficiency, or vitamin B_{12} deficiency. Patients with these disorders are at increased risk for severe hematologic toxicity. It is also given with caution to patients who have recently received cytotoxic drugs or radiation therapy because zidovudine may induce myelosuppression. Because of the risk for myelosuppression, patients with dental disease are also given zidovudine with caution.

Zidovudine should be used with caution in patients with hepatic or renal disease. The drug is metabolized in the liver to an inactive metabolite. In patients with impaired hepatic function, zidovudine can accumulate. Both zidovudine and its inactive metabolite are excreted in the urine. Zidovudine can accumulate in patients with renal impairment, causing an increased risk for toxicity.

Adverse Effects

Zidovudine may cause the serious adverse effects associated with all NRTIs, which are listed in Table 46.2. GI symptoms include nausea and vomiting, diarrhea, abdominal pain, dyspepsia, and anorexia. Esophageal ulceration also has occurred. Several central nervous system (CNS) effects have been reported, including headache, seizures, somnolence, paresthesias, agitation, restlessness, and insomnia. Other adverse effects that have been described include nail discoloration, rash, and an alteration in taste.

TABLE 46.2	Potential Life-Threatening and Serious Adverse Effects of Antiretroviral Drug Classes
Class	**Effects**
Nucleoside/nucleotide reverse transcriptase inhibitors (NRTIs)	Bone marrow suppression
	Fatigue
	Hepatic steatosis
	Hepatotoxicity
	Lactic acidosis with hepatic steatosis
	Muscle pain and wasting
	Pancreatitis
	Peripheral neuritis
Nonnucleoside reverse transcriptase inhibitors (NNRTIs)	Hepatotoxicity
	Skin rash
	Stevens-Johnson syndrome
	Toxic epidermal necrosis
Protease inhibitors (PIs)	Cardiovascular effects
	Fat maldistribution
	GI intolerance
	Elevated liver enzymes/hepatotoxicity
	Hyperlipidemia
	Hyperglycemia
	Osteonecrosis
	Uncontrolled bleeding in hemophiliacs
Entry inhibitors	Injection site reactions
	Pneumonia
	Hypersensitivity reaction
Chemokine co-receptor antagonist	Cough
	Pyrexia
	URI
	Rash
	Musculoskeletal symptoms
	Abdominal pain
Integrase inhibitors	Nausea
	Diarrhea
	headache
	Muscle enzyme elevation

In addition, zidovudine has several Black Box warnings:

- Hematologic toxicities, including granulocytopenia and severe anemia, may occur due to its bone marrow toxicity. Signs of granulocytopenia, such as predisposition to a recurring infection, can develop in 6 to 8 weeks, and signs of anemia, such as fatigue, can develop in 2 to 4 weeks. Discontinuing the drug usually resolves the granulocytopenia and anemia. Although zidovudine actually can produce an increased platelet count, drug-induced thrombocytopenia can occur as well. Initial increases in platelet count usually occur within 1 to

2 weeks of initiation of therapy and can continue for 4 to 7 weeks.

- Prolonged zidovudine use has been associated with symptomatic myopathy. Because myopathy also may be a component of HIV infection, it may be overlooked as an adverse effect. Discontinuation of the drug may lead to some improvement, but rapid worsening can occur when it is readministered. Cardiomyopathy also has been reported.
- Lactic acidosis and severe hepatomegaly with steatosis, including fatalities, may occur with the NRTIs alone or in combination with other medications, HAART included. Although the actual incidence of these adverse effects is low, mortality is extremely high. Patients may complain of fatigue, nausea, vomiting, abdominal pain, weight loss, or dyspnea. Evaluation shows lactic acidosis with elevated levels of creatine phosphokinase (CPK), alanine aminotransferase (ALT), lactate dehydrogenase, or all three; abdominal computed tomography scans and liver biopsy often show steatosis. The initial clinical manifestations of lactic acidosis are variable and may include nonspecific GI symptoms without dramatic elevation of hepatic enzymes and, in some cases, dyspnea. All NRTIs have been implicated, although these effects occur most frequently with stavudine, didanosine, lamivudine, and emtricitabine.

Drug Interactions

The most important drug interaction with zidovudine is with ganciclovir, a medication use to treat cytomegalovirus retinitis, a late opportunistic infection seen with HIV infection, which may induce life-threatening hematologic toxicity. Other drugs that interact with zidovudine include acetaminophen, interferon beta-1b, probenecid, rifampin, trimethoprim, and valproic acid.

Table 46.3 presents a list of drugs that interact specifically with zidovudine. Additionally, Table 46.4 presents drugs with overlapping toxicities, including zidovudine.

Assessment of Relevant Core Patient Variables

Health Status

Assess the patient for hypersensitivity to zidovudine and for early pregnancy. Also assess the patient for pre-existing hepatic or renal dysfunction. Review the patient's current pharmacotherapies for drugs that are potentially myelosuppressive, nephrotoxic, or directly toxic to red blood cells. Any positive findings should be communicated to the prescriber.

Before starting therapy, perform a complete physical examination. Documenting this baseline status is important because drug therapy may be discontinued or modified

TABLE 46.3	Agents That Interact with P Zidovudine	
Interactants	**Effect and Significance**	**Nursing Management**
acetaminophen	Enhanced nonhepatic or renal clearance of zidovudine (ZDV) may occur. This may result in subtherapeutic levels of ZDV.	Limit frequency of acetaminophen administration. Discuss dosage adjustment with health care provider.
atovaquone	Atovaquone inhibits metabolism of zidovudine, resulting in increased zidovudine serum concentration.	Monitor for zidovudine adverse effects or toxicity. Monitor CBC.
food	Rate and extent of ZDV absorption may be decreased by fatty meals.	Administer ZDV at least 1 h before meals.
ganciclovir	Although mechanism of action is unclear, ganciclovir in combination with ZDV may induce life-threatening hematologic toxicity.	Verify order with health care provider prior to administration.
interferon beta-1b	Interferon beta may inhibit the glucuronidation of ZDV. This may increase ZDV serum concentrations and induce toxic effects.	Monitor ZDV serum concentration levels. Discuss dosage adjustment of ZDV with health care provider.
methadone	Concurrent use may increase zidovudine serum concentration.	Monitor for zidovudine adverse effects or toxicity. Monitor CBC.
probenecid	Probenecid appears to inhibit ZDV glucuronidation. This may increase ZDV serum concentration levels and induce toxic effects.	Monitor for systemic symptoms, such as malaise, myalgia, and fever. Discuss dosage adjustment of ZDV with health care provider.
rifampin/rifabutin	Rifampin may increase hepatic metabolism of ZDV, resulting in decreased serum concentration.	Discuss dosage adjustment of ZDV with health care provider.
trimethoprim	Pharmacologic effects of ZDV may be increased in patients with impaired hepatic function who receive trimethoprim.	Monitor ZDV serum concentration. Discuss dosage adjustment of ZDV with health care provider.
valproic acid	First-pass glucuronide metabolism of ZDV may be decreased.	Discuss dosage adjustment of ZDV with health care provider when starting, changing, or stopping valproic acid.

TABLE 46.4 HIV-Related Drugs with Overlapping Toxicities

Bone Marrow Suppression	Peripheral Neuropathy	Pancreatitis	Nephrotoxicity	Hepatotoxicity	Rash	Diarrhea	Ocular Effects
amphotericin B	didanosine	cotrimoxazole	acyclovir	azithromycin	abacavir	atovaquone	cidofovir
cidofovir	isoniazid	didanosine	adefovir	clarithromycin	amprenavir	clindamycin	didanosine
cotrimoxazole	linezolid	lamivudine	aminoglycosides	delavirdine	atazanavir	darunavir	ethambutol
cytotoxic chemotherapy	stavudine	(children)	amphotericin B	efavirenz	atovaquone	fosamprenavir	linezolid
drugs	zalcitabine	pentamidine	cidofovir	fluconazole	cotrimoxazole	lopinavir/	rifabutin
dapsone		ritonavir	foscarnet	isoniazid	dapsone	ritonavir	voriconazole
flucytosine		stavudine	indinavir	itraconazole	darunavir	nelfinavir	
ganciclovir		zalcitabine	pentamidine	ketoconazole	delavirdine	ritonavir	
hydroxyurea			tenofovir	neviparine	efavirenz	tipranavir	
interferon-alfa				NRTIs	fosamprenavir		
linezolid				PIs	neviparine		
peginterferon-alfa				rifabutin	sulfadiazine		
primaquine				rifampin	tipranavir		
pyrimethamine				voriconazole	voriconazole		
ribavirin							
rifabutin							
sulfadiazine							
trimetrexate							
valganciclovir							
zidovudine							

based on changes from baseline. Laboratory tests may include a CBC, chemistry profile, liver and renal function tests, CD4 cell count, drug resistance testing and plasma HIV RNA measurement.

Life Span and Gender

Assess the patient for pregnancy and breast-feeding. Women who are taking zidovudine and become pregnant should remain on the drug. However, if the patient is not taking zidovudine at the time of conception, it is given antenatally after 14 weeks' gestation and throughout the rest of pregnancy, intravenously during the intrapartum period, and to the newborn for the first 6 weeks of life. In women who have not received antiretroviral therapy during pregnancy, intravenous (IV) zidovudine during labor can reduce the risk of transmitting HIV to the neonate. Box 46.6 describes general considerations for the management of HIV during pregnancy.

The risk of lactic acidosis is increased in women taking zidovudine, and they should be monitored closely for signs and symptoms. Presumptive symptoms of pregnancy can mimic early symptoms of lactic acidosis (nausea, vomiting, fatigue, and anorexia); thus, the patient should be scheduled for periodic serum electrolyte monitoring and liver function tests, especially during the last trimester of pregnancy.

To prevent adverse effects of zidovudine in the neonate, zidovudine should not be given during lactation. In addition, HIV-positive women are advised not to breast-feed in order to avoid potential postnatal transmission to an infant who may not be infected.

Children younger than 15 months should have HIV infection confirmed by PCR test. HIV antibody test findings in

infants may reflect maternal antibodies, not the infant's own antibodies.

Lifestyle, Diet, and Habits

It is important to assess the patient's understanding of HIV transmission and to explain that despite drug therapy, the patient can still transmit HIV to others. In addition, assess the adherence issue. Even when zidovudine is taken exactly as directed, resistance may develop. However, resistance develops much more quickly when serum concentrations are suboptimal, which can be caused by imperfect adherence: either missing doses during the day or using the drug intermittently.

Assess the patient's typical dietary habits. Although zidovudine is taken without regard to meals, avoidance of fatty foods is important because these foods decrease the drug's absorption. Outline a high-carbohydrate, moderate-protein, low-fat diet.

It is also important to investigate whether the patient has a problem or a potential problem with substance abuse. HIV infection is highly prevalent among IV drug abusers. Once the diagnosis of HIV infection is made, some patients may see no reason to change their behavior because it is already "too late." The advent of HAART significantly altered the prognoses of HIV from debilitating and ultimately fatal to a disease to a chronic condition that can be managed with judicious care. Explain the toll drug abuse takes on the body and the need for the patient to establish a healthy lifestyle.

Gently question the patient's sexual lifestyle. Explain that unsafe sex may result in transmission of HIV to others, re-infection with another strain, or co-infection with other sexually transmitted and or blood borne diseases.

Box 46.6	HIV MANAGEMENT DURING PREGNANCY

The goal of antiretroviral therapy during pregnancy is to preserve the health of both mother and child.

Clinical Situation	Recommendation Woman	Recommendation Infant
HIV-infected woman who is receiving HAART and becomes pregnant	• Continue current HAART regimen if successfully suppressing viremia, except avoid use of EFV or other potentially teratogenic drugs in the first trimester and drugs with known adverse potential for mother. • HIV antiretroviral drug resistance testing is recommended if the woman has detectable viremia on therapy. • In general, if woman requires treatment, antiretroviral drugs should not be stopped during the 1st trimester. • Continue HAART regimen during intrapartum period (ZDV given as continuous infusion during labor while other antiretroviral agents are continued orally and postpartum. • Schedule cesarean delivery at 38 weeks gestation if plasma HIV RNA remains greater than 1,000 copies/mL near the time of delivery.	• ZDV for 6 weeks started within 6 to 12 hours after birth
HIV-infected pregnant woman who is antiretroviral naïve and has indications for antiretroviral therapy.	• HIV antiretroviral drug resistance testing is recommended prior to the initiation of therapy and if suboptimal viral suppression after initiation of HAART. • Initiate HAART regimen. • For women who require immediate initiation of therapy for their own health, treatment should be initiated as soon as possible, including in the 1st trimester. • Continue HAART regimen during intrapartum period (ZDV given as continuous infusion during labor while other antiretroviral agents are continued orally and postpartum. • Schedule cesarean delivery at 38 weeks gestation if plasma HIV RNA remains greater than 1,000 copies/mL near the time of delivery	• ZDV for 6 weeks started within 6 to 12 hours after birth

HIV-infected pregnant woman who is antiretroviral naïve and does NOT require treatment for her own health.	• HIV antiretroviral drug resistance testing is recommended prior to the initiation of therapy and if suboptimal viral suppression after initiation of HAART.
	• HAART is recommended for prophylaxis of perinatal transmission in women who do not require treatment for their own health.
	  • Consider delaying HAART initiation until after 1st trimester is completed.
	  • Avoid use of EFV or other potentially teratogenic drugs in the 1st trimester and drugs with known adverse potential for mother.
	  • Use of ZDV is recommended as a component of antiretroviral regimen when feasible
	• Use of DDV prophylaxis alone is controversial but may be considered for those women with plasma HIV RNA levels less than 1,000 copies/mL on no therapy.
	• Continue HAART regimen during intrapartum period (ZDV given as continuous infusion during labor while other antiretroviral agents are continued orally and postpartum.
	• Evaluate need for continued therapy postpartum; discontinue HAART unless has indications for continued therapy.
	• Schedule cesarean delivery at 38 weeks gestation if plasma HIV RNA remains greater than 1,000 copies/mL near the time of delivery
		• ZDV for 6 weeks started within 6 to 12 hours after birth

HIV-infected pregnant woman who has not received antiretroviral therapy during pregnancy	• ZDV: continuous infusion during labor OR • ZDV given as a continuous infusion during labor, plus single dose NVP at onset of labor. Consideration should be given to adding 3Tc during labor and maternal ZDV/3TC for 7 days postpartum, which may reduce development of NVP resistance OR • ZDV: continuous infusion during labor	• ZDV: for 6 weeks started within 6 to 12 hours after birth • Single dose NVP plus ZDV for 6 weeks. OR • ZDV in combination with additional drugs in the infant. Consultation with a pediatric HIV specialist is recommended.

Adapted from Public Health Service Taskforce. (2009). Recommendations for use of antiretroviral drugs in pregnant HIV-1 infected women for maternal health and interventions to reduce perinatal HIV-1 transmission in the United States. Retrieved from *http://aidsinfo.nih.gov/ContentFiles/PerinatalGL.pdf*

Be aware of the patient's economic status. Many patients do not have insurance or other resources to obtain this drug. Patients may qualify for medical assistance through county, state, or federal funds, pharmaceutical drug programs, or local health departments through the AIDS Drug Assistance Program (ADAP). Refer patients with financial problems to the hospital or clinic social worker.

Environment

Zidovudine is administered most frequently in an outpatient setting. Because HIV infection is treated routinely with complicated polytherapy, assess the patient's ability to understand complex instructions. Be explicit—in both spoken and written language—concerning the instructions for taking which drug at what time of day.

IV zidovudine, which can be given in any setting, is stable for 24 hours at room temperature and for 48 hours when refrigerated. The drug should be infused over 1 hour. Before infusion, examine the solution for particulate matter and discoloration. If either is present, the solution should not be administered. All preparations of zidovudine should be protected from light once prepared as well as during infusion.

Nursing Diagnoses and Outcomes

- Acute Pain related to headache from drug effects
  Desired outcome: The patient will self medicate with over the counter remedies such as nonsteroidal anti-inflammatory drugs (NSAIDS), and or practice non-pharmacological pain relief to alleviate the headache.
- Ineffective Protection related to anemia and granulocytopenia
  Desired outcome: The patient will remain free of opportunistic diseases related to blood dyscrasias.
- Imbalanced Nutrition: Less than Body Requirements, related to GI distress
  Desired outcome: The patient will self medicate with over the counter remedies to control transient GI symptoms and will contact the provider for persistent GI complaints
- Disturbed Sleep Pattern: Insomnia related to CNS adverse effects
  Desired outcome: The patient will obtain adequate sleep throughout drug therapy.
- Disturbed Thought Processes related to adverse CNS effects
  Desired outcome: The patient will remain oriented and able to communicate effectively with others.
- Diarrhea related to adverse drug effects
  Desired outcome: The patient will avoid dehydration and contact the prescriber if diarrhea persists.
- Risk for Injury related to adverse drug effects
  Desired outcome: The patient will remain injury free throughout therapy.

Planning and Intervention

Maximizing Therapeutic Effects

Administer zidovudine 1 hour before meals. Also, make sure the patient receives 600 mg/d in divided doses—200-mg tablets three times daily or 300-mg tablets twice daily. Make sure the patient is on a low-fat diet.

Minimizing Adverse Effects

Intramuscular injections should be cautiously administered to patients receiving zidovudine; they may cause bleeding, bruising, or hematomas because of thrombocytopenia secondary to zidovudine-induced depression of bone marrow function.

Providing Patient and Family Education

- Emphasize that zidovudine does not cure HIV. Encourage the patient to take precautions to avoid exposing others to blood and body fluids and the use of latex condoms during sex.
- Explain the importance of adhering to the therapeutic regimen. The instructions should be clear and preferably in writing and at the patient's reading comprehension level.
- Explain the importance of periodic blood monitoring to ensure the efficacy of therapy and early recognition of adverse effects associated with AZT.
- It is important to advise patients about potential adverse effects, especially the Black Box warnings. Stress the importance of contacting the prescriber if signs of anemia or depressed bone marrow function appear, such as bleeding, easy bruising, or fatigue. Also explain that adverse effects, such as GI distress or headache, may resolve spontaneously after 3 to 4 weeks of therapy. Headaches can be treated with NSAIDs. Persistent problems should be reported to the prescriber.
- Instruct patients to advise the prescriber if any other drugs are ordered by another prescriber. Explain that many drugs may alter the way zidovudine works, and other drugs may increase the risk of adverse effects from zidovudine therapy.
- Advise patients to postpone any dental work if myelosuppression is suspected.
- Instruct patients with sleep disturbance to attempt relaxation techniques or warm baths to facilitate sleep.
- Explain the importance of contacting the prescriber if patients have difficulty thinking or experience memory problems.

Ongoing Assessment and Evaluation

Perform a physical examination at each visit with the patient who is taking zidovudine. Laboratory data should be obtained ideally every 2 to 4 weeks. Once HIV RNA levels are undetectable and the CD4 count is stable and the patient is clinically stable, follow-up visits should ideally occur every other month.

Monitor for signs and symptoms of adverse effects of lactic acidosis, anemia, depressed bone marrow function, or nephrotoxicity. Also monitor for signs of myelosuppression or myalgias. Symptoms of myalgia include proximal muscle weakness and elevations of creatinine kinase values.

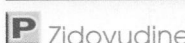

MEMORY CHIP

P Zidovudine

- Used for management of HIV and AIDS
- Major contraindications: hypersensitivity, first 14 weeks of pregnancy
- Most common adverse effects: nausea, headache, rash, fever, and abdominal pain
- Most serious adverse effects: anemia, granulocytopenia, and thrombocytopenia; suppression of bone marrow function; lactic acidosis; and hepatomegaly with steatosis
- Maximizing therapeutic effects: Administer 1 hour before meals.
- Minimizing adverse effects: Avoid IM injections because of thrombocytopenia.
- Most important patient education: signs and symptoms of anemia and importance of notifying the prescriber immediately
- **Black box warning: Neutropenia and severe anemia, myopathy with prolonged use, and potential for lactic acidosis and hepatomegaly.**

Monitor for the need to change pharmacotherapy such as intolerance to the regimen, or unwanted results of serological markers, such as a declining CD4 count and or an elevation in the HIV viral load. Remember that blood analysis may be necessary to determine whether changes in therapy are needed because of sub-optimal therapy or, because the patient may remain asymptomatic with the medications associated toxicity such as with mild anemia associated with bone marrow suppression or upward fluctuation of liver enzymes above the upper limits of normal with hepatotoxicity.

The patient should have a stable CD4 count and a declining or undetectable HIV RNA count throughout therapy. The patient should be free of opportunistic infections and signs of anemia or depressed bone marrow function and other known toxic effects of the therapy.

Drugs Closely Related to P Zidovudine

Abacavir Sulfate

Abacavir sulfate (ABC, Ziagen) is an analogue of guanine. Like zidovudine, it must be converted to its active form, carbovir triphosphate, to be effective. It may be substantially more potent than some other reverse transcriptase inhibitors. Abacavir is available in tablet and suspension forms. It has excellent bioavailability and widespread distribution, including the cerebrospinal fluid (CSF). Abacavir plus Lamivudine (Epzicom) is a combination of an NNRTI and an NRTI in one pill and given once a day. Trizivir is co-formulation of three antiretrovirals that include abacavir and zidovudine, and lamivudine that is given twice a day. This formulation combines two NRTIs and one NRTI. Several Black Box warnings are associated with abacavir:

- Serious and sometimes fatal hypersensitivity reactions may occur. This multiorgan clinical syndrome is characterized by two or more groups of the following signs and symptoms: (1) fever; (2) rash; (3) GI symptoms such as nausea, vomiting, diarrhea, or abdominal pain; (4) constitutional symptoms such as generalized malaise, fatigue, or achiness; and (5) respiratory symptoms such as dyspnea, cough, or pharyngitis.
- Hypersensitivity may occur. Monitor the patient for a rash. Most antiretroviral drugs may cause a rash, but the rash caused by abacavir may signal hypersensitivity to the drug.
- The drug should be discontinued as soon as hypersensitivity reaction is suspected
- Any product containing abacavir should be permanently discontinued if hypersensitivity cannot be ruled out, even when other diagnoses are possible. More severe symptoms, which may include life-threatening hypotension and death, can occur within hours of restarting abacavir.
- Lactic acidosis may occur, as with zidovudine.

Check for the completion of HLA-B5701 testing. Inform the provider if the test is positive because abacavir is contraindicated in those patients. Document abacavir as an allergy in the patient's chart if the HLA-B5701 test is positive.

Instruct the patient to refrain from drinking alcohol. Alcohol increases the plasma levels of abacavir by about 40%, which increases the risk of adverse effects. Abacavir can be taken with or without food. It is a pregnancy category C drug. Recommendations during pregnancy are similar to those for zidovudine.

Didanosine

Didanosine (ddI, Videx, Videx EC) was approved in 1991 as a first-line drug for treating HIV infection. The pharmacokinetics of didanosine are similar to those of zidovudine. However, its active metabolite, dideoxyadenosine triphosphate, has a much longer half-life, which allows twice-daily dosing. Like other NRTIs, it is renally excreted, so patients with renal insufficiency should receive a reduced dose.

Didanosine is available in two formulations. In its buffered versions, didanosine decreases gastric pH, thus affecting the absorption of other drugs, such as the fluoroquinolones, dapsone, indinavir, and azole antifungals. This buffering agent also complicates the timing of administration for other antiretroviral drugs and may cause diarrhea. Didanosine can be taken at the same time as other NRTIs, nevirapine, and efavirenz. However, delavirdine and indinavir should be taken at least 1 hour before didanosine, whereas lopinavir/ritonavir and atazanavir should be taken 2 hours before or 1 hour after didanosine. As an enteric-coated capsule, didanosine is taken on an empty stomach (1 hour before or 2 hours after a meal) because it is inactivated by the stomach acid.

The adverse effect profile of didanosine includes GI problems similar to those seen with zidovudine as well as peripheral neuropathy. Didanosine has two Black Box warnings: Fatal and nonfatal pancreatitis can occur. Prior episodes of pancreatitis, active alcohol abuse, or coadministration of other drugs that may cause pancreatitis further increases the risk of pancreatitis. Didanosine should be discontinued at the first signs or symptoms of pancreatitis, such as anorexia, nausea, vomiting, and abdominal pain.

Lactic acidosis can occur, especially among pregnant women who receive a combination of didanosine and stavudine with other antiretroviral combinations..

Didanosine should not be given with drugs that have overlapping toxicities (see Table 46.4). Didanosine should not be given concurrently with tenofovir because this combination may increase the risk of adverse effect. Didanosine is a pregnancy category B drug.

Emtricitabine

Emtricitabine (FTC, Emtriva) is a derivative of lamivudine that must be converted into emtricitabine triphosphate to be active. It is available in combination with tenofovir and efavirenz (Atripla) and in a two–drug, one-pill combination with tenofovir (Truvada). Like lamivudine, emtricitabine is also active against HBV. However, it is not FDA-approved for this use, and there is a Black Box warning that the safety and efficacy of emtricitabine has not been established for the treatment of HBV. Additional Black Box warnings include:

- Lactic acidosis may occur with hepatomegaly and severe steatosis, especially among women.
- Severe acute exacerbations of HBV may occur when emtricitabine is discontinued. Hepatic function should be monitored closely with both clinical and laboratory follow-up for several months after discontinuation of tenofovir in HIV/HBV-coinfected patients.
- Anti-HBV therapy may be needed. Initiation of anti-HBV therapy may be indicated after discontinuation of emtricitabine.

The most common adverse effects associated with emtricitabine are headache, diarrhea, nausea, and rash. Hyperpigmentation on the palms, soles, or both has been observed in nonwhite patients. Because emtricitabine is so similar to lamivudine, patients with HIV that is resistant to lamivudine are unlikely to benefit from emtricitabine treatment. Emtricitabine is approved for patients older than 18 years. The benefit of emtricitabine is its once-daily dosing with or without food. Because it is renally excreted, patients with renal insufficiency should receive a reduced dose. Emtricitabine is not known to interact with CYP450 metabolism and may have limited drug to drug interaction. Emtricitabine is a pregnancy category B drug. Recommendations during pregnancy are similar to those for zidovudine.

Lamivudine

Lamivudine (3TC, Epivir) is an analogue of cytidine, a natural nucleoside, and it must be converted to its active form, lamivudine triphosphate, to be effective. It is available as an individual drug or in the combination products Combivir, with AZT, Epzicom with abacavir, and Trizivir with AZT and abacavir. Lamivudine is approved for use in patients 3 months of age and older. This drug should always be used in conjunction with other antiretroviral agents and should not be used alone to manage HIV infection. In addition to its indication for HIV infection, lamivudine is used as the drug Epivir-HBV in low dose in managing hepatitis B.

Black Box warnings for lamivudine include:

- Like the other NRTIs, lactic acidosis can occur.
- The Epivir-HBV formulation and dosage may not be sufficient to treat HIV infection. Patients with HIV infection should receive only appropriate preparations in proper dosages.
- Severe acute exacerbations of HBV have been reported in HBV/HIV-coinfected patients on discontinuation of lamivudine-containing products. Hepatic function should be monitored for several months after discontinuation.
- Anti-HBV treatment may be needed. Initiation of anti-HBV therapy may be appropriate.

The most common adverse effect of lamivudine is nausea. Also, pancreatitis has been observed with pediatric administration of lamivudine. The drug is renally excreted; therefore, patients with substantial renal impairment should be given reduced doses. Because food decreases the rate but not the extent of oral absorption, lamivudine may be administered with or without food. Lamivudine is a pregnancy category C drug. Recommendations during pregnancy are similar to those for zidovudine. Additionally, lamivudine may be used in combination with zidovudine in women who did not receive zidovudine therapy throughout their pregnancy.

Stavudine

Stavudine (d4T, Zerit) is another analogue of thymidine that is converted to its active form, stavudine triphosphate. Absorption and serum concentrations are not affected by meals, and its half-life enables twice-daily dosing. Stavudine is excreted by the kidneys; therefore, a reduced dose should be considered for patients with decreased renal function.

Stavudine is generally well tolerated. A major clinical adverse effect is peripheral neuropathy and as such should not prescribed with other medications with overlapping and additive toxicities, such as didanosine, INH, or Rifampin. The drug should be discontinued in patients with symptoms of neuropathy, such as tingling, burning, pain, or numbness in the distal extremities. It should not be combined with zidovudine or any combination product containing zidovudine. Stavudine is also known to cause lipoatrophy, clinically manifesting as loss of buccal fat and or thinning of the extremities. Finally, Stavudine is associated with higher rate of lactic acidosis, lipodystrophy, and disorders of lipid metabolism among all the NRTIs and for these reasons is not recommended as part of the initial treatment of HIV. Stavudine is a pregnancy category C drug. It is important to remember that pregnant women taking stavudine in combination with didanosine and other antiretroviral agents have an increased risk of developing lactic acidosis. Black Box warnings for stavudine are the same as for didanosine.

Tenofovir

Tenofovir disoproxil fumarate (TDF, Viread) is the only nucleotide analogue reverse transcriptase inhibitor that is approved by the FDA. In 2008 Tenofovir was approved by the FDA in the treatment of HBV. Nucleotide analogues differ from nucleoside analogues because they are chemically preactivated and therefore require less processing in the body for them to become active. Tenofovir is a once-daily medication that is taken without regard to meals. Adverse effects include asthenia, headache, diarrhea, nausea, vomiting, and flatulence. Tenofovir is also renally excreted; thus, a dosage adjustment is necessary in patients with renal insufficiency. Serious cases of acute renal failure have been observed with patients on Tenofovir. Monitor renal function, urinalysis and electrolytes. Black Box warnings are the same as for emtricitabine.

© NONNUCLEOSIDE REVERSE TRANSCRIPTASE INHIBITORS (NNRTIS)

The **nonnucleoside reverse transcriptase inhibitors (NNRTIs)** comprise the second class of drugs used to treat HIV infection. NNRTIs affect only HIV-1; they do not inhibit reverse transcriptase in HIV-2. Although NNRTIs still affect reverse transcriptase, they have a different mechanism of action than NRTIs. Unlike NRTIs, NNRTIs are not incorporated into viral DNA. Instead, they inhibit a specific site on the reverse transcriptase that is required to carry out the process of DNA synthesis; this results in the inability to convert viral RNA into DNA. The NNRTIs are less toxic because they are not structurally similar to natural nucleosides or nucleotides; thus, they have less of an effect on the body's natural enzymes. The prototype NNRTI is efavirenz (Sustiva). Table 46.5 presents a summary of NNRTIs.

Nursing Management of the Patient Receiving ℗ Efavirenz

Core Drug Knowledge

Pharmacotherapeutics

Efavirenz is indicated for use in treating HIV-1 infection in combination with other antiretroviral drugs. It is the preferred component of an NNRTI based HAART for the initial treatment of HIV, except during pregnancy, or high risk for pregnancy due to its high teratogenic potential. Atripla is co-formulation of tenofovir, emtricitabine, and efavirenz rolled into one drug and is the HAART preferred option for the initial treatment of HIV infection. It is a formulation of 2 NRTIs combined with one NRRTI with the tremendous advantage of once a day dosing. Resistant virus emerges rapidly when efavirenz is administered as monotherapy or in combination with other NNRTIs.

Pharmacokinetics

Efavirenz is absorbed readily after oral administration. A high-fat meal significantly increases the bioavailability of efavirenz as well as the potential for adverse effects. Peak plasma concentrations occur within 3 to 5 hours. Efavirenz is approximately 99% protein bound. It is distributed widely in the body, crosses the blood–brain barrier and placenta, and enters breast milk. Efavirenz is metabolized by the P-450 system and excreted in urine and feces.

Pharmacodynamics

Efavirenz inhibits HIV reverse transcriptase. It binds directly to the active site on reverse transcriptase, resulting in the inability to change viral RNA into DNA.

TABLE 46.5	Summary of Selected © Nonnucleoside Reverse Transcriptase Inhibitors		
Drug (Trade) Name	**Route and Dosage Range**	**Pharmacokinetics**	**Special Considerations**
℗ efavirenz (EFV, Sustiva)	*Adult and adolescent >40 kg:* PO, 600 mg daily *Child 32.5–40 kg:* PO, 400 mg daily *Child 25–32.5 kg:* PO, 350 mg daily *Child 20–25 kg:* PO, 300 mg daily *Child 15–20 kg:* PO, 250 mg daily *Child 10–15 kg:* PO, 200 mg daily	*Onset:* Rapid *Duration:* 24 h $t_{1/2}$: 40–55 h	Take on an empty stomach, preferably at bedtime. Administer at least 1 h apart from Videx or antacids. Assess for pregnancy: potentially teratogenic. Monitor for potential interactions with other antiretroviral medications.
delavirdine mesylate (DLV, Rescriptor)	*Adult and adolescent:* PO, 400 mg 3×/d	*Onset:* Rapid *Duration:* 8 h $t_{1/2}$: 5.8 h	No food restrictions Administer at least 1 h apart from Videx or antacids.
nevirapine (NVP, Viramune)	*Adult and adolescent:* PO, 200 mg daily for 14 d, then 200 mg 2×/d *Child >8 y:* PO, 4 mg/kg daily for 14 d, then 4 mg/kg 2×/d; max: 200 mg daily *Child and infant >2 mo–8 y:* PO, 7 mg/kg daily for 14 d, then 7 mg/kg 2×/d; max: 200 mg daily	*Onset:* Rapid *Duration:* 12 h $t_{1/2}$: 25–30 h	No food restrictions
rilpivirine (Edurant)	*Adult PO*: 5 mg daily *Child:* not recommended	*Onset:* 3–4 h *Duration:* unknown $t_{1/2}$: 34–55 h	Administer with meals. Avoid administration with protein drinks

Contraindications and Precautions

Efavirenz is contraindicated for patients with hypersensitivity to any of its components. It is also contraindicated for patients taking the benzodiazepines midazolam or triazolam, ergot derivatives, or voriconazole.

Efavirenz is used cautiously in patients with concomitant use of alcohol or psychoactive drugs because they increase the risk of CNS adverse effects. Patients with a history of psychiatric disorders also have an increased risk of psychiatric adverse effects and therefore this medication should be cautiously used with them. Efavirenz is metabolized by the liver; thus, patients with hepatic impairment are more likely to have increased serum concentrations of efavirenz. The drug should be used with caution in patients with a history of hepatitis B or C; they have an increased risk of hepatotoxicity. Efavirenz is also used with caution in patients with elevated cholesterol or triglycerides because it can cause these lipid disorders.

Efavirenz is a pregnancy category D drug and is contraindicated during pregnancy.

Adverse Effects

More than 50% of patients who take efavirenz have CNS adverse effects such as dizziness, impaired concentration, insomnia, abnormal dreams, and hallucinations which is described as "spacey," "high," or "confused." Therefore, it is best to administer the medication at night to negate these CNS side effects. Also, the patient should be forewarned about cautious driving or not driving at all during the first week of taking the medication and until the body is acclimated to its side effects. These symptoms start within the first 2 days of therapy and generally abate between weeks 1 and 4. Rash is another common adverse effect. The severity of the rash can be mild to severe. Most rashes present as maculopapular skin eruptions or pruritic erythema. Rarely, erythema multiforme, Stevens-Johnson syndrome, or toxic epidermal necrolysis may occur and maybe severe and life threatening.

Other adverse drug effects include hyperlipidemia, lipodystrophy (defective fat metabolism leading to abnormal body fat distribution), GI distress, and hepatotoxicity. In rare circumstances, efavirenz may induce seizures and psychiatric disorders such as severe depression, suicidal ideation, aggressive behavior, and paranoid or manic reactions. Psychiatric adverse effects occur more frequently in patients with a prior history of psychiatric disorders.

Drug Interactions

Efavirenz interacts with drugs that are metabolized by P-450 CYP3A4. It induces the metabolism of many drugs, such as voriconazole, resulting in a reduction of their serum concentration level. Although efavirenz decreases the serum concentration of voriconazole, it in turn increases the serum concentration of efavirenz, resulting in decreased efficacy of voriconazole and increased risk of adverse effects caused by efavirenz. Conversely, efavirenz inhibits the metabolism of drugs such as benzodiazepines and ergot derivatives, leading to dangerously elevated serum concentrations of these drugs.

Efavirenz may decrease the effectiveness of oral contraceptives. Table 46.6 presents these drug–drug interactions.

Assessment of Relevant Core Patient Variables

Health Status

Assess the patient for hypersensitivity to efavirenz and for pregnancy or lactation. Also, assess the patient for pre-existing hepatic dysfunction or lipid abnormalities. Review the patient's current drug therapy for other drugs that may react with efavirenz, or those with overlapping toxicities. Communicate positive findings to the prescriber.

Before the initiation of therapy, perform a complete physical examination. It is important to document this baseline status because drug therapy may be discontinued or modified based on changes from baseline. Laboratory tests should include CBC, complete metabolic profile, lipid panel, liver function tests, CD4 cell count, and plasma HIV RNA measurements.

Life Span and Gender

Assess the patient for pregnancy. Efavirenz is a pregnancy category D drug and considered teratogenic during all trimesters. Women of childbearing age should use birth control methods other than hormonal contraceptives because efavirenz decreases the effectiveness of birth control pills. Almost 40% of children develop a rash. Monitor children closely and report any rash to the health care provider.

Lifestyle, Diet, and Habits

As with other anti-HIV drugs, resistance to efavirenz is more likely when the drug is taken inconsistently. Therefore, assess the patient's understanding of the importance of taking the drug as directed. Also, the patient who abuses drugs or alcohol is more likely to experience CNS or psychiatric adverse effects. Advise the patient to refrain from their use. Assess for use of herbal remedies such as St. John's wort. Instruct the patient to refrain from its use because it decreases the serum concentration of efavirenz. Assess for the use of garlic; it may also decrease the serum concentration of efavirenz.

Assess the patient's financial status because efavirenz is expensive. Refer those without insurance to social services. These patients may qualify for medical assistance through county, state, or federal funds or receive their drugs from local health departments.

Environment

Efavirenz is administered most frequently in an outpatient setting, always as polytherapy. Therefore, assess the patient's ability to understand complex instructions. It is important that the instructions be explicit—both spoken and written—concerning which drug to take at which time of day.

Nursing Diagnoses and Outcomes

- Risk for Injury related to CNS adverse effects
  Desired outcome: The patient will remain free from injury and contact the health care provider if symptoms should occur

TABLE 46.6	Agents That Interact with P Efavirenz	
Interactants	**Effect and Significance**	**Nursing Management**
benzodiazepines	Efavirenz inhibits metabolism of benzodiazepines, resulting in potential toxicity.	Monitor for sedation. Monitor for incoordination. Monitor vital signs, especially respiratory rate.
cyclosporine	Efavirenz may decrease serum concentration of cyclosporine.	Monitor for signs of transplant organ rejection. Discuss dosage adjustment of cyclosporine with health care provider.
ergot derivatives	Efavirenz interferes with hepatic metabolism of ergot derivatives, resulting in potential ergotism.	Monitor for peripheral vasospasm. Monitor for extremity ischemia.
lipid-lowering drugs	Efavirenz may increase serum concentration of these drugs, resulting in increased risk of adverse effects or toxicity.	Monitor for rhabdomyolysis and myopathies.
methadone	Efavirenz may decrease serum concentration of methadone	Monitor for signs of opiate withdrawal.
oral contraceptives	Efavirenz increases hepatic metabolism of estrogenic and progestational components of oral contraceptives	Assess for pregnancy. Instruct patient to use another form of birth control.
protease inhibitors	Efavirenz may decrease serum concentration of protease inhibitors.	Monitor T-cell count. Monitor viral load. Monitor for opportunistic diseases. Discuss dosage adjustment of protease inhibitor with health care provider.
rifamycins	Rifamycins increase metabolism of efavirenz, resulting in decreased serum concentration.	Same as for protease inhibitors
St. John's wort	St. John's wort may decrease serum concentration of efavirenz.	Same as for protease inhibitors
thiazolidinediones	Thiazolidinediones may decrease serum concentration of efavirenz.	Same as for protease inhibitors
voriconazole	Coadministration decreases efficacy of voriconazole as well as increases serum concentration of efavirenz.	These drugs should not be coadministered. Verify order with health care provider.

- Disturbed Thought Processes related to CNS adverse effects
  Desired outcome: The patient will remain oriented and able to communicate effectively with others.
- Ineffective Protection related to drug-related rash
  Desired outcome: The patient will report any rash to the prescriber.
- Imbalanced Nutrition: Less than Body Requirements, related to GI distress
  Desired outcome: The patient will maintain adequate weight and nutrition and notify the health care provider about persistent GI symptoms.

Planning and Intervention

Maximizing Therapeutic Effects
Administer efavirenz once a day, preferably at bedtime. For missed doses, it is important that the patient take the drug as soon as remembered unless it is time for the next dose. Efavirenz must be given concurrently with other antiretroviral medications.

Minimizing Adverse Effects
Administer efavirenz on an empty stomach. Food, especially high-fat food, increases the bioavailability of efavirenz, resulting in an increased risk of developing adverse effects. Also, administering efavirenz at bedtime decreases the severity of CNS adverse effects. Coordinate serial laboratory testing for liver function. Liver function tests should be evaluated prior to initiation of therapy and periodically thereafter. Periodic lipid studies are also important.

Providing Patient and Family Education
- Emphasize that efavirenz does not cure HIV. Encourage the patient to take precautions to avoid exposing others to blood and body fluids and the use of latex condoms during sex.
- Explain the importance of adherence to drug therapy. Make sure the instructions are clear and in writing.
- Explain the importance of periodic blood monitoring to ensure the efficacy of therapy and assessment of potential adverse effects.
- Explain the potential CNS adverse effects. Encourage patients to continue the efavirenz because these symptoms generally abate. Instruct patients to refrain from activities that require concentration if they are experiencing these adverse effects.

- Advise patients experiencing depression, anxiety, or behavior changes and those feeling paranoid or manic to contact the health care provider immediately.
- Inform patients that one of the most common adverse reactions to efavirenz is rash. Instruct patients to contact the health care provider if the skin becomes ulcerated or denuded.
- Instruct patients to monitor for signs of hepatic dysfunction, such as fatigue, jaundice, and nausea or vomiting. Advise them to contact the health care provider immediately if signs of hepatic dysfunction occur.
- Instruct patients to advise their prescriber if any other drugs are ordered by another prescriber. It is important to explain that many drugs may alter the way efavirenz works and that other drugs may increase the risk of adverse effects from efavirenz therapy.
- Instruct patients with GI distress to eat small, frequent meals. For persistent symptoms and weight loss, patients should contact the prescriber.
- Explain to women of childbearing age the importance of using contraceptive measures other than hormonal contraceptives. Instruct female patients to contact the health care provider immediately if they become pregnant while taking efavirenz.
- Caution patients that they may experience changes in their physical appearance. Lipodystrophy may cause increased fat in the upper back, neck, breast, and trunk and loss of fat from the legs, arms, and face.

Ongoing Assessment and Evaluation

Coordinate periodic examinations and blood monitoring in patients receiving efavirenz to assess for potential progression of HIV disease, treatment failure, the emergence of resistance, or development of adverse effects. CD4 cell counts and HIV RNA should be assessed every 3 months. The patient should have a stable CD4 cell count and a declining or undetectable HIV RNA count throughout therapy. Monitor for the need to change pharmacotherapy.

Monitor for CNS adverse effects. Remind the patient to refrain from activities that require mental alertness if he or she experiences these adverse effects. Check for lipid abnormalities. Monitor for a diffuse, maculopapular, or erythematous rash. Refer the patient to his or her health care provider immediately if the rash is accompanied by aching joints or muscles; redness, blistering, peeling, or loosening of skin; unusual tiredness or weakness; or fever; these are symptoms of Stevens-Johnson syndrome. Monitor for signs of liver dysfunction. Coordinate periodic liver function tests.

Drugs Closely Related to P Efavirenz
Delavirdine

Delavirdine mesylate (DLV, Rescriptor) was approved by the FDA in 1997. It is indicated for combined use with NRTIs. Unlike efavirenz and nevirapine, delavirdine is a potent inhibitor of CYP3A4. As a result, concurrent administration

---

CRITICAL THINKING SCENARIO

Ms. M. Williams is a 24-year-old female diagnosed of HIV about 5 years ago. She has been a transient, moved to several states and cities but has since settled down and now is at the Clinic for a second visit. Her CD4 was 250/mm³, her viral load is 75,000 copies/mL. The remainders of her laboratory values are within the normal limits. After her consultation with her doctor, she asked if she can talk to you since she has several questions about Atripla, the medication that the provider prescribed. She is puzzled since she has to take only one pill a day when many of her friends who are also infected takes several pills daily. She also said that she heard something about pregnancy but missed a great portion of what the provider said because she got distracted. Also, she asked if she could take it during the day and confided, but did not tell her doctors, that she wants to skip a dose or two to give her body a chance to "rest."

1. What patient education will you provide Ms. Williams about Atripla, its drug classes, their mechanism of action?
2. What patient teaching will you provide her about pregnancy? About taking the medications during the day and its implication? Why will you recommend that she takes the medications during her time of sleep?
3. What will tell Ms. Williams about taking a medication holiday? What are its potential implications?

---

of other CYP3A4 drugs may increase their serum drug concentrations, resulting in an increased risk for adverse effects and potential drug toxicity. Delavirdine may inhibit the metabolism of several medications that may result in a clinically important elevation of their plasma concentration. These drugs include amphetamines; anticoagulants (warfarin); anti-infectives (clarithromycin, dapsone, rifabutin, and saquinavir); sedative hypnotics (alprazolam, midazolam, triazolam); cardiovascular agents (nifedipine, quinidine); ergot alkaloids and derivatives; HMG-CoA reductase inhibitors (atorvastatin, cerivastatin, fluvastatin); immunosuppressive agents (dexamethasone, cyclosporine, sirolimus, tacrolimus); methadone; and sildenafil. Drugs known to decrease the

---

MEMORY CHIP

P Efavirenz

- Used for the management of HIV infection and AIDS
- Major contraindication: hypersensitivity and taking midazolam or triazolam, ergot derivatives, or voriconazole
- Most common adverse effects: dizziness, impaired concentration, insomnia, abnormal dreams, hallucinations, and rash
- Most serious adverse effects: Stevens-Johnson syndrome, hepatotoxicity, and psychiatric disorders
- Maximizing therapeutic effects: Administer with other antiretroviral agents—never as monotherapy.
- Minimizing adverse effects: Administer at bedtime to decrease CNS adverse effects.
- Most important patient education: Explain the importance of laboratory follow-up to monitor for hepatotoxicity and lipid abnormalities.

bioavailability of delavirdine include antacids, proton pump inhibitors, histamine-2 blockers, anticonvulsants such as carbamazepine, phenobarbital, or phenytoin, and St. John's Wort. Drugs know to significantly increase the plasma concentration of delavirdine include clarithromycin, fluoxetine, ketoconazole, and rifabutin or rifampin.

Adverse reactions associated with delavirdine include rash, which may spontaneously resolve, increased liver enzyme levels, and headache. Delavirdine is a pregnancy category C drug; however, it is not recommended for use during pregnancy.

Nevirapine

Nevirapine (Viramune), the first NNRTI on the market, is also indicated for the treatment of HIV-1. Like efavirenz, resistance emerges rapidly when nevirapine is administered as monotherapy or in combination with other NNRTIs. The drug is lipophilic, which means that it can easily pass through the blood–brain barrier so its concentration in the CSF is greater than that of the other NNRTIs. Unfortunately, that same lipophilic property allows nevirapine to pass through the placental barrier as well as enter breast milk. Although it is a pregnancy category C drug, it is contraindicated during pregnancy.

Nevirapine has several Black Box warnings:

- Severe, life threatening and in some cases fatal hepatotoxicity, particularly in the first 18 weeks, has been reported in patients treated with nevirapine. In some cases, patients presented with non-specific prodromal signs or symptoms of hepatitis and progressed to hepatitis. These events are often associated with rash.
- Female gender and patients with higher CD4 counts at initiation of therapy place patients at increased risk.
- Women with CD4 counts greater than 250 cells/mm³, including pregnant women receiving nevirapine in combination with other antiretrovirals for the treatment of HIV infection, are at the greatest risk.
- Hepatotoxicity associated with the use of this agent can occur in both genders, all CD4 counts, and at any time during treatment.
- Patients with signs or symptoms or hepatitis, or increased transaminases combined with rash or other systemic symptoms, must discontinue the drug and seek medical evaluation immediately.
- Severe, life-threatening skin reactions (sometimes fatal) have occurred during therapy.
- Cases include Stevens-Johnson syndrome, Toxic Epidermal Necrolysis (TEN), and hypersensitivity reactions characterized by rash, constitutional findings, and organ dysfunction.
- Patients developing signs or symptoms of severe skin reactions or hypersensitivity must discontinue product and seek medical attention immediately.
- Transaminase levels should be checked immediately for all patients who develop a rash within the first 18 weeks of treatment. The 14-day lead-in period with nevirapine 200 mg daily dosing has been observed to decrease the incidence of rash and must be followed.

- Patients must be monitored intensively during the first 18 weeks to detect signs and symptoms of life-threatening skin/hepatic reactions.
- Extra vigilance is warranted during the first 6 weeks of therapy, which is the period of greatest risk of these events.
- Do not start nevirapine following severe hepatic, skin, or hypersensitivity reactions.
- In some cases, hepatic injury has progressed despite discontinuation of treatment.

Like efavirenz, nevirapine may cause rash. Instructions for patients with a rash are the same as for efavirenz recipients. Unlike efavirenz, nevirapine does not generally cause CNS or psychiatric symptoms. Other common adverse effects of nevirapine therapy include fever, headache, nausea, and vomiting.

Nevirapine and efavirenz have similar drug interactions. Other than the requirement of dose escalation during the first 2 weeks of treatment, patient management for nevirapine is the same as that for efavirenz.

Etravirine (Intelence, TMC-125)

Etravirine received accelerated approval by the FDA in January 2008. It is approved for treatment-experienced adults with HIV resistance to other HAART medications, including other NNRTIs. It has not been approved for use in treatment naïve **(never taken HIV therapy)** patients because of insufficient data due to its accelerated approval. Like other NNRTIs, it is not approved for monotherapy.

While there are no contraindications to its use, etravirine is used cautiously in patients receiving many other medications because it is a substrate of cytochrome CYP 450 enzyme system, as well as inducer of CYP3A4, and inhibitor of CYP2CO and CYP2C19 resulting in many potentially serious drug-drug interactions. These drugs include other HAART medications (especially Kaletra), antibiotics, antifungals, heart medications, antiseizure medications, cholesterol lowering medications, erectile dysfunction medications, and herbal medications such as St. John Wart. It is a pregnancy category B; it is not known whether it passes into breast milk.

Rash, nausea, diarrhea, are predictable side effects of NNRTIs, including etravirine. Other possible side effects include vomiting, abdominal pain, tiredness, tingling or pain in hands or feet, numbness, headache and high blood pressure. Laboratory abnormalities include increased serum cholesterol, triglycerides, and transaminitis especially in patients with hepatitis B or C co-infection.

Administer etravirine after a meal, not on an empty stomach. It must be swallowed whole. If your patient is unable to swallow, dissolve the tablet in a glass of water.

Rilpivirine (Edurant)

Rilpivirine is the newest FDA-approved antiretroviral drug. It is used in combination with other antiretroviral drugs for the treatment of HIV-1 infection in adults who are treatment naïve. Like delavirdine, rilpivirine is primarily metabolized by cytochrome P-450 CYP3A and has similar drug-drug interactions that result in either an significant increase or decrease in its plasma concentration. The most common adverse drug reactions to rilpivirine include depression, insomnia, headache and rash. Rilpivirine is Pregnancy Category B because animal reproduction studies have not shown a risk to the animal fetus but adequate and well-controlled trials in pregnant women have not been conducted. Therefore, rilpivirine should be used during pregnancy only if the potential benefit justifies the potential risk to the fetus.

Ⓒ PROTEASE INHIBITORS

Protease inhibitors (PIs) are the third major class of drugs used in treating HIV infection and AIDS. Their arrival has changed the opinion of experts as to the ultimate fatality of HIV and AIDS. The PIs represent the most potent anti-HIV drugs. However, their potency and activity vary widely among individual patients.

As with the other classes of antiretrovirals, PIs should not be used as monotherapy. Cross-resistance may occur within the PI class; however, it does not extend to NRTIs or NNRTIs. All of the PIs have the potential to cause serious adverse effects such as hyperlipidemia, lipodystrophy and lipoatrophy (Box 46.7), hyperglycemia, osteopenia or osteoporosis, hepatic dysfunction, and increased bleeding in patients with hemophilia. Saquinavir (Invirase), the first FDA-approved PI, is the prototype PI. Table 46.7 presents a summary of protease inhibitors.

Nursing Management of the Patient Receiving Ⓟ Saquinavir

Core Drug Knowledge

Pharmacotherapeutics

Saquinavir mesylate is an agent for treating HIV infection in adults. It is approved for use in combination with two reverse transcriptase inhibitors. Combination therapy enables reduced dosage and helps to limit the incidence of adverse events. Saquinavir demonstrates activity against both HIV-1 and HIV-2 and is effective in acutely and chronically infected cells.

Pharmacokinetics

Saquinavir is only about 4% bioavailable after dosing, because of a combination of poor absorption and extensive first-pass metabolism. It is always combined with ritonavir because ritonavir significantly inhibits saquinavir's metabolism, resulting in an increased serum concentration of saquinavir. This is called synergistic boosting.

Metabolism occurs in the liver and is affected by the P-450 enzyme system; the isozyme CYP3A4 is responsible for about 90% of the initial biotransformation of saquinavir. The metabolites of saquinavir have not been identified and appear to play little part in antiviral activity. The serum half-life of saquinavir is 1 to 2 hours. Renal elimination of saquinavir is negligible; only 1% is excreted in urine, whereas 88% is excreted in feces.

Pharmacodynamics

Saquinavir is a competitive inhibitor of HIV protease, an enzyme required for HIV replication. During the later stages of the HIV growth cycle, integrated DNA is translated into polyproteins to become mature budding viral particles. Protease is responsible for packaging these polyproteins into mature virions. Virions produced without protease are immature, rendering the virus noninfectious. PIs also inhibit replication of HIV in the macrophages, which are major reservoirs of HIV.

Contraindications and Precautions

Saquinavir is contraindicated for patients with hypersensitivity to any of its components. The drug is not approved for use in infants, children, or adolescents younger than 16 years.

Saquinavir should be used with caution in patients with pre-existing hepatic dysfunction because the drug is largely metabolized by the liver. It should also be used cautiously

---

BOX 46.7 FOCUS ON RESEARCH

Lessening Lipoatrophy

Mest, D. R., & Humble, G. (2006). Safety and efficacy of poly-ʟ-lactic acid injections in persons with HIV-associated lipoatrophy: The U.S. experience. *Dermatologic Surgery*, 32(11):1336–1345.

The Study

The researchers evaluated the quantifiable improvement in HIV-infected patients with facial wasting (lipoatrophy) after serial injections of poly-ʟ-lactic acid (PLLA) as well as the long-term safety and durability of the material. Patients underwent up to six treatment sessions with injectable PLLA, and after completion of the treatment, they were followed for 12 months. Quantifiable improvement was evaluated by measuring the increase in total cutaneous thickness, using skin calipers. In addition, before-and-after photographs were taken, and patient-satisfaction questionnaires were completed throughout the study period.

Results showed a mean increase in skin thickness of 65.1% compared with baseline values. This correction was maintained throughout the 12-month follow-up period (68.8% at 6 months and 73% at 12 months). Patient satisfaction was 4.5/5 at the end of treatment and increased to 4.8/5 at 12 months. No serious adverse events were reported. The researchers concluded that PLLA is a safe and well-tolerated treatment option for HIV-associated lipoatrophy.

Nursing Implications

Advise patients of the safety and efficacy of the PLLA treatment. Be sensitive to the changes in appearance that HIV-infected patients who receive HAART may experience. Keep abreast of new treatments to boost the self-esteem of these patients. Advise the patient that PLLA injections may induce the appearance of small bumps under the skin in the treated area. Generally, these bumps are not visible, and they may be noticed only when pressing on the treated area. Advise the patient that other injection-related events at the site of injection, such as bleeding, tenderness, discomfort, redness, bruising, or swelling, may occur.

TABLE 46.7	Summary of Selected Ⓒ Protease Inhibitors		
Drug (Trade) Name	**Route and Dosage Range**	**Pharmacokinetics**	**Special Considerations**
Ⓟ saquinavir mesylate (SQV, Invirase)	*Adult and adolescent:* PO, five 200-mg hard gel capsules PLUS 100 mg ritonavir 2×/d	*Onset:* Rapid *Duration:* 8 h $t_{1/2}$: 1–2 h	Administer within 2 h of a meal. Must be dosed with ritonavir.
amprenavir (APV, Agenerase)	*Adult and adolescent >13 y weighing >50 kg:* PO, 1,200 mg 2×/d *Adolescent and child 4–16 y weighing <50 kg:* PO, 20 mg/kg 2×/d or 15 mg/kg 3×/d Oral Solution *Adult and adolescent >13 y weighing >50 kg:* PO, 1,400 mg (93.3 mL) 2×/d *Child 4–16 y:* PO, 22.5 mg/kg 2×/d or 17 mg/kg 3×/d *Child <4 y:* Safe and effective dosage has not been established.	*Onset:* Rapid *Duration:* 8–12 h $t_{1/2}$: 7.1–10.6 h	No food restrictions, except high-fat meals Advise patient to avoid supplemental vitamin E.
atazanavir sulfate (ATV, Reyataz)	*Adult:* PO, Treatment-naive: Two 200-mg capsules once daily Treatment-experienced: Two 150-mg capsules PLUS one 100-mg ritonavir capsule once daily *Child:* Safe and effective dosage has not been established.	*Onset:* Rapid *Duration:* 24 h $t_{1/2}$: 7 h	Administer with food. Administer 2 h before or 1 h after Videx.
darunavir (Prezista)	*Adult:* PO, two 300-mg tablets PLUS one 100-mg ritonavir capsule 2 ×/d *Child:* Safe and effective dosage has not been established.	*Onset:* Slow *Duration:* Unknown $t_{1/2}$: 15 h	Administer with food.
fosamprenavir calcium (FPV, Lexiva)	*Adult:* PO, Treatment-naive patients without ritonavir: Two 700-mg tablets 2×/d Treatment-naive patients with ritonavir: Two 700-mg once daily with ritonavir 200 mg once daily Protease inhibitor–experienced patients: One 700-mg tablet with ritonavir 100 mg 2×/d *Child:* Safe and effective dosage has not been established.	*Onset:* Rapid *Duration:* 12–24 h $t_{1/2}$: 7.7 h	No food restrictions
indinavir sulfate (IDV, Crixivan)	*Adult and adolescent:* PO, two 400-mg capsules 3×/d *Child:* PO, 350–500 mg/m² q8h has been used; available data inadequate for optimal dosing in pediatric population	*Onset:* Rapid *Duration:* 8 h $t_{1/2}$: 1.5–2 h	Administer 1 h before or 2 h after a meal. May be taken with a light snack Advise the patient to drink at least 1.5 L of water daily. Administer 1 h apart from Videx.
nelfinavir mesylate (NFV, Viracept)	*Adult and adolescent:* PO, 750 mg 3×/d or 1,250 mg 2×/d *Child 2–13 y:* PO, 20–30 mg/kg (max: 750 mg/dose) 3×/d	*Onset:* Rapid *Duration:* 8 h $t_{1/2}$: 3.5–5 h	Administer with food.
ritonavir (RTV, Norvir)	*Adult and adolescent >16 y:* PO, six 100-mg tablets 2×/d *Adolescent and child 2–16 y:* PO, 400 mg/m², not to exceed 600 mg, 2×/d	*Onset:* Rapid *Duration:* 12 h $t_{1/2}$: 3–5 h	Mostly used for boosting other drugs Administer with food. Administer 2½ h before or after didanosine. Refrigeration recommended for the capsules
tipranavir (Aptivus)	*Adult:* PO, two 250-mg capsules PLUS two 100-mg ritonavir capsules 2×/d	*Onset:* slow *Duration:* Unknown $t_{1/2}$: 4.8–6 h	Administer with food.
Combination Drugs			
lopinavir/ritonavir (Kaletra)	*Adult and adolescent >45 kg:* PO, 533 mg lopinavir/133 mg ritonavir (4 capsules or 6.5 mL) 2×/d *Adult and adolescent >40 kg:* PO, 400 mg lopinavir/100 mg ritonavir (3 capsules or 5 mL) 2×/d	*Onset:* Rapid *Duration:* 12 h $t_{1/2}$: 5–6 h	No food restrictions Must be swallowed whole

in patients with elevated triglyceride or cholesterol levels because fat redistribution and hyperlipidemia are adverse effects associated with the use of PIs. Saquinavir is also used with caution in patients with diabetes because it causes hyperglycemia. Some patients with hemophilia type A or B have experienced bleeding episodes during saquinavir therapy. Although a direct causal relation has not been established, these patients should be monitored closely.

Saquinavir is a pregnancy category B drug.

Adverse Effects

The most common adverse effects of saquinavir are nausea, diarrhea, stomach discomfort, insomnia, and headache. As previously mentioned, the drug may induce hyperglycemia, resulting in loss of glycemic control in patients with diabetes. Prediabetic patients may need to start antidiabetic medications. Saquinavir is also associated with increased bone loss. Use of calcium and vitamin D supplements reduces the occurrence of osteopenia and osteoporosis.

HIV-positive patients with hemophilia (type A or B) may be at increased risk for bleeding. Episodes of spontaneous skin hematomas and hemarthrosis, in some cases requiring additional doses of factor VIII, have been reported.

As a class, PIs also have been associated with an unusual adverse reaction involving the deposition of fatty-like tissue at the base of the posterior neck ("buffalo hump") and the abdominal area ("protease paunch"). The syndrome is associated with peripheral lipodystrophy, central adiposity, female breast enlargement, hyperlipidemia, and insulin resistance. Although the long-term consequences of fat redistribution are unknown, substantial increases in triglycerides or cholesterol are of concern because of the possible association with cardiovascular events and pancreatitis.

Like other antiretroviral drugs, saquinavir may cause hepatotoxicity. The risk of this condition is highest in patients with pre-existing liver dysfunction and those with a history of hepatitis B or C.

Drug Interactions

Like nevirapine, saquinavir interacts with drugs that are metabolized by P-450 CYP3A4. Saquinavir inhibits the metabolism of many drugs, resulting in elevated serum levels of these drugs, and it can be inhibited by other drugs, resulting in elevated saquinavir levels. Conversely, saquinavir induces the metabolism of some drugs, and its metabolism is induced by several drugs. Table 46.8 presents these complex drug–drug interactions.

Assessment of Relevant Core Patient Variables

Health Status

Assess the patient for hypersensitivity to saquinavir. Also, assess for pre-existing hepatic dysfunction, diabetes mellitus, hyperlipidemia, or hemophilia. Patients receiving rifampin or rifabutin for TB should delay the use of saquinavir until rifampin or rifabutin has been deleted from the treatment regimen. Review the patient's current drug therapy for other drugs that may interact with saquinavir or

have overlapping toxicities. Communicate positive findings to the prescriber.

Before therapy begins, perform a complete physical examination. Document the patient's baseline status because drug therapy may be discontinued or modified based on changes from baseline. Laboratory tests should include CBC, complete metabolic profile, liver function tests, lipid profile, CD4 cell count, and plasma HIV RNA measurement. Some health care providers may also request a bone density evaluation.

Life Span and Gender

Assess the patient for pregnancy or lactation. In female patients receiving HAART when they conceive, therapy should be continued throughout the pregnancy. If a patient is not receiving therapy when the conception occurs, the patient may consider delaying HAART until after 10 to 14 weeks of gestation. It is unknown whether saquinavir is excreted into breast milk. However, HIV-positive women are advised not to breast-feed, to avoid potential postnatal transmission to an infant who may not be infected.

Note the patient's age before administering saquinavir. Saquinavir has not been studied in patients younger than 16 years or older than 65 years.

Lifestyle, Diet, and Habits

Assess the patient's ability and willingness to adhere to drug therapy. Adherence to the saquinavir drug regimen is crucial. Viral load may increase dramatically when saquinavir is not taken as directed, and as with other anti-HIV drugs, resistance is more likely when drugs are taken inconsistently. The development of viral resistance to this PI may eliminate other drugs in this class from the therapeutic strategy for the patient, because cross-resistance to other PIs does occur. Vigorously discourage nonadherence and drug holidays.

Assess dietary habits. Because of the potential for hyperlipidemia, limit high-fat and high-cholesterol foods. Assess alcohol consumption because of the increased risk of hepatic injury. Advise the patient to refrain from taking saquinavir with grapefruit or pomegranate juice because they inhibit the metabolism of saquinavir. Assess the use of garlic because it may lower saquinavir levels.

As with other antiretroviral agents, discuss potential substance abuse with the patient. Explain how a healthy lifestyle complements pharmacotherapy of HIV infection.

Assess the patient's financial status. Refer patients with financial problems to the hospital or clinic social worker. Patients may qualify for medical assistance through county, state, or federal funds or receive their drugs from local health departments.

Environment

Saquinavir is administered most frequently in an outpatient setting. HIV infection is treated routinely with complicated polytherapy. Therefore, assess the patient's ability to understand complex instructions. It is important that the instructions be explicit—both spoken and written—concerning

TABLE 46.8	Agents That Interact with ℗ Saquinavir	
Interactants	**Effect and Significance**	**Nursing Management**
amiodarone	Saquinavir may inhibit metabolism of amiodarone.	Monitor for QT prolongation. Monitor for arrhythmias.
azole antifungal agents	Azole antifungal agents may inhibit metabolism of saquinavir.	Monitor for saquinavir toxicity.
benzodiazepines	Saquinavir may inhibit metabolism of benzodiazepines.	Monitor for sedation. Ensure safety. Monitor vital signs, especially respiratory rate.
carbamazepine	Coadministration of these drugs may increase serum concentration level of carbamazepine and decrease serum concentration level of saquinavir.	Monitor CBC. Monitor for rash, seizures, and hepatotoxicity. Monitor T-cell count and viral load. Monitor for opportunistic infections.
cimetidine	Saquinavir may inhibit first-pass metabolism of saquinavir.	Monitor for adverse effects or toxicity of saquinavir.
clarithromycin	Coadministration of these drugs may increase serum concentration of saquinavir and decrease serum concentration of clarithromycin.	Monitor for increased adverse effect or toxicity of saquinavir. Monitor for treatment failure of clarithromycin.
cyclosporine	Coadministration of these drugs may increase serum concentration levels of both cyclosporine and saquinavir.	Monitor for adverse effects of both drugs.
diltiazem	Saquinavir may inhibit metabolism of diltiazem.	Monitor for arrhythmias, bradycardia, hypotension, and CHF.
ergot derivatives	Saquinavir may inhibit metabolism of ergot derivatives.	Verify order with health care provider because coadministration is contraindicated.
felodipine	Saquinavir may inhibit metabolism of felodipine.	Monitor for edema. Monitor for orthostatic hypotension.
fentanyl	Saquinavir may inhibit metabolism of fentanyl.	Monitor for sedation. Ensure safety. Monitor vital signs, especially respiratory rate.
HMG-CoA reductase inhibitors	Saquinavir may inhibit metabolism of HMG-CoA reductase inhibitors.	Monitor for rhabdomyolysis. Monitor for myalgias.
levothyroxine	Saquinavir may inhibit metabolism of levothyroxine.	Monitor for signs of hyperthyroidism.
methadone	Saquinavir may inhibit metabolism of methadone.	Monitor for pain relief. Monitor for opiate withdrawal.
ranolazine	Saquinavir may inhibit metabolism of ranolazine.	Verify order with health care provider because coadministration is contraindicated.
pimozide	Saquinavir may inhibit metabolism of pimozide.	Verify order with health care provider because coadministration is contraindicated. Monitor for life-threatening arrhythmias.
rifamycins	Coadministration of these drugs may increase serum concentration level of rifamycins and decrease serum concentration level of saquinavir.	Monitor for adverse effects and toxicity of rifamycins. Monitor for decreased efficacy of saquinavir.
risperidone	Saquinavir may inhibit metabolism of risperidone.	Monitor for decreased LOC, lethargy, ataxia.
sildenafil	Saquinavir may inhibit metabolism of sildenafil.	Monitor for severe hypotension. Monitor for cardiac arrhythmias. Ensure safety.

(Continued)

TABLE 46.8	Agents That Interact with ℗ Saquinavir *(continued)*	
Interactants	**Effect and Significance**	**Nursing Management**
tacrolimus	Saquinavir may inhibit metabolism of tacrolimus.	Monitor renal function. Monitor tacrolimus levels. Discuss dosage adjustment with health care provider.
trazodone	Saquinavir may inhibit metabolism of trazodone.	Monitor for nausea, dizziness, hypotension.
St. John's wort	St. John's wort induces metabolism of saquinavir, resulting in decreased efficacy.	Monitor for opportunistic infections. Advise patient to refrain from use of St. John's wort.
warfarin	Saquinavir may inhibit metabolism of warfarin.	Monitor PT and INR. Monitor for signs of bleeding or bruising.

which drug to take at which time of the day. Saquinavir tablets and capsules should be stored at room temperature.

Nursing Diagnoses and Outcomes

- Acute Pain related to headache from adverse drug effect
  Desired outcome: The patient will self-medicate with analgesics such as acetaminophen.
- Imbalanced Nutrition: Less than Body Requirements, related to GI distress
  Desired outcome: The patient will maintain body weight and report any persistent symptoms affecting nutritional status to the prescriber.
- Disturbed Thought Processes related to adverse CNS effects
  Desired outcome: The patient will remain oriented and able to communicate effectively with others.
- Diarrhea related to adverse GI effects
  Desired outcome: The patient will avoid dehydration and report persistent diarrhea to the prescriber.
- Risk for injury related to hepatotoxicity.
  Desired outcome: The patient will recognize the symptoms of hepatotoxicity and contact the health care provider immediately.

Planning and Intervention

Maximizing Therapeutic Effects
Administer saquinavir tablets or capsules within 2 hours after eating a full meal. Administer ritonavir with each dose of saquinavir.

Minimizing Adverse Effects
Give small, frequent meals if GI distress is problematic. Administer acetaminophen for complaints of headache. Encourage a regular exercise program to offset fat redistribution. Encourage a low-fat, low-cholesterol diet.

Providing Patient and Family Education
- Emphasize that saquinavir does not cure HIV. Encourage the patient to take precautions to avoid exposing others to blood and body fluids and the use of latex condoms during sex.
- Explain the importance of adherence to drug therapy. As previously mentioned, it is important to make sure that the instructions are clear and in writing.

- Explain the importance of periodic clinical and blood monitoring to ensure the efficacy of therapy and to monitor for possible adverse effects.
- Advise patients about potential adverse effects. Also, explain that adverse effects, such as GI distress or headache, may spontaneously resolve after 3 to 4 weeks of therapy. Tell patients that persistent problems should be reported to the prescriber.
- Teach patients the signs and symptoms of diabetes. Question patients about polyuria, polydipsia, and polyphagia at each visit. Monitor patients' weight. Advise patients with diabetes to monitor blood glucose frequently.
- Teach patients the signs of hepatotoxicity. Advise patients to contact the health care provider if symptoms such as yellowing of the skin or eyes, nausea, abdominal pain or discomfort, unusual bleeding/bruising, or severe fatigue occur.
- Teach patients with hemophilia to monitor for bleeding, especially in joints.
- Instruct patients to advise the prescriber if any other drugs are ordered by another prescriber. Explain that many drugs may alter the way saquinavir works and that other drugs may increase the risk of adverse effects from saquinavir therapy.
- Instruct patients to use over-the-counter antidiarrheal agents if diarrhea occurs. If diarrhea is persistent, patients should contact the prescriber.
- Instruct patients to develop good eating habits and an exercise plan that decreases the risks associated with fat redeposition. Teach patients about foods that are rich in calcium and vitamin D and low in fat and cholesterol.

Ongoing Assessment and Evaluation

Patients who take saquinavir should have periodic examinations and blood monitoring, which are important to assess for potential progression of the disease, treatment failure, or the emergence of drug resistance or an adverse reaction to the therapy. CD4 cell counts and HIV RNA load should be assessed every 3 months. The patient should have a stable CD4 count and a declining or undetectable HIV RNA load. In addition, the patient should have a stable lipid

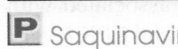

MEMORY CHIP

P Saquinavir

- Used for the management of HIV infection and AIDS
- Major contraindications: hypersensitivity, age less than 16 years
- Most common adverse effects: diarrhea, abdominal discomfort, and nausea and vomiting
- Most serious adverse effects: cardiovascular events and pancreatitis resulting from fat redistribution
- Maximizing therapeutic effects: Administer within 2 hours of a high-fat, high-calorie meal.
- Minimizing adverse effects: small, frequent meals to decrease GI distress
- Most important patient education: Refrain from taking any medication that is not prescribed by the health care provider treating the patient for HIV infection.

panel. Monitor for the need to change pharmacotherapy. The patient should be free of opportunistic infections and adverse effects associated with saquinavir.

Monitor patients with hemophilia for signs of bleeding and for clinical signs, particularly those evident in laboratory test results, if necessary. It also is important to monitor patients for hepatic dysfunction. For patients with pre-existing hepatic disorders, monitor liver function test results.

Evaluate the patient for fat redistribution and hypertriglyceridemia or hypercholesterolemia. If these adverse effects occur, check for cardiovascular events and pancreatitis. Potential interventions include dietary modifications or discontinuation of PIs.

Obtain periodic hemoglobin A1C tests in patients with diabetes, and monitor other patients for signs of diabetes. Coordinate periodic bone density testing.

Drugs Closely Related to P Saquinavir

Atazanavir (Reyataz)

Atazanavir is a new PI for treating HIV infection. As a new drug, it has similarities to and differences from other PIs. Like other PIs, it should be used in combination with other antiretroviral drugs.

Atazanavir differs from other PIs in three ways: it is the first drug in its class to be given once daily and this low pill burden may strongly and positively affect compliance; it does not appear to have a substantial adverse effect on lipoprotein concentrations such as low density lipoprotein, triglycerides, total cholesterol, and may positively affect patients with high cardiovascular risk and or problems with lipodystrophy; and it has a unique chemical structure that alters its resistance profile. If the patient's virus is resistant to other PIs, the virus may also be resistant to atazanavir. However, when resistance develops initially to atazanavir, the resistance may or may not be conferred to other PIs.

Atazanavir should be taken orally with a low-calorie, low-fat snack or meal to enhance absorption. Atazanavir requires an acidic gastric pH for dissolution. Proton pump inhibitors,

H2 antagonists, or antacids may impair its absorption. Do not administer those drugs within 2 hours of atazanavir. Monitor for efficacy of atazanavir when the patient is receiving any drug that alters gastric pH.

The most common adverse effects of atazanavir are rash, nausea, diarrhea, vomiting, headache, and abdominal pain. It may also increase bilirubin levels, resulting in jaundice. An elevation of indirect bilirubin signals a medication associated abnormality and is inconsequential; on the other hand, an elevation of direct bilirubin infers a liver injury.

Atazanavir has been associated with prolonging the PR interval, resulting in asymptomatic first-degree heart block. It should be used with caution in patients with pre-existing rhythm disturbances and in patients receiving other medications that cause PR-interval prolongation such as atenolol or diltiazem.

Drug–drug interactions of atazanavir are similar to those of saquinavir. Specific drug classes that should be avoided without the approval of the prescriber include PIs, antimigraine medications, antidysrhythmics, and antipsychotics

Atazanavir is not approved for children younger than 16 years. It is a pregnancy category B drug, and recommendations for its use during pregnancy are the same as those for saquinavir.

Darunavir

Darunavir (Prezista) is a PI approved for use in treatment-experienced patients such as those with HIV-1 infection that has been resistant to more than one PI. The risks and benefits of darunavir have not been studied in treatment-naive or pediatric patients. Because darunavir is used in patients who have already experienced resistance to other PIs, genotypic or phenotypic studies are recommended prior to use. Like saquinavir, darunavir must be administered with ritonavir and food. Administration with food increases the bioavailability by approximately 30%.

Darunavir contains a sulfonamide moiety and cannot be used in patients with a sulfa allergy. It is contraindicated in patients taking ergot derivative, pimozide, and the benzodiazepines midazolam and triazolam because of potentially fatal drug–drug interactions. Darunavir should not be taken by patients who take antiepileptics, rifampin, 3-hydroxy-3-methylglutaryl coenzyme A reductase inhibitors, or St. John's wort, although the interactions are not potentially fatal. The most common adverse effects are diarrhea or constipation, abdominal pain, and vomiting. Other drug–drug interactions, precautions, and adverse effects are similar to those with saquinavir. Darunavir is a pregnancy category B drug.

Fosamprenavir

Fosamprenavir (Lexiva) is a prodrug of amprenavir, the active metabolite. Fosamprenavir is metabolized by P-450 3A4 isoenzyme and as such may alter the concentrations of other drugs metabolized by this pathway, including rifapentine or rifampin, oral contraceptives, ergot derivates, astemizole, bepridil, simvastatin or lovastatin, pimozide, and midazolam or triazolam. Review the mediation administration record

(MAR) for these drugs and notify the primary provider immediately if other providers order any of these medications. Fosamprenavir should be used with caution in patients with sulfonamide allergy. Since fosamprenavir is metabolized by the liver, monitor patients with hepatic impairment closely. Common adverse effects include rash, appetite loss, headaches, malaise, diarrhea, nausea, and vomiting. Additional adverse effects include numbness/tingling around the mouth (perioral paresthesias). Very often, these adverse effects improve within a few months/weeks of starting fosamprenavir. Fosamprenavir may increase triglycerides. Assess cholesterol, and triglyceride levels prior to initiation of therapy and periodically throughout therapy.

Fosamprenavir is taken twice a day in combination with ritonavir by patients who have previous experience with PIs. It may be taken once daily by PI-naive patients. Fosamprenavir may be taken with or without food. Fosamprenavir is not approved for children younger than 18 years. It is a pregnancy category C drug; recommendations for it use during pregnancy are the same as those for saquinavir.

Indinavir

Indinavir (Crixivan) is another oral PI indicated for treating HIV infection. When indinavir is the only PI in the HAART cocktail, it is given three times a day. It can be given twice a day if given with other PI drugs. It should be taken on an empty stomach for best absorption.

Indinavir may induce serious adverse effects such as kidney stones, elevated liver enzymes, and worsening of pre-existing thrombocytopenia. To decrease the potential for kidney stones, instruct the patient to drink at least 1 to 2 L of water a day especially during hot days or episodes of diarrhea. Patients with pre-existing hepatic dysfunction or thrombocytopenia should be monitored closely, and appropriate laboratory testing should be scheduled regularly.

Self-limiting common adverse effects include nausea, headache, fatigue, abdominal pain, vomiting, rash, and dry skin. Other potential adverse effects include paronychia, severely dry skin, or cracked lips.

Drug–drug interactions are similar to those for saquinavir. Drugs to be avoided include rifamycins, benzodiazepines, ergotamines, and drugs for erectile dysfunction. Additionally, instruct the patient to avoid St. John's wort, garlic, and high doses of vitamin C.

Indinavir is not approved for children. It is a pregnancy category C drug; recommendations for its use during pregnancy are the same as those for saquinavir.

Nelfinavir

Nelfinavir (Viracept) is another oral PI. One benefit of Viracept is that resistance that develops to nelfinavir does not always confer resistance to other PIs. Nelfinavir is taken twice daily with a large snack or meal.

The major adverse effect of nelfinavir is diarrhea, which may be controlled with loperamide or other antidiarrheals. Other interventions for nelfinavir-induced diarrhea include twice-daily calcium tablets, probiotics such as yogurt, and soluble fiber supplements. Nelfinavir also is associated with elevations in ALT, aspartate aminotransferase, and CPK levels.

Drug interactions are similar to those with saquinavir.

Nelfinavir is approved for use in children. It is a pregnancy category B drug, and recommendations for its use during pregnancy are the same as those for saquinavir.

Ritonavir

Ritonavir (RTV, Norvir) is an oral PI used to treat HIV infection. It is available as a capsule or oral suspension. It is formulated with lopinavir as Kaletra as fixed combination medication. Low-dose ritonavir is frequently prescribed in combination with another PI to "boost" the anti-HIV effect of the other PI. Ritonavir is the only PI approved for this "boosting" effect. At a full dose, and lone PI, ritonavir is not recommended because of its persistent and long-term adverse effects.

Taking ritonavir within 2 hours of a meal increases its absorption and decreases nausea. Patient management for this PI is similar to that for saquinavir.

Adverse effects are most likely to occur at the beginning of therapy and affect women more frequently than they affect men. They include headache, nausea, vomiting, diarrhea, and tingling or numbness around the mouth. Ritonavir may induce kidney failure in patients with pre-existing renal dysfunction or patients taking nephrotoxic drugs. A Black Box warning concerns coadministration of ritonavir with certain nonsedating antihistamines, sedative hypnotics, antidysrhythmics, and ergot derivatives; serious or life-threatening drug-drug interactions may occur because of its inhibition of P-450 CYP3A and CYP2D6 as well as inducer of other hepatic enzymes.

Ritonavir is available as an oral solution; however, it has a very bitter taste. It may be combined with chocolate milk or Ensure to mask its taste, as long as it is given within 1 hour of mixing. Ritonavir solution is kept at room temperature, but the oral capsules should be kept refrigerated.

Ritonavir is approved for use in children older than 2 years. It is a pregnancy category B drug.

Tipranavir

Tipranavir (Aptivus) is another PI indicated for use in treatment-experienced patients or with patients with HIV-1 infections that are resistant to multiple PIs. All current PIs are theoretically less able to adapt their shape to inhibit protease with minor structural changes, which is the hallmark of mutations. Aptivus is structurally different and as such is more amenable to alterations in these binding site. This flexibility at the binding site is the reason it is thought to be effective against multiple PI resistant viruses. It is not recommended on treatment naïve patients because of insufficient data.

Genotypic or phenotypic testing is recommended prior to treatment. Like darunavir, it is administered with ritonavir and food to increase its efficacy. Patient management for tipranavir is similar to that for saquinavir.

Tipranavir contains a sulfonamide moiety and cannot be used in patients with a sulfa allergy. It is contraindicated for patients with moderate to severe hepatic insufficiency as well as for patients who take amiodarone, flecainide, propafenone, quinidine, ergot derivatives, pimozide, midazolam, and triazolam because of the risk of life-threatening drug–drug interactions. Tipranavir decreases platelet aggregation. It is given cautiously to patients who are at risk for bleeding from trauma, surgery, or other medical conditions, or those taking drugs known to decrease platelet aggregation such as antiplatelets or anticoagulants The most common adverse effects involve the GI system and include nausea, vomiting, and diarrhea. Also, tipranavir may elevate cholesterol and triglycerides. Assess baseline lipid parameters prior to administration and intermittently throughout therapy.

Tipranavir has two Black Box warnings related to the drug's association with the following:

- Intracranial hemorrhage (fatal and nonfatal) when given in combination with ritonavir
- Clinical hepatitis and hepatic decompensation, including some fatalities, when given in combination with ritonavir. Extra vigilance is warranted in patients with chronic hepatitis B or C coinfection, because these patients have an increased risk of hepatotoxicity.

Other drug–drug interactions, precautions, and adverse effects are similar to those for saquinavir. Tipranavir is a pregnancy category C drug. It should be used during pregnancy only if the benefits outweigh the risks of therapy.

Lopinavir/Ritonavir

Lopinavir/ritonavir (Kaletra) is a relatively new PI for adults and children 6 months and older. It is available in tablet and oral liquid formulations. The tablet may be taken with or without food.

One of the most important attributes of this drug combination is its potency. Because of the addition of ritonavir, lopinavir reaches high serum levels.

Lopinavir/ritonavir is contraindicated in patients who have hypersensitivity to either component and in patients with polyoxyethylated castor oil hypersensitivity. The medication should be given cautiously to patients with pre-existing hepatic disease because it is associated with the development of hepatic dysfunction. The most common adverse effects reported are diarrhea, shortness of breath, nausea, abdominal pain, headache, and vomiting.

Lopinavir/ritonavir can cause multiple drug–drug interactions, which are similar to those of saquinavir. Because ritonavir suppresses a liver enzyme used to break down dozens of drugs, it may boost the blood levels of street drugs such as Ecstasy (3,4-methylenedioxymethamphetamine [MDMA]) or heroin.

The DHHS 2008 Guideline recommends lopinavir/ritonavir as a preferred option of a PI based initial HAART.

It is a pregnancy category C drug, and recommendations for its use during pregnancy are the same as those for saquinavir. The once a day lopinavir/ritonavir combination is not recommended during pregnancy because of lower drug exposure during pregnancy and may need increase dose in third trimester of pregnancy.

INTEGRASE INHIBITORS

The integrase inhibitor raltegravir (Isentress) is the prototype for the newest class HAART therapy approved for the management of HIV disease. The enzyme integrase is a key component that allows the converted HIV viral DNA to enter the host cell DNA to begin producing genetic material for new viruses and raltegravir is the first of its kind to block or inhibit this very crucial step. Table 46.9 presents an overview of raltegravir.

Nursing Management of the Patient Receiving P Raltegravir

Core Drug Knowledge

Pharmacotherapeutics

Raltegravir is approved for use as part of combination HAART for patients with HIV strains that are resistant to multiple antiretroviral regimens and experiencing ongoing viral replication while receiving HAART. In July, 2009, raltegravir received approval for use in treatment naïve adult patients.

Pharmacokinetics

Raltegravir has a half life of approximately 9 hours. It is primarily metabolized in the liver and excreted out of the body by way of feces and urine. It does not require a dose adjustment for gender, renal impairment, or mild to moderate liver impairment.

Pharmacodynamics

Raltegravir is a HIV virus integrase strand transfer inhibitor. By blocking the integrase enzyme the reverse transcribed HIV DNA cannot enter into to the host CD4 cell chromosomes. When this integration does not take place the replication process is disrupted, thus the viral life cycle is not completed and viral replication is terminated

Contraindications and Precautions

There are no known contraindications for raltegravir. It is used cautiously in patients receiving other medications that can cause muscle problems, such as lipid-lowering agents, due to the increased risk for myopathy and rhabdomyolysis.

TABLE 46.9	Overview of P Raltegravir		
Drug	**Route and Dosage Range**	**Pharmacokinetics**	**Special Considerations**
P raltegravir (RAL, Isentress)	*Adult* PO: 400 mg 2×/d	*Onset:* rapid *Duration:* unknown *T ½:* 9 h	No food restrictions Do not administer as monotherapy

Adverse Effects

Common adverse effects include diarrhea, nausea, abdominal distension and pain, flatulence, headache, and fatigue. Serious adverse effects include Stevens-Johnson syndrome, depression, and suicidal tendencies. Rarely, elevated liver enzyme levels and pancreatic amylase have occurred. Also, abnormal elevation in muscle enzymes has been observed. Raltegravir is a pregnancy class C.

Drug Interactions

Raltegravir interacts with many of the HAART medications with either an increase or decrease in serum raltegravir levels. However, only tipranavir requires a dose adjustment. In addition, there are substantial interactions with rifampin and proton pump inhibitors. Table 46.10 presents these interactions.

Assessment of Relevant Core Patient Variables

Health Status

Raltegravir initially received approval for treatment experience patients. It is also now approved as an earlier treatment option for treatment naïve patients.

Life Span and Gender

Assess the patient for pregnancy and breast feeding. Raltegravir is a Class C drug and there are no well controlled clinical studies conducted among pregnant patients. As such, raltegravir should only be used if the potential benefits of the medication outweigh the potential risk to the fetus. Clinical studies of raltegravir have not included sufficient numbers of patients aged 65 and over to see how they respond to therapy compared to the younger subjects. Monitor the elderly carefully due to decreased renal, liver, cardiac output, and concomitant disease and other drug therapy found among the older patients.

Lifestyle, Diet, and Habits

Raltegravir can be given with or without food. Like other antiretroviral drugs, instruct the patient that it does not prevent or cure HIV and AIDS. Explain the importance of practicing safe sex with latex condom barriers and abstention from a risky lifestyle.

Environment

Assess the patient for apprehensiveness regarding introduction of a new class of drugs such as raltegravir. The lack of familiarity and paucity of post approval information related to a new drug and new class of drugs maybe disconcerting and intimidating for the patient. Similarly, adverse effects of the medication gathered through the clinical trial phase of the drug may bring apprehensiveness on the part of the patient. A discussion of the benefit-risk of the medication is important.

Nursing Diagnoses and Outcomes

- **Nursing Diagnosis:** Imbalanced Nutrition: Less than Body Requirements, related to GI distress
  Desired Outcome:
  The patient will self medicate with over the counter remedies to control transient GI symptoms and will contact the provider for persistent GI complaints.
- **Nursing Diagnosis:** Acute Pain related to headache from drug effects
  Desired Outcome:
  The patient will self medicate with over-the-counter remedies such as nonsteroidal anti-inflammatory drugs (NSAIDS), and or practice non-pharmacological pain relief to alleviate the headache.

Planning and Intervention

Maximizing Therapeutic Effects

Administer raltegravir with or without food. Offer small frequent meals for patients with GI distress. Ensure that raltegravir is administered twice daily. Ensure raltegravir is not used as monotherapy.

Minimizing Adverse Effects

Monitor patients receiving other drugs that are strong inducers of uridine diphosphate glucuronosyltransferase, such as rifampin, for treatment failure.

Providing Patient and Family Education

- Emphasize that zidovudine does not cure HIV. Encourage the patient to take precautions to avoid exposing others to blood and body fluids and the use of latex condoms during sex.
- Instruct patient when a missed dose occur to take it as soon as he/she remembers it, and if not remembered it until the next dose, to skip the dose and take it at the next scheduled dose.
- Explain the importance of consistent use of raltegravir to avoid potential resistance to the drug.

TABLE 46.10	Agents that Interact with P Raltegravir	
Interactants	**Effect and Significance**	**Nursing Management**
Proton Pump Inhibitors (PPI)	PPI drugs decrease the metabolism of raltegravir resulting in an increased serum concentration and increased risk for raltegravir toxicity.	Monitor for raltegravir toxicity.
Rifampin	Rifampin increases the metabolism of raltegravir resulting in subtherapeutic serum concentration.	Verify order with provider: generally not given together. Monitor for efficacy of raltegravir.

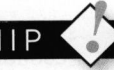

MEMORY CHIP

P Raltegrvir

- Used for the management of HIV infection and AIDS
- Major contraindication: none
- Most common adverse effects: GI distress, headache, fatigue
- Most serious adverse effect: Depression, suicide ideation
- Maximizing therapeutic effect: Offer small frequent meals if GI distress present
- Minimizing adverse effects: Monitor for drug–drug interactions
- Most important patient education: Advise women of childbearing age to contact provider immediately should pregnancy occur

---

- Instruct the patient to use OTC medications for common adverse effects such as headache or diarrhea and small, frequent meals for GI complaints. Encourage the patient to advise the provider if these symptoms are severe and persistent.
- Instruct women of child-bearing age to advise the provider immediately should she become pregnant.

Ongoing Assessment and Evaluation

Coordinate periodic examinations and blood monitoring in patients receiving raltegravir to assess for potential progression of HIV disease, treatment failure, the emergence of resistance, or development of adverse effects. CD4 cell counts and HIV RNA should be assessed every 3 months. Monitor for the need to change pharmacotherapy. Monitor for opportunistic diseases such as *Pneumocystis jiroveci*, mycobacterium avium complex, or varicella zoster. The patient should have a stable CD4 cell count and a declining or undetectable HIV RNA count throughout therapy.

© ENTRY INHIBITORS

Entry inhibitors are also known as **fusion inhibitors.** Before enfuvirtide's approval, anti-HIV drugs affected the virus inside the infected cell. This class of drugs inhibits HIV from binding to, fusing with, and entering the human cell by binding with a region of HIV envelope glycoprotein gp41 and preventing the viral fusing with the target cell membrane. The prototype fusion inhibitor is enfuvirtide (Fuzeon). Table 46.11 presents a summary of selected entry inhibitors.

Nursing Management of the Patient Receiving P Enfuvirtide

Core Drug Knowledge

Pharmacotherapeutics

Enfuvirtide is approved for managing HIV infection in patients who have experienced treatment failure with drugs from each existing class of antiretrovirals or who have proved unable to tolerate previous antiretroviral regimens. It is not recommended for initial treatment protocols. Enfuvirtide is expensive ($20,000 a year), hard to manufacture, and the complexity of its administration will likely reserve it as part of **salvage therapy** (a treatment for people who are nonresponsive to or cannot tolerate other available therapies).

Pharmacokinetics

Enfuvirtide is a subcutaneous injection that must be reconstituted prior to administration. It can be injected into the arms, upper thigh, or abdomen and reaches plasma concentration within 8 hours. Enfuvirtide is not excreted; it is catabolized by tissue recycling of amino acids.

Pharmacodynamics

Enfuvirtide binds to the gp41 protein on the surface of HIV. This protein is considered to be the "key" used by HIV to bind onto and enter cells. By blocking gp41, enfuvirtide blocks the HIV from entering the cell. Unfortunately, resistance to enfuvirtide has emerged. Resistance to enfuvirtide does not induce resistance to NRTIs, NNRTIs, or PIs. Conversely, resistance to NRTIs, NNRTIs, or PIs does not induce resistance to enfuvirtide.

Contraindications and Precautions

Enfuvirtide should not be used in patients with hypersensitivity to any of its components, including mannitol. Enfuvirtide is associated with the development of bacterial

TABLE 46.11	Summary of Selected Entry Inhibitors		
Drug	**Route and Dosage Range**	**Pharmacokinetics**	**Special Considerations**
P enfuvirtide (ENF, Fuzeon, T-20)	*Adult and Child > 16y* SQ: 90 mg 2×/d *Child 6–16 y* SQ: 2 mg/kg 2×/d maximum dose 90 mg 2×/d Child < 6 y: not approved	*Onset:* slow *Duration:* unknown $t_{1/2}$: 3.2–4.4 h	Assess for lung disease and pregnancy. Advise provider if positive. Rotate sites regularly. Use reconstituted drug within 24 h.
maraviroc (Selzentry)	*Adult PO:* 150–600 mg 2×/d *Child:* not approved	*Onset:* slow *Duration:* unknown $t_{1/2}$: 14–18 h	No food restrictions Monitor for rash, eosinophilia, and elevated IgE levels and hepatotoxicity Monitor for reactivation of previous opportunistic infections

pneumonia; thus, it should be used with caution in patients with risk factors that predispose them to infection. Such risk factors include pre-existing pulmonary dysfunction, smoking, or use of IV drugs; patients with low CD4 or high viral load counts are also predisposed to infection.

Enfuvirtide is a pregnancy category B drug.

Adverse Effects

The major adverse effect of enfuvirtide is injection-site reaction but they are normally mild and do not require discontinuation of the therapy. This reaction occurs in 95% of the patients using enfuvirtide. Reactions include itchy rash and red, swollen, puffy, or hardened skin. Patients using the thigh for injection are more likely than others to have cysts or nodules form.

In addition to injection site reactions, enfuvirtide may induce anorexia, nausea, weight loss, fatigue, anxiety, headache, insomnia, peripheral neuropathy, and infections such as sinusitis, herpes simplex, influenza, and conjunctivitis. Patients receiving enfuvirtide are more likely than others to acquire bacterial pneumonia and lymphadenopathy, although a direct correlation with the drug has not yet been established.

Drug Interactions

Drug–drug interactions have not yet been identified. Patients may take rifamycins safely with enfuvirtide.

Assessment of Relevant Core Patient Variables

Health Status

Review the patient's HIV history and treatment plan carefully. Evaluate the patient's potential for adherence with self-administration of a subcutaneous medication and for the ability to follow aseptic guidelines. Assess the patient's dexterity and vision. Filling the syringe and looking for viable injection sites requires coordinated hand and eye effort.

Life Span and Gender

Assess the patient for pregnancy or lactation; as previously stated, enfuvirtide is a pregnancy category B drug. In female patients receiving HAART when they conceive, therapy should be continued throughout the pregnancy. If a patient is not receiving therapy when the conception occurs, the patient may consider delaying HAART until after 10 to 12 weeks of gestation. It is unknown whether enfuvirtide is excreted into breast milk. However, HIV-positive women are advised not to breast-feed, to avoid potential postnatal transmission to an infant who may not be infected.

Note the patient's age before administering enfuvirtide because this drug is not approved for patients younger than 6 years.

Lifestyle, Diet, and Habits

Teach the patient to avoid risk factors that predispose them to infection. Such factors include smoking and IV drug use. Instruct the patient to eat a healthy diet to optimize immune system function.

Be aware of the patient's economic status. The cost of enfuvirtide is prohibitive. In fact, it is so expensive that not all insurers have added enfuvirtide to their formularies. Also, complex manufacturing of the drug may not insure a steady uninterrupted supply.

Environment

Enfuvirtide is most frequently self-administered by the patient at home. Enfuvirtide powder is stored at room temperature. Once the drug is reconstituted, it should remain in the vial, not the syringe, and should be refrigerated. Advise the patient to remove the refrigerated solution and allow it to return to room temperature before administration.

Nursing Diagnoses and Outcomes

- Pain related to injection site reactions and headache
  Desired outcome: *The patient will self-medicate with analgesics such as acetaminophen.*
- Risk for Infection related to drug adverse effect
  Desired outcome: *The patient will recognize symptoms associated with infections such as pneumonia, sinusitis, herpes simplex, influenza, and conjunctivitis and will contact the prescriber immediately for appropriate intervention.*
- Imbalanced Nutrition: Less than Body Requirements, related to anorexia and nausea
  Desired outcome: *The patient will maintain optimal body weight and nutrition throughout therapy.*
- Risk for Injury related to insomnia and peripheral neuropathy
  Desired outcome: *The patient will remain injury free throughout therapy.*

Planning and Intervention

Maximizing Therapeutic Effects

Reconstitute the enfuvirtide with sterile water, and then allow the solution to sit until the powder dissolves completely, which may be as much as 45 minutes. When two doses of medication are prepared from the vial, the second dose should be refrigerated in the vial, not in a syringe. After adding the diluent, tap the vial for several seconds and then roll between hands to allow for full absorption.

Administer subcutaneous enfuvirtide at 12-hour intervals. Rotate the site of administration to optimize absorption. Avoid injecting into the umbilicus, moles, scars, bruises, or areas that could be irritated by a belt or waistband, or areas experiencing an injection-site reaction.

Minimizing Adverse Effects

Use aseptic technique when reconstituting or administering enfuvirtide. Monitor the patient for early signs of infection in areas of skin where an injection site reaction occurs. Also, monitor for signs of systemic infections, such as sinusitis or pneumonia.

Providing Patient and Family Education

- Emphasize that enfuvirtide does not cure HIV. Encourage the patient to take precautions to avoid exposing others to blood and body fluids and the use of latex condoms during sex.

• Emphasize the importance of aseptic technique when reconstituting and administering enfuvirtide.

• Teach patients and families how to use the enfuvirtide convenience pack correctly. Be sure to explain the different types of syringes (the 3-mL syringe is used to reconstitute the powder, and the 1-mL syringe is used to administer the solution).

• Explain how to inject air into the vial in order to withdraw the solution.

• Teach patients to read the barrel of the syringe (to measure 1.1 mL of solution for administration) accurately.

• Teach patients the correct areas of the body for subcutaneous injection of enfuvirtide (upper arms, upper thigh, and abdomen).

• Teach patients to avoid injecting into the umbilicus, moles, scars, bruises, or areas that could be irritated by a belt or waistband, or areas of skin where an injection site reaction has occurred.

• Explain the potential for injection-site reactions and the need to rotate the injection site to ensure appropriate drug absorption.

• Teach patients healthy lifestyle choices to decrease the potential for infections, especially the need to avoid recreational drugs and tobacco products.

• Teach patients the signs of infection and advise them to contact the prescriber if such signs occur.

Ongoing Assessment and Evaluation

Assess the patient taking enfuvirtide for signs of infectious disorders such as pneumonia, sinusitis, herpes simplex, influenza, and conjunctivitis. Assess for anorexia, nausea, weight loss, fatigue, anxiety, headache, insomnia, and peripheral neuropathy.

Monitor for the need to change pharmacotherapy. It is important to remember that changes in therapy may have to be based on blood analysis because the patient may remain asymptomatic.

MEMORY CHIP

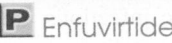 Enfuvirtide

• Used for the management of HIV infection and AIDS
• Major contraindication: hypersensitivity
• Most common adverse effects: injection-site reactions
• Most serious adverse effect: bacterial pneumonia
• Maximizing therapeutic effect: Rotate injection sites to increase absorption.
• Minimizing adverse effects: Use aseptic technique to administer subcutaneous injection.
• Most important patient education: Teach to reconstitute and administer subcutaneous injections.

The patient should have a stable CD4 count and a declining or undetectable HIV RNA load throughout therapy. The patient should be free of opportunistic infections.

Drugs Significantly Different Than Enfuvirtide
CCR5 Inhibitors

Maraviroc (Selzentry) is a new type of oral entry inhibitor approved by the FDA in 2008. In HIV replication, a protein on the virus (gp120) attaches to a primary receptor which in turn allows binding to a co-receptor, resulting in viral entry into the cell. Only two co-receptor variants, known as CCR5 and CXCR4, are used by all HIV strains. Most viruses predominantly use the CCR5 co-receptor, especially in treatment-naive patients. Maraviroc blocks the CCR5 co-receptor. Once it does this, HIV cannot successfully bind with the surface of CD4 cells, thus preventing the virus from infecting healthy cells. Maraviroc exclusively targets CCR5 co-receptor. It does not work on CCR4 receptors, or dual CCR4/CCR5 tropism. It is hypothesized that blocking the CCR5 co-receptor might stimulate a conversion to HIV that uses the alternative CXCR4 co-receptor. In addition to causing resistance to maraviroc, this may be linked to more rapid disease progression. Ideally, assays should be able to detect coreceptor tropism before maraviroc is used. However, current test are not yet available. Maraviroc is a substrate of CYP3A and P-glycoprotein (Pgp). The recommended dose is 300 mg twice daily; however, the dose must be adjusted for patients receiving other CYP3A inducers or inhibitors. Patients receiving CYP3A inhibitors (PIs, delavirdine, ketoconazole, itraconazole, and clarithromycin) require a lower dose. Patients receiving CYP3A inducers (efavirenz, rifampin, carbamazepine, phenobarbital, and phenytoin) require a higher dose because the faster clearance will result in subtherapeutic levels of maraviroc.

Common adverse effects include cough, pyrexia, upper respiratory infections, rash, musculoskeletal symptoms, abdominal pain, and dizziness. There is a black box warning regarding the risk for hepatoxicity, which may be preceded by symptoms of a systemic allergic reaction such as rash, eosinophilia, and elevated IgE levels. Contact the provider immediately if any of these symptoms occur.

Cardiovascular events, such as acute myocardial ischemia or infarction, have been observed in patients receiving maraviroc, although its connection to this adverse effect has not been identified. Maraviroc may induce postural hypotension, especially in patients receiving antihypertensive medications.

Finally, since maraviroc interferes with CCR5 co-receptors found in immune cells, the patient may experience some form of unintended infection, or reactivation of an infection such as PCP, mycobacterium, or cytomegalovirus infection.

Maraviroc is a pregnancy category B drug.

POSTEXPOSURE PROPHYLAXIS

Postexposure prophylaxis (PEP) may be either occupational (as for health care providers) or nonoccupational. Although the incidence of workplace needle stick exposure has decreased due to education, needle disposal, and engineering changes, the exposure risk is still a significant concern. For the purposes of this text, only occupational PEP will be discussed.

PEP decreases, but does not eliminate, the risk of seroconversion (the development of HIV) after a single exposure. Exposure is defined as a needle stick or cut with a sharp object or contact of mucous membranes or nonintact skin with blood, tissue, or other potentially infectious body fluids (Box 46.8). In terms of rate of exposure, nurses top the list, followed by physicians, phlebotomists, and non laboratory technicians. The risk of seroconversion is low and is estimated to 3 out of 100 without prophylaxis. It is estimated that the risk of seroconversion is reduced by 80% when PEP is administered in a timely fasion. The risk of seroconversion increases with exposure to a larger quantity of blood from the HIV-infected patient (source patient). For example, a needle stick with a needle visibly contaminated with the patient's blood or an exposure after a procedure that involved a needle being placed directly in a vein or artery would increase the risk of seroconversion. The depth of the needle penetration, the placement of the needle, vein or artery in the contact person, and a high viral load are considered high-risk injury. Low-risk injuries, on the other hand, are those that are superficial in depth and the source person has a low viral load. This high versus low risk injury has implications affecting how the exposure is addressed.

PEP is recommended when the source patient is HIV positive. PEP is generally offered to the health care provider if the HIV status of the source is unknown. Ideally, PEP should start within 1 to 2 hours after exposure and no more than 72 hours later. It is thought that PEP effectiveness is lessened if given 24 to 36 hours post-exposure. PEP is continued for 4 weeks, unless the source patient is found to be HIV negative. Approximately one-third of health care providers who start PEP do not complete the regimen because adverse effects to the drugs are significant. For example, efavirenz has the major disadvantage of CNS toxicity which may be is acceptable to someone who requires lifetime treatment, but may be problematic to a health care professional who needs to continue to function at a high cognitive level even though it is a relatively short therapy of at least 4 weeks. It is important to remember that not every health care provider's exposure requires PEP.

There are many variables to consider prior to the initiation of PEP, and the guidelines are complex and well beyond the scope of this text. Currently, the simplified recommendations for occupational PEP are one of the following:

- Basic regimen:
- zidovudine + lamivudine, available as Combivir, or
- zidovudine + emtricitabine, or
- tenofovir + lamivudine, or
- tenofovir + emtricitabine (Truvada)
- Expanded regimen:
- basic regimen + lopinavir/ritonavir (Kaletra)

Remember, these regimens are the simplified version of PEP. There are many alternative regimens, based on specific variables. Laboratory follow-up is essential. Testing for HIV antibodies should be done at 6 weeks, 12 weeks, and 6 months after exposure.

For further information about PEP the information is available online: http://www.cdc.gov/mmwr/preview/mmwrhtml/rr5011a1.htm#tab4. Also, the National Clinician Post Exposure Prophylaxis Hotline telephone number is 888 448 4911 and it has a web site: http://www.ucdf.edu/hivcntr.

Box 46.8	BODY FLUIDS THAT CAN TRANSMIT HIV INFECTION

Potentially Infectious Fluids
blood
cerebrospinal fluid
synovial fluid
pleural fluid
peritoneal fluid
pericardial fluid
amniotic fluid
Noninfectious Fluids (unless they are visibly bloody)
feces
nasal secretions
saliva
sputum
sweat
tears
urine
vomitus

PROPHYLAXIS FOR OPPORTUNISTIC INFECTIONS

The advent of HAART has led to dramatic decline of opportunistic infections because of the improved health of the patient as well as the rise of his or her CD4. However, a patient with HIV infection still has an increased risk for a multitude of opportunistic infections. These opportunistic infections are a significant contributor of mortality and mortality among patients afflicted with HIV.

Many of these diseases must be treated on an individual basis, and routine prophylaxis is not recommended. However, for several diseases there are recommendations for prophylaxis to avoid initial infection (outlined in Table 46.12). In addition to these opportunistic infections, immunocompromised patients are more vulnerable than immunocompetent patients to certain conditions of the mouth (Box 46.9).

TABLE 46.12	Prophylaxis to Prevent First Episode of Opportunistic Disease		
Infection	**Indication**	**First Choice**	**Alternative**
Pneumocystis jiroveci pneumonia	CD4 count <200/mm³ or oropharyngeal candidiasis	Sulfamethoxazole-trimethoprim (SMZ-TMP), 1 DS tablet daily	SMZ-TMP 1 DS tablet 3×/week dapsone, 50 mg bid or 100 mg daily **or** dapsone, 50 mg daily, plus pyrimethamine, 50 mg weekly, and leucovorin, 25 mg, weekly **or** dapsone, 200 mg, plus pyrimethamine, 75 mg, plus leucovorin, 25 mg, weekly **or** aerosolized pentamidine, 300 mg, monthly **or** atovaquone, 1,500 mg daily **or** atovaquone 1,500 mg daily plus pyrimethamine 25 mg and leucovorin 10 mg daily
Mycobacterium tuberculosis	Tuberculin skin test (TST) reaction >5 mm **or** contact with person with active tuberculosis, regardless of TST result	Isoniazid, 300 mg, plus pyridoxine, 50 mg daily for 9 mo **or** isoniazid, 900 mg, plus pyridoxine, 100 mg 2×/wk for 9 mo	Rifampin, 600 mg daily **or** Rifabutin (dose adjusted based on concomitant HAART)
Toxoplasma gondii	Immunoglobin G antibody to *Toxoplasma* and CD4 count of <100/mm³	SMZ-TMP, 1 double strength daily	SMZ-TMP, 1 single strength daily **or** dapsone, 50 mg daily, plus pyrimethamine, 50 mg, and leucovorin, 25 mg, weekly **or** dapsone, 200 mg, plus pyrimethamine, 75 mg, and leucovorin, 25 mg, weekly **or** atovaquone, 1,500 mg, with or without pyrimethamine, 25 mg, plus leucovorin, 10 mg, daily
Disseminated Mycobacterium avium complex	CD4 count <50/cell/µL Must rule out active infection	Azithromycin, 1,200 mg weekly **or** clarithromycin, 500 mg twice daily **or** Azithromycin 600 mg 2×/wk	Rifabutin, 300 mg daily
Streptococcus pneumoniae infection	CD4 count <200 cells/µL and no receipt of pneumococcal vaccine in past 5 years	23-valent PPV 0.5mL IM every 5 y	None
Influenza A and B	All HIV positive patients	Inactivated influenza vaccine annually	None
Histoplasma Capsulatum infection	CD4 count <150 cells/µL and occupational exposure or living in area of hyperendemic histoplasmosis	Itraconazole 200 mg daily	None
Coccidiomycosis	CD4 count <250 cells/µL and positive IgM or IgG test in a patient from a disease endemic area	Fluconazole 200 mg daily Itraconazole 200 mg 2×/d	None
Varicella-zoster virus (VZV)	Substantial exposure to chickenpox or shingles for patients who have no history of either condition or, if available, negative antibody to VZV	Varivax, 2 doses 3 mo apart	Vaccinate all household contacts

Adapted from Guidelines for preventing opportunistic infections among HIV-infected persons. (2009). *Morbidity and Mortality Weekly Report, Apr 10;58(RR-4):1-207;*

Box 46.9 ORAL HEALTH CARE FOR IMMUNOCOMPROMISED PATIENTS

Both immunocompetent and immunocompromised patients may have oral health problems. A few conditions are seen only in immunocompromised patients. Conditions that are seen in both populations may cause more problems in immunocompromised patients than in others. These conditions include:

- Dental caries
- Dry mouth
- Periodontal disease
- Human papillomavirus (HPV)
- Oral candidiasis (thrush)
- Aphthous stomatitis (canker sores)
- Herpes simplex virus
- Hairy leukoplakia
- Opportunistic tumors

Teach the HIV-positive patient the importance of having dental examinations twice yearly. Other suggestions may include:

- Regularly brushing and flossing the teeth and gums
- Using artificial saliva products
- Sucking on sugar-free citrus candies
- Engaging in safe oral-sex practices
- Seeking treatment for aphthous ulcers rather than allowing them to self-heal
- Not smoking
- Limiting alcohol use

Pneumocystis Jiroveci Pneumonia

Pneumocystic jiroveci pneumonia (PCP) is a type of pneumonia that affects immunosuppressed patients. In the past, PCP was responsible for serious illness and death among patients with HIV and AIDS. Since the use of HAART began, morbidity and mortality related to PCP have dramatically decreased. Patients should start prophylactic therapy for PCP when their CD4 cell counts are less than 200/cells/µL or when they have a history of oropharyngeal candidiasis. If the CD4 cell count increases to at least 200/ cells/µL, prophylaxis may be discontinued.

The drug treatment of choice is sulfamethoxazole-trimethoprim (SMZ-TMP). Patients who experience non–life-threatening adverse drug effects should continue SMZ-TMP therapy if clinically feasible. If SMZ-TMP cannot be tolerated, alternative prophylactic regimens include dapsone, dapsone plus pyrimethamine, aerosolized pentamidine, or atovaquone. Unfortunately, these alternatives are not as effective as SMZ-TMP. For additional information on SMZ-TMP, see Chapter 42. Pentamidine is discussed in Chapter 47.

Tuberculosis

Patients with a diagnosis of HIV infection should have a baseline tuberculin skin test (TST). Depending on the progression of infection at the time of diagnosis, the TST results may be a false negative whereby the immunocompromised patient is unable to mount an immune response to the test. Clinical evaluation for the potential of TB is needed to determine whether anergy testing should be done at this time.

All HIV-positive patients who have positive TST results (induration exceeding 5 mm) should undergo chest radiography. For patients with positive TST findings and normal chest x-ray findings, prophylaxis with INH and pyridoxine maybe initiated and continued for 9 months, or 6 months, or 12 months, given daily or twice a week depending on institutional policy. Alternative therapies include rifampin or rifabutin daily for 4 months.

Any HIV-positive patients who are in close contact with people who have active TB should be started on prophylaxis therapy with isoniazid regardless of their TST results. Infants of HIV-positive mothers should have a TST between 9 and 12 months. These children should be retested every 2 to 3 years. Additional information on isoniazid can be found in Chapter 43.

Toxoplasma gondii

Patients infected with HIV should be tested for IgG antibody to *Toxoplasma* soon after the diagnosis of HIV infection to detect latent infection with *T. gondii*. Patients harboring toxoplasmosis are at risk for cerebral abscesses and severe morbidity and mortality. The vast majority of patients are positive.

Prophylaxis should be initiated for patients with IgG antibody to *Toxoplasma* and a CD4 cell count of less than 100 cells/µL. The drug of choice is SMZ-TMP. If the patient is unable to tolerate SMZ-TMP, he or she may receive alternative prophylaxis, including dapsone plus pyrimethamine plus leucovorin weekly, or atovaquone with or without pyrimethamine plus leucovorin daily.

Counsel patients to avoid raw or undercooked meat, particularly undercooked pork, lamb, and venison. It also is important to caution patients to wash their hands after touching raw meat, after gardening, and after changing a cat's litter box. Patients with cats should be advised to change the litter box daily.

Disseminated *Mycobacterium avium* Complex

Prophylaxis for disseminated *Mycobacterium avium* complex (MAC) should be initiated when the patient's CD4 cell count falls below 50 cells/µL. The drugs of choice are azithromycin once or twice weekly or clarithromycin twice-daily. Clarithromycin, however, has several drug interactions, including with PIs. In addition to MAC protection, these drugs also offer protection against respiratory bacterial infections.

For patients who cannot tolerate azithromycin or clarithromycin, rifabutin is the alternative drug. It is important to remember that rifabutin interacts with almost all anti-HIV agents; therefore, it should be administered cautiously. Additional information on azithromycin and clarithromycin is located in Chapter 40.

Streptococcus pneumoniae

Streptococcus pneumoniae is very common in the community, and there is no effective way to limit exposure to these bacteria. For patients with a CD4 cell count of at least 200 cells/μL, pneumococcal vaccine should be administered. For patients with a CD4 cell count of less than 200 cells/μL, pneumococcal vaccine may be administered, but the humoral response is likely to be diminished.

Influenza Virus

Every HIV-positive patient should receive annual influenza virus prophylaxis. The preferred drug is inactivated trivalent influenza virus vaccine, one dose annually.

Histoplasma capsulatum

Histoplasma capsulatum is the organism that causes the most common fungal respiratory infections in the world. Most infections are mild; however, approximately 10% of these infections cause serious complications, including inflammation of the pericardium and fibrosis of major blood vessels (see Chapter 44). Prophylaxis is recommended for patients who live in an endemic geographic area and have a CD4 count less than 150 cells/μL. Itraconazole is the drug of choice.

Varicella-Zoster Virus

Prophylaxis against varicella-zoster virus (VZV) is recommended for patients who have no antibodies to VZV and for patients who have been substantially exposed to either chickenpox or shingles. Patients should receive Varivax, 2 doses given 3 months apart. In patients experiencing an active VZV outbreak, treatment centers on antiviral drugs such as acyclovir, valacyclovir, or famciclovir. Information on these drugs is located in Chapter 45.

Hepatitis B

HIV-positive patients should be tested for antibodies to HBV. If the patient tests negative, the hepatitis B vaccine should be administered. This vaccine is administered in three doses, with the second dose given 1 month after the initial dose and the last dose given 6 months after the initial dose.

Hepatitis A

HIV-positive patients should be tested for antibodies to hepatitis A virus. If the patient is negative or has chronic hepatitis C, the hepatitis A vaccine should be administered. This vaccine is administered in two doses.

Cytomegalovirus

Cytomegalovirus (CMV) is found universally throughout all geographic locations and socioeconomic groups and infects between 50% and 85% of adults in the United States by 40 years of age. In the general population, the infection may go unnoticed; however, in the immunocompromised population, CMV may cause infection in many organs of the body,

especially in the retina of the eye (see Chapter 45). Patients who are CMV antibody positive and have a CD4 cell count of less than 50 cells/μL should receive ganciclovir, 1 g three times daily.

CHAPTER SUMMARY

- HIV infection and AIDS are chronic diseases affecting the immune system.
- HIV infection is diagnosed by positive results on EIA, ELISA, WB, rapid HIV, oral HIV, or PCR tests.
- HIV infection is monitored by CD4 cell count and HIV RNA load.
- Genotypic and phenotypic resistance assays are available to assess patterns of resistance to HAART.
- Pharmacotherapy should be considered for all symptomatic patients. For asymptomatic patients, drug therapy should be considered when the CD4 cell count is less than 200 cells/μL or any CD4 count if opportunistic infection is present.
- Resistance develops to all classes of anti-HIV agents, especially when the therapeutic regimen is not followed.
- Absorption of individual anti-HIV agents is enhanced by administration either with food or on an empty stomach (while fasting).
- All anti-HIV drugs may produce adverse effects that decrease the patient's quality of life.
- Most anti-HIV drugs have numerous drug–drug interactions that may increase or decrease their effectiveness. Many antiretroviral drugs have Black Box warnings.
- Anti-HIV agents include NRTIs, PIs, NNRTIs, integrase inhibitors, entry inhibitors, and CCR5 inhibitors.
- Antiretroviral therapy may be given throughout pregnancy or during the intrapartum and postpartum periods.
- Not all occupational exposures to HIV require PEP. However, PEP is recommended when the source patient is HIV positive.
- Opportunistic diseases develop as HIV infection progresses. Many opportunistic diseases have recommended prophylactic regimens.

QUESTIONS FOR STUDY AND REVIEW

1. How is HIV infection diagnosed?
2. Why do patients with HIV infection have an increased risk for opportunistic diseases?
3. What information is gained from CD4 cell counts and viral load counts?
4. What is the rationale for highly active antiretroviral therapy (HAART)?
5. Which adverse effects of zidovudine (AZT, ZDV) therapy may indicate a need to stop therapy?
6. Before initiation of zidovudine therapy, what laboratory tests should be completed?
7. What assessments and interventions apply to lifestyle, diet, and habits for the patient taking zidovudine?
8. How do PIs inhibit HIV replication?

9. How do NNRTIs differ in action from NRTIs?

10. How does the action of the entry inhibitors affect the ability of HIV to replicate?

11. Why is opportunistic disease prophylaxis necessary?

12. What is the mechanism of action for raltegravir?

NEED MORE HELP?

Chapter 46 of the Study Guide to Accompany *Drug Therapy in Nursing*, 4th Edition, contains additional NCLEX-style questions and other learning activities to reinforce your understanding of the concepts presented in this chapter. For additional information or to purchase the study guide, visit thePoint.

REFERENCES

Bartlett, J. (2009). *The stages and natural history of HIV infection*. Retrieved from www.uptodate.com

Brown, K. C., Paul, S., Kashuba, A. D. (2009). Drug interactions with new and investigational antiretrovirals. *Clinical Pharmacokinetics*, 48(4):211–241.

Coffey, S., & Peiperl, D. (2009). *Overview of Antiretroviral Drugs*, Retrieved from http://hivinsite.ucsf.edu/InSite?page=kb-00&doc=ar-drugs

Colson, A., & Sax, P. (2009). *Primary HIV 1 Infection: Pathogenesis, epidemiology, and clinical manifestations*. Retrieved from www.uptodate.com

Croom, K. F., Dhillon, S., Keam, S. J. (2009). Atazanavir: A Review of its Use in the Management of HIV-1 Infection. *Drugs*, 69(8):1107–1140.

Facts and Comparisons. (2010). *Drug facts and comparisons*. Philadelphia, PA: Lippincott Williams & Wilkins.

Ford, N., Lee, J., Andrieux-Meyer, A, (2011). Safety, efficacy, and pharmacokinetics of rilpivirine: systematic review with an emphasis on resource-limited settings. Retrieved June 3, 2011 from http://www.dovepress.com/safety-efficacy-and-pharmacokinetics-of-rilpivirine-systematic-review—peer-reviewed-article-HIV

Guidelines for Prevention and Treatment of Opportunistic Infections in HIV Adults and Adolescents. (2009). *Morbidity and Mortality Weekly Report*, April 10;58:RR-4.

Guidelines for the Use of antiretroviral agents in HIV-1 Infected Adults and Adolescents. (2008). Retrieved at http://aidsinfo.nih.gov/contentfiles/AdultandAdolescentGL.pdf

HIV/AIDS Update. (2009). Isentress (Raltegravir) Indication Extended for the Treatment of HIV-1 Infection in Treatment-Naive Patients. Retrieved from http://www.thebodypro.com/content/art52641.html

Hughes, A., & Nelson, M. (2009). HIV entry: new insights and implications for patient management. *Current Opinion in Infectious Diseases*, 22(1):35–42.

Karch, A. M. (2010). *Nursing Drug Guide*. Philadelphia, PA: Lippincott Williams & Wilkins.

Koda-Kimbal, M. A, Young, L. Y., Kradian, W. A., et al. (2008). *Applied Therapeutics: The Clinical Use of Drugs*. Philadelphia, PA: Lippincott Williams & Wilkins.

Kojic, E. M., & Carpenter, C. J. (2009). *Initiating Antiretroviral Therapy*. Retrieved from http://hivinsite.ucsf.edu/InSite?page=kb-00&doc=ar-drugs

McKeage, K., Perry, C. M., & Keam, S. J. (2009). Darunavir: a review of its use in the management of HIV infection in adults. *Drugs*, 69(4):477–503.

Micromedex Healthcare Series. Retrieved from *http://thomsonhc.com*

Osmond, D. H. (2009). *Epidemiology of HIV in the United States*. Retrieved from http://hivinsite.ucsf.edu/InSite?page=kb-00&doc=kb-01-03

Raltegravir (MK-0518, Isentress) package insert. Retrieved from http://www.merck.com/product/usa/pi_circulars/i/isentress/isentress_pi.pdf

Sayana, S., & Khanlou, H. (2009). Maraviroc: a new CCR5 antagonist. *Expert Review of Antiinfective Therapy*, 7(1):9–19.

Schiller, D. S., & Youssef-Bessler M. (2009). Etravirine: a second-generation nonnucleoside reverse transcriptase inhibitor (NNRTI) active against NNRTI-resistant strains of HIV. *Clinical Therapeutics*, 31(4):692–704.

Shafer, R. W. (2009). *Genotypic Testing for HIV-1 Drug Resistance*. Retrieved from http://hivinsite.ucsf.edu/InSite?page=kb-00&doc=kb-03-02-07

Shey, M., Kongnyuy, E. J., Shang. J., & Wiysonge, C. S. (2009). A combination drug of abacavir-lamivudine-zidovudine (Trizivir) for treating HIV infection and AIDS. *Cochrane Database of Systematic Reviews*, (3):CD005481.

Tatro, D. S. (2009). *Drug interaction facts*. Philadelphia, PA: Lippincott Williams & Wilkins.

U.S. Department of Health and Human Services. (2009). Recommendations for Use of Antiretroviral Drugs in Pregnant HIV-1 Infected Women for Maternal Health and Interventions to Reduce Perinatal HIV-1 Transmission in the United States.

Wilkin, T., Glesby, M., & Gulick, R. M. (2009). *Changing Antiretroviral Therapy: Why, When, and How*. Retrieved from http://hivinsite.ucsf.edu/InSite?page=kb-00&doc=kb-03-02-06

Wohl, D. (2008). HIV Journal View: *Top10 HIV Clinical Developments of 2008*: 1–38. February 27, 2009, http://www.thebodypro.com/content/art50584.html

Drugs Treating Parasitic Infections

Learning Objectives

At the completion of this chapter the student will:

1. Describe the guidelines that govern the choice of antiparasitic drugs.
2. Identify core drug knowledge about drugs used to treat parasitic infections.
3. Identify core patient variables relevant to drugs used to treat parasitic infections.
4. Relate the interaction of core drug knowledge and core patient variables to drugs used to treat parasitic infections.
5. Generate a nursing plan of care from the interactions between core drug knowledge and core patient variables for drugs used to treat parasitic infections.
6. Describe nursing interventions to maximize therapeutic actions and minimize adverse effects for drugs used to treat parasitic infections.
7. Determine key points for patient and family education for drugs used to treat parasitic infections.
8. Explain the hygiene measures needed to prevent parasitic reinfection.

Key Terms

amebiasis
arthropods
cestodes
ectoparasites
giardiasis

helminths
malaria
nematodes
parasite
Pneumocystis jiroveci pneumonia

pneumonia
protozoa
toxoplasmosis
trematodes
trichomoniasis

Drugs Treating Parasitic Infections

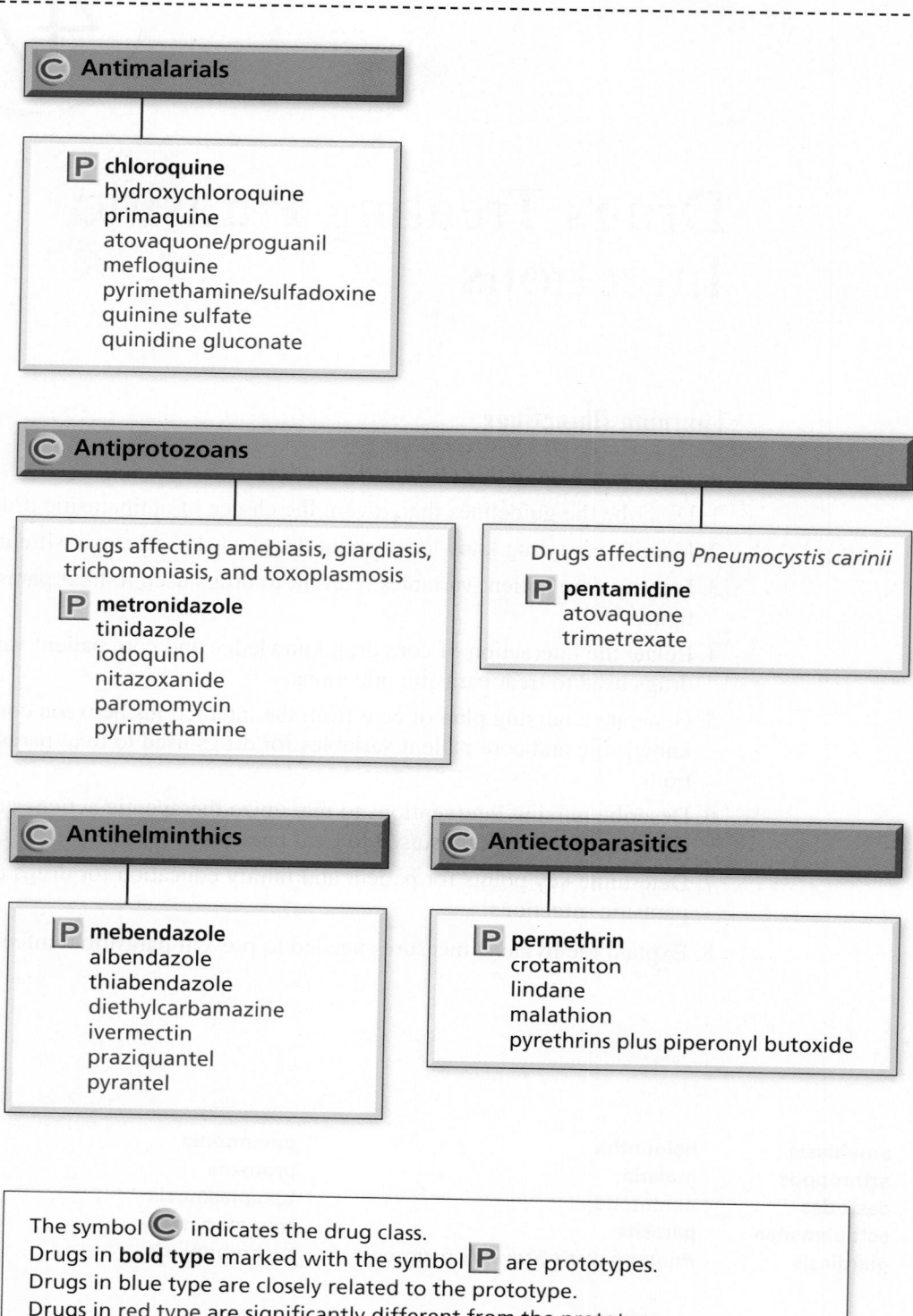

C Antimalarials

P **chloroquine**
hydroxychloroquine
primaquine
atovaquone/proguanil
mefloquine
pyrimethamine/sulfadoxine
quinine sulfate
quinidine gluconate

C Antiprotozoans

Drugs affecting amebiasis, giardiasis, trichomoniasis, and toxoplasmosis

P **metronidazole**
tinidazole
iodoquinol
nitazoxanide
paromomycin
pyrimethamine

Drugs affecting *Pneumocystis carinii*

P **pentamidine**
atovaquone
trimetrexate

C Antihelminthics

P **mebendazole**
albendazole
thiabendazole
diethylcarbamazine
ivermectin
praziquantel
pyrantel

C Antiectoparasitics

P **permethrin**
crotamiton
lindane
malathion
pyrethrins plus piperonyl butoxide

The symbol **C** indicates the drug class.
Drugs in **bold type** marked with the symbol **P** are prototypes.
Drugs in blue type are closely related to the prototype.
Drugs in red type are significantly different from the prototype.
Drugs in black type with no symbol are also used in drug therapy; no prototype.

A parasite is an organism that must live on other organisms to survive. The parasitic diseases are commonly grouped according to the type of organism that causes them: helminths, arthropods, or unicellular organisms, such as **protozoa.** Protozoan infections include malaria, amebiasis, giardiasis, *Pneumocystis carinii* pneumonia, toxoplasmosis, and trichomoniasis. **Helminths** (worms) are grouped into three categories: **nematodes** (roundworms), **trematodes** (flukes), and **cestodes** (tapeworms). **Ectoparasites** are vectors of disease, such as ticks, mosquitoes, and biting flies, and other parasites that infect external body surfaces. **Arthropods** include mites (scabies), chiggers, lice (pediculosis), and fleas.

Pharmacologic intervention for parasitic infections must be specific not only to the type of parasite but also to the appropriate stage of its life cycle. Some parasites have simple life cycles, and some have extremely complex life cycles. Thus, many parasitic diseases are treated with a combination of drugs to eradicate all stages of the parasite.

This chapter discusses the appropriate drug or drugs used to eradicate the most common parasitic diseases. Antiparasitic drugs are divided into four drug families: antimalarials, antiprotozoan drugs, anthelminthic drugs, and antiectoparasitic drugs. The antiprotozoan drugs used in treating *Pneumocystis carinii* pneumonia (PCP), a common complication of AIDS, are discussed separately within the antiprotozoan drug class section.

Prototypes presented in the chapter (and their target diseases) include chloroquine (malaria), metronidazole (protozoal infections), pentamidine isethionate (PCP), mebendazole (helminthic infections), permethrin (scabies), and malathion (pediculosis). In addition to explaining how these drugs work, this chapter discusses nursing management related to evaluating the patient's condition, administering antiparasitic drugs, monitoring the patient's response, and teaching the patient and family about antiparasitic therapy.

PATHOPHYSIOLOGY

Malaria

Malaria is caused by protozoan parasites of the genus *Plasmodium.* Four species of *Plasmodium* produce disease in humans—*P. falciparum, P. vivax, P. ovale,* and *P. malariae. P. falciparum* is the most widespread and dangerous of the four. Because *P. falciparum* can destroy up to 60% of circulating red blood cells (RBCs) and induce serious adverse complications such as toxic encephalopathy, it is fatal in about 1% of all cases. That 1% accounts for more than 95% of all malaria-caused deaths worldwide.

The complex life cycle of *Plasmodium* species begins when a female *Anopheles* mosquito bites a human whose blood contains the sexual forms of the malaria parasite (gametocytes). Within the now-infected mosquito, the gametocyte completes a maturation process and becomes a sporozoite that is stored in the salivary glands of the mosquito. When the mosquito next feeds, it inoculates another human host with the sporozoites.

Once the sporozoites are in the human host, the asexual portion of the life cycle begins. The first stage of asexual development, the exoerythrocytic phase, occurs in the liver. During this phase, the form of the *Plasmodium* is called a tissue schizont. At the end of the phase, the *Plasmodium,* now in a form called a merozoite, is released from the liver into the bloodstream.

The second stage of asexual development, the erythrocytic phase, begins when the merozoites are released into the bloodstream. The merozoites invade the erythrocytes and develop into erythrocytic schizonts. They, in turn, develop more merozoites within the red blood cells. At the end of this phase, the RBCs rupture, releasing the merozoites and pyrogenic substances into the bloodstream, where the merozoites invade new RBCs. The release of merozoites into the bloodstream initiates malarial symptoms of fever, shivering, joint pain, and headache. With *P. vivax* and *P. ovale,* merozoites may reinvade the liver tissue and develop a dormant hepatic stage (hypnozoite), which is responsible for subsequent relapses.

The cycle of invasion, multiplication, and RBC rupture is repeated many times. After a few cycles, some of the asexual parasites develop into sexual forms (gametocytes), which remain in the bloodstream. When a mosquito bites a human with gametocytes in the blood, the cycle begins again (Figure 47.1). Because of its complex life cycle, malaria is frequently treated with combination drug therapy.

Parasitic Diseases

Amebiasis

Amebiasis is most frequently caused by the microorganism *Entamoeba histolytica,* which is passed from host to host by ingestion of fecally contaminated food or water. It also is transmitted by vectors such as flies. Amebic disease is present worldwide, but it is most common in those tropical areas where crowded living conditions and poor sanitation exist. Africa, Latin America, Southeast Asia, and India have substantial health problems associated with this disease. In the United States, amebiasis is more common among homosexual men than it is in other populations.

Ingested in its cyst form, the microorganism has thick walls that are resistant to stomach acids. In the intestine, the cysts change into a sexually active organism called a trophozoite. The trophozoite produces active amebiasis. The active disease organisms may remain in the intestine (intestinal amebiasis), or the trophozoites may penetrate the intestinal wall and produce abscesses in other tissues and organs (extraintestinal amebiasis). Symptoms may be mild or severe. Mild symptoms include mucoid diarrhea, flatulence, fatigue, weight loss, and colicky abdominal pain. Severe disease may be marked with frequent foul-smelling stools tinged with mucus and blood, fever to 105°F, tenesmus (painful but unsuccessful straining to defecate), generalized abdominal tenderness, and vomiting.

PHYSIOLOGY

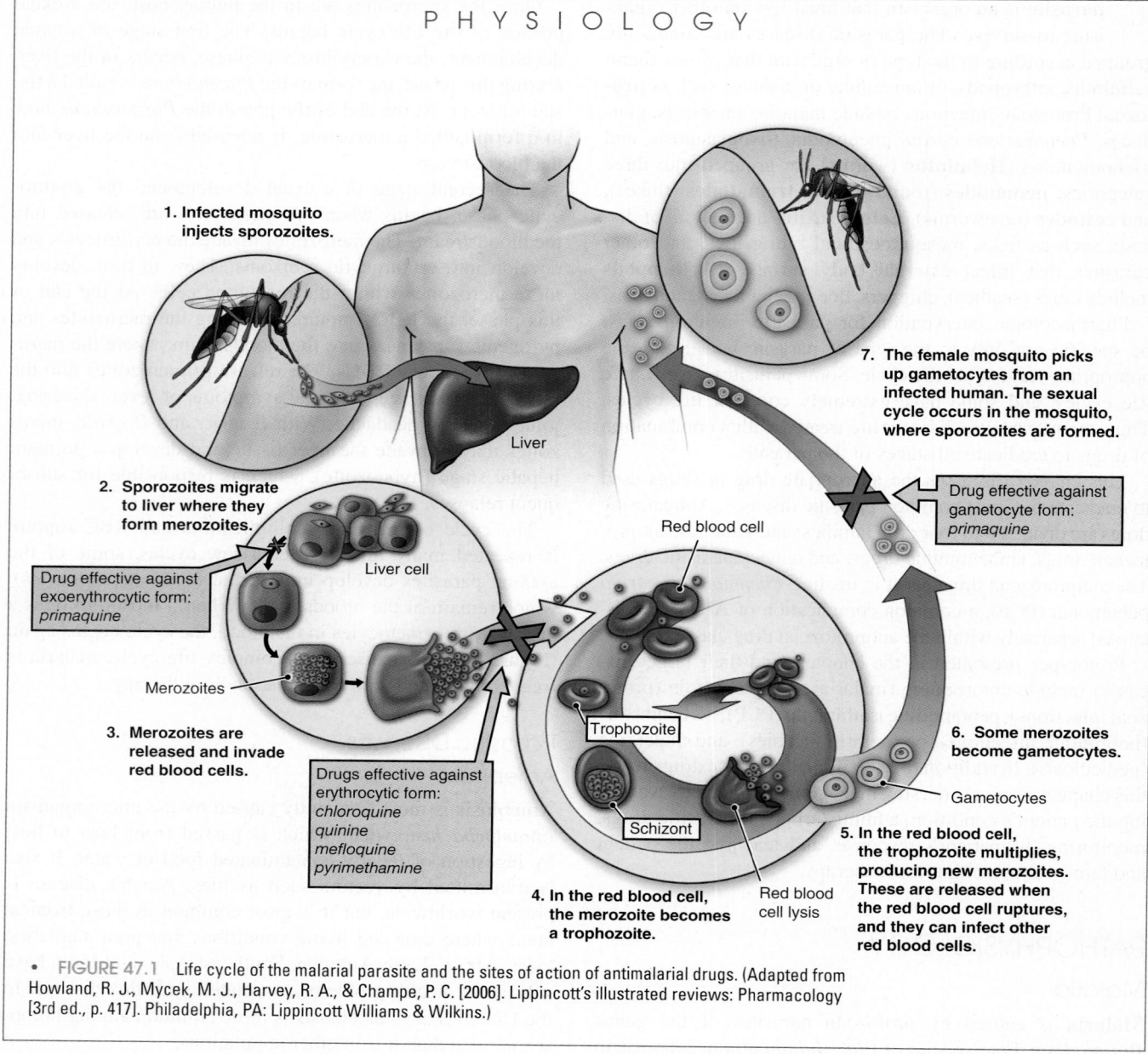

1. Infected mosquito injects sporozoites.

2. Sporozoites migrate to liver where they form merozoites.

Drug effective against exoerythrocytic form: *primaquine*

Liver cell

Liver

Merozoites

3. Merozoites are released and invade red blood cells.

Drugs effective against erythrocytic form:
*chloroquine
quinine
mefloquine
pyrimethamine*

4. In the red blood cell, the merozoite becomes a trophozoite.

Red blood cell

Trophozoite

Schizont

Red blood cell lysis

Red blood cell

5. In the red blood cell, the trophozoite multiplies, producing new merozoites. These are released when the red blood cell ruptures, and they can infect other red blood cells.

6. Some merozoites become gametocytes.

Gametocytes

7. The female mosquito picks up gametocytes from an infected human. The sexual cycle occurs in the mosquito, where sporozoites are formed.

Drug effective against gametocyte form: *primaquine*

• **FIGURE 47.1**   Life cycle of the malarial parasite and the sites of action of antimalarial drugs. (Adapted from Howland, R. J., Mycek, M. J., Harvey, R. A., & Champe, P. C. [2006]. Lippincott's illustrated reviews: Pharmacology [3rd ed., p. 417]. Philadelphia, PA: Lippincott Williams & Wilkins.)

Cryptosporidiosis

Cryptosporidiosis ("crypto") is a diarrheal disease caused by *Cryptosporidium parvum*. It is found in soil, food, water, or surfaces that have been contaminated with infected human or animal feces. Transmission is fecal–oral, and cryptosporidiosis may be acquired by several mechanisms: swallowing recreational water (from swimming pools, hot tubs, jacuzzis, fountains, lakes, rivers, springs, ponds, or streams) contaminated with sewage or feces from humans or animals; eating uncooked contaminated foods, including raw vegetables and fruits; or swallowing *C. parvum* picked up from surfaces (such as bathroom fixtures, changing tables, diaper pails, or toys) contaminated with feces from an infected person. Symptoms include nausea, vomiting, diarrhea, dehydration, weight loss, stomach cramps or pain, and fever. In immunocompetent persons, symptoms last for 1 to 2 weeks. Immunocompromised patients may experience more severe symptoms, sometimes leading to life-threatening illness.

Giardiasis

Giardiasis is a common disease caused by a flagellated protozoan, *Giardia lamblia*. It is transmitted by fecal contamination. Hikers who drink unfiltered water or travelers to foreign countries where the water supply is impure are most susceptible. Animal reservoirs for the parasites include beavers and dogs.

Giardiasis is more prevalent in children than in adults, possibly because many individuals seem to have a lasting immunity after infection. The disease is common in children's day-care centers, especially those in which diapering is done. This disease also afflicts many homosexual men, both HIV-positive and HIV-negative individuals, presumably as a result of sexual transmission.

The disease affects only the intestinal system, resulting in acute or chronic diarrhea and possibly malabsorption syndrome. The acute phase may last days to weeks; however, the chronic phase may last years. Symptoms include diarrheal, soft, or steatorrheal stools with mucus but without blood. Abdominal cramps, vomiting, flatulence, and weight loss also may occur.

Trichomoniasis

Trichomoniasis is an infection of the vagina caused by the parasite *Trichomonas vaginalis*. Both sexual partners are generally infected, although both may not be symptomatic. Symptoms of trichomoniasis include a thin, yellow, frothy, and malodorous discharge. The vagina may be inflamed, and the woman may also have a "strawberry" cervix, which is very friable and bleeds easily.

Toxoplasmosis

Toxoplasmosis is caused by a parasite found in a variety of animals, especially cats and birds. Infection results from ingesting oocysts from cat feces, ingesting cysts in raw or undercooked meat, congenital transmission, or transmission during blood transfusion.

In adults, the disease is usually mild with symptoms such as fever, malaise, headache, lymphadenopathy, and sore throat. However, toxoplasmosis is very dangerous to immunocompromised patients. The infection may affect the lungs, heart, and liver, but usually it affects the brain. Patients may succumb to meningoencephalitis.

Congenital toxoplasmosis may result in damage to the eyes (retinochoroiditis) and brain (encephalitis) of the fetus or other congenital anomalies.

Pneumocystis jiroveci Pneumonia

An opportunistic lung infection, **Pneumocystis jiroveci pneumonia** (PCP), formerly known as *Pneumocystis carinii* pneumonia, is caused by a phylogenetic fungal species. This particular species is not found in nonhuman hosts. Most people have been exposed to *Pneumocystis jiroveci* because it is in our environment; however, a healthy immune system keeps the fungus from causing illness within the host. In patients with depressed immunity, *Pneumocystis jiroveci* pneumonia causes serious illness.

Patients with the highest risk for the development of PCP include those with a T-cell count below 200; those with oral thrush or unexplained fevers lasting more than 2 weeks, regardless of T-cell count; and those who have previously been infected with PCP.

The symptoms of PCP develop slowly. They include weakness, fever, chest tightness, shortness of breath, dry cough, and weight loss. As the disease progresses, patients have symptoms similar to those of adult respiratory distress syndrome. Historically, PCP has had an exceptionally high mortality rate. Fortunately, with current prophylaxis and treatment options, death occurs in about 10% of cases of PCP.

Helminthic Infections

Intestinal Nematode Infections

The common intestinal nematodes are the giant roundworm, pinworm, threadworm, whipworm, and pork roundworm.

Ascariasis (Giant Roundworm)

Ascariasis is endemic in areas known for poor hygiene or sanitation and those where human feces are used as fertilizer. Ascariasis is transmitted by ingesting fecally contaminated foods or drinks. Once ingested, the worm eggs migrate to the small bowel, where they hatch, releasing larvae. The motile larvae migrate from the small bowel to the heart and lungs, to the esophagus, and back to the small bowel. They can survive up to 5 years and reach a length of 30 cm. Symptoms include low-grade fever, nonproductive cough, blood-tinged sputum, wheezing, dyspnea, and substernal pain.

Enterobiasis (Pinworm)

Enterobius vermicularis is the most common helminthic infection in the United States. Children are infected more frequently than adults. Transmission occurs by contact with eggs in food, water, or bed linens. Adult worms inhabit the cecum and adjacent bowel areas. Female worms migrate through the anus to the perianal skin and deposit large numbers of eggs, especially at night. In a few hours, infection can be transmitted to others or remain in the host. The most common symptoms are rectal itching and vulvar itching.

Strongyloidiasis (Threadworm)

Strongyloidiasis results from infection with *Strongyloides stercoralis*. The infection is potentially serious in adults because the worm can multiply within the host. In its filariform larvae cycle, the parasites penetrate the skin from soil, enter the bloodstream, and travel to the lungs. From the lungs, they escape the alveoli and ascend the bronchial tree to the glottis, where they are swallowed and propelled to the small intestine to mature into adult threadworms. The mature worm embeds itself in the mucosa, where eggs are laid and hatched. The larvae disseminate into the lungs and most other tissues, causing local inflammation and granulomas. Symptoms include skin reactions, such as inflammation, petechiae, and urticaria, and intestinal reactions, such as diarrhea, abdominal pain, and flatulence. Pulmonary symptoms include dry cough, throat irritation, dyspnea, wheezing, and hemoptysis. Hyperinfection syndrome caused by intense dissemination of larvae to the lungs and other tissues can result in complications, such as pleural effusion, pericarditis, and myocarditis. Additional problems include perforation of the colon and peritonitis, gram-negative septicemia, and shock leading to death.

Trichuriasis (Whipworm)

Trichuriasis infection is acquired by ingesting egg-contaminated soil on hands or food. Human-to-human transmission is not possible. Worms attach to the mucosa of the large intestine by means of their anterior whip-like end. Symptoms include abdominal cramps, tenesmus, diarrhea, flatulence, nausea, vomiting, and weight loss.

Trichinosis (Pork Roundworm)

Trichinella spiralis is the parasite that causes trichinosis. The infection is transmitted by ingesting encysted larvae in inadequately cooked meat, especially pork. Gastric juices liberate the encysted larvae, which migrate to the intestines, where they mature, mate, and produce eggs that hatch into new larvae. These larvae are distributed through the body and enter skeletal muscle tissues, producing an inflammatory response. Eventually, the larvae become re-encysted and remain within the tissues. Symptoms include diarrhea, cramps, and malaise. As the infection progresses, patients may experience muscle pain, tenderness, fever, periorbital and facial edema, and conjunctivitis.

Blood and Tissue Nematode Infections

Filarial infections are among the more serious and debilitating helminthiases associated with blood and tissue nematodes. There are two forms of filarial infections. The first form is caused by two microbes, *Wuchereria bancrofti* and *Brugia malayi*. Both microbes are transmitted by mosquitoes.

Bancroftian filariasis also is known as elephantiasis because the helminths migrate to the lymphatic system, causing lymphadenopathy and resultant edema of the extremities. Brugian filariasis also affects the lymphatic system. In this infection, microfilariae are produced and circulated in the bloodstream.

The second type of filariasis also is known as onchocerciasis or river blindness. The adult helminths reside in subcutaneous nodules and migrate to the eye, causing ocular lesions and eventual loss of vision.

Cestode Infections

Cestodes cause taeniasis infections. Tapeworm infections are transmitted in contaminated raw or improperly cooked fish (*Diphyllobothrium latum*), beef (*Taenia saginata*), and pork (*Taenia solium*). The adult tapeworm consists of a head (scolex) that attaches to the intestinal wall and segments called proglottids. The proglottids contain tapeworm eggs and are expelled in feces. Beef and fish tapeworms do not cause serious illness. Pork tapeworms, however, produce larvae that enter the bloodstream and invade other body tissues. Symptoms include nausea, vomiting, diarrhea, fatigue, hunger, and dizziness.

Trematode Infections

Trematodes cause schistosomiasis, which is a leading cause of morbidity and mortality from parasitic diseases. The vector of schistosomiasis is a specific snail; humans acquire this parasite by drinking or contacting contaminated water. There are three major types of schistosomes. Each migrates to a specific part of the human host and produces clinical symptoms specific to each type.

Ectoparasitic Infections

Common ectoparasitic infections include scabies and pediculosis (lice).

Scabies

Scabies is a skin inflammation caused by a mite, *Sarcoptes scabiei*. The mite is barely visible with the naked eye and is transmitted by contact with an infected individual or infested bedding. Characteristic lesions consist of generalized excoriations with small pruritic vesicles, pustules, and burrows. The infestations occur on the sides of the fingers and the palms, wrists, and elbows and around the axillae. The head and neck are usually spared in adults. Diagnosis is made by identifying the parasite or its ova or feces microscopically. Treatment includes all family members and close contacts, which helps prevent reinfestation.

Pediculosis

Pediculosis is also known as lice. Pediculosis infestations occur on the scalp (pediculosis capitis), trunk (pediculosis corporis), or pubic areas (pediculosis pubis). Each year, approximately 6 to 12 million children between the ages of 3 and 12 years are infested with head lice. Transmission is by direct contact with lice, particularly those on hats, combs, and body hair. Symptoms include pruritus with excoriation, nits on hair shafts, and lice on skin or clothes.

C ANTIMALARIAL DRUGS

Drug therapy for malaria comprises three distinct types: suppressive therapy (prophylaxis), treatment of an acute attack (clinical cure), and prevention of a relapse (radical cure). Some drugs may be used in more than one type of therapy. Drug therapy is guided by three factors: the identity of *Plasmodium* species (laboratory confirmation necessary), the clinical status of the patient, and the geographic area where the infection was acquired (Figure 47.2).

Most cases of malaria, especially in the United States, are considered uncomplicated and are generally treated with oral antimalarial drugs. Patients with symptoms such as impaired consciousness/coma, severe normocytic anemia, renal failure, pulmonary edema, acute respiratory distress syndrome, circulatory shock, disseminated intravascular coagulation, spontaneous bleeding, acidosis, hemoglobinuria, jaundice, and repeated generalized convulsions have severe malaria and are treated with parenteral drugs.

Chloroquine (Aralen) is the prototype antimalarial drug. Table 47.1 presents a summary of selected antimalarial drugs.

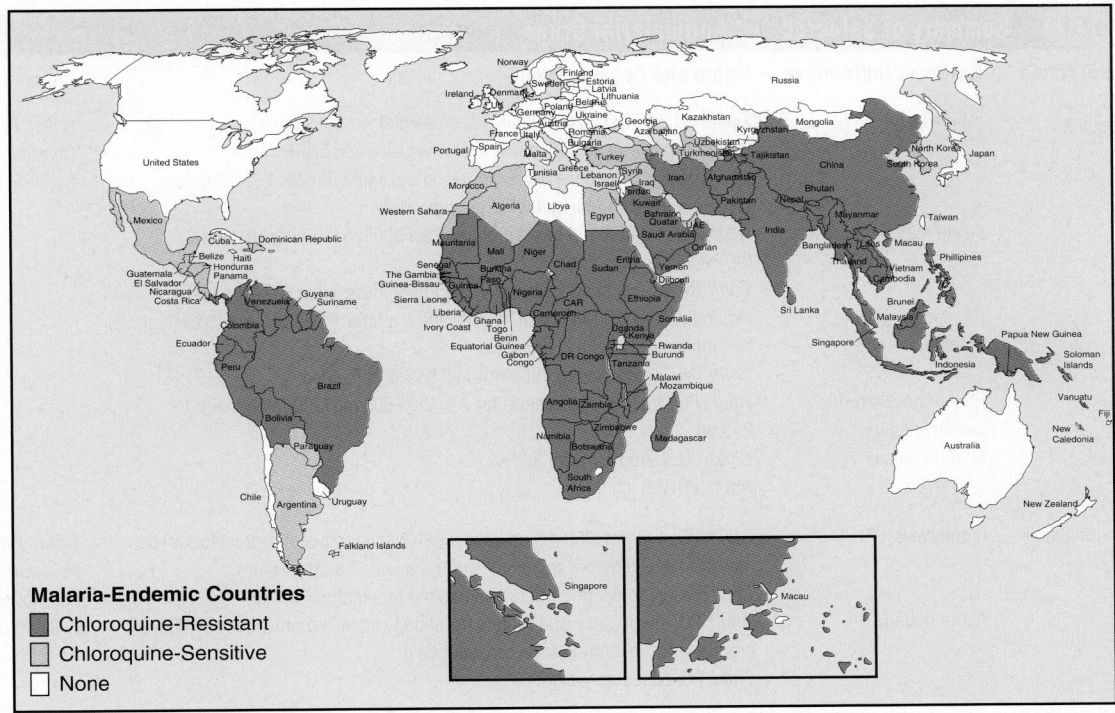

- FIGURE 47.2 Malaria-endemic countries. (Source: Centers for Disease Control and Prevention, *http://www. cdc.gov/malaria/.*)

Nursing Management of the Patient Receiving [P] Chloroquine

Core Drug Knowledge

Pharmacotherapeutics

Chloroquine is indicated to suppress or treat acute attacks of malaria caused by *P. vivax, P. malariae, P. ovale,* and susceptible strains of *P. falciparum.* It does not prevent relapses because it is not effective against exoerythrocytic forms of the parasite. Also, it does not prevent infections caused by *P. vivax* or *P. malariae* when administered as a prophylactic. In addition to its use in treating malaria, chloroquine also is used to treat extraintestinal amebiasis, rheumatoid arthritis, and systemic lupus erythematosus.

Pharmacokinetics

Chloroquine is absorbed rapidly and completely from the gastrointestinal (GI) system. The drug concentrates in the erythrocytes (RBCs), liver, spleen, kidney, lung, melanin-containing tissues, and leukocytes (white blood cells). It penetrates the central nervous system (CNS) and crosses the placenta. Although chloroquine action peaks rapidly, its half-life is between 70 and 120 hours. About 70% of chloroquine is excreted unchanged by the kidneys. Any unabsorbed drug is excreted in feces. Small amounts of chloroquine have been detected in urine for months and even years after treatment stops.

Pharmacodynamics

Chloroquine, a 4-aminoquinoline, is classified as a blood schizonticide. In treating malaria, its direct effects are on the parasite. Chloroquine is taken up by plasmodia residing within the RBCs of the human host. Chloroquine is thought to increase blood pH and upset phospholipid metabolism in the parasite, thereby interrupting the synthesis of ribonucleic acid (RNA) and deoxyribonucleic acid (DNA). In patients with rheumatoid arthritis, chloroquine antagonizes histamine and serotonin, thereby inhibiting prostaglandin synthesis. The result is an anti-inflammatory effect. The drug's action in treating amebiasis is unknown.

Contraindications and Precautions

Chloroquine is contraindicated for patients with a hypersensitivity to any 4-aminoquinoline, such as hydroxychloroquine. Chloroquine also is contraindicated for patients with pre-existing eye disease because the drug can cause corneal opacities, keratopathy, or retinopathy. Retinopathy can lead to blindness and can progress even after the drug is discontinued.

Chloroquine is used with caution in patients with various pre-existing disorders. In patients with psoriasis or porphyria, chloroquine has precipitated severe attacks. Because chloroquine concentrates in the liver, it can produce toxic effects in patients with hepatic disease or alcoholism or in patients using other hepatotoxic drugs concurrently. The drug should be given with caution to patients with GI disorders, blood dyscrasias, dental disease, and neurologic disorders. Patients with these conditions may have exacerbations of disease because of the actions and potential adverse effects of chloroquine. Chloroquine has a black box

TABLE 47.1	Summary of Selected ⒼAntimalarial Drugs		
Drug (Trade) Name	**Selected Indications**	**Route and Dosage Range**	**Pharmacokinetics**
℗ chloroquine (Aralen)	Prophylaxis	*Adult:* PO, 500 mg (300-mg base) once a week on the same day for 1–2 wk before exposure and continuing until 4 wk after exposure *Child:* PO, 5 mg/kg base once a week on the same day for 1–2 wk before exposure and continuing 4 wk after exposure	*Onset:* Rapid *Duration:* 1 wk t₁/₂: 3–5 d
	Acute malaria attack	*Adult:* PO, 1 g (600-mg base) initially, then 500 mg (300-mg base) at 6, 24, and 48 h *Child:* PO, 10-mg base/kg initially, then 5-mg base/kg at 6, 24, and 48 h	
	Extraintestinal amebiasis	*Adult:* IM, 160–200-mg base initially and 6 h later if needed; not to exceed 800 mg base/d *Child:* IM, 5-mg base/kg initially and 6 h later if needed	
	Rheumatoid arthritis/ systemic lupus erythematosus	*Adult:* PO, 1 g (600-mg base)/d for 2 d, then 500 mg (300-mg base)/d for 2–3 wk *Child:* PO, 10 mg/kg/d for 2-3 wk *Adult:* PO 150 mg daily	
atovaquone/proguanil (Malarone)	Prophylaxis	*Adult:* PO, 1 tablet (250 mg atovaquone/100 mg proguanil hydrochloride) per day; start 1–2 d before travel and continue until 7 d after return. *Child:* Based on weight; not recommended for children <11 kg	*Onset:* Rapid *Duration:* Unknown t₁/₂: atovaquone, 2–3 d; proguanil, 12–21 h
	Acute malaria	*Adult:* PO, single dose of 4 tablets (total daily dose, 1 g atovaquone/400 mg proguanil hydrochloride)for 3 consecutive d *Child:* PO, based on weight	
Hydroxychloroquine (Plaquenil Sulfate)	Prophylaxis	*Adult:* PO, 310-mg base/wk on the same day each week, beginning 1–2 wk before exposure and continuing for 4 wk after leaving the malaria area *Child:* 5-mg base/kg/wk, then the same dosage regimen as for adults	*Onset:* Rapid *Duration:* Unknown t₁/₂: 50 d
	Acute malaria attack	*Adult:* PO, initial dose (day 1), 620-mg base; dose 2 (6 h after dose 1), 310 mg; dose 3 (day 2), 310 mg; dose 4 (day 3), 310 mg *Child:* PO, same as for adult in the following amounts, respectively: 10 mg/kg base, 5 mg/kg, 5 mg/kg, 5 mg/kg	
mefloquine (Lariam)	Prophylaxis	*Adult:* PO, 250 mg weekly beginning 1–2 wk before exposure and continuing for 4 wk after exposure *Child:* PO, based on weight, starting 1–2 wk before exposure and for 4 wk after exposure	*Onset:* Delayed *Duration:* Unknown t₁/₂: 3 wk
	Acute malaria attack	*Adult:* PO, 750 mg initially, followed by 500 mg 6–12 h after initial dose *Child:* PO, 15 mg/kg initially, followed by 10 mg/kg 6–12 h after initial dose	
primaquine	Prophylaxis in special circumstances	*Adult:* PO, 30 mg daily beginning 1–2 d before exposure until 7 d after return *Child:* PO, 0.5 mg/kg beginning 1–2 d before exposure until 7 d after return *Adult:* PO, 30 mg base for 14 d *Child:* PO, 0.5 mg/kg base for 14 d	*Onset:* Rapid *Duration:* Unknown t₁/₂: 3.7–9.6 h
pyrimethamine/ sulfadoxine (Fansidar)	Suppression of malaria (used in conjunction with quinine) Toxoplasmosis	*Adult:* PO, 25 mg pyrimethamine/500 mg sulfadoxine (fixed dose), 2–3 tablets on the last day of quinine dosing *Child:* PO, Age 9–14 y: 2 tablets Age 4–8 y: 1 tablet Age <4 y: 1/2 tablet	*Onset:* Unknown *Duration:* Unknown t₁/₂: 56–148 h
quinine	Chloroquine-resistant malaria Chloroquine-sensitive malaria	*Adult:* PO, 650 mg q8h, for 5–7 d *Child:* PO, 25 mg/kg/d in divided doses q8h for 5–7 d *Adult:* PO, 600 mg q8h for 5–7 d *Child:* PO, 10 mg/kg/d in divided doses q8h for 5–7 d	*Onset:* Varies *Duration:* Varies t₁/₂: 4–5 h
quinidine gluconate	Severe *P. falciparum*	*Adult and child:* IV, 6.25 mg base/kg over 1–2 h, then 0.0125 mg base/mg/min for at least 24 h or 15 mg base/kg infused over 4 h, followed by 7.5 mg base/kg infused over 4 h, q8h, starting 8 h after the loading dose	*Onset:* Rapid *Duration:* 6–8 h t₁/₂: 6–7 h

warning that it should be administered only for malaria and extraintestinal amebiasis.

Chloroquine is a pregnancy category C drug. It should be given with extreme caution to infants and children because of potentially fatal toxicities.

Adverse Effects

Potential adverse effects of chloroquine may affect the cardiovascular, GI, hematologic, integumentary, and neurologic systems. The most common adverse effects are hypotension, cardiac changes reflected on an electrocardiogram (ECG), nausea, vomiting, diarrhea, and abdominal pain.

Infrequent but important potential adverse effects include blurred vision, difficulty focusing, changes in accommodation, irreversible retinal damage, tinnitus and reduced hearing in patients with pre-existing auditory damage, headaches or psychic stimulation, convulsive seizures, and neuromyopathy.

Potential adverse hematologic effects include agranulocytosis, aplastic anemia, pancytopenia, neutropenia, and thrombocytopenia. Potential integumentary effects are pruritus, skin discoloration, skin eruption, and hair bleaching or loss.

Patients who exhibit signs of toxicity may complain of headache, drowsiness, visual disturbances, nausea, or vomiting. Cardiovascular collapse, convulsions, and respiratory or cardiac arrest may rapidly follow. Patients suspected of experiencing toxicity should go to an emergency department.

Drug Interactions

Chloroquine may interact with cimetidine, penicillamine, cyclosporine, and methotrexate. With aluminum and magnesium-containing antacids, its absorption is decreased. Most patients remember any prescription drugs they are taking, but they may forget to mention over-the-counter (OTC) drugs, such as cimetidine or antacids. Therefore, it is important to remember to assess the patient's use of OTC drugs as well. See Table 47.2 for more information.

Assessment of Relevant Core Patient Variables

Health Status

Before administering chloroquine, assess for anemia, porphyria, psoriasis, ocular disease, neurologic disorders, liver and kidney diseases, and other conditions that contraindicate using the drug or that require close monitoring. Next, review the patient's drug history to identify substances that may interact with chloroquine and advise the patient to consult with the prescriber before taking any OTC drugs.

Because chloroquine may affect the eyes, arrange for the patient to have a complete baseline ophthalmologic examination, including visual acuity, slit-lamp, and funduscopic examinations. Similarly, because chloroquine may affect reflexes, muscle strength, and hearing, perform a physical examination and document baseline measurements of these factors. Additional baseline data include laboratory results related to liver function, kidney function, and complete blood count (CBC).

Life Span and Gender

In general, chloroquine may be administered to children to prevent or treat malaria. However, careful monitoring is needed because of the drug's potential for fatal toxicity in children. Assess the adult female patient for pregnancy or lactation. Breast-feeding women need to know that chloroquine enters breast milk. Although chloroquine is assigned to pregnancy category C, most prescribers believe the benefits of chloroquine therapy outweigh the risks associated with malaria.

TABLE 47.2	Agents That Interact with P Chloroquine	
Interactants	Effect and Significance	Nursing Management
aluminum/magnesium antacids	Antacids containing aluminum or magnesium may decrease absorption and therapeutic effect of chloroquine; antacid activity may also be decreased.	Administer doses of chloroquine and antacids containing aluminum or magnesium at least 2 h apart.
cimetidine	Metabolism of chloroquine may be decreased, resulting in elevation of chloroquine serum concentration.	Monitor for possible chloroquine toxicity.
cyclosporine	Chloroquine may inhibit metabolism of cyclosporine, resulting in elevated cyclosporine serum concentration.	Monitor for signs of nephrotoxicity.
methotrexate	Chloroquine reduces the bioavailability of methotrexate.	Monitor for decreased efficacy of methotrexate.
penicillamine	Serum levels of penicillamine may be increased. This may induce hematologic, renal, or skin reactions to penicillamine.	During concurrent use of penicillamine and chloroquine, monitor patient closely for adverse effect to penicillamine. Avoid concurrent use if possible.

Lifestyle, Diet, and Habits

Determine the patient's willingness or ability to arrange activities and lifestyle to accommodate weekly therapy for suppression.

Environment

It is important to ensure that the patient understands the need for prophylactic drug therapy. People traveling to areas where malaria is endemic should begin drug prophylaxis 2 weeks before the trip begins and continue therapy for 4 to 6 weeks after returning. In addition to taking pharmacologic prophylaxis, the patient should implement activities, such as using insect repellent, protective clothing, and netting, that decrease exposure to disease-bearing mosquitoes.

Nursing Diagnoses and Outcomes

• Acute Pain related to headache and itching resulting from drug therapy
Desired outcome: *The patient will use acetaminophen and take soothing oatmeal baths to relieve drug-related discomforts.*
• Risk for Deficient Fluid Volume related to drug-induced fluid losses from nausea, vomiting, diarrhea, and anorexia
Desired outcome: *The patient will maintain adequate hydration despite the effects of drug therapy and minimize GI upset by taking the drug with food.*
• Ineffective Protection related to possible agranulocytosis, aplastic anemia, neutropenia, and thrombocytopenia resulting from drug therapy
Desired outcome: *The patient will report signs and symptoms of blood abnormalities (bruising, unexplained fatigue) to the prescriber immediately.*
• Disturbed Sensory Perception, Auditory and Visual related to potential tinnitus, hearing loss, retinopathy, and blurred vision related to drug therapy
Desired outcome: *The patient will report problems with hearing or vision to the prescriber immediately.*
• Risk for Injury: Cardiovascular Toxicity, Neuromyopathy, or Seizures related to drug therapy
Desired outcome: *The patient will remain free of injury throughout therapy with chloroquine.*

Planning and Intervention

Maximizing Therapeutic Effects

The patient taking chloroquine on a weekly basis for prophylaxis should take the drug on the same day each week, usually by mouth. An intramuscular (IM) injection is given when the oral route is not possible. In such situations, the nurse or patient injects the drug into a large muscle mass, making sure to aspirate to avoid hitting a blood vessel. The IM route is unsuitable for children because of the risk for toxic effects. For children, the bitter-tasting tablets may be pulverized and mixed with a pleasantly flavored preparation, such as chocolate syrup or grape jam.

Minimizing Adverse Effects

The patient may take chloroquine with meals to minimize GI discomfort. After taking the drug, the patient may need to change positions slowly to minimize symptoms of dizziness or light-headedness, which signify a hypotensive response. The patient who experiences pruritus (itching) may be soothed by an oatmeal bath because antihistamines are ineffective in such cases. To relieve a headache, the patient may take acetaminophen. Patients with blood dyscrasias or myelosuppression should postpone dental work or other procedures that increase the risk for infection. Patients with these disorders have a higher risk for infection. Double-check pediatric doses to prevent toxicity.

Providing Patient and Family Education

• Teach patients how to take chloroquine to prevent or treat malaria.
• Prophylactic chloroquine therapy should begin about 1 to 2 weeks before entering the malarial area and should continue for 4 to 6 weeks after leaving the area.
• Tell patients to wear cover-up clothing as a barrier to mosquitoes (Box 47.1).
• Explain that if a fever develops within 2 months after a trip to a malarial area, the patient should notify the health care provider immediately.
• Point out potential adverse effects of chloroquine. For example, chloroquine use may discolor urine (red or brown). In addition, itching, nausea, vomiting, dizziness, and headaches may occur. Periodic ophthalmologic and audiometric examinations should be scheduled by patients taking prolonged therapy because the drug can cause vision and hearing problems. Instruct patients to contact the prescriber immediately if fever, sore throat, easy bruising, unusual fatigue, or problems with hearing or eyesight develop.
• Caution patients to avoid alcohol while taking chloroquine.
• Caution patients to notify the prescriber if nausea, vomiting, or diarrhea is persistent.

BOX 47.1 COMMUNITY BASED CONCERNS

Stop Malaria Before It Starts!

• In addition to prophylactic pharmacotherapy instructions, include the following when educating the patient about malaria:
• Be sure to use mosquito netting. Check for holes in the net.
• Always sleep in screened areas. Spray the area with permethrin-containing insecticide before the sun sets.
• Wear protective clothing. Use 30-mL DEET (N,N-diethyl metatoluamide) in 250 mL of water to impregnate cotton garments.
• Minimize nocturnal exposure; long-sleeved clothing and long pants should be worn outdoors after sunset.
• DEET insect repellents should be applied to exposed skin. Refined lemon eucalyptus oil also may be used on the skin but is not as effective.

Ongoing Assessment and Evaluation

Monitor patients taking chloroquine for episodes of misty or foggy vision, difficulty reading and complaints that words tend to disappear, and visual field changes (e.g., seeing half an object, light flashes or streaks, or pigmentation changes). Evaluate the patient's gross hearing, reflexes, and muscle strength throughout therapy. In addition, assess for irritability, excitability, and personality or behavioral changes and signs and symptoms of anemia and hepatic or renal dysfunction. Symptomatic patients or patients at high risk for hemolytic anemia should have periodic blood analyses. Institute seizure precautions as needed.

Drugs Closely Related to 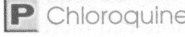 Chloroquine

Hydroxychloroquine

Hydroxychloroquine (Plaquenil Sulfate) is very similar to chloroquine but is less toxic. Although it may be used to treat malaria, it is used more commonly to treat rheumatoid arthritis and lupus erythematosus. Higher dosages are needed for treating rheumatoid arthritis.

The pharmacokinetics and pharmacodynamics of hydroxychloroquine are the same as those of chloroquine, except that it is unknown whether it enters breast milk. Because the drugs are so similar and chloroquine does enter breast milk, the safest course is to refrain from its use in patients who are breast-feeding.

Hydroxychloroquine has the same extensive adverse effect profile as chloroquine. Like chloroquine, the most common adverse effects of hydroxychloroquine affect the GI tract. Patients should take hydroxychloroquine with food to minimize these effects.

Primaquine

Primaquine is an 8-aminoquinoline. It is classified as a tissue schizonticide. The exact mechanism of action is uncertain,

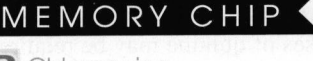

MEMORY CHIP

P Chloroquine

- Used primarily for malaria; secondarily for amebiasis, rheumatoid arthritis, and lupus
- Major contraindications: pre-existing eye diseases
- Most common adverse effects: hypotension, nausea, vomiting, diarrhea, and abdominal pain
- Most serious adverse effects: retinopathy and aplastic anemia
- Maximizing therapeutic effects: Administer medication on the same day each week.
- Minimizing adverse effects: Administer with meals to decrease potential GI effects.
- Most important patient education: Begin prophylaxis 2 weeks before entering any area where malaria is endemic and continue for 4 to 6 weeks after leaving the area.
- **Black box warning: Administer only for treatment of malaria and extraintestinal amebiasis**

although it is believed to interfere with the function of plasmodial DNA. Primaquine is the only tissue schizonticide available for the radical cure of *P. vivax* and *P. ovale* infection (killing dormant plasmodium in the liver). In addition to destroying exoerythrocytic (tissue) forms, primaquine prevents the development of erythrocytic (blood) forms, which cause relapses in *P. vivax* infection. Primaquine also is gametocidal for all four *Plasmodium* species.

Because of its potential toxicity, primaquine is not used as a first-line drug, except in cases of chloroquine-resistant malaria. Toxicity may occur when primaquine is given concurrently with other antimalarial drugs, such as quinacrine.

Primaquine is contraindicated for patients with known sensitivity. Patients with iodoquinol hypersensitivity may have cross-sensitivity to primaquine. Patients must be tested for glucose-6-phosphate dehydrogenase (G6PD) deficiency and have a documented G6PD level in the normal range before using primaquine. Those with pre-existing hematologic conditions secondary to G6PD deficiency are at risk for developing hemolytic anemia and methemoglobinemia.

Symptoms such as dark urine, anorexia, pallor, unusual tiredness or weakness, and back, leg, or abdominal pain may indicate that the patient is developing hemolytic anemia. Bluish fingernails, lips, or skin; dizziness; breathing difficulty; or unusual tiredness or weakness may indicate methemoglobinemia. This adverse effect occurs most frequently with high-dose therapy. If any of these adverse reactions occur, primaquine treatment must be discontinued immediately.

Drugs Significantly Different From **P** Chloroquine

Artemether/lumefantrine

Artemether/lumefantrine (Coartem) is the newest drug approved for the treatment of malaria in the United States. It is approved for treatment of uncomplicated *P. falciparum* disease, but not for prevention. Artemether/lumefantrine is prescribed based on weight and is given over 3 days for a total of 6 doses: an initial dose, second dose after 8 hours, and then twice daily for the following 2 days. It should be administered with food to increase its absorption. Precautions for its use include patients with a history of QT prolongation, or those taking QT-prolongation drugs, and patients taking drugs using the same metabolic pathway (CYP3A4), such as antiretroviral agents. Artemether/lumefantrine should not be given within 1 month of halofantrine treatment. Adverse effects such as headache, anorexia, dizziness, asthenia, arthralgia, and myalgia occur commonly in adults. The most common adverse effects in children are pyrexia, cough, vomiting, anorexia, and headache. It is a pregnancy category C.

Atovaquone/Proguanil

Atovaquone/proguanil (Malarone) is used for the treatment of uncomplicated *P. falciparum* disease. The advantage of atovaquone/proguanil is that it is effective in regions where resistance to other antimalarial drugs has developed. Another unique feature of atovaquone/proguanil is that it is not metabolized. It is eliminated by biliary excretion.

Atovaquone/proguanil therapy should be started 1 or 2 days before entering a malaria-endemic area and continued daily during the stay and for 7 days after return. It should be taken at the same time each day with food or milk to increase its bioavailability. In the event of vomiting, a repeat dose should be taken within 1 hour of dosing.

Among adults who receive atovaquone/proguanil for the treatment of malaria, adverse effects can include abdominal pain, nausea, vomiting, and headache. Among pediatric patients, vomiting and itching have been reported. This drug combination should not be used in infants less than 11 kg, pregnant women, women breast-feeding infants less than 11 kg, or patients with severe renal impairment (creatinine clearance less than 30 mL/min).

Mefloquine

Mefloquine (Lariam), a 4-quinolinemethanol derivative, is related chemically to quinine. Mefloquine is used for chloroquine-resistant and multidrug-resistant *P. falciparum*. Mefloquine prevents erythrocytic parasites from replicating but has no action on exoerythrocytic parasites. Its mechanism of action is unknown, but it may work by raising intravascular pH in parasite acid vesicles, causing death.

Despite its variable absorption, mefloquine is given orally because it is irritating to tissues. It is distributed widely, crosses the placenta, and may enter breast milk. It is highly bound to plasma proteins and concentrates in blood erythrocytes.

Mefloquine is contraindicated in persons with known hypersensitivity to the drug. It is also contraindicated in patients with seizure disorders, depression, acute anxiety disorder, or other psychiatric disturbances. Mefloquine is contraindicated during pregnancy because it is potentially teratogenic and embryotoxic.

The adverse effects of mefloquine when used in suppressive therapy are GI disturbance, headache, insomnia, abnormal dreams, visual disturbances, and dizziness. Psychiatric symptoms such as acute anxiety, depression, restlessness, or confusion may also occur during prophylaxis, but they are more frequent when the drug is given for acute malaria. When these symptoms occur while the patient is taking mefloquine as prophylaxis, the drug must be discontinued and an alternative drug substituted.

Several important drug–drug interactions can occur with mefloquine. Concurrent use of beta blockers, quinine, or quinidine can result in ECG abnormalities or cardiac arrest. Coadministration with chloroquine or quinine increases the risk of seizure activity. Concurrent use with valproic acid may decrease valproic acid concentrations, resulting in loss of seizure control.

Quinine Sulfate

Quinine sulfate has been used to treat malaria for more than 170 years. In combination with an adjunctive drug, quinine sulfate is the drug of choice for treatment against chloroquine-resistant plasmodia. Quinine is substantially more toxic than chloroquine. It is active against the asexual erythrocytic forms of *Plasmodium*. It does not provide a radical cure for malaria because it is not effective against exoerythrocytic forms of malaria.

Although the exact mechanism of action is unknown, quinine elevates the pH of parasitic acid vesicles and may upset molecular transport and phospholipase activity. Quinine is administered orally and distributes widely into the liver, lungs, kidneys, and spleen, with some distribution into the cerebrospinal fluid (CSF). Although it crosses the placenta and enters breast milk, the American Academy of Pediatrics considers quinine compatible with breast-feeding.

Quinine should not be used in patients with a known allergy to quinidine. Patients with quinidine hypersensitivity may have cross-sensitivity to quinine. Quinine is a pregnancy category X drug. Quinine can cause congenital malformation and has been associated with stillbirths. In addition to the potential effects on the fetus, quinine stimulates the release of insulin and may induce hypoglycemia in pregnant women.

In addition, quinine should be used cautiously in patients with G6PD deficiency, myasthenia gravis, or cardiac arrhythmias. Patients with G6PD deficiency have a higher than usual risk for developing hemolytic anemia. Quinine produces neuromuscular blockade and can exacerbate muscular weakness and cause respiratory distress and dysphagia in myasthenic patients. Patients with cardiac arrhythmias may be at risk for developing quinine-induced dysrhythmias. Patients treated with quinine have shown prolonged Q-T intervals.

Quinine should not be used for patients with optic neuritis or tinnitus because it can exacerbate these conditions. Even at therapeutic dosages, quinine may cause cinchonism (tinnitus, headache, nausea, vertigo, and vision impairment).

Quinine can cause several important drug–drug interactions. High doses of quinine can affect the clearance of digitalis glycosides and require dosage adjustment to avoid digoxin toxicity. Alkalinization of the urine by acetazolamide can decrease the renal clearance of quinine, resulting in an increased risk for toxicity. Conversely, rifampin has been shown to substantially accelerate quinine clearance and reduce its half-life. Higher doses of quinine may be required in patients who are receiving rifampin. Quinine can increase the hypoprothrombinemic (anticoagulant) effects of warfarin. The patient should be closely monitored for signs and symptoms of bleeding. Additionally, the possibility of cinchonism is increased if quinine and quinidine are administered concomitantly. Finally, quinine should not be used concomitantly with mefloquine because additive cardiac effects can produce arrhythmias and seizures.

Quinidine Gluconate

Quinidine gluconate is the only parenteral antimalarial drug in the United States. It is actually an antiarrhythmic drug that also slows or destroys the parasites in the red blood cells. Parenteral therapy is indicated for patients with life-threatening *P. falciparum* malaria who have symptoms such as impaired consciousness, severe normocytic anemia, renal failure, pulmonary edema, acute respiratory distress syndrome, circulatory shock, disseminated intravascular coagulation, spontaneous bleeding, acidosis, hemoglobinuria, jaundice, generalized seizures, and/or parasitemia more than 5%.

Quinidine gluconate has not been generally used in the United States; newer, less toxic antiarrhythmic drugs have been developed. It is contraindicated for patients with pre-existing arrhythmias and myasthenia gravis. Because of the potential for cardiotoxicity, the drug is contraindicated for patients who have received 40 mg/kg of quinine in the preceding 48 hours or those who have received mefloquine within the preceding 12 hours.

Quinidine gluconate is administered in an intensive care setting. Continuous cardiac monitoring, blood pressure monitoring, and glucose monitoring are imperative. It is necessary to watch for hypotension and widening of the QRS complex or lengthening of the QTc interval. When the patient's parasitemia is less than 1% and the patient is able to tolerate oral medication, treatment is completed with oral quinine for 3 days (if exposure occurred in Africa or South America) and 7 days (if exposure occurred in Southeast Asia).

Several potential drug interactions, especially with other drugs that alter cardiac rhythm, are associated with quinidine gluconate.

Antibacterials

Doxycycline, tetracycline, and clindamycin are antibacterial agents used in combination with quinine or quinidine to treat malaria. Doxycycline is also used to prevent malaria in chloroquine-resistant areas. These three drugs are discussed in Chapter 40.

C ANTIPROTOZOAN DRUGS

Antiprotozoan drugs are used to treat many human infections, including amebiasis, giardiasis, trichomoniasis, toxoplasmosis, and opportunistic infections such as PCP. The most frequently used drugs are metronidazole, iodoquinol, pentamidine, and atovaquone. Some drugs are effective for many types of infections, whereas others are effective for only one or two types of infections (Box 47.2). Because of an increase in the past decade in protozoan infections in the United States, many new antiprotozoan drugs are being developed. Several drugs are obtainable only from the Centers for Disease Control and Prevention (CDC) in Atlanta, Georgia.

• DRUGS AFFECTING AMEBIASIS, GIARDIASIS, TRICHOMONIASIS, AND TOXOPLASMOSIS

Metronidazole (Flagyl) is the prototype antiprotozoan drug for treating amebiasis, giardiasis, and trichomoniasis. In addition to its antiprotozoan effects, metronidazole has antibacterial effects and is extremely effective against the anaerobic bacteria that cause intra-abdominal infections and *Helicobacter pylori*, which is a cause of peptic ulcer disease. For a summary of selected antiprotozoal drugs, see Table 47.3.

Box 47.2 DRUGS FOR PROTOZOAN DISEASES

	Amebiasis	Cryptosporidiosis	Giardiasis	Pneumocystis jiroveci	Trichomoniasis	Toxoplasmosis
atovaquone				X		
dapsone				X		
furazolidone			X			
iodoquinol	X		X			
metronidazole	X		X		X	
nitazoxanide		X	X			
paromomycin	X					
pentamidine				X		
primaquine				X		
pyrimethamine						X
SMP-TMZ				X		
quinacrine			X			
tinadazole	X		X		X	

Nursing Management of the Patient Receiving P Metronidazole
Core Drug Knowledge
Pharmacotherapeutics

Metronidazole is a synthetic antibacterial and antiprotozoan drug in a class called nitroimidazoles. As an antiprotozoan drug, it is the drug of choice for the treatment of trichomoniasis, amebiasis, and giardiasis. As an antibacterial drug, it is extremely effective against anaerobic infections. It also is useful in treating Crohn disease, antibiotic-associated diarrhea, and rosacea.

Pharmacokinetics

Metronidazole can be administered orally, intravenously, and topically. About 90% of metronidazole is absorbed orally, with food delaying but not interfering with absorption. Minimal amounts of metronidazole are absorbed systemically when it is used as an intravaginal drug. Both intravenous (IV) and oral metronidazole are distributed widely into most body tissues and fluids, including CSF. Metronidazole is metabolized in the liver and is a substrate of CYP3A4.

Pharmacodynamics

Metronidazole has no direct effects on the human body. It is taken up readily by anaerobic organisms and cells. Its selectivity for anaerobic bacteria results from the ability of these organisms to reduce metronidazole to its active form intracellularly because the electron transport proteins necessary

TABLE 47.3	Summary of Selected © Antiprotozoal Drugs		
Drug (Trade) Name	**Selected Indications**	**Route and Dosage Range**	**Pharmacokinetics**
P metronidazole (Flagyl)	Bacterial prophylaxis	*Adult:* IV, 15 mg/kg 1 h before surgery, then 7.5 mg/kg q6h ×2	*Onset:* PO, varies; IV, immediate
	Anaerobic bacterial infection	*Adult:* IV, 15 mg/kg loading dose followed by 7.5 mg/kg every 6 h for 7–10 d; not to exceed 4 g/d	*Duration:* Unknown
		Child: PO/IV, 7.5 mg/kg q48h	$t_{1/2}$: 6–8 h
	Amebiasis	*Adult:* PO, 500–750 mg 3×/d for 7–10 d	
		Child: PO/IV, 35–50 mg/kg/d in 3 doses for 5–7 d	
	Giardiasis	*Adult:* PO, 250 mg 3×/d for 5–7 d	
		Child: PO 15 mg/kg/d in 3 doses for 5-7 d	
	Trichomoniasis	*Adult:* PO, 2 g at one time or 500 mg 2×/d for 7 d	
		Child: PO 15/mg/kg/d in 3 doses for 7 d	
	Bacterial vaginosis	*Adult:* PO, 750 mg extended release daily for 7 d; pregnant females: 500 mg 2×/d or 250 mg 3×/d for 7 d	
	Antibiotic-associated pseudomembranous colitis	*Adult:* PO, 500 mg 3×/d for 7–14 d	
		Child: PO, 30 mg/kg/d, divided, 4×/d for 7–10 d	
P pentamidine (NebuPent, Pentam 300)	PCP	*Adult and child:* Inhalational, 300 mg once every 4 wk with Respigard nebulizer; IM/IV 4 mg/kg once daily for 14 d by deep IM injection or IV infusion over 60 min	*Onset:* Inhalation, rapid; IM, slow *Duration:* 6–8 wk $t_{1/2}$: 6.5–9.5 h
atovaquone (Mepron)	PCP	*Adult:* PO, 750 mg, tid for 21 d	*Onset:* Varies *Duration:* 3–5 d $t_{1/2}$: 2–3 d
iodoquinol (Yodoxin)	Amebiasis	*Adult:* PO, 650 mg tid before meals for 20 d	*Onset:* Minimal absorption
		Child: PO, 40 mg/kg/d in 3 divided doses before meals for 20 d, not to exceed 1.95 g/d	*Duration:* Unknown $t_{1/2}$: Unknown
nitazoxanide (Alinia)	Cryptosporidiosis or giardiasis	*Adult:* PO, 500 mg 2×/d for 3 d	*Onset:* Unknown
		Child 1–3 y: PO, 5 mL oral suspension q12h with food for 3 d	*Duration:* Unknown
		Child 4–11 y: PO, 10 mL oral suspension q12h with food	$t_{1/2}$: 1–1.6 h
		Child >12 y: PO, 500 mg q12h with food or 25 mL oral suspension q12h with food	
paromomycin (Humatin)	Amebiasis	*Adult and child:* PO, 25–35 mg/kg body weight daily, administered in 3 divided doses with meals, for 5–10 d	*Onset:* Unknown *Duration:* Unknown $t_{1/2}$: Unknown
pyrimethamine (Daraprim)	Toxoplasmosis	*Adult:* PO, initially 50–75 mg daily for 1–3 wk, then 25 mg daily for 4–5 wk with 1g of sulfadiazine, q6h	*Onset:* Unknown *Duration:* Unknown
		Child: PO, 1 mg/kg daily in 2 equally divided doses for 2–4 d, then 0.5 mg/kg daily for 4 wk, with 100 mg sulfadiazine daily, divided in 4 doses	$t_{1/2}$: 4 d
tinidazole (Tindamax)	Trichomoniasis	*Adult:* PO, 2 g as a single dose	*Onset:* Unknown
	Giardiasis	*Adult:* PO, 2 g as a single dose	*Duration:* Unknown
		Child >3 y: PO, 50 mg/kg as a single dose	$t_{1/2}$: 12–14 h
	Intestinal amebiasis	*Adult:* PO, 2 g daily for 3 d	
		Child >3 y: PO, 50 mg/kg daily for 3 d	
	Amebic liver abscess	*Adult:* PO, 2 g daily for 3–5 d	
		Child >3 y: PO, 50 mg/kg daily for 3–5 d	
trimetrexate (NeuTrexin)	Moderate to severe PCP not responding to other therapies; **must be given concurrently with leucovorin**	*Adult:* IV, 45 mg/m² daily over 60–90 min for 21 d **Leucovorin:** PO/IV, 20 mg/m2 4×/d; if IV, give over 5–10 min. Continue leucovorin for 3 d after the last dose of trimetrexate.	*Onset:* PO, 3 d; IV, immediate *Duration:* 12 wk $t_{1/2}$: 11–20 h

for this reaction are found only in anaerobic bacteria. Metronidazole acts against anaerobic bacteria by inhibiting DNA synthesis, which causes bacterial cell death.

Contraindications and Precautions
Major precautions are taken when using metronidazole in patients who are alcohol dependent or pregnant. Metronidazole enters fetal circulation rapidly. A theoretical risk remains for the fetus. Most prescribers prefer to postpone using metronidazole, a pregnancy B category drug, until after the first trimester. The drug also enters breast milk.

Because of the capacity for a disulfiram-like interaction (i.e., nausea, vomiting, headache, and chest pain), ingestion of metronidazole and alcohol should be separated by at least 1 day. Patients with hepatic dysfunction should be monitored for toxicity resulting from decreased clearance and possible accumulation of metronidazole. Dosage reduction may be necessary for patients with severe hepatic dysfunction. Because metronidazole can cause leukopenia, the drug should be used with caution in patients with active or previous depression of bone marrow function. Metronidazole carries a black box warning because it has been found to be carcinogenic in rodents.

Adverse Effects
The most common adverse effects of metronidazole are nausea and vomiting, dry mouth (xerostomia), altered sense of taste (dysgeusia), anorexia, and abdominal pain. Other consequences of xerostomia include periodontal disease and dental caries. Some patients report discolored (reddish brown) urine while taking metronidazole.

Other common adverse effects include CNS effects, such as dizziness, light-headedness, and headache. CNS toxicity has occurred and is exhibited as ataxia, mood changes, encephalopathy, or clumsiness. High dosages and prolonged use of metronidazole are associated with peripheral neuropathy and seizures.

As noted previously, patients receiving metronidazole who drink alcoholic beverages may experience disulfiram-like adverse effects. The flavor of alcoholic beverages may be altered as well.

Vaginal candidiasis occurs in some women because metronidazole can suppress natural bacteria, leading to an overgrowth of *Candida* organisms. Candidal overgrowth may also occur in the mouth. Symptoms include glossitis, stomatitis, and furry tongue.

IV metronidazole contains 28 mEq of sodium per gram of metronidazole, which may promote water retention and exacerbate pre-existing chronic heart failure (CHF) or peripheral edema. Oral preparations of the drug do not contain this large amount of sodium and can be used without jeopardy. Thrombophlebitis can occur from administration of IV metronidazole and is characterized as pain, redness, and swelling at the injection site. The potential for this adverse effect can be minimized by avoiding prolonged use of indwelling IV catheters.

Less common potential adverse effects include visual impairment, photophobia, and ocular motility disorders. Rare reports of optic neuritis have occurred. Additionally, using metronidazole may lead to blood dyscrasias and leukopenia. Pancreatitis is another serious, but rare, adverse reaction.

Drug Interactions
Metronidazole interferes with the metabolism of ethanol (alcohol), resulting in disulfiram-like effects, such as nausea, vomiting, and abdominal cramps. Patients taking disulfiram have reported psychotic reactions with concomitant use of metronidazole. Table 47.4 lists additional drugs that interact with metronidazole.

Assessment of Relevant Core Patient Variables

Health Status
Before administering metronidazole, assess the patient for potential medical conditions that contraindicate use or require close monitoring, such as alcoholism, cardiac disease, dental disease, hepatic disease, seizure disorders, and depressed bone marrow function.

Perform a baseline neurologic assessment because metronidazole may cause CNS toxicity or exacerbate peripheral neuropathy and seizure disorders. In addition, a baseline visual acuity assessment may be necessary. Other important assessments include liver function tests, because metronidazole is metabolized in the liver, and a CBC, particularly for patients with a history of depressed bone marrow function or severe anemia. Review the patient's drug history to identify drugs that may interact with metronidazole.

Life Span and Gender
Assess women for possible pregnancy because metronidazole, a pregnancy category B drug, is not recommended in the first trimester. Metronidazole enters breast milk and is not recommended for use in children or infants.

Lifestyle, Diet, and Habits
Determining the patient's typical intake of alcohol is important. Caution patients to refrain from alcohol ingestion for 48 hours after completing metronidazole therapy. They should also be reminded that because many OTC products contain alcohol, they should avoid using them without consulting their health care providers.

Environment
Be aware of the setting in which metronidazole will be administered. Hospitalized patients usually receive metronidazole by IV infusion. Monitor the patient's cardiovascular and respiratory status frequently because IV metronidazole may promote fluid retention, leading to an exacerbation of CHF or peripheral edema. Also, monitor the IV site frequently for signs of thrombophlebitis.

Nursing Diagnoses and Outcomes

- Risk for Deficient Fluid Volume: Anorexia, nausea, vomiting, and diarrhea related to drug administration
  Desired outcome: The patient will maintain adequate hydration throughout therapy.
- Risk for Disturbed Sensory Perception: Drug-induced dizziness, vertigo, syncope, and ataxia
  Desired outcome: The patient will compensate for sensory-perceptual disturbances by moving slowly and carefully to prevent accidents and asking for help with ambulation as needed.
- Disturbed Thought Processes: Acute confusional state related to potential disulfiram-like interaction
  Desired outcome: The patient will refrain from alcohol consumption for 48 hours after completing drug therapy.
- Risk for Injury: Potential teratogenic effects related to drug administration
  Desired outcome: The patient will act to prevent conception while taking metronidazole.

Planning and Intervention

Maximizing Therapeutic Effects

To avoid reinfection, patients taking metronidazole for *Trichomonas* infection need to understand that their sexual partners must be treated at the same time. To avoid early cessation of therapy, advise the patient that the drug may discolor the urine and reassure the patient that this discoloration is harmless.

Minimizing Adverse Effects

Because some patients downplay their intake of ethanol or neglect to mention they take disulfiram because of the social stigma attached to alcoholism, emphasize the importance of potential adverse effects resulting from the interaction of ethanol and metronidazole.

To minimize possible GI irritation, metronidazole may be administered with meals. Suggest to patients who experience dry mouth that they may use sugar-free hard candies or ice chips to moisten the mouth. Sugar-containing products

TABLE 47.4	Agents That Interact with P Metronidazole	
Interactants	Effect and Significance	Nursing Management
amiodarone	Metronidazole may inhibit metabolism of amiodarone, resulting in increased risk of adverse effects or toxicity.	Monitor for QT interval prolongation and torsade de pointes.
anticoagulants	Hepatic metabolism of anticoagulants may be decreased by metronidazole, resulting in enhanced effects of anticoagulant. This may induce hemorrhage.	Monitor patients more frequently, and teach them to recognize signs and symptoms of bleeding. Notify the prescriber, who may need to prescribe a lower dose of anticoagulant.
barbiturates	Barbiturates may induce faster elimination of metronidazole, resulting in therapeutic failure of metronidazole.	Observe for treatment failure in patients receiving a barbiturate concurrently with metronidazole. Notify the prescriber, who may need to prescribe a higher dose of metronidazole.
busulfan	Coadministration may result in increased serum busulfan level.	Monitor for signs of veno-occlusive disease and hemorrhagic cystitis.
carbamazepine	Metronidazole may inhibit metabolism of carbamazepine, resulting in increased risk of adverse effects or toxicity.	Monitor carbamazepine level. Monitor for signs of toxicity. Monitor CBC, liver and renal status.
cyclosporine	Metronidazole may inhibit metabolism of cyclosporine, resulting in increased risk of adverse effects or toxicity.	Monitor cyclosporine level. Monitor for nephrotoxicity.
disulfiram	Coadministration of disulfiram and metronidazole may result in acute psychosis or confusional state. Mechanism of the interaction is unclear.	Monitor patients closely for signs of confusion or acute psychosis. Discontinue both agents if symptoms occur. Avoid coadministration.
ethanol	Metronidazole can inhibit alcohol dehydrogenase and other alcohol-metabolizing enzymes. This can lead to an accumulation of drug in the blood and the development of disulfiram-like side effects.	Caution patient to avoid ethanol during therapy and 1–2 d after therapy stops.
hydantoins	Metronidazole may inhibit metabolism of hydantoins, resulting in an increased risk of adverse effects or toxicity.	Monitor for signs of hydantoin toxicity.
lithium	Coadministration may result in increased serum lithium level.	Monitor for signs of lithium toxicity.
tacrolimus	Coadministration may result in increased serum tacrolimus level.	Monitor for signs of toxicity or transplant rejection.

tend to promote dental caries in dry mouth, an environment that is already friendly to decay-causing organisms. Infuse IV metronidazole slowly over 1 hour.

Providing Patient and Family Education

- Create teaching plans that focus on explaining the potential adverse effects (such as GI upset, altered taste, discolored urine), adapting to adverse effects (taking drug with meals to relieve GI upset), and identifying which effects to report to the prescriber. For example, candidal overgrowth, ataxia, easy bruising, or bleeding may represent adverse effects that require immediate intervention.
- Discuss the importance of refraining from ethanol or disulfiram use during metronidazole therapy.
- For patients taking metronidazole for giardiasis, stress the importance of treating sex partners simultaneously for trichomonal infections and of having follow-up stool examinations.
- Emphasize the need for birth control measures for women taking metronidazole long-term.

Ongoing Assessment and Evaluation

When administering IV metronidazole, monitor for thrombophlebitis and signs of edema or CHF. When administering oral metronidazole, monitor all patients for signs of oral candidiasis (white spots in the mouth) and women for symptoms of vaginal candidiasis. In addition, monitor for signs and symptoms of peripheral neuropathy (numbness and tingling of the extremities) and CNS toxicity (mood changes and irritability).

For patients on prolonged therapy, arrange for periodic CBCs and liver function tests as well as tests for visual acuity. Remind the patient to schedule frequent dental checkups.

For patients with giardiasis, arrange for testing of three stool specimens, taken several days apart. Three negative stool test results indicate successful metronidazole therapy.

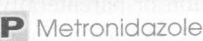

MEMORY CHIP

P Metronidazole

- Used for *Trichomonas vaginalis,* amebiasis, giardiasis, and anaerobic infections
- Major contraindications: alcohol dependency and pregnancy
- Most common adverse effects: nausea, vomiting, xerostomia, and dysgeusia
- Most serious adverse effect: blood dyscrasias
- Maximizing therapeutic effects: Treat both partners at the same time.
- Minimizing adverse effects: Assess alcohol intake closely.
- Most important patient education: Reinforce the need to refrain from alcohol intake during therapy.
- **Black box warning: Carcinogenic in rodents – avoid unnecessary use.**

Drug Closely Related to Metronidazole

Tinidazole (Tindamax) is another nitroimidazole drug with the same indications as metronidazole. The drug has a longer half-life, which means that it may be given less frequently. Adverse effects are similar to metronidazole; however, tinidazole is generally better tolerated.

Tinidazole is also a substrate of CYP3A4 and may interact with drugs that inhibit or induce this substrate. Like metronidazole, tinidazole interacts with alcohol. Advise the patient to refrain from drinking alcohol while taking tinidazole.

Drugs Significantly Different From **P** Metronidazole

Iodoquinol

Iodoquinol (Yodoxin) is an oral antiprotozoan agent used to treat intestinal amebiasis. It exerts its action directly in the large intestine, although the exact mechanism of this action is unknown. Iodoquinol is active against both the trophozoite and encysted forms of the parasite. It can be used alone in mild cases or in asymptomatic carriers. In more severe cases, it should be used in combination with metronidazole or tinidazole.

Adverse effects associated with iodoquinol include mild GI disturbances, skin disorders, discoloration of hair and nails, thyroid enlargement, fever, chills, headache, vertigo, and malaise. Neurotoxicity may induce optic neuritis, optic atrophy, and peripheral neuropathy.

Protein-bound serum iodine levels may increase during iodoquinol treatment, and therapy may therefore interfere with certain thyroid function tests. These effects may persist for up to 6 months after therapy discontinues.

Nitazoxanide

Nitazoxanide (Alinia) is used to treat diarrhea in adults and children caused by *G. lamblia* or *C. parvum*. These conditions are also sometimes referred to as traveler's diarrhea. The drug has also been shown to be as effective as metronidazole in the treatment of *Clostridium difficile* colitis. Nitazoxanide works by interfering with the pyruvate:ferredoxin oxireductase (PFOR) enzyme-dependent electron transfer reaction that is essential to anaerobic energy metabolism. Nitazoxanide is used cautiously in patients who are immunocompromised and those with liver or kidney disease because it is not known how nitazoxanide will affect these conditions. Common adverse effects are GI distress, headache, and vomiting. The effects, if any, on the developing fetus are unknown. Until more information is available, nitazoxanide should be used during pregnancy only if the maternal condition justifies the potential risk to the fetus. Teach the patient with diabetes to increase the frequency of blood glucose monitoring, because 5 mL of nitazoxanide suspension contains 1.48 g of sucrose. Teach the patient to discard any opened suspension remaining after 7 days.

Paromomycin

Paromomycin (Humatin) is not an antiprotozoan drug; it is an oral aminoglycoside antibiotic with broad-spectrum antibacterial and amebicidal activity. Paromomycin is used for extraintestinal amebiasis and cestode infestation. It is absorbed poorly from the GI tract and thus is used only for intestinal forms of amebiasis and helminths.

Adverse GI effects of paromomycin include anorexia, nausea, vomiting, gastric burning and pain, abdominal cramps, and diarrhea. Because of its antibacterial action, an overgrowth of nonsusceptible organisms, including fungi, may occur. The only important drug–drug interaction with paromomycin occurs with succinylcholine. When given in combination, paromomycin may potentiate the neuromuscular effects of succinylcholine.

Pyrimethamine

Pyrimethamine (Daraprim) is a folic acid antagonist that blocks the protozoal enzyme dihydrofolic reductase, thereby blocking the parasite's folic acid metabolism. It is used in combination with sulfadiazine for the treatment of toxoplasmosis.

After oral administration, pyrimethamine is distributed mainly into the kidneys, lungs, liver, and spleen, with concentrations in blood erythrocytes. It crosses the placenta and enters breast milk. Metabolism produces several unidentified metabolites that all are excreted in the urine. Urine excretion of this agent can persist for up to 30 days.

Pyrimethamine should be used cautiously in patients with anemia, folate deficiency, and suppressed bone marrow function. It is used cautiously in patients with pre-existing anemia because folic acid antagonism can potentiate anemias, especially megaloblastic anemia. Suppression of bone marrow function may result in myelosuppression, leading to leukopenia, agranulocytosis, or thrombocytopenia. Some clinicians routinely prescribe folic acid when treating toxoplasmosis because higher doses of pyrimethamine are necessary. Routine CBCs are also prudent. High doses of pyrimethamine may precipitate seizures.

In addition, pyrimethamine should be used with extreme caution during the first 14 to 16 weeks of pregnancy. Possible interference with folic acid metabolism could cause birth defects. If its use cannot be avoided, concurrent use of folinic acid is recommended. Use during breast-feeding should be avoided because the drug may interfere with the infant's folic acid metabolism.

Several adverse effects of pyrimethamine may occur. Common GI complaints include anorexia, nausea, vomiting, abdominal pain, and diarrhea. As with other antimalarials, taking the medication with food may decrease these symptoms. Potential dermatologic reactions include urticaria, toxic epidermal necrolysis, exfoliative dermatitis, and Stevens-Johnson syndrome. Pyrimethamine should be discontinued at the first sign of rash. CNS effects include weakness, ataxia, tremor, and, rarely, respiratory failure. In patients with pre-existing seizure disorders, pyrimethamine may precipitate seizures, especially in those on high-dose therapy.

Drug–drug interactions include the potential for the development of blood dyscrasias if pyrimethamine is used with other bone marrow depressants or folate antagonists. Bone marrow function may be more likely to be depressed with sulfonamide combination therapy. Other drugs that can interact with pyrimethamine in this manner include carbamazepine, clozapine, chloramphenicol, phenothiazines, procainamide, antiretroviral agents, antineoplastic agents, or antithyroid agents. Folic acid (vitamin B_9) can interfere with the action of pyrimethamine and therefore should not be used concomitantly with pyrimethamine.

• Drugs Affecting *Pneumocystis jiroveci* Pneumonia

Drugs used to treat PCP include pentamidine isethionate, atovaquone, primaquine, and sulfamethoxazole-trimethoprim (SMZ-TMP). SMZ-TMP, the drug of choice, is not an antiprotozoan drug but an antibiotic (see Chapter 42). Patients at high risk for PCP (low T-cell count or high viral load) and unable to take SMZ-TMP are maintained on a prophylactic dosage of pentamidine, atovaquone, or dapsone. The prototype antiprotozoan drug for prophylaxis and treatment of PCP is pentamidine isethionate (Pentam). Table 47.5 presents an overview of pentamidine.

Nursing Management of the Patient Receiving P Pentamidine Isethionate
Core Drug Knowledge
Pharmacotherapeutics
Historically, pentamidine was used only for trypanosomiasis (African sleeping sickness) and leishmaniasis. Currently, pentamidine is an important therapeutic drug for prophylaxis and treatment of PCP.

Pharmacokinetics
Pentamidine is absorbed readily and binds to body tissues. It is sequestered in the liver and kidneys and eliminated unchanged by the kidneys. Pentamidine can be detected in the urine up to 8 weeks after therapy has ended.

Pharmacodynamics
Pentamidine is administered by inhalation or parenterally. Its mechanism of action is unclear, but it appears to interfere with nucleotide, phospholipid, and protein synthesis of the parasite. It causes local tissue damage when given intramuscularly and is therefore usually given intravenously. For prophylaxis, pentamidine is delivered by inhalation through an aerosol device to the alveoli where *P. carinii* lodges.

Contraindications and Precautions
Pentamidine is contraindicated for use in patients with a history of an anaphylactic reaction to it. However, once the diagnosis of PCP is established, no absolute contraindications apply. The drug is given with caution to patients with asthma; hematologic disorders; cardiac, hepatic, and renal diseases; and diabetes mellitus.

TABLE 47.5 Overview of Pentamidine

pentamidine (NebuPent, Pentam)	Pneumocystis Jiroveci prophylaxis	Adult and child: IV 3–4 mg/kg/d for 21 d Adult and child >5 y: Aerosolized: 300 mg monthly with Respirgard II nebulizer;	Onset: Inhalation, rapid; IM, slow IV: rapid Duration: 6–8 wk $t_{1/2}$: 6.4–9.4 h

Adverse Effects

Sudden severe effects may develop after a single dose of pentamidine. Patients should be lying down and monitored closely during administration. Equipment for emergency resuscitation should be readily available.

The most frequent adverse effects from pentamidine are cough and bronchospasm, especially in patients with asthma. Another frequent adverse reaction to pentamidine is a sudden, severe hypotension.

Thrombocytopenia, leukopenia, and anemia are potential hematologic problems; arrhythmias, tachycardia, torsades de pointes, or other adverse cardiac effects may occur as well. Pentamidine is toxic to pancreatic cells. When receiving IV pentamidine, patients with diabetes mellitus can become acutely hypoglycemic immediately after the infusion. Additionally, pentamidine may precipitate pancreatitis. Pentamidine also can cause elevations in aspartate transaminase (AST), alanine transaminase (ALT), bilirubin, and alkaline phosphatase. Patients with pre-existing hepatic diseases are more vulnerable to these effects. Pentamidine can cause azotemia and acute renal insufficiency as well.

Drug Interactions

Concomitant use of other drugs associated with suppression of bone marrow function, electrolyte imbalance, pancreatitis, or nephrotoxicity may cause additive effects. Pentamidine also may interact with drugs that have similar adverse effects (Table 47.6).

Assessment of Relevant Core Patient Variables

Health Status

Assess for concurrent drug use that is potentially nephrotoxic. Obtain and review baseline measurements. These measurements include vital signs (especially blood pressure), CBC, hepatic and renal function values, and glucose and amylase levels.

Closely monitor administration of aerosolized pentamidine to patients with a history of asthma because the drug may induce bronchospasm and acute asthma.

Lifestyle, Diet, and Habits

It is important to assess lifestyle because patients at risk for PCP and diseases associated with compromised immune function include IV drug abusers, men who have sex with men, and people with multiple sex partners.

Immunocompromised patients may be taking multiple drugs, placing them at risk for potential hematologic, renal, and hepatic toxicities. Because pentamidine also may affect these systems, monitor patients closely for adverse effects.

Environment

Note the environment in which pentamidine will be administered. Many patients receive IV or aerosolized pentamidine therapy at home.

Nursing Diagnoses and Outcomes

- Ineffective Protection: Risk for drug-induced leukopenia, thrombocytopenia, and anemia
  Desired outcome: The patient will report any signs and symptoms of blood abnormalities (i.e., unusual fatigue, fever and infection, and bruising).
- Risk for Deficient Fluid Volume related to drug-induced nausea, vomiting, and anorexia
  Desired outcome: The patient will remain adequately hydrated throughout therapy.
- Risk for Injury: Hypoglycemia, hyperglycemia, or acute renal failure related to drug therapy and bronchospasm, cough, hypotension, or cardiovascular complications related to drug administration
  Desired outcome: The patient will remain free of injury or complications related to pentamidine administration.

Planning and Intervention

Maximizing Therapeutic Effects

Protect IV pentamidine from the light and use it within 24 hours of preparation. Do not mix it with other drugs because of incompatibilities, and do not mix it with saline solutions because a precipitate will form. When administering pentamidine by inhalation, give a bronchodilator before treatment to reduce bronchospasm and increase drug effectiveness.

Minimizing Adverse Effects

Administer pentamidine with the patient lying down. Obtain baseline vital signs initially, and monitor them continuously during the infusion and then every 2 hours after the infusion until blood pressure stabilizes. Do not give IM injections to patients receiving pentamidine because the injections may cause bleeding, bruising, or hematomas as a result of thrombocytopenia secondary to pentamidine-induced depression of bone marrow function. Do not administer pentamidine at bedtime because hypoglycemia may occur at a time when the patient cannot respond to the symptoms.

TABLE 47.6 Agents that Interact with P Pentamidine

Interactants	Effect and Significance	Nursing Management
Bone Marrow Suppressants		
antineoplastic agents azathioprine carbamazepine clozapine cotrimoxazole phenothiazines zidovudine	Concomitant use of bone marrow suppressants and pentamidine has the potential to cause additive hemotoxicity.	Monitor for sore throat, easy bruising, or bleeding. Monitor CBC and platelet counts.
Diuretics		
loop diuretics thiazide diuretics	Diuretics and pentamidine can produce similar toxicities.	Monitor for hypokalemia, hypomagnesemia, and pancreatitis. Monitor serum electrolyte and amylase levels.
Drugs That May Cause Nephrotoxicity		
aminoglycosides amphotericin B cyclosporine vancomycin	Drugs associated with nephrotoxicity and pentamidine have the potential for causing additive renal toxicity.	Monitor for nephrotoxicity, hypokalemia, hypomagnesemia, and bone marrow depression.
Drugs That May Cause Pancreatitis		
azathioprine didanosine estrogens furosemide tetracycline valproic acid	Drugs associated with pancreatitis and pentamidine have the potential for causing additive pancreatic toxicity.	Monitor for signs of pancreatitis. Monitor amylase levels.

Take appropriate respiratory precautions to protect health care staff from contact with organisms, such as mycobacteria, that may be aerosolized if the patient coughs.

Providing Patient and Family Education

• Make sure that patients and families understand the therapeutic and adverse effects of pentamidine and the importance of monthly treatments for PCP prophylaxis. In addition, they need to realize that PCP infection is still possible despite pentamidine prophylaxis.

• Urge patients to contact the prescriber if fever or respiratory difficulties occur. Other conditions that necessitate contact with the prescriber include nausea, vomiting, or diarrhea that does not subside; persistent urinary frequency, inability to void, continual hunger and thirst, or unexplained weight loss; and abdominal pain, leg cramps, fever, sore throat, unexplained bruising, or extreme fatigue.

• Emphasize the need for small, frequent meals despite the patients' anorexia.

Ongoing Assessment and Evaluation

For hospitalized patients receiving pentamidine, monitor blood urea nitrogen, serum creatinine, serum calcium, and blood glucose levels; CBC and platelet counts; and liver function test results (including bilirubin, alkaline phosphatase, AST, and ALT levels) on a daily basis. Arrange for the scheduling of ECGs at regular intervals throughout therapy. It is important to measure daily fluid intake and output.

Drugs Significantly Different From Pentamidine

Atovaquone

Oral atovaquone (Mepron) is indicated for the acute treatment of mild to moderate *P. carinii* in patients who are intolerant to cotrimoxazole (SMZ-TMP). Atovaquone is approximately equivalent to IV pentamidine, but less effective than cotrimoxazole, for treating PCP.

Atovaquone is unique among agents used to manage PCP because it can kill *Pneumocystis* organisms rather than merely inhibiting their growth. Besides *Pneumocystis,* atovaquone is active against other protozoans, including *Plasmodium* species, *T. gondii, E. histolytica, T. vaginalis, Leishmania* species, and microsporidia. The antiprotozoan activity of atovaquone is probably related to its ability to selectively inhibit mitochondrial electron transport, leading to inhibition of pyrimidine synthesis.

Atovaquone is absorbed poorly from the GI tract. It is a highly lipophilic compound; thus, administering it with a

MEMORY CHIP

P Pentamidine

- Used for prophylaxis and management of PCP
- Major contraindication: previous anaphylactic reactions to the drug
- Most common adverse effects: cough and broncho-spasm
- Most serious adverse effects: cardiac abnormalities, renal failure, and suppression of bone marrow function
- Maximizing therapeutic effects: Protect from light and administer within 24 hours of preparation.
- Minimizing adverse effects: Monitor blood pressure throughout administration.
- Most important patient education: Contact the health care provider if fever or respiratory difficulties occur; PCP may occur despite prophylactic treatment.

Box 47.3 WHICH DRUG FOR WHICH WORM?

	Ascariasis	Enterobiasis	Filarial	Schistosomiasis	Strongyloidiasis	Taeniasis	Trichuriasis	Trichinosis
albendazole	X	X	X		X	X	X	X
diethylcarbamazine		X						
ivermectin	X		X		X		X	
mebendazole	X	X	X				X	X
niclosamide						X		
praziquantel				X		X		
pyrantel		X						

fatty meal improves its absorption. Because many patients who are treated with atovaquone have advanced HIV infection, distinguishing adverse effects caused by atovaquone from those caused by underlying medical conditions is often difficult. No life-threatening effects have yet been attributed to atovaquone.

Trimetrexate

Trimetrexate (NeuTrexin) is a parenteral drug used for moderate to severe PCP for immunocompromised patients who are not candidates for SMZ-TMP. Additionally, the agent is an off-label drug for the treatment of colorectal cancer. To avoid serious, life-threatening adverse effects, leucovorin **must** be given concurrently with trimetrexate and continued for 3 days after the completion of trimetrexate therapy.

Contraindications to trimetrexate include anemia, a low platelet count, or a low white blood cell count because the drug may cause these adverse effects. It is also contraindicated for patients with mouth or stomach ulcers and liver or kidney dysfunction because it may make these conditions worse.

The most common adverse effects of trimetrexate include abdominal pain or tenderness, black tarry stools, blood in urine or stools, clay-colored stools, dark urine, decreased appetite, fever and sore throat, headache, itching, loss of appetite, nausea and vomiting, pinpoint red spots on skin, skin rash, swelling of feet or lower legs, unusual bleeding or bruising, unusual tiredness or weakness, and jaundice.

Trimetrexate has many drug–drug interactions. Prior to administration, a careful history of current drug therapy is necessary. The patient should be advised to refrain from receiving any vaccines during therapy. During therapy, the CBC, as well as renal and hepatic function tests, should be monitored at least two times a week.

C ANTHELMINTHIC DRUGS

As discussed previously, helminthic infections result from cestodes, nematodes, and trematodes. The most commonly used anthelminthic drugs are mebendazole, albendazole,

thiabendazole, niclosamide, pyrantel pamoate, diethylcarbamazine, oxamniquine, and praziquantel. Box 47.3 summarizes which drugs are used to treat the various types of helminths.

Of all the drugs in the class, the prototype for treating most helminths is mebendazole (Vermox). Mebendazole is indicated to treat infection with cestodes and nematodes, such as pinworm, whipworm, common roundworm, common hookworm, and American hookworm. It also is used to treat enterobiasis. Mebendazole is usually the drug of choice in helminthic infections because mixed infections are common. Table 47.7 presents a summary of selected anthelminthic drugs.

Nursing Management of the Patient Receiving **P** Mebendazole

Core Drug Knowledge

Pharmacotherapeutics

Mebendazole is an oral, broad-spectrum, synthetic anthelminthic drug. It is particularly effective against susceptible GI nematodes, such as whipworms, pinworms, hookworms, and giant roundworms. Mebendazole is considered a drug of choice for treating infections caused by these nematodes.

Pharmacokinetics

Mebendazole is absorbed minimally from the GI tract because of substantial first-pass metabolism. It is metabolized to an inactive metabolite. Approximately 10% of the drug is excreted unchanged in the urine, and the remainder is excreted in the feces.

Pharmacodynamics

Direct pharmacodynamics occurs in the parasite. Mebendazole is a broad-spectrum anthelminthic, available in chewable tablets. It selectively damages cytoplasmic microtubules in the absorptive and intestinal cells of the helminth but not in those of the host. This microtubular deterioration is irreversible and leads to disruption of absorptive

TABLE 47.7 Summary of Selected 🅒 Anthelminthic Drugs

Drug (Trade) Name	Selected Indications	Route and Dosage Range	Pharmacokinetics
🅟 mebendazole (Vermox)	ascariasis or trichuriasis infection	*Adult and child: 2:* PO, 100 mg bid for 3 consecutive d or 500 mg once	*Onset:* <2 h
	Enterobiasis	*Adult and child:* PO, 100 mg;; repeat in 2 wk	*Duration:* 48 h
	Filarial infection	*Adult and child:* PO 100 mg 2× d for 30 d	$t_{1/2}$: 3–9 h
	Trichinosis infection	*Adult and child:* PO 200–400 mg 3×/d for 3 d then 400–500 mg/d for 10 d	
albendazole (Albenza)	Pinworm	*Adult and child:* 400 mg; repeat in 2 wk	*Onset:* Rapid
	Hookworm, giant roundworm	*Adult and child:* 400 mg once only	*Duration:* Unknown
	Chinese liver fluke	*Adult and child:* 10 mg/kg for 7 d	$t_{1/2}$: 8–12 h
	Neurocysticercosis	*Adults >60 kg:* 3 cycles of 400 mg 2×/d for 28 d, with 14 d between cycles	
		Adults <60 kg: 15 mg/kg/d, as scheduled above	
	Hydatid disease	*Adult:* PO, 400 mg 2×/d for 8–30 d	
diethylcarbamazine (Hetrazan)	Ascariasis	*Adult:* PO, 13 mg/kg/d for 7–10 d	*Onset:* 1 h
		Child: PO, 6–10 mg/kg tid for 7–10 d	*Duration:* Variable
	Filariasis	*Adult:* PO, 6–10 mg/kg tid for 3–4 wk	$t_{1/2}$: 8 h
ivermectin (Stromectol)	Onchocerciasis	*Adult and child >15 kg:* PO, 150 mcg/kg 1 h after breakfast	*Onset:* Well absorbed
	Strongyloidiasis	*Adult and child >15 kg:* PO, 200 mcg/kg 1 h after breakfast	*Duration:* Unknown
	Scabies	*Adult and child >15 kg:* PO, 150–200 mcg/kg	$t_{1/2}$: 16–35 h
praziquantel (Biltricide)	Schistosomiasis	*Adult:* PO, 60 mg/kg in three equally divided doses as a 1-d treatment, with 4–6 h between doses	*Onset:* Rapid
		Child: Safety and efficacy not established	*Duration:* Unknown
	Clonorchiasis and opisthorchiasis	*Adult:* PO, 75 mg/kg in three equally divided doses as a 1-d treatment	$t_{1/2}$: 0.8–1.5 h
		Child: Safety and efficacy not established	
pyrantel pamoate (Antiminth)	Pinworm and round-worm infections	*Adult:* PO, 11 mg/kg as a single dose; maximum dose, 1 g	*Onset:* Poorly absorbed
		Child >2 y: PO, same as adults	*Duration:* Unknown
		Child <2 y: Safety and efficacy not established	$t_{1/2}$: Unknown
thiabendazole (Mintezol)	Enterobiasis	*Adult <150 lb and child >30 lb:* PO, 10 mg/kg per dose >150 lb PO, 1.5 g/dose; maximum daily dose, 3 g, 2 doses/d for 1 d; repeat in 7 d to reduce risk of reinfection	*Onset:* Rapid
			Duration: 24 h
			$t_{1/2}$: 1.2 h

and secretory functions of the cells that are essential to the helminth's survival. Efficacy varies, depending on pre-existing diarrhea and GI transit time, degree of infection, and helminth strains.

Contraindications and Precautions
Mebendazole is contraindicated in patients with hypersensitivity to the drug, and it is used with caution in patients with inflammatory bowel disease or hepatic disease and during pregnancy, especially during the first trimester. In patients with Crohn disease or ulcerative colitis, drug absorption—and therefore the risk for toxicity—is increased. Mebendazole is metabolized primarily by the liver and can accumulate in patients with hepatic impairment, increasing the risk of adverse effects. Mebendazole is a pregnancy category C drug, and because it is not known

whether mebendazole is excreted in breast milk, the drug is used with caution in breast-feeding mothers. It has not been evaluated for use in children younger than 2 years old.

Adverse Effects
Because of its poor absorption, mebendazole rarely causes systemic toxicity, except in patients with diseases that increase absorption of drugs from the bowel. Transient abdominal pain, diarrhea, dizziness, headache, and fever are common. However, these symptoms may result from expulsion of worms rather than from the drug. Other reported adverse effects include blood abnormalities, such as leukopenia, thrombocytopenia, and eosinophilia. Integumentary effects include pruritus, rash, and flushing. In the renal system, hematuria and crystalluria are possible. In addition, mebendazole may elevate liver enzyme levels.

Drug Interactions

Mebendazole may interact with antiepileptic drugs, such as carbamazepine and the hydantoins. Although the mechanism of interaction is unknown, mebendazole's pharmacologic effects may be decreased, resulting in failure to eradicate the helminth. However, no special precautions appear necessary. If an interaction is suspected, dosage may have to be increased.

Assessment of Relevant Core Patient Variables

Health Status

Assess the patient for medical conditions that contraindicate or require close monitoring during therapy. Additional assessments should be made to prepare for potential drug interactions. Collect helminth specimens to ensure that mebendazole will be therapeutic. A baseline CBC is needed because mebendazole may cause blood abnormalities.

Monitor patients with a history of Crohn disease or ulcerative colitis closely. Patients in whom the bowel lumen is no longer intact may absorb mebendazole in toxic quantities.

Life Span and Gender

Assess for pregnancy and lactation, and determine the age of the patient, before administering mebendazole. Laboratory studies of mebendazole demonstrate birth defects in animals. Therefore, it should not be given during pregnancy. The drug is in pregnancy category C. Because it has not been adequately tested in children younger than 2 years of age, it should not be given to them or to breast-feeding women.

Environment

Evaluate the patient's close contacts because helminthic infections are highly contagious. Ideally, all family members are treated simultaneously, and care is taken to disinfect clothing and bedding.

Nursing Diagnoses and Outcomes

- Acute Pain related to headache, abdominal discomfort, rash, and perianal itching from drug therapy
  Desired outcome: *The patient will adopt measures to help tolerate therapy, including taking acetaminophen for headache, taking with food if GI distress occurs, and applying cream if indicated to sooth perianal itching.*
- Risk for Deficient Fluid Volume related to drug-induced diarrhea
  Desired outcome: *Unless contraindicated, the patient will maintain fluid intake to prevent dehydration.*

Planning and Intervention

Maximizing Therapeutic Effects

If necessary, crush and mix anthelminthic tablets with applesauce or other food. Chewing the drug offers the greatest effectiveness, as does taking the drug with fatty foods, such as milk, cheese, or ice cream. All family members and close patient contacts should be treated at the same time to avoid reinfection.

Minimizing Adverse Effects

Give mebendazole with small, frequent meals if GI distress occurs. Recommend soothing oatmeal baths to relieve pruritus or rash, because antihistamines are not effective. Relaxation techniques or acetaminophen may be used to manage headaches or constant GI distress. Unless contraindicated, increase fluid intake to at least eight 8-oz glasses of fluid daily to minimize the potential for crystalluria.

Providing Patient and Family Education

- Provide information about potential adverse drug effects, such as anemia and other blood problems signaled by sore throat, fever, and fatigue. In addition, stress the importance of contacting the prescriber if serious adverse effects occur. Explain that minor adverse effects, such as itching, may be relieved with oatmeal baths.
- Instruct women of childbearing age to contact the health care provider immediately should pregnancy occur while taking mebendazole.
- Urge patients to follow the instructions of the prescriber; printed directions may be given if appropriate.
- To prevent treatment failure, encourage patients to complete the full course of drug therapy.
- To prevent future infections, urge patients to wear shoes and wash all fruits and vegetables well before eating. Moreover, it is important to teach patients about hygiene (such as laundering infested bed linens and undergarments daily) and other measures that help prevent reinfection.

Ongoing Assessment and Evaluation

Evaluation of nursing care of patients taking mebendazole includes monitoring to ensure that the helminth has been eradicated and for complications of therapy, such as dehydration in instances of severe nausea and vomiting; sore throat, fever, and easy bruising; and hematuria or crystalluria. Ensure that periodic CBC counts and liver function tests are performed in patients at risk for hematologic or hepatic effects and in patients on long-term therapy.

Drugs Closely Related to P Mebendazole
Albendazole

Albendazole (Albenza) is used in the management of multiple parasites. Approved uses include hydatid disease (echinococcosis), *Gnathostoma* infection, and neurocysticercosis (pork tapeworm). Off-label uses include infestations of hookworm, pinworm, roundworm, and Chinese liver fluke.

Adverse effects to albendazole are generally mild. They include nausea, headaches, and fever. More serious potential adverse effects include elevation of liver transaminases and neutropenia. Obtain a baseline CBC and liver function tests, and arrange for periodic repeat laboratory testing throughout therapy.

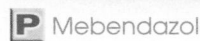

P Mebendazole

- Used for management of helminthic infections
- Major contraindication: hypersensitivity
- Most common adverse effects: abdominal pain, diarrhea, dizziness, and headache
- Most serious adverse effect: blood dyscrasias
- Maximizing therapeutic effects: Treat all family members at the same time.
- Minimizing adverse effects: small, frequent meals to decrease GI effects
- Most important patient education: Wash all clothing and bed linens at the same time the whole family is being treated.

Like mebendazole, albendazole is considered teratogenic. Follow the same precautions and patient teaching as for mebendazole.

Thiabendazole

Thiabendazole (Mintezol) is a vermicidal drug related structurally to mebendazole. It has more limited usefulness than mebendazole because of its potential toxicity. The precise mechanism of action is not clear. It inhibits specific enzymes in the helminth and is used to treat pinworm, roundworm, threadworm, and hookworm infections.

Because thiabendazole is better absorbed than mebendazole from the bowel, adverse effects are more common than with mebendazole. It is used with caution in children weighing less than 15 kg, in patients with hepatic or renal dysfunction, and in patients with severe dehydration, malnutrition, or anemia.

Drugs Significantly Different From P Mebendazole
Diethylcarbamazine

Diethylcarbamazine (Hetrazan) is the only drug currently used for suppressing and curing bancroftian and brugian filariasis. It works in two ways. First, it decreases muscular activity in the microfilariae and eventually paralyzes them. Second, it causes changes in the microfilarial surface that make the parasite more susceptible to the host's immune responses.

Common adverse effects include nausea and vomiting, anorexia, and headache. Another reaction, caused by the dying parasite, is characterized by severe itching, papular rash, tachycardia, and intense headache.

Ivermectin

Ivermectin (Stromectol) is an oral drug used in managing onchocerciasis or strongyloidiasis. Although it is not approved to treat lice and scabies, ivermectin has been used successfully to treat these conditions. Ivermectin therapy for ectoparasites is used only when treatment with topical agents fails.

Ivermectin works by binding to glutamate-gated chloride ion channels in muscle and nerve cells of the parasite. This binding results in hyperpolarization of the cell, leading to paralysis and death of the parasite.

The most common adverse effects of ivermectin are pruritus and dizziness. Ivermectin may induce a mild to severe Mazzotti reaction when administered for onchocerciasis. This reaction is an inflammatory response to the death of microfilariae; it does not occur when treating strongyloidiasis. Symptoms include itching, rash, headache, joint pain, swollen lymph nodes, fever, tachycardia, vertigo, and hypotension.

Ivermectin should not be used during pregnancy or by women who breast-feed. It should be given cautiously to patients with severe illness such as hepatic, cardiovascular, renal, or pulmonary diseases.

Pyrantel

Like mebendazole, pyrantel pamoate (Antiminth) is used to treat pinworm and roundworm infections. Unlike mebendazole, pyrantel pamoate exhibits a selective depolarizing neuromuscular blocking action that causes spastic paralysis of worms.

Pyrantel is administered as an oral suspension that is absorbed poorly from the GI tract. Because of its poor absorption, it is well tolerated by patients older than 2 years. It is metabolized in the liver and excreted mainly in feces and secondarily in urine.

Pyrantel is used with caution in patients who have liver dysfunction, anemia, or both and in patients who are malnourished or dehydrated. Its safety has not been proved during pregnancy or for children younger than 2 years of age. Pyrantel and piperazine are mutually antagonistic and should not be given together because each blocks the other's activity.

Praziquantel

Praziquantel (Biltricide) is used in treating infection with schistosomes: flukes and tapeworms. It increases the helminths' permeability to calcium, thereby causing contracture and paralysis of the helminth.

Adverse effects are minimal; the most common include malaise, headache, dizziness, and abdominal discomfort. Patients should be warned not to drive a car or operate machinery on the day of treatment and the day after. Praziquantel did not exhibit mutagenicity, carcinogenicity, or teratogenicity in animal trials. However, prescribers advise breast-feeding women to refrain from nursing on the day of treatment and for 72 hours thereafter.

C ANTIECTOPARASITIC DRUGS

Antiectoparasitic drugs include permethrin, lindane, crotamiton, malathion, pyrethrins plus piperonyl butoxide and benzyl alcohol 5%. These are topical drugs with local action. Although they can eradicate the parasite, they have minimal effect on the pruritus that frequently accompanies ectoparasitic infections. Resistance is problematic with all of the topical drugs, even those that require a prescription. The use of

TABLE 47.8   Summary of Selected Ⓒ Antiectoparasitic Drugs

Drug (Trade) Name	Selected Indications	Route and Dosage Range	Pharmacokinetics
Ⓟ permethrin (Elimite, Nix)	Scabies	*Adult and child:* Topical cream, apply to clean, dry skin from the neck to the toes and rub in well; leave on skin for 8–12 h; wash skin well.	*Onset:* 10 min *Duration:* Unknown $t_{1/2}$: 16 h
	Pediculosis	*Adult and child:* Topical lotion, apply to the affected site and leave on for 10 min; rinse thoroughly.	
crotamiton (Eurax)	Scabies	*Adult:* Apply 10% preparation to the affected skin. Massage gently into skin until completely absorbed. Repeat as needed.	*Onset:* Unknown *Duration:* Unknown $t_{1/2}$: Unknown
lindane (Kwell, Scabene)	Scabies and pediculosis	*Adult and child:* Topical cream, apply to clean, dry skin from the neck to the toes and rub in well; leave on skin for 8–12 h; wash skin well. *Adult and child:* Topical shampoo, wash and dry the hair and allow to cool; apply shampoo to dry hair and rub into scalp; allow shampoo to remain in place for 4 min; use enough water to work up a good lather; rinse thoroughly and towel dry; use a fine-toothed comb when hair is thoroughly dry.	*Onset:* Rapid *Duration:* 3 h $t_{1/2}$: 18 h
malathion (Ovide)	Pediculosis	*Adult and child >6 y:* Apply approximately 30 mL and leave in place for 8–12 h; rinse thoroughly.	*Onset:* Rapid *Duration:* 2 d–2 wk $t_{1/2}$: 8–48 h

hot air (Louse Buster) is a nonchemical, effective treatment for lice and has the added benefit that lice cannot become resistant to it. However, this is a pharmacology text, and permethrin will be discussed as the prototype antiectoparasitic drug. Table 47.8 presents a summary of selected antiectoparasitic drugs.

Nursing Management of the Patient Receiving Ⓟ Permethrin

Core Drug Knowledge

Pharmacotherapeutics

Permethrin is a topical scabicide and pediculicide. For lice, it is available OTC as a 1% cream (Nix). Scabies should be treated with the 5% prescription cream (Elimite).

Pharmacokinetics

Permethrin is applied topically. A small amount may be systemically absorbed, especially from abraded or denuded skin. It is excreted as inactive metabolites through the kidneys.

Pharmacodynamics

Direct effects of permethrin occur in the parasite. Permethrin disrupts the parasite's nerve cell membrane, resulting in paralysis and death. Permethrin also exhibits residual ovicidal activity for approximately 2 days. Generally, 70% to 80% of eggs are eradicated after one application.

Contraindications and Precautions

Permethrin should not be used in patients who have had previous hypersensitivity reactions to household insecticides because it contains similar substances. It is a pregnancy category B drug.

Adverse Effects

Common adverse effects include burning, itching, numbness, rash, redness, stinging, swelling, or tingling of the scalp. Pruritus, edema, and erythema caused by the parasite can be exacerbated during therapy. Inhaling substantial quantities of permethrin can aggravate bronchial asthma.

Drug Interactions

No drug–drug interactions are known to occur with permethrin.

Assessment of Relevant Core Patient Variables

Health Status

Evaluate the extent of infection. Lice that are visible in the eyebrows or eyelashes should not be treated by the patient at home.

Life Span and Gender

Permethrin is not approved for use in children younger than 2 years of age. Whether this pregnancy category B drug enters breast milk is unknown; however, the American Academy of Pediatrics recommends discontinuing breast-feeding during therapy.

Lifestyle, Diet, and Habits

Determine the patient's use of creams, ointments, or oils. Caution the patient not to use them during permethrin therapy.

Environment

Because permethrin is routinely used at home, the patient needs to clearly understand how to use the drug properly. Explain that the infection may take up to 2 weeks to resolve.

HOME CARE CONCERNS IN ANTIECTOPARASITIC THERAPY

After treatment and recovery from status epilepticus, your patient, J. Colone, is discharged home on phenytoin (Dilantin) therapy. One of your assignments as a student nurse is to accompany the visiting nurse who will visit with Mr. Colone to assess his progress. When you arrive, you are surprised to learn that the whole family is being treated for head lice. Examine your concerns about Mr. Colone's current situation. In addition to teaching him about drug therapy, what other points will you emphasize in the teaching plan? What is especially important for Mr. Colone to know?

Nursing Diagnosis and Outcome

• Risk for Impaired Skin Integrity: Rash and pruritus related to drug therapy
  Desired outcome: *The patient will self-medicate with OTC diphenhydramine.*

Planning and Intervention

Maximizing Therapeutic Effects

Permethrin is for external use only, and encourage the patient to use it exactly according to directions. Prior to application, wash the hair with a nonconditioning shampoo. Apply the cream to the scalp and leave in place for 10 minutes. Rinse thoroughly with cool water. Because head louse eggs hatch in 5 to 11 days, apply a second treatment in 10 days.

Minimizing Adverse Effects

Tell the patient to follow the directions for using permethrin carefully to avoid potential adverse effects. Keep the drug out of the reach of children, who may ingest it accidentally.

Providing Patient and Family Education

• Emphasize the potential adverse effects of permethrin and the importance of contacting the provider should any such effects occur.
• Provide directions for using permethrin correctly. It is important to cover the following teaching points for use with scabies:
• Thoroughly wash and dry the skin.
• Massage the cream into the skin from the head to the soles of the feet, paying special attention to creases in the skin, hands, feet, underarms, and groin, and between fingers and toes.
• Scabies rarely infests the scalp of adults, although the hairline, neck, side of the head, and forehead may be infested in older people and in infants. Treat infants on the scalp, side of the head, and forehead.
• Leave the permethrin cream on the skin for 8 to 14 hours.
• Wash off by taking a shower.
• Change into clean clothes.
• It is important to cover the following teaching points for treatment against lice:

• Shampoo the hair and scalp using a nonconditioning shampoo.
• Rinse thoroughly and towel-dry the hair and scalp.
• Allow hair to air-dry for a few minutes.
• Shake the permethrin lotion well before applying.
• Wet the hair and scalp thoroughly with the permethrin lotion. Be sure to cover the areas behind the ears and on the back of the neck also. Allow the lotion to remain in place for 10 minutes.
• Rinse the hair and scalp thoroughly with cool water and dry with a clean towel.
• Remove nits only after the hair is completely dry.
• Instruct the patient how to eliminate nits (tiny, white, oval-shaped eggs of the adult louse, which lodge on hair close to the scalp):
• Buy a good metal lice or nit comb.
• Choose a well-lit area in the home to use as a lice-picking station.
• Comb through the hair a section at a time, using metal clips to divide sections—and a magnifying glass if one is handy.
• Remove lice and nits from the comb with a tissue after each stroke, or rinse the comb in sudsy hot water between strokes.
• Continue combing for at least 30 strokes or until the scalp and hair are nit free. Hand-pick any remaining nits.
• Repeat the procedure in 10 days.
• Additional information to reduce the potential for reinfection includes:
• Machine wash all clothing (including hats, scarves, and coats), bedding, towels, and washcloths in very hot water and dry them by using the hot cycle of a dryer for at least 20 minutes. Clothing or bedding that cannot be washed should be dry cleaned or sealed in an airtight plastic bag for 2 weeks.
• Shampoo all wigs and hairpieces.
• Wash all hairbrushes and combs in very hot soapy water (above 130°F) for 5 to 10 minutes and do not share them with other people.
• Clean the house or room by thoroughly vacuuming upholstered furniture, rugs, and floors.
• Wash all toys in very hot soapy water (above 130°F) for 5 to 10 minutes.
• Place all stuffed animals in sealed plastic bags for about a month. (Lice live only about 25 days.)

Ongoing Assessment and Evaluation

After-treatment evaluations consist of monitoring for signs of successful treatment (eradication) or failure (reinfection).

Drugs Closely Related to P Permethrin

Benzyl Alcohol

Benzyl alcohol 5% lotion is the newest drug approved by the FDA for the treatment of lice. It has a unique mechanism of action. Lice breathe though a system of spiracles that close

MEMORY CHIP

P Permethrin

- Used for scabies and pediculosis
- Major contraindications: hypersensitivity to household insecticides
- Most common adverse effects: skin irritation and pruritus
- Maximizing therapeutic effects: Apply only as directed.
- Minimizing adverse effects: Keep out of reach of children.
- Most important patient education: To minimize the risk for systemic absorption, do not leave on the scalp or body for longer than the recommended time.

upon contact with most liquids. This allows the lice to go into "suspended animation" and survive for hours without respiration. Benzyl alcohol prevents lice from closing their spiracles, thereby asphyxiating them within ten minutes. Adverse effects include itching, redness, or irritation. Advise the patient to ensure an adequate amount of lotion to completely cover the affected area and leave in place for 10 minutes. A second treatment is done 1 week later.

Crotamiton

Crotamiton (Eurax) is a prescription scabicidal and antipruritic drug used for treating *S. scabiei* (scabies) and relieving pruritus. The drug can be used with caution during pregnancy, and the only contraindication to its use is hypersensitivity. Pediatric safety has not been established. Crotamiton should not be applied in the eyes or around the mouth because it may cause irritation. It should not be applied to acutely inflamed skin or raw or weeping surfaces until the acute inflammation resolves. The only potential adverse reaction is rash.

Crotamiton should be applied from the chin to the toes after taking a routine bath or shower. A second application is advisable 24 hours later. A cleansing bath should be taken 48 hours after the last application. Clothing and bed linens should be changed the second day. Contaminated clothing and bed linen may be dry cleaned or washed in very hot water.

Lindane

Lindane (Kwell) is is highly effective; however, its use is highly controversial. In fact, many states have banned it as a pharmaceutical because of its potential for neurotoxicity.

In March 2003, the Food and Drug Administration (FDA) approved a Black Box warning stating that lindane be used only in patients who cannot tolerate first-line treatment with safer medications to treat lice or scabies infestation or in whom such treatment has failed. Lindane is contraindicated for patients with known seizure disorders and for individuals with known hypersensitivity. CNS toxicity may precipitate seizures. Lindane should not be used where skin rash, abrasion, or inflammation exists because such use can enhance systemic absorption and increase the possibility of CNS toxicity. Lindane also is contraindicated for children younger than 2 years of age, who have more permeable skin than

adults do, and may therefore be at high risk for systemic absorption and resultant neurotoxicity. Caution should be used in administering this drug to children between 2 and 10 years of age, because the risk for toxicity is greater in this age group than in others.

Lindane is a pregnancy category C drug. It is not recommended for use while breast-feeding because it is secreted into breast milk. An alternative form of infant feeding should be used for at least 2 days after using lindane.

Malathion

Malathion (Ovide) is an organophosphate insecticide commonly known to the public as an aerosolized insecticide that is sprayed over vegetation. It was originally approved by the FDA in 1989, then removed from the market, and then reintroduced in 1999. It is used to manage human lice infections that are resistant to permethrin, although many providers feel it should be the first-line treatment.

Malathion works by enabling acetylcholine to overstimulate cholinergic receptor sites, which leads to rapid insect death. It is not recommended for children under the age of 6 years and is contraindicated for use in infants because their scalp is more permeable and allows more absorption. The topical formulation contains isopropyl alcohol, making it flammable. For that reason, it should not be used in proximity to any heat source, such as electric rollers, curling irons, and especially cigarettes, pipes, lighters, matches, and other smoking-related items.

If ingested, malathion is a poison. The most serious symptom of organophosphate poisoning is respiratory distress, including potential respiratory arrest. Other respiratory symptoms include rhinorrhea, chest tightness, and wheezing. In addition to affecting the respiratory system, organophosphate poisoning can induce gastrointestinal peristalsis, diarrhea or fecal incontinence, and abdominal pain or cramps. It can also cause miosis, loss of ocular accommodation, blurred vision, and ocular pain. In the cardiovascular system, potential symptoms include bradycardia or hypotension. CNS symptoms include confusion, drowsiness or lethargy, and seizures. The patient may also experience weakness or muscle paralysis. Atropine and pralidoxime are the antidotes to organophosphate poisoning.

Malathion is a pregnancy category B drug; whether it is excreted into breast milk is unknown.

Pyrethrins Plus Piperonyl Butoxide

Pyrethrins plus piperonyl butoxide (Rid) constitute an OTC medication for treating both lice and scabies. It is available in liquid, gel, and shampoo forms. Pyrethrins are absorbed through the exoskeletons of arthropods and block nerve impulse transmissions from the parasite's nervous system, resulting in its paralysis and death. Piperonyl butoxide has little or no insecticidal activity but inhibits the enzymes responsible for metabolism of pyrethrins in arthropods; this increases the insecticidal activity of pyrethrins by 2 to 12 times.

Patients should be instructed to use enough medication to cover the affected hairy area and adjacent areas and to wash the medication off their hands after application. The medication is left on the affected area for exactly 10 minutes, and then the area should be washed with warm water and soap or regular shampoo. The drug should not be used near the eyes, mouth, nose, or vagina. If accidental contact with the eyes occurs, patients should thoroughly rinse the eyes for at least 5 minutes.

Pyrethrins plus piperonyl butoxide are contraindicated for patients who are allergic to either ragweed or chrysanthemums. Pyrethrin is a pregnancy category C drug. Piperonyl butoxide's pregnancy category is unknown.

CHAPTER SUMMARY

- Parasites include protozoa, helminths, and arthropods.
- Helminths include cestodes, nematodes, and trematodes.
- Arthropods include ectoparasites, such as scabies and lice.
- Pharmacologic intervention for parasites must be specific not only to the type of parasite but also to the stage of its life cycle.
- Chloroquine is the prototypical antimalarial drug. Additional drugs used in treating malaria include hydroxychloroquine, mefloquine, primaquine, atovaquone/proguanil, pyrimethamine/sulfadoxine, and quinine.
- Metronidazole is the prototypical antiparasitic drug. Additional antiprotozoan drugs include tinidazole, iodoquinol, paromomycin, and pyrimethamine.
- PCP occurs most often in immunocompromised patients. Drug treatment for PCP includes pentamidine, atovaquone, trimetrexate, and SMZ-TMP.
- Mebendazole is the prototypical anthelminthic drug. However, the choice of anthelminthic therapy depends on the type of helminth. Other anthelminthic drugs include albendazole, thiabendazole, pyrantel, diethylcarbamazine, and praziquantel.
- Permethrin is the prototypical antiectoparasitic drug. Drugs closely related to permethrin include benzyl alcohol, crotamiton, lindane, malathion, and pyrethrins plus piperonyl butoxide.

QUESTIONS FOR STUDY AND REVIEW

1. Why should patients who undergo chloroquine therapy continue to have their eyes examined after completing therapy?
2. Why is chloroquine used cautiously in children?
3. What baseline evaluations should be done for a patient on long-term antimalarial therapy?
4. Why would a patient with alcoholism need to be monitored closely during antiparasitic therapy?
5. Why should you take respiratory protective measures during the administration of inhaled pentamidine?
6. How can you intervene to minimize potential severe adverse effects from the administration of pentamidine?
7. Why is mebendazole contraindicated for women who are pregnant?

NEED MORE HELP?

Chapter 47 of the Study Guide to Accompany *Drug Therapy in Nursing*, 4th Edition, contains NCLEX-style questions and other learning activities to reinforce your understanding of the concepts presented in this chapter. For additional information or to purchase the study guide, visit thePoint.

REFERENCES

Centers for Disease Control and Prevention. (2009). Malaria Treatment. Retrieved July 19, 2009 from http://www.cdc.gov/malaria/pdf/treatmenttable.pdf

Centers for Disease Control and Prevention. (2009). Lice. Retrieved July 20, 2009 from http://www.cdc.gov/lice/head/treatment.html

Coartem Monograph. (2009). Novartis Pharmaceuticals. Retrieved July 20, 2009 from http://www.coartem.com/

Diamantis, S. A., Morrell, D. S., Burkhart, C. N. (2009). Treatment of Head Lice. *Dermatologic Therapy*, 22(4):273–278.

Drugs for Parasitic Infections. (Updated 2009). *The Medical Letter on Drugs and Therapeutics*, September, 2007;(Suppl):1–15.

Facts and Comparisons. (2010). *Drug facts and comparisons*. Philadelphia, PA: Lippincott Williams & Wilkins.

Getting the Bugs Out. (2009). *Child Heath Alert*, May;27:2.

Johnstone, P. P., & Strong, M. (2008). *Scabies*, ii,1707.

Karch, A. M. (2010). *Nursing Drug Guide*. Philadelphia, PA: Lippincott Williams & Wilkins.

Keiser, J., Utzinger, J. (2009). Food-borne trematodiasis, *Clinical Microbiology Reviews*, 22(3):466–483.

Keiser, J., & Utzinger, J. (2008). Efficacy of current drugs against soil-transmitted helminth infections: systematic review and meta-analysis. *JAMA*, 299(16):1937–1948.

Koda-Kimbal, M. A., Young, L. Y., Kradian, W. A., et al. (2008). *Applied Therapeutics: The Clinical Use of Drugs*. Philadelphia, PA: Lippincott Williams & Wilkins.

Leoung, G. S. (2006). Pneumocystosis and HIV. Retrieved July 22, 2009 from http://hivinsite.com/InSite?page=kb-05-02-01

Micromedex Healthcare Series. Retrieved from *http://thomsonhc.com*

Rosen, M. J. (2008). Pulmonary Complications of HIV infection. *Respirology*, 13(2):181–190.

Sinclair, D., Zani, B., Donegan, S., et al. (2009). Artemisinin-based combination therapy for treating uncomplicated malaria. *Cochrane Database of Systematic Reviews*, (3):CD007483.

Tatro, D. S. (2009). *Drug interaction facts*. Philadelphia, PA: Lippincott Williams & Wilkins.

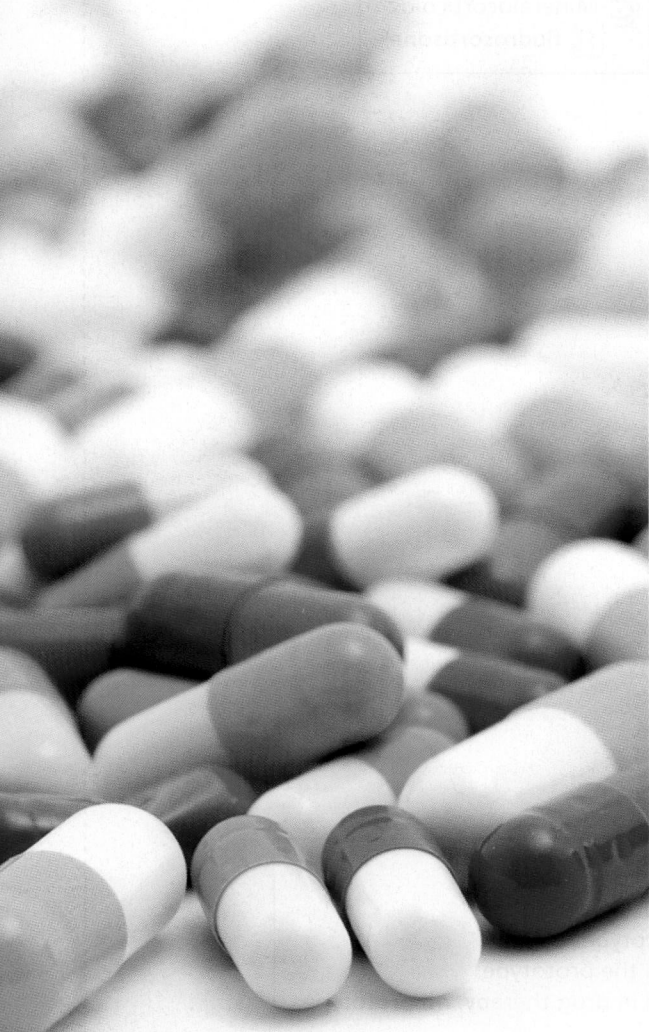

UNIT 11
Endocrine Drugs

48

Drugs Affecting Corticosteroid Levels

Learning Objectives

At the completion of this chapter the student will:

1. Describe the physiologic effects of and clinical indications for mineralocorticoids and glucocorticoids.

2. Discuss complications associated with glucocorticoids.

3. Discuss nursing interventions to maximize therapeutic and minimize adverse effects for drugs that affect corticosteroid hormone levels and have anti-inflammatory action.

4. Describe the most frequently encountered adverse effects associated with the glucocorticoids and mineralocorticoids.

5. Identify dosing strategies that may minimize glucocorticoid-related adverse effects.

6. Determine key points for patient and family education for drugs that affect corticosteroid hormone levels and have anti-inflammatory action.

7. Discuss the clinical indications of drugs referred to as steroid hormone antagonists.

Key Terms

Addison disease	cortisol	mineralocorticoid
addisonian crisis	Cushing syndrome	salt-losing adrenogenital syndrome
adrenal insufficiency	glucocorticoid	steroid hormone inhibitors
aldosterone	hyperaldosteronism	

Drugs Affecting Corticosteroid Levels

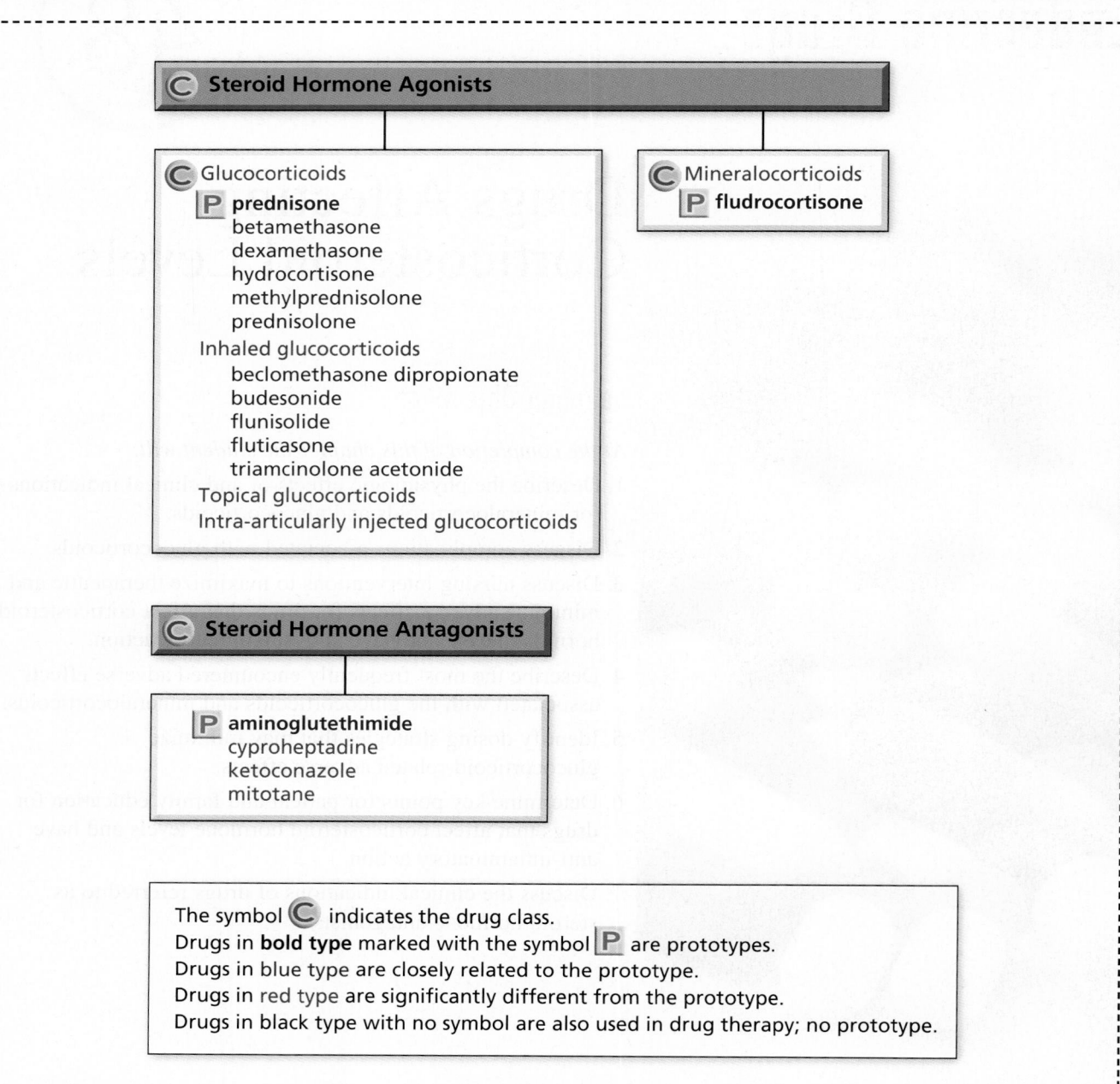

© Steroid Hormone Agonists

© Glucocorticoids
P **prednisone**
betamethasone
dexamethasone
hydrocortisone
methylprednisolone
prednisolone
Inhaled glucocorticoids
beclomethasone dipropionate
budesonide
flunisolide
fluticasone
triamcinolone acetonide
Topical glucocorticoids
Intra-articularly injected glucocorticoids

© Mineralocorticoids
P **fludrocortisone**

© Steroid Hormone Antagonists

P **aminoglutethimide**
cyproheptadine
ketoconazole
mitotane

The symbol © indicates the drug class.
Drugs in **bold type** marked with the symbol P are prototypes.
Drugs in blue type are closely related to the prototype.
Drugs in red type are significantly different from the prototype.
Drugs in black type with no symbol are also used in drug therapy; no prototype.

Synthetic corticosteroids are used for replacement therapy to maintain adequate levels of hormones in patients with inadequate adrenal function and diminished natural corticosteroid production. Corticosteroids are also used for their anti-inflammatory properties by reducing irritation and swelling; antiallergenic by minimizing and or preventing the body's response to allergens; and immunosuppressive effects by decreasing the body's harmful response to diseases that affect the immune system (Box 48.1).

The benefits derived from chronic use of corticosteroids, also known as steroids in lay terminology, are often accompanied by a number of risks (adverse effects). Corticosteroid complications vary from mild to life threatening and are a function of the dosage, route of administration, and duration of therapy and results from the body's altered natural endogenous production of corticosteroid during the course of receiving exogenous corticosteroid therapy. With this in mind, the benefit–risk of corticosteroid therapy requires careful deliberation. Furthermore, the use of the smallest dose, the shortest treatment duration, and as necessary, gradual dose tapering prior to its discontinuance are important considerations.

Box 48.1 THERAPEUTIC USES FOR THE CORTICOSTEROIDS

Glucocorticoid and Mineralocorticoid Effects at Physiologic Doses

Adrenocortical insufficiency
Adrenogenital syndrome (salt-losing)

Glucocorticoid Effects at Supraphysiologic (Pharmacologic) Doses

Acute allergic conditions (e.g., bronchial asthma, serum sickness)
Acute spinal injury
Cerebral edema
Collagen diseases, rheumatic disorders (e.g., systemic lupus erythematosus, acute rheumatic carditis)
Dermatologic diseases (e.g., seborrheic dermatitis, severe psoriasis)
Gastrointestinal diseases (e.g., Crohn disease, intractable sprue, ulcerative colitis)
Hematologic disorders (e.g., autoimmune hemolytic anemia, thrombocytopenia)
Hepatic diseases (e.g., liver cirrhosis with ascites)
Joint inflammation (e.g., bursitis)
Meningitis
Neoplastic diseases (e.g., leukemias, lymphomas)
Nephrotic syndrome
Ocular disorders (e.g., allergic conjunctivitis, chorioretinitis, iritis, keratitis)
Organ transplantations
Respiratory diseases (e.g., interstitial pulmonary fibrosis, pulmonary emphysema with bronchial edema)
Thyroiditis

PHYSIOLOGY

The hormones of the endocrine system are important messengers in the communication between cells. The nervous system, adrenal glands, and other endocrine glands contribute to homeostasis, thus allowing physical and emotional adaptation to internal and external changes.

There are two adrenal glands, one at the top of each kidney. Each gland is composed of two distinct parts—the medulla and the cortex.

The medulla and cortex are crucial to metabolism, the body's stress response, and fluid and electrolyte balances. The adrenal medulla synthesizes and secretes catecholamines—epinephrine and norepinephrine. These hormones are important in counteracting short-term stress.

The adrenal cortex is involved primarily in the synthesis and secretion of **glucocorticoids** and **mineralocorticoids** (collectively referred to as the corticosteroids or corticoids) from plasma-derived, low-density lipoproteins and high-density lipoproteins (cholesterol). Corticosteroids are characterized by mineralocorticoid and glucocorticoid effects, depending on the predominant pharmacologic action of the agent. Adrenal corticosteroids exert effects on almost every organ in the body. Their pharmacologic actions are generally an extension of their physiologic effects. Their primary actions include carbohydrate, protein, and fat metabolism; electrolyte and water metabolism; cardiovascular functions; and immune effects. The zona reticularis region of the adrenal cortex produces and secretes other steroid hormones, including adrenal androgens, progesterone, and the estrogens.

Glucocorticoids

The glucocorticoids acquired their name from their role in glucose metabolism; they increase blood glucose concentrations by:

- Stimulating gluconeogenesis and glucose secretion by the liver
- Increasing the hepatic sensitivity to the gluconeogenic actions of glucagon and catecholamines
- Decreasing glucose uptake and utilization by peripheral tissue
- Increasing proteolysis and decreasing protein synthesis in muscles to support the gluconeogenesis activities

Glucocorticoids exert potent and diverse actions on glucose, protein, and bone metabolism and possess anti-inflammatory, antiallergenic, and immunosuppressant actions. Metabolic effects of glucocorticoids include gluconeogenesis, mobilization of amino acids from protein in striated muscle, protein catabolism, fat synthesis and lipolysis, and hepatic enzymatic activities that convert amino acids to glucose, with most of the excess glucose stored in the liver as glycogen. The metabolic effects of the glucocorticoids result in the following:

- An increase in circulating amino acid levels
- An overall depletion of muscle protein
- A negative nitrogen balance
- A mobilization of fatty acids, converting cell metabolism from using glucose for energy to using fatty acids for energy

Other physiologic effects of the glucocorticoids include:

- An antagonistic effect on antidiuretic hormones to maintain water balance
- A lowering of the threshold for electrical excitation in the brain
- A reduction in the amount of new bone synthesis

In addition, glucocorticoids have actions that allow the body to cope effectively with physiologic or psychological stress (e.g., overwhelming illness or trauma). For example, the natural glucocorticoid **cortisol** sensitizes the arterioles to norepinephrine for vasopressor effects and allows epinephrine and glucagon to activate gluconeogenesis and glycogenolysis.

Hypothalamic corticotropin-releasing factor (CRF) stimulates the release of pituitary adrenocorticotropic hormone (ACTH). The hypothalamic-pituitary-adrenal (HPA) axis regulates and stimulates cortisol synthesis release by the adrenal cortex. Each of these substances is regulated by a complex feedback loop because the production of each substance is regulated by the plasma concentrations of the other two. Glucocorticoid, androgen, and estrogen secretion depend on adrenocortical stimulation by ACTH from the anterior pituitary. CRF controls ACTH release into the bloodstream (Figure 48.1).

Three factors are important in regulating ACTH secretion:

- Circulating cortisol levels
- Stress levels
- Circadian (diurnal) rhythms

Pituitary production of ACTH is very sensitive to suppression by exogenous glucocorticoids. Long-term or chronic administration may result in adrenocortical atrophy and its subsequent reduction in the secretory ability to produce these hormones.

Mineralocorticoids

The mineralocorticoids (**aldosterone** is the most prevalent naturally occurring mineralocorticoid) exert a major influence on regulating potassium, sodium, and water balance. Mineralocorticoids are produced in the outer layer of cells of the adrenal cortex (zona glomerulosa). Numerous systemic factors affect the synthesis and secretion of aldosterone. Angiotensin II is the most potent of these factors. In the distal renal tubules, aldosterone promotes the reabsorption of sodium into the blood in exchange for potassium secreted into the renal tubules for urinary excretion.

Several mechanisms control aldosterone levels:

- Extracellular sodium and potassium levels—when serum sodium levels are low or potassium levels are high, aldosterone levels rise.
- Renal renin release—a reduction in renal blood flow increases aldosterone levels by the renin-angiotensin-aldosterone system.
- Pituitary ACTH—the glucocorticoid hormones produced in the adrenal cortex have mineralocorticoid effects.

Sex Steroids

The adrenal cortex produces small amounts of sex steroids (e.g., testosterone and estrogens) and some weak anabolic

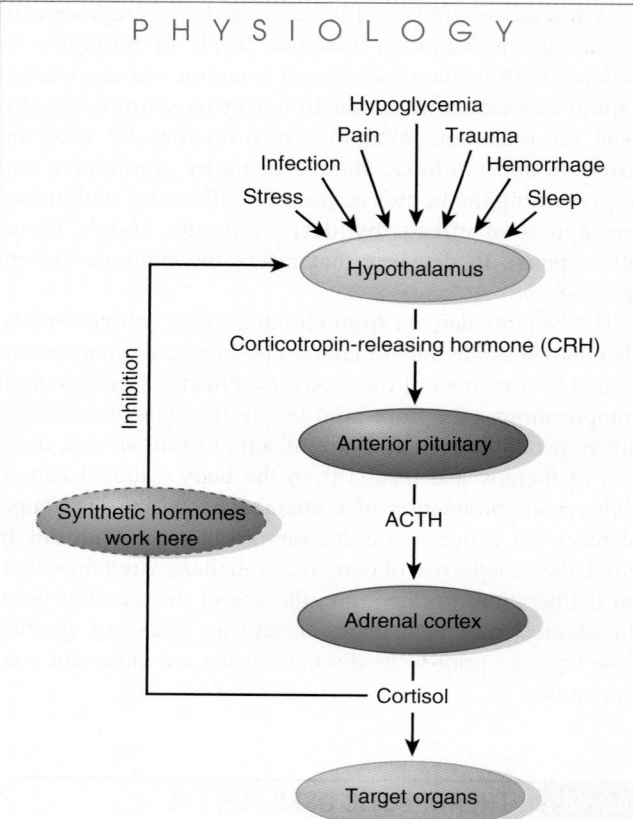

PHYSIOLOGY

• FIGURE 48.1   The hypothalamic-pituitary-adrenal (HPA) feedback system regulates and stimulates cortisol synthesis and release by the adrenal cortex. Each hormone in the HPA axis is influenced by a complex feedback loop because synthesis of one substance is regulated by plasma concentrations of the others. For instance, secretion of glucocorticoid, androgen, and estrogen depends on adrenocortical stimulation by adrenocorticotropic hormone (ACTH) from the anterior pituitary. Corticotropin-releasing factor, produced by the hypothalamus, controls ACTH release into the bloodstream. Circulating cortisol levels, stress, and circadian rhythms are also important in regulating ACTH secretion. ACTH in turn regulates cortisol release. The objectives of replacement and pharmacologic drug therapy involve maintaining balance in the HPA feedback system.

androgens (e.g., dehydroepiandrosterone and androstenedione). These hormones are produced by the adrenal glands in males and females. The amounts are usually insignificant compared with the hormone amounts secreted by the gonads. However, under certain conditions (e.g., tumors, cushingoid effects), their excess may cause a substantial endocrine imbalance. These gonadal hormones are discussed in depth in Chapters 53 and 54.

PATHOPHYSIOLOGY

Adrenal Insufficiency

There are two forms of **adrenal insufficiency**—primary and secondary. Primary adrenal insufficiency (**Addison disease**) results from the destruction of the adrenal cortex caused by infection or hemorrhage, which results in hyposecretion of all adrenocortical hormones—most importantly, the glucocorticoid *cortisol* and the mineralocorticoid *aldosterone*.

Characteristics of Addison disease include those related to glucocorticoid deficiency, such as hypoglycemia, anorexia, nausea, vomiting, flatulence, diarrhea, hyperpigmentation of skin, anxiety, depression, and loss of mental acuity; and those related to mineralocorticoid deficiency, such as fluid and electrolyte imbalance, orthostatic hypotension, hyponatremia, hyperkalemia, general malaise, muscle weakness, muscle pain, and cardiac arrhythmias.

The major complication of Addison disease is a sudden, life-threatening exacerbation called **addisonian crisis** (adrenal crisis). The patient experiences severe hypotension, hyponatremia, dehydration, hyperkalemia, and hyperthermia in the absence of another cause. A stressor is often the trigger for an addisonian crisis. These physiologic responses are initially treated with standard resuscitative therapy (e.g., vasopressors, plasma expanders). When the source of these symptoms is adrenal hypofunction, the treatment includes immediate replacement of adrenocortical hormone (e.g., intravenous [IV] hydrocortisone [Solu-Cortef]), salt, and fluids to restore normal blood volume and blood pressure.

In secondary adrenal insufficiency, the deficiency of cortisol secretion is secondary to insufficient secretion of ACTH by the anterior pituitary. Little or no alteration in aldosterone secretion occurs. Thus, glucocorticoid insufficiency occurs without affecting mineralocorticoid levels. The most common cause of secondary adrenal insufficiency is long-term treatment of nonendocrine disorders with pharmacologic doses of glucocorticoid drugs. Because it bypasses the negative feedback loop, this treatment results in gradual loss of adrenal and pituitary hormonal reserves and some degree of atrophy of the ACTH-secreting cells of both the pituitary and the adrenal cortex. Sudden withdrawal of the glucocorticoid drug may result in secondary adrenal insufficiency, manifested clinically by acute adrenal insufficiency. HPA axis suppression resulting from glucocorticoid therapy may last for as long as 1 year after drug therapy has been discontinued.

A patient receiving pharmacologic doses of glucocorticoids for more than 2 weeks may have some degree of HPA axis suppression. Prevention of secondary adrenal insufficiency following prolonged administration of glucocorticoid drugs can be avoided by "weaning" the patient from the drug over weeks or months.

Cushing Syndrome

Cushing syndrome is a rare disorder resulting from increased adrenocortical secretion of cortisol, resulting in chronic elevation in glucocorticoid and adrenal androgen hormones. Mineralocorticoid hormone levels are usually not affected because increased ACTH production is usually the causative agent. Cushing syndrome may be caused by any one of the following sources:

- ACTH-dependent adrenocortical hyperplasia
- Tumor
- ACTH-secreting tumor
- Long-term administration of large doses of any steroid that is a potent glucocorticoid (iatrogenic Cushing syndrome)

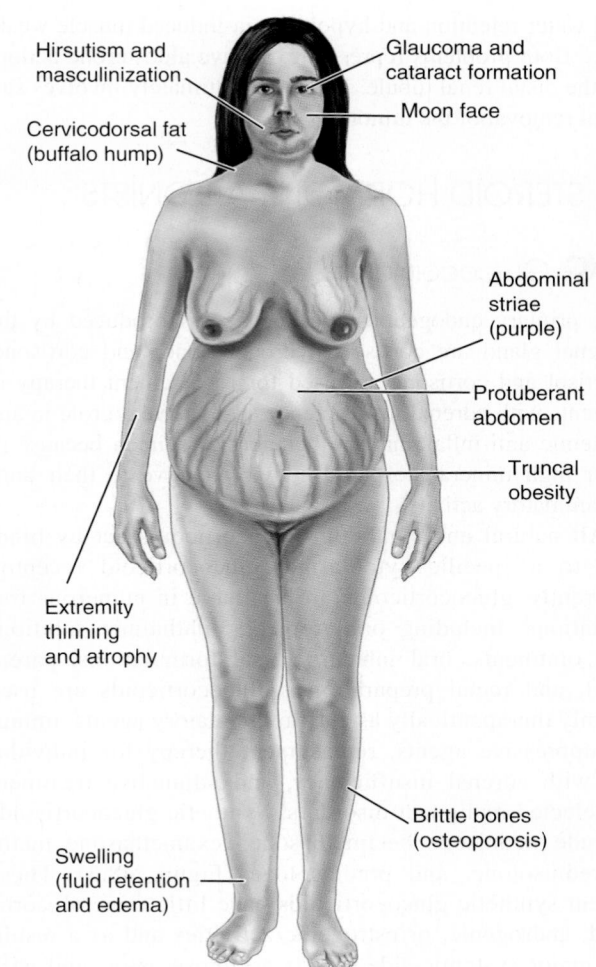

- FIGURE 48.2 Cushingoid characteristics.

The term *cushingoid* refers to the variable number of the physiologic changes associated with Cushing syndrome (Figure 48.2).

Salt-Losing Adrenogenital Syndrome

Salt-losing adrenogenital syndrome, a congenital condition, is characterized by an inherited enzymatic interference with the normal biosynthesis of glucocorticoids and mineralocorticoids. The resulting low levels of these corticosteroids stimulate the body's feedback mechanism to produce large amounts of corticotropin (ACTH). The adrenal glands are only able to respond to the increased ACTH by increasing their production of adrenal androgens. Consequently, testosterone levels are abnormally high, which results in masculinization.

Hyperaldosteronism

Hyperaldosteronism is another abnormality of adrenal hormone production. Certain tumors of the adrenal cortex produce excessive amounts of aldosterone (or occasionally another mineralocorticoid). Two problems occur as a result of hyperaldosteronism: hypertension secondary to sodium and water retention and hypokalemia-induced muscle weakness. Both problems represent excessive aldosterone actions on the distal renal tubule. Treatment ultimately involves surgical removal of the tumor.

Ⓒ STEROID HORMONE AGONISTS

• Ⓒ GLUCOCORTICOIDS

The primary endogenous glucocorticoids produced by the adrenal gland are cortisol (hydrocortisone) and cortisone. Cortisol and cortisone are used for replacement therapy in patients with adrenal insufficiency. They have no role in any systemic anti-inflammatory therapeutic regimen because of their high mineralocorticoid activity relative to their anti-inflammatory activity.

All natural and synthetic glucocorticoids act by binding to a specific cytoplasmic glucocorticoid receptor. Currently, glucocorticoids are available in numerous formulations, including oral, topical, ophthalmic solutions and ointments, oral inhalers, nasal formulations, parenteral, and rectal preparations. Glucocorticoids are used mainly therapeutically as anti-inflammatory agents, immunosuppressive agents, replacement therapy for individuals with adrenal insufficiency, and adjunctive treatment in selected malignant disorders. Synthetic glucocorticoids include prednisone, betamethasone, dexamethasone, methylprednisolone, and prednisolone (Figure 48.3). These potent synthetic glucocorticoids have little mineralocorticoid, androgenic, or estrogenic activities and as a result, the major systemic side effects are those associated with

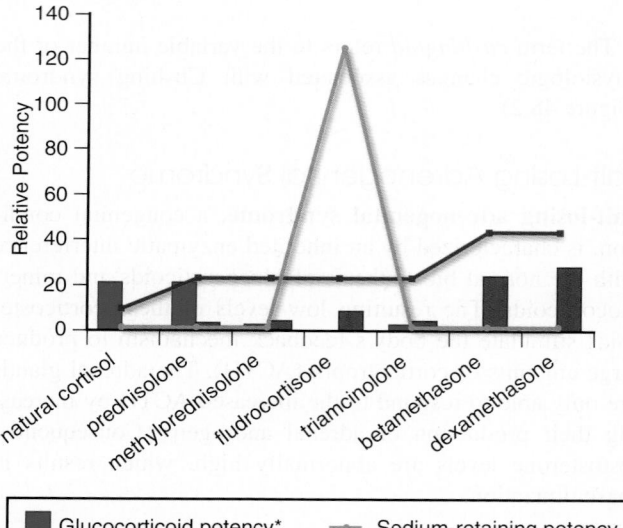

*Glucocorticoid activity signifies the stimulation of glucose formation, a reduction in its utilization, and the promotion of its storage as glycogen.

• FIGURE 48.3 Comparison of glucocorticoids.

hypothalamic-pituitary-adrenal function suppression. Table 48.1 presents a summary of selected glucocorticoids.

A common adverse effect of synthetic glucocorticoids administered in high doses for anti-inflammatory and immunosuppressant effects (combined or separately) is suppression of the HPA axis and may lead to secondary adrenal insufficiency. This effect appears within days of beginning glucocorticoid therapy. The time needed for the HPA axis to recover depends on the type of glucocorticoid given, the dose and frequency of administration (daily dosing or alternate-day dosing), and the duration of treatment. Occasionally, the patient's HPA axis remains permanently suppressed by glucocorticoid anti-inflammatory therapy. Consequently, the corticosteroid therapy reverts to replacement therapy.

Abrupt discontinuation of a glucocorticoid following prolonged administration may result in acute adrenal insufficiency because of a lack of both exogenous and endogenous glucocorticoids. To prevent acute adrenal insufficiency, exogenously administered glucocorticoids must be withdrawn gradually (tapered) so that the HPA axis can resume secretion of cortisol at a normal level and rate.

Prednisone (Deltasone, Prednicot), a synthetic analogue of cortisone, is the prototype glucocorticoid. It is four times more potent than naturally occurring cortisol; thus, its results are longer acting and have a more potent anti-inflammatory effect. Prednisone and its derivatives are the most commonly used glucocorticoids for the treatment of inflammatory conditions and a variety of autoimmune diseases.

Nursing Management of the Patient Receiving Ⓟ Prednisone

Core Drug Knowledge

Pharmacotherapeutics

Prednisone is used for both its anti-inflammatory effects and immunosuppressive effects. It may be used as replacement therapy for adrenal insufficiency; however, hydrocortisone is preferred because of its glucocorticoid and mineralocorticoid activity. Therapeutic uses of prednisone are extensive and include anti-inflammatory treatment for conditions such as asthma, allergies, rheumatoid arthritis, inflammatory bowel disease (such as ulcerative colitis), skin disorders, and neoplasms (such as leukemia and lymphoma); for other inflammatory conditions such as tendonitis or bursitis; and increasingly for acute gout on patients intolerant of, or poor candidate for, NSAIDs. Prednisone is also used for its immunosuppressive effects to prevent organ transplant rejection, cerebral edema, and spinal cord injuries. Prednisone also has unlabeled investigational use such as adjunctive treatment for pneumocystis jiroveci, autoimmune hepatitis, and as adjunct for pain management of immunocompetent patients with herpes zoster.

Prednisone may be used as either short- or long-term therapy. Short-term therapies include during acute allergic reactions, during periods of acute exacerbation of chronic diseases such as chronic obstructive pulmonary disease,

TABLE 48.1 Summary of Selected ⓒ Glucocorticoids

Drug (Trade) Name	Selected Indications	Route and Dosage Range	Pharmacokinetics
P prednisone (Deltasone, Prednicot)	Adrenal insufficiency Inflammatory disorders Multiple sclerosis, relapsing Pneumocystis pneumonia Nephrotic syndrome Asthma	*Adult and Child:* PO, 4–5 mg/m² daily *Adult:* PO, 5–60 mg daily *Child:* PO, 0.05–2 mg/kg daily *Adult:* PO, 200 mg daily ×7 d, then 80 mg every other day ×1 mo *Adult:* PO, 40 mg daily ×5 d, then 20 mg daily *Child:* PO, 2 mg/kg daily *Child:* PO, 1–2 mg/kg daily	*Onset:* Varies *Duration:* 1–1.5 d $t_{1/2}$: 3.5 h
betamethasone (Celestone)	Anti-inflammatory Adrenal Insufficiency	*Adult:* PO, 0.6–7.2 mg/d *Child:* PO, 62.5–250 mcg/kg in 3 divided doses *Child:* PO, 17.5 mcg/kg in 3 divided doses	*Onset:* Varies *Duration:* 3 d $t_{1/2}$: 36–54 h
betamethasone sodium phosphate	Anti-inflammatory Adrenal insufficiency	*Adult:* IM, IV, up to 9 mg *Child:* IM, 20.8–125 mcg/kg every 12–24 h *Child:* IM, 5.8–8.75 mcg/kg daily	
betamethasone sodium phosphate/betamethasone acetate (Celestone Soluspan)	Anti-inflammatory Prevention of respiratory distress syndrome in preterm infants Intralesional, intrabursal, intra-articular	*Adult:* IM, 0.5–9 mg *Adult:* IM, 12 mg daily ×2–3 d before delivery *Adult:* IL, 0.25–2 mL	
dexamethasone (Decadron)	Adrenocortical insufficiency Suppression test Cerebral edema Anti-inflammatory	*Adult:* PO, 0.5–9 mg daily *Child:* PO, 23.3 mcg/kg in 3 divided doses *Adult:* PO, 2 mg every 6 h ×2 d *Adult:* IM, IV, 10 mg IV then 4 mg IM every 6 h *Adult:* PO, 0.5–9 mg daily *Child:* PO, 83.3–333.3 mcg/kg	*Onset:* Oral, slow; IM, IV, rapid *Duration:* 2–3 d $t_{1/2}$: 110–210 min
hydrocortisone (Cortef)	Adrenal insufficiency Anti-inflammatory Congenital adrenal hyperplasia	*Adult:* PO, 25–30 mg daily in divided doses *Child:* PO, 0.5–0.7 mg/kg daily in divided doses *Adult:* PO, 20–240 mg daily in divided doses *Child:* PO, 2.5–10 mg/kg daily in divided doses *Child:* PO, 20–25 mg/m2 daily in divided doses	*Onset:* Oral, 1–2 h; IM, rapid; IV, immediate *Duration:* 1–1.5 d $t_{1/2}$: 80–120 min
hydrocortisone sodium succinate (Solu-Cortef)	Acute adrenal insufficiency Anti-inflammatory Status asthmaticus Shock	*Adult:* IV: 100 mg every 6–8 h *Child:* IV, 1–2 mg/kg once, then 25–150 mg daily in divided doses *Adult:* IM, IV, 20–240 mg daily in divided doses *Child:* IM, IV, 1–5 mg/kg every 12–24 h *Adult:* IV, 300–400 mg divided every 6 h *Child:* IV, 4–8 mg/kg once, then 2 mg/kg every 6 h *Adult:* IV, 200–300 mg, divided, every 6–8 h ×5–10 d	
methylprednisolone (Medrol)	Anti-inflammatory	*Adult:* PO, 2–60 mg/d *Child:* PO, 0.5–0.7 mg/kg daily	*Onset:* IM, IV, rapid *Duration:* IM, 1–5 wk; IV, unknown $t_{1/2}$: 78–188 min
methylprednisolone acetate (Depo-Medrol)	Anti-inflammatory Congenital adrenal hyperplasia Multiple sclerosis exacerbation Interarticular/interlesional	*Adult:* IM, 40–20 mg every 1–4 wk *Adult:* IM, 40 mg every 2 wk *Adult:* IM, 160 mg daily ×7 d, then 64 mg every other day ×1 mo *Adult:* IM/IL, 4–80 mg every 1–5 wk	

(Continued)

TABLE 48.1 Summary of Selected C Glucocorticoids (continued)

Drug (Trade) Name	Selected Indications	Route and Dosage Range	Pharmacokinetics
methylpred-nisolone sodium succinate (Solu-Medrol)	Anti-inflammatory	*Adult*: IM, IV, 10–250 mg every 4 h *Child*: IM, IV, 0.5–1.7 mg/kg daily, divided, every 6–12 h	
	Aplastic anemia Lupus nephritis	*Adult*: IV, 1 mg/kg daily ×4 *Adult*: IV, 1 g daily ×3 d *Child*: IV, 30 mg/kg every other day ×6 doses *Adult*: IM, IV, 100–250 mg every 4 h	
	Shock Spinal cord injury	*Adult*: IV, 5.4 mg/kg/h daily *Child*: IV, 30 mg/kg over 15 min, then 5.4 mg/kg daily	
	Status asthmaticus	*Adult and Child*: IM, IV, 2 mg/kg once, then 0.5–1 mg/kg every 6 h	
prednisolone acetate (Orapred, Orapred [ODT])	Adrenal insufficiency Anti-inflammatory	*Adult and Child*: IM, IV, 4–5 mg/m^2 daily *Adult*: IM, IV: 5–60 mg/d *Child*: IM, IV, 1–2 mg/kg/d, divided up to 4×/d	*Onset*: Rapid *Duration*: IV, 1.5 d; IM, 4 wk $t_{1/2}$: 3.5 h
	Intra-articular Multiple sclerosis exacerbation Asthma exacerbation	*Adult*: IL, 2–30 mg every 3 d to every 3 wk *Adult*: IM, IV 80 mg every other day ×7 d *Child*: IV, 1–2 mg/kg every 6 h ×2 d	

asthma, or ulcerative colitis, and at the beginning of treatment for a chronic condition to manage symptoms until other drugs become effective. Long-term high-dose or low-dose therapy may be indicated, depending on the underlying condition (e.g., transplantation) or disease (e.g., rheumatoid arthritis) being treated (see Table 48.1).

Pharmacokinetics

Prednisone, like other glucocorticoids, is absorbed readily from the gastrointestinal (GI) tract because of its lipophilic nature. Glucocorticoids also are absorbed at a moderate rate from the synovial and the conjunctival spaces and very slowly through the skin. Consequently, topical administration is used for a localized action. Excessive and prolonged local application of certain drugs may result in enough absorption to cause systemic effects. In contrast to oral dosage forms, injectable preparations (e.g., esters, suspensions) have greatly altered onsets and durations of action; they are, however, absorbed slowly and completely. Prednisone—inactive on its own—must be metabolized in the liver into pharmacologically active prednisolone. Prednisolone is excreted in the urine, crosses the placenta, and enters the breast milk.

Metabolic factors can increase or decrease the levels of prednisone in the blood. The liver and kidney are the major sites of glucocorticoid inactivation. Drugs that are cyproheptadine inducers (e.g., phenobarbital, phenytoin, rifampin) may accelerate the hepatic biotransformation of glucocorticoids. Conditions such as hypothyroidism may cause the hepatic metabolism to be decreased.

Pharmacodynamics

Prednisone has primarily glucocorticoid activity, although some mineralocorticoid activity is present and more apparent when the drug is administered in high doses (see Figure 48.3). Prednisone may cause salt and water retention, resulting in edema and hypertension. Prednisone affects virtually all body cells but not in the same way. Anti-inflammatory effects include retardation of the migratory polymorphonuclear leukocytes, suppression of tissue repair and granulation, reduction in the erythrocyte sedimentation rate, decrease in fibrinogenesis, and diminished C-reactive protein. However, prednisone does not affect antigen-antibody reactions or immediate hypersensitivity reactions.

Its immunosuppressant effects are attributable to suppression of phagocytosis, decrease in the number of circulating eosinophils and lymphocytes, suppression of delayed hypersensitivity reactions, decrease in antigen–antibody tissue reactions, and a decrease in plasma immunoglobulins.

The effects of glucocorticoid on carbohydrate, fat, and protein metabolism are responsible for both the beneficial and adverse results. The normal physiologic action of systemic glucocorticoids, including prednisone, is increased gluconeogenesis and decreased glucose use. These actions provide for glucose production (and energy) during periods of stress or decreased carbohydrate intake (Box 48.2).

Contraindications and Precautions

Contraindications to prednisone use are a hypersensitivity to the drug and systemic fungal infections or administration of live virus or live attenuated vaccines with immunosuppressive doses of prednisone. It may enhance the adverse effects and/or diminish the effectiveness of a live vaccine, or may bring about vaccine-associated infection. Precautions include closely monitored use for individuals with sensitivity to additives such as tartrazine or sulfites, because they may develop severe allergic or anaphylactic

Box 48.2 PHARMACODYNAMIC EFFECTS OF GLUCOCORTICOIDS

Metabolic

- Increased glycogenolysis and gluconeogenesis
- Increased protein catabolism and decreased protein synthesis
- Decreased gastrointestinal absorption of calcium
- Decreased secretion of thyroid-stimulating hormone (TSH)
- Decreased activity and formation of osteoblasts

Anti-inflammatory (systemic and local effects)

- Decreased production of prostaglandins, cytokines, and interleukins
- Decreased proliferation and migration of lymphocytes and macrophages

reactions to some preparations. Caution is also necessary in patients with hypertension, myasthenia gravis, GI disorders, diabetes mellitus, osteoporosis, cataract, glaucoma, increased intra-ocular pressure, peptic ulcer, and renal insufficiency because the actions of the drug may increase the risk of the complications of these disorders, and or exacerbate or induce these conditions.

Prednisone is a pregnancy category C drug. It is secreted in breast milk and may suppress growth or cause other adverse effects in nursing infants.

Adverse Effects

Treatment with prednisone may produce adverse effects. These effects include the central nervous system (CNS) stimulation with anxiety, mood swings, insomnia, and headache. GI complaints include nausea, vomiting, increased appetite, weight gain, and dyspepsia. Prednisone should be used with caution for patients at risk for gastrointestinal perforation, such as those with diverticulitis, ulcerative colitis, and peptic ulcer. Endocrine changes of menstrual irregularities, alteration with glucose regulation and production leading to hyperglycemia, and suppression of pituitary ACTH release (after 2 to 3 days) are common with continued prednisone use. In addition, dermatologic and integumentary adverse effects include acne, suppression of skin test reactions, and delayed healing of wounds. Other effects of continued prednisone use include muscle weakness, prolonged, or exacerbation, or increased susceptibility to infections (especially those due to herpes virus, varicella virus, and *Candida* and *Mycobacterium* species), suppression and/or masking of physiologic responses to infection; also sodium and fluid retention, fatigue, and malaise. Caution should be exercised for patients at risk for congestive heart failure. Similarly, corticosteroids have been associated with myocardial rupture following acute infarction. Also, use of prednisone may enhance hepatic impairment for patients with cirrhosis.

Administration of prednisone produces a negative feedback effect on the HPA axis; this effect results in the suppression of endogenous cortisol production. Suppression of ACTH release and cortisol secretion has been shown to occur with 50 mg/day of oral prednisone for as few as 5 days. Although long believed to be important, high doses and long-term use of glucocorticoids are no longer thought to be reliable predictors of a probable HPA axis deficiency. There appears to be considerable patient variability in responses to dosages and duration of therapy. Acute adrenal insufficiency caused by HPA axis suppression following drug withdrawal is one of the most serious complications of prednisone therapy (Box 48.3).

Adverse reactions occur with long-term administration of supraphysiologic (pharmacologic) doses of prednisone. Cushingoid characteristics include redistribution of fat deposits (e.g., buffalo hump, moon face, and truncal obesity). Signs of protein catabolism, such as loss of muscle mass and thinning of the extremities, muscle aches, and weakness may also develop. Visual acuity may be affected by the development of cataracts and glaucoma. Hyperlipidemia and thrombus formation also may occur. Other adverse effects from long-term therapy (doses above 5 mg/d) include undesired dermatologic responses of acne, hirsutism, delayed wound healing, skin atrophy, tearing, and striae. Women and the elderly of both genders are more prone to these effects.

A clinically important adverse effect of long-term or high-dose prednisone therapy is osteoporosis due to its association with increased bone mineral density loss putting the patient at increased risk for fracture, which is often considered to be a major limitation of long-term prednisone therapy. Long-term prednisone therapy (doses over 7.5 mg/d) enhances calcium loss and increases parathyroid hormone levels. Calcium loss from bone substance resorption decreases bone mineral density, thereby promoting an osteoporotic condition that increases the risk for hip, pelvic, rib, or vertebral fractures.

Substantial bone effects (e.g., suppression of bone growth) may occur when corticosteroid drugs are used in long-term or intermittent treatment of a variety of diseases. The bones most often affected are the vertebrae, ribs, and long bones, although all bones are at risk. A high incidence of vertebral compression fractures exists in both male and female patients who receive extended prednisone treatment.

There appears to be a direct correlation between the extent of bone loss and the duration of prednisone therapy; research suggests that the majority of bone loss occurs within the first 3 to 12 months, with a slowing of bone loss thereafter. Although alternate-day therapy has been shown to delay some of the adverse effects of long-term prednisone therapy, it does not appear to decrease the risk of osteoporosis. The prevalence of osteoporosis is difficult to assess when corticosteroids are used in diseases in which the risk of osteoporosis is already increased (e.g., rheumatoid arthritis and renal disease).

Finally, glucose tolerance is affected by prednisone. This reaction occurs in as many as 15% of individuals on long-term therapy. The risk for iatrogenic diabetes mellitus

Central Nervous System Problems

- Emotional lability
- Anxiety
- Paresthesias
- Seizures
- Increased intracranial pressure with papilledema
- Insomnia
- Psychosis
- Paradoxical suicidal depression
- Aggravation of preexisting psychiatric disorders

Endocrine/Metabolic Problems

- Antagonistic effects on insulin, parathyroid, and thyroid hormones
- Glucose intolerance
- Hirsutism
- Suppression of HPA axis
- Hyperglycemia
- Hyperlipidemia
- Iatrogenic diabetes
- Obesity
- Increased serum lipids
- Increased serum triglycerides (in transplant and asthmatic patients and those with organ transplantation treated with >5 mg/d of prednisone)
- Protein wasting
- Amenorrhea
- Postmenopausal bleeding

Cardiovascular Problems

- Thromboembolism (fat embolism)
- Arrhythmias secondary to K+ alterations
- Hypertension
- CHF

Gastrointestinal Problems

- Fatty liver infiltrates
- Pancreatitis
- Increased appetite (which leads to weight gain)
- Ulcerative esophagitis

- Nausea and vomiting
- Peptic ulceration with perforation or hemorrhage

Fluid and Electrolyte Problems

- Fluid retention
- K+ loss (hypokalemia)
- Na+ retention (hypernatremia)
- Ca++ loss (hypocalcemia)

Hematologic and Immunologic Problems

- Altered inflammatory response
- Eosinopenia
- Leukocytosis
- Opportunistic infections
- Leukopenia

Musculoskeletal Problems

- Aseptic necrosis (femur, humerus head)
- Growth failure
- Myopathy
- Osteopenia
- Osteoporosis

Ophthalmic Problems

- Increased intraocular pressure
- Cataracts
- Glaucoma
- Exophthalmos

Integumentary Problems

- Acne
- Ecchymoses
- Petechiae
- Skin atrophy
- Striae purpura
- Subcutaneous fat atrophy

General Problems

- Cushingoid characteristics
- Withdrawal syndrome

increases with age, obesity, a previous history of glucose intolerance, and a family history of diabetes. Even low-dose therapy can impair glucose tolerance in patients with type 1 and 2 diabetes. Patients with diabetes may need changes in diet or hypoglycemic therapy (e.g., insulin, oral drugs) to maintain control of blood sugar.

Drug Interactions

Major interactions may occur between prednisone and a variety of drugs. Prednisone also causes some interactions with laboratory measurements. Urine glucose and serum cholesterol levels may be increased. Serum levels of K+ may be decreased. Triiodothyronine (T_3), thyroxine (T_4), thyroid iodine-131 (I-131) uptake, and protein-bound iodine concentrations may be decreased, making it difficult to monitor

the therapeutic response of patients receiving the drugs for thyroiditis or assessing patients for thyroid dysfunction. Prednisone also may produce a false-positive result in some tests for systemic bacterial infections. In addition, reactions to skin tests may be suppressed. Prednisone alters glucose tolerance tests. Patients with diabetes should be monitored closely and adjustments in dosage of insulin or oral anti-diabetic drugs made accordingly. Table 48.2 lists drugs that interact with prednisone.

Assessment of Relevant Core Patient Variables

Health Status

Before administering prednisone, review the patient's drug history for use of prescription, over-the-counter (OTC),

TABLE 48.2	Agents That Interact with P Prednisone	
Interactants	**Effect and Significance**	**Nursing Management**
anticholinesterases	Corticosteroids antagonize the effects of anticholinesterases in patients with myasthenia gravis, resulting in profound muscle depression.	Monitor patient's muscle strength. Ensure safety.
azole antifungal agents	Prednisone clearance possibly decreased	Monitor for increased adverse effects of prednisone.
barbiturates	Barbiturates induce hepatic metabolism of prednisone, resulting in subtherapeutic serum concentrations of prednisone.	Monitor for exacerbation of presenting symptoms. Discuss dosage adjustment of prednisone with health care provider.
hydantoins	Hydantoins induce hepatic metabolism of prednisone, resulting in subtherapeutic serum concentrations of prednisone.	Monitor for exacerbation of presenting symptoms. Discuss dosage adjustment of prednisone with health care provider
oral anticoagulants	Anticoagulant dose requirements possibly reduced; conversely, prednisone may oppose the anticoagulant action.	Monitor PT/INR. Monitor for signs of bruising or bleeding. Monitor for signs of hypercoagulability.
oral contraceptives/estrogens	Possible increased prednisone half-life and concentration and decreased clearance	Monitor for corticosteroid adverse effects. Discuss dosage adjustment of prednisone with health care provider.
potassium-depleting agents (diuretics)	May increase depletion of potassium	Observe patients for muscular and systemic effects of hypokalemia.
rifamycins	Rifamycins induce hepatic metabolism of prednisone, resulting in subtherapeutic serum concentrations of prednisone.	Avoid coadministration if possible. Monitor for exacerbation of presenting symptoms. Discuss dosage adjustment of prednisone with health care provider.
salicylates	Prednisone stimulates the metabolism of salicylates, resulting in decreased serum salicylate levels, and may decrease their effectiveness.	Monitor for effectiveness of salicylates.
tacrolimus	Prednisone may decrease tacrolimus serum concentration.	Monitor for signs of transplant rejection.
theophylline	Alterations in the pharmacologic activity of either agent are possible.	Monitor for theophylline toxicity. Discuss dosage adjustment of theophylline with health care provider.
warfarin	Prednisone may reduce warfarin dose requirements. Conversely, prednisone may occasionally induce a hypercoagulable state that could oppose warfarin action.	Monitor PT/INR closely, especially when starting or stopping prednisone therapy. Discuss potential dosage adjustments with the health care provider.

and herbal medications and recreational drugs. In addition, it is important to review the patient's medical history for GI problems. Assess the patient's nutritional status, weight control, and disease or trauma history to correlate risk for fall and fracture. Perform a complete physical examination and review current laboratory data. In addition, muscle strength and body proportions should be observed, as should patterns of hair growth and distribution. Depending on the findings, further testing (e.g., hepatic and renal function studies) may be indicated. Throughout therapy, continue to assess the patient for signs of adrenal insufficiency.

Life Span and Gender
Determine whether the patient is pregnant or lactating, because prednisone is a pregnancy category C drug and enters breast milk. Growth suppression can occur in children receiving prolonged prednisone therapy. Growth suppression is proportional to the duration, dose, and frequency of prednisone administered. Divided daily doses are more growth inhibiting than a single daily dose.

Assess the age of the patient. Elderly patients are more prone to adrenal suppression from prolonged prednisone administration. They may require lower doses because of physiologic changes resulting from aging, such as decreased muscle mass and plasma volume or impairment of hepatic or renal functions. Monitor blood pressure, blood glucose, and electrolyte levels regularly.

Lifestyle, Diet, and Habits

Assess the patient's typical diet. The patient's diet plan should include low sodium and high potassium. A diet that controls carbohydrate and calorie intake is important (unless contraindicated) because of the increased gluconeogenesis, decreased glucose use, increased appetite, and weight gain effects of pharmacologic glucocorticoid therapy. Encourage increased protein intake to decrease the risk of protein deficiency.

Assess the patient's typical daily activities and fall risk. The weak muscles and easily fatigued state characteristic of unintentional glucocorticoid excess secondary to therapy predispose the patient to accidents such as a fall injury. With this in mind, assessment and discussion of environmental elements that may predispose the patient to a fall injury and implementation of necessary preventive measures are warranted. Osteoporosis and vertebral-compression effects of prolonged, thus, excessive glucocorticoid therapy may make bone fractures more likely. It is important to encourage passive and active range-of-motion exercises, and anaerobic forms of exercises such as weightlifting and resistance training may help to offset the tendency toward muscle weakness and atrophy. Similarly, medications such as calcium, vitamin D, and bisphophonates, e.g., Fosamax, may help prevent and/or arrest the risk of glucocorticoid-induced osteoporosis. Physical or occupational therapy referrals may be necessary.

Nursing Diagnoses and Outcomes

- **Excess Fluid Volume** related to sodium and water retention secondary to corticosteroid therapy
  Desired outcome: The patient will relate causative factors and methods of preventing edema and exhibit decreased peripheral and sacral edema.
- **Risk for Infection or Risk for Injury** related to anti-inflammatory, immunosuppressive, dermatologic, and metabolic effects of chronic corticosteroid therapy
  Desired outcome: The patient will demonstrate knowledge of risk factors associated with potential for infection or injury and will practice appropriate precautions for prevention.
- **Imbalanced Nutrition: More than Body Requirements** related to increased appetite secondary to corticosteroid medications
  Desired outcome: The patient will maintain a healthy weight, discuss current nutritional needs, and discuss the effects of exercise on weight control.
- **Altered Body Image** related to cushingoid characteristics or physical changes secondary to glucocorticoid therapy
  Desired outcome: The patient will verbalize and demonstrate acceptance of appearance (grooming, dress,

posture, presentation of self), verbalize and demonstrate increased positive feelings, and demonstrate healthy adaptation and coping skills.

Planning and Intervention
Maximizing Therapeutic Effects

Hormone production by the adrenal gland is influenced by many factors. Normal cortisol production follows a diurnal cycle. Levels peak in the early morning hours (6 AM to 8 AM) and decline throughout the day with a second, lower peak in the late afternoon (4 PM to 6 PM). Cortisol secretion increases in response to stress (physical or emotional) and low endogenous glucocorticoid levels. Thus, the most opportune time for administration of daily doses or alternate-day doses of glucocorticoids is early in the morning.

When prednisone is prescribed for replacement therapy, teach the patient about:

- Signs and symptoms of glucocorticoid imbalances
- Monitoring the response to therapy
- Drug schedule
- Identifying factors that increase adrenal stress (e.g., physical illness, injury, trauma, or emotional upset)
- Stress management
- Dosage changes during periods of stress or illness
- Prevention of injury and infection
- Drug interactions

Alert the patient that following intra-articular injection, the injected joint should not be overused. Weight-bearing joints, such as the knee, should be rested 24 to 48 hours after the injection.

Minimizing Adverse Effects

Monitor the patient, especially the surgical patient, carefully for signs of infection, because prednisone's immunologic activity may mask the symptoms of infection. Advise the patient to stay away from those with cold or flu-like symptoms or situations that increase the risk of exposure to potential infections. Emphasize the importance of adherence to the drug regimen, especially the adverse consequences of stopping therapy abruptly, such as the danger of adrenal insufficiency, without consultation with their health provider. Administration of prednisone can lead to peptic ulcer disease, as can the use of other anti-inflammatory drugs. Therefore, teach the patient to reduce gastric irritation from prednisone use by consuming milk (unless contraindicated), food, or appropriately timed taking of nonsystemic antacids (e.g., Al^+, Ca^{2+}, or Mg^+ salts), taken 2 hours before or after prednisone dose, or by using adjunct antiulcer drug therapy (e.g., H_2-receptor antagonists, proton pump inhibitors) when taking the medication. Caffeine, alcohol, and products containing aspirin interact with prednisone, increasing the secretion of gastric acid irritating the gastric mucosa and leading to an increased risk of GI bleeding.

Altered growth and development is a risk with systemic glucocorticoid therapy. Inhaled glucocorticoids may cause hoarseness, fungal infections, throat irritation, and dry mouth. Teach the patient to rinse the mouth or brush the teeth following use of the inhaled steroids to minimize the risk for oral, laryngeal, or pharyngeal fungal infections. Carefully monitor patients who are transitioning from systemic prednisone to an inhaled glucocorticoid. When systemic glucocorticoids are withdrawn too quickly after beginning inhalation therapy, a corticosteroid withdrawal syndrome (e.g., malaise, myalgia, nausea, headache, and low-grade fever) and asthma relapse may develop.

Alternate-day administration (glucocorticoids given every other day instead of daily) of long-term, systemic glucocorticoids has been used to lessen the suppression of the hypothalamus, the anterior pituitary, and the rate of bone loss. However, alternate-day dosing does not minimize the risk of osteoporosis or cataract formation. Intermediate-acting glucocorticoids, such as prednisone, are most appropriate for alternate-day therapy. Ensure that the change from daily to alternate-day administration does not occur abruptly, because this abrupt change may cause signs and symptoms of adrenal insufficiency (e.g., fatigue, nausea, vomiting, and hypotension) on the days between doses.

When a patient receiving ongoing corticosteroid therapy requires surgery, review the preoperative orders to ensure a dose of a rapid-acting corticosteroid has been added to the patient's daily dose of corticosteroid. If not, obtain the order from the prescriber. To promote recovery after the stress of surgery, an increased dose of steroid should be continued postoperatively in decreasing doses over several days, returning to the patient's baseline dose of corticosteroid.

Providing Patient and Family Education
- Discuss taking the drug exactly as prescribed.
- Discuss not stopping the drug abruptly because of the risk of acute adrenal insufficiency.
- Discuss dealing with missed doses and the dosing strategy (Box 48.4).
- Discuss the purpose of the medication therapy and the need for maintaining therapy.
- Teach that prednisone replacement therapy is used to treat the chronic, lifelong conditions of adrenal cortical insufficiency.
- Provide emotional support and assistance in the grieving process over loss of health and loss of control, as needed (PRN).
- Advise patients to wear a medical identification device with the diagnosis and drug therapy clearly indicated.
- Emphasize the importance of patients' notifying all health care providers about glucocorticoid therapy when seeking medical treatment.
- Discuss the adverse effects of drug therapy and identify symptoms that should be reported to the prescriber.
- Discuss alterations in appearance that may cause disturbances in self-concept from long-term therapy.

BOX 48.4 COMMUNITY BASED CONCERNS

Home Dosing Strategies

One Dose Every Other Day
If a dose is missed, take the missed dose as soon as possible. If the medication is remembered the same morning, take it and then go back to the regular dosing schedule.

If the dose is remembered several hours late, then wait and take it the following morning. Skip the next day and start the regular dosing schedule the day after.

One Dose Every Day
If a dose is missed, take the missed dose as soon as possible, then go back to the regular schedule.
If the missed dose is not remembered until the next day, skip it and do not double the next dose.

Several Doses Every Day
If a dose is missed, it is important to take the missed dose as soon as possible, then go back to the regular schedule.
If the missed dose is not remembered until the next dose is due, double the next dose.

Periods of Stress, Illness, Injury, or Surgery
Make sure that the directions for dosage adjustment are clearly indicated on the drug label.

- Discuss strategies to deal with the changes that occur (e.g., truncal obesity, acne, hair growth, stretch marks, thinning of extremities, weight gain, or "buffalo hump" may be camouflaged with loose clothing).
- Discuss bone health (supplemental daily intake of 1,500 mg of oral calcium and 510 IU of vitamin D, or bisphosphonates, is recommended).
- Teach how to identify signs and symptoms of acute adrenal insufficiency, including symptoms of anorexia, hypoglycemia, lethargy, malaise, nausea, psychological despondency, restlessness, and weakness, and to report symptoms to the prescriber.
- Discuss the importance of rest, sleep, and health-maintenance behaviors.
- Teach ways to avoid infection and how to recognize signs of infection.
- Discuss self-medication for minor illnesses handled at home (e.g., flu with vomiting and diarrhea) that may require dosage adjustments, medical intervention, or hospitalization.
- Provide patients and their caregivers with written instructions on what to do on sick days.
- Discuss safety issues and fall preventions. Emphasize the possible occurrence of osteoporosis and encourage patients and caregivers to report all bone pain.
- Evaluate the safety of the home environment. Stress the importance of reporting bone pain, because aseptic necrosis or pathologic fractures may occur spontaneously.
- Explain the importance of serial ophthalmologic examination and may include continued screening for cataract, glaucoma, intraocular pressure, and or eye infections.

Ongoing Assessment and Evaluation

During prednisone therapy, the patient must be monitored for therapeutic drug response, adverse drug reactions, and indications of drug toxicity. Monitor for periods of stress (e.g., trauma, surgery, or severe illness) in order to coordinate medication adjustment of prednisone dosage to avoid drug-induced adrenal insufficiency. Assess for appropriate healing of all wounds and infections during and after hospitalizations or minor surgery because prednisone delays wound healing and increases the risk for infection. Common indicators of infection (including temperature elevation, erythema, and leukocytosis) are repressed because corticosteroids block the inflammatory responses. Also, assess for changes in energy level, activity level, and appetite as indicators of infection.

Glucocorticoids cause an increase in gluconeogenesis and a decrease in glucose utilization, causing hyperglycemia to occur. Monitor patients for the development of iatrogenic diabetes mellitus. Patients with existing diabetes may require an adjustment in therapy to maintain glucose control. Prophylactic antitubercular drug therapy may be required in infected persons because high glucocorticoid levels are likely to reactivate encapsulated tuberculosis.

Maintain vigilance in assessing patients receiving long-term therapy with prednisone (and other glucocorticoids). Adrenal suppression may occur, whereas effects of endogenous glucocorticoid hormones on the body may be exaggerated. Indications of adrenal suppression include anorexia, diarrhea, fluid and electrolyte imbalances (especially decreased Na^+, decreased glucose, and increased K^+), fatigue, nausea, vomiting, and weight loss. If fluid volume deficit occurs, it is important to assess for hypotension, pyrexia, tachycardia and tachypnea, dry skin, and dry mucous membranes. Also, assess for adverse reactions from prednisone (and other glucocorticoids), such as changes in mood or affect (e.g., agitation, depression, euphoria, and insomnia), edema, muscle weakness, nausea, vomiting, and weight gain.

While caring for a patient on glucocorticoid therapy, monitor specific laboratory tests results. Actual serum levels of cortisol and ACTH may be determined by a 24-hour urine collection. Electrolytes are measured with a metabolic panel. Lymphocyte levels (primarily T_4) should decrease when glucocorticoids are being used for immunosuppressive effects. In addition, monitor patients receiving digoxin or other digitalis-based drugs for toxicity.

Evaluate for the effectiveness of the therapy and assess signs and symptoms that precipitated the use of glucocorticoid drugs. When prednisone is used as replacement therapy, the patient should report an increased state of health (e.g., absence of fatigue, hypoglycemia, hypovolemia, and weakness) and a feeling of well-being. When prednisone is used for chronic inflammatory conditions (e.g., rheumatoid arthritis), the patient should experience less pain and discomfort and increased joint mobility.

MEMORY CHIP

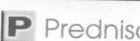 **Prednisone**

- Anti-inflammatory or immunosuppressive therapy
- Hepatic dysfunction may impair prednisone conversion into active prednisolone.
- Prednisone may cause HPA axis suppression if given for more than 2 weeks and then withdrawn too abruptly, placing the patient at risk for acute adrenal insufficiency.
- Major contraindications: hypersensitivity to prednisone; systemic fungal infections
- Most common adverse effects: CNS complaints of euphoria, headache, and vertigo; GI complaints of nausea, vomiting, increased appetite, weight gain, and dyspepsia
- Most serious adverse effect: acute adrenal insufficiency due to HPA axis suppression following prednisone withdrawal
- Maximizing therapeutic effects: Administer prednisone according to established schedule (preferably one that follows the normal diurnal pattern of cortisol secretion); increase the dosage in times of stress to prevent drug-induced adrenal insufficiency.
- Minimizing adverse effects: Give prednisone with meals and/or antacids.
- Most important patient education: Advise the patient to wear medical identification so that any emergency medical personnel will know about this drug therapy.

CRITICAL THINKING SCENARIO

CONCERNS RAISED BY METHYLPREDNISOLONE AND OTHER GLUCOCORTICOIDS

Mr. Vito, 62 years old, is admitted to the emergency department with acute respiratory distress related to chronic obstructive pulmonary disease. Emergency treatment consists of respiratory inhalation therapy and IV methylprednisolone sodium succinate (Solu-Medrol), after which Mr. Vito is transferred to the telemetry unit. The nursing history that accompanies him discloses that he has type 2 diabetes that is controlled by diet and oral antidiabetic drugs.

1. Discuss assessment data needed to ensure safe administration of methylprednisolone to Mr. Vito, identifying any condition that represents a need for particularly cautious drug administration.

2. Define any concerns related to respiratory therapy and diabetes control. As Mr. Vito recovers, plans are made for him to begin long-term, anti-inflammatory corticosteroid therapy. At discharge, he will be on a tapering dose of oral prednisone and a beclomethasone (Vanceril) inhaler as needed.

3. Identify any important assessments that should be done to ensure safe administration of prednisone. In addition, propose important points to include in a patient education program.

Drugs Closely Related to P Prednisone

Betamethasone

Betamethasone (Celestone) is available as an oral, effervescent, or extended-release tablet, or as a syrup. Betamethasone sodium phosphate/betamethasone acetate (Celestone Soluspan) is a solution for intramuscular (IM) administration when the oral form cannot be given. Clinical uses and adverse effects are similar to those for dexamethasone and methylprednisolone (see below). In addition, betamethasone sodium phosphate/betamethasone acetate may be used to prevent respiratory distress syndrome in premature infants. Betamethasone dipropionate combined with calcipotriene or clotrimazole is available as a lotion or ointment for disorders of the skin.

Dexamethasone

Dexamethasone (Decadron) exhibits essentially no mineralocorticoid activity and maximal anti-inflammatory activity with a prolonged plasma half-life (see Figure 48.3). Indications are similar to those for prednisone; however, it is most frequently used in short-term situations that require maximum anti-inflammatory activity (e.g., cerebral edema and septic shock) or as replacement therapy, or as an anti-emetic. Also, it is used for steroid-responsive ophthalmologic inflammatory conditions, such as allergic conjunctivitis, iritis, and also for symptomatic treatment of corneal injuries associated with trauma, such as thermal or chemical burns, and also foreign body eye penetration. Dexamethasone is also used to diagnosis Cushing disease (idiopathic adrenocortical hyperfunction). Patients are given a dexamethasone suppression test. In normal patients, dexamethasone suppresses the release of ACTH, resulting in a decreased release of cortisol. In patients with Cushing disease, there is little or no change in the release of cortisol. Off-label uses of dexamethasone include acute mountain sickness, bacterial meningitis, bronchopulmonary dysplasia in preterm infants, diagnosis of depression, hirsutism, and for antiemetic purposes. Contraindications, adverse effects, drug–drug interactions, and patient management are similar to those for prednisone.

Hydrocortisone

Hydrocortisone (Cortef) is structurally identical to natural cortisol. It is available in many forms, including oral tablets, rectal cream or enema, ophthalmic drops, and topical cream, lotion, gel, ointment, spray, and even a stick. Hydrocortisone sodium succinate (Solu-Cortef, A-Hydrocort) is administered parenterally for acute adrenal insufficiency or when oral administration is not possible for other indications. Because of its glucocorticoid and mineralocorticoid activity, as well as its salt-retaining properties, hydrocortisone is the treatment of choice for adrenal insufficiency replacement therapy. The drug is bound reversibly to corticosteroid-binding albumin and globulin. It is metabolized by the liver and excreted in the urine. Rectal preparations of hydrocortisone (Anusol HC, Colocort) are absorbed as much as 50% and used as adjunctive therapy in patients with ulcerative colitis

and other steroid-responsive conditions. Contraindications to rectal preparations are systemic fungal infections, recent ileocolostomy or intestinal anastomoses, abscess, obstruction, peritonitis, and perforation. Contraindications, adverse effects, drug–drug interactions, and patient management of oral hydrocortisone are similar to those for prednisone. In addition, its intramuscular injection is contraindicated on patients with idiopathic thrombocytopenia purpura (ITP).

Methylprednisolone

Methylprednisolone (Medrol) and its derivatives, methylprednisolone acetate (Depo-Medrol) and methylprednisolone sodium succinate (Solu-Medrol), are synthetic glucocorticoids characterized by potent anti-inflammatory and immunosuppressive effects. These drugs have little mineralocorticoid activity and usually are not used to manage adrenal insufficiency unless a more potent mineralocorticoid is administered concomitantly.

Methylprednisolone is administered orally, whereas methylprednisolone sodium succinate may be given by IM or IV injection. Methylprednisolone acetate may be administered by IM, intra-articular, intralesional, or soft-tissue injection. Avoid IM injections of acetate to deltoid area due to high incidence of subcutaneous atrophy because of its low solubility and sustained IM effect. Also, avoid injections on areas with acute local infection. As in prednisone therapy, systemic methylprednisolone must be discontinued gradually or changed to an oral form of a glucocorticoid to prevent acute adrenal insufficiency. Contraindications, adverse effects, drug-drug interactions, and patient management are similar to those for prednisone.

Prednisolone

Prednisolone sodium phosphate (Pediapred, Orapred) is primarily a glucocorticoid. It is available for parenteral and ophthalmic administration. Prednisolone has indications similar to those for prednisone, although it is not approved for adrenal insufficiency. Non–Food and Drug Administration (FDA)-approved uses include breast cancer, malignancy-induced fever, primary intracranial tumor, nerve injury due to leprosy, multiple myeloma, and prostate cancer. Prednisolone acetate (Pred Forte, Pred Mild) is an ophthalmologic drug for inflammatory disorders of the eye. For a comparison of glucocorticoids, see Figure 48.3.

Inhaled Glucocorticoids

Beclomethasone, budesonide, flunisolide, fluticasone, and triamcinolone acetonide constitute a class of pulmonary and intranasal steroids possessing enhanced topical anti-inflammatory activity and low systemic potency. Inhaled glucocorticoids are metabolized in the lung before they are absorbed, thereby reducing their systemic effects. These drugs are relatively equal in potency and clinical effectiveness and are thought to have variable systemic activity and complications. The intranasal and inhaled glucocorticoids are covered in depth in Chapters 48 and 49.

Topical Glucocorticoids

Topical steroids are effective therapy for a variety of inflammatory skin conditions. They are ranked according to their potency, from very high to very low (Table 48.3). Available formulations include lotions, creams, solutions, ointments, gel, or foams. Ointments are often preferred, are most potent because of its occlusive effect as they facilitate steroid absorption and penetration by trapping the moisture in the epidermis. However, its greasy effect may not enhance patient's compliance. Lotions are best for hairy and large surface areas and provide coolness and drying effect that is excellent for moist dermatoses or pruritus. Foams, on the other hand, are readily and easier to apply especially on an inflamed skin and scalp. It is the most cosmetically acceptable and thus increases compliance, but tend to be more expensive. Topical steroids are best applied when skin is moist, such as after taking a bath.

The primary therapeutic effects of the topical corticosteroids are their nonspecific anti-inflammatory activity on most causes of inflammation, including chemical, immunologic, mechanical, and microbiologic etiologies. When the glucocorticoids are applied to inflamed skin, they inhibit the migration of macrophages and leukocytes into the area by reversing the vascular dilation and permeability. The clinical result is a decrease in edema, erythema, and pruritus.

Topical application of corticosteroids rarely produces systemic effects. Topical steroids may be absorbed systemically if applied to the nasal mucosa or large areas of abraded skin, inhaled excessively for prolonged periods, or used in large doses. Optic and otic steroid preparations are not absorbed systemically.

Adverse effects with topical application are usually milder and more transient than those seen after systemically administered steroids. However, adrenal function may be suppressed when potent topical agents are used in large amounts for long periods especially when the skin surface is denuded or when occlusive dressings are used. Occlusive dressings substantially increase percutaneous absorption, increasing the risk for local adverse effects (e.g., skin atrophy) and systemic adverse effects. Increased skin temperature, hydration, and application to skin with a thin surface layer also enhance absorption. Duration of potent topical corticosteroid should not exceed 3 weeks, but is alright for persistent small areas. Intermittent treatment is preferable over continuous therapy to avoid tachyphylaxis. Also, weaker form of topical steroids should be used on intertriginous areas, the face, and genitalia as they are most susceptible to corticosteroid-induced atrophy and telangiectasia.

Intra-articularly Injected Glucocorticoids

Intra-articular injection produces localized effects for symptomatic relief of joint pain and increase joint mobility. Patients receiving this form of the drug need to be cautioned to allow time for the treated area to heal, about 24 to 48 hours. The pain-induced limitation may be eliminated, but overusing the joint may still aggravate the active inflammatory process. Frequent intra-articular injections may damage joint tissues.

TABLE 48.3	Comparative Potency of Topical Glucocorticosteroids					
Very High Potency	High Potency	High/Medium Potency	Medium Potency	Medium/Low Potency	Low Potency	Lowest Potency
betamethasone dipropionate augmented (0.05% G,O) clobetasol (0.05% C,G,F, L,O,S) halobetasol (0.05% C,O)	amcinonide (0.1% O) betamethasone dipropionate augmented (0.05% C,L) betamethasone dipropionate (0.05% O) desoximetasone (0.25% C,O; 0.05% G) diflorasone (0.05% O) diflorasone emollient (0.05% C,O) fluocinonide (0.05% C,G, O,S) halcinonide (0.1% C) mometasone (0.1% O)	amcinonide (0.1% C,L) betamethasone dipropionate (0.05% C) betamethasone valerate (0.1% O) desoximetasone (0.05% C) diflorasone (0.05% C,L) fluocinonide emollient (0.05% C) fluticasone (0.005% O) halcinonide (0.1% O,S) triamcinolone (0.1% O, 0.5% C, aerosol)	betamethasone valerate (0.12% F) clocortolone (0.1% C); fluocinolone (0.025% O) flurandrenolide (0.05% O) hydrocortisone valerate (0.2% O) mometasone (0.1% C,L) prednicarbate (0.1% O) triamcinolone (0.1% C,O)	betamethasone dipropionate (0.05% L) betamethasone valerate (0.1% C) desonide (0.05% O) fluocinolone (0.025% C, 0.01% Shmp) flurandrenolide (0.05% C) fluticasone (0.05% C,L) hydrocortisone butyrate (0.1% C,O,S) hydrocortisone valerate (0.2% C) prednicarbate (0.1% C) triamcinolone (0.025% O; 0.1% L)	alclometasone (0.05% C,O) betamethasone valerate (0.1% L) desonide (0.05% C,F,G,L) fluocinolone (0.01% C,S) triamcinolone (0.025% C,L; 0.1% C)	hydrocortisone (0.5%,1% C,L,O; 2.5% C,L,S) methylprednisolone (0.25% O)

C, cream; F, foam; G, gel; L, lotion; O, ointment; S, solution; Shmp, shampoo.

• MINERALOCORTICOIDS

Aldosterone, the naturally occurring mineralocorticoid, is expensive and requires parenteral administration. Therefore, fludrocortisone (Florinef Acetate) is the prototype exogenous mineralocorticoid. This adrenal corticosteroid has both high mineralocorticoid and glucocorticoid activity (its glucocorticoid potency is 15 times greater than that of hydrocortisone). However, when used as replacement therapy in adrenocortical deficiency, its therapeutic effect is the mineralocorticoid activity.

Nursing Management of the Patient Receiving P Fludrocortisone

Core Drug Knowledge

Pharmacotherapeutics

Fludrocortisone is used for partial replacement therapy for primary and secondary adrenocortical insufficiency in Addison's disease and for treating salt-losing adrenogenital syndrome.

Pharmacokinetics

Orally administered, fludrocortisone is absorbed readily from the GI tract, with peak concentration in 1.7 hours. It is metabolized in the liver and excreted by the kidney. Plasma half-life is approximately 3.5 hours, but biologic half-life ranges from 18 to 36 hours. Fludrocortisone crosses the placenta and is secreted in breast milk. The usual adult dosage is 0.1 mg/day (range, 0.1 mg three times a week, up to 0.2 mg/day). See Table 48.4.

Pharmacodynamics

Fludrocortisone acts on the distal renal tubule to enhance the reabsorption of sodium and to increase the urinary excretion of both potassium and hydrogen ions. In small oral doses, the mineralocorticoid effects of fludrocortisone predominate: urinary excretion of potassium, marked sodium retention, and a rise in blood pressure as a result of the physiologic effects of these electrolyte levels. Larger doses of fludrocortisone result in predominance of glucocorticoid effects such as endogenous adrenal cortical secretion, thymic activity, and corticotropin excretion.

Contraindications and Precautions

Fludrocortisone hypersensitivity, systemic fungal infections, and conditions not requiring intense mineralocorticoid activity are contraindications to use. Fludrocortisone is a pregnancy category C drug, and it should be used cautiously during lactation because it is secreted into breast milk. Safety and efficacy are not established in children. It should also be used cautiously in patients with cardiovascular disease because it can elevate sodium and fluid levels.

Adverse Effects

In small oral doses, fludrocortisone produces marked sodium retention and increased urinary potassium excretion, causing a rise in blood pressure. In larger doses, fludrocortisone inhibits endogenous adrenal cortical secretion and pituitary corticotropin excretion. It promotes the deposition of liver glycogen. It induces negative nitrogen balance when protein intake is inadequate. Adverse effects usually occur when the dosage is too high or when the drug is withdrawn too rapidly. Cardiovascular adverse effects may include edema, hypertension, chronic heart failure, and cardiomegaly. Dermatologic adverse effects may include bruising, diaphoresis, urticaria, or allergic skin rash. Hypokalemic alkalosis may occur. Additionally, fludrocortisone may cause adverse effects similar to those seen with the glucocorticoids.

Drug Interactions

Fludrocortisone interacts with many of the same drugs as prednisone because of its high glucocorticoid activity. The drugs with which fludrocortisone interacts include barbiturates, hydantoins, rifampin, anticholinesterases, and salicylates. Table 48.5 lists agents that interact with fludrocortisone.

Assessment of Relevant Core Patient Variables

Health Status

Review the patient's history for pre-existing conditions that require cautious use of fludrocortisone (e.g., diabetes mellitus, hypertension, osteoporosis, or impaired renal function).

Report any positive findings to the health care provider. Before administering fludrocortisone, assess the patient's fluid and electrolyte balance, nutritional status, and weight control history. Depending on the patient's condition before drug administration, assess appropriate laboratory or diagnostic tests to manage the adverse events associated with fluid and electrolytes (particularly hypertension).

Life Span and Gender

Determine whether the patient is pregnant or lactating, because fludrocortisone is a pregnancy category C drug, which means that safety for use during pregnancy has not been established. If fludrocortisone is given during pregnancy, observe the newborn for signs of adrenocortical insufficiency because of adrenal suppression.

TABLE 48.4 Overview of P Fludrocortisone			
Drug (Trade) Name	Selected Indications	Route and Dosage Range	Pharmacokinetics
P fludrocortisone	Adrenal insufficiency	Adult PO: 0.1–0.2 mg daily Child: safety and efficacy not established.	Onset: gradual Duration: 18–36 h $t_{1/2}$: 3.5 h

TABLE 48.5   Agents That Interact with P Fludrocortisone

Interactants	Effect and Significance	Nursing Management
Anticholinesterases	Corticosteroids antagonize the effects of anticholinesterases in patients with myasthenia gravis, resulting in profound muscle depression.	Monitor patient's muscle strength. Ensure safety.
Barbiturates	Barbiturates induce hepatic metabolism of prednisone, resulting in subtherapeutic serum concentrations of prednisone.	Monitor for exacerbation of presenting symptoms. Discuss dosage adjustment of prednisone with health care provider.
Hydantoins	Hydantoins induce hepatic metabolism of prednisone, resulting in subtherapeutic serum concentrations of prednisone.	Monitor for exacerbation of presenting symptoms. Discuss dosage adjustment of prednisone with health care provider.
Oral anticoagulants	Anticoagulant dose requirements possibly reduced; conversely, prednisone may oppose the anticoagulant action.	Monitor PT/INR. Monitor for signs of bruising or bleeding. Monitor for signs of hypercoagulability.
Rifamycins	Rifamycins induce hepatic metabolism of prednisone, resulting in subtherapeutic serum concentrations of prednisone.	Avoid coadministration if possible. Monitor for exacerbation of presenting symptoms. Discuss dosage adjustment of prednisone with health care provider.
Salicylates	Prednisone stimulates the metabolism of salicylates, resulting in decreased serum salicylate levels, and may decrease their effectiveness.	Monitor for effectiveness of salicylates.

Fludrocortisone is secreted in breast milk. Therefore, use caution when giving it to lactating women. It is important to note the patient's age before administering fludrocortisone. Monitor growth and development of infants and children on long-term therapy.

Lifestyle, Diet, and Habits

Assess the patient's diet because fludrocortisone-mediated sodium retention and potassium loss are affected by food choices. Teach the patient about foods that are low in sodium or high in potassium.

Environment

Fludrocortisone may be given in any setting, including the home environment.

Culture and Inherited Traits

Traditional foods and herbal and home remedies consumed by patients of various ethnic or cultural groups may be high in sodium. For example, Chinese foods are traditionally prepared with high-sodium soy sauce and monosodium glutamate (MSG). Many other preserved and fermented foods are high in sodium. Take a complete dietary history, including usual dietary intake, food preferences and intolerances, and use of home remedies. This information allows you to assess the patient's risk of weight gain or edema and also provides the knowledge to use when teaching the patient, family, and caregivers.

Nursing Diagnoses and Outcomes

- Excess Fluid Volume related to mineralocorticoid-induced sodium and water retention

Desired outcome: The patient will relate causative factors and methods of preventing fluid retention and exhibit decreased peripheral and sacral edema.
- Risk for Infection or Risk for Injury related to immunosuppressive effects of chronic corticosteroid therapy
Desired outcome: The patient will demonstrate knowledge of risk factors associated with potential for infection and will practice appropriate precautions for prevention.
- Risk for Injury related to adrenocortical insufficiency
Desired outcome: The patient will demonstrate knowledge of risk factors associated with potential for injury and will practice appropriate precautions for prevention.

Planning and Intervention

Maximizing Therapeutic Effects

Assess for drugs that may interact with fludrocortisone and decrease its efficacy. These drugs include barbiturates, cholestyramine, oral contraceptives, and salicylates. As with prednisone, evaluate the need for an increased dose of fludrocortisone during times of injury, stress, or infection, or during surgery.

Minimizing Adverse Effects

Monitor blood pressure, fluid balance, signs of edema, serum electrolyte status, and serum renin activity. Patients with a history of renal or cardiovascular dysfunction are at risk for adverse effects from fludrocortisone. Review the importance of following a diet high in potassium-rich foods in order to prevent potassium loss and low sodium intake to reduce the risk for hypertension, weight gain, and edema.

MEMORY CHIP

P Fludrocortisone

- Fludrocortisone is given for adrenal insufficiency (Addison disease)
- Fludrocortisone may cause HRA axis suppression if given for more than 2 weeks and withdrawn too abruptly; abrupt withdrawal places the patient at risk for acute adrenal insufficiency.
- Major contraindications: hypersensitivity to fludrocortisone; conditions not requiring intense mineralocorticoid activity
- Most common adverse effects: sodium retention and increased urinary potassium excretion
- Most serious adverse effects: chronic heart failure, cardiomegaly, and hypokalemic alkalosis
- Maximizing therapeutic effects: Increase the dosage in times of stress to prevent drug-induced adrenal insufficiency.
- Minimizing adverse effects: Monitor fluid balance.
- Most important patient education: Eat potassium-rich foods and moderate sodium intake.

Providing Patient and Family Education

- Instruct patients to adhere to drug therapy as prescribed, stressing the importance of regular follow-up visits with the prescriber.
- Encourage patients to wear a medical identification bracelet stating their medical condition and the specific drug therapy.
- Teach patients to report unusual weight gain, lower extremity edema, muscle weakness, and severe or continuing headache.
- Teach patients to monitor blood pressure.
- Schedule follow-up appointments to monitor serum electrolytes (including calcium) regularly to prevent fludrocortisone overdosage.
- Help patients develop a low-sodium and high-potassium dietary plan.
- Teach patients to weigh themselves daily; any sudden weight increase indicates fluid retention.
- Teach signs and symptoms for self-monitoring adverse effects to drug therapy.

Ongoing Assessment and Evaluation

Monitor for edema, weight gain, hypertension, cardiac arrhythmias, or muscular weakness that may develop because of fludrocortisone's sodium-retaining effects. Potassium supplementation may be necessary related to

potassium loss. Periods of stress (e.g., those related to trauma, surgery, or severe illness) may require medication adjustment of mineralocorticoid and glucocorticoid dosage to avoid drug-induced adrenal insufficiency.

Assess the patient for adverse reactions to fludrocortisone, including fluid retention (e.g., increased blood pressure, sudden weight gain), ankle edema, and respiratory crackles. Additionally, monitor for acute adrenal insufficiency or characteristic adverse glucocorticoid reactions. Fludrocortisone replacement therapy is effective when the patient exhibits a normal blood pressure, and fluid and electrolyte balance is within normal limits. The patient should be able to explain the importance of self-monitoring for adverse effects.

C STEROID HORMONE ANTAGONISTS

Steroid hormone antagonists, otherwise known as adrenal **steroid hormone inhibitors,** act to inhibit or suppress the steroidogenesis by the adrenal cortex, thus controlling the symptoms of Cushing syndrome. Drugs within this class include aminoglutethimide, cyproheptadine, ketoconazole, mifepristone, and mitotane. Aminoglutethimide, which suppresses adrenal cortical function, is the prototype steroid hormone antagonist.

Nursing Management of the Patient Receiving P Aminoglutethimide

Core Drug Knowledge

Pharmacotherapeutics

Aminoglutethimide is used to treat hypercortisolism (Cushing syndrome). It does not affect the underlying pathology of the hypercortisolism and is used for a short period (less than 3 months) until more definitive therapy (e.g., surgery or pituitary radiation) can be initiated. Non-FDA-approved uses include advanced breast cancer in postmenopausal women and metastatic prostate cancer.

Pharmacokinetics

Aminoglutethimide is well absorbed orally and is bound minimally to plasma proteins. Its plasma half-life of 5 to 9 hours (initially, 11 to 16 hours) decreases following 1 to 2 weeks of therapy because of its action as a hepatic enzyme inducer. Aminoglutethimide crosses the placenta and is secreted in breast milk. It is excreted in the urine. The usual adult dosage for Cushing syndrome is 250 mg every 6 hours, up to a maximum of 2 g/d (see Table 48.6).

TABLE 48.6	Overview of P Aminoglutethimide		
Drug (Trade) Name	Selected Indications	Route and Dosage Range	Pharmacokinetics
P aminoglutethimide	Cushing syndrome	Adult PO: 250 mg every 6 h to a maximum of 2 g/d Child: Safety and efficacy not established	Onset: gradual Duration: unknown T ½: 11–16 h
	Breast cancer	Adult PO: 250 mg 2×/d for 2 wk then increase to 250 mg 4×/d. Given in combination with hydrocortisone.	

Pharmacodynamics

Aminoglutethimide inhibits enzymatic conversion of cholesterol to pregnenolone, which is the first step in steroid syntheses pathway. This reduces the synthesis of all adrenal steroids. The decrease in adrenal steroids induces a compensatory increase in secretion of ACTH, necessitating coadministration of hydrocortisone to maintain aminoglutethimide's effect. Aminoglutethimide also blocks the aromatase enzyme, which decreases estrogen production from androgens in peripheral tissues.

Contraindications and Precautions

Hypersensitivity to glutethimide (a nonbarbiturate sedative-hypnotic) or aminoglutethimide is a contraindication for use. A pregnancy category D drug, aminoglutethimide is used cautiously during pregnancy.

Adverse Effects

Common adverse reactions to aminoglutethimide include drowsiness, dizziness, skin rash, nausea, and anorexia. These effects usually disappear spontaneously within 1 to 2 weeks of therapy. Aminoglutethimide may suppress aldosterone production by the adrenal cortex, resulting in hypotension and compensatory tachycardia. Additional adverse effects include headache, myalgias, and blood dyscrasias such as granulocytosis, leukopenia, neutropenia, and pancytopenia. Rarely, elevated liver enzymes or hepatotoxicity may occur.

Drug Interactions

Drug interactions with aminoglutethimide occur because of its action as an enzyme inducer. Aminoglutethimide interacts with coumarin, warfarin, other oral anticoagulants, theophylline, digoxin, medroxyprogesterone, and dexamethasone. Table 48.7 lists agents that interact with aminoglutethimide.

Assessment of Relevant Core Patient Variables

Health Status

Review current laboratory data because hypothyroidism and hematologic abnormalities may occur with aminoglutethimide use. These tests include a CBC, serum electrolyte levels, thyroid function studies, kidney and liver function, glucose tolerance test results, electrocardiogram, x-ray films of spine and chest, and tuberculin skin test results. Assess the patient's history of prescription, OTC, recreational, or illicit drug use; GI upset; ulcers; or epigastric pain. Also assess nutritional status, weight control, concurrent disease, and trauma history. Include orthostatic vital signs in the physical assessment. Observe muscle strength and body proportions as well as hair growth and distribution patterns. Throughout therapy, continue to assess for signs of adrenal insufficiency.

Life Span and Gender

Determine whether the patient is pregnant. Aminoglutethimide is a pregnancy category D drug and should be avoided during pregnancy. It is unknown whether it is secreted in breast milk; safety in lactation and safety and efficacy in children have not been established. It is important to note the patient's physical condition and age before administering aminoglutethimide. Geriatric patients may have increased sensitivity to CNS effects and may become lethargic.

Lifestyle, Diet, and Habits

Assess the patient's typical daily activities. Dizziness and drowsiness may occur with aminoglutethimide use, and caution when performing activities requiring alertness and concentration is necessary until drug effects are known. It also is important to determine the patient's alcohol intake because alcohol potentiates aminoglutethimide's effect.

Environment

Aminoglutethimide may be given in any setting, including the home environment.

Nursing Diagnoses and Outcomes

- Risk for Injury related to CNS effects of hypotension and sedation, endocrine effects of hypothyroidism, or hematologic effects of agranulocytosis, leukopenia, and thrombocytopenia

TABLE 48.7	Agents That Interact with P Aminoglutethimide	
Interactants	Effect and Significance	Nursing Management
oral anticoagulants	Aminoglutethimide increases warfarin metabolic clearance, reducing action of warfarin.	Monitor PT/INR. Monitor for signs of bruising or bleeding. Discuss dosage adjustment of warfarin with health care provider.
corticosteroids	Aminoglutethimide may induce loss of dexamethasone-induced adrenal suppression, resulting in unsuccessful chemical adrenalectomy.	Doses of dexamethasone higher than usually required may be necessary. Discuss substituting hydrocortisone for dexamethasone with health care provider.
theophyllines	Aminoglutethimide is a potent inducer of hepatic enzymes responsible for the metabolism of theophylline.	Monitor serum theophylline levels. Monitor respiratory status. Discuss dosage adjustment of theophylline with health care provider.

Desired outcome: The patient will remain injury free during aminoglutethimide therapy.

- Imbalanced Nutrition: Less than Body Requirements related to adverse effects of anorexia and nausea
Desired outcome: There will be no change or an improved nutritional status.

- Disturbed Body Image related to hirsutism and masculinization (in females)
Desired outcome: The patient will identify and incorporate methods for camouflaging the adverse hormonal effects of aminoglutethimide therapy.

Planning and Intervention

Maximizing Therapeutic Effects

Advise the patient to carry medical identification and to inform health care professionals that aminoglutethimide is being taken. It is important to remind the patient that an injury, infection, or illness may cause adrenocortical insufficiency, and the patient may require a medication dose adjustment.

Minimizing Adverse Effects

Suppression of aldosterone production may cause orthostatic or persistent hypotension. Teach the patient to change positions slowly and to avoid situations or environments that enhance hypotension (e.g., consumption of alcohol, overheated areas) to decrease the risk of accidental injury from postural hypotension.

Providing Patient and Family Education

- Discuss the adverse reactions of aminoglutethimide, including dizziness or drowsiness, nausea, anorexia, headache, orthostatic hypotension, and hirsutism.
- Caution patients about driving or performing other tasks that requires alertness, coordination, or physical dexterity until the effects of the drug are known.
- Teach patients that small, frequent meals of bland foods may reduce the symptoms of nausea.
- Teach patients to change positions slowly to reduce fall risk caused by orthostatic hypotension.
- Teach patients to report skin rash, severe drowsiness or dizziness, headache, or severe nausea.
- Teach patients to avoid pregnancy, alcohol consumption, and overheated environments while taking this drug.

Ongoing Assessment and Evaluation

Continuously assess for adrenal insufficiency because adjustment of the aminoglutethimide dose may be necessary. Monitor blood pressure and assess for hematologic abnormalities and physical and mental changes associated with hypothyroidism. Thyroid hormone replacement may be necessary.

Nursing management of aminoglutethimide therapy is considered successful when the patient sustains a reduced plasma cortisol level. The patient should be able to state the importance of self-monitoring for adverse effects and of reporting symptoms to the prescriber.

MEMORY CHIP

P Aminoglutethimide

- Used to treat adrenocortical hormone excess (Cushing syndrome); it suppresses adrenal cortical function
- Major contraindication: hypersensitivity to glutethimide
- Most common adverse effects: drowsiness, skin rash, nausea, headache, myalgia, and anorexia
- Most serious adverse effects: orthostatic hypotension and tachycardia
- Maximizing therapeutic effects: Provide supplemental doses of steroids during times of injury, infection, or illness.
- Minimizing adverse effects: Help the patient change positions slowly to decrease the risk of injury related to orthostatic hypotension.
- Most important patient education: Take the drug with small, frequent meals to lessen GI effects; do not drive or perform other tasks that require alertness, coordination, or physical dexterity until the effects of the drug are known.

Drugs Significantly Different From P Aminoglutethimide

Cyproheptadine

Cyproheptadine (Periactin) is a potent serotonin and cholinergic antagonist that inhibits secretion of ACTH from pituitary microadenoma cells. It is used for treatment of ACTH hypersecretion and Cushing syndrome secondary to pituitary disorders. Remission of Cushing syndrome usually occurs 1 to 3 months after beginning therapy.

Ketoconazole

Ketoconazole (Nizoral) is an antifungal that strongly inhibits all gonadal and adrenal steroid hormone synthesis. It is used in conjunction with surgery or radiation to inhibit glucocorticoid synthesis. The dose required for adrenal suppression is much higher than when ketoconazole is used as an antifungal agent. Ketoconazole is also discussed in Chapter 44.

Mitotane

Mitotane (Lysodren) is an adrenal cytotoxic agent, although it can cause adrenal inhibition without cellular destruction. It is used for palliative treatment of inoperable adrenal cortical carcinoma. Its biochemical action is unknown, but it reduces production of adrenal steroids and is thought to modify the peripheral metabolism of steroids and directly suppress the adrenal cortex. Approximately 40% of oral mitotane is absorbed; it is primarily stored in fat and undergoes hepatic metabolism. It is excreted in the urine and feces. Its blood levels, detectable for up to 10 weeks after discontinuation of therapy because of the drug's lipophilic nature, does not appear to be related to therapeutic or toxic effects. This may require that the patient be tapered to the usual replacement dose for several weeks after the patient is cured or mitotane is discontinued.

Mitotane is assigned to pregnancy category C. Reliable contraceptive measures are recommended during therapy.

Precautions include concomitant drug therapy, hepatic enzyme induction, and the probability that adrenal insufficiency may develop. Adverse reactions include GI distress such as nausea, diarrhea, vomiting, lethargy and somnolence, transient skin rashes, and hypercholesterolemia and hypouricemia. It is also hepatotoxic and requires monitoring of serum alkaline phosphatase concentration. The drug has a black box warning that the drug be used under the supervision of a physician experienced in the use of cancer chemotherapeutic agents. Also, the drug should temporarily be discontinued following shock or severe trauma as adrenal suppression is its prime action.

CHAPTER SUMMARY

- Corticosteroids affect every body system and have the potential to cause severe adverse effects. Prolonged high-dose corticosteroid therapy increases the incidence of disabling and lethal effects.
- Glucocorticoids occupy an important role in the pharmacologic management of various inflammatory diseases despite the numerous complications that may occur from therapy. Uses of the corticosteroids include replacement, anti-inflammatory, and immunosuppressive therapies. Glucocorticoids are used as replacement therapy in Addison disease, as pharmacologic anti-inflammatory drugs for serious inflammatory disorders and autoimmune diseases, and for a chemotherapeutic effect in certain malignant neoplasms.
- Glucocorticoids are potentially useful in many situations when used with caution. To prevent or manage adverse effects, the nurse, the patient, and the family need a clear understanding of the drugs' actions and uses.
- Glucocorticoids used therapeutically are usually synthetic analogues of the naturally occurring adrenal corticosteroid cortisol, also known as cortisone. The prototype glucocorticoid is prednisone.
- Some patients are at high risk for the serious adverse or toxic effects of the glucocorticoids. Use precautions to avoid viral infections and live virus vaccines. Use with caution in children, pregnant or lactating women, and patients with diseases and disorders, such as cardiovascular disease, renal impairment, peptic ulcer disease, diabetes mellitus, osteoporosis, and treatment-resistant infections.
- Adverse effects, also known as cushingoid effects or characteristics, may be debilitating and life threatening. Cushingoid effects occur with long-term high dosages of systemic glucocorticoids.
- Acute adrenal insufficiency (addisonian crisis) may occur after abrupt withdrawal of pharmacologic dosages of glucocorticoids. A patient experiencing acute adrenal insufficiency is in a potentially life-threatening situation because of the multiple body systems involved.
- During steroid therapy, the underlying disease or condition and its extent suggest the therapeutic goals that direct the nursing care. Patient and family education is fundamental to nursing management.

- Mineralocorticoids are essential for fluid, sodium, and potassium homeostasis.
- Fludrocortisone is the prototype mineralocorticoid. It is used therapeutically with a glucocorticoid for treating patients with adrenocortical insufficiency (Addison disease).
- Episodes of acute stress (e.g., surgery or trauma) may require a dosage adjustment of the corticosteroids to prevent acute adrenal insufficiency.
- Aminoglutethimide, an adrenal steroid inhibitor, suppresses adrenal cortical function. It is used for disorders chiefly characterized by adrenocortical hormone excess (Cushing syndrome).

QUESTIONS FOR STUDY AND REVIEW

1. What are the main effects of glucocorticoids on metabolism?
2. What are the physiologic changes that occur as a result of untreated acute and chronic adrenal insufficiency (Addison disease)?
3. What is Cushing syndrome? What is the physiologic effect of chronic pharmacologic dosage of glucocorticoids? How is Cushing syndrome different from "cushingoid" characteristics?
4. What are the three major actions of the adrenal steroids?
5. What are the two major clinical uses of adrenal steroids?
6. Why should glucocorticoid therapy never be stopped suddenly in a patient who has been receiving long-term therapy?
7. What are the advantages and disadvantages of glucocorticoid alternate-day therapy?
8. What drug interactions commonly occur with glucocorticoids?
9. What is the major clinical use of fludrocortisone? What steroid characteristics does it possess?
10. What patient teaching should be done with patients taking fludrocortisone?
11. What is the major clinical indication for use of the adrenal steroid inhibitors? Name the prototype adrenal steroid inhibitor. Explain its function.

NEED MORE HELP?

Chapter 48 of the Study Guide to Accompany *Drug Therapy in Nursing*, 4th Edition, contains NCLEX-style questions and other learning activities to reinforce your understanding of the concepts presented in this chapter. For additional information or to purchase the study guide, visit the**Point**.

REFERENCES

Facts and Comparisons. (2010). *Drug facts and comparisons*. Philadelphia, PA: Lippincott Williams & Wilkins.

Furst, D., & Saag, K. Glucocorticoid withdrawal. December 20, 2006. http://www.uptodate.com/online/content/topic.do?topicKey=treatme/5199&selectedTitle=8%7E150&source=search_result

Hillel, R. Pathogenesis and clinical features of glucocorticoid-induced osteoporosis. April 22, 2009. http://www.uptodate.com/online/content/topic.do?topicKey=bone_dis/14430&selectedTitle=15%7E150&source=search_result

Karch, A. M. (2010). *Nursing Drug Guide*. Philadelphia, PA: Lippincott Williams & Wilkins.

Koda-Kimbal, M. A, Young, L. Y., Kradian, W. A., et al. (2008). *Applied Therapeutics: The Clinical Use of Drugs*, Philadelphia, PA: Lippincott Williams & Wilkins.

Micromedex Healthcare Series. Retrieved from *http://thomsonhc.com*

Nieman, L. K. Pharmacologic use of glucocorticoids, Jun 16, 2009, http://www.uptodate.com/online/content/topic.do?topicKey=adrenal/12178&selectedTitle=1%7E150&source=search_result

Neman, L. Treatment of adrenal insufficiency in adults. October 16, 2009. http://www.uptodate.com/online/content/topic.do?topicKey=adrenal/4402&selectedTitle=32%7E150&source=search_result

Saag, K., & Furst, D. Major side effects of systemic glucocorticoids. July 26, 2009. http://www.uptodate.com/online/content/topic.do?topicKey=treatme/6535&selectedTitle=13%7E150&source=search_result

Saag, K., Furst, D., & Barnes, P. Major side effects of inhaled glucocorticoids. September 25, 2009. http://www.uptodate.com/online/content/topic.do?topicKey=asthma/16423&selectedTitle=21%7E150&source=search_result

Tatro, D. S. (2009). *Drug interaction facts*. Philadelphia, PA: Lippincott Williams & Wilkins.

49

Drugs Affecting Blood Glucose Levels

Learning Objectives

At the completion of this chapter the student will:

1. Discuss the importance of diabetes in terms of prevalence and costs.

2. Compare the characteristics of type 1, type 2, and gestational diabetes; describe their pathophysiologic processes.

3. Explain the current principles of insulin therapy, which guide care of the diabetic patient.

4. Identify core drug knowledge and core patient variables for the various insulins and for the oral antidiabetic drugs.

5. Identify the peak action time for the four types of insulin and determine when a hypoglycemic episode is most likely to occur with the use of each type.

6. Generate a nursing plan of care from the interactions between core drug knowledge and core patient variables for drugs that affect blood glucose.

7 Describe nursing interventions to maximize therapeutic effects and minimize adverse effects for the drugs that lower blood glucose.

8. Describe treatment for hypoglycemia and hyperglycemia

9. Determine key points for patient and family education for insulin and the oral antidiabetic drugs that affect blood glucose levels.

Key Terms

basal insulin	glycogenolysis	nonketotic hyperglycemia
correctional insulin	glycosylated hemoglobin	prandial insulin
dawn phenomenon	hyperglycemia	Somogyi effect
diabetes mellitus	hypoglycemia	supplemental insulin
diabetic ketoacidosis	insulin	type 1 diabetes
gestational diabetes mellitus	lipodystrophy	type 2 diabetes
gluconeogenesis	metabolic syndrome	

Drugs Affecting Blood Glucose Levels

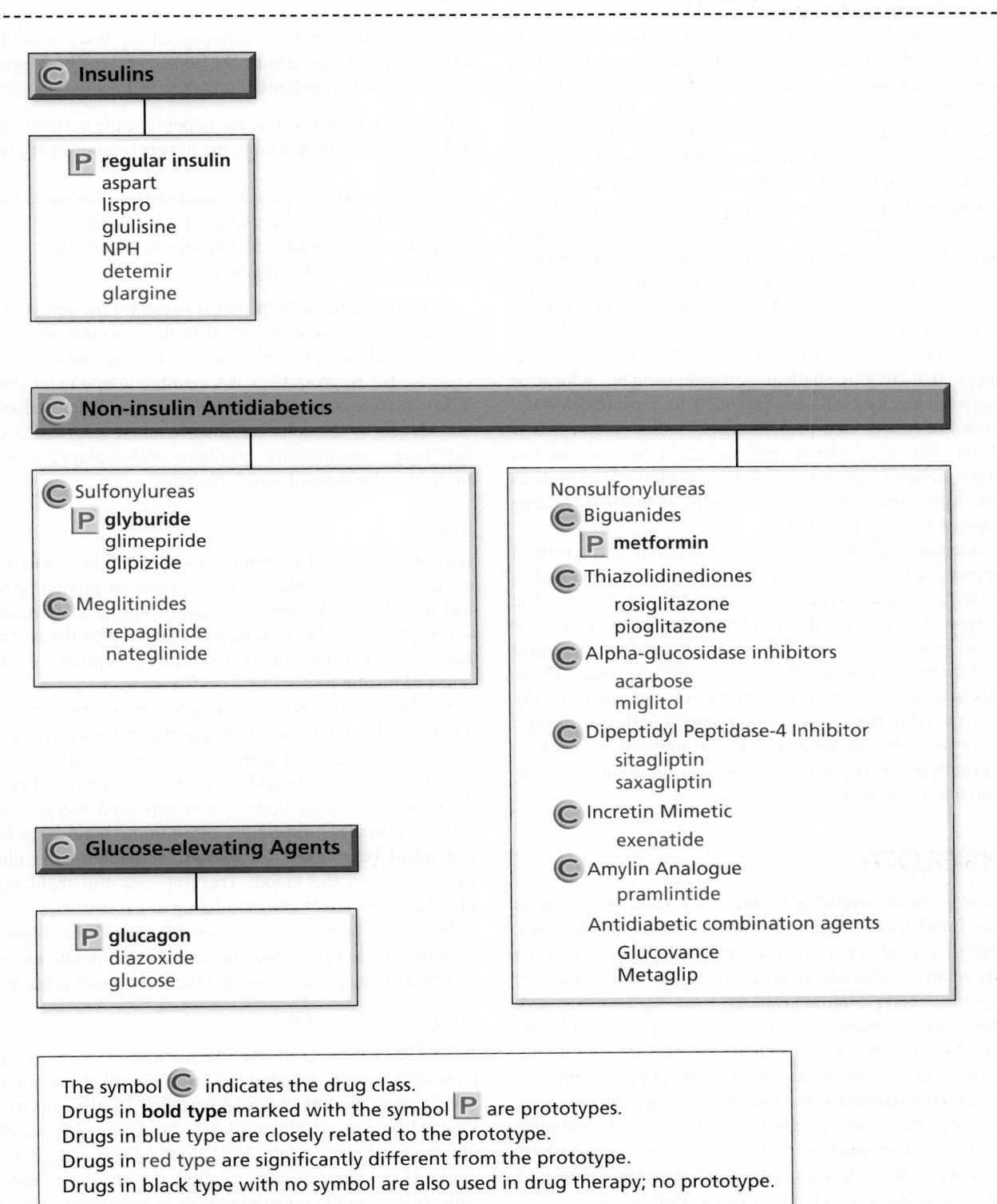

C Insulins

P regular insulin
aspart
lispro
glulisine
NPH
detemir
glargine

C Non-insulin Antidiabetics

C Sulfonylureas
P glyburide
glimepiride
glipizide

C Meglitinides
repaglinide
nateglinide

Nonsulfonylureas
C Biguanides
P metformin
C Thiazolidinediones
rosiglitazone
pioglitazone
C Alpha-glucosidase inhibitors
acarbose
miglitol
C Dipeptidyl Peptidase-4 Inhibitor
sitagliptin
saxagliptin
C Incretin Mimetic
exenatide
C Amylin Analogue
pramlintide
Antidiabetic combination agents
Glucovance
Metaglip

C Glucose-elevating Agents

P glucagon
diazoxide
glucose

The symbol **C** indicates the drug class.
Drugs in **bold type** marked with the symbol **P** are prototypes.
Drugs in blue type are closely related to the prototype.
Drugs in red type are significantly different from the prototype.
Drugs in black type with no symbol are also used in drug therapy; no prototype.

Diabetes mellitus is a common chronic disease that affects 23.6 million people in the United States, or 7.8% of the population (CDC, 2007). Although an estimated 17.9 million people are diagnosed with diabetes, 5.7 million are unaware they have the disease (CDC, 2010a). Approximately 5% to 10% of Americans diagnosed with diabetes have type 1 (lack of endogenous insulin), whereas 90% to 95% have type 2 (diminished insulin effectiveness) (CDC, 2010a). In the United States, diabetes is the sixth leading cause of death by disease, although it is believed to be underreported as a cause of death (Heron, Hoyert, Murphy, et al. 2009; CDC, 2010a).

People with diabetes are at increased risk for cardiovascular disease (hypertension, heart disease, stroke), kidney failure, blindness, nervous system disease, extremity amputations, dental disease, and complications of pregnancy. These morbidities add to the cost of care for diabetes. In 2007, the total annual economic cost of diabetes was estimated to be $174 billion (CDC, 2010a). Diabetes has serious consequences that require patient self-management education and continuing medical care provided by an interdisciplinary team of health care professionals. Although research is exploring how to correct the pathologies in the pancreas that produce diabetes (e.g., transplantation of islets of Langerhans cells), at this time, diabetes is normally controlled by drug therapy and cannot be cured.

Exogenous insulins (manufactured versions of the protein hormone that helps regulate the use of sugar and other carbohydrates) are used to replace deficient intrinsic insulins. The prototype insulin is regular insulin. There are several other types of insulin. Oral antidiabetic drugs are used to control type 2 diabetes, in which there is insulin resistance. These agents belong to several chemical classes, but can generally be considered in two groups: sulfonylureas and nonsulfonylureas (also known as antiglycemics or antihyperglycemics). The prototype sulfonylurea is glyburide; the prototype nonsulfonylurea is metformin.

PHYSIOLOGY

Glucose is made available to the body from food that is ingested and from the production of glucose by the liver. Unable to store or synthesize glucose, the brain depends on a steady supply of glucose from the circulation and extracts its energy on a nearly continuous basis.

Three body systems are involved in the regulation and use of glucose—the liver, pancreas, and skeletal muscle tissue. The liver synthesizes its own glucose supply (a process called **gluconeogenesis**) in addition to storing and releasing glucose that has been converted from dietary carbohydrates. Normally, the liver releases some of its stored or synthesized glucose when blood levels are low and stops producing and releasing glucose when blood levels are high.

The pancreas is both an exocrine and endocrine gland. Its exocrine pancreatic function is to produce digestive enzymes. Its endocrine function is to synthesize and secrete peptide hormones—insulin, glucagon, and somatostatin—by the islets of Langerhans. The islets of Langerhans are cellular structures that lie in the interstitial tissue of the pancreas and are richly innervated by adrenergic and cholinergic nerves. Insulin, glucagon, and somatostatin play an important role in regulating the metabolic activities of the body as well as in regulating and maintaining the homeostasis of blood glucose. The islets of Langerhans contain the following types of cells:

- Beta cells, which secrete the hypoglycemic hormone insulin
- Alpha cells, which secrete the hyperglycemic hormone glucagon
- Delta cells, which release somatostatin, a hormone that inhibits both glucagon and insulin secretion
- F cells, which synthesize and secrete pancreatic polypeptides used in digestion

The muscle tissue is the target organ for the action of insulin; it contains the majority of insulin receptor sites. When insulin binds with receptor sites on the skeletal muscle, glucose is able to cross over the membrane and enter the cell. When muscle tissue has fewer available receptor sites than are needed by the cells for glucose entry, a condition called insulin resistance occurs. Insulin resistance plays a major role in the development of type 2 diabetes.

Insulin

Insulin is a small protein, consisting of two polypeptide chains, which is synthesized as a precursor protein (proinsulin) that then undergoes enzymatic splitting to form insulin and peptide C—both of which are secreted by the pancreatic beta cells. Measurement of circulating C peptide provides an index of insulin levels.

Insulin secretion is regulated tightly by a coordinated interaction of blood glucose levels, gastrointestinal (GI) and pancreatic hormones, and autonomic neurotransmitters. Insulin secretion is most commonly triggered by high blood glucose. Glucose is one of the body's most important energy sources, and some tissues—especially those in the brain—are highly dependent on glucose for energy, particularly the glucose extracted from the blood. Therefore, careful regulation of blood glucose levels and cellular uptake is essential.

Numerous hormones are involved in regulating blood glucose levels. However, two hormones—insulin and glucagon, secreted by the pancreas—exert the most direct influence.

Functions of Insulin

Insulin has a number of important actions. Primarily, it regulates carbohydrate metabolism, but it also plays an important role in metabolizing fats and proteins. Insulin and its analogues lower blood glucose levels by stimulating peripheral glucose uptake, especially by skeletal muscle and fat. Insulin works at specific receptors to allow the glucose to enter the cells. It is normally released rapidly in response to elevations of circulating glucose. Insulin resistance leads to an inappropriately elevated hepatic glucose output and impaired glucose uptake by the muscle tissue. In the liver, insulin has several functions; it promotes the uptake and storage of glucose in the form of glycogen, promotes the conversion of excess glucose into fat, and suppresses hepatic gluconeogenesis (production of glucose) and **glycogenolysis** (breakdown of glycogen to glucose). Most tissues in the body need insulin so that glucose can enter their cells (Figure 49.1). However, the tissues of the brain, nerves, intestine, liver, retina, erythrocytes, and renal tubules do not.

Insulin Synthesis and Release

The plasma glucose level is the single most important factor in controlling the rate of insulin synthesis and release. Other factors that directly or indirectly influence insulin release or its action include blood levels of sugars (fructose, sucrose, and others), levels of free fatty acids, growth hormone, thyroid-stimulating hormone,

glucagon, sympathetic and parasympathetic stimulation, adrenocorticotropic hormone, and cortisol.

Stimulated by plasma glucose levels, insulin secretion occurs in two phases. During the first phase, insulin secretion peaks after 1 to 2 minutes and is short lived. Delayed onset and a longer duration of action characterize the second phase. The exact mechanism by which glucose stimulates insulin release is not fully understood.

Blood glucose levels may be influenced by several factors other than insulin secretion. Any of the following can cause changes in blood glucose levels:

- Stress or illness
- Secretion of insulin-antagonistic hormones (counter-regulatory hormones) that affect glucose metabolism

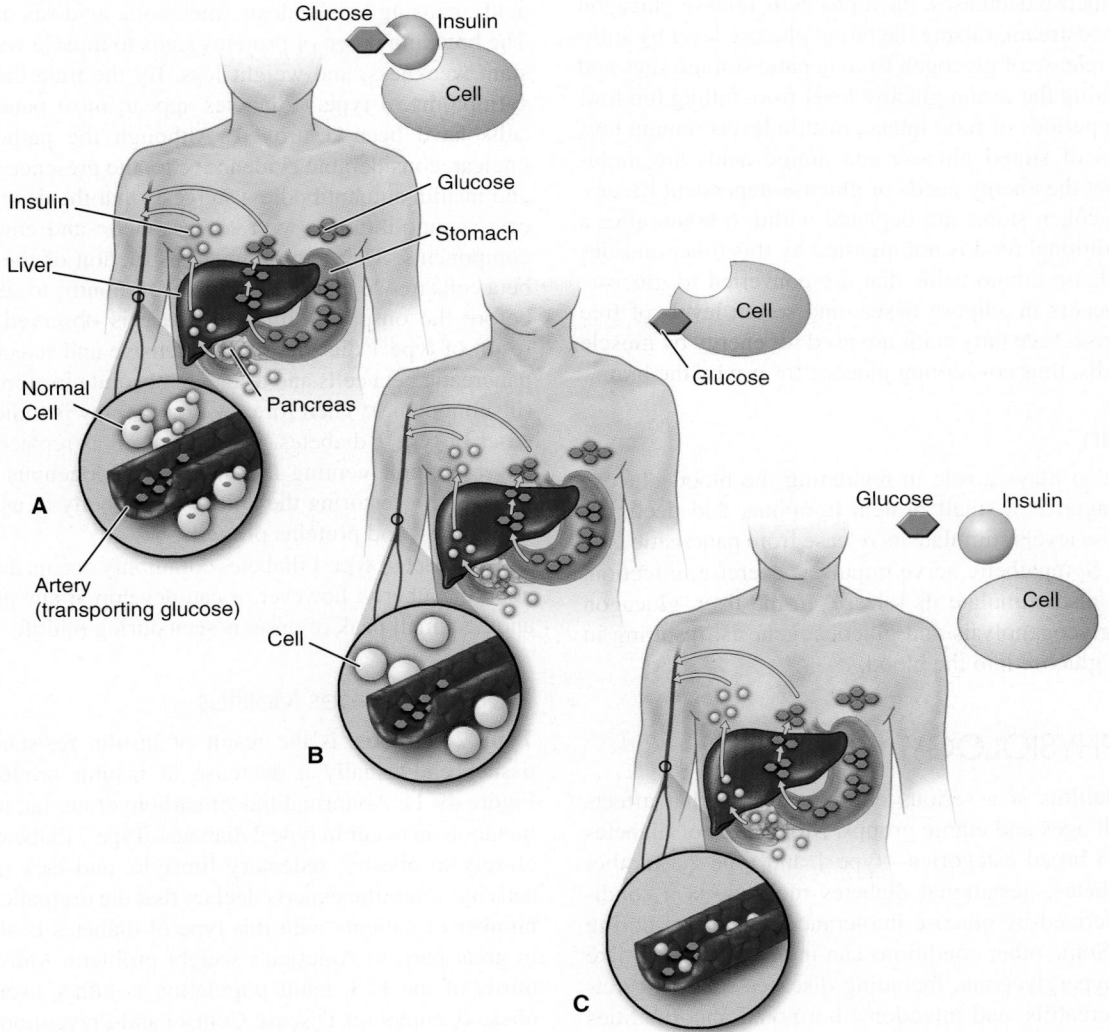

• FIGURE 49.1 **(A)** Normally, glucose is made available to the body from the food that is ingested and from glucose production by the liver. Insulin secreted by beta cells in the pancreas binds to the skeletal muscle cells, allowing glucose to cross the plasma membrane and enter the cell. As depicted in the enlargement, insulin provides the key that unlocks the cellular membrane to allow glucose to enter. **(B)** In type 1 diabetes, the pancreas does not produce insulin, so glucose cannot refuel the cells. Without insulin (the key), glucose is unable to enter the cell. **(C)** In type 2 diabetes, insulin is produced by the pancreas but it does not work properly and the glucose is not absorbed by the cell. Both types of diabetes have the same result: failure of glucose to be absorbed into the cells, leading to hyperglycemia.

(e.g., cortisol, epinephrine, growth hormone, glucagon, and somatostatin)
- Rates of hepatic synthesis of glucose (gluconeogenesis) or conversion of glycogen to yield glucose (glycogenolysis)
- Presence and levels of insulin antibodies
- Use of glucose by peripheral cells or tissues
- Number of cellular insulin receptors

In response to postprandial elevations of blood glucose levels (those that occur after a meal), insulin is released into the bloodstream by the beta cells. A prompt increase in insulin release occurs so that absorbed carbohydrates are transported rapidly to the liver and other tissues where carbohydrates are stored or used, preventing the serum glucose level from rising too much. As a result, blood glucose levels decline, and the stimulus for insulin secretion is suppressed. When the level of serum glucose decreases, the alpha cells release glucagon into the bloodstream, raising the blood glucose level by stimulating the release of glycogen from hepatic storage sites and thus preventing the serum glucose level from falling too low.

Between periods of food intake, insulin levels remain low, and sources of stored glucose and amino acids are mobilized to meet the energy needs of glucose-dependent tissues. Hepatic glycogen stores are depleted within 6 hours after a meal. If additional food is not ingested by this time, muscles begin to release amino acids that are converted to glucose. Lipolysis occurs in adipose tissue, and serum levels of free fatty acids rise. Free fatty acids are used for energy by muscle and liver cells, thus conserving glucose for use by the brain.

Glucagon

Glucagon also plays a role in regulating the blood glucose level. Glucagon is a small protein hormone, and declining blood glucose levels stimulate its release from pancreatic islet alpha cells. Sympathetic nerve impulses, exercise, infection, and trauma also stimulate its release. In the liver, glucagon stimulates glycogenolysis and gluconeogenesis, resulting in a release of glucose into the blood.

PATHOPHYSIOLOGY

Diabetes mellitus is a serious chronic disease that affects people of all ages and ethnic groups. Most cases of diabetes fall into two broad categories—type 1 and type 2. Another type of diabetes, gestational diabetes mellitus, is a condition characterized by glucose intolerance with onset during pregnancy. Some other conditions can induce a diabetes-like state with hyperglycemia, including diseases such as carcinomas, pancreatitis, and infections; hormonal abnormalities such as acromegaly and Cushing syndrome; drugs such as corticosteroids; and genetic defects of the beta cell. A different type of diabetes, termed diabetes insipidus, is a metabolic disorder in which high amounts of dilute urine are formed because of deficient production of antidiuretic hormone (ADH) or inability of the kidney tubules to concentrate urine (see Chapter 53). This type of diabetes does not alter blood glucose levels and is not treated by insulin or oral antidiabetic drugs. For simplicity, this text will use the term *diabetes* to refer to diabetes mellitus.

Type 1 Diabetes Mellitus

Type 1 diabetes is an autoimmune disorder characterized by the destruction of the insulin-secreting beta cells in the pancreas, leading to absolute insulin deficiency (see Figure 49.1). The body's reserve of insulin is depleted, resulting in **hyperglycemia** (abnormally high blood glucose). Because the circulating glucose is not accessible to the cells, the body mistakenly interprets this to mean that there is not enough glucose and thus initiates two other processes to gain energy: breaking down lipids and breaking down proteins. The increase in lipid metabolism leads to an increase in ketoacids, causing ketoacidosis (metabolic acidosis of diabetes). The breaking down of proteins leads to muscle wasting, constant weakness, and weight loss. By the time the signs and syfmptoms of type 1 diabetes appear, most pancreatic beta cells have been destroyed. Although the pathogenesis is unclear, considerable evidence (e.g., the presence of islet cell and insulin autoantibodies) suggests that the destructive process is autoimmune, with some genetic and environmental components. The autoimmune destruction of the pancreatic beta cells may occur over a period of months to several years before the onset of clinical disease is observed. The final result of type 1 diabetes is an extensive and selective loss of pancreatic beta cells and a state of absolute insulin deficiency (insulinopenia). Therefore, insulin therapy is indicated in all cases of type 1 diabetes. Insulin is used as replacement therapy by supplementing the deficient endogenous levels and temporarily restoring the ability of the body to use carbohydrates, fats, and proteins properly.

The onset of type 1 diabetes commonly occurs during childhood or puberty; however, it can develop at any age. In fact, another small peak of onset is seen during midlife.

Type 2 Diabetes Mellitus

Type 2 diabetes is the result of insulin resistance by the tissues and usually a decrease in insulin production (see Figure 49.1). Abnormalities of carbohydrate, fat, and protein metabolism occur in type 2 diabetes. Type 2 diabetes is linked closely to obesity, sedentary lifestyle, and lack of physical activity; scientific experts declare that the dramatic rise in the number of patients with this type of diabetes is attributable, in great part, to America's weight problem. More than two thirds of the U.S. adult population is either overweight or obese (Centers for Disease Control and Prevention, 2010b)

No appreciable loss of pancreatic beta cells or cellular activity from the islets occurs in type 2 diabetes. Plasma concentrations of insulin are essentially normal or may even be increased because the pancreas tries to overcome the resistance by producing more insulin; because the peripheral tissue is resistant to insulin, the insulin does not enter the cells but stays in the bloodstream.

Historically, type 2 diabetes was rare in children, adolescents, and young adults. However, this is no longer the case because type 2 diabetes is increasing in these younger age groups as the childhood population becomes increasingly overweight. Almost one in five American children is overweight (American Obesity Association, 2010c). Type 2 diabetes is now seen as an emerging epidemic in the pediatric population. Obesity and diabetes are also risk factors for cardiovascular disease, and as the incidence of diabetes increases in the pediatric population so does the risk for cardiovascular disease.

Race also appears to be a risk factor for developing type 2 diabetes. Type 2 diabetes occurs in a disproportionately higher prevalence in some racial groups in the United States, including African Americans, Hispanic Americans, and Native Americans. Other factors (besides obesity, race/ethnicity, and impaired glucose metabolism) are associated with type 2 diabetes, including older age, family history of diabetes, and history of gestational diabetes.

Insulin resistance can be considered the primary defect in type 2 diabetes. An insulin-resistance syndrome known as **metabolic syndrome** (or Syndrome X) is a precursor to the development of type 2 diabetes. This syndrome is a combination of conditions, namely insulin resistance with a compensatory hyperinsulinemia to maintain glucose homeostasis; obesity (especially abdominal or visceral obesity); dyslipidemia characterized by high triglycerides, low high-density lipoproteins (HDLs), or both; prothrombotic state (e.g., high fibrinogen or plasminogen activator inhibitor); proinflammatory state (e.g., elevated high-sensitivity C-reactive protein in the blood); and hypertension (130/85 mm Hg or greater). Approximately 33% to 35% of American adults have metabolic syndrome (American Heart Association, 2010d). The focus of these signs and symptoms is an increasing inability to use insulin. Hyperlipidemia linked to insulin abnormalities leads to atherosclerotic plaques in the vessels. Metabolic syndrome increases the risk of cardiovascular disease. Patients with undiagnosed type 2 diabetes (which is fairly common) are at greatly increased risk for coronary heart disease, stroke, and peripheral vascular disease.

In many cases, type 2 diabetes can be controlled with weight reduction, age-appropriate physical activity, dietary modifications, and oral drug therapy or injections of insulin.

Table 49.1 compares type 1 with type 2 diabetes.

TABLE 49.1	Comparison of Type 1 and Type 2 Diabetes Mellitus	
Patient Characteristics	Type 1 (Absolute Insulin Deficiency)	Type 2 (Relative Insulin Deficiency)
Age at onset	Usually before 20 y; onset sudden	Usually after 40 y with incidence increasing as age and weight increase; gradual onset; may occur in youth
Incidence	5%–10%	90%–95%
Body weight	Usually thin/underweight or normal weight	Usually overweight/obese
Endogenous insulin production/activity	Significantly decreased/absent	Slightly decreased; normal or may be increased; insulin effects reduced by inadequate tissue (receptor) response
Insulin receptors/resistance	Normal receptors/no resistance	Decreased or defective receptors/definite insulin resistance
Dietary modifications	Necessary	Beneficial for blood glucose and weight control
Exogenous insulin requirement	Required for all patients with type 1 diabetes	May be necessary for patients with type 2 diabetes
Clinical signs/symptoms	Hyperglycemia, significant polyphagia/ polydipsia/ polyuria, weight loss	Hyperglycemia, fatigue, weakness, mild polyphagia/polydipsia/polyuria, fungal infections (especially skin, vaginal), blurred vision
Complications		
Acute—ketoacidosis	Likely	Unlikely; may occur in the presence of severe illness/stress
Chronic—microvascular and macrovascular disorders	Frequent	Frequent
Etiology/genetic susceptibility	Not fully known; related to human leukocyte antigen (HLA-DR3, HLA-DR4), proposed beta-cell destruction by viral infection or autoimmune process	Not fully known; strong familial component
Clinical management	Insulin injections, dietary controls, exercise regimen	Weight reduction, dietary controls, exercise regimen, oral drug therapy, insulin

Gestational Diabetes Mellitus

Gestational diabetes mellitus (GDM) occurs when a woman's pancreatic function is not sufficient to overcome the insulin resistance created by the anti-insulin hormones secreted by the placenta (e.g., estrogen, prolactin, cortisol, and progesterone), as well as the increased fuel consumption needed for the mother and the fetus. Diagnosis and treatment are essential because the severe hyperglycemia that can result is associated with increases in the incidence of preeclampsia, fetal macrosomia (i.e., large infants), birth trauma, and perinatal mortality. GDM complicates approximately 4% of all pregnancies in the United States (American Diabetes Association, 2010). This rate may be much higher in certain populations, such as Asians, Hispanics, Native Americans, and Pacific Islanders, than in the general population. If the patient is at high risk for GDM (from obesity or because of GDM in a previous pregnancy for example) and is found to be positive for diabetes on initial screening when entering prenatal care these patients are now considered to have "overt diabetes" rather than GDM (American Diabetes Association, 2010). Treatment for GDM may include diet, exercise, and insulin. One research study of 958 pregnant women with mild gestational diabetes (an abnormal OGTT but a fasting glucose of 95 mg/dL or less) found that treating mild GDM with diet and if needed insulin (as opposed to standard prenatal care) decreased the incidence of excessive weight of the newborn (over 4,000 g), shoulder dystocia, cesarean delivery, and hypertensive disorders (gestational hypertension and preeclampsia). Rates of stillbirth or perinatal deaths were not altered by treatment (Landon et al., 2009). Generally, glucose regulation in GDM returns to normal following delivery, although 5% to 10% of women with a history of GDM are found to have type 2 diabetes. The long-term risk of developing type 2 diabetes also exists; women who have had GDM have a 20% to 50% chance of developing diabetes within the next 5 to 10 years (CDC, 2010).

Other Causes of Diabetes Mellitus

Some other factors, some endogenous some exogenous, may cause the person to develop diabetes. Endogenous sources which may produce diabetes mellitus include genetic defects in Beta cell function or insulin action or diseases of the pancreas such as cystic fibrosis. Exogenous causes of diabetes include surgical removal of the pancreas, or ingestion of certain drugs or chemicals (example: glucocorticoid steroids) (American Diabetes Association, 2010).

Criteria for Diabetes Mellitus Diagnosis

Four criteria are used to diagnose diabetes:

1. Plasma glucose = 126 mg/dL after fasting for 8 hours, or
2. Plasma glucose = 200 mg/dL during an oral glucose tolerance test (OGTT) in which 75 g of glucose dissolved in water is ingested or
3. An A1C level of ≥6.5%. (A1C is a blood test that measure long term mean glucose 6 is equal to a mean plasma glucose level of 126) or

4. Symptoms of diabetes and hyperglycemia or hyperglycemic crisis (plasma glucose ≥200 mg/dL at any time of day, regardless of time since last meal,)

Between the fasting and the oral glucose tolerance tests, the preferred screening and diagnostic test is measuring the fasting plasma glucose (FPG) because it is less expensive and easier to perform than the OGTT. The OGTT is more sensitive and more specific than the FPG, yet it is poorly reproducible and rarely used in clinical practice. A random screening is more likely to vary because of dietary intake and is not conclusive by itself. If a random screening is unexplainably elevated, a fasting specimen is ordered to confirm or disprove the diagnosis of diabetes.

A1C blood tests measure the average blood glucose level from the last 2 to 3 months. This test is being used more and more frequently in diagnosis of diabetes. Hemoglobin molecules react with glucose molecules and form glycosylated hemoglobin. This process is increased when blood glucose levels are elevated, such as in diabetes. Because this reaction of glucose with hemoglobin will last the life of the red blood cell it is possible to determine a patient's blood glucose level over time as opposed to a "snap shot view" that measures the level at a given time. Because the glucose molecule is attached to the hemoglobin molecule the lab test is sometimes referred to as an HbA1C.

When a patient's blood glucose levels are higher than normal but do not meet the criteria for diabetes they are at increased risk for developing diabetes (this was formerly termed prediabetes). Under guidelines established by the American Diabetes Association (ADA), an FPG of less than 100 mg/dL is normal, and 100 to 125 mg/dL is considered Impaired Fasting Glucose and a risk for diabetes. Impaired Glucose Tolerance where 2 hour OGTT readings are 140 to 199 mg/dl is also considered a risk factors. IFG and IGT are associated with obesity (especially abdominal or visceral obesity), dyslipidemia with high triglycerides and/or low HDL cholesterol, and hypertension. Elevated A1C of 5.7%–6.4% (normal is 6% or less) may also be recognized as a high risk for future diabetes. Chronic elevated glucose is almost always a precursor to type 2 diabetes, unless lifestyle modifications are instituted (American Diabetic Association, 2010).

Complications of Diabetes

The consequences of uncontrolled diabetes are serious and can result in acute or chronic complications.

Acute Complications

Hyperglycemia is an abnormally high concentration of glucose in the circulating blood. According to the ADA guidelines, hyperglycemia is a fasting plasma glucose value of more than 126 mg/dL. The classic signs of hyperglycemia include excessive urination (polyuria) and excessive thirst (polydipsia) caused by the osmotic pull of glucose. Other symptoms include fatigue, dry or itchy skin, poor wound healing, and vision changes (often blurred vision).

Diabetic ketoacidosis and **nonketotic hyperglycemia,** also known as hyperosmolar hyperglycemic nonketotic syndrome, are two serious acute complications of diabetes that greatly contribute to the morbidity and mortality among patients with diabetes. These disorders are extreme manifestations of impaired carbohydrate regulation that can occur in diabetes.

Diabetic ketoacidosis occurs primarily in type 1 diabetes. It occurs when ketone production by the liver outpaces ketone loss through the kidneys. Lack of insulin is usually the cause of the ketone imbalance. The onset of diabetic ketoacidosis is slow and gradual. The major metabolic imbalances present in diabetic ketoacidosis are hyperglycemia, ketosis, and metabolic acidosis. Glucose levels are more than 250 mg/dL and can potentially be more than 1,000 mg/dL. These elevated glucose levels can cause loss of consciousness. Other symptoms that may occur include osmotic diuresis, dehydration, electrolyte imbalance, tachycardia, acetone smell to the breath (sometimes referred to as a fruity breath), and hypotension. Treatment for diabetic ketoacidosis is regular insulin administered by intravenous (IV) infusion and IV replacement of fluids and electrolytes.

Nonketotic hyperglycemia also has a slow, gradual onset, but unlike diabetic ketoacidosis, it occurs primarily in type 2 diabetes. In nonketotic hyperglycemia, insulin is present, but it is not as effective as it should be. This circulating insulin prevents the formation of ketones yet is ineffective in moving the glucose from the blood into the cells. The two primary factors that contribute to nonketotic hyperglycemia are the body's increased resistance to insulin and high dietary carbohydrate consumption. The symptoms of nonketotic hyperglycemia are severe hyperglycemia (glucose level, greater than 600 mg/dL), hyperosmolarity of the blood (≥310 mOsm/L), and dehydration. The severe hyperosmolarity pulls water out of cells, including brain cells, causing neurologic changes such as altered reflexes (presence of Babinski sign), grand mal seizures, aphasia, hyperthermia, visual hallucinations, and hemiparesis. Nonketotic hyperglycemia may initially be misdiagnosed as stroke because of the overlap of some of the neurologic changes. Treatment involves careful rehydration and drug therapy to lower blood glucose.

Two types of fasting hyperglycemia can occur in diabetics receiving insulin treatment: the **dawn phenomenon** and the **Somogyi effect** (Figure 49.2). In the dawn phenomenon, blood glucose levels are at their highest between 5 AM and 6 AM. The release of growth hormone overnight is believed to produce this increase in blood glucose. Dawn phenomenon is treated by providing larger doses of intermediate-acting insulin at bedtime to prevent early-morning elevations of glucose. The Somogyi effect also produces early-morning hyperglycemia, but the precipitating factor is actually a hypoglycemic event sometime after midnight. The body compensates for the low blood glucose by using counter-regulatory hormone release, directing the liver to release glucose to restore the glucose level to normal. When the body overcompensates, rebound hyperglycemia occurs. The Somogyi effect is treated

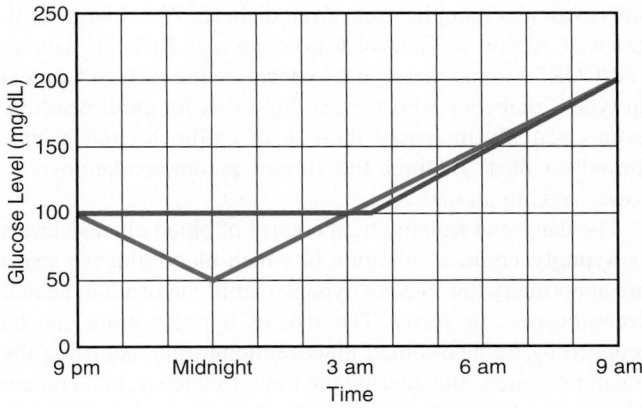

● FIGURE 49.2 Blood glucose levels characteristic of unusual phenomena: the Somogyi effect (*red line*) and the dawn phenomenon (*blue line*). In the Somogyi effect, the blood glucose dips around midnight but rises significantly in the morning before breakfast. In the common problem known as the dawn phenomenon, the blood glucose level is stable until about 3 AM but begins rising after dawn. These kinds of problems illustrate why diabetic drug dosages are tailored to meet the individual patient's needs. They present the health care practitioner with challenges and opportunities to mix insulins and adjust dosage regimens to benefit the patient.

by lowering the insulin dose, increasing dietary intake at bedtime, or both. The patient's exercise habits should also be evaluated to determine the appropriate balance between calorie intake and insulin needs.

Chronic Complications

The chronic complications of diabetes are usually classified as microvascular or macrovascular, according to the type of blood vessel damage that underlies the problem. Among the macrovascular chronic complications are atherosclerotic vascular disease, myocardial infarction, and cerebrovascular accident. Among the microvascular complications are cataracts, glaucoma and blindness from retinopathy, lower-extremity infections and gangrene, foot ulcers and Charcot joints resulting in amputation, renal failure from nephropathy and gastroparesis, and sexual dysfunction as a result of autonomic neuropathy.

Chronic complications can be prevented by a closer control of chronic glucose levels; the lab value that measures this is the hemoglobin A_{1C} level. Lowering the hemoglobin A_{1C} has been associated with a reduction of microvascular and neuropathic complications of diabetes, and it may also lower macrovascular disease. Current clinical guidelines recommend that the target hemoglobin A_{1C} is around or below 7 (American Diabetes Association, 2010). Reducing A1C to one percentage point greater than normal has been found to reduce microvascular and neuropathic complications of type 1 and type 2 diabetes. Research that studied the effect of lowering A1c closer to 6 (normal) has been mixed. Two large clinical trials that examined type 1 diabetics: Diabetes Control and Complications Trial (1993) and Association of glycaemia with macrovascular and microvascular complications of type 2 diabetes (UKPDS) (Stratton et al., 2000) showed that reducing the A1C closer to 6 further reduces the risk of microvascular complications from diabetes. Yet, a large clinical trial Action to Control Cardiovascular Risk in diabetes (ACCORD) found that trying to decrease the A1C to 6 or less in type 2 diabetics who were at high risk for cardiovascular events actually increased the risk of cardiovascular events. Based on these findings the current recommendation is to lower A1C to around 7.

The danger of keeping tight control of blood glucose levels is **hypoglycemia,** a condition in which blood glucose levels are abnormally low. Severe hypoglycemia can result in altered consciousness or coma. The risk of hypoglycemia can be reduced by frequent blood glucose monitoring, adjusting the insulin regimen, and altering the time, frequency, and content of the patient's meals. Recent research suggests that achieving appropriate glycemic control can be particularly challenging when patients have limited access to health care (Box 49.1).

In addition to controlling glucose levels, chronic cardiovascular complications can be minimized by treating hypertension with a goal being less than 130/80, treating hyperlipidemia (In individuals without overt CVD, the primary goal is an LDL cholesterol less than 100 mg/dL, in those with overt CVD, a lower LDL cholesterol goal of less than 70 mg/dl from using statin drug therapy) encouraging weight loss and exercise (150 minutes of moderate exercise per week), and encouraging dietary changes to include a low fat low sodium foods. Aspirin therapy (75 to 162 mg/d) can be used a primary prevention for coronary vascular disease in those with increased cardiovascular risk. A similar dosing of aspirin can also be used as secondary prevention for those with diabetes who have a history of CVD (American Diabetic Association, 2010).

Diabetic Therapy

The treatment for type 1 diabetes includes two different insulin regimens. The nonphysiologic regimen does not mimic normal beta-cell secretion and is ideal for those newly diagnosed patients who still produce some endogenous insulin and have not progressed to complete beta-cell failure. This regimen includes one or two daily injections of long-acting insulin. The physiologic regimen, used in complete beta-cell failure when glucose control cannot be achieved with the non-physiologic regimen, attempts to mimic normal insulin secretion, consisting of basal and prandial insulin. **Basal insulin** is the continuous secretion that maintains glucose homeostasis, that is, the body's baseline level of insulin. **Prandial insulin** is the insulin secretion stimulated in response to meals. A regimen that meets both basal and prandial needs combines quick-onset, short-duration insulin with slower-onset, longer-duration insulin. Typically, this mixed basal and prandial regimen includes giving intermediate- to long-acting insulin (such as NPH or glargine) daily and short-acting (regular) or rapid-acting (aspart or lispro) insulin before each meal. Meal timing and consistency are very important to avoid hypoglycemic episodes. The physiologic regimen has several variations. Overall, the main goal of this therapy is to avoid hypoglycemic episodes and improve hemoglobin A_{1C} levels yet maintain a simple regimen to which the patient can adhere.

Hospitalized patients with type 1 diabetes who are not eating regularly should be receiving other forms of nutrition such as IV fluids with dextrose, total parenteral nutrition, or partial parenteral nutrition, tube feedings, in addition to some oral feedings. They need to receive enough glucose to prevent

---

BOX 49.1 FOCUS ON RESEARCH

Diabetes Case Management Among Low-Income Ethnic Minority Populations

Jovanovic, L., Wollitzer, A. O., Gorke, K., et al., The California Med-Cal Type 2 Diabetes Study Group. (2004). Closing the gap: Effect of diabetes case management on glycemic control among low-income ethnic minority populations. *Diabetes Care*, 27(1):95–103.

The Study

A primary objective of diabetes management is to improve glycemic control. When normal glycemic control can be achieved in patients with diabetes, microvascular and macrovascular complications are reduced. Therefore, it is cost effective to monitor glycemic control by measuring hemoglobin A_{1C} levels periodically and by self-monitoring blood glucose daily. However, research indicates that many patients with diabetes have poor glycemic control. In particular, disparities exist among low-income ethnic minority populations relative to other groups. Barriers to care include high cost of glucose monitoring strips and medications, lack of English language skills, and poor cultural sensitivity of health care providers.

In this study, 362 participants were randomized into two groups: a control group that continued to receive usual care from their primary care provider, and an intervention group that received individualized education from registered nurses and dietitians. The intervention group was assessed for diet, exercise, and self-care behaviors, and strategies to improve self-care education and management were used throughout the

study in this group. The strategies considered the patient's level of education, literacy, and functional understanding and also his or her treatment goals, general health status, cultural beliefs, and support network. All interactions occurred in a clinic setting or by telephone; appointments were monitored and were rescheduled if missed. Transportation issues were also addressed to ensure visits were completed. Both groups had similar mean hemoglobin A_{1C} levels at baseline. During the 2 years of study, a progressive reduction in hemoglobin A_{1C} levels was seen in both groups; however, the reduction in the intervention group was significantly greater at each time ($p < 0.01$). By the end of the study, the mean difference from baseline in hemoglobin A_{1C} levels in the intervention group was 0.87 greater than that in the control group. The authors conclude that diabetes case management, added to primary care, substantially improves glycemic control.

Nursing Implications

Registered nurses play a vital role in patient education and diabetic management for people with diabetes. Diabetes management can help reduce disparities among low-income ethnic populations but also can improve diabetic health status in all populations. You need a clear understanding of drug therapies and management strategies for diabetes to ensure that patients receive high-quality, accurate patient education that will lead to better control of their diabetes

starvation ketosis and hypoglycemia; usually 5 to 10 g of glucose/hour is sufficient. Some insulin coverage is also necessary, so that this essential glucose can enter the cells. The term *nutritional dose* (as opposed to prandial dose) may be used in these circumstances. In addition to the basal and prandial doses, patients with diabetes who are ill and hospitalized may also require some **correctional** (or **supplemental**) **insulin** doses to correct any elevations in blood glucose, with the goal of keeping the blood glucose close to normal at all times, because the physiologic stress of illness increases glucose levels. Some medications can also increase glucose levels. Preprandial glucose levels greater than 110 mg/dL should be treated with a correctional dose of short-acting or rapid-acting insulin (in addition to their normal prandial dose). The correctional dose is administered before the meal. In contrast, the prandial dose may be given either before the meal, or if it is adjusted based on precise amount eaten, immediately after eating. The goal for non-critically ill hospitalized patients is a pre-meal glucose level of less than 140 mg/dL.

When a patient is critically ill and in an intensive care unit control of blood glucose levels warrants special treatment goals as patients have been found to have better hospital outcomes if their glucose is better controlled. However, intensive controlling of glucose levels have been found to increase mortality rates (Griesdale, de Souza, van Dam, et al., 2009) Critically ill patients may receive IV insulin infusions when their glucose levels are greater than 180 mg/dL which should be titrated to maintain their glucose levels between 140 and 180) instead of subcutaneous (SC) injections.

Patients who are at risk for diabetes are treated with lifestyle modifications (e.g., weight reduction, exercise, diet modification). If they have other significant risk factors, they may also be treated with oral antidiabetic drugs. The first line of treatment for diagnosed type 2 diabetes consists of oral antidiabetic agents in addition to lifestyle modifications. Starting insulin therapy is recommended if hemoglobin A_{1C} approaches 8% despite optimal oral therapy. The best regimen uses bedtime long-acting basal insulin (such as NPH or glargine) while continuing one or two daytime oral antidiabetic medications. Because of the insulin resistance associated with type 2 diabetes, the patient may require large doses of exogenous insulin; therefore, the goal of therapy is to lower the hemoglobin A_{1C} level, not the insulin dose. Patients with type 2 diabetes require insulin if they become pregnant, have major surgery, or experience severe trauma, infections (including gangrene), fever, hepatic or renal dysfunction, and hyperthyroidism or other endocrine dysfunction. Table 49.2 presents a summary of selected antidiabetic drugs.

Ⓒ INSULINS

Synthetic insulin (exogenous; i.e., not produced within a person's body) acts in the same manner as endogenously produced insulin. Sources of exogenous insulin historically included pork and beef pancreas, but now only recombinant DNA technology or genetic engineering is used to create human-like insulin. Modifying the amino acid sequence of the human insulin molecule has resulted in new, rapid-acting insulin analogues, such as aspart, lispro, or glulisine (produced by rDNA technology). Human-sourced insulin is considered the standard therapy.

Insulin is available as rapid-, short- (also known as "regular"), intermediate-, and long-acting types. Type usually refers to the action time of a particular product, which includes the onset, peak, and duration of effects. Some insulins are injected separately, whereas others may be mixed together in a syringe. Other insulins are available premixed in standard concentrations in one vial.

The potency of insulin is expressed in the *United States Pharmacopeia* (USP) or international units. The standard concentrations of insulins are solutions of 100 U/mL. A 500 U/mL of regular insulin is also available. The numbers after the "U" indicate the number of units per milliliter (e.g., U-100). A special insulin syringe that has been calibrated to 100 U/mL is used to administer insulin; markings show the units. The standard insulin syringe measures up to a maximum of either 50 or 100 U of insulin, and some very-low-dose syringes hold a maximum of 25 U. Regular (U-100) and NPH insulins are sold as over-the-counter (OTC) drugs, but other forms require a prescription. Consequently, the type of insulin—as well as injection technique, presence of insulin antibodies, site of injection, and individual patient response differences—can all affect the onset, peak, degree, and duration of insulin activity.

Short-acting regular insulin is the prototype insulin. Regular insulin is sold OTC under the trade names Novolin-R and Humulin-R; the R stands for regular. There are also longer-acting insulins. Combinations of some of these drugs also exist.

Nursing Management of the Patient Receiving Ⓟ Regular Insulin

Core Drug Knowledge

Pharmacotherapeutics

Insulin therapy is indicated for all patients with type 1 diabetes and for those patients with type 2 diabetes whose hyperglycemia cannot be controlled properly by diet, exercise, weight reduction, oral antidiabetic drugs, or a combination of these interventions. Regular insulin is used only to correct a current glucose elevation or an expected rise after eating, it is not used to control the glucose level all day (i.e., basal dosing) due to its short duration of action (see pharmacokinetics below). Regular insulin is also indicated for patients with hyperkalemia because an infusion of glucose and insulin produces a shift of potassium into cells and lowers serum potassium levels. Like all insulins, regular insulin is administered subcutaneously. It can also be administered intravenously and subcutaneously through an implantable insulin pump.

Subcutaneous insulin therapy for type 1 diabetes frequently consists of daily injections of mixtures of short-acting regular

TABLE 49.2 Summary of Selected Antidiabetic Drugs

Drug (Trade) Name	Selected Indications	Route and Dosage Range	Pharmacokinetics
C Insulins			
Short Acting			
P regular insulin (Humulin R, Novolin R)	**All insulin preparations,** types 1 and 2 diabetes mellitus	**All insulin preparations** *Adult and child:* SC, dosages determined and adjusted depending on plasma glucose, diet, activity, and health status	*Onset:* 0.5–1 h *Duration:* 8–12 h $t_{1/2}$: Varies with preparation
Rapid Acting			
insulin lispro (Humalog)			*Onset:* 0.25 h *Duration:* 6–8 h $t_{1/2}$: 1 h
insulin aspart (Novolog)			*Onset:* 5–10 min *Duration:* 3–5 h $t_{1/2}$: 1.5 h
Intermediate Acting			
isophane insulin suspension, NPH (Humulin N, NPH Iletin I, *Canadian:* Novolin ge)			*Onset:* 1–1.5 h *Duration:* 18–24 h $t_{1/2}$: Unknown
Long Acting			
glargine (Lantus)			*Onset:* 1 h *Duration:* 24 h $t_{1/2}$: Unknown
Combination			
isophane insulin suspension (NPH) and insulin injection (70% NPH and 30% regular insulin) (Novolin 70/30)			*Onset:* 30 min *Duration:* 24 h $t_{1/2}$: Unknown
50% lispro protamine suspension and 50% lispro (Humalog Mix 50/50)			*Onset:* 15 min *Duration:* 10–12 h $t_{1/2}$: Unknown
70% aspart protamine suspension and 30% aspart (Novolog Mix 70/30)			*Onset:* 15 min *Duration:* Up to 24 h $t_{1/2}$: Unknown
C Oral Antidiabetics			
C Sulfonylureas			
P glyburide (Diabeta)	**All oral antidiabetics,** type 2 diabetes mellitus	*Adult:* PO, initially 2.5–5 mg with breakfast; maintenance, 1.25–20 mg/d *Child:* Safety and efficacy not determined	*Onset:* 1–2 h *Duration:* 16–24 h $t_{1/2}$: 10 h
glipizide (Glucotrol)		*Adult:* PO, initially 5 mg before breakfast; then increase in increments of 2.5–5 mg, not to exceed 15 mg/d *Child:* Safety and efficacy not determined	*Onset:* 1–3 h *Duration:* 10–24 h $t_{1/2}$: 2–4 h
chlorpropamide (Diabenese;)		*Adult:* PO, 200–500 mg/d; maximum dose, 750 mg/d	*Onset:* 1 h *Duration:* 24–60 h $t_{1/2}$: 36 h
Meglitinides			
repaglinide (Prandin)		*Adult and child:* PO, 0.5–4 mg before meals; maximum dose, 16 mg/d	*Onset:* Rapid *Duration:* Unknown $t_{1/2}$: 1 h
nateglinide (Starlix)		*Adult and child:* PO, 120 mg tid (60 mg tid if HbA$_{1c}$ is near therapeutic goal), 1–30 min before meals	*Onset:* Rapid *Duration:* Unknown $t_{1/2}$: 1.5 h

TABLE 49.2   Summary of Selected Antidiabetic Drugs *(continued)*

Drug (Trade) Name	Selected Indications	Route and Dosage Range	Pharmacokinetics
C **Biguanide** **P** metformin (Glucophage)		*Adult:* 500–2,000 mg/d in divided doses *Child:* Safety and efficacy not determined	*Onset:* 2–2.5 h *Duration:* 10–16 h $t_{1/2}$: 1.5–6.2 h
C **Alpha-Glucosidase Inhibitors** acarbose (Precose)		*Adult:* PO, 50–100 mg tid with the first bite of each main meal *Child:* Safety and efficacy not determined	*Onset:* <30 min *Duration:* 4–6 h $t_{1/2}$: 2 h
miglitol (Glyset)		*Adult and child:* PO, initial dose of 25 mg tid at first bite of meal; may start at 25 mg/d if GI effects are severe. Maintenance dose of 50 mg/tid; maximum dose of 100 mg tid	*Onset:* Rapid *Duration:* Unknown $t_{1/2}$: 2 h
C **Thiazolidinediones** rosiglitazone (Avandia)		*Adult and child:* PO, 4 mg/d as single dose or divided into two doses; may increase to maximum of 8 mg/d after 8 wk	*Onset:* Rapid *Duration:* Unknown $t_{1/2}$: 3–4 h
C **Amylin analogue** pramlintide (Symlin)		*Adult:* type 2 diabetes: SC, initially 60 mcg; increase to 120 mcg; type 1 diabetes: SC, initially 15 mcg; increase to 30–60 mcg	*Onset:* Rapid *Duration:* about 3 h $t_{1/2}$: 48 min
C **Dipeptidyl peptidase-4 (DPP-4) enzyme inhibitor** sitagliptin (Januvia)		*Adult:* PO, 100 mg once daily *Child:* Safety and efficacy not established	*Onset:* Unknown *Duration:* 24 h $t_{1/2}$: 12.4 h
C **Incretin Mimetic** exenatide (Byetta)		*Adult:* SC, 5 mcg twice daily, no more than 60 min before a meal; may increase up to 10 mcg twice daily *Child:* Safety and efficacy not established	*Onset:* <1 h *Duration:* 5 h $t_{1/2}$: 2.4 h
P **Glucose-Elevating Agent**			
P glucagon (GlucaGen)	Reverse severe hypoglycemia resulting from insulin overdosage	*Adult and child (>20 kg):* SC, IM, IV, 1.0 mg; dose may be repeated once or twice *Child (=20 kg):* 0.5 mg	*Onset:* IM, 8–10 min; IV, 1 min *Duration:* IM, 19–32 min; IV, 9–20 min $t_{1/2}$: 3–10 min

insulin with intermediate-acting insulins; multiple doses of regular insulin before each meal (i.e., prandial) in association with one or two daily doses of long-acting insulin may also be used. Combining the two types of insulin allows for rapid adjustment to elevated glucose levels as well as for prolonged control, such as all day or overnight. Some premixed combinations are also available.

Regular insulin may be used on a correctional (or supplemental) basis (previously termed "sliding scale"). When administered as a correctional dose, it is given in addition to basal insulin (with a long-acting preparation) or in additions to regimens of basal insulin and prandial insulin. In correctional doses, the number of units of regular insulin administered is based on blood glucose levels, according to guidelines provided in a specific medication order. Correctional insulin may be used before meals and at bedtime or every 4 to 6 hours if a patient is receiving continuous total parenteral nutrition. Correctional insulin is ordered frequently for hospitalized diabetic patients when insulin needs may be greatest, for example, with fever, infection, or internal stress, or after surgery or trauma.

Pharmacokinetics

Regular insulin, like all insulins, is destroyed by gastric acids and cannot be given orally. The SC route usually produces slow, steady absorption. The rate of absorption is affected by the site of administration. The most rapid absorption occurs when administration is into the abdominal SC layer (as much as 50% faster than other routes). The next most rapid is into the arm, followed by the thigh, and finally the buttocks.

When regular insulin is given by IV infusion, some of the drug—usually between 20% and 30%—is absorbed into the plastic tubing set. Up to 80% loss has occasionally been reported. Close monitoring of the therapeutic effect is necessary because it is not possible to determine the exact amount that will be lost and never received by the patient.

Regular insulin has a quick onset and a short duration of action; therefore, it can be administered to a patient several times a day. In comparison to regular insulin, some other forms of insulin have slower onsets but longer durations of action, although insulin analogues have a more rapid onset (see Table 49.2). Insulin deteriorates if exposed to excessive heat or light. Regular insulin is stable at room temperature for 1 month. For longer storage, place insulin in the refrigerator.

Insulin is filtered at the glomerulus, with most of the dose (98%) reabsorbed in the proximal renal tubule. Slightly more than half of the reabsorbed insulin is metabolized and excreted; the remaining insulin is returned to the venous blood. Renal function impairment occurs commonly in diabetic patients because of vascular insufficiency. Renal function impairment reduces the amount of insulin excreted, thus reducing the amount of insulin required.

Pharmacodynamics

Insulin is the principal hormone required for proper glucose use in normal metabolic processes. Most of the body's cells require insulin to facilitate entry of glucose. Insulin's effects are tissue specific; it facilitates membrane transport of glucose (and some other amino acids and ions) into muscle, adipose, and connective tissue cells and into leukocytes. Nerve tissues, erythrocytes, kidney epithelium (tubules), and cells of the brain, intestines, liver, and retina do not require insulin to absorb glucose.

Injected insulin mimics the effect of endogenous insulin. Serum glucose level is regulated by insulin control over the metabolism of carbohydrates, fats, and proteins. At the cellular level, insulin increases the cell membrane permeability to glucose, amino acids, and fatty acids and maintains a constant glucose level by changing glycogen into glucose. In addition, insulin converts excess glucose into glycogen and promotes the storage of fat by combining alpha-glycerophosphate (a product of glucose metabolism) with fatty acids to form triglycerides. Consequently, one effect of insulin on metabolism is weight gain.

Contraindications and Precautions

Regular insulin is contraindicated in times of hypoglycemia or if the patient has any sensitivity to any of its components. When changing the type of insulin (e.g., from short acting to rapid acting or to intermediate acting, or vice versa), caution should be used and the patient monitored carefully for hypoglycemia or hyperglycemia, either of which may occur as the body adjusts to the different pharmacokinetics of the preparation.

Insulin is a pregnancy category B drug.

Adverse Effects

Hypoglycemia, the most common adverse effect of insulin therapy, may result from an excessive insulin dose or from increased physical activity without eating. Hypoglycemia is a substantial drop in blood glucose level (to less than 70 mg/dL) that may result from excessive insulin entering the bloodstream or from insufficient glucose levels to meet tissue demands. The earliest signs of hypoglycemia are neurologic in nature because the brain uses only glucose for fuel. They include fatigue and malaise, trembling, irritability, headache, nausea, numbness, paresthesias, muscle weakness, blurred vision, confusion, and ultimately convulsions, stupor, coma, and death. Hypoglycemia may cause increased sympathetic activity and manifest as hunger, tachycardia, sweating, and nervousness.

Repetitive SC injections into the same injection site can cause disturbances in fat metabolism. This adverse effect, known as **lipodystrophy,** can present as either as lipoatrophy or lipohypertrophy. In lipoatrophy, SC fat breaks down because of repeated insulin injections into the same site and causes a depression in the skin; in lipohypertrophy, there are additional lipid deposits at a particular site, causing a spongy area. Both forms of lipodystrophy may delay insulin absorption, adversely affecting pharmacotherapeutics.

Drug Interactions

Table 49.3 lists important drug interactions with insulin.

Assessment of Relevant Core Patient Variables

Health Status

Assess patients for allergies and for immunocompromised states and determine whether the patient has been receiving daily insulin, either as a lifelong therapy or as short-duration

TABLE 49.3	Agents that Interact with P Regular Insulin		
Interactants		**Effect and Significance**	**Nursing Management**
acetazolamide, AIDS antivirals, calcitonin, corticosteroids, diazoxide, diltiazem, thiazide diuretics, dobutamine, epinephrine, estrogens (including oral contraceptives), isoniazid, lithium carbonate, morphine sulfate, niacin, phenothiazines, phenytoin, nicotine, thyroid hormones		Decreased hypoglycemic effect of insulin	Monitor plasma glucose and A₁c levels. Observe for hyperglycemic complications.
ACE inhibitors, alcohol, beta blockers, calcium, chloroquine, clofibrate, guanethidine, lithium carbonate, MAO inhibitors, mebendazole, octreotide, pentamidine, phenylbutazone, pyridoxine, salicylates, sulfinpyrazone, sulfonamides, tetracyclines		Increased hypoglycemic effect of insulin	Monitor blood glucose level. Observe for hypoglycemic complications.

therapy (such as that needed during acute infections). When the patient has been receiving regular insulin at home, determine the type, amount, and usual time of administration, who administers it, and what sites are used. Also, determine the frequency of hypoglycemic reactions and how the patient or family handles these reactions. This information helps the health care team assess knowledge, usual practices, and teaching needs.

Complete a thorough history and physical assessment from which to establish a baseline. Solicit current drug history, including information on all prescription and OTC drugs, from the patient or family. A careful review of this information may identify drugs that can alter the action of insulin. Drugs taken for other disorders (e.g., thiazide diuretics, corticosteroids, and estrogens) may cause hyperglycemia, which complicates diabetic control and requires higher dosages of an antidiabetic medication or insulin.

Assess for complications related to diabetes, such as neuropathy, nephropathy, or retinopathy, and for the patient's ability to perform psychomotor skills such as self-monitoring of blood glucose or self-injection of insulin.

Assess the integumentary system and inquire into the patient's general health practices, especially in regard to the skin. For example, assess for lipoatrophy or lipohypertrophy at injection sites, color and temperature of the lower extremities, presence of calluses and ulcers on feet, delayed healing of wounds, and signs of peripheral neuropathy.

It is important to obtain baseline and periodic assessments of blood glucose levels, blood cell counts, electrolytes (especially potassium), blood lipid levels (e.g., cholesterol and triglycerides), and hemoglobin A_{1C} levels. Assess the patient's knowledge of diabetes and basics of self-care.

Patients who are critically ill and hospitalized in an intensive care unit require close assessment of their glucose levels.

Life Span and Gender

Assess the patient for pregnancy. Human insulin is preferred for use during gestation as opposed to an oral antidiabetic drug (both in gestational diabetes and in women who have diabetes before becoming pregnant). Human insulin is also recommended for women with diabetes who are considering pregnancy. Insulin is a pregnancy category B drug. Inquire about breast-feeding status. Although the hormone does not pass into breast milk, lactation may decrease insulin requirements despite the increase in caloric intake necessitated by it.

Adjust care to meet the patient's chronologic and developmental age. Assess infants and toddlers carefully to avoid hypoglycemic episodes, which could have harmful effects on the developing brain and spinal column. With adolescents, monitor growth spurts, which can cause a substantial increase in insulin requirements. Also, assess the adolescent's acceptance of and actual adherence to therapy. Adolescents with type 1 or 2 diabetes may resist medication, especially insulin injections. They may delay or omit their insulin dosages to fit in socially or to control their weight.

With older adults, assess for changes in the management and control of diabetes and glucose levels. Changes in the diet and activity level of elderly patients pose challenges to control of blood glucose levels. Examples of these changes include ill-fitting dentures, difficulty chewing and swallowing, decreased ability and interest in cooking, age-related changes in taste perception, reluctance to change long-established eating patterns, limited finances, and reliance on others for meals. Furthermore, decreased motor coordination and visual acuity may impair patients' ability to perform self-monitoring of blood glucose levels and self-injection of insulin. Older adults may have impaired vision, decreased motor coordination, or other health problems that affect their ability to perform tasks needed for diabetic control, such as fingersticks, self-administration of insulin, and managing diet and exercise.

Lifestyle, Diet, and Habits

An assessment of psychosocial aspects of diabetes, such as role changes and financial concerns, may help ascertain the patient's ability to cope with a chronic illness that involves major changes in lifestyle.

Exercise increases the permeability of the cell membrane to glucose, decreasing the need for insulin to transport glucose into the cell. Therefore, determine the activity and exercise patterns of the patient, which can be accomplished by asking about the patient's usual activity level, occupation, amount and type of recreational activities, and daily exercise patterns. Also, assess the patient's typical eating habits because these also alter the individual response to regular insulin.

The patient's typical alcohol intake is also a factor because consuming alcohol may cause hypoglycemia or hyperglycemia. Alcohol has no nutritional value, although if consumed, it must be included in the fat allowances of the diabetic diet plan. A patient taking insulin and consuming alcohol may need to adjust the insulin dosage because alcohol potentiates the hypoglycemic effect of insulin. Also, assess for the use of dietary supplements and herbal products because they may alter glucose production or storage or interact with insulin.

Environment

Note the environment in which regular insulin will be administered. Insulin is most commonly self-administered by the patient in the home. Proper needle disposal is a growing concern because of the large number of patients administering medications with syringes in the home care setting. Current Environmental Protection Agency (EPA) guidelines recommend that syringes, lancets, and other sharp objects be placed in a hard plastic or metal container with a screw-on or other tight-fitting lid. Patients should check local regulations regarding sharps disposal. For information on patients who use an insulin pump at home, see Box 49.2. Insulin given by intravenous infusion should be done in a critical care setting.

BOX 49.2 COMMUNITY BASED CONCERNS

Understanding How an Insulin Infusion Pump Works

Patients who have type 1 diabetes and require frequent insulin injections throughout the day to control their elevated blood glucose levels may have their insulin delivered by an insulin pump. An insulin pump is a small (2- × 3-in), precise computerized device that consists of a reservoir filled with insulin. The reservoir is connected by an infusion set (a thin plastic tube) to a subcutaneous (SC) catheter or needle. The catheter is changed every 2 to 3 days. An insulin pump can be programmed to deliver a basal infusion of insulin (microdoses; about 0.1 U) 24 hours a day. Continuous delivery of insulin helps maintain blood glucose concentrations between meals and overnight. Insulin dosing adjustments require little or no patient effort. When the patient eats, a predetermined prandial bolus dose of insulin is delivered that is matched to the estimated caloric intake. The bolus mode requires the patient to determine the dose and push a button to administer insulin before or after each meal. Pump devices help patients achieve tighter blood glucose control, thus minimizing potential complications. The pumps have an alarm system that alerts the patient if insulin delivery is interrupted. Some patients may find the pump complicated to use. The individual needs to be very motivated and adherent to therapy. The pump is not automatic; the user must decide how much insulin to give.

Some combinations of pumps and glucose monitors are available. A combination of a glucose monitor and an insulin pump with a dose calculator is manufactured by Medtronic MiniMed, Inc., and Becton Dickinson. The combination of these two products allows for better interchange of data between the two. Glucose values are automatically sent to the insulin pump, thus preventing possible errors that can result when the patient inputs the glucose data manually into the pump. The software that ac companies this glucose monitor–insulin pump also allows for transfer of data to a personal computer fitted with the appropriate software program.

Nursing Diagnoses and Outcomes

- Deficient Knowledge related to insulin pharmacotherapeutics
  Desired outcome: The patient (or family) will state brand, type, onset, peak, duration, and dose of insulin.
- Risk for Nonadherence to Self-Care related to the complexity and chronic nature of the insulin regimen.
  Desired outcome: The patient will adhere to the treatment regimen and communicate an understanding of the insulin regimen and its importance (i.e., demonstrate techniques for administering insulin and verbalize recommendations for site rotation, storage of insulin, and disposal of syringes).
- Potential Complication: Hypoglycemia related to administration of too much insulin.
  Desired outcome: The patient will assess for and report signs and symptoms of hypoglycemia and if an episode should occur will implement the appropriate treatment.
- Pain related to insulin injections and self-monitoring blood glucose testing via fingerstick.
  Desired outcome: The patient will state two nonpharmacologic methods used to control pain and will demonstrate proper subcutaneous injection and fingerstick techniques to minimize pain.

Planning and Intervention

Maximizing Therapeutic Effects

Store opened vials of regular insulin at room temperature. Extra supplies are stored in the refrigerator, but not the freezer. Extreme temperatures (less than 28C or greater than 308C) should be avoided to prevent loss of maximum function.

Administer regular insulin with an insulin syringe into an appropriate subcutaneous site. Regular insulin is administered about 30 to 60 minutes before eating. To promote regular absorption, one anatomic area should be selected for regular insulin injections (e.g., the abdomen). Serial locations within that anatomic area are chosen to rotate the exact injection site. This practice is sometimes called intra-site rotation. Do *not* rotate injection sites by using the arm one day, the stomach the next day, and the thigh the next day because this practice will substantially change the absorption of the insulin and the blood glucose levels of the patient. If the patient routinely receives regular insulin in the morning and in the evening, one anatomic area may be selected for each time of day (e.g., use the abdomen for all morning injections and the thighs for all evening injections).

Frequent monitoring of blood glucose by fingersticks and periodic determinations of hemoglobin A_{1C} levels help determine the therapeutic effect of insulin and overall consistency of diabetic control. Such monitoring also provides the necessary data to change the insulin regimen (if necessary) so that maximal effects are achieved. When supplemental doses are based on a current glucose level obtained from a glucometer, it is important that the reading achieved with the measurement is accurate. Calibrate the glucometer per manufacturer recommendations or hospital protocol, and perform quality control checks per protocol. Use the appropriate technique for obtaining the specimen. Assess for physiologic conditions, which may cause inaccurate bedside blood glucose readings. See Box 49.3 for factors that may alter glucometer accuracy.

Most diabetic patients (those at home and those in the hospital) can have their glucose levels effectively controlled with subcutaneous injections. Some patients at home may use an implantable subcutaneous insulin pump to administer their insulin. A review of the literature (Misso, Egberts, Page, et al., 2010) found that continuous subcutaneous insulin infusion (via an insulin pump) may provide better control of glucose levels than multiply subcutaneous injections in a day. Subcutaneous infusion pumps did not appear to provide any benefit in reducing non severe hypoglycemic events.

When a patient receives regular insulin intravenously, carefully monitor blood sugar levels to account for varying absorption of the drug into the plastic tubing. Patients who are hospitalized and critically ill will require insulin by drip infusion if their glucose level exceeds 180 mg/dL. The infusion should be titrated to achieve a blood glucose level between 140 and 180 mg/dL. Avoiding significant hyperglycemia promotes positive outcomes for the patient.

Box 49.3 FACTORS THAT ALTER THE ACCURACY OF BEDSIDE BLOOD GLUCOSE RESULTS

As regular insulin or the rapid-acting analogues are frequently dosed based on the current blood glucose level, an accurate reading is essential. Errors in glucometer readings have two sources: users or intrinsic patient factors.

Common User Errors:

- Inadequate meter calibration or meter maintenance
- Inadequate quality control testing
- Using a test strip that does not match the meter code or that has expired
- Poor technique in performing a fingerstick
- Insufficient size of blood droplet
- Poor technique in applying blood droplet to test strip
- Failure to record result in patient chart
- Inability to correctly interpret medication order and administer the appropriate amount of insulin based on current glucose level

Potential Patient Factors:

- Low hematocrit (falsely higher readings)
- High hematocrit (falsely lower readings)
- Shock and dehydration (falsely lower readings)
- Hypoxia (either falsely higher or falsely lower readings)
- Hyperbilirubinemia, severe lipemia (falsely higher readings)
- Sodium fluoride as specimen additive (falsely lower readings)
- Use of these drugs: acetaminophen overdose, ascorbic acid, dopamine, fluorescein, mannitol, salicylate (either falsely higher or falsely lower readings)

Minimizing Adverse Effects

Avoid administering cold insulin to help limit local irritation (e.g., lipodystrophy) at the injection site. Injection-site rotation also helps prevent lipodystrophy. Prevention is especially important in infants and children.

Assess the current blood sugar level of the patient before administering regular insulin. Caution is necessary if the blood glucose level is below 70 mg/dL before administration. Usually, the dose is withheld until the blood sugar level has risen to normal levels (at least 70 mg/dl). Consult with the physician or nurse practitioner before administering regular insulin if the blood sugar is low. Regular insulin can be used in a prandial dose where a set number of prescribed units are administered when the patient eats. Regular insulin could also be used for correctional doses, where the blood glucose is monitored before meals and bedtime, and the number of units of regular insulin given is according to the degree of glucose detected. The patient should receive a basal dose of a long acting insulin (NPH, glargine, or determir, described below) in addition to receiving prandial doses and/or correctional doses. Use of regular insulin as a correctional dose without a basal insulin should be avoided for most diabetic patients as this method creates recurring episodes of hyperglycemia

which lead to poorer patient outcomes (American College of Endocrinology and American Diabetes Association Consensus Statement on Inpatient Diabetes and Glycemic Control, 2006).

Determining the correct dose of insulin for a patient requires adjustments based on the individual patient's needs. Much like Goldilocks who was looking for something "just right," the correct insulin dose will prevent hyperglycemia but avoid hypoglycemia. Each of these can be dangerous to the patient. Severe hypoglycemia is an acute life threatening event. Hyperglycemia contributes to poor outcomes for the hospitalized patient and long term sequela, such as cardiovascular disease, for the diabetic at home. The nurse must monitor the patient closely for hypoglycemic reactions, especially near the peak action time of the insulin (see Table 49.2). Reassess the patient's blood glucose level if signs or symptoms of hypoglycemia occur. The fear of hypoglycemia may prevent nurses and other health care providers from treating diabetes appropriately. To minimize this risk explicit guidelines should be developed and followed so that the appropriate treatment for hypoglycemic episodes occurs (American College of Endocrinology and American Diabetes Association Consensus Statement on Inpatient Diabetes and Glycemic Control, 2006). Treat hypoglycemic episodes by following the institutional guidelines or by administering one of the following: 4 ounces of juice or a regular soda (not diet), 4 oz of water with four sugar packets (i.e., 4 teaspoons), or 8 oz of low fat milk if the patient is hypoglycemic and able to swallow. Administer 50% IV dextrose or glucagon if the hypoglycemic patient is not able to swallow.

If the regular insulin dose is too low for the patient's current metabolic needs, hyperglycemia may occur. Monitor the patient for signs and symptoms of hyperglycemia and re-evaluate blood glucose levels as appropriate. If the patient has frequent hyperglycemia the nurse should consult with the physician or nurse practitioner concerning adjusting the basal insulin dose.

When drawing up insulin, always have the dose double-checked by another nurse to prevent accidental overdosage, because insulins are very potent. A small dose produces a big effect and could cause serious and even life-threatening consequences to the patient. Read labels very carefully, because many forms of insulin have similar-sounding trade names. *When referring to insulins, use generic names rather than trade names.*

Use special consideration when caring for infants and toddlers with type 1 diabetes. Infants and toddlers require low dosages of insulin to maintain a goal serum glucose level of 100 to 200 mg/dL. Hypoglycemia may occur because of unpredictable food intake and activity levels in preschool-aged children. The brain and spinal column do not develop normally without an adequate and available source of glucose. Therefore, hypoglycemia must be avoided in infants and young children because it can have potentially damaging effects on growth and development.

Box 49.4 PATIENT AND FAMILY EDUCATION COMMON TO DIABETIC DRUG THERAPY

In addition to receiving routine medical care provided by health care professionals, patients and their families need to be educated on important topics of self-management and drug therapy for diabetes if their management is going to be successful. People with diabetes need to understand:

- What diabetes is and why treatment is necessary
- How to administer and store insulin
- How and when to test their blood glucose
- How and when to take oral medications if they have type 2 diabetes

Emphasize that drug therapy is not a substitute for diet control, exercise, and weight loss. The patient must understand the balance among exercise, diet, and drug therapy, realizing that changes in dietary intake and exercise will result in a change in drug therapy.

Caution the patient against consuming alcohol because of its hypoglycemic or hyperglycemic effects with insulin and other antidiabetic drugs, and because of the possibility of a disulfiram-like reaction when alcohol is combined with some sulfonylureas.

Teach the patient to recognize and report symptoms of hypoglycemia (e.g., fatigue, excessive hunger, diaphoresis, and numbness or tingling of extremities), or hyperglycemia (e.g., excessive thirst or urination, urinary glucose, or ketones) to the health care team.

Teach the patient and the family to treat symptoms of hypoglycemia by taking 4 oz of juice or non diet soda, 4 oz of water with 4 teaspoons of sugar in it, 8 oz of non fat milk,. If the patient is receiving acarbose or miglitol for type 2 diabetes they cannot take a dietary sugar but should take glucose tablets

Teach the patient to notify the prescriber when his or her blood sugar is consistently outside of the set parameters (too high or too low), so that changes in the drug regimen can be made.

Encourage the patient to carry some type of medical identification (e.g., a Medic Alert bracelet) and to inform all health care providers of current drug therapy.

Providing Patient and Family Education

In addition to the information provided within this section, which is specific to insulin therapy, see Box 49.4.

DISCUSSING DIET

- Emphasize the importance of eating the prescribed diet after insulin dosing. Warn patients that hypoglycemia may occur from omission of a meal or from altered absorption of food if a meal is postponed.
- Counsel patients not to take any nonprescription or OTC preparations, including herbs or alcohol, without first consulting the prescriber, because these substances may interact with regular insulin and alter its effectiveness.

UNDERSTANDING ACTIVITY AND REST

Emphasize that changing the daily exercise or activity pattern will vary the hypoglycemic effect from insulin. If patients are more active than usual, they will use more glucose, thus lowering the available glucose for insulin to act on. The molecules of insulin administered in the ordered dose each have the pharmacodynamic ability to move a certain number of molecules of glucose. If less glucose is available in the bloodstream than is usual for that particular patient, when insulin moves the set number of glucose molecules into the cells, hypoglycemia will result. Therefore, the patient may need to eat more to offset the glucose burned by exercising. If the increase in exercising is a permanent change, the insulin dose may need to be adjusted.

RECOGNIZING THE ROLE OF STRESS

- Teach patients and families that stress, both physiologic (e.g., from illness, surgery, and trauma) and psychological (e.g., from death in the family, divorce, and job changes), may change insulin requirements because the hormones released in stressful situations are antagonistic to insulin.

- In cases of stress, urge patients to consult the prescriber to see whether a change is needed in the insulin dosage or regimen.

MONITORING THE BLOOD GLUCOSE LEVEL

- Most patients with diabetes learn to test their own blood to measure the level of circulating glucose. Various kits and devices are commercially available for this task.

ADMINISTERING INSULIN

- Most patients with type 1 diabetes administer their own insulin with disposable needle and syringe injection devices or with a special injection pen device. Teach patients to use aseptic technique, select the appropriate type of insulin, mix insulin properly (if necessary), administer insulin correctly by SC injection (see Chapter 3 on injection technique), rotate sites serially in an anatomic location (intrasite rotation), and store insulin carefully (Box 49.5). If an acute infection is present or resistance to infection is impaired, the needles should not be reused.
- Manufacturers of disposable syringes recommend a single use. However, some patients prefer to reuse a syringe until its needle becomes dull, usually up to three or four times. Reuse reduces the cost of injections, which may be important for patients with limited financial resources. Most insulin preparations have bacteriostatic additives that inhibit the growth of bacteria commonly found on the skin. If reuse is planned, the needle must be carefully recapped by the patient after each use. Aseptic technique should be followed. The patient who reuses a syringe should be taught to inspect the skin around the injection sites for unusual redness or signs of infection.
- Teach patients thoroughly about safe insulin administration. Needles or syringes should never be shared with anyone

Box 49.5 INSULIN ADMINISTRATION

American Diabetes Association Guidelines for Preparing and Administering a Subcutaneous Dose of Insulin

- Check the type of insulin and the expiration date.
- Inspect the solution for visible changes (e.g., solid clumps) that indicate deterioration of the drug.
- If possible, verify Dose, Expiration date, Concentration, and Type with another individual (nurse if in health care setting).
- Wash hands.
- Cleanse injection site and insulin vial by wiping with alcohol.
- If using suspension (cloudy solution), roll gently between palms of hands to resuspend the insulin.
- Inject an amount of air into the vial (each vial, if using two) that is equal to the dose of insulin.
- When mixing two types of insulin in one syringe, the short-acting clear insulin should be drawn into the syringe first.
- Eliminate air bubbles from the syringe to ensure an accurate dose.
- Injection sites—in their order of rapidity of absorption—include the (1) abdomen (excluding 2 inches around the umbilicus), (2) subcutaneous tissue of the upper arm, (3) anterior and lateral aspects of the thigh, and (4) buttocks.*
- Insulin injections are made into SC tissue, so it is not necessary to aspirate for blood routinely before injecting the insulin.
- The needle angle during the injection (45 to 90 degrees) should be individualized to avoid IM injection; the needle length is usually 5/8 inches. Gently pinch a skin fold to determine the angle that will deliver an SC injection.

Other Considerations

- Insulin vials in current use may be stored at room temperature; avoid exposure to direct sunlight and high temperatures. Some potency of product may be lost after 30 days.
- Spare insulin vials should be stored in the refrigerator. No potency is lost when stored in the refrigerator.

- Prefilled syringes:
  - Are stable up to 30 days when stored in the refrigerator.
  - Filled with an insulin suspension (cloudy solution) should preferably be stored with the needle pointed up (vertical position) to avoid clumping of suspended insulin molecules in the needle.
  - Insulins that cannot be mixed with any other type of insulin: glargine and detemir
- Injection pens:
  - Are unique because they combine the insulin container and the syringe into a single modular unit.
  - Are available in a variety of types and styles (e.g., prefilled single use or reusable), but generally, they have a characteristic design— the patient must attach a needle, prime the pen, dial the dose, and depress a plunger to deliver the dose.
  - Add lifestyle flexibility (because pens are pocket sized and easy to carry) and confidentiality (because some look like fountain pens, not a medical device) and may lead to improved glycemic control.
  - Many of the rapid-acting insulins come in insulin pens.
- Adaptive equipment—several products are available for patients with diabetes who are visually or functionally impaired. Some of the commonly used assistive devices include:
  - Syringe magnifiers to enlarge the measurements on the syringe barrel.
  - Needle guides to help direct the needle into the vial stopper.
  - Vial stabilizers mounted on a surface to hold the vial in place during needle insertion.
  - Insertion aids add bulk to the syringe for patients unable to hold a small syringe.
  - Dose-measuring devices assist the visually impaired patient to draw up the recommended insulin dosage into a syringe.
  - "Talking" blood glucose meters produce audible test results with tactile guides for test strip insertion.

*Site selection affects absorption; it is recommended that site rotation for insulin injection take place within the same anatomic area.

else because this practice may cause transmission of blood-borne infections (e.g., hepatitis B or C, or HIV infection).
- Nearly as important as learning about injection techniques is learning about safe and proper disposal of insulin injection equipment. The EPA recommends that insulin needles and lancets be discarded whole in opaque, puncture-resistant containers to avoid the hazards of exposed or broken needles and that the lid be taped on tightly before the container is put in the trash. For example, a plastic milk container or a coffee can is preferable to a glass jar, which can break.

EXPLAINING OTHER SAFETY MEASURES
- Encourage patients to wear diabetic identification, such as a MedicAlert bracelet, so that appropriate treatment can be given if complications, such as diabetic coma, occur away from home.
- Also, caution patients that changing the kind of insulin normally used may affect blood glucose control and

should be done only under the supervision of the health care professional.
- Advise patients always to carry a spare vial of each type of insulin used and to pay attention to the expiration date stamped on the vial.

Ongoing Assessment and Evaluation

It is important to evaluate the technical skills (e.g., insulin injection) that will be used by the patient for self-care at home. Specific assessment and evaluation criteria may include the patient's stated willingness to adhere to recommended drug therapy and management techniques for diabetes and may also include blood glucose levels that remain within normal limits as specified by the prescriber.

Fasting blood glucose and hemoglobin A_{1C} levels are valuable in monitoring the patient's response to therapy.

Nursing management of drug therapy is considered successful if the patient experiences few episodes of hypoglycemia or hyperglycemia, demonstrates the ability to correctly perform the technical tasks necessary for managing diabetes at home, follows the ADA diet and incorporates it into his or her lifestyle, incorporates an exercise regimen to attain or maintain normal body weight, and recognizes situations in which knowledge deficit may require the guidance of a diabetes health care professional for additional information or follow-up care.

Drugs Closely Related to Regular Insulin

Rapid-acting Insulins: Aspart, Lispro, and Glulisine

Three rapid-acting insulins that are analogues of rapid-acting regular insulin are now available: aspart (NovoLog), lispro (Humalog), and glulisine (Apidra). The use of these drugs is becoming preferred over the use of regular insulin. Like regular insulins, these are clear insulins. Caution should be used so as not to confuse the trade names for aspart and lispro with the trade names for regular insulin. These rapid-acting insulins may be used in type 1 diabetes (in combination with an intermediate- or long-acting insulin), or in type 2 diabetes, where glucose control cannot be achieved solely from oral therapy. Compared with regular insulin, the pharmacodynamically rapid-acting (rDNA) insulins have a faster onset of glucose-lowering activity, an earlier peak glucose-lowering effect, and a shorter duration of action after SC administration. The rapid onset of action allows patients more flexibility in taking insulin and preparing and consuming meals. All rapid-acting insulins are well suited for use in implantable pumps because their short duration of action mimics endogenous insulin more closely than regular insulin. These insulins are also used as either prandial doses or supplemental doses when combined with a basal dose of an intermediate- or long-acting insulin. Unlike regular insulin, these rapid-acting insulins should be administered closer to the time a meal is started because of their onset of action. The pharmacologic and pharmacokinetic features of these analogues are quite similar. To compare pharmacokinetics of various insulins, see Table 49.4. These newer analogues are less likely to cause hypoglycemia than human formulations of regular or NPH (Moghissi, 2010). Other adverse effects and patient education are similar to those for regular insulin with the exception of the timing of the dose. All of the rapid-acting insulins are sold by prescription, in contrast to regular insulin, which may be obtained OTC.

In patients with type 1 diabetes, insulin lispro is used in regimens that include a longer-acting insulin. However, in patients with type 2 diabetes, lispro may be used without a longer-acting insulin when used in combination therapy with an oral antidiabetic drug. It may also be used in adults and children older than three years of age. Lispro is administered no more than 15 minutes before a meal; in some situations (e.g., when a patient needs to adjust a prandial dose based on how much is eaten), it may be administered immediately after a meal (Magee & Clement, 2004). This insulin analogue produces a smaller postprandial glucose increase than regular insulin. Lispro is administered subcutaneously, either by direct injection (via needle and syringe or special injector pen) or by infusion via an insulin pump—never intravenously. It *can be* mixed with NPH insulin for administration in a syringe but *cannot* be mixed with NPH for SC administration via an external insulin pump. Lispro is a pregnancy category B drug.

MEMORY CHIP

P Regular Insulin

- Used primarily to treat type 1 diabetes mellitus; only type of insulin used for intravenous administration, in external insulin pumps, and for "sliding scale" coverage for hypoglycemia
- Most common adverse effect: hypoglycemia
- Most serious adverse effects: anaphylaxis and hypersensitivity
- **Patient safety alert: Sound-alike names for various types of insulin and the high potency of insulins are both common sources of medication errors**
- Maximizing therapeutic effects: Protect insulin from excessive heat and light to avoid deterioration.
- Minimizing adverse effects: Use the same type and brand of syringe to avoid dosage errors; rotate injection sites to prevent tissue damage; have second nurse check dose; read labels carefully.
- Most important patient education: thorough teaching regarding dosage, administration techniques for subcutaneous injection, delivery devices, diet and exercise, and capillary blood glucose testing; wear medical alert tag identifying diabetic condition treated with insulin to alert emergency medical personnel

---

TABLE 49.4 Pharmacokinetics of Insulins

Nurses should be familiar with the onset, peak, and duration of insulins, because this affects the time of administration and the time to assess the patient for therapeutic and adverse effects.

| Insulin | Number of Hours | | |
	Onset	Peak	Duration
Regular (short-acting)	0.5–1	2–3	8–12
lispro (rapid-acting)	0.25	0.5–1.5	3–4
aspart (rapid-acting)	0.15	0.75–1.5	3–5
glulisine (rapid-acting)	0.3	1.5	Up to 5.3
50% lispro protamine suspension and 50% lispro (mixed intermediate-acting and rapid-acting)	0.25	0.75–2	10–12
70% aspart protamine suspension and 30% aspart (mixed intermediate-acting and rapid-acting)	0.15	1–4	Up to 24
NPH (intermediate-acting)	1–1.5	4–12	18–24
Levemir (long-acting)	Unknown	3–14	5.7–23.2
70% NPH with 30% regular (mixed-acting)	0.5–1	2–12	24
glargine (long-acting)	1	—	24

Aspart should be administered just before starting a meal, no more than 5 to 10 minutes before eating. This insulin analogue can be given intravenously or subcutaneously, either via needle and syringe, via special injection pen (NovoLog FlexPen), or by infusion via an external insulin pump. Aspart can be mixed with NPH in one syringe (draw up the aspart first, then the NPH) and administered subcutaneously. However, aspart–NPH mixtures should not be subcutaneously administered via an insulin pump. Aspart is a pregnancy category B drug, and it is approved for use in children 6 years of age and older.

Glulisine is almost identical to lispro in terms of its pharmacokinetics, clinical indications, and adverse effects. It also is administered subcutaneously and as an SC infusion via an insulin pump. No other insulins should be mixed with it for SC infusion. Glulisine should be administered within 15 minutes of the start of a meal. Unlike regular insulin and the other rapid-acting insulins, glulisine is a pregnancy category C drug and is not approved for use in children.

Drugs Significantly Different From P Regular Insulin

Insulin is available in a variety of forms, with the different forms made by adding protamine, zinc, or isophane with a buffer. These modifications delay the absorption of the insulin from a subcutaneous site, resulting in a later onset of action, peak action, and an extended duration of action. Thus, insulin preparations may be rapid-, short-, intermediate-, or long-acting, depending on whether an additive is mixed into the insulin. Drugs significantly different from regular insulin are NPH (a suspension of isophane), detemir, glargine, and the human insulin Exubera. To compare pharmacokinetics of these insulins, see Table 49.4.

Preparations of Aspart or Lispro with Protamine

Some forms of the rapid-acting insulins, aspart or lispro, are available as mixtures with protamine added to the drug. This provides some rapid action as well as some prolonged action from the insulin. Mixtures of insulins always list the longer-acting component first. The aspart combination is sold under the trade name of NovoLog Mix 70/30 and contains 70% aspart protamine and 30% aspart. The lispro combination is sold under the name Humalog Mix 75/25 or Humalog Mix 50/50 and contains 75% lispro protamine and 25% lispro, or 50% lispro protamine and 50% lispro, respectively. The similarity of the trade names compared with each other and regular insulin (Novolin or Humulin), as well as with each other, makes these combination insulins extremely easy to confuse; and this is a major source of drug errors (Paparella, 2006). *To avoid confusion, the drugs should be referred to by their generic names, not their trade names.*

NPH

Although the full chemical name of NPH (Humulin N) insulin is Neutral Protamine Hagedorn insulin, it is known and referred to in clinical practice as NPH. Protamine is added to insulin to create NPH insulin and lengthen its duration of action. Onset of action is 1 to 1.5 hours, peak action occurs in 4 to 12 hours, and duration of action is up to 24 hours. The N on the label signifies NPH. NPH differs from regular insulin primarily in terms of duration of action, appearance, and frequency of administration. It is considered intermediate acting. Cloudy in appearance, NPH is now the only insulin that is not clear. NPH is administered once or twice daily via SC injection, never by IV infusion or SC insulin pump. It is never used for supplemental coverage. Because NPH insulin is a suspension and tends to separate inside the vial, it must be mixed by rolling the vial between the palms of both hands before withdrawing the mixture into the insulin syringe. Excessive agitation should be avoided to prevent damaging the additive used to create a long-term drug action.

NPH insulin is the most widely used intermediate-acting insulin. Occasionally, a white precipitate (flocculus) may appear as frosting that adheres to the vial. This effect, called flocculation, occurs for unknown reasons, although vigorous mixing of the vial is thought to contribute. Flocculation decreases the potency of the insulin; if it is present, the insulin should be discarded. NPH insulin may be mixed with regular insulin; premixed solutions of NPH and regular insulin are also available in ratios of 70/30 (sold as Novolin 70/30 or Humulin 70/30) and 50/50 (sold as Humulin 50/50). The proportion of insulin for these preparation means that for every 100 U of insulin, there are 70 of NPH and 30 of regular insulin, or 50 of NPH and 50 of regular insulin, respectively. Use of premixed insulin is especially useful for patients who are visually impaired or have difficulty with fine motor skills and may reduce the number of errors that might occur using the standard mixing technique. A limitation of the premixed solutions is that the patient's insulin requirements must match the fixed ratio of the premixed preparations.

Nursing interventions specific for intermediate-acting insulin include observing patients for adequate nutritional intake and monitoring for hypoglycemia during mid to late afternoon (after an early-morning dose), because the lengthy peak action time produces additional risks for hypoglycemic reactions. The onset of hypoglycemia with the intermediate-acting insulin is insidious and more prolonged. Adverse effects, nursing actions, and patient education are also similar to those for regular insulin.

Detemir

Detemir (Levemir) is a long-acting insulin that differs from human insulin by slight chemical modification (deletion of one amino acid and addition of one fatty acid chain). These changes cause the insulin particles to be more slowly absorbed from the SC injection site than NPH insulin and to distribute to the target sites in the peripheral tissues more slowly, preferring to be highly protein bound once absorbed. Detemir is used in the treatment of type 1 and type 2 diabetes. The drug is administered once or twice a day by SC injection. Detemir cannot be administered intravenously or subcutaneously via insulin infusion pumps. It should not be mixed with any other insulins, because this will decrease its effectiveness. Unlike NPH, detemir is a clear insulin, similar to regular insulin.

Caution must be used not to confuse detemir for regular insulin. Detemir comes in a multidose vial and in cartridges to use with an injection pen. This insulin provides glycemic control similar to that of NPH, with a slightly greater reduction in FPG. Detemir may be associated with less weight gain and a lower risk of nocturnal hypoglycemia than NPH.

Glargine

Insulin glargine (rDNA) is characterized by a chemical structure that regulates its release from the SC tissue into the circulation, providing a relatively constant glucose-lowering effect with no pronounced peak of action over a 24-hour period. Glargine, unlike NPH, is a clear insulin, similar to regular insulin in its appearance. Extreme caution must be used not to confuse glargine for regular insulin because serious adverse effects, including hypoglycemia, can occur. Glargine must not be diluted or mixed with any other insulin or solution because its onset of action may be delayed, and the solution will become cloudy. Insulin glargine is administered subcutaneously once daily at bedtime. This timing of administration is unique for glargine. Patients who have previously received twice-daily injections of NPH insulin may be switched over to glargine's once-daily regimen under medical supervision. The initial dose of glargine is usually 20% less than the previous NPH dose. Taking one injection daily instead of two may be viewed as an improvement in quality of life for some patients. Adverse effects, administration techniques, and patient education are similar to those for regular insulin.

NON-INSULIN ANTIDIABETIC MEDICATIONS

Until the mid-1990s, the sulfonylurea drugs were the only class of antidiabetic agents available to manage type 2 diabetes. Currently, five chemical classes of oral antidiabetic agents are available for treating type 2 diabetes, and two classes of subcutaneous antidiabetic agents. For simplicity, they are grouped here, based on chemical composition, into sulfonylureas and nonsulfonylureas.

● C SULFONYLUREAS

The sulfonylureas consist of first- and second-generation drugs. The terms *first generation* and *second generation* are applied to groups of drugs that are in the same class but are developed at different times and have some different characteristics. The first-generation drugs are the original group of drugs in the class, and the second-generation drugs are those that are developed to overcome recognized limitations of the first generation. For example, second-generation sulfonylurea drugs have fewer drug interactions than those in the first generation. The first-generation sulfonylureas—acetohexamide, chlorpropamide, tolazamide, and tolbutamide—are rarely used today. Glyburide (Diabeta), a second-generation drug, is the prototype sulfonylurea hypoglycemic. See Table 49.2 for a summary of selected sulfonylureas.

Nursing Management of the Patient Receiving P Glyburide
Core Drug Knowledge
Pharmacotherapeutics

Glyburide is a potent second-generation oral sulfonylurea that is indicated as an adjunctive treatment to lower blood glucose levels in patients with type 2 diabetes in whom hyperglycemia cannot be controlled by diet and exercise alone.

Combination administration of a sulfonylurea and insulin has been used with some success in patients with type 2 diabetes whose disease is difficult to control with diet and sulfonylurea therapy alone. One such method is the "BIDS" system—*B*edtime *I*nsulin (usually NPH) in combination with a *D*aytime (morning only or morning and evening) *S*ulfonylurea. Temporary use of insulin in addition to glyburide may be necessary during periods of physiologic stress (e.g., from systemic infection, trauma, surgery, or fever); stress can induce alterations in glucose regulation that can be controlled only with exogenously administered insulin.

Pharmacokinetics

Administered orally, glyburide is absorbed rapidly and completely from the GI tract. The onset of action occurs within 2 hours, with a maximal decrease in serum glucose occurring within 3 to 4 hours. Like other second-generation sulfonylureas, glyburide is highly protein bound by non-ionic binding, which differs from the ionic protein binding observed with first-generation sulfonylureas. Therefore, first-generation sulfonylureas are more likely to be displaced by drugs that competitively bind to proteins (e.g., warfarin), resulting in greater hypoglycemic response.

Glyburide is metabolized completely in the liver by the CYP3A3/4 isoenzyme to two metabolites, both of which are only weakly active. Both unchanged drug and metabolites are excreted equally in the urine and feces. The elimination half-life of the drug is 10 hours, and the duration of action is 24 hours in patients with normal renal function.

There are two forms of glyburide—micronized and non-micronized. The two forms differ in absorption, onset of action, and delivery system, and consequently also differ in their bioavailability. Patients transferring to micronized glyburide from conventional glyburide or other oral antidiabetic agents should have their dosages adjusted.

Pharmacodynamics

The hypoglycemic action of glyburide results from the stimulation of pancreatic beta cells, leading to increased insulin secretion. Glyburide, like other sulfonylureas, is ineffective in type 1 diabetes, in which no endogenous release of insulin occurs, and in severe cases of type 2 diabetes, in which the release of insulin is severely impaired. Glyburide also reduces the glucose output from the liver by decreasing liver glycogenolysis (breakdown of glycogen stored in liver into glucose) and gluconeogenesis (formation of glycogen from fatty acids and proteins rather than from carbohydrates).

Glyburide also increases insulin sensitivity at cellular sites. These mechanisms lower blood glucose levels.

Contraindications and Precautions

Glyburide is contraindicated in patients with a known hypersensitivity to sulfa drugs because the sulfonylureas are related chemically to the antimicrobial sulfonamides (although they do not demonstrate any antimicrobial activity). Glyburide should not be used in type 1 diabetes and should be used cautiously in individuals with renal or hepatic disease.

Glyburide is a pregnancy category B drug.

Adverse Effects

Glyburide and other sulfonylureas are generally well tolerated. The primary adverse effect associated with glyburide (and the other sulfonylureas) is hypoglycemia. Renal or hepatic insufficiency may elevate drug blood levels, and hepatic insufficiency may also diminish gluconeogenic capacity. Both effects increase the risk of serious hypoglycemic reactions. In addition to excessive dosage, other factors that result in hypoglycemia include altered hepatic metabolism and renal excretion, improper diet, excessive physical activity, ingestion of alcohol (more of a problem with first-generation sulfonylureas), or concomitant use of more than one glucose-lowering drug. The hypoglycemia

CRITICAL THINKING SCENARIO

UNEXPECTED HYPOGLYCEMIA

At the beginning of your 7 am shift, Mr. B., an 81-year-old African American male, is unresponsive when brought to the emergency department by ambulance. He is accompanied by his wife. She states she was unable to wake him up this morning. Mr. B. is found to have a serum glucose level of 8 mg/dL. One amp of D_{50} (50% dextrose) is administered, and his glucose level increases to 40 mg/dL and is closely monitored. He becomes responsive, alert, and oriented. Mr. B. has a past medical history of hypertension, chronic heart failure (CHF), and end-stage renal disease, for which he undergoes hemodialysis three times a week. He does not have diabetes, and there is no family history of diabetes, although his wife has type 2 diabetes. He and his wife are able to care for one another and live in their own home. Throughout your 12-hour shift, you continue to administer amps of D_{50} after checking his blood glucose every hour. His blood sugar continues to fluctuate and remains low, never getting above 60 mg/dL. A computed tomography scan of his head is negative, and his cardiac enzymes are also negative, indicating there has been no heart damage. After all of the fluid is administered, you notice crackles in the bases of his lung, leading to fluid overload and exacerbation of his CHF. By the end of your shift, you start a continuous infusion of D_{50} at 75 mL/h while continuing to check his blood glucose levels every hour. Without the D_{50}, Mr. B.'s blood glucose will drop.

1. After analyzing all of this information, how do you account for Mr. B.'s symptoms?

2. What further information might be helpful to fully assess Mr. B.'s condition?

induced by glyburide and other sulfonylureas, although typically mild, may occasionally be severe and require immediate re-evaluation and adjustment of the drug dosage and the patient's lifestyle (e.g., diet and activity). Elderly, debilitated, or malnourished patients and those with adrenal or pituitary insufficiency are particularly susceptible to the hypoglycemic action of glucose-lowering drugs.

Glyburide may also cause GI effects, including anorexia, nausea, vomiting, heartburn, and a metallic taste in the mouth. Sulfonylurea drugs like glyburide result in weight gain, which may be a problem for some patients with diabetes who are already overweight. Signs of allergic reactions to glyburide therapy can include maculopapular rash, urticaria, pruritus, and erythema. These reactions are usually mild, but if they persist or become severe, the drug should be discontinued. Photosensitivity reactions also may occur with sulfonylureas. Rarely, blood dyscrasias occur (e.g., leukopenia, thrombocytopenia, pancytopenia, agranulocytosis, aplastic anemia, hemolysis) that may lead to hemolytic anemia. These effects typically subside once the drug is stopped, assuming the condition is detected early after its onset; if undetected and untreated, these conditions may progress and be fatal.

Hyponatremia and the syndrome of inappropriate secretion of antidiuretic hormone (SIADH) have occurred in patients receiving sulfonylureas. As the medication stimulates ADH release, the normal feedback mechanism that controls ADH release is overridden, making the kidneys more permeable to water. This effect results in an increased plasma volume and dilutional hyponatremia. Signs and symptoms of SIADH include water intoxication characterized by mental confusion, nausea, anorexia, dizziness, decreased sodium concentration, increased urinary osmolality, and decreased serum osmolality.

Research performed in the 1970s demonstrated a higher rate of cardiovascular death in patients who received a first-generation sulfonylurea than patients treated with placebo or diet plus insulin. Although the question has always lingered concerning second-generation sulfonylurea drugs, a recent review of the literature indicates that glyburide or other second-generation sulfonylureas cause no cardiovascular effects of any clinical consequence (Riveline, Danchin, Ledru, et al., 2003). Recent comparisons of sulfonylureas with other antidiabetic drugs (pioglitazone and metformin) have shown similar cardiovascular outcomes with all treatments (Belcher, Lambert, Edwards, et al., 2005).

Drug Interactions

As with other first- and second-generation sulfonylureas, a synergistic drug interaction occurs between glyburide (which stimulates insulin release) and the "insulin sensitizers" metformin and rosiglitazone (which improve tissue use of insulin). Hypoglycemia may occur. A disulfiram-like reaction (see Chapter 5) may occur when glyburide or other sulfonylureas are administered with alcohol. This disulfiram-like reaction is characterized by facial flushing

TABLE 49.5 — Agents that Interact with P Glyburide

Interactants	Effect and Significance	Nursing Management
antacids (MG+ salts)	Increased glyburide serum levels due to increased glyburide absorption	Monitor blood glucose level for hypoglycemia.
sulfonamides, chloramphenicol, phenylbutazone, salicylates, clofibrate, anticoagulants, fluconazole, H_2 antagonists (e.g., cimetidine), MAOIs, probenecid, sulfonamides, tricyclic antidepressants	Increased risk for hypoglycemia	Monitor blood glucose level for hypoglycemia. Teach patient to recognize signs of hypoglycemia, and to carry food with sugar to eat if necessary.
diazoxide, beta blockers, cholestyramine, hydantoins, thiazide diuretics, rifampin	Decreased hypoglycemic effect	Monitor blood glucose level for hyperglycemia. Monitor A_{1c} levels.
digitalis	Increased serum digitalis levels	Monitor serum digitalis levels and heart rate and rhythm. Observe for symptoms of digitalis toxicity.
alcohol	Disulfiram-like reaction with some sulfonylureas; may cause hypoglycemia or hyperglycemia	Avoid concomitant use.

and occasional breathlessness but without the nausea, vomiting, and hypotension seen with a true alcohol–disulfiram reaction. A number of drug interactions are possible because these drugs are metabolized by the CYP3A3/4 system. Table 49.5 lists drugs that interact with glyburide.

Concomitant use of some alternative therapies (e.g., juniper berries, ginseng, garlic, fenugreek, coriander, dandelion root, or celery) increases the risk of hypoglycemia.

Assessment of Relevant Core Patient Variables

Health Status

Assessments to be made before therapy with glyburide are similar to those necessary with insulin. Because glyburide undergoes hepatic metabolism and renal excretion, impairment in these functions can result in elevated serum concentrations of glyburide and increase the risk of hypoglycemia. Therefore, assess renal and hepatic function. To detect or prevent possible adverse drug interactions, additional assessments should include a review of all other drugs—prescription and OTC, including herbal products and dietary supplements—used by the patient. If hypoglycemic reactions occur, it is important to determine their frequency and how the patient or family handles these reactions. This information helps assess knowledge, usual practices, and teaching needs.

Life Span and Gender

Assess the patient for pregnancy or lactation. Glyburide is in pregnancy category B. Animal reproduction studies have shown adverse fetal effects with glyburide; thus, insulin is recommended instead to maintain blood glucose levels during pregnancy. Prolonged severe neonatal hypoglycemia may occur if glyburide is administered near the time of delivery. Whether glyburide is excreted in breast milk is unknown; however, some first-generation sulfonylureas are excreted in breast milk. Because of the possibility of hypoglycemia in breast-fed infants, lactating women should avoid use of glyburide.

Note the age of the patient before administering glyburide. The drug's safety and efficacy have not been established in children. Although the Food and Drug Administration has not approved any of the oral antidiabetic drugs for use in children with type 2 diabetes, they are frequently prescribed by physicians who treat this population. Elderly patients may be more susceptible to the hypoglycemic effects of glyburide because of age-related decline in renal function that slows down the drug excretion. Rapid and prolonged hypoglycemia (less than 12 hours), despite hypertonic glucose injections, has been reported. Hypoglycemic reactions may be more difficult to recognize in elderly individuals because they may be obscured by other pathologies or drug therapies.

Lifestyle, Diet, and Habits

It is a good idea to assess the patient's willingness or ability to adhere to strict drug therapy. Tell the patient to take the pills daily and at the same time each day. Note the patient's weight and typical alcohol consumption before therapy is initiated. An obese patient (those more than 20% over ideal body weight) may not respond to glyburide. Concomitant alcohol use increases the rate of glyburide metabolism and may cause a disulfiram-like reaction. Also, assess for use of herbs that might interact with glyburide.

Environment

Be aware of the environment in which glyburide will be administered. Glyburide is most commonly self-administered by the patient in the home setting.

Nursing Diagnoses and Outcomes

• Ineffective Health Maintenance related to glyburide-induced nausea, vomiting, abdominal pain, and disulfiram-like reaction secondary to alcohol ingestion
Desired outcome: *The patient will follow American Diabetes Association dietary guidelines and avoid consuming alcohol.*

- Imbalanced Nutrition: More than Body Requirements, related to weight gain secondary to glyburide/sulfonylurea therapy
  Desired outcome: *The patient will follow American Diabetes Association dietary guidelines and not experience a weight gain.*
- Ineffective Protection related to leukopenia secondary to bone marrow depression associated with glyburide use
  Desired outcome: *The patient will be free from infection while taking glyburide.*

Planning and Intervention

Maximizing Therapeutic Effects

Administer glyburide before breakfast or the first main meal of the day in order to stimulate insulin production. In addition, glyburide should be stored in a tightly capped container at room temperature.

Minimizing Adverse Effects

Monitor the patient's blood glucose levels periodically throughout therapy to detect hypoglycemia. Assess blood glucose levels most closely at the start of therapy and whenever the dose is increased. Because older adults are more sensitive to the hypoglycemic effects of glyburide, administer the drug cautiously at a reduced dosage until the effects on the patient are known. More frequent monitoring of blood glucose levels may be required with older adults.

Monitor patients with renal and hepatic impairment for signs of adverse effects. General blood work should also be monitored periodically throughout therapy to detect blood dyscrasias.

Providing Patient and Family Education

In addition to general teaching on diabetes and diabetic management (see Box 49.4), teach specific information about glyburide.

- Teach patients and families the signs and symptoms of hypoglycemia (irritability, confusion, nervousness, weakness, hunger), which is a common adverse effect of glyburide. They should know to treat hypoglycemia with a small amount of quickly absorbed carbohydrate, such as a hard candy, orange juice, or a teaspoon of sugar.
- Alert patients and families to the signs and symptoms of out-of-control diabetes, such as hyperglycemia, polydipsia, polyphagia, and polyuria. Persistent hyperglycemia may indicate a need to adjust the glyburide dose or some other aspect of the therapeutic regimen, such as diet.
- Teach patients to avoid alcohol while using glyburide.
- It is important to caution patients to avoid OTC medications and herbal or dietary supplements without first consulting the prescriber. Drug interactions may occur; for example, cough syrups containing alcohol and sugar may cause an unintended effect.
- Provide patients with oral and written information about amount and timing of the doses to be taken.

MEMORY CHIP

P Glyburide

- Oral hypoglycemic that stimulates insulin release and increases peripheral tissue sensitivity to insulin effects; used as adjunct with dietary restrictions to treat type 2 diabetes mellitus; is available commercially, combined with metformin, to manage type 2 diabetes (e.g., Glucovance)
- Major contraindications: severe hepatic or renal impairment; allergy to sulfa drugs
- Most common adverse effects: nausea, epigastric fullness, heartburn
- Most serious adverse effect: hypoglycemia
- **Life span alert: Older adults may be at greater risk for hypoglycemia related to drug accumulation from age-related decline in hepatic and renal functions.**
- Maximizing therapeutic effects: Daily dosage of greater than 10 mg should be divided into two doses and taken 30 minutes before the meal.
- Minimizing adverse effects: Avoid taking glyburide with certain alternative dietary therapies, supplements, or herbs because of increased risk for hypoglycemia.
- Most important patient education: signs and symptoms of out-of-control diabetes, such as hyperglycemia, polydipsia, polyphagia, and polyuria; dietary restrictions for serum glucose control and weight loss

Ongoing Assessment and Evaluation

Interview the patient and family and observe for therapeutic and adverse responses to glyburide and adherence to prescribed treatments. When assessing the success of nursing management, be alert for adverse drug effects (especially hypoglycemia) and appropriately refer the patient to the prescriber for re-evaluation of pharmacotherapy if pertinent symptoms are identified. Blood tests monitoring glucose levels (e.g., fasting, 2-hour postprandial, and hemoglobin A_{1C}) are as important as they are for patients taking exogenous insulin. Review the patient's hepatic and renal function periodically, particularly if he or she has pre-existing liver or kidney impairment. Drug therapy with glyburide is considered effective if blood glucose levels are controlled and the patient does not experience appreciable adverse effects.

Drugs Closely Related to **P** Glyburide

There are two other second-generation sulfonylurea drugs, glipizide (Glucotrol or Glucotrol XL) and glimepiride (Amaryl). Glipizide has a slight variation from glyburide in the recommended time of administration. Because the absorption of glipizide is delayed by approximately 40 minutes when taken with food, it is more effective when given approximately 30 minutes before a meal. Like glyburide, glipizide and the other sulfonylureas may be taken with food. Glipizide is a pregnancy category C drug, unlike glyburide, which is in category B. Otherwise, glipizide is very similar to glyburide.

Glimepiride is much like glipizide, with two major differences: it is metabolized in the liver via the CYP2C9 pathway, and it is excreted via two routes, fecal and renal.

Drugs Significantly Different From P Glyburide

The meglitinides, consisting of repaglinide and nateglinide, are significantly different from the prototype glyburide. These drugs act similarly to the sulfonylureas but have a different chemical structure.

Repaglinide

Repaglinide (Prandin), which belongs to the meglitinide class, is an oral hypoglycemic agent. This class shares many of the pharmacologic actions and adverse effects of the sulfonylureas. In lowering blood glucose levels, repaglinide has a mechanism of action much like that of the sulfonylureas. Similar to glyburide, it stimulates the secretion of insulin from the pancreatic beta cells by binding to the beta cell sites. In contrast to the sulfonylureas, this agent is absorbed rapidly and undergoes minimal renal excretion, making it suitable for elderly patients or others with decreased kidney function. Peak action occurs within 1 hour of ingestion; the drug is metabolized completely in 3 to 4 hours. Administered orally before each meal, repaglinide is effective in lowering postprandial glucose levels, as the amount of insulin released from the pancreas increases during and just after a meal, mimicking the normal blood glucose response to eating. Because of its rapid elimination in contrast to the sulfonylureas, repaglinide does not cause the beta cells to continuously release insulin for long periods of time. Therefore, insulin levels return to normal before the next meal. The number of meals eaten is equivalent to the number of doses taken; for example, if a meal is missed, the corresponding dose of medication also is skipped. Conversely, a dose is added when an extra meal or large snack is taken. Weight gain (up to three kg in three months) occurred more frequently from repaglinide compared to metformin. (see below for discussion of metformin) (Black, Donnelly, McIntyre et al. 2007)

Nateglinide

Nateglinide (Starlix) is a meglitinide that may be used alone or in combination therapy with metformin. It lowers blood glucose by stimulating insulin secretion from the pancreas within 20 minutes following oral administration; the extent of pancreatic insulin release is glucose dependent and diminishes at low glucose levels. Used before meals, it causes a rapid rise in plasma insulin, with peak levels occurring within 1 hour and a fall to baseline by 4 hours. Nateglinide is metabolized predominantly by the CYP450 system and is rapidly and completely eliminated renally. Nateglinide is a category C drug and is contraindicated in pregnancy and lactation. It should be used with caution in chronic hepatic disease, and its safety and efficacy in children is not established. Although hypoglycemia occurs infrequently, it is the most common adverse reaction. Drug interactions that potentiate the hypoglycemic effect of nateglinide include nonsteroidal anti-inflammatory drugs, salicylates, and nonselective beta-adrenergic blockers. Drug interactions that reduce the hypoglycemic effect of nateglinide include thiazides, corticosteroids, thyroid products,

and sympathomimetics. Like repaglinide, weight gain (up to three kg in three months) occurred more frequently from nateglinide compared to metformin. (see below for discussion of metformin) (Black, Donnelly, McIntyre et al. 2007)

• NONSULFONYLUREAS

The nonsulfonylurea antidiabetics comprise three different classes grouped by their chemical structure: biguanides, thiazolidinediones, and alpha-glucosidase inhibitors. However, more commonly, these drugs are considered by their mode of action, which is either improving insulin action or delaying the digestion of carbohydrates; thus, the terms *antiglycemic* or *antihyperglycemic* may also be used. Metformin (Fortamet, Glucophage), a biguanide, works by improving insulin action and is the prototype drug.

Nursing Management of the Patient Receiving P Metformin

Core Drug Knowledge

Pharmacotherapeutics

Metformin is used as an adjunct to diet and exercise to lower blood glucose in type 2 diabetes (see Table 49.2) and is usually the drug of first choice to use in type 2 diabetes. Metformin is not a hypoglycemic agent because it does not stimulate insulin secretion; rather, it is an antihyperglycemic or "insulin sensitizer" agent. Metformin works by suppressing hepatic glucose production (reducing glyconeogenolysis) while enhancing insulin sensitivity in adipose and skeletal muscle tissue, increasing glucose uptake into those cells. As a result, insulin resistance is lessened. Metformin is ineffective if patients are without some residual functioning pancreatic islet cells.

In addition, metformin lowers triglyceride levels and total and low-density lipoprotein (LDL) cholesterol levels, and it promotes weight loss. Metformin may be used with a sulfonylurea or with insulin to control glucose levels in type 2 diabetes. When it is necessary to give insulin as well as an oral antihyperglycemic, metformin combined with insulin appears to be the best regimen for most patients with type 2 diabetes because this combination has resulted in fewer hypoglycemic episodes, lower insulin doses, and less weight gain than other combinations of sulfonylureas and insulin.

Pharmacokinetics

Administered in oral tablet form, metformin is absorbed slowly but incompletely from the GI tract; this incomplete absorption results in a bioavailability of only 50% to 60%. Food slightly delays and decreases the extent of its absorption. The absorbed drug is distributed rapidly into peripheral body tissues and fluids, and peak serum levels are achieved in 2 to 3 hours after administration. Metformin does not bind to plasma proteins and does not undergo hepatic metabolism. Metformin is excreted mostly unchanged by the kidneys; 90% of the absorbed drug is eliminated renally within the first 24 hours, with a plasma elimination half-life of 6.2 hours. Half-life is longer in patients with impaired renal function.

Pharmacodynamics

Metformin decreases hepatic glucose production, decreases intestinal absorption of glucose, and improves insulin sensitivity by increasing peripheral glucose uptake and use in skeletal muscle and adipose tissue through increased transport of glucose across the cell membrane.

Unlike the sulfonylureas, metformin rarely causes hypoglycemia when used alone because it does not stimulate insulin secretion. In fact, insulin secretion remains unchanged, whereas fasting insulin levels and day-long plasma insulin response may actually decrease. In addition, metformin lowers triglyceride levels and promotes weight loss. Metformin lowers fasting and postprandial hyperglycemia. Full therapeutic effect from a given dose takes up to 2 weeks to occur; thus, when the dose is being titrated upward, increases should occur no more frequently than every 1 to 2 weeks.

Contraindications and Precautions

Metformin is contraindicated in patients with hepatic disease, alcoholism, acute or chronic metabolic acidosis, chronic heart failure, clinical situations that predispose to hypoxemia, and renal impairment (creatinine clearance, less than 40 mL/min) because these conditions may predispose the patient to lactic acidosis. This risk of lactic acidosis is highlighted in a Black Box warning for metformin.

Metformin is a pregnancy category B drug.

Adverse Effects

Minor but common side effects of metformin include GI disturbances such as anorexia, nausea and vomiting, weight loss, abdominal discomfort, dyspepsia, flatulence, diarrhea, and a metallic taste sensation. These adverse effects tend to decline with continued use and can be minimized by initiating therapy with lower doses of metformin. Hypoglycemia can occur if metformin is combined with a sulfonylurea drug or with insulin.

Serious adverse effects are rare and usually occur in individuals with impaired renal or hepatic function. Lactic acidosis is listed in the drug label information as a very rare serious, potentially lethal adverse effect. Lactic acidosis is a metabolic complication characterized by an increased anion gap, elevated blood lactate levels, decreased blood pH, and electrolyte disturbances. The onset of lactic acidosis is often subtle and presents with nonspecific symptoms such as malaise, myalgias, respiratory distress, increasing somnolence, and nonspecific abdominal distress Hypothermia, hypotension, and bradyarrhythmias may be present with more marked acidosis. However, despite its black box warning, a recent "review from all known comparative and observational studies lasting at least one month found no cases of fatal or nonfatal lactic acidosis in 70,490 patient-years of metformin use, Average lactate levels measured during metformin treatment were no different than for placebo or for other medications used to treat diabetes" (Salpeter, Greyber, Pastemak, et al., 2010). It appears that the cases of lactic acidosis noted during original drug trials were related to normal occurrence of this condition in the general population and not secondary to the drug itself. Other rare, serious adverse effects associated with metformin include blood dyscrasias such as aplastic anemia, agranulocytosis, and thrombocytopenia.

Drug Interactions

Metformin, which improves insulin use, interacts synergistically with the sulfonylureas, which stimulate insulin production. This interaction causes hypoglycemic adverse effects. Metformin may react with contrast media used for radiographic procedures. Table 49.6 lists drugs that interact with metformin.

Assessment of Relevant Core Patient Variables

Health Status

Assessments to be made before therapy with metformin are similar to those necessary with insulin. Assess current health status, including diet, activity, medication, any adverse effects from medications, and methods used for monitoring blood glucose. Ensure that the patient receiving metformin has periodic renal and hepatic function tests. Metformin's half-life is prolonged and its excretion is decreased in patients with impaired renal function, especially those with decreased creatinine clearance. Impaired hepatic function

TABLE 49.6 Agents That Interact with P Metformin

Interactants	Effect and Significance	Nursing Management
cimetidine	Increased risk for hypoglycemia	Monitor blood glucose levels.
sulfonylureas	Synergistic reaction between metformin and sulfonylurea that improves insulin use; may increase risk for hypoglycemia	Monitor blood glucose levels. Observe for hypoglycemic complications.
glucocorticoids, alcohol	Increased risk of lactic acidosis	Monitor serum lactate levels.

may increase the risk of lactic acidosis. Also, ensure that the patient has periodic blood tests, because blood dyscrasias are rare but possible. Assess the patient's weight during therapy, because weight loss—a beneficial side effect for overweight patients with type 2 diabetes—may occur. Monitor lipid levels because metformin decreases LDL cholesterol; again, this result is usually a positive effect for the patient with diabetes.

Life Span and Gender

Assess whether the patient is pregnant or breast-feeding. Metformin is in pregnancy category B. Animal studies demonstrate metformin excretion into breast milk, but studies in lactating women have not been performed. It is important to determine the age of the patient before administering metformin. Safety and efficacy in children have not been established. Age-related changes in renal function account for altered pharmacokinetics; metformin should be used cautiously in elderly patients because of the prevalence of decreased renal function in this age group. In general, elderly patients are better able to tolerate lower doses of metformin.

Lifestyle, Diet, and Habits

Ask patients about their typical diet and exercise habits and about alcohol intake. Hypoglycemia is more common when metformin is administered concomitantly with other oral hypoglycemic agents, if caloric intake is deficient, or if the patient exercises strenuously. Caution patients against excessive alcohol intake while taking metformin because alcohol use increases the risk of lactic acidosis. Concurrent use with chromium, garlic, gymnema, or alcohol may increase the risk for hypoglycemia.

Environment

Note the environment in which metformin will be administered. Metformin is an oral drug that is easily self-administered in the home setting.

Culture and Inherited Traits

In controlled clinical studies of metformin in individuals with type 2 diabetes, the antihyperglycemic effect was comparable among whites, African Americans, and Hispanics.

Nursing Diagnosis and Outcome

• Risk for Imbalanced Nutrition: Less than Body Requirements, related to anorexia secondary to adverse GI effects of weight loss, diarrhea, and anorexia from metformin

Desired outcome: *The patient will ingest daily nutritional requirements in accordance with activity level and metabolic needs and relate the importance of good nutrition.*

Planning and Intervention

Maximizing Therapeutic Effects

Administer metformin twice a day, with the morning and evening meals. The dosage is individualized on the basis of both effectiveness and tolerance. FPG and hemoglobin A_{1C} (**glycosylated hemoglobin**) are used to identify the minimum effective dose of metformin, when used either as monotherapy or in combination with a sulfonylurea or insulin. Adherence with the recommended diabetic diet and daily exercise help in the control of type 2 diabetes, when used in conjuncture with metformin.

Metformin is frequently prescribed with other oral antidiabetic drugs, especially a sulfonureas drug. When patients have difficulty achieving control on oral medication, an insulin can be added to the drug thereapy. Recent research that examined the A1C level of patients who received metformin and a sulfonureas drug and one of three insulin regimens: aspart twice a day, aspart with each meal, or basal detemir once or twice a day. Patients who received either the prandial (mealtime) dose with aspart or the basal dose of detemir were more likely to achieve an A1C level of 6.5% or less than those who received aspart twice a day. Using basal dosing of detemir created fewer hypoglycemic episodes and allowed for less weight gain than the other methods (Holman, Farmer, Davies, et al for the 4-T study group, 2009).

Minimizing Adverse Effects

Adverse GI effects during initiation of metformin therapy appear to be dose related. Taking the drug at mealtimes and using gradual dosage increments minimize these effects. Because it is excreted renally, metformin should be withheld temporarily when patients undergo any procedure using iodinated contrast dye, which is also excreted renally. Lower doses are usually indicated in older adults to prevent adverse effects. If the patient is having any surgical procedure (except for minor procedures), metformin should be temporarily withheld until oral intake has resumed and renal function has returned to normal.

Providing Patient and Family Education

• Teach patients to take metformin with meals, morning and evening.
• Emphasize that patients should not use alcohol while taking metformin.
• Advise patients not to take any OTC preparations, including dietary and herbal supplements, without first consulting the prescriber.
• For general teaching, see Box 49.4.

Ongoing Assessment and Evaluation

Monitor blood glucose levels (fasting and hemoglobin A_{1C}) throughout metformin therapy. Periodic screening for hematologic changes is recommended during therapy because blood dyscrasias may occur. Metformin therapy is effective when glucose levels are controlled and the patient does not experience any important adverse effects (see also the "Ongoing Assessment and Evaluation" section in the "Insulin" discussion).

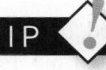

Drugs Closely Related to P Metformin

Drugs closely related to metformin are the thiazolidinediones, including rosiglitazone and pioglitazone. These drugs also enhance the effectiveness of insulin.

C Thiazolidinediones: Rosiglitazone and Pioglitazone

The pharmacodynamic actions of the thiazolidinedione oral antihyperglycemic drugs are similar to those of the biguanides; they are antihyperglycemics and "insulin sensitizers." Thiazolidinedione antidiabetic drugs include rosiglitazone (Avandia) and pioglitazone (Actos). Rosiglitazone and pioglitazone are both indicated as an adjunct to diet and exercise to lower blood glucose in patients with type 2 diabetes. They are prescribed in combination with a sulfonylurea, metformin, or insulin when adequate glycemic control is not achieved."Although these drugs are quite effective in helping to maintain normal blood glucose levels, the class of drugs has been dogged, almost since first brought to market, with concerns that they may create serious adverse effects. The first drug in this class troglitazone was taken off the market in March 2000 after it was found in post-marketing use to cause acute liver failure"(Aschenbrenner, 2011). Thiazolidinedione drugs cause weight gain.Weight gain is important to note, because this adverse effect differentiates this class from metformin, which causes weight loss. Both drugs are absorbed rapidly after oral administration.

Rosiglitazone

Rosiglitazone, while an effective antidiabetic drug, now has limitations as to its use. The restrictions limit the initiation of rosiglitazone to second line therapy for those who have not been able to achieve glycemic control from other antidiabetic drugs and in whom the drug appears to be a medical necessity. Patients who were prescribed rosigllitazone prior to the label changes in 2011 may also continue to receive the drug, if they choose. All patients must receive documented education concerning potential risks from the therapy (Aschenbrenner, 2011).

The restrictions are based on meta-analysis of clinical trials that indicate rosiglitazone may potentially increase the risk of myocardial infarction and other cardiovascular events. Unfortunately, these clinical trials were never designed to assess cardiovascular risk, so this makes it difficult to accurately draw conclusions about the findings from these trials. Other clinical trials did not find that there was an increased risk of myocardial infarction from rosiglitazone. Uncontrolled diabetes is in itself a risk factor for cardiovascular disease and this complicates the interpretation of some of the clinical trial findings. More research must be done to determine conclusively what effects rosiglitazone have on the cardiovascular system. (Aschenbrenner, 2011).

One large multicentered clinical trial that examined the risks of rosiglitazone was the RECORD trial (Rosiglitazone Evaluated for Cardiac Outcomes and Regulation of Glycaemia in Diabetes) RECORD examined the effect of adding rosiglitazone to oral monotherapy with either metformin or a sufuonureas drug compared to receiving combination therapy with metformin and a sulfonureas This trial found that the addition of rosiglitazone increases the risk of heart failure (most likely due to the increase in fluid retention) as well as increasing the risk of upper and distal lower limb fractures, mostly in women. Rosiglitazone's effect on myocardial infarction is inconclusive from this study, although cardiovascular morbidity or mortality from all sources did not increase (Home, Pocock, Beck-Nielsen, et al., for RECORD study team, 2009). The findings from this trial contributed to the FDA's decision to include a black box warning stating that rosiglitazone may increase the risk of congestive heart failure, most likely from fluid retention, and that it may increase the risk of myocardial infarction.

Rosiglitazone is highly protein bound and undergoes hepatic metabolism through the P-450 system. Rosiglitazone is metabolized by P-450 2C8 and 2C9. These are not major pathways for most other drugs; therefore, drug interactions are minimal. Rosiglitazone is excreted in the urine and feces. The elimination half-life of rosiglitazone is much shorter than the half-life of pioglitazone (3 to 4 hours, compared with 16 to 24 hours).

Rosiglitazone should not be given to patients with symptomatic heart failure(based on the black box warning) or those with active liver disease or increased serum transaminase or aminotransferase levels (ALT or AST more than 2.5 times the upper limits of normal) (based on the earliest drug in this class increasing the risk of hepatic failure). Patients treated with these drugs should undergo periodic monitoring of liver enzymes. Hepatic enzymes should be measured before therapy begins. In patients with normal baseline liver enzymes, liver enzymes should be monitored every 2 months for the first 12 months and periodically thereafter. Rosiglitazone therapy is generally well tolerated despite its black box warnings; the few adverse effects include fluid retention (while it may be significant enough to exacerbate CHF or to induce it in susceptible individuals, generally it is a minor effect), headache, and weight gain (likely from fluid retention). Plasma volume expansion may occur with rosiglitazone therapy. As a result, small decreases in hemoglobin, hematocrit, and neutrophil counts (within the normal range) have occurred

Triglyceride levels can significantly increase with rosiglitazone therapy. HDLand LDL cholesterol will also increase from baseline levels.

The assessment of current health status for rosiglitazone is the same as for metformin. Particular attention to hepatic function blood tests is needed because of the risk of hepatotoxicity. It is necessary to emphasize the importance of follow-up blood work and to teach patients to report signs of early liver impairment (e.g., nausea, vomiting, malaise, and dark urine). Premenopausal, anovulatory women with diabetes taking rosiglitazone are at risk for resuming ovulation with drug therapy and so are at risk for pregnancy. Female patients should be counseled to consider an alternative method of contraception or be referred to their prescribers to discuss a dosage increase in the oral contraceptive. Rosiglitazone is a pregnancy category C drug.

Pioglitazone

Pioglitazone is very similar in action to rosiglitazone. At this time there is still unrestricted access to prescribing pioglitazone, unlike for rosiglitazone. The decision to allow unrestricted access to the other drug in the same class, pioglitazone, is considered controversial even among FDA officials and should not be construed by providers that pioglitazone is without risk. Rosiglitazone and pioglitazone have never been tested head to head in a clinical trial comparing cardiovascular risk from each drug. The FDA's decision to encourage the use of pioglitazone before the use of rosiglitazone was based on data that some scientists believe is without strong scientific basis (Parks, 2010).

Like rosiglitazone, however, pioglitazone carries a black box warning that it may cause congestive heart failure from fluid retention.

Like rosiglitazone, pioglitazone is highly protein bound and undergoes hepatic metabolism through the P-450 system, although they are metabolized by different isoenzymes. Pioglitazone is metabolized hepatically by P-450 2C8 and 3A4. Isoenzyme 3A4 is an important pathway for metabolism of some drugs; therefore, drug interactions can occur. Drugs that are metabolized by CYP3A4, such as erythromycin, calcium channel blockers, cortical steroids, cyclosporine, the statins, tacrolimus, triazolam, and trimetrexate, may have their metabolism impaired by pioglitazone, and caution should be used. Drugs that inhibit CYP3A4, such as ketoconazole, appear to increase the metabolism of pioglitazone. Additionally,

pioglitazone is metabolized by the P-450 isoenzyme 1A1 via extrahepatic pathways. Like rosiglitazone,pioglitazone is excreted in the urine and feces. The elimination half-life of pioglitazone is much longer than that for rosiglitazone (16 to 24 hours compared with 3 to 4 hours).

Like rosiglitazone, pioglitazone should not be given to patients with symptomatic heart failure or those with active liver disease or increased serum transaminase or aminotransferase levels (ALT or AST more than 2.5 times the upper limits of normal). Monitoring for liver adverse effects is identical. Pioglitazone therapy has the same adverse effects as rosiglitazone, except pioglitazone may cause its own unique adverse effects as animal and human research indicates that it may increase the risk of bladder cancer.

Pioglitazone will also alter lipid levels. Triglyceride levels were significantly decreased with pioglitazone therapy and (while significantly increased with rosiglitazone therapy). Although both these drugs increase HDL cholesterol, pioglitazone provides significantly greater increases from the baseline. Both pioglitazone and rosiglitazone also increase LDL cholesterol, but mean changes from baseline are significantly less with pioglitazone.

The assessment of current health status for rosiglitazone and pioglitazone is the same as for metformin. Hepatic function needs to be assessed and monitored for pioglitazone as done for rosiglitazone. Similarly to those taking rosiglitazonen, premenopausal, anovulatory women with diabetes taking pioglitazone are at risk for resuming ovulation with drug therapy and so are at risk for pregnancy. Female patients should be counseled to consider an alternative method of contraception or be referred to their prescribers to discuss a dosage increase in the oral contraceptive. Pioglitazone is a pregnancy category C drug. Pioglitazone has been found to increase a woman's risk of fractures in distal upper limbs (forearm, hand, and wrist) or distal lower limbs (foot, ankle, fibula, and tibia) (Food and Drug Administration MedWatch, 2007). It is necessary to assess the risk of fracture when initiating therapy with pioglitazone in women, as well as the risk of falls, which may increase the risk of fractures.

Drugs Significantly Different From P Metformin

C Alpha-Glucosidase Inhibitors: Acarbose and Miglitol

Alpha-glucosidase inhibitors provide yet a different mechanism of action for patients with type 2 diabetes. These medications do not enhance insulin secretion, nor are they insulin sensitizers like metformin. Rather, the antihyperglycemic activity results from a substantial reduction in postprandial glucose levels. Alpha-glucosidase inhibitors slow down enzymes needed to digest carbohydrates; specifically, they inhibit alpha-glucosidase enzymes in the brush border of the small intestine and inhibit pancreatic alpha-amylase. Pancreatic alpha-amylase hydrolyzes complex starches to oligosaccharides in the lumen of the small intestine, whereas the membrane-bound intestinal alpha-glucosidases hydrolyze oligosaccharides, trisaccharides, and disaccharides to glucose and other monosaccharides in the small intestine. Inhibition of these enzyme systems reduces the rate of digestion of complex carbohydrate. Less glucose is absorbed because the carbohydrates are not broken down into glucose molecules. In patients with diabetes, the short-term effect of these drug therapies is to decrease current blood glucose levels; the long-term effect is a small reduction in the hemoglobin A_{1C} level. Alpha-glucosidase inhibitors are an ideal alternative therapy for patients with type 2 diabetes who have mild to moderate hyperglycemia and who are at risk for hypoglycemia or lactic acidosis (see Table 49.2).

Acarbose (Precose) and miglitol (Glyset), two alpha-glucosidase inhibitors, effectively lower postprandial serum glucose when administered alone or in combination with insulin, metformin, or a sulfonylurea. Both these drugs should be administered orally with the first bite of food. The drugs differ in their metabolism and excretion. Acarbose undergoes exclusive metabolism within the GI tract—principally by intestinal bacteria but also by digestive enzymes. An active metabolite is created that produces the therapeutic effects of acarbose. Little of the active metabolite is absorbed; only about 35% of the dose is converted and then absorbed. Miglitol, on the other hand, does not undergo any metabolism, so the therapeutic effect comes directly from the drug. The elimination half-life of acarbose and miglitol is about 2 hours. Acarbose is eliminated through the kidneys and the GI tract, whereas miglitol is eliminated unchanged by renal excretion.

Acarbose and miglitol are contraindicated in patients with diseases of the bowel (e.g., inflammatory bowel disease, absorptive disorders, colonic ulceration, and history of bowel obstruction). They should be used cautiously in patients with hiatal hernia or other conditions that might be exacerbated by increased formation of gas, which is an adverse effect of acarbose. The drugs are also contraindicated in patients with chronic liver diseases and substantial renal impairment (serum creatinine, greater than 2 mg/dL). Acarbose and miglitol are in pregnancy category B. They are excreted into breast milk and should not be given to lactating women.

Adverse effects of acarbose and miglitol are primarily GI in nature and include flatulence, diarrhea, and abdominal distention. These effects occur because the delay in carbohydrate absorption increases fermentation and formation of intestinal gases.

Assessments to be made before starting therapy with the alpha-glucosidase inhibitors are similar to those necessary with insulin. In addition, 1-hour postprandial blood glucose and serum transaminase levels should be obtained as baseline data. It is necessary to stress the importance of notifying the health care team if unusual fatigue or muscle pain, difficulty breathing, GI distress, dizziness, light-headedness, or irregular heartbeat occurs, because these symptoms may indicate the onset of lactic acidosis, which is often insidious. Initial education of the patient should involve telling him or her that acarbose and miglitol inhibit the absorption of regular cane

sugar (such as in candy or orange juice). The most important difference between these drugs and insulin or metformin therapy is that if a hypoglycemic reaction occurs, *the patient must not use cane or table sugar products because the sugar will not be absorbed.* It should be emphasized that he or she should use oral glucose tablets instead to increase blood glucose levels. (See Box 49.4.)

C Dipeptidyl Peptidase-4 Inhibitor

Sitagliptin (Januvia) and saxagliptin (Onglyza) are antidiabetic drugs that works in a unique way to lower blood glucose in type 2 diabetes. Saxagliptin is more potent, but not more effective. Both sitagliptin and saxagliptin are dipeptidyl peptidase-4 (DPP-4) enzyme inhibitors, which work by protecting the endogenous incretin hormones and enhancing their actions. Incretin hormones (glucose-dependent insulinotropic polypeptide and glucagon-like peptide-1) are released in response to glucose elevations that occur after a meal to maintain normal levels of glucose. These incretin hormones increase insulin synthesis and its release from pancreatic beta cells by intracellular signaling pathways. Glucagon-like peptide-1 also lowers glucagon secretion from the pancreas, thus reducing hepatic glucose production. However, incretin hormones are metabolized rapidly by the special enzyme DPP-4, leading to a decrease of insulin production and an increase in glucagons levels. As the result of sitagliptin's and saxagliptin's inhibition of the breakdown of incretin hormones by DPP-4, incretin hormone activity is more pronounced; therefore, insulin release continues and glucagon levels decrease. Both of these factors result in lower blood glucose levels. Incretin hormones function only when the blood glucose level is high. Because of this, sitagliptin and saxagliptin only rarely cause hypoglycemia if they are used in monotherapy.

The most common adverse effects are central nervous system (CNS)–related (headache), GI (abdominal pain, diarrhea, nausea), and respiratory (nasopharyngitis, upper respiratory infections). Saxagliptin may also cause peripheral edema and urinary tract infections. Infections from all causes increase significantly with sitagliptin for an unknown reason. No long term data regarding the drug's effect on the immune function is currently available (Richter, Bandeira-Echtler, Bergerhoff, et al. 2008). Both drugs are pregnancy category B drugs.

The only known drug interaction with sitagliptin is with digoxin. Coadministration increases digoxin levels, but no dose adjustment is recommended. However, the patient should be monitored for any adverse effects from this combination. It is unknown what effect sitagliptin will have on cardiovascular disease in diabetics (Richter, Bandeira-Echtler, Bergerhoff, et al. 2008).

Saxagliptin has a drug interaction with the following drugs: atazanavir, clarithromycin, indinavir, itraconazole, ketoconazole, nefazodone, nelfinavir, ritonavir, saquinavir, and telithromycin. All of these drugs will increase the circulating level of saxagliptin.

C Incretin Mimetic

Exenatide (Byetta) is a synthetic incretin mimetic. By mimicking the actions of incretin hormones, the drug decreases blood glucose levels, helping them to return to normal. Exenatide works at the glucagon-like peptide-1 receptors and produces effects similar to glucagon-like peptide-1. However, all observed pharmacodynamic effects of exenatide have not been consistent with those of glucagon-like peptide-1, suggesting that the drug may also produce some actions via functionally different receptors not yet identified. Actions of exenatide include enhancement of insulin secretion in the presence of glucose, decrease in glucagon secretion, slowing of gastric emptying, reduction of food intake, promotion of beta-cell proliferation and neogenesis, reduction in adiposity, and insulin-sensitizing effects (this was seen only in animal models; natural exendin-4 was first isolated from the saliva of *Heloderma suspectum* [Gila monster]). Exenatide is a gene product that is distinct from glucagon-like peptide-1. Although it shares more than half of the amino acid sequence with that found in mammalian glucagon-like peptide-1, exenatide is not an analogue of, or a modified form of, glucagon-like peptide-1. Unlike endogenous glucagon-like peptide-1, exenatide is relatively resistant to degradation by dipeptidyl peptidase-4; thus it has a longer half-life.

Exenatide is used as an adjunct in treating patients with type 2 diabetes (i.e., those who are taking metformin, a sulfonylurea, a thiazolidinedione, a combination of metformin and a sulfonylurea, or a combination of metformin and a thiazolidinedione but have not achieved adequate glycemic control). It reduces hemoglobin A_{1C}, fasting plasma glucose, and body weight. Weight loss is probably related to slower gastric emptying.

Exenatide is administered by subcutaneous injection up to one hour before breakfast and dinner. It should always be given before a meal, not afterward. The dose does not need to be adjusted based on size of meal or amount of exercise. Because weight loss is expected from exenatide therapy, the dose should not be decreased based on weight. Exenatide is not an insulin and must not be confused with an insulin, although it is administered subcutaneously. The drug comes in a special prefilled injection "pen," and the lancets must be purchased separately. Until the injection pen is used for the first time, it should be kept refrigerated; after first use, it may be kept at room temperature.

Hypoglycemia can occur, especially if exenatide is given in combination with a sulfonylurea drug. Other common adverse effects are GI (diarrhea, indigestion, nausea, vomiting); immunologic (antibody development); and neurologic (dizziness, headache, nervousness). Serious adverse effects are rare but include anaphylaxis; pancreatitis; and acute renal failure, which may be related to dehydration from severe vomiting and diarrhea. Acute renal failure is reversible with appropriate treatment. Exenatide is a pregnancy category C drug. Because exenatide slows gastric emptying, drugs that require absorption at a certain rate in order to achieve a therapeutic level may be effected by exenatide use. For this reason,

if the patient is taking birth control pills or antibiotics, he or she should be taught to take these medications at least one hour before taking exenatide. Exenatide may also slow the absorption of acetaminophen, so this drug should also be taken 1 hour prior to exenatide. Exenatide, when coadministered with lovastatin, an antihyperlipidemic, may decrease lovastatin's bioavailability and possibly decrease the lipid-lowering ability of lovastatin. Lipid serum levels should be monitored, and the dose should be adjusted if necessary.

C Amylin Analogue

Pramlintide (Symlin) is an antihyperglycemic used as an adjunct in the treatment of type 1 and type 2 diabetes when glucose levels cannot be controlled by insulin therapy. It is an analogue of endogenous amylin and sometimes is classified as an amylinomimetic. Endogenous amylin is secreted, like insulin, from the pancreatic beta cells in response to food intake. Amylin affects the rise of postprandial glucose levels by slowing gastric emptying without altering overall absorption of nutrients. Amylin also suppresses glucagon secretion so that the liver does not release glucose. Amylin has an additional role in suppressing feelings of hunger. Amylin, similar to insulin, is absent or deficient in patients with diabetes. Like endogenous amylin, pramlintide delays gastric emptying, prevents a postprandial rise in plasma glucagon, and promotes feelings of satiety so that the patient eats less. Pramlintide is *not* an insulin, but like the prototype metformin, it is used as a supplement to insulin therapy. Unlike the prototype metformin, it is administered subcutaneously immediately before meals. Pramlintide should be administered using an insulin syringe, but it should never be mixed in the same syringe as insulin. The abdomen or the thighs are the preferred injection sites because absorption is erratic in the arms.

An adverse effect of pramlintide is hypoglycemia; this appears to be a drug interaction with any insulin the patient is receiving. Pramlintide carries a Black Box warning that hypoglycemia can occur. When hypoglycemia is significant it will occur within 3 hours after administration of pramlintide. Because of this risk, any dose of a short-acting insulin also administered before a meal should be decreased by 50% initially when beginning pramlintide therapy.

GI complaints, including nausea, vomiting, anorexia, and abdominal pain, are also fairly common adverse effects of pramlintide. Because of these adverse effects, patients who require drugs that stimulate gastrointestinal motility should *not* be considered for pramlintide therapy. Central nervous system adverse effects include headache, dizziness, and fatigue. Allergic reactions are also possible. Pramlintide is a pregnancy category C drug.

Effectiveness of pramlintide therapy is assessed by control of daily blood glucose levels and improved hemoglobin A_{1C} values.

Antidiabetic Combination Agents: Glucovance and Metaglip

Glucovance and Metaglip are both combination antidiabetic agents consisting of a sulfonylurea and a biguanide. Glucovance is a combination of glyburide and metformin, and Metaglip is a combination of glipizide and metformin. Both are indicated as an adjunct to diet and exercise to improve glycemic control. They are also indicated as a second-line therapy when initial treatment with a sulfonylurea or metformin does not result in adequate glycemic control in type 2 diabetes. For patients taking Glucovance who require additional therapy, a thiazolidinedione can be added. Both medications are administered once or twice daily with meals to avoid hypoglycemia (largely because of glyburide or glipizide) and to reduce GI side effects (largely because of metformin). These agents are not recommended for use during pregnancy or in children. Careful consideration is needed in the elderly population and those with renal function impairment. One of the advantages of a combined drug is that it helps to promote adherence to drug therapy because the patient has to take fewer pills daily. For other information, please refer to the individual prototype drugs (see Table 49.2).

Ⓒ GLUCOSE-ELEVATING AGENTS

Glucagon is a hyperglycemic polypeptide hormone produced by the alpha cells of the pancreatic islets of Langerhans. Its physiologic effect is generally the opposite of that of insulin. Glucagon is the body's first line of defense against hypoglycemia. Whether endogenous or exogenous, it reduces the effectiveness of insulin and some commonly used drugs.

The main stimulus to glucagon secretion is a decrease in intracellular glucose concentrations that usually occurs as a result of a drop in serum blood sugar. Patients with diabetes have been shown to have high levels of glucagon, although the cause-and-effect relationship is uncertain. Theoretically, glucagon imbalances could contribute to many of the diabetic patient's problems with glucose metabolism.

Nursing Management of the Patient Receiving Ⓟ Glucagon
Core Drug Knowledge
Pharmacotherapeutics
Most commonly, glucagon (GlucaGen) is used in unconscious patients with diabetes to reverse the severe hypoglycemia resulting from insulin overdosage. Glucagon is effective in hypoglycemia only if liver glycogen is available. It is administered by the intramuscular (IM), IV, or SC route. Glucagon also is used to induce intestinal relaxation before radiographic examinations. Off-label uses for glucagon include treatment for propranolol (beta-adrenergic antagonist) overdose and cardiovascular emergencies.

Pharmacokinetics
Glucagon has a plasma half-life of 3 to 10 minutes (see Table 49.2). The hormone undergoes hepatic metabolism and is excreted in urine and bile.

Pharmacodynamics
Glucagon increases blood glucose levels by stimulating glycogenolysis in the peripheral tissues, exerts a positive inotropic and chronotropic effect on the heart (increasing heart

contraction and heart rate, respectively) by increasing cyclic adenosine monophosphate, and relaxes the GI smooth muscle. After parenteral injection of glucagon, the maximum hyperglycemic effect occurs within 30 minutes. The duration of action is about 1 to 2 hours. GI smooth muscle relaxation occurs within 15 minutes and lasts for approximately 30 minutes. The mechanism by which glucagon relaxes GI smooth muscle is not known.

Contraindications and Precautions
A hypersensitivity to glucagon contraindicates its use. Glucagon causes insulin release and is contraindicated in cases of insulinoma (also known as hyperinsulinism) related to a tumor of the functional islet cells. It causes catecholamine release and is contraindicated in pheochromocytoma. Glucagon is a pregnancy category B drug. It should be used cautiously in pregnancy and lactation.

Adverse Effects
Glucagon may cause hypotension, respiratory distress, nausea and vomiting, hypersensitivity reactions of urticaria, and hypokalemia in overdosage.

Drug Interactions
Glucagon increases the hypoprothrombinemic effect of oral anticoagulants and may cause bleeding. The interaction appears to be dose related.

Assessment of Relevant Core Patient Variables
Health Status
Assess the patient's blood sugar levels and level of consciousness. After emergency use of glucagon, assess the patient's level of adherence to the therapeutic regimen and the patient's level of understanding of the disease and its treatment.

Life Span and Gender
Note whether the patient is pregnant or breast-feeding. Glucagon, a pregnancy category B drug, crosses the placental barrier and enters breast milk. However, emergency use overshadows concerns regarding breast-feeding.

Lifestyle, Diet, and Habits
Review the patient's adherence to the diabetic treatment plan. It is important to assess whether the patient is administering the insulin and monitoring blood glucose correctly, and whether he or she is adhering to the prescribed dietary and exercise regimens. Adherence to the treatment plan helps prevent episodes of hypoglycemia.

Environment
Be aware of the environment in which glucagon will be administered. Glucagon is usually administered as an emergency treatment. Although it most frequently is administered in an acute care setting, it may be administered in extended care settings or in the home. Home use is limited to patients at high risk for experiencing severe hypoglycemia when a family member or caregiver can be taught how to assess for hypoglycemia and administer the drug.

Nursing Diagnosis and Outcome

- **Risk for Injury** related to hypotension from the adverse effects of glucagons
  Desired outcome: *Substantial hypotension will not result from glucagon treatment.*

Planning and Intervention

Maximizing Therapeutic Effects

Glucagon is dispensed in a powder form and must be reconstituted to a concentration of 1 mg/mL using the diluent supplied by the manufacturer. Use reconstituted glucagon immediately, although refrigerated solution may be kept for 48 hours. If the solution is not clear after dilution, discard it. A dose of 0.5 to 1.0 mg is usually effective. Reconstitute doses exceeding 2 mg with sterile water and use them immediately. Administer an additional dose if the patient's response is inadequate or incomplete after 20 minutes.

Minimizing Adverse Effects

Administer supplemental carbohydrates as soon as possible once consciousness has been achieved to restore liver glycogen and prevent secondary hypoglycemia.

Providing Patient and Family Education

- Emphasize to patients and family members measures to prevent hypoglycemic reactions from insulin (reasonable uniformity from day to day with regard to diet, insulin, and exercise; routine blood glucose self-monitoring; and carrying sugar, candy, or other readily absorbable carbohydrate so that it may be taken at the first warning of hypoglycemia).
- Teach family members the importance of quick intervention if severe hypoglycemia occurs, to prevent CNS damage.
- Instruct family members in the proper technique for emergency administration of glucagon, if appropriate.

Ongoing Assessment and Evaluation

Blood glucose levels should be monitored before, during, and after glucagon administration, and the patient's emergency supply of glucagon should be restored (if appropriate) as soon as possible. Survival and return to normal function are signs of effective nursing management.

Drugs Significantly Different From P Glucagon

Diazoxide

Administered orally, diazoxide (Proglycem) produces a prompt, dose-related increase in blood glucose levels. Its hyperglycemic effects occur because it inhibits insulin release from the pancreas and has an extrapancreatic effect. Its clinical indications are hyperinsulinism caused by an inoperable islet cell cancer, islet cell hyperplasia, or an extrapancreatic cancer. Diazoxide administered intravenously will quickly lower blood pressure in a hypertensive emergency. See Chapter 28 for a discussion of this use of the drug.

MEMORY CHIP

P Glucagon

- Glucose-elevating agent that accelerates hepatic glyconeogenesis, increasing blood glucose levels
- Major contraindications: insulinoma and pheochromocytoma
- Most common adverse effects: nausea, vomiting, generalized allergic reactions, including urticaria, respiratory distress, and hypotension
- Most serious adverse effect: hypokalemia
- Maximizing therapeutic effects: Use the diluent provided in preparation of glucagons for parenteral injection (SC, IM, or IV). Reconstituted glucagons should be clear, watery, and used immediately. Any unused portion should be discarded. Provide supplemental carbohydrates as soon as possible after drug injection to restore liver glycogen and prevent secondary hypoglycemia.
- Minimizing adverse effects: Teach the patient and family members preparation and administration techniques for glucagons before an emergency arises.
- Most important patient education: Teach the patient and family members measures to prevent hypoglycemic reactions due to insulin; convey importance of early recognition and treatment of hypoglycemic episodes.

Diazoxide is absorbed rapidly. Onset of action occurs within 1 hour. It is highly protein bound (more than 90%), has an 8-hour duration of effect, and has a half-life that ranges from 24 to 36 hours. Diazoxide undergoes hepatic metabolism and renal elimination. Diazoxide is in pregnancy risk category C.

The most common adverse effects from oral dosing are sodium and fluid retention, hyperglycemia, and glycosuria. In some patients, chronic heart failure may develop secondary to sodium and fluid retention.

Other adverse effects can include dizziness and weakness, GI discomfort (e.g., nausea, vomiting, anorexia, abdominal pain, and constipation), and taste alterations.

The usual dosage of diazoxide (adult or child) is 3 to 8 mg/kg/d divided into two or three doses every 8 or 12 hours. Infants and newborns may be given 8 to 15 mg/kg/d every 8 to 12 hours. The total daily dose is divided equally, and administration times also are evenly spaced within the 24-hour day.

Glucose

Glucose, a monosaccharide, is absorbed directly from the intestine, resulting in a rapidly increased blood glucose concentration. It is indicated for managing hypoglycemia. The dosage is 10 to 20 g orally, repeated in 10 minutes if necessary. An occasional adverse effect is nausea. Glucose is not absorbed from the buccal mucosa. It must be swallowed to be effective. It should be used with caution in children younger than 2 years of age. IV glucose (dextrose) is also used to treat hypoglycemia. Solutions with a concentration of 25% dextrose are used in neonates and infants, and solutions of 50% dextrose are used in other age groups.

CHAPTER SUMMARY

- Diabetes is primarily a disorder of carbohydrate metabolism, although it is associated with derangements of protein and fat metabolism and a series of vascular disorders.
- The patient with type 1 diabetes has an absolute insulin deficiency, cannot maintain a normal blood glucose level, and depends on exogenous insulin for survival. Combinations of short- or rapid-acting and longer-acting insulins may be administered to fully manage and control glucose levels. Basal and preprandial doses may be required to control glucose levels. During times of physiologic stress, when glucose levels are elevated (such as after surgery), the patient with diabetes may also require additional correctional doses of short-acting or rapid-acting insulins. Critically ill patients may need to receive an insulin drip to maintain glucose levels as close to normal as possible.
- The patient with type 2 diabetes has a developed insulin resistance. Although insulin is produced, it is not effective in moving glucose into the cells. Oral antidiabetic agents are used to improve glucose control. Occasionally, this patient may also need insulin to achieve glucose balance during times of stress, such as illness, or to achieve maximum control of blood sugar.
- All insulins manage hyperglycemia by promoting cellular glucose uptake and metabolism. Insulins vary in peak, onset, and duration of action; they are similar in absorption, distribution, metabolism, and excretion.
- Hypoglycemia is the most common adverse effect of insulin therapy. Severe hypoglycemia may produce loss of consciousness and is termed insulin shock.
- Regular insulin has a quick onset and peak, and a short duration of therapy. Because of these pharmacokinetic features, it can be used multiple times a day, usually before meals and at bedtime. Regular insulin can be used in addition to long-acting insulin. The dose of regular insulin is often variable and based on the current blood glucose reading. This approach is known as correctional or supplemental dosing (previously referred to as sliding-scale insulin).
- Rapid-acting insulins, lispro, aspart, and glulisine, have a more rapid onset of action than regular insulin. When administered subcutaneously, they are administered closer to the time of a meal than regular insulin. These insulins can also be administered by an insulin pump. When used as prandial doses, they may be administered immediately after a meal if the dose varies, depending on the amount and type of food eaten.
- Intermediate-acting insulins, such as NPH and detemir, have a slower onset with a peak effect occurring later than with regular insulin. Their effects also last longer than those of regular insulin. These longer-acting insulins are normally assigned a standard daily dosage that the patient takes once or twice a day. Intermediate-acting insulins may be used in combination with regular insulin or rapid-acting insulins to meet both the current and long-term glucose levels of the patient. NPH can be mixed in a syringe with other insulins, but detemir cannot be mixed with any other insulin. Intermediate- or long-acting insulins are not administered by the IV route or by SC insulin pumps, or used as correctional-dose insulin. NPH is a suspension, and it is the only insulin that appears cloudy.
- Long-acting glargine does not create the peak and trough in blood insulin levels that NPH does. It has a more flat, sustained effect, which lasts for 24 hours. It is taken subcutaneously once daily at bedtime.
- Combinations of NPH and regular insulins or rapid-acting insulins as well as rapid-acting insulins and protamine are available. The trade names of these products are very similar and may cause medication errors. Avoiding referring to these drugs by their trade names minimizes the risk of serious medication errors.
- Insulins are very potent (a small dose creates a big effect). When drawing up insulin, the dose should always be double-checked by another nurse to prevent accidental overdosage, which could cause serious, even life-threatening, consequences to the patient.
- Nursing care of the patient receiving insulin therapy calls for balancing diet, exercise, and insulin requirements; preventing and monitoring for complications of therapy; and teaching the patient how to do the same.
- Glyburide is the prototype oral antidiabetic sulfonylurea drug. It is used to treat type 2 diabetes. It works by stimulating insulin release from the beta cells of the pancreas and by reducing glucose output from the liver. It also increases the sensitivity of the peripheral cells to insulin. The patient must make some endogenous insulin for glyburide to work. The most common adverse effect is hypoglycemia.
- Other antidiabetic drugs work in different ways than the sulfonylureas. Metformin is the prototype for these drugs. Metformin decreases intestinal absorption of glucose and improves insulin sensitivity in type 2 diabetes. It rarely causes hypoglycemia when used alone.
- Alpha-glucosidase inhibitors (acarbose and miglitol) inhibit enzymes needed to digest carbohydrates; thus, they produce a slower postprandial rise in glucose in type 2 diabetes. Because of how they work, if hypoglycemia does occur during their use, do not use dietary sugars (orange juice, cane sugar) but use glucose tablets.
- The thiazolidinedione oral antihyperglycemic drugs rosiglitazone and pioglitazone are similar to those of the biguanides; they are antihyperglycemics and "insulin sensitizers" and are used in type 2 diabetes. Both drugs carry a black box warning that they may induce or exacerbate heart failure. Rosiglitazone now carries a black box warning that it may increase the risk of myocardial infarction. Its use is now restricted to those who cannot be controlled on other anti diabetic therapy.
- Sitagliptin is a dipeptidyl peptidase-4 (DPP-4) enzyme inhibitor; it works by enhancing the action of endogenous incretin hormones. Incretin hormones are released in response to glucose elevations that occur after a meal in

order to maintain normal levels of glucose. These incretin hormones increase insulin synthesis and its release from pancreatic beta cells by intracellular signaling pathways as well as lowering glucagon secretion from the pancreas. Sitagliptin may be used as monotherapy or in combination with other oral antidiabetic drugs to treat type 2 diabetes.

- Exenatide is an incretin mimetic drug and is used as an adjunct in treating patients with type 2 diabetes. Administered subcutaneously, it increases insulin synthesis, lowers glucagon secretion, slows gastric emptying, and promotes weight loss. Exenatide is not an insulin, and care must be used not to confuse it with insulin.
- Pramlintide is an analogue of endogenous amylin, a hormone secreted like insulin from pancreatic beta cells. It is used as a subcutaneous supplement to insulin therapy in patients with type 1 or type 2 diabetes who have not been able to achieve sufficient glucose control on insulin alone. It is not an insulin and cannot be mixed with an insulin. Like endogenous amylin, pramlintide delays gastric emptying, prevents postprandial rise in plasma glucagon, and promotes feelings of satiety so that the patient eats less. Adverse effects that can occur include hypoglycemia and GI distress.
- Glucagon is a protein made by the pancreas that is used for emergency treatment of severe hypoglycemia. It regulates the rate of glucose production through glycogenolysis, gluconeogenesis, and lipolysis.
- The management of type 1 and type 2 diabetes has become more complicated in recent years because of the variety of new drugs available to control elevated glucose levels, but these new therapies mean that patients who have previously been unsuccessful in controlling their glucose levels may be able to achieve glucose control. Long-term glucose control is important, as it prevents the serious sequelae that accompany uncontrolled diabetes.

QUESTIONS FOR STUDY AND REVIEW

1. What effect does insulin have on blood glucose levels?
2. What effect does glucagon have on glucose metabolism? What effect does it have on the effect of insulin?
3. How do the characteristics of type 1 and type 2 diabetes compare?
4. Why can insulin not be given orally?
5. What effect would be expected from too much insulin? How would this effect be recognized?
6. Why is regular insulin often combined with a longer-acting insulin?
7. Which insulins are used to provide supplemental doses (insulin dose based on current blood glucose level)?
8. What is the difference between NPH and glargine insulins?
9. What is the most common adverse effect of glyburide, a sulfonylurea oral antidiabetic drug?
10. How does acarbose produce its therapeutic effect?
11. What patient and family education should be given if the patient is prescribed glucagons for emergency home use?

NEED MORE HELP?
Chapter 49 of the Study Guide to Accompany *Drug Therapy in Nursing*, 4th Edition, contains NCLEX-style questions and other learning activities to reinforce your understanding of the concepts presented in this chapter. For additional information or to purchase the study guide, visit thePoint.

REFERENCES

American College of Endocriniology and American Diabetes Association consensus statement on inpatient diabetes and glycemic control: A call to action. (2006). *Diabetes Care,* 29(8):1955–1962. Retrieved from http://care.diabetesjournals.org/content/29/8/1955.full

American Diabetes Association. (2010a). Standards of medical care in diabetes: 2010. Retrieved from *http://care.diabetes-journals.org/content/33/Supplement_1/S11.full#sec-63*

American Diabetes Association. (2010b). Gestational diabetes. Retrieved from *http://www.diabetes.org/diabetes-basics/gestational/what-is-gestational-diabetes.html*

American Obesity Association. (2010c). Obesity in youth. Retrieved from *http://www.obesity.org/information/child-hood_overweight.asp*

American Heart Association. (2010d). Statistical Fact Sheet – Risk Factors 2010 update. Metabolic syndrome-statistics. http://www.americanheart.org/downloadable/heart/1260809371480FS15META10.pdf

Aschenbrenner, D. S. (2011). Drug Watch. Safety update: restricted access to rosiglitazone. *American Journal of Nursing;,* 111(1):26–27.

Belcher, G., Lambert, C., Edwards, G., et al. (2005). Safety and tolerability of pioglitazone, metformin, and gliclazide in the treatment of type 2 diabetes. *Diabetes Research and Clinical Practice,* 70(1):53–62.

Black, C., Donnelly, P., McIntyre, L., et al. (2007). Meglitinide analogues for type 2 diabetes mellitus. *Cochrane Database of Systematic Reviews* 2007, (2):CD004654

Centers for Disease Control and Prevention. (updated 2010a). National diabetes fact sheet, United States, 2003. Retrieved from *http://www.cdc.gov/diabetes/pubs/general.htm*

Centers for Disease Control and Prevention. (2010b). Obesity and overweight. http://www.cdc.gov/nchs/fastats/overwt.htm. Page last update January 18, 2010.

Food and Drug Administration MedWatch. (2007). Safety alert: Actos (pioglitazone). Retrieved from *http://www.fda.gov/med-watch/safety/2007/safety07.htm#Actos*

Griesdale, D. E., de Souza, R. J., van Dam, R. M., et al. (2009). Intensive insulin therapy and mortality among critically ill patients: a meta-analysis including NICE-SUGAR study data. *CMAJ,* 180:821–827.

Heron, M. P., Hoyert, D. L., Murphy, S. L., et al. (2009). Deaths: final data for 2006. National Vital Statistics Reports vol 57, number 14. April 17, 2009. National Center for Health Statistics. Online at: http://www.cdc.gov/nchs/data/nvsr/nvsr57/nvsr57_14.pdf

Holman, R. R., Farmer, A. J., Davies, M. J., et al. for 4-T Study Group. Three-year efficacy of complex insulin regimens in type 2 diabetes. *New England Journal of Medicine,* 361(18):1736–1747. Epub 2009 Oct 22.

Home, P. D., Pocock, S. J., Beck-Nielsen, H., et al. for RECORD Study Team. (2009). Rosiglitazone evaluated for cardiovascular outcomes in oral agent combination therapy for type 2 diabetes (RECORD): a multicentre, randomised, open-label trial. *Lancet.* 373(9681):2125–2135. Epub 2009 Jun 6.

Landon, M. B., Spong, C. Y., Thom, E., et al. (2009). A multi-center, randomized trial of treatment for mild gestational diabetes. *New England Journal of Medicine*, 361(14):1339–1348.

Misso, M. L., Egberts, K. J., Page, M., et al. (2010). Continuous subcutaneous insulin infusion (CSII) versus multiple insulin injections for type 1 diabetes mellitus. *Cochrane Database of Systematic Reviews*, (1):CD005103.

Moghissi, E. S. (2010). Addressing hyperglycemia from hospital admission to discharge. *Current Medical Research and Opinion*, 26(3):589–598.

Paparella, S. (2006). Avoiding errors with insulin therapy. *Journal of Emergency Nursing*, 32(4):325–328.

Parks, M. H., Food and Drug Administration. Memo dated Aug 19, 2010 to Curtis J Rosebraugh, MD, MPH, Director, Office of Drug Evaluation 2. Subject: Recommendations on marketing status of Avandia® (rosiglitazonemaleate) and the required post-marketing trial, Thiazolidinedione Intervention and Vitamin D Evaluation (TIDE) following the July 13 and 14, 2010 public advisory committee meeting - 8/19/2010. http://www.fda.gov/downloads/Drugs/DrugSafety/PostmarketDrugSafetyInformationforPatientsandProviders/UCM226235.pdf

Richter, B., Bandeira-Echtler, E., Bergerhoff, K., & Lerch, C. (2008). Dipeptidyl peptidase-4 (DPP-4) inhibitors for type 2 diabetes mellitus. *Cochrane Database of Systematic Reviews*, (2):CD006739.

Riveline, J. P., Danchin, N., Ledru, F., et al. (2003). Sulfonylureas and cardiovascular effects: From experimental data to clinical use. Available data in humans and clinical applications. *Diabetes Metabolism*, 29(3):207–222.

Salpeter, S. R., Greyber, E., Pasternak, G. A., Salpeter, E. E. (2010). Risk of fatal and nonfatal lactic acidosis with metformin use in type 2 diabetes mellitus. *Cochrane Database of Systematic Reviews*, (4):CD002967.

Stratton, I. M., Adler, A. I., Neil, H. A., et al. (2000). Association of glycaemia with macrovascular and microvascular complications of type 2 diabetes (UKPDS 35): prospective observational study. *British Medical Journal*, 321:405–412.

Turkoski, B. B. (2006). Diabetes and diabetes medications. *Orthopedic Nursing*, 25(3):227–231.

50

Drugs Affecting Pituitary, Thyroid, Parathyroid, and Hypothalamic Function

Learning Objectives

At the completion of this chapter the student will:

1. Identify drugs commonly used for pituitary hypofunction and hyperfunction, thyroid hypofunction and hyperfunction, and parathyroid hypofunction and hyperfunction.

2. Identify core drug knowledge about drugs affecting the pituitary gland and its hormones, the thyroid gland and its hormones, and the parathyroid glands and their hormones.

3. Identify core patient variables relevant to drugs affecting the pituitary gland and its hormones, the thyroid gland and its hormones, and the parathyroid glands and their hormones.

4. Generate a nursing plan of care from the interactions between core drug knowledge and core patient variables for drugs affecting the pituitary gland and its hormones, the thyroid gland and its hormones, and the parathyroid glands and their hormones.

5. Describe nursing interventions to maximize therapeutic and minimize adverse effects for drugs affecting the pituitary gland and its hormones, the thyroid gland and its hormones, and the parathyroid glands and their hormones.

6. Determine key points for patient and family education for drugs affecting the pituitary gland and its hormones, the thyroid gland and its hormones, and the parathyroid glands and their hormones.

Key Terms

acromegaly	gigantism	Paget disease
bone resorption	Graves disease	syndrome of inappropriate antidiuretic hormone
cretinism	hyperthyroidism	thyroid crisis
diabetes insipidus	hypothyroidism	thyrotoxicosis
effector hormones	myxedema coma	tropic hormones

Drugs Affecting Pituitary, Thyroid, Parathyroid, and Hypothalamic Function

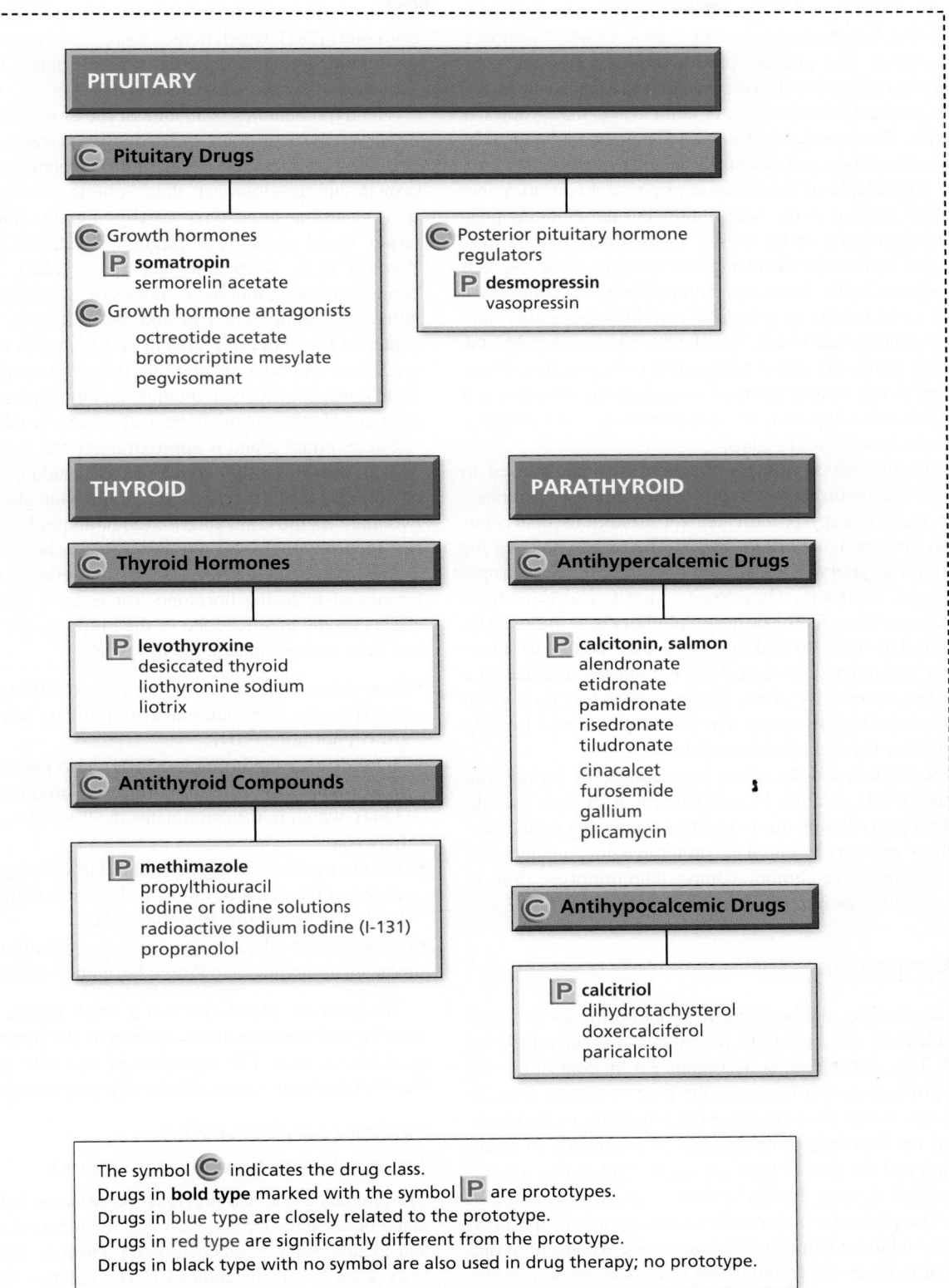

PITUITARY

C Pituitary Drugs

C Growth hormones
   P **somatropin**
     sermorelin acetate
C Growth hormone antagonists
   octreotide acetate
   bromocriptine mesylate
   pegvisomant

C Posterior pituitary hormone regulators
   P **desmopressin**
     vasopressin

THYROID

C Thyroid Hormones

P **levothyroxine**
  desiccated thyroid
  liothyronine sodium
  liotrix

C Antithyroid Compounds

P **methimazole**
  propylthiouracil
  iodine or iodine solutions
  radioactive sodium iodine (I-131)
  propranolol

PARATHYROID

C Antihypercalcemic Drugs

P **calcitonin, salmon**
  alendronate
  etidronate
  pamidronate
  risedronate
  tiludronate

  cinacalcet
  furosemide
  gallium
  plicamycin

C Antihypocalcemic Drugs

P **calcitriol**
  dihydrotachysterol
  doxercalciferol
  paricalcitol

The symbol C indicates the drug class.
Drugs in **bold type** marked with the symbol P are prototypes.
Drugs in blue type are closely related to the prototype.
Drugs in red type are significantly different from the prototype.
Drugs in black type with no symbol are also used in drug therapy; no prototype.

The endocrine system works with the central nervous system (CNS) to integrate and regulate all aspects of body function, including energy metabolism, growth and development, sexual development, fluid and electrolyte balance, muscle and adipose tissue distribution, and inflammation and immune responses. This system has three major components: glands, hormones, and receptors. The glands—pineal, pituitary, thyroid, parathyroid, thymus, adrenal, pancreas, and gonads (ovaries and testes)—are specialized organs or cell clusters that synthesize hormones. Hormones are substances that are manufactured by a dedicated cell type and that, released into the circulation, produce a physiologic or biochemical response. Most hormones are always present in the body fluids, but the amounts present vary, depending on the body's needs. Receptors are molecules that initiate specific changes in a target cell in response to stimulation by the hormones. Homeostasis is accomplished through coordination of glandular activities that either suppress or stimulate hormones. Specific disorders occur when the endocrine glands are either hyperactive or hypoactive. Drugs discussed in this chapter are used to manage the disorders that occur from either hyperactivity or hypoactivity of the pituitary, thyroid, and parathyroid glands.

Agents that affect pituitary function are mainly used to mimic or antagonize the effect of the pituitary hormones. Replacement therapy is indicated for conditions that occur from an underactive pituitary gland. The prototype drug for the anterior pituitary is somatropin (Genotropin, Humatrope, Norditropin, Nutropin, Omnitrope, Saizen, and Serostim). The prototype drug for the posterior pituitary is desmopressin.

Agents that affect thyroid function are used either to antagonize an overactive thyroid gland or to replace hormones as a result of an underactive gland. The prototype drug for thyroid replacement is levothyroxine. The prototype drug for treating an overactive thyroid is methimazole.

Serum calcium and phosphate are regulated by parathyroid hormone (PTH), vitamin D, and calcitonin. Agents used to regulate serum calcium do so by either increasing or decreasing serum calcium levels. The prototype drug to decrease serum calcium is calcitonin, salmon. The prototype drug to increase serum calcium is calcitriol.

PHYSIOLOGY

To remain healthy, the body ensures that hormones are present in adequate concentrations in the areas in which they are needed. This distribution is accomplished by controlling the rate of production of a hormone, the time of release from its storage site, the speed of clearance from the body, or the breakdown of the hormone. Both the rate of production of many hormones and the time of their release is regulated by a negative feedback system. In this system, when sensors detect a change in a particular hormone level, the amount of hormone secreted is adjusted to maintain homeostasis. When a hormone is present in excessive amounts, the sensors decrease production and prevent further release of that hormone, so that levels remain within an appropriate range. Conversely, an increase in

levels of a particular hormone stimulates the feedback system to decrease the amount produced and released. For example, if thyroid hormone levels increase, sensors in the hypothalamus or anterior pituitary gland detect the increase. This interaction triggers a reduction in secretion of thyroid-stimulating hormone (TSH), which in turn causes a decrease in the release of thyroid hormone from the thyroid gland. The combined sequence of events maintains homeostasis.

The hypothalamus is an area of the brain that exerts direct effects on the neurologic and endocrine systems (Figure 50.1), including temperature regulation, catecholamine secretion, growth and development, fluid volume regulation, perspiration, gastrointestinal (GI) activity, appetite and thirst regulation, blood pressure, respiration, regulation of basic body rhythms (e.g., sleep and menstrual cycles), and complex behavioral and emotional reactions (e.g., sexual behavior and defensive reactions of fear and rage). It is the coordinating center of the endocrine system and produces hormones that are stored and later secreted by the pituitary gland. To promote homeostasis, the hypothalamus transmits stimuli to the pituitary gland, causing hormonal release or inhibition.

The pituitary gland is approximately the size of a pea and rests in the bony sella turcica (Turkish saddle) under a layer of dura mater at the base of the brain. This gland consists of two main regions: the anterior (adenohypophysis) and posterior (neurohypophysis) pituitary lobes, which are connected to the hypothalamus by a stalk of neurosecretory fibers. Groups of releasing hormones (or factors) have controlling effects on the anterior lobe of the pituitary. These hormones and their actions include the following:

- Growth hormone–releasing hormone (GHRH), also known as sermorelin, stimulates anterior pituitary release of growth hormone (GH).
- Thyroid-releasing hormone (TRH), also known as protirelin, stimulates the anterior pituitary to produce thyrotropin (TSH), which in turn stimulates the thyroid to produce thyroxine.
- Gonadotropin-releasing hormone (GnRH) controls the release of the gonadotropins: follicle-stimulating hormone (FSH) and luteinizing hormone (LH).
- Corticotropin-releasing factor (Xerecept) stimulates release of adrenocorticotropic hormone (ACTH).

The pituitary gland also has a small region between the anterior and posterior lobes, known as the intermediate lobe (pars intermedia). The hormones of this lobe stimulate synthesis of melanin, which affects skin pigmentation.

Pituitary Gland Function
Anterior Lobe of the Pituitary Gland

The pituitary gland was previously considered to be the master gland because its hormones control the function of many cells and glands, such as glucocorticoid hormone levels (ACTH), body growth and metabolism (GH), function of the thyroid gland (TSH), gonadal function (FSH and LH), and milk production and breast growth (prolactin). The hypothalamus is

PHYSIOLOGY

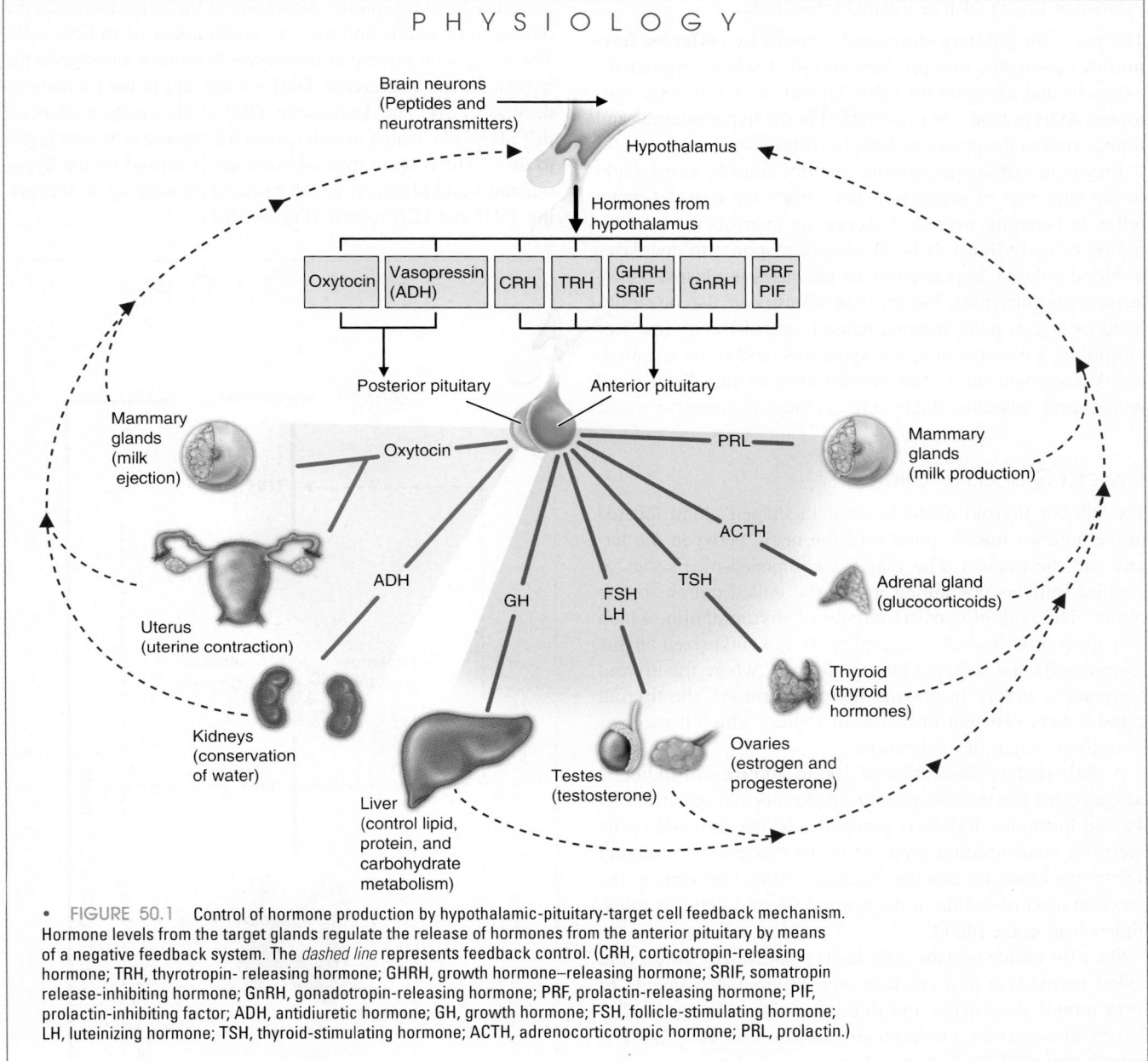

• FIGURE 50.1 Control of hormone production by hypothalamic-pituitary-target cell feedback mechanism. Hormone levels from the target glands regulate the release of hormones from the anterior pituitary by means of a negative feedback system. The *dashed line* represents feedback control. (CRH, corticotropin-releasing hormone; TRH, thyrotropin- releasing hormone; GHRH, growth hormone–releasing hormone; SRIF, somatropin release-inhibiting hormone; GnRH, gonadotropin-releasing hormone; PRF, prolactin-releasing hormone; PIF, prolactin-inhibiting factor; ADH, antidiuretic hormone; GH, growth hormone; FSH, follicle-stimulating hormone; LH, luteinizing hormone; TSH, thyroid-stimulating hormone; ACTH, adrenocorticotropic hormone; PRL, prolactin.)

now recognized as the coordinating center of the brain that stimulates the pituitary gland to release specific hormones when indicated. The first five hormones listed are **tropic hormones,** which means that they stimulate other organs or glands to secrete substances that are hormonally active. Secretion varies with physiologic activity (such as exercise) or with the time of day. Various drugs, the CNS, hypothalamic hormones, some diseases, and hormones of the peripheral endocrine system affect their synthesis and release. Prolactin acts directly on breast tissue to stimulate milk production.

GH does not have a specific target gland. Its rate of production in adulthood is almost equal to that of childhood. GH is necessary for linear bone growth. It regulates cellular metabolism, facilitates protein synthesis, enhances amino acid

transport across cell membranes (which stimulates an anabolic effect), decreases the rate of carbohydrate use in cells, increases the rate of fatty acids for fuel, and maintains or increases blood glucose levels in both children and adults. Many of the effects of GH depend on the production of insulin-like growth factor-1 (IGF-1), which is mainly produced by the liver.

GH is the most apparent of the pituitary hormones. Its secretion is regulated by two hypothalamic hormones: GHRH (GH-releasing hormone), which increases the release of GH; and somatostatin, which inhibits GH release. GH secretion fluctuates over a 24-hour period, with peak levels occurring during sleep stages 3 and 4 (1 to 4 hours after the onset of sleep). GH is also released during periods of hypoglycemia, stress, exercise, and excitement, and in response to levodopa and arginine.

Posterior Lobe of the Pituitary Gland

The posterior pituitary stores and secretes two **effector hormones** (hormones that produce an effect when stimulated): oxytocin and vasopressin (also known as antidiuretic hormone [ADH]). Both are synthesized in the hypothalamus and transported to the posterior lobe for future use.

Oxytocin stimulates uterine smooth muscle contraction in the later part of pregnancy and causes the milk let-down reflex in lactating women. Vasopressin controls the concentration of body fluids. It is released in response to decreases in blood volume, hypotension, or increases in plasma osmolarity (concentration). Vasopressin release can also be stimulated by stress, pain, trauma, nausea, use of tranquilizers or morphine, a positive-pressure apparatus, and some anesthetics. Vasopressin alters the permeability of the distal renal tubules and collecting ducts in the kidneys to conserve water.

Thyroid Gland Function

The bilobar thyroid gland is a shield-shaped gland located in the anterior middle portion of the neck, between the larynx and the trachea. The gland is composed of a series of circular follicles containing a material called colloid in the center. The colloid consists largely of thyroglobulin, which is a glycoprotein–iodine complex. It is synthesized in the thyroid cells and secreted into the follicle, where the thyroid hormone is stored. In making thyroid hormone, the thyroid gland is very efficient in its use of iodide, which it receives from food, water, or medications.

A daily dietary absorption of 100 to 200 mcg of iodide is adequate for the thyroid gland to make normal quantities of thyroid hormone. Iodide is pumped into the follicular cells against a concentration gradient in the process of removing it from the blood for storage. Because of this mechanism, the concentration of iodide in the normal thyroid gland is much higher than in the blood.

Once the iodide is in the follicle, it is oxidized by an enzyme called peroxidase in a reaction with a tyrosine molecule to form monoiodotyrosine and diiodotyrosine. Thyroxine (T_4) is formed when two diiodotyrosine residues are coupled. Triiodothyronine (T_3) is formed when a monoiodotyrosine and a diiodotyrosine are coupled. Collectively, these two hormones are referred to as thyroid hormone. When thyroid hormone is needed, T_4 and T_3 are released into the bloodstream. Once in the bloodstream, both $_4$ are more than 99% bound to thyroid-binding globulin and other plasma proteins for transport. The three major thyroid-binding proteins are thyroid hormone-binding globulin, thyroxine-binding prealbumin, and albumin. Some medications, systemic diseases, and congenital diseases can affect either the amount of binding protein in the blood or the binding ability of the hormone.

The hypothalamic-pituitary-thyroid feedback system regulates secretion of thyroid hormone. The hypothalamus produces TRH, which controls the release of TSH from the anterior pituitary gland. TSH increases the release of thyroid hormone from the follicles into the bloodstream and thyroglobulin breakdown, which increases thyroid activity. This increased activity

activates the iodide pump. Activation of the pump increases the oxidation of iodide and the size and number of follicle cells. The increase in thyroid hormone levels sends a message to the hypothalamus to decrease TRH release and to the pituitary to decrease TSH. The decrease in TRH levels causes a decrease in TSH levels, which in turn causes the thyroid hormone levels to drop. The drop in thyroid hormone is sensed by the hypothalamus and pituitary, which respond by once again increasing TRH and TSH release (Figure 50.2).

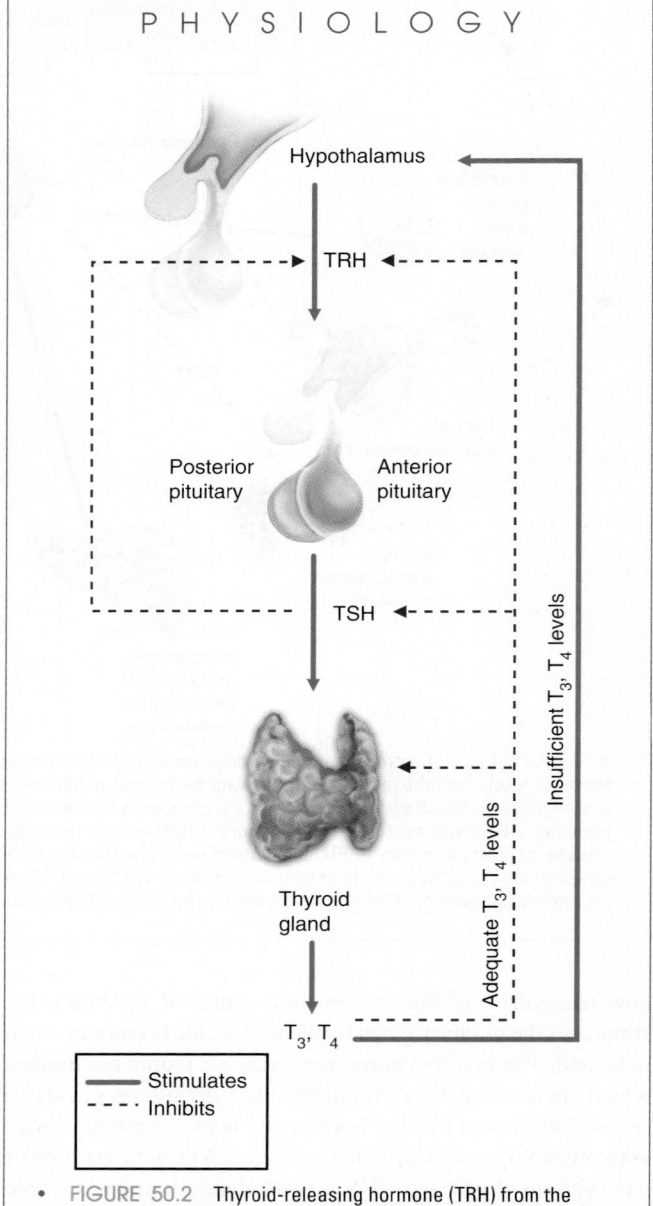

PHYSIOLOGY

— Stimulates
- - - Inhibits

• FIGURE 50.2 Thyroid-releasing hormone (TRH) from the hypothalamus stimulates the anterior pituitary to release thyroid-stimulating hormone (TSH). TSH stimulates the thyroid gland to release T_3 and T_4. It also inhibits the hypothalamus from releasing TRH and the anterior pituitary from releasing more TSH. The release of T_3 and T_4 from the thyroid gland inhibits TRH release from the hypothalamus, TSH release from the pituitary, and further T_3 and T_4 release from the thyroid gland. Falling T_3 and T_4 levels will stimulate the hypothalamus to release TRH, and the process repeatedly continues to maintain effective hormone levels.

TABLE 50.1 Effect of Thyroid Hormones

Target Physiologic Process or Body System	Primary Effects
Carbohydrate metabolism	Increases cellular glucose uptake Increases gluconeogenesis and glycolysis Increases GI carbohydrate absorption Increases insulin secretion
Cardiovascular system	Increases heart rate, cardiac output, arterial pressure
Central nervous system	Increases mental processes Increases activity in spinal cord areas controlling muscle tone
Fat metabolism	Increases fat metabolism, including lipid mobilization from fat tissues and free fatty acid oxidation
GI function	Increases appetite, food absorption, digestive enzyme secretions, GI motility
Growth metabolism	Accelerates growth (in children) Accelerates food use for energy, speeds protein synthesis and catabolism, excites mental processes Increases other endocrine gland functions

Thyroid hormones control cellular metabolism and promote normal growth and development. They regulate heat and energy production, blood volume, cardiac output, oxygen consumption, and metabolism of fats, carbohydrates, and proteins (Table 50.1). All major organs are affected by disorders of the thyroid gland.

The thyroid gland also produces calcitonin, which maintains the serum calcium level by preventing release of calcium from the bone.

Parathyroid Gland Function

The four tiny, highly vascular parathyroid glands work together as a single gland to produce PTH, which helps to regulate serum calcium and phosphate. These glands are located on the dorsal surface of the thyroid. In the healthy individual, plasma calcium concentration is maintained within narrow limits.

PTH affects three target organs: bone, kidneys, and GI tract. The primary storage site for calcium is in the bone. The major controlling factor for PTH secretion is serum calcium. When serum calcium levels are low, the parathyroid gland stimulates the release of PTH. Release of this hormone promotes increased bone resorption, which increases the serum calcium level. PTH also activates vitamin D in the kidney, which boosts absorption of phosphate and calcium from the GI tract. When serum calcium levels are elevated, PTH secretion decreases. Magnesium and phosphate levels also affect PTH secretion.

PATHOPHYSIOLOGY

Pituitary Gland Dysfunction

Pituitary dysfunction may occur from many causes, such as congenital defects, developmental abnormalities, acute or chronic inflammation, invasive tumors, circulatory disturbances (infarction or hemorrhage), surgery, radiation therapy, injury (head trauma), or infection. These conditions may cause either a decrease or increase in hormonal secretions. A single hormone or multiple hormones may be affected.

Anterior Pituitary Gland Dysfunction

Conditions of anterior pituitary dysfunction include growth hormone deficiency and excess.

Growth Hormone Deficiency

Several forms of GH deficiency can occur in children, including idiopathic and congenital. Idiopathic is the most common. Children with idiopathic GH deficiency have adequate somatotropes but inadequate GHRH, leading to short stature or dwarfism. Those with congenital GH deficiency have a normal birth length but are noted to have a decreased growth rate within the first year or two of life.

Adults with GH deficiency also fit into two categories: those who manifest GH deficiency as children, and those who develop GH deficiency in adulthood secondary to a pituitary tumor or its treatment. Aging can cause decreases in GH levels (termed somatopause); the effects of decreasing GH levels in the elderly are being investigated. It is unclear whether GH replacement for somatopause is beneficial, however metabolic disorders that affect mobility, energy levels and socialization, and cardiovascular mortality are all associated with GH deficiency in adults.

Growth Hormone Excess

When GH excess occurs before puberty and the fusion of the epiphysis of the long bones, linear skeletal growth is accentuated and causes **gigantism.** Gigantism is an uncommon condition, caused by excessive secretion of GH by somatotrope adenomas. These children have normal body proportions but grow to be 7 ft or taller.

Acromegaly is the term used to describe excessive GH secretion that occurs in adulthood, after puberty and the closure of the epiphyseal plate. This is an uncommon condition with an annual incidence estimated at three to four cases per 1 million people. The most common cause of acromegaly is somatotrope adenoma. It can also be caused by hypothalamic or some nonendocrine tumors (such as small cell lung cancer). Because the epiphysis of the long bones has closed, these people cannot grow taller, but soft tissues continue to grow. As a result, small bones of the feet and hands and membranous bones of the skull and face enlarge. This enlargement causes the hands and feet to grow and gives the face coarse features, such as a broadening nose, slanting forehead, and protruding jaw. All body organs are affected, leading to an enlarged heart, hypertension, accelerated atherosclerosis, peripheral neuropathies, and muscle weakness.

Posterior Pituitary Gland Dysfunction

Two major disorders that arise from posterior pituitary gland dysfunction are **diabetes insipidus** (DI) and **syndrome of inappropriate antidiuretic hormone** (SIADH). DI is caused by either a deficiency in or a decreased response to ADH. SIADH is caused from excessive ADH secretion secondary to a failure of the negative feedback system responsible for its release and inhibition. Most disorders of the posterior pituitary gland are secondary to lymphoma, metastatic cancer, septicemia, or disseminated intravascular coagulation.

Diabetes Insipidus

Increases in plasma osmolarity or decreases in blood volume stimulate the release of ADH. ADH is produced in the kidney, causing areas of the collecting duct to become more permeable to water and allowing water reabsorption to increase. Increased water reabsorption increases both plasma osmolarity and blood volume.

DI occurs when there is either a decreased response to ADH (termed nephrogenic DI), or a deficiency in the synthesis or release of ADH (termed central or neurogenic DI). In either case, the person is unable to concentrate urine at times when water is restricted and often excretes large amounts of urine (as much as 3 to 20 L/d). Excessive thirst accompanies the large amount of urine output. As long as the thirst mechanism is normal and fluids are replenished, fluid levels are not altered. However, if the person with DI is unable to communicate a need for water or does not have access to fluids, hypertonic dehydration and increased serum osmolality occur. Nephrogenic DI may have a genetic cause or may occur secondary to lithium ingestion, chronic hypercalcemia, or potassium depletion. Neurogenic DI may occur following surgery near the hypothalamus or from head injury. DI can be an acute or chronic problem.

Syndrome of Inappropriate Antidiuretic Hormone

SIADH is a condition in which ADH secretion continues, regardless of decreased serum osmolarity, which causes dilutional hyponatremia and marked water retention. It results from a failure of the negative feedback system that regulates the release and inhibition of ADH. SIADH may be chronic (secondary to tumors or CNS disorders) or acute (secondary to stress, pain, or surgery). A variety of drugs can also cause SIADH (Box 50.1). Clinical manifestations seen in SIADH (as a result of the dilutional hyponatremia) include lethargy, anorexia, muscle cramps, nausea, vomiting, seizure, coma, and death.

Thyroid Gland Dysfunction

Thyroid function alterations can occur from a hyperfunctioning or hypofunctioning gland, which are malfunctions that may be caused by either a congenital defect or by a problem that occurs later in life. Dramatic changes in patterns of

Box 50.1 DRUGS THAT MAY CAUSE SYNDROME OF INAPPROPRIATE ANTIDIURETIC HORMONE SECRETION (SIADH)

carbamazepine (Tegretol)
chlorpropamide (Diabinese)
clofibrate (Atromid-S)
cyclophosphamide (Cytoxan)
isoproterenol (Isuprel)
morphine
oxytocin (Pitocin)
phenothiazines
prostaglandins
thiazide diuretics
tricyclic antidepressants
vasopressin
vincristine (Oncovin)

growth and development, and in functions of the cardiovascular, respiratory, GI, neuromuscular, skeletal, and reproductive systems, can result.

An increase in the size of the thyroid gland (goiter) can occur in hyperthyroid, euthyroid, and hypothyroid states. Goiters may be toxic or nontoxic. Toxic goiters cause signs of extreme hyperthyroidism or thyrotoxicosis, described later in this section. The amount of thyroid gland enlargement is proportional to the extent and/or duration of thyroid deficiency. Some goiters grow so large that they can cause difficulty breathing or swallowing. Table 50.2 compares the clinical manifestations of hypothyroidism and hyperthyroidism.

Hypothyroidism

Congenital **hypothyroidism** is present at birth, and acquired hypothyroidism occurs later in life as a result of either a primary or secondary disorder of the hypothalamus or pituitary gland.

Untreated congenital hypothyroidism (which affects approximately 1 out of every 5,000 infant births) can have devastating effects, such as mental retardation and impaired physical growth. Congenital hypothyroidism occurs from abnormal biosynthesis of thyroid hormone, deficient TSH hormone, or an absence of the thyroid gland. **Cretinism,** the term used for the condition of untreated hypothyroidism, does not apply to the normally developing infant, born with hypothyroidism, who receives thyroid hormone replacement therapy soon after birth. Fortunately, a very effective screening test for hypothyroidism is readily available. A drop of blood is taken from the infant's heel and analyzed for thyroid hormones and TSH, and treatment can be instituted immediately if hypothyroidism is detected.

Hypothyroidism that is evident in older children and adults occurs as a result of either dysfunction or destruction of the thyroid gland (primary hypothyroidism) or of impaired hypothalamic or pituitary function (secondary hypothyroidism). Primary hypothyroidism may result from surgical removal of the thyroid gland (thyroidectomy) or from radiation, which ablates the gland. Certain drugs (e.g., lithium carbonate, used for manic depression, and propylthiouracil and methimazole, which are antithyroid drugs) can block hormone synthesis causing hypothyroidism with a goiter. Thyroid hormone production can be blocked by drugs containing iodine (e.g., kelp tablets, radiographic contrast media, and cough syrups containing iodide). Thyroid problems are also being reported

TABLE 50.2	Clinical Comparison of Hypothyroidism and Hyperthyroidism	
Body System	**Clinical Picture of Hypothyroidism**	**Clinical Picture of Hyperthyroidism**
Central nervous system	General slowing of mental processes Lethargy Neuropathies	Emotional lability Hyperkinesia Nervousness
Cardiovascular system	Decreased peripheral vascular resistance, heart rate, stroke volume, cardiac output, pulse pressure ECG changes: bradycardia, increased PR interval, flat T wave, low voltage Low-output congestive heart failure Pericardial effusion	Increased peripheral vascular resistance, heart rate, stroke volume, cardiac output, pulse pressure High-output congestive heart failure Increased inotropic and chronotropic effects Angina Arrhythmias
EENT	Enlarged tongue Eyelid drooping Periorbital edema Puffy, nonpitting face	Diplopia (Graves disease) Exophthalmos (Graves disease) Periorbital edema Retraction of upper lid with wide stare
Gastrointestinal system	Decreased appetite Decreased frequency of bowel movements Ascites	Increased appetite Increased frequency of bowel movements Hypoproteinemia
Hematopoietic system	Decreased erythropoiesis Anemia	Increased erythropoiesis Anemia
Metabolic system	Decreased basal metabolic rate with slight positive nitrogen balance Delayed degradation of insulin with increased insulin sensitivity Increased cholesterol and triglycerides Decreased hormone degradation Decreased requirements for fat- and water-soluble vitamins Decreased drug detoxification	Increased basal metabolic rate with negative nitrogen balance Hyperglycemia Increased free fatty acids Decreased cholesterol and triglycerides Increased hormone degradation Increased requirements for fat- and water-soluble vitamins Increased drug detoxification
Musculoskeletal system	Stiffness and muscle fatigue Decreased deep tendon reflexes Increased alkaline phosphatase, LDH, AST	Weakness and muscle fatigue Increased deep tendon reflexes Hypercalcemia Osteoporosis
Renal system	Impaired water excretion Decreased renal blood flow Decreased glomerular filtration rate	Mild polyuria Increased renal blood flow Increased glomerular filtration rate
Reproductive system	Hypermenorrhea Infertility* Decreased libido* Men: impotency, oligospermia decreased gonadal steroid metabolism*	Women: menstrual irregularities decreased fertility, decreased gonadal steroid metabolism*
Respiratory	Pleural effusions Hypoventilation Hypercarbia	Dyspnea Decreased vital capacity
Skin	Pale, cool, puffy skin (myxedema) Dry, brittle hair Brittle nails Cold intolerance	Warm, moist, diaphoretic skin Fine, thin hair Heat intolerance

*Both men and women

from the use of the antiarrhythmic medication amiodarone, because of its high iodine content. In the United States, the use of iodized salt and other dietary iodide sources has decreased the incidence of iodine deficiency, which causes hypothyroidism and goiter. The major cause of goiter and hypothyroidism is Hashimoto thyroiditis, an autoimmune disorder that damages the thyroid. This is a condition that affects females to males at a 5:1 ratio.

Clinical manifestations of hypothyroidism can vary widely. Subclinical hypothyroidism can cause nonspecific complaints. Overt manifestations of hypothyroidism occur as a result of decreased cellular metabolism secondary to thyroid hormone deficiency and myxedematous involvement of the body tissues. These manifestations include lethargy, hypoactive reflexes, weight gain, anxiety, impaired memory, constipation, hypotension, bradycardia, intolerance to cold, loss of hair, decreased sexual function, menstrual irregularities, infertility, edema of the hands, feet, and face, pale and rough skin, thickened tongue, and husky voice.

Hyperthyroidism

An excessive amount of thyroid hormone in the peripheral tissues results in **hyperthyroidism,** or **thyrotoxicosis.** Patients with hyperthyroidism exhibit signs and symptoms of overactive cellular metabolism of all body systems, tachycardia, palpitations, hypertension, increased body temperature, heat intolerance, weight loss, amenorrhea, and goiter (see Table 50.2). These manifestations result from increased oxygen consumption and increased sympathetic nervous system activity. Graves disease, the most common cause of hyperthyroidism, is accompanied by goiter and exophthalmos (bulging of the eyeballs). Other causes of hyperthyroidism include thyroid gland adenoma, multinodular goiter, and ingestion of excessive thyroid hormone.

Graves disease is an autoimmune disorder that arises from sustained overactivity of the thyroid gland, caused by thyroid-stimulating antibodies and growth of the entire thyroid gland (goiter). Infiltrative ophthalmopathy (exophthalmos) occurs in as many as 50% of all patients with Graves disease Skin lesions (dermopathy) may also occur. Patients with exophthalmos appear to have protruding eyes. Even with treatment, once exophthalmos exists, it remains essentially unchanged. Vision loss (secondary to involvement of the optic nerve) and corneal ulceration (secondary to the eyelids not closing tightly) also occur.

An extreme, life-threatening form of thyrotoxicosis is called **thyroid crisis** (also known as thyroid storm). It is seen in patients who are not adequately treated for their hyperthyroidism or who are undiagnosed. Thyroid crisis is frequently precipitated by infection (usually respiratory), diabetic ketoacidosis, stress, manipulation of a hyperactive thyroid gland during thyroidectomy, or emotional or physical trauma. Manifestations of thyroid crisis include severe CNS effects (e.g., restlessness, agitation, or delirium), extreme cardiovascular effects (e.g., angina, heart failure, or tachycardia), and high fever. Treatment must be implemented immediately; it includes administration of methimazole (MMI), beta blockers, corticosteroids, fluids and electrolytes, measures to control hyperthermia, and oxygen.

Parathyroid Gland Dysfunction

PTH is secreted by the parathyroid glands. This hormone is a major regulator of serum calcium and phosphate. A decrease in serum calcium concentration is the dominant regulator of PTH, with a response rate of just a few seconds. A decrease in phosphate causes an indirect effect on PTH by combining with calcium and decreasing serum calcium concentrations. Magnesium also affects the secretion, synthesis, and action of PTH; severe and prolonged hypomagnesemia can have a marked effect on the inhibition of PTH levels. Hypocalcemia can cause tetany, convulsions, muscle spasm, and neuromuscular excitability. Hypercalcemia has been associated with life-threatening cardiac dysrhythmias, CNS abnormalities, renal damage, and soft tissue calcification. For these reasons, maintaining calcium at the desired level is important. Table 50.3 summarizes disorders of bone and calcium metabolism.

TABLE 50.3	Disorders of Bone and Calcium Metabolism	
Disorders	**Examples**	**Management**
Hypocalcemia	• Inadequate dietary intake of Ca++ and/or vitamin D • Malabsorption caused by vitamin D lack or end-organ resistance • Hypoparathyroidism, pseudohypoparathyroidism • Renal failure	• Treatment with calcium and vitamin D compounds
Hypercalcemia	• Hyperparathyroidism • Hypervitaminosis D • Neoplasia • Hyperthyroidism • Immobilization	• Treatment with fluids, low-calcium diet, calcitonin, bisphosphonates, glucocorticoids, loop diuretics
Impaired bone remodeling	• Osteoporosis	• Treatment with bisphosphonates, calcitonin, calcium, estrogen (female)

Hypoparathyroidism

Hypoparathyroidism (inadequate PTH levels) can be either inherited or acquired. This condition is characterized by hypocalcemia and frequently by hypophosphatemia. As stated previously, hypocalcemia can cause tetany, convulsions, muscle spasm, and neuromuscular excitability. Acquired hypoparathyroidism occurs most commonly as a result of surgery in the neck, but this adverse outcome has become less common with the advent of improved surgical techniques and the increased use of nonsurgical therapy. Lack of PTH can cause vitamin D deficiency, leading to osteomalacia (softening and bending of the bones) in adults and rickets (skeletal deformities) in children.

Hyperparathyroidism

Hypersecretion of PTH leads to hyperparathyroidism. Primary hyperparathyroidism is most common in women older than 50 years and is caused by an adenoma, a carcinoma of the parathyroid gland, or hyperplasia. Hyperparathyroidism causes excessive levels of calcium in both serum (hypercalcemia) and urine (hypercalciuria). Urine phosphate levels are also high, and serum phosphate levels are normal to low. Potential complications of these imbalances include nervous system complaints, pancreatitis, peptic ulcers, kidney stones, severe osteoporosis and osteopenia, and pathologic bone fractures. These complications can be remembered by the rhyme, "moans, groans, stones, and bones." Secondary hyperparathyroidism occurs primarily in persons with renal failure, but it can also occur with multiple myeloma, bone metastasis, and Paget disease. Regardless of the cause, hyperparathyroidism is characterized by deposits of calcium salts in body tissues and bone decalcification. In primary hyperparathyroidism, the severity of hypercalcemia reflects the quantity of hyperfunctioning tissue. Excessive quantities of PTH stimulate transport of calcium into the serum from the kidneys, bones, and intestines. Nephrolithiasis (formation of kidney stones) can occur secondary to calcium deposits in the soft tissues of the kidney.

The influence of PTH on the cells of the bones is very strong and causes them to release calcium into the serum. Under normal conditions, the amount of calcium in the bones remains at a constant level, but in the presence of too

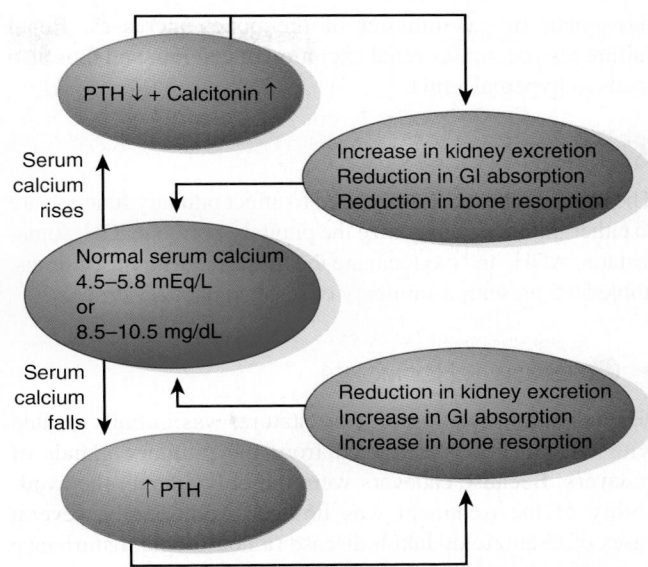

• FIGURE 50.3 Regulation of serum calcium. Parathyroid hormone (PTH) and calcitonin regulate normal serum calcium. As serum calcium rises, PTH is inhibited by calcitonin. The kidney then excretes more calcium, the GI system absorbs less, and a reduction in bone resorption occurs. As serum calcium falls, PTH is secreted and raises the calcium level by decreasing the amount of calcium lost in the kidney, increasing the amount absorbed in the GI tract, and increasing bone resorption.

much PTH, the bones release their calcium into the bloodstream at a high rate, resulting in osteopenia and osteoporosis (Figure 50.3). PTH also influences the lining of the intestine to absorb more calcium from the diet (Table 50.4).

Secondary hyperparathyroidism is caused most often by corticotropin-releasing factor and hyperphosphatemia. There is an inverse relationship between the glomerular filtration rate and serum phosphate levels: as the glomerular filtration rate decreases, serum phosphate levels increase. In turn, this increase decreases serum calcium levels, and this drop then stimulates secretion of PTH.

As the serum calcium level rises, neuromuscular irritability decreases, because of the sedative effect of serum calcium on the body. Hypercalcemia is commonly associated with hyperparathyroidism, but it can also occur secondary to neoplastic disease or immobilization, during which

TABLE 50.4	Actions of Parathyroid Hormone (PTH) and Vitamin D	
	PTH	Vitamin D (and Metabolites)
Bone	• High doses—calcium and phosphate resorption increased • Low doses—may increase bone formation	• Increased calcium and phosphate resorption by calcitriol • Increased bone formation
Kidney	• Decreased calcium excretion • Increased phosphate excretion	• Calcium and phosphate excretion may be decreased by calciferol and calcitriol.
Intestine	• Increased calcium and phosphate absorption by increased calcitriol production	• Increased calcium and phosphate absorption by calcitriol
Effect on serum levels	Serum calcium is increased and serum phosphate is decreased	Serum calcium and serum phosphate are both increased

movement of calcium out of the bones increases. Renal failure also decreases renal excretion of calcium and thus also leads to hypercalcemia.

PITUITARY DRUGS

The primary effects of drugs used to affect pituitary function are to either mimic or antagonize the pituitary hormone. GH, somatostatin, ADH, and oxytocin are the most frequently used drugs. Table 50.5 presents a summary of selected pituitary drugs.

• GROWTH HORMONES

GH deficiency, leading to short stature, was initially treated with GH injections extracted from the pituitary glands of cadavers. Because cadavers were the only source, the availability of the treatment was limited. Additionally, several cases of Creutzfeldt-Jakob disease (a neurologic disturbance that progresses to coma and death, caused by encephalopathy)

secondary to an infectious agent in the GH put an end to this practice. Presently, synthetic human GH (rhGH), produced from recombinant DNA, is available. Although rhGH therapy is very expensive, it has been shown to be effective in treating children and adolescents with GH deficiencies. Somatropin (Humatrope) is the prototype rGH discussed in this chapter (see Table 50-5). Somatropin is produced by many pharmaceutical laboratories, and each preparation has a different trade name. They do not all share the same Food and Drug Administration (FDA) indications.

Nursing Management of the Patient Receiving P Somatropin
Core Drug Knowledge
Pharmacotherapeutics
Somatropin is a recombinant DNA formulation of GH (rGH) that has an amino acid sequence identical to that of pituitary-derived GH. It is used as long-term replacement

TABLE 50.5 Summary of Selected Pituitary Drugs

Drug (Trade) Name	Selected Indications	Route and Dosage Range
Growth Hormones		
P somatropin (Humatrope) Genotrope, Norditropin, Nutropin Omnitrope Saizen Serostim Tev-Tropin Zorbtive	Treatment of growth failure from growth-hormone deficiency or chronic renal failure (prior to transplant) Turner syndrome AIDS wasting syndrome Treatment (long-term) of growth failure in children Short stature of Turner syndrome (orphan use) Short-bowel syndrome	Dosing is dependent on specific type of growth hormone and on individual patient requirements.
Growth Hormone Antagonists		
octreotide acetate (Sandostatin)	Acromegaly (reduce growth hormone levels), severe diarrhea	*Adult*: SC, 50–600 mcg bid–qid *Child*: Safety and efficacy not established
bromocriptine mesylate (Parlodel)	Acromegaly Parkinson disease (idiopathic) Suppression of physiologic lactation following parturition Hyperprolactinemia	*Adult*: PO, 1.25–30 mg/d *Adult*: PO, 2.5–100 mg/d; efficacy for >2 y not established *Adult*: PO, 2.5 mg bid × 14–21 d *Adult*: PO, 5–10 mg/d
Posterior Pituitary Hormone Regulators		
desmopressin (DDAVP, Stimate*)	Neurogenic diabetes insipidus	*Adult:* Intranasal, 0.1–0.4 mL/d daily or bid, 1 spray (300 mg)/nostril; SC, IV, 0.5–1.0 mL/d bid; PO, 0.05 mg bid *Child, 3 mo–12 y:* Intranasal, 0.05–0.3 mL/d qd or bid, 1 spray (300 mg)/nostril; SC, IV, 0.5–1.0 mL/d bid; PO, 0.05 mg bid (*dosage adjusted according to water turnover pattern*)
	Primary nocturnal enuresis	*Adult and child >6 y:* Intranasal, 20–40 mcg at bedtime
Vasopressin (Pitressin)	Neurogenic diabetes insipidus Abdominal distention Antiflatulent effect for abdominal roentgenography	*Adult*: IM, SC, intranasal; 5–10 U repeated bid to tid *Adult*: IM, 5–10 U repeated q3–4h *Adult*: IM, SC, 10 U at 2 h and 10 U 30 min before procedure *Child*: Decrease dosage proportionately
	Ventricular fibrillation, ventricular tachycardia	*Adult*: IV, 40 U

therapy for children who have growth failure because of inadequate endogenous GH secretion and those with short stature caused by Turner syndrome. Somatropin stimulates linear growth in such patients, resulting in an increase in skeletal growth. Therefore, it is given for short stature only when the epiphyses are not closed. Somatropin is also indicated for use in patients with idiopathic short stature (non–GH-deficient short stature). The American Association of Clinical Endocrinologists and Growth Hormone Research Society defines short stature as height more than 2 standard deviations (SDs) below the mean for sex and age. Patients more than 2.25 SD below the mean for sex and age are treated with somatropin.

Pharmacokinetics
Somatropin is well absorbed and distributed. The absolute bioavailability of somatropin is 75% and 63% after subcutaneous (SC) and intramuscular (IM) administration, respectively. GH localizes to the liver and kidney. It is filtered by the glomerulus in the kidney, reabsorbed in the proximal tubule, and broken down within renal cells into amino acids. A portion of the breakdown products is returned to the systemic circulation. Intravenous (IV) somatropin has a mean half-life of 0.36 hours, whereas SC- and IM-administered somatropin doses have mean half-lives of 3.8 and 4.9 hours, respectively. The longer half-life of SC and IM administration is attributable to slower absorption from the injection site. The liver and kidney are the major elimination organs for exogenously administered GH. Caution must be used in administering somatropin to patients with severe hepatic and renal function because reduced clearance occurs.

Pharmacodynamics
Treatment with GH has powerful effects on growth and metabolism. It stimulates cell growth and cellular mitosis, facilitates cellular uptake of amino acids for protein synthesis, and promotes use of fatty acids for energy. These effects are caused indirectly by an increase in IGF-1, an intermediary peptide. In vitro and clinical testing has demonstrated that somatropin is equivalent therapeutically to GH of pituitary origin in adults.

Contraindications and Precautions
Somatropin is contraindicated for growth promotion in children with closed epiphyses. It is also contraindicated in patients with intracranial tumors until the antimalignancy treatment is completed. Somatropin is not indicated for patients with acute critical illness due to complications following open heart or abdominal surgery, multiple accidental trauma, or acute respiratory failure because of an increased risk of mortality with these conditions.

Pediatric patients with endocrine disorders, including GH deficiency, are more likely to develop slipped-capital epiphysis. For this reason, if a pediatric patient taking GH begins to limp or complain of hip or knee pain, the patient must be evaluated. Patients with a history of scoliosis who are being treated with GH are at elevated risk for developing more severe scoliosis, which occurs more frequently if rapid growth occurs. Patients with Turner syndrome have an increased risk of otitis media or hearing disorders. They are also at a greater risk for cardiovascular disorders (aortic aneurysm, stroke, and hypertension). Somatropin is a pregnancy category C drug. It should be given only when clearly needed because it is not known whether it can cause fetal harm or is excreted in breast milk. Cautious use also is advised in patients with diabetes because insulin resistance resulting in hyperglycemia may develop. Some product formulations contain diluent preservatives that may cause hypersensitivity.

Adverse Effects
Adverse effects with high-dose somatropin include headache, hypertension, joint and back pain, peripheral edema, muscle aches, and rhinitis. Many of these adverse effects occur initially and then resolve spontaneously or in response to dosage adjustments. Others include hypothyroidism, hyperglycemia, glycosuria, and pain at the injection site. Recurrent growth of an intracranial tumor also may occur. Leukemia has occurred in a small number of children receiving somatropin or somatrem, but its relation to therapy is uncertain.

A small percentage of patients (approximately 2%) may develop antibodies to the rGH protein molecule. However, GH antibody–binding capacities (2 mg/L) have not been associated with any growth reduction.

Drug Interactions
GH reduces the activity of hepatic mixed-function oxidases. This reduction may alter the metabolism of many drugs (Table 50.6). Glucocorticoid or other corticosteroid therapy may inhibit the growth-promoting effect of rGH. Patients with coexisting ACTH deficiency may need their glucocorticoid replacement dosages adjusted carefully to avoid an inhibitory effect on growth. Therefore, patients should be monitored closely if this combination must be used. Use of somatropin with anabolic steroids, androgens, estrogens, or thyroid hormones may accelerate epiphyseal maturation.

Assessment of Relevant Core Patient Variables
Health Status
Before administering somatropin, review the patient's record to determine whether it can be administered safely. A physical assessment establishes baseline data from which to monitor the effects of the drug. This assessment should include height and weight measurements, bone age determinations, thyroid function tests, blood glucose tests, and levels of GH. Monitor these data, and review them periodically during treatment. If the growth rate does not meet or exceed the pretreatment rate by at least 2 cm/y, consider nonadherence to therapy, antibody formation, malnutrition, or hypothyroidism as possible causes. X-rays of the hip and funduscopic examination are recommended before starting and periodically during the course of GH therapy.

TABLE 50.6 Agents That Interact with P Somatropin

Interactants	Effect and Significance	Nursing Management
Antiarrhythmics disopyramide dofetilide	Somatropin induces metabolism of antiarrhythmics.	Monitor antiarrhythmic drug levels. Monitor for cardiac arrhythmias. Discuss adjustment of antiarrhythmic drugs with health care provider.
anti-impotence drugs sildenafil tadalafil vardenafil	Somatropin induces metabolism of anti-impotence drugs.	Instruct patient of potential drug interaction.
antipsychotic drugs clozapine pimozide	Somatropin induces metabolism of some antipsychotic drugs.	Monitor antipsychotic drug levels. Monitor for psychotic symptoms. Discuss adjustment of antipsychotic drugs with health care provider.
antiseizure drugs carbamazepine felbamate tiagabine	Somatropin induces metabolism of some antiseizure drugs.	Monitor for seizure activity. Ensure safety. Monitor antiseizure drug levels. Discuss adjustment of antiseizure drugs with health care provider.
corticosteroids	Corticosteroids have antagonistic effect on GH.	Monitor GH levels. Monitor for efficacy of GH. Discuss adjustment of GH with health care provider.
Hormones oral contraceptives hormone replacement testosterone	Somatropin induces metabolism of certain hormones.	Advise patient to use other form of birth control. Monitor for signs of estrogen deficiency. Monitor for signs of testosterone deficiency. Discuss adjustment of hormonal drugs with health care provider.
hypoglycemic drugs acarbose insulins metformin meglitinides nateglinide repaglinide sitagliptin sulfonylureas thiazolidinediones	Somatropin induces metabolism of many oral and parenteral hypoglycemic drugs.	Monitor blood glucose. Monitor Hb A$_{1c}$. Monitor for signs of hyperglycemia. Discuss adjustment of hypoglycemic drugs with health care provider.
Immunosuppressants cyclosporine sirolimus tacrolimus	Somatropin induces metabolism of some immunosuppressant drugs.	Monitor for signs of transplant rejection. Monitor immunosuppressant drug levels. Discuss adjustment of immunosuppressant drugs with health care provider.
methadone	Somatropin induces metabolism of methadone.	Monitor for pain. Monitor for opioid withdrawal. Discuss adjustment of methadone with health care provider.
warfarin	Somatropin induces metabolism of warfarin	Monitor PT/INR. Monitor for signs of thromboembolism. Discuss adjustment of warfarin with health care provider.

Observe patients with diabetes or glucose intolerance closely during somatropin therapy. Evaluate individuals with GH deficiency secondary to an intracranial lesion regularly for progression or recurrence of the underlying disease process. Assess individuals routinely for any malignant transformation of skin lesions. Monitor those with growth failure secondary to chronic renal insufficiency regularly for progression of renal osteodystrophy progression, because slipped capital femoral epiphysis or avascular necrosis of the femoral head may be seen in children with advanced renal osteodystrophy. Whether these problems are affected by GH therapy is uncertain. Examine the injection site for pain and swelling.

Life Span and Gender

It is important to assess whether the patient is pregnant or breast-feeding. Somatropin is classified in pregnancy category C and should be given to a pregnant or lactating woman only if use is clearly indicated. It is not known whether somatropin is excreted in breast milk. Available data suggest that rGH clearances are similar in adults and children. Treatment with GH requires a long-term regimen. Children receiving this drug need continual monitoring, and once therapy has begun, measure and record the patient's height and weight at regular intervals. Question pediatric patients about hip or knee pain at each visit.

Lifestyle, Diet, and Habits

Adherence to the drug regimen is imperative; therefore, evaluating the patient's ability and willingness to adhere is important. Actual somatropin dosage is individualized to each patient. SC injections each evening are most effective because nightly injections mimic the natural hormone surge that occurs after sleep. Stimulation of growth is most effective when treatment begins early and injections are continued until the epiphyses close. Response to treatment tends to decrease with time.

Environment

Assess the setting in which somatropin will be administered, the ability of the patient or caregiver to administer the drug properly, and the patient's and family's financial situation. Most often, it is necessary to instruct the patient or caregiver in the proper way to reconstitute and administer the medication according to the manufacturer's instructions because it is frequently given in the home. Also, tell the patient to refrigerate the drug following reconstitution. The drug is very expensive, and some insurance companies resist covering the cost of treatment. In such cases, sources of financial support may have to be solicited. Health care visits are decreased if parents or caregivers administer the injections, but regular visits to the physician must still occur to monitor blood and urine samples, make bone age determinations, and track growth rate. Regular follow-up health care is necessary.

Nursing Diagnoses and Outcomes

- Delayed Growth and Development related to deficiency of GH secretion
  Desired outcome: The patient will demonstrate an increase in linear growth.
- Imbalanced Nutrition: More (or Less) than Body Requirements, related to endocrine changes and rapid changes in height and weight
  Desired outcome: The patient will receive adequate nutrition for growth appropriate to age and need.
- Impaired Tissue Integrity related to pain and swelling at injection site
  Desired outcome: The patient will not experience pain and swelling at the injection site.
- Altered Comfort related to headache, joint, and muscle discomfort secondary to somatropin effects
  Desired outcome: The patient will describe measures to improve comfort.

Planning and Intervention

Maximizing Therapeutic Effects

Hypothyroidism may develop during somatropin therapy and, if untreated, may prevent an optimal response. For this reason, it is essential to perform periodic thyroid function tests and initiate thyroid hormone replacement therapy if indicated. Glucocorticoid replacement dosage must be carefully adjusted in patients with coexisting ACTH deficiency to avoid an inhibitory effect on growth. Inform patients who require dialysis in a daytime ambulatory setting of the need to take their doses before bedtime. Patients who require chronic cycling peritoneal dialysis should receive their doses of somatropin in the morning, after the dialysis is completed.

Minimizing Adverse Effects

GH therapy may induce insulin resistance; thus, it is important to monitor the patient closely for glucose intolerance. Children being treated with rGH for growth failure secondary to chronic renal insufficiency may develop problems of renal osteodystrophy (generalized bone changes resembling osteomalacia and rickets). Slipped capital femoral epiphyses or avascular necrosis of the femoral head can also occur in these patients. Although it is uncertain whether these problems are a direct result of GH therapy, x-rays of the hip should be obtained before initiating GH therapy. Be alert for the development of a limp or complaints of hip or knee pain, and tell parents to do the same. Slipped capital femoral epiphysis may occur more frequently in patients with endocrine disorders or in patients undergoing rapid growth. Pain and discomfort related to headache, bone, and muscle discomfort can be treated with appropriate analgesics and environmental controls.

Sudden growth spurts and changes in growth and development, coupled with potential thyroid changes and insulin resistance, may cause nutritional imbalance that can complicate the desired effect of the GH. Consider nutritional assessment and appropriate replacement of necessary nutrients.

Providing Patient and Family Education

- Explain that this drug is replacing an important hormone (GH) that is necessary for normal growth and development.
- Explain to patients and their families that the drug can be given only by injection. Teach patients, family members, or caregivers how to reconstitute and administer the drug. Review injection site rotation to maximize therapeutic effect and avoid problems of lipodystrophy. Periodic review of injection technique is important to ensure effectiveness and decrease adverse effects.
- Instruct patients to refrigerate the reconstituted solution. Vials are stable for up to 14 days if reconstituted with diluent or bacteriostatic water for injection. If sterile water is used, only one dose of somatropin can be used, and the unused portion must be discarded.

• Alert patients with diabetes to the fact that insulin resistance may develop. Instruct these patients to monitor blood sugar closely and to report variations to their health care team.

• Instruct patients or their families to report any adverse drug effects and emphasize the importance of reporting a limp or any hip or knee pain as soon as possible. Slipped capital femoral epiphysis may occur more frequently in patients with endocrine disorders or in patients undergoing rapid growth.

Ongoing Assessment and Evaluation

In patients taking somatropin, evaluate thyroid function at regular intervals because hypothyroidism compromises rGH drug effects. Additionally, it is important to be alert for signs of glucose intolerance because insulin resistance may develop and disrupt diabetes control. As with all protein pharmaceuticals, a small percentage of patients may develop antibodies to the protein. Evaluate adherence to the prescribed treatment program, assess thyroid status, and test for GH antibodies in any patient who fails to respond to therapy. Stress the importance of follow-up appointments and periodic analysis of thyroid function, glucose tolerance, and GH levels to evaluate the effectiveness of the drug and possible development of adverse effects. Therapy is considered effective when anticipated growth occurs. The patient and family should demonstrate appropriate drug administration technique, acknowledge the importance of monitoring for adverse effects, and show understanding of when to report findings to the health care team (Box 50.2).

BOX 50.2 COMMUNITY BASED CONCERNS

Children Receiving Growth Hormone (somatropin)

As a nurse educating patients and families about the use of growth hormone (GH) therapy, you should include the following information:

• GH is indicated for children with inadequate endogenous GH secretion and for those with short stature caused by Turner syndrome.
• GH is not clearly indicated for children who are born to a short family but whose parents want them to be taller.
• GH is not indicated for children with closed epiphyses.
• GH therapy requires long-term commitment from the patient; treatment generally lasts 3 to 9 years.
• Although GH may be covered in part by insurance, the cost of treatment can be as much as $50,000 annually.
• GH is given as a daily SC injection, usually in the evening, because this timing mimics the natural hormone surge that occurs after sleep.
• Parents or other caregivers are taught how to administer the injections, but regular physician visits are mandatory during treatment to monitor bone age determinations, growth rate, and blood and urine samples.
• Insulin resistance may develop in a diabetic patient taking GH; therefore, blood sugar in these patients must be closely monitored.

Drugs Closely Related to P Somatropin

Other Somatropin Preparations

Commercially available drug preparations of somatropin include Genotropin, Genotropin MiniQuick, Norditropin, Nutropin, Omnitrope, Saizen, Serostim, Tev-Tropin, and Zorbtive. Most are powders that need reconstitution. They differ in the amounts of rGH international units contained in the vial, whether vials are single or multiple dose, what diluents are used (some diluents are preservative free), and FDA-approved indications.

Genotropin is approved for use in both children and adults with GH deficiency. It is also approved for long-term management of growth failure in pediatric patients born small for gestational age who fail to complete "catch-up growth" by 2 years of age, and those with growth failure due to Prader-Willi syndrome. This syndrome is a complex genetic disorder that includes short stature, incomplete sexual development, mental retardation or learning disabilities, behavior problems, low muscle tone, and an involuntary urge to eat constantly, which leads to obesity.

Nutropin is indicated for long-term treatment of growth failure stemming from inadequate endogenous GH secretion, for growth failure associated with chronic renal insufficiency (until renal transplant), idiopathic short stature and for short stature related to the chromosomal disorder, Turner syndrome. Turner syndrome exclusively affects females and is characterized in part by short stature and incomplete sexual development. Nutropin is also indicated for adults with growth hormone deficiency who developed GH deficiency as a result of pituitary disease, hypothalamic disease, surgery, radiation, or trauma.

Serostim is indicated for concomitant use with antiviral therapy for HIV-associated cachexia (wasting syndrome) to increase lean muscle mass and body weight. Serostim is in pregnancy category B.

MEMORY CHIP

P Somatropin

• Genetically engineered (recombinant DNA) human growth hormone used for long-term treatment of children with deficient endogenous growth hormone
• Major contraindications: closed epiphyses and cranial lesions
• Most common adverse effects: joint and muscle pain
• Most serious adverse effects: development of antibodies to growth hormone, hypothyroidism, and insulin resistance
• Maximizing therapeutic effects: Reconstitute drug according to manufacturer's directions.
• Minimizing adverse effects: periodic testing of glucose tolerance, thyroid function, and presence of growth hormone antibodies
• Most important patient education: proper preparation and storage of medication; proper SC or IM injection technique

Zorbtive is approved for use in patients with short-bowel syndrome receiving specialized nutritional support.

Norditropin, Tev-Tropin, and Saizen are used for the long-term treatment of children with inadequate endogenous GH secretion. Omnitrope is used in both children and adults with GH deficiency.

Sermorelin Acetate

Sermorelin acetate (Geref) is another drug used in the diagnosis and management of GH deficiency. It is also known as growth-releasing hormone and GHRH. Sermorelin directly stimulates the pituitary gland to release GH. It is given cautiously in patients with growth deficiency due to intracranial lesions and those older than 65 years of age. Adverse effects to sermorelin include injection site reactions, flushing, and antibody development. Sermorelin is a pregnancy category C drug and is not recommended for women who breast-feed.

Drugs Significantly Different From
P Somatropin

GH antagonists decrease GH secretion. Almost all conditions of GH hypersecretion are caused by pituitary tumors and are usually treated by radiation therapy or surgery. Pharmacotherapy for GH excess includes two groups of drugs: the somatostatin analogues (octreotide acetate) and the dopamine agonists (bromocriptine) (see Table 50.5). Hypothalamic somatostatin (from the hypothalamus) is an effective GH inhibitor, but it is rarely used because of its short initial half-life (1 to 3 minutes) and its multiple effects on many secretory systems (e.g., it inhibits the release of gastrin, glucagon, insulin).

Octreotide Acetate

Octreotide acetate (Sandostatin) is a more potent inhibitor than somatostatin of growth hormone, insulin, and glucagon. It also suppresses LH response to GnRH (gonadotropin-releasing factor), inhibits the release of serotonin, gastrin, and pancreatic polypeptide, and decreases visceral blood flow and the secretion of TSH. Octreotide is highly effective in treating both children and adults with excess GH, and it has replaced bromocriptine as the most commonly used agent for acromegaly. It is indicated to reduce GH blood levels and IGF-1 (somatomedin C) levels in patients with acromegaly, who either cannot be treated surgically or have an inadequate response to surgery or irradiation of the pituitary. The goal of treatment is to reduce blood levels of GH and IGF-1. GH is reduced to normal ranges in 50% of patients treated with octreotide acetate; IGF-1 is reduced to normal ranges in 50% to -60% of patients. Adjunctive therapy with octreotide acetate is beneficial for patients who have been treated with pituitary irradiation, as it takes several years for the maximal benefit of this treatment to be realized.

Other indications for octreotide include treating diarrhea and flushing symptoms associated with metastatic carcinoid tumors and profuse and watery diarrhea that can occur with vasoactive intestinal peptide tumors (VIPomas) as well as esophageal varices. In single doses, the drug has been shown to decrease bile secretion and to inhibit gallbladder contractility in normal volunteers. Those with acromegaly have an increased incidence of biliary tract abnormalities if this medication is used for extended periods of time (one year or longer). Off-label uses include AIDS-associated diarrhea, breast cancer, insulinomas, small bowel fistulas, Cushing syndrome, dumping syndrome after gastrectomy, and graft-versus-host disease–induced diarrhea.

The elimination half-life of octreotide from the plasma is 1.7 hours, with approximately 32% of the dose excreted unchanged in the urine. During clinical trials in elderly patients there was a significant increase in the half-life of the drug (46%) and a significant decrease in clearance (26%); therefore, dose adjustment may be necessary in these patients. In patients with severe renal failure requiring dialysis, octreotide half-life is increased, which also necessitates adjusting the maintenance dose.

Individuals with acromegaly may experience either hypoglycemia (3%) or hyperglycemia (16%) during octreotide therapy. This effect may result in overt diabetes mellitus or require dosage changes for insulin or other hypoglycemic agents.

Adverse effects of octreotide include GI discomfort (diarrhea, loose stools, abdominal discomfort, and nausea), headache, and sinus bradycardia or other cardiac arrhythmias. Decreased glucose tolerance may also occur. Octreotide therapy may cause acute cholecystitis, cholestatic jaundice, biliary tract obstruction, or pancreatitis. More frequently, it causes cholelithiasis in patients requiring therapy for 12 months or more. Dietary fat absorption may be altered in some patients. Periodic fecal fat and serum carotene determinations should be performed to help assess possible drug-induced fat malabsorption. It is vital to stress the importance of reporting icterus (jaundice), dark urine, or clay-colored stools to the health care team immediately, as well as any abdominal pain, edema, chest pain, shortness of breath, or fainting.

When octreotide is administered concomitantly with cyclosporine, it may decrease blood levels of cyclosporine and cause rejection of transplanted organs. Octreotide is associated with alterations in nutrient absorption and may have an effect on oral medications. Drug and food interactions include altered absorption of dietary fats, decreased vitamin B_{12} levels, and abnormal Schilling test results. (The Schilling test is done to diagnose pernicious anemia.)

For prolonged storage, unused octreotide should be protected from light and stored in the refrigerator. If refrigerated, the solution should be allowed to warm to room temperature before administration. At room temperature, octreotide is stable for 14 days if protected from light. Octreotide is usually administered subcutaneously but can also be delivered through a continuous subcutaneous infusion. Because it is most often given subcutaneously, the patient and family should be taught details of sterile technique, injection-site rotation, and signs of infection for which to watch. The patient receiving octreotide therapy requires long-term follow-up and regular evaluation for signs of acromegaly and other endocrine dysfunction (e.g., thyroid or insulin resistance), which may require dosage adjustment. The importance of regular follow-up visits with the health care provider should be emphasized. Responsiveness to octreotide therapy may be evaluated by assessing GH and IGF-1 serum levels.

Bromocriptine Mesylate

Bromocriptine mesylate (Parlodel) is a semisynthetic ergot alkaloid that inhibits prolactin secretion. In the majority of patients with acromegaly, it also lowers elevated blood levels of GH. It can be used alone or as an adjunct to irradiation. In some children, bromocriptine and octreotide used in combination have proved successful. Bromocriptine, a dopamine receptor agonist, is also used to treat Parkinson disease, prolactin-secreting adenomas and dysfunctions associated with hyperprolactinemia including infertility, amenorrhea, and hypogonadism. Dopamine agonists inhibit GH secretion in some patients with acromegaly, although the opposite effect occurs in healthy individuals. Dopamine increases somatostatin release from the hypothalamus. This effect may explain the GH-inhibiting properties of bromocriptine. Off-label uses for bromocriptine include treating neuroleptic malignant syndrome, cocaine addiction, and cyclical mastalgia (pain in the breast). Bromocriptine is administered orally. It has a substantial hepatic first-pass effect; 28% of an oral dose is absorbed from the GI tract. Bromocriptine undergoes first-pass metabolism, and only a small percentage (6%) of the absorbed dose reaches the systemic circulation unchanged. Plasma half-life is 6 to 8 hours. Bromocriptine is highly bound (90% to 96%) to serum albumin and is metabolized in the liver before being excreted in the feces and urine. The most common adverse reactions include nausea, headache, dizziness, drowsiness, and fatigue, but serious reactions including seizures, stroke, hallucination, and syncope have also been reported. Contraindications include sensitivity to ergot alkaloids, severe ischemic heart disease, or peripheral vascular disease. This medication is pregnancy category B.

Pegvisomant

Pegvisomant (Somavert) is a genetically engineered GH receptor antagonist that has selective affinity for the GH receptor. It reduces IGF-1 levels and improves the clinical symptoms of GH excess. Pegvisomant is considered second-line treatment. It is given as a subcutaneous injection once a day. Pegvisomant is given cautiously to patients with pre-existing hepatic dysfunction, diabetes mellitus, and those over the age of 65 (clinical studies did not include enough subjects over 65 to determine whether they react differently to this medication than younger subjects). It is a pregnancy category B drug and is not approved for use in children. Patients receiving pegvisomant need baseline hepatic function tests prior to initiation of therapy and

periodically thereafter because it may cause hepatotoxicity. Patients with a history of diabetes mellitus require determination of the baseline hemoglobin A_{1C} level and close monitoring of blood glucose levels. Adverse effects include injection site reactions, chest pain, hypertension, and peripheral edema.

C POSTERIOR PITUITARY HORMONE REGULATORS

The posterior pituitary stores two hormones that are produced in the hypothalamus: vasopressin (also known as ADH), which controls the concentration of body fluids; and oxytocin, which stimulates uterine contractions and causes the milk let-down reflex.

Desmopressin and vasopressin are synthetic analogues of the naturally occurring posterior pituitary hormone, vasopressin, that are used to treat DI. In pharmacologic doses, oxytocin can be used to induce or improve uterine contractions during labor. Oxytocin is discussed in depth in Chapter 52. The prototype posterior pituitary hormone is desmopressin acetate (see Table 50.5). It is the preferred treatment for most individuals with chronic DI because it has a longer duration of action, a more specific antidiuretic action, and an antidiuretic-to-pressor ratio significantly greater than that of vasopressin.

Nursing Management of the Patient Receiving P Desmopressin

Core Drug Knowledge

Pharmacotherapeutics

Desmopressin (DDAVP, Stimate, Minirin) may be administered intranasally, orally, or parenterally (IV or SC route) to manage central DI and for temporary polyuria and polydipsia following surgery in the pituitary region or head trauma. Primary nocturnal enuresis and episodes of spontaneous or trauma-induced bleeding are also effectively managed with intranasal desmopressin. Parenteral desmopressin maintains homeostasis in hemophilia A and von Willebrand disease (type I). It is ineffective for treating nephrogenic DI.

An off-label use for intranasal desmopressin is treating chronic autonomic failure characterized by nocturnal polyuria, morning postural hypotension, and overnight weight loss. Individualized dosage is necessary to maintain normal urine volume.

Pharmacokinetics

Desmopressin provides prompt onset of antidiuretic action with a long duration after administration because it has biphasic half-lives of 7.8 and 75.5 minutes for the fast and slow phases, respectively. The injectable form has an antidiuretic effect 10 times that of an equivalent dose of intranasal desmopressin. The half-life of the nasal spray is approximately 3.5 hours. Plasma concentrations of the nasal spray are highest 40 to 45 minutes after dosing. Desmopressin is metabolized rapidly by the liver and excreted by the kidneys.

Pharmacodynamics

The naturally occurring posterior pituitary hormone, vasopressin (ADH), and its synthetic analogue (desmopressin) interact with V1 and V2 receptors. V1 receptors have a pressor response, whereas V2 receptors have both an antidiuretic and hemostatic response. General vasoconstriction by smooth muscle contraction of most blood vessels occurs with the binding of the V1 receptors. At higher concentrations, ADH interacts with these receptors. This vasoconstriction is marked in the portal vessels, somewhat less in cerebral, coronary, peripheral, and pulmonary vessels, and slightly in intrahepatic vessels. GI motility and tone are also enhanced. V2 receptors are found on renal tubule cells. They mediate antidiuresis by stimulating the increase of water permeability and resorption in the renal collecting tubules. Release of and increase in circulating levels of factor VIII and von Willebrand factor occur with the binding of the V2 receptors. These proteins are involved in blood coagulation.

Contraindications and Precautions

The only contraindication to desmopressin use is hypersensitivity. Intranasal delivery may be inappropriate if the patient has an impaired level of consciousness. Use with caution in patients with coronary artery insufficiency or those who are hypertensive because high intranasal doses of desmopressin may elevate the blood pressure slightly. Caution should also be used in patients who are predisposed to thrombus formation, because of reports of thrombotic events, such as thrombosis, acute cerebrovascular thrombosis, or myocardial infarction (MI), although such reports are rare. Use with caution in patients with conditions associated with fluid and electrolyte imbalance, such as cystic fibrosis or renal or cardiovascular diseases, because these patients are especially prone to hyponatremia. When administered to either pediatric or geriatric individuals, fluid intake should be adjusted downward to limit the risk of hyponatremia and water intoxication.

Desmopressin is in pregnancy category B.

Adverse Effects

Most adverse effects of desmopressin are mediated through the V1 receptor acting on vascular and GI smooth muscle. Adverse reactions are mild and infrequent and are often resolved with dosage reduction. Possible reactions for intranasal or parenteral administration include mild abdominal pain and cramps, transient headache, nasal congestion, nausea, rhinitis, and facial flushing. Injection of desmopressin is associated with local erythema, burning, pain, or swelling. Changes in blood pressure (either a slight elevation or a transient fall) with a compensatory heart rate increase have also been reported infrequently. Oral administration of tablets for 12 to 44 months has shown a transient increase in aspartate aminotransferase (AST); however, the elevated AST returned to normal range despite continued use of the medication. The major

V2 receptor–mediated adverse effect is water intoxication. Rare severe allergic reactions have been reported with desmopressin.

Drug Interactions

Although desmopressin pressor activity is very low, large intranasal or parenteral doses (greater than 0.3 mcg/kg) should be used cautiously with other pressor agents because of the potential for additive or synergistic effects. Carbamazepine, chlorpromazine, and nonsteroidal anti-inflammatory drugs (NSAIDs) enhance the antidiuretic response to vasopressin; thus, these drugs may potentiate the effects of desmopressin.

Assessment of Relevant Core Patient Variables

Health Status

Assess for pre-existing health conditions that require cautious use of desmopressin. Perform a baseline assessment, including measurements of weight, serum and urine osmolality, and serum sodium to allow determination of the effectiveness of the drug. Careful monitoring for cardiac reactions during desmopressin treatment is also important. Posterior pituitary agonists should be used with caution in patients with vascular disease, especially coronary artery disease, because changes in blood pressure can occur. Desmopressin should also be used cautiously in patients with conditions associated with fluid and electrolyte imbalances, such as cystic fibrosis, because these patients are prone to hyponatremia and water intoxication while taking this drug. Early signs include confusion, drowsiness, listlessness, and headache.

Life Span and Gender

Determine whether the patient is pregnant or breast-feeding. Desmopressin is a pregnancy category B medication. Although there are several publications describing the use of desmopressin to manage diabetes insipidus during pregnancy, no adequate and well-controlled studies have determined its safety and efficacy for use during pregnancy and lactation. It is unknown whether this drug is excreted in human milk. Thus, use in pregnancy and lactation should occur only when the potential benefits outweigh the potential hazards to the fetus or infant.

Clinical trials have demonstrated that desmopressin is an effective agent in both adults and children and has few side effects. Safety and efficacy of parenteral desmopressin in children (less than 12 years of age) or intranasal desmopressin in infants (less than 3 months of age) have not been established. Infants and children require careful fluid intake restriction to prevent possible hyponatremia and water intoxication, which can cause seizures.

Lifestyle, Diet, and Habits and Environment

Assess the patient's lifestyle in terms of work, rest patterns, leisure activities, and use of social or recreational drugs. Decreased plasma volume, pain, stress, sleep, exercise, and use of certain drugs (e.g., barbiturates, nicotine, morphine, and vincristine) are all factors that stimulate the secretion of ADH.

Nursing Diagnoses and Outcomes

- Risk for Fluid Volume Excess related to administration of desmopressin, secondary to diabetes insipidus
  Desired outcome: The patient will not demonstrate signs and symptoms of water intoxication and will maintain urine specific gravity within a normal range.
- Risk for Ineffective Therapeutic Regimen Management related to lack of knowledge of diabetes insipidus, disease management, and signs and symptoms of complications
  Desired outcome: The patient will describe the disease process, causes, and factors contributing to symptoms and the regimen for disease or symptom control, relate intent to practice health behaviors needed or desired to control disease and prevent complications, and report less anxiety from fear of the unknown and loss of control.

Planning and Intervention

Maximizing Therapeutic Effects

Establish baseline values for weight, blood pressure, electrolytes, and urine specific gravity. Individualize the dosage of desmopressin according to the diurnal pattern of water elimination, control of nocturia, and adequate duration of sleep. During long-term therapy, periodically assess the condition of nasal passages. Inappropriate administration may lead to nasal ulceration and, as a consequence, subsequent administered doses may be inadequate.

Protect ADH solutions from agitation and temperature extremes (excessive heat or freezing). To maintain potency, it is important to refrigerate nasal and parenteral solutions of desmopressin.

Minimizing Adverse Effects

Assess the patient for pre-existing cardiovascular or renal disorders and monitor patients carefully for cardiac reactions from desmopressin. The very young and elderly require careful fluid intake restriction to prevent possible water intoxication and hyponatremia. Limit fluid intake 1 hour before and 8 hours after the dose. Desmopressin therapy should be temporarily interrupted during acute illness, febrile episodes, hot days and other conditions that require increased water intake.

When administering the drug by IV infusion, ensure patency of venous access, preferably in a large vein, and use an infusion-control device. This precaution decreases the chance of extravasation.

Providing Patient and Family Education

- Provide information about antidiuretic drugs, including action, use, adverse effects, and drug interactions that may occur. Emphasize to patients and families that sudden changes in weight, pulse rate, and blood pressure may indicate serious fluid imbalance.
- Alcohol can alter the therapeutic response to desmopressin. Caution patients against consuming alcohol during therapy. Many over-the-counter (OTC) products contain alcohol, so it is important to discuss the need to read drug labels before taking any OTC medications. Also, advise patients to carry appropriate medical identification to alert medical personnel in case of an emergency.
- Review with patients and families or caregivers the proper administration technique for nasally administered dosage forms. Intranasal preparations are administered through a flexible nasal catheter that measures the appropriate dose. After the drug is drawn into the catheter, one end is placed in the mouth and the other end in the nose. Patients should then blow into the catheter to deposit the drug into the nasal passageways. Proper technique lessens nasal irritation that may occur. Nasal congestion may impair absorption when desmopressin is administered intranasally.
- Stress the importance of taking desmopressin as directed and to consult the health care provider before discontinuing its use.

Ongoing Assessment and Evaluation

Instruct patients taking desmopressin to monitor urine specific gravity and intake and output as well as to weigh themselves daily to determine drug efficacy. Decreased urine output and thirst are signs of therapeutic drug response. If desmopressin is being used for abdominal distention, it is important to assess bowel sounds and the presence or absence of flatus. During prolonged therapy, electrocardiographic (ECG) studies should be monitored as well as fluid and electrolyte status.

MEMORY CHIP

P Desmopressin

- Synthetic analogue of human ADH; for treatment of neurogenic diabetes insipidus
- Major contraindication: presence of hemophilia A with factor VIII levels 5% or less
- Most common adverse effects: localized erythema with intranasal administration; burning pain with parenteral injection
- **Life span alert: Infants, children, and the elderly require careful fluid intake restriction to prevent possible hypo-natremia and water intoxication.**
- Maximizing therapeutic effects: Keep solutions (nasal, parenteral) refrigerated.
- Minimizing adverse effects: Monitor urine volume/osmolality, plasma osmolality; patients with conditions associated with fluid/electrolyte imbalances are prone to hyponatremia.
- Most important patient education: Inform patients that medication bottle accurately delivers 25 to 50 doses and any solution remaining after 25 to 50 doses should be discarded because the amount delivered thereafter may be substantially less than prescribed. The remaining solution should not be transferred to another bottle.

Drug Closely Related to 🅿 Desmopressin Vasopressin

Synthetic vasopressin (Pitressin) is effective for treating DI resulting from a partial or complete deficiency in production and secretion of posterior pituitary ADH. It also may be used to prevent or treat postoperative abdominal distention and to facilitate abdominal radiography. According to the American Heart Association Advanced Cardiac Life Support Guidelines (AHA, 2005) a single dose of vasopressin (40 units IV) may be used to replace the first or second dose of epinephrine in the management of pulseless ventricular tachycardia or ventricular fibrillation.

An off-label use of vasopressin is managing bleeding esophageal varices. Following SC, IM, or IV injection, synthetic vasopressin aqueous solution has a plasma half-life of 10 to 20 minutes. The duration of antidiuretic activity is 2 to 8 hours. Vasopressin is metabolized rapidly by the liver and is excreted by the kidneys.

Use of vasopressin is contraindicated in patients with hypersensitivity or chronic nephritis with increased levels of blood urea nitrogen (BUN). Vasopressin is in pregnancy category C. Its effect on lactation is unknown. The literature reports that vasopressin, when used during pregnancy in doses sufficient for an antidiuretic effect, is not likely to produce tonic uterine contractions that could be harmful to the fetus or threaten the continuation of the pregnancy.

THYROID DRUGS

Thyroid hormones influence essentially every organ system in the body. They have numerous biological effects, including stimulation of the basal metabolic rate, which affects protein, carbohydrate, and lipid metabolism. Thyroid hormones are essential for normal growth and development throughout the entire life cycle. Like most endocrine glands, the thyroid glands can secrete too much hormone (hyperthyroidism) or too little hormone (hypothyroidism).

Thyroid disorders involve an alteration in the quantity of thyroid hormone secretion, enlargement of the thyroid gland (goiter), or both and are classified as either hyperthyroidism or hypothyroidism.

The prevalences of hyperthyroidism (thyrotoxicosis) and hypothyroidism are similar—approximately 2% of women and 0.2% of men are affected. Increasing age is associated with an increase in the incidence of hypothyroidism. Six percent of women and 2.5% of men older than 60 years have TSH levels greater than twice the upper limit of normal. Hypothyroidism may be mistaken for the normal aging process.

🅒 THYROID HORMONES

The only treatment for hypothyroidism is lifelong replacement of thyroid hormones that are adequate to meet the individual's metabolic needs. A number of pharmacologic preparations of endogenous thyroid hormone, including levothyroxine, desiccated thyroid, liothyronine sodium, and liotrix can completely correct hypothyroidism. The preferred treatment, and prototype drug, for hypothyroidism is levothyroxine (T_4; Levothroid, Synthroid), and it is used almost universally. Table 50.7 presents a summary of selected thyroid hormones.

Nursing Management of the Patient Receiving 🅿 Levothyroxine

Core Drug Knowledge

Pharmacotherapeutics

Levothyroxine is used as replacement therapy in hypothyroidism of any etiology, except transient hypothyroidism during

TABLE 50.7	Summary of Selected 🅒 Thyroid Hormones		
Drug (Trade) Name	Selected Indications	Route and Dosage Range	Pharmacokinetics
🅿 levothyroxine (T_4 L-thyroxine; Synthroid, Levothroid)	Replacement therapy for hypothyroidism, including cretinism	*Adult:* PO, 50–200 mcg/d *Child:* PO, 0–6 mo, 8–10 mcg/kg/d; 6–12 mo, 6–8 mcg/ kg/d; 1–5 y, 5–6 mcg/kg/d; 6–12 y, 4–5 mcg/kg/d; >12 y, 2–3 mcg/kg/d	*Onset:* Slow *Duration:* 3 wk $t_{1/2}$: 2–7 d
	Emergency treatment of myxedema coma	*Adult:* IV, 400 mcg initially	
liothyronine (T3; Cytomel, Triostat)	Same as above	*Adult:* PO, 25 mcg/d; increase q1–2wk by 12.5–25 mcg; maintenance, 25–75 mcg/d *Child (and elderly adult):* PO, 5–50 mcg/d	*Onset:* Varies *Duration:* 3–4 d $t_{1/2}$: 1–2 d
liotrix (T4 and T3; Thyrolar)	Same as above	*Adult:* PO, 15–30 mg/d; increase q2wk to maximum of 60–120 mg/d	*Onset:* Slow *Duration:* 3 wk $t_{1/2}$: 2–7 d
thyroid desiccated (T3 and T4; Armour Thyroid)	Same as above	*Adult:* PO, 300 mg/d initially; increase by 15 mg q2–3wk; maintenance, 60–120 mg/d *Child:* PO, 1.2–6 mg/kg/d, depending on age	*Onset:* Slow *Duration:* 3 wk $t_{1/2}$: 2–7 d

the acute phase of subacute thyroiditis. It also can be used for pituitary suppression of TSH in treating and preventing euthyroid goiter, in managing hypothyroidism secondary to thyroid cancer, and in treating **myxedema coma.** Levothyroxine also may be used in conjunction with antithyroid drugs to treat thyrotoxicosis and to prevent goiter formation, hypothyroidism, and thyrotoxicosis during pregnancy.

Pharmacokinetics
The absorption of levothyroxine from the GI tract varies from 48% to 79% of the administered dose. Absorption is increased during fasting states. Excessive fecal loss has been found with malabsorption syndromes. Levothyroxine must be converted to T_3 for its clinical effects. When the drug is taken orally, the onset of effect occurs very slowly, with the peak effect occurring in 1 to 3 weeks. When the drug is administered intravenously to treat myxedema, the onset of effect is 6 to 8 hours, with a peak effect in 24 to 48 hours. Levothyroxine has a half-life of 6 to 7 days. Levothyroxine is metabolized in the liver and excreted in the bile. It crosses the placenta and enters breast milk.

Pharmacodynamics
Levothyroxine acts as a replacement for natural thyroid hormone. Increased oxygen consumption, respiration, heart rate, growth and maturation, and speed of fat, protein, and carbohydrate metabolism occur secondary to increases in the basal metabolic rate.

Contraindications and Precautions
Contraindications include hypersensitivity, thyrotoxicosis uncomplicated by hypothyroidism, acute MI complicated by hypothyroidism or in patients with uncorrected adrenal insufficiency. The metabolic stimulating effects of levothyroxine could worsen the MI, cause arrhythmias, and lead to further complications and thyroid hormones may precipitate an acute adrenal crisis.

Levothyroxine is a pregnancy category A drug. It is safe for maintaining and regulating thyroid function during pregnancy but should be used with caution in lactating women because it crosses into breast milk and can affect the infant's thyroid-pituitary balance. Levothyroxine should also be used with caution in patients with coronary artery disease or coronary insufficiency because the resulting increase in basal metabolic rate may aggravate angina pectoris caused by the increased myocardial oxygen demand. Use of levothyroxine in cardiovascular disease should be initiated at a low dosage and titrated upward gradually. Its use in patients with concomitant DI, diabetes mellitus, or adrenal insufficiency (Addison disease) exacerbates the intensity of their symptoms. An appropriate adjustment in therapy for these concomitant diseases is necessary. For individuals with myxedema, it is necessary to begin treatment at low doses with gradual increases, because they are particularly sensitive to thyroid preparations.

Adverse Effects
Adverse effects observed with the use of levothyroxine are related to therapeutic overdosage. These include hypertension, tachycardia, arrhythmias, anxiety, headache, nervousness, GI irritation, sweating, and heat intolerance. Long-term use in women has been shown to lead to increased bone resorption and decreased bone density. Patients with sensitivity to lactose may show intolerance because lactose is used in the manufacture of this product. There is no well-documented evidence of allergic reactions to thyroid hormones. In children, partial hair loss may occur in the first few months of therapy. There is a black box warning that levothyroxine is not appropriate for obesity or weight loss. Large doses may cause serious or life-threatening toxicity especially when given concurrently with sympathomimetic or anorectic drugs.

Drug Interactions
Levothyroxine interacts with many drugs. Many drugs interfere with its absorption, resulting in decreased serum concentration. Coadministration with levothyroxine should be separated by several hours. In addition, many drugs increase the metabolism of levothyroxine, decreasing the efficacy of levothyroxine. It is necessary to assess the patient for signs of hypothyroidism and discuss potential dosage adjustments with the health care provider. Table 50.8 lists the drugs that interact with levothyroxine.

Assessment of Relevant Core Patient Variables
Health Status
Before administering levothyroxine, review the patient's record to determine whether the drug can be administered safely. Perform a baseline physical examination to monitor the effects of the drug. Skin color, temperature, texture, and presence of any lesions should be noted to monitor for any reactions and to assess thyroid hormone effectiveness. Note muscle tone, weight, temperature, blood pressure, pulse, and respirations to assess for the desired therapeutic effects of levothyroxine and to monitor for toxic or adverse effects. Thyroid function tests, ECGs, and serum laboratory analyses must be completed to monitor appropriate dosage and response to the drug.

Individuals with known cardiac problems should begin drug therapy with smaller doses of thyroid hormone replacement, because of the cardiac stimulant effect of levothyroxine. Carefully monitor the individual for angina and cardiac arrhythmias.

Life Span and Gender
Determine the patient's age before administering levothyroxine. Geriatric patients should start with a low dosage of thyroid hormone replacement. Gradual increases prevent serious cardiovascular and neurologic adverse effects. If the pulse rate is greater than 100 bpm, withhold the levothyroxine dose. Closely monitor elderly patients who are also receiving beta blockers or digitalis glycosides, because of the increased risk of toxic effects. In both premenopausal and postmenopausal women, long-term levothyroxine therapy has been associated with decreased

TABLE 50.8	Agents That Interact with 🅿 Levothyroxine	
Interactants	**Effect and Significance**	**Nursing Management**
beta-adrenergic blockers	Actions of beta blockers possibly blocked as patient returns to euthyroid state	Assess for decreased beta-blocking action. Discuss dosage alteration of beta blockers with health care provider.
cholestyramine	Cholestyramine binds with thyroid hormones in gut, decreasing its absorption.	Administer 4–6 h apart. Monitor TSH when patients start or stop cholestyramine therapy.
conjugated estrogens	Serum-free thyroxine concentration may be decreased, increasing serum thyrotropin concentration and need for levothyroxine.	Obtain serum thyrotropin concentrations ~12 wk after starting estrogen.
digitalis glycosides	Reduced serum levels of digitalis and decreased therapeutic effects	Evaluate serum digoxin levels. Discuss dosage alteration of digoxin with health care provider.
HMG-CoA reductase inhibitors	HMG-CoA reductase inhibitors may increase or decrease efficacy of thyroid hormones.	Monitor TSH. Monitor for signs of hypo- or hyperthyroidism. Discuss dosage alteration of thyroid hormones with health care provider.
Imatinib	Imatinib may increase metabolism of thyroid hormones.	Monitor TSH. Monitor for signs of hypothyroidism. Discuss dosage alteration of thyroid hormones with health care provider.
iron salts	Iron salts may decrease the absorption of thyroid hormones.	Administer 12 h apart. Monitor TSH. Monitor for signs of hypothyroidism.
protease inhibitors	Protease inhibitors decrease glucuronosyl transferase activity of levothyroxine, resulting in increased T_3/T_4 levels.	Monitor patients with PI therapy for signs of hyperthyroidism. Discuss dosage alteration of thyroid hormones with health care provider.
raloxifene	Raloxifene may decrease absorption of thyroid hormones.	Monitor TSH. Monitor for signs of hypothyroidism. Discuss dosage alteration of thyroid hormones with health care provider.
rifamycins	Rifamycins may increase thyroid metabolism, resulting in a hypothyroid state.	Monitor TSH when patients start or stop rifamycin therapy. Discuss dosage alteration of thyroid hormones with health care provider.
sucralfate	Sucralfate decreases the absorption of levothyroxine.	Administer at least 8 h apart. Monitor TSH. Monitor for signs of hypothyroidism.
theophylline	Hypothyroid states induce decreased theophylline clearance, and hyperthyroid states induce decreased theophylline clearance.	Monitor TSH. Euthyroid does not affect theophylline clearance. Discuss dosage alteration of theophylline with health care provider.
warfarin	Thyroid hormones increase anticoagulant effect of warfarin. The mechanism is unknown.	Monitor PT/INR closely. Monitor for bruising or bleeding. Discuss dosage alteration of warfarin with health care provider.

bone density in the spine and hip. A basal bone density measurement and monitoring for osteoporosis would be beneficial.

Monitor children maintained on levothyroxine for growth and development and for toxic effects. Additionally, adjust the dosage as the child grows.

Because pregnant patients who are receiving thyroid hormone replacement may require a dosage increase during pregnancy, assess the patient for pregnancy.

Thyroid hormone deficiency may have an adverse effect on fetal nervous system development and on the outcome of the pregnancy. Levothyroxine is in pregnancy category A.

Lifestyle, Diet, and Habits

Assess the patient's ability to adapt to a long-term drug regimen. Patients maintained on levothyroxine most often take the drug for life. Levothyroxine is best taken as a single

CRITICAL THINKING SCENARIO

LEVOTHYROXINE AND WEIGHT CONTROL

A woman comes to the clinic and asks for a prescription for thyroid hormone. She has tried multiple diets without success and is convinced that she must have a "glandular" problem. She tells you that she read that thyroid hormone is an effective way to lose weight because it increases your metabolism, and she wants to try it. After obtaining thyroid function tests, it is determined that this patient has normal thyroid function.

1. Think about the problems that could occur if thyroid replacement hormone is given to a euthyroid patient. Outline the normal controls of thyroid activity, and predict what could happen.

2. Develop a patient education tool to explain this situation to the patient, and propose other ways of dealing with her weight problem.

---

daily dose before breakfast. Assist the patient to establish a routine for taking the medication.

Assess the patient's intake of grapefruit juice. Excessive grapefruit juice may delay the absorption of levothyroxine.

Caution the patient to avoid changing from one brand of this drug to another without first consulting the pharmacist or prescriber. Products manufactured by different companies may not be equally effective, and bioavailability differences have occurred with different preparations of levothyroxine.

Environment

Know the environment where the drug will be administered. Most often, levothyroxine is taken at home as an oral drug. IV levothyroxine is administered only for myxedema coma. It is used for short-term therapy until the patient is able to take the oral drug.

Nursing Diagnoses and Outcomes

- Imbalanced Nutrition: More than Body Requirements, related to dietary intake in excess of metabolic demands secondary to hypothyroidism
  Desired outcome: The patient will maintain normal body weight, describe reasons why weight gain may occur, discuss nutritional needs related to age, lifestyle, and diagnosis, and discuss the effects of exercise and diet on weight control.
- Risk for Injury related to adverse drug reactions
  Desired outcome: The patient will not experience adverse reactions to thyroid hormone replacement.
- Risk for Injury related to pre-existing health status that requires cautious use of a thyroid agent
  Desired outcome: The patient will not experience complications of pre-existing health conditions linked to the prescribed thyroid hormone replacement therapy. Such complications include coronary artery disease, angina, myocardial infarction, and hypertension secondary to

increased metabolic demands on the heart, and acute adrenal crisis secondary to increased tissue demand for adrenal hormones.
- Knowledge Deficit related to thyroid dysfunction and the necessity for thyroid hormone replacement
  Desired outcome: The patient and family will express an accurate understanding of the teaching regarding the disease process and the prescribed thyroid hormone replacement therapy. An example includes avoidance of myxedema coma from interrupted drug therapy.

Planning and Intervention

Maximizing Therapeutic Effects

Replacement therapy is a lifelong occurrence. Levothyroxine is absorbed best when taken once a day on an empty stomach, preferably before breakfast. During drug therapy, monitor cardiovascular response and serum thyroid function to determine the appropriate dosage and response to levothyroxine. Monitor children regularly to assess the need to change dosage to allow for appropriate growth and development. If the patient is on other medications, it is important to monitor the response to these drugs and to levothyroxine, especially as the patient achieves a euthyroid state. Offer support and encouragement to deal with the need for lifelong therapy.

Minimizing Adverse Effects

Young adults without evidence of coronary artery disease can begin a full replacement dose of levothyroxine. Older individuals and those with (or at risk for) coronary artery disease, atrial arrhythmias, or both should begin with a low dose (e.g., 25 to 50 mcg/d), which can be slowly titrated to the target dosage.

Check adrenal function in hypothyroid patients because some of these individuals also have adrenal insufficiency. Without appropriate glucocorticoid replacement, thyroid administration in these individuals can precipitate an acute adrenal crisis because thyroid agents increase tissue demand for adrenal hormones.

Thyroid agents may potentiate the hypo-prothrombinemic effect of oral anticoagulants by increasing the catabolism of vitamin K. Administering thyroid agents to diabetic patients may increase the dosage requirement of insulin or oral agent.

Providing Patient and Family Education

- Explain to patients and their families that this drug is a hormone that is being used to replace the thyroid hormone that their body is not able to produce. Tell them that this hormone is responsible for regulating the body's metabolism. Explain to patients that they will most likely need to take levothyroxine for life and that it should be taken every day, preferably in the morning before breakfast.
- Explain that although this drug causes few adverse effects, patients should report any increase in the symptoms of thyroid dysfunction, such as weight changes,

nervousness, skin changes, lethargy, and sleeplessness, or any skin rash or lesions.

- Advise patients to avoid OTC drugs and to check with the prescriber if they feel that an OTC medication is needed. Many OTC drugs contain ingredients that interfere with thyroid function, and patients may want to obtain a medical identification tag or card so that people taking care of them in an emergency are aware that they are taking a thyroid replacement drug.
- Educate patients to keep this drug out of the reach of children.
- Stress the importance of notifying the health care provider if manifestations of hyperthyroidism (e.g., headache, nervousness, chest pain, palpitations, increased pulse rate, diarrhea, diaphoresis, or heat intolerance) occur.

Ongoing Assessment and Evaluation

In patients taking levothyroxine, monitor serum thyroid hormone levels periodically. As a patient reaches a euthyroid state, reassess the potential for drug interactions and the need to adjust the dosage of other drugs appropriately. It is important to monitor pulse rate and rhythm as well as respiratory rate to assess the effect of the thyroid hormone on these systems and the possible need for dosage adjustment. Medications are administered to the patient with hypothyroidism very cautiously because of altered metabolism and excretion and depressed metabolic rate and respiratory status.

Long-term use of levothyroxine may decrease hip and spine bone density in women. Measure bone density before beginning levothyroxine therapy to establish a baseline and then monitor it routinely.

Thyroid hormones may increase blood glucose levels, necessitating adjustment in doses of insulin or oral hypoglycemic agents for patients with diabetes. Patients with hypothyroidism have an increased susceptibility to all hypnotic and sedative agents, analgesics, and anesthetics. These drugs, even in small doses, may induce profound somnolence lasting far longer than anticipated. Respiratory depression is likely as a result of the decreased respiratory reserve and alveolar hypoventilation that occur with hypothyroidism.

As the patient moves from a hypothyroid to a euthyroid state, the body's response to many drugs may be altered. Closely monitor patients taking multiple drugs as they return to a euthyroid state and adjust dosages of the other drugs as needed. For example, the actions of some beta-adrenergic blockers may be impaired. Serum digitalis levels may be reduced, reducing the therapeutic effect of digitalis glycosides. Theophylline clearance is altered. Nursing management of drug therapy is considered effective if the patient adheres successfully to drug therapy, can recognize various signs and symptoms of hypothyroidism, and seeks appropriate attention from the health care team.

Drugs Closely Related to 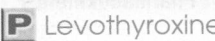 Levothyroxine

Desiccated Thyroid

Desiccated thyroid (Armour Thyroid) is composed of desiccated (dried) animal thyroid glands. It is much less pure, stable, and predictable than synthetic preparations of thyroid hormone. The active thyroid hormones (T_4 and T_3) are available in their natural states and at their natural ratios. Although these preparations are the least expensive, their standardization by iodine content or bioassay is inexact. Optimal dosage is determined by the patient's clinical response and laboratory findings. Therapy is instituted using low doses, with increments that depend on cardiovascular status. The usual starting dose is 30 mg, with increments of 15 mg every 2 to 3 weeks. Patients with long-standing myxedema are started at a lower dose (15 mg/d), particularly if cardiovascular impairment is suspected. The drug dosage should be reduced if angina occurs.

Liothyronine Sodium

Liothyronine sodium (Cytomel [oral form]; Triostat [parenteral form]) is a synthetic form of the natural thyroid hormone T_3. It has the pharmacologic activities of the natural hormone. Its short duration of activity enables quick dosage adjustment and facilitates control of overdosage. Patients who are allergic to thyroid extract derived from pork or beef can be safely treated with this medication. Liothyronine injection is for IV use only and should be stored between 2°C and 8°C (36°F to 46°F).

Liotrix

Liotrix (Thyrolar) is a uniform mixture of synthetic T_4 and T_3 in a 4:1 ratio by weight. Optimal dosage is determined by patient's clinical response and laboratory findings.

MEMORY CHIP

P Levothyroxine

- Synthetic thyroid hormone replacement
- Major contraindications: acute myocardial infarction, thyrotoxicosis; use cautiously in hypoadrenalism
- Most common adverse effects: symptoms of hyperthyroidism, alopecia with initial therapy (particularly in children)
- Maximizing therapeutic effects: Monitor drug response carefully at the start of therapy; administer oral drug as a single daily dose before breakfast.
- Minimizing adverse effects: Monitor cardiac response, as increased basal metabolic rate may exacerbate angina pectoris.
- Most important patient education: Have patient wear medical ID (tag or bracelet) to alert emergency medical personnel of drug therapy.
- **Black box warning: Not for use for obesity or weight loss.**

• Ⓒ ANTITHYROID COMPUNDS

Hyperthyroidism is treated with thyroid-hormone antagonist drugs, surgery, or radioactive iodine. The purpose of treatment is to reduce the amount of functional thyroid tissue. The antithyroid agents used clinically to manage hyperthyroidism include methimazole, propylthiouracil, iodide or iodine solutions (Lugol solution), radioactive iodine (I-131), and propranolol. Methimazole (MMI) is the prototype antithyroid compound. Table 50.9 presents a summary of selected antithyroid agents.

Nursing Management of the Patient Receiving Ⓟ Methimazole (MMI)
Core Drug Knowledge
Pharmacotherapeutics

MMI is used for palliative treatment of hyperthyroidism, as an adjunct in preparation for surgery (thyroidectomy) or radioactive iodine therapy, or to manage thyrotoxic crises. Additionally, if thyroidectomy is contraindicated or otherwise not advised, MMI is the drug of choice.

Pharmacokinetics

MMI is readily absorbed from the GI tract. Onset of action is slow, and it requires an average of 5.8 weeks to lower T_4 levels to normal. The half-life of MMI is 5 to 13 hours. It is metabolized in the liver and excreted in the urine. MMI is usually preferred over propylthiouracil (PTU), another thionamide, because it reverses hyperthyroidism more quickly and has fewer adverse effects. MMI can be administered in single or divided doses, whereas PTU must be given in three equal doses at approximately 8-hour intervals.

Pharmacodynamics

MMI inhibits the synthesis of thyroid hormones (T_4 and T_3); hence, new T_3 and T_4 are not produced. It neither inactivates existing thyroxine and triiodothyronine that are stored in the thyroid nor interferes with the effectiveness of thyroid hormones given as tablets or by injection. Some clinical evidence suggests that the thionamide drugs have immunosuppressant effects. Thus, they are beneficial for suppressing the immune-mediated hyperthyroidism of Graves disease.

Contraindications and Precautions

MMI is contraindicated with any known hypersensitivity to antithyroid drugs. The drug is in pregnancy category D. It is contraindicated during pregnancy and nursing because the drug crosses the placenta and is excreted in breast milk.

Adverse Effects

Most adverse effects are minor, but some major ones can occur. Up to 15% of people taking an antithyroid drug experience minor adverse effects. Both MMI and PTU can cause hives, itching, rash, fever, arthralgia, joint swelling, vertigo, drowsiness, nausea and vomiting, and altered taste sensation. The nausea and vomiting may depend on the amount of the drug ingested with each dose. For this reason, spreading large total daily doses out over the day may reduce these side effects. If adverse effects occur with one drug, frequently the same effects will occur if the patient switches to the other drug.

Major adverse effects include agranulocytosis, which affects only 0.2% to 0.5% of all people taking antithyroid medication. If this adverse effect occurs, it usually does so within the first 3 months of treatment. Agranulocytosis resolves within a few days when treatment is discontinued. Hepatotoxicity, aplastic anemia, and vasculitis are other rare complications. Most people recover fully when the drug is stopped.

Drug Interactions

A hyperthyroid state *increases* the pharmacologic effects of beta-blocking agents and theophylline. As MMI becomes

TABLE 50.9	Summary of Selected Ⓒ Antithyroid Drugse		
Drug (Trade) Name	**Selected Indications**	**Route and Dosage Range**	**Pharmacokinetics**
Ⓟ methimazole (Tapazole)	Treatment of hyperthyroidism Amelioration of hyperthyroidism before thyroidectomy, radioactive iodine	*Adult:* PO, 15 mg/d for mild hyperthyroidism; 30–40 mg/d for moderate hyperthyroidism; 60 mg/d for severe hypothyroidism *Child:* PO, 0.4 mg/kg/d; maintenance, 1/2 initial dose	*Onset:* 1 wk *Duration:* Weeks $t_{1/2}$: 5–13 h
propylthiouracil (PTU)	Treatment of hyperthyroidism Attain euthyroid state before thyroidectomy, radioactive iodine therapy	*Adult:* Initial dose, PO, 300–900 mg/d; maintenance, PO, 100–150 mg/d *Child:* PO, 6–10 y, 50–150 mg/d; ≥10 y, 150–300 mg/d; maintenance, based on response	*Onset:* 10–21 d *Duration:* Weeks $t_{1/2}$: 1–2 h
sodium iodide I-131 (Iodotope, Sodium iodide I-131 [therapeutic])	Treatment of hyperthyroidism, thyroid cancer	*Adult:* PO, hyperthyroidism, 4–10 mCi; thyroid cancer, 50 mCi; then 100–150 mCi as needed	*Onset:* Rapid *Duration:* Unknown $t_{1/2}$: 7.61 d
strong iodine solution (Lugol solution, Thyro-Block)	Treatment of hyperthyroidism	*Adult:* PO, 2–6 drops tid for 10 d before surgery	*Onset:* 24–48 h *Duration:* 6 wk $t_{1/2}$: Unknown

effective and the patient becomes more euthyroid, these drugs have a greater effect on the body, necessitating a decrease in their dosage. A hyperthyroid state *decreases* the vitamin K–dependent clotting factors. As the patient becomes more euthyroid, the clotting factors increase and the dose of warfarin is less effective. In rare circumstances, the efficacy of warfarin is increased by an unknown mechanism and the patient has an increased risk of bleeding. It is necessary to monitor prothrombin time/international normalized ratio (PT/INR) levels closely whenever MMI is administered to a patient taking warfarin. Conversely, a hypothyroid state *increases* serum digoxin levels. As the patient becomes more euthyroid, the risk of digoxin toxicity increases.

Assessment of Relevant Core Patient Variables
Health Status
Before administering MMI, review the patient's record to determine whether the drug can be administered safely. Perform a physical examination before starting drug therapy to establish a baseline for monitoring the drug's effects. Note skin color, temperature, texture, and presence of any lesions to assess for allergic reactions and thyroid hormone effectiveness. It also is important to review liver and kidney function tests, because MMI is metabolized in the liver and excreted in the urine. Perform a complete blood count (CBC) with differential as a baseline for potential hematologic changes that can occur during therapy. In addition, perform baseline thyroid function tests to monitor the effect of the drug on thyroid function.

Life Span and Gender
Determine whether the patient is pregnant or breast-feeding. Antithyroid agents are in pregnancy category D. They readily cross the placenta and can induce goiter and cretinism in the developing fetus. Fortunately, in many pregnant women, thyroid dysfunction decreases as the pregnancy proceeds. This decrease enables reduction of the thionamide dose. If thionamide therapy is necessary during pregnancy, PTU is preferred because it crosses the placenta to a lesser extent than MMI. Patients receiving antithyroid preparations during the postpartum period should use formula preparations to feed their infants.

Note the patient's age before administering MMI. Hepatotoxicity has occurred in some pediatric patients. Monitor children closely to ensure that thyroid function is maintained and that growth and development proceed normally. Dosage adjustment may be required with prolonged use.

Lifestyle, Diet, and Habits
Assess the patient's ability to adapt to a long-term drug regimen because patients taking MMI may require prolonged therapy to achieve the full effect. The drug can be taken once daily or in divided doses every 8 hours around the clock. Help the patient establish a schedule that causes the least interference with the patient's sleep pattern. Drowsiness and vertigo are potential adverse effects of this drug. Therefore, caution the patient to avoid driving or performing tasks that require precision and alertness if these effects occur.

Environment
Know the environment where MMI will be administered. It is usually given in the home. It is necessary to teach patients the importance of taking the drug as prescribed and the necessity of making special arrangements in their schedules and routines to facilitate this need.

Nursing Diagnoses and Outcomes
- Imbalanced Nutrition: Less than Body Requirements, related to increased metabolic demands secondary to hypothyroidism
  Desired outcome: The patient will describe reasons why weight loss may occur and discuss nutritional needs related to age, lifestyle, and diagnosis.
- Risk for Injury related to blood dyscrasias (e.g., granulocytosis) or to drowsiness and vertigo secondary to adverse reactions of PTU
  Desired outcome: The patient will demonstrate no adverse hematologic reactions to thyroid therapy (e.g., hypoprothrombinemia or bleeding), identify factors that increase the risk from injury (e.g., from CNS side effects), and relate intentions to practice and use safety measures to prevent injury.
- Nonadherence related to long-term use of the antithyroid agent and need to take the prescribed medication frequently
  Desired outcome: The patient will describe the reasons for the therapeutic regimen, identify barriers to adherence, and identify the behaviors that must change to facilitate adherence.

Planning and Intervention
Maximizing Therapeutic Effects
If the patient is unable to take MMI once daily, ensure that the drug is being administered appropriately (three equal doses at 8-hour intervals) to maintain serum concentration. Encourage fluid intake of 3 to 4 L/day unless contraindicated. MMI can be given with meals to minimize GI irritation.

Minimizing Adverse Effects
During drug therapy, arrange for periodic blood tests to monitor for hematologic and thyroid functions. Also, encourage frequent, small meals to alleviate GI symptoms and to help maintain nutrition while the patient is taking MMI. Encourage the patient to avoid driving or performing hazardous tasks if drowsiness or vertigo occurs. Monitor the patient's bone marrow function. It is important to obtain a baseline assessment of the CBC with a differential. Emphasize the importance of regular follow-up care and monitoring of bone marrow, CBC, and thyroid functions at intervals determined by the physician.

Providing Patient and Family Education

- Explain to patients and their families that this agent is an antithyroid drug that blocks the production and activity of the thyroid hormone responsible for regulating the body's metabolism, that is, the speed with which the body's cells burn energy. This drug will most likely have to be taken for a prolonged time to achieve the desired effect.

- If the drug is taken in divided doses, instruct patients to take them every 8 hours around the clock. Work with patients and families to establish a schedule that causes the least interference with sleep.

- Adverse effects of this drug include vertigo and drowsiness. Advise patients to avoid driving or performing hazardous tasks while taking this drug and to take extra precautions to prevent falls and injuries.

- Other adverse effects include nausea, vomiting, and epigastric distress. Encourage patients to eat small, frequent meals to maintain nutrition and alleviate some of the discomfort associated with these adverse effects.

- Advise patients that they will have periodic blood tests while taking this drug to monitor its effectiveness and possible adverse effects. Stress the need to report fever, sore throat, unusual bleeding or bruising, and headache to the health care team.

- Review the signs and symptoms of hepatotoxicity with patients. Assure them this adverse effect is rare but needs to be reported if any symptoms occur.

- Instruct patients to keep this drug, and all other medications, out of the reach of children.

Ongoing Assessment and Evaluation

Monitor serum thyroid hormone levels periodically to evaluate the effectiveness of MMI and to assess the need for replacement thyroid hormone because the thyroid gland is suppressed. With continued antithyroid therapy, an insidious goitrogenic hypothyroidism may appear. Alert the patient to watch for signs of this adverse effect, such as decreased cardiac rate, intolerance to cold, and weight gain. Thyroid function tests, used to evaluate drug therapy, should be measured routinely (every 4 to 6 weeks). Periodically review the signs of hypothyroidism and hyperthyroidism with the patient and significant others. Review the signs and symptoms of hepatotoxicity and the importance of contacting the health care provider if any symptoms occur. As the patient reaches a euthyroid state, assess the need for dosage adjustment with drugs affected by metabolic rate and activity. Therapy is considered successful when normal thyroid status is maintained, and the patient can explain and demonstrate self-monitoring techniques.

Drug Closely Related to ℗ Methimazole

Propylthiouracil (PTU) is a thionamide with characteristics similar to those of MMI. Adverse effects are also similar and include pruritus, rash, urticaria, arthritis, fever, abnormal taste, nausea, and vomiting. Serious complications, such

as agranulocytosis, are dose dependent. Serum aminotransferase concentrations increase transiently in up to one third of patients taking PTU. Well-documented hepatotoxicity is equally divided between PTU and MMI.

Drugs Significantly Different From ℗ Methimazole

Iodide or Iodine Solutions (Lugol Solution, Thyro-Block (tablets))

Iodine is the oldest of the antithyroid drugs. Low doses of iodine are needed in the body to form thyroid hormone. However, high doses tend to inhibit thyroid function. A hyperfunctioning thyroid gland responds to iodine by promptly inhibiting the release of hormone. Iodine helps firm the thyroid gland by reducing its size and vascularity. This effect helps prevent postoperative hemorrhage and the surgical complication of thyroid storm.

Potassium iodide, or occasionally strong iodine solution, is used preoperatively to reduce the vascularity of the gland before thyroidectomy and, alone or in combination with the beta blocker, propranolol, to manage thyrotoxic crisis (thyroid storm), usually in conjunction with other antithyroid agents (e.g., MMI). When used preoperatively, potassium iodide is administered 10 to 14 days before surgery.

Chronic toxicity may occur when potassium iodide is given in large doses or over a long duration. Chronic toxicity is usually dose dependent and is manifested as a metallic taste, burning in the mouth and throat, sore teeth and gums, increased salivation, and eye irritation with swollen eyelids. Gastric irritation is common, and diarrhea may occur. When the drug is discontinued, the clinical manifestations of toxicity generally subside spontaneously within a few days.

Hypersensitivity reactions to iodides may cause angioedema, cutaneous and mucosal hemorrhage, and clinical signs (e.g., fever, arthralgia, lymphadenopathy, and eosinophilia) resembling serum sickness.

Prolonged use or excessive doses of iodides may result in thyroid gland hyperplasia, thyroid adenoma, goiter, and severe hypothyroidism.

Concomitant use of lithium salts, other iodides, or antithyroid agents and potassium iodide may result in an additive or synergistic hypothyroid effect. If these drugs are used together, the patient should be monitored closely for signs and symptoms of hypothyroidism. Simultaneous use of potassium iodide and potassium-containing drugs or potassium-sparing diuretics may result in hyperkalemia.

Cautious initial administration of potassium iodide is recommended because some individuals are markedly sensitive to iodides. Persons at highest risk are those with goiter or autoimmune thyroid disease (Hashimoto thyroiditis). Some commercially available formulations of potassium iodide contain sodium bisulfite, a sulfite that may cause allergic-type reactions, including anaphylaxis and life-threatening asthmatic episodes, in susceptible individuals. It is necessary to question the patient carefully about the presence of goiter, autoimmune thyroid disease, or asthma, because this sensitivity occurs more frequently in asthmatic individuals.

Iodine-131

I-131 (radioactive iodine) is used to treat hyperthyroidism and well-differentiated thyroid carcinoma. While destroying thyroid tissue, it exposes only the thyroid tissue to the altering radiation, eliminates the problems of surgery, and enables outpatient treatment. Most patients treated with radioactive iodine become euthyroid and then require lifelong replacement therapy with thyroid hormones.

The total amount of I-131 needed to achieve clinical remission of hyperthyroidism without destroying the entire gland varies widely. The usual dosage range to treat hyperthyroidism is 4 to 10 millicuries (mCi). The usual dosage for ablation of normal thyroid tissue (in thyroid carcinoma) is 50 mCi, with subsequent therapeutic doses of 100 to 150 mCi.

The exposure level around a patient treated with I-131 depends on the administered dose, the time elapsed following treatment, and the amount absorbed by thyroid tissue. Hospital radiation-safety protocols (based on the U.S. Nuclear Regulatory Commission [NRC] regulations for radiopharmaceutical therapy) must be strictly followed during the hospitalization. Radioactive iodine therapy is considered safe. Some individuals, particularly the elderly, may be treated with antithyroid drugs before I-131 therapy to minimize the risk of exacerbating the hyperthyroidism.

I-131 has orphan-drug status for detection of hepatocellular carcinoma, hepatoblastoma, and alpha-fetoprotein–producing germ-cell tumors; detection of tumors that produce human chorionic gonadotropin; adrenal cortical imaging; and B-cell lymphomas and leukemias. It also has orphan-drug status as a diagnostic adjunct in pheochromocytoma.

I-131 is absorbed readily from the GI tract and distributed primarily within the extracellular fluid of the body. It is trapped and rapidly converted by the thyroid to protein-bound iodine. It is then concentrated by the stomach and salivary glands and excreted within several days by the kidney. The physical half-life of I-131 is 8.04 days.

I-131 is in pregnancy category X. It is contraindicated for women who are or may become pregnant because it crosses the placenta and can cause permanent damage to the fetus' thyroid gland. It is also contraindicated for lactating women because iodine is excreted in breast milk. Another contraindication to therapy is pre-existing vomiting because if the patient vomits during the first few hours after therapy, the vomitus will be highly radioactive. I-131 is seldom used in patients younger than 30 years of age unless circumstances preclude other treatment.

The immediate adverse reactions following I-131 treatment for hyperthyroidism are usually mild. More severe reactions occur following larger doses, such as those used in thyroid carcinoma. Severe reactions include depression of the hematopoietic system (acute leukemia, depressed bone marrow function, anemia, leukopenia, and thrombocytopenia). Signs of radiation sickness may also occur. Manifestations may include nausea and vomiting, tachycardia, chest pain, itching skin, hives, rash, chromosomal abnormalities, acute thyroid crisis, and death. Tenderness and swelling around the neck area, pain on swallowing, sore throat, and cough may occur 72 hours after treatment. These manifestations usually respond to treatment with analgesics.

The uptake of I-131 is affected by recent intake of iodine in any form and by thyroid and antithyroid agents. Antithyroid therapy (e.g., methimazole) of a severely hyperthyroid patient is usually discontinued 3 to 4 days before I-131 is administered.

Fears of radiation-induced genetic damage, leukemia, and neoplasia have shaped this practice, although these fears have not been realized during several decades of clinical experience. Studies indicate that the risk for infertility and birth defects following I-131 treatment is not increased if pregnancy is avoided for at least 1 year following treatment.

Patients with Graves disease may be given an antithyroid drug, such as MMI, for several months preceding radiotherapy in order to establish a euthyroid state. I-131 dosing is then based on the ability of the abnormal thyroid tissue to absorb and eliminate I-131.

Patients should be questioned regarding previous medication and procedures involving radiographic contrast media because the uptake of I-131 is affected by recent intake of these agents. Patients should be reassured that they will not be isolated from other household members. Instead, they should be cautioned to avoid prolonged, close contact with others, particularly children and pregnant women, for about 1 week following therapy with I-131.

Household contamination is not a great risk, but saliva and urine may be contaminated for several days following treatment. Patients and families should be provided with both verbal and written instructions specific to their living situations. Patients should be instructed to sleep alone, to avoid close personal contact with family members, and to drink liberal amounts of fluids for 2 days after treatment. Eating utensils should be washed thoroughly with soap and water after every meal. The importance of handwashing should be emphasized. Typically, the toilet is the most contaminated item because most of the I-131 dosage is excreted in the urine. The NRC recommends an annual radiation dose limit of 100 mrem for the general public. This limit excludes exposure to family members of outpatients receiving radiation, however. Hyperthyroid patients treated with I-131 typically emit only low levels of radiation beyond a 1-meter distance (approximately 3.3 ft). It is necessary to make certain that household members understand they can minimize their exposure by staying 1 meter or more away from the patient for the first few days. Anxious household members should understand that exposure from diagnostic x-rays (typically, 10–2,000 mrem) is considerably greater than exposure that results from minimal contact with the patient.

Patients should be advised that temporary thinning of the hair may occur 2 to 3 months after treatment. Patients and families should be educated about the signs and symptoms of hypothyroidism, which may occur following I-131 therapy.

Propranolol

Propranolol (Inderal), a beta-adrenergic blocker, is commonly used intravenously in treating thyroid storm to minimize the excessive cardiac stimulation that results from the catecholamine activity. Therefore, it controls the symptoms but does not alter the disease. Propranolol is discussed in depth in Chapter 13.

PARATHYROID DRUGS

• C ANTIHYPERCALCEMIC, CALCIUM-REGULATOR DRUGS

Antihypercalcemic drugs do not directly affect the parathyroid gland or PTH but rather inhibit bone resorption of calcium. These agents are frequently used in the treatment of **Paget disease,** which is an idiopathic disease characterized by chronic bone inflammation that results in thickening, softening, and bowing of the affected bones. Many people with Paget disease are not symptomatic because only small areas of the bones are involved. However, individuals with symptomatic disease experience bone pain and deformity, fractures, spinal cord compression, or cranial and spinal cord entrapment. Because vascularity of the bone is increased, high-output chronic heart failure may be evident. When a large mass of bone is involved, urinary hydroxyproline excretion may increase secondary to the breakdown of the collagen-containing bone matrix. Serum alkaline phosphatase also increases, secondary to increased bone formation. Antihypercalcemic drugs decrease the rate of bone turnover, with a resultant decrease in both urinary hydroxyproline excretion and serum alkaline phosphatase.

Calcitonin is a polypeptide hormone secreted by the thyroid gland. Commercially available calcitonin drugs are calcitonin, salmon and calcitonin, human. Both are derived synthetically and are used when the hypercalcemia is related to hyperparathyroidism. The prototype calcium-regulator drug is calcitonin, salmon. Table 50.10 presents a summary of selected antihypercalcemic drugs.

Nursing Management of the Patient Receiving P Calcitonin, Salmon

Core Drug Knowledge

Pharmacotherapeutics

Calcitonin, salmon (Miacalcin) is indicated for treatment of symptomatic Paget disease of the bone (osteitis deformans), postmenopausal osteoporosis, and hypercalcemia. The actions of this synthetic polypeptide of 32 amino acids are very similar to those of the hormone secreted by the parafollicular cells of the thyroid gland but with a greater potency per milligram and longer duration of action. It inhibits **bone resorption** (pathologic or physiologic loss or destruction of bone tissue, which can occur as a result of neoplasm, hyperparathyroidism, osteoporosis, or prolonged immobility). Calcitonin also increases the excretion of calcium, sodium, and phosphorus by the kidney, thereby lowering serum calcium levels. Intranasal calcitonin increases spinal bone mass in postmenopausal women with established osteoporosis, but has not been shown to be effective early in menopause.

Calcitonin, human (Cibacalcin) is a synthetic form of the hormone produced by the human thyroid gland. Calcitonin, human is also used to treat Paget disease. It must be administered subcutaneously up to three times a week. It should be discontinued once symptoms are relieved.

Pharmacokinetics

Calcitonin can be administered subcutaneously, intramuscularly (for Paget disease, postmenopausal osteoporosis, and hypercalcemia), or intranasally (for postmenopausal osteoporosis). It is rapidly metabolized, primarily in the kidneys, by conversion to smaller inactivated fragments. A small amount of unchanged hormone and its inactive metabolites are excreted in the urine. Half-life is 1.2 hours. Calcitonin does not cross the placenta. Whether it passes to breast milk and cerebrospinal fluid has not been determined.

Pharmacodynamics

In mammals, calcitonin is a polypeptide hormone that is secreted by the parafollicular cells of the thyroid gland. Calcitonin, salmon is a synthetic polypeptide with essentially the same actions as calcitonin. It plays a role in the regulation of calcium and bone metabolism and has direct renal effects and actions on the GI tract. Single injections of calcitonin cause a transient but marked inhibition of bone resorption. With prolonged use, a persistent, smaller decrease occurs in the rate of bone resorption. This decrease is associated with a decreased number of osteoclasts and a

TABLE 50.10	Summary of Selected **C** Antihypercalcemic Drugs		
Drug (Trade) Name	**Selected Indications**	**Route and Dosage Range**	**Pharmacokinetics**
P calcitonin, salmon (Calcimar, Miacalcin Nasal Spray, Miacalcin)	Treatment of Paget disease Postmenopausal osteoporosis with calcium and vitamin D Emergency treatment of hypercalcemia	*Adult:* Paget disease, initial dose, SC or IM, 100 IU/d; maintenance, 50 IU/d or qod; postmenopausal osteoporosis, SC or IM, 100 IU/d; hypercalcemia, SC or IM, 4 IU/kg q12h, may increase to 8 IU/kg q6h *Child:* Safety and efficacy not established	*Onset:* 15 min *Duration:* 8–24 h $t_{1/2}$: 1.2 h
cinacalcet (Sensipar)	Secondary hypertension in patients on renal dialysis Parathyroid cancer	*Adult:* PO, 30 mg/d, increase gradually to maximum 180 mg/d *Adult:* PO, 30 mg bid up to 90 mg qid	*Onset:* Unknown *Duration:* Unknown $t_{1/2}$: 30–40 h
alendronate (Fosamax)	Treatment of Paget disease in patients at risk for complications	*Adult:* Osteoporosis, PO, 70 mg/wk or 10 mg/d; Paget disease, PO, 40 mg/d for 6 mo *Child:* Safety and efficacy not established	*Onset:* Slow *Duration:* Days $t_{1/2}$: Unknown
etidronate (Didronel)	Treatment of Paget disease Heterotropic ossification Hypercalcemia resulting from malignancy	*Adult:* Paget disease, PO, 5–10 mg/kg/d up to 6 mo or 11–20 mg/kg/d not to exceed 3 mo; Heterotropic ossification, PO, 20 mg/kg/d, total; treatment not to exceed 4 mo; Hypercalcemia, IV, 7.5 mg/kg/d × 3 d. May repeat with at least 7-d interval between courses of tx. Follow with oral dose of 20 mg/kg/d not to exceed 3 mo.	*Onset:* Slow *Duration:* 6 h; 6 h (serum) $t_{1/2}$: 90 d
furosemide (Lasix)	Promotes renal excretion of calcium	*Up to 100 mg IV*	*Onset:* 5 min *Duration:* 2 h $t_{1/2}$: 2 h
gallium nitrate (Ganite)	Treatment of malignancy-related hypercalcemia	*Adult:* IV, 200 mg/m2/d for 5 consecutive d *Child:* Safety and efficacy not established	*Onset:* Slow *Duration:* 3–4 d $t_{1/2}$: Unknown
pamidronate (Aredia)	Treatment of hypercalcemia resulting from malignancy Paget disease Osteolytic bone lesions Postmenopausal osteoporosis	*Adult:* Hypercalcemia, IV, 60–90 mg over 24 h; Paget disease, IV, 30 mg/d over 4 h for 3 d; osteolytic bone lesions, IV, 90 mg over 4 h each mo *Child:* Safety and efficacy not established	*Onset:* Rapid *Duration:* 72 h $t_{1/2}$: 1.6 h, then 27.3 h
plicamycin (Mithracin)	Hypercalcemia and hypercalciuria in symptomatic patients associated with advanced neoplasms	Base dose on body weight. Use ideal weight if patient has abnormal fluid retention. 25 mcg/kg/d for 3 or 4 d; may repeat at intervals of ≥1 wk to maintain serum and urinary calcium excretion at normal levels.	*Onset:* Rapid *Duration:* Unknown $t_{1/2}$: Unknown
risedronate (Actonel)	Treatment of Paget disease Prevention of bone loss in postmenopausal women	*Adult:* PO, 30 mg/d for 2 mo *Adult:* PO, 5 mg/d or 35 mg/wk	*Onset:* Rapid *Duration:* Unknown $t_{1/2}$: 480 h
tiludronate (Skelid)	Treatment of Paget disease	*Adult:* PO, 400 mg/d for 3 mo *Child:* Safety and efficacy not established	*Onset:* 2 h *Duration:* Days $t_{1/2}$: 150 h

reduction in their resorptive activity. Endogenous calcitonin, in conjunction with PTH, has been shown to regulate blood calcium in animal studies. High blood calcium levels increase secretion of calcitonin, which inhibits bone resorption. This effect returns the blood calcium to normal.

Contraindications and Precautions
In calcitonin, salmon, there is a risk for allergic reaction to the salmon antigens. For this reason, if a person is suspected to have sensitivity to calcitonin or has multiple allergies, skin testing is recommended. The skin test consists of administering 0.1 mL of a 10-IU/mL solution subcutaneously on the inner aspect of the forearm. The appearance of a wheal or mild erythema, usually within 15 minutes, indicates a positive reaction. No serious allergic-type reactions have been reported with the nasal spray. Use caution when administering calcitriol to patients with renal dysfunction or upper GI disease.

Calcitonin is in pregnancy category C.

Adverse Effects

Adverse effects are generally infrequent and mild. GI disturbances are most evident at the start of treatment and tend to decrease with continued use. Other adverse effects include injection site reactions, dermatologic effects of skin rash and flushing of the face and hands, and nasal irritation or rhinitis (if using the nasal spray).

Rare but serious allergic-type reactions, such as anaphylaxis, have been reported with injectable calcitonin, salmon. People who are allergic to fish products are at a greater risk for anaphylaxis.

Drug Interactions

If calcitonin, salmon is taken with calcium supplements, antacids, or vitamin D, there is a risk of hypercalcemia, and therapeutic effect is decreased. Advise patients against using OTC vitamin and mineral preparations and antacids, because many of these products contain calcium. Concurrent administration of theophylline may increase bone resorption. Formal studies to evaluate drug interactions with the nasal spray have not been done.

Assessment of Relevant Core Patient Variables

Health Status

Before administering calcitonin, review the patient's record to determine whether calcitonin can be administered safely. Perform a physical examination to establish a baseline from which to monitor the drug's effects. It is important to evaluate bone pain, muscle tone, bowel sounds, renal function tests, and serum calcium levels. While collecting a thorough health history, ask about bone disease, endocrine disorders, kidney stones, or ulcer diseases. Also, obtain a complete drug history, including use of prescription and OTC drugs. Thiazide diuretics and excessive ingestion of vitamin D can cause hypercalcemia.

Include the family history because primary hyperparathyroidism occurs in a number of familial syndromes. Perform a nasal examination before nasal calcitonin administration and repeat it if the patient experiences nasal complaints.

Life Span and Gender

Calcitonin is in pregnancy category C. Assess for pregnancy and lactation. Whether calcitonin is excreted in human milk is unknown. For this reason, nursing is not recommended while the patient is on this drug. No studies have been conducted with pregnant women, but in animal studies, decreased fetal birth weights have been shown. In one large study utilizing the nasal spray, subjects greater than 65 years of age had a higher incidence of rhinitis, erythema, excoriation, and irritation. Most were mild, however greater sensitivity of the older population must be considered.

Lifestyle, Diet, and Habits and Environment

Long-term treatment with calcitonin occurs in the home or community. Monitor the patient's responses to detect adverse effects or previously unrecognized effects of the drug. Abnormal serum calcium levels and signs of allergy may occur.

Take a thorough health history to identify factors relating to the cause of hyperparathyroidism, such as vitamin D intoxication, hyperphosphatemia, and osteolytic bone metastases. Obtain a broad database about the patient for comparison during therapy; for example, record dietary practices, visible bone deformities that may interfere with activities, allergic tendencies, emotional lability, and lethargy.

Nursing Diagnoses and Outcomes

• Imbalanced Nutrition: Less than Body Requirements, related to GI effects of drug therapy
  Desired outcome: *The patient will relate the importance of good nutrition and ingest daily nutritional requirements in accordance with activity level and metabolic needs.*
• Pain, Acute or Chronic related to complications of calcium or phosphate imbalances (e.g., renal stones, pathologic fractures, and osteoporosis)
  Desired outcome: *The patient will practice pain relief measures to avoid or manage the pain.*

Planning and Intervention

Maximizing Therapeutic Effects

Be aware of the proper dosages of calcitonin, salmon. For postmenopausal osteoporosis, the recommended intranasal dose of calcitonin is 200 international units, in alternating nostrils each day. This practice decreases nasal irritation. An adequate diet and supplemental calcium carbonate (1.5 g daily), plus vitamin D intake (400 U daily), is essential. SC and IM injections of 100 international units per day are also available.

For Paget disease, it is necessary to give the drug by injection. The recommended starting dose is 100 international units per day SC (preferred for outpatient administration) or IM. Arrange for periodic measurement of serum alkaline phosphatase and 24-hour urinary hydroxyproline in order to measure drug effect. Decrease in bone pain and normalization of biochemical abnormalities usually occur within the first few months of treatment, if they are going to occur. When normalization does occur, 50 international units per day or every other day is often sufficient to maintain clinical and biochemical improvement.

For hypercalcemia, the recommended starting dose is SC or IM injection of 4 international units per kilogram every 12 hours. If adequate response does not occur within 2 days, an increase to 8 international units per kilogram every 12 hours is expected. If this dosage is inadequate, it can be further increased to 8 international units per kilogram every 6 hours. If the volume is greater than 2 mL, IM injection is preferred.

Minimizing Adverse Effects

Watch for nausea, which is the most common adverse effect with SC or IM administration. It is most evident at the initiation of treatment and tends to decrease or disappear with continued administration. Rotate injection sites to minimize local inflammatory reactions from SC and IM injections. Rhinitis, nasal crusts, and dryness are the most common adverse effects of nasal calcitonin. Alternating nostrils daily is recommended. Nasal symptoms, including rhinitis, crusting, dryness, and erythema were reported less frequently with the nasal spray than with the placebo.

Providing Patient and Family Education
- Instruct patients or family members in sterile SC and IM injection technique.
- For nasal forms of the drug, teach patients how to activate the pump and instruct them to evaluate the mucous membranes daily.
- This drug is designed to decrease the level of calcium in the blood. Calcium is needed for many of the body's activities, and it is important to keep the blood calcium levels in an effective range.
- Explain that adverse effects are usually mild but may include GI upset with nausea, vomiting, and epigastric discomfort or local inflammation. The drug should be taken once a day at the same time each day. If GI upset occurs, suggest small, frequent meals to maintain nutrition and decrease the unpleasant effects of the drug. Explaining that these adverse effects usually decrease with continued use may promote adherence.
- Starting therapy may exacerbate Paget disease–associated bone pain. It is important to assure patients that such exacerbation is usually transient. Teach patients the following ways to manage bone pain associated with Paget disease:
  - Nonnarcotic analgesics (e.g., NSAIDs, cytochrome-C-oxidase-2 [COX-2] inhibitors)
  - Applications of heat
  - Massage
  - Bracing
  - Guided imagery
  - Relaxation techniques
  - Biofeedback
  - Meditation
- Instruct patients to report twitching, muscle pain, severe diarrhea, or dark urine.
- Instruct patients to keep this drug, and all other medications, out of the reach of children.
- Alert patients and family members that skeletal deformities (e.g., bowed tibia or femur, kyphosis, or barrel-shaped chest) are not corrected by treatment. You can teach patients to camouflage deformities using clothing (e.g., slacks for women, tunic-style tops, and loosely fitted apparel).

Ongoing Assessment and Evaluation

Calcitonin can cause the serum calcium level to drop, resulting in tetany and cardiac arrhythmias. In addition, antibodies may form after several months of therapy, causing resistance to the drug and decreased therapeutic effects. Monitor the calcium level and clinical response in those receiving long-term therapy.

Nursing management of drug therapy is judged effective when calcium levels are maintained within a normal range. The patient should express the importance of self-monitoring for adverse effects and of reporting significant effects to the prescriber.

Drugs Closely Related to Calcitonin, Salmon

Bisphosphonates

The bisphosphonates are calcium-regulator drugs closely related to calcitonin. The major pharmacologic action of this class of drugs is to inhibit normal and abnormal bone resorption. Reduction of abnormal bone resorption is responsible for therapeutic benefit in hypercalcemia. Bisphosphonate drugs are recommended for long-term management of hypercalcemia to increase bone resorption of calcium, in treating and preventing osteoporosis in postmenopausal women, and in managing Paget disease.

Patients taking bisphosphonates should be cautioned that the expected benefits of the drug are obtained only when each tablet is taken upon arising in the morning with a full glass of plain water (6 to 8 oz) and at least 30 minutes before ingesting any other medications, food, or beverages. Taking bisphosphonates with juice or coffee markedly reduces absorption (especially of alendronate). After taking the drug, the patient must stay in an upright position for 30 minutes to facilitate drug delivery to the stomach and prevent esophageal irritations. Patients must be instructed not to take this medication at bedtime or before arising for the day. Sucking on or chewing these medications can cause oropharyngeal ulceration. Supplemental calcium and vitamin D must also be administered for the bisphosphonates to be effective. Weight-bearing exercise and modifying certain behavioral factors (e.g., cigarette smoking and alcohol consumption)

MEMORY CHIP

Calcitonin, Salmon
- Calcium regulator used to treat postmenopausal osteoporosis, Paget disease, hypercalcemia
- Major contraindication: hypersensitivity to fish products
- Most common adverse effects: nausea, vomiting, and diarrhea
- **Life span alert: *Children—safety and efficacy not established.***
- Maximizing therapeutic effects: Store unopened bottle (nasal drug formulation) in the refrigerator between 36° and 43°F; once the pump has been activated, store at room temperature.
- Minimizing adverse effects: Periodically examine urine sediments of patients on chronic therapy; coarse granular casts and renal tubular epithelial cell casts result from therapy and may cause renal calculi.
- Most important patient education: With intranasal dosing, alternate nostrils daily; notify health care provider if significant nasal irritation occurs.

may aid in diminishing bone resorption. Bisphosphonates are very effective when given as a once-a-week medication. If a dose is missed, the patient should be instructed to take the missed dose on the morning after it is remembered and then resume taking the medication on the regularly chosen day. Chapter 52 discusses bisphosphonates in detail.

Drugs Significantly Different From P Calcitonin, Salmon

Cinacalcet

Cinacalcet (Sensipar) an oral calcimimetic agent, is the first approved agent in this drug class. It is indicated to treat patients with secondary hyperparathyroidism caused by chronic kidney disease and patients with hypercalcemia associated with parathyroid carcinoma. Cinacalcet directly reduces PTH levels while lowering calcium and phosphorus levels. This action is consistent with the National Kidney Foundation Disease Outcomes Quality Initiative clinical practice guidelines for bone metabolism and disease in chronic kidney disease. In a clinical trial reported by the manufacturer, cinacalcet was shown to reduce high serum calcium levels in patients with parathyroid carcinoma. Nearly 500 patients develop this rare condition annually, and the FDA designated cinacalcet as an orphan drug.

Furosemide

Furosemide (Lasix) is a loop diuretic that promotes renal excretion of calcium. Dosage of up to 100 mg may be given intravenously. Adverse effects include dehydration, hypokalemia, hyperuricemia, hypomagnesemia, and hypochloremic alkalosis. Fluid balance, blood pressure, pulse, and serum electrolytes must be carefully monitored when furosemide is administered. Furosemide is discussed in depth in Chapter 27.

Gallium

Gallium (Ganite) inhibits calcium resorption from bone and reduces bone turnover, effects that result in a lowered serum calcium level. Gallium is indicated for treating cancer-related hypercalcemia. It is administered intravenously over a 5-day period to patients who are symptomatic and do not respond to conventional treatment. This drug carries a substantial risk of severe renal insufficiency, especially if it is administered concomitantly with other nephrotoxic agents (e.g., amphotericin B or aminoglycosides). Renal function tests must be monitored closely for any sign of renal toxicity. It is crucial to maintain adequate hydration in patients receiving gallium and to monitor serum electrolytes closely.

Plicamycin

Plicamycin (Mithracin) is an antineoplastic, antihypercalcemic agent that is indicated for hypercalcemia secondary to neoplasms. It has been reported to be effective in treating Paget disease; however, it has not been approved by the FDA for this use. This medication is for IV administration only, and it is highly recommended that it be given only under the supervision of a qualified physician experienced in the use of chemotherapeutic agents. The patient must be hospitalized during administration because of the possibility of severe reactions.

When plicamycin is used for Paget disease, the dose should be about 10% of that used for cancer treatment. Adverse effects are much less common with this use, because of the lower dose. The dosage is based on body weight; ideal body weight should be used if the individual has abnormal fluid retention. Extravasation may cause local irritation and cellulitis at injection sites. Plicamycin blocks the hypercalcemic action of pharmacologic doses of vitamin D, acts on osteoclasts, and blocks the action of PTH. Plicamycin inhibition of DNA-dependent RNA synthesis renders osteoclasts unable to respond fully to PTH with the biosynthesis necessary for osteolysis. Decreases in serum phosphate levels and urinary calcium excretion accompany the lowering of serum calcium concentrations. The drug is cleared rapidly from blood within the first 2 hours; excretion also is rapid (90% in the first 24 hours after injection). Contraindications to plicamycin use are thrombocytopenia, coagulation disorders, impaired bone marrow function, and pregnancy. The drug is in pregnancy category X. The most common adverse effects include GI symptoms (anorexia, nausea, vomiting, diarrhea, and stomatitis). Electrolyte disturbances and depression of serum calcium, phosphorus, and potassium levels may occur. Calcium supplements are sometimes needed during plicamycin therapy.

• C ANTIHYPOCALCEMIC DRUGS

Vitamin D compounds regulate absorption of calcium and phosphate from the small intestine, reabsorption of phosphate from the renal tubules, and mineral resorption in bone. Vitamin D is considered a hormone, although it is not a natural human hormone. The commonly used term "vitamin D" refers to both ergocalciferol (D_2) and cholecalciferol (D_3). Vitamin D_2, a plant vitamin, is predominantly used to fortify milk and cereals, and it can substitute for D_3.

Vitamin D metabolites control intestinal absorption of dietary calcium, tubular reabsorption of calcium by the kidney, and mobilization of calcium from the skeleton, in conjunction with PTH. They act directly on bone cells (osteoblasts) to stimulate skeletal growth and on the parathyroid glands to suppress PTH synthesis and secretion. Vitamin D is also involved in magnesium metabolism.

Vitamin D works together with PTH and calcitonin to regulate calcium homeostasis. It functions as a hormone. Hypoparathyroidism is treated primarily with vitamin D. If necessary, dietary supplements of calcium are also given. Patients with hypoparathyroidism have deficient levels of PTH, which result in hypocalcemia. Vitamin D stimulates calcium absorption from the intestine and restores the serum calcium to a normal level. It is a fat-soluble vitamin derived from natural sources (fish liver oils) or from conversion of provitamins. In humans, natural supplies of vitamin D depend on ultraviolet (UV) light for conversion to vitamin D_3 or vitamin D_2. Following exposure to UV light, vitamin D_3 must then be

TABLE 50.11 Summary of Selected Ⓒ Antihypocalcemic Drugs

Drug (Trade) Name	Selected Indications	Route and Dosage Range	Pharmacokinetics
P calcitriol (Calcijex, Rocaltrol)	Management of hypocalcemia in chronic renal dialysis Hypoparathyroidism Predialysis	*Adult:* 0.25 mcg/d; may increase by 0.25 mcg/d at 4–8-wk intervals *Hypoparathyroidism:* 0.25 mcg/d. *Adult and child ≥6 y:* usually respond to 0.5–2 mcg/d. *<6 y:* 0.25–0.75 mcg	*Onset:* 2–6 h *Duration:* 3–5 d $t_{1/2}$: 3–6 h
dihydrotachysterol (DHT, Hytakerol)	Treatment of hypoparathyroidism; postoperative or idiopathic tetany	*Adult and child >3 y:* 0.25 mcg/d *Adult:* PO, 0.75–2.5 mg/d initially; maintenance, PO, 0.2–1.75 mg/d to maintain serum calcium levels	*Onset:* 10–24 h *Duration:* 3–5 d $t_{1/2}$: 16 d
doxercalciferol (Hectorol)	Reduction of elevated parathyroid hormone levels in the management of secondary hyperparathyroidism in patients undergoing chronic renal dialysis	10 mcg administered three times a week at dialysis; initial dose adjusted as needed to lower blood PTH to 15- to 300-pg/mL range. Increase dosage at 8-wk intervals by 2.5 mcg, to maximum recommended dose of 20 mcg 3×/wk at dialysis, for a total of 60 mcg/wk.	*Onset:* 10–24 h *Duration:* 3–5 d $t_{1/2}$: 32–37 h
paricalcitol (Zemplar)	Prevention and treatment of secondary hyperparathyroidism associated with chronic renal failure	Initially, 0.04–0.1 mcg/kg (2.8 to 7 mcg); dose may be increased by 2–4 mcg at 2–4-wk intervals, to maximum of 0.24 mcg/kg (16.8 mcg), administered as a bolus every other day during dialysis.	*Onset:* 10–24 h *Duration:* 16 d $t_{1/2}$: 15 h

converted to its active forms by the liver and kidneys. Vitamin D is hydroxylated by the hepatic microsomal enzymes to calcifediol. It is further hydroxylated in the kidney to calcitriol and doxercalciferol. Calcitriol (1,25-dihydroxyvitamin D_3, Rocaltrol [capsules, solution], Calcijex [parenteral]) is believed to be the most active form of vitamin D in stimulating intestinal calcium and phosphate transport, and it is the prototype antihypocalcemic drug. Table 50.11 presents a summary of selected antihypocalcemic drugs.

Nursing Management of the Patient Receiving **P** Calcitriol

Core Drug Knowledge

Pharmacotherapeutics

Clinical indications for calcitriol include management of hypocalcemia and resulting bone disease in patients on chronic renal dialysis; management of secondary hyperparathyroidism and metabolic bone disease in predialysis patients with moderate to severe chronic renal failure (creatinine clearance, 15 to 55 mL/min); and management of hypocalcemia and its clinical manifestations in patients with hypoparathyroidism (postsurgical, idiopathic, or pseudohypoparathyroidism). Off-label uses for calcitriol (oral) include increasing bone mass and preventing fractures in patients with osteoporosis, and (topical) decreasing severity of psoriatic lesions.

Pharmacokinetics

Calcitriol can be administered orally or intravenously. It is rapidly absorbed from the small intestine, with a peak effect occurring in 3 to 6 hours. Absorption is reduced with liver or biliary disease because bile is essential for adequate absorption. Vitamin D is chiefly stored in the liver but is also found in fat, muscle, skin, and bones. Calcitriol is 99% bound in blood. It is transported in blood by an alpha-globulin vitamin D–binding protein. Vitamin D is converted to calcifediol in the liver and then to doxercalciferol in the kidney. The half-life of calcitriol is 5 to 8 hours. Its pharmacologic activity persists for 3 to 5 days. The half-life increases at least twofold in patients with chronic renal failure and in hemodialysis patients. The primary route of vitamin D excretion is in the bile, but a small percentage is found in the urine.

Pharmacodynamics

Vitamin D is a fat-soluble vitamin derived from natural sources (fish liver oils) or from conversion of provitamins, 7-dehydrocholesterol, and ergosterol. In humans, natural supplies of vitamin D depend on UV light for conversion of 7-dehydrocholesterol to vitamin D_3 or ergosterol to vitamin D_2. Following exposure to UV light, vitamin D_3 is converted to the active form of vitamin D, calcitriol, in the liver and kidneys. Calcitriol is believed to be the most active form of vitamin D_3. It stimulates intestinal calcium and phosphate transport. Calcitriol is a fat-soluble vitamin that helps to regulate calcium homeostasis, bone growth, and maintenance. It increases calcium absorption from the intestine, thereby increasing serum calcium levels. It decreases alkaline phosphatase and possible PTH levels.

Biologically active vitamin D metabolites control the intestinal absorption of dietary calcium, the tubular reabsorption of calcium by the kidney, and, in conjunction with

PTH, the mobilization of calcium from the skeleton. They act directly on bone cells (osteoblasts) to stimulate skeletal growth and on the parathyroid glands to suppress PTH synthesis and secretion. Vitamin D also is involved in magnesium metabolism.

Contraindications and Precautions

Excessive doses of calcitriol can cause hypercalcemia and hypercalciuria. For these reasons, it is important to monitor serum calcium twice a week during initial dosing. In dialysis patients, decreased serum alkaline phosphatase levels often precede hypercalcemia. An abrupt increase in calcium intake, usually from dietary sources, may trigger hypercalcemia. If hypercalcemia develops, it is necessary to discontinue calcitriol immediately. During periods of hypercalcemia, daily serum calcium and phosphate levels must be determined. When calcium levels return to normal, calcitriol can be readministered at a daily dose 0.25 mcg lower than initially used. Patients on digitalis therapy are at an increased risk for cardiac arrhythmias; thus, calcitriol must be given cautiously. Chronic hypercalcemia can lead to generalized vascular calcification, nephrocalcinosis, and other soft-tissue calcifications. Chronic hypercalcemia may be associated with a transient increase in serum creatinine levels in patients with normal renal function. It is important for these patients to pay careful attention to factors that may lead to hypercalcemia. Patients with end-stage renal disease are unable to adequately synthesize calcitriol, the active hormone formed from the precursor vitamin D. Resultant hypocalcemia and secondary hyperparathyroidism are major causes of the metabolic bone disease of renal failure.

Some vitamin D products contain tartrazine, which may cause allergic-type reactions (including bronchial asthma) in susceptible individuals. Although the incidence of this sensitivity is low, it is frequently seen in patients with aspirin hypersensitivity. Products containing tartrazine are identified in product listings on the label.

Calcitriol therapy should always be started at the lowest possible dose and increased only with careful monitoring of serum calcium levels. During periods when the medication is adjusted, serum calcium levels should be monitored twice a week. Once the optimal dose is determined, serum calcium levels require monthly monitoring.

Calcitriol is in pregnancy category C.

Adverse Effects

Adverse effects are similar to those encountered with vitamin D excess. Early signs include weakness, headache, nausea and vomiting, dry mouth, constipation, and bone pain. Late signs include polyuria, polydipsia, and weight loss; elevated BUN, AST, and alanine aminotransferase (ALT); and cardiac arrhythmias, hypertension, and dehydration.

Drug Interactions

There are very few significant drug–drug interactions with calcitriol. Hypermagnesemia is a risk if calcitriol is taken with magnesium-containing antacids. If both drugs must be taken, they should be spaced 2 to 4 hours apart. Patients on chronic renal dialysis should not take both types of medications. Calcitriol may decrease the efficacy of verapamil. Monitor the cardiovascular status of the patient if the drugs are given concurrently. A possible risk of hypercalcemia occurs in some patients when thiazide diuretics and calcitriol are combined. Table 50.12 lists drugs that interact with calcitriol.

TABLE 50.12	Agents That Interact with P Calcitriol	
Interactants	**Effect and Significance**	**Nursing Management**
Cholestyramine, ketoconazole, mineral oil, phenytoin, pheno-barbital, thiazide diuretics	Decreased pharmacologic effects of vitamin D Intestinal absorption of vitamin D may be reduced. Ketoconazole may inhibit both synthetic and catabolic enzymes of calcitriol. Absorption of vitamin D is reduced with prolonged use of mineral oil. Hypoparathyroid patients on vitamin D may develop hypercalcemia due to thiazide diuretics. Endogenous synthesis of calcitriol will be inhibited; higher doses of calcitriol may be necessary with concurrent administration of phenytoin and phenobarbital.	Assess the patient for management of concurrent disease states. Assess the patient for evidence of therapeutic effects of interacting drugs. Check for therapeutic serum levels (if applicable) of interacting drugs.
Mg++-containing antacids, digitalis glycosides, verapamil	Increased pharmacologic effects from interaction with vitamin D Hypermagnesemia may develop in patients on chronic renal dialysis. Hypercalcemia in patients on digitalis may precipitate cardiac arrhythmias.	Assess the patient for control of concurrent disease states. Evaluate patient for evidence of therapeutic effects of interacting drugs. Measure therapeutic serum levels (if applicable) of interacting drugs. Monitor cardiac rhythm and function.

Assessment of Relevant Core Patient Variables

Health Status

A thorough health history is necessary to identify any factors that relate to the cause of hypoparathyroidism. Before administering calcitriol, review the patient's record to determine whether calcitriol can be safely administered. Caution should be used when administering the drug to patients with renal stones.

Before beginning drug therapy, perform a physical examination including skin color, temperature, orientation, and status of mucous membranes to establish a baseline from which to monitor the effects of the drug. Determine serum levels of calcium, phosphorus, magnesium, alkaline phosphatase, and renal and liver function to establish a baseline from which to measure drug activity and adverse effects.

Life Span and Gender

Assess the patient for pregnancy or breast-feeding. Calcitriol is in pregnancy category C. No adequate, well-controlled studies have been performed in pregnant women. The drug should be used during pregnancy only if the potential benefits outweigh the potential hazards to the fetus. Vitamin D may be excreted in breast milk; therefore, breast-feeding should be avoided when taking calcitriol. Safety of vitamin D in amounts greater than 400 international units per day is not established.

The safety and efficacy of calcitriol given to pediatric patients undergoing dialysis have not been studied but are based on adult patients. Dosing guidelines have not been established for patients with hypoparathyroidism who are younger than 1 year of age or for those younger than 6 years of age with pseudohypoparathyroidism. Long-term calcitriol therapy is well tolerated by pediatric patients who are not undergoing dialysis. Pediatric doses should be individualized and monitored closely.

Calcitriol should be used with caution in elderly patients, especially those with coronary disease, renal function impairment, and arteriosclerosis. Dosage for elderly patients should start at the low end of the dosing range, because they have a greater risk of decreased renal, hepatic, or cardiac function.

Lifestyle, Diet, and Habits

Calcitriol is generally given in the home setting. IV doses can be given following dialysis to increase calcium levels. Evaluate vitamin D ingested in fortified foods, dietary supplements, and other concomitantly administered drugs. It may be necessary to limit dietary vitamin D and its derivatives during treatment.

Patients receiving calcitriol are likely to experience multiple GI effects. Small, frequent meals may help alleviate some of these symptoms. A bowel-training program may be needed if constipation is a problem. Closely monitor nutritional status.

Nursing Diagnoses and Outcomes

• Imbalanced Nutrition: Less than Body Requirements related to reduced absorption of fat-soluble vitamins, including calcitriol, in the presence of a very low-fat diet
  Desired outcome: The patient will ingest a nutritionally balanced diet to allow for normal absorption of fat-soluble vitamins.

• Imbalanced Nutrition: More than Body Requirements, related to drug–vitamin interaction of vitamin D and calcium supplements
  Desired outcome: The patient will identify sources of dietary vitamin D and calcium, consume these foods in moderation, and refrain from consuming vitamin or dietary supplements containing vitamin D and calcium.

• Acute Pain related to headache and general discomfort secondary to drug effects
  Desired outcome: The patient will not experience undue pain and discomfort as a result of drug therapy.

Planning and Intervention

Maximizing Therapeutic Effects

Calcitriol capsules should be swallowed whole, rather than crushed or chewed. Eating a balanced diet and getting exposure to sunlight usually satisfies normal vitamin D requirements. Caution the patient and family to avoid using vitamin supplements as a substitute for a balanced diet. Monitor serum calcium levels before and during drug therapy because adequate dietary calcium is necessary for a clinical response to vitamin D therapy. Begin therapy at the lowest possible dose, with dosage increases made only after careful analysis of the serum calcium. Adjust the dosage as soon as clinical improvement is seen. It is essential to estimate the daily dietary calcium intake and adjust that intake as indicated. Patients with normal renal function taking calcitriol should maintain an adequate fluid intake to avoid dehydration because the range between therapeutic and toxic doses is narrow. When high therapeutic doses are used, frequent serum and urinary calcium, phosphate, and BUN determinations are necessary.

The recommended initial IV dose of calcitriol injection (Calcijex) is 1 to 2 mcg administered every other day (approximately three times/week). Doses may be increased slowly at 2 to 4 week intervals if a satisfactory response is not detected. While titrating the medication, serum calcium and phosphorous levels should be monitored twice weekly. If hypercalcemia occurs, Calcijex should be discontinued immediately until levels return to the appropriate range, then a lower dose should be administered.

Serum calcium levels should be maintained between 9 and 10 mg/dL.

Minimizing Adverse Effects

Chronic dialysis patients should avoid magnesium-containing antacids while taking these drugs. Arrange for small, frequent meals to alleviate GI discomfort and to provide adequate nutrition. Monitor bowel function and begin a bowel-training program as appropriate. Provide analgesics as appropriate to decrease discomfort and pain related to drug effects.

Providing Patient and Family Education

• Explain to patients and their families that this drug is a form of vitamin D and that it is being used to increase the patient's low calcium levels. Calcium is needed for many of the body's activities, and it is important to keep calcium levels in the blood in an effective range.

• Discuss the possible adverse effects of the drug, including GI upset with nausea, vomiting, and epigastric upset. Advise patients to eat small, frequent meals to maintain nutrition and decrease some of the unpleasant side effects of the drug.

• Advise patients to monitor noise, temperature, and light and to take prescribed analgesics as needed to decrease discomfort of the headache, muscle ache, and irritability that are common adverse effects of the drug.

• Instruct patients to report lethargy, weight loss, severe bone pain, excessive urine output, or constipation.

• Instruct patients to keep this drug, and all other medications, out of the reach of children.

Ongoing Assessment and Evaluation

Dosage adjustment is required for patients taking calcitriol as soon as clinical improvement occurs. Therapy should be started at the lowest possible dose, with increases made after careful monitoring of the serum calcium. It is important to estimate daily dietary calcium intake and adjust the intake when indicated. Patients with normal renal function taking calcitriol should avoid dehydration by maintaining adequate fluid intake. The range between therapeutic and toxic doses is narrow. When high therapeutic doses are used, it is especially important to chart the progress with frequent determinations of urinary calcium, phosphate, and BUN and to chart serum calcium, phosphate, magnesium, and alkaline phosphatase levels. Monitor 24-hour urinary calcium and phosphate levels. These laboratory determinations are especially important in hypoparathyroid and dialysis patients. Serum calcium levels should be maintained between 9 and 10 mg/dL.

Nursing management in drug therapy is considered effective when calcium levels are maintained within a normal range and when the patient recognizes and expresses the importance of self-monitoring for adverse effects and takes responsibility for reporting significant adverse effects to the health care provider.

Drugs Closely Related to [P] Calcitriol
Dihydrotachysterol

Dihydrotachysterol (DHT) is a vitamin D derivative that is indicated for treating postoperative tetany (acute, chronic, and latent), idiopathic tetany, and hypothyroidism. Off-label,

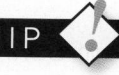

MEMORY CHIP

[P] Calcitriol

• Vitamin D; management of hypocalcemia and resultant bone disease in patients undergoing chronic renal dialysis

• Major contraindications: hypercalcemia, hypervitaminosis D, malabsorption syndrome, and decreased renal function

• Most common adverse effects: weakness, headache, somnolence, nausea, vomiting, dry mouth, constipation, muscle or bone pain, and metallic taste

• Most serious adverse effect: chronic hypercalcemia can lead to generalized vascular calcification, nephrocalcinosis, and other soft tissue calcifications

• **Life span alert: Use caution in elderly patients, especially those with coronary disease, renal function impairment, and arteriosclerosis.**

• Maximizing therapeutic effects: Patients with normal renal function taking calcitriol should maintain adequate fluid intake and avoid dehydration; periodically monitor serum calcium, phosphate, magnesium, alkaline phosphatase, and 24-hour urinary calcium and phosphate, especially in hypoparathyroid and dialysis patients.

• Minimizing adverse effects: Maintain serum calcium levels between 9 and 10 mg/dL.

• Most important patient education: Adequate dietary calcium is necessary for a clinical response to vitamin D therapy; compliance with dosage instructions, diet, phosphate-binder use, and calcium supplementation is essential; avoid use of nonprescription drugs, including magnesium-containing antacids.

it is used for familial hypophosphatemia and renal osteodystrophy. DHT mobilizes bone calcium and stimulates intestinal calcium absorption in the absence of PTH. It also increases the excretion of phosphate from the kidneys. It exerts a slow but persistent effect and can be used for long periods. The beginning dose is 0.8 to 2.4 mg/d for several days, followed by a maintenance dose of 0.2 to 1.0 mg/d to maintain normal serum calcium levels. It can be supplemented with 10 to 15 mg of oral calcium gluconate or calcium lactate daily if needed. Toxicity is manifested by symptoms of hypercalcemia. It is important to monitor standard hypercalcemia-related metabolic parameters (e.g., serum levels of calcium, phosphate, magnesium, and potassium) carefully.

Doxercalciferol

Doxercalciferol (Hectorol), a vitamin D analogue, is indicated to treat hyperparathyroidism secondary to renal failure. It can be administered intravenously or orally and has a mean half-life of 32 to 37 hours. Doxercalciferol is a prohormone of vitamin D that undergoes hepatic conversion to active vitamin D. Hyperphosphatemia lessens its effectiveness. Decreased absorption may occur when it is combined with agents known to interfere with the absorption of fat-soluble vitamins (e.g., cholestyramine and mineral oil). Adverse effects include edema, headache, dizziness, malaise, nausea, and vomiting.

Paricalcitol

Paricalcitol (Zemplar) is a parenterally administered synthetic vitamin D analogue used for hyperparathyroidism secondary to renal failure. It has a mean half-life of 15 hours. Paricalcitol suppresses PTH levels in patients with chronic renal failure. It may also reduce serum total alkaline phosphatase levels. Effective therapy with paricalcitol requires a dietary regimen of calcium supplementation and phosphorus restriction. Phosphate-binding compounds may be needed. Excessive use of aluminum-containing compounds should be avoided.

CHAPTER SUMMARY

- A combination of neural and endocrine systems, originating in the hypothalamus, regulates CNS, autonomic nervous system, and endocrine functions.
- The hypothalamus produces two hormones—oxytocin and vasopressin—that are stored in and released from the posterior lobe of the pituitary gland. The hypothalamus releases a series of stimulating and inhibiting factors to promote the release of stimulating hormones from the anterior pituitary gland. These stimulating hormones affect several other endocrine glands.
- The anterior lobe of the pituitary gland produces growth hormone (GH), a hormone important for the regulation of growth and development. Release of GH is determined by inhibiting and releasing factors and by chemical signals for growing tissue.
- The thyroid gland is a bilobar gland located in the neck around the trachea. This vascular gland uses dietary iodine to produce two thyroid hormones (T_3 and T_4). These hormones affect the way many body cells utilize energy and maintain metabolism. These hormones are regulated by a balance between TRH, TSH, and the thyroid hormone levels.
- The parathyroid glands are four very small groups of tissue located on the back of the thyroid gland. These cells produce parathyroid hormone (PTH), the most important regulator of serum calcium levels in the body. PTH stimulates osteoclasts to release calcium from the bone, increases intestinal absorption of calcium, and increases calcium resorption from the kidneys. It also stimulates cells in the kidney to produce calcitriol, the active form of vitamin D, which stimulates intestinal transport of calcium into the blood. Calcium is a vital anion that is used in many of the body's metabolic processes, including membrane transport processes, conduction of nerve impulses, muscle contraction, and blood clotting. To be effective, the serum levels of calcium must be maintained between 9 and 11 mg/dL.
- The GH somatropin is an example of a drug used to replace a pituitary hormone. It is given by injection to children with GH deficiency, to some adults with GH deficiency, and to girls with Turner syndrome.
- Release of GH is blocked by octreotide, bromocriptine, and GH-inhibiting factor (somatostatin). These drugs can be used to treat acromegaly and must be given by injection.

- Vasopressin (or ADH) is administered by injection or intranasally in order to regulate water loss when levels of ADH are low or absent. Vasopressin blocks the release of water in the nephron and increases vascular volume while decreasing osmolarity. The dosage of this drug is determined by patient response and water balance.
- Thyroid hormone is given to replace low levels of thyroid hormone resulting from surgery, radiation, autoimmune disorders, inadequate iodine in the diet, malignancies, or pituitary-hypothalamic disorders. Levothyroxine (T_4) is the most commonly used thyroid hormone because of its predictability and reliability.
- Patients treated with thyroid hormone need lifelong therapy. They should be monitored for nutritional balance related to changes in metabolism and should be evaluated periodically for the effectiveness of other maintenance drugs as the patient reaches normal thyroid function and metabolism changes.
- Drugs used to block thyroid function include the thionamides—methimazole (MMI) and propylthiouracil (PTU)—and iodine preparations. The thionamides block the coupling of iodine to the thyroid hormone, whereas the iodine preparations prevent formation of thyroid hormone by blocking iodine uptake. I-131 is used in diagnostic imaging to isolate areas of increased thyroid gland activity or in one large dose to cause thyroid gland destruction by beta ray emission. Patients effectively treated with antithyroid drugs will need to be monitored for hypothyroidism and the need for thyroid hormone replacement.
- Hypercalcemia is treated with calcitonin (a thyroid hormone that counters the action of PTH), the bisphosphonates, and gallium. These drugs are used to treat any condition characterized by increased calcium levels or bone resorption, such as postmenopausal osteoporosis, Paget disease, and hypercalcemia associated with malignancy.
- Hypocalcemia is treated with vitamin D derivatives. Vitamin D compounds regulate the following processes: absorption of calcium and phosphate from the small intestine, mineral resorption in bone, and reabsorption of phosphate from the renal tubules. Working with PTH and calcitonin to regulate calcium homeostasis, vitamin D actually functions as a hormone. Patients receiving vitamin D products need to be cautioned about using OTC multiple-vitamin preparations and should be encouraged to increase dietary intake of calcium.

QUESTIONS FOR STUDY AND REVIEW

1. What is the importance of calcium balance, and how is it maintained in the body?
2. How do the hypothalamus and pituitary glands interact to help maintain homeostasis in the body?
3. What are the special educational needs of the patient and family when somatropin is used to replace deficient GH?
4. List the signs and symptoms of hypothyroidism.

5. A patient with malignancy-induced severe hypercalcemia is admitted with a serum calcium level of 18 mg/dL. The patient is given IV gallium as an emergency treatment. What special precautions need to be observed with the use of this drug?

6. An order is written for calcitonin, salmon to treat hypercalcemia. Before administering the drug, the patient assessment reveals a history of allergy to animal products. What steps should you take before administering the drug?

NEED MORE HELP?

Chapter 50 of the Study Guide to Accompany *Drug Therapy in Nursing*, 4th Edition, contains NCLEX-style questions and other learning activities to reinforce your understanding of the concepts presented in this chapter. For additional information or to purchase the study guide, visit the**Point**.

REFERENCES

American Heart Association. (2005). Guidelines for cardiopulmonary resuscitation and emergency cardiovascular care. Retrieved from *http://circ.ahajournals.org/cgi/content/full/112/24_suppl/IV-1 on July 28, 2010.*

Ayuk, J. & Sheppard, M. C. (2006). *Postgraduate medical journal,* 82(963):24–30. Retrieved from http://www.pubmedcentral.nih.gov/articlerender.fcgi?artid=2563724; May 17, 2009.

Barbesino, G. (2010). Drugs Affecting Thyroid Function, *Thyroid,* 20(7):763–770.

Bromocriptine mesylate (parlodel): Retrieved May 24, 2009 from: http://www.fda.gov/medwatch/safety/2005/Nov_PI/Parlodel_PI.pdf

DDAVP: Retrieved May 29, 2009 from: http://www.fda.gov/medwatch/SAFETY/2003/03NOV_PI/DDAVP_Tablets_PI.pdf

Facts and Comparisons. (2010). *Drug facts and comparisons.* Philadelphia, PA: Lippincott Williams & Wilkins.

Frindik, J. P., & Kemp, S. F. (2010). Managing idiopathic short stature: role of somatropin (rDNA origin) for injection. *Biologics,* 4:147–155.

Kazuna, T., Nobuyuki A., Sumihisa K., et al. Benefit of short-term iodide supplementation to antithyroid drug treatment of thyrotoxicosis due to Graves' disease. *Clinical endocrinology.* Retrieved May 10, 2009 from http://www3.interscience.wiley.com/cgi-bin/fulltext/122682360/PDFSTART

Karch, A. M. (2010). *Nursing Drug Guide.* Philadelphia, PA: Lippincott Williams& Wilkins.

Koda-Kimbal, M. A., Young, L. Y., Kradian, W. A., et al. (2008). *Applied Therapeutics: The Clinical Use of Drugs (9th Ed.).* Philadelphia, PA: Lippincott Williams& Wilkins.

Melmed, S. (2010). Treatment of acromegaly. *UpToDate.* Retrieved from http://www.uptodate.com/online/content/topic.do?topicKey=pituitar/2085&selectedTitle=3~67&source=search_result on July 26, 2010.

Miacalcin (Calcitonin-salmon). Retrieved May 15, 2009 from: http://www.fda.gov/medwatch/SAFETY/2006/Jan_PI/Miacalcin_PI.pdf

Micromedex Healthcare Series. Retrieved from *http://thomsonhc.com.*

Nutropin AQ info: http://www.rxlist.com/nutropin-aq-drug.htm Rx list: the internet drug

Octreotide acetate info: Retrieved May 24, 2009 from: http://www.fda.gov/medwatch/SAFETY/2005/Sep_PI/Sandostatin_PI.pdf

Papavasiliou, K. A., Kirkos, J. M., Kapetanos, G. A., et al. (2007). Potential influence of hormones in the development of slipped capital femoral epiphysis: A preliminary study. *Journal of Pediatric Orthopaedics,* 16(1):1–5.

Pegvisomant info: Retrieved May 24, 2009 from: http://www.fda.gov/medwatch/safety/2008/Aug_PI/Somavert_PI.pdf

Porth, C. M. (2008). Pathophysiology: *Concepts of altered health states* (8th Ed.). Philadelphia, PA: Lippincott Williams & Wilkins.

Quarles, L. D., & Cronin, R. E. (2010). Management of secondary hyperparathyroidism and mineral metabolism abnormalities in dialysis patients, *Up To Date.* Retrieved from http://www.uptodate.com/online/content/topic.do?topicKey=dialysis/34199&selectedTitle=3~7&source=search_result on July 26, 2010.

Ross, D. S. (2010). Treatment of hypothyroidism. In U*pToDate.* Retrieved from http://www.uptodate.com/online/content/topic.do?topicKey=thyroid/2117&selectedTitle=3~150&source=search_result on July 26, 2010

Silverberg, S. J., & Fuleihan, G. H. (2010). Management of primary hyperparathyroidism, *Up To Date.* Retrieved from http://www.uptodate.com/online/content/author.do?topicKey=bone_dis%2F5677 on July 26, 2010.

Somatropin injection info: Retrieved May 24, 2009 from: http://www.medicinenet.com/somatropin-injection/index.htm

Tatro, D. S. (2011). *Drug Interaction Facts: the authority on drug interactions.* Philadelphia, PA: Lippincott Williams & Wilkins.

Drugs Affecting Men's Health and Sexuality

Learning Objectives

At the completion of this chapter the student will:

1. Identify common health problems of men that are treated with drug therapy.

2. Identify core drug knowledge about drugs that affect men's health and sexuality.

3. Identify core patient variables relevant to drugs that affect men's health and sexuality.

4. Relate the interaction of core drug knowledge and core patient variables for drugs that affect men's health and sexuality.

5. Generate a nursing plan of care from the interactions between core drug knowledge and core patient variables for drugs that affect men's health and sexuality.

6. Describe nursing interventions to maximize therapeutic and minimize adverse effects of drugs that affect men's health and sexuality.

7. Determine key points for patient and family education related to drugs that affect men's health and sexuality.

Key Terms

androgens
benign prostatic hypertrophy

erectile dysfunction
follicle-stimulating hormone

luteinizing hormone
male pattern baldness

Drugs Affecting Men's Health and Sexuality

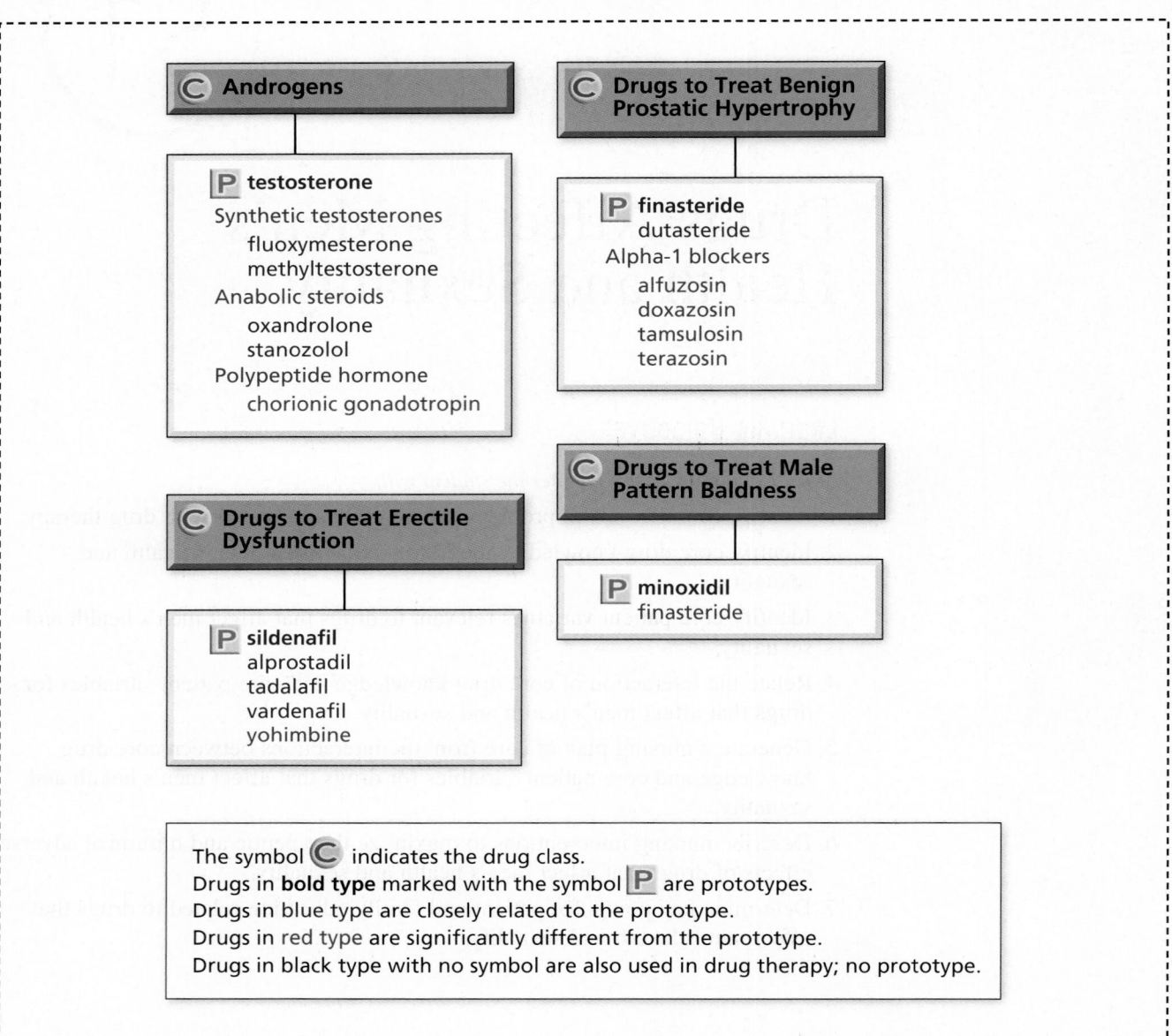

C Androgens

P testosterone
Synthetic testosterones
    fluoxymesterone
    methyltestosterone
Anabolic steroids
    oxandrolone
    stanozolol
Polypeptide hormone
    chorionic gonadotropin

C Drugs to Treat Benign Prostatic Hypertrophy

P finasteride
    dutasteride
Alpha-1 blockers
    alfuzosin
    doxazosin
    tamsulosin
    terazosin

C Drugs to Treat Erectile Dysfunction

P sildenafil
alprostadil
tadalafil
vardenafil
yohimbine

C Drugs to Treat Male Pattern Baldness

P minoxidil
finasteride

The symbol **C** indicates the drug class.
Drugs in **bold type** marked with the symbol **P** are prototypes.
Drugs in blue type are closely related to the prototype.
Drugs in red type are significantly different from the prototype.
Drugs in black type with no symbol are also used in drug therapy; no prototype.

Men's health and sexuality differ from women's. Men, over their lifetime, experience unique health problems. Some of these may be directly related to deficiencies of the male sex hormone testosterone; others may be indirectly related to changing hormone levels. Additionally, cardiovascular (e.g., peripheral vascular disease, ischemic heart disease), neurologic (e.g., neuropathies), and endocrine (e.g., diabetes mellitus) system changes are responsible for other health problems in men.

This chapter discusses drug therapy used to treat problems specific to men, including: insufficient testosterone, erectile dysfunction (ED), benign prostatic hypertrophy (BPH), and male pattern baldness, with emphasis on prototype drugs such as sildenafil for treating ED; finasteride for treating BPH; and minoxidil for treating male pattern baldness. The prototype male sex hormone, testosterone, will also be discussed.In addition, this chapter briefly discusses prostatic cancer. Chapters 56 and 57 present a fuller discussion of the drugs used to treat prostate cancer.

PHYSIOLOGY

Hormones

Androgens are naturally occurring or synthetic steroidal compounds that produce the masculinizing and tissue-building properties of testosterone, the main male sex hormone. Other androgens include dihydrotestosterone, androstenedione, and dehydroepiandrosterone. During puberty, the pituitary gland secretes large volumes of **follicle-stimulating hormone** (FSH) and **luteinizing hormone** (LH). The predominant effect of FSH is forming sperm cells. LH in males stimulates the interstitial cells of the testes, which produce approximately 95% of the body's testosterone. Interstitial cell development is also influenced by interstitial cell-stimulating hormone (ICSH). Therefore, increased production of ICSH stimulates production of testosterone.

Testosterone is responsible for the normal growth and development of the male sex organs. Testosterone is also responsible for development and maintenance of the male secondary sexual characteristics: hair distribution (beard, pubic area, chest, and axillae); all hair related to secondary sex characteristics; hair texture and color (more deeply pigmented, heavier, and sometimes more curly); laryngeal enlargement and vocal cord thickening (resulting in voice deepening); and alterations in body musculature and fat distribution.

Testosterone causes retention of sodium, potassium, and phosphorus as well as decreased urinary excretion of calcium. Sodium retention may lead to fluid retention. Testosterone also has multiple effects on bone. It stimulates the growth of skeletal muscle tissue and enhances the growth of long bones in prepubescent boys—the growth spurt of adolescence. The ossification (hardening) of the epiphyseal growth plates, which stops the growth of the long bones, occurs with prolonged elevation of testosterone levels. Testosterone also is reported to stimulate the production of red blood cells by enhancing the production of erythropoietin-stimulating factor.

The adult male produces approximately 7 to 8 mg of testosterone daily. In women, the adrenal cortex and the ovaries secrete androgens, including testosterone, although in much smaller amounts than are found in men.

Penis

The male penis has a dermal layer of smooth muscle, under which is loose connective tissue. This pliable connective tissue allows the skin of the penis to move without distorting the underlying structures. This important characteristic enables the penis to become erect. Beneath the connective tissue is a dense network of elastic fibers that encircle the internal structures of the penis. Most of the shaft of the penis is composed of three cylindrical columns of erectile tissue, each of which consists of a maze of vascular channels incompletely separated by partitions of elastic connective tissue and smooth muscle fibers. In the non-aroused state, the arterial branches are constricted, and the muscular partitions are tense, so that blood flow into the erectile tissue is restricted.

The parasympathetic system innervates the penile arteries. Normal erection involves the release of nitric oxide, secondary to sexual stimulation, in the erectile tissue of the penis. The nitric oxide activates an intermediary enzyme that boosts cyclic guanosine monophosphate (cGMP), a substance that mediates the action of certain hormones. By some unknown mechanism, cGMP stimulates smooth muscle, producing relaxation and an inflow of blood into the erectile tissue.

Urethra and Prostate

Passing through the penis is the urethra, which in men transports both urine and semen. The prostate gland is a small, muscular, rounded organ that encircles the proximal portion of the urethra as it leaves the urinary bladder (Figure 51.1). The ejaculatory duct joins the urethra in the prostate. The prostate gland is very small until puberty, when it begins to grow as a result of hormonal changes. The growth of the prostate gland slows after age 20 years but continues throughout the rest of a man's life. The primary hormone in prostate cells that affects growth of the prostate is dihydrotestosterone. A special enzyme, 5-alpha reductase, converts testosterone to dihydrotestosterone.

PATHOPHYSIOLOGY

Hormonal Problems

If a male is deficient in endogenous sex hormones, he does not experience normal sexual development. The primary sex organs do not mature, secondary sexual characteristics do not develop, reproduction is not possible, and the normal growth spurt of adolescence does not happen. If the level of endogenous hormones drops after puberty has occurred and the sexual organs and reproductive system have matured, secondary sexual characteristics may diminish. Ability to reproduce, despite developed organs, is diminished, and the man may not create enough sperm to impregnate a woman.

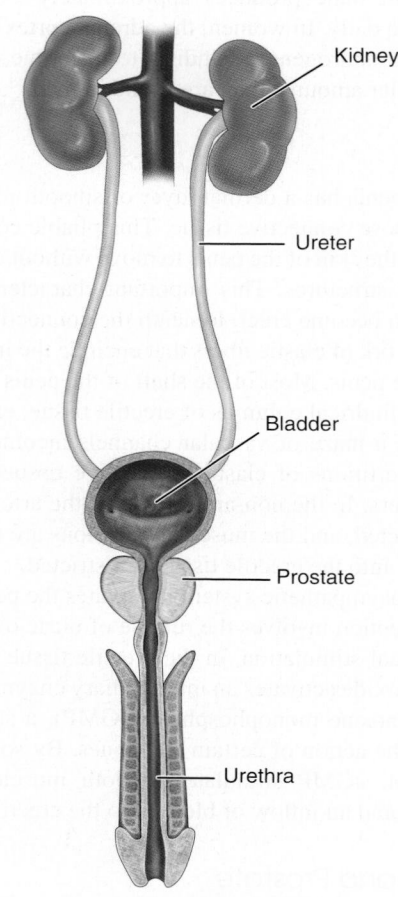

• FIGURE 51.1 Normal urine flow.

Erectile Dysfunction

Erectile dysfunction (ED), a subjective complaint of being unable to attain or sustain an erection to satisfactorily complete sexual activity, is highly prevalent, affecting more than 18 million men in the United States. However, in spite of increased awareness and effective drug therapies, ED continues to be under-diagnosed, under-treated, and can have an adverse affect on an individual's self-esteem (Ellsworth & Kirshenbaum, 2008). As men become older they are more likely to have erectile dysfunction The problem may be temporary or chronic, and may be caused by certain drug therapies, alcohol use, trauma, or illness that affects either the autonomic nervous system or the central nervous system (CNS). Physiologic causes such as cardiovascular disease and diabetes are highly correlated with erectile dysfunction. Risk factors for heart disease such as hypertension, smoking, inactivity, and high cholesterol levels are also closely related to erectile dysfunction (Selvin, Burnett, & Platz, 2007;). Severe stress, emotional problems, depression, anxiety, or fear of impaired performance may all result in sexual dysfunction. In almost 90% of men older than 50 years of age, the cause of erectile dysfunction is organic; in most younger men, the cause is psychogenic.

Benign Prostatic Hypertrophy

Prostatic enlargement that is not caused by cancer is called **benign prostatic hypertrophy or hyperplasia** (BPH). BPH occurs spontaneously in men as they age, and the incidence rises after age 40 years. By age 80, approximately 90% of men have BPH (Rosenberg, Miner, Riley & Staskin, 2010).

The exact cause of BPH is not well understood; however, as a man ages, the prostate increases in size via cellular proliferation and expansion. Because of its location, the increase in size of the prostate causes constriction of the urethra and impairs the flow of urine (Figure 51.2). This mechanical component of BPH is the basis for therapies aimed at reducing the volume of the prostate in an attempt to decrease symptoms directly related to this obstruction. An additional component of BPH relates to insufficient relaxation of smooth muscle near the prostate and neck of the bladder during urination. Activation of alpha-adrenergic receptors leads to contraction of this smooth muscle. Blocking or inhibiting this response is the goal of alpha-adrenergic blockers which enhance relaxation of the bladder neck (Rosenberg, Miner, Riley, & Staskin, 2010). Although testosterone levels fall with aging, levels of DHT (the primary hormone in the prostate) remain fairly constant. DHT is the hormone primarily responsible for prostate growth. Additionally, the small amount of estrogen in the man may also affect prostate growth because decreasing testosterone levels no longer offset the effects of estrogen.

BPH first affects the urethra as the enlarged prostate tightens around it. The pressure of the gland against the urethra is like a clamp on a garden hose, making passage of fluid more difficult (see Figure 51.2). The man has difficulty initiating a stream or stopping the flow of urine (dribbling). Over time, this pressure on the urethra from the prostate causes the man's bladder to thicken. Initially, the bladder is irritable and

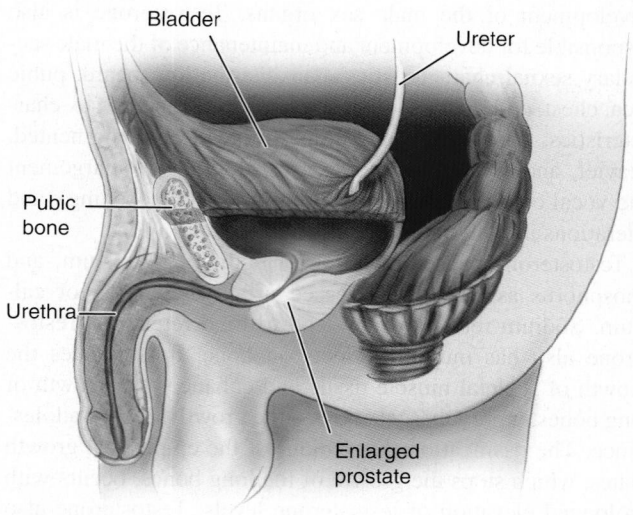

• FIGURE 51.2 Urine flow with benign prostatic hypertrophy.

contracts even when it contains only a small amount of urine, resulting in frequent urination and nocturia. As the prostate continues to place pressure on the bladder, the bladder weakens, resulting in poor contraction during urination. Eventually, the bladder can no longer empty completely, causing urinary retention. Urinary tract infections may result. Complete inability to void may also occur.

Male Pattern Baldness

The adult has two major types of hair: vellus hair and terminal hair. *Vellus hair* is the fine "peach fuzz" located over much of the body surface. *Terminal hair* is heavy, more deeply pigmented, and sometimes curly. It is located mostly on the head. Hair follicles may alter the structure of the hair on the body in response to circulating hormones. In men, decreasing levels of sex hormones can affect the scalp, causing a shift from terminal hair to vellus hair production beginning at the temples and the crown of the head. Changes in the receptors for testosterone and other male sex hormones may also induce hair loss.

Male pattern baldness, also called androgenetic alopecia, is baldness of the vertex of the scalp. Women may also have hair loss related to decreased sex hormone levels, but it differs from hair loss in men in that the loss is diffuse or may involve thinning of the frontoparietal areas.

Prostate Cancer

Prostate cancer is a malignant metastasizing cancer and the second most common cause of cancer death in men. One in 6 men in the United States will develop prostate cancer, and 1 in 33 will die from it. As men become older, their risk of developing prostate cancer increases. Compared with white men, the incidence of prostatic cancer is more common in African American men and less common in Hispanic, Asian, Pacific Islander, and Native American men. Until recently, there was no scientific consensus on effective strategies to reduce the risk of prostate cancer; however, a combined panel of experts from the American Society of Clinical Oncology and the American Urological Association, after reviewing multiple studies, developed evidence-based recommendations for prostate cancer chemoprevention. These guidelines suggest that men who have regular PSA screenings and are asymptomatic may benefit from 7 years of 5-alpha-reductase inhibitors for the prevention of prostate cancer and are encouraged to discuss this option with their healthcare provider (Kramer, Hagerty, Justman, et al., 2009).

Prostate cancer is not caused by BPH. It usually originates in one of the secretory glands. As the cancer grows, it produces a nodular lump on the surface of the prostate. During a digital rectal examination, this lump can be palpated through the rectal wall. If diagnosis is not made until after the cancer has metastasized, the prognosis for survival decreases because metastasis can rapidly involve the lymphatic system, lungs, bone marrow, liver, or adrenal glands.

Treatment of prostate cancer varies for each affected man. Treatment options include the following:

- Watchful waiting—monitoring the prostate cancer by performing a prostate-specific antigen (PSA) test and digital rectal exam regularly, and treating the cancer only if and when it causes symptoms or shows signs of growing
- Surgical intervention—radical prostatectomy (removal of the prostate)
- Internal radiation therapy—brachytherapy (surgical placement of small radioactive pellets inside or near the cancer to destroy cancer cells)
- External radiation therapy—destruction of cancer cells by directing radiation at the prostate
- Cryotherapy—placement of a special probe inside or near the prostate cancer to freeze and destroy the cancer cells
- Hormonal therapy—using antiandrogen antineoplastics and gonadotropin-releasing hormone analogues, which keep prostate cancer cells from growing. (Drugs used to treat prostate cancer are discussed in Chapters 56 and 57.)

© ANDROGENS

The prototype male sex hormone is testosterone. When testosterone is administered exogenously as a drug, it may be given in different forms. These differences may relate to the onset or duration of action or to the route of administration (oral, buccal, parenteral, topical, transdermal, and subdermal implants).

Table 54.1 provides a summary of selected drugs used to treat men's health problems.

Nursing Management of the Patient Receiving Ⓟ Testosterone
Core Drug Knowledge
Pharmacotherapeutics
In males, testosterone is used as replacement therapy for hypogonadism associated with low or no endogenous testosterone (see Table 51.1). Boys with low or no testosterone before puberty need testosterone treatment to develop secondary sexual characteristics and must continue it after puberty to maintain them. Men who develop a deficiency of testosterone after puberty require testosterone to maintain sexual characteristics. Testosterone may also be given to males with delayed puberty (puberty that is expected to occur but much later than normal) to stimulate the onset of puberty. These patients must be carefully selected and have a clear familial pattern of delayed puberty that is not secondary to a pathologic disorder. Brief treatment with conservative doses may be justified if these patients are having serious emotional problems as a result of delayed puberty. Testosterone is also used in treating erectile dysfunction and male climacteric symptoms when these conditions are secondary to androgen deficiency.

In women 1 to 5 years after menopause, testosterone may be used as secondary treatment to slow the growth of advanced, inoperable metastatic breast cancer.

TABLE 51.1 Summary of Selected Drugs Used to Treat Men's Health Problems

Drug (Trade) Name	Selected Indications	Route and Dosage Range	Pharmacokinetics
C Androgens			
P Testosterone			
testosterone (short-acting; Histerone)	*Males:* replacement therapy in hypogonadism, delayed puberty, impotence secondary to androgen deficiency	*Male:* hypogonadism (initiation of puberty), IM, 40–50 mg/m²/dose/mo or 50–400 mg/dose q2–4wk; androgen replacement, IM, 25–50 mg 2–3×/wk	*Onset:* Slow *Duration:* 1–3 d $t_{1/2}$: 10–100 min
testosterone (long-acting; Delatestryl)	*Males:* replacement therapy in hypogonadism, delayed puberty *Females:* palliation of inoperable breast cancer	*Adult:* hypogonadism (initiation of puberty), IM, 50–200 mg q2–4wk; androgen replacement, IM, 50–400 mg q2–4wk *Female:* IM, 200–400 mg q2–4wk	*Onset:* Slow *Duration:* 2–4 wk $t_{1/2}$: Up to 8 d
testosterone, transdermal (Androderm, Testim)	*Males:* primary hypogonadism, hypogonadotropic hypogonadism	*Adult:* Patch, 4–6 mg/d applied to scrotal skin (Testoderm); 5 mg/d applied to nonscrotal skin (Androderm)	*Onset:* Rapid *Duration:* 24 h $t_{1/2}$: 10–100 min
Drugs to Treat Erectile Dysfunction			
P sildenafil (Viagra)	Erectile dysfunction	PO: usual dose, 50 mg once daily; may use 25–100 mg, based on effectiveness and tolerance	*Onset:* <30 min *Duration:* up to 4 h $t_{1/2}$: 4 h
sildenafil (Revatio)	Pulmonary hypertension	PO: 20 mg 3×/d, with or without food	Same as above
tadalafil (Cialis)	Erectile dysfunction	PO, 10 mg or 20 mg once daily	*Onset:* <30 min *Duration:* Up to 36 h
vardenafil (Levitra)	Erectile dysfunction	PO, 2.5–20 mg once daily, with recommended starting dose of 10 mg	*Onset:* 15–30 min *Duration:* Up to 4 h
alprostadil (Caverject, Edex, Muse)	Erectile dysfunction	Intracavernosal injection: initial dose, 2.5 mcg; titrate upward, first by another 2.5 mcg, then by 5–10 mcg, until desired effect achieved; give no more than 3×/wk. Intraurethral: 125–1,000 mcg; use smallest effective dose (no more than 2 doses in 24 h)	*Onset:* 5–20 min *Duration:* 1 h $t_{1/2}$: 40–60 min *Onset:* 30–60 min *Duration:* Unknown $t_{1/2}$: Unknown
Drugs to Treat Benign Prostatic Hypertrophy (BPH)			
P finasteride (Proscar, Propecia)	BPH Male pattern baldness	PO: 5 mg/d PO: 1 mg/d	*Onset:* <2 h *Duration:* 24 h $t_{1/2}$: 6 h
C Alpha-1 Blockers tamsulosin (Flomax)	BPH	PO: 0.4 mg/d about 30 min after the same meal daily	*Onset:* Varies *Duration:* 24 h $t_{1/2}$: 9–13 h
Drugs to Treat Male Pattern Baldness			
P minoxidil (Rogaine, Minoxidil for Men)	Male pattern baldness	Topically: to affected area of scalp, 1 mL bid	*Onset:* ≥4 mo *Duration:* 3–4 mo after discontinuing effective dosing $t_{1/2}$: Unknown

Testosterone is available as an oral drug (Android, methyltestosterone, Testred); as a buccal extended-release tablet (Striant); as a parenteral drug (Delatestryl, Depo-Testadiol, Depo-Testosterone); as a topical drug (AndroGel); as a transdermal (Androderm, Testim), and as an implantable pellet (Testopel).

Pharmacokinetics

Natural testosterone undergoes a high first-pass effect and is not used orally. The form of testosterone that is used orally is a synthetic androgen that is less extensively metabolized and has a longer half-life than natural testosterones. The synthetic androgens are also available as buccal tablets. They are absorbed directly into the bloodstream, bypassing the gastrointestinal (GI) tract and the first-pass effect. These buccal androgens have approximately twice the potency of oral androgens. Peak serum level from buccal administration occurs in 1 hour, compared with 2 hours for oral administration. Testosterone esters are less polar than free testosterone. Testosterone esters in oil are given intramuscularly. These testosterone esters are slowly absorbed, allowing for dosing intervals of 2 to 4 weeks.

In the plasma, testosterone is about 98% bound to a specific testosterone-estradiol–binding globulin. The amount of binding globulin in the plasma determines the relative percentages of free and bound testosterone. The concentration of free testosterone determines half-life. Inactivation of testosterone occurs mostly in the liver. The conjugates and metabolites of testosterone are eliminated in the urine and feces. Testosterone crosses the placenta and enters the breast milk.

Pharmacodynamics

The effects of exogenous testosterone on males are the same as the effects of endogenous testosterone. In females, the drug causes masculinization. In addition, increased testosterone levels in women slow the growth of advanced breast cancers, which are estrogen dependent.

Contraindications and Precautions

Testosterone is contraindicated for patients with serious cardiac, hepatic, or renal disease because edema with or without chronic heart failure (CHF) may be a complication in these patients. It is also contraindicated in those people hypersensitive to the drug and in men with carcinomas of the breast or prostate. Testosterone is not normally used in premenopausal women, but it is nonetheless designated as a pregnancy category X drug because it causes masculinization of the genitalia in the female fetus.

Caution must be used when administering testosterone to the following patients:

- Young males with delayed puberty, because of testosterone's adverse effect on bone maturation
- Males with pre-existing gynecomastia (breast enlargement) because testosterone may compound the problem
- Elderly men because they may be at increased risk for BPH and prostate cancer
- Patients with BPH because they may develop acute urethral obstruction
- Patients with acute intermittent porphyria (a group of disorders that result from a disturbance in the metabolism of porphyrins, nitrogen-containing organic compounds in protoplasm) because androgens have precipitated attacks of this condition
- Patients with a history of myocardial infarction (MI) or coronary artery disease (CAD) because testosterone may promote hypercholesterolemia

Adverse Effects

Most adverse effects are related to high doses of the drug. In males, the most common adverse effects include gynecomastia, excessive frequency and duration of penile erections, decreased ejaculatory volumes, and oligospermia (low sperm count).

In females, the most common adverse effects are androgenic and include amenorrhea and other menstrual irregularities (if given before menopause), inhibition of gonadotropin secretion, and virilization, including deepening of the voice and clitoral enlargement. Clitoral enlargement is not reversible after therapy ends.

Other effects related to the actions of testosterone on the body may occur. They include hypercalcemia, particularly in immobile patients and patients with metastatic breast cancer; retention of sodium, chloride, water, potassium, calcium, and inorganic phosphates; hypercholesterolemia; and edema. In addition, rash, acne, seborrhea, and hirsutism may occur. Prostatic hypertrophy, prostatic cancer, and urethral obstruction are also possibilities. Other potential adverse effects include hepatitis (which can be life threatening), hepatocellular carcinoma (with prolonged use of high doses), premature closing of the long bones, dizziness, headache, sleep disorders, fatigue, changes in libido, and polycythemia (excess of red blood cells).

Drug Interactions

No important drug interactions are associated with natural testosterone. With the synthetic forms, anticoagulation effect is increased if anticoagulants are given with either fluoxymesterone or methyltestosterone. Coadministering methyltestosterone and imipramine may result in paranoia-like symptoms.

Assessment of Relevant Core Patient Variables

Health Status

Assess for existing serious heart, kidney, or liver disease, which are contraindications for therapy, and screen for established hypersensitivity to testosterone. Determine whether male patients have carcinoma of the breast or prostate, which is a contraindication, or whether they have gynecomastia or BPH, because these conditions require precautions. Assessing for a history of MI, CAD, or acute intermittent porphyria is important because all these factors require caution in use of testosterone. Because of testosterone's effects on bone growth, only people with expert training and knowledge of the drug and its effects on bone growth should prescribe it.

Life Span and Gender

Carefully consider age-related assessment data for problems possibly related to the use of testosterone. When testosterone is used in prepubescent boys to treat hypogonadism or delayed onset of puberty, premature closure of the long bones may lead to stunted growth. Caution also is necessary when testosterone is used in elderly men. Testosterone is not normally used in

BOX 51.1 COMMUNITY BASED CONCERNS

Athletes and Testosterone

Nurses perform a significant service when they teach patients or community groups about pitfalls of unorthodox drug use:

- Athletes have used and abused testosterone and anabolic steroids in an effort to increase muscle mass. These drugs have not been shown to be effective for this purpose.
- Serious potential adverse effects include early closure of epiphyseal growth plates, which stunts normal growth; edema (with or without CHF); and male gynecomastia.
- Increase in weight and muscle size is partially the result of water retention.

premenopausal females because it is likely to produce masculinization. If a woman is prescribed testosterone, assess the patient for pregnancy. Testosterone is a pregnancy category X; it causes masculinization of the female fetus, as characterized by clitoromegaly, abnormal vaginal development, and fusion of the genital folds to form a scrotum-like structure. These effects are most likely to occur if testosterone is given during the first trimester. If large amounts of the drug are given to a male fetus, adverse effects also are possible. It is not known whether testosterone crosses into breast milk, but testosterone is rarely used in young women.

Lifestyle, Diet, and Habits

Although anabolic steroids are abused more frequently to enhance athletic performance, testosterone has also been abused for this purpose. This use is not a safe and effective one for this drug. Verify that the patient is not abusing testosterone (Box 51.1).

Environment

Testosterone may be administered in any setting.

Nursing Diagnoses and Outcomes

- Delayed Growth and Development related to potential for early epiphyseal closure secondary to drug therapy
  Desired outcome: *The patient will attain normal height while receiving drug therapy.*
- Ineffective Sexuality Patterns related to effect of drug therapy
  Desired outcome: *The male patient will develop normal male sexual organs and characteristics. The female patient will not experience excessive masculinization during therapy.*
- Excess Fluid Volume related to potential effects of drug therapy
  Desired outcome: *The patient will not experience enough increase in fluid volume to become edematous during drug therapy.*
- Potential Complication: Hypercalcemia related to drug therapy, immobility, breast cancer
  Desired outcome: *The patient will not develop hypercalcemia.*

Planning and Intervention

Maximizing Therapeutic Effects

Administer the drug at regular intervals to maintain therapeutic testosterone levels. Adjust the dose upward per order when giving testosterone to treat hypogonadism and induce puberty. At the end of the growth spurt, the patient should remain on a maintenance dose.

Some nursing actions specific to the route of administration can maximize the therapeutic effect of testosterone. Do not place transdermal patches on the scrotum. Rather, place them on clean, dry skin on the arm, back, or upper buttocks. The skin area should not be oily, damaged, or irritated. The patient wears these patches for 24 hours and then replaces them. Apply topical preparations to clean, dry, intact skin of the shoulder, upper arm, or abdomen, *not* to the genitals.

Either the nurse or the patient places buccal tablets between the gum and the cheek. The tablets should be allowed to dissolve; they should never be swallowed.

For suspensions, agitate the vial to mix the drug thoroughly before drawing it into a syringe and administering it intramuscularly.

Minimizing Adverse Effects

When prepubescent boys undergo testosterone therapy, radiographs should be taken every 6 months to assess bone age. Radiographs help document bone maturation and the effect of testosterone on the epiphyseal centers.

Some nursing actions can minimize the adverse effects of testosterone. Monitor serum cholesterol levels and liver function periodically. Check hemoglobin and hematocrit levels periodically for polycythemia during treatment with high doses. Monitor serum and urine calcium levels in women receiving testosterone for disseminated breast cancer. In women receiving testosterone for palliative treatment of metastasized breast cancer, monitor the disease progression closely because occasionally the drug may accelerate the disease process.

When administering testosterone by intramuscular injection, inject deep into the gluteal muscle to prevent inflammation and pain at the administration site. Never administer the drug intravenously.

When administering transdermal testosterone, rotate sites of application, with at least 1 week between applications to the same area to minimize localized reactions. Discard used transdermal patches by folding them and putting them into trash in an appropriate manner or flush them down the toilet. Active drug remains after use, so accidental application or ingestion of patches by children would be dangerous.

Assess for signs of adverse effects and contact the prescriber if adverse effects are noted, especially severe masculinization in women or edema or jaundice in either sex. Dosage adjustments or cessation of therapy may be indicated.

Providing Patient and Family Education

- Teach patients and families the rationale for use of the drug, including therapeutic effects and potential adverse effects.

- Instruct patients and families about proper administration technique. If drug administration is intramuscular, teach patients how to safely dispose of needles and syringes. If administration is transdermal, teach patients how to dispose of used patches. If administration is buccal, teach patients to place the tablet between gum and cheek and not to swallow it. Remind these patients not to eat, drink, or smoke while the tablet is in place, because doing so will alter absorption of the drug.
- Review the importance of scheduling and keeping follow-up appointments for radiographs and blood tests.
- Alert patients to notify the prescriber if swelling of the extremities (edema), jaundice, or prolonged painful erection develops. Women should notify the prescriber if they develop hoarseness, deepening of the voice, menstrual irregularities, acne, or facial hair growth.

Ongoing Assessment and Evaluation

Throughout testosterone therapy monitor for adverse effects as well as blood test results. Assess bone growth regularly, as noted previously. In men, therapy is considered effective if development of male sex organs and male sexual characteristics occurs normally, or if patients maintain secondary male sexual characteristics without adverse effects. In women with breast cancer, testosterone therapy is considered effective if discomfort from the malignant tumor is minimized and the disease advances no further.

Drugs Closely Related to P Testosterone

Synthetic Testosterones

Fluoxymesterone (Halotestin) is a synthetic testosterone derivative with significant androgen activity. Synthetic fluoxymesterone is similar to the endogenous form; it suppresses testosterone release and spermatogenesis. It also inhibits the secretion of luteinizing hormone and follicle-stimulating hormone through a negative feedback mechanism. Fluoxymesterone is approved for use as an adjunct treatment for breast cancer in women who are more than 1 year but less than 5 years postmenopausal. It has palliative (not curative) effects in tumors that are androgen hormone responsive but recurrent and metastasized. Fluoxymesterone is also approved for use in adults and children with delayed puberty and hypogonadotropic hypogonadism.

Methyltestosterone (Android) is a synthetic derivative of testosterone. Its uses include delay in male sexual development and/or puberty, hypogonadotropic hypogonadism, primary hypogonadism, and metastasis from inoperable metastatic (to the skeletal system) breast cancer in women who are 1 to 5 years postmenopausal.

Anabolic Steroids

The anabolic steroids are derived from testosterone and, like testosterone, have both anabolic and androgenic effects. Unlike testosterone, these drugs have anabolic effects that are much stronger than their androgenic effects. In fact, their two

MEMORY CHIP

P Testosterone

- Used as hormone replacement therapy in male hypogonadism that is associated with low or absent endogenous testosterone
- Major contraindication: serious cardiac, hepatic, or renal disease, because edema with or without CHF may be a complication
- Most common adverse effects: gynecomastia, excessive frequency and duration of penile erections, decreased ejaculatory volumes, and oligospermia; masculinization in females
- Most serious adverse effect: life-threatening hepatitis
- **Life span alert: Pregnancy category X drug; prepubescent boys may have premature closing of long bones.**
- Maximizing therapeutic effects: Administer at regular intervals; place transdermal patches appropriately on skin.
- Minimizing adverse effects: radiographs every 6 months to determine bone maturation and the effect on the epiphyseal growth centers when treating prepubescent boys; safe disposal of used transdermal patches
- Most important patient education: Notify health care provider if swelling of the extremities (edema), jaundice, or painful, continued erection develops.

---

major actions are to promote body tissue-building processes and reverse catabolic or tissue-depleting processes. Anabolic steroids are also used to control metastatic breast cancer in women.

Oxandrolone (Oxandrin), given orally, is an adjunct for weight gain in adults and children who have lost weight as a result of chronic infection, surgery, or severe trauma as well as in patients who fail to gain or maintain weight without definite pathophysiologic reasons. The drug is also used to offset protein catabolism after prolonged corticosteroid use. Its anabolic activity is approximately six times that of methyltestosterone in human subjects following oral administration. Oxandrolone stimulates protein synthesis in skeletal muscle without affecting protein breakdown, resulting in net anabolism. The increase in protein synthesis is accomplished by increased intracellular reutilization of amino acids.

Oxandrolone is effective in increasing weight gain in HIV-associated weight loss (AIDS-related wasting syndrome) but is associated with significant increases in transaminases and low-density lipoproteins (LDLs) as well as decreases in high-density lipoproteins (HDLs). This remains an off-label use of the drug.

Stanozolol (Winstrol), another anabolic steroid, is used prophylactically to decrease the frequency and severity of attacks of hereditary angioedema (characterized by episodic edema of the abdominal viscera, extremities, face, and airway). It also has the ability to decrease HDL and increase LDL cholesterols, sometimes markedly. Stanozolol carries a Black Box warning concerning its ability to increase cholesterol levels.

Serious adverse effects common to both oxandrolone and stanozolol include peliosis hepatitis (in which blood-filled cysts replace normal liver cells and sometimes spleen cells, a condition that can be associated with liver failure), liver tumors (possibly malignant), and blood lipid changes associated with an increased risk of atherosclerosis (resulting from the previously mentioned decreased HDLs and sometimes increased LDLs). Stanozolol and oxandrolone carry Black Box warnings for these adverse effects. In females, masculinization effects similar to those effects produced by (short-acting) testosterone occur with use of anabolic steroids. Like testosterone, anabolic steroids are in pregnancy category X because of the possibility of fetal masculinization.

An abuse or addiction syndrome has been recognized with the chronic use of anabolic steroids to improve athletic performance (see Box 51.1). The use of these drugs to improve athletic performance is questionable because of the possibility of serious adverse effects, which may be irreversible.

Drug Significantly Different From

Testosterone

Chorionic gonadotropin is virtually identical to luteinizing hormone, which is produced in the pituitary gland. However, this drug has a small amount of follicle-stimulating hormone activity as well. Chorionic gonadotropin exerts its actions primarily on the ovaries and testes. In the ovaries, it works with follicle-stimulating hormone to produce a mature ovum, and it stimulates the corpus luteum to produce progesterone. In the testicles, it stimulates the production of androgen, leading to the development of male secondary sex characteristics, and it may stimulate testicular descent if there are no anatomic abnormalities preventing descent. Chorionic gonadotropin is used in the treatment of cryptorchidism (undescended testes in boys), in the treatment of hypogonadotropic hypogonadism in men, and to induce ovulation in women with fertility problems. It is discussed further in the chapter on women's health and sexuality (Chapter 52).

Drugs Used To Treat Erectile Dysfunction

Agents to treat erectile dysfunction work to mimic the body's natural methods of achieving an erection. Sildenafil (Viagra) is a cGMP-specific phosphodiesterase type 5 (PDE5) inhibitor. This drug class is considered the standard first-line therapy for erectile dysfunction (Ellsworth & Kirshenbaum, 2008).

Nursing Management of the Patient Receiving P Sildenafil

Core Drug Knowledge

Pharmacotherapeutics

Sildenafil is used to treat erectile dysfunction. It is administered orally, usually 1 hour before sexual activity. Sildenafil is effective only with accompanying sexual stimulation. A large percentage of men with diabetes and cardiovascular risk factors also have erectile dysfunction. The drug has been shown to be effective and well tolerated in men with erectile dysfunction, diabetes, and at least one other cardiovascular risk factor. In controlled studies, men with known heart disease who were taking sildenafil or one of the other PDE5 inhibitors, did not experience increased cardiac discomfort or increased ischemia during stress testing (Ellsworth & Kirshenbaum, 2008). Sildenafil is effective in erectile dysfunction after a radical prostatectomy, but only if either a bilateral or unilateral nerve-sparing procedure has been performed. It may be effective in men younger than 55 years of age if one nerve is not cut (unilateral sparing).

Sildenafil, sold under the trade name of Revatio, is also used as treatment for pulmonary arterial hypertension (PH) (Box 51.2). When given for PH, sildenafil is dosed differently; it is administered three times a day, with or without food. The RELAX trial, funded by the National Institutes of Health, is currently studying the potential for the use of sildenafil for the treatment of diastolic heart failure (Desai, 2009).

BOX 51.2 FOCUS ON RESEARCH

New Indications for Sildenafil

Blanco, I., Gimeno, E., Munoz, P. A., et al. (2010). Hemodynamic and gas exchange effects of sildenafil in patients with chronic obstructive pulmonary disease and pulmonary hypertension. *American Journal of Respiratory and Critical Care Medicine*, 181(3):270–278.

The Study

The researchers studied the hemodynamic and gas exchange effects of sildenafil in patients with COPD-associated pulmonary hypertension (PH). Eleven patients were randomly assigned to 20 mg, and nine patients to 40 mg, of sildenafil. Pulmonary hemodynamics and gas exchange, including ventilation-perfusion (V(A)/Q) relationships, were assessed at rest and during exercise, before and 1 hour after sildenafil administration. Both doses of sildenafil equally decreased the mean pulmonary arterial pressure (PAP) at rest and during exercise (–6 mm Hg at rest; –11 mm Hg during exercise). In addition, during rest, PaO_2 decreased –6 mm Hg because of increased perfusion in units with low V/Q ratios. PaO2 and V/Q relationships remained stable during exercise. The researchers concluded sildenafil improves pulmonary hemodynamics at rest and during exercise in patients with COPD-associated PH. Sildenafil also inhibited hypoxic vasoconstriction, which impairs arterial oxygenation at rest.

Nursing Implications

There are few effective drugs for the management of pulmonary hypertension (PH) and most have significant contraindications and precautions that preclude their use. Sildenafil (Revatio) is a new dosage formulation made specifically for the management of PH. Studies are now being conducted that will assess its use in COPD and heart failure patients. It is important for the nurse to remain updated on the off-label use of drugs and how to manage the patient appropriately.

Pharmacokinetics

Sildenafil is rapidly absorbed. Maximum plasma concentrations are reached within 30 to 120 minutes of oral dosing when taken on an empty stomach (the most frequent peak time is 60 minutes). When taken with a high-fat meal, absorption is delayed, so that approximately 60 extra minutes are needed to reach peak plasma levels. A high-fat meal also reduces peak serum concentrations by 29%.

Sildenafil is metabolized by two hepatic microsomal isoenzymes. The primary isoenzyme involved in metabolism is CYP3A4. A second isoenzyme, with a more minor effect on metabolism, is CYP2C9. Through these pathways, sildenafil is converted into an active metabolite that is further metabolized. The metabolite has pharmacologic properties similar to the parent drug and accounts for about 20% of sildenafil's pharmacologic effect. The metabolite of sildenafil is excreted primarily in the stool and to a small extent in the urine. Men older than 65 years have a reduced sildenafil clearance and elevated free plasma concentrations that are about 40% greater than in younger men.

Pharmacodynamics

Sildenafil inhibits PDE type 5, the isoenzyme that metabolizes cGMP. The decreased metabolism of cGMP allows it to remain active longer, increasing smooth muscle relaxation and inflow of blood. These circumstances allow for an improved and more sustained erection. Because sildenafil works at the end of a cascade of events that produce erection, starting with sexual stimulation releasing nitric oxide, in normal doses sildenafil is not effective without sexual stimulation. Men must continue sildenafil treatment to maintain improvement in erectile function. Use of sildenafil improves erectile function and also self-esteem, confidence, and satisfaction in a man's personal relationship. Studies suggest improved erectile quality leading to more satisfying sexual experiences can have a positive impact on psychosocial quality of life (Ellsworth & Kirshenbaum, 2008).

When sildenafil is used to treat pulmonary arterial hypertension, it stabilizes patients clinically, as well as improving their exercise capacity and the function of the right ventricle (Ramani & Park, 2010). The drug causes vasodilation of the pulmonary vascular bed, and to a lesser degree, vasodilation in the systemic circulation.

Contraindications and Precautions

Sildenafil is contraindicated if the patient is currently using nitrates because its vasodilating effects potentiate the hypotensive effects of nitrates. Sildenafil is also contraindicated if the patient has hypersensitivity to any component of the tablet.

The American College of Cardiology and the American Heart Association recommend caution when sildenafil is prescribed to patients who have coronary ischemia, CHF, or hypotension, or to those patients with a history of MI, cerebrovascular accident (stroke), or life-threatening arrhythmias within the past 6 months. These professional groups also recommend that any patients with strong cardiac risk factors or known cardiac disease should undergo an exercise stress test before beginning any treatment for erectile dysfunction.

Adverse Effects

Adverse effects from sildenafil are generally transient and mild to moderate in nature. The most common adverse effects are facial flushing, headache, nasal congestion, and heartburn. Other adverse effects are diarrhea, urinary tract infections, blue-tinged vision and light sensitivity, blurred vision, dizziness, and rash.

A rare adverse effect of sildenafil has been reported: nonarteritic anterior ischemic optic neuropathy, in which the patient has a sudden loss of vision in one or both eyes that is occasionally permanent. It is believed that other comorbidities, considered risk factors for nonarteritic anterior ischemic optic neuropathy, are the underlying cause of this problem, but this has not been determined conclusively. In the few post-marketing reports, most of the patients who developed this adverse effect had underlying anatomic or vascular risk factors (low cup-to-disc ratio, age older than 50 years, diabetes, hypertension, coronary artery disease, hyperlipidemia, and smoking).

Although some cardiovascular system–related deaths of patients taking sildenafil have been reported since the drug has been on the market, research and statistical analysis have found that sildenafil is not responsible for causing an excessive number of cardiovascular deaths. The anecdotal reports of deaths are believed to be caused by pre-existing cardiac risk factors (e.g., hypertension, diabetes mellitus, smoking, and depression) and the cardiovascular "work" or effort involved in sexual intercourse. However, based on these incidents, precautions must be used with patients who have known cardiovascular problems because they may have greater risk for cardiovascular adverse effects from sildenafil (see Contraindications and Precautions, above).

Overdosing produces adverse effects similar to those effects associated with normal dosing but at an increased rate of incidence. Standard supportive measures for drug overdose should be used. Renal dialysis is not helpful because little of the drug is excreted renally.

Drug Interactions

The CYP3A4 isoenzyme and, to a lesser degree, the CYP2C9 isoenzyme mediate sildenafil metabolism. Any drug that inhibits these systems may produce a drug interaction with sildenafil and decrease its clearance, raising plasma levels as a result. Strong CYP3A4 inhibitors (e.g., ketoconazole, itraconazole, erythromycin, and cimetidine) have been shown to increase the plasma levels of sildenafil as much as 200%. Any drug that induces CYP3A4, such as rifampin, will therefore probably increase the metabolism of sildenafil and subsequently decrease plasma levels of sildenafil. However, this association has not been definitively proved. As previously discussed, nitrates interact with sildenafil, increasing both vasodilation and hypotension. Table 51.2 lists drugs that interact with sildenafil.

TABLE 51.2	Drugs That Interact with P Sildenafil	
Interactants	**Effect and Significance**	**Nursing Management**
Nitrates	Sildenafil potentiates the vasodilating effect of nitric oxide from nitrates, resulting in a significant and potentially fatal decrease in blood pressure (BP).	Teach patient that he should not use any nitrate while taking sildenafil.
Azole antifungal agents	Azole antifungal agents inhibit the metabolism of sildenafil. Elevated plasma levels of sildenafil may increase risk for adverse effects	Monitor for adverse effects; a decreased dose may be indicated; consider starting dose of 25 mg.
macrolides	Macrolide antibiotics inhibit the metabolism of sildenafil. Elevated plasma levels of sildenafil may increase risk for adverse effects	Monitor for adverse effects; a decreased dose may be indicated; consider starting dose of 25 mg.
Protease Inhibitors	Protease inhibitors inhibit the metabolism of sildenafil. Elevated plasma levels of sildenafil may result in severe and potentially fatal hypotension.	Advise the patient of the risk for hypotension. Encourage the patient to refrain from use.
Serotonin Reuptake Inhibitors	SSRIs inhibit the metabolism of sildenafil. Elevated plasma levels of sildenafil may increase risk for adverse effects	Monitor for adverse effects; a decreased dose may be indicated; consider starting dose of 25 mg.

A drug–food interaction occurs when a patient takes sildenafil with a high-fat meal, delaying the rate of absorption and reducing peak serum levels.

Assessment of Relevant Core Patient Variables

Health Status

Review the patient's medication history to determine whether the patient is taking nitrates, because nitrate use is a contraindication for use of sildenafil. Assess for any of the cardiovascular problems that require cautious use of sildenafil: coronary ischemia, CHF, or hypotension; or a history of MI, cerebrovascular accident, or life-threatening arrhythmias within the past 6 months. Verify that the patient is not allergic to any component of sildenafil. Assess also for hepatic cirrhosis, which decreases metabolism of sildenafil and increases blood level of active sildenafil. Such patients may need a decreased dose. Although only a small portion of sildenafil is excreted renally, severe renal impairment does increase the maximum blood concentration of the drug. A decreased dose may also be indicated in this situation. Finally, assess for a history of nonarteritic anterior ischemic optic neuropathy, because this may increase the patient's risk of developing this adverse effect from sildenafil.

Life Span and Gender

Inquire about the patient's age. Men aged 65 years or older show increased circulating levels of sildenafil, which is most likely the result of decreased metabolism from normal age-related changes in the liver. These patients may require a decreased dose. Sildenafil is not approved for use in women.

Lifestyle, Diet, and Habits

A high-fat meal eaten before the use of sildenafil decreases the rate of absorption and reduces the maximum blood level achieved by drug therapy by about 29%. If the patient states that the drug is not always effective, assess his dietary intake. Decreasing dietary fat may increase the effectiveness of the drug therapy without a need for an increased dose.

Environment

Sildenafil is self-administered in the home.

Culture and Inherited Traits

Although most research on sildenafil has been performed on white men, the drug has also been studied in Asian men and found to be effective and well tolerated in this population.

Nursing Diagnoses and Outcomes

- Sexual Dysfunction related to erection dysfunction
  Desired outcome: Use of sildenafil will allow the patient to experience normal expression of sexuality.
- Risk for Injury related to adverse effects of drug therapy
  Desired outcome: The patient will not experience adverse effects from sildenafil, or effects will be mild, transient, and well tolerated.

Planning and Intervention

Maximizing Therapeutic Effects and Minimizing Adverse Effects

Nursing strategies to maximize the therapeutic effects and minimize the adverse effects of sildenafil are related to the patient education that is provided.

Providing Patient and Family Education

- Tell patients that sildenafil is not effective without sexual stimulation and arousal.
- Teach patients to take sildenafil about 1 hour before sexual activity.
- Instruct patients not to take nitrates (e.g., nitroglycerin, isosorbide) while taking sildenafil.
- Inform patients that sexual activity increases the risk of cardiovascular problems, including MI, for people with known cardiovascular risks. If patients experience any

CRITICAL THINKING SCENARIO

EFFECTIVENESS OF SILDENAFIL

Joe Rosenbaum is 64 years old and takes sildenafil for erectile dysfunction. He returns to the clinic for follow-up. On assessment, you learn that the drug therapy appears to be effective and that Mr. Rosenbaum is tolerating it well without apparent adverse effects. You ask whether he has any other concerns or questions. He hesitates, and then laughingly says, "The only thing is, this pill doesn't seem to be as helpful if we've gone out to a restaurant for dinner. I guess it likes my wife's cooking better." What questions might you ask Mr. Rosenbaum to help determine a possible cause of this variation in sildenafil's effectiveness?

symptoms of cardiovascular problems during sexual intercourse (e.g., angina, dizziness, nausea), they must stop the sexual activity. They should discuss any such problems with the prescriber.
- Tell patients to avoid high-fat meals before using sildenafil.
- Instruct patients that if vision loss occurs, they should discontinue the drug and notify the physician or nurse practitioner as soon as possible.

Ongoing Assessment and Evaluation

Sildenafil therapy is considered if the patient reports decreased problems with erectile dysfunction, or if the pulmonary arterial hypertension is controlled.

Drugs Closely Related to 🅟 Sildenafil

Two Food and Drug Administration (FDA)–approved drugs closely related to the prototype sildenafil are vardenafil and tadalafil, which are also PDE5 inhibitors. All three of these PDE5 inhibitors have a similar action and efficacy; however, slight differences exist—primarily related to their duration of action. Sildenafil should be taken approximately one hour before anticipated sexual activity, while tadalafil has a much longer duration and can be taken if sexual activity is anticipated within 36 hours. Another drug closely related to sildenafil is the injectable drug alprostadil.

MEMORY CHIP

🅟 Sildenafil

- Used to treat erectile dysfunction in men
- Major contraindication: current use of nitrates
- Most common adverse effects: facial flushing, headache, nasal congestion, and heartburn
- Most serious adverse effect: may increase risk of cardiovascular death in patients with current cardiovascular problems
- Most important patient education: Sexual stimulation and arousal are needed for drug effectiveness; take 1 hour before engaging in sexual activity.

Vardenafil

Vardenafil (Levitra) treats erectile dysfunction similarly to sildenafil, as another PDE5 inhibitor. Like sildenafil, it is taken orally 1 hour before intercourse for best results. Vardenafil is metabolized by the P-450 system, primarily CYP3A4 and CYP2C isoforms. Patients who take other drugs that inhibit CYP3A4, such as ritonavir, may have elevated blood levels of vardenafil, although no specific recommendations to decrease the dose of vardenafil exist. Coadministering vardenafil with alpha blockers can produce severe hypotension and is contraindicated. Nitrate use is also contraindicated for vardenafil, as it is for sildenafil. The contraindications and adverse effects of vardenafil are similar to those of sildenafil. The incidence of visual disturbances is somewhat less with vardenafil than with sildenafil.

Tadalafil

The third cGMP drug for treating erectile dysfunction is tadalafil (Cialis). Like the other two drugs in this class, sildenafil and vardenafil, tadalafil works by blocking the degradation of cyclic guanosine monophosphate. Like the other drugs, tadalafil should not be taken within 48 hours of taking nitrates, such as nitroglycerine, because substantially lower blood pressure and possibly death may result. Nitroglycerine use is a contraindication for taking tadalafil, as it is for all drugs in this class. Additionally, tadalafil should not be taken with alpha blockers, other than tamsulosin (given for BPH), because the same drug interaction may occur. Adverse effects are similar to the other drugs in the class.

The major advantage of tadalafil is that it has a longer duration of action than the other two drugs used to treat erectile dysfunction. Improved ability to achieve and sustain an erection can occur as soon as 30 minutes after taking tadalafil and as long as 36 hours after taking the drug.. This longer duration may be an advantage for those patients who feel that the need to take the drug within 60 minutes of desired sexual activity produces emotional anxiety.

Alprostadil

A drug closely related to sildenafil is alprostadil (Caverject, Edex, Muse), which is also used to treat erectile dysfunction. It is used in men who have failed to respond to sildenafil or for whom sildenafil is contraindicated. Unlike sildenafil, which is administered orally, alprostadil is administered by injection into the dorsal lateral aspect of the proximal third of the penis, or by intraurethral pellets. Alprostadil produces various pharmacologic effects; the most important are relaxation of smooth muscle, vasodilation of the arteries in the erectile tissue, and inhibition of platelet aggregation. Erection is achieved by the combination of relaxation of smooth muscles in the penis and vasodilation. An erection should occur within 5 to 20 minutes after administration. Unlike sildenafil, sexual arousal is not a prerequisite to the effectiveness of alprostadil.

Alprostadil is also given intravenously as palliative treatment for infants with patent ductus arteriosus until surgery can be performed. Off-label uses of alprostadil include pulmonary hypertension, Raynaud disease, peripheral vascular disease, and fulminant hepatic failure due to viral hepatitis.

Absorption of alprostadil occurs from the urethra with both forms of administration. With the intraurethral technique, urination should precede drug administration. The residual urine then disperses the medicated pellet, allowing absorption through the urethral mucosa. Little alprostadil enters the general circulation. Alprostadil is rapidly converted to compounds that are further metabolized before excretion. Metabolism occurs in the first pass through the lung by way of enzymatic oxidation, and almost all the drug is metabolized. This finding accounts for the very low systemic concentration of alprostadil. Excretion of the metabolites occurs primarily through the kidneys.

Contraindications to alprostadil use are those conditions that might predispose the patient to priapism (erection lasting more than 6 hours), including sickle cell anemia or trait, multiple myeloma, and leukemia. Alprostadil is also contraindicated in patients with anatomic deformations of the penis (e.g., angulation, cavernosal fibrosis) or penile implants (intracavernosal placement), if sexual activity is inadvisable or contraindicated for the man, and for sexual intercourse with a pregnant woman unless a condom is used, because vasodilation from the drug's action may be harmful to the fetus. The most common adverse effect for both routes of administration is penile pain, which is usually mild or moderate. The most common adverse effects that are solely related to intraurethral administration are urethral pain and burning. Vaginal burning, itching, or both can occur in the female partner of the man using intraurethral alprostadil. Other adverse effects that may occur with intracavernosal administration are penile fibrosis, hematoma at the injection site, prolonged erection, and penile rash or edema. Priapism may occur, although it is not common. The pharmacodynamics of alprostadil may lead to hemodynamic changes, such as decreased blood pressure and increased heart rate, although these changes are not clinically important.

Patient education on the administration technique is important. Assess the patient's technique before the patient uses the drug on his own at home.

Drug Significantly Different From P Sildenafil

Yohimbine

Yohimbine (Aphrodyne, Dayto Himbin, Yocon, Yohimex), although recognized as a drug by the FDA, has no FDA-approved indications. It is actually an herbal preparation. It is the principal alkaloid of the bark of the *Corynanthe yohimbe* tree. Clinical trials show that it has a modest benefit in treating erectile dysfunction, particularly in psychogenic erectile dysfunction, but results of the trials are not always statistically significant. Since the development of sildenafil and the other PDE5 inhibitors, its use is not generally recommended (American Urological Association, 2005/2006).

Yohimbine is taken orally, three times a day. It is an alkaloid with chemical similarities to the drug reserpine. Yohimbine is believed to have properties similar to *Rauwolfia* alkaloids. It is primarily an alpha-2 adrenergic blocker of presynaptic alpha-2 receptors, which causes release of norepinephrine. It affects the peripheral autonomic nervous system by increasing parasympathetic (cholinergic) activity and by decreasing sympathetic (adrenergic) activity, thus producing erection. Yohimbine has a stimulating effect on mood and may increase anxiety, although mostly at high doses. Yohimbine is contraindicated in renal disease. All major adverse effects occur in the CNS (e.g., nervousness, irritability, tremor, dizziness, headache, and skin flushing). Reportedly, the drug exerts no appreciable influence on cardiac stimulation. Its exact effect on blood pressure is not known.

Drugs To Treat Benign Prostatic Hypertrophy

As discussed earlier, 5-alpha reductase (specifically type II) converts testosterone into the androgen 5-alpha dihydrotestosterone (DHT). Alpha-1 blockers are also used in treating BPH, either alone or as combination therapy with a 5-alpha reductase; the combination therapy has been found to be more effective than alpha blockers alone (American Urological Association, 2003). Because the prostate gland depends on DHT for growth, interference with this process is helpful in treating BPH. Surgical intervention is another option. Transurethral resection of the prostate is the most common surgical intervention, although a prostatectomy or radical prostatectomy may be performed.

The prototype drug for treating BPH is finasteride (Proscar). Alpha-blockers are discussed briefly in this chapter related to their use in BPH; additional information about these drugs can be found in Chapters 13 and 26.

Nursing Management of the Patient Receiving P Finasteride

Core Drug Knowledge

Pharmacotherapeutics

Finasteride is used to treat BPH and androgenetic alopecia (male pattern baldness); the dose used for male hair loss is much smaller than that used for BPH (see Table 51.1). Two separate trade names are used to differentiate these preparations. Proscar is the trade name of finasteride used in BPH. Propecia is the trade name of finasteride used for male pattern baldness. The therapeutic effect for BPH is seen within 6 to 12 months of treatment, although it sometimes occurs earlier. Daily usage for more than 3 months is needed to see therapeutic effects when treating baldness. The therapeutic effects are reversed for both BPH and hair loss if the patient stops drug therapy.

Pharmacokinetics

Finasteride is well absorbed after oral administration. Food does not affect its absorption. Finasteride is highly protein bound, at a rate of about 90%. It is extensively metabolized in the liver through oxidative pathways. The inactive metabolites are excreted in the bile and feces.

Pharmacodynamics

Finasteride specifically inhibits the steroid 5-alpha reductase and consequently blocks the peripheral conversion of testosterone to DHT. Increased DHT contributes to increased size of the prostate and subsequently, to the symptoms associated with urethral obstruction. Finasteride leads to lowered serum and tissue DHT concentrations, reducing prostatic DHT by as much as 90% and circulating levels of DHT by between 60% and 80%. Finasteride also decreases DHT prostate-specific antigen levels by between 41% and 71%. As noted earlier, by blocking the conversion of testosterone to DHT, the goal of finasteride therapy is to reduce the volume of the prostate in an attempt to decrease symptoms directly related to this obstruction. These changes improve BPH-related symptoms, increase maximum urinary flow rates, and decrease prostate size.In men with male pattern hair loss, DHT is found in increased amounts in the scalp. Finasteride decreases scalp and serum DHT concentrations in these men. Finasteride does not appear to affect body hair.

Contraindications and Precautions

Finasteride is contraindicated in women and children. It is a pregnancy category X drug because it causes abnormalities of the external genitalia in the male fetus. Because of these risks, pregnant women or women who may become pregnant should not handle crushed or broken finasteride tablets. Finasteride is also contraindicated if hypersensitivity to the drug or any of its components exists. Caution should be used if the patient has impaired liver function, because finasteride is metabolized extensively in the liver.

Adverse Effects

Finasteride is generally well tolerated; adverse effects are usually mild and transient. Adverse effects, which occur in less than 4% of patients taking finasteride, include erectile dysfunction, decreased libido, and decreased volume of ejaculate. Sexual adverse effects resolved with continued treatment in more than 60% of patients who reported these effects. Overdose of finasteride has not been associated with adverse effects.

Drug Interactions

Finasteride decreases PSA levels by about 50%. A decrease in PSA level occurs even if the patient has prostate cancer. This reduction does not suggest a beneficial effect of finasteride on prostate cancer but rather an effect of the drug.

Assessment of Relevant Core Patient Variables

Health Status

Before administering the drug, verify that the patient has the clinical indications for receiving finasteride. Assess patients with BPH for prostate cancer before beginning therapy and periodically throughout therapy.

Life Span and Gender

Finasteride is not given to women or children.

Lifestyle, Diet, and Habits

Assess the patient for use of alternative medications, such as herbs.

Environment

Be aware of the environment in which the medication will be administered. Finasteride may be administered in any environment but is most frequently self-administered in the home.

Nursing Diagnoses and Outcomes

• Risk for Sexual Dysfunction related to drug therapy
  Desired outcome: *If the patient experiences sexual dysfunction, it will resolve with continued drug therapy.*
• Impaired Urinary Elimination related to BPH
  Desired outcome: *Following drug therapy with finasteride, the patient will have no or fewer lower urinary tract symptoms from BPH.*

Planning and Intervention

Maximizing Therapeutic Effects

No specific actions maximize the therapeutic effects of finasteride.

Minimizing Adverse Effects

Adverse effects are a concern for the female nurse as well as the patient. The drug is in pregnancy category X. If you are pregnant or a female and in your childbearing years do not handle crushed or broken finasteride tablets, because absorption is more likely to occur in these circumstances.

When the drug is given at home, teach the patient and family how to handle the drug to minimize risks.

Providing Patient and Family Education

• Teach patients about the rationale for drug use.
• Teach patients about possible adverse effects of the drug (impotence and decreased libido), and inform patients that these effects are usually transient.
• Tell patients that the volume of ejaculate may decrease with the use of finasteride but that this effect does not interfere with normal sexual function.
• Teach patients and their families that female family members who are pregnant or capable of having children must not handle broken or crushed finasteride.

Ongoing Assessment and Evaluation

Monitor the patient for improvement in BPH-related symptoms and increased ease of urination. If finasteride is used for male pattern baldness, increased hair growth and decreased hair loss indicate effectiveness. Throughout therapy, monitor men with BPH for prostate cancer and check PSA levels. Carefully evaluate any man on finasteride whose PSA levels increase; this development may be related to nonadherence to the drug regimen or to prostate cancer.

MEMORY CHIP

P Finasteride

- Used to treat BPH and male pattern baldness
- Major contraindication: use in women and children
- Most common adverse effects: altered sexual function (effects are mild and transient)
- **Life span alert: pregnancy category X**
- Most important patient education: Women who are or may become pregnant should not handle crushed or broken tablets.

Drug Closely Related To C Finasteride

Dutasteride (Avodart) is a 5-alpha reductase inhibitor like finasteride. Preliminary data from a 2-year study comparing dutasteride and finasteride indicated greater decreases in serum dihydrotestosterone with dutasteride after 24 weeks of treatment (at least 95% versus 70%). Compared with finasteride, dutasteride has a much longer systemic half-life (5 weeks versus 6 to 8 hours). It is metabolized through the P-450 isoenzyme 3A4 pathway, so it is likely to cause drug interactions with drugs also metabolized through this pathway. Otherwise, dutasteride is similar to finasteride.

Drugs Significantly Different From P Finasteride

Drugs significantly different from finasteride are the alpha-1 blockers, which include terazosin (Hytrin), doxazosin (Cardura), tamsulosin (Flomax), and alfuzosin (Uroxatral). As mentioned earlier, an additional component of BPH relates to insufficient relaxation of smooth muscle near the prostate and neck of the bladder during urination. Activation of alpha-adrenergic receptors leads to contraction of this smooth muscle. Blocking or inhibiting this response is the goal of these alpha-adrenergic blockers which enhance relaxation of the bladder neck (Rosenberg, Miner, Riley, & Staskin, 2010).

Each of the alpha-adrenergic blockers has been found to be equally effective in treating BPH. Larger doses generally provide additional therapeutic effects. All alpha-adrenergic receptor antagonists may work similarly, but the FDA has approved only terazosin, doxazosin, tamsulosin, and alfuzosin for this use. Alpha-1 blockers have a rapid onset of action, producing a therapeutic response within weeks (regardless of the presence of prostatic enlargement or bladder outlet obstruction). In contrast, finasteride takes longer to achieve therapeutic effects and alleviates only those symptoms associated with a large prostate.

Terazosin and doxazosin are alpha-1 blockers that are also used to treat hypertension (see Chapter 26 for more information). Alfuzosin and tamsulosin are used only to treat BPH.

Terazosin is a little more likely to cause cardiovascular adverse effects than doxazosin. Terazosin has the least hepatic metabolism of any of these drugs.

Tamsulosin is similar to finasteride in that neither drug lowers blood pressure and therefore neither is associated with the cardiovascular adverse effects (e.g., dizziness, postural hypotension) that are linked with the other alpha blockers. However, both are associated with an increased risk of sexual dysfunction; tamsulosin is associated with ejaculatory dysfunction, and finasteride is associated with decreased libido and erectile dysfunction. Alfuzosin hydrochloride (Uroxatral) is known outside of the United States as Oxatral OD. Compared with terazosin and doxazosin, it has a low incidence of possible adverse effects such as postural hypotension, syncope, and sexual side effects. This medication is dosed as a once-daily extended-release formula. It is metabolized through the P-450 3A5 pathway and so has many potential drug interactions. Alfuzosin is a pregnancy category B drug, whereas the others are in pregnancy category C.

DRUGS TO TREAT MALE PATTERN BALDNESS

At present, the FDA has only approved two drugs to treat male pattern baldness: the prototype drug, minoxidil (Rogaine, Minoxidil for Men) (see Table 51.1) and finasteride (Propecia), which is significantly different from minoxidil, as previously noted.

Nursing Management of the Patient Receiving P Minoxidil

Core Drug Knowledge

Pharmacotherapeutics

Minoxidil is used topically to treat androgenetic alopecia. Although men primarily use minoxidil, women also may use it. Minoxidil is effective in male pattern baldness of the vertex and in women with diffuse hair loss or thinning of the frontoparietal areas. It is not effective in patients who have predominantly frontal hair loss. Topical minoxidil is available as an over-the-counter (OTC) medication.

Pharmacokinetics

Topical minoxidil is poorly absorbed from normal intact scalp. Decreased integrity of the epidermal barrier from conditions such as inflammation, excoriations of the scalp, scalp psoriasis, or severe sunburn may increase systemic absorption. These abnormal scalp conditions may increase absorption enough to pose a risk for increased adverse effects.

Pharmacodynamics

The exact mode of action for topical minoxidil is unknown; however, it seems to increase the length of the anagen phase and possibly has a positive effect on the blood supply to the hair follicle (Feinstein, 2010). Oral minoxidil was originally developed as a peripheral vasodilator used in treating hypertension, and hair growth was considered an adverse effect of the drug (see Chapter 26 for more information on peripheral vasodilators used in hypertension). Topical applications require at least 4 months of twice-daily application before the patient can expect evidence of hair growth. About 60% of patients who use minoxidil experience hair growth.

Patients who respond to drug therapy need to continue the drug to maintain therapeutic effects. Reports indicate that the balding process resumes fairly soon after drug therapy is stopped.

Contraindications and Precautions

The only contraindication to topical minoxidil is hypersensitivity to any component of the drug. Topical minoxidil is classified as a pregnancy category C drug because no adequate and well-controlled studies in pregnant women have been conducted. Thus, women must avoid using it during pregnancy. Safety and efficacy in children younger than 18 years have not been established.

Adverse Effects

The most common adverse effects of topical minoxidil are irritant dermatitis and allergic contact dermatitis. Other dermatologic effects are eczema, local erythema, pruritus, dry skin and scalp flaking, and exacerbated hair loss. Systemic absorption can cause the adverse effects associated with orally administered minoxidil, including edema, chest pain, increased or decreased blood pressure, and increased or decreased pulse. Oral minoxidil carries a Black Box warning for its appropriate use and its potential for serious cardiac events in patients with preexisting cardiovascular disorders.

Topical minoxidil contains alcohol. Burning or irritation may develop if the drug gets into the eyes, mouth, or mucous membranes or onto sensitive skin. Overdose has not been reported with topical applications of minoxidil.

Drug Interactions

Topical minoxidil should not be used with other topical agents (e.g., corticosteroids, retinoids, petrolatum) known to enhance cutaneous drug absorption.

Assessment of Relevant Core Patient Variables

Health Status

Verify that the patient has male pattern baldness and does not have predominantly frontal hair loss, because topical minoxidil is not effective for frontal hair loss. If the drug is given to women, the hair loss must be diffuse or identified as thinning of the frontoparietal area for therapy to be effective. Ensure that the patient has a normal, healthy scalp before and throughout therapy. A non-intact scalp promotes systemic absorption, and adverse effects may be more prominent, especially in patients with a history of heart disease. Monitor these patients closely for any problems with tachycardia or fluid retention.

Life Span and Gender

Topical minoxidil is used primarily in men, although it may be used in women. In female patients, assess for pregnancy and intention to become pregnant because use of minoxidil in pregnancy is to be avoided. Minoxidil is a pregnancy category C drug. Ensure that the patient is older than 18 years of age because the drug's safety in children has not been established.

Environment

Be aware of the environment in which minoxidil will be administered. Topical minoxidil is self-administered in the patient's home.

Nursing Diagnoses and Outcomes

- Situational Low Self-Esteem related to hair loss
  Desired outcome: *The patient's self-esteem will improve, related to hair growth from drug therapy.*
- Risk for Injury related to adverse effects of drug therapy
  Desired outcome: *The patient will not experience adverse effects of drug therapy.*

Planning and Intervention

Maximizing Therapeutic Effects

Nursing actions to maximize the therapeutic effect are related to patient education.

Minimizing Adverse Effects

Nursing actions to minimize the adverse effects are related to patient education.

Providing Patient and Family Education

- Teach patients receiving topical minoxidil the purpose and possible adverse effects of the drug.
- Teach patients to administer the drug using this technique:
  1. Dry the hair and scalp before application.
  2. Apply 1 mL to the total affected area of the scalp twice daily, once in the morning and once at night.
  3. Wash hands after applying the drug.
- Advise patients not to use minoxidil with other topical medications on the scalp.
- Caution patients not to apply minoxidil if the scalp is irritated or sunburned, because these conditions may increase the risk of adverse effects.
- Advise patients not to try to make up for any missed doses but to simply resume the normal administration schedule instead.
- Teach patients not to use more than the prescribed amount twice a day.

MEMORY CHIP

P Minoxidil (topical)

- Used topically to promote growth of hair in male pattern baldness
- Use for 4 months or more required to see effect
- Is an over-the-counter drug
- Most common adverse effects: irritation and dermatitis at application site
- Most serious adverse effects: edema and tachycardia
- Most important patient education: Use bid; do not increase dosage or frequency; do not use if scalp is irritated or sunburned.

• Advise patients that twice-daily use for 4 months or longer may be needed to see results. Fine, soft, colorless hair that is barely visible may be the first hair to grow. Over time, the new hair will become the same color and thickness as the other hair on the scalp.

• Keep medication out of the eyes and mouth; avoid applying it to sensitive skin on the face. If accidental exposure occurs, flush the area with large amounts of cool tap water. Consult with the prescriber if irritation continues.

• If no response to treatment occurs in 4 months or more, consult with the physician about the appropriateness of continuing therapy.

Ongoing Assessment and Evaluation

Assess the patient's scalp periodically to determine whether irritation has developed. The patient usually checks his own scalp during therapy. Topical minoxidil treatment is effective when hair growth has occurred with no adverse effects.

CHAPTER SUMMARY

• Testosterone is the main male sex hormone. Insufficient testosterone prevents the growth spurt of adolescence and the development of secondary male sex characteristics. Lack of testosterone after development of secondary sex characteristics causes those characteristics to diminish.

• Exogenous testosterone is used when endogenous levels are low. Exogenous testosterone causes the same effects on the body as endogenous testosterone.

• One problem affecting male sexuality is erectile dysfunction. This problem may result from multiple factors, such as stress, adverse effects of drug therapy, and cardiovascular or neurologic impairments.

• When erectile dysfunction is a recurring problem, drug therapy may be used. Sildenafil and the other PDE5 inhibitors have the advantage of being very effective oral drugs. However, they are effective only in conjunction with sexual stimulation; they are not aphrodisiacs.

• PDE5 inhibitor drugs are the first-line drug treatment for erectile dysfunction. Because they cause vasodilation, significant hypotension can occur if they are taken with nitrates or alpha-1 blockers, which also cause vasodilation and hypotension.

• Sildenafil is also used in the treatment of pulmonary arterial hypertension and under study for the management of diastolic heart failure.

• A common problem of the older man is BPH. The exact cause of BPH is unknown, although excessive growth of the prostate is believed to be caused primarily by elevated levels of DHT (the primary hormone in the prostate cells). Overgrowth of the prostate places pressure on the urethra and the bladder, resulting in lower-urinary-tract symptoms.

• Drug therapy is one type of treatment for BPH. Drug therapy for BPH includes finasteride or dutasteride, which decreases the size of the prostate over time, and alpha-1 blockers, which relax the smooth muscle of the bladder and decrease difficulties in voiding.

• Male pattern baldness is another men's health issue. This problem may be related to changing testosterone levels or alterations in the male sex hormone receptors.

• Topical minoxidil can be effective in promoting hair growth for male pattern baldness. This drug is available OTC. Women may also use minoxidil.

QUESTIONS FOR STUDY AND REVIEW

1. What effects does testosterone have on the male?
2. What is the main risk when administering testosterone to induce the growth spurt of puberty?
3. How does sildenafil act to help the man achieve an erection?
4. Why should women not handle broken or crushed finasteride?
5. Topical minoxidil is poorly absorbed into the systemic circulation. What is the advantage of this factor?

NEED MORE HELP?

Chapter 51 of the Study Guide to Accompany *Drug Therapy in Nursing*, 4th Edition, contains NCLEX-style questions and other learning activities to reinforce your understanding of the concepts presented in this chapter. For additional information or to purchase the study guide, visit thePoint.

REFERENCES

American Urological Association. (2005; updated 2006). Guidelines on the management of erectile dysfunction: Diagnosis and treatment recommendations. Retrieved from *http://www.auanet.org/guidelines/main_reports/edmgmt/chapter1.pdf*

Centers for Disease Control and Prevention. Prostate cancer. Retrieved June 20, 2010, from *http://www.cdc.gov/cancer/prostate/index.htm*

Colucci, W. S. (2010). Treatment of acute decompensated heart failure: Components of therapy, Up To Date. Retrieved from http://www.uptodate.com/online/content/topic.do?topicKey=hrt_fail/10223&selectedTitle=10~110&source=search_result on July 30, 2010.

Desai, A. (2009). Sildenafil for the treatment of heart Failure Access Medicine from McGraw-Hill, 2009-01-13 Retrieved July 17, 2010, from *http://www.Medscape.com*

Ellsworth, P., & Kirshenbaum, E. (2010). Current concepts in the Evaluation and management of Erectile Dysfunction. *Urological Nursing, 28*(5):357–369.

Facts and Comparisons. (2010). *Drug facts and comparisons.* Philadelphia, PA: Lippincott Williams & Wilkins.

Feinstein, R. P. (2010). Androgenic Alopecia: Treatment and Medication. Retrieved from: http://www.medscape.com

Kramer, B. S., Hagerty, K. L., Justman, S., et al. (2009). Use of 5 alpha-reducatase inhibitors for prostate cancer chemoprevention: American Society of Clinical Oncology/American Urological Association 2008 Clinical Practice Guideline. *The Journal of Urology,* (181):1642–1657.

National Cancer Institute, U. S. National Institutes of Health. Prostate Cancer Treatment (PDQ) Health Professional Version.

National Cancer Institute, U. S. National Institutes of Health. Prostate Cancer Treatment (PDQ) Health Professional Version. Retrieved July 20, 2010, from http://www.cancer.gov/cancertopics/pdq/treatment/prostate/HealthProfessional

Porth, C. M. (2008). *Pathophysiology: concepts of altered health states* (8th Ed.). Philadelphia, PA: Lippincott Williams & Wilkins.

Ramani, G. V., & Park, M. H. (2010). Update on the clinical utility of sildenafil in the treatment of pulmonary arterial hypertension. *Drug Design, Development, and Therapy*, 4:61–70.

Rosenberg, M. T., Miner, M. M., Riley, P. A., & Staskin, D. R. (2010). STEP: Simplified Treatment of the enlarged Prostate. *International Journal of Clinical Practice*, 64(4):488–496.

Rosenberg, M. T., Adams, T. A., McBride, J. N., Roberts, J. N., & McCallum, S. W. (2009). Improvement in duration of

erection following Phosphodiesterase Type 5 Inhibitor Therapy with Vardenafil in Men with erectile dysfunction: The ENDURANCE Study. *International Journal of Clinical Practice*, 63(1):27–34.

Selvin, E., Burnett, A. L., & Platz, E. A. (2007). The prevalence and risk factors for erectile dysfunction in the US. *American Journal of Medicine*, 120(2):151–157.

Spark, R. F. (2010). Treatment of male sexual dysfunction, Up to Date. Retrieved from http://www.uptodate.com/online/content/topic.do?topicKey=r_endo_m/6961&selectedTitle=3~150&source=search_result on July 30, 2010.

Tatro, D. S. (2011). *Drug interaction facts: the authority on drug interactions*. Philadelphia, PA: Lippincott Williams & Wilkins.

52

Drugs Affecting Women's Health and Sexuality

Learning Objectives

At the completion of this chapter the student will:

1. Identify core drug knowledge about drugs that affect women's health and sexuality.

2. Identify core patient variables relevant to drugs that affect women's health and sexuality.

3. Relate the interaction of core drug knowledge to core patient variables for drugs that affect women's health and sexuality.

4. Compare the risks and benefits of hormone replacement therapy in postmenopausal women.

5. Generate a nursing plan of care from the interactions between core drug knowledge and core patient variables for drugs that affect women's health and sexuality.

6. Describe nursing interventions to maximize therapeutic effects and minimize adverse effects of drugs that affect women's health and sexuality.

7. Determine key points for patient and family education for drugs that affect women's health and sexuality.

Key Terms

estrogen	menopause	progestin
follicle-stimulating hormone	osteoporosis	proliferative phase
gonadotropin-releasing hormone	Paget disease	secretory phase
luteinizing hormone		

Drugs Affecting Women's Health and Sexuality

C Estrogens

P **conjugated estrogen**
synthetic conjugated estrogens
contraceptives
clomiphene
gonadotropins
menotropins
human chorionic gonadotropin
gonadotropin-releasing hormones
gonadotropin-releasing hormone antagonists
synthetic androgens

C Bisphosphonates

P **alendronate**
etidronate
ibandronate
tiludronate
pamidronate
risedronate
zoledronic acid
calcitonin, salmon
raloxifene
teriparatide

C Progestins

P **progesterone**
contraceptives
medroxyprogesterone
norethindrone
norethindrone acetate
megestrol
mifepristone

C Contraceptives

oral contraceptives
emergency oral contraceptives
transdermal contraceptives
vaginal ring contraceptive
implanted contraceptives
intrauterine system contraceptives

The symbol C indicates the drug class.
Drugs in **bold type** marked with the symbol P are prototypes.
Drugs in blue type are closely related to the prototype.
Drugs in red type are significantly different from the prototype.
Drugs in black type with no symbol are also used in drug therapy; no prototype.

The female sex hormones are responsible for the normal development and maintenance of adult female sexual characteristics. If endogenous hormone levels are insufficient, sexual characteristics fail to develop. If endogenous levels are low after female sexual characteristics develop, the woman may be unable to become pregnant or maintain a pregnancy. If levels of sex hormones become low enough, masculinization may occur. Additionally, research has shown that low levels of female sex hormones contribute to some common women's health problems. This chapter presents the use of female sex hormones as replacement drug therapy when endogenous levels are absent or insufficient. It discusses two classes of female sex hormones: estrogens and progestins. The prototype estrogen is conjugated estrogen (Premarin), and the prototype progestin is progesterone (Prometrium, Progesterone).

This chapter also discusses bisphosphonates, the drugs used in treating osteoporosis, a common health problem in postmenopausal women. The prototype bisphosphonate is alendronate (Fosamax).

PHYSIOLOGY

The female sex hormones are responsible for producing female sexual characteristics, developing the female reproductive system, and maintaining pregnancy. The two types of female sex hormones are **estrogen** and **progestin.** Both are steroidal compounds that the ovaries begin to secrete at puberty and that the placenta secretes during pregnancy. The adrenal cortex also secretes estrogen and progestin, but in much smaller amounts.

Estrogen

The female body produces six different estrogens but only three in substantial amounts: estradiol, estrone, and estriol. Estradiol is the most potent and the major estrogen secreted by the ovaries. In addition to promoting and maintaining female organs and secondary sexual characteristics (e.g., distribution of body hair, high-pitched voice), estrogen affects the release of pituitary gonadotropins, causes capillary dilation, and promotes fluid retention. It also enhances protein anabolism, promotes thinning of cervical mucus, inhibits or facilitates ovulation, and prevents postpartum breast pain. Estrogen also maintains the tone and elasticity of the urogenital structures and stimulates growth of axillary and pubic hair and pigmentation of the nipples and genitals.

Estrogen promotes growth during the adolescent growth spurt; continued elevated levels of estrogen terminate growth by stimulating closure of the epiphyses of the long bones. Closure occurs because estrogen stimulates the osteoblasts in the bone to produce bone faster than the epiphyseal cartilage can expand. Because estrogens cause a faster epiphyseal closure than androgens, women are generally shorter than men by adulthood. Estrogen indirectly contributes to strengthening the skeleton by conserving calcium and phosphorus and encouraging bone formation. After puberty, estrogen is important in maintaining normal bone density and composition. The organic and mineral components of bone are continuously being recycled and renewed throughout life; this process is called bone remodeling.

Progestin

Progestins, which include progesterone and its derivatives, are the other female sex hormones. Progesterone is the primary endogenous progestin. The progestins change the proliferative endometrium into a secretory endometrium. Through positive feedback, they also inhibit or facilitate secretion of pituitary gonadotropins. Doing so either prevents follicular maturation and ovulation or promotes maturation for the primed follicle. Progestins also inhibit spontaneous uterine contractions and contractions of other smooth muscles throughout the body. They may also demonstrate some anabolic or androgenic activity.

Menstrual Cycle

Much secretion of the female sex hormones is cyclic, and these cyclic changes constitute the menstrual cycle. **Gonadotropin-releasing hormone** (GnRH), which is secreted by the hypothalamus and then perfused throughout the anterior pituitary, stimulates the release of **follicle-stimulating hormone** (FSH) and **luteinizing hormone** (LH). During puberty, the pituitary gland secretes large volumes of FSH and LH to initiate and establish the menstrual cycle. These hormones stimulate the development of the ovarian follicles and the release of the ovum from the mature follicle (Figure 52.1). As the follicles grow, they produce estrogen. Estrogen increases the vascularity of the uterine lining, preparing it for implantation of a fertilized egg. This phase of the menstrual cycle is termed the **proliferative phase.** The rapidly rising estrogen levels further stimulate GnRH, encouraging further release of LH. The high levels of LH trigger the rupture of the mature follicle, and ovulation occurs.

After ovulation, the follicle is transformed into the corpus luteum, which secretes progesterone and estrogen. This phase is known as the **secretory phase** of the menstrual cycle. In response to the rising levels of estrogen and progesterone, the endometrial glands continue to grow, the arteries of the endometrium become spiraled, and the endometrium prepares for implantation of a fertilized egg. When estrogen and progesterone have reached critical levels, they create negative feedback, directly preventing further release of GnRH and indirectly preventing the release of FSH and LH. If fertilization does not occur, the corpus luteum disintegrates, estrogen and progesterone levels fall, and the endometrial tissue sloughs off in the menses. As the levels of estrogen and progesterone continue to decline, GnRH is again secreted, reinitiating the process. If fertilization occurs, the corpus luteum remains and continues to secrete estrogen and progesterone until the placenta takes over at approximately 10 weeks

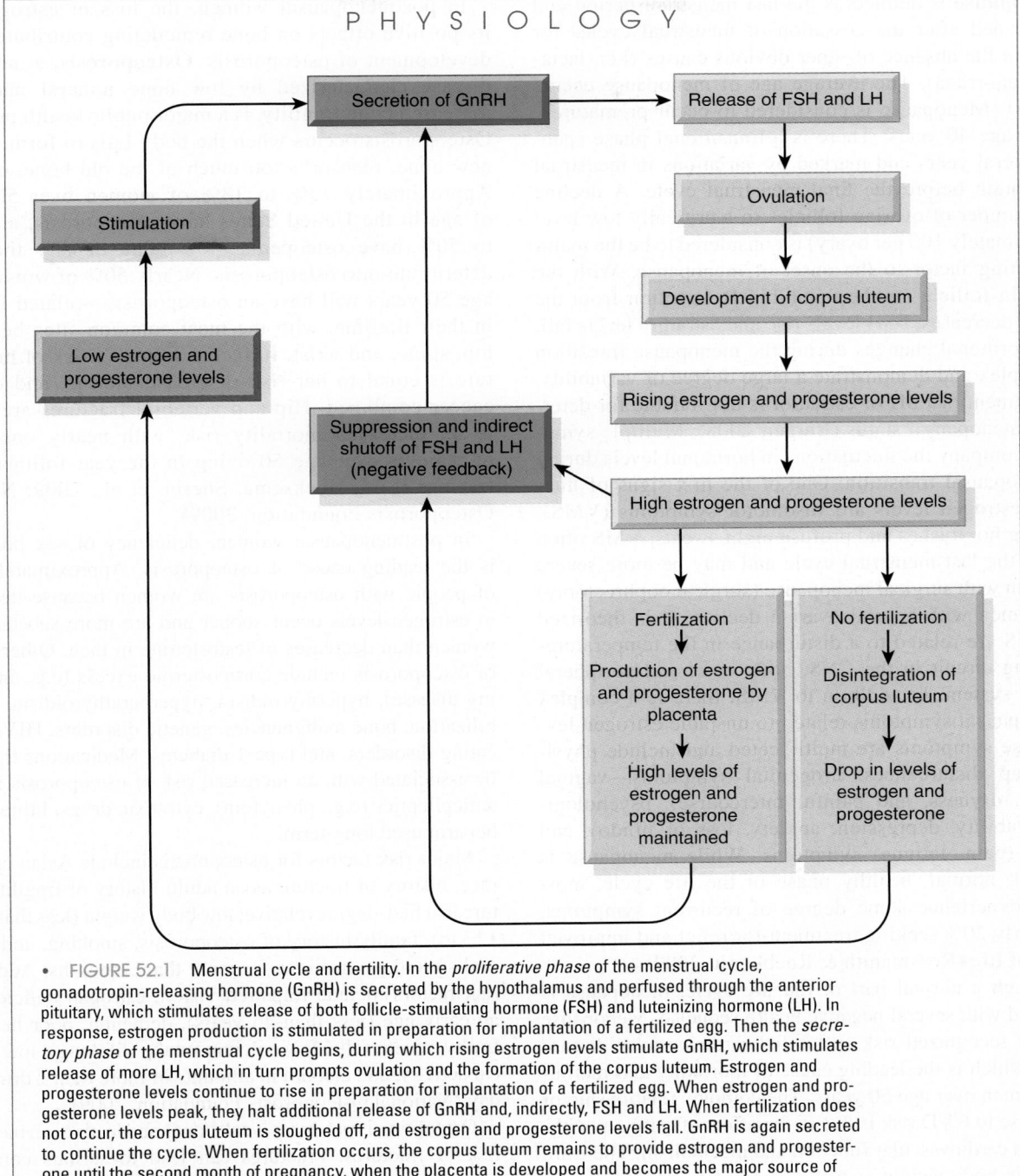

PHYSIOLOGY

• FIGURE 52.1 Menstrual cycle and fertility. In the *proliferative phase* of the menstrual cycle, gonadotropin-releasing hormone (GnRH) is secreted by the hypothalamus and perfused through the anterior pituitary, which stimulates release of both follicle-stimulating hormone (FSH) and luteinizing hormone (LH). In response, estrogen production is stimulated in preparation for implantation of a fertilized egg. Then the *secretory phase* of the menstrual cycle begins, during which rising estrogen levels stimulate GnRH, which stimulates release of more LH, which in turn prompts ovulation and the formation of the corpus luteum. Estrogen and progesterone levels continue to rise in preparation for implantation of a fertilized egg. When estrogen and progesterone levels peak, they halt additional release of GnRH and, indirectly, FSH and LH. When fertilization does not occur, the corpus luteum is sloughed off, and estrogen and progesterone levels fall. GnRH is again secreted to continue the cycle. When fertilization occurs, the corpus luteum remains to provide estrogen and progesterone until the second month of pregnancy, when the placenta is developed and becomes the major source of estrogen and progesterone to maintain the pregnancy.

gestation and becomes the major source of estrogen and progesterone to maintain the pregnancy.

PATHOPHYSIOLOGY

If a woman is deficient in endogenous sex hormones, she does not experience normal sexual development. The primary sex organs do not mature, secondary sexual characteristics do not develop, reproduction is not possible, and the normal growth spurt of adolescence does not happen. If levels of endogenous hormones drop after puberty has occurred and the sexual organs and reproductive system have matured, secondary sexual characteristics may diminish. The ability to reproduce is diminished, despite the presence of developed organs, and the woman may be unable to carry a pregnancy to term.

Menopause is defined as the last menstrual period and is confirmed after the cessation of menstrual cycles for 1 year, in the absence of other obvious causes (i.e., lactation amenorrhea). The average age of menopause occurs at age 51. Menopause is considered to occur prematurely prior to age 40 years. There is a transitional phase spanning several years and marked by variations in menstrual cycle length before the final menstrual cycle. A decline in the number of ovarian follicles to a critically low level (approximately 100 per ovary) is considered to be the major contributing factor to the onset of menopause. With the decline in follicle numbers, inhibin B secretion from the follicles decreases, FSH levels rise and estradiol levels fall. These hormonal changes during the menopause transition are complex and demonstrate a large degree of variability. Measurement of FSH or estradiol is not reliable for determining menopausal status (Burger, 2008). Multiple symptoms accompany the fluctuations in hormonal levels during the menopausal transition. One of the first signs of fluctuating estrogen levels are vasomotor symptoms (VMS), including hot flushes and profuse night sweats. VMS often precede the last menstrual cycle and may be more severe in women with surgical menopause (surgical oophrectomy) than women with natural ovarian decline. It is theorized that VMS are related to a disturbance in the temperature-regulating circuit in the CNS, body core, and peripheral vascular system. In addition to VMS, there is a complex of menopausal symptoms related to unstable estrogen levels. These symptoms are multifaceted and include physical (sleep disturbances, urogenital symptoms—vaginal thinning, dryness, and painful intercourse), psychological (irritability, depression, anxiety, loss of libido), and somatic (pain, fatigue) symptoms. While menopause is a natural, normal, healthy phase of the life cycle, most women experience some degree of recurrent symptoms, with nearly 20% seeking treatment for relief and improved quality of life (Rossmanith & Ruebberdt, 2009).

Although a normal part of the life cycle, menopause is associated with several negative health sequelae. Menopause is a well recognized risk factor for cardiovascular disease (CVD), which is the leading cause of morbidity and mortality in women over age 50 years. The complex relationship of menopause to CVD risk is due to the effect of estrogen withdrawal on cardiovascular function and metabolism. There are changes in body weight as well as body fat distribution to a more android pattern. Changes in body weight are associated with insulin resistance, sodium and fluid retention, abnormal plasma lipid levels, increased blood pressure, and vascular inflammation (Rosano, Vitale, Maazzi, & Volterrani, 2007). This combination of risk factors (abdominal obesity, dyslipidemia, glucose intolerance, and hypertension), known as metabolic syndrome, is common in postmenopausal women, with estimates that nearly 40% of postmenopausal women meet criteria for the disorder. Metabolic syndrome may be an important link to postmenopausal cardiovascular disease (Kaaja, 2008).

In postmenopausal women, the loss of estrogen and its positive effects on bone remodeling contribute to the development of osteoporosis. **Osteoporosis,** a metabolic disease characterized by low bone mineral mass and increased bone fragility, is a major public health problem. Osteoporosis occurs when the body fails to form enough new bone, reabsorbs too much of the old bone, or both. Approximately 13% to 18% of women over 50 years of age in the United States have osteoporosis, and 37% to 50% have osteopenia—low bone density that may deteriorate into osteoporosis. Nearly 50% of women over age 50 years will have an osteoporosis—related fracture in their lifetime, with the most common sites being the hip, spine, and wrist. In fact, a woman's risk of hip fracture is equal to her risk of breast, uterine, and ovarian cancer combined. Hip and vertebral fractures are linked to an increased mortality risk, with nearly one-fourth of patients over age 50 dying in the year following the fracture (Lim, Hoeksema, Sherin, et al., 2009; National Osteoporosis Foundation, 2009).

In postmenopausal women, deficiency of sex hormones is the leading cause of osteoporosis. Approximately 80% of people with osteoporosis are women because decreases in estrogen levels occur sooner and are more substantial in women than decreases of testosterone in men. Other causes of osteoporosis include corticosteroid excess (e.g., in Cushing disease), hyperthyroidism, hyperparathyroidism, immobilization, bone malignancies, genetic disorders, HIV/AIDS, eating disorders, and type 1 diabetes. Medications that may be associated with an increased risk of osteoporosis include antiepileptics (e.g., phenytoin), cytotoxic drugs, lithium, and heparin used long-term.

Major risk factors for osteoporosis include Asian or white race, history of fracture as an adult, history of fragility fracture in a first-degree relative, low body weight (less than about 127 lb), family history of osteoporosis, smoking, and use of oral steroid medications for more than 3 months. Additional risk factors include impaired vision, estrogen deficiency at an early age (less than 45 years), dementia, poor health or frailty, recent falls, low calcium intake (lifelong), low physical activity, and alcohol in amounts of more than 2 drinks per day (National Osteoporosis Foundation, 2009).

Osteoporosis produces weak bones and leads to an increased risk of fractures. Fractures can lead to serious complications, including pain, loss of mobility, complications related to immobility, and death. Bone changes in postmenopausal women may also be related to decreased physical activity. Heavily stressed bones, such as those used in regular weight-bearing exercise (e.g., walking, running), are stronger and thicker than bones not subjected to these ordinary stresses, which become thin and brittle. Moderate physical activity and weight bearing are essential for bone remodeling.

Nonpharmacologic interventions to reduce fracture risk from osteoporosis can be recommended to the general population. These include an adequate intake of calcium and vitamin D, lifelong participation in regular weight-bearing and muscle-strengthening exercise, avoidance of tobacco use, identification and treatment of alcoholism, and treatment of other risk factors for fracture. A recent analysis of data from the Framingham Osteoporosis Study found that 41.1% of women and 17% of men 50 years of age and older met the 2008 National Osteoporosis Foundation Guidelines recommending pharmacologic treatment of osteoporosis (Berry, Kiel, Donaldson, et al., 2010).

Ⓒ ESTROGENS

Estrogens are available in many chemical formulations, including conjugated estrogens, synthetic conjugated estrogens, esterified estrogens, estradiol, estropipate, ethinyl estradiol, and estradiol acetate. The many different types of exogenous estrogen differ somewhat in terms of indications, route of administration, and pharmacokinetics. Routes of administration may be oral, intramuscular (IM), transdermal, or topical (as vaginal creams). Most of these estrogens are used for correction of low endogenous estrogen or in birth control products combined with progestins. The prototype estrogen is conjugated estrogen (Premarin). Table 52.1 provides a summary of selected estrogens.

Nursing Management of the Patient Receiving Ⓟ Conjugated Estrogen

Core Drug Knowledge

Pharmacotherapeutics

Conjugated estrogen is used primarily in hormone replacement therapy (HRT) in female hypogonadism, female castration, and primary ovarian failure. Estrogen replacement therapy is also used in menopausal women to treat moderate to severe vasomotor responses (hot flashes). Other uses in menopause include treating atrophic vaginitis, vaginal dryness, painful intercourse, mood swings, and loss of tone in genitourinary muscles. *Menopausal symptoms should be treated with as small a dose as possible for as short a time as possible*. It should not be considered life-long therapy. Although estrogen is approved for use in postmenopausal women who have evidence of bone loss (osteoporosis) and has been shown to reduce further bone loss and to improve bone density, it is *not* currently recommended as a first-line treatment for this condition because of complications arising from estrogen use. Other drugs to help promote bone density are safer and should be used first (Mitchner & Harris, 2009). (See the discussion of alendronate later in this chapter; also

TABLE 52.1 — Summary of Selected Ⓒ Estrogens

Drug (Trade) Name	Selected Indications	Route and Dosage Range	Pharmacokinetics
Ⓟ conjugated estrogen (Premarin)	Hormone replacement therapy	*Adult:* PO, 0.3–0.625 mg/d cyclically (3 wk on, 1 wk off)	*Onset:* Slow *Duration:* 24 h $t_{1/2}$: Unknown
estradiol, transdermal (Vivelle, Estraderm, Climara)	Female hypogonadism Vasomotor symptoms associated with menopause Hormone replacement therapy	*Adult:* 0.025–0.05 mg applied to skin once or twice weekly (brand dependent)	*Onset:* Slow *Duration:* 3–7 d $t_{1/2}$: Unknown
estradiol, oral (Estrace)	Hormone replacement therapy Inoperable breast cancer Prostatic cancer	*Adult:* PO, 1–2 mg/d *Adult:* PO, 10 mg tid *Adult:* PO, 1–2 mg tid	*Onset:* Slow *Duration:* Unknown $t_{1/2}$: Unknown
estradiol valerate in oil (Delestrogen)	Hormone replacement therapy Prostate cancer	*Adult:* IM, 10–20 mg q4wk *Adult:* IM, 30 mg q1–2wk	*Onset:* Slow *Duration:* 4 wk $t_{1/2}$: Unknown
Selected Nonestrogens			
clomiphene (Clomid, Milophene)	Ovulatory failure	*Adult:* PO, 50–100 mg/d for 5 d	*Onset:* 5–8 d *Duration:* 6 wk $t_{1/2}$: 5 d
menotropins (Pergonal, Humegon)	Ovulation stimulation Spermatogenesis stimulation	*Adult:* IM, 75 IU/d for 7–12 d; follow with HCG *Adult:* IM, 75–150 IU 3∞/wk; pretreat and cotreat with HCG	*Onset:* Slow $t_{1/2}$: Unknown *Duration:* Months
chorionic gonadotropins (Choron, Pregnyl)	Hypogonadotropic hypogonadism (males) Ovulation stimulation Spermatogenesis stimulation	*Adult:* 500–4,000 USP 3∞/wk *Adult:* 5,000–10,000 USP 1 d after last menotropin dose *Adult:* Pretreatment, IM, 5,000 IU 3∞/wk for 4–6 mo; cotreatment, 2,000 IU 2∞/wk with menotropins	*Onset:* Unknown *Duration:* Unknown $t_{1/2}$: Unknown after pretreatment with menotropins

see Table 52.3). Conjugated estrogen is also used to treat abnormal uterine bleeding resulting from hormonal imbalance with no organic pathology. Additionally, conjugated estrogen is used as palliative therapy in advanced prostatic cancer, in men with metastatic breast cancer, and in selected women with breast cancer who do not have an estrogen-dependent tumor. General consensus holds that estrogen replacement therapy should *not* be used in postmenopausal women in an attempt to prevent cardiovascular disease or complications. Recent research however suggests that the timing of estrogen treatment may be a factor. There may be potential cardiovascular benefits with earlier initiation of therapy after menopause, specifically in women between 50 and 59 years. Continued research is needed to address this issue (Gungor, Kalelioglu, & Turfanda, 2009; Palacios, 2008).

Pharmacokinetics

Absorption from the gastrointestinal (GI) tract is complete. Estrogen binds to specific receptor proteins in tissues that are responsive to estrogen (female genital organs, breasts, hypothalamus, pituitary). Metabolism occurs primarily in the liver. While circulating through the liver, estrogen is degraded to less active estrogenic compounds. Some estrogens are excreted into the bile and then reabsorbed from the intestines and returned to the liver. The estrogen conjugates are water soluble and are excreted through the kidneys, with minimal resorption. Conjugated estrogen crosses the placenta and enters breast milk.

Pharmacodynamics

Estrogen given to females with insufficient endogenous estrogen (hypogonadism) stimulates the development of the female sex organs and secondary female sexual characteristics. Estrogen also stimulates the long-bone growth spurt of adolescence; when circulating estrogen reaches a certain level, it triggers closure of the epiphyseal plates to stop growth. Other actions of estrogen include facilitating or inhibiting ovulation (depending on dose), increasing fluid retention, facilitating protein anabolism, conserving calcium and phosphorus, stimulating bone formation, and maintaining tone and elasticity of urogenital structures.

The use of hormonal replacement therapy (HRT) for postmenopausal symptoms is controversial. Some symptoms occur due to declining ovarian function, while other may be related to more complex life changes and aging. In 2005, the National Institute of Health published a Consensus and State-of-the-Science statement evaluating the current evidence on HRT. Evidence was supportive for relief of vasomotor symptoms (hot flashes and night sweats) as well as for vaginal dryness and painful intercourse. There was insufficient support for the role of HRT in mood symptoms, cognitive disturbances, somatic symptoms, urinary incontinence, sexual dysfunction, or quality of life. Recently, additional research has focused new light on the role of HRT demonstrating that it may alleviate some postmenopausal symptoms, improve quality of life, and provide chemoprevention of some co-morbid conditions when used within the first 5 years of cessation of menses. A recent systematic review by Canerelli and colleagues (2007) found beneficial effects for type II diabetes, cardiovascular disease, osteoporosis, and colorectal cancer when used within a therapeutic window early in menopause and for a limited time. The protective effect for colon cancer is not demonstrated with estrogen therapy alone (Boursi & Arber, 2007; Schindler, 2007).

Contraindications and Precautions

There are also substantial risks associated with HRT. The Women's Health initiative (WHI), a randomized controlled clinical trial of over 16,000 postmenopausal women, was stopped early when the risks exceeded the benefits of treatment. Specifically, women assigned to the HRT arm of the trial had significantly higher risk of cardiovascular disease, stroke, venous thromboembolism, and breast cancer than those assigned to the placebo group (Rossouw, Anderson, Prentice, et al., 2002). In 2003, based on the findings of the WHI, the FDA issued a black box warning to be included on the labeling of HRT products stating the medication increases the risk of cardiovascular events, including stroke, memory loss, and dementia. Additionally, therapy should only be prescribed for the shortest duration possible consistent with treatment goals.

Estrogen is contraindicated in patients with breast cancer because it stimulates the growth of breast cancer cells. However, it may be used in appropriately selected patients receiving treatment for metastatic disease. For a discussion of the role of hormones in cancer, see Chapter 37. Estrogen is also contraindicated in the following conditions:

- Estrogen-dependent neoplastic diseases
- Undiagnosed abnormal genital bleeding
- Active thrombophlebitis or thromboembolic disorders
- History of thrombophlebitis, thrombosis, or thromboembolic disorders associated with previous estrogen use (except when used in treating breast or prostatic malignancy)
- Known or suspected pregnancy (estrogen is a pregnancy category X drug because of known adverse effects on the developing fetus)

Conjugated estrogen should be administered with caution to breast-feeding women because estrogen has been shown to decrease the quantity and quality of breast milk and may be excreted into it. Its safety and efficacy in children have not been established. Cautious use must be observed in patients with incomplete bone growth because of the epiphyseal closure that accompanies estrogen use. Caution also is necessary in patients for whom some degree of fluid retention may cause complications, such as those with epilepsy, migraine headaches, cardiac dysfunction, or renal dysfunction. Caution should also be used in patients with renal insufficiency or metabolic bone diseases associated with hypercalcemia.

Adverse Effects

Postmenopausal estrogen use has been associated with some serious and important adverse effects, and estrogen now carries several Black Box warnings related to these adverse effects. Although postmenopausal women are more at risk for cardiovascular disease and MI than premenopausal women, recent landmark research from the WHI trial indicates that estrogen given to postmenopausal women in combination with progestin significantly increases the risk of stroke and coronary heart disease (CHD) in all subgroups examined (Focus on Research Box 52.1); when used without progestin, estrogen was found to also increase the risk of stroke, but had no major effect on CHD (Hsia, Langer, Manson, et al., for the Women's Health Initiative Investigators, 2006). A recent review of the women involved in this study found that prehypertension was present in more than one third of participants and that prehypertension was associated with more cardiovascular complications (MI, stroke, heart failure, and cardiovascular death), regardless of race (Hsia, Margolis, Eaton, et al., 2007).

Findings from the WHI also indicate that estrogen-progestin combinations increase the incidence of breast cancers, and that when cancer is detected, it is at a more advanced stage than if the woman were not taking HRT. Additionally, it is more likely that a woman receiving estrogen-progestin will have an abnormal mammogram. Estrogen with progestin, therefore, may stimulate breast cancer growth and hinder breast cancer diagnosis (Chlebowski, Hendrix, Langer, et al., 2003). However, a Black Box warning on the estrogen labeling now states that it may increase the risk of invasive breast cancer in postmenopausal women. Findings from the WHI study also indicate that estrogen with progestin appears to increase the risk of ovarian cancer, although it does not have this effect on endometrial cancer (Anderson, Judd, Kaunitz, et al., 2003). Estrogen given alone is known to increase the risk of endometrial cancer and carries a Black Box warning to this effect. The progestin in combination therapy has a positive effect on the endometrium, offsetting any increase in risk for endometrial cancer from estrogen.

The branch of the WHI study that examined the use of estrogen alone continued until March 2004, when it was stopped a year early. Final data analysis shows that, like combination HRT, estrogen replacement appears to increase the risk of stroke and probably for dementia or mild cognitive impairment but decreases the risk of hip fracture. Estrogen, alone or in combination with a progesterone, carries a Black Box warning not to use it to prevent dementia. Unlike combination HRT, estrogen alone did not appear to have any effect (positive or negative) on heart disease and did not increase the risk of breast cancer (Stefanick, Anderson, Margolis, et al., Women's Health Initiative Investigators, 2006).

The adverse effects that have been found in postmenopausal women treated with HRT cannot be generalized to premenopausal women, because premenopausal women were not included in the clinical trials. However, it has been concluded that hormones found in birth control pills do not increase cardiovascular risk unless the dose of estrogen is high. Most forms of oral contraceptives now have low doses of estrogen.

Most other adverse effects of estrogen therapy are related to the effect of estrogen on the body and may be dose related. Common adverse effects include breakthrough bleeding, changes in menstrual flow, dysmenorrhea, premenstrual-like syndrome, headache, nausea, vomiting, bloating, abdominal cramps, chloasma (dark, patchy pigmentation to skin), and photosensitivity. Less common adverse effects include cholestatic jaundice, colitis, acute pancreatitis, steepened corneal curvature, intolerance to contact lenses, migraine headaches, dizziness, mental depression, pain at injection site, edema, changes in libido, and breast tenderness, enlargement, or secretion.

The use of estrogen during early pregnancy may have teratogenic effects on the fetus. Use of conjugated estrogen in patients with breast cancer and bone metastases may cause severe hypercalcemia. Estrogen use increases the risk of thrombosis formation (thrombophlebitis and thromboembolism) in all women receiving the drug, regardless of age.

Drug Interactions

No important drug interactions are associated with conjugated estrogen.

Assessment of Relevant Core Patient Variables

Health Status

Before the patient begins estrogen therapy, assess her blood pressure (for hypertension) and breasts (for masses). If the patient is prehypertensive, this may increase the risk of cardiovascular complications (Hsia, Margolis, Eaton, et al., Women's Health Initiative Investigators, 2007). The patient should also undergo a pelvic examination and a Papanicolaou test to rule out cervical cancer. It is important to determine whether the patient has breast cancer, undiagnosed genital bleeding, active thrombophlebitis or thromboembolic disorders, or a history of thrombophlebitis, thrombosis, or thromboembolic disorders associated with previous estrogen use (except in the palliative treatment of breast or prostate cancer). These conditions are contraindications to use of conjugated estrogen.

Assess whether the patient has a personal or family history of breast cancer, a history of benign breast tumors, early menarche, a first pregnancy late in life, or never having been pregnant. These factors are thought to increase the risk of breast cancer with estrogen replacement therapy.

It is also important to determine whether the patient has a metabolic bone disease associated with hypercalcemia or renal insufficiency, because these conditions mandate cautious use of estrogen. Determine whether the patient has a condition that might be adversely affected by fluid retention, such as epilepsy, migraine headaches, cardiac dysfunction, or renal insufficiency.

BOX 52.1 FOCUS ON RESEARCH

Summary of Findings from the Women's Health Initiative

Anderson, G. L., Judd, H. L., Kaunitz, A. M., et al., Women's Health Initiative Investigators. (2003). Effects of estrogen plus progestin on gynecologic cancers and associated diagnostic procedures: The Women's Health Initiative randomized trial. *Journal of the American Medical Association,* 290(13):1739–1748.

Chlebowski, R. T., Hendrix, S. L., Langer, R. D., et al., Women's Health Initiative Investigators. (2003). Influence of estrogen plus progestin on breast cancer and mammography in healthy postmenopausal women: The Women's Health Initiative Randomized Trial. *Journal of the American Medical Association,* 289(24):3243–3253.

Curb, J. D., Prentice, R. L., Bray, P. F., et al. (2006). Venous thrombosis and conjugated equine estrogen in women without a uterus. *Archives of Internal Medicine,* 166(7):772–780.

Hsia, J., Langer, R. D., Manson, J. E., et al., for the Women's Health Initiative Investigators (2006). Conjugated equine estrogens and coronary heart disease: The Women's Health Initiative. *Archives of Internal Medicine,* 166(3):357–365.

Manson, J. E., Hsia, J., Johnson, K. C., et al., Women's Health Initiative Investigators. (2003). Estrogen plus progestin and the risk of coronary heart disease. *New England Journal of Medicine,* 349(6):523–534.

Shumaker, S. A., Legault, C., Rapp, S. R., et al., Women's Health Initiative Memory Study Investigators. (2003). Estrogen plus progestin and the incidence of dementia and mild cognitive impairment in postmenopausal women. The Women's Health Initiative Memory Study: A randomized controlled trial. *Journal of the American Medical Association,* 289(20):2651–2662.

Stefanick, M. L., Anderson, G. L., Margolis, K. L., et al., Women's Health Initiative Investigators. (2006). Effects of conjugated equine estrogens on breast cancer and mammography screening in postmenopausal women with hysterectomy. *Journal of the American Medical Association,* 295(14):1647–1657.

Wassertheil-Smoller, S., Hendrix, S. L., Limacher, M., et al., Women's Health Initiative Investigators. (2003). Effect of estrogen plus progestin on stroke in postmenopausal women. The Women's Health Initiative: A randomized trial. *Journal of the American Medical Association,* 289(20):2673–2684.

The Study

The Women's Health Initiative (WHI) was a large, multicenter, randomized clinical trial of almost 27,000 postmenopausal women between the ages of 50 and 79 years. The women were divided into two groups: those without a uterus who received just estrogen (10,739), and those with a uterus who received estrogen with progestin (16,608). The primary goal of the trial was to determine whether estrogen or estrogen-progestin hormone replacement therapy (HRT) was cardioprotective for postmenopausal women. The chief outcome criterion was the incidence of CHD (nonfatal MI or death caused by CHD). The study was designed to follow the women for up to 13 years. However, both arms of the study were prematurely stopped because the data indicated that the overall risks of continuing the study exceeded any benefits that could be obtained.

When estrogen was administered alone, the researchers concluded that the women had:

- Increased risk of stroke
- Increased risk of deep venous thrombosis, especially within the first two years of use, but this risk elevation was less than that for women taking estrogen plus progestin.
- No overall protection from MI or coronary death. Although there was a slight trend of lower CHD in this group, in general it did not have any effect (positive or negative) on the overall risk of CHD.
- No increase in incidence of breast cancer, but abnormal or suspicious mammograms were more prevalent, increasing the need for short-term follow-up.
- No difference in colorectal cancer
- Decreased risk of hip fractures

When estrogen was administered with progestin, the researchers concluded that the women had:

- Increased risk of stroke
- Increased risk of CHD within the first year of hormone therapy use, including the risk of MI

- Increased (double) risk of venous thrombosis. Venous thrombosis is more likely if risk factors for venous thrombosis (older age, overweight or obese, and genetic variations of factor V Leiden) were present
- Neither increased nor decreased risk of pulmonary artery disease
- Increased risk of breast cancer. When breast cancer was determined, the stage at which breast cancer was diagnosed was more advanced if the woman had been on HRT. This finding suggests that HRT not only stimulates breast cancer growth but also may make its diagnosis more difficult.
- Increased risk of ovarian cancer but not endometrial cancer.
- Decreased risk of colorectal cancer
- Decreased risk of hip fractures

From the main study, 4,532 of the women were also recruited to participate in a study (WHI Memory Study) to evaluate the effect of HRT on memory and cognitive processes. The findings from these women showed that, contrary to previous thinking, HRT increased the risk of dementia, including Alzheimer disease, and did not prevent mild cognitive impairment.

All of these findings caused the researchers to conclude that postmenopausal estrogen alone or plus progestin conferred greater risks than benefits and that this therapy should generally be avoided.

Nursing Implications

The results of the WHI study dramatically changed the thinking in the medical community about the use of HRT in postmenopausal women. Although postmenopausal women are known to be at a substantially higher risk for coronary heart disease, and estrogen is known to reduce low-density lipoprotein (LDL) cholesterol, a cardiovascular risk factor, exogenous hormone therapy with estrogen or estrogen and progestin is obviously not the answer, as was previously thought. Couple this information with the knowledge that HRT increases the risk of Alzheimer disease, breast cancer (in combination), and ovarian cancer (in combination), and the therapy now appears to pose too great a risk compared to its known benefits (e.g., increasing postmenopausal bone density and slightly improving sleep). How is it possible that the scientific thinking could switch from encouraging women to use HRT to avoiding its use as much as possible?

First, understand that science and the state of knowledge on any topic are constantly evolving. As more is learned through research, different recommendations about therapy may be indicated. Second, the WHI was an exceedingly large study, much larger than any previous studies, some of which had a few thousand participants. The larger the number of participants in a clinical drug study, the more likely adverse effects of drug therapy will be identified. Similarly, the larger the trial, the more likely that findings regarding drug efficacy (whether the drug is found effective or not) are valid and can be applied to a larger population. Here, although the study was initially intended to prove a positive effect, the data pool was large enough to show there was too much risk for any small benefit that could be achieved.

It is important to understand how clinical trials are conducted and how their results modify practice. Patients often hear of an outcome from a trial reported in the general media. The report may not accurately or completely represent the facts from the clinical trial. Patients can become fearful, angry, or confused as to why medical advice regarding a particular drug therapy may change. Nurses should be able to discuss the facts of these studies with patients to help them sort out and understand the findings in relation to their own health.

Life Span and Gender

Check the patient's age. The use of parenteral conjugated estrogen in premature infants has been associated with the development of a fatal "gasping syndrome" because of the benzyl alcohol in the preparation. Assess whether long-bone growth has been completed. If the patient is prepubescent, monitor growth throughout therapy to prevent premature closing of the epiphyses.

Assess for pregnancy, which is a contraindication for therapy (estrogen is pregnancy category X). Use of conjugated estrogen during pregnancy may promote congenital defects, including heart and limb-reduction defects. Male fetuses exposed to conjugated estrogen through maternal use may develop genitourinary structural problems and, later, abnormal semen. Use of estrogen to treat threatened or habitual miscarriage has not been proved effective. Also, assess the patient's menopausal or postmenopausal status. If the patient is menopausal, assess for severity of symptoms.

Environment

Conjugated estrogen may produce photosensitivity. Patients who are outdoors frequently need to take precautions against the sun's ultraviolet rays until tolerance to the drug is determined. Be aware of the environment in which estrogen will be administered. Oral conjugated estrogen may be administered in any setting, including in the home by the patient. Parenteral conjugated estrogen (IM or intravenous [IV]) is administered in a hospital setting.

Nursing Diagnoses and Outcomes

• Ineffective Sexuality Patterns related to therapy for female hypogonadism or lack of intrinsic estrogen
  Desired outcome: *The patient will develop normal sex organs and secondary sexual characteristics while using estrogen drug therapy.*
• Risk for Delayed Growth and Development related to intrinsic estrogen deficiency and early hypophysis closing from estrogen replacement therapy
  Desired outcome: *The patient will achieve normal growth and development while using drug therapy.*
• Decisional Conflict related to comparison of risks and benefits of postmenopausal estrogen replacement therapy
  Desired outcome: *The patient will make an informed decision about estrogen replacement therapy after comparing personal risks and benefits.*

Planning and Intervention

Maximizing Therapeutic Effects

Several nursing actions are geared toward maximizing the therapeutic effects of estrogen. Administer conjugated estrogen cyclically (3 weeks of daily administration followed by 1 week off) to simulate the normal cycling of endogenous estrogen when given due to low intrinsic levels of the hormone. Give it on a daily basis for carcinomas, postpartum breast engorgement, and treatment of severe menopausal symptoms. Refrigerate the drug before reconstitution (IV or IM use); after reconstitution, the solution can remain refrigerated for up to 60 days. Do not use the solution if it darkens or if precipitation occurs.

Minimizing Adverse Effects

To minimize adverse effects of estrogen therapy, monitor for signs of thrombophlebitis and thromboembolus. In women with a uterus, the combination of estrogen and progestin should always be used to minimize the risk of endometrial cancer. The estrogen dosage should remain as low as possible to minimize the chances for development of ovarian cancer or breast cancer, but still achieve the desired therapeutic effects. HRT should be limited to treating only those menopausal women who have substantial menopausal symptoms. The dose and the duration of therapy should be minimized in menopausal women to decrease the risk of cancer, stroke, and CHD. Applying estrogen topically to urogenital structures may decrease the risk of systemic adverse effects, compared with risk of oral preparations, when it is used to treat the symptoms of menopause. Do not administer IV conjugated estrogen with other agents. (An exception is in emergencies in which a separate drug infusion has already been started. In such cases, inject the drug into the IV tubing as close to the angiocatheter insertion site as possible.) Protect the patient from ultraviolet light until it is determined whether the patient experiences photosensitivity.

Providing Patient and Family Education

• Teach patients and their families about the therapeutic purpose of estrogen. Provide and clarify information on risks and benefits of postmenopausal therapy, so that patients can make an informed choice regarding drug therapy.
• Provide instruction on how to take the estrogen, either cyclically or daily, depending on the clinical indication for the drug.
• Instruct patients about the signs and symptoms of thrombophlebitis and thromboembolism (pain in groin or calves, sharp chest pain or sudden shortness of breath, sudden severe headache, dizziness or fainting, vision or speech disturbance, weakness or numbness in arm or leg). Urge patients to notify the physician or nurse practitioner at once if these signs or symptoms occur.
• Teach patients to notify the physician or nurse practitioner if any of the following signs or symptoms occurs: abnormal vaginal bleeding, missed menstrual period or suspected pregnancy, lumps in the breast, severe abdominal pain, yellowing of the skin or eyes, or severe depression.
• Teach patients to avoid prolonged exposure to the sun and to use sunblock and appropriate clothing in the sun, because photosensitivity may occur.
• In addition, emphasize to patients the importance of returning for follow-up care and physical examinations while receiving estrogen therapy.

CRITICAL THINKING SCENARIO

INDIVIDUAL DECISIONS ABOUT HORMONE REPLACEMENT THERAPY

Sue Rosario is 46 years old and is undergoing menopause. She reports that she hasn't slept well in the past 3 months because she awakens two or three times a night with such severe episodes of sweating that she has to get up and change her night clothes because they are soaked in perspiration. She states she is having trouble focusing at work, where she is a computer software engineer, because she is fatigued. Additionally, she often has severe hot flashes and episodes of sweating at work, which further impair her ability to be productive. Her physician has ordered her a course of HRT to treat the menopausal symptoms. She discusses with you her concerns about taking HRT. She says, "I heard these drugs cause you to have a heart attack. Isn't this drug too dangerous to take?"

1. How will HRT be helpful to Sue at this time?
2. What points will you include in your patient education to help Sue understand the risks and benefits of HRT in her situation? Include what precautions should be used to minimize any risk she might incur.

Ongoing Assessment and Evaluation

If the patient is a prepubescent girl, evaluate for normal sexual development with estrogen therapy and monitor the patient's growth as appropriate. It is essential to check for evidence of early epiphyseal closure. Monitor the postmenopausal woman for development of endometrial cancer (when estrogen is used alone) and ovarian or breast cancer (when estrogen is used in combination with progestin), as well as for cardiovascular complications. Therapy is considered effective when normal growth and sexual development occur, the symptoms of menopause are controlled, and the patient does not show any serious adverse effects from the drug therapy.

Drugs Closely Related to P Conjugated Estrogen

Contraceptives are combinations of estrogen and progesterone and are discussed later in the chapter. Synthetic conjugated estrogens, such as Cenestin, are very similar to conjugated estrogen. The major difference is that Cenestin is made of nine synthetic estrogen components obtained from plant material, whereas conjugated estrogen is derived from the urine of a pregnant mare. Cenestin is approved only for short-term use in treating vasomotor symptoms of menopause. It is administered orally.

Drugs Significantly Different From P Conjugated Estrogen

Clomiphene

Clomiphene (Clomid, Milophene, Serophene) is an ovulation stimulant. This nonsteroidal agent promotes ovulation by indirectly increasing the output of the pituitary

MEMORY CHIP

P Conjugated Estrogen

- Used as hormone replacement when premenopausal endogenous levels of estrogen are low
- Used in combination with progesterone in contraceptives
- Used to treat moderate to severe symptoms of menopause (small dose, short duration of therapy)
- Major contraindications: most breast cancers, estrogen-dependent cancers, thrombophlebitis or thromboembolic disorders (active or history of), undiagnosed abnormal genital bleeding; do **not** use to prevent cardiovascular events or to prevent dementia
- Most common adverse effects: menstrual cycle problems (breakthrough bleeding, changes in menstrual flow, dysmenorrheal, premenstrual-like syndrome, headache, nausea, vomiting, bloating, abdominal cramps, chloasma, and photosensitivity)
- Most serious adverse effects (when used alone): thromboembolic events, increased risk for stroke, increased risk for dementia or mild cognitive impairment, increased risk for endometrial cancer
- Most serious adverse effects (when used with progestin): increased risk for stroke, increased risk for coronary heart disease, increased risk for breast and ovarian cancers
- **Life span alert: pregnancy category X drug**
- Maximizing therapeutic effects: Administer cyclically or daily, depending on clinical indication.
- Minimizing adverse effects: Administer with progestin if the woman has a uterus, to reduce risk of endometrial cancer; monitor for thrombophlebitis or thromboembolism; minimize dose and duration of therapy (in postmenopausal women); monitor bone growth for early epiphyseal growth plate closure (in prepubescent girls).
- Most important patient education: benefits and risks of postmenopausal HRT; report signs and symptoms of thrombophlebitis or thromboembolism at once.

gonadotropins. Clomiphene binds to estrogenic receptors, preventing estrogen from binding. The hypothalamus and pituitary gland interpret this development as indicative of low estrogen levels and respond by increasing secretion of LH, FSH, and gonadotropins, thus stimulating ovulation. Clomiphene is used in treating ovulatory failure in patients who want to become pregnant and have a fertile partner. Use of clomiphene increases the chance of multiple pregnancies, although most births are single births. Clomiphene therapy is not effective in primary pituitary or ovarian failure. Clomiphene is administered orally. Hot flashes are the most common adverse effect; they are usually not severe and disappear after treatment stops.

Gonadotropins and Menotropins

The gonadotropins are preparations of FSH and include follitropin alpha, follitropin beta, and urofollitropin. Follitropin alpha and follitropin beta are human FSH preparations made using recombinant DNA technology. Urofollitropin is an FSH preparation extracted from the urine of postmenopausal women. Menotropins (Humegon, Menopur, Pergonal), purified preparations also made from the urine of postmenopausal women, are biologically standardized for FSH and LH activity. All of these drugs stimulate ovarian follicular growth in women who do not have primary ovarian failure yet do not experience an endogenous surge in LH level. They must be administered in conjunction with, but slightly before, human chorionic gonadotropin (HCG) to induce ovulation (see below for discussion of HCG). HCG is administered after it has been determined by laboratory analysis that sufficient follicular development has occurred. The gonadotropins are also used in follicle stimulation for women being treated with assisted reproduction technologies, such as in vitro fertilization. Urofollitropin is used to induce ovulation in women with polycystic ovary disease who are unresponsive to clomiphene therapy. Menotropins with HCG are also given to men with primary or secondary hypogonadism to stimulate spermatogenesis.

Overstimulation of the ovary occurs in approximately 20% of women receiving therapy with gonadotropins, resulting in mild to moderate uncomplicated ovarian enlargement with or without abdominal distention or pain. A more severe condition, ovarian hyperstimulation syndrome, may occur and result in severe ovarian enlargement, abdominal pain and distention, nausea, vomiting, diarrhea, dyspnea, and oliguria. Ascites, pleural effusion, hypovolemia, electrolyte imbalance, hemoperitoneum, and thromboembolic events may also occur.

Use of follitropins is associated with multiple births, including triplets, quadruplets, and quintuplets. The incidence of multiple births is about 12% with follitropin alpha, 8% with follitropin beta, and 21% with urofollitropin. Singleton births still outnumber multiple births, however. Follitropin alpha and urofollitropin are administered by subcutaneous (SC) injection, follitropin beta is administered by SC or IM injection, and menotropins are administered by IM injection. All gonadotropins are in pregnancy category X. Adverse effects include vascular and pulmonary complications, ovarian enlargement, ovarian cysts, nausea, headaches, and sensitivity reactions.

Human Chorionic Gonadotropin

HCG (A.P.L., Follutein, Gonic, Pregnyl) is a polypeptide hormone that stimulates the interstitial cells to produce androgens in male patients. In women, it can substitute for LH to trigger ovulation. It is used to induce ovulation in females after pretreatment with follitropins or menotropins. It is also used to treat prepubertal cryptorchidism not resulting from anatomic obstruction and to treat hypogonadism in males. HCG is administered by IM injection. It is a pregnancy category X drug. Adverse effects include headache, irritability, edema, precocious puberty, and ovarian hyperstimulation syndrome. Choriogonadotropin alfa is a DNA derived form of human chorionic gonadotropin and acts as endogenous HCG acts.

Gonadotropin-Releasing Hormones

Gonadorelin acetate (Lutrepulse, Canadian only) is a synthetic GnRH used to induce ovulation in women with primary hypothalamic amenorrhea. The hypothalamus releases endogenous GnRH in a pulsating manner. As discussed in the Physiology section of this chapter, GnRH also helps synthesize and promote the release of FSH and LH. FSH and LH stimulate the gonads to produce steroids necessary for reproductive processes. Gonadorelin acetate works similarly. It is administered by a special pump, a Lutrepulse pump, through an IV line. Gonadorelin acetate may cause multiple pregnancies, ovarian hyperstimulation syndrome, and anaphylaxis.

Nafarelin acetate (Synarel) is a potent agonistic analogue of GnRH and stimulates the release of FSH and LH from the pituitary. Repeated dosing abolishes the stimulatory effect on the pituitary gland and leads to decreased secretion of FSH and LH. Therefore, tissues and body functions that depend on gonadal steroids for their maintenance become inactive. Nafarelin acetate is used to treat endometriosis and central precocious puberty of children of both sexes. When used in children with precocious puberty, nafarelin causes the LH and sex steroid hormone levels to remain at prepubertal levels. This effect arrests development of secondary sexual characteristics and slows linear growth and skeletal maturation. Nafarelin acetate is a pregnancy category X drug. It is administered as a nasal spray. Adverse effects are hypoestrogenic (hot flashes, decreased libido, vaginal dryness) and androgenic (acne, myalgia, reduced breast size, edema) effects. An additional adverse effect is nasal irritation.

Gonadotropin-Releasing Hormone Antagonist

Ganirelix inhibits the premature LH surges in women undergoing controlled ovarian hyperstimulation as part of treatment for infertility. It suppresses natural gonadotropin secretion. When gonadotropin is suppressed, LH and FSH secretion by the pituitary are suppressed—LH more so than FSH. After starting FSH therapy on day 2 or 3 of the menstrual cycle, begin daily SC injections of ganirelix. Continue with therapy until the day that HCG is to be administered, as determined by follicular development. Ganirelix is packaged in a container with a natural rubber stopper and should not be given to patients with latex allergies. It is a pregnancy category X drug and causes resorption of fetal contents if administered to a pregnant woman. Confirm that the patient is not pregnant before administering this drug.

Synthetic Androgens

Androgen-estrogen combination drugs are indicated for treating moderate to severe vasomotor symptoms associated with menopause (e.g., hot flashes) if estrogen use alone has been ineffective. Effects are similar to those of each hormone individually. See Chapter 54 for a discussion of the effects of testosterone.

Danazol (Danocrine) is a synthetic androgen with weak, dose-related androgenic effects. Its similarities to testosterone are limited. Danazol suppresses pituitary ovarian response by inhibiting pituitary gonadotropins. It is used to treat endometriosis because it inactivates and atrophies the normal and ectopic endometrial tissue. It is also used in treating fibrocystic breast disease when pain and tenderness are severe enough to warrant suppression of ovarian function. Danazol is also used prophylactically for hereditary angioedema. Three off-label uses include treatment of precocious puberty, gynecomastia, and menorrhagia.

Adverse effects are mostly androgenic and hypoestrogenic (flushing, sweating, vaginitis, nervousness, emotional lability); they also include hepatic dysfunction. Like testosterone, danazol can cause masculinization in the female fetus.

C PROGESTINS

Progestins consist of progesterone and its derivatives. Through stimulation or inhibition, they regulate secretion of pituitary gonadotropins, which in turn regulate development of the ovarian follicle. Progestins also inhibit spontaneous uterine contractions. The prototype progestin is progesterone (Prometrium, Crinone). Table 52.2 provides a summary of selected progestins.

Nursing Management of the Patient Receiving P Progesterone

Core Drug Knowledge

Pharmacotherapeutics

Progesterone helps produce normal menstrual cycles in patients with amenorrhea and stops dysfunctional uterine bleeding. These seemingly opposite uses are possible because of the timing of drug administration and the drug's pharmacodynamics (see Table 52.2). Progesterone is also added to postmenopausal HRT to decrease the risk of endometrial cancer from estrogen therapy. It may be added cyclically (i.e., for so many days in every cycle) or daily. The exact dose and the preferred number of days the drug is given in a month (if dosing is cyclic) are still unknown,

and research continues in this area. Progesterone may be administered intramuscularly (for dysfunctional uterine bleeding and for amenorrhea), orally (for endometrial hyperplasia or amenorrhea), or by vaginal gel (for amenorrhea). One form of progesterone can be administered by the intrauterine route for contraception (see Drugs Closely Related to Progesterone, later in chapter).

Pharmacokinetics

Progesterone is absorbed rapidly, whether administration is oral or by IM injection. Hepatic transformation is rapid; metabolites are present in the bloodstream for several days. Nonmetabolized progesterone and the metabolites of progesterone are excreted in the urine. Progesterone crosses the placenta and enters breast milk.

Pharmacodynamics

Exogenous progesterone affects the body in ways similar to endogenous progesterone. When the ovarian follicle creates the corpus luteum, progesterone is produced. Progesterone changes the endometrium from its proliferative phase into its secretory stage. When levels of progesterone (in combination with estrogen) are high enough, a signal is sent to the pituitary gonadotropins to stop producing FSH and LH, thus preventing further ovulation. Progesterone is necessary to increase endometrial receptivity for implantation of an embryo. Once the embryo is implanted, progesterone helps maintain the pregnancy. If pregnancy does not occur, the corpus luteum disintegrates, progesterone levels fall, the pituitary gonadotropins are stimulated, and more FSH and LH are produced, causing ovulation again. Progesterone also inhibits spontaneous uterine contractions and contractions of other smooth muscles in the body, but because of its potential teratogenic effects, its use to prevent spontaneous abortion (miscarriage) is not recommended. Progesterone

TABLE 52.2	Summary of Selected C Progestins		
Drug (Trade) Name	**Selected Indications**	**Route and Dosage Range**	**Pharmacokinetics**
P progesterone (Prometrium)	Endometrial hyperplasia, prophylaxis Amenorrhea	*Adult:* 200 mg/d for 12 d *Adult:* PO, 400 mg/d for 10 d	*Onset:* Within 1 h *Duration:* Unknown $t_{1/2}$: About 16 h
medroxyprogesterone (Provera, Depo-Provera [IM])	Amenorrhea Abnormal uterine bleeding Contraception Inoperable recurrent endometrial or renal cell cancer	*Adult:* PO, 5–10 mg/d for 5–10 d *Adult:* IM, 150 mg q3mo *Adult:* IM, 400 mg–1g every week	*Onset:* <2 h *Duration:* Unknown $t_{1/2}$: 50 d
megestrol (Megace)	Breast cancer, palliative Endometrial cancer, palliative Appetite enhancement in AIDS patients	*Adult:* PO, 400–800 mg/d	*Onset:* Unknown *Duration:* Unknown $t_{1/2}$: Unknown
Letonogestrel implants (Implanon)	Prevention of pregnancy	*Adult:* Insertion of a single sterile rod containing 68 mg of etonogestrel	*Onset:* Slow *Duration:* Up to 3 y $t_{1/2}$: Unknown

has demonstrated beneficial effects in the prevention of preterm birth prior to 32 weeks gestation in women with singleton pregnancies who have a history of preterm delivery. Additionally, a systematic review identified decreased perinatal death, respiratory distress syndrome, and necrotizing enterocolitis in the neonate (Rode, Langhoff-Roos, Andersson, et al., 2009).

Progesterone decreases the risk of endometrial cancer in postmenopausal women receiving estrogen. Progesterone, when combined with estrogen, increases bone mineral density and reduces the risk of fracture (Cauley, Robbins, Chen, et al., 2003). However, the risks of therapy outweigh these benefits in treating osteoporosis.

Contraindications and Precautions

Progesterone is contraindicated in patients with hypersensitivity to progestins. It should not be prescribed to prevent cardiovascular disease (a Black Box warning). Progesterone is also contraindicated for patients with thrombophlebitis, thromboembolic disorder, cerebral hemorrhage, or a history of any of these conditions. Further contraindications include impaired liver function or disease, carcinoma of the breast or genital organs, undiagnosed vaginal bleeding, or missed abortion. Progesterone is a pregnancy category B drug. However, there have been case reports of fetal abnormalities in male and female infants, including masculinization of the female fetus during the first four months of pregnancy. Additionally, because progesterone causes uterine relaxation, if the pregnancy is due to a fertilized defective ovum, the body takes longer to respond with a spontaneous abortion; this can increase the risk of complications to the mother. For these reasons, progesterone should be avoided during the first four months of pregnancy. It passes into breast milk, but the concentration is believed to be too low to affect the nursing infant. The American Academy of Pediatrics has determined that progesterone is usually compatible with breast feeding.

Caution should be used in patients with pathologies that may be adversely affected by fluid retention (epilepsy, migraine headaches, asthma, cardiac dysfunction, or renal dysfunction). Patients who have a history of depression should be observed carefully for signs of this disorder while taking progesterone. Photosensitivity may occur with use of this drug. As mentioned with regard to conjugated estrogen, the benzyl alcohol that some progesterone products contain may produce a fatal gasping syndrome if given to premature infants.

Adverse Effects

Research from the WHI indicates that progesterone may increase the risk of breast and ovarian cancer when given in combination with estrogen to postmenopausal women (Chlebowski, Hendrix, Langer, et al., 2003; Anderson, Judd, Kaunitz, et al., 2003). All estrogens and progesterones now carry a Black Box warning related to this adverse effect. The WHI also found that postmenopausal

women who received these hormones had an increased risk of MI, stroke, pulmonary embolus, and deep vein thrombosis; progesterone carries a Black Box warning for these effects also. A post-hoc analysis of the WHI study recently demonstrated an increased rate of death from lung cancer in the combined HRT group, although incidence rates for lung cancer were similar in both the HRT and placebo groups (Chlebowski, Schwartz, Wakalee, et al., 2009).

When it is used alone, common adverse effects of progesterone include menstrual disorders (breakthrough bleeding, spotting, change in flow, amenorrhea, changes in cervical secretions), breast tenderness, changes in weight, and nausea, mental depression, and changes in mood. Uncommon but serious adverse effects include MI, thromboembolic disorders, sudden partial or complete loss of eyesight, and cholestatic jaundice. Progesterone is irritating at the injection site; the aqueous form is especially painful.

Drug Interactions

No known drug interactions are associated with progesterone. However, progesterone may affect results of the following laboratory tests: hepatic function, coagulation (decrease in prothrombin and factors VII, VIII, IX, and X), thyroid, metyrapone, and endocrine function.

Assessment of Relevant Core Patient Variables

Health Status

Assess for conditions that contraindicate use of progesterone: a history of or current thrombophlebitis, thromboembolic disorder, and cerebral hemorrhage; impaired liver function or disease; depression; and undiagnosed vaginal bleeding. Before progesterone treatment, a complete physical examination is required, including assessment of the breasts and pelvic organs. A Papanicolaou test should be performed. Assess the patient's menstrual cycles for irregularities. All vaginal bleeding should be diagnosed carefully before therapy starts.

Life Span and Gender

Assess the patient for pregnancy or intention to become pregnant because progesterone, which is in pregnancy category B, is associated with genital and congenital abnormalities when exposure occurs in the first four gestational months. Genital abnormalities include masculinization of the genital organs in the female fetus and hypospadias in the male fetus. Congenital abnormalities include congenital heart defects and limb-reduction defects. If the patient is in the later stages of pregnancy, progesterone might be used to halt premature labor. Assess whether the patient is breast-feeding, because progesterone's effects on the infant are unknown. Progesterone may be added to postmenopausal HRT.

Environment

Caution patients about exposure to ultraviolet light. Be aware of the environment in which progesterone will be administered. Progesterone may be administered in any environment, including the home, if the patient or family member has learned to administer an IM injection correctly.

Nursing Diagnoses and Outcomes

- Disturbed Body Image related to potential breakthrough bleeding, spotting, changes in menstrual flow, weight gain, or breast tenderness secondary to adverse effects of drug therapy
  Desired outcome: The patient will not experience substantial adverse effects from drug therapy to alter body image.
- Risk for Injury related to loss of vision, onset of thrombotic disorders, and depression secondary to adverse effects of drug therapy
  Desired outcome: The patient will not suffer an injury related to adverse effects of drug therapy.

Planning and Intervention

Maximizing Therapeutic Effects

The dosing schedule varies, depending on the clinical indication for using progesterone. In treating amenorrhea, the drug should be administered for 6 to 8 consecutive days. For treating dysfunctional uterine bleeding, the drug should be administered daily for 6 days. The best dosing schedule when progesterone is used in HRT is currently unknown.

Minimizing Adverse Effects

Take steps to minimize the adverse effects of progesterone therapy. To avoid risk for injury to the fetus, do not administer the drug to any woman who is in the first 4 months of pregnancy. In postmenopausal women, use the minimum effective dose to decrease risk of endometrial cancer while limiting any increased risk of breast or ovarian cancer. It is essential to assess throughout therapy for signs and symptoms of breast or ovarian cancer. Do not give progesterone to patients with a history of or active thrombophlebitis, thromboembolic disorders, breast cancer, ovarian cancer, or cerebral hemorrhage because these conditions are possible adverse effects of therapy. Discontinue therapy at the first sign of any of these conditions. Carefully monitor patients who may be adversely affected by fluid retention; therapy also must be discontinued if excessive fluid retention places patients at risk for their primary disease or disorder.

Providing Patient and Family Education

- Instruct patients and their families on the therapeutic and adverse effects of progesterone.
- Teach patients how to perform breast self-examination.
- Teach patients to notify the prescriber if they suspect that they are pregnant or if sudden loss of vision, severe headache, or numbness in an arm or leg occurs.
- Inform patients who are using the vaginal gel form of progesterone that it is the only intravaginal therapy they should be using. If they require other intravaginal therapy, administration should be at least 6 hours before or after progesterone gel. If indicated, discuss with patients how to time self-administration of intravaginal therapies.

Ongoing Assessment and Evaluation

Monitor premenopausal women taking progesterone for return of normal menstrual flow and cessation of abnormal bleeding. If amenorrhea or dysfunctional uterine bleeding is corrected without adverse effects, the drug therapy has been effective. Assess postmenopausal women throughout progesterone therapy for signs or symptoms of breast or ovarian cancer. Combination therapies of estrogen and a progestin (e.g., progesterone) are effective in the postmenopausal woman if they relieve symptoms while avoiding serious adverse effects.

Drugs Closely Related to P Progesterone
Medroxyprogesterone, Norethindrone, and Norethindrone Acetate

Other progestins are medroxyprogesterone (Depo-Provera, Provera), norethindrone (Ortho Micronor, Nor-QD), and norethindrone acetate (Aygestin).

Medroxyprogesterone, a derivative of progesterone, has androgenic and anabolic effects. Medroxyprogesterone is used to treat abnormal uterine bleeding, endometrial

---

MEMORY CHIP

P Progesterone

- Used to treat amenorrhea to help produce normal menstrual cycles, to stop dysfunctional uterine bleeding, or as part of postmenopausal HRT to decrease risk of endometrial cancer
- Used alone or in combination with estrogen in contraceptives
- Major contraindications: thrombophlebitis, thromboembolic disorder, cerebral hemorrhage (current or history of), breast or genital organ cancer, undiagnosed vaginal bleeding, and missed abortion
- Most common adverse effects: menstrual irregularities (breakthrough bleeding, spotting, change in menstrual flow, amenorrhea, changes in cervical secretions), breast tenderness, changes in weight, and nausea
- Most serious adverse effects (when used alone): MI, thromboembolic disorders, sudden loss of sight, gallbladder disorders
- Most serious adverse effects (when used with estrogen): increased risk for stroke, increased risk of coronary heart disease, increased risk of breast and ovarian cancers
- **Life span alert: pregnancy category B drug**
- Maximizing therapeutic effects: Dosing schedule will vary based on clinical indication for drug.
- Minimizing adverse effects: Minimize dose and duration of therapy in postmenopausal women.
- Most important patient education: Premenopausal women should report serious adverse effects at once; postmenopausal women should perform breast self-examination.

hyperplasia prophylaxis, pain from endometriosis, and amenorrhea and is a progestin-only contraceptive. Off-label uses include treatment of breast cancer, endometrial cancer, and renal cell cancer. Medroxyprogesterone can be administered orally, intramuscularly, and subcutaneously. Long-term use may increase bone loss. If the drug is used in adolescence or early adulthood, when bone mass is being stored for adult use, it may increase the risk of osteoporosis and osteoporotic fractures later in life.

Norethindrone, a synthetic progestin, is used as a progestin-only contraceptive. Norethindrone acetate (Aygestin), the acetic acid ester of norethindrone, is not used as a contraceptive but as treatment for abnormal uterine bleeding, amenorrhea, and endometriosis. These two drugs differ in terms of potency; norethindrone acetate is approximately twice as potent as the parent drug (norethindrone).

Other Forms of Progesterone

Other closely related drugs are forms of progesterone used alone or in combination with estrogens as contraceptives. These are described below under the section titled Contraceptives.

Drugs Significantly Different From P Progesterone

Megestrol

Megestrol (Megace) is a progestin-like progesterone and shares many of progesterone's qualities and characteristics. The two drugs differ mostly in their pharmacotherapeutic effects. Unlike progesterone, megestrol is used as palliative treatment for patients with advanced breast or endometrial cancer (tablet form) or to increase appetite in patients with AIDS (suspension form), cancer–related anorexia-cachexia syndrome, and severe malnutrition. Exactly how megestrol increases appetite in patients with AIDS who have anorexia and cachexia is unknown. The resulting weight gain is not related to water retention. Megestrol is not used as part of HRT in postmenopausal women. Its contraindications are similar to those of progesterone. Safety and efficacy of megestrol acetate therapy in children have not been established.

Mifepristone

Mifepristone (Mifeprex) is used to end an early pregnancy (defined as 49 days or less from the start of the last menstrual period). It competes with progesterone for binding at the progesterone-receptor sites and is a progesterone antagonist. Mifepristone inhibits the activity of endogenous and exogenous progesterone, resulting in termination of pregnancy. Mifepristone also has antiglucocorticoid and weak antiandrogenic effects. Compensatory elevation of adrenocorticotropic hormone and cortisol levels have been observed in some patients. Animal studies have indicated some antiandrogenic effects with large doses, but no studies have been done on this effect in humans. Mifepristone is rapidly absorbed. It is highly protein bound and is metabolized by the CYP3A4 pathway in the liver. Most mifepristone is excreted in the feces.

Mifepristone, although effective for most women who use it, may result in an incomplete medical abortion, necessitating surgical intervention. Mifepristone may also fail to initiate an abortion or produce substantial vaginal bleeding; either of these events may also require a surgical procedure. Between 1% and 5% of women require a surgical procedure related to one of these problems. For this reason, the FDA has established very specific and unique requirements in the United States for the use of mifepristone. Although it is a prescription drug, mifepristone is not available in pharmacies. Instead, it is distributed directly to physicians, who can determine the duration of a patient's pregnancy through menstrual history and clinical examination and are able to detect an ectopic pregnancy. Ultrasonographic scanning should be used if the duration of pregnancy is uncertain or if ectopic pregnancy is suspected. Physicians must be able to provide surgical intervention in cases of incomplete abortion or severe bleeding, or they must have pre-established plans for providing such care through others. Some states allow nurse practitioners or nurse midwives who work closely with physicians to be authorized prescribers of mifepristone.

Drug therapy with mifepristone should not be used if the patient cannot return or is unwilling to return to the physician's office for two follow-up visits. It also should not be administered to patients who do not have adequate access in the following 2 weeks to medical facilities equipped for emergency treatment of incomplete abortion, blood transfusion, and emergency resuscitation. The prescriber must give the patient the FDA-written Medication Guide for mifepristone and discuss the information thoroughly. The Medication Guide contains FDA-approved information written especially for patients. Medication Guides accompany drugs that the FDA has determined to pose a serious risk; appropriate patient education reduces the risk. The patient should be instructed to bring the Medication Guide with them if they need to go to an emergency department so that other providers realize that they have received mifepristone for an abortion. The patient must sign an agreement before receiving treatment.

After the patient meets all the baseline requirements, she swallows three tablets of mifepristone in the physician's or other provider's office. This visit is considered day 1. At day 3, the woman returns to the provider's office to determine whether she is still pregnant. If medical abortion is incomplete, the woman takes two tablets of misoprostol. (Misoprostol is a different drug, a synthetic prostaglandin E_1 analogue. Although it is used to prevent gastric ulcers resulting from the use of nonsteroidal anti-inflammatory drugs [NSAIDs], it also is known to have abortifacient properties, by producing uterine contractions. See Chapter 50 for more information on the antiulcer properties of misoprostol.) It is recommended that the labeled routes and timing of administration of the misoprostol tablets be followed exactly; off-label uses (including intravaginal placement of the misoprostol tablets) have been associated with sepsis (see below).

In clinical trials, about 44% of women who took misoprostol following mifepristone expelled the products of conception within 4 hours; approximately 63% expelled them within 24 hours after the misoprostol dose. The patient returns to the provider's office at day 14 to verify complete ending of the pregnancy. Although bleeding itself is not proof that the pregnancy has been terminated, lack of bleeding indicates that the therapy was ineffective in causing a medical abortion. If the pregnancy has not been completely terminated, surgical intervention to end the pregnancy is recommended. Pregnancies that are carried to term after use of mifepristone may result in fetal deformities.

Contraindications for using mifepristone are a pregnancy that has lasted longer than 49 days since the start of the last menstrual period; confirmed or suspected ectopic pregnancy; intrauterine device in place (which must be removed before drug therapy begins); chronic adrenal failure; concurrent long-term corticosteroid therapy; bleeding disorders or use of anticoagulant drugs; allergy to mifepristone, misoprostol, or other prostaglandins; and inherited porphyrias (rare inherited disturbances in porphyrin metabolism that may cause hemolytic anemia and splenomegaly).

The most common adverse effects of mifepristone are heavy vaginal bleeding, abdominal pain, and uterine cramping. Most women have vaginal bleeding or spotting for 9 to 16 days after ending the pregnancy; some women bleed for 30 days or more. Prolonged heavy bleeding may indicate an incomplete abortion. Vaginal bleeding may be severe enough to warrant blood transfusion, treatment with vasoconstrictor or uterotonic drugs, surgical intervention, or IV fluids.

Case reports of deaths from sepsis have been reported and are highlighted in a Black Box warning for mifepristone. The patients who have died have all had the same unusual but very serious bacterial infections (e.g., *Clostridium sordellii*). Patients with sepsis may present with atypical findings: without fever, with or without abdominal pain, and without other signs of infection. However, what is present is an elevated white blood cell count with a marked shift to the left, tachycardia, hemoconcentration, and general malaise. The FDA recommends that all providers of medical abortion and emergency department health care providers should investigate the possibility of sepsis in patients who are undergoing medical abortion and present with nausea, vomiting, or diarrhea and weakness with or without abdominal pain, and without fever or other signs of infection *more than 24 hours after taking misoprostol*. To help identify those patients with a hidden infection, obtain a complete blood count. If infection is suspected it is recommended that immediate treatment with an antibiotic that will treat anaerobic bacteria, such as *Clostridium sordellii*, be started (FDA Public Health Advisory, 2006). Nausea, vomiting, and diarrhea may occur initially after taking the mifepristone; this should not be confused with their occurrence 24 hours later after drug administration, which can indicate sepsis.

Specific drug or food interactions with mifepristone have not been studied; however, because the CYP3A4 pathway metabolizes this drug, other drugs that are metabolized by or inhibit metabolism from this pathway may produce a drug interaction.

Mifepristone does not prevent subsequent pregnancies. The patient should resume contraception after verifying that the pregnancy has been completely eliminated or before resuming sexual activity.

CONTRACEPTIVES

Contraceptives are forms of estrogen and progesterone, usually in combination. They are administered orally and by a number of other routes (Box 52.2).

● C ORAL CONTRACEPTIVES

The oral contraceptives are closely related to both estrogen and progestin because they contain varying amounts of these drugs in combination. A very few oral contraceptives contain progestins only. Oral contraceptives are given to prevent pregnancy; the patient's cultural beliefs may affect their use because some cultures and religions do not support interference with reproduction. Combination oral contraceptives inhibit ovulation by suppressing the gonadotropins FSH and LH. In addition, oral contraceptives alter the quality of cervical and other mucus in the female genital tract (inhibiting sperm penetration) and change the characteristics of the endometrium (reducing the likelihood of implantation). These drug effects may also assist in preventing pregnancy.

Oral contraceptives differ in the type and relative strength (potency) of their components and the relative dominance of estrogen or progesterone activity. Their ultimate effect is related to combined activity. Progestin-only oral contraceptives prevent pregnancy in a way that is not clearly understood. They are known to alter the cervical mucus and exert a progestational effect on the endometrium, which apparently produces cellular changes that render the endometrium hostile to implantation of a fertilized egg. In some patients, the effects of progestin also prevent ovulation.

BOX 52.2   COMMUNITY BASED CONCERNS

Contraceptives and Sexually Transmitted Diseases

Women who use any of the hormonal contraceptives are protected against pregnancy. Pregnancy can also be prevented with over-the-counter preparations that are spermicides, although they are not as effective in preventing pregnancy as the hormonal contraceptives are. None of these contraceptives protect women from sexually transmitted diseases, such as syphilis, gonorrhea, chlamydia, or HIV. Barrier protection from a condom is needed to prevent the transmission of the bacteria or viruses that cause these diseases. Condoms may be used with any of the other contraceptives. After ejaculation, care must be taken not to allow the semen to spill out of the condom during withdrawal of the penis from the vagina.

The three types of combination oral contraceptives are as follows:

- Monophasic: the dose of estrogen and progestin remains the same throughout the entire cycle.
- Biphasic: the amount of estrogen remains the same, but the amount of progestin rises in the second half of the cycle.
- Triphasic: estrogen amounts remain the same or may vary throughout the cycle, whereas progestin varies throughout the cycle.

Some serious adverse effects may occur with oral contraceptive use. These effects are usually related to high doses of estrogen in the drug. Oral contraceptives should be prescribed with the smallest effective dose of estrogen possible; thus, high-dose estrogen formulations are prescribed infrequently, usually only when a lower dose has been ineffective. Dose-related serious adverse effects include thromboembolism, stroke, MI, hepatic lesions, and gallbladder disease. The risk of cardiovascular and cerebrovascular effects is substantially increased in women age 35 years or older with other risk factors (e.g., smoking, uncontrolled hypertension, hypercholesterolemia, elevated low-density lipoprotein [LDL] cholesterol, obesity, and diabetes). Mortality rates associated with circulatory disease have been shown to increase substantially in smokers older than 35 years and in nonsmokers older than 40 years.

In addition, a decrease in glucose tolerance has been observed in a small percentage of patients on estrogen-progestin combination drugs; the mechanism appears to be related to estrogen dose. Elevated blood pressure may be related to the use of oral contraceptives and is believed to result from estrogen and progesterone effects. Other adverse effects are related to the dosage of estrogen and progestin and reflect the individual adverse effects of these drugs. Lower doses minimize these effects, which include breakthrough bleeding (transitory), spotting, amenorrhea during and after treatment, breast tenderness, nausea and vomiting (usually transitory), steepening of the corneal curvature, contact lens intolerance, weight gain or loss, edema, migraine, elevated triglyceride levels, and depression.

An important nursing intervention is teaching about signs and symptoms of potential complications of estrogen and progestin contraceptives. The nurse can use the acronym ACHES to guide patient instruction: A (abdominal pain—severe: may be related to hepatic problems or gallbladder disease), C (chest pain—severe: may be due to cardiovascular event, MI, pulmonary embolism), H (headache—severe: may be due to hypertension or CVA), E (eye problems—visual loss or blurring: may be related to CVA or hypertension), and S (severe pain in calf or thigh: may be DVT).

Oral contraceptives are known to interact with the penicillins and the tetracyclines (both classes of antimicrobials). This drug interaction decreases the level of circulating hormones, and contraceptive failure may result. Although the interaction is well documented with these classes of antimicrobials, it can potentially occur with other antimicrobials as well. Women should be cautioned about this potential lack of effectiveness and encouraged to use another form of birth control while they are taking a penicillin or a tetracycline. There is a drug interaction between oral contraceptives and St. John's wort, an over-the-counter (OTC) herb used as an antidepressant, which induces the P-450 system, specifically the CYP3A isoenzymes. Although studies on this subject are small and may be considered inconclusive, St. John's wort appears to increase the metabolism of the oral contraceptives, allowing breakthrough bleeding, follicle growth, and ovulation with unplanned pregnancies (Hu, Yang, Ho, et al., 2005; Murphy, Kern, Stanczyk, et al., 2005). Patients should be cautioned that they may experience some breakthrough bleeding if they use this combination. They should also be counseled to use a second form of birth control if they use St. John's wort while taking oral contraceptives. Patients may not always receive accurate information about the risk of a drug interaction between oral contraceptives and St. John's wort. They may purchase St. John's wort OTC (perhaps in a health food store), or their health care providers may not know of the interaction (Sarino, Dang, Dianat, et al., 2007).

For greatest effectiveness, the woman should take the oral contraceptive every day at the same time, such as with a particular meal or at bedtime. Packets have either 21 or 28 pills. The last 7 pills in the 28-day pack are inert and do not contain hormones; they are a different color from the active pills. If the woman is using a 21-pill pack, she takes one pill daily for 21 days and then no pill for 7 days. If she is using the 28-day pack, she takes one pill every day. The advantage of this regimen is that the risk of forgetting to take an active pill is minimized if taking a pill every day is routine. Patients may follow one of several regimens for beginning a cycle. The patient should refer to the package insert with each preparation.

Another form of oral combination contraceptive is now available for women. Femcon Fe (Ovcon 35) is the first chewable oral contraceptive tablet. It is spearmint flavored. To guarantee that the entire dose reaches the stomach, the woman should drink a glass of water after chewing and swallowing the tablet. The contraceptive tablet can also be swallowed whole. Ovcon comes in 28-day packs, with 21 active pills and 7 inert pills.

The newest combination oral contraceptives (termed extended-cycle contraception) contain both the progesterone levonorgestrel and an estrogen. Two of these drugs (Seasonale and Seasonique) are taken daily for 84 days, followed by either 7 days of inert pills or 7 days of a pill that has only a low-dose estrogen, depending on the brand. The menstrual period occurs only once every 3 months. Another of these drugs, Lybrel is taken continuously with no breaks for a menstrual cycle. Initial breakthrough bleeding or spotting may occur more often with these extended-cycle contraceptives than with normal monthly cycling versions.

If the woman misses one dose of an oral contraceptive, she should take the next dose as soon thereafter as possible; a woman may take two tablets on the same day. If a woman misses two doses of active pills, she should make up two missed pills over 2 days. If she misses three consecutive pills, she may not have adequate birth control protection, and she should also use a nonhormonal backup contraceptive. At that point, if she is receiving monthly cycle packs, she has two choices for how to proceed. She can either begin a new cycle pack as soon as she realizes that she has missed 3 days' worth of pills, or she can wait until it has been 7 days since she last took a pill and then begin a new cycle pack. She should use another form of birth control as a backup for at least the first 7 consecutive days after starting a new cycle pack and preferably for the entire new cycle. If she is using one of the extended-cycle contraceptives and misses three pills, she should not attempt to make up the pills but should finish the pack on the normal daily schedule. She should use backup contraception at this time. If she misses one of the inert pills in the monthly or Seasonale pack, or one of the low-estrogen (last 7) pills in a Seasonique pack, she does not have to make up these pills.

If a woman misses a menstrual period while on any form of oral contraceptive, she should be evaluated for pregnancy. Oral contraceptives should be withheld until pregnancy is ruled out because of possible damage to the fetus if the woman takes the drug during early pregnancy. Because there is no regular menstrual period with Lybrel, it may be difficult to determine whether unintended pregnancy has occurred. To prevent this, Lybrel is started during the first 24 hours of a menstrual period.

Mothers who do not breast-feed may begin use of oral contraceptives 4 to 6 weeks after delivery even if they have not resumed spontaneous menstrual periods. Oral contraceptives are not recommended in breast-feeding women, although they may be used carefully if absolutely necessary.

Emergency Oral Contraceptives

Emergency oral contraceptives are used to prevent pregnancy after unprotected sexual intercourse or a known or suspected contraceptive failure (such as a condom breaking). Currently, the only available emergency oral contraceptive is a progestin-only product (levonorgestrel) known by its trade name of Plan B. In Plan B, levonorgestrel prevents pregnancy in the same manner as when it is taken as a daily oral contraceptive, that is, *by preventing ovulation*. If the woman is already pregnant when she takes Plan B, the drug does *not* cause a spontaneous abortion. The first dose should be taken as soon as possible after intercourse; the drug is most effective if taken within 24 hours of unprotected sex but may be taken up to 72 hours after the event. The second dose is taken 12 hours after the first. Plan B One Step has the advantage of only requiring one pill. Both forms of emergency contraception are effective in preventing pregnancy when taken as directed. Emergency contraceptive pills are not used for routine contraception.

Plan B and Plan B One Step are unique in that the same formula is available as an over-the-counter (OTC) drug for women 18 years of age and older and as a prescription drug for those younger than 18 years of age. (The FDA recently approved sale without a prescription to young women 17 years of age, but it will take some time before this takes effect.) Because of its dual status, there are some unique limitations regarding how it can be sold. Plan B is sold only behind a pharmacy counter, unlike other OTC drugs, such as aspirin, which are offered for sale not only in the aisles of a pharmacy, but in convenience stores and gas stations, among other places. Proof of age is required to buy the drug OTC. Pharmacists in some states (Alaska, California, Hawaii, Maine, Massachusetts, New Hampshire, New Mexico, Vermont, and Washington) can provide emergency contraception to women younger than 17 without a prescription.

Nurses providing contraceptive counseling to patients should include information about how to access emergency contraception if it is needed and that the effectiveness of the drug is improved the sooner it is taken after unprotected sex. Keeping an emergency dose of the drug allows the drug to be taken as quickly as possible after unprotected sex. Information related to how it works and its general safety should be emphasized. After taking Plan B (or Plan B One Step), the woman should experience a menstrual period at the normal expected time (Aschenbrenner, 2006).

• OTHER COMBINATION CONTRACEPTIVES

Transdermal Contraceptives

The norelgestromin/ethinyl estradiol transdermal system (Ortho Evra) is similar to oral contraceptives in that it is a combination of a progestin and an estrogen. Unlike oral contraceptives, the combination of hormones is administered topically from a patch that releases the drugs. Its efficacy in preventing pregnancy and adverse effects are similar to those of oral contraceptives. Like 21-day cycle packs of oral contraceptives, the transdermal system is designed to be used for 3 weeks and then not used for 1 week, creating a 4-week cycle. A new patch is applied weekly on the same day of the week for three consecutive weeks. During the fourth week, no patch is applied. Menstruation begins during this week, when the woman is not wearing a patch.

The first time a woman uses the norelgestromin/ethinyl estradiol transdermal system, she should start it after her menstrual period begins. She can choose to apply the first patch either the day her period starts or the following Sunday. If she chooses the Sunday after the start of her period, she needs to use backup contraception for the first week of her first cycle (unless there is no delay in starting the method because the start of the menstrual period is on a Sunday). Directions for applying the patch are as follows:

• Choose a site to apply the patch on clean, dry, intact, healthy skin on the buttocks, abdomen, upper outer arm, or upper torso. Do not place on the breasts. The patch should be placed so that it will not be rubbed by tight clothing.
• Avoid using makeup, creams, lotions, powders, or other topical products on the site where the patch will be placed.

- Peel apart the foil pouch that contains the patch and open flat. Grasp a corner of the patch and gently remove it from the pouch.
- Using a fingernail, lift one corner of the patch, removing both the patch and the plastic liner from the foil liner.
- Peel away half of the clear plastic protective liner. Care should be taken to avoid touching the sticky surface of the patch.
- Apply the sticky surface of the patch to the skin and then remove the other half of the backing.
- Press down on the patch with the palm for 10 seconds to guarantee that the edges stick well to the skin.
- Change the patch weekly, using a new location for each patch. Before discarding the used patch, fold it in half so that it sticks to itself and seals in any active hormone remaining in the patch.

If the patch comes off and remains off for less than 24 hours, it can be reapplied if still sticky, or it can be replaced with a new patch. If the patch has been off for more than 24 hours, a new 4-week cycle must be started immediately and the "Day 1" patch from a new packet applied. Backup contraception should be used for the first week of the new cycle. If a woman forgets to replace a patch at the start of a new cycle (the end of week 4), she should apply the new week "Day 1" patch as soon as she remembers and use backup contraception for the first week. Birth control is not guaranteed if more than 7 days elapse without wearing a patch. In that case, backup birth control is needed.

If the woman forgets to change the patch for up to 48 hours at the end of week 1 or 2, she should change the patch as soon as she remembers. No backup contraception is needed in this situation. If more than 48 hours have elapsed, she should stop the current cycle and start a new 4-week cycle. Backup contraception should be used for the first week. If she forgets to remove the patch at the end of the third week, she should remove it as soon as possible. The first patch of the next cycle should be applied on the usual patch-change day.

Vaginal Ring Contraceptive

The etonogestrel/ethinyl estradiol vaginal ring (NuvaRing) is another combination of progestin and estrogen used for contraception. It has actions and adverse effects similar to those of the norelgestromin/ethinyl estradiol transdermal system. It is inserted into the vagina by the woman, left in place for 3 weeks, and then removed for 1 week. The drug is absorbed through the mucous membranes of the vagina and into the vascular system. Exact placement of the ring inside the vagina is not critical for effective birth control. The ring is removed by hooking the index finger under the forward rim of the ring or by grasping the rim between the index and middle fingers and pulling it out. Removed rings should be wrapped in the foil pouch and discarded in the trash; they should not be flushed down the toilet. Menstruation follows after the ring is removed, usually 2 or 3 days later.

Implanted Contraceptives

Implanon, an implantable contraceptive containing the progestin etonogestrel, was approved in the United States in 2006. It consists of a single, flexible plastic rod, about the size of a matchstick, implanted under the skin on the arm. It is effective for up to 3 years. Implanon prevents pregnancy by inhibiting ovulation through suppression of the lutenizing hormone surge, thickening the cervical mucus, and thinning the endometrium. It is more than 99% effective in preventing pregnancy. Prior to insertion, a negative pregnancy test must be documented. Insertion should be done within the first few days of the menstrual cycle and a backup form of contraception, such as condoms, should be used for the first 7 days. Irregular bleeding is the most common side effect, especially during the first 3 months of use. Implanon must be removed at the end of 3 years, at which time a new rod can be inserted if desired. Contraindications to use include current pregnancy, undiagnosed vaginal bleeding, history of or current breast cancer, liver tumors, active liver disease, thromboembolic disorders, chronic use of cytochrome P-450 3A4 inducing medications, or sensitivity to etonogestrel. Two small studies of lactating women suggest that use of Implanon does not interfere with breastfeeding and has no untoward effects on the infant. It is recommended that Implanon not be inserted until 6 weeks postpartum in women who are breastfeeding (Adams & Beal, 2009).

Intrauterine System Contraceptive

Intrauterine progesterone inserts (Levonorgestrel-releasing intrauterine system: LNG-IUS) are T-shaped units filled with 52 mg of levonorgestrel, with low doses administered directly into the uterine cavity. This form of contraception is recommended for women who have already had a child and are in a monogamous relationship. The insert is positioned in the uterine cavity by a health care provider and remains in place for up to 5 years; after 5 years it must be replaced. The mechanism of action is localized to the uterine cavity, resulting in glandular atrophy, leucocyte infiltration, and marked thinning of the endometrium. The progesterone also may thicken cervical mucus and inhibit ovulation. The LNG-IUS is highly effective and its contraceptive effect is immediately reversible after removal (Fantasia, 2008).

The LNG-IUS has additional non-contraceptive benefits due to decreased menstrual blood loss, and has been used as a treatment for menorrhagia due to fibroids. Adverse effects of the intrauterine progesterone inserts include some that are similar to all progesterone products and some that are unique to the route of administration; the latter may be severe. They include increased risk of pelvic inflammatory disease, increased risk of ectopic pregnancy (if there was a previous history of this condition), and enlarged ovarian follicles. Bleeding changes are likely, with most women having lighter menstrual periods after their uterus has adjusted to having the device. IUDs are contraindicated in pregnancy, active pelvic inflammatory disease, recent history of postpartum endometritis or septic abortion, uterine abnormalities, or a history of sexually transmitted diseases.

C BISPHOSPHONATES

The bisphosphonate drug class affects normal and abnormal bone resorption. The prototype is alendronate (Fosamax). The other bisphosphonates are closely related to alendronate. Table 52.3 provides a summary of selected drugs used to treat bone resorption.

Nursing Management of the Patient Receiving P Alendronate

Core Drug Knowledge

Pharmacotherapeutics

Alendronate is used to treat and prevent osteoporosis in postmenopausal women. Alendronate is also approved to treat men who have osteoporosis. Other uses are treating glucocorticoid-induced osteoporosis (in men and women) and treating patients with **Paget disease.** Paget disease is an idiopathic bone disease characterized by chronic, focal areas of bone destruction complicated by concurrent excessive bone repair. The result is thick but weak bones that may fracture or bend under stress. Off-label uses include treating osteoporosis from Crohn disease and treating hypercalcemia of malignancy. Alendronate is given orally, except for hypercalcemia of malignancy, for which it is administered as an intravenous infusion.

Alendronate is also available in a combination tablet containing cholecalciferol, a vitamin D preparation. It is sold under the trade name Fosamax Plus D.

Pharmacokinetics

Alendronate is absorbed orally. Food and beverages other than plain water can decrease its absorption and bioavailability by about 40%. After absorption, alendronate is stored in the skeleton and does not appear to be metabolized. It is excreted in the urine as it is slowly released from the skeleton.

Pharmacodynamics

The major action of alendronate is to inhibit both normal and abnormal bone resorption. Alendronate is a highly selective and potent inhibitor of bone resorption, which occurs following recruitment, activation, and polarization of osteoclasts. The exact mechanism of antiresorptive action is not fully understood but may be related to the inhibition of hydroxyapatite crystal dissolution or the drug's action on bone-resorbing cells. Reduction of abnormal bone resorption is responsible for reductions in serum calcium and phosphate concentrations. Alendronate greatly increases bone-mineral density in patients with osteoporosis. Evidence of increased bone-mineral density is seen after 3 months of use and continues throughout therapy. Alendronate thus appears to reverse the progression of osteoporosis.

TABLE 52.3	Summary of Selected C Drugs Used to Treat Bone Resorption		
Drug (Trade) Name	Selected Indications	Route and Dosage Range	Pharmacokinetics
P alendronate (Fosamax)	Treat/prevent postmenopausal osteoporosis	PO, 10 mg/d	*Onset:* Slow *Duration:* Days $t_{1/2}$: Unknown
	Paget disease	PO, 40 mg/d for 6 mo	
etidronate (Didronel)	Paget disease	PO, 5–10 mg/kg/d not to exceed 6 months	*Onset:* Slow for PO, rapid for IV
	Hypercalcemia of malignancy	IV, 7.5 mg/kg/d for 3 successive d diluted in at least 250 mL sterile normal saline	*Duration:* Days $t_{1/2}$: 6 h in plasma; >90 d in bone
pamidronate (Aredia)	Paget disease	IV, 30 mg diluted in 500 mL normal saline or 0.45% saline, infuse over 4 h for 3 consecutive d	*Onset:* Rapid *Duration:* Days
	Hypercalcemia of malignancy	IV, 60–90 mg as a single-dose infusion diluted in 1 L normal saline, 0.45% saline, or 5% dextrose. Infuse 60 mg over 4 h, 90 mg over 24 h	$t_{1/2}$: 28 h ± 7 h Terminal elimination from bone up to 300 d (in animal studies)
	Breast cancer with bone metastases	IV, 90 mg over 4 h every 3–4 wk in at least 500 mL	
risedronate (Actonel)	Paget disease	PO, 30 mg/d for 2 mo	*Onset:* Rapid *Duration:* Days $t_{1/2}$: Multiphasic, 1.5 to 220 h
tiludronate (Skelid)	Paget disease	PO: 400 mg active tiludronate/d (comes in 240 mg tablets each with 200 mg active drug) for 2 mo	*Onset:* Rapid *Duration:* Unknown $t_{1/2}$: Unknown

Contraindications and Precautions

Alendronate is contraindicated if the patient is hypocalcemic or hypersensitive to the drug or any of its components. It is also contraindicated if the patient has any abnormalities of the esophagus that delay esophageal emptying, such as stricture or inability of the esophagus to relax. Alendronate should not be used if the patient is unable to stand or sit upright for at least 30 minutes. The drug is not recommended for patients with severe renal insufficiency, which can cause increased accumulation of alendronate in the bone. Alendronate is a pregnancy category C drug. Animal studies show increases in maternal and fetal hypocalcemia and deaths; no studies have been done on pregnant women. Alendronate is used in pregnancy only if benefits outweigh risks. Although it is unknown whether alendronate enters breast milk, based on the fetal risks determined from results of animal studies, the drug should not be given to breast-feeding mothers. Its safety and efficacy in children have not been established.

Spontaneous osteonecrosis of the jaw has been reported primarily in cancer patients who have received bisphosphonates as a component of their therapy, but it has also occurred in postmenopausal women with other types of diagnoses. Symptoms include nonhealing extraction socket or an exposed jawbone. A dental examination with appropriate preventive dentistry should be considered before treatment with bisphosphonates. Invasive dental procedures should be avoided during treatment.

Adverse Effects

When given to treat osteoporosis, the most common adverse effect of alendronate is abdominal pain; musculoskeletal pain is also fairly common. Other adverse effects are flatulence, acid regurgitation, esophageal ulcer, abdominal distention, gastritis, headache, rash, and erythema (rare). GI irritation is more likely to occur if the patient does not take the drug with a full glass of water, or if the patient lies down after taking the drug. When given to treat Paget disease, alendronate increases the risk for upper GI symptoms; otherwise, the adverse effects are similar to those for osteoporosis.

Overdose of alendronate produces hypocalcemia, hypophosphatemia, and upper GI adverse effects. Administering milk or antacids to bind with the alendronate may be helpful in counteracting the effects of overdose, but dialysis is not beneficial. Otherwise, care is directed at treating the symptoms of overdosage.

Drug Interactions

Drug interactions are known to occur between alendronate and some other drugs. Because of potential interactions, the patient is advised to wait at least 30 minutes after taking alendronate before taking any other drug. Table 52.4 lists drugs that interact with alendronate. All food and beverages interfere with the absorption of alendronate, by as much as 60%. For this reason the drug must be taken at least 30 minutes before any other food or beverage.

Assessment of Relevant Core Patient Variables

Health Status

Assess whether the patient has hypocalcemia or other disturbances in mineral metabolism, such as phosphate or vitamin D deficiency. These imbalances must be corrected before starting drug therapy with alendronate, because alendronate may cause additional slight decreases in serum calcium and phosphate levels. Verify that the patient has a clinical indication for use of alendronate (e.g., treating or preventing osteoporosis or Paget disease) before beginning therapy. Also, assess for a family history of osteoporosis, which increases a woman's risk of developing osteoporosis. Assess for severe renal insufficiency as well because this condition may necessitate a dose reduction.

Life Span and Gender

Alendronate is used in postmenopausal women to treat or prevent osteoporosis; it may be used as treatment for all patients with Paget disease. Assess the patient for pregnancy or intention to become pregnant, because alendronate is a pregnancy category C drug. Also, assess the patient's lactation status, because administration to breast-feeding mothers must be avoided. Use of this drug in children requires caution because its safety and efficacy for this age group have not been established. Older adults require no precautions or dosage adjustments.

TABLE 52.4	Agents That Interact with Ⓒ Alendronate	
Interactants	**Effect and Significance**	**Nursing Management**
ranitidine	IV ranitidine doubles alendronate's bioavailability. Clinical significance is unknown.	Monitor for therapeutic and adverse effects.
calcium supplements, antacids	Products with calcium and other multivalent ions interfere with absorption of alendronate.	Separate doses of alendronate and calcium or antacids by 2 h.
aspirin	Coadministration increases risk of adverse effects in upper gastrointestinal system.	Monitor for adverse effects. If severe adverse effects develop, discontinue aspirin.

Lifestyle, Diet, and Habits

Review the patient's normal eating habits, because all food and beverages (e.g., coffee, orange juice, and mineral water) will decrease absorption of alendronate. Verify that the patient's diet contains adequate intake of calcium and vitamin D. Patients who have a history of eating disorders, such as excessive dieting, have an increased risk of osteoporosis. Assess for normal weight-bearing exercise, which helps prevent osteoporosis. Also, ask the patient about smoking and alcohol consumption because these factors increase the risk of osteoporosis.

Environment

Be aware of the setting in which alendronate will be administered. Alendronate is normally self-administered in the home, although it could be given in any setting.

Culture and Inherited Traits

Asian and white women are at increased risk of osteoporosis.

Nursing Diagnoses and Outcomes

- Risk for Injury related to fractures from osteoporosis or Paget disease
  Desired outcome: The patient using drug therapy will have no fractures.
- Potential Complication: Electrolyte Imbalance related to drug therapy with alendronate
  Desired outcome: The patient will not experience electrolyte imbalance.
- Potential Complication: Altered GI Function related to adverse effects of drug therapy with alendronate
  Desired outcome: The patient will experience either no or minimal adverse effects.

Planning and Intervention

Maximizing Therapeutic Effects

Nursing actions to maximize therapeutic effects are related to patient education. Assist patients in identifying a time in their normal routine when it will be appropriate to take alendronate.

Minimizing Adverse Effects

To minimize adverse effects from hypocalcemia, take measures to correct pre-existing hypocalcemia before treatment. Monitor electrolyte levels throughout therapy as indicated. Other actions to minimize adverse effects are related to patient education.

Providing Patient and Family Education

- Teach patients to take alendronate at least 30 minutes before eating, drinking any beverage other than plain water, or taking any other medication. Patients should swallow the medicine with 6 to 8 oz (180 to 240 mL) of plain water, which improves absorption of the drug.
- Instruct patients not to lie down for at least 30 minutes after swallowing alendronate, to decrease adverse GI effects.
- Encourage patients to take supplemental calcium and vitamin D if dietary intake is inadequate to meet the needs of the bones. However, calcium or vitamin D decreases absorption of alendronate if either is taken at the same time as alendronate. Instruct patients to take alendronate at least 1 hour before taking calcium or vitamin D.
- Encourage patients to make lifestyle changes that benefit bone health, such as engaging in weight-bearing exercise (including walking as tolerated and permitted by the patient's physical condition), limiting or stopping cigarette smoking, and limiting or stopping alcohol use.

Ongoing Assessment and Evaluation

Verify throughout therapy that the patient is not experiencing hypocalcemia or other adverse effects from alendronate therapy. Therapy is effective when adverse effects are absent or minimal, bone mass density increases, and bone resorption and bone formation decrease.

Drugs Closely Related to ℗ Alendronate

Ibandronate

Ibandronate (Boniva) is another bisphosphonate that is approved for use in treating postmenopausal osteoporosis. It is administered orally once monthly or intravenously as an IV push over 15 to 30 seconds once every 3 months. Its pharmacologic characteristics are similar to those of the prototype. A large, randomized controlled, 12-month trial comparing ibandronate to alendronate—the MOTION (Monthly Oral Therapy with Ibandronate for Osteoporosis Intervention) study—found that 150-mg ibandronate is clinically comparable to 70-mg alendronate for bone mineral density response, reduction of bone turnover, and GI tolerability (Emkey, Delmas, Bolognese, et al., 2009). A recent meta-analysis found that adherence to bisphosphonate therapy was better with weekly rather than daily regimens, and this improved compliance with therapy results in a reduction of fracture risk (Cramer, Gold, Silverman, & Lewiecki, 2007).

MEMORY CHIP

℗ Alendronate

- Used to treat or prevent osteoporosis in postmenopausal women, and other sources of osteoporosis; also used to treat Paget disease
- Prevents bone resorption
- Major contraindication: hypocalcemia
- Most common adverse effects: GI problems
- Most serious adverse effect: hypocalcemia (uncommon)
- **Life span alert: used in postmenopausal women**
- Most important patient education: Take medication at least 30 minutes before eating, drinking, or taking other medication; take with plain water only. Do not lie down after taking the medication.

Risedronate

Risedronate (Actonel), a bisphosphonate, is approved for used in postmenopausal osteoporosis (treatment or prevention) as well as osteoporosis in men, osteoporosis from corticosteroids, and Paget disease. For postmenopausal osteoporosis, it is given orally once weekly. In some regimens it is prescribed in combination with oral calcium carbonate tablets; the risedronate is given one day per week and the calcium carbonate is given the other 6 days of the week.

Etidronate, Tiludronate, Pamidronate, and Zoledronic Acid

The other bisphosphonates are etidronate (Didronel), tiludronate (Skelid), pamidronate (Aredia), and zoledronic acid (Zometa). They all act primarily on bone to prevent bone resorption. Unlike alendronate, they are not used to treat or prevent osteoporosis; their therapeutic indication is for treatment of Paget disease. Additional indications are as follows:

- Etidronate—(1) treatment or prevention of heterotropic ossification (formation of bone in an abnormal location) after total hip replacement or spine injury; (2) hypercalcemia of malignancy
- Pamidronate—(1) hypercalcemia of malignancy; (2) breast cancer or multiple myeloma in conjunction with standard chemotherapy
- Zoledronic acid—(1) bone metastasis; (2) hypercalcemia of malignancy; (3) multiple myeloma; (4) prophylaxis of osteopenia secondary to androgen-deprivation therapy in prostate cancer. The FDA recently approved IV administration of zoledronic acid as a once-a-year treatment for postmenopausal osteoporosis and every 2 years to prevent osteoporosis in postmenopausal women with osteopenia (In Brief, 2010).

Pharmacokinetics, pharmacodynamics, and adverse effects of all of these drugs are similar to those of alendronate.

Drugs Significantly Different From
P Alendronate

Raloxifene

Like alendronate, raloxifene (Evista) is prescribed to prevent osteoporosis in postmenopausal women. It reduces resorption of bone and decreases overall bone turnover. Unlike alendronate, however, raloxifene works as a selective estrogen-receptor modulator. Raloxifene is actually an estrogen antagonist at some sites because it blocks estrogen from attaching itself to the estrogen-receptor sites. At other estrogen-receptor sites, it produces estrogen-like effects. These effects include increasing bone-mass density and decreasing levels of total and LDL cholesterol. Raloxifene does not share estrogen's effects on the uterus or the breasts because it is an antagonist at these receptor sites.

Raloxifene is rapidly absorbed after oral dosing and can be administered any time of the day without regard to meals.

It has extensive first-pass metabolism, although the P-450 pathways do not appear to metabolize it. The metabolites that are formed have a long half-life. The drug is highly protein bound. Raloxifene is excreted in the feces. It may cause fetal harm if given to pregnant women. It is a pregnancy category X drug, and its use is therefore contraindicated in pregnant women. Raloxifene is also contraindicated if the woman has a history of or active venous thromboembolic events (deep vein thrombosis, pulmonary embolism, retinal vein thrombosis). Caution should be used if raloxifene is coadministered with other highly protein-bound drugs, such as lidocaine, diazoxide, or diazepam. Raloxifene may decrease the binding of these drugs, which results in more free and active drug. When coadministered with warfarin, the anticoagulant, a 10% decrease in the prothrombin time (PT) may occur. If patients are receiving oral anticoagulation with warfarin, the prothrombin time or international normalized ratio should be closely monitored with the addition and withdrawal of treatment with raloxifene. Coagulation parameters should also be reassessed periodically during concurrent therapy. Adjustments of the warfarin dose may be necessary in order to maintain the desired level of anticoagulation. Cholestyramine greatly decreases the absorption of raloxifene (by about 60%); cholestyramine and raloxifene should not be administered concurrently. If both therapies are necessary, administration of the drugs should be spread out as much as possible.

Common adverse effects of raloxifene are hot flashes and leg cramps. Raloxifene increases the risk of venous thromboembolic events, especially during the first 4 months of treatment. To minimize this risk, patients should discontinue use of raloxifene at least 72 hours before an expected prolonged immobilization (e.g., a planned surgical event requiring immobilization or bed rest). Raloxifene also should be discontinued throughout periods of prolonged immobilization and bed rest. Patients should resume raloxifene therapy only when fully ambulatory. If patients are traveling, advise them to avoid prolonged sitting in the same position.

Teach patients to take supplemental calcium and vitamin D if their dietary intake is inadequate. As with alendronate, the patient should be encouraged to do weight-bearing exercises and to decrease alcohol consumption and cigarette smoking to promote bone density.

Calcitonin, Salmon

Calcitonin, salmon (Fortical) is a calcium regulator. It is a potent synthetic polypeptide hormone that has effects similar to those of calcitonins of mammalian origin. It reduces the number of osteoclasts and prevents resorptive activity of the bone, resulting in a reduced bone turnover rate. It also temporarily improves bone formation by increasing osteoblastic activity. Calcitonin, salmon is used in the treatment of hypercalcemia and Paget disease as well as in postmenopausal osteoporosis. It does not appear to be as effective as alendronate for treating osteoporosis. See Chapter 53 for further information.

Teriparatide

Teriparatide (Forteo) is a recombinant human parathyroid hormone. Like alendronate, it is approved for use in post-menopausal osteoporosis. When administered once daily, teriparatide stimulates new bone; however, it has been found to increase the bone mass density at the spine, but not at the hip or femoral neck, unless given in combination with alendronate. Teriparatide needs to be administered subcutaneously. See Chapter 53, which discusses parathyroid hormones.

CHAPTER SUMMARY

- Women need adequate levels of sex hormones to develop and maintain the sexual and reproductive organs, create and maintain the secondary sexual characteristics, induce and stop the growth spurt of adolescence, and achieve and maintain pregnancy.
- Estrogen and progestin are the primary female sex hormones.
- Estrogen causes capillary dilation, promotes fluid retention, enhances protein anabolism, contributes to strengthening the skeleton, and maintains normal bone density and composition.
- Progestins are composed of progesterone and its derivatives. They regulate, through stimulation or inhibition, the secretion of pituitary gonadotropins. This secretion, in turn, regulates the development of the ovarian follicle. Progestins also inhibit spontaneous uterine contractions.
- Decreased levels of female sex hormones (primarily estrogen) that result from menopause increase the risk for cardiovascular disease and osteoporosis. Cardiovascular disease is the primary cause of death in postmenopausal women. Osteoporosis affects women more than men because male sex hormones (testosterone) decline more gradually and at a later age than estrogen in women.
- Postmenopausal hormone replacement therapy (HRT) carries substantial risks. Research has found that the risk of coronary artery disease and stroke increases substantially with the use of postmenopausal hormones. An adverse effect on cognition and a greater risk of Alzheimer disease also exist.
- Use of HRT should be limited to menopausal women who have considerable vasomotor symptoms. The dose and the length of time therapy is administered should be kept to a minimum. Postmenopausal HRT should never be administered to prevent cardiovascular events.
- Most contraceptives are combinations of estrogen and progestin, although some contain progestin only. They prevent pregnancy. They may have serious adverse effects, but these effects are usually related to higher doses of estrogen in the drugs. Contraceptives should be prescribed with the smallest effective dose of estrogen possible. Contraceptives are available in various forms and routes of administration: oral tablets, transdermal patches, vaginal inserts, uterine inserts, and subcutaneous implants.
- The bisphosphonates, like alendronate, are used to treat or prevent osteoporosis by increasing bone mineral density and decreasing the risk of fractures. These drugs are preferred to estrogen therapy for treatment or prevention of postmenopausal osteoporosis because, unlike estrogens, they do not have negative effects on the cardiovascular system or on cognition. Because these drugs have interactions with food, beverages, and other drugs that impair their absorption, and because a flat position after taking the drug significantly increases the risk of GI irritation, patient education about the timing of the drug dosage is extremely important.

QUESTIONS FOR STUDY AND REVIEW

1. Explain why progesterone can be used to treat amenorrhea and abnormal uterine bleeding.
2. What are the serious adverse effects that may result from estrogen therapy?
3. What is the benefit of using the selective estrogen receptor modulator raloxifene instead of conjugated estrogen to treat postmenopausal osteoporosis?
4. What teaching points regarding missed pills would you review with a patient who is starting oral contraceptives?
5. What unique instructions about drug administration do you need to give to a patient who is to receive alendronate for osteoporosis?

NEED MORE HELP?

Chapter 52 of the Study Guide to Accompany *Drug Therapy in Nursing*, 4th Edition, contains NCLEX-style questions and other learning activities to reinforce your understanding of the concepts presented in this chapter. For additional information or to purchase the study guide, visit the**Point**.

REFERENCES

Adams, K., & Beal, M. W. (2009). Implanon: A review of the literature with recommendations for clinical management. *J Midwifery Womens Health*, 54(2):142–149.

Anderson, G. L., Judd, H. L., Kaunitz, A. M., et al., Women's Health Initiative Investigators. (2003). Effects of estrogen plus progestin on gynecologic cancers and associated diagnostic procedures: The Women's Health Initiative randomized trial. *Journal of the American Medical Association*, 290(13): 1739–1748.

Aschenbrenner, D. S. (2006). Drug Watch: Over-the-counter access to emergency contraception. *American Journal of Nursing*, 106(11):34–36.

Berry, S. D., Kiel, D. P., Donaldson, M. G., et al. (2010). Application of the National Osteoporosis Foundation Guidelines to postmenopausal women and men: the Framingham Osteoporosis Study. *Osteoporosis International*, 21:53–60.

Boursi, B., & Arber, N. (2007). Current and future clinical strategies in colon cancer prevention and the emerging role of chemoprevention. *Current Pharmaceutical Design*, 13(22): 2274–2282.

Burger, H. (2008). The menopausal transition – Endocrinology. *The Journal of Sexual Medicine*, 5:2266–2273.

Canderelli, R., Leccesse, L. A., & Miller, N. L. (2007). Benefits of hormone replacement therapy in postmenopausal women. *Journal of the American Academy of Nurse Practitioners,* 19(12):635–641.

Cauley, J. A., Robbins, J., Chen, Z., et al., Women's Health Initiative Investigators. (2003). Effects of estrogen plus progestin on risk of fracture and bone mineral density: the Women's Health Initiative randomized trial. *Journal of American Medical Association,* 290(13):1729–1738.

Chlebowski, R. T., Hendrix, S. L., Langer, R. D., et al., Women's Health Initiative Investigators. (2003). Influence of estrogen plus progestin on breast cancer and mammography in healthy postmenopausal women: The Women's Health Initiative Randomized Trial. *Journal of the American Medical Association,* 289(24):3243–3253.

Chlebowski, R. T., Schwartz, A. G., Wakelee, H., et al., (2009). Oestrogen plus progestin and lung cancer in postmenopausal women (Women's Health Initiative trial): a post-hoc analysis of a randomsed controlled trial. *Lancet,* 374(9697):1243–1251.

Cramer, J. A., Gold, D. T., Silverman, S. L., & Lewiecki, E. M. (2007). A systematic review of persistence and compliance with bisphosphonates for osteoporosis. *Osteoporosis International,* 18(8):1023–1031.

Curb, J. D., Prentice, R. L., Bray, P. F., et al. (2006). Venous thrombosis and conjugated equine estrogen in women without a uterus. *Archives of Internal Medicine,* 166(7):772–780.

Emkey, R., Delmas, P. D., Bolognese, M., et al. (2009). Efficacy and tolerability of once-monthly oral Ibandronate (150 mg) and once-weekly oral Alendronate (70 mg): Additional results from the monthly oral therapy with Ibandronate for Osteoporosis Intervention (MOTION) study. *Clinical Therapeutics,* 31(4):751–761.

Fantasia, H. C. (2008). Options for intrauterine contraception. *JOGNN,* 37(3):375–383.

FDA Public Health Advisory. (2006, March 17). Sepsis and medical abortion update. Retrieved from *http://www.fda.gov/cder/drug/advisory/mifeprex200603.htm*

Gungor, F., Kalelioglu, I., & Turfanda, A. (2009). Vascular effects of estrogen and progestins and risk of coronary artery disease: Importance of timing estrogen treatment. *Angiology,* 60(3):308–317.

Hays, J., Ockene, J. K., Brunner, R. L., et al., Women's Health Initiative Investigators. (2003). Effects of estrogen plus progestin on health-related quality of life. *New England Journal of Medicine,* 348(19):1839–1852.

Hsia, J., Langer, R. D., Manson, J. E., et al. Women's Health Initiative Investigators (2006). Conjugated equine estrogens and coronary heart disease: The Women's Health Initiative. *Archives of Internal Medicine,* 166(3):357–365.

Hsia, J., Margolis, K. L., Eaton, C. B., et al., Women's Health Initiative Investigators. (2007). Prehypertension and cardiovascular disease risk in the Women's Health Initiative. *Circulation,* 115(7):852–860.

Hu, Z., Yang, X., Ho, P. C., et al. (2005). Herb-drug interactions: A literature review. *Drugs,* 65(9):1239–1282.

In Brief. (2010). Biennial IV zoledronic acid (Reclast) for prevention of osteoporosis. *Obstetrics and Gynecology,* 115(1):178–179.

Kaaja, R. J. (2008). Metabolic syndrome and the menopause. *Menopause International,* 14(1):21–25.

Lim, L. S., Hoeksema, L. J., Sherin, K., et al. (2009). Screening for osteoporosis in the U.S. adult population: ACPM position statement on preventive practice. *American Journal of Preventive Medicine,* 36(4):366–375.

Manson, J. E., Hsia, J., Johnson, K. C., et al., Women's Health Initiative Investigators. (2003). Estrogen plus progestin and the risk of coronary heart disease. *New England Journal of Medicine,* 349(6):523–534.

Mitchner, N. A., & Harris, S. T. (2009). Current and emerging therapies for osteoporosis. *The Journal of Family Practice,* 58(10):S45–S49.

Murphy, P. A., Kern, S. E., Stanczyk, F. Z., et al. (2005). Interaction of St. John's wort with oral contraceptives: Effects on the pharmacokinetics of norethindrone and ethinyl estradiol, ovarian activity and breakthrough bleeding. *Contraception,* 71(6):402–408.

National Institutes of Health. (2005). NIH State-of-the-Science conference statement on management of menopause-related symptoms. Retrieved from http://consensus.nih.gov/2005/2005MenopausalSymptomsSOS025html.htm

National Osteoporosis Foundation. (2007). Physician's guide to prevention and treatment of osteoporosis. Retrieved from *http://www.nof.org/professionals/clinical.htm*

Palacios, S. (2008). Advances in hormone replacement therapy: Making the menopause manageable. *BMC Women's Health,* 8:22–26.

Rapp, S. R., Espeland, M. A., Shumaker, S. A., et al., WHIMS Investigators. (2003). Effect of estrogen plus progestin on global cognitive function in postmenopausal women. The Women's Health Initiative Memory Study: A randomized controlled trial. *Journal of the American Medical Association,* 289(20):2663–2672.

Rode, L., Langhoff-Roos, J., Andersson, C., et al. (2009). Systematic review of progesterone for the prevention of preterm birth in singleton pregnancies. *Acta Obstetricia et Gynecologica Scandinavica,* 88(11):1180–1189.

Rosano, G. M. C., Vitale, C., Marazzi, G., & Volterrani, M. (2007). Menopause and cardiovascular disease: The evidence. *Climacteric,* 10(Suppl 1):19–24.

Rossouw, J. E., Anderson, G. L., Prentice, R. L., et al. (2002). Risks and benefits of estrogen plus progestin in healthy postmenopausal women: Principal results from the Women's Health Initiative randomized controlled trial. *JAMA,* (288):321–33.

Rossmanith, W. G. & Ruebberdt, W. (2009). What causes hot flushes? The neuroendocrine origin of vasomotor symptoms in the menopause. *Gynecologicla Endocrinology,* 25(5):303–314.

Sarino, L. V., Dang, K. H., Dianat, N., et al. (2007). Drug interaction between oral contraceptives and St. John's wort: Appropriateness of advice received from community pharmacists and health food store clerks. *Journal of the American Pharmaceutical Association,* 47(1):42–47.

Schindler, A. E. (2007). Long-term use of progestogens: Colon adenoma and colon carcinoma. *Gynecological Endocrinology,* 23(S1):42–44.

Shumaker, S. A., Legault, C., Rapp, S. R., et al., WHIMS Investigators. (2003). Estrogen plus progestin and the incidence of dementia and mild cognitive impairment in postmenopausal women. The Women's Health Initiative Memory Study: A randomized controlled trial. *Journal of the American Medical Association,* 289(20):2651–2662.

Stefanick, M. L., Anderson, G. L., Margolis, K. L., et al., Women's Health Initiative Investigators. (2006). Effect of conjugated equine estrogens on breast cancer and mammography screening in postmenopausal women with hysterectomy. *Journal of the American Medical Association,* 295(14):1647–1657.

Wassertheil-Smoller, S., Hendrix, S. L., Limacher, M., et al., Women's Health Initiative Investigators. (2003). Effect of estrogen plus progestin on stroke in postmenopausal women. The Women's Health Initiative: A randomized trial. *Journal of the American Medical Association,* 289(20):2673–2684.

53

Drugs Affecting Uterine Motility

Learning Objectives

At the completion of this chapter the student will:

1. Identify core drug knowledge about drugs that affect uterine motility.
2. Identify core patient variables relevant to drugs that affect uterine motility.
3. Relate the interaction of core drug knowledge to core patient variables for drugs that affect uterine contraction.
4. Generate a nursing plan of care from the interactions between core drug knowledge and core patient variables for drugs that affect uterine motility.
5. Describe nursing interventions to maximize therapeutic effects and minimize adverse effects for drugs that affect uterine motility.
6. Determine key points for patient and family education for drugs that affect uterine motility.

Key Terms

| antepartum | oxytocics | tachysystole |
| intrapartum | postpartum | tocolytics |

Drugs Affecting Uterine Motility

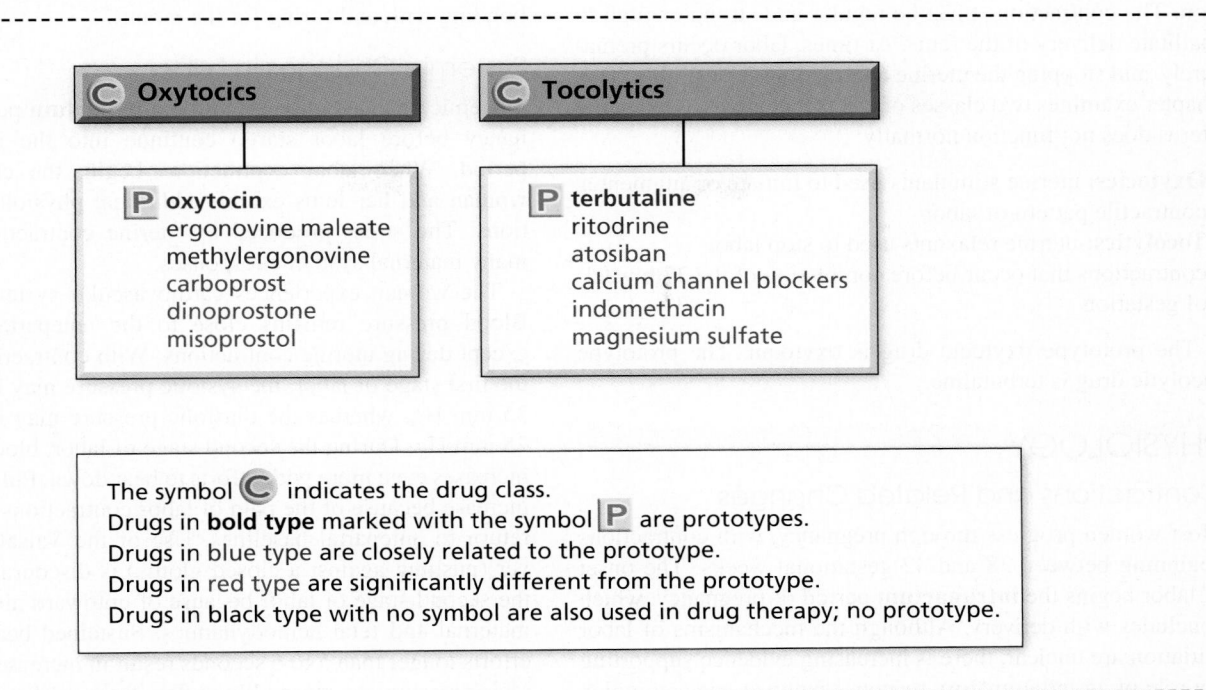

Oxytocics

P oxytocin
ergonovine maleate
methylergonovine
carboprost
dinoprostone
misoprostol

Tocolytics

P terbutaline
ritodrine
atosiban
calcium channel blockers
indomethacin
magnesium sulfate

The symbol **C** indicates the drug class.
Drugs in **bold type** marked with the symbol **P** are prototypes.
Drugs in blue type are closely related to the prototype.
Drugs in red type are significantly different from the prototype.
Drugs in black type with no symbol are also used in drug therapy; no prototype.

For labor and delivery of the fetus, normal uterine function is necessary. Normal uterine function consists of labor contractions beginning between 38 and 42 weeks of gestation. The contractions must be regular and strong enough to facilitate delivery of the fetus. At times, labor occurs prematurely, and stopping the uterine contractions is desirable. This chapter examines two classes of drugs that are used when the uterus does not function normally:

- **Oxytocics:** uterine stimulants used to initiate or augment a contractile pattern of labor
- **Tocolytics:** uterine relaxants used to stop labor contractions that occur before completion of the 37th week of gestation

The prototype oxytocic drug is oxytocin. The prototype tocolytic drug is terbutaline.

PHYSIOLOGY

Contractions and Related Changes

Most women progress through pregnancy, with contractions beginning between 38 and 42 gestational weeks. The onset of labor begins the **intrapartum** period of pregnancy, which concludes with delivery. Although the mechanisms of labor initiation are unclear, there is increasing evidence supporting the role of an inflammatory response pathway via a complex interplay of fetal and maternal signals. Pro-inflammatory cytokines released from the myometrium, cervix, and fetal membranes increase the expression of cyclooxygenase-2 (COX2) and prostaglandins, which stimulate uterine contractility. Prostaglandins also interact with oxytocin. Endogenous oxytocin stimulates the release of prostaglandins and prostaglandins increase the number of oxytocin receptors. Oxytocin does not initiate labor, but it is important in maintaining labor (Jabbour, Sales, Catalano, & Norman, 2009; Vidaeff & Ramin, 2008). Oxytocin is a hormone that is produced in the hypothalamus, stored in the posterior pituitary, and released into the circulatory system. Once the pituitary releases oxytocin, oxytocin binds to cell membrane receptors on target tissues, primarily the uterine myometrium (muscle cells), the decidua (lining of the gravid uterus), and the mammary epithelium. Although circulating oxytocin levels are unchanged before labor, there may be an increase in myometrial sensitivity to oxytocin prior to labor. Recent research suggests that this increased sensitivity may be related to a functional progesterone withdrawal and estrogen activation (Vidaeff & Raamin, 2008). If the number of oxytocin receptors is limited, the response of the uterus to oxytocin will be diminished. Pretreatment with prostaglandins, which increase the number of oxytocin receptors, results in an increased uterine response to exogenous oxytocin in labor. Oxytocinase, produced by the placenta, rapidly degrades oxytocin, which allows circulating oxytocin to restimulate the oxytocin receptors.

Endogenous oxytocin also has some vasopressive effects (causing vascular constriction) and antidiuretic effects (causing increased water resorption from the glomerular filtrate).

Oxytocin is also necessary for the let-down of breast milk. Additionally, oxytocin is believed to have an intricate role in the creation and maintenance of maternal behavior (e.g., bonding with and caring for the infant).

Systemic Changes in Labor

Systemic changes initiated in the **antepartum** period (pregnancy before labor starts) continue into the intrapartum period. When labor contractions begin, the childbearing woman and her fetus exhibit additional physiologic alterations. The stress produced by uterine contractions affects many maternal systemic responses.

The woman experiences cardiovascular system changes. Blood pressure remains close to the antepartal baseline, except during uterine contractions. With contractions during the first stage of labor, the systolic pressure may increase by 35 mm Hg, whereas the diastolic pressure may increase by 25 mm Hg. During the second stage of labor, blood pressure increases even more with efforts to bear down. Pulse rate may increase because of the pain of labor contractions but should return to antepartal baselines. Use of the Valsalva maneuver (pushing against a closed glottis) is discouraged during the second stage of labor because of untoward alterations in maternal and fetal hemodynamics. Sustained bearing-down efforts longer than 5 to 6 seconds result in increased intrathoracic pressure, decreased blood flow from the lower extremities, decreased maternal cardiac output and blood pressure, decreased placental blood flow, fetal acidosis, non-reassuring fetal heart patterns, neonatal academia, and lower APGAR scores. Evidence-based practice recommendations support the use of open-glottis pushing to avoid these physiologic alterations in second stage (Roberts & Hansen, 2007). Immediately after birth, cardiac output increases to 80% above prelabor values; within the first hour after delivery, cardiac output slowly returns to normal. Most childbearing women adapt to these cardiovascular changes successfully.

During the intrapartum period, the woman experiences respiratory system changes because oxygen demand and consumption increase. Uterine contractions cause the respiratory rate to increase above pregnancy rates. This hyperventilation causes the level of $PaCO_2$ to fall; consequently, respiratory alkalosis develops.

As labor progresses, the contracting uterus increases muscular activity and oxygen requirements, which produces a mild metabolic acidosis. This mild metabolic acidosis continues, so that during the second stage of labor and by the time of birth, the acid-base imbalance remains because metabolic acidosis is uncompensated by respiratory alkalosis. The acid-base imbalances created by labor are quickly reversed after delivery because respiratory rates return to prepregnancy values and lactic acid production decreases. By 24 hours after birth, acid-base status is similar to prepregnancy levels.

The major labor adaptation in the hemopoietic system is the development of leukocytosis above pregnancy levels. The childbearing patient's white blood cell count may be between 25,000 and 30,000 mm^3. Although an elevated white blood cell count is normally considered a sign of infection, laboratory assessment that shows an elevation of the white blood cells in the woman who has just delivered must not routinely be considered a sign of infection. This leukocytosis most likely results from labor stress, heavy exertion, and healing of the opened placental site.

Profuse perspiration and hyperventilation alter fluid and electrolyte balance during labor. Generally, healthy women having uncomplicated vaginal deliveries do not require intravenous (IV) fluids during labor. Clear liquid intake during labor does not increase maternal complications and modest amounts should be encouraged, according to a recent ACOG committee opinion (ACOG, 2009). IV fluids, including a preload bolus, are needed prior to regional analgesia (i.e., epidural) to mitigate the resulting maternal hypotension and subsequent insufficient placental perfusion and non-reassuring fetal heart tracings.

The renal system compensates for this decreased oral intake and increased water loss in part by excreting urine that is more concentrated. Also, the increasing uterine muscular activity leads to a breakdown of proteins and the presence of a trace of protein in the urine. As the fetal head descends in the pelvis, it extends pressure against the bladder walls and the urethra. The woman may not be sensitive to bladder filling. Regional anesthesia also alters bladder sensation and results in an inability to void. Overfilling of the bladder results in loss of uterine tone and ineffective labor contractions.

The gastrointestinal (GI) system experiences a reduction of gastric motility and absorption of solid foods during labor. Gastric emptying time is prolonged, and more than 25 mL of gastric contents remain in the stomach regardless of when the woman consumed her last meal. Narcotic analgesia or the use of epidural opioids further delays gastric emptying. Gastric acidity increases, and more than 50% of laboring women have a gastric pH below 2.5. This may be related to fasting in labor, which increases the concentration of hydrochlric acid. Most circulating blood shifts away from the GI system to more vital maternal organs during labor.

The healthy fetus can progress through a normal labor and delivery with no adverse effects. The labor process produces a stressful physiologic state in the fetus with each contraction, but fetal compensatory mechanisms generally allow the fetus to respond successfully to those events.

Fetal acid-base status in labor depends on the maternal contractile pattern and the fetus's ability to compensate for contraction-produced decreases in oxygen. Oxygen/carbon dioxide exchange between the mother and the fetus occurs primarily between contractions, when the blood flow is not impeded. In women who are laboring efficiently, the contractions occur at intervals that allow the intervillous spaces in the placenta to refill with oxygenated blood between contractions; this refilling maintains an adequate oxygen supply to the fetus. The healthy fetus thus maintains a pH above 7.25. The indicators of fetal well-being and adequate fetal compensation during labor are a Category I tracing consisting of (1) a baseline rate of 110 bpm to– 160 bpm, (2) moderate

variability, (3) absence of late or variable declerations. Accelerations and early decelerations may be absent or present (Macone, Hankins, Spong, Hauth, & Moore, 2008).

PATHOPHYSIOLOGY

Occasionally, uterine function proceeds abnormally, causing failure of labor to occur or failure of labor to progress. The two main categories of obstetric situations that require drug administration to initiate the onset of contractions include labor that does not begin at term and a pregnancy that is detrimental to the patient or her fetus.

Stimulation of uterine contractions using drugs before spontaneous labor has started is called induction of labor. Elective inductions for non-medical reasons should not be performed prior to 39 weeks gestation, to minimize complications from prematurity. Specific maternal and fetal conditions that may require induction of labor include the following:

• Gestational or chronic hypertension
• Post-term gestation
• Pre-eclampsia or eclampsia
• PROM at term
• PPROM near term with pulmonary maturity
• Severe intrauterine growth restriction

Before induction is initiated, the patient's cervix is assessed using the Bishop scoring system, and the fetus is assessed for evidence of maturity. The Bishop scale is a prelabor scoring system used to assist in predicting patient success if labor is induced. The system consists of five assessment parameters:

1. Cervical dilation
2. Cervical effacement
3. Fetal station
4. Cervical consistency
5. Cervical position

Each parameter is scored on a scale of 0 to 3. The higher the score, the greater is the likelihood that induction will lead to a vaginal delivery. The favorable cervix is described as one that is anterior, soft, at least 50% effaced, and 2 cm dilated, with the fetal station at +1 or lower. Induction is more likely to be successful if the score is 9 or greater in nulliparas or 5 or greater in multiparas.

Drugs may be administered to increase uterine contractions if labor is spontaneous but its patterns are dysfunctional, particularly when labor patterns are not strong or rhythmic enough to effect delivery. This type of labor needs augmentation with drug therapy that increases uterine contractions.

Another obstetric event usually requiring drug therapy is premature labor. The parturitional (child-birthing) process is now known to begin long before clinically detected preterm labor. If labor begins before completion of the 37th gestational week, drug therapy may be used to stop the uterine contractions and prolong the pregnancy. None of the currently used drug therapies, including IV fluid hydration, appears to alter the fundamental process of preterm parturition. The goal of tocolytic drug therapy, covered later in this chapter, is to secure some additional time before delivery to administer drugs to the mother. Delaying delivery allows other drugs, which help to promote fetal respiratory function, to be administered and allows time to transfer the mother, if necessary, to a hospital capable of providing acute medical care to the mother and neonatal intensive care to the newborn. During this short but crucial interval, corticosteroids are administered to improve neonatal outcomes. Corticosteroid administration significantly reduces the risk for neonatal death, respiratory distress syndrome, and intraventricular hemorrhage, a risk factor for cerebral palsy. These effects of corticosteroids are greatest if the pregnancy is prolonged for at least 24 hours; the benefits continue for at least 7 days. (See Chapter 48 for a complete discussion of corticosteroids.)

C OXYTOCICS

Oxytocic drugs are synthetic forms of the endogenous posterior pituitary hormone oxytocin. They produce uterine contractions and milk ejection for breast-feeding. The prototype oxytocic drug is oxytocin (Pitocin). Table 53.1 provides a summary of selected uterine motility drugs.

Nursing Management of the Patient Receiving P Oxytocin

Core Drug Knowledge

Pharmacotherapeutics

Oxytocin is given by IV drip infusion to initiate or augment (improve) labor contractions when important fetal or maternal reasons to do so exist. Indications for labor induction were previously listed. Augmentation of labor with oxytocin is done when hypotonic uterine dysfunction exists, resulting in a protracted labor. IV oxytocin may also be used to treat incomplete or inevitable spontaneous abortion during the second trimester Evidence-based practice calls for the administration of oxytocin by IV drip infusion or intramuscularly (IM) in the third stage of labor to decrease the risk of postpartum hemorrhage.

Oxytocin is considered a high-alert medication that has substantial implications for patient safety. Labor nurses are primarily responsible for management of oxytocin administration. Evidence-based strategies to prevent errors and harms must be in place. Based on recommendations by Simpson & Knox (2009), these processes include the following:

- Standardized order sets and protocols which start induction or augmentation at 1 mU/min and increase by 1– to 2 mU/min every 30 to 60 min based on maternal-fetal response;
- Standard concentrations prepared by the pharmacy
- Standard definition of uterine tachysystole as a contraction frequency of more than 5 in 10 minutes or a series of single contractions lasting 2 minutes or more.
- Standard treatment of oxytocin-induced uterine tachysystole.

The desired contractile pattern consists of one contraction every 2 to 3 minutes, with durations of 40 to 90 seconds per contraction and, an intensity of 40 to 90 mm Hg for internal uterine monitoring, or strong to palpation for external monitoring. Conservative, specific protocols are currently recommended to improve maternal and neonatal outcomes. High-dose regimens for pitocin administration are not supported due to increased adverse events and a lack of improved perinatal outcomes (Clark, Simpson, Knox, & Garite, 2009).

Currently, research is ongoing about an unusual, off-label use of oxytocin: the infusion of oxytocin as a treatment for autism or Asperger syndrome. No labeled use of oxytocin exists for children or men.

Pharmacokinetics

Onset of action occurs almost immediately after IV administration. It is distributed throughout the extracellular fluid and has a plasma half-life of 1 to 6 minutes. Steady-state plasma levels are reached in approximately 40 minutes with continuous IV infusion, during which maximum uterine contraction occurs (see Table 53.1). Physiologic steady state is achieved when no further uterine response to increased oxytocin infusion occurs because the receptor sites are already bound with oxytocin and are temporarily unavailable. Elimination is through the liver, kidneys, and mammary glands and by the enzyme oxytocinase.

Pharmacodynamics

Synthetic, exogenous oxytocin has the same effects on the body as natural, endogenous oxytocin. It stimulates uterine contractions and milk let-down for breast-feeding. Although the endogenous hormone has a known effect on milk production, exogenous oxytocin is not administered for this purpose.

Response to oxytocin therapy has three phases (see Figure 53.1):

1. Incremental phase: uterine activity increases evenly as the dose of oxytocin increases.
2. Stable phase: uterine activity remains constant even if the oxytocin dose increases, because the myometrial receptor sites are already fully bound with oxytocin. Because the sites are full, they cannot be receptive to more effects from the oxytocin. As half-life and elimination of oxytocin occur, the uterus again has open receptors and is responsive to increases in oxytocin levels. The uterus shifts periodically between the incremental and stable phases.
3. Tachysystole: if this third phase of uterine response to oxytocin occurs, it indicates adverse effects from the drug. If the dose continually increases, the frequency of contractions will increase, but the uterine pressure will decrease so that the contractions are less effective. The result is tachysystole, with uterine fibrillation and prolonged contraction. Tachysystole is a pattern of more than 5 contractions in 10 minutes, averaged over

TABLE 53.1 **Summary of Selected ⒸUterine Motility Drugs**

Drug (Trade) Name	Selected Indications	Route and Dosage Range	Pharmacokinetics
Ⓒ Oxytocics			
Ⓟ oxytocin (Pitocin)	Antepartum: to induce or augment uterine contractions Postpartum: to control postpartum bleeding or hemorrhage (parenteral)	*Adult:* IV (induction or augmentation of labor), 1 mU/min via infusion pump; increase by this amount every 30–60 min; do not exceed 20 mU/min; IV (treatment of incomplete or spontaneous abortion), infusion of 30 U oxytocin with 500 mL Lactated Ringers solution, (concentration: 1 mL/h = 1 milliunit/min.); IV drip (control of postpartum uterine bleeding), add 10–40 U to 1,000 mL Lactated Ringers solution and run at a rate to control uterine atony; IM, 10 U after delivery of placenta as evidence-based practice to reduce risk of postpartum hemorrhage.	*Onset:* IV, immediate; IM, 3–5 min *Duration:* IV, 60 min; IM, 2–3 h $t_{1/2}$: 1–6 min
ergonovine maleate (Ergotrate Maleate)	Prevention and treatment of postpartum and postabortal hemorrhage due to uterine atony	*Adult:* IM, 0.2 mg (severe bleeding may require repeat dosing q2–4h); IV, 0.2 mg in emergency situations	*Onset:* IM, 7–8 min; IV, immediate *Duration:* IM, 3 h; IV, 45 min $t_{1/2}$: 0.5–2 h
methylergonovine (Methergine)	Routine management after delivery of the placenta Treatment of postpartum atony and hemorrhage; subinvolution of the uterus	*Adult:* IM, 0.2 mg after delivery of the placenta, after delivery of the anterior shoulder, or during puerperium; may be repeated q2–4h; IV, same dosage as IM, infused slowly over at least 60 sec (monitor BP very carefully because severe hypertensive reaction can occur); oral, 0.2 mg tid or qid daily in the puerperium for up to 1 wk. Typically administered every 6 hours for 24 h for uterine atony not responsive to oxytocin.	*Onset:* IM, 2–5 min; IV, immediate; oral, 5–10 min *Duration:* IM, 3 h; IV, 1–3 h; oral, 3 h $t_{1/2}$: 30 min
Ⓒ Tocolytics			
Ⓟ terbutaline sulfate (Brethine)	Unlabeled use: inhibition of premature labor	*Adult:* IV, initially 10 mg/min; titrate upward to a maximum of 80 mg/min; maintain at minimum effective dosage for 4 h Use is restricted to 48–72 h maximum	*Onset:* IV, unknown *Duration:* IV, unknown; $t_{1/2}$: Unknown
ritodrine	Management of preterm labor in selected patients at ≥20 wk gestation	*Adult:* IV, 0.05 mg/min initially; gradually increase by 0.05 mg/min q10min until desired result is attained; usual effective dosage between 0.15 and 0.35 mg/min, continued for at least 12 h after uterine contractions cease	*Onset:* Rapid *Duration:* Unknown $t_{1/2}$: 1.7–2.6 h
Ⓒ Others			
carboprost (Hemabate)	Termination of pregnancy at 13–20 wk Evacuation of the uterus in instance of missed abortion or intrauterine fetal death in the second trimester Postpartum hemorrhage due to uterine atony that does not re-spond to conventional methods	*Adult:* IM (abortion), 250 mcg at 1.5–3.5-h intervals; may be increased to 500 mcg; do not exceed 12-mg total dose or continuous administration over 2 d; IM (postpartum hemorrhage), 250 mcg as one dose; multiple doses at 15–90-min intervals may be used; do not exceed a total dose of 2 mg	*Onset:* 15 min *Duration:* Unknown $t_{1/2}$: 8 h
dinoprostone (Prostaglandin E₂)	Termination of pregnancy at 12–20 wk Evacuation of the uterus in missed abortion or intrauterine fetal death up to 28 wk gestational age Management of nonmetastatic gestational trophoblastic disease (benign hydatidiform mole) Initiation of cervical ripening before induction of labor	*Adult:* Intravaginally (abortion), one suppository (10 mg); additional suppositories may be given at 3–5-h intervals; intravaginal gel (cervical ripening), 0.5 mg, repeated if no response in 6 h	*Onset:* 10 min *Duration:* 2–3 h $t_{1/2}$: 2.5–5 min
magnesium sulfate	Unlabeled use: inhibition of premature labor; seizure prevention and control in preeclampsia and eclampsia	*Adult:* IM, 4–5 g of a 50% solution q4h as necessary; IV, 4 g of a 10%–20% solution; do not exceed 1.5 mL/min of a 10% solution; IV infusion, 4–5 g in 250 mL 5% dextrose; do not exceed 3 mL/min	*Onset:* IV, immediate; IM, 60 min *Duration:* IV, 30 min; IM, 3–4 h $t_{1/2}$: Unknown

P H Y S I O L O G Y

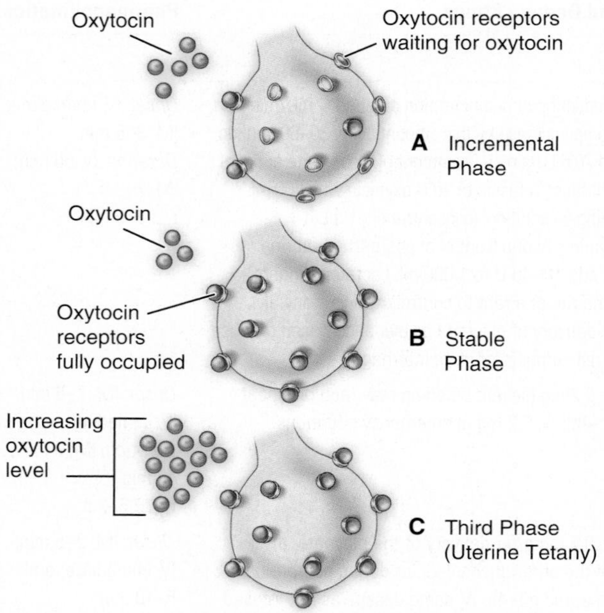

• FIGURE 53.1 Phases of oxytocin activity. Oxytocic drug therapy is usually initiated to mimic the role of natural oxytocin in prompting or augmenting labor. Oxytocin undergoes three phases of activity. (A) In the incremental phase, oxytocin levels rise, and oxytocin receptors are stimulated, producing increased intensity and frequency of uterine contractions. (B) In the stable phase, receptor sites are occupied with oxytocin, so no further oxytocin effects occur until a receptor site opens again. (C) In the third phase—uterine tetany tachysystole —oxytocin levels continually rise. Uterine contractions increase in number while the force of the contractions decreases. In such instances, the uterus experiences hyperstimulation tachysystole.

a 30-minute window, or a series of single contractions lasting 2 minutes or more.

Oxytocin therapy also has vasopressive and antidiuretic effects. Oxytocin affects the cardiovascular system by initially decreasing blood pressure. With prolonged oxytocin administration, baseline blood pressure may increase by 30%. Cardiac output and stroke volume also increase. Oxytocin doses of 15 milliunits/min or above have antidiuretic effects when administered over a prolonged period; the antidiuretic effect seems to reach its maximal effect at 45 milliunits/min. Antidiuresis appears to be initiated by the direct action of oxytocin on the kidney and not as a result of any stimulation of the release of antidiuretic hormone (i.e., syndrome of inappropriate secretion of antidiuretic hormone). Fatal water intoxication has occurred with the use of oxytocin, although the antidiuretic effects are weak. Additionally, oxytocin increases the water permeability of the nephron, which causes more water retention than sodium reabsorption and in turn leads to water intoxication and dilutional hyponatremia. Symptoms of water intoxication affect primarily the central nervous system

(CNS) and musculoskeletal systems. CNS effects range from headache, fatigue, nausea, and anorexia to lethargy, confusion, disorientation, agitation, vomiting, seizures, and coma. Musculoskeletal symptoms may include cramps and weakness. Cardiovascular effects, such as tachycardia and hypotension, can also occur.

Oxytocin and vasopressin are known to play a role in social and repetitive behaviors. A small study of adults with autism or Asperger disorder who were administered oxytocin infusions showed a significant reduction in repetitive behaviors after the infusion, compared with placebo (Hollander, Novotny, Hanratty, et al., 2003). Oxytocin has also been linked to social recognition; the administration of oxytocin to individuals with autism appears to facilitate comprehension of the emotions behind speech (Hollander, Novotny, Hanratty, et al., 2003; Hollander, Bartz, Chaplin, et al., 2007).

Contraindications and Precautions

Oxytocin is contraindicated in cephalopelvic disproportion (fetal head relative to maternal pelvis) and with unfavorable fetal positions or presentations that must be converted before delivery (such as transverse lie). It is also contraindicated in the following conditions:

• Obstetric emergencies in which the benefit-to-risk ratio for either mother or fetus favors cesarean section
• Fetal distress without signs of imminent delivery
• Prolonged use in uterine inertia or severe preeclampsia
• Tachysystolic uterine patterns
• Failure of uterine activity to achieve satisfactory progress
• Contraindication to vaginal delivery (e.g., invasive cervical carcinoma, active genital herpes, cord presentation or prolapse, total placenta previa, vas previa)
• Hypersensitivity to the drug

Oxytocin must be administered very cautiously if cyclopropane anesthesia is used, because maternal sinus bradycardia with abnormal atrioventricular rhythms and hypotension may result. Water intoxication is possible with oxytocin use and should be considered if oral fluids or large doses of IV fluids are given in addition to oxytocin infusion. Overstimulation of the uterus, which may be hazardous to the mother or fetus, can occur with oxytocin administration, even with proper administration and supervision.

Adverse Effects

Adverse effects of oxytocin are dose related and take two forms: maternal and fetal. The most common maternal adverse effects are nausea, vomiting, uterine tachysystole and cardiac arrhythmias. Less common but potentially fatal are severe water intoxication and hyponatremia. Other maternal adverse effects are spasm and rupture of the uterus (usually from excessive doses or hypersensitivity to the drug), postpartum hemorrhage, subarachnoid hemorrhage, and pelvic hematoma. The most common fetal adverse effect is bradycardia. Other adverse fetal effects are premature ventricular contractions and other arrhythmias, impaired fetal oxygenation, permanent brain or CNS damage and death (from excessive uterine motility), low Apgar scores 5 minutes after birth, neonatal jaundice, and retinal hemorrhage.

When administered intrapartally for induction or augmentation of labor, oxytocin does not cause fetal structural defects or congenital anomalies but may be responsible for fetal CNS depression. Such CNS depression severely compromises the neonate's ability to successfully adapt to the extrauterine environment.

Overdosage depends on uterine hyperactivity. Uterine tachysystole (greater than 5 contractions within 10 minutes or a series of single contractions lasting 2 minutes or more) or a resting tone of 15 to 20 mm Hg or more between contractions can cause tumultuous labor, uterine rupture, cervical and vaginal lacerations, postpartum hemorrhage, uteroplacental hypoperfusion, deceleration of FHR, fetal hypoxia, fetal hypercapnia, or fetal demise. These fetal effects occur as a result of uteroplacental hypoperfusion, a state in which the placenta does not have time to recover and be refilled with oxygenated blood. The lack of oxygenated blood creates a state of fetal hypoxia. The greatest drop in fetal oxygen saturation occurs 90 seconds after a contraction, and the fetus needs an additional 90 seconds to recover. In women who are laboring efficiently, intervals occur between the contractions that allow the fetus to be reoxygenated. In tachsystole from oxytocin therapy, no insufficient rest occurs between contractions. Fetal oxygen desaturation begins within 5 minutes of excess uterine contractions. With continued insult, anaerobic glycolysis, metabolic acidosis, and direct fetal myocardial depression results. The fetal heart rate tracing will demonstrate late decelerations with absent or minimal variability; a pattern associated with abnormal fetal acid-base balance (Simpson & Knox, 2009). Recovery of the fetus from oxytocin-induced hypoxia therefore requires cessation of oxytocin administration.

Water intoxication with convulsions may occur if large doses of oxytocin (40 to 50 milliunits/min) are given for a long time. Treatment consists of discontinuing the drug, restricting fluid intake, initiating diuresis, administering IV hypertonic saline solutions, correcting electrolyte imbalance, controlling convulsions cautiously with barbiturates, and following general nursing measures to care for an unconscious patient.

Drug Interactions
If oxytocin is given at the same time as sympathomimetic drugs (those drugs that stimulate the sympathetic nervous system), the vasopressor effect may be increased. A possible consequence is postpartum hypertension.

Assessment of Relevant Core Patient Variables
Health Status
Assess, or verify that the physician or nurse midwife has assessed, the patient's pelvic adequacy before beginning oxytocin therapy. Determine or confirm with the physician

or nurse midwife that the fetal position is favorable for vaginal delivery. Assess for fetal distress and for conditions that would contraindicate vaginal delivery (e.g., invasive cervical carcinoma, active genital herpes, cord presentation or prolapse, total placenta previa, vas previa). Assess contractions for tachysystolic patterns or for contractions that should be successful in advancing labor but are not.

Assess whether the patient's cervix is favorable for induction (Bishop score of 5 or greater in multiparas and 9 or greater in primiparas). Before and throughout therapy, assess maternal vital signs, length of contractions, time between contractions, FHR, fetal movement, and fluid status. Assessment of FHR patterns and uterine activity is documented every 15 minutes in the active phase of the first stage of labor and every 5 minutes in the pushing phase of the second stage of labor. This assessment is performed by an RN providing care to not more than two induction patients (AWHONN, 2008).

Life Span and Gender
Before oxytocin is administered, assess the duration of the pregnancy. Oxytocin is not used during the first trimester except in cases of spontaneous or induced abortion.

Lifestyle, Diet, and Habits
Consider the patient's risk of water intoxication if the patient is receiving large amounts of fluids by either intravenous or oral route, or in the patient with impaired renal excretion (i.e., severe preeclampsia).

Environment
Be aware of the environment in which oxytocin will be administered. Oxytocin is administered only in a hospital labor and delivery suite where the patient and fetus can be continually monitored.

Nursing Diagnoses and Outcomes
- Risk for Fetal or Maternal Injury related to uterine hypertonicity secondary to oxytocin therapy
  Desired outcome: *The mother and fetus will progress through labor and delivery without injury during oxytocin therapy.*
- Excess Fluid Volume related to drug-induced water intoxication and altered electrolyte levels
  Desired outcome: *The patient's fluid status will remain normal during oxytocin therapy.*

Planning and Intervention
Maximizing Therapeutic Effects
Assess cervical ripening using the Bishop scoring system before oxytocin therapy starts. If the cervix is not ripe, PGE_2 gel may need to be instilled or vaginal doses of misoprostol given at least 4 hours before administering oxytocin. (For further discussion of these drugs, see the section on Drugs Significantly Different From Oxytocin.) Specific orders from the prescriber are required for administering either of these drugs. A protocol may also be required.

Standard concentrations of oxytocin in lactated Ringers IV solution should be prepared by the pharmacy to decrease risk of errors. Simpson (2009) recommends a pharmacy preparation of 30 U in 500 mL of LR yielding 1 mL/h = 1 mU/min. Use an infusion pump for precise administration of oxytocin.

Start the infusion at 0.5 to 1 milliunits/min and increase the dose by 1 to 2 milliunits/min every 30 to 60 minutes based on the maternal-fetal response until the desired contractile pattern is achieved. If labor is progressing at 1 cm/hour, oxytocin dosage does not need to be increased (Simpson & Knox, 2009). One research study found that once the patient achieves cervical dilation of 5 cm or more (active labor), there is no advantage in continuing oxytocin infusion at all; discontinuing the infusion did not result in significantly longer duration of the second phase of labor (Daniel-Spiegel, Weiner, Ben-Shlomo, et al., 2004).

If oxytocin is being used to control postpartum hemorrhage, the timing of the dose may be important. One small study found that if oxytocin was injected immediately after birth of the infant, there was less postpartum hemorrhage than if the drug was administered after the placenta had been delivered (Huh, Chelmow, & Malone, 2004).

Minimizing Adverse Effects

Piggyback the diluted oxytocin solution into a primary IV line, which also supplies a physiologic electrolyte solution. Doing so makes it possible to discontinue the solution immediately if adverse maternal or fetal effects occur. An infusion pump is continuously used throughout therapy to prevent overdosage.

Use of drugs that stimulate uterine activity requires close monitoring of the patient and fetus throughout administration of the oxytocin. Assess maternal vital signs, FHR, and contractile pattern before each increase in the infusion rate. If maternal vital signs show hypertension or substantial changes, if the FHR decreases, or if fetal movement stops, notify the prescriber immediately. Once the dose is stabilized during induction, check maternal vital signs at least every 4 hours.

The FHR monitor continuously records the patient's uterine contraction pattern. If the dose of oxytocin remains unchanged, assess FHR and uterine activity every 15 minutes during the active phase of stage one labor and every 5 minutes during the second stage of labor (Simpson & Knox, 2009).

Assess for evidence of tachysystole. Tachysystole occurs when there are 5 or more contractions within 10 minutes or contractions lasting 2 minutes or longer. Labor and delivery units should have a standardized procedure if a tachysystolic labor pattern develops from the oxytocin infusion. Simpson and Knox (2009) recommend a standard course of action based on fetal response. If there is a reassuring FHR: (1) place the mother in a lateral position, (2) provide an IV fluid bolus of 500 mL lactated Ringers, (3) if uterine activity has not returned to normal after 10 minutes, decrease oxytocin rate by half, and (4) if uterine activity has not returned to normal after 10 minutes more, discontinue oxytocin until normal uterine activity resumes and notify the provider. If there is a non-reassuring (Category II or III) FHR: (1) discontinue the oxytocin, (2) reposition the mother into a lateral position, (3) provide an IV fluid bolus of 500 mL lactated Ringers, (4) provide oxygen at 10 L/min via non-rebreather facemask, (5) give 0.25 mg terbutaline subcutaneously, and (6) notify the provider

The appropriate dose for restarting oxytocin after hyperstimulation is unknown. Simpson and Knox (2009) delineate a standardized protocol to decrease errors. Based on the physiology of contractions and the pharmacokinetics of oxytocin, it has been suggested that if the oxytocin has been discontinued for less than 20- to 30 minutes, if the fetal status is reassuring and the contractions no longer meet the definition of tachysystole, the oxytocin may be restarted at no more than half the previous rate. If the oxytocin was discontinued for more than 30- to 40 minutes, essentially all the circulating exogenous oxytocin has been metabolized. Restart at the initial rate.

Making these assessments in the intrapartum period is challenging and raises issues of nursing conduct and patient safety. If you have a professional difference of opinion with the physician or nurse midwife about whether the patient is experiencing tachysystole or whether the oxytocin should be slowed or stopped, use the appropriate chain of command in the institution to seek appropriate assistance for the patient. Failure to continue to seek care for a patient when necessary may legally be considered negligence on your part if the patient or fetus has an adverse outcome from oxytocin therapy (Simpson & Knox, 2009). A review of malpractice claims showed that the best ways to avoid litigation regarding oxytocin use include the following: accurate interpretation of FHR tracings, adoption and following of well-designed policies for the administration of oxytocin, using the chain of command, and comprehensive and objective documentation of the patient's response to oxytocin (Greenwald & Mondor, 2003).

Assess the patient's fluid intake and urinary output and urge the patient to urinate at least every 2 hours throughout oxytocin therapy. Assess for signs of water intoxication, including anorexia, nausea, vomiting, headache, confusion, muscle cramps, hypotension, and tachycardia.

Providing Patient and Family Education

- Educate the patient and family about the rationale for oxytocin use, the desired effects, and the potential adverse effects of oxytocin therapy (important).
- Explain that the patient and fetus will be monitored closely to determine the effectiveness of the therapy and to detect any early signs of adverse effects.

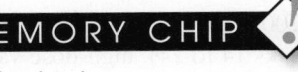

MEMORY CHIP

P Oxytocin

- Used to induce labor or to augment labor
- Works similarly to endogenous oxytocin by attaching to oxytocin receptors and stimulating them
- Major contraindications: conditions that require cesarean section; hypermotility of the uterus
- Most common adverse effects: maternal—nausea, vomiting, uterine hypertonicity, and cardiac arrhythmias; fetal—bradycardia
- Most serious adverse effects: maternal—uterine rupture, water intoxication (uncommon); fetal—demise, hypoxia, permanent brain damage, death
- **Life span alert: used in third trimester of pregnancy**
- **Patient safety alert: Oxytocin can cause maternal and fetal death, most commonly associated with overdosage of the drug.**
- Maximizing therapeutic effects: Administer when the cervix has ripened; titrate the dose upward slowly, based on the frequency of contractions and uterine response.
- Minimizing adverse effects: Assess mother and fetus carefully throughout therapy for adverse effects and poor fetal tolerance; stop the infusion if hypertonicity or fetal compromise occurs.
- Most important patient education: purpose of drug; rationale for frequent assessment

Ongoing Assessment and Evaluation

Throughout induction, monitor continually for evidence of adverse maternal or fetal effects. Oxytocin drug therapy is considered effective when labor progresses predictably, no maternal or fetal adverse effects occur, vaginal delivery happens without complications, and the postpartum period is uneventful.

Drugs Closely Related to P Oxytocin

Ergonovine maleate and methylergonovine, ergot derivatives, are two additional oxytocic drugs. Unlike oxytocin, they are primarily used to prevent postpartum or postabortal hemorrhage.

Ergonovine Maleate

Ergonovine maleate (Ergotrate), when used after placental delivery, increases the strength, duration, and frequency of uterine contractions and decreases uterine bleeding. Ergonovine maleate exerts its effects by acting as a partial agonist or antagonist at the alpha-adrenergic, dopaminergic, and tryptaminergic receptors. Ergonovine maleate may also be used to treat migraine headache (an off-label use of this drug), although it is less effective for this condition than the drug ergotamine.

Onset of action is rapid, although it varies by route of administration. IM injection is the preferred method. IV injection is confined to emergencies, such as excessive uterine bleeding, because of the higher incidence of adverse effects that

accompany IV administration. Uterine contractions continue for 3 or more hours after IM injection. Ergonovine maleate promotes a higher uterine tone than oxytocin and therefore is not recommended for routine use before the delivery of the placenta. As with oxytocin, hypertension and headache may occur with use of ergonovine maleate. The principal manifestations of serious overdosage of ergonovine maleate are convulsions (acute overdosage) and gangrene of the fingers and toes (chronic overdosage). Other symptoms of overdosage include nausea, vomiting, diarrhea, hypertension or hypotension, weak pulse, dyspnea, loss of consciousness, numbness and coldness of extremities, tingling, chest pain, hypercoagulability, confusion, excitement, delirium, hallucinations, and coma.

Methylergonovine

Methylergonovine (Methergine) also has substantial effects on uterine tone. It acts directly on the smooth muscle of the uterus and induces a rapid and sustained tetanic uterotonic effect, which shortens the third stage of labor and reduces blood loss. Excretion is rapid and appears to be both renal and hepatic. IM use of methylergonovine is considered routine management after delivery of the placenta, although it may also be administered after the delivery of the anterior shoulder if full obstetric supervision is available. It is given orally three or four times a day immediately postpartum for a maximum of 1 week. Hypertension, sometimes with seizures or headache, is the most common adverse effect. Other adverse effects are hypotension, nausea, vomiting, dizziness, tinnitus, transient chest pain, hematuria, thrombophlebitis, water intoxication, hallucinations, leg cramps, nasal congestion, diarrhea, diaphoresis, palpitations, and dyspnea. Signs of acute overdosage include nausea, vomiting, abdominal pain, numbness, tingling of the extremities, and increase in blood pressure.

Drugs Significantly Different From P Oxytocin

Carboprost

Carboprost (Hemabate) is a prostaglandin used to induce abortion in pregnancies of 13 to 20 weeks' duration. Prostaglandins stimulate the myometrium of the pregnant uterus to contract in a manner similar to that of labor. The exact mechanisms of action of carboprost are unknown. Carboprost may also be used to control postpartum hemorrhage resulting from uterine atony that has not responded to oxytocin and IM ergot preparations. Carboprost is contraindicated in the following conditions: acute pelvic inflammatory disease; active cardiac, pulmonary, renal, or hepatic disease; and hypersensitivity to the agents. Carboprost is administered intramuscularly.

Carboprost also stimulates the smooth muscle of the GI tract, which may be responsible for the nausea, vomiting, and diarrhea that sometimes accompany its use. Nausea is the most common adverse effect. Other possible adverse effects are cardiovascular (arrhythmia, chest pain), CNS related (headache, flushing, anxiety, hot flashes, paresthesia, dizziness, weakness), genitourinary (endometritis, uterine rupture, uterine or vaginal pain), and respiratory (coughing, dyspnea). Other miscellaneous adverse effects include chills and shivering, backache, blurred vision, breast tenderness, diaphoresis, eye pain, muscle cramps, fever, rash, and leg cramps.

Dinoprostone

Dinoprostone (Prepidil, Cervidil) has two major uses. Dinoprostone given as a vaginal suppository (Prostin E2) is used to terminate pregnancies of 12 to 20 weeks. It is usually reserved for evacuating the uterus in managing incomplete spontaneous abortion or intrauterine fetal death up to 28 weeks. It is also used in managing nonmetastatic gestational trophoblastic disease (benign hydatidiform mole).

Dinoprostone in a gel form (PGE_2 gel; Prepidil) or a vaginal insert (Cervidil) is used as an agent for cervical ripening at term when induction of labor is indicated. In most patients, treatment with dinoprostone changes the consistency, dilation, and effacement of the cervix.

The liver appears to be the primary site of metabolism for dinoprostone. Metabolites are excreted renally.

Misoprostol

Misoprostol (Cytotec) is a synthetic PGE_1 analogue. It produces uterine contractions. It also has antisecretory and mucosal protective properties. Although the only approved uses of misoprostol are to prevent gastric ulcers induced by therapy with nonsteroidal anti-inflammatory drugs (NSAIDs) and after mifepristone use in medical abortion (see Chapter 52), many research studies have demonstrated that misoprostol is safe and effective in producing cervical ripening and initiating labor. Although still an off-label use, the FDA removed pregnancy as an absolute contraindication to misoprostol use in 2002.

Multiple studies have indicated that misoprostol is more effective than PGE_2 in achieving vaginal deliveries within 24 hours of administration with no difference in serious maternal or neonatal outcomes. There is conflicting data about cesarean delivery rates, with a trend toward fewer C-sections for failure to progress, but more C-sections for non-reassuring fetal heart tracings in the misoprostol group (Allen & O'Brien, 2009).

The best dose for induction of labor in pregnant women at term is still debatable; some studies support low oral doses (25 to 50 mcg), and others find no difference between low-dose and high-dose vaginal protocols (up to 200 mcg) (Ewert, Powers, Robertson, et al., 2006). Recent research studies found the drug to be effective in inducing labor in women at term who experienced prelabor rupture of their amniotic membranes, although not all studies concurred (Lin, Nuthalapaty, Carver, et al., 2005; Wing, Guberman, & Fassett, 2005). One study has shown that misoprostol has similar risks compared with oxytocin for causing contraction abnormalities (hypertonus, hyperstimulation) and maternal and neonatal complications (when used to induce labor in women at term with premature rupture of membranes) (Lin,

Nuthalapaty, Carver, et al., 2005). When used to induce labor in midterm pregnancies (weeks 14 to 24), high-dose vaginal misoprostol shortens the labor induction compared with a low-dose regimen of vaginal misoprostol with oxytocin infusion (Nuthalapaty, Ramsey, Biggio, et al., 2005).

Misoprostol should not be used in patients with a previous cesarean delivery or prior major uterine surgery, to prevent uterine rupture. There is insufficient data to support the use of miesoprostol in the active management of third stage of labor to prevent postpartum hemorrhage or in the treatment of postpartum hemorrhage (Allen & O'Brien, 2009).

C TOCOLYTICS

Drugs that inhibit uterine activity are classified as tocolytics. Preterm labor is the medical complication requiring the administration of tocolytics. Tocolytics are used when true labor begins after 20 weeks' gestation and usually before completion of the 34th gestational week. While late preterm neonates (34 –to 37 weeks gestation) have significantly more medical problems than full term infants, the major morbidities—respiratory distress, intraventricular hemorrhage, and necrotizing enterocolitis—are rare by 34 weeks gestation. Although the use of tocolytic drugs can stop preterm labor, they have not been found to have an effect on perinatal or neonatal outcomes. The use of tocolytics stops labor for 24 to 48 hours (and occasionally for up to 7 days), which affords additional time before delivery for the mother to receive corticosteroids. During that interval, the corticosteroids can exert a therapeutic effect on the fetal lungs so that they are prepared for life outside the uterus. If necessary, the mother can also be transferred to another facility during that time.

Currently, several drugs are used for their tocolytic properties, including beta agonists, such as terbutaline and ritodrine, and in the United States, magnesium sulfate. A new drug class, the oxytocin antagonists, works directly on the uterine receptors in treating preterm labor. Calcium channel blockers, especially nifedipine, have also been found to be effective in treating preterm labor. Prostaglandin inhibitors, such as indomethacin, have been used as tocolytic agents, but their use is limited to pregnancies less than 32 weeks gestation due to concern about premature closure of the fetal ductus arteriosis and effects on amniotic fluid volume (i.e., oligohydramnios) (Haas, et al., 2009). Thus far, the FDA has approved only ritodrine for use as a tocolytic. However, despite its approval and proven short-term effectiveness, this drug is seldom used to treat preterm labor. Discontinuation rates because of reported maternal adverse effects may be as high as 38%, contributing to the obstetric community's lack of confidence in ritodrine and a general view that ritodrine therapy is unsafe. However, clinical trials have shown that adverse effect profiles are actually very similar among beta agonists, and there may be no sufficient rationale for choosing one over another (Chan, Cabrol, Ingemarsson, et al., 2006). Terbutaline is a drug that acts similarly to ritodrine.

Although using terbutaline to control preterm labor is an off-label use, the drug has been widely used for this purpose. Because of its use, the prototype tocolytic for this chapter is terbutaline (Brethine).

Research on tocolytics has produced mixed results, with some studies showing that all of the tocolytics are equally effective in stopping preterm labor, some showing that a particular drug is better than other drugs, and some indicating that none of the drugs are very effective (Tan, Devendra, Tan, et al., 2006). Although tocolytics are accepted as effective over the short term (delaying delivery by 24 hours up to 7 days), research has not found them to be effective in delaying delivery over the long term. A recent meta-analysis of 58 studies including women between 28 and 32 weeks gestation, demonstrated that tocolytics are superior to placebo at delaying delivery for 48 hours and for 7 days, but not at delaying delivery until 37 weeks (Haas, Imperiale, Kirkpatrick, et al., 2009). Thus, the efficacy of all tocolytic drugs remains unclear, which is one reason for the continued controversy surrounding their use.

Nursing Management of the Patient Receiving P Terbutaline

Core Drug Knowledge

Pharmacotherapeutics

The labeled uses of terbutaline include treatment of asthma and bronchospasm, although it is rarely used in the treatment of asthma (see Chapter 35 Table 35.3, for more information on this use). Although the drug label for terbutaline specifically states that the drug should not be used to control preterm labor, terbutaline has been used off-label to control preterm labor in pregnancies of 20 weeks to 34 weeks. Some disagreement exists as to what the earliest gestational age to use terbutaline should be, and some authorities believe drug therapy should be started later than 20 weeks, if used at all. Recent Food and Drug (FDA) label changes for terbutaline (FDA, 2011) restrict the use of terbutaline to a maximum 48 to 72 hours given either by cutaneous subinjection or intravenous infusion. The drug must be administered in an inpatient setting. Using terbutaline to control preterm labor, although widespread, is still considered controversial by many experts, who believe that the effectiveness of the drug for this use has never been clearly demonstrated by positive perinatal or neonatal outcomes. Perscribing practices for terbutaline are likely to change based on the recent revised labeling of the drug from the FDA.

When terbutaline is administered to control preterm labor it should be used concomitantly with corticosteroids, which are effective in preventing respiratory complications in the premature newborns. Terbutaline prolongs delivery long enough for the corticosteroids to take effect. Like other tocolytic therapy, terbutaline therapy has not been found to be effective long term when used on a maintenance basis to prevent premature labor and its use in this manner is now contraindicated on the label (FDA, 2011) (Box 53.1).

BOX 53.1 FOCUS ON RESEARCH

Tocolytic Therapy: A meta-analysis and decision analysis.

Haas, D. M., Imperiale, T. F., Kirkpatrick, P. R., Klein, R. W., Zollinger, T. W., & Golichowski, A. M. (2009). Tocolytic therapy: A meta-analysis and decision analysis. *Obstetrics & Gynecology*, 113(3):585–594.

The Study
A meta-analysis of 58 randomized controlled trials of tocolysis was conducted to determine the optimal first-line tocolytic agent for treatment of preterm labor. Results demonstrated that all tocolytic agents were superior to placebo or control groups for delaying delivery for at least 48 hours and 7 days. Calcium-channel blockers were superior for delaying delivery to 37 weeks gestation. No statistically significant differences were found for neonatal outcomes, including respiratory distress syndrome or neonatal survival. A decision analysis found that prostaglandin inhibitors yielded the best tolerance and delayed delivery. Extrapolating to clinical implications, if 1,000 women were treated for preterm labor, 80 of those treated with prostaglandin inhibitors would deliver within 48 hours compared to 182 to 416 for other tocolytic treatments. The authors concluded that prostaglandin inhibitors may be the best first-line tocolytic agent before 32 weeks gestation to delay delivery for 48 hours and 7 days; calcium-channel blockers may be superior for delaying delivery until 37 weeks gestation.

Nursing Implications
Preterm birth, defined as a delivery prior to 37 completed weeks gestation, is a significant cause of neonatal morbidity and mortality in the United States. Current practice involves interventions to delay birth as long as possible to mitigate neonatal risk. Decisions about which treatments to use for prevention of preterm labor are made by the provider and are based on multiple fetal and maternal factors. Risks and benefits of therapy for both mother and fetus must be carefully considered in this decision process. Nurses are often faced with the task of explaining and clarifying these issues for patients and families. This can pose a dilemma when treatments have been shown to be ineffective or dangerous in achieving outcomes (i.e., bedrest for preterm labor). Patients may also have questions about which medication is the best to use. A meta-analysis of many trials is helpful because the sample size can be larger when several studies are considered as one and this yields the highest level of evidence for practice. Nurses can work with interdisciplinary evidence-based practice teams to bring the latest evidence to the bedside to achieve the best possible outcomes.

Intervention should begin as soon as a diagnosis of preterm labor is established and contraindications are ruled out. Conservative therapy (e.g., bed rest and lying on the left side), although lacking evidence to support its effectiveness, may be tried first and may also be used simultaneously with drug therapy. If terbutaline therapy is necessary, the drug is administered subcutaneously, or intravenously.

Some research, although quite limited, supports treating uterine tachysystole with tocolytics as a means of intrauterine resuscitation. A critical review of the literature by de Heus and colleagues (2008) found that the best available evidence supports the use of beta-adrenergic agonists such as terbutaline or ritodrine, although the dosage remains unclear.

Pharmacokinetics
Aspects of its pharmacokinetics are not well known.

Pharmacodynamics

Terbutaline is a beta-receptor agonist (stimulant) that selectively prefers the beta-2 receptors over beta-1 receptors. Stimulation of these receptors inhibits contractility of uterine smooth muscle and provides bronchial dilation, vasodilation, and hepatic glycogenolysis and gluconeogenesis, among other effects (for a full discussion of the effects from beta-2 receptor stimulation, see Chapter 13). Although terbutaline prolongs pregnancy, it has not been found to decrease the incidence of premature births or have any effect on perinatal or neonatal outcomes.

Contraindications and Precautions

Terbutaline now carries a black box warning that it should not be used for longer than 48–72 hours as it increases the risk of serious maternal cardiovascular events (including increased heart rate, cardiac arrhythmias, pulmonary edema, and myocardial ischemia), transient hyperglycemia, hypokalemia, and maternal death. Use of terbutaline in outpatient settings (such as via infusion pumps) is now contraindicated. Oral use of terbutaline is also now contraindicated as it has not been found to be effective in preventing or treating preterm labor and it has the same safety concerns.

Terbutaline is contraindicated before the 20th week of pregnancy because the impetus for a spontaneous abortion may be related to genetic fetal defects.

Terbutaline is also contraindicated in the following conditions, in which continuing the pregnancy is hazardous to the mother or fetus:

- Antepartum hemorrhage that requires immediate delivery
- Eclampsia and severe preeclampsia
- Intrauterine fetal death
- Chorioamnionitis (inflammation of the amniotic membranes)
- Maternal cardiac disease
- Pulmonary hypertension
- Maternal hyperthyroidism
- Uncontrolled maternal diabetes mellitus

Additional contraindications include pre-existing maternal medical conditions that would be seriously affected by the pharmacologic properties of a beta agonist such as terbutaline. Examples include hypovolemia, cardiac arrhythmias associated with tachycardia or digitalis toxicity, uncontrolled hypertension, and pheochromocytoma (a hypertension-producing tumor of the adrenal glands). Hypersensitivity to any component of the drug is also a contraindication. Precautions that apply to the use of terbutaline include controlled diabetes, controlled hypertension, and bronchial asthma already being treated with beta agonists. Terbutaline is a pregnancy category C drug.

Adverse Effects

Terbutaline is a potent drug that may produce serious, even fatal, adverse effects in the woman and the fetus. The adverse effects are related to the other effects of beta stimulants on the body, including beta-1 stimulation effects, because although terbutaline is relatively selective for beta-2 receptors, some stimulation of beta-1 receptors still occurs. These maternal adverse effects include tachycardia, palpitations, hypotension, cardiac arrhythmias, electrocardiographic changes, dyspnea, nervousness, tremor, transient hyperglycemia, hypokalemia (occurring possibly through intracellular shunting), pulmonary edema, cerebral and myocardial ischemia, nausea, and vomiting. Maternal deaths have occurred. Fetal and neonatal effects include increased FHR and neonatal hypoglycemia. Of these adverse effects, tachycardia (maternal and fetal), cardiac arrhythmias, palpitations, and tremor (maternal) are probably the most common, and pulmonary edema and cerebral and myocardial ischemia are the most serious. Cardiac arrhythmias are also potentially serious.

In instances of overdose, the drug should be discontinued, and an appropriate beta blocker, such as propranolol, should be given as an antidote.

Drug Interactions

Additive effects may occur if terbutaline is administered with other beta stimulants. Coadministration of terbutaline and beta blockers decreases the effectiveness of terbutaline. Table 53.2 lists drugs that interact with terbutaline.

Assessment of Relevant Core Patient Variables

Health Status

Determine whether the patient has any conditions that contraindicate therapy or require cautious use of terbutaline. These conditions may include cardiac arrhythmias

TABLE 53.2	Agents That Interact with P Terbutaline	
Interactants	**Effect and Significance**	**Nursing Management**
Beta blockers	Will compete with terbutaline for the same receptors, thereby preventing terbutaline from having its effect	Give as antidote if overdosage of terbutaline; otherwise, not recommended to be coadministered.
Beta-2 agonists; other sympathomimetic drugs	Increased effects at other beta receptors; may significantly increase blood pressure	Avoid coadministration if possible; monitor patient's BP carefully if coadministration is essential.
Halothane, cyclopropane (halogenated hydrocarbon anesthetics)	Increases the risk for cardiac arrhythmias	Monitor patient carefully if this combination must be used.

associated with tachycardia, uncontrolled hypertension, pheochromocytoma, diabetes, or bronchial asthma already being treated with beta agonists. Assess the patient's pulse rate and blood pressure. A baseline electrocardiogram (ECG) should be performed to rule out undiagnosed maternal heart disease before beginning terbutaline infusion. Determine whether the patient is taking beta blockers.

Life Span and Gender

Ask whether the woman's pregnancy is 20 weeks' gestation or more, because pregnancy of less than 20 weeks is a contraindication. Terbutaline is a pregnancy category C drug.

Environment

Be aware of the environment required to administer terbutaline. Terbutaline given to control a current episode of preterm labor must be given in a hospital labor and delivery suite where the mother and fetus can be monitored while the IV solution or the continuous SC solution is infused. Terbutaline is contraindicated in the outpatient setting.

Nursing Diagnoses and Outcomes

- Risk for Injury to mother from adverse effects of drug therapy
  Desired outcome: *No adverse effects will occur from drug therapy.*
- Risk for Injury to infant stemming from premature delivery or adverse effects from drug therapy
  Desired outcome: *Drug therapy will prevent premature delivery of infant and will not cause adverse effects to the newborn.*
- Excess Fluid Volume, pulmonary edema, related to potential adverse effects of drug therapy
  Desired outcome: *The patient's fluid volume will remain within normal limits.*

Planning and Intervention

Maximizing Therapeutic Effects

Begin drug therapy as soon as possible after preterm labor is diagnosed and the order to start therapy has been received. Terbutaline therapy is usually given by the IV route. Administer the prescribed glucocorticoid steroids with the terbutaline to promote fetal lung development.

Minimizing Adverse Effects

Monitor the patient's pulse rate and blood pressure closely throughout therapy. Have the patient lie on her left side during infusion to help minimize the risk of hypotension and promote circulation to the fetus. Closely monitor the patient's fluid status and avoid fluid overload. Related measures include monitoring intake and output of fluids, assessing peripheries for edema, and auscultating breath sounds for rales and rhonchi every hour. If pulmonary edema develops, discontinue drug administration and notify the prescriber or nurse midwife immediately. Seek orders to manage the edema by diuretic therapy.

BOX 53.2   COMMUNITY BASED CONCERNS

Teaching About Drugs That Affect Uterine Function

Prenatal teaching should include the following:

- Signs of preterm labor
- Rationale for not giving tocolytics to stop preterm labor before 20 weeks' gestation (spontaneous abortion may be related to fetal defects)
- Rationale regarding use of oxytocin (these should focus on medical indications, not convenience of delivery)

If the patient demonstrates signs of adverse effects, such as palpitations, tachycardia, hypotension, or nervousness, the dosage of terbutaline should be decreased. Ensure that a beta blocker such as propranolol is available as an antidote in case of overdosage. If the patient is diabetic or receives potassium-depleting diuretics, monitor the serum glucose and potassium levels carefully. Administer terbutaline infusions through an IV infusion controller or pump to keep the dosage rate accurate. Because of the risk of pulmonary edema, avoid diluting terbutaline with saline (0.9% sodium chloride solution or lactated Ringer's solution) and Hartmann's solution; use a dextrose solution instead.

Providing Patient and Family Education

- Educate the patient and family about the therapeutic and adverse effects of the drug.
- Explain to the patient the rationale for lying on her left side.
- Instruct the patient to notify you or another health care provider immediately if she experiences swelling in her hands or feet, shortness of breath, palpitations, or chest pain.

For more on patient and family education, see Box 53.2.

Ongoing Assessment and Evaluation

Monitor the maternal heart rate, FHR, and maternal blood pressure and fluid status throughout terbutaline therapy. Drug therapy is considered effective when the premature contractions decrease in intensity and frequency, the woman and fetus do not experience adverse effects, and premature birth is avoided for at least 24 hours so that administered corticosteroids can exert their beneficial effects.

CRITICAL THINKING SCENARIO

MATERNAL MONITORING AND TERBUTALINE

Susan Hartmann, who is 30 weeks pregnant, has diabetes that is well controlled with glyburide, an oral antidiabetic agent. She begins preterm labor, and terbutaline is ordered for her.

1. Discuss which laboratory values you would monitor most closely if you were her nurse.
2. Explain the rationale for your choices.

MEMORY CHIP !

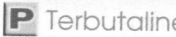 Terbutaline

- Used off-label to control preterm labor after 20 weeks' and up to 34 weeks' gestation; allows time for administered corticosteroids to be effective in newborn
- Beta-2 receptor agonist (stimulant); antidote: beta blockers
- Major contraindications: oral use for prevention or treatment; use in outpatient settings via infusion pumps; before the 20th week of pregnancy; when continuing the pregnancy is hazardous to the woman or fetus; pre-existing maternal medical conditions that would be seriously affected by the pharmacologic properties of a beta agonist
- Most common adverse effects: maternal and fetal tachycardia; maternal palpitations, cardiac arrhythmias, tremor
- Most serious adverse effects: maternal—multiple serious cardiovascular problems; death
- Maximizing therapeutic effects: Administer as soon as preterm labor is diagnosed and order is written for drug therapy.
- Minimizing adverse effects: Monitor maternal pulse rate, blood pressure, fluid status, and fetal heart rate; decrease infusion rate if adverse effects (excessive beta stimulation) are present.
- Most important patient education: Drugs to control preterm labor help buy time for other drug therapy to have an effect in preventing complications in the newborn.
- **Black box warning: IV and injectable use is limited to 48 to 72 hours in a hospital setting; oral doses should not be used at all**

Drug Closely Related to 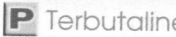 Terbutaline

Ritodrine is a beta agonist, like terbutaline. Unlike terbutaline, it is labeled to treat preterm labor. Frequently perceived by clinicians to cause more adverse effects than terbutaline, ritodrine appears to have a similar (and potentially serious) adverse effect profile to other beta agonists and similar (although limited) efficacy (Chan, Cabrol, Ingemarsson, et al., 2006; Tan, Devendra, Tan, et al., 2006). Ritodrine's, as well as other beta agonists', place in therapy is still debatable in the literature. It is infrequently used.

Drugs Significantly Different From 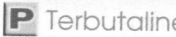 Terbutaline

Magnesium Sulfate

Magnesium is a trace mineral involved in many chemical reactions in the body. Therefore, the pharmacotherapeutics of magnesium sulfate are diverse, and more potential therapeutic uses are under consideration. Oral magnesium sulfate preparations are used in laxatives and antacids (see Chapters 50 and 51). Oral and IV forms of magnesium sulfate are often given to correct electrolyte imbalances (hypomagnesemia). IV magnesium effectively suppresses ventricular ectopy and is a first-line therapy for torsades de pointes, a variation on ventricular tachycardia that can progress to fibrillation and be

fatal. It may also be useful in treating patients with chronic heart failure or acute myocardial infarction. Magnesium sulfate is used to control hypertension, encephalopathy, and convulsions in children with acute nephritis. IV magnesium may be useful in treating asthma and chronic lung disease that have been unresponsive to conventional therapy with beta agonists.

Magnesium sulfate is used frequently for treating or preventing seizures associated with preeclampsia, eclampsia, and pregnancy-induced hypertension. Its effectiveness in preventing seizures in eclampsia is well accepted and documented. The onset of eclamptic seizures can be antepartum, intrapartum, or postpartum. Magnesium sulfate is the drug of choice for intrapartum or postpartum eclampsia, and it prevents furthers convulsions (Sibai, 2005). It is more controversial when used in women with preeclampsia or hypertension to prevent progression to eclampsia and seizures. Some research supports the use of magnesium sulfate in mild preeclampsia 12 hours postpartum (Ehrenberg & Mercer, 2006), but other clinical trials indicate that although the drug is effective, it has an adverse effect profile (respiratory difficulties and postpartum hemorrhage) and should probably be avoided in mild preeclampsia (Duley, Henderson-Smart, & Meher, 2006). One very large clinical trial (Magpie Trial) found no long-term differences among children at age 18 months who were exposed to maternal magnesium sulfate for preeclampsia before birth, compared with children who were not exposed to maternal magnesium sulfate before birth (i.e., their mothers had preeclampsia but they received a placebo). This study also found no difference in long-term complications for women treated with magnesium sulfate (Magpie Trial Follow-Up Study Collaborative Group, 2007a, 2007b).

Magnesium sulfate has been used as a tocolytic, although North American use of the drug in this manner is considered an anomaly, as other countries do not use magnesium sulfate as a tocolytic (Grimes & Nanda, 2006). As with terbutaline, use as a tocolytic is off-label. The effectiveness of magnesium sulfate as a tocolytic remains controversial, although it is widely used in the United States for this purpose. Some practitioners believe that magnesium sulfate appears to inhibit myometrial contractility but does not prolong pregnancy significantly. It can help prevent labor long enough to allow corticosteroids to be administered to the mother to protect the infant's lungs. But reviews of current research do not support this belief; instead, these findings state that magnesium sulfate is not effective in delaying birth or preventing preterm birth. In addition, magnesium sulfate carries a serious risk of adverse effects to the infant, including an increased risk of fetal death. For these reasons, some experts have begun to call for abandoning the use of magnesium sulfate as a tocolytic (Crowther, Hiller, & Doyle, 2002; Pryde, Janeczek, & Mittendorf, 2004; Grimes & Nanda, 2006). However, a recent Cochrane Review by Doyle and colleagues (2009) clearly supports the use of antenatal magnesium sulfate for neuroprotection of the fetus and significantly reduces the risk of cerebral palsy.

The mechanism of action of magnesium sulfate makes it particularly suitable for use in complications of pregnancy. Magnesium sulfate acts as a CNS and muscular depressant, producing peripheral neuromuscular blockade. It prevents or controls convulsions by blocking neuromuscular transmission and by decreasing the amount of acetylcholine freed at the end plate by the motor nerve impulse. Secondarily, magnesium sulfate relaxes smooth muscle and decreases blood pressure. This effect may be related to its antagonistic effect on calcium, which prevents calcium influx into the cells for cellular contraction.

Although magnesium sulfate is a pregnancy category A drug (which means that it does not cause fetal structural defects), its use still carries some risk to the fetus because the drug may cause other adverse effects. Magnesium sulfate may also cause adverse effects in the mother. Adverse effects are related to how the drug works and are usually associated with elevated serum levels or magnesium intoxication (Table 53.3). A serum level of 10 to 12 mg/dL is associated with toxicity (normal levels without any infusion of magnesium sulfate are 1.8 to 3 mg/dL). The most common maternal adverse effects are:

- Headache
- Hyporeflexia
- Weakness
- Thirst
- Flushing
- Burning at infusion site

The most life-threatening maternal adverse effects are:

- Circulatory collapse
- Respiratory depression
- Pulmonary edema
  The most common fetal and neonatal adverse effects are:
- Heart rate changes
- Neonatal hypotonia
- Neonatal respiratory depression (possibly serious)

Other maternal adverse effects from magnesium toxicity are sweating, hypotension, flaccid paralysis, hypothermia,

and cardiac depression. IV infusion, especially for prolonged periods (more than 24 hours), may produce hypermagnesemia in the newborn, including neuromuscular or respiratory depression. Overdosage produces a sharp drop in the blood pressure, respiratory paralysis, and ECG changes (increased PR interval, increased QRS complex, and prolonged QT interval). Heart block and asystole may also occur. Serum levels need to be monitored closely when the patient is receiving magnesium sulfate to prevent overdosage and adverse effects from therapy. Calcium gluconate antagonizes the effects of magnesium toxicity and is the antidote for overdose.

Magnesium sulfate may be administered by the IM or IV route or by IV infusion (see Table 53.1). An IV pump should be used to regulate the flow of magnesium sulfate infusion. Dosing is accomplished with a loading dose followed by a maintenance dose. The IV route is preferred for initial stabilization; after that, an oral dose may be used for maintenance. The goal is to maintain a therapeutic serum level without causing adverse effects. The therapeutic level varies, depending on the clinical indication for the therapy. It is 5 to 8 mg/dL in preterm labor and 4 to 8 mg/dL in pregnancy-induced hypertension. These levels are higher than would normally be found in the serum but are the elevations required to produce a therapeutic effect.

In addition to using an IV pump, several other nursing actions can minimize adverse effects. It is necessary to assess for signs of magnesium toxicity by monitoring the serum magnesium levels and the patient's clinical response to drug administration. Continuous maternal cardiac monitoring and continuous fetal monitoring should be used while the patient is receiving IV magnesium sulfate. The patient should be placed on bed rest in the left lateral recumbent position to prevent hypotension and to maximize blood flow to the fetus. The patient must receive nothing orally to eat or drink (i.e., remain NPO) during stabilization to help prevent nausea and vomiting. With each change in dose, it is necessary to document uterine activity, cervical changes, and maternal-fetal responses. Safety measures or seizure precautions should be implemented if the drug is used to prevent or treat seizures associated with pregnancy-induced hypertension. Finally, calcium gluconate should always be kept at the bedside to use as an antidote if magnesium toxicity occurs.

Calcium Channel Blockers

Because calcium channel blockers prevent muscle contractility, they have been studied for their possible use as tocolytics. The calcium channel blocker that is used most often as a tocolytic is nifedipine. Research has shown that calcium channel blockers, like nifedipine, are as effective, if not more effective, in preventing preterm labor as the more traditionally used beta agonists, like terbutaline. Calcium channel blockers may be the best first-line tocolytic for delaying birth until 37 weeks gestation (Haas, et al., 2009). Calcium channel blockers do not induce the same adverse effects in the mother or infant as the beta agonists (Pryde, Janeczek, & Mittendorf, 2004), and they are effective in reducing blood pressure and

TABLE 53.3	Correlation of Serum Levels and Effects of Magnesium Sulfate	
Serum Level (mEq/L)	Effect
1.5–3	Normal level
4–7	Therapeutic level for preeclampsia/eclampsia/convulsions
7–10	Loss of deep tendon reflexes, hypotension, loss of consciousness
13–15	Respiratory paralysis
16–25	Cardiac conduction altered (lengthened PR interval, QRS widening, prolonged QT interval, arrhythmias)
25	Cardiac arrest

preventing recurrent elevations when used to treat hypertension in pregnancy (Duley, Henderson-Smart, & Meher, 2006). Long-term follow-up of children exposed to either the beta agonist ritodrine or the calcium channel blocker nifedipine showed no postnatal differences in terms of psychosocial and motor functioning (Houtzager, Hogendoorn, Papatsonis, et al., 2006). Calcium channel blockers are discussed in depth in Chapter 31 as well as in Chapter 28.

Atosiban

A new drug class, the oxytocin antagonists, works directly on the uterine receptors in treating preterm labor. These drugs do not seem to cause the maternal and fetal adverse effects seen with the beta agonists and are equally effective as, but not more effective than, the beta agonists. A recent Cochrane Review (Papatosonis, Flenady, & Liley, 2009) concluded that there was insufficient evidence to support the use of this class of drugs for preterm birth prevention.

Indomethacin

Indomethacin is an NSAID that suppresses uterine activity by inhibiting prostaglandin synthesis. It is effective in stopping premature labor for 48 hours and up to 7 days (Haas, et al., 2009). This may be related to a decreased adverse side-effect profile when compared to beta-memetics and magnesium sulfate. Typically used prior to 32 weeks gestation, newer evidence suggests that indomethacin may be used safely up to 34 weeks gestation (Blumenfield & Lyell, 2009). For information about the other uses of indomethacin, see Chapter 25.

CHAPTER SUMMARY

- Drug therapy may be used when labor does not occur at term, does not bring about delivery effectively, or begins preterm.
- Oxytocin is given by IV drip infusion to initiate or augment (improve) labor contractions when important fetal or maternal reasons to do so exist. It is also used to control postpartum bleeding or hemorrhage.
- Response to oxytocin therapy has three phases: the incremental phase, the stable phase, and hyperstimulation. The hyperstimulation phase is undesirable and indicates that administration of oxytocin has been excessive.
- Adverse effects of oxytocin are dose related.
- You need an accurate understanding of the physiology involved in producing contractions, the core drug knowledge (most specifically the pharmacokinetics, pharmacodynamics, and adverse effects of oxytocin), and the relevant core patient variables to be able to make sound professional judgments in managing patients receiving oxytocin therapy.
- You are responsible for determining the maternal and fetal response to oxytocin therapy (frequency of contractions, progress of labor, and fetal tolerance) and for titrating the dose, per the physician's or nurse midwife's orders, based on this assessment.

- You must stop the infusion of oxytocin if tachysystole occurs.
- Tocolytic drugs are used to stop preterm labor. Although they are effective for short-term use, they have not decreased the number of preterm births, neonatal morbidity, or neonatal mortality. Tocolytic drugs do help prolong labor long enough to allow administration of corticosteroids and to transfer the mother (if necessary) to an institution that has facilities for premature infants.
- Terbutaline is a beta-receptor agonist (stimulant) that attaches to receptors in the uterine smooth muscle. Stimulation of these receptors inhibits contractility of uterine smooth muscle. Terbutaline decreases the intensity and frequency of uterine contractions and is used off-label to control premature labor. Its use is limited to 48 to 72 hours via injection or infusion in an inpatient setting due to the risk of serious maternal cardiovascular events and deaths. Oral terbutaline should not be used to treat or prevent preterm labor.
- Dose-related maternal and fetal tachycardia and changes in maternal blood pressure can occur in patients receiving terbutaline. Adverse effects reflect stimulation of the beta receptors.
- Magnesium sulfate infusions depress the CNS and cause muscle relaxation. Magnesium sulfate is the drug of choice to treat preeclampsia and seizures in eclampsia and is used off-label to stop preterm labor. Adverse effects, particularly respiratory depression, are related to high levels of the drug in the blood. Recent research demonstrates a neuroprotective effect of magnesium sulfate for the fetus.
- Drugs that alter uterine motility are potentially dangerous to the woman and fetus. Infusions of these drugs should be regulated with IV controllers or pumps. These patients need close monitoring for signs of adverse effects throughout therapy.

QUESTIONS FOR STUDY AND REVIEW

1. Why should you titrate oxytocin slowly upward, with dosage adjustments every 40 to 60 minutes?
2. Define the three phases of oxytocin response.
3. Which adverse effect of oxytocin is most dangerous to the pregnant woman?
4. What nursing assessments should be made to minimize adverse effects from oxytocin?
5. How does terbutaline stop preterm labor?
6. If the patient develops tachycardia, palpitations, and nervousness while on terbutaline infusion, what action should you take?
7. List the reasons that magnesium sulfate may be prescribed during pregnancy.
8. State the antidote to magnesium sulfate overdosage.
9. What are the most common maternal, fetal, and neonatal adverse effects from infusion of magnesium sulfate?

NEED MORE HELP?

Chapter 53 of the Study Guide to Accompany *Drug Therapy in Nursing*, 4th Edition, contains NCLEX-style questions and other learning activities to reinforce your understanding of the concepts presented in this chapter. For additional information or to purchase the study guide, visit thePoint.

REFERENCES

ACOG Practice Bulletin No. 107: Induction of labor. *Obstetrics and Gynecology*, 114(2):386–397.

Allen, R., & O'Brien, B. M. (2009). Uses of misoprostol in obstetrics and gynecology. *Rev Obstet Gynecol*, 2(3):159–168.

AWHONN Position Statement. (2008). Fetal Heart Monitoring.

Balestreieri-Martinez, B. (2009). Complications in obstetric anesthesia: Nursing's role to anticipate, recognize, and respond. *J Perinat Neonat Nurs*, 23(1):23–30.

Blumenfield, Y. J., & Lyell, D. J. (2009). Prematurity Prevention: The role of acute tocolysis. *Current Opinion in Obstetrics and Gynecology*, 21(2):136–141.

Chan, J., Cabrol, D., Ingemarsson, I., et al. (2006). Pragmatic comparison of beta 2-agonist side effects within the Worldwide Atosiban Versus Beta Agonists Study. *European Journal of Obstetrics, Gynecology, and Reproductive Biology*, 128 (1–2):135–141.

Clark, S. L., Simpson, K. R., Knox, G.E., et al. (2009). Oxytocin: New perspectives on an old drug. *Am J Obstet Gynecol*, 200(35e):1–35.

de Heus, R., Mulder, E. J. H., Derks, J. B., & Visser, G. H. A. (2008). Acute tocolysis for uterine activity reduction in term labor: A review. *Obstetrical & Gynecological Survey*, 63(6):383–388.

Daniel-Spiegel, E., Weiner, Z., Ben-Shlomo, I., et al. (2004). For how long should oxytocin be continued during induction of labour? *British Journal of Obstetrics and Gynaecology*, 111(4):331–334.

Dodd, J. M., Crowther, C. A., Dare, M. R., et al. (2006). Oral betamimetics for maintenance therapy after threatened preterm labour. *Cochrane Database of Systematic Reviews*, (1):CD003927.

Doyle, L. W., Crowther, C. A., Middleton, P., Marret, S., & Rouse D. Magnesium sulphate for women at risk of preterm birth for neuroprotection of the fetus. *Cochrane Database of Systematic Reviews*, (1):CD004661.

Duley, L., Henderson-Smart, D. J., & Meher, S. (2006). Magnesium sulphate and other anticonvulsants for women with pre-eclampsia. *Cochrane Database of Systematic Reviews*, (3):CD001449.

Ehrenberg, H. M., & Mercer, B. M. (2006). Abbreviated postpartum magnesium sulfate therapy for women with mild preeclampsia: A randomized controlled trial. *Obstetrics and Gynecology*, 108(4):824–825.

Ewert, K., Powers, B., Robertson, S., et al. (2006). Controlled–release misoprostol vaginal insert in parous women for labor induction: A randomize controlled trial. *Obstetrics and Gynecology*, 108(5):1130–1137.

Food and Drug Administration. (1997, 13 November). Letter: Subcutaneous terbutaline via pump. Retrieved from *http://www.fda.gov/medwatch/SAFETY/1997/terbut.htm*

Food and Drug Administration.(2011, 17 February). FDA Drug Safety Communication: New warnings against use of terbutaline to treat preterm labor. Retrieved from http://www.fda.gov/Drugs/DrugSafety/ucm243539.htm

Gilbert, W. M. (2006). The cost of preterm birth: the lost cost versus the high value of tocolysis. *BJOG* 113(Suppl 3):4–9.

Grimes, D. A., & Nanda, K. (2006). Magnesium sulfate tocolysis: Time to quit. *Obstetrics and Gynecology*, 108(4):986–989.

Haas, D. M., Imperiale, T. F., Kirkpatrick, P. R., Klein, R. W., Zollinger, T. W., & Golichowski, A. M. (2009). Tocolytic therapy: A meta-analysis and decision analysis. *Obstetrics & Gynecology*, 113(3):585–594.

Hollander, E., Bartz, J., Chaplin, W., et al. (2007). Oxytocin increases retention of social cognition in autism. *Biological Psychiatry*, 61(4):498–503.

Hollander, E., Novotny, S., Hanratty, M., et al. (2003). Oxytocin infusion reduces repetitive behaviors in adults with autistic and Asperger's disorders. *Neuropsychopharmacology*, 28(1):193–198.

Houtzager, B. A., Hogendoorn, S. M., Papatsonis, D. N., et al. (2006). Long-term follow up of children exposed in utero to nifedipine or ritodrine for the management of preterm labour. *British Journal of Obstetrics and Gynaecology*, 113(3):324–331.

Huh, W. K., Chelmow, D., & Malone, F. D. (2004). A double-blinded randomized controlled trail of oxytocin at the beginning versus the end of the third stage of labor for prevention of postpartum hemorrhage. *Gynecologic and Obstetric Investigation*, 58(2):72–76.

Institute for Clinical System Improvement. (2005). Health care guideline: Management of labor. *http://www.icsi.org/labor/labor__management_of__full_version__2.html*

Jabbour, H. N., Sales, K. J., Catalano, R. D., & Norman, J. E. (2009). Inflammatory pathways in female reproductive health and disease. *Reproduction*, 138:903–919.

Lam, F., & Gill, P. (2005). β-agonist tocolytic therapy. *Obstetrics & Gynecology Clinics of North America*, 32(3):457–484.

Lapaire, O., Schneider, M. C., Stotz, M., et al. (2006). Oral misoprostol vs intravenous oxytocin in reducing blood loss after emergency cesarean delivery. *International Journal of Gynaecology and Obstetrics*, 95(1):2–7.

Lin, M. G., Nuthalapaty, F. S., Carver, A. R., et al. (2005). Misoprostol for labor induction in women with term premature rupture of membranes: a meta-analysis. *Obstetrics and Gynecology*, 106(3):593–601.

Macones, G. A., Hankins, D. V., Spong, C. Y., Hauth, J., & Moore, T. (2008). The 2008 National Institute of Child Health and Human Devlopment workshop report on electronic fetal monitoring: Update on definitions, interpretation, and research guidelines. *JOGNN*, 37(5):510–515.

Magpie Trial Follow-Up Study Collaborative Group. (2007a). The Magpie Trial: a randomised trial comparing magnesium sulphate with placebo for pre-eclampsia. Outcome for children at 18 months. *British Journal of Obstetrics and Gynaecology*, 114(3):289–299.

Magpie Trial Follow-Up Study Collaborative Group. (2007b). The Magpie Trial: a randomised trial comparing magnesium sulphate with placebo for pre-eclampsia. Outcome for women at 2 years. *British Journal of Obstetrics and Gynaecology*, 114(3):300–309.

Maharaj, D. (2009). Eating and drinking in labor: Should it be allowed? *EJOG*, 146(1):3–7.

Mendelson, C. R. (2009). Minireview: Fetal-maternal hormonal signaling in pregnancy and labor. *Molecular Endocrinology*, 23(7):947–954.

Mozurkewich, E., Chilimigras, J., Koepke, E., Keeton, K., & King, V. J. (2009). Indications for induction of labour: a best-evidence review. *BJOG*, 116(5):626–636.

Nand, K., Cook, L. A., Gallo, M. F., et al. (2002). Terbutaline pump maintenance therapy after threatened preterm labor for preventing preterm birth. *Cochrane Database of Systematic Reviews*, (4):CD003933.

Nuthalapaty, F. S., Ramsey, P. S., Biggio, J. R., et al. (2005). High-dose vaginal misoprostol versus concentrated oxytocin plus low-dose vaginal misoprostol for midtrimester labor induction: A randomized trial. *American Journal of Obstetrics and Gynecology,* 193(3 Pt 2):1065–1070.

Oral intake during labor. (2009). ACOG Committee Opinion No. 441. American College of Obstetricians and Gynecologists. *Obstet Gynecol,* (114):714.

Pacheco, L. D., Rosen, M. P., Gei, A. F., et al. (2006). Management of uterine hyperstimulation with concomitant use of oxytocin and terbutaline. *American Journal of Perinatology,* 23(6):377–380.

Papatsonis, D., Flenady, V., Liley, H. (2009). Maintenance therapy with oxytocin antagonists for inhibiting preterm birth after threatened preterm labour. *Cochrane Database of Systematic Reviews,* (1):CD005938.

Roberts, J., Hanson, L. (2007). Best practices in second stage labor care: Maternal bearing down and positioning. *J Midwifery Womens Health,* 52(3):238–245.

Rossignol, D. A. (2009). Novel and emerging treatments for autism spectrum disorders: A systematic review. *Ann Clin Psychiatry,* 21(4):213–236.

Sibai, B. M. (2005). Diagnosis, prevention, and management of eclampsia. *Obstetrics and Gynecology,* 105(2):402–410.

Simpson, K. R., & Know, G. E. (2009). Oxytocin as a high-alert medication: implications for perinatal patient safety. *MCN,* 34(1):8–15.

Tan, T. C., Devendra, K., Tan, L. K., et al. (2006). Tocolytic treatment for the management of preterm labour: A systematic review. *Singapore Medical Journal,* 47(5):361–366.

Thornton, J. G. (2005). Maintenance tocolysis. *British Journal of Obstetrics and Gynaecology,* 112(Suppl 1):118–121.

Vidaeff, A. C., & Ramin, S. M. (2008). Potential biochemical events associated with initiation of labor. *Current Medicinal Chemistry,* 15(6):614–619.

Wing, D. A., Guberman, C., & Fassett, M. (2005). A randomized comparison of oral mifepristone to intravenous oxytocin for labor induction in women with prelabor rupture of membranes beyond 36 weeks' gestation. *American Journal of Obstetrics and Gynecology,* 192(2):445–451.

UNIT 12

Immune System and Cancer Chemotherapy Drugs

54

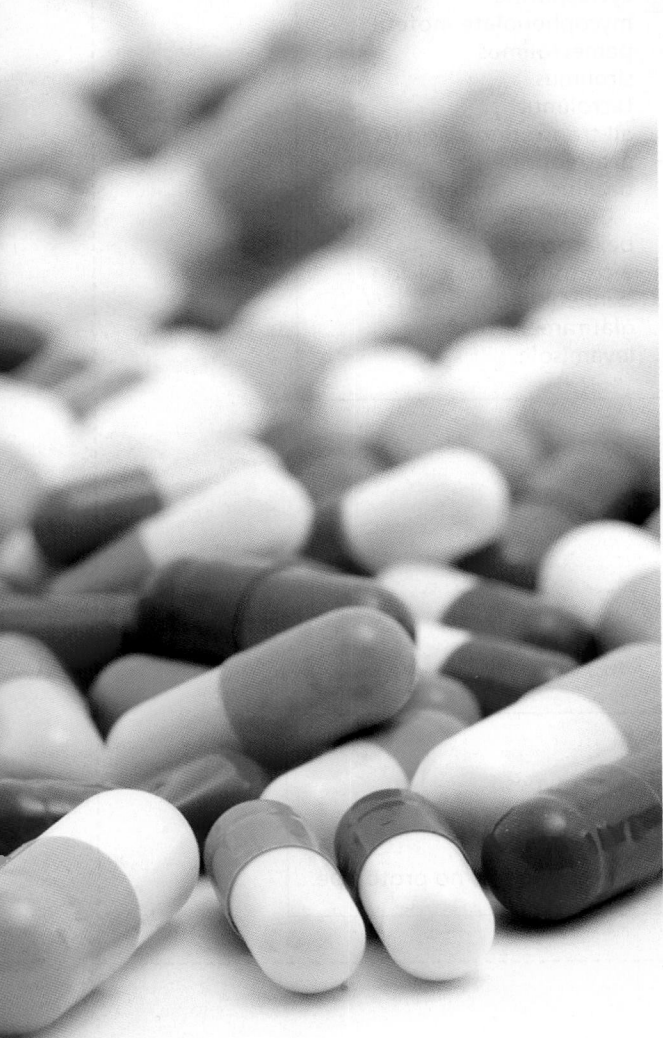

Drugs Affecting the Immune Response

Learning Objectives

At the completion of this chapter the student will:

1. Identify core drug knowledge about drugs that affect the biologic responses.
2. Relate the interaction of core drug knowledge to core patient variables for drugs that affect biologic responses.
3. Generate a nursing plan of care from the interactions between core drug knowledge and core patient variables for drugs that affect biologic responses.
4. Describe nursing interventions to maximize therapeutic effects and minimize adverse effects for drugs that affect the immunologic system.
5. Determine key points for patient and family education for drugs that affect the immune system.

Key Terms

angiogenesis, anti-angiogenesis	complement	lymphokines
autoimmune disease	cytokines	retinoids
biologic modulator	interleukins	rexanoids
cellular immune response	immune modulators	vascular endothelial growth factor (VEGF)
chemotaxis	immunotoxins	

Drugs Affecting the Immune Response

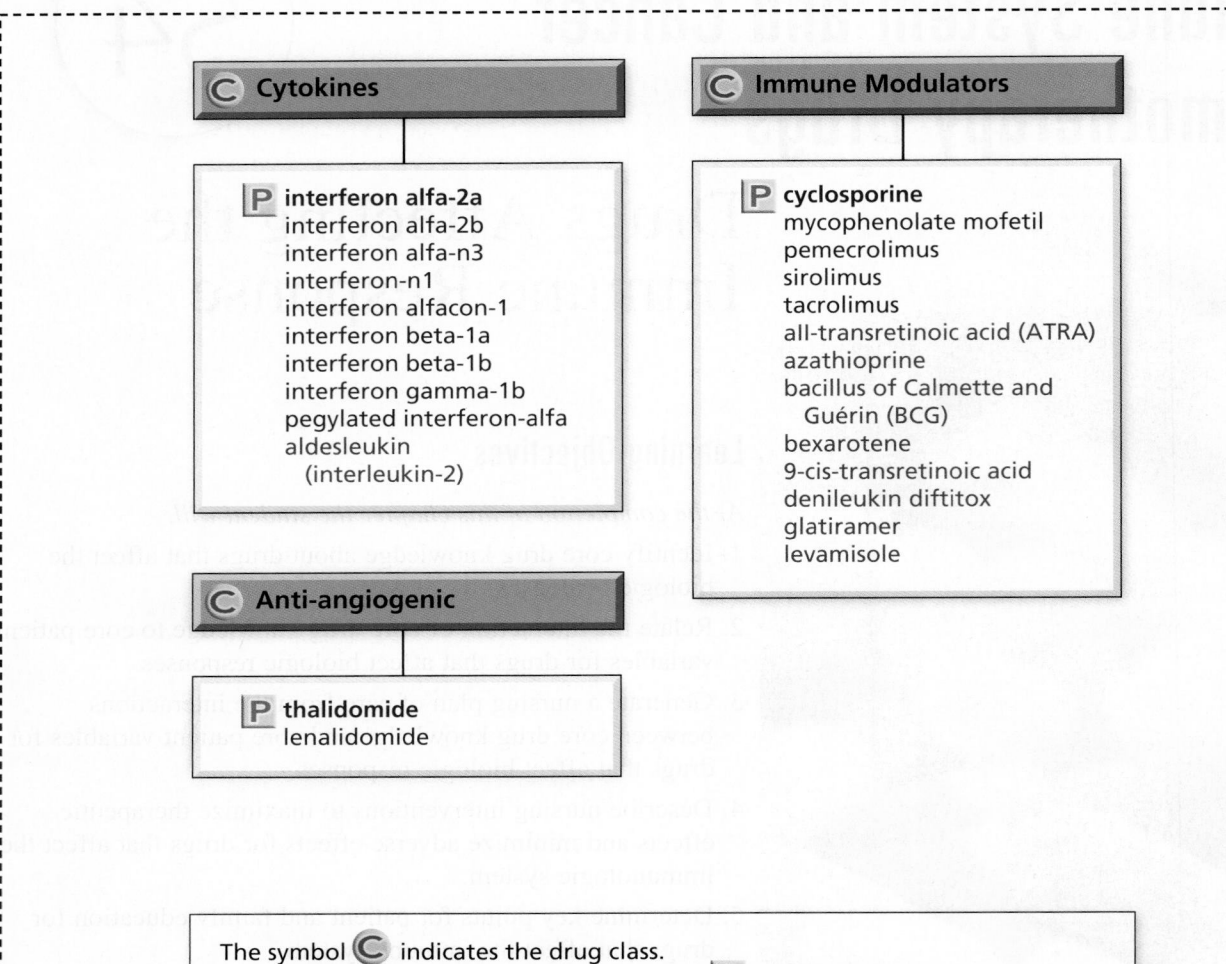

C Cytokines

P interferon alfa-2a
interferon alfa-2b
interferon alfa-n3
interferon-n1
interferon alfacon-1
interferon beta-1a
interferon beta-1b
interferon gamma-1b
pegylated interferon-alfa
aldesleukin
    (interleukin-2)

C Immune Modulators

P cyclosporine
mycophenolate mofetil
pemecrolimus
sirolimus
tacrolimus
all-transretinoic acid (ATRA)
azathioprine
bacillus of Calmette and
    Guérin (BCG)
bexarotene
9-cis-transretinoic acid
denileukin diftitox
glatiramer
levamisole

C Anti-angiogenic

P thalidomide
lenalidomide

The symbol **C** indicates the drug class.
Drugs in **bold type** marked with the symbol **P** are prototypes.
Drugs in blue type are closely related to the prototype.
Drugs in red type are significantly different from the prototype.
Drugs in black type with no symbol are also used in drug therapy; no prototype.

Biologic modulators, or biologic modifiers, are a group of biopharmaceuticals that are naturally occurring proteins used to alter the body's immunologic responses (Polovich, Whiteford, and Olsen, 2009). The use of biologic modulators is also called biologic therapy. The rapid growth of these therapies has been attributed to two major biologic advances. In the 1970s, refinement of recombinant DNA technology enabled researchers to produce large quantities of active biologic molecules outside the body and then administer them systemically. More recently, advancements in defining tumor-specific molecular targets have enhanced development of targeted cytotoxic agents (Beijnen & Schellens, 2010). Agents are classified by their specific biologic mechanism of activity and by whether they stimulate or suppress immune processes. Some stimulate specific immunologic activity to combat unique antigens (substances that induce formation of antibodies). Moreover, some agents may at once stimulate some parts of the immune system and depress other parts of the immune system.

This chapter discusses three classifications of agents used to alter biologic responses: cytokines, immune modulators, and anti-angiogenic agents. Active and passive antibody-conferred vaccinations are addressed in Appendix E rather than in this chapter (appendices are located online at thePoint.).

Cytokines are immunologic toxins produced by white blood cells (WBCs, also called leukocytes) in response to foreign antigens such as microorganisms, transplanted tissue, or malignant cells. The prototype cytokine is interferon alfa-2a (Roferon-A).

The **immune modulators** are a group of several agents with distinctly different structures that alter T-cell or B-cell activity. The prototype is cyclosporine (Sandimmune, Neoral, SangCya). As this area of pharmacology develops and broadens in scope, more specific types of agents are appearing. For the purposes of this text, polypeptide antibiotics also known as calcineurins used as immunosuppressives, immunoconjugates, retinoid-like agents, bacillus calmette Guerin (BCG), and miscellaneous immune modulators such as levamisole are grouped together; however, it is conceivable that in the future, they will be separated into discrete groups. Research is now being conducted to determine whether other essential cell proteins, nutrients, and growth factors (e.g., dendritic cells, enzyme or proteosome inhibitors) can be manipulated to provide a clinical benefit (Buchsel & DeMeyer, 2006; Wu & Lanier, 2003; Cho & Bhardwaj, 2003; Luo & Prestwich, 2002; Polovich et al., 2009). **Anti-angiogenesis** drugs are a new form of biologic therapy that block blood vessel development. Recent knowledge of the molecular process of carcinogenesis has led to recognition of the importance of vascularity to the growth and metastasis of some tumors (Cook & Figg, 2010). Anti-angiogenetic agents target VEGF and other secondary angiogenesis mechanisms. Small molecules that inhibit angiogenesis via tyrosine kinase pathways such as sunitinib, sorafenib, and the monoclonal antibody bevacizumab are included in Chapter 55. The most representative example of a general anti-angiogenic biologic

agent is thalidomide Another agent similar to thalidomide is lenalidomide. Pamalidomide is another agent in this class that is still underinvestigation (Lacy, & Rajkumar, 2010).

The body of knowledge about the components and actions of the immune system is developing daily. As researchers make new discoveries and better understand biologic interactions, they will find more ways to modify immune systems and treat a variety of viral, autoimmune, hematologic, and neoplastic disorders.

PHYSIOLOGY

The immune system is composed of hematopoietic cells and multiple hematologic-immunologic production and storage sites. Hematopoietic physiology and pharmacologic agents are described in greater detail in Chapter 33. The reticulo-endothelial system includes immunologically active tissue and cells found in the lymph system, spleen, liver, lungs, gastrointestinal (GI) tract, and brain. An integrated immune response involving hematopoietic cells and immune tissues provides the body's nonspecific and specific response to invasion by antigens identified as nonself. The essential components of the immune system are hematopoietic cells, barrier defenses, the nonspecific immune response, the specific immune response, and immunity. Leukocytes (or WBCs) are key components of all immune system responses. (See Chapter 33 for an overview of hematopoiesis and a discussion of leukocytes' primary actions relating to combating invasion by microbes and establishing an initial barrier and inflammatory response.) This chapter will focus on pharmacologic agents that affect other aspects of the immune response.

Specific Immune Responses

If an invader gets past the barrier and nonspecific immune systems and enters the tissues or bloodstream, a specific immune response involving lymphocytes is initiated (Figure 54.1). Bone marrow stem cells develop into two types of lymphocytes: T lymphocytes, or T cells, and B lymphocytes, or B cells. These T and B lymphocytes may also differentiate into specialized cells, such as natural killer cells and lymphokine-activated killer cells, which have been identified as the cells that aggressively attack and destroy neoplastic cells. Because research in the area of lymphocyte identification is relatively new, other lymphocytes not yet identified may also take part in the immune response.

T cells are "programmed" in the thymus gland to develop into at least three different cell types. Effector or cytotoxic T cells are found in various areas of the body and aggressively attack nonself cells by releasing chemicals called **lymphokines.** These chemicals either directly destroy a foreign cell or mark it for destruction by phagocytes and elicit an inflammatory response. This effect is termed the **cellular immune response.** Foreign or nonself cells have different membrane-identifying antigens called histocompatibility

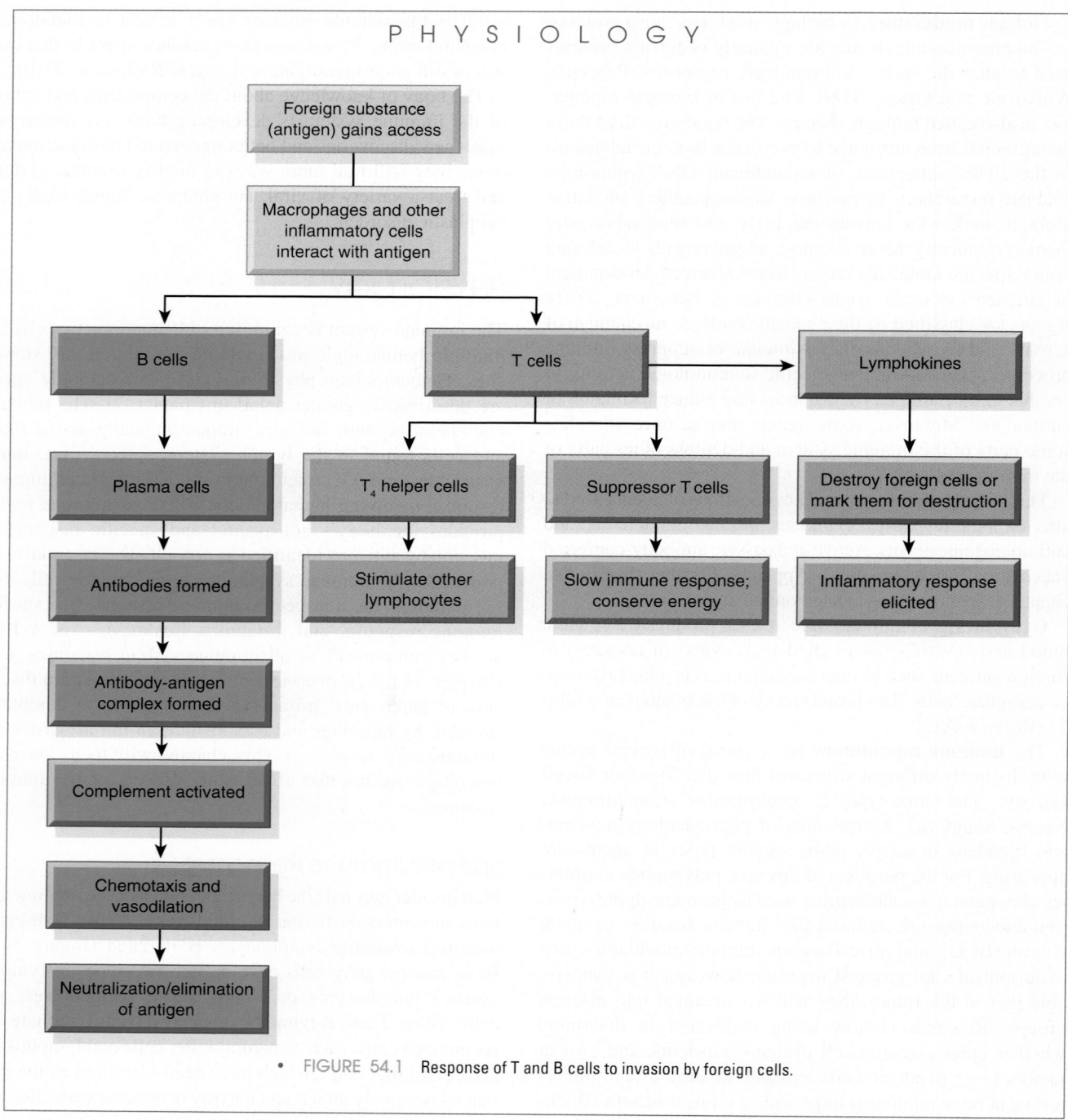

PHYSIOLOGY

- FIGURE 54.1 Response of T and B cells to invasion by foreign cells.

leukocyte antigens (HLAs). Helper T cells respond to the chemical indicators of immune activity and stimulate other lymphocytes to be more aggressive and responsive. Suppressor T cells respond to rising levels of chemicals associated with an immune response and suppress or slow the reaction. The balance between these two systems permits a rapid response that destroys invaders immediately, followed by a slowing reaction if the invasion continues. This slowing conserves energy and the components of the immune and inflammatory reaction.

B lymphocytes are found in reticuloendothelial tissue throughout the body and responsible for develop of antigen-specific antibodies to target foreign cells. The antibody response system and agents that target antigen-antibody receptors are included in the Targeted Therapies Chapter 55.

Chemical factors also play an important role in the specific immune reaction, acting as communicators within the immune system to coordinate the immune response. For example, interferons are chemicals secreted by cells that have been invaded by viruses and possibly other stimuli.

They prevent viral replication and suppress malignant cell replication and tumor growth. **Interleukins** are chemicals secreted by active WBCs to influence other WBCs. Interleukin-1 (lymphocyte-activating factor) stimulates T cells to initiate an immune response. Interleukin-2 (T-cell growth factor) is released from active T cells to stimulate the production of more T cells and to increase the activity of B cells, cytotoxic cells, and natural killer cells. Interleukin-2 also causes fever, arthralgia, myalgia, and slow-wave sleep-energy-conserving measures that help the body fight off invaders.

Several other factors released by lymphocytes and basophils have been identified. These include B-cell growth factor, macrophage-activating factor, macrophage-inhibiting factor, platelet-activating factor, eosinophil-chemotactic factor, and neutrophil-chemotactic factor. The presence or absence of these factors can influence the immune response.

The thymus gland, located in the mediastinal cavity, also releases a number of types of hormones that circulate in the body to stimulate and communicate with T cells. Thymosin, a thymus hormone, is important in the maturation of T cells and cell-mediated immunity. Research is currently under way to evaluate the use of exogenous thymosin in treating certain leukemias and melanomas.

Immunity

Immunity to a pathogen is achieved when the body has formed antibodies, which protect the body from developing an illness. Vaccines are used to stimulate an active immunity to commonly encountered antigens that could cause serious illness with first exposure. These vaccines are discussed in Appendix E. Sera are used to provide preformed antibodies, or passive immunity, in situations of acute exposure that could prove serious. In other words, giving an antibody permits an immediate immune response, whereas giving an antigen would require time to produce antibodies and a later response against illness. Several drugs discussed in this chapter are used to affect immune system recognition or reaction to nonself proteins.

PATHOPHYSIOLOGY

Pathophysiologic conditions requiring drug therapy with immune modulators are varied and are related to a dysfunction in any part of the immune response. Four abnormal conditions can weaken the immune system and stimulate the immune response: neoplasms, viral invasion, autoimmune disease, and transplant rejection (Dillman, 2011). Neoplasms result from the growth of mutant cells that escape the normal surveillance of the immune system. Viral invasion of a cell changes the cell's membrane and antigenic presentation. In autoimmune disease, the body responds to specific self-antigens by producing antibodies against self-cells (autoantibodies). Organ transplantation weakens the immune system as the body reacts to the introduction of foreign cells. Three types of biotherapy agents are used to combat immune dysfunction: cytokines, immune modulators, and anti-angiogenesis agents. Table 54.1 provides a summary of selected biotherapy agents that affect the biologic response to immune dysfunction.

ⓒ CYTOKINES

Cytokines are chemical mediators released by WBCs in response to antigenic invasion of the blood or tissues. Cytokines serve to enhance and accelerate the inflammatory and specific responses that will destroy the invading antigen. Cytokines are generally proinflammatory, but many also have antiviral, antiproliferative, and antineoplastic properties. Interferons and interleukins are cytokines produced by activated lymphocytes. The prototype is interferon alfa-2a (Roferon-A). Drugs in the same class as interferon alfa-2a include interferon alfa-2b, interferon alfa-n3, interferon-n1, interferon alfacon-1, interferon beta-1a, and interferon beta-1b. Interferon alpha is also available in a pegylated form (Pegasys, Peg-Intron). A drug that is significantly different from interferon alfa-2a is aldesleukin (also known as IL-2). One must recognize that these cytokines have considerable differences from the prototype in both actions and adverse effects.

The interferons available for pharmacologic use are produced by recombinant DNA technology from harvested human or animal WBCs. As stated, the prototype is interferon alfa-2a, produced by recombinant DNA technology using *Escherichia coli* bacteria.

Nursing Management of the Patient Receiving ⓟ Interferon Alfa-2a

Core Drug Knowledge

Pharmacotherapeutics

Interferon alfa-2a is licensed to treat hairy cell leukemia in selected patients 18 years and older, AIDS-related Kaposi sarcoma in selected patients 18 years and older, chronic myelogenous leukemia in chronic-phase Philadelphia chromosome–positive patients, chronic hepatitis, and metastatic renal cell carcinoma, and it is used as adjuvant therapy after resection of high-risk malignant melanoma or in patients with metastatic malignant melanoma. Substantial antineoplastic activity has been noted when this agent has been used to treat superficial bladder cancer, carcinoid tumors, cutaneous T-cell lymphoma, and low-grade non-Hodgkin's lymphoma (see Table 54.1). It has also been widely used to treat select viral diseases such as hepatitis C, condylomata acuminata, cutaneous warts, and cytomegalovirus. It is normally given by subcutaneous (SC) or intramuscular (IM) administration, although intravenous (IV) administration is preferred in some regimens.

Pharmacokinetics

Interferon alfa-2a must be given by injection. If given intramuscularly, it is absorbed rapidly with peak effects in 3.8 hours; if given subcutaneously, absorption is slower, with peak effects in 7.3 hours. IV infusion may be intermittent or continuous. The drug is metabolized in the liver and kidneys

TABLE 54.1 | **Summary of Selected Biotherapy Agents**

Drug (Trade) Name	Selected Indications	Route and Dosage Range	Pharmacokinetics
C Cytokines			
P interferon alfa-2a (Roferon-A)	Hairy cell leukemia in patients >18 years, AIDS-related Kaposi sarcoma (KS), chronic myelogenous leukemia (CML)	Hairy cell leukemia: *Adult:* IM/SC, 3 million IU/d for 16–24 wk, then 3 million IU 3×/wk AIDS-related KS: IM/SC, 36 million IU/d for 10–12 wk, then 36 million IU 3×/wk CML: IM/SC, 1 million IU/d Chronic hepatitis C: 3–9 million units IM or SC 3×/wk for 3–12 mo *Child for any disorder:* safety and efficacy not established	*Onset:* IM, rapid; PO, slow *Duration:* Unknown $t_{1/2}$: 3.7–8.5 h
interferon alfa-2b (Intron A)	Hairy cell leukemia, intra-lesional treatment of condylomata acuminata, AIDS-related KS, malignant melanoma (adjuvant therapy with interleukin-2, or alone for localized disease), chronic hepatitis (non A/ non B/C)	Hairy cell leukemia: IM/SC, 2 million units/m² 3×/wk Condylomata acuminata: intralesionally, 1 million IU/lesion 3×/wk AIDS-related KS: IM/SC, 30 million IU/m² 3×/wk Malignant melanoma: IV, 20 million IU/m² for 4 wk, maintenance 10 million IU/m² 3×/wk for 48 wk Chronic hepatitis: IM/SC, 3 million IU/m² 3×/wk Pegylated interferon used for treatment of hepatitis is usually administered as a weekly IM injection of 180 mcg. *Child, for any disorder:* Safety and efficacy not established	*Onset:* IM/SC/IV, rapid *Duration:* IM/SC, 3–12 h; IV, end of infusion $t_{1/2}$: 2–3 h
interferon beta-1b (Betaseron)	Decrease exacerbations in relapsing or remitting multiple sclerosis (MS)	*Adult:* SC, 0.25 mg qod, discontinue if disease is unremitting longer than 6 mo *Child, for any disorder:* Safety and efficacy not established	*Onset:* Slow *Duration:* Hours $t_{1/2}$: 8 min–4.3 h
IL-2	Metastatic renal cell carcinoma or malignant melanoma; adjuvant therapy with IFN alfa-2a for high risk of recurrence of malignant melanoma	Metastatic renal cell and malignant melanoma: *Adult:* IV, short infusion, 600,000 IU/kg every 8 h for a total of 14 doses, separated into two 5-d cycles with 9-d rest between *Child:* Safety and efficacy not established	*Onset:* 5 min *Duration:* 180–240 min $t_{1/2}$: 85 min
C Immune Modulators			
P cyclosporine (Sandimmune IV and oral Neoral oral)	Prophylaxis of organ rejection in kidney, liver, heart, and bone marrow transplantation; solid organ transplantation regimen is concomitant with that of corticosteroids	*Adult and child:* PO, 15 mg/kg/d initially within 4–12 wk of transplantation, continued for 1–2 wk, then tapered by 5%/wk to maintenance level of 5–10 mg/kg/d; IV, 1/3 of PO dose, given 4–12 h before transplantation and infused over 2–6 h; switch to PO form as soon as possible	*Onset:* PO, varies; IV, rapid *Duration:* 24–36 h $t_{1/2}$: 17.9 h
all-transretinoic acid (ATRA, Tretinoin, Vesanoid)	Induction therapy for acute promyelocytic leukemia; topical therapy for acne vulgaris, used investigationally for other skin disorders	Promyelocytic leukemia: *Adult:* PO, 45–60 mg/m²/d in evenly divided doses bid, to be continued for 30–90 d until complete remission is achieved Acne vulgaris: Topical cream (0.1%, 0.05%, 0.025%), gel (0.025%, 0.01%), or liquid (0.05%), applied once daily at bedtime to areas of skin where acneiform lesions appear	*Onset:* 1–2 h *Duration:* Approximately 2–3 wk $t_{1/2}$: 0.5–2 h
levamisole (Ergamisol)	Adjunct to fluorouracil for adjuvant postoperative treatment in surgically resected colorectal carcinoma, or with metastatic disease	*Adult:* PO, 50 mg q8 h for 3 d in conjunction with fluorouracil 450 mg/m²/d for 5 d starting 7–30 d after surgery, or when presenting for treatment; maintenance dose is the same, but given every 2 wk during 1×/wk FU therapy	*Onset:* Varies *Duration:* Unknown $t_{1/2}$: 3–4 h
azathioprine (Imuran)	Adjunct therapy with corticosteroids or cyclosporine for prevention of allograft rejection in renal, heart, and lung transplantation	Transplantation: *Adult and child:* PO/IV, 3–5 mg/kg as a single dose on the day of organ transplantation; PO maintenance, 1–2 mg/kg/d Rheumatoid arthritis: *Adult:* PO, 1 mg/kg/d as a single or double dose; may be increased to 2.5 mg/kg/d	*Onset:* PO, varies; IV, immediate *Duration:* 6–8 h $t_{1/2}$: 5 h
C Anti-angiogenic Agents			
P thalidomide (Thalomid)	Used with dexamethasone for primary or secondary multiple myeloma; or used with bortezimid or prednisone or melphalan and prednisone for multiple myeloma Treatment of erythema nodosum leprosy	*Adult:* PO, 200 mg daily with other identified antineoplastic agents on days 1–4, 9–12, and 7–20 every 28 d. Most patients receive four of these 28 d cycles. *Adult:* PO, 100–300 mg/d	*Onset:* Unknown *Duration:* Unknown $t_{1/2}$: 5–7 h

with a half-life of 3.7 hours to 8.5 hours. Direct lesional injection or instillation (as in the bladder) is indicated for some disorders. Interferon alfa-2a crosses the placenta and may be secreted in breast milk. It is excreted in the urine.

Pharmacodynamics

Interferon alfa-2a inhibits the growth of tumor cells, prevents these cells from multiplying, and modulates the host immune response to help protect the body from tumor cells. It blocks specific viral infection by preventing viral replication in the body.

Contraindications and Precautions

Caution should be used when administering interferon alfa-2a to patients with pancreatitis, hepatic or renal disease, depressed bone marrow function, cardiac disease or a history of cardiac disease, or compromised central nervous system (CNS) function.

In addition, interferon alfa-2a is a pregnancy category C drug, so its use during pregnancy may be risky to the fetus. It should also be avoided during lactation and in patients with known allergies to interferon or its components.

Adverse Effects

The most common adverse effects of interferon alfa-2a are dizziness, confusion, lethargy, flu-like symptoms, anorexia, nausea, and changes in taste. Depression, anxiety, and suicidal ideation have been reported in a substantial number of cases. Disease processes that exacerbate these symptoms warrant careful monitoring. Hypothyroidism may occur in up to 10% of the patients treated with interferon alfa-2a. Long-term therapy increases the risk of this complication. Other adverse effects include hypotension or hypertension, edema, arrhythmias, depression of bone marrow function, increased liver enzymes, rash, dry skin, partial alopecia, and glucose intolerance.

Drug Interactions

An increased risk of theophylline toxicity occurs when theophylline is administered concomitantly with interferon alfa-2a. This effect is caused by a decrease in theophylline clearance through the liver. Monitor patients to evaluate theophylline levels and adjust their theophylline dosages appropriately. Interferon alfa-2a can also cause increased effects and toxicity when combined with other neurotoxic, hematotoxic, and cardiotoxic drugs. Neurologic and hematologic toxicity has been particularly problematic for patients with HIV who receive concomitant antiretroviral therapy. Renal toxicity is more likely if interferon alfa-2a is given with IL-2 than if either is given alone. Anyone receiving drugs with overlapping toxicities must be carefully monitored. Table 54.2 lists drugs that interact with interferon alfa-2a.

Assessment of Relevant Core Patient Variables

Health Status

Before administering interferon alfa-2a, review the patient's record to see whether the drug is contraindicated. Cardiovascular, pulmonary, and neurologic disorders may escalate the adverse effects of this agent. Patients with depression are at particular risk of suicidal ideation and should be screened prior to initiation of therapy. Glucose intolerance is a common effect of interferon alfa therapies, and patients with diabetes mellitus are at particular risk of hyperglycemic crises. Assess and monitor patients with borderline thyroid function carefully for potential hypothyroidism. Perform a complete physical examination to establish a baseline for monitoring therapy. Next, record the patient's weight, temperature, skin condition, orientation, reflexes, pulse, and blood pressure. Because bone marrow depression and liver damage can be very serious, obtain a complete blood count (CBC) and hepatic profile at least monthly during therapy (Rieger & Khari, 2001).

Life Span and Gender

Determine whether the patient is pregnant or lactating, because interferon alfa-2a is a pregnancy category C drug, and the drug enters breast milk. Assess the age of the patient because the drug is not approved for patients who are younger than 18 years.

Lifestyle, Diet, and Habits

Assess whether the patient consumes alcohol or other nonprescribed mood-altering drugs that might increase the neurotoxicities of this agent.

Environment

Be aware of the environment in which the drug will be administered. Interferon alfa-2a may be given at home or in a clinic. If it is given at home, the patient needs a refrigerator so that the reconstituted drug can be stored. Explore with the patient any factors in the home setting that may affect adherence to drug therapy.

TABLE 54.2	Agents That Interact with P Interferon Alfa-2a	
Interactants	**Effect and Significance**	**Nursing Management**
theophylline/aminophylline	Decreased theophylline clearance in patients with hepatitis. This may raise theophylline levels.	Monitor theophylline levels. If they increase significantly, dosage adjustments may be required.
cimetidine	May amplify the effects of interferon when used in treating melanoma; significance unknown	Monitor effects of interferon.
vinblastine	Enhances interferon toxicity in some patients	Monitor for adverse effects of interferon.

Nursing Diagnoses and Outcomes

- Risk for Infection related to possible suppression of bone marrow function, injections
  Desired outcome: The patient will be protected from exposure to infection and will remain infection free.
- Altered Nutrition: Less than Body Requirements, related to GI effects and flu-like symptoms
  Desired outcome: The patient will maintain nutritional status.
- Risk for Injury related to CNS changes from drug therapy
  Desired outcome: The patient will not sustain injury while on drug therapy.
- Potential for Maladaptive Coping related to fatigue, mental status changes from medication
  Desired outcome: Patient shows effective coping strategies and acceptance of therapy independently or with the assistance of mental health professionals.
- Activity Intolerance attributed to treatment-related fatigue, flu-like syndrome
  Desired outcome: Activity intolerance is mediated, and no therapy break is required.

Planning and Intervention

Maximizing Therapeutic Effects

Following the manufacturer's guidelines for reconstitution and storage increases the therapeutic effectiveness of the drug. Obtaining baseline blood counts and chemistries before therapy and at least monthly during therapy helps direct therapy and ensures accurate dosage and treatment guidelines. Other nonpharmacologic strategies, such as adequate sleep and proper nutrition, may assist patients in coping with therapy and enhance their immunologic function.

Minimizing Adverse Effects

Most clinical experts recommend premedicating patients with drugs such as acetaminophen or diphenhydramine to reduce the flu-like adverse effects and administering interferon injections in the late evening to allow patients to sleep through most of the adverse effects. Encourage the patient to rest if he or she is experiencing fatigue with drug therapy. Observe how the patient and family members use sterile technique, perform the injection, and rotate injection sites. Advise the patient to avoid crowds and people with known infections and to wash and treat injuries immediately to prevent infection. Warn the patient that interferon alfa-2a can cause confusion and dizziness, making falls and injury a risk. Consequently, stress the need for adequate lighting, bedside rails, assistance with walking, and avoidance of dangerous activities and driving. Severe GI effects may warrant a nutritional consultation, and small, frequent meals or nutritional supplements may be prescribed. Unusual, but potentially life-threatening autoimmune disorders, infectious disease, ischemic organ failure, and neuropsychiatric conditions may occur and should become part of routine assessment of patients receiving treatment.

Providing Patient and Family Education

- Explain that interferon alfa-2a inhibits the growth of tumor cells.
- Teach patients or family members how to reconstitute the powder into a solution and to date and refrigerate the reconstituted solution.
- For maximum therapeutic effects, advise patients to use reconstituted solution within 30 days and to mark drug days on the calendar so that the drug is taken when prescribed.
- Teach patients and families to administer the drug, use sterile technique, and rotate injection sites. Review injection technique periodically to ensure effectiveness and decrease adverse effects.
- Advise any women of childbearing age to whom this drug is prescribed to use barrier contraception to avoid pregnancy.
- If patients have pre-existing infectious or autoimmune diseases, they may be exacerbated and life-threatening in the context of interferon therapy. Advise patients to report these symptoms immediately.
- Because hypotension can occur for several days after drug administration, advise patients to slowly move from a sitting to standing position and to avoid operating machinery or driving while adjusting to the therapy's adverse effects.
- Tell patients of the Black Box warning of potential neuropsychiatric effects, and advise them to contact their health care provider if they experience severe emotional distress, extreme sadness, or depression, or if they or family perceive that they are confused.
- Teach patients to avoid infection and injury, maintain good nutrition, get regular blood tests and medical follow-up care, and watch for adverse effects.
- Emphasize the importance of calling the prescriber if fever, chills, sore throat, unusual bleeding or bruising, chest pain, palpitations, or changes in mental status occur.

Ongoing Assessment and Evaluation

Monitor the patient's CBC and white cell differential and liver and renal function before interferon alfa-2a therapy and at least monthly during therapy to gauge the drug's effectiveness and to check for adverse effects.

Drugs Closely Related to P Interferon Alfa-2a

Drugs in the same class as interferon alfa-2a are interferon alfa-2b (Intron-A), interferon alfa-n3 (Alferon N), interferon-n1 (Wellferon), interferon alfacon-1 (Infergen), interferon beta-1a (Avonex), interferon beta-1b (Betaseron), and interferon gamma-1b (Actimmune). These agents differ from the prototype in terms of their specific cellular actions and therefore indications but are similar in molecular structure, mechanism of action, and adverse effects. Pegylated interferon-alfa is also available (Pegasys, Peg-Intron). With its longer half-life of approximately 72 hours, only one injection per week

MEMORY CHIP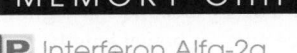

P Interferon Alfa-2a

- Inhibits growth of tumor cells, prevents their multiplication, and heightens the host immune response to help protect the body from tumor cells. Blocks specifically viral infection by preventing viral replication
- Used to treat some types of leukemia, AIDS-related Kaposi sarcoma, and various cancers
- Most common adverse effects: dizziness, confusion, lethargy, flu-like symptoms, anorexia, nausea, and altered taste
- Most serious adverse effects: depression and suicidal ideation
- **Life span alert: Generally, avoid during pregnancy and breast-feeding.**
- Maximizing therapeutic effects: Reconstitute and store following manufacturers' instructions.
- Minimizing adverse effects: Premedicate patient with other drugs to reduce the flu-like adverse effects.
- Most important patient education: Teach patients about the importance of avoiding infection.
- **Black box warning: Interferon-alfa-2a has been associated with serious or fatal neuropsychiatric, autoimmune, ischemia and infectious disorders. Patients must be closely monitored and withdrawal of medication is indicated with persistently severe or worsening signs and symptoms. Symptom resolution will occur in many, but not all cases of toxicity.**

---

is necessary, rather than three. The pegylated form has a limited adverse-effect profile; however, myelosuppression and thrombocytopenia have been reported more frequently in patients receiving the pegylated form than the prototype interferon. Enveloping interferon in a liposomal molecule prolongs its clinical effects and slows its clearance.

Drug Significantly Different From
P Interferon Alfa-2a

Interleukins are cytokines produced by T cells to communicate between WBCs. Aldesleukin (Proleukin) is approved for treating metastatic renal cell carcinoma and metastatic malignant melanoma, although many additional indications are emerging. The agent's immunostimulatory effects have been useful to stabilize helper T-cell counts in HIV disease and for bone marrow engraftment protection after bone marrow transplantation, and its antiviral effects have been promising in treating hepatitis.

Aldesleukin has been administered subcutaneously, intravenously, and intralesionally. It is paradoxically more potent when given by continuous infusion than by bolus injections, and the adverse effect profile is widely variable because of dose ranges from 20,000 IU daily after bone marrow transplantation to 72,000,000 IU daily for treating metastatic renal cell carcinoma or melanoma. The drug may be contraindicated in lactating patients or those with known allergies to aldesleukin. A Black Box warning cautions against its use in patients with abnormal thallium stress tests or abnormal pulmonary function tests and in those with organ homografts.

In the Black Box warning is a statement that mild lethargy during administration can rapidly progress to coma, even after discontinuation of the agent. Coadministration of radiographic iodinated IV contrast material has been associated with atypical hypersensitivity reactions. The drug should be used cautiously in patients with renal, liver, or CNS impairment.

Aldesleukin has an adverse effect profile very similar to that of high-dose interferon, but effects are potentially more acute in onset and severe in intensity. Even severe adverse effects resolve when the agent is discontinued, although hepatic, endocrine, and neurologic effects can persist for months after the conclusion of therapy. Concomitant administration of corticosteroids is not recommended, based on preclinical data suggesting that steroids may nullify the immunostimulatory effects of this agent (Cuaron & Thompson, 2001).

C IMMUNE MODULATORS

Immune modulators appear to act directly on the function of T cells and B cells, stimulating or suppressing the immune response. Lymphocytic modulators are divided into subcategories according to their primary chemical structure and pharmacologic properties. Immune modulators may suppress or stimulate immune function. Some of these agents stimulate certain functions of the cell response and suppress others.

In this text, the prototype immune modulator is the immune suppressant cyclosporine (Sandimmune, Neoral). Cyclosporine is in the subclass of polypeptide antibiotics, although they are currently known as calcineurin inhibitors. This classification recognizes the precise mechanism of action that is inhibition of calcineurin, an essential nuclear substance responsible for T-lymphocytic activity (van Rossum et al., 2010). Drugs that are also immune modulators and calcineurin inhibitors and are represented by the prototype include tacrolimus, sirolimus, pimecrolimus, and mycophenolate mofetil. Drugs that are also immune modulators but are significantly different from cyclosporine are the retinoids (all-transretinoic acid [ATRA], 9-cis-transretinoic acid, acitretin, alitretinoin, bexarotene, and isotretinoin); levamisole; azathioprine; glatiramer; BCG; and denileukin diftitox. These drugs have a variety of immunologic actions and targets, making many of them more a group of miscellaneous agents rather than members of the same category.

The calcineurin inhibitors are a group of agents that were developed as antibiotics but were determined to be too toxic to hematopoietic cells for that use. What has evolved is a group of agents that destroy cells in the G_0 or G_1 phase of cell cycling, a long phase that is common for all lymphocytes. This is achieved by blocking nucleic mechanisms of T cell receptor activation and calcineurin activity that normally upregulates IL-2. The first drug of this class to be licensed for use was cyclosporine. Immune modulators that act as immune suppressants block the normal effects of the immune system in the body. This action is beneficial in organ transplantation, in which the body destroys foreign tissue, and in autoimmune diseases, in which the body destroys its own cells.

Nursing Management of the Patient Receiving P Cyclosporine

Core Drug Knowledge

Pharmacotherapeutics

Cyclosporine is used as an adjunct treatment to prevent rejection in solid organ transplantation and to prevent graft-versus-host disease in allogeneic bone marrow or stem cell transplants. Adjunct therapy with corticosteroids is recommended. Cyclosporine is also used as second line treatment of rheumatoid arthritis and various other blistering disorders or connective tissue diseases (Amor, Ryan, & Mentor, 2010). The two brands of the drug are different, and dosage adjustment may be required for patients who switch. Other labeled uses (for the Neoral form only) include severe rheumatoid arthritis and extensive, refractory psoriasis. Topical cyclosporine is commonly used for treatment of severe eczema, erythematosis nodosum, and atopic dermatitis (Gallini et al., 2011). Opthmalmic solution of cyclosporine (Restasis) is used for chronic dry eyes. Unlabeled uses include treating alopecia areata, biliary cirrhosis, Crohn's disease, ulcerative colitis, dermatomyositis, Graves disease, lupus nephritis, multiple sclerosis, myasthenia gravis, nephrotic syndrome, pemphigus, polymyositis, and pulmonary sarcoidosis. It is used with corticosteroids to prevent rejection in kidney, liver, and heart transplantation and to treat chronic rejection in patients previously taking other immunosuppressants. The drug is being studied for use in pancreas, liver, kidney, bone marrow, and heart and lung transplantation. Sandimmune formulations are available as soft gelatin capsules, an oral solution, and as an IV solution. The IV form should be administered at one third of the oral dose. Neoral formulations are available as soft gelatin capsules and as an oral solution.

Pharmacokinetics

The absorption of cyclosporine from the GI tract is incomplete and variable; the lipid formulation has improved absorption characteristics. The absolute bioavailability of oral cyclosporine varies widely among patients. Factors that affect bioavailability include food, enterohepatic recirculation, and the type of assay used to measure levels. Ingesting conventional cyclosporine (Neoral) with food high in fat may increase bioavailability. Sandimmune and Neoral are not bioequivalent and cannot be exchanged one for another without dose adjustments. Sandimmune capsules and oral solution have decreased bioavailability compared with Neoral. Cyclosporine is extensively metabolized by the cytochrome P-450 enzyme system in the liver, and to a lesser degree in the GI tract and the kidneys. Many metabolites have been identified in the bile, feces, blood, and urine. Fortunately, these metabolites contribute little to drug toxicity. Excretion is primarily biliary, with less than 6% excreted in the urine. Neither dialysis nor renal failure substantially alters cyclosporine clearance. Children often need a larger oral dose, probably because of the limited absorptive area of their intestines. Patients with malabsorption may have difficulty achieving therapeutic levels with oral use. The IV dose is not significantly related to age, body surface area, or bowel length.

Pharmacodynamics

Cyclosporine is a potent immunosuppressant that is produced as a metabolite by the fungus *Beauveria nivea*. It suppresses some humoral immunity, but to a greater extent, it suppresses cell-mediated immune reactions. The exact mechanism of action is not known, but experimental evidence suggests that cyclosporine acts by specific, reversible inhibition of immunocompetent T lymphocytes that target their cytotoxic effects to lymphocytes in the G_0 and G_1 phases of the cell cycle. The helper T cell is the main target, but the suppressor T cell may also be suppressed. It also inhibits lymphokine production and release, including IL-2 or T-cell growth factor. Cyclosporine does not suppress bone marrow function.

Contraindications and Precautions

Cyclosporine that is injected (Sandimmune) is contraindicated in patients with hypersensitivity to polyoxyethylated castor oil. Oral cyclosporine (Neoral) should not be used concomitantly with psoralen UV A range or UV B light therapy in patients with psoriasis. It is assigned to pregnancy category C and is used during pregnancy only if the potential benefit justifies the possible risk to the fetus. It readily crosses the placenta and is secreted in breast milk.

Adverse Effects

Cyclosporine is associated with a substantial risk of nephrotoxicity. A form of chronic, progressive cyclosporine-associated nephrotoxicity is characterized by deterioration in renal function and morphologic changes in the kidney, which may persist even if the drug is discontinued. Additional manifestations of drug-related renal dysfunction include: hyperkalemia, hypercalciuria, or hypomagnesemia. Oversuppression of the immune system can increase susceptibility to infection, and in the Black Box warning; it is recommended that the drug be administered only under the direction of a prescriber with specialized knowledge of immunosuppressive therapy. Hepatotoxicity is also possible. Liver and renal function tests should be monitored closely. If a severe reaction occurs, dosage should be decreased, or the drug should be discontinued.

The most common adverse effects of cyclosporine are renal dysfunction, tremor, hirsutism, hypertension, and gum hyperplasia. The risk of malignancy in recipients of cyclosporine is higher than in the healthy population but similar to that of patients receiving immunosuppressive therapies. Lymphoproliferative and skin malignancies are most commonly reported. Other, less common adverse effects primarily involve the CNS and include confusion, lethargy, headache, ataxia, blurred vision, depression, encephalopathy, and convulsions. Studies have associated these symptoms with low cholesterol, low magnesium, aluminum overload, high-dose methylprednisolone, nephrotoxicity, and hypertension. Miscellaneous adverse effects include brittle nails, pruritus, anorexia, gastritis, hiccups, mouth sores, swallowing difficulty, pancreatitis, constipation, hypomagnesemia, anemia, conjunctivitis, hearing loss, edema, tinnitus, thrombocytopenia, joint pain, night sweats, hyperkalemia, and hyperuricemia. An uncommon, but serious and potentially life-threatening adverse effect associated with cyclosporine and other similar drugs is posterior reversible encephalopathy syndrome (PRES) that occurs in the vertebral basilar circulatory system. The disorder is associated with hypertension, but is unclear if the hypertension precipitates the ischemic brain injury, or if it is a protective reflection of compensation by the brain for the physiologic process of injury (Kim et al., 2011; Zhang, 2010).

Drug Interactions

Concomitant use of medications that affect the hepatic microsomal enzymes (P-450 system) requires monitoring and dose adjustment of cyclosporine. Drugs that can produce nephrotoxicity have an increased risk for producing renal dysfunction when used concomitantly with cyclosporine. Administering oral cyclosporine (Neoral) within 30 minutes of consuming food, particularly a high-fat meal, may decrease levels. Patients should not take cyclosporine with grapefruit juice unless instructed to do so; trough concentrations may be increased. Table 54.3 lists drugs that interact with cyclosporine.

Assessment of Relevant Core Patient Variables

Health Status

Before administering cyclosporine, review the patient's record to see whether the drug is contraindicated. If it can be administered safely, perform a physical examination to establish a baseline for monitoring therapy. Assess the patient's skin color, temperature, and texture, and note the appearance of any lesions to monitor for allergic reactions and signs of rejection. Assess vital signs, because hypertension is the most common adverse effect associated with cyclosporine administration. The associated hypertension is believed to be vasospastic in nature; therefore, calcium channel blockers are the antihypertensive treatment of choice. Hepatic function should be reviewed because the drug is metabolized primarily by the liver. Renal function should be evaluated because nephrotoxicity is a fairly common and irreversible adverse effect of the drug. Many now advocate changing to another immunosuppressive agent as soon as possible after engraftment or symptom resolution to minimize the risk of chronic renal insufficiency or loss of graft (Chapman, 2011). A CBC and differential should be done as a baseline for potential hematologic changes that might occur during therapy. Acute tremors, seizures, mental status changes, or visual disturbances are indicative of neurologic toxicities. These toxicities usually are related to high serum blood cyclosporine levels and are an indication to discontinue the medication.

Life Span and Gender

Assess whether female patients are of childbearing age, because the drug is in pregnancy category C. Children may require higher doses of medications because of decreased drug absorption.

Lifestyle, Diet, and Habits

Determine whether the patient is frequently in crowds, where he or she could be exposed to infection. Assess whether the patient has a lifestyle that involves frequent sun exposure. Determine whether the patient eats a high-fat diet because doing so increases the bioavailability of one form of the drug (Sandimmune) but decreases the bioavailability of another form (Neoral).

TABLE 54.3 Agents That Interact with P Cyclosporine

Interactants	Effect and Significance	Nursing Management
rifampin, phenytoin, phenobarbital	Decrease plasma concentrations of cyclosporine; may decrease therapeutic effectiveness of cyclosporine	Monitor for effectiveness of cyclosporine.
azithromycin, clarithromycin, diltiazem, erythromycin, fluconazole, itraconazole, ketoconazole, nicardipine, verapamil, and grapefruit juice	Increases the concentrations of cyclosporine through altering metabolism; may increase risk of adverse effects	Monitor for adverse effects of cyclosporine.
aminoglycosides, amphotericin B acyclovir, SMZ-TMP, melphalan, ketoconazole, diclofenac, naproxen, sulindac, cimetidine, ranitidine, tacrolimus	These nephrotoxic drugs may increase cyclosporine nephrotoxicity.	Monitor for signs of nephrotoxicity; dosage adjustment may be required.
HMG-CoA reductase inhibitors (atorvastatin, cerivastatin, fluvastatin, lovastatin, simvastatin)	Increased risk of myositis, rhabdomyolysis, and acute renal failure from cyclosporine	Monitor for adverse effects carefully. The HMG-CoA reductase inhibitor may need to be stopped if serious adverse effects occur.
nifedipine	Increased risk of gingival hyperplasia.	Provide good oral hygiene to minimize risk of gingival hyperplasia.

Environment

Be aware of the environment in which cyclosporine will be given. Cyclosporine is usually started in the hospital after solid organ or bone marrow transplantation and then continued at home. Explore with the patient any factors in the home setting that might affect adherence to drug therapy. For special teaching when the drug is used at home, see Box 54.1.

Nursing Diagnoses and Outcomes

- Risk for Infection related to suppression of the immune system
  Desired outcome: The patient will be protected from exposure to infection, and infections will be prevented or decreased.
- Altered Perfusion related to hypertension caused by the medication
  Desired outcome: Blood pressure will remain within normal limits or be controlled to normal limits with anti-hypertensive medications.
- Altered Renal Function related to nephrotoxic and hypertensive effects of the medication

---

BOX 54.1 COMMUNITY BASED CONCERNS

Cyclosporine at Home

Patients who receive cyclosporine at home need to have the following points emphasized in their teaching:

- Take this drug at the same time every day and consistently in relation to meals to maximize the immunosuppressive activity of the drug.
- Do not substitute an oral preparation of one form of cyclosporine for another without making dosage adjustments. Be familiar with the form you take and check each prescription refill to make sure you have the same product.
- Measure oral solutions using the dosing syringe provided with the medication, not a household teaspoon or tablespoon. Do not rinse the syringe with water either before or after measuring a dose because any water that is accidentally mixed into the drug will cause a variation in the dose provided.
- To improve the flavor, mix the cyclosporine with orange or apple juice (preferably at room temperature). Avoid using grapefruit juice because it interacts with the P-450 system and changes drug metabolism. (Sandimmune can be mixed with milk or chocolate milk, but the combination of Neoral and milk is unpalatable.)
- Use a glass container, not plastic, to prevent possible chemical interactions.
- Stir the oral solution into the diluent and drink immediately, all at once. Do not allow the drug to sit in the diluent.
- After drinking the medication and diluent, pour more of the same type of diluent into the glass to rinse it. Drink this glass also to ensure that you have received the entire dose.
- Inform your health care provider if you are taking any of the following medications, which may interfere with cyclosporine absorption or blood levels: drugs for irregular heart rhythms, medications to prevent or treat fungal infection, antibiotics, seizure medications, medications to treat tuberculosis, agents to treat HIV infection, lipid-lowering medications, or heart disease–related platelet-blocking agents.

Desired outcome: The patient will be monitored closely for deterioration in renal function, and permanent renal damage will be prevented.
- Altered Mental Status related to neurotoxic effects of cyclosporine (tremors, seizures, mental status changes, visual defects)
  Desired outcome: The patient will maintain normal orientation, reasoning ability, and motor activity.
- Deficient Knowledge related to multiple drug interactions and adverse effects
  Desired outcome: The patient will be instructed in potential drug interactions, including both prescription and over-the-counter medications. The patient will be instructed in potential adverse effects of medications and the need for close monitoring after discharge.

Planning and Intervention

Maximizing Therapeutic Effects

Ensure that cyclosporine therapy is started soon after transplantation. Medication should be administered as prescribed and according to recommendations to ensure therapeutic drug levels. Although cyclosporine can be given intravenously, the oral form should be used as soon as possible. It can be mixed with juice (other than grapefruit juice) to increase palatability but should not be refrigerated. Drug levels should be appropriately monitored to ensure adequate dosing. The metabolism of this agent is significantly variable, particularly in the oral form, and it warrants a warning in the prescriber's information suggesting the need for specialized laboratory support and drug level monitoring (Box 54.2). Cyclosporine should not be taken with foods, particularly those that are high in fat.

Minimizing Adverse Effects

Arrange for periodic blood tests to monitor for renal, hepatic, and hematologic effects of the medication. The drug should be held, and the physician should be notified, if signs of toxicity occur. Avoid mixing the drug with grapefruit juice. The patient should be protected from exposure to infection; immediate action must be taken at the first sign of infection. Assess patients for adverse CNS effects, and monitor vital signs, watching for hypertension.

Providing Patient and Family Education

- Teach patients how to take the oral form of this agent to maximize absorption and maintain stable blood levels.
- Caution patients not to discontinue taking this drug without consulting with their prescribers.
- Discuss with women of childbearing age the potential adverse effects on the fetus (most commonly, premature birth).
- Teach patients receiving cyclosporine to avoid exposure to infection by avoiding crowds and to promptly report injuries or signs of infection.
- Advise patients to avoid sun exposure to decrease the risk of skin malignancies.
- Ensure patients have blood drawn for medication levels and electrolyte panels to detect potential sub or supra

BOX 54.2 FOCUS ON RESEARCH

Blood Levels of Cyclosporine Drawn Peripherally or From a Central Access Device

Senner, A. M., Johnston, K., & McLachlan, A. J. (2005). A comparison of peripheral and centrally collected cyclosporine A blood levels in pediatric patients undergoing stem cell transplant. *Oncology Nursing Forum, 32*(1):73–77.

The Study

This prospective, comparative study of 14 pediatric patients in a university hospital in Australia was designed to compare trough serum blood levels of cyclosporine. The researchers compared 71 paired blood samples drawn from a peripheral line and from a central venous catheter.

The study found that when blood levels were drawn from a central venous catheter lumen not used for cyclosporine administration, they correlated well with peripherally drawn levels. All patients in the study were receiving intermittent infusion cyclosporine, and it is advisable to generalize these findings to a similar clinical situation.

Nursing Implications

Cyclosporine doses are based on trough blood levels. Pediatric patients have variable rates of metabolism and clearance of medications, making it exceptionally challenging to ensure reliable laboratory test results. The accuracy of these levels is essential to ensure protection from rejection with minimal toxicities. Inaccurate blood levels may lead either to underdosing of cyclosporine, which is associated with an increased risk of rejection, or overdosing of cyclosporine, which may cause hypertension, nephrotoxicity, or thromboembolic events.

---

therapeutic drugs levels, hyperkalemia, or hypomagnesemia that may require dose adjustment or supportive measures.

Ongoing Assessment and Evaluation

Cyclosporine is an agent with many drug interactions, issues of bioavailability, and considerable adverse effects. It is important to follow cyclosporine serum drug levels and have the dose adjusted appropriately to achieve maximal immune suppression without excess adverse effects. There is some debate whether trough, two-hour post dose or four-hour post dose levels are most accurate, so clinicians should establish institutional standards and perform levels in a consistent manner (Einollahi & Teimoori, 2011).

MEMORY CHIP

Cyclosporine

- Immunosuppressant that inhibits T-lymphocytes by causing cytotoxicity during the G_0 and G_1 phase.
- Used as an adjunct treatment to prevent rejection in solid organ transplantation and to prevent graft-versus-host disease in allogeneic bone marrow or stem cell transplant recipients.
- Major contraindication: hypersensitivity to polyoxyethylated castor oil
- Most common adverse effects: renal dysfunction, tremor, hirsutism, hypertension, and gum hyperplasia.
- Most serious adverse effects: renal toxicity and hepatic toxicity
- **Life span alert: Children may need higher doses; therapy usually avoided during pregnancy.**
- Maximizing therapeutic effects: Start as soon after transplantation as possible.
- Minimizing adverse effects: Monitor blood work.
- Most important patient education: Teach patients about the importance of preventing infection.
- **Black box warning: This medication produces extreme immune suppression and only prescribers experienced in management of patient who have medical conditions requiring therapeutic immune suppression and in facilities which are equipped to evaluate and treat serious life-threatening infections if they should occur. Monitoring for secondary malignancies should also be incorporated into the patient's plan of care.**

Drugs Closely Related to P Cyclosporine

Tacrolimus

Tacrolimus (Prograf) is a calcineurin inhibitor more similar to cyclosporine than any other agent. It is administered both orally and intravenously, and more recently a topical form of the medication is available for serious dermatologic disorders. It causes potent T-lymphocytic destruction. The variability of absorption and clearance necessitates serum blood level monitoring with dosage adjustment. Like cyclosporine, the most common adverse reactions are nephrotoxicity, neurotoxicity, and a risk of developing diabetes. Hypertension is also common and may be dose-related. The incidence of dysrhythmias and left ventricular hypertrophy with heart failure, microangiopathic anemia, and pulmonary fibrosis are higher with tacrolimus than with cyclosporine. Tacrolimus is rarely used as initial therapy because of its potency of immunosuppression and additional myelosuppressive properties that affect granulocytes and platelets. Interactions with antiretroviral protease inhibitors and phenobarbital are common, and the assistance of pharmacists familiar with the interactions can reduce the potential for serious toxicities.

Sirolimus

Sirolimus (Rapamycin, Rapamune) is a macrolide antibiotic much like cyclosporine and tacrolimus in terms of its structure and function, but it works later in the immune activation pathway, directly blocking the effects of interleukin-2. This agent is rarely used as rejection prevention therapy for this reason but may be used to treat acute or chronic rejection. Sirolimus has less nephrotoxicity and neurotoxicity than either cyclosporine or tacrolimus, but is noted for its propensity for hepatotoxicity and arthralgias. Hyperlipidemia and hypercholesterolemia occur with this agent but not with cyclosporine or tacrolimus.

Pemecrolimus

A topical immune suppressive used for treatment of dermatologic conditions such as atopic dermatitis, eczema, or psoriasis, this agent is only known for its added risk for infection (Sehgal & Pahwa, 2007).

Mycophenolate Mofetil

Mycophenolate mofetil (CellCept), a semisynthetic ester created from a mold, is a prodrug for mycophenolic acid. It has direct and selective destruction of actively replicating lymphocytes. This selectivity means that mycophenolate is usually given in combination with at least one other immunosuppressive agent. This agent is available in only an oral form, and patients must be advised of food and drug interactions. They should take it on an empty stomach and avoid antacids within one hour of consuming the drug. Patients receiving around the clock proton pump inhibitors may have erratic absorption and inconsistent drug levels. The most common adverse effect is GI toxicity in the form of nausea, vomiting, and diarrhea. Bone marrow suppression is also common. However, unlike many other immunosuppressives, mycophenolate is not mutagenic and is not associated with secondary malignancies.

Drugs Significantly Different From P Cyclosporine

Retinoids

The **retinoids** are a group of naturally occurring compounds that are derivatives of preformed (dietary) vitamin A or provitamin A carotenoid. Preformed vitamin A is primarily found in food substances, and the provitamin A group involves precursors of retinol. Retinol has long been recognized for its importance in vision, growth, reproduction, and epithelial cell differentiation. We now know that retinoids exert most of their effects through their influence on gene expression (Rieger, 2001; Yousefi & Azizzadeh, 2010). They are essential for controlling growth and differentiation of normal cells during embryonic development. Because of their ability to influence differentiation of some cells while arresting development of others, they have become an important part of chemoprevention protocols aimed at preventing cancer in high-risk individuals (Tang & Gudas, 2011). Retinoids are known to enhance humoral and cell-mediated immune responses as well. Bexarotene is used to treat cutaneous lymphoma such as mycosis fungoides (Abbott et al., 2009). There are two major families of nuclear retinoid receptors: the RAR receptors and the RXR receptors. Because the RAR receptors must first bind with RXR receptors before activating gene expression, it is thought that agents targeting RXR receptors may have greater immunologic antitumor activity (Tang & Gudas, 2011). The agent that has been used the longest and most extensively is all-transretinoic acid (ATRA). Other similar retinoids include 9-cis-transretinoic acid (panretinide) and bexarotene. Retinoids used for severe dermatologic conditions include acitretin, alitretinoin, and isotretinoin (Gallini et al., 2011). Some are only available in topical form, but alitretinoin may also be administered systemically by the oral route. These agents capitalize upon the epidermal effects, producing skin sloughing without other systemic effects or mutagenicity. Promising **rexanoids** (synthetic retinoids) still in investigational trials include 13-cisretinoic acid, tazarotene, and TAC-101 (Tang & Gudas, 2011).

All-Transretinoic Acid

This natural retinol metabolite is licensed for treating acute progranulocytic leukemia refractory to or relapsed from anthracycline chemotherapy; some unlabeled uses include treating myelodysplasia and providing chemoprevention against cervical dysplasia and precancerous skin lesions. The pharmacokinetics of ATRA (Tretinoin, Vesanoid) are poorly defined. For its licensed use, ATRA is given intravenously as an infusion. Chemoprevention protocols use oral formulations, and some research protocols use a topical formulation (Tang & Gudas, 2011).

Like all retinoids, ATRA is teratogenic and in pregnancy category D; this classification precludes pregnancy during therapy and for an undefined period afterward. Egg or sperm banking before therapy is recommended for patients of childbearing age.

Acute hypervitaminosis A toxicity is a commonly described phenomenon with treatment doses of this agent. CNS symptoms prevail and include drowsiness, irritability, headache, and vomiting. More common are the dermatologic symptoms that include alopecia, dry desquamation, pruritus, and increased pigmentation. Constitutional symptoms are arthralgia, hepatosplenomegaly, and eye irritation. Symptoms are not usually life threatening and resolve 1 to 4 weeks after the conclusion of therapy. Other major toxicities of retinoids are hypercholesterolemia, hypothyroidism, teratogenesis, visual disturbances, and hyperleukocytosis (Abbott et al., 2009).

Hyperleukocytosis with fever, respiratory distress, pulmonary infiltrates, and fluid retention are the characteristics of a syndrome called retinoic acid syndrome, which occurs in 20% to 30% of patients receiving therapy for progranulocytic leukemia (Rogers & Yang, 2011). It so closely mimics infection and sepsis that it may be difficult to differentiate from them. High-dose steroids and leukapheresis have been used to supplement supportive care, to help resolve the symptoms without discontinuing therapy. ATRA has no known drug interactions.

9-Cis-Transretinoic Acid

Like ATRA, 9-cis-transretinoic acid (Panretinide, isomer ATRA) is a naturally occurring retinol derivative that acts on several sites. It is licensed for topical treatment of Kaposi sarcoma lesions. Administration guidelines and adverse effects are similar to those of ATRA except for the absence of retinoic acid syndrome, which is unique to ATRA. This retinoid is taken with food to enhance its bioavailability (Schmitt-Hoffmann et al., 2011).

Bexarotene

Bexarotene (Targretin gel), a naturally occurring retinol derivative, is available in both a systemic and topical form to treat cutaneous T-cell lymphoma (mycosis fungoides) (Abbott et al., 2009). This agent is also used to treat acne (Accutane).

Levamisole

Levamisole (Ergamisol) is used as an adjunctive therapy in patients being treated with fluorouracil (Adrucil) after surgical resection of colon cancer. It may also be included in the regimen to manage early stage disease. The exact mechanism of synergy is unclear, but therapy responses are nearly doubled when the two agents are administered concomitantly (Bese et al., 2005). Levamisole restores depressed immune function, stimulating antibody formation, enhancing T-cell response, and potentiating monocyte and macrophage activity. Levamisole is readily absorbed when given orally. An interesting phenomenon has emerged in recent years since illicit cocaine has become commonly contaminated with levamisole. Patients using large amounts of contaminated cocaine develop neutropenia or thrombocytopenia thought to be related to the effects of levamisole (ref). This is termed levamicoke syndrome (Van Wieren et al., 2010).

Levamisole is assigned to pregnancy category C and should also be avoided with lactation. Common adverse effects include dizziness, headache, depression, paresthesias, changes in taste, nausea, stomatitis, diarrhea, dermatitis, alopecia, fatigue, fever, arthralgia, myalgia, and infection. Depression of bone marrow function is a potentially serious but infrequent complication.

Increased phenytoin (Dilantin) levels and phenytoin toxicity can occur if this drug is combined with levamisole. Patients on this combination should be monitored closely and have their phenytoin levels checked regularly, with changes in dosage made as appropriate. Because disulfiram (Antabuse)–like reactions can occur if levamisole is combined with alcohol, patients should be warned not to drink alcohol.

Azathioprine

Azathioprine (Imuran) is an intravenously infused antimetabolite that splits into a precursor, mercaptopurine. It is a unique antimetabolite agent because it is exclusively an immunosuppressant and not an antineoplastic. Because of its action, it is highly mutagenic and has been associated with the development of secondary malignancies, resulting in reduced use as safer and equally effective immunosuppressive regimens have been identified. It is indicated as part of a multidrug regimen to prevent rejection in renal transplantation and to treat rheumatoid arthritis not responsive to conventional management. Unlabeled uses include treating Crohn's disease and myasthenia gravis and preventing rejection after cardiac transplantation. Notable drug interactions occur with allopurinol, angiotensin-converting enzyme inhibitors, and anticoagulants. The most common and severe adverse event is infection, although GI distress may be great enough to warrant limiting the dose. Azathioprine is given cautiously with other immunosuppressants because of increased risk of infection, and dose reduction is necessary in hepatic dysfunction.

Glatiramer

Glatiramer acetate (Copaxone) is a synthetic copolymer of essential amino acids. It suppresses the specific immune processes involved in the pathogenesis of multiple sclerosis and reduces the frequency of relapses. Although the exact mechanism of action is unknown, it is thought to act by modulating T-cell autoimmune responses to myelin. The drug is given by daily SC injections and must be reconstituted and used immediately. A set of postinjection reactions—including chest pain, palpitations, anxiety, dyspnea, and urticaria—occurs in about 10% of patients with injection and is usually transient. Transient chest pain separate from the postinjection reaction has also been reported by about 20% of patients, but the symptom is self-limiting and not associated with other life-threatening symptoms. This drug may interfere with normal immune function while blocking the mechanism that causes multiple sclerosis; therefore, the patient should be protected from infection and injury. Photosensitivity is also common, necessitating use of sunscreen and protective clothing when outdoors.

Bacillus of Calmette and Guérin (BCG)

BCG in the form of ImmuCyst is a suspension of an attenuated strain of *Mycobacterium bovis* that has been used as immunoadjuvant since the 1960s. TheraCys is live BCG. This agent in either of its forms is currently licensed to treat carcinoma in situ of the urinary bladder with or without papillary tumors (Uchida, Yonou, Hayashi, et al., 2007; Babjuk et al., 2011), although its unlabeled uses also include hematologic malignancies and non-pulmonary tuberculosis (Triccas, 2010). It has been given intradermally, although it is more frequently administered intravenously or instilled into the bladder. Acting as a nonspecific immunomodulatory agent, it stimulates both nonspecific and specific immune responses, although the precise mechanism of action is not known (Shintani et al., 2007).

Denileukin Diftitox

Denileukin diftitox (Ontak) (diphtheria toxin and IL-2) is an **immunotoxin** that combines an inactivated microbe (diphtheria toxin) and a cytokine (IL-2); it is licensed for treating persistent or relapsed cutaneous T-cell lymphoma whose malignant cells express the CD25 component of the IL-2 receptor (Manoukian & Hagemeister, 2011). It is administered at either 9 mg/kg/day or 18 mg/kg/day for a 5-day course every 21 days (Lansigan, Stearns, & Foss, 2010). Denileukin diftitox is administered over at least 15 minutes while observing the patient for infusion-related reactions such as fever, chills, urticaria, or respiratory distress. Although no clear guidelines exist regarding the length of treatment, most individuals receive approximately four cycles of therapy. Two acute reactions have been reported with this agent: acute hypersensitivity and a flu-like syndrome complex (Lansigan, Stearns, & Foss, 2010). Acute hypersensitivity reactions within hours of infusion are common (67%) (Lansigan, Stearns, & Foss, 2010). These reactions may be prevented by administering acetaminophen or diphenhydramine, although many clinicians also administer nonsteroidal anti-inflammatory agents or corticosteroids to these patients. A more delayed flu-like syndrome often has the typical fever and chills, but also GI distress, myalgias, and asthenia. In addition to these hypersensitivity toxicities, vascular leak syndrome with weight gain, edema, hypoalbuminemia, and hypotension occurs in up to 27% of patients. This agent has not been studied and established safe for administration to children or to women who are lactating or pregnant.

Nursing Management of the Patient Receiving **P** Thalidomide

Core Drug Knowledge

Pharmacotherapeutics

Thalidomide (Thalomid), used for many years for various purposes, has immunomodulatory, anti-inflammatory, and anti-angiogenic properties. It is believed that thalidomide's most promising features for treating malignancy lie in its "anti-angiogenesis" properties, yet its actions on autoantibodies have also made it a useful agent for treating autoimmune diseases and organ transplant rejection. Some of its immunomodulatory activities include antiproliferative and pro-apoptosis functions (Prommer, 2010). Immune suppression properties vary considerably between individuals and seem to be based on suppression of tumor necrosis factor-alpha production and macrophage function, and down-regulation of tumor cell-surface adhesion molecules responsible for leukocyte migration.

Licensed uses for thalidomide include treating cutaneous manifestations of erythema nodosum leprosum (a complication of leprosy treatment), rheumatoid arthritis, multiple myeloma, bone marrow transplantation, and chronic graft-versus-host disease refractory to standard therapy. There are several reports of its effective use for severe aphthous ulcers of the oropharynx, esophagus and stomach, myelodysplastic syndrome, follicular non-Hodgkin's lymphoma, diffuse large cell lymphoma, and refractory psoriasis (Eichholz, Merchant, & Gaya, 2010; Li, Gill, & Lentzsch, 2010).

Pharmacokinetics

Thalidomide has immunomodulatory, anti-inflammatory, and anti-angiogenic properties. Its mechanism of action is not fully understood. It is not hepatically metabolized to a large extent and appears to undergo nonenzymatic hydrolysis in plasma into multiple metabolites.

Pharmacodynamics

This is an oral agent available in 50, 100, 150, and 200 mg capsules. Bioavailability is poorly defined due to poor aqueous solubility; however, once in solution, reportedly 90% is bioavailable. The mean time to peak blood concentrations is 2.9 to 5.7 hours, indicating that thalidomide is slowly absorbed in the gastrointestinal tract. This feature makes it difficult to plan a time of administration that will not be impaired by food or antacids. Administering thalidomide with a high-fat meal does not seem to alter the onset of absorption, but does prolong the time to peak serum concentration.

Thalidomide's mean protein binding capacity is 55% to 66%, and it is found well distributed throughout the body, inclusive of excrement such as semen. The exact metabolic route for thalidomide distribution and excretion is not well understood but it is thought to be hydrolyzed without significant secondary metabolites. The mean half-life is 5 to 7 hours, and all drug is absent from the urine at the end of 48 hours. The effects of renal impairment have not been well studied, but appear to not influence excretion, so thalidomide is not dose adjusted for renal insufficiency. The same is true for hepatic impairment.

Contraindications and Precautions

The most significant contraindication for use of thalidomide is the unwillingness or inability to ensure that the individual receiving the drug will not get pregnant or impregnate another person. This agent is highly teratogenic and informed consent and signed agreement to avoid pregancny is required before prescription of the drug.

Absolute contraindications include only pregnancy, based on the fetal risk for birth defects or death. Relative contraindications considered based on a therapeutic risk-benefit ratio include the presence of pre-existing peripheral neuropathy or venous thromboembolism. These serious and common adverse effects may become life-threatening or highly morbid when combined with other pre-existing risks.

Precaution is advised before prescribing thalidomide in patient with pre-existing seizure disorders or bradycardia as these are significant medical problems of themselves, and the addition of thalidomide has been noted to increase their incidence. The prescribing information also suggests that during ongoing therapy, the medication should be withheld if the absolute neutrophil count falls below 750 mg/dL.

During therapy, close monitoring for neurologic changes and skin reactions is advised with prompt discontinuation when present. These symptoms can progress to severe and irreversible complications, which may be abrogated by immediate discontinuation of the drug.

Adverse effects

Common adverse effects include thrombotic problems, drowsiness, photosensitivity, and peripheral neuropathies (Prommer, 2010). The incidence of VTE is as high as 22.7% in patients with multiple myeloma receiving thalidomide in conjunction with dexamethasone, while the same population receiving only dexamethasone had an incidence of only 4.9% with VTE (Celgene Corporation, 2010). Skin disorders, GI distress, secretory disorders (e.g., decreased lacrimation, dry mouth), and fluid retention have also been reported with some frequency. Dose-related tremors occur in about 35% of patients (Prommer, 2010). Patients taking thalidomide are advised to immediately report neurologic symptoms because toxicity may be reversible only if the agent is promptly stopped.

Drug Interactions

High-fat meals or snacks taken with thalidomide may prolong the time to peak drug concentrations, so this medication should be taken orally with water, preferably at bedtime and at least two hours after the evening meal. Table 54.4 presents a summary of agents that interact with thalidomide.

TABLE 54.4	Agents That Interact with P Thalidomide	
Interactant	**Effect and Significance**	**Nursing Management**
docetaxel	Concurrent use of docetaxel and thalidomide may result in an increased risk of venous thromboembolism	Assess for co-administration; discuss with prescriber to determine necessity if ordered; assess for thromboembolism if co-administered; use appropriate nursing interventions and seek orders for thromboembolism prophylaxis
dexamethasone acefurate	Concurrent use may result in increased risk of developing toxic epidermal necrolysis	Assess for co-administration; discuss with prescriber to determine necessity if ordered; assess for trashes and skin alterations
darbepoetin alfa	When used in patients who have myelodysplastic syndromes the likelihood of blood clots may increase	Assess closely for indication of blood clots; notify prescriber if symptoms present
midazolam	Concurrent use may result in increased midazolam metabolism and clearance	Assess for potential decreased effectiveness of midazolam
cyclosporine	Concurrent use may result in increased cyclosporine A metabolism and clearance	Assess for potential decreased effectiveness of cyclosporine

Assessment of Relevent Core Patient Variables

Health Status

Limited data are available to inform the use of thalidomide in patients with comorbid health conditions, but information suggests that no dosage adjustment is required for patients with renal or hepatic impairment.

Life Span and Gender

As a result of its early use in pregnant women and the resulting severe birth defects, it is classified as a pregnancy category X drug. It is possible that severe birth defects can occur with only one dose. In the United States, it is marketed under a special distribution program called "System for Thalidomide Education and Prescribing Safety," which means that it is a restricted drug that may be prescribed only by registered individuals. Male and female patients who are prescribed thalidomide must receive oral and written instructions about the need to use two methods of contraception; they must use the contraception for 1 month before starting thalidomide, during treatment, and for 1 month after stopping thalidomide. Periodic pregnancy testing is required while receiving thalidomide. Breast-feeding must also be avoided.

The safety of this drug in children has not been established and is therefore considered unsafe in children below the age of 18 years. No special precautions have been identified for the elderly. No gender or race-based differences in bioavailability or metabolism have been identified.

Lifestyle, Diet and Habits

Patients receiving thalidomide must be aware of the significant influence that adverse effects may have on their personal and private life. The physical effects may influence their energy level, ability to eat foods they like, and safety to independently perform activities of daily living. Drowsiness may interfere with their ability to work, operate machinery, or drive a vehicle. When taking thalidomide, the patient must time their medication to be between meals despite their sensations of nausea, and refrain from taking antacids. More personally, since thalidomide is teratogenic, patients are advised to implement stringent birth control measures that may influence their intimate relationships.

Environment

Thalidomide should be stored at room temperature and protected from light. These capsules may be administered in the hospital, clinic or home care setting. Assurance that the patient is competent to remember when and how to take the medication is essential. It is important for healthcare providers to offer information and supplies to implement chemotherapy safety precautions for family at home.

Nursing Diagnosis and Outcomes

- Altered nutrition due to persistent nausea or vomiting.
  Desired outcome: Absence of nausea or vomiting.
- Altered sensory perception related to peripheral neuropathy
  Desired outcome: Absence of fall or injury due to altered perception
- Altered elimination related to constipation
  Desired outcome: Normal bowel habits maintained.
- Altered mental status due to severe drowsiness
  Desired outcome: Patient verbalizes no distress related to drowsiness and able to maintain desired level of ADLs.
- Potential altered circulation due to risk for venous thromboembolism
  Desired outcome: Absence of venous thromboembolism or other hypercoagulability syndromes.
- Potential risk for infection due to immunosuppressive effects
  Desired outcome: Absence of infection.

Planning and Intervention

Maximizing Therapeutic Effects

Patients receiving thalidomide will achieve the greatest benefit from therapy when they have a complete understanding of when is best to take their medication for best absorption. This may be challenging and require review of their other medications and meal planning. Thalidomide is such a dangerous drug if not taken properly, that a pillbox and system for pill counting to ensure proper administration is usually implemented. Most patients find that taking their thalidomide at night-time is the most effective way to ensure there is no interruption of absorption and to compensate for the drowsiness that is often encountered. If this is the plan, ensure measures are taken to reduce the patient's fall risk due to orthostasis. Thalidomide is prescribed in conjunction with other medications for treatment of multiple myeloma, and administration of the thalidomide should follow the prescribed combination therapy plan as closely as possible to ensure optimum tumor response. Some new data also suggests that some of the disorders that are treated may benefit from a lower dose maintenance therapy, but these are still under investigation except with erythema nodosum leprosum.

Minimizing Adverse Effects

Ensuring that preventive measures for the most common and severe adverse effects will enhance the ability to continue therapy without dose-limiting toxicities. Compression stockings, and planned exercise can reduce the risk of VTE, although many patients will also receive prophylactic anticoagulation. Blood counts are monitored carefully and infection prevention precautions are implemented even with limited neutropenia. Proper health maintenance to boost the immune system includes adequate rest, nutritional meal planning, and maintaining activities of daily living. Infection prevention strategies such as avoiding crowds, careful food selection, avoidance of soil exposure and excellent personal hygiene are employed even before neutropenia occurs. Neutropenia lower than 750 cells/mm^3 is an indication for holding the medication. Precautions to prevent pregnancy are essential and must be followed, and constantly evaluated by the healthcare team to reduce the risk of injury to the fetus. Precautions are recommended for a month prior to starting treatment until one month after the conclusion of therapy. During therapy, healyhcare providers should frequently interview patients about the sexual practices and reinforce the need for contraception. Patients are usually placed on a "bowel regimen" of stool softeners (docusate [Colace]) with mild laxatives (Senna) unless constipation occurs despite this regimen. The next progression is to Miralax, and anticholinergic medications such as lomotil or irritants such as magnesium citrate are reserved for refractory constipation. It is unclear whether peripheral neuropathies from thalidomide can be prevented, but frequent assessment for hand and feet sensory changes may provide early detection. There is some evidence that supplemental Vitamin E may reduce this adverse effect, but it has not been tested in patients

Mrs. Jones is a 45 year old moderately obese (Height 64 inches, weight 200 pounds, BMI 34) woman who recently presented to the primary care provider with hip and back pain, fatigue, and persistent nausea. Upon physical exam and diagnostic evaluation she was found to have multiple myeloma, stage III, IgG subtype.

She works as a hygienist at a pediatric dentist's office, is married, and has two teen-age boys aged 14 years and 15 years. Denies smoking and rare alcohol intake.

Physical Exam Findings:
- Neurologically intact and excellent cognition
- No tenderness in spine or joints
- Heart rate 110/min and regular, lungs clear
- Pulses normal bilaterally in upper and lower extremities
- 1+ edema bilateral lower extremities
- Conjunctiva and mucous membranes pale

Past Medical History:
- Hypertension for 2 years
- Life-long severe upper respiratory allergies to grasses and trees
- Intermittent irritable bowel syndrome

Medications:
- Lisinopril (ACE inhibitor) once daily
- HCTZ (thiazide diuretic) twice daily
- Omeprezole (proton pump inhibitor) twice daily
- Laxatives and immodium as needed for gastrointestinal distress

CBC: Hgb 7.9 g/dL (baseline 12.7 g/dL)

Metabolic Panel:
- BUN 22 mg/dL; creatinine 2.4 mg/dL (baseline 1.3 mg/dl); calcium 10.5 mg/dl; albumin 3.5 g/dL
- CrCl 42 mL/min
- Total protein 12.6 g/dL (baseline 8.0 g/dL)

B2M: 8.0 g/mL

Urinalysis:
- 2+ proteinuria
- Glucose >1,000 mg/dL
- No increased leukocytes, no casts

Skeletal x-ray: Acute fracture of l,2 and three skeletal lytic lesions
Bone marrow biopsy: 30% plasma cells

Impressions:
Treatment plan: Bortezomib, thalidomide and dexamethasone for four months to be followed by hematopoietic stem cell transplant

1. Before starting therapy, what mandated patient counseling and consent must occur?
2. Mrs. Jones has compromised renal function, with a creatinine clearance of <50mL/min. Do we need to alter the dose or administration procedures for thalidomide?
3. Based upon her occupation, what adverse effect(s) would we want to alter her to based upon her specific risks?
4. Based upon her past medical history and current medications, what unique concerns may be present related to initiation of thalidomide?

receiving thalidomide. Patients should consult their health-care provider for taking any of the available recommended complementary therapies to abrogate any symptom. Other symptoms are managed supportively as they arise.

Providing Patient and Family Education

This drug's administration is only permitted in circumstances in which there is not a viable alternative therapy and the patient or health care proxy can be educated about its teratogenic risks. Females must receive both oral and written warning about the risks of thalidomide to fetuses and the importance of using two simultaneous forms of birth control and acknowledge in writing her understanding and agreement to these precautions. Males must acknowledge in writing a similar understanding and agreement to perform contraceptive measures appropriate to men. These measures are in place from one month prior to starting therapy until one month after conclusion of treatment.

From the onset of therapy, safety measures are reinforced and patients are advised to implement preventive measures for thromboemboembolic events and monitor for their occurrence. They are advised to remain as active as possible, consume one quart or more of water daily and if advised by their healthcare provider implement mechanical prophylaxis measues such as compression stockings or sequential compression devices. Many of these patients have additional thromboembolic risks and may be prescribed prophylactic anticoagulation. This may involve education regarding self-administration techniques, food monitoring, frequent blood assessment, and bleeding precautions. Due to the complexities of their risks and the prophylactic regime, these patients are often referred to an anticoagulation clinic for management of their anticoagulation and ongoing education.

Safety measures also extend to protection from injury related to altered sensation if peripheral neuropathies occur. Patients should be taught to protect their hands and feet from excessive temperatures and other trauma. They should reduce the temperature of their home water heater, wear gloves and socks when appropriate, spend more time in supportive footwear and remove injury risks such as loose rugs or low-standing tables from their home, keeping clear walking pathways.

Ongoing Assessment and Evaluation

Patients receiving thalidomide will be monitored closely by health care providers who are "certified" by the S.T.E.P.S. program to prescribe and counsel patients receiving thalidomide. During visits, serum laboratory tests for toxicity (e.g., neutropenia) are drawn, and medication validation is performed and include pill counts and assessment for medications or over the counter products that may interfere with contraception. Healthcare providers will also assess the patient's risk for venous thromboembolism and institute prophylactic measures if additional risk factors occur. The patient must be interviewed for resolvable adverse effects such as constipation, or signs and symptoms of dose-limiting toxicities such as neuropathies.

MEMORY CHIP

P Thalidomide

- Anti-angiogenic agent that has immunomodulatory, anti-inflammatory, and anti-angiogenic properties thought to be related to suppression of tumor necrosis factor alpha production and down-regulation of surface adhesion molecules involved in leukocyte migration.
- Used as primary therapy for newly diagnosed or relapsed multiple myeloma, myelodysplastic syndrome, follicular and diffuse large cell lymphoma, erythema nodosum leprosy, and refractory rheumatoid arthritis.
- Major contraindications: it is essential for patients receiving thalidomide to avoid becoming pregnant or impregnating another for four weeks prior to and after concluding therapy due to the certain teratogenic effects of the medication.
- Most common adverse effects: drowsiness, neutropenia, constipation, peripheral neuropathies and venous thromboembolism.
- Most serious adverse effects: human teratogenecity
- **Life span alert: Teratogenecity is of such high risk that and male or female of childbearing age must be enrolled in the S.T.E.P.S. counseling always use contraception with a latex condom while on therapy and for four weeks after treatment conclusion. Additionally, consult the prescriber who is counseling the patient on the S.T.E.P.S. program for any medication changes that may influence the efficacy of contraception.**
- Maximizing therapeutic effects: High fat meals or snacks taken with thalidomide may prolong the time to peak drug concentrations, so this medication should be taken orally with water, preferably at bedtime and at least two hours after the evening meal.
- Minimizing adverse effects: Use cautiously with medications that also cause somnolence, peripheral neuropathies or neutropenia, as these effects will be enhanced by combination agents with these adverse effects.
- Most important patient education: The most important patient educations with thalidomide is the importance of effective contraception and prevention of pregnancy. The teratogenic effects are well-documented and consistent. Patients are also advised to monitor for the presence of drowsiness or sedation and modify their activities accordingly, and drink plenty of fluids or take mild laxatives to reduce the incidence or severity of constipation. Since many patients experience a safety risk due to drowsiness, peripheral neuropathies or neutropenia, precautions to prevent injury are emphasized.
- **Black box warning: This medication is teratogenic and should never be administered to an individual who is or could become pregnant. Black box warning provide extensive advisement to prevent infection and avoid medications that could interfere with contraception. The risk for venous thromboembolism is as high as 22.7% and also outlines in the black box warning. Clinicians should be observant for signs and symptoms of venous thromboembolism and provide concurrent prophylactic anticoagulation.**

Drugs Closely Related to **P** Thalidomide
Lenalidomide

Lenalidomide is a thalidomide analogue with similar pharmacokinetic properties to the native drug thalidomide. It is licensed with dexamethasone for second-line treatment of multiple myeloma, but has been administered concurrently with bortezimib, prednisone, melphalan, and cyclophosphamide (Zeldis et al., 2010). Lenalidomide is also licensed for treatment of transfusion dependent, low-to-intermediate risk myelodysplastic syndrome (MDS) with a deletion of 5 g abnormality. Like thalidomide, this agent also has a black box warning related to its teratogenic effects and requires patient counseling, consent, and agreement to not become pregnant or impregnate another. It is also associated with neutropenia and venous thromboembolism when administered concomitantly with dexamethasone. Other notable unique adverse effects include fatigue, gastrointestinal distress, peripheral edema and thrombocytopenia. Patients with MDS also experiences pruritis, nasopharyngitis, and arthralgias. This medication is oral, and administered 25 mg daily days 1–21 every 28 days for multiple myeloma and 10 mg once daily for MDS. The starting dose of lenalidomide is reduced by 50% for patients with renal insufficiency or on dialysis. The only significant interaction is with digoxin, where digoxin levels may increase while receiving lenalidomide. Patients receiving lenalidomide are carefully monitored and taught similar key points as with thalidomide.

CHAPTER SUMMARY

- The immune system is a complex system of cells and chemical mediators that prevents foreign pathogens or cells from invading the body.
- WBCs are active in the surveillance and initiation of inflammatory reactions to specific stimuli. WBCs include neutrophils, which digest foreign material; basophils, which release chemicals to initiate the immune response; mast cells, which are located in the skin and the respiratory and GI tracts; macrophages, which release chemicals to initiate the immune response; and eosinophils, which seem to be active in allergic reactions.
- Lymphocytes include T cells, which are important in modifying the immune response and in protecting the body from nonself cells, and B cells, which produce antibodies to specific antigens. The antibodies stimulate an immune and inflammatory reaction to the antigen and cause its destruction.
- Interferons are produced by WBCs in response to viral invasion and other stimuli. They block viral replication and inhibit tumor cell growth. Interferons are used to treat various malignant and viral diseases.
- Interleukins are chemicals secreted by active WBCs to influence other WBCs.
- Immune modulators may restore depressed immune function, stimulate immune function, stimulate antibody formation, or enhance T-cell response.
- Drugs that suppress the immune system are used to block T-cell activity in organ transplant patients when the immune system tries to destroy the foreign cells, and to treat autoimmune diseases when the immune system is mistakenly trying to destroy self cells.
- The most significant adverse effects of calcineurin inhibitors are hypertension, nephrotoxicity, and neurotoxicity.
- Retinoids alter cell proliferation and differentiation and are used in treatment of leukemia, but resistance is common.
- Patients taking drugs that modify the immune system need protection against infection, injury, and neoplasms because their susceptibility is increased.
- These drugs often cause adverse GI effects; therefore, efforts must be made to maintain nutritional status. A nutritional consultation, supplemental feedings, and small, frequent meals are often necessary.
- Anti-angiogenic agents act by interfering with tumor necrosis factor and development of new blood vessels, and are among the most teratogenic and mutagenic agents used as therapeutic medications.
- Anti-angiogenic require patient monitoring for dose-limiting somnolence, peripheral neuropathy, venous thromboembolism, or neutropenia.

QUESTIONS FOR STUDY AND REVIEW

1. What effects do cytokines have on the immune response?
2. What are interferons and interleukins?
3. Why are interferons used against malignant cells?
4. How do the adverse effects of IL-2 differ from those of interferons?
5. What are the labeled indications for cyclosporine?
6. What are the dose-limiting toxicities of cyclosporine?
7. What are the most common toxicities of the family of retimoid agents?
8. Name two clinical indications for administrations of bacillus calmette Guerin (BCG).
9. What is the most common toxicity limiting clinical use of thalidomide?
10. What special precautions and consenting procedures are required prior to administration of thalidomide?

NEED MORE HELP?

Chapter 54 of the Study Guide to Accompany *Drug Therapy in Nursing*, 4th Edition, contains NCLEX-style questions and other learning activities to reinforce your understanding of the concepts presented in this chapter. For additional information or to purchase the study guide, visit thePoint.

REFERENCES

Abbott, R. A., Whittaker, S. J., Morris, S. L., et al. (2009). Bexarotene therapy for mycosis fungoides and Sézary syndrome. *The British Journal of Dermatology,* 160(6):1299–1307.

Amor, K. T., Ryan, C., Menter, A. (2010). The use of cyclosporine in dermatology: part 1. *Journal of the American Academy of Dermatology,* 63(6):925–946.

Babjuk, M., Oosterlinck, W., Sylvester, R., et al. (2011). EAU guidelines on non-muscle-invasive urothelial carcinoma of the bladder, the 2011 update. *European Urology*, 59(6): 997–1008.

Buchsel, P. C., & DeMeyer, E. S. (2006). Dendritic cells in tumor immunotherapy. *Clinical Journal of Oncology Nursing*, 10(5):629–640.

Buzaid, A. C., & Atkins, M. (2001). Practical guidelines for the management of biochemotherapy-related toxicity in melanoma. *Clinical Cancer Research*, 7(9):2611–2619.

Chapman, J. R. (2011). Chronic calcineurin inhibitor nephrotoxicity—lest we forget. *American Journal of Transplantation*, 11:693–697.

Cho, H. J., & Bhardwaj, N. (2003). Against the self: Dendritic cells versus cancer. *Acta Pathologic, Microbiologica, et Immunologica Scandinavica [APMIS]*, 111(7–8):805–817.

Cuaron, L., & Thompson, J. (2001). The interferons. In P. T. Rieger (Ed.), *Biotherapy: A comprehensive overview* (2nd ed., pp. 125–194). Boston, MA: Jones and Bartlett.

Dereure, O. (2003). Skin reactions related to treatment with anti-cytokines, membrane receptor inhibitors and monoclonal antibodies. *Expert Opinion on Drug Safety*, 2(5):467–473.

Dillman, R. O. (2011). Cancer immunotherapy. *Cancer Biotherapy and Radiopharmaceuticals*, 26(1):1–64.

Einollahi, B., & Teimoori, M. (2011). Cyclosporine trough monitoring. *Iranian Journal of Kidney Diseases*, 5(3):211–212.

Fu, M. R., Anderson, C. M., McDaniel, R., et al. (2002). Patients' perceptions of fatigue in response to biochemotherapy for metastatic melanoma: A preliminary study. *Oncology Nursing Forum*, 29(6):961–966.

Gallini, P. C., Maza, A., Montaudié, H., et al. (2011). Evidence-based recommendations on conventional systemic treatments in psoriasis: systematic review and expert opinion of a panel of dermatologists. *Journal of the European Academy of Dermatology and Venereology*, 25(Suppl 2):2–11.

Gemmill, R., & Idell, C. S. (2003). Biological advances for new treatment approaches. *Seminars in Oncology Nursing*, 19(3):162–168.

Kahan, B. D., Kirken, R. A., & Stepkowski, S. M. (2003). New approaches to transplant immunosuppression. *Transplantation Proceedings*, 35(5):1621–1623.

Kim, M. U., Kim, S. Y., Son, S. M., et al. (2011). A case of tacrolimus-induced encephalopathy after kidney transplantation. *Korean Journal of Pediatrics*, 54(1):40–44.

Lansigan, F., Stearns, D. M., & Foss, F. (2010). Role of denileukin diftitox in the treatment of persistent or recurrent cutaneous T-cell lymphoma. *Cancer Management and Research*, 2:53–59.

Luo, Y., & Prestwich, G. D. (2002). Cancer-targeted polymeric drugs. *Current Cancer Drug Targets*, 2(3):209–226.

Malaguarnera, M., Ferlito, L., Gulizia, G., et al. (2001). Use of interleukin-2 in advanced renal carcinoma: Meta-analysis and review of the literature. *European Journal of Clinical Pharmacology*, 57(4):267–273.

Manoukian, G., & Hagemeister, F. (2009). Denileukin diftitox: a novel immunotoxin. *Expert Opinion on Biological Therapy*, 9(11):1445–1451.

Polovich, M., Whitford, J. M., & Olsen, M. (2010). Chemotherapy and biotherapy guidelines and recommendations for practice (3rd ed.). Pittsburgh, PA: Oncology Nursing Society.

Prommer, E. E., Twycross, R., & Mihalyo, M. (2010). Thalidomide. *Journal of Pain and Symptom Management*, Oct 20, epub ahead of print.

Rieger, P. T. (2001). Patient management. In P. T. Rieger (Ed.), *Biotherapy: A comprehensive overview* (2nd ed., pp. 461–506). Boston, MA: Jones and Bartlett.

Rieger, P. T., & Khuri, F. R. (2001). The retinoids. In P. T. Rieger (Ed.), *Biotherapy: A comprehensive overview* (2nd ed., pp. 407–430). Boston, MA: Jones and Bartlett.

Rogers, J. E., & Yang, D. (2011). Differentiation syndrome in patients with acute promyelocytic leukemia. *Journal of Oncology Pharmacy Practice*, March 7, epub ahead of print.

Schmitt-Hoffmann, A. H., Roos, B., Sauer, J., et al. (2011). Influence of food on the pharmacokinetics of oral alitretinoin (9-cis retinoic acid). *Clinical and Experimental Dermatology*, 36(Suppl 2):18–23.

Sehgal, V. N., & Pahwa, M. P. (2007). Pimecrolimus, yet another intriguing topical immunomodulator. *The Journal of Dermatological Treatment*, 18(3):147–150.

Senner, A. M., Johnston, K., & McLachlan, A. J. (2005). A comparison of peripheral and centrally collected cyclosporine A blood levels in pediatric patients undergoing stem cell transplant. *Oncology Nursing Forum*, 32(1):73–77.

Shintani, Y., Sawada, Y., Inagaki, T., Kohjimoto, Y., Uekado, Y., & Shinka, T. (2007). Intravesical instillation of bacillus Calmette-Guerin for superficial bladder cancer: Study of the mechanism of bacillus Calmette-Guerin immunotherapy. *International Journal of Urology*, 14(2):140–146.

Tang, X. H., & Gudas, L. J. (2011). Retinoids, retinoic acid receptors, and cancer. *Annual Review of Pathology*, 6:345–364.

Triccas, J. A. (2010). Recombinant BCG as a vaccine vehicle to protect against tuberculosis. *Bioengineered Bugs*, 1(2):110–115.

Uchida, A., Yonou, H., Hayashi, E., et al. (2007). Intravesical instillation of Bacille Calmette-Guerin for superficial bladder cancer: Cost effectiveness analysis. *Urology*, 69:275–279.

Van Wieren, A., Kapoor, M., Rao, P., et al. (2010). A new low for an old high: neutropenia induced by levamisole-adulterated cocaine. *Medicine and Health, Rhode Island*, 93(10):320–321.

Yousefi, B., & Azizzadeh, F. (2010). The histopathalogical effects of retinoic acid on the tissues. *Pakistan Journal of Biological Sciences*, 13(19):927–936.

Zeldis, J. B., Knight, R., Hussein, M., et al. (2011). A review of the history, properties, and use of the immunomodulatory compound lenalidomide. *Annals of the New York Academy of Sciences*, 1222:76–82.

Zhang, H. L. (2011). Tacrolimus leukoencephalopathy—is it posterior reversible encephalopathy syndrome? *Pediatric Neurology*, 44(3):359–362.

55

Targeted Therapies

Learning Objectives

At the completion of this chapter the student will:

1. Understand the goals of treatment and the strategies used in targeted therapy.
2. Identify the internal and external molecular targets which are inhibited by drugs in this category.
3. Differentiate mechanisms of action and adverse effects between targeted therapies and traditional chemotherapy drugs.
4. Explain the differences in classifications of monoclonal antibodies: conjugated and nonconjugated, murine derived and human derived.
5. Identify the different routes of administration for the various targeted therapies.
6. Identify core drug knowledge about targeted drugs.
7. Identify core patient variables relevant to targeted drugs.
8. Relate the interaction of core drug knowledge to core patient variables for targeted drugs.
9. Generate a nursing plan of care from the interactions between the core drug knowledge and core patient variables for targeted drugs.
10. Describe nursing interventions to maximize therapeutic effects and minimize adverse effects targeted drugs.
11. Determine key points for patient and family education for targeted drugs.

Key Terms

Epidermal growth factor receptor (EGFR, also known as HER1)
HER2/neu receptor
Monoclonal antibodies
Polyclonal antibodies

Small molecule inhibitors
Tyrosine kinase
Mammalian target of rapamycin (mTOR) inhibitor

Vascular endothelial growth factor (VEGF)

Targeted Therapies

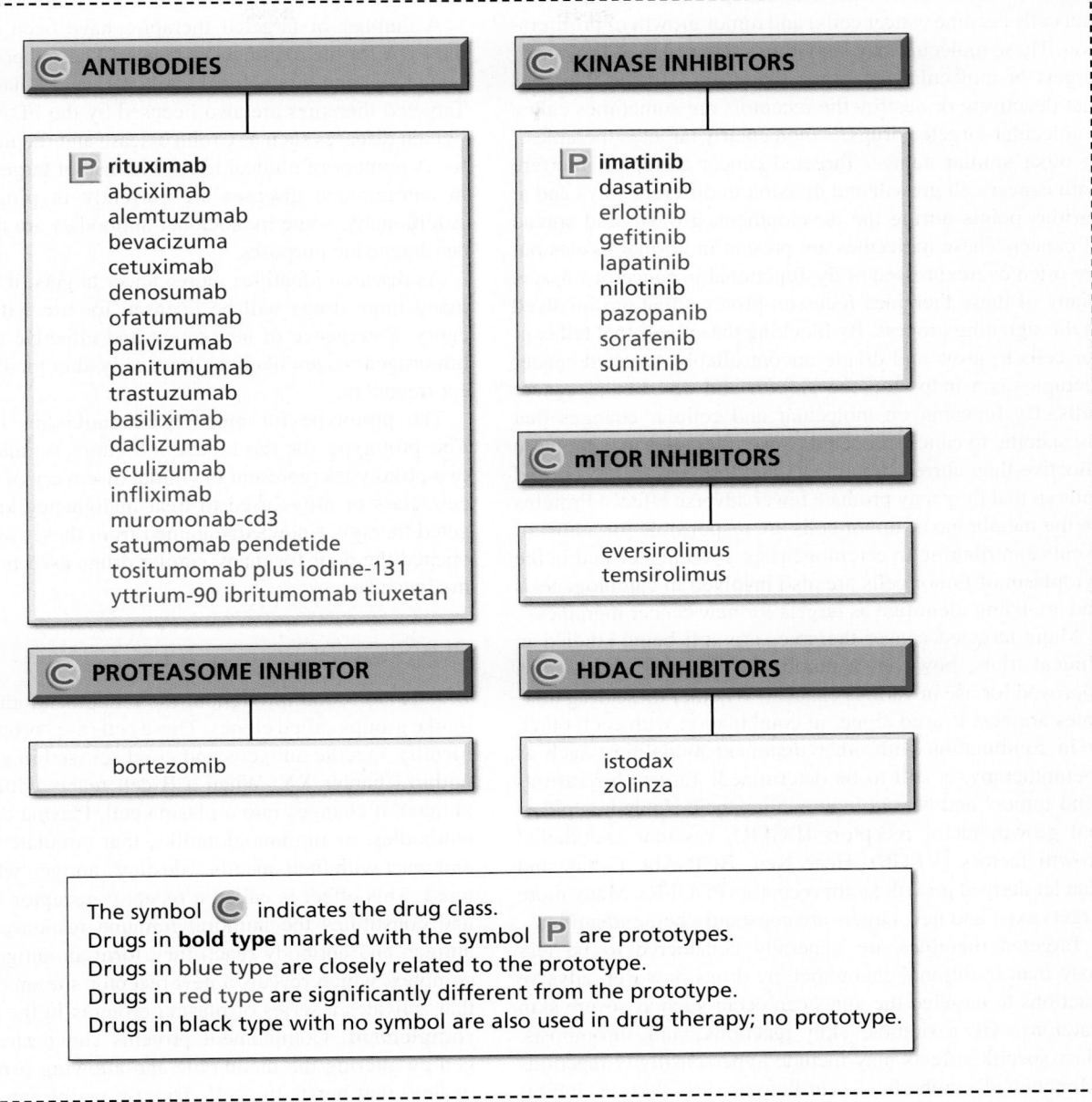

C ANTIBODIES

P rituximab
abciximab
alemtuzumab
bevacizuma
cetuximab
denosumab
ofatumumab
palivizumab
panitumumab
trastuzumab
basiliximab
daclizumab
eculizumab
infliximab
muromonab-cd3
satumomab pendetide
tositumomab plus iodine-131
yttrium-90 ibritumomab tiuxetan

C KINASE INHIBITORS

P imatinib
dasatinib
erlotinib
gefitinib
lapatinib
nilotinib
pazopanib
sorafenib
sunitinib

C mTOR INHIBITORS

eversirolimus
temsirolimus

C PROTEASOME INHIBTOR

bortezomib

C HDAC INHIBITORS

istodax
zolinza

The symbol **C** indicates the drug class.
Drugs in **bold type** marked with the symbol **P** are prototypes.
Drugs in blue type are closely related to the prototype.
Drugs in red type are significantly different from the prototype.
Drugs in black type with no symbol are also used in drug therapy; no prototype.

Targeted cancer therapies are new types of drugs used to treat cancer. Targeted cancer therapies interfere with specific extracellular and intracellular molecules and receptor sites involved in carcinogenesis (the process by which normal cells become cancer cells) and tumor growth or proliferation. These molecules are sometimes referred to as molecular targets or molecular receptors; therefore, targeted therapies that deactivate or destroy the receptors are sometimes called "molecular-targeted drugs," "molecularly targeted therapies," or other similar names. Targeted cancer therapies interfere with cancer cell growth and division in different ways and at various points during the development, growth, and spread of cancer. These molecules are present in normal tissues but are often overexpressed or dysfunctional in cancerous tissue. Many of these therapies focus on proteins that are involved in the signaling process. By blocking the signals that tell cancer cells to grow and divide uncontrollably, targeted cancer therapies can help stop the growth and division of cancer cells. By focusing on molecular and cellular changes that are specific to cancer, targeted cancer therapies may be more effective than current treatments and less harmful to normal cells so that they may produce fewer adverse effects. Proteins on the membrane of tumor cells are responsible for a host of events contributing to carcinogenesis. Proteins located in the cytoplasm of tumor cells are also involved in carcinogenesis and are being identified as targets for new cancer therapies.

Many targeted cancer therapies are still being studied in clinical trials; however, a number of these drugs are now approved for use in various cancers. Whether these drug therapies are best if used alone, in combination with each other, or in combination with other treatment modalities, such as chemotherapy, is still to be determined. Targets for various solid tumors and hematologic malignancies include; epidermal growth factor receptors (EGFR), vascular endothelial growth factors (VEGF), Her2 Neu, BCR-Abl, C-Kit, and platelet derived growth factor receptor (PDGFR). Many more targets exist and new targets are constantly being identified.

Targeted therapies are generally considered to be less toxic than traditional chemotherapy drugs however, adverse reactions to targeted therapies can occur such as severe skin reactions, GI toxicities, skin reactions, and thrombosis. Class specific effects may include hypersensitivity reactions (Monoclonal antibodies), cardiotoxicities (kinase inhibitors), and vasculitis (kinase inhibitors). Drugs considered targeted therapies are often metabolized by cytochrome P-450 enzymes. This may increase the risk of drug interactions and patients should be carefully evaluated and monitored to avoid problems.

Two other important considerations with targeted therapies include cost and patientadherance. These therapies tend to be costly and careful analysis of cost benefit ratio must be considered. Patient adherance with the oral targeted therapy regimens is an important area of interest. Tumor resistance to targeted therapies has occurred in select tumor types and is an area of concern and investigation, with particular attention to resistance emergence related to consistent regimen adherence. Traditional treatments for cancer in particular have been administered by the health care provider intravenously in a hospital or clinic setting making it easier to ensure correct dosing and timing of therapy is followed.

A number of targeted therapies have been approved by the FDA for the treatment of cancer. These therapies include polyclonal and monoclonal antibodies and kinase inhibitors. Targeted therapies are also licensed by the FDA for nonmalignant diseases such as Crohn disease and rheumatoid arthritis. A number of clinical trials with use of targeted therapies in autoimmune diseases are currently in progress (REF). Additionally, some monoclonal antibodies are used for cancer diagnostic purposes.

As research identifies more cancer targets, it is likely that many more drugs will be licensed for use within this category. Emergence of new target and effective disruption in tumorogenesis are likely to drastically alter the future of cancer treatment.

The prototype for monoclonal antibodies is rituximab. The prototype for the kinase inhibitors is imatinib. These two prototyoes represent the initial discovery of this exciting new class of drugs used to treat malignancy known as targeted therapy. Knowledge gained from these two prototypes opened the door for many similar drugs used in a variety of malignancies.

PHYSIOLOGY

B cells are found throughout the reticuloendothelial system in like groups called clones. These cells are "programmed" to identify specific antigens and are discussed in greater detail within Chapter XX. When a B cell reacts with its specific antigen, it changes into a plasma cell. Plasma cells produce antibodies, or immunoglobulins, that circulate in the body and react with their specific "destiny" antigen when encountered. This effect is called a receptor–receptor site reaction and constitutes the humoral immune response. When the antigen and antibody react, they form an antigen–antibody complex, which reveals a new receptor site on the antibody that activates a series of plasma proteins in the body called **complement.** Complement proteins can destroy the antigen by altering the membrane and allowing osmotic inflow of fluid that bursts the cell. These proteins can also induce **chemotaxis** (attraction of phagocytic cells to the area) and increase the activity of phagocytes. In addition, they can release histamine, which causes vasodilation, increases blood flow to the area, and brings together all the components of the inflammatory reaction to destroy the antigen. Direct cytotoxicity may also occur when a receptor site is occupied by a ligand other than the normal one. This mechanism is capitalized upon by monoclonal antibody therapy that is intended to disrupt that cell's normal function, growth and replication.

The initial formation of antibodies, called the primary response, takes several days. However, once the response is activated, the B cells form memory cells that, in turn, produce antibodies that are released immediately whenever the antigen is encountered. This process is a lifelong reaction called active immunity. B cells cluster in areas where they are most likely to encounter their specific antigen. For example, airborne antigens meet B cells in the tonsils and upper respiratory tract. Experts believe that most B cells are programmed genetically and are formed before birth. The introduction of a new and unusual antigen can result in widespread disease because the body is unable to recognize the foreign protein and mount an immune response.

PATHOPHYSIOLOGY

Pathophysiologic conditions requiring drug therapy with targeted agents are usually related to abnormal cell surface markers or molecular pathways. The molecular activities governing differentiation, proliferation, and cell death are often impaired in the cells of patients with disease. When the specific surface marker or molecular pathway of fault in a disease is known, it has become possible to administer targeted agents to disrupt or modify that process, redirecting cell activity. In some therapies such as the antineoplastic agents, the goal is to induce cell death, or apoptosis. For others, it may be to redirect the signal transduction or recreate messenger RNA in order to alter the final cell activity. This chapter discussed the monoclonal antibodies that target surface markers and the tyrosine kinase inhibitors that affect internal cell processes for treatment of malignancies, autoimmune disease, transplanted tissue, and other specific pathophysiologic disorders. Table 55.1 provides a summary of selected targeted agents that affect the external and internal molecular signals.

Ⓒ ANTIBODIES

The earliest antibody preparations were general agents directed toward destruction of lymphoid cells (antilymphocyte globulins). They were derived from animals (horses and rabbits) that were injected with human thymocytes (the thymus gland is the source of T cells in humans) and RBCs; the injections stimulated the animal to produce nonspecific immunoglobulin G (IgG) antibodies. The most common preparations were equine antithymocyte globulin (ATG, Atgam), antilymphocyte globulin (ALG), and antilymphocyte serum (ALS). These polyclonal antibodies are so named because they react to more than one antigen. The term *antilymphocyte immunoglobulin* (ALG; lymphocyte immune globulin) implies a product raised against all lymphocytes, and anti thymocyte immunoglobulin (antithymocyte gammaglobulin; antithymocyte globulin; ATG) implies specificity for T cells. Despite what appear to be substantial differences in levels of immune suppression, in clinical practice, these agents show few differences in action and only ATG is currently available. These agents have historically been administered to graft recipients, so that the foreign antibodies directly attack the host's T cells and reduce their circulating number.

Because these agents are derived from nonhuman sources, they have caused the production of atypical antibodies, and individuals easily become resistant to their beneficial effects. Because of production shortages, difficulties in purification, and scientific advances in specific antibody development, these agents are now rarely used and not discussed in detail within this chapter. Instead, targeted antibodies called monoclonal antibodies are used, which suppress one cell subtype or receptor site. Monoclonal antibodies can react with specific tumor receptor sites for diagnosis or treatment of malignancy. As the body of knowledge regarding specific cellular defects with particular diseases grows, so does our ability to develop cell-targeted antibody therapy for abnormal cells, genes, or receptor sites.

Antibody therapy has rapidly progressed in recent years, with increasingly greater specificity of the newly developed agents. Monoclonal antibodies target specific receptor sites of cells, causing varied immunologic effects depending on the cell to which they attach themselves. Each monoclonal antibody has a defined "destiny" target that is expressed on cells and predict the clinical indication. Abiximab (ReoPro) targets the platelet, interfering with platelet aggregation and used extensively in cardiology to reduce coronary thrombus after interventional procedures; whereas trastuzumab is attracted to the her-2-neu receptor that is overexpressed in certain patients with breast cancer. Clinical indications are based upon which diseases are characterized by the presence of unique antigens. Monoclonal antibodies may be created from animal antibodies (almost always murine fused), animal-human antibodies (chimeric), mostly human (humanized), or totally human antibodies. Monoclonal antibodies are named based upon their origin; murine are –momab, chimeric antibodies end in-iximab, humanized are –zumab, and fully human antibodies end with –tumumab (Polovich et al., 2009). The nonhuman antibodies produce more allergic and rejection reactions, caused by human antimurine antibodies (HAMA), which can contraindicate future therapy with a specific monoclonal antibody or any other with a murine component. These antibody responses manifest as allergic or anaphylactic reactions in patients receiving the antibody product. Monoclonal antibodies also may directly target a cell receptor, paralyzing the usual actions by that receptor and its ligands. Alternatively, they can be conjugated, meaning combined with another substance such as radiation or toxic drug that then produces indirect cell destruction as the conjugate infiltrates the cell (Polovich et al., 2009). Because of the rapidly developing practice of using antibodies to target tumor cell receptor sites, the antibody prototype is the monoclonal antitumor antibody called rituximab (Rituxan). Monoclonal antibodies available for use as immunosuppressants are considered significantly different from the prototype, as are the monoclonal antibodies fused to radioactive substances, or those used to highlight a cell for diagnostic purposes. All antibodies can produce allergic reactions, and most administration guidelines suggest premedicating the patient with acetaminophen and diphenhydramine and

TABLE 55.1	Summary of Selected Targeted Agents		
Drug (Trade) Name	**Selected Indications**	**Route and Dosage Range**	**Pharmacokinetics**
ⓒ **Monoclonal Antibodies**			
Ⓟ rituximab (Rituxan)	Relapsed or refactory low-grade or follicular CD20-positive B-cell non-Hodgkin's lymphoma, or multiple myeloma, refractory rheumatoid arthritis	*Adult:* IV, 375 mg/m2 once weekly for four doses *Child:* Safety and efficacy not established	*Onset:* Unknown *Duration:* 3–6 mo after completion of treatment $t_{1/2}$: 59.8 h after first dose, and 174 h after fourth dose
muromonab CD (Orthoclone OKT3)	Acute allograft rejection in renal transplantation, steroid-resistant acute allograft rejection in liver, lung, cardiac, and bone marrow transplantation	*Adult:* IV (bolus only: <1 min), 5 mg/d with diagnosed rejection *Child:* Safety and efficacy not established	*Onset:* Minutes *Duration:* 7 d $t_{1/2}$: 47–100 h
trastuzumab (Herceptin)	All women with breast cancer that overexpresses the her2 neu receptor. It may also be administered with adjuvant chemotherapy in women without active disease, but who are at risk of relapse.		*Onset:* Slow *Duration:* Days $t_{1/2}$: 2–9 d
bevacizumab (Avastin)	In combination for initial treatment of colorectal cancer; in combination with chemotherapy for management of metastatic or relapsed colorectal cancer, metastatic non-small-cell lung cancer, metastatic breast cancer, metastatic renal cell carcinoma. Given as a single agent for refractory ovarin cancer or glioblastoma multiforme.	*Always administered as IV infusion over 90 min first week, then if tolerated, over 60 min in subsequent dose.* *For initial treatment of colorectal cancer:* 5 mg/kg or 10 mg/kg with irinotecan, fluorouracil, and leukovorin. *For metastatic colorectal cancer:* 10 mg/kg with oxaliplatin, flourouracil and folinic acid. *Non-small-cell lung cancer:* IV infusion 15 mg/kg every 3 wk. *Breast cancer:* 10 mg/kg every 14 d in conjunction with paclitaxel. *Ovarian cancer:* 15 mg/kg every 3 wk. *Renal cell carcinoma:* 10 mg/kg every 2 wk in conjunction with interferon alia. *Glioblastoma multiforme:* 10 mg/kg every 3 wk *Pediatric solid tumors:* 10 mg/kg in combination with chemotherapy or 15 mg/kg every 28 d.	*Onset:* Slow *Duration:* 100 d $t_{1/2}$: 20 d
cetuximab (Erbitux)	As a single agent or in combination with irinotecan for treatment of metastatic colorectal cancer where KRAS wild-type cytogenetics are verified; as a single agent or in combination with radiation therapy for locally invasive squamous cell carcinoma of the head and neck	Initial loading IV dose of 400 mg/kg over 120 min (not exceeding 5 mL/min), followed by IV weekly 250 mg/kg administered over 60 min. In all circumstances, patients are observed for an additional 60 min for infusion reactions.	*Onset:* 3–12 h *Duration:* 24 h to 3 wk $t_{1/2}$: 75–188 h
ⓒ **Kinase Inhibitors**			
Ⓟ imatinib (Gleevec)	Philadelphia positive (PH+) CML: gastrointestinal stromal tumor	PO 400–800 mg daily	*Onset:* Unknown *Peak:* 2–4 h *Duration:* Unknown
dasatinib (Sprycel)	PH+ CML	PO 140 mg daily	*Onset:* Unknown *Peak:* Unknown *Duration:* Unknown
nilotinib (Tasigna)	PH+ CML	PO 300–400 mg BID	*Onset:* Unknown *Peak:* 3 h *Duration:* Unknown
erlotinib (Tarceva)	Non-small cell lung cancer and pancreatic cancer	PO 100–150 mg daily	*Onset:* Unknown *Peak:* 4 h *Duration:* Unknown

Drug (Trade) Name	Selected Indications	Route and Dosage Range	Pharmacokinetics
gefitinib (Iressa)	Non-small cell lung cancer	PO 200 mg daily	Onset: Unknown Peak: 3–7 h Duration: Unknown
lapatinib (Tykerb)	Breast cancer	PO 1250–1500 mg daily	Onset: Unknown Peak: 4 h Duration: Unknown
sorafenib (Nexavar)	Hepatocellular and renal carcinoma	PO 400 mg BID	Onset: Unknown Peak: 3 h Duration: Unknown
sunitinib (Sutent)	GIST, renal carcinoma, pancreatic neuroendocrine tumors	PO 37.5–50 mg daily	Onset: Unknown Peak: Unknown Duration: Unknown
pazopanib (Votrient)	Renal carcinoma, pancreatic neuroendocrine tumors, subependymal giant cell astrocytoma associated with tubous sclerosis		Onset: Unknown Peak: Unknown Duration: Unknown
temsirolimus (Torisel)	Renal cell carcinoma	IV 25 mg once weekly	Onset: Unknown Peak: Unknown Duration: Unknown
eversirolimus (Afinitor)	Renal carcinoma, pancreatic neuroendocrine tumors, subependymal giant cell astrocytoma associated with tubous sclerosis	PO 10 mg daily	Onset: Unknown Peak: 1–2 h Duration: Unknown
bortezomib (Velcade)	Multiple myeloma, mantle cell lymphoma	IVP 1.3 mg/m2	Onset: Unknown Peak: Unknown Duration: Unknown
zolinza (Vorinostat)	Cutaneous T-cell lymphoma	PO 400 mg once daily	Onset: Unknown Peak: Unknown Duration: Unknown
istodax (Romidepsin)	Cutaneous T-cell lymphoma	IV 14 mg/m2 day 1, 8, 15 repeated every 28 d	Onset: Unknown Peak: Unknown Duration: Unknown $t_{1/2}$: 3 h

TABLE 55.1 Summary of Selected Targeted Agents (continued)

having emergency equipment, corticosteroids, and adrenaline (epinephrine) readily available. All antibody products also carry the risk of cross-reactivity with other vaccine products, necessitating careful consideration before administering any other antibody or vaccine to these patients after monoclonal antibody therapy.

Nursing Management of the Patient Receiving [P] Rituximab

Core Drug Knowledge

Pharmacotherapeutics

Rituximab has historically been used to treat CD20-positive B-cell malignancies such as B-cell leukemias, chronic lymphocytic leukemia, non-Hodgkin's lymphoma, and some multiple myeloma. Since the recognition of CD20 positivity among all B-cell malignancies, the application of rituximab exceeds the specific licensed indications. Recent research advances have demonstrated the activity of CD20 positive cells in autoimmune diseases, reflected in new licensed indication for treatment of rheumatoid arthritis, and use with other therapy-refractory autoimmune disorders (Perosa et al., 2010).

Pharmacokinetics

Rituximab binds to the B-lymphocytes which are expressing CD20 surface marker, and because of individual tumor variability, the blood concentrations and duration of action will vary as well. Our greatest experience with this agent is with non-Hodgkin's lymphoma, and pharmacologic information is based upon these patients. Rituximab is given as a slow IV infusion at 375 mg/m² weekly for 4 to 8 weeks, with a possible additional 4 weeks for responsive patients. Although initially used as a single agent therapy, Rituximab is now usually given in conjunction with standard chemotherapy regimens. The serum half-life is 59.8 hours after the first infusion (375 mg/m²) and 174 hours after the fourth infusion, although the drug is detectable for 3 to 6 months after treatment is completed. The actual drug infusion is calculated based on the total dose the patient is to receive, not exceeding 50 mg/h for the first half-hour of the initial infusion. If no reactions are apparent after 30 minutes, the dose may be escalated every 30 minutes by 50 mg/h until a maximum infusion rate of 400 mg/h is reached. All subsequent infusions begin at 100 mg/h and can be escalated by 100-mg/h increments every 30 minutes until the maximum infusion rate of 400 mg/h is reached. The average infusion time for routine periodic rituximab when the patient has no history of reactions is about 90 minutes. Patients with large cell lymphoma receive this agent concomitant with chemotherapy, but with nonprogressing low grade lymphoma, it is given at the conclusion of chemotherapy cycles. Prolonged maintenance therapy for patients with responding tumors is currently under investigation (Vidal et al., 2009).

- In chronic lymphocytic leukemia, rituximab is administered as a loading dose of 375 mg/m² prior to fludarabine and cyclophosphamide on the same day, then 500 mg/m² at the beginning of cycles 2 to 6 (Biogen Idec, Inc and Genentech, Inc, 2010).
- Recently, rituximab has been licensed in combination with methotrexate for treatment of rheumatoid arthritis. It is administered as two- 1,000 mg IV infusions separated by two week, given every 24 weeks or based upon clinical evaluation. In this setting, the prescribed premedications are only methylprednisilone 100 mg or equivalent corticosteroid given 30 minutes prior to rituximab infusion.

See also Table 55.1, summary of selected targeted agents.

Pharmacodynamics

Rituximab is a type of monoclonal antibody that binds specifically to the CD20 antigen found on the surface of normal and malignant B lymphocytes and causes cell lysis. The CD20 antigen is expressed in more than 90% of B-cell non-Hodgkin's lymphoma cells but not on normal bone marrow cells, pre-B cells, or other normal tissues. The CD20 antigen is also expressed excessively in patients with specific autoimmune disorders. One section of the drug binds to CD20 antigen and another section of the drug calls other immune activators to assist in cell lysis. Cell lysis is possibly caused by complement-dependent cytotoxicity or antibody-dependent cytotoxicity (Biogen Idec, Inc. & Genentech, Inc., 2010). Decreased IgG and IgM serum levels are evident for 5 to 11 months after the last infusion. This direct cytotoxicity is believed to be the mechanism of acute tumor lysis syndrome that may occur 24–72 hours after administration. It is viewed as a positive clinical sign of antitumor activity but can cause fatal electrolyte disturbances and renal failure if not closely monitored and treated. The significance of this complication has resulted in a special warning label on the product prescribing information (see below).

Contraindications and Precautions

The only contraindication to rituximab therapy is type 1 hypersensitivity or anaphylaxis to murine proteins or any components of the product. Severe and fatal reactions

within 24 hours of rituximab infusion have been reported, most often with the first infusion. A Black Box warning to observe for reactions is included in the prescribing information. Safety in children or in pregnant or lactating women has not been tested. Experience with older adults has developed considerably since the initial licensing and thought to produce good clinical effects without excessive toxicity (Barni et al., 2008).

Adverse Effects

Infusion-related effects reportedly occur in 80% of patients within 30 minutes to 2 hours after beginning the first rituximab infusion, although only 7% have severe reactions (Biogen-Idec, Inc and Genentech, Inc, 2010). Although reactions are less common with subsequent infusions (40%), its severity is unchanged. With several years experience in administration of this agent and perfection of pre-medication regimens, recent reaction rates may be less frequent, but literature updating these data were not available. Reactions may be related to dose because most of the reaction dissipates when the infusion rate is slowed or interrupted. The most common infusion-related reactions include fever, flushing, chills, and rigors. Other reported symptoms include nausea, urticaria, fatigue, headache, pruritus, bronchospasm, dyspnea, hypotension, angioedema, dyspnea, rhinitis, vomiting, flushing, pain at disease sites, and throat swelling (Castells, 2008). Mucocutaneous reactions associated with the allergic response can be severe. Respiratory distress and hypotension are reportedly more common when tumors are larger than 10 cm. As many as 16% of patients experience asthenia on retreatment. Other possible effects include tachycardia, arrhythmias, anorexia, peripheral edema, dizziness, and depression. Bone marrow effects such as leukopenia, thrombocytopenia, and anemia can be present for up to 30 days after the last dose. A rare but potentially fatal neurologic adverse effect called progressive multifocal leukoencephalopathy that can cause seizures, coma, or death is associated with rituximab infusion (Ram et al., 2009). Initially it was thought to occur only in conjunction with JC virus (a type of human polyomavirus); but now it has been reported in a greater variety of patients without this risk factor (Perosa, 2010).

About 1% of patients develop antibodies to human antimurine or chimeric antibodies, producing severe allergic reactions and limiting their future treatment with any antibody (Biogen Idec, Inc and Genentech, Inc, 2010).

Drug Interactions

Concomitant vaccines of any type are not recommended because of theorized potential interactions; no research has been done on these potential interactions (Biogen Idec, Inc and Genentech, Inc, 2010).

Assessment of Relevant Core Patient Variables

Health Status

Assess for pre-existing cardiac and respiratory problems. Rituximab should be used cautiously in patients with

RITUXIMAB FOR TREATMENT OF NON-HODGKIN'S LYMPHOMA

James Miller is a 54-year-old man recently diagnosed with low-grade follicular lymphoma. Physicians consider his tumor pathology and decide that the best therapy is an outpatient biochemotherapy regimen of rituximab with cyclophosphamide, doxorubicin, Oncovin, and prednisone (R-CHOP). He has been instructed to make certain he has a driver to take him home the day he receives the biochemotherapy. Before starting chemotherapy, extensive laboratory tests (CBC, serum metabolic panel with magnesium, phosphate, uric acid) and diagnostic tests (chest and abdomen computed tomography, bone marrow aspiration, and MUGA scan of the heart) are performed to assess baseline organ function. Adequate renal function is confirmed. You obtain the necessary premedications: diphenhydramine and a 5-HT$_3$ blocker antiemetic. The dexamethasone that is usually administered with chemotherapy can be omitted, because the patient is receiving corticosteroids with his regimen. However, you know that additional follow-up doses of corticosteroids should be prescribed.

1. When starting the rituximab infusion, what rate is set, and how quickly and in what increments is the rate titrated?
2. What are symptoms of rituximab-related infusion reaction?
3. How is an infusion reaction managed?
4. How long after infusion of rituximab is it possible for a reaction to occur?
5. Will this patient be able to receive future doses of rituximab if he has an infusion reaction?

---

pre-existing cardiac conditions such as arrhythmias or coronary artery disease because ventricular tachycardia, supraventricular tachycardia, angina, hypotension, and hypertension are potential adverse effects, which are all most often associated with infusion reaction syndrome. Interstitial pneumonitis and alveolar hemorrhage have been reported infrequently, but require careful monitoring in high risk patients with pre-existing pulmonary disease or tumors larger than 10 cm in size (Heresi et al., 2008).

Assess for other concurrent drug therapy use before giving rituximab. Rituximab has such potential for infusion reactions that concomitantly administering other agents that may cause severe allergic or anaphylactic reactions should be avoided during infusion and within 2 hours before or after infusion. Agents to avoid include amphotericin, blood products, or first doses of antibiotics.

Consider the serum lactate dehydrogenase (LDH) level, which often reflects the severity and extensiveness of tumor burden. Patients with high LDH values are at highest risk for developing tumor lysis syndrome.

Life Span and Gender
Consider the patient's age. Rituximab is not recommended for use in children or in pregnant or lactating women.

Experience with elderly patients is limited; thus, careful evaluation for contraindications is strongly recommended before starting therapy with this agent.

Environment
Be aware of the environment in which rituximab will be administered. Rituximab is usually given in the ambulatory care oncology clinic, although patients with specific risk factors for cardiac or pulmonary adverse effects may be admitted to the hospital for the first dose.

Nursing Diagnoses and Outcomes

• Altered Comfort related to fever, chills, or headache
Desired outcome: *Symptoms will be abrogated with premedications or relieved with mild analgesics or antipyretics.*
• Potential Altered Cardiac Output related to drug infusion
Desired outcome: *Cardiac symptoms will not occur.*
• Potential Alteration in Nutrition (fluids and electrolytes) because of cytotoxicity and tumor lysis syndrome
Desired outcome: *Normal fluid and electrolyte balance will be maintained throughout the treatment period.*
• Potential Impaired Oxygenation caused by infusion-related adverse effects
Desired outcome: *The patient will maintain a normal breathing pattern, oxygen saturation will be adequate, and adventitious breath sounds will be absent.*

Planning and Intervention
Maximizing Therapeutic Effects
Mix rituximab in normal saline or dextrose solutions in a plastic bag, not in a glass container. The antibody sticks to glass, diminishing the amount of drug administered.

Minimizing Adverse Effects
Because infusion-related adverse effects are common, many clinicians administer premedications to reduce their severity. Premedications often include antipyretics (e.g., acetaminophen) and antihistamines (e.g., diphenhydramine and ranitidine). If patients experience infusion-related adverse effects, stop rituximab until symptoms resolve, then restart it at half the dose that produced adverse effects. Subsequent infusions should begin slowly and can be escalated in the same manner, with temporary discontinuation if infusion effects recur. Patients are usually observed in the ambulatory area for several hours after the initial dose (Chung, 2008).

For patients with hypertension, all antihypertensive agents are usually held for 12 hours before rituximab administration and for 12 to 24 hours afterward. Patients with cardiac or pulmonary risk factors should have continuous cardiac monitoring and frequent vital sign assessment. Stop the infusion at the first sign of adverse effects, which may worsen before resolving. To reduce the risk of recurrence, medications such as nitrates or magnesium can be administered. After symptoms have resolved, resume the infusion at a slower infusion rate, with continuous monitoring.

Providing Patient and Family Education

- Teach patients and families about the purpose of the drug and common adverse effects. Instruct patients to notify the prescriber if they begin to experience adverse effects.
- Assure patients that they will be closely monitored while receiving rituximab. Doing so may require prolonged visits in the clinic, even after the infusion is complete, or frequent follow-up visits after initial therapy to permit monitoring clinical and laboratory parameters for tumor lysis syndrome.
- Ambulatory patients returning home after therapy including rituximab are advised to consume large amounts of water to enhance renal excretion of tumor lysis products as well as to report any unusual symptoms or decreased voiding.
- Because immunologic effects persist for many weeks or months, instruct patients to use birth control for 12 months after completing treatment and to avoid breast-feeding for the same amount of time.

MEMORY CHIP

P Rituximab

- Binds specifically to CD20 antigen on the surface of malignant B lymphocytes and causes cell lysis.
- Used in non-Hodgkin's lymphoma
- Major contraindication: Patients with hepatitis C, major infection, JC virus, renal dysfunction, or cardiac dysrhythmias, may experience worsening of their condition while receiving rituximab. It is administered cautiously to these patients. Live vaccines are contraindicated for patients receiving rituximab.
- Most common adverse effects: infusion-related effects (fever, flushing, chills, and rigors)
- Most serious adverse effects: respiratory distress and hypotension (more common when tumors are larger than 10 cm)
- **Life span alert: Use birth control during therapy and for 1 year afterward and avoid breast-feeding during this time; use with caution in older adults.**
- Maximizing therapeutic effects: Administer in saline or dextrose stored in plastic bags, not glass.
- Minimizing adverse effects: Premedicate patient with other drug therapies.
- Most important patient education: Instruct patient to notify nurse of adverse effects.
- **Black box warning: Fatal infusion reactions have been reported and it is unclear if this relates to hypersensitivity or acute tumor lysis. When acute reactions including angioedema, hypotension, bronchospasm, or respiratory distress occur, the infusion should be immediately stopped and supportive measures instituted. In some cases, rituximab may be resumed after additional premedications and slowed infusion rate. Severe mucocutaneous reactions such as Stevens-Johnson syndrome have been reported. Severe skin reactions warrant immediate discontinuation of the drug. Progressive multifocal leukoencephalopathy (PML) is a rare but potentially fatal neurologic infiltration with lymphocytes. Neurologic symptoms indicate the need to discontinue the drug until diagnostic tests can validate PML.**

Ongoing Assessment and Evaluation

Given the high rate of infusion reactions after the first dose, patients require premedication and close monitoring of vital signs for all rituximab infusions, unless no reactions have occurred.

Drugs Closely Related to P Rituximab

Monoclonal antibodies that are considered closely related to rituximab are those that target a specific receptor site overexpressed by tumors. These agents vary widely in their clinical effects and adverse effects and trastuzumab, bevacizumab, cetuximab, panitumumab, alemtuzumab, and ofatumumab.

Trastuzumab

Trastuzumab (Herceptin) is a humanized monoclonal antibody that targets cells overexpressing the HER2 protein. This protein is overexpressed in as many as 25% to 30% of breast cancers (Murphy & Fornier, 2010). Patients are tested at the time of diagnosis or disease recurrence for amplification of HER2/neu or p185-HER2 protein. Trastuzumab is indicated in all patients with HER2-expressing tumors, even after total tumor resection, who are receiving adjuvant therapy. Patients whose breast cancer cells overexpress this protein then are clinically evaluated for eligibility based on their ability to tolerate the expected adverse effects. A focused cardiopulmonary physical examination, in addition to a test of cardiac function (echocardiogram or MUGA scan), screens patients for adequate cardiovascular reserve or for lung diseases that predispose the patient to adverse effects that have been defined as potentially life threatening in the Black Box warning in the prescribing information. Patients treated previously or concurrently with anthracyclines (e.g., doxorubicin, epirubicin), cyclophosphamide, or radiation to the chest have enhanced risk for the most common cardiac toxicity—chronic heart failure (CHF). CHF with or without persistent cardiomyopathy occurs most commonly as reversible CHF that occurs hours to days after a dose of trastuzumab. Although usually self-limiting, it is a relative indication for discontinuing trastuzumab therapy, especially if independent risk factors such as older age, heavy pretreatment with anthracyclines, or chest irradiation are present (Fiuza, 2009). Pulmonary toxicity may overlap with cardiac symptoms, making it difficult to tell which is which. Infusion-related allergic reactions and cases of acute lung injury have been known to occur. Taxanes have also been reported to increase serum blood levels of trastuzumab that may enhance toxicities. Other clinical effects include suppression of bone marrow function (especially anemia and leukopenia), diarrhea, and rare nephrotic syndrome or acute pneumonitis/respiratory distress syndrome.

Trastuzumab is administered as an initial loading dose of 4 mg/kg over 90 minutes, with subsequent weekly doses of 2 mg/kg over 30 minutes. The clinical benefit of prolonged therapy (beyond planned chemotherapy dosing) is currently being studied to ascertain whether disease-free survival can be extended, because patients who overexpress the HER2 protein have a high risk of relapse (Iwata, 2009).

Bevacizumab

Early in 2004, the Food and Drug Administration (FDA) approved licensing of bevacizumab (Avastin), the first monoclonal antibody to target the natural protein VEGF that is responsible for stimulation of new blood vessel formation. Although new blood vessels are important for all cell growth, malignant cells are notoriously more dependent on a large blood supply for their survival. Technically a monoclonal antibody, bevacizumab was the first agent licensed specifically for its antiangiogenesis properties. It is a humanized monoclonal antibody that binds to VEGF so that it is unable to attach to its receptor site on cells. Bevacizumab is licensed for use as a single agent or in combination with chemotherapy for refractory or metastatic tumors of the colon/rectum, kidney, nonsmall cell lung, and glioblastoma. Intravitreal bevacizumab application for treatment of chronic progressive macular degeneration has shown promise in improving vision, but is not yet commercially available for this use (Schmucker et al, 2010).

Bevacizumab is administered at a dosage of 5 mg/kg over 90 minutes for two weeks in initial treatment of metastatic colorectal cancer. It may also be administered as 10 mg/kg every two weeks or 15 mg/kg every three weeks. Dosages in other solid tumor malignancies range from 10 mg/kg every two weeks inc onjunction with chemotherapy to 15 mg/kg every three weeks for refractory glioblastoma. The drug is light sensitive and should be covered during administration. As with all monoclonal antibodies, allergic reactions have been reported, and careful monitoring during the initial minutes of the infusion is recommended.

The most common adverse effects of bevacizumab have been asthenia, headache, hypertension, anorexia, mouth sores, diarrhea, minor bleeding, leukopenia, and proteinuria. Hypertensive crises and thromboembolic events have occurred with a frequency rate of 2% to 18%, so this agent is rarely used in patients with a previous history of uncontrolled hypertension, or central nervous system metastases that may bleed (Mir, Mouthon, Alexandre, et al., 2007; Zangari et al, 2009). In patients with non-small-cell lung cancer, life-threatening hemoptysis has occurred, warranting a special warning to prescribers. Bevacizumab may also be contraindicated for use in other patients at high risk for life-threatening hemorrhage. A few isolated reports have also described the occurrence of nasal septal perforation with bevacizumab, although the incidence is less than 1%. Serious but infrequent complications described in a Black Box warning in the prescribing information include intestinal perforation and wound dehiscence. Patients with a higher risk of this complication or those with abdominal pain should not receive bevacizumab. Wound dehiscence has also occurred, even outside the context of leukopenia, so the agent is not recommended for use within 28 days before or after a surgical procedure (Hapani, et al., 2009).

Cetuximab

Cetuximab (Erbitux) is a chimeric monoclonal antibody, licensed early in 2004, that targets the EGRF site of both malignant and normal tissues. Competitive binding of this site with this monoclonal antibody can deprive cells of cytokines and ligands that are necessary for cellular growth and metabolism. Certain tumor cells overexpress EGFR, often connoting a poorer prognosis, and are more reliant on activation of this receptor, thus making them prone to apoptosis when the receptor is blocked. The downstream effects of EGFR competitive binding include inhibition of cell differentiation and proliferation, inhibitions of endothelial growth factors such as VEGF, inhibition of matrix metalloproteinases (MMPs), and induction of apoptosis that enhances mutant cell death (Lurje & Lenz, 2009; Martinelli et al., 2009). As our understanding of the biology of this drug has advanced, we have recognized that there are two different presentations of the k-ras gene- kras- wild-type and k-ras mutant. Patients with k-ras wild-type gene have a significantly higher clinical response rate to EGFR inhibition, and the drug labeling now reflects that patients with metastatic colorectal cancer should have k-ras tumor testing, and only be offered therapy with cetuximab if their tumor is k-ras wild-type (Fakih, 2010).

The FDA has licensed cetuximab for use (1) as a single agent, (2) in combination with irinotecan to treat colorectal cancer previously refractory or intolerant to irinotecan, and (3) as either a single agent or in combination with radiation therapy in patients with locoregional squamous cell carcinoma of the head and neck (Imclone, Inc & Bristol-Myers Squibb, 2010). Antitumor response rates in heavily pretreated patients with colorectal cancer approximate 20%. EGRF is also overexpressed in multiple other solid tumor malignancies, but studies to date have not shown adequate clinical response to warrant new indications for this agent. Although the colorectal cancer indication stipulates that patients must overexpress EGRF receptor tumors, immunohistochemistry testing in these patients is no longer required because response rates have not been associated with receptor status. Patients with squamous cell head and neck cancer have demonstrated a 10% to 15% response to cetuximab as a single agent, and significantly enduring (~30-month) responses of 30% to a cetuximab–radiation combination.

Cetuximab is administered as a 2-hour loading dose of 400 mg/m², followed by a 1-hour weekly infusion of 250 mg/m², and is well tolerated by most recipients. When given with radiation therapy, the first dose is administered a week before the start of radiotherapy. The most common adverse effect, occurring in 85%–90% of patients, is an acne-like rash with dry or cracking skin that can be a dose-limiting toxicity if it becomes infected (Tan & Chan, 2009). A severe infusion-related reaction with bronchospasm, stridor, urticaria, and hypotension has been reported in 3% of patients except in specific geographic regions where the severe reaction rate may be as high as 25% (Chung, 2008). Potentially fatal interstitial lung disease has been reported, but occurrence is extremely infrequent (Peerzada et al, 2010; Hoag et al, 2009). Significant hypomagnesemia that begins within two weeks of starting treatment and may persist for up to 8 weeks after treatment conclusion has been recognized as a manifestation of renal tubular injury (Imclone, Inc & Bristol-Myers Squibb, 2010). Safety of this agent in children, pregnant or lactating women, and the elderly has not been established. An in-line filter is used for administration.

Panitumumab

Panitumumab (Vectibix) is a fully human monoclonal antibody that binds to the ligand-binding site of the extracellular domain of the EGFR, causing effects similar to cetuximab (Martinelli et al., 2009). This agent has been licensed for use in patients with metastatic colorectal cancer that has progressed on or following fluoropyrimidine-, oxaliplatin-, and irinotecan-containing regimens. This agent is administered as 6 mg/kg diluted in 100 mL and given intravenously over sixty minutes every two weeks. Infusional reactions are rare because of the human origin of this antibody, although other adverse effects of EGFR inhibition such as rash, hypomagnesemia, and interstitial pneumonitis are similar to those seen with other EGFR antagonists.

Alemtuzumab

Alemtuzumab (Campath 1-H) is humanized monoclonal antibody directed against the CD52 cell surface antigen of the lymphocytic cells of patients with B- and T-cell chronic lymphocytic leukemia (CLL). This medication is indicated as single-agent first-line therapy all patients with CLL having 17p deletion in at least 20% of the malignant cell line, or for patients over 70 years of age even without 17p deletion. It is also acceptable second-line therapy in alkylating-agent or fludarabine-refractory chronic leukemias or low-grade lymphoma because many of these diseases are histopathologically difficult to differentiate from one another (Hallek et al, 2008). It is administered as a daily 2-hour infusion with dose escalation until toxicity is reached; then therapy is begun three times weekly on alternate days. The first dose is 3 mg, and when this dose is tolerated with minimal toxicity, the dose is increased to 10 mg daily, until tolerated. Once 10 mg per day is tolerable, the patient is given the planned maintenance dose of 30 mg three times a week for a 12-week course (Bayer Healthcare Pharmaceuticals, 2009). More recent studies with a broader range of hematologic malignancies, including the peripheral T-cell lymphomas and adult T-cell leukemia, have shown equivalent efficacy with reduced adverse effects when this agent is administered subcutaneously in the same dose and frequency of administration (Moccia & Ghielmini, 2008). The most common adverse effects are related to lymphopenia and infections associated with suppressed lymphocytes (e.g., *Pneumocystis jerivichi* or *cytomegalovirus*). Prophylactic trimethoprim-sulfamethoxazole DS twice daily three times per week is used to protect against *pneumocystis jirovechi*, and famciclovir 250 mg twice daily is taken as herpes virus prophylaxis. Patients are at risk for cytomegalovirus (CMV), but the approach to prophylaxis varies with the patient's past

history of CMV, and their total lymphocyte count. Other bone marrow components may also be suppressed, and infusion-related allergic reactions may also occur, although they are less frequent with SC administration. Injection site erythema and edema are transient, becoming less severe after a few weeks. Lymphocyte counts can be monitored weekly to determine the need to discontinue therapy early, and many patients receive antimicrobial prophylaxis against viruses (acyclovir) or *Pneumocystis* species (e.g., sulfamethoxazole-trimethoprim) (Morrison, 2009).

Ofatumumab

Ofatumumab (Arzerra™) is a fully human monoclonal antibody licensed by the FDA in 2009, and indicated for fludarabine-resistant CD20 positive chronic lymphocytic leukemia. Its use in rituximab-refractory non-hodgkins lymphoma has also shown considerable promise (Zhang, 2009). It binds to a variable epitope of the CD20 molecule, creates direct antibody cytotoxicity through complement activation, and disassociates more slowly, perhaps conferring benefit even rituximab does not control CD20 growth. It appears to even have affinity for cells that have low CD20 expression (Ostenborg, 2010). Like other monoclonal antibodies causing infusional reactions and antibody-induced cytotoxicity, patients receive premedication with acetaminophen, diphenhydramine, and corticosteroids 30 minutes prior to administration, and gradual infusion rate escalation as tolerated. It is administered as progressive dose escalation starting at 300 mg for the initial dose, followed one week later at 2000 mg weekly for seven doses, then 2000 mg every four weeks for four doses (GlaxoSmithKline, 2010). The most common adverse effects are related to leukocyte suppression, with fever, and infectious complications leading the list. Other reported adverse effects include: rash, nausea, and diarrhea.

Abciximab

Abciximab (ReoPro) is a monoclonal antibody and is actually a fragment called the Fab fragment. Unlike the prototype, rituximab, it does not have an antitumor function. It binds to a glycoprotein receptor on human platelets and inhibits their aggregation, leading to reduced hemostasis. The circulating half-life after IV bolus injection is 30 minutes, although clinical effects are evident for about 48 hours. In some patients, antiplatelet activity persists for up to 10 days. Many patients receive a 6- to 12-hour continuous IV infusion after the initial bolus to maintain optimal antiplatelet activity. Abciximab is used with a number of cardiovascular conditions, such as ischemic heart disease, or after percutaneous coronary interventions in which antiplatelet activity is desired. It is administered as an IV infusion before planned procedures or at the onset of unstable angina. It may be contraindicated in patients with a recent history of stroke, major surgery or trauma, GI or genitourinary bleeding, vascular deformities, or uncontrolled hypertension. The primary adverse effect associated with abciximab is increased risk of bleeding.

Palivizumab

Palivizumab (Synagis) is a monoclonal antibody like rituximab; unlike rituximab, it has a unique function. This monoclonal antibody has been developed by recombinant DNA technology to be directly cytotoxic to the respiratory syncytial virus (RSV), reducing the number of viral organisms in the lower respiratory tract. It is administered as prophylaxis in neonates at high risk for developing life-threatening pulmonary disease if infected with RSV (e.g., premature infants, children with cystic fibrosis). Its use in treating confirmed RSV infection has not been established. It is contraindicated in adults in whom serious illness with RSV infection has not been documented. It is administered as a monthly IM injection given fall through spring and has a half-life of 18 to 20 days. The reconstituted drug does not contain a preservative and should be administered within 6 hours of reconstitution. Common adverse effects include infection with other organisms, worsening respiratory symptoms, GI upset, hepatic dysfunction, injection site erythema, and flu-like syndrome. The serum blood levels of alanine aminotransferase and aspartate transaminase may be elevated as a consequence of treatment with this agent.

Denosumab

Denosumab (Xgeva) is a new monoclonal antibody licensed late in 2010 that binds to the RANK ligand that is a transmembrane protein essential to formation and function of the osteoclasts. Its similarity to rituximab is in its affinity for a specific transmembrane receptor, but it produces a very different clinical effect. Osteoclasts are known for their activity in dermineralizing and weakening bone. This process is upregulated in patients with solid tumors and bone metastases and multiple mveloma with bone involvement. Administration of denosumab as a 120 mg subcutaneous injection monthly has been shown to reduce the time to skeletal related events such as pathologic fractures. This agent is a pregnancy category C and has not been tested in children. The most common adverse effects are fatigue, nausea, hypophosphatemia and hypocalcemia. Uncommonly osteonecrosis of the jaw and immunogenicity due to antibodies against this protein have occurred (Henry et al., 2011).

Drugs Significantly Different From
P Rituximab

Monoclonal antibodies significantly different from rituximab include muromonab-CD3, infliximab, basiliximab, and daclizumab. These drugs are significantly different because unlike the prototype rituximab, which targets the B lymphocytes, they target T lymphocytes to produce therapeutic immune suppression or have attached molecules such as radioactive substances, chemotherapy agents, or toxins.

Muromonab-CD3

Muromonab-CD3 (Orthoclone OKT3) is used to prevent allograft rejection in patients who have undergone renal transplantation and to treat steroid-resistant acute allograft rejection in heart and liver transplants. Muromonab-CD3 is a murine monoclonal antibody to the T3 complex of T cells. It acts on the T cell as an antigen and disables it. Muromonab-CD3 is available only for IV use.

Muromonab-CD3 is assigned to pregnancy category C. It is contraindicated in patients with known allergies to the drug or any murine product and in cases of fluid overload. It should be used cautiously in patients with fever (give antipyretics before drug administration) and in those previously on muromonab-CD3, because serious reactions can occur.

The most common adverse effects of muromonab-CD3 are nausea, vomiting, diarrhea, tremor, fever, chills, dyspnea, and chest pain. Potentially serious adverse effects include acute pulmonary edema and cytokine-release syndrome (flu-like symptoms progressing to shock).

Muromonab-CD3 combined with other immunosuppressants poses a serious risk of infection and lymphoma. To decrease this risk, the dosage of other immune suppressants should be reduced and then returned to previous levels 3 days before muromonab-CD3 treatment is finished. Encephalopathy and CNS effects are risks when muromonab-CD3 is combined with indomethacin (Indometh); therefore, this combination should be avoided.

Daclizumab

Daclizumab (Zenapax) saturates a subunit of the IL-2 receptor (Tac subunit), thus inhibiting IL-2–mediated cellular responses known to be important in allograft rejection. It is indicated as part of a three- or four-drug regimen for prophylaxis of acute organ rejection in adults receiving their first cadaveric kidney transplant. It is currently undergoing human trials for prevention and treatment of allograft rejection with other solid-organ and bone marrow transplants. It is dosed at 1 mg/kg and administered within 24 hours before transplantation, then every 14 days for a total of 5 doses. It effectively binds at the Tac subunit for as much as 120 days when the serum levels are 5 to 10 mg/mL. It has the same precautions and gender and age recommendations as basiliximab. Immunosuppression is the most important adverse effect; however, as with other immunosuppressive monoclonal antibodies, GI distress is common. Hypertension is agent specific and reported in both children and adults.

Basiliximab

Basiliximab (Simulect) is a monoclonal antibody that is an IL-2 receptor antagonist. It acts by binding to and blocking the CD25 antigen receptor site; this site is active in the cellular immune response involved in allograft rejection. Basiliximab is licensed as part of an immunosuppressive regimen that includes cyclosporine with or without corticosteroids for preventing organ transplantation rejection in patients undergoing renal transplantation. More effective immunosuppression without significant rejection or need for prolonged immunosuppressive therapy has led to increased use of this agent in these patients (McKeage & McCormack, 2010). It is administered as an IV infusion over 20 to 30 minutes, 2 hours before transplantation surgery and 4 days after surgery. The average duration of immunosuppressive IL-2 receptor blockade activity is 36 days. Readministration after initial therapy with basiliximab has not been studied, but excess immunosuppression or hypersensitivity reactions are projected. Pediatric patients in whom it has been used have demonstrated slower renal clearance, although no appreciable differences have been noted between adults and the elderly. This agent has not been tested with pregnant or lactating women, because IL-2 is known to cross the placenta, and great risk to the fetus has been suspected. The most common adverse effects relate to the infection risk associated with the immunosuppressive regimen; however, GI symptoms such as nausea, vomiting, and diarrhea have also commonly occurred (McKeage & McCormack, 2010). Occasional reports of headache, tremors, insomnia, and electrolyte disorders warrant careful assessment within 48 hours of therapy.

The following three agents are monoclonal antibodies attached to radioactive substances that attach to tumor cells and either target them for recognition on scan or enhance tumor-specific cell lysis. All agents require special handling procedures appropriate to radiopharmaceutical use by professionals. Reasonable limitations on exposure of bodily fluids with others are advised, although all radiolabeled monoclonal antibodies emit beta rather than gamma emissions; hence, fewer precautions are necessary. Patients may be advised to wash their dishes or clothes separately, or to flush the toilet two times after use, or to use condoms for sexual relations (Hendrix, 2004). These measures are suggested to avoid exposing family members to the small amount of radioactive substance that may be emitted.

Infliximab

Infliximab (Remicade) is a monoclonal antibody, a chimeric human-murine IgG antibody that acts by blocking tumor necrosis factor (TNF). It is licensed for treating moderate to severe Crohn's disease. Its safety and efficacy have not been established in children or in pregnant or lactating women, or beyond three doses. It is also licensed for use with methotrexate to treat rheumatoid arthritis in patients who do not respond to methotrexate alone. In studies with this disease, more than 50% of patients achieved clinical remission, with a tolerable toxicity profile. Infliximab is administered once as a short IV infusion; in severe Crohn's disease, it is readministered on a monthly basis for a total of three doses. Because of its low toxicity profile, many allogeneic bone marrow transplantation protocols have been established to evaluate the efficacy of this agent in this population. The most common adverse effect is an infusion-related allergic-type reaction that includes fever, chills, pruritus, dyspnea, chest pain, and hypotension. Skin reactions such as rash, eczema, dry skin, acne, sweating, and flushing are also common. Autoimmune antibodies that produce a lupus-like syndrome have been reported and warrant discontinuing the drug. Infliximab is incompatible with polyvinyl chloride tubing and should be mixed in glass bottles and administered through polyethylene line infusion sets.

Eculizumab

Eculizumab (Solirus) is a chimeric monoclonal antibody that binds to the complement protein C5, inhibiting cleavage of the a and b components, preventing formation of C5b-9 that causes the hemolysis of paroxysmal nocturnal hemoglobinemia (PNH). Eculizumab is indicated for patients with PNH and refractory, persistent hemolysis (Alexion Pharmaceuticals, 2009). It is administered as a 600 mg 35 minute infusion weekly for the first 4 weeks, followed by 900 mg every 2 weeks until disease exacerbation or unacceptable toxicity is reached. The most serious adverse effect of therapy is meningococcal infection, so patients are advised to receive meningococcal vaccination at least two weeks prior to starting therapy. Other adverse effects include headache, nasopharyngitis, back pain, fatigue and nausea. Adverse effects are well tolerated. Since it is unclear that ecuclizumab therapy alters thrombotic risk, anticoagulation therapy should be continued as prior to treatment.

Satumomab Pendetide

Indium-111 (^{111}In) satumomab pendetide (OncoScint CR/OV) is a murine monoclonal antibody that is unlike the prototype because it is bound to indium and targets tumor-associated glycoprotein but does not have properties that initiate cell lysis. This agent is used during lymphoscintigraphy to detect microscopic extrahepatic colorectal or ovarian cancer, although tumor types (e.g., breast, non–small cell lung, esophageal, gastric, pancreatic cancers) have also shown some sensitivity to its actions. It is not indicated as a screening tool for any of these diseases. After IV injection, serial nuclear scans detect the distribution of this radiolabeled monoclonal antibody. It is eliminated by natural metabolic pathways, with about 10% cleared through the kidneys over approximately 56 hours, but in some cases, it can be detectable for up to 120 hours. This agent has not been studied in children or in pregnant or lactating women, and it is therefore not recommended for use in these groups. Data are limited, but no clear contraindication exists for using this agent in the elderly. Preparation to administer this agent includes a laxative or enema to prevent nuclear localization in stool within the colon that could interfere with interpretation of the scans performed after injection of the antibody. Common adverse effects are similar to those for other monoclonal antibodies, but because satumomab pendetide is a murine-based product, allergic and late antibody reactions may also occur.

Tositumomab Plus Iodine-131

Tositumomab plus ^{131}I (Bexxar) is a murine antibody directed against the CD20 antigen found on the surface of normal and malignant B lymphocytes. It is indicated to treat CD20-positive follicular non-Hodgkin lymphoma that has relapsed after chemotherapy and has been refractory to rituximab. Because most of the tositumomab plus ^{131}I is renally cleared, serum blood urea nitrogen (BUN) and creatinine levels are checked before administration, and creatinine clearance is calculated if renal function is potentially impaired. Treatment with this radiolabeled monoclonal antibody involves a two-step plan involving a dosimetric step, in which a priming dose of 450 mg tositumomab is administered intravenously over 1 hour, followed by administration of ^{131}I tositumomab (5 millicurie [mCi] [131]I combined with 35 mg tositumomab) intravenously over 20 minutes. Whole-body scans for biodistribution must be obtained within 1 hour of the end of infusion of ^{131}I tositumomab and before the patient voids. This process is repeated once between days 2 and 4, with scans after the patient voids, and again on day 6 to 7. These serial scans verify biodistribution of the monoclonal antibody carrier before a therapeutic dose of radiation is administered. At about the seventh day, tositumomab is again administered as a 450-mg dose, followed this time by ^{131}I and tositumomab, 35 mg, designed to deliver 75 cGy of whole-body radiation.

Because hypothyroidism is a common clinical effect with tositumomab plus ^{131}I, all eligible patients must receive thyroid-blocking agents from 24 hours before the dosimetric dose until 14 days after the therapeutic dose, to protect against permanent thyroid destruction (Estes & Clapp, 2004). Prolonged myelosuppression has been reported, particularly if the patient's disease involves the bone marrow. Consequently, baseline and weekly CBCs are monitored for bone marrow tolerance. As with other murine proteins, severe or persistent hypersensitivity reactions may occur. The safety of future vaccines and antibody therapy may be compromised in the patient who receives this drug, because of the creation of antimurine antibodies (Estes & Clapp, 2004). This therapy is not recommended for children and pregnant or lactating women.

Yttrium-90 Ibritumomab Tiuxetan

[90]Y ibritumomab tiuxetan (Zevalin) is licensed as a two-step therapy similar to tositumomab, but rituximab is used as the monoclonal antibody carrier. In the dosimetric phase, rituximab is administered as a 250-mg/m² dose by IV infusion with a graduated infusion rate, as is done routinely with this agent. Four hours after the administration of rituximab, ^{111}In ibritumomab tiuxetan is administered intravenously over 10 minutes (dose of 5 mCi [1.6 mg total antibody dose]). Imaging for biodistribution is performed within the first 2 to 24 hours, between 48 and 72 hours, and optionally between 90 and 120 hours after the infusion. Initially, it was recommended that if biodistribution is acceptable, a therapeutic infusion should be administered between days 7 and 9, with the rituximab dose unchanged, but the ^{111}In ibritumomab tiuxetan administered as 0.4 mCi/kg (14.8 megabecquerels/kg [actual body weight of ^{90}Y ibritumomab tiuxetan; maximum dose is 32 mCi, or 1184 MBq]). More recent studies have shown that the dosimetry step is unnecessary in heavily pretreated patients, and patients may safely move straight to therapeutic doses. Infusion-related reactions are prevented by administering premedications. The most common adverse reactions involve suppression of bone marrow function and its clinical effects. Infection and bleeding caused by leukopenia or thrombocytopenia are more common when the

patient's disease involves the bone marrow. Patients are cautioned to implement radiation precautions for 3 days after tositumomab is administered.

C KINASE INHIBITORS

Kinase inhibitors include tyrosine kinase inhibitors, mTOR inhibitors proteasome inhibitors, and histone deacetylase inhibitors. They work on a specific type of cell involved in cancer reproduction. Extracellular tumor targets include: epidermal growth factor receptor (EGFR), vascular endothelial growth factor (VEGF-1, 2 and 3), platelet-derived growth factor beta (PDGF-beta), and transforming growth factor alfa (TGF-alfa). Intracellular tumor targets that have been identified include: platelet-derived growth factor (PDGF-alfa), hypoxia-inducible factor (HIF), c-Raf, b-Raf, and transforming growth factor (TGF).

Tyrosine kinase inhibitors are small molecules that prevent signal transduction, usually by interfering with binding of ATP. They vary in their affinity for various receptors and consequently have differing spectra of activity and adverse effects. Intracellular tyrosine kinase pathways branching from the RTK receptor include the RAS and RAF pathways and the P13K-Akt pathway. The P13K-Akt pathway is commonly mutated in malignancy (Ciuffreda et al., 2010). The prototype kinase inhibitor is imatinib (Gleevec).

Agents that can be inhibit multiple growth pathways are thought to have multiple anti-tumor effects, and may not only destroy tumor cells through their extracellular targets, but also target activities known to give rise to malignant transformation (Wood & Manchen, 2007). These agents are classified as multikinase inhibitors. The two multikinase inhibitors currently FDA licensed are sorafenib and sunitinib, both for primary or secondary treatment of metastatic renal cell carcinoma. They are discussed as drugs significantly different from the prototype.

Drug–drug interactions can be unpredictable and complicated with these drugs. Health care professionals need to be knowledgeable about the clinical pharmacokinetics of these drugs when prescribing and administering to minimize complications. More detailed information is described with each individual drug in this chapter.

Nursing Management of the Patient Receiving P Imatinib

Core Drug Knowledge

Pharmacotherapeutics

Imatinib is a "small molecule" tyrosine kinase inhibitor. "Small-molecule" drugs block specific enzymes and growth factor receptors involved in cancer cell growth. These drugs are also called signal-transduction inhibitors. Imatinib mesylate is an oral drug licensed by the FDA to treat GI stromal tumor (a rare cancer of the GI tract), Philadelphia chromosome positive chronic myeloid leukemia (CML) and acute lymphoblastic leukemia (ALL).

Pharmacokinetics

Imatinib is well absorbed and has a mean absolute bioavailability of 98% after oral administration with an elimination half life of about 18 hours. Imatinib is primarily eliminated in the feces as metabolites. Dose adjustments may be necessary for hepatic impairement, renal impairment, neutropenia, thrombocytopenia, and severe fluid retention.

Pharmacodynamics

Imatinib mesylate inhibits bcr-abl tyrosine kinase which is created by the Philadelphia chromosome abnormality. This drug induces apoptosis in bcr-abl positive cell lines as well as fresh leukemic cells from Philadelphia chromosome positive CML. It is also an inhibitor of platelet-derived growth factor, c-kit, and stem cell factor (SCF).

Contraindications and Precautions

Imatinib may be associated with edema. Patients should be weighed regularly and assessed for signs of fluid retention that could be severe (e.g. pleural or pericardial effusions or ascites). The risk of edema increases with higher doses of Imatinib and age greater than 65 years. Imatinib is associated with myelosuppression and a complete blood count should be used to monitor patients on a regular basis. Combining Imatinib with chemotherapy can result in an increase in these toxicities. Gastric irritation can occur with Imatinib. The drug should be taken with food and water to minimize this problem. Imatinib is a pregnancy category D drug. Caution should be taken when Imatinib is administed with strong CYP3A4 inhibitors. CYP3A4 inhibitors may decrease metabolism and increase concentrations of imatinib. Concomitant warfarin administration should be avoided in patients receiving this drug. Grapefruit juice should also be avoided as it may increase concentrations of imatinib.

Adverse Effects

As previously mentioned the most common toxicities associated with Imatinib are fluid retention which is treated by holding (or discontinuing if severe) the drug or administering diuretics. Another significant toxicity is myelosuppression. The severity of myelosuppression is related to the stage of the patient's disease in chronic myelogenous leukemia patients and usually occurs in the first few months of therapy. Severe congestive heart failure and left ventricular dysfunction have been reported most commonly in patients with comorbid conditions or risk factors. Hypothyroidism can be exacerbated in patients who are on levothyroxine replacement or those who have had a thyroidectomy. TSH levels should be closely monitored in these cases. Gastrointestinal bleeding can occur and is associated with gastric intestinal stromal tumor (GIST) sites that become friable and necrotic as they are destroyed. Patients taking imatinib may also experience muscle cramps, rashes and fatigue while on this therapy.

Drug Interactions

CYP3A4 inhibitors may decrease metabolism and increase concentrations of imatinib. CYP3A4 inducers may decrease concentrations of imatinib. Enzyme-inducing anti-epileptic drugs such as carbamazepine, phenytoin, fosphenytoin and Phenobarbital can reduce the AUC of imatinib. Acetaminiphen levels may be increased if taken concurrently with imatinib. See also Table 55.2.

Assessment of Relevant Core Patient Variables

Health Status

A thorough history and physical exam should be conducted to monitor for fluid retention, myelosuppression and cardiac toxicities during treatment. Patient's home medications, including any over the counter or complimentary therapies, should be screened on an ongoing basis to avoid drug interactions.

Life Span and Gender

Imatinib can cause fetal harm when administered to women who are pregnant. Imatinib is introduced into breast milk as an active metabolite. Breast feeding while on imatinib is not recommended. The safety of imatinib has been established in children over the age of 2 years. Patients over the age of 65 in clinical trials demonstrated similar toxicities with the exception of a higher incidence of edema.

Lifestyle, Diet, and Habits

Discuss the importance of monitoring for edema or other signs of severe fluid retention or cardiac abnormalities.

TABLE 55.2	Agents That Interact with Imatinib	
Interactants	**Effect and Significance**	**Nursing Management**
carbamazepine, phenytoin, fosphenytoin, phenobarbital	Reduces the AUC	
acetaminophen	Imatinib may increase acetaminophen levels	Monitor for increased liver toxicity. Ensure acetaminophen maximum dose allowed is not exceeded.
warfarin	Metabolized by CYP3A4	Avoid use in patients receiving imatinib. Utilize low molecular weight or standard heparin instead.

Note: CYP3A4 inducers decrease imatinib C_{max} and AUC. CYP3A4 inhibitors increase imatinib C_{max} and AUC.

Patients may need to modify their medication regimes to ensure optimal imatinib absorption or reduced interference of other drugs by imatinib.

Environment

Because imatinib is an oral drug patients can self administer this therapy as outpatients. Patient compliance should be monitored closely during treatment. Home safety to ensure other members of the family are not exposed to this hazardous agent may include instructions to not share eating utensils, store medications in a safe place, or double flush the toilet after use.

Nursing Diagnoses and Outcomes

- Risk for edema related to adverse effects of imatinib
  Desired outcome: *The patient will be absent of edema. The patient will state reportable signs and symptoms of edema or severe fluid retention.*
- Risk for Infection and Bleeding related to depression of bone marrow function
  Desired outcome: *Bone marrow recovery will be attained; rare and mild myelosuppression might occur. The patient will verbalize and also implement self-care measures to prevent infection.*

Planning and Intervention

Maximizing Therapeutic Effects

Imatinib should be taken orally with food and a large glass of water. Doses between 400 and 600 mg should be administered once daily. Doses of 800 mg should be administered in divided doses of 400 mg twice daily. This is important to decrease iron exposure as the tablet coating contains iron. For patients who cannot take oral tablets, the tablet(s) can be placed in 50 mL of juice or water and stirred until dissolved. The suspension must be taken orally immediately after tablet is disintegrated.

Minimizing Adverse Effects

Assess for signs of fluid overload and heart failure (e.g., weight gain, dyspnea, shortness of breath, edema, fatigue). Prevent exposure to people with infections. Evaluate for infection if a low grade fever (greater than 100.5°) develops. Assess complete blood count on a regular basis. Severe hepatic impairement requires dose reductions of imatinib by at least 25%. Renal impairment defined as CrCL 20 to 39 mL/min, should be dose reduced by 50%. Doses greater than 600mg are not recommended for mild renal impairment (CrCL 40 to 59 mL/min. Imatinib may be held or dose reduced for hematologic toxicities at the discretion of the provider consider disease state and goals of therapy.

Providing Patient and Family Education

- Discuss signs and symptoms of edema and severe fluid retention. Teach importance of routine weight assessment and reporting weight gain.
- Teach patients to report any rash or pruritis and how to implement supportive care measures for management.

- Stress the importance of regular laboratory tests to monitor for toxicities
- Teach patients measures to avoid infection resulting from myelosuppression and signs and symptoms to report that might indicated the presence of an infection (e.g., temperature greater than 100.5, redness, pain, drainage from any site, or chills.
- Instruct the patient to notify the provider for any gastrointestinal pain or bleeding.
- Discuss with patients and their significant others both reproductive goals and birth control.
- Discuss the importance of avoiding any new medications such as over the counter medications or complimentary therapies until discussing in detail with provider.

Ongoing Assessment and Evaluation

Patients should be closely monitored to ensure compliance with this oral therapy. Fluid retention should be assessed for at each visit and diuretics administered if necessary.

Drugs Closely Related to Imatinib

Dasatinib (Sprycel)

Dasatinib is also approved for Philadelphia chromosome positive CML and for Philadelphia chromosome positive acute lymphocytic leukemia (ALL). Dasatinib works similarly to imatinib and is used for patients who are refractory to imatinib. Dasatinib should be used with caution in patients who have QT prolongation. The impact of this adverse effect can be reduced by providing electrolyte replacement to ensure the serum potassium level is greater than 4.0mEq/L and the magnesium is greater than 2.0 mEq/L. Antacids and H2 antagonists may decrease dasatinib concentrations.

MEMORY CHIP

P Imatinib

- A tyrosine kinase inhibitor that targets special mechanisms of cancer cell growth. Used in the treatment of GI stromal tumor, Philadelphia chromosome positive chronic myeloid leukemia, and acute lymphoblastic leukemia.
- Most common adverse effects: fluid retention and myelosuppression
- Most serious adverse effects: heart failure and left ventricular dysfunction
- Maximizing therapeutic effect: take orally with food and a large glass of water
- Minimizing adverse effects: assess for fluid overload and heart failure; monitor complete blood count regularly
- Most important patient education: teach to monitor for signs/symptoms of fluid overload (e.g., weight gain, dyspnea, shortness of breath, edema); teach to avoid infections and report any low grade fever (greater than 100.5°)

Nilotinib (Tasigna)

Nilotinib is indicated for newly diagnosed Ph+ CML. The mechanism of action is similar to other drugs in this category. Nilotinib and dasatinib are also used in patients who show resistance to one of the other drugs in this category. Nilotinib has a black box warning related to QT prolongation and sudden deaths. Hypokalemia and hypomagnesemia should be corrected prior to administering nilotinib. Drugs that prolong QT interval and CYP34A inhibitors should be avoided. Patients should avoid food 2 hours before and 1 hour after taking nilotinib. Nilotinib should be taken with water only, twice daily and capsules should not be opened.

Drugs Significantly Different from Imatinib

Many of the other tyrosine kinase inhibitors primarily work by inhibiting the cellular action of growth factors. Other kinase inhibitors include drugs such as erlotinib (Tarceva), gefitinib (iressa), lapatinib (Tykerb), sunitinib (Sutent), sorafenib (Nexavar), pazopanib (Votrient). These drugs work in various solid tumors including; breast, lung and renal cancer.

Erlotinib (Tarceva)

Erlotinib is indicated for non-small cell lung cancer and advanced, unresectable, metastatic pancreatic cancer in combination with gemcitabine. Erlotinib inhibits EGFR. Erlotinib tablets should be taken on an empty stomach at least one hour before or two hours after food. The most common adverse effects include mild to moderate rashes, mucositis, fatigue, nausea, vomiting, infection, dyspnea and diarrhea. Cigarette smoking decreases erlotinib plasma concentrations and should be avoided. Corneal ulceration or perforations have been reported in patients receiving erlotinib. Abnormal eyelash growth and kerititis have been observed. A rare but potentially life threatening toxicity of erlotinib is interstitial lung disease and pneumonitis.

Gefitinib (Iressa)

Gefitinib is licensed by the FDA for the continued treatment in responding patients with locally advanced or metastatic non–small-cell lung cancer after failure of platinum and docetaxel failures. Currently the optimal use of gefitinib is under investigation. It appears that in non-small cell lung cancer patients that have EGFR mutations this drug may provide benefit, investigation is currently underway. Being a non-smoker, having a bronchioloalveolar carcinoma and being female has been found to be associated with EGFR mutations. (Marchetti, et al., 2005). Gefitinib is only available in the United States through a mail order pharmacy using an access program developed by the pharmaceutical company that makes the drug. This drug targets the epidermal growth factor receptor, which is overproduced by many types of cancer cells. The most significant toxicity with gefitinib is interstitial lung disease which can be fatal. Patients present with acute onset of dyspnea, which may be associated with cough, or low grade fever. If interstitial disease is diagnosed gefitinib should be discontinued. Gefitinib is administered once daily as a tablet with or without food. See Box 55.1.

Lapatinib (Tykerb)

Lapatinib has a unique dual action and blocks tyrosine kinase receptor for epidermal growth factor receptor and HER2 receptors. Lapatinib is approved for use in advanced or metastatic breast cancer whose tumor overexpress HER2 in combination with Xeloda (capecitabine). Lapatinib should be taken once daily at least one hour before or one hour after a meal. Capecitabine is to be taken with food or within 30 minutes of taking food. Adverse effects include decreases in left ventricular ejection fraction, hepatotoxicity, severe diarrhea, interstitial lung disease and pneumonitis. Other toxicities are similar to the prototype drug. A rare but potentially life threatening toxicity of erlotinib is interstitial lung disease and pneumonitis.

BOX 55.1 FOCUS ON RESEARCH

Gefitinib First Line for Patients with Advanced Non-Small-Cell Lung Cancer with Egfr Mutations Shows Improved Progression-Free Survival when Compared to Standard Chemotherapy.

Maemondo, M., Inoue, A., Kobayashi, K., et al. (2010). Gefitinib or Chemotherapy for Non-Small-Cell Lung Cancer with Mutated EGFR. N Engl J Med, 363:2380–2388.

The Study

230 patients with metastatic, non-small-cell lung cancer and EGFR mutations with no prior history of receiving chemotherapy were randomized to receive gefitinib or carboplatin-paclitaxel. The primary end point of this study was progression-free survival. Additionally they studied overall survival, response rate and toxicities. The interim analysis demonstrated that progression free survival was significantly longer in the group that received gefitinib compared to the group that received chemotherapy (10.8 months versus 5.4 months). The median overall survival was 30.5 months in the gefitinib group and 23.6 months in the chemotherapy group. The gefitinib study group experienced rash (71.1%) nad elevated aminotransferase levels (55.3%) and the chemotherapy group experienced neutropenia (77%), anorexia (56.6%), sensory neuropathy (54.9%), and anemia (64.6%). One patient who received gefitinib experienced fatal interstitial lung disease.

This study demonstrates the importance of identifying specific populations of patients who respond to therapies, determining factors that improve sensitivity and selecting those who are more likely to benefit from a drug therapy than others. This allows for a more focused approach while minimizing the risk of administering unnecessary treatments to nonresponders which increases the likelihood of toxicities.

Sorafenib (Nexavar)

Sorafenib is indicated for unresectable hapatocellular carcinoma and advanced renal cell carcinoma. Toxicities of sorafenib are similar to sunitinib. Sorafenib tablets are administered twice daily without food (1 hour before or 2 hours after a meal). Drug interactions with UGT1A1, UGT1A9, CYP2B6, CYP2C8 and CYP3A4 substrates can occur increasing the drug AUC. Other drugs that increase sorafenib AUC when administered concurrently include doxorubicin, docetaxel, and fluorouracil. Immunosuppression, hypertension, hand and foot syndrome, diarrhea and fatigue are also common toxicities. Rarely cardiac toxicity has been reported. Additional laboratory values that can be affected include amylase, lipase, (both increase) and phosphorous (decreases).

Sunitinib

Sunitinib (sutent) is licensed for GIST after disease progression or intolerance to imatinib and for patients with advanced renal cell cancer. Sunitinib is given orally in capsules. Sunitinib is primarily metabolized by the cytochrome P-450 enzyme, CYP3A4 and is eliminated via the feces and urine (60% and 16 % of the administered dose, respectively). The terminal half life of sunitinib is 40 hours. Sunitinib may be taken with or without food. Dosage forms are 12.5, 25, and 50 mg capsules. Sunitinib inhibits multiple tyrosine kinases including VEGF, SCF, PDGFR, FLT-3. This causes inhibition of the growth of tumor cells and pathologic angiogenisis. Sunitinib can cause prolonged QT intervals and hypokalemia and hypomagnesemia should be corrected. Electrocardiograms should be monitored before and during treatment. The most frequent adverse effects are fatigue, diarrhea, nausea, mucositis, dyspepsia, abdominal pain, constipation, hypertension, congestive heart failure, rash, hand-foot reaction, skin discoloration, taste changes and bleeding. Bleeding characterized by tumor related hemorrhage has been reported. Thrombolytic events may occur with sunitinib and patients should be thoroughly assessed for deep vein thrombosis/pulmonary embolism and be instructed on reportable signs and symptoms. Skin discoloration can occur secondary to the yellow coloring in the capsules. Depigmentation of the hair and skin can occur with sunitinib. Blood pressure should be measured prior to and weekly during Sunitinib therapy due to the risk of hypertension. Pre-existing hyprtension should be resolved prior to starting therapy to help ensure that the full treatment can be administered without dose-limiting hypertension. Baseline assessment of thyroid function should be performed and treatment initiated if necessary as sunitinib can cause thyroid dysfunction.

Pazopanib (Votrient)

Pazopanib is indicated for the treatment of renal cell carcinoma. Hepatic impairment can occur and pazopanib is not recommended in patients with severe hepatic impairement. Toxicities are similar to the prototype drug however; additional side effects include arterial thrombotic events and protenuria. Pazopanib is administered orally once daily with food (at least 1 hour prior or 2 hours after a meal). The dose should not exceed 800 mg. Tablets should not be crushed due to the potential for rapid systemic absorption. Doses should be reduced for hepatic impairment. Discontinue at least 7 days prior to surgery due to the potential for decreased wound healing. Safety of pazopanib in pediatric patients has not been established.

© MTOR-I INHIBITORS

A significant receptor on the P13K-Akt arm of intracellular kinase leads to the mammalian target of rapamycin (mTOR) pathway that enhances cell division. When this agent binds with the KBP-12 protein, a complex is formed that inhibits mTOR signaling, and enzymes responsible for cell cycle regulation, cell motility and angiogenesis are impaired. Some early research suggests that inhibition of cell motility may reduce metastatic potential or rate (Zhou & Huang, 2010). The mTOR pathway is also essential for fat and lipid metabolism, influencing metabolic regulation of these essential nutrients. This target is also highly expressed in lymphocytes, and has been the focus of the transplant immunosuppressive rapamycin, hence serious immunosuppression is associated with medications in this class. Drugs in this class are noted for risk for opportunistic infections and idiopathic pneumonitis. There are currently two licensed agents classified as mTOR inhibitors. (Feldman & Shokat, 2010).

MTOR-I Inhibitors: Temsirolimus, Eversirolimus
Temsirolimus (Torisel)

Temsirolimus (Torisel™) was the first mTOR inhibitor to be licensed by the FDA in 2007 as treatment for advanced or metastatic renal cell carcinoma. In a comparison trial to standard therapy with interferon, it offered more than double the objective response rate and a longer duration of response. It is less clear where this agent is placed in therapy options for newly diagnosed disease due to availability of two multikinase inhibitors and another mTor inhibitor. It is administered as an initial dose of 25 mg infused over 30 to 60 minutes once a week until disease progression or unacceptable toxicity is experienced. Premedication 30 minutes prior to therapy with 25 to 50 mg diphenhydramine or its equivalent is recommended (Abraham, 2007). If infusion reaction occurs, corticosteroids with redosing of diphenhydramine may be administered and the infusion resumed at a slower rate (Wyeth Pharmaceuticals, 2010). Concomitant use of known inducers of the P-450 3A4 metabolic pathway should be avoided, or the dose of temsirolimus increased to 50 mg. If inhibitors of CYP 3A4 are administered, temsirolimus may be dose-reduced to 12.5 mg. Medication and over the counter remedies should be assessed frequently to quickly detect those that may interfere with temsirolimus blood levels. Like other anti-angiogenic agents, this medication should not be administered to patients during the perioperative period. Although not specifically recommended in prescribing information, other agents' precautions suggest a 28 day period before or after surgical intervention. Common adverse effects include: infection, rash, fatigue, oral mucositis, edema, nausea, loss of appetite, and renal impairment. Because of its effects on metabolism, hyperglycemia and hyperlipidemia commonly occur during therapy and necessitate frequent ongoing laboratory monitoring of glucose and triglycerides. Although rare, interstitial lung disease and idiopathic bowel perforation can occur and require prompt assessment of distressing respiratory or gastrointestinal symptoms. Temsirolimus administered concomitantly with sunitinib demonstrated dose-limiting toxicities and is not recommended (Wyeth, Inc, 2010).

Eversirolimus (Afinitor)

Everolimus (Afinitor™) is the first oral mTor Inhibitor available and was licensed in 2009 for treatment of advanced renal cell carcinoma after treatment with sorafenib and sunitinib. Patients who have progressive disease while on or within 6 months of the multikinase inhibitors are eligible to receive everolimus (Coppin, 2010). This agent inhibits the mTOR pathway in two distinct locations producing reduced cell proliferation, cell division, metabolism and angiogenesis. It is similar to temsirolimus in both action and adverse effect provide. Administered as a once a day 10 mg oral agent, it is essential to provide thorough patient and family education regarding conscientious administration and follow-up with providers as well as home chemotherapy safety.

OTHER INHIBITORS

The discovery of additional mutagenesis pathways are contributing greatly to our knowledge of malignant disease and its therapeutic targets. Other licensed targeted therapies that inhibit cellular processes include proteasome inhibitors and histone deacetylase inhibitors. A proteasome inhibitor is bortezomib (velcade) and the histone deacetylase inhibitors include zolinza (vorinostat) and Istodax (Romidepsin). Each has unique targets and limited clinical indications at present, but it is anticipated that more will be licensed for use in the upcoming years.

Ⓒ PROTEASOME INHIBITORS

Bortezomib (Velcade)

The first apoptosis-inducing drug to be approved by the FDA was bortezomib (Velcade), which is indicated for treatment of multiple myeloma in both up-front and relapsed disease (Stadtmauer, 2010). It has also been licensed for treatment of refractory mantle cell lymphoma that have progressed after at least one other treatment. Apoptosis-inducing drugs cause cancer cells to undergo apoptosis (cell death) by interfering with proteins involved in the process. Bortezomib causes

cancer cells to die by blocking enzymes called proteasomes, which help to regulate cell function and growth. Proteosomes in normal cells are also temporarily inhibited, but unlike malignant cells, they resume normal function within 72 hours. This medication should not be given to anyone who has a history of hypersensitivity to boron or mannitol. Bortezimib is administered 1.3 mg/m^2 as a 3 to 5 second IV push twice a week for two weeks in a row, followed by 10 days rest. It is important to space the twice weekly injections by at least 72 hours to allow for normal cell recovery. Each cycle comprises a total of 21 days, and up to eight cycles may be prescribed. This agent has been commonly associated with drowsiness, gastrointestinal distress, bone pain, peripheral neuropathy and bone marrow suppression. The platelet count nadirs around day 11, and the white blood cell count decreases shortly after. Anemia is a later and more chronic adverse effect. Less common but serious adverse events include hepatic dysfunction, hypotension, interstitial pneumonitis, and heart failure exacerbation. The most common causes of dose-reduction due to toxicity is due to bone marrow suppression, peripheral neuropathy, posterior reversible leukoencephalopathy (PRES), or hepatic failure. This medication interacts with the Cytochrome P-450 metabolic pathway, and all medications should be reviewed with each patient encounter (Millennium Pharmaceuticals, Inc, 2009).

Ⓒ HDAC INHIBITORS

Zolinza (Vorinostat)

Zolinza (vorinostat) is a drug in a new category of targeted drugs called histone deacetylase inhibitors (HDAC). Currently Zolinza is approved for refractory cutaneous T-cell lymphoma however, it is being studied in clinical trials for many different tumor types.

Zolinza is eliminated primarily through metabolism. Less than1 % of the drug was found excreted in the urine in clinical studies. The mean terminal half life was approximately 2 hours. Zolinza was not evaluated in patients with liver abnormalities. Furthermore Zolinza is not an inhibitor of CYP drug metabolizing enzymes making it less susceptible to drug interactions.

Zolinza works by inhibiting histone deacetylases. Vorinostat is thought to induce cell-cycle arrest and apoptosis and inhibit angiogenesis. It may also improve NK cell-mediated tumor immunity. The mechanism of action has not been fully characterized.

Zolinza is a category D drug and should not be given in women who are breast feeding. This drug has not been fully studied in patients with liver or renal impairment and thus should be used with caution in these populations. QT prolongation can occur and electrolytes should be monitored at baseline and ongoing. Gastrointestinal disturbances such as nausea, vomiting, anorexia, and diarrhea may occur and appropriate symptom management may be necessary. Pulmonary embolism or deep vein thrombosis were reported in clinical trials. Hyperglycemia was observed in patients receiving

Zolinza. Myelosuppression is an adverse effect with Zolinza. Thrombocytopenia and gastrointestinal bleeding can occur in patients who are on valproic acid concurrently. Prolongations of prothrombin time and international normalized ratio (INR) have been noted in patients receiving coumarin derivative anticoagulants in conjunction with Zolinza.

Baseline electrocardiogram should be evaluated prior to initiation of Zolina therapy. Contraception should be utilized to prevent fetal harm during treatment with Zolinza. Carefully assess a complete blood cell count, serum creatinine and electrolytes prior to and during treatment to monitor for toxicities. Zolinza is taken once daily with food. Capsules should not be opened or broken. Patients should be instructed to drink at least 2 liters of fluid per day to prevent dehydration. Assess patients for nausea and vomiting that may affect intake and increase the risk of dehydration. Before administering Zolinza ensure that electrolytes and complete blood counts are reviewed to ensure results do not preclude administration of the drug.

Assess QT interval and electrolytes prior to and during therapy. Hyperglycemia may occur in as many as 40% of patients. High risk patients include those with preexisting diabetes and treatment or modifications to existing diabetes treatment may be necessary. Antiemetics may be indicated for nausea and vomiting. Diarrhea should be treated after an infectious source is ruled out.

Istodax (Romidepsin)

Istodox is also approved for cutaneous T-cell lymphoma however, it is administered intravenously over 4 hours. The most common adverse reactions are nausea, fatigue, myelosuppression, vomiting, and anorexia, QT prolongation, and lymphopenia. Strong CYP3A4 inhibitors may increase concentrations of Istodax and should be avoided. Potent CYP3A4 inducers may decrease concentrations and should be avoided. Concurrent warfarin administration can prolong prothrombin time and INR.

CHAPTER SUMMARY

- The humoral immune system involves the interaction between cell surface antigens of B-lymphocytes and antibody formation. The antibodies stimulate an immune and inflammatory reaction to the antigen and cause its destruction.
- Antibodies can be used to target malignant cell clones, to modify T or B lymphocytes, or to alter normal cell effects. Antibodies are usually monoclonal, and attach to a specific destiny antigen to alter the normal actions of that cell.
- Current licensed monoclonal antibodies originate from murine antibodies, modified part-murine (chimeric) antibodies, or humanized antibodies.
- Hypersensitivity reactions are common with monoclonal antibody therapy. Antibodies without murine proteins produce fewer adverse effects and less risk for eliciting human antimurine antibodies (HAMAs) that preclude future therapy with other antibodies.

- Targeted therapies cause antineoplastic effects by selectively blocking a specific extracellular or intracellular receptor or metabolic pathway. Nurses administering these targeted antineoplastic agents understand how these targeted receptors and pathways cause tumor cell death.
- Subtypes of the targeted therapies have some common class effects based upon their similar targets.
- Several agents in the class of targeted therapies are oral. Patients should receive extensive education on taking oral therapy correctly and implementing chemotherapy protective strategies for their family and friends when at home.
- Many oral targeted therapies are metabolized by the CYP3A4 pathway and have a large number of drug-drug interactions to consider when planning nursing care.
- These drugs often cause adverse GI effects; therefore, efforts must be made to maintain nutritional status. A nutritional consultation, supplemental feedings, and small, frequent meals are often necessary.

QUESTIONS FOR STUDY AND REVIEW

1. What are the intracellular tumor targets for kinase inhibitors?
2. List two important considerations for patient taking kinase inhibitors.
3. How do targeted therapies differ from traditional chemotherapy treatments?
4. Why are drug interactions significant with many of the kinase inhibitors?

NEED MORE HELP?
Chapter 55 of the Study Guide to Accompany *Drug Therapy in Nursing*, 4th Edition, contains NCLEX-style questions and other learning activities to reinforce your understanding of the concepts presented in this chapter. For additional information or to purchase the study guide, visit thePoint.

REFERENCES

Abraham, J. (2007). Temsirolimus for advanced renal cell carcinoma. *Community Oncology*, 4:476–479.

Ciuffreda, L., Di Sanza, C., Incani, U. C., Miella, M. (2010). The mTOR pathway: a new target in cancer therapy. *Curr Cancer Drug Targets*, 10(5):484–495.

Coppin, C. (2010). Everolimus: the first approved product for patients with advanced renal cell cancer after sunitinib and/or sorafenib. *Biologics*, 4:91–101.

Feldman, M. E., & Shokat, K. M. (2010). New Inhibitors of the PI3K-Akt-mTOR Pathway: Insights into mTOR Signaling from a New Generation of Tor Kinase Domain Inhibitors (TORKinibs). *Curr Top Microbiol Immunol*, June 12 E pub ahead of print.

Fiuza, M. (2009). Cardiotoxicity associated with trastuzumab treatment of HER-2+ breast cancer. *Adv Ther*, (Suppl 1): S9–S17.

Gurcan, H. M., Keskin, D. B., Stern, J. N., Nitzberg, M. A., Shekhani, H., & Ahmed, A. R. (2009). A review of the current use of rituximab in autoimmune diseases. *Int Immunopharmacol*, 9(1):10–25.

Halle, K., Cheson, B. D., Catovsky, D., et al. (2008). Guidelines for the diagnosis and treatment of chronic lymphocytic leukemia: a report from the International Workshop on Chronic Lymphocytic Leukemia updating the National Cancer Institute-Working Group 1996 guidelines. *Blood,* 111:5446–5456.

Hapani, S., Chu, D., & Wu, S. (2009). Risk of gastrointestinal perforation in patient with cancer treated with bevacizumab: a meta-analysis. *Lancet Oncol,* 10(6):559–568.

Hendrix, C. (2004). Radiation safety guidelines for radioimmunotherapy with yttrium 90 ibritumomab tiuxetan. *Clinical Journal of Oncology,* 8(1):31–34.

Heresi, G. A., Farver, C. F., & Stoller, J. K. (2008). Interstitial pneumonitis and alveolar hemorrhage complicating use of rituximab: case report and review of the literature. *Respiration,* 76(4):449–553.

Hill, A. (2008). Update on eculizumab for the treatment of paroxysmal nocturnal hemoglobinuria. *Clin Adv Hematol Oncol,* 6(7):499–500.

Hoag, J. B., Azizi, A., Doherty, T. J., Lu, J., Willis, R. E., & Lund, M. E. (2009). Association of cetuximab with adverse pulmonary events in cancer patients: a comprehensive review. *J Exp Clin Cancer Res,* 28:113.

Iwata H. (2009). Neo(adjuvant) trastuzumab treatment: current perspectives. *Breast Cancer,* 16(4):288–294.

Kimura, F. (2007). Molecular target drug discovery. *Intern Med,* 46(2):87–89.

Lurje, G., Lenz, H. J. (2009). EGFR signaling and drug discovery. *Oncology,* 77(6):400–410.

Martinelli, E., DePalma, R., Orditura, M., DeVita, F., & Ciardiello, F. (2009). Anti-epidermal growth factor receptor monoclonal antibodies in cancer therapy. *Clin Exp Immunol,* 158(1):1–9.

McKeage, K., & McCormack, P. L. (2010). *BioDrugs,* 24(1): 55–76.

Millennium Pharmaceuticals, Inc. Bortezimib (Velcade™). Full Prescribing Information, Cambridge, MA, 2009.

Mir, O., Mouthon, L., Alexandre, J., Mallion, J., Deray, G., Guillevin, L., & Goldwasser, F. (2007). Bevacizumab-induced cardiovascular events: A consequence of cholesterol emboli syndrome? *Journal National Cancer Institute,* 99(1):85–86.

Mishra, B. K., & Parikh, P. M. (2006). Targeted therapy in oncology. Retrieved from *http:/www.medind/nic.in/maa/+06/i2/ maat06i2p169. pdf*

Moccia, A., Ghielmini, M. (2008). Monoclonal antibodies for the treatment of hematologic malignancies: schedule and maintenance therapy. *Semin Hematology,* 45(2):75–84.

Morris, V. A. (2009). Infectious complications in patients with chronic lymphocytic leukemia: pathogenesis, spectrum of infection, and approaches to prophylaxis. *Clin Lymphoma Myeloma,* 9(5):365–370.

Murphy, C. G., & Fornier, M. (2010). HER-2 positive breast cancer beyond trastuzumab. *Oncology,* 24(5):410–415.

Osterborg, A. (2010). Ofatumumab, a human anti-CD20 monoclonal antibody. *Expert Opin Biol Ther,* 10(3):439–449.

Pal, S., Figlin, R., & Reckamp, K. (2010). Targeted therapies for non-small cell lung cancer: an evolving landscape. *Molecular Cancer Therapeutics.* 9(7):0F1–0F13.

Peerzada, M. M., Spiro, T. P., & Daw, H. A. (2010). Pulmonary toxicities of biologics: a review. *Anticancer Drugs,* 21(2): 131–139.

Perosa, F., Prete, M., Racanelli, V., & Dammacco, F. (2010). CD20-depleting therapy in autoimmune diseases: from basics to research to the clinic. *J Intern Med,* 267(3):260–277.

Polovich, M., Whitford, J. M., & Olsen, M. (2009). *Chemotherapy and biotherapy: Guidelines and recommendations for practice.* Oncology Nursing Society. Pittsburgh, PA: Oncology Nursing Press.

Ram, R., Ben-Bassat, I., Shpilberg, O., Polliack, A., & Raanani, P. (2009). The late adverse events of rituximab therapy-rare but there! *Leuk Lymphoma,* 50(7):1083–1095.

Schilsky, R., Allen, J., Benner, J., Sigal, E., & McClellen, M. (2010). Commentary: Tackling the challenges of developing targeted therapies for cancer. *The Oncologist,* 15:484–487.

Schmucker, C., Ehlken, C., Hnsen, L. L., Antes, G., Agostini, H. T., & Leigemann, M. (2010). Intravitreal bevacizumab (AvastinTM) vs. ranibizumab (LucentisTM) for the treatment of age-related macular degeneration: a systemic review. *Curr Opin Ophthalmol,* 21(3):218–226.

Shabason, J., Tofilon, P., & Camphausen, K. (2010). HDAC Inhibitors in Cancer Care. *Oncology.* 24(2):180–185.

Shih, T., & Lindley, C. (2006). Bevacizumab: An angiogenesis inhibitor for the treatment of solid malignancies. *Clinical Therapeutics,* 28(11):1779–1802.

Stadtmauer, E. A. (2010). Tailoring initial treatment for newly diagnosed, transplantation-eligible multiple myeloma. *Oncology,* 24(3):7–13.

Vidal, L., Gafter-Gvili, A., Leibovici, L., & Shpilberg, O. (2009). Rituximab as maintenance therapy for patients with follicular lymphoma, The Cochrane Library, 2: At www.mcw.interscience.wiley.com/cochrane/CIsysrev/Articles/CD0065521/frame.html, Accessed 6/27/10.

Yarbro, C. H., Frogge, M. H., Goodman, M., et al. (Eds.). (2011). *Cancer nursing: Principles and practice* (7th ed). Boston, MA: Jones and Bartlett.

Zangari, M., Fink, L. M., Elice, F., Zhan, F., Adsock, D. M., & Tricot, G. J. (2009). Thrombotic events in patients with cancer receiving antiangiogenesis agents. *J Clin Oncol,* 27(29): 4865–4873.

Zhang, B. (2009). Ofatumumab. *MAbs,* 1(4):326–331.

Zhou, H., & Huang, S. (2010). mTOR signaling in cancer cell motility and metastasis. *Crit Rev Eukaryot Gene Expr,* 20(1):1–16.

Drugs That Are Cell Cycle–Specific

Learning Objectives

At the completion of this chapter the student will:

1. Understand the goals of treatment and the strategies used in chemotherapy.
2. Identify the phases of the cell life cycle and describe what happens at each phase.
3. Differentiate a normal from a malignant cell.
4. Explain the difference between a cell cycle–specific and a cell cycle–nonspecific chemotherapeutic agent.
5. Identify the different routes of administration for the various chemotherapeutic agents.
6. Describe precautions and practices to ensure safety, minimize exposure, and deal with untoward effects of chemotherapy to the patient, health care provider, and the environment.
7. Identify core drug knowledge about cell cycle–specific drugs.
8. Identify core patient variables relevant to cell cycle–specific drugs.
9. Relate the interaction of core drug knowledge to core patient variables for cell cycle–specific drugs.
10. Generate a nursing plan of care from the interactions between the core drug knowledge and core patient variables for cell cycle–specific drugs.
11. Describe nursing interventions to maximize therapeutic effects and minimize adverse effects for cell cycle–specific drugs.
12. Identify the potential effects of herbal medicine on chemotherapy.
13. Determine key points for patient and family education for cell cycle–specific drugs.

Key Terms

adjuvant therapy
cell cycle
cell cycle–nonspecific
cell cycle–specific
chemotherapy
consolidation therapy
cytokinesis
first-order kinetics
G_0 phase

G_1 phase
G_2 phase
generation time
growth fraction
induction therapy
intensification
irritant
maintenance

mitosis (M) phase
nadir
neoadjuvant therapy
palliative therapy
radiation recall
salvage therapy
synthesis (S) phase
vesicant

Drugs That Are Cell Cycle–Specific

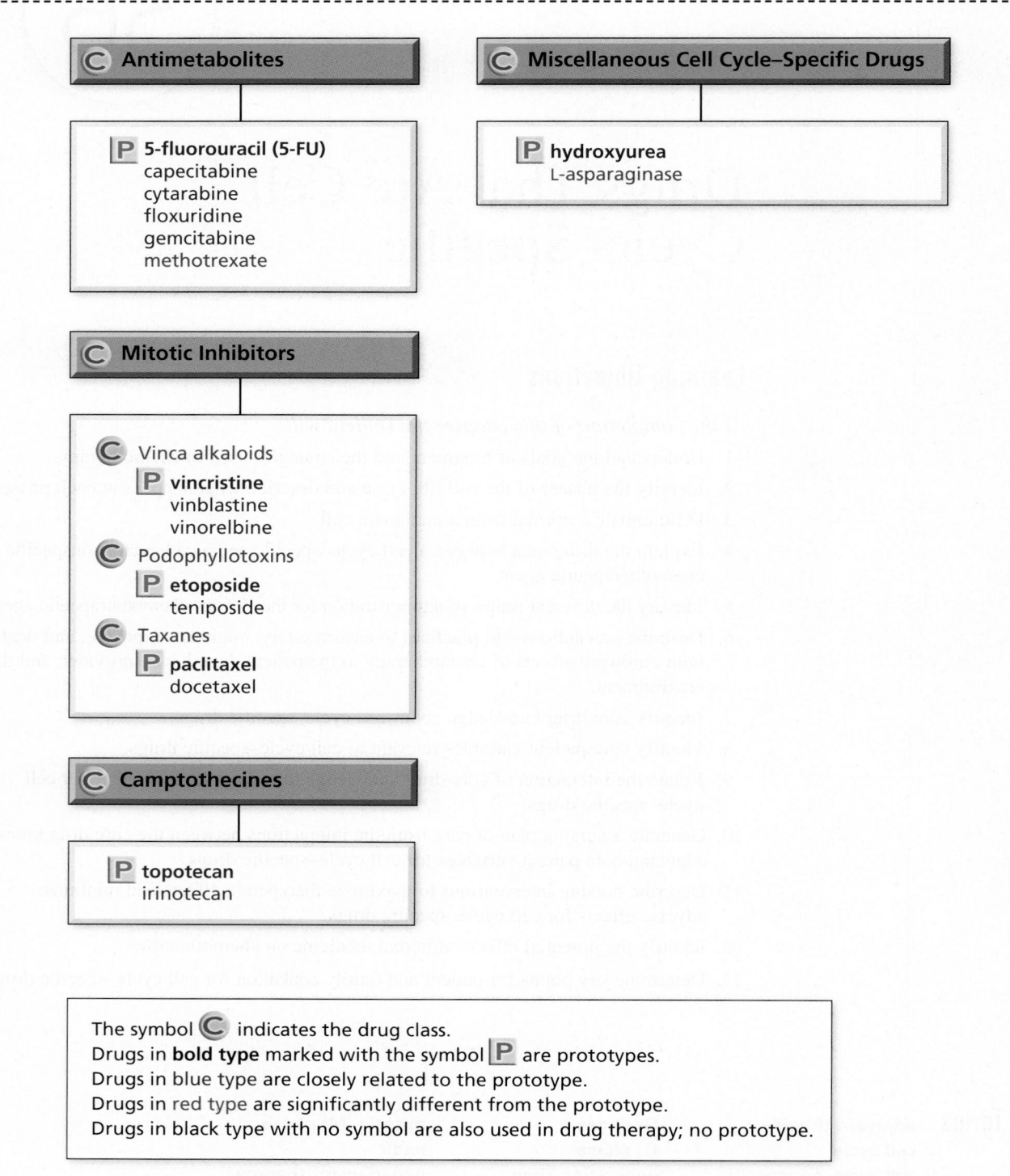

Ⓒ Antimetabolites

Ⓟ **5-fluorouracil (5-FU)**
capecitabine
cytarabine
floxuridine
gemcitabine
methotrexate

Ⓒ Miscellaneous Cell Cycle–Specific Drugs

Ⓟ **hydroxyurea**
L-asparaginase

Ⓒ Mitotic Inhibitors

Ⓒ Vinca alkaloids
 Ⓟ **vincristine**
 vinblastine
 vinorelbine
Ⓒ Podophyllotoxins
 Ⓟ **etoposide**
 teniposide
Ⓒ Taxanes
 Ⓟ **paclitaxel**
 docetaxel

Ⓒ Camptothecines

Ⓟ **topotecan**
irinotecan

The symbol Ⓒ indicates the drug class.
Drugs in **bold type** marked with the symbol Ⓟ are prototypes.
Drugs in blue type are closely related to the prototype.
Drugs in red type are significantly different from the prototype.
Drugs in black type with no symbol are also used in drug therapy; no prototype.

ancer remains the second leading cause of death in the U.S., behind heart disease, despite improvements in 5-year survival rates. Between 1984 and 1986, the five-year relative survival estimate was 53%. The latest estimates for the years between 1996 and 2002 showed improvement to 66%. According to estimates by the American Cancer Society, almost 1.5 million new cases of cancer will be diagnosed in the United States in 2009, and more than 500,000 people will die from the disease in that same year. This translates to almost 1,500 deaths each day from cancer.

Today, the treatment options for cancer include more choices than ever before. Novel agents that function differently from the familiar cancer regimens of radiation, chemotherapy, surgery, and biotherapy have generated a lot of research initiatives and hopes for cure. However, chemotherapy remains a vital part of the cancer armamentarium. **Chemotherapy** is the term that describes the use of cytotoxic agents (substances that are toxic to cells) that inhibit the growth, development, and proliferation of malignant cells. Sometimes the term *antineoplastic* is used instead of the term *chemotherapy*. Chemotherapy dates back to the 1500s, when heavy metals were used to treat cancers. Severe toxicities and few cures were reported. Since then, a vast spectrum of chemotherapeutic drugs has been discovered to achieve the goals of chemotherapy: cure, control, and palliation.

Unlike two other methods of treating cancer, surgery and radiation, chemotherapy produces a systemic effect. The chemotherapeutic drugs are transported by the bloodstream throughout the body, although most of these drugs do not cross the blood–brain barrier and therefore cannot reach the central nervous system (CNS).

Chemotherapy plays an important role in cancer therapy. It is the primary treatment for some cancers (Box 56.1) and serves as an adjunct to the other treatment methods.

Chemotherapeutic agents may be administered as single agents or in combination regimens. They are used in the following treatment strategies:

- **Adjuvant therapy:** This therapy involves a short course of high-dose drug therapy (usually with a combination of drugs) administered after radiation or surgery to destroy residual tumor cells or micrometastases and prevent recurrence.
- **Induction therapy:** This term refers to the start of chemotherapy. As commonly used in treating hematologic cancers, induction consists of high-dose drug therapy (usually with a combination of drugs) given to induce a complete response when initiating a curative regimen.
- **Consolidation therapy:** This strategy consists of chemotherapy given after induction therapy has achieved a complete remission; the regimen is repeated to increase the probability of cure or to prolong patient survival.
- **Intensification:** After complete remission is achieved, the same agents used for induction therapy are given at higher (intensified) doses, or different drugs are given (also at high doses) to improve the chances of cure or longer remission.
- **Maintenance:** This therapy involves using low-dose cytotoxic drugs, singly or in combination, on a long-term basis in patients who are in complete remission, to delay regrowth of residual cancer cells.
- **Neoadjuvant therapy:** Chemotherapy is administered to reduce the tumor burden before surgery or radiation, to improve the outcomes of these methods by shrinking the tumor.
- **Palliative therapy:** This therapy involves the use of chemotherapeutic drugs to control symptoms, provide comfort, and improve the patient's quality of life if cure is not achievable.

Box 56.1 ROLE OF CHEMOTHERAPY IN VARIOUS CANCERS

Primary Treatment

Chemotherapy is the primary treatment for the following localized cancerous neoplasms:

- Burkitt's lymphoma
- CNS lymphomas
- Hodgkin's disease (of childhood and some adult stages)
- Embryonal rhabdomyosarcoma
- Wilms' tumor
- Small-cell lung cancer
- Large-cell lymphomas

Future as a Primary Treatment

Chemotherapy holds promise as a future primary treatment for the following cancers:

- Breast cancer
- Esophageal cancer
- Non–small-cell lung cancer

- Nasopharyngeal cancer and other cancers of the head and neck
- Pancreatic cancer
- Prostate cancer
- Cervical carcinoma
- Gastric carcinoma

Treatment Before Surgery

Sometimes chemotherapy is the treatment used to shrink a tumor so that surgery can be less extensive and therefore less mutilating. Some cancers for which chemotherapy is used as a pretreatment include the following:

- Soft-tissue sarcomas
- Laryngeal cancer
- Anal carcinoma
- Bladder cancer
- Breast cancer
- Osteogenic sarcoma

• **Salvage therapy:** This strategy involves the use of a potentially curative high-dose drug regimen given to a patient whose symptoms have recurred or whose treatment by another regimen has failed.

Nurses need to be equipped with a clear knowledge of cell physiology, cancer pathophysiology, routes of administration for chemotherapeutic drugs, safety guidelines for handling chemotherapeutic drugs, classifications of antineoplastic drugs, and the therapeutic and adverse effects (toxicities) of antineoplastic drugs so that patients' needs can be anticipated early. Armed with this knowledge and set of skills, the nurse will be able to assist the patient in navigating the often overwhelming challenges that the various treatment options offer. It is important to offer the best education for the patient and family so that the patient can be managed well within any clinical setting and be able to participate in his or her care and adhere to a treatment regimen with a clear understanding of the goals and expectations of treatment.

PHYSIOLOGY

Knowledge of cellular kinetics and the life span of the **cell cycle** is needed to understand how chemotherapy works. The cell is the basic structure of the human organism.

Normally, cell growth is strictly regulated. The process by which a cell replicates itself, forming two identical daughter cells, is called cell division. Cell division, which is rare, occurs only to replace worn-out or dying cells and as part of the process of wound healing. Cell death is controlled, and when cells die, they are replaced in an orderly fashion. However, in cancer, the mechanisms for cell growth are disrupted, resulting in uncontrolled proliferation of cells. The time span over which a cell reproduces is called the cell cycle. The cell cycle has five phases: G_0, G_1, S, G_2, and M. All cells, whether normal or abnormal, progress through the different phases of the cell cycle. The complete cycle is illustrated in Figure 56.1.

The cell cycle is the cornerstone of cell cycle division and proliferation. Both normal and malignant cells undergo this process, which can last for approximately 25 to 30 hours. In the first phase, the **Gap 0 (G_0) phase** (also known as the resting phase), a cell can stay in a dormant or latent state for months or even years until stimulated to move forward in the cycle. Because certain cells divide more rapidly than others, some rest in the G_0 phase for a brief period, whereas others bypass the G_0 phase and directly enter the second phase, the **Gap 1 (G_1) phase,** if the body needs a certain cell immediately. During the G_1 phase, the cell increases in size and synthesizes ribonucleic acid (RNA) and the proteins needed for deoxyribonucleic

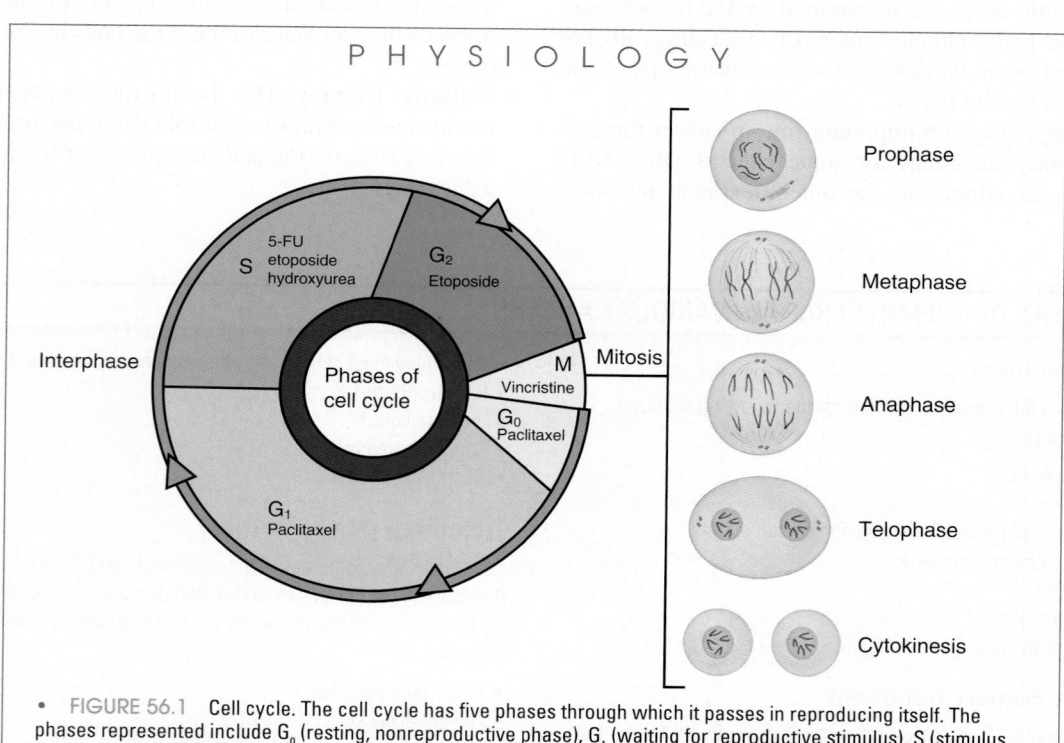

• FIGURE 56.1 Cell cycle. The cell cycle has five phases through which it passes in reproducing itself. The phases represented include G_0 (resting, nonreproductive phase), G_1 (waiting for reproductive stimulus), S (stimulus received; DNA and RNA assembled), G_2 (mitotic spindles constructed and RNA synthesized), and M (mitosis; cell division). Antineoplastic drugs with actions that occur in a particular phase of the cycle are known as cell cycle–specific drugs. Among these drugs are 5-fluorouracil, which affects the S phase of the cell cycle; vincristine, which affects the M phase (mitosis); etoposide, which affects the S and G_2 phases; paclitaxel, which affects the G_0 and possibly the G_1 phases; and hydroxyurea, which affects the S phase.

TABLE 56.1	Administration Routes for Antineoplastic Drugs			
Route	Advantages	Disadvantages	Potential Complications	Nursing Implications
Oral	Ease of administration	Inconsistency of absorption Redosing issues if the patient has emesis	Drug-specific complications (e.g., drug–herb–diet interactions)	Evaluate compliance with medication schedule. Teach patient handling techniques, drug-specific diet considerations.
Subcutaneous, intramuscular	Ease of administration Decreased side effects	Requires adequate muscle mass and tissue for absorption (may require more than 1 injection, based on the maximum recommended safe volumes for injections) Pain	Infection, bleeding	Evaluate platelet count Use smallest needle gauge possible. Prepare injection site with an antiseptic solution. Assess injection site for signs and symptoms of infection.
IV	Consistent absorption Required for vesicants	Sclerosing of veins over time	Infection, phlebitis, extravasation, tissue necrosis (vesicants)	Check for blood return before, during, and after administration of chemotherapy agentss Mandatory with vesicants..
Intra-arterial*	Increased dose directly to tumor with decreased systemic toxic effects	Requires surgical procedure or special radiography for device placement	Bleeding, embolism	Monitor for signs and symptoms of bleeding. Monitor partial thromboplastin time, prothrombin time.
Intrathecal,* intraventricular	More consistent drug levels in cerebrospinal fluid Bypass blood–brain barrier	Requires lumbar puncture or surgical placement of reservoir or implanted pump for drug delivery	Headaches, confusion, lethargy, nausea and vomiting, seizures (increased intracranial pressure)	Observe site for signs of infection. Monitor functioning of reservoir or pump. Assess patient for headache or signs of increased intracranial pressure.
Intraperitoneal*	Direct exposure of intra-abdominal metastases to drug	Requires placement of Tenckhoff catheter or intraperitoneal port	Abdominal pain, abdominal distention, bleeding, ileus, intestinal perforation, infection	Warm chemotherapy solution to body temperature. Check patency of catheter or port. Instill solution according to protocol—infuse, dwell, and drain or use continuous infusion.
Intrapleural	Sclerosing of pleural lining to prevent recurrence of effusions	Requires insertion of a thoracotomy tube	Pain, infection, fever	Monitor for complete drainage (or minimal drainage <100 mL/d optimal) from pleural cavity before instillation of drug. Following instillation, clamp tubing and reposition patient q10–15 min for 2 h (or as ordered). Attach tubing to suction for 18 h (or as ordered). Assess patient for pain, fever, or anxiety. Provide analgesic, antipyretic, and emotional support.
Intravesicular	Direct exposure of bladder surfaces to drug	Requires insertion of Foley catheter	Urinary tract infections, cystitis, bladder contracture, urinary urgency, allergic drug reactions	Maintain sterile technique when inserting Foley catheter. Instill solution, clamp catheter for 1 h, and unclamp to drain (or as ordered).

*Note: Specialized nursing education may be required for certain administration methods. Refer to individual state nurse practice acts and agency policies and procedures.

Data from: Polovich, M, Whitfor, J., Olsen, M. (2009). *Chemotherapy and biotherapy guidelines and recommendation for practice*. Oncology Nursing Society. Pittsburgh, PA: Oncology Nursing Press.

Recommendations to Minimize Exposure During Preparation, Transport, Disposal, and Storage of Chemotherapeutic Agents

To minimize exposure during preparation, transportation, disposal, and storage of chemotherapeutic agents, adhere to the following recommendations:

1. Prepare these in a primary engineering control (PEC), such as a biologic safety cabinet (BSC). These cabinets contain high-efficiency particulate air filters that pull and filter air away from the face of the person preparing the drug. It is recommended that these cabinets remain functioning 24 hours a day, 7 days a week, that they be vented to the outside, that they be cleaned daily with a 70% alcohol solution, and that they be serviced according to manufacturer's recommendations to ensure adequate performance.

2. During drug preparation, wear disposable, lint-free, long-sleeved, nonabsorbent gowns made with a low-permeability fabric. The gowns should have a solid front with tight-fitting elastic at the wrists and back closure to prevent skin exposure.

3. Use disposable, powder-free latex gloves that have been tested for use with hazardous drugs. Double gloving is recommended activities such as drug preparation, administration and handling of body excreta of patients who have received these drugs within a 48-hour period. Personnel who have latex allergy should use alternative products made with nitrile. Change gloves when soiled, torn, or punctured. Change gloves every 30 minutes when in continuous use.

4. Wear a mask with face shield whenever there is a possibility of splashing. Wear a NIOSH-approved mask when cleaning up spills.

5. Use a plastic absorbent pad to cover the work surface preparation area so that any droplet contamination is absorbed.

6. Prime IV lines for chemotherapy administration with a compatible non hazardous solution before the actual drug administration. Do not prime with the chemotherapy drug unless the infusion device has an in-line prime function to reduce the risk of aerosolization.

7. If more than a negligible amount of air exists in the syringe, return to the preparation area for removal of air using the BSC. Carefully connect and disconnect IV tubing containing antineoplastic drugs, and remove syringes from IV lines used for IV push administration. Remove empty chemotherapy bags or bottles when completed, leaving the spike intact, and dispose of in an approved hazardous waste container. Consider the use of a closed system transfer device when preparing and administering chemotherapy (e.g. Phaseal ®).

8. Use a needleless delivery system or Luer-Lok connection to prevent accidental disconnection.

9. Wash hands before and after handling antineoplastic agents to protect from exposure to hazardous drugs.

10. Never store food or beverages in a refrigerator used for chemotherapy storage, to reduce the risk of food contamination.

11. Avoid eating, drinking, applying cosmetics, or chewing gum in the vicinity of drug preparation/administration, to prevent ingestion of chemotherapy/hazardous materials.

12. Transport chemotherapeutic drugs in sealed bags to prevent spilling. Spill kits should be readily available to personnel who have been properly instructed in chemotherapy handling and exposure procedures.

13. Institute standard precautions when handling the blood, vomitus, stool, or bed linens of a patient who has received chemotherapy within the past 48 hours. Wear personal protective equipment, including mask with face shield if splashing may occur.

14. Flush the toilet with the lid down and flush twice after disposing of body fluids from patients who have received cytotoxic agents within the past 48 hours. Although this practice is not research based, this may be helpful for minimizing exposure of others from residual chemotherapy not effectively removed with low-flow toilets.

15. Cover the toilet with a waterproof shield or pad before flushing to reduce the risk of aerosolization of chemotherapeutic agents.

16. Dispose of all chemotherapy waste in impervious, leak-proof containers dedicated for chemotherapy waste and not used for other hospital waste.

17. Instruct patients who receive chemotherapy at home to label drugs to indicate hazardous content and to store the drugs in areas where proper temperature will be maintained and where children cannot reach them.

18. All equipment contaminated with antineoplastic drugs must be disposed of in distinctly labeled hazardous waste receptacles or cleaned per institutional guidelines. These chemotherapy wastes should be disposed of in Environmental Protection Agency–approved landfill waste sites or incinerators.

Management of Chemotherapy Spills

To manage spills of chemotherapeutic agents, adhere to the following recommended sequence:

1. Post a sign immediately to warn people away from the exposed area.
2. Don two pairs of powder-free gloves, a disposable gown, and eye protection.
3. Wear a NIOSH-approved respirator.
4. Place an absorbent pad over the spill to contain it.
5. Pick up glass fragments with a scoop and dispose of them in a puncture-proof container.
6. Clean the area with a detergent three times, from the least contaminated to the most contaminated areas.
7. Rinse the absorbed spill area with clean water. Repeat the washing and rinsing.

8. Dispose of all cleanup equipment according to institutional policy for chemotherapuetic waste.
9. Document the spill according to institutional policy. The following data should be included in the documentation: name of chemotherapy agent and approximate volume spilled, how spill occurred, procedures followed to contain and clean up spill, and names of people who were exposed and of those who were notified of spill.

To expedite the handling of a spill and to minimize undue patient and employee exposure, well-equipped chemotherapy spill kits and staff trained in the proper procedure for cleaning spills should be readily available.

Measures for Accidental Exposure to Chemotherapy

To manage accidental exposure to chemotherapy, implement the following measures:

1. Eye contact: Immediately rinse the affected eye or eyes with copious amounts of water for no less than 15 minutes. Seek emergency treatment per institutional policy.
2. Skin contact: Immediately wash the area with soap and water. Refer to Material Safety Data Sheets (MSDS) for specific agents.
3. Clothing contact: Immediately remove the contaminated clothing; if skin contact occurred, wash all such areas with soap and water. Place soiled clothing in a plastic bag until it is laundered, and then wash it twice, separately from all other clothing. After laundering the clothing twice, put the machine through a separate wash-rinse cycle.
4. Bed linen contact: Immediately remove the linens and place them in a contaminated linen receptacle; then clean the mattress using a 70% alcohol solution. Once the alcohol dries, the bed may be remade with clean linens.
5. Complete institutional reporting and documentation requirements.

CLASSIFICATION OF ANTINEOPLASTIC DRUGS

Antineoplastic drugs are classified according to their mode of action and the phase of the cell cycle in which the drug is active. However, rapidly dividing cells are the most sensitive to these drugs. Chemotherapeutic drugs that are most effective during a particular phase of the cycle are known as **cell cycle–** (or cell phase) **specific**, whereas drugs that act independently of a specific cell cycle (or cell phase) are **cell cycle–nonspecific.** This classification is not absolute; the cytotoxic effects of the drugs likely involve more than one mechanism. Multiple intracellular sites might be affected, and the drugs' effects might not be confined to specific cycle events.

This chapter discusses the cell cycle–specific group of drugs (Table 56.2). Chapter 37 discusses the cell cycle–nonspecific group of drugs and targeted therapy. The cell cycle–specific drugs consist of the antimetabolites (prototype, 5-fluorouracil

[5-FU]) and mitotic inhibitors. These drugs exert the greatest killing effect on tumors when given as a continuous infusion or in divided doses with a short cycle. The mitotic inhibitors are subdivided into the vinca alkaloids (prototype, vincristine), the podophyllotoxins (prototype, etoposide), and the taxanes (prototype, paclitaxel). Another category of cell cycle–specific drugs is called camptothecines (prototype, topotecan). A miscellaneous group of antineoplastic drugs, such as the prototype drug hydroxyurea and L-asparaginase, is also discussed in this chapter.

Ⓒ ANTIMETABOLITES

Antimetabolites are synthetic products that mimic the naturally produced metabolites, purines, pyrimidines, and folates that are essential for DNA and RNA synthesis. When the cell uses antimetabolites instead of the naturally occurring metabolites, cell death results. Because antimetabolites exert their cytotoxic activity during the S phase of the cell's life cycle, they are most effective against tumors that have a high **growth fraction.** The growth fraction of a tumor is the fraction of its cell population that is in any active phase of the cell cycle. Relatively quiescent tumors found in organs such as the pancreas and the uterus have low growth fractions, whereas rapidly proliferating tumors, such as those of the gastrointestinal (GI) mucosal epithelium and the hair follicles, have high growth fractions.

The prototype antimetabolite drug is 5-fluorouracil (5-FU, Adrucil), a pyrimidine antagonist that is a mainstay in chemotherapy.

Nursing Management of the Patient Receiving Ⓟ 5-Fluorouracil

Core Drug Knowledge

Pharmacotherapeutics

The drug 5-FU interferes with DNA synthesis and, to a lesser extent, inhibits the formation of RNA. It has proved to be clinically effective against a wide spectrum of solid tumors, particularly malignant GI tumors. It is indicated for the palliative management of carcinoma of the colon, breast, liver, ovary, pancreas, rectum, head and neck, and stomach. It has been used in combination with cisplatin, irinotecan, oxaliplatin, bevacizumab and most often with leucovorin, which potentiates the action of 5-FU.

Dosage adjustments (see Table 56.2) are imperative for patients who develop severe toxicities. Patients must be monitored closely throughout therapy.

In addition to being administered intravenously (the most common route), 5-FU is given by intra-arterial infusion into the hepatic artery through a surgically implanted pump. The goal of this type of delivery is to supply a high concentration of the antineoplastic drug directly to the tumor and surrounding area while sparing the normal tissues from toxic effects. A topical form of 5-FU is also available and has been curative for basal cell carcinomas and other malignant skin cancers.

TABLE 56.2 ● **Summary of Selected** ● **Cell Cycle–Specific Antineoplastic Drugs**

Drug (Trade) Name	Selected Indications	Route and Dosage Range	Pharmacokinetics
● **Antimetabolites**			
▶ 5-fluorouracil (5-FU, Adrucil)	Carcinoma of colon, rectum, stomach, pancreas, breast, and ovary; hepatocellular carcinoma	*Adult:* IV, 12–15 mg/kg daily for 4 d/wk (maximum daily dose: 800 mg), then 6 mg/kg on days 6, 8, 10, and 12; maintenance, repeat first course q30 d Bolus, 400 mg/m² with irinotecan or oxaliplatin, followed by 2,400–3,000 mg/m² 22-h infusion on days 1, 2, 15, and 16 *or* 2400 mg/m² 46-h infusion on days 1 and 15	*Onset:* IV, immediate *Duration:* IV, 6 h $t_{1/2}$: IV, 18–20 min
	Skin cancer, superficial basal cell cancer	*Adult:* Topical, apply sufficient drug to cover affected area bid	*Onset:* Minimal absorption in topical use *Duration:* Unknown $t_{1/2}$: Unknown
capecitabine (Xeloda)	Metastatic colon cancer, breast cancer	*Adult:* PO, 1,250 mg/m² bid for 2 wk q21–28 d for 8 cycles or 1,000 mg/m² in combination with oxalipla-tin for 2 wk q21–28 d. Lower doses may be used for esophagogastric or gastric cancers in combination with epirubicin, oxaliplatin or cisplatin.	*Onset:* Rapid (food decreases absorption) *Duration:* Unknown $t_{1/2}$: 30–60 min
cytarabine (Ara-C)	Acute myelocytic leukemia, acute lymphocytic leukemia (ALL), Hodgkin's and non-Hodgkin's lymphoma, CNS leukemia	*Adult:* IV, 100 mg/m²/d by continuous infusion for 7 d; then 100 mg/m² q12h for 1–3 wk; high dose induction therapy, 3 g/m(2) IV infused over 1–3 hr every 12 hr for 2–6 d, intrathecal, 20–30 mg/m² (higher dose up to 75 mg/m² may be used to treat CNS disease). A liposomal cytarabine, DepoCyt can also be used at a dose of 50mg.	*Onset:* Rapid *Duration:* 12–18 h $t_{1/2}$: 1–3 h
floxuridine (FUDR)	Gastrointestinal (GI) adenocarcinoma with metastasis to liver, gallbladder, or bile ducts	*Adult:* Intra-arterial only, 0.1–0.6 mg/kg/d	*Onset:* Immediate *Duration:* 3 h $t_{1/2}$: 20 h
fludarabine (Fludara)	Chronic lymphocytic leukemia, non-Hodgkin's lymphoma (investigational)	*Adult:* IV, 25 mg/m²/d for 5 d, q28d	*Onset:* Rapid *Duration:* Unknown $t_{1/2}$: 10 h
6-mercaptopurine (Purinethol)	Acute leukemia, chronic myelogenous leukemia (CML)	*Adult and child:* PO (induction and consolidation), 2.5 mg/kg/d; maintenance, 1.5–2.5 mg/kg/d	*Onset:* Varies *Duration:* Unknown $t_{1/2}$: 20–50 min
methotrexate (Mexate, Folex)	Hodgkin's lymphoma, non-Hodgkin's lymphomas; acute lymphoblastic and myelocytic leukemia; CNS metasta-sis; carcinoma of ovary, lung, cervix, testicle, breast; sarcomas; epidermoid carcinoma of head and neck	*Adult:* Trophoblastic neoplasms, PO/IM, 3–5 cycles of 15–30 mg/d for 5 d; leukemia maintenance, IV, 2.5 mg/kg q14 d or 15 mg/m² PO/IM 2×/wk; lymphoma, PO, 10–25 mg/d *High dose:* 8,000–12,000 mg/m² q2–4wk-only with urine alkalinization and leukovorin.	*Onset:* PO, varies; IV, rapid *Duration:* Unknown $t_{1/2}$: 2–4 h (high dose, 8–15 h)
6-thioguanine (Tabloid)	Acute myelocytic leukemia, chronic granulocytic leukemia	*Adult:* PO, 1–3 mg/kg/d	*Onset:* Slow *Duration:* 8 h $t_{1/2}$: 11 h
● **Vinca Alkaloids**			
▶ vincristine (Oncovin)	ALL, Hodgkin and non-Hodgkin lymphoma, CML, sarcomas, breast and small-cell lung cancers	*Adult:* IV, 1.4 mg/m²/wk *Child:* 2.0 mg/m²/wk; • Maximum single dose of 2 mg is seldom exceeded. INTRATHECAL ADMINISTRATION OF VINCRISTINE IS FATAL; vincristine is for intravenous use only	*Onset:* Varies *Duration:* Not available $t_{1/2}$: 5 min, then 2–3 h, then 85 h
vinblastine (Velban)	Hodgkin's disease, lymphocytic and histiocytic lymphomas, mycosis fungoi-des, advanced testicular cancer, breast cancer, squamous cell carcinoma of head and neck, Kaposi sarcoma	*Adult:* IV, 0.1 mg/kg to 6 mg/m² weekly; continuous infusion, 1.4–1.8 mg/d for 5 d • INTRATHECAL ADMINISTRATION OF VINCRISTINE IS FATAL; vincristine is for intravenous use only	*Onset:* Slow *Duration:* Unknown $t_{1/2}$: 3.7 min, then 16 h, then 24.8 h

TABLE 56.2 **Summary of Selected Ⓒ Cell Cycle–Specific Antineoplastic Drugs** *(continued)*

Drug (Trade) Name	Selected Indications	Route and Dosage Range	Pharmacokinetics
vinorelbine (Navelbine)	Non–small-cell lung cancer, breast cancer combination with cisplatin	*Adult:* IV, 30 mg/m² weekly • INTRATHECAL ADMINISTRATION OF VINCRISTINE IS FATAL; vincristine is for intravenous use only	*Onset:* Slow *Duration:* Unknown $t_{1/2}$: 22–66 h
Ⓒ Podophyllotoxins			
Ⓟ etoposide (VePesid)	Refractory testicular tumors Small-cell lung cancer Other cancers	*Adult:* IV, testicular cancer, 50–100 mg/m²/d for 5 d q3–4wk or 100 mg/m² on days 1, 3, and 5 *Adult:* IV, 35 or 50 mg/m²/d for 5 d q3–4wk *Adult:* PO, twice the IV dose *Higher doses are used for acute leukemia treatment and as a preparatory regimen for stem cell transplantation.*	*Onset:* IV, 30 min; PO, 30–60 min *Duration:* IV/PO, 20–30 h $t_{1/2}$: 4–11 h
teniposide (VM-26, Vumon)	Childhood acute lymphoblastic leukemia	*Adult:* IV, 165 mg/m² with cytarabine 300 mg/m² 2×/wk for 8 or 9 doses	*Onset:* 30 min *Duration:* Unknown $t_{1/2}$: 5 h
Ⓒ Taxanes			
Ⓟ paclitaxel (Taxol)	Metastatic carcinoma of the breast, ovary; small-cell lung cancer, Kaposi;s sarcoma	*Adult:* IV, 135–200 mg/m² over 3–24 h q3 wk *Low-dose:* 80 mg/m² over 1 h *Kaposi's sarcoma-* 135 mg/m(2) IV over 3 h every 3 wk; OR 100 mg/m(2) IV over 3 hr every 2 wk;	*Onset:* Rapid *Duration:* 6–12 h $t_{1/2}$: 5.3–17.4 h
docetaxel (Taxotere)	Breast, gastric, non-cmall cell lung cancer, head and neck cancer, metastatic prostate cancer	*Adult:* IV, 60–100 mg/m² q3 wk	*Onset:* Unknown *Duration:* Unknown $t_{1/2}$: 11 h
Ⓒ Camptothecines			
Ⓟ topotecan (Hycamtin)	Metastatic carcinoma of the ovary, cervical cancer, non small cell lung cancer.	*Adult:* IV, 1.5 mg/m² for 5 d q3 wk	*Onset:* Unknown *Duration:* Unknown $t_{1/2}$: 3 h
irinotecan (Camptosar, CPT-11)	Metastatic carcinoma of the colon or rectum in patients whose disease has progressed or recurred after 5-FU therapy. Also used investigationally in many other cancer types at lower doses.	*Adult:* IV, 125 mg/m²/wk for 4 wk, then 2 wk rest. Dosage varies by protocol.	*Onset:* Unknown *Duration:* Unknown $t_{1/2}$: 6 h
Ⓒ Miscellaneous			
Ⓟ hydroxyurea (Hydrea)	CML, malignant melanoma, inoperable carcinoma of ovary, squamous cell carcinoma of head and neck, sickle cell disease.	*Adult:* PO, for CML, 20–30 mg/kg as continuous therapy; for solid tumors, 80 mg/kg q3d or 20–30 mg/kg/d, 15 mg/kg daily for sickle cell disease- based on blood counts.	*Onset:* Varies *Duration:* 18–20 h $t_{1/2}$: 2–3 h
L-asparaginase (Elspar)	ALL, used investigationally for CLL, Hodgkin's lymphoma, lymphosarcoma	*Adult:* IV/IM, 200 IU/kg for 28 d; dosage varies with protocol	*Onset:* IM, varies; IV, 30–40 min *Duration:* Unknown $t_{1/2}$: 8–30 h

*Note: Antineoplastic drug dosages are calculated specifically for each patient based on his/her body surface area (BSA). The BSA is calculated from height and weight measurements and determined by using an institutionally approved BSA formula (e.g., Mosteller's formula = square root of [height in cm multiplied by weight in kg/3,600]) or an electronic conversion calculator. The Oncology Nursing Society does not recommend the use of a nomogram because of inaccuracy that can occur from distortion due to the copying of nomograms and difficulty of reading these charts. (need a disclaimer here about dosage ranges?)

Pharmacokinetics

After infusion, 5-FU distributes into tumors, intestinal mucosa, bone marrow, liver, and tissues throughout the body. It diffuses readily across the blood–brain barrier and distributes into cerebrospinal fluid (CSF) and brain tissue. The drug is extensively metabolized in the liver and excreted by the kidneys and lungs. The mean half-life of elimination from plasma is about 16 minutes, with a range of 8 to 20 minutes. The clearance of 5-FU is substantially lower in women than in men, whereas age has no appreciable effect on clearance in either gender. There is increased interest in pharmacokinetic dose adjustments when administering 5-FU due to the variability person to person when based soley on BSA. This approach used in the future may assist with minimizing toxicities while administering the maximum dose needed to reach therapeutic levels.

Pharmacodynamics

During the S phase, 5-FU exerts its maximum cytotoxic effects. It acts as a "false" antimetabolite, causing a thymine deficiency. This deficiency deprives the cell of DNA and RNA, which are essential for cell division and growth. The result is unbalanced growth and death of the cell. The deprivation of DNA and RNA is most marked in rapidly growing cells because these cells take up 5-FU at a faster rate.

Contraindications and Precautions

5-FU is a pregnancy category D drug. Whether it is excreted in human milk is not known, so caution should be exercised by women who are breast-feeding. The drug has demonstrated carcinogenic and mutagenic properties. The use of 5-FU is contraindicated in patients with poor nutritional status, depressed bone marrow function, and any known serious infection. The drug should not be administered to patients who have a known sensitivity to the drug. Patients with familial pyrimidinemia, an enzyme deficiency (dihydropyrimidine dehydrogenase enzyme deficiency), should not receive 5-FU because of the potential for severe neurotoxicity due to the inability to metabolize 5-FU.

Adverse Effects

Serious adverse effects of 5-FU include myelosuppression (evidenced by anemia, leukopenia, and thrombocytopenia), which is the dose-limiting side effect of 5-FU. The **nadir** is the period during which the maximum cytotoxic effect of the drug is exerted on the bone marrow, causing the lowest blood cell count. The white blood cell (WBC) nadir occurs within 10 to 14 days after the drug is given; recovery is within 21 days.

Cardiotoxicity is also an important rare but severe adverse effect of 5-FU. Cardiac events occur during the first 72 hours of the initial treatment cycle, manifested by angina, palpitations, sweating, and/or syncope. Electrocardiogram (ECG) changes, arrhythmias, pulmonary edema, myocardial infarction, (rarely) cardiac arrest, and severe but reversible cardiogenic shock have been noted with this drug.

Patients may also develop an acute cerebellar syndrome characterized by headache, disorientation, and nystagmus; this condition may persist after the drug is discontinued. Photophobia and ocular changes, such as increased lacrimation and blurred vision, may occur as well.

Other dose-dependent toxicities that can be mild to severe include nausea, vomiting, anorexia, diarrhea, and stomatitis. GI ulceration and hemorrhage can lead to death. Cutaneous changes can also occur: alopecia (hair loss; thinning of the hair); hyperpigmentation of the skin, hands, and vein along the site of infusion; brittle and cracking nails; maculopapular rash; and painful, erythematous desquamation and fissures of the palms and soles. Palmar–plantar erythrodysesthesia, also known as hand–foot syndrome, is also possible; symptoms include pain, swelling, numbness, tingling, and redness of the hands or feet.

Because 5-FU is known for its toxicity, patients who are at increased risk for these toxicities should be monitored vigilantly; for example, death from toxicity, anaphylaxis, angina, or thrombophlebitis can result even in patients who are relatively healthy. Patients with familial pyrimidinemia, an enzyme deficiency (dihydropyrimidine dehydrogenase enzyme deficiency), should not receive 5-FU because of the potential for severe neurotoxicity due to the inability to metabolize 5-FU.

Drug Interactions

A number of drug- drug interactions have been observed with 5-FU. A careful review of all of the patients medications should be done prior to starting 5-FU and periodically. Examples of drugs that cause interactions include; warfarin, phenytoin, and tamoxifen. 5-FU is incompatible with diazepam, droperidol, metoclopramide, ondansetron, and other chemotherapeutic drugs such as cytarabine, gallium nitrate, and vinorelbine. Leucovorin calcium may enhance the toxicity of 5-FU. Some drug–laboratory test interferences can occur with 5-FU administration, such as increased excretion of 5-hydroxyindoleacetic acid (5-HIAA); plasma albumin levels may decrease as a result of protein malabsorption. Table 56.3 lists drugs that interact with 5-FU.

Assessment of Relevant Core Patient Variables

Health Status

Before treatment begins, assess the patient's hematologic profile and document baseline neurologic status. Asses liver function prior to administration. Because GI alterations may occur with 5-FU dosing, check the patient's oral mucosa, bowel elimination patterns, and dietary habits. Review the patient's drug and hypersensitivity history, especially to 5-FU. Because of potential cutaneous changes, assess the condition of the patient's skin, nails, and hair. Monitor patients with a pre-existing cardiac disease closely.

Life Span and Gender

Explore the reproductive goals of the patient and assess women of childbearing age for pregnancy and lactation.

TABLE 56.3 Agents That Interact with P 5-Fluorouracil

Interactants	Effect and Significance	Nursing Management
thiazide diuretics: hydrochlorothiazide, chlorothiazide, chlorthalidone, benzthiazide, metolazone	Possible blood abnormalities	Notify physician for possible dose modification. Monitor hematopoietic status of patient.
cimetidine	Increased pharmacologic effect of 5-fluorouracil (5-FU)	Same as above.
leucovorin	Potentiates toxicity of 5-FU	Same as above.

Chemotherapy with 5-FU may cause fetal harm when administered to pregnant women. The drug has been found to be carcinogenic and mutagenic, and it can impair fertility. It is not known whether 5-FU is excreted in the breast milk; therefore, breast-feeding may be hazardous. Compare the benefits and risks to children. The safety and efficacy of 5-FU in children are not established.

Lifestyle, Diet, and Habits
One adverse effect of 5-FU is skin sensitivity to the sun. Ask the patient whether he or she engages in activities that cause undue exposure to the sun and what methods of sun protection are used. Assess the patient's feelings regarding hair loss—the major visible reminder that the patient is undergoing chemotherapy—and consider its effect on the patient's sexuality and body image. The possibility and actuality of hair loss can be very distressing, particularly if the patient has an active social and work life. Because of 5-FU's deleterious effects on the GI mucosa, obtain information on normal dietary intake and eating patterns, which might necessitate dietary modifications.

Environment
5-FU is given in both inpatient and ambulatory care settings. In some situations, 5-FU may be given as a continuous infusion through an ambulatory pump in the home setting. In these instances, explore whether the patient or significant other is ready to take on this responsibility and knows how to troubleshoot problems with the pump, should they arise.

Nursing Diagnoses and Outcomes
- Risk for Infection related to drug-induced suppression of bone marrow function
  Desired outcome: The patient will be free from infection and exercise caution to avoid exposure to sources of infection.
- Risk for Injury: Bleeding related to drug-induced suppression of bone marrow function
  Desired outcome: The patient will recover adequate hematologic status and learn to recognize, monitor, and manage situations that might induce bleeding.
- Imbalanced Nutrition: Less than Body Requirements, related to drug-induced nausea, vomiting, mucositis, and diarrhea

Desired outcome: The patient will maintain adequate nutrition with good emetic control and less frequent passage of stools. Patient will state proper oral mucosa care and self-care measures to manage pain or discomfort in the GI mucosa.
- Disturbed Body Image related to loss of cutaneous integrity, as evidenced by alopecia and changes in skin and nails
  Desired outcome: The patient will develop coping strategies (use of wigs, hair covering) to enhance appearance that may be distorted because of hair loss. In addition, cutaneous integrity will be sustained.
- Disturbed Sensory Perception related to ocular changes, photophobia, and cerebellar ataxia
  Desired outcome: The patient will be free from adverse effects resulting from oculomotor dysfunction.

Planning and Intervention
Maximizing Therapeutic Effects
Do not exceed the 800-mg maximum daily dose of 5-FU. Reduce the dose if the patient has impaired liver function or poor nutritional status. Protect the drug from light and inspect it for precipitates before infusion. Make sure that the solution is stored at controlled temperature. If a precipitate caused by low-temperature storage occurs, restabilize the solution by heating it to 140°F, shaking it vigorously, and allowing it to cool down to body temperature before administration. A slight discoloration may occur during storage, which does not affect the potency and safety of 5-FU.

Minimizing Adverse Effects
Monitor the patient closely. hematologic and GI toxicities can be fatal despite dosage reductions. A WBC differential count should be obtained before each drug course. Treatment should be withheld if laboratory test values are below safe levels (e.g., absolute neutrophil count (ANC) less than 1,500 and platelets less than 100K). Carefully monitor patients with pre-existing cardiac conditions. Do not administer to patients with familial pyrimidinemia because of the risk of severe neurotoxicity.

If any of the following conditions occur, immediately notify the prescriber and consider discontinuing the drug:

- Mucositis (e.g., Stomatitis, esophagopharyngitis and perirectal cellulitis) (first visible sign)
- Leukopenia (WBC count less than 1,500 cells/mm^3)
- Thrombocytopenia (platelet count less than 100,000 cells/mm^3)

- Intractable vomiting
- Diarrhea
- GI ulceration and bleeding
- Bleeding from any site

Providing Patient and Family Education
Follow the guidelines described in Box 56.2.

- Explain that 5-FU requires special precautions to prevent chemotherapy from coming into accidental contact with patients or others.
- Give troubleshooting instructions if an alternative access device or an ambulatory infusion device is used at home.

BOX 56.2 COMMUNITY BASED CONCERNS

General Patient and Family Education for Chemotherapy

The nurse plays a pivotal role in providing adequate information to assist the patient/family with the new roles so that treatment outcomes will be achieved. After diagnosis, the treatment modality is discussed and chosen. For most cancers, chemotherapy is a significant benefit. The talking points for the nurse when called on to educate patients, irrespective of the type of chemotherapeutic agent used, include:

- Instruct patient about the significant side effects and reportable signs and symptoms of the chemotherapeutic agent(s).
- Emphasize self-management measures to be undertaken to prevent or decrease the side effects:
  - Practice good personal hygiene, wash hands frequently, and avoid sources of infection.
  - Maintain dietary intake of food and fluids. Refer to dietician for consultation.
  - Avoid trauma or injury and potential sources of bleeding by shaving with an electric razor, avoiding aspirin and other nonsteroidal anti-inflammatory drugs, and avoiding unnecessary injections, use of rectal thermometers, and venipunctures.
  - Check urine, stool, skin for signs of bleeding.
  - Practice good oral hygiene; use soft toothbrush, noncommercial (i.e., non-alcohol-based) mouthwashes, and lubricants.
  - Schedule appointments for blood tests and follow-up visits for chemotherapy and related medications.
- If the patient goes to other physicians, dentists, or another health care provider, patient should inform them of chemotherapy treatment.
- Teach patients the importance of relaxation techniques and other forms of complementary medicine from which they might benefit.
- Refer to other agencies and support groups as appropriate. Provide patient with a list of these resources.
- Instruct patients in the importance of maintaining a balance between rest and exercise to minimize fatigue.
- Explain to patient that some side effects of treatment are reversible and are thus not a sign of disease progression.
- If a patient is using chemotherapy drugs at home, teach the patient how to properly handle, store, and dispose of the agents and related materials.
- Encourage and support patient to accept a "new" baseline, especially in activities and responsibilities, imposed by demands of disease and treatment. Encourage patients to learn how to delegate and ask for assistance with activities of daily living.

Patients should also know whom to call and how to reach that person, in case of problems.

- Explain that nausea and vomiting may occur 3 to 6 hours after drug therapy is administered; provide an appropriate antiemetic regimen. The metallic taste of the drug may be minimized by sucking on hard candy.
- Instruct patients to observe the stools and notify the prescriber if stools are black or if blood is visible. Instruct the patient to notify the prescriber for loose stools including freqnecy and amount.
- Mouth sores may develop 5 to 8 days after drug administration. Offer helpful strategies such as practicing daily oral hygiene after meals and at bedtime, using a salt, baking soda and water rinse (1½ teaspoons of baking soda, 1 tsp salt to 1 quart of water), brushing with a soft toothbrush, avoiding alcohol containing mouthwashes, and gently flossing with unwaxed dental floss if the patient currently flosses. If bleeding occurs, flossing should be stopped until bleeding subsides.
- Caution patients not to use aspirin or any pain-relieving drugs containing aspirin without consulting the prescriber, to decrease the risk of bleeding following 5-FU therapy.
- Teach patients to self-assess for signs and symptoms of potential infection, check temperature, and report temperature spikes higher than 100.5°F.
- Suggest that patients apply moisturizer to the lips and to avoid irritating, very hot, cold, or spicy foods and beverages. Bland, cool, soft foods, such as yogurt, custards, gelatins, and puddings, may be less irritating.
- Help patients to understand that drug therapy produces photosensitivity. Instruct the patient to avoid the sun or protect the skin by applying a sunscreen (skin protection factor [SPF] = 15) and wearing protective clothing year round.
- Encourage patients to express their concerns about the effects of cutaneous changes on body image and assist in developing strategies to minimize the emotional impact. Offer cosmetic strategies, such as wearing nail polish to cover darkened, dry, brittle nails and using wigs, hats, and scarves to protect the scalp and prevent heat loss..
- Instruct patients to notify the physician if confusion or any visual disturbances occur.
- Advise women of childbearing potential about the possibility of harm to the fetus and about methods of contraception.

Ongoing Assessment and Evaluation

The main adverse effects of 5-FU therapy are alterations in the patient's hematopoietic system and GI functions. Therefore, monitor the patient's complete blood counts (CBCs) closely during each drug administration cycle to make sure that bone marrow recovery has occurred before another dose of the drug is given. Likewise, assess the patient's nutritional status. Stomatitis or other problems related to the gastric mucosa should be kept under control to avoid putting the patient at risk for poor nutrition.

MEMORY CHIP

P 5-Fluorouracil

- Indicated for treating carcinoma of the colon, rectum, breast, stomach, and pancreas
- Major contraindications: poor nutritional status, decreased bone marrow reserve, or a potentially serious infection
- Most common adverse effects: mucositis, diarrhea, alopecia and other cutaneous changes, such as photo-sensitivity and increased pigmentation of the skin
- Dose-limiting effects: mainly on the bone marrow, manifested by myelosuppression, and the gastrointestinal mucosa, causing nausea, vomiting, diarrhea, and stomatitis
- **Life span alert: Advise women of child-bearing age of the potential for harm to the fetus so that they practice contraception. It is not known whether the drug is excreted in breast milk; therefore, explain that breast-feeding is not advised.**
- Maximizing therapeutic effects: Potentiate antineoplastic activity of 5-FU by the addition of reduced folates, such as leucovorin calcium.
- Minimizing adverse effects: Monitor CBC and assess for signs and symptoms of myelosuppression, which include infection and bleeding.
- Most important patient education: Teach patient good oral care and to monitor for signs and symptoms of mucositis and infection. Advise patient of the possibility of transient alopecia, which will reverse after chemotherapy is finished.

Drugs Closely Related to **P** 5-Fluorouracil

The other drugs in the antimetabolite category are listed in Table 56.2, which includes specific disease indications and routes of administration.

Cytarabine

Cytarabine (Ara-C) is commonly used in hematologic malignancies. It is associated with a unique toxicity termed chemical keratitis, which is usually treated with dexamethasone eye drops. Ara-C given in high doses as a bolus infusion can cause cerebellar toxicitiess. Cerebellar checks must be completed at baseline and prior to each bolus dose of Ara-C so that changes can be detected early and the drug can be discontinued. Ara-C given in high doses as a continuous infusion is associated with pulmonary toxicity, and nurses must carefully monitor fluid status, weight, and lung sounds and administer diuretics to maintain patients at a specified goal weight.

Floxuridine

Floxuridine (FUDR) is an analogue of 5-FU. FUDR is most commonly administered directly into the liver through a hepatic arterial pump for patients with colorectal or GI cancer and liver metastasis. Special training is required prior to administering chemotherapy through a hepatic arterial pump.

Gemcitabine

Gemcitabine (Gemzar) causes myelosuppression, most notably thrombocytopenia. It is important to note that infusion times longer than 60 minutes can cause increased toxicities. In addition, Gemcitabine causes a skin rash in about 20% of patients. Gemcitabiner should be reconstituted with normal saline only.

Capecitabine

Capecitabine (Xeloda) is the oral prodrug of 5-FU, which means that when capecitabine is taken orally, it converts to 5-FU in the body. Despite its oral administration, capecitabine is as efficacious as 5-FU (Box 56.3). The most common dose-limiting adverse effect is hand-and-foot syndrome. Development of this syndrome requires stopping of the drug until resolution, with subsequent dose modifications.

BOX 56.3 FOCUS ON RESEARCH

Capecitabine Results in Superior Response Rate, Improved Safety Profile, and Improved Convenience

Van Cutsem, E., Hoff, P. M., Harper, P., Bukowski, R. M., Cunningham, D., Dufour, P., et al. (2004). Oral capecitabine vs intravenous 5-fluorouracil and leucovorin: Integrated efficiency data and novel analysis from two large randomized, phase III trials. *British Journal of Cancer*, 90: 1190–1197.

The Study

This trial involved a total of 1207 patients with metastatic colorectal cancer who were randomized to treatment with standard therapy of 5-fluorouracil (5-FU) and leucovorin (5-FU/LV) versus oral capecitabine (OX). Treatment involved either of the following:

1. Capecitabine, 1,250 mg/m^2 twice daily on days 1 to 14, every 21 days
2. Leucovorin, 20 mg/m^2, followed by 5-FU, 425-mg/m^2 IV bolus, on days 1 to 5 every 28 days.

OX showed a statistically significant superior response rate compared to 5-FU/LV ($p < 0.0002$). Even in patients with poor prognostic indicators, subgroup analysis showed that OX demonstrated superior effects. Patients were treated for up to 48 weeks or until disease progression. Capecitabine resulted in a superior response rate and equivalent time to progression and overall survival. In addition, this study demonstrated the improved safety profile of the drug. It had a significantly lower rate of diarrhea (47.7% versus 58.2%), stomatitis (24.3% versus 61.6%), nausea (37.9% versus 47.6%), and alopecia (6% versus 20.6%). The only adverse effect that occurred significantly more frequently was hand-and-foot syndrome (53.5% versus 6.2%).

The results of this study support the use of capecitabine as first-line monotherapy for advanced colorectal cancer. Capecitabine offers patients an effective oral treatment, which can be administered on an outpatient basis. This study also showed that fewer patients required hospitalization related to adverse effects (11.6% versus 18%; $p < 0.005$).

Drug Significantly Different From P 5-Fluorouracil

Methotrexate (MTX) is a folate antimetabolite that induces folate depletion, leading to the inhibition of purine synthesis and arrested DNA, RNA, and protein synthesis. MTX is indicated in managing Hodgkin's disease; trophoblastic neoplasm; acute leukemia; meningeal leukemia; breast carcinoma; head, neck, and lung neoplasms; Burkitt lymphoma; CNS lymphomas, osteosarcoma; lymphosarcoma; and mycosis fungoides. It may be given in a variety of doses and schedules through various routes of administration. A small portion is metabolized in the liver; the drug is excreted in the urine mostly as unchanged drug. Because MTX is secreted by the renal tubules, certain drugs that follow the same pathway, such as salicylates, sulfonamides, phenytoin, and penicillin, may compete with MTX excretion, resulting in accumulation and increased toxicity. Therefore, these drugs should be discontinued 2 days before and restarted 2 days after MTX therapy. Adverse effects are similar to 5-FU, with the exception of neurotoxicity (at high doses) and acute hepatotoxicity manifested by elevated liver enzyme levels. With high-dose regimens, the following important considerations should be undertaken:

• Emetogenic potential is moderate (30% to 90% frequency of emesis) with doses greater than 250 mg/m^2; make sure that an appropriate antiemetic regimen is initiated.
• Monitor urine specific gravity, urine output, and urinary pH. Administer sodium bicarbonate and hydrate the patient to maintain urinary alkalinization (pH >7) and urinary output of more than 100 mL/h.
• Obtain orders for leucovorin rescue. Leucovorin is given to bypass the inhibitor action of MTX and supplies the form of folic acid needed by the normal cells for DNA synthesis. Leucovorin is usually initiated 24 to 36 hours after MTX, according to a prescribed schedule based on serum MTX and creatinine levels. No doses of leucovorin should be missed, because missed doses may increase toxicity.
• Monitor MTX blood levels for at least 72 hours until the nontoxic level of less than 0.1 micromolar is reached.

Like 5-FU, MTX is a pregnancy category X drug. MTX is discussed in depth in Chapter 25.

C MITOTIC INHIBITORS

The mitotic inhibitors (also known as plant alkaloids) interfere with the formation of the mitotic spindle, causing metaphase arrest. They are primarily known as M-phase active drugs, but they may also have some activity in the G$_2$ and S phases. These drugs are the vinca alkaloids, the podophyllotoxins, and the taxanes.

• C VINCA ALKALOIDS

Vinca alkaloids are extracts of the periwinkle plant *Vinca rosea*. They bind to microtubular proteins, which are key to formation of the mitotic spindle in dividing cells. This binding arrests mitosis and eventually causes cell death. The vinca alkaloids act mainly in the M phase. However, high doses of the vinca alkaloids vincristine (Oncovin, Vincasar PFS) and vinblastine (Velban, VLB) can also disrupt RNA and protein synthesis. The prototype vinca alkaloid is vincristine.

Nursing Management of the Patient Receiving P Vincristine
Core Drug Knowledge
Pharmacotherapeutics

The major clinical use of vincristine is in the treatment of acute lymphoblastic leukemia. It is used in combination therapy for Hodgkin's and non-Hodgkin's lymphomas, sarcoma, breast cancer, small-cell lung cancer, rhabdomyosarcoma, neuroblastoma, and Wilms' tumor. The recommended dosage of vincristine for an adult is discussed in Table 56.2. For children weighing less than 10 kg or with body surface areas of less than 1 square meter, the dose is 0.05 mg/kg/wk.

Pharmacokinetics

Following IV administration, vincristine binds extensively to both the plasma proteins and the blood elements, particularly the platelets. Its penetration across the blood–brain barrier is poor. Vincristine is metabolized by the hepatic system, and 70% of the drug is excreted in the bile or feces. A small fraction is excreted in the urine.

Pharmacodynamics

The mechanism of action of vincristine is attributed to mitotic inhibition, which arrests cell division in the metaphase stage of mitosis. The drug interferes with a protein called tubulin, which is required for formation of microtubules and the mitotic spindle. The depolymerized tubulin proteins do not allow the spindle proteins to assemble, and cell division is halted in the metaphase.

Contraindications and Precautions

Neurotoxicity from vincristine may be more pronounced in patients with underlying neurologic problems. Vincristine is contraindicated in patients with the demyelinating form of Charcot-Marie-Tooth syndrome, a neurologic disease characterized by absence of deep tendon reflexes. Because liver disease may alter the elimination of vincristine, dosage modifications may be needed in patients with elevated bilirubin levels. Care must be taken to prevent accidental contamination of the eyes, especially when the drug is administered intravenously under severe pressure, because the drug can cause severe eye irritation, including corneal ulceration if it splashes into the eye. If eye contamination occurs, the eyes must be washed immediately and thoroughly.

Vincristine is administered by IV routes only. Given intrathecally, vincristine may be fatal. The drug can be delivered through a side port of a free-flowing IV line to allow dilution. It can also be given by continuous infusion, but only through a central venous access device with positive blood return. Vincristine is a **vesicant.** Vesicants are drugs that may cause substantial tissue damage, including tissue

Box 56.4 MANAGING PERIPHERAL EXTRAVASATION

Extravasation is the inadvertent infiltration of the chemotherapeutic drug into the subcutaneous tissues surrounding the site of infusion. Vesicant drugs can cause severe damage depending on the tissue infiltrated, the amount of drug the tissue absorbed, and the length of the tissue's exposure to the infiltrated drug.

Extravasation over joint spaces, tendons, or neuromuscular bundles increases the risk of tissue damage and therefore should be avoided as areas for infusion of vesicants. When a drug extravasates, the patient typically complains of pain, burning, or discomfort and possible swelling at the injection site. There may be leaking around the injection site of the drug. Sometimes pain might be a delayed reaction with other signs, such as reddening of the skin and blistering, which may progress to severe tissue involvement. The best approach when dealing with vesicants is prevention of extravasation.

The nurse should be familiar with the institutional policies for managing extravasation. Although specific protocols for managing extravasation may vary among health care settings, general guidelines for managing extravasation include the following:

- Stop the infusion immediately.
- Attempt to aspirate residual drug in the intravenous cannual and tissues.
- Apply warm or cold compresses as indicated to the extravasation site, and if prescribed, administer the appropriate antidote to minimize any tissue damage.
- Notify the health care provider.
- Rest and elevate the affected extremity for 48 hours.
- Apply a sterile dressing that allows the extravasation area to remain visible. Avoid any pressure to the site.
- Obtain a photograph of the site for baseline comparisons.
- Document the following in the patient's medical record per institutional guidelines: date and time of extravasation, name of drug, approximate volume of infiltrate, needle gauge, site of extravasation, symptoms reported by the patient and assessed by the nurse, nursing measures implemented, name of health care provider notified, patient education provided, and nurse's signature.
- Consult physician regarding need for referral to plastic surgeon, if appropriate.

Ensure patient has appropriate follow up to monitor site.

necrosis, when accidental infiltration occurs. Therefore, extravasation precautions should be exercised during their infusion (Box 56.4). Vincristine carries a Black Box warning related to the risk of extravasation.

Vincristine is a pregnancy category D drug.

Adverse Effects

The most common dose-limiting adverse effects with vincristine are neurologic, including motor, sensory, and autonomic neuropathies. Signs and symptoms of these neurologic deficits include loss of deep tendon reflexes, numbness and tingling of the hands and feet, foot drop, myalgias, weakness, and jaw pain. Constipation, which is a forerunner of paralytic ileus, can be serious and bothersome to the patient. The neurotoxic signs and symptoms appear weeks or months after drug administration and are long lasting and slow to resolve. The severity of the neurotoxicity is related to the cumulative dose of the drug.

Drug Interactions

The toxicity of vincristine may be potentiated by drugs that act on the peripheral nervous system. Vincristine has been reported to increase the uptake of high-dose MTX by cancer cells. When given concomitantly with digoxin, vincristine may decrease serum digoxin levels and, consequently, the effects of digoxin. Mitomycin used together with vincristine may cause acute pulmonary reactions. Table 56.4 presents drug interactions with vincristine.

Assessment of Relevant Core Patient Variables

Health Status

Give careful consideration to administering vincristine to patients with pre-existing neuromuscular disease or to those who are taking other neurotoxic drugs. Clinical evaluation, including a thorough history and physical examination, may be needed for dose adjustments. Also take into account concurrent use of drugs that cause constipation, such as narcotic analgesics and cholinergic drugs.

Life Span and Gender

Vincristine may affect sexual function. Explore the patient's sexual patterns. Assess women of childbearing age for pregnancy and lactation. Vincristine may cause fetal harm; therefore, pregnant patients should be apprised of this possibility if the drug is used in pregnancy. Whether vincristine is excreted in breast milk is unknown. Because of the potential for adverse effects in breast-feeding infants, the patient should decide either to stop breast-feeding or to stop drug therapy. Note the patient's age and developmental status. Vincristine therapy may cause azoospermia and amenorrhea in postpubertal patients, although recovery occurs after therapy is completed. Risk of potential motor and sensory dysfunction (peripheral neuropathies) associated with

TABLE 56.4 Agents That Interact with P Vincristine

Interactants	Effect and Significance	Nursing Management
digoxin	Decreased serum level and therapeutic effect	Monitor digoxin level.
methotrexate (MTX)	Increased cellular uptake of MTX when given sequentially	Notify physician for dosage modification. Monitor for signs and symptoms of neurotoxicity.

vincristine is greater in patients with liver dysfunction, with advanced age, and with cumulative doses of vincristine.

Lifestyle, Diet, and Habits

Before drug administration, determine the patient's sensory, motor, and perceptual functions, because of the potential dysfunctions associated with vincristine. Consider bowel elimination patterns and food and fluid intake.

Environment

Vincristine may be given in an inpatient or ambulatory care setting.

Nursing Diagnoses and Outcomes

- Disturbed Sensory Perception related to perceptual neuropathies, as evidenced by absent deep tendon reflexes, numbness, weakness, and myalgias
  Desired outcome: The patient will be able to function safely without injury. Optimal sensory and perceptual function will be maintained.
- Risk for Constipation related to adverse effects of vincristine
  Desired outcome: The patient will have a regular bowel elimination pattern and will pass soft stools. The patient will state self-care measures if he or she is unable to pass stool.
- Risk for Infection and Bleeding related to depression of bone marrow function
  Desired outcome: Bone marrow recovery will be attained; rare and mild myelosuppression might occur. The patient will verbalize and also implement self-care measures to prevent infection.
- Impaired Skin Integrity related to potential for vesicant extravasation
  Desired outcome: The skin will remain intact, without cutaneous breakdown. The patient and health care provider will be able to recognize signs and symptoms of suspected extravasation and initiate prompt measures that will prevent further tissue damage.
- Disturbed Body Image related to drug-induced hair loss
  Desired outcome: The patient will develop strategies to cope with hair loss and changes in physical appearance.
- Ineffective Sexuality Patterns: Impotence related to adverse effects of vincristine
  Desired outcome: The patient will state understanding that this effect of the drug is reversible and will exhibit behavior changes that will result in more satisfying sexual functioning.

Planning and Intervention

Maximizing Therapeutic Effects

The drug is light sensitive; therefore, protect it from light. Also, refrigerate it. Give an initial bolus through a new and patent free-flowing IV access, noting patient's response during and after drug instillation. If the drug is given as a continuous infusion, a central line should always be used.

Minimizing Adverse Effects

The occurrence of peripheral neuropathies is a major concern with vincristine therapy. Its toxicity to the nerve fibers can induce severe motor, sensory, and autonomic deficits. Conduct a neurologic evaluation of the patient before each cycle to assess for major changes. Report any changes in perceptual or sensory functioning and consult the oncologist immediately regarding dosage modifications or discontinuation of the drug.

Because vincristine has vesicant properties, careful attention should be given to prevent extravasation (see Box 56.4). Anyone administering vesicants must be thoroughly familiar with appropriate antidotes and protocols for the use of vesicants (Table 56.5).

Make sure that every patient is prescribed stool softeners to prevent constipation.

Providing Patient and Family Education

Follow the guidelines described in Box 56.2.

- Discuss and explain precautionary measures to the patient to lessen further insult to the cutaneous systems.
- Advise patients to promptly report problems resulting from the IV infusion—for example, pain, burning, redness, swelling, or blistering at the infusion site.
- Instruct patients and caregivers to observe and monitor the infusion site for early extravasation and cutaneous reactions.
- Teach patients and caregivers how to care for suspected extravasation at home until medical attention can be obtained, if needed.
- Discuss methods for coping with adverse effects, such as a metallic taste sensation during drug administration, nausea or appetite loss, or constipation accompanied by cramping.
- Encourage patients to maintain adequate nutrition. A high-fiber diet and plenty of fluids should be consumed to help relieve constipation. Stool softeners, laxatives, or both should be given for severe constipation. The usual constipation regimen consists of Colace, 100 mg once a day; and Senokot, two tablets at bedtime.
- Instruct patients to avoid injury related to altered sensory and perceptual changes manifested by muscle weakness and neuropathy, numbness of the fingers and toes, tingling sensation, or absence of deep tendon reflexes. These changes may be temporary or permanent.
- Review with patients strategies for taking care of hair and skin, because thinning or loss of hair may occur 2 or 3 weeks after treatment. Teach patients techniques to provide gentle care by avoiding heat or chemical irritants and wearing wigs or hair coverings. Educate patients that hair will regrow within a few months after therapy stops.
- Emphasize to patients and caregivers the importance of scheduling and keeping appointments for laboratory tests and medical checkups.
- Explore with patients and their significant others sexuality issues and discuss strategies for maintaining sexual

TABLE 56.5	Common Vesicants and Known Antidotes	
Vesicant	**Antidote**	**Nursing Management**
vincristine (Oncovin, Vincasar PFS) vinblastine (Velban) Etoposide if in large volumes of concentrated solutions	Hyaluronidase	Stop infusion of drug. Inject antidote locally to extravasation site subcutaneously. Apply warm compress to extravasation site for 15–20 min at least 4 times a day for 24–48 h.
vinorelbine (Navelbine) mechlorethamine hydrochloride (nitrogen mustard)	Isotonic sodium thiosulfate	Stop infusion of drug. Rapid administration of antidote is crucial. Prepare antidote as prescribed. The solution should be 1/6 molar. 2 mL solution for each mL of vesicant extravasated. Give four 1-mL SC injections in a clockwise pattern around site using a new 25 guage needle at each site. Apply ice for 6–12 h following antidote injection.
Others: cisplatin (Platinol) (>20 mL of 0.5-mg/mL solution), dactinomycin (Actinomycin), daunorubicin (Cerubidine), doxorubicin (Adriamycin), epirubicin (Ellence), idarubicin (Idamycin), fluorouracil (5-FU, rare vesicant potential), mitomycin (Mitomycin-C), mitoxantrone (Novantrone)	Isotonic sodium thiosulfate Dimethyl sulfoxide (DMSO)	Rapid administration of antidote is crucial. Apply ice pack for 15–20 min at least four times a day for the first 24 h. Teach patient how to prevent infection. Protect from sunlight. For anthracylines: remove ice pack at least 15 minutes prior to administration of Totect ®. Administer Totect ® IV over 1–2 h in a large vein in an area other than the extravasated area, preferably the opposite arm. See Totect ® package insert for detailed administration guidelines.

health. Reassure patients that impotence, should it occur, is usually reversible after drug therapy is discontinued.

Ongoing Assessment and Evaluation

Acute elevation of uric acid may occur during induction of remission for patients with leukemia. Measure uric acid levels during the first week of treatment and undertake measures to prevent the occurrence of uric acid nephropathy. Assess the patient's bowel function and motor and sensory functions daily.

Drugs Closely Related to P Vincristine

Vinblastine

Vinblastine (Velban) is another vinca alkaloid derived from the periwinkle plant. Although its chemical structure, pharmacokinetics, and mechanism of action are similar to those of vincristine, this drug has markedly more clinical indications than vincristine does. Similar to vincristine in its efficacy in treating lymphomas, vinblastine is also used for chemotherapy in testicular carcinoma, Kaposi sarcoma, choriocarcinoma, squamous cell cancer of the head and neck, and breast cancer.

The toxicity profile of vinblastine differs from that of vincristine. The dose-limiting toxicity of vinblastine is myelosuppression, whereas that of vincristine is neurotoxicity. Neurotoxicity occurs less frequently with vinblastine; however, with high doses, this adverse effect can occur. The mildly myelosuppressive action of vincristine makes it more

attractive than vinblastine for combination chemotherapy. Vinblastine is considered a vesicant.

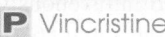

MEMORY CHIP

P Vincristine

- Primarily indicated for acute leukemia and for other cancers such as Hodgkin's disease, breast cancer, neuroblastoma, and multiple myeloma
- Major contraindications: demyelinating form of Charcot-Marie-Tooth syndrome
- Most common adverse effect: tissue necrosis if the drug, which is a vesicant, accidentally extravasates
- Most serious adverse effects: neurotoxic deficits manifested by paresthesias, myalgias, loss of deep tendon reflexes, and jaw pain. Paralytic ileus as evidenced by constipation may also occur.
- **Life span alert: Caution elderly patients regarding the potential for motor and sensory deficits that may compromise their safety and sensory acuity. Vincristine may cause fetal harm or risk to mothers who are breast-feeding. Apprise patients of these side effects.**
- **Patient safety alert: Vincristine is fatal if given intrathecally.**
- Maximizing therapeutic effects: The drug is light sensitive; protect it from light. Infuse it slowly over approximately 1 minute.
- Minimizing adverse effects: Always assess bowel elimination pattern because of the danger of paralytic ileus.
- Ensure good vascular access and monitor for signs and symptoms of extravasation.
- Most important patient education: Instruct the patient to obtain a prescription for a prophylactic stool regimen.

Vinorelbine

Vinorelbine (Navelbine) is a semisynthetic vinca alkaloid active against breast, cervical, and non–small-cell lung cancer. This drug's toxicity profile is similar to that of vinblastine and vincristine and involves myelosuppression (WBCs) and neurotoxicity. In addition to its vesicant properties, vinorelbine is also considered an irritant that can cause aching, tightness, and phlebitis with or without inflammation. It is important to flush peripheral lines with at least 125 mL of normal saline following administration to reduce irritation to the vein.

• Ⓒ PODOPHYLLOTOXINS

The podophyllotoxins were isolated from the mandrake plant (May crab apple). Examples of drugs in this group are etoposide (VP-16) and teniposide (VM-26), both of which are semisynthetic derivatives extracted from the American mandrake, *Podophyllum peltatum*. They are also known as epipodophyllotoxins. They act in the premitotic, G_2, and S phases and interfere with the topoisomerase II enzyme reaction. The prototype podophyllotoxin is etoposide.

Nursing Management of the Patient Receiving Ⓟ Etoposide

Core Drug Knowledge

Pharmacotherapeutics

Etoposide is used in combination therapy for refractory testicular tumors and small-cell lung cancer. It is also effective in treating Hodgkin's and non-Hodgkin's lymphomas, acute lymphocytic leukemia (ALL), breast cancer, and multiple myeloma. Etoposide is usually administered intravenously but is also available in an oral formulation (see Table 56.2). The recommended dose for oral use is twice the IV dose rounded to the nearest 50 mg.

Pharmacokinetics

Etoposide binds to serum albumin and becomes extensively bound to tissues. It is predominantly excreted in the urine and to a lesser extent in the bile. About 30% of the drug is excreted unchanged. The drug's half-life is 4 to 11 hours.

Pharmacodynamics

Etoposide acts by inhibiting a DNA enzyme called topoisomerase II, causing breaks in the double strands of protein-linked DNA. This action inhibits DNA synthesis in the S and G_2 phases so that cells do not enter mitosis and prophase.

Contraindications and Precautions

Etoposide should not be given to patients with a known hypersensitivity to the drug or teniposide, the other podophyllotoxin derivative. Etoposide should never be administered by IV push or rapid IV infusion because doing so can cause hypotension. It should be infused over 30 to 60 minutes or longer, depending on the volume of the infusion. If the patient is taking warfarin concomitantly with etoposide, the patient's prothrombin time should be monitored closely.

Etoposide is a pregnancy category D drug and should not be used in pregnant women.

Adverse Effects

Hypersensitivity or anaphylaxis-like reactions manifested by hypotension, chills, fever, facial flushing, bronchospasm, dyspnea, and tachycardia can occur during an etoposide infusion. However, these signs are not related to any cardiorespiratory pathology but rather to the rapid infusion of the drug itself. They can be ameliorated by stopping the infusion and giving the patient IV fluids, corticosteroids, antihistamines, and volume expanders as ordered.

The major dose-limiting effect of etoposide is myelosuppression, manifested primarily by granulocytopenia, which reaches a nadir in 7 to 14 days; the platelet nadir is 9 to 16 days after parenteral administration. Recovery is noted in 20 days. When etoposide is given orally, the nadir granulocyte counts occur between 21 and 28 days, with recovery in 35 days. Etoposide carries a Black Box warning relating to myelosuppression; resulting infection or bleeding may occur. The other adverse effects of note are mild to moderate nausea and vomiting, which can be controlled by antiemetics. GI toxicities are more pronounced with the oral form of the drug. Hepatic toxicity, shown by elevated liver enzyme levels, results from administering higher than recommended doses. Etoposide is also associated with the development of secondary malignancies.

Drug-induced alopecia is reversible when the drug is discontinued. Although rare, patients who have had radiation therapy may develop **radiation recall,** which is characterized by an erythematous rash in the irradiated area. This condition may progress to desquamation, vesicle formation, and permanent hyperpigmentation of the affected area.

Etoposide is classified as an **irritant.** As such, it may produce pain, aching, tightness, urticaria, or redness, with or without inflammation along the path of the vein (phlebitis) into which the drug is infusing. Apply warmth for local care. If a large amount of concentrated solution extravasates, treat as for a vincristine extravasation. Unlike vesicants, irritants do not generally cause tissue damage.

Drug Interactions

Etoposide has a synergistic effect with cisplatin. It is incompatible with gallium nitrate and MTX. Table 56.6 presents more information about these interactions.

Assessment of Relevant Core Patient Variables

Health Status

Assess the patient for prior extensive myelosuppressive chemotherapy or irradiation to marrow-bearing areas of the skeleton. Knowing such a history is important so that dose reduction can be considered, if indicated, to avoid the potential for more severe myelosuppression. Obtain the patient's CBC before and during etoposide therapy. Monitor the patient's renal and hepatic functions, so that dose adjustments may be made in case these systems malfunction.

TABLE 56.6 Agents That Interact with P Etoposide		
Interactants	Effect and Significance	Nursing Management
warfarin	Increases prothrombin time (PT)	Monitor PT closely. Monitor for signs of increased bleeding.
gallium-nitrate and methotrexate	Incompatible combinations	Avoid combined therapy.

Life Span and Gender

Document the age and gender of the patient. The safety and efficacy of etoposide have not been established in children. Explore the patient's sexual patterns and reproductive goals. Assess women of childbearing age for pregnancy. This drug has mutagenic, carcinogenic, and teratogenic properties. Secondary malignancies have been reported with the use of this drug.

Lifestyle, Diet, and Habits

Alopecia affects 20% to 90% of patients who receive etoposide. Explore with the patient the likely effect of therapy on sexuality and body image. Hair loss could be complete and may be more distressing for socially active, working patients.

Environment

Etoposide can be given in an acute care or ambulatory setting where the necessary clinical support is available in case hypotension or an anaphylactic reaction develops.

Nursing Diagnoses and Outcomes

- Risk for Injury related to etoposide-induced hypotension or anaphylactic reaction
  Desired outcome: The patient will not experience hypotension or anaphylactic reaction.
- Risk for Infection related to bleeding resulting from suppression of bone marrow function
  Desired outcome: The patient will recover adequate hematologic function. The patient will undertake self-care measures to prevent infection and bleeding.
- Imbalanced Nutrition: Less than Body Requirements, related to nausea, vomiting, and anorexia from drug therapy
  Desired outcome: The patient will maintain proper nutritional status and good emetic control.
- Disturbed Body Image related to drug-induced alopecia
  Desired outcome: The patient will implement coping strategies to alleviate feelings associated with loss of hair.
- Sexual Dysfunction related to disease process and drug therapy
  Desired outcome: The patient will increase knowledge about the effects of chemotherapy on sexual function and will continue functioning without interfering with sexual patterns and reproductive goals.
- Impaired Skin Integrity resulting from irritation to infusion site and possible radiation recall
  Desired outcome: The patient's skin will remain intact without breakdown from irritant chemotherapy. Patient will demonstrate competence in wound management if radiation recall occurs.

Planning and Intervention

Maximizing Therapeutic Effects

The stability of etoposide depends on the concentration. At a concentration of 0.2 mg/mL, etoposide is stable in a glass container for 96 hours and in plastic for 48 hours. (To prevent crystallization, dilute it in 5% dextrose for injection or in 0.9% sodium chloride solution to reach a final concentration of 0.2 to 0.4 mg/mL.)

Minimizing Adverse Effects

Because of dose-limiting myelosuppression, monitor WBC counts before chemotherapy and at the expected WBC nadir. Observe the patient receiving etoposide therapy closely for hypotension or anaphylactic reactions. Give the drug by slow infusion, never by rapid infusion, over 30 to 60 minutes and possibly longer, depending on the volume of the infusion. Cardiopulmonary resuscitation equipment should be present at the patient's bedside. During drug administration, help allay the patient's fears about possible anaphylactic reactions by staying with the patient and infusing the solution slowly through a patent IV line to prevent hypotension and chemical phlebitis. Apply warm compresses to the affected site. Monitor the patient's hepatic and renal function before and during therapy. Assess for signs and symptoms of infection and teach the patient to monitor and self-report the same. If the oral formulation of etoposide is given, also give the patient adequate antiemetics.

Providing Patient and Family Education

Follow the guidelines described in Box 56.2.

- Focus education for patients receiving etoposide on the importance of minimizing risks related to infection and injury, which are major concerns of patients with cancer.
- Discuss what to expect during the infusion (e.g., metallic taste, which may last a while but can be relieved by sucking on hard candy). If the oral formulation is used, the drug should be taken on a full stomach.
- Explain to patients that an allergic reaction may occur during infusion or after it and that this reaction is signaled by facial flushing, shortness of breath, or feeling faint.
- Help patients explore ways to manage adverse effects of mild nausea, loss of appetite, and mouth sores, which may develop in 4 to 7 days.
- Offer helpful oral hygiene practices, such as brushing the teeth at least four times daily with a soft brush and avoiding commercial mouthwashes containing alcohol, which can be irritating to the mucous lining.

- Provide nutritional guidelines, such as taking antiemetics as prescribed, eating many small meals rather than a few full meals, and avoiding highly seasoned food.
- Explain the importance of regular laboratory examinations, such as blood tests at certain intervals, to detect any decreases in blood counts (usually within 1 to 2 weeks after treatment).
- Stress guidelines for avoiding infection resulting from suppressed bone marrow function.
- Demonstrate methods to cope with hair loss and tingling in the hands and feet.
- Teach patients how to avoid injury resulting from drug-related neuropathy.
- Instruct the patient to contact the prescriber about serious adverse effects, such as a temperature higher than 100.5°F, excessive vomiting, painful mouth sores with inability to eat or drink for 24 hours, black stools, or uncontrolled bleeding.
- Discuss with patients and their significant others both reproductive goals and birth control because of the possible mutagenic and teratogenic properties of the drug.

Ongoing Assessment and Evaluation

Before each dose of etoposide therapy, check the WBC and platelet counts; platelet levels less than 50,000 cells/mm³ or an absolute neutrophil count less than 500 cells/mm³ may necessitate withholding the drug until the bone marrow recovers sufficiently.

Drug Closely Related to P Etoposide

Teniposide (VM-26, Vumon) and etoposide possess basic similarities in their pharmacologic makeup, toxicities, and clinical applications. The chemical structures of etoposide and teniposide differ only by the substitution of a methyl group (etoposide) for the thenylidene (teniposide) on the glucopyranoside sugar.

For teniposide administration, only nondiethylhexylphthalate (non-DEHP) containers, such as glass or polyolefin plastic containers, can be used. This precaution prevents DEHP from leaching out of polyvinyl containers and into the solution. Administration with heparin is contraindicated because heparin causes a precipitate to form.

C TAXANES

The taxanes arrest mitosis by promoting the formation of abnormal spindle fibers and mitotic asters. Paclitaxel (Taxol), the first drug in this category, was isolated from the bark of the Pacific yew, *Taxus brevifolia*. Because the demand for this drug exceeded the supply of bark available, a semisynthetic form was developed. Docetaxel (Taxotere) is the other taxane, a semisynthetic derivative of the European yew, *Taxus baccata*. Both taxanes have similar structures and pharmacologic

MEMORY CHIP

P Etoposide

- Indicated for the treatment of testicular carcinoma, small-cell and non–small-cell lung cancer
- Major contraindications: known hypersensitivity to etoposide or to any podophyllotoxin derivative
- **Patient safety alert: The most common adverse effect is hypersensitivity or anaphylaxis evidenced by orthostatic hypotension, chills, dyspnea, or bronchospasm (wheezing) when given rapidly.**
- Dose-limiting effect: myelosuppression
- **Life span alert: Radiation recall may occur. The safety and efficacy of VP-16 have not been established in children.**
- Maximizing therapeutic effects: Always infuse slowly (over 30 to 60 minutes or slower), never by IV push.
- Minimizing adverse effects: Monitor results of complete blood count before chemotherapy and at expected nadir, approximately 10 to 14 days after the drug dose. Monitor for signs and symptoms of myelosuppression, which include infection and bleeding.
- Most important patient education: Forewarn the patient that the infusion causes a metallic taste. Advise the patient that sucking on hard candy may alleviate the metallic taste.

properties: long half-lives, substantial hepatic metabolism, biliary excretion, and large volumes of distribution. These drugs are given intravenously. They differ somewhat in their toxicity profile, particularly in the nonhematologic adverse effects. The prototype taxane is paclitaxel. Paclitaxel protein-bound (Abraxane) is a newer drug in this category that is free of solvents. Premedication for hypersensitivity is not required. Side effects are similar to the other drugs in this category.

Nursing Management of the Patient Receiving P Paclitaxel

Core Drug Knowledge

Pharmacotherapeutics

The most important cytotoxic activity of paclitaxel has been in treating ovarian and breast cancers. It is approved for use after failure of first-line or subsequent therapy in metastatic ovarian cancer. In breast cancer, it is given to patients who have metastatic breast cancer that has progressed or relapsed during anthracycline-based therapy. It is also used for adjuvant treatment of node-positive breast cancer, administered sequentially to standard doxorubicin-containing combination chemotherapy. Clinical studies have shown that it is effective against a diverse range of solid tumors that are refractory to conventional chemotherapy. It has recently been approved for second-line treatment of AIDS-related Kaposi sarcoma. Several administration regimens are used, such as 1-, 3-, 6-, and 24-hour infusions with varying doses.

Pharmacokinetics

Paclitaxel crosses the placenta and enters breast milk. The liver is the principal organ responsible for paclitaxel metabolism. The drug is excreted into the bile; less than 10% of the intact drug is excreted in the urine.

Pharmacodynamics

Paclitaxel inhibits the normal dynamic reorganization of the microtubular network during interphase and mitosis. Microtubules are cellular elements that appear to play an important role in the initiation of DNA synthesis, mitosis, and other cellular functions. The interference with the microtubules prevents depolymerization, which triggers apoptosis, or cell death, in rapidly dividing cells. It also prevents transition from the G_0 phase to the S phase by blocking cellular response to protein growth factors.

Contraindications and Precautions

Patients who have a history of hypersensitivity to drugs formulated in Cremophor EL—an excipient used as a vehicle for paclitaxel because the drug is not water soluble—should not be challenged with paclitaxel because of the possibility of a hypersensitivity reaction, including anaphylaxis. Paclitaxel is a pregnancy category D drug. Taxanes are not used in children.

Adverse Effects

Paclitaxel carries a Black Box warning related to the risk of anaphylaxis and risk of severe hypersensitivity reaction. About 10% of patients experience a hypersensitivity reaction. In nearly 80% of patients, this reaction occurs during the first 20 minutes of the infusion and happens on the first or second exposure to the drug. Whether the hypersensitivity reaction is caused by the drug itself or by Cremophor EL is debated. The manifestations of this anaphylactoid reaction are dyspnea, hypotension, tachycardia, wheezing, and chest pain.

Myelosuppression, especially risk of severe neutropenia, is also included in the Black Box warning for paclitaxel. Neutrophils reach nadir at day 11, and platelets reach nadir by day 8. Fever is associated with low WBC counts. Neurotoxicity is another important problem, which generally begins 2 or 3 days after infusion. Patients complain of numbness, tingling, and pain in the hands and feet, which may progress to painful paresthesias, loss of deep tendon reflexes, arthralgia, and diffuse myalgia. The GI manifestations are mucositis, diarrhea, mild nausea and vomiting, and elevated liver enzyme levels. The cutaneous reactions are alopecia, facial flushing, and chemical phlebitis.

Paclitaxel has irritant properties. It also appears to be cardiotoxic: bradyarrhythmias, including heart block, have been reported. Severe conduction abnormalities have been observed in less than 1% of patients receiving paclitaxel, in some cases necessitating pacemaker insertion.

Drug Interactions

The most substantial drug interaction is between paclitaxel and cisplatin. When given in combination, they can cause synergistic myelosuppression and neurotoxicity. Table 56.7 presents other drugs that might have substantial interactions with paclitaxel. Additionally, paclitaxel infusion must be administered in glass, or in polyolefin or polypropylene containers with polyethylene-lined administration sets. Polyvinyl chloride containers and tubing cause the plasticizer DEHP to leach into the fluid and should not be used. An in-line filter of 0.22 microns should also be used because particulates can form.

Assessment of Relevant Core Patient Variables

Health Status

Before administering the first dose of paclitaxel, ensure that baseline CBC, ECG, and vital signs are recorded. Assess the patient's hepatobiliary function, particularly serum bilirubin levels. Patients with existing neuropathies resulting from diabetes mellitus or alcohol ingestion could experience potentiated neurotoxicity resulting from paclitaxel administration. Investigate hypersensitivity to other drugs with a Cremophor EL base.

Life Span and Gender

Assess women of childbearing age for pregnancy and lactation. This drug is believed to be embryotoxic; therefore, its use should be avoided in pregnancy. It may be excreted in milk; breast-feeding should be stopped during paclitaxel therapy. The clinical efficacy of the taxanes in children has not been evaluated.

Lifestyle, Diet, and Habits

Discuss the impact of alopecia and other adverse effects on the patient's sexuality, body image, and activities of daily living. Alopecia, which may include loss of eyebrow, eyelash, pubic, and axillary hair, may be devastating to a patient who leads an active social life. Similarly limiting are the neurotoxic effects of pain, burning, sensory loss,

TABLE 56.7	Agents That Interact with P Paclitaxel	
Interactants	Effect and Significance	Nursing Management
quinidine, cyclosporine, quinine, verapamil	Reversal of multidrug resistance	Administer medications as ordered.
cisplatin (CDDP)	Myelosuppression more severe when CDDP is given before paclitaxel	Give paclitaxel first when these two drugs are ordered sequentially.
ketoconazole	Inhibits metabolism of paclitaxel	Monitor for paclitaxel toxicity.

paresthesia, and loss of deep tendon reflexes. These symptoms might be more pronounced in patients with a history of alcohol abuse.

Environment

Paclitaxel may be administered on either an inpatient or outpatient basis. Severe reactions—manifested by hypotension, bronchospasm, tachycardia, and chest pain—can occur and are most common with the first or second infusion. In any setting where the drug is given, stay with the patient for the first 20 minutes and continue to closely monitor throughout the infusion. Resuscitation equipment and adequate supportive drugs should always be present, so that prompt intervention can be implemented if necessary.

Nursing Diagnoses and Outcomes

- Risk for Injury related to hypersensitivity or anaphylactic reactions from paclitaxel
  Desired outcome: The patient will not suffer any injury resulting from a hypersensitivity reaction to paclitaxel.
- Risk for Infection and bleeding related to depressed bone marrow function
  Desired outcome: The patient will be free from infection and bleeding, evidenced by normal vital signs and recovery from neutropenia and anemia, demonstrated by blood counts.
- Disturbed Sensory Perception related to neuropathy
  Desired outcome: The patient will be able to function safely within limitations of lessened perceptual and sensory acuity caused by paclitaxel.
- Imbalanced Nutrition: Less than Body Requirements, related to drug-induced nausea, vomiting, and diarrhea
  Desired outcome: The patient will maintain adequate nutritional intake and be able to gain adequate control over emesis and diarrhea.
- Impaired Skin Integrity and Disturbed Body Image related to drug-induced alopecia
  Desired outcome: The patient will state understanding that the loss of hair is reversible and will initiate strategies to minimize body image distortion stemming from alopecia.

Planning and Intervention

Maximizing Therapeutic Effects

Store diluted paclitaxel in glass bottles or plastic bags and administer with polyethylene-lined administration sets using an in-line 0.22-micron filter. Do not allow the undiluted concentrate to come in contact with polyvinyl chloride equipment or devices. When paclitaxel is used to treat breast cancer, it should be part of a multidrug regimen that includes doxorubicin. Paclitaxel may be used as part of combination therapy with cisplatin to treat certain types of cancer, such as non–small-cell lung cancer. The cytotoxicity from these two drugs is sequence dependent; for optimal results, give paclitaxel first.

Minimizing Adverse Effects

Measure and closely monitor the patient's baseline vital signs during the first 20 minutes of the paclitaxel infusion, and continue monitoring the patient for the first hour. Stay with the patient because most hypersensitivity reactions occur within the first 20 minutes of the first and second infusions. If the reaction is mild, patients can be rechallenged after the clinical manifestations have subsided. To prevent severe reactions, premedication is mandatory. Give premedication consisting of corticosteroids (dexamethasone), diphenhydramine, and an H_2-antagonist (e.g., cimetidine) at least a half hour before the paclitaxel infusion. Current experience indicates that longer infusions and an adequate premedication regimen, such as the one mentioned previously, minimize the hypersensitivity effect. If a severe hypersensitivity reaction or anaphylaxis occurs, discontinue the drug immediately and institute supportive measures (Box 56.5). Under these circumstances, the patient should not be rechallenged.

Ensure that baseline neutrophil counts are checked prior to paclitaxel infusion. The use of growth factors are often used to accelerate bone marrow recovery and prevent severe WBC nadir from occurring. Give filgrastim subcutaneously

---

Box 56.5 MANAGING A GENERALIZED HYPERSENSITIVITY REACTION AND ANAPHYLAXIS

Hypersensitivity or anaphylactic-like reactions manifested by hypotension, chills, fever, facial flushing, bronchospasm, dyspnea, and tachycardia can occur during a chemotherapeutic infusion. Hypersensitivity reactions usually occur within the first 10 to 15 minutes of the first infusion, but they may also happen during a later cycle, even after an uneventful first infusion. Because hypersensitivity reactions can be life threatening, the nurse needs to know what to do should one occur:

1. Stop the infusion immediately.
2. Stay with the patient.
3. Call for medical support.
4. Maintain a good IV line with normal saline solution.
5. Administer emergency drugs as prescribed: Adults: 1:1,000 (1 mg/mL) 0.2 to 0.5 mL IM or subcutaneously every 5 minutes as needed to control symptoms and increase blood pressure Pediatrics: 0.01 mg/kg (maximum 0.3 mg) IM or subcutaneously every 5 minutes as needed to control symptoms and increase blood; diphenhydramine, 50 mg IV; hydrocortisone 50 mg IV.
6. Place the patient in a supine position.
7. Measure vital signs every 2 to 5 minutes until they stabilize.
8. Maintain a patent airway, and administer oxygen as needed.
9. Provide emotional support to the patient and family.
10. Document all nursing measures and patient responses.
11. Consult with the health care provider about a change in treatment plans or the need to rechallenge the patient. If the drug needs to be given, the following measures should be implemented: desensitization with the health care provider's support, a premedication regimen, prolongation of infusion time or an increase in the volume of diluent and, if appropriate, substitution of a similar drug.

at a dose of 5 mcg/kg every day for 10 days, starting 24 hours after the completion chemotherapy.

Providing Patient and Family Education
Follow the guidelines described in Box 56.2.

- The first treatment is usually stressful for patients and families because of the fear of the possible anaphylactic reaction. Reassure patients that the health care team will be present during the first 20 minutes of the infusion, when most of these reactions occur. Teach patients to report the first symptoms of hypersensitivity/anaphylaxis, so that supportive measures can be undertaken.
- Explain drug delivery methods; for example, say that an IV drug can be given as a continuous infusion or intra-abdominally by a catheter placed in the abdomen.
- Review premedication regimens for preventing allergic reactions, including regimens for dexamethasone (Decadron), diphenhydramine (Benadryl), and an H_2-antagonist.
- Discuss medications to relieve adverse effects (nausea, joint pain, body aches), such as acetaminophen (Tylenol) or ibuprofen (Motrin, Advil) for pain.
- Offer methods to enhance appearance when alopecia occurs, such as wearing wigs and hats.
- Explain signs and symptoms of peripheral neuropathy, such as numbness, tingling in the hands and feet, impairment of fine motor skills, and difficulty in ambulating, and explore their potential effects on the patient's activities of daily living; for example, suggest moving carefully to avoid injury.
- Discuss measures to alleviate fatigue by getting rest, sleep, and exercise; pacing activities; and obtaining help with activities and chores of daily living.
- Explain how to self-administer a prescribed drug (e.g., granulocyte colony-stimulating factor [G-CSF]) by subcutaneous (SC) injection to minimize a severe drop in WBC count.
- Review the danger signs of infection and blood abnormalities that should be reported, such as a temperature higher than 100.5°F.
- Explain the importance of oral hygiene and careful nutrition to relieve the discomfort of mouth sores.

Ongoing Assessment and Evaluation

Depression of bone marrow function, primarily neutropenia, is a dose-limiting toxicity of paclitaxel. Monitor the patient's CBCs frequently. Patients should not be given subsequent courses until the neutrophils reach a level exceeding approximately 1,500 cells/mm³ and platelets recover to above 100,000 cells/mm³. Perform cardiac monitoring during subsequent drug administration to ensure that patients do not develop severe cardiac abnormalities.

Drug Closely Related to P Paclitaxel

Docetaxel (Taxotere) is the only other drug in the taxane family. It is used in patients with locally advanced or metastatic breast

MEMORY CHIP

P Paclitaxel

- Indicated for patients who breast and ovarian cancer, Kapos;s sarcoma, and non-small cell lung cancer.
- Major contraindications: hypersensitivity to Cremophor El, baseline neutropenia of less than 1,500/mm³, pregnancy and lactation
- Most common adverse effects: nausea, vomiting, alopecia, and joint pains
- Dose-limiting effect: depression of bone marrow function, particularly neutropenia
- **Patient safety alert: Most serious adverse effects are severe hypersensitivity reactions (anaphylaxis), which occur during the first 10 to 15 minutes of drug infusion.**
- Maximizing therapeutic effects: Use glass or polyolefin containers, non-DEHP administration sets, and in-line filtration for drug administration.
- Minimizing adverse effects: Administer paclitaxel first when given in combination with cisplatin or carboplatin to prevent profound myelosuppression. Premedicate patients with a corticosteroid, diphenhydramine, and an H_2-antagonist IV 60 minutes before paclitaxel to avoid anaphylactic reactions.
- Most important patient education: If the physician prescribes the corticosteroid premedication regimen to be started at home, ensure that patient understands the importance of complying with the dosing schedule and will have enough medications (dexamethasone) at home.

---

carcinoma after disease progression with an anthracycline-based therapy or relapse during anthracycline-based adjuvant treatment. It is approved for the treatment of patients with head and neck malignancies, ovarian cancer, and non–small-cell lung cancer that is locally advanced or has metastasized and has not responded to cisplatin. The Food and Drug Administration has just approved docetaxel in combination with prednisone for patients with hormone-refractory prostate cancer. An adverse effect unique to docetaxel administration is fluid retention syndrome. This syndrome is manifested by edema, weight gain, and third-space fluid retention. The fluid retention is cumulative and is believed to be caused by increased capillary permeability and by the vehicle used to increase docetaxel's solubility, Tween 80. Prophylactic measures include the use of corticosteroids, such as dexamethasone, 8 mg orally twice daily for 5 days, before docetaxel, with or without H_1- and H_2-receptor antagonists given intravenously 30 minutes before the drug; these measures appear to be effective in reducing the fluid retention. Other measures include the use of diuretics, such as spironolactone or furosemide, if ordered by the prescriber.

C CAMPTOTHECINES (TOPOISOMERASE-I INHIBITORS)

Topoisomerase-I is a nuclear enzyme needed for maintaining DNA structure during replication, transcription, and translation of genetic materials. Inhibition of this enzyme causes single-stranded DNA breaks and, subsequently, cell death. Topoisomerase-I inhibitors are the newest category of cell cycle–specific agents, semisynthetic agents derived from the Chinese tree *Camptotheca acuminata*. The parent compound, camptothecin, was isolated in 1966 and was found to have antitumor activity in animal models. However, further testing was not pursued because of unpredictable toxicities, such as hemorrhagic cystitis and myelosuppression. In the early 1980s, inhibition of topoisomerase-I activity was found to be an important anticancer strategy. The prototype is topotecan hydrochloride (Hycamtin).

Nursing Management of the Patient Receiving P Topotecan

Core Drug Knowledge

Pharmacotherapeutics

Topotecan HCl (Hycamtin), a semisynthetic derivative of camptothecin, was approved in 1996 to treat patients with metastatic ovarian cancer after failure of initial or subsequent chemotherapy. It has also demonstrated clinical efficacy in treating small-cell lung cancer and ALL. It is administered intravenously.

Pharmacokinetics

The half-life of topotecan is about 3 hours. The drug has minimal protein binding, which may contribute to its ability to cross the blood–brain barrier. Topotecan is metabolized in the liver. The drug is primarily excreted by the kidneys, with approximately 30% to 40% excreted unchanged. Renal clearance is an important determinant of topotecan elimination.

Pharmacodynamics

Topotecan inhibits the activity of topoisomerase-I, an enzyme involved in gene transcription and DNA replication. This enzyme causes nicks and breaks along DNA strands, relieving stresses that build up as the DNA molecule unwinds in preparation for cell division and protein synthesis. Normally, the nicks would then be repaired by topoisomerase-I. Topotecan, by attaching to the enzyme, prevents it from repairing the nicks in the DNA, and the cell is unable to repair them efficiently.

Contraindications and Precautions

Topotecan is myelosuppressive and is contraindicated in patients who have poor bone marrow reserves. It should only be administered when the baseline neutrophil count is at least 1,500 cells/mm^3 and the platelet count is at least 100,000 cells/mm^3. It is a pregnancy category D drug. Whether the drug is excreted in human milk is unknown. It should not be administered to patients who are pregnant or breast-feeding.

Adverse Effects

The dose-limiting toxicity of topotecan is myelosuppression, especially neutropenia (listed as a Black Box warning), with a median time to nadir of 11 days. Thrombocytopenia

is also dose-limiting in some regimens; median time to nadir is 15 days, with resolution after 5 days. Growth factor support has not been necessary for most patients. The nonhematologic adverse effects are nausea and vomiting, which are usually relieved with the appropriate antiemetic regimen. Other GI adverse effects are diarrhea and abdominal pain, which are managed symptomatically. Headache is a common neurologic complaint. Alopecia, fever, and flu-like symptoms have also been reported.

Drug Interactions

No known interactions with other drugs occur that might affect the potency of topotecan. Concomitant use of topotecan and cisplatin or other cytotoxic drugs worsens myelosuppression; concomitant use of G-CSF can prolong neutropenia.

Assessment of Relevant Core Patient Variables

Health Status

Assess the adequacy of the patient's bone marrow reserve. Because severe neutropenia is most common with the first course of treatment, topotecan should be given only to patients who have a baseline neutrophil count of at least 1,500 cells/mm^3 and a platelet count of at least 100,000 cells/mm^3.

Life Span and Gender

Explore the patient's reproductive goals. Topotecan is in pregnancy category D. Assess women of childbearing age for pregnancy and lactation. Because it is not known whether the drug is excreted in human milk, this drug should not be administered to patients who are pregnant or breast-feeding. The safety and efficacy of topotecan have not been established in children.

Lifestyle, Diet, and Habits

Assess the patient's activities of daily living, including rest and exercise patterns. Fatigue is frequently reported. Obtain information on the patient's normal dietary intake to plan necessary antiemetic measures.

Environment

Topotecan is usually given in an ambulatory setting. There are no acute risks that necessitate inpatient hospitalization. Clinical trials are currently in progress with an oral form of the drug. Home therapy, an attractive alternative, will make drug administration convenient and cost effective for the patient.

Nursing Diagnoses and Outcomes

• Risk for Infection and Bleeding related to depression of bone marrow function
  Desired outcome: *The patient will be free from infection and bleeding evidenced by normal vital signs and recovery from neutropenia and anemia, as shown in the blood counts.*
• Imbalanced Nutrition: Less than Body Requirements, related to drug-induced nausea, vomiting, and stomatitis

Desired outcome: *The patient will maintain adequate nutritional intake and be able to gain adequate control of emesis and diarrhea.*

- Disturbed Body Image related to alopecia
Desired outcome: *The patient will develop strategies to minimize body image distortion from loss of hair.*
- Altered Self-Image related to fatigue
Desired outcome: *The patient will understand the etiology of fatigue and will implement fatigue management strategies that will minimize level of fatigue.*

Planning and Intervention

Maximizing Therapeutic Effects

A minimum of 4 courses (topotecan, 1.5 mg/m^2 intravenously for 5 days, given every 21 days) is recommended because the median time to response, as shown in three ovarian cancer clinical trials, was 9 to 12 weeks and median time to response in four small-cell lung cancer trials was 5 to 7 weeks. Protect unopened vials of the drug from light, and keep them at a controlled temperature of 68°F to 79°F. Use reconstituted solutions immediately.

Minimizing Adverse Effects

Because of dose-limiting myelosuppression, monitor WBC counts before chemotherapy and at the expected nadir. If the nadir is especially low, hematopoietic growth factors such as G-CSF may be given to decrease the depth and duration of the nadir. However, these substances should not be given concomitantly with topotecan, because doing so prolongs the duration of the neutropenia. Growth factors should be administered 24 hours after the last dose of topotecan.

Providing Patient and Family Education

Follow the guidelines described in Box 56.2.

- Advise patients of ways to lessen the fatigue level by conserving energy; engaging in moderate exercise and activity; observing good sleep hygiene; and talking to the physician about other possible underlying causes. Emphasize that fatigue is a side effect rather than a sign of disease progression or treatment failure.
- Teach patients to eat small and frequent meals and take antiemetics if needed. Emphasize good oral hygiene.
- Review the signs and symptoms of infection and bleeding and instruct patients about which ones should be reported to a prescriber.
- If G-CSF injections are necessary, ensure that patients or caregivers know how to administer the drug.
- Reassure patients that alopecia is a reversible process and teach them techniques for enhancing their appearance.

Ongoing Assessment and Evaluation

Undertake frequent monitoring of the patient's blood counts when subsequent topotecan therapy is planned. Neutrophil recovery to more than 1,000 cells/mm^3, platelet count to more than 100,000 cells/mm^3, and hemoglobin levels of 9.0 mg/dL are safe parameters to maintain for follow-up cycles.

MEMORY CHIP

Ⓟ Topotecan

- Approved for use in patients with ovarian, small-cell lung, and cervical cancer
- Major contraindications: severe depression of bone marrow function, particularly when the neutrophil count is less than 1,500 cells/mm^3; known hypersensitivity to the drug or its components
- Most common adverse effects: nonhematologic adverse events including nausea and vomiting, diarrhea or constipation, alopecia, and fatigue
- Most serious adverse effect: depression of bone marrow function, particularly neutropenia
- Maximizing therapeutic effects: A minimum of four courses (1.5 mg/m^2 intravenously for 5 days given every 21 days) is recommended, because the median time to response as shown in three ovarian cancer clinical trials was 9 to 12 weeks, and median time to response in four small-cell lung cancer trials was 5 to 7 weeks.
- Minimizing adverse effects: To minimize severe neutropenia, reduce subsequent doses. Growth factor support may be necessary for neutrophil recovery.
- Most important patient education: Teach the patient the importance of careful monitoring of blood counts and the avoidance of risk factors that might expose patient to sources of bleeding and infection.

Drug Closely Related to Ⓟ Topotecan

Irinotecan (CPT-11) is the second topoisomerase-I inhibitor. First synthesized in Japan in 1984, it was found to have activity against many tumor models, both in vitro and in animals. This drug is effective in treating metastatic carcinoma of the colon or rectum that has recurred or progressed following therapy with 5-FU; more recently, it has been useful as first-line therapy in combination with 5-FU and leucovorin in metastatic colon or rectal cancer. Irinotecan is also used in small-cell and non-small cell lung cancer and ovarian cancer.

The principal adverse effects associated with irinotecan are GI and hematologic. Diarrhea occurs early and late in treatment and can be dose limiting, depending on the time of onset. Early-onset diarrhea, which happens within 24 hours of drug administration, is thought to be caused by inhibition of anticholinesterase by irinotecan. It is characterized by sweating, flushing, abdominal cramping, hyperlacrimation, and sudden diarrhea. It responds to IV or SC injection of atropine, 0.25 to 1.0 mg. Late-onset diarrhea, which can be dose limiting, usually occurs between days 5 and 12 of the treatment cycle but can happen as early as day 2. Management of the diarrhea consists of giving loperamide, as a 4-mg first dose and then after each loose stool, up to 16 mg each day. Most patients also experience nausea and vomiting, which can be ameliorated with suitable antiemetic therapy. Other toxicities include leukopenia, anemia, and neutropenia, alopecia, and fatigue.

Irinotecan is usually given in an ambulatory setting, with follow-up telephone calls to patients to ensure proper

CRITICAL THINKING SCENARIO

IMPLEMENTING IRINOTECAN THERAPY

Mr. J is a 65-year-old patient with colon cancer whose disease has progressed after 5-FU therapy. He was started on irinotecan monotherapy at a starting dose of 125 mg/m² administered by IV. The patient will return each week for 4 consecutive weeks. He will have a 2-week rest period between cycles. Diarrhea is a principal adverse effect. What are the important nursing considerations to review regarding this problem?

control of side effects, particularly diarrhea, which can cause nutritional deficits. For colon cancer, the initial dose of irinotecan is 125 mg/m² given intravenously over 90 minutes every week for 4 consecutive weeks, followed by a 2-week rest period.

MISCELLANEOUS CELL CYCLE–SPECIFIC DRUGS

Several antineoplastic drugs, which are believed to be cell cycle–specific but have unclear modes of action, are classified in the miscellaneous group. Hydroxyurea and L-asparaginase are in this category. Hydroxyurea (Hydrea) is the prototype miscellaneous cell cycle–specific drug discussed in this chapter.

Nursing Management of the Patient Receiving P Hydroxyurea

Core Drug Knowledge

Pharmacotherapeutics

Hydroxyurea is used in managing hematologic cancers, such as acute myelogenous leukemia or chronic myelogenous leukemia particularly in the presence of hyperleukocytosis. It is also used in other hematologic conditions, such as essential thrombocytopenia, polycythemia vera, and sickle cell. It is used in combination chemotherapy or with radiation and has shown some clinical efficacy against renal cancer, malignant melanoma, ovarian cancer, head and neck tumors, and prostate cancer. It is given orally (see Table 56.2) until the WBC count falls to 50,000 cells/mm³, after which dosage is reduced gradually or discontinued.

Pharmacokinetics

Hydroxyurea is well absorbed from the GI tract. It penetrates the blood–brain barrier, achieving peak levels in the CSF within 3 hours. About 50% of the drug is metabolized in the liver, excreted in the urine as urea, and eliminated in the respiratory tract as carbon dioxide. The remainder is excreted intact in the urine.

Pharmacodynamics

The exact mechanism of action of hydroxyurea remains unestablished. It is a potent inhibitor of the enzyme ribonucleotide reductase, and it causes inhibition of DNA without inhibiting RNA or protein synthesis. It is S-phase specific and may hold other cells in the G_1 phase of the cell cycle.

Contraindications and Precautions

Hydroxyurea is contraindicated in patients with severe anemia, severely depressed bone marrow function with WBC count of less than 1,500 cells/mm³, or platelet count less than 100,000 cells/mm³; an exception is patients being treated for blast crisis of acute leukemia. Megaloblastosis unrelated to vitamin B_{12} or folic acid deficiency is often seen during chronic hydroxyurea therapy. Because the drug is excreted in the urine, it should be used with caution in patients with marked renal problems. Renal function should be monitored carefully; reduced dosing may be necessary in patients with impaired renal function.

Adverse Effects

Hydroxyurea is a pregnancy category D drug. The major toxicity of hydroxyurea is dose-related myelosuppression. Leukopenia is common, with an onset of 10 days. Thrombocytopenia and anemia are less common and have a later onset. CNS effects, such as drowsiness, headache, dizziness, hallucinations, and disorientation, have been reported with high-dose therapy. GI problems, such as nausea, vomiting, diarrhea, and stomatitis, are less common. Combined therapy with radiation can increase the severity and incidence of side effects. If the reactions are severe, interruption of treatment might be indicated; this action is rarely necessary. Increases in serum uric acid, blood urea nitrogen (BUN), and creatinine levels have been noted.

A Black Box warning for cutaneous vasculitic toxicities (vasculitic ulcerations and gangrene) associated with the use of hydroxyurea has been issued. These toxicities have predominantly occurred in patients receiving hydroxyurea for myeloproliferative disorders who have a history of prior or concurrent therapy with interferon. Hydroxyurea also has a Black Box warning related to the risk of second malignancies, because it is a known mutagenic and possible carcinogenic drug.

Drug Interactions

No important drug interactions with hydroxyurea are known to exist.

Assessment of Relevant Core Patient Variables

Health Status

Before treatment, assess the patient's hematologic profile, including a CBC and, if indicated, a bone marrow biopsy, especially if the patient has previously received antineoplastic or radiation therapy. Ask the patient about adverse effects from these treatments. Order tests to determine adequate renal and hepatic function.

Life Span and Gender

Elderly patients may be more sensitive than young patients to the drug; dose reductions may be indicated. The dosage regimens for children have not been established. Assess women of childbearing age for pregnancy and lactation. Hydroxyurea has shown teratogenic effects in animals and may be mutagenic. Therefore, women should be cautioned about possible fetal harm if they are or may become pregnant.

Lifestyle, Diet, and Habits

Because hydroxyurea is an oral formulation, ensure that the patient will adhere to the dosing schedule at home and will incorporate this schedule into his or her daily activities. No dietary restrictions apply to the ingestion of hydroxyurea.

Environment

Hydroxyurea is self-administered at home. No emergency adverse effects of the drug are known that might require hospitalization. Patients taking long-term hydroxyurea therapy should be monitored closely because of the possibility of severe depression of bone marrow function. If appropriate, assess the home for potential sources of infection and bleeding risk (Box 56.6).

BOX 56.6 COMMUNITY BASED CONCERNS

Home Therapy with Hydroxyurea

Some patients receive hydroxyurea (Hydrea) at home. They need to learn about safe, effective self-care. Some considerations to cover in patient education include the following:

- Because hydroxyurea is taken PO, problems with swallowing capsules can present difficulties. To counteract swallowing problems, hydroxyurea capsules can be mixed with applesauce, water, or juice and swallowed in liquid form.
- Taken in large doses, hydroxyurea may cause moderate drowsiness; patients should be cautioned to prevent injury.
- Early side effects of nausea, vomiting, diarrhea, and loss of appetite may interfere with drug effectiveness. Antiemetic medications should be taken as prescribed. In some cases, taking hydroxyurea before bedtime helps to decrease nausea.
- The health care provider should be notified if foods or liquids cannot be retained for more than 24 hours after taking hydroxyurea.
- If the physician recommends blood testing, appointments should be scheduled so that the blood count can be monitored closely. A temporary decrease may occur within 7 to 14 days after treatment, but the blood counts will recover. (blood counts will drop more significantly with higher dose therapy such as for acute leukemia),
- Ways to prevent infection include avoiding people who have colds or any infection during the drug therapy period and avoiding injury, such as cuts from razor blades or kitchen knives.
- The health care provider should be notified if a severe skin rash or facial redness develops, although a less severe rash may occur in 1 to 2 weeks after treatment.
- Because hydration is important for therapeutic effect, the patient should drink plenty of fluids to prevent any problems with kidney function.
- Proper handling of cytotoxic agents, particularly avoidance of contact with skin and crushing tablets, should be observed.

Nursing Diagnoses and Outcomes

- Risk for Infection and Bleeding related to suppressed bone marrow function
  Desired outcome: The patient will recover adequate hematologic function. Patient will undertake self-care measures to prevent infection and bleeding.
- Imbalanced Nutrition: Less than Body Requirements, related to nausea and vomiting, anorexia, stomatitis, and hepatic dysfunction
  Desired outcome: The patient will maintain a proper nutritional state and good emetic control. The patient will maintain intact oral mucosa and practice a good oral hygiene regimen. The patient will have normal hepatic function.
- Disturbed Sensory Perception: Drowsiness, disorientation, confusion, or headache related to adverse effects of drug therapy
  Desired outcome: The patient will be free from injury. The patient will maintain sensory acuity and orientation to time and environment.
- Ineffective Sexuality Patterns related to effects of hydroxyurea
  Desired outcome: The patient will increase knowledge about the effects of chemotherapy on sexual function and will initiate behaviors that will not interfere with sexual patterns and reproductive goals.

Planning and Intervention

Maximizing Therapeutic Effects

When hydroxyurea is given concomitantly with irradiation, give hydroxyurea 1 week before initiating radiation therapy. It can then be continued during radiotherapy and given indefinitely. The maximum therapeutic radiation dosage indicated for the clinical condition should be given. Modifying the radiation dosage is not usually necessary with concurrent hydroxyurea administration, as long as the patient is closely monitored and does not experience severe adverse effects.

Minimizing Adverse Effects

The dosage of hydroxyurea should be based on the patient's actual or ideal weight, whichever is less. Hydroxyurea therapy may be interrupted if the WBC count falls below 1,500 cells/mm^3 or the platelet count falls below 100,000 cells/mm^3, except in a patient with blast crisis of acute leukemia. Anemia does not necessitate interrupting hydroxyurea therapy because whole blood replacement can be given. Dose modifications may be indicated in patients who have received prior radiation therapy or other cytotoxic drugs. Assess the patient's renal function because hydroxyurea can impair renal tubular function, an event manifested by elevated uric acid, BUN, and creatinine levels. Because tumor lysis can occur, the patient may need to be pretreated to prevent this complication.

Providing Patient and Family Education
Follow the guidelines described in Box 56.2.

- Before initiating drug therapy, review the common side effects of hydroxyurea with the patient and caregiver.
- Emphasize the importance of monitoring blood counts, particularly the WBC and platelets, at the prescribed intervals.
- If patients will be managed from home, teach self-care measures to prevent risks of infection and bleeding. Also, instruct patients on which signs and symptoms to report when they become pronounced. For more information, see Box 56.6.
- Instruct patient not to crush hydroxyurea tablets due to hazardous exposure potential.
  Instruct patient to perform oral care as previously described to prevent oral mucositis.

Ongoing Assessment and Evaluation

Throughout therapy with hydroxyurea, assess the patient for signs of bleeding disorders and infection. Closely monitor CBCs to make sure that they are within safe treatment parameters. If the patient is receiving concomitant radiation therapy, check the oral mucosa to ensure that severe reactions, which can cause pain and difficulty with food intake, do not compromise the patient. Because radiation recall may occur with concomitant treatment, dermatologic changes should be reported to the prescriber and managed appropriately.

MEMORY CHIP

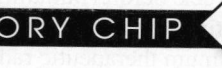 Hydroxyurea

- Indicated for managing acute leukemia with blasts. Also indicated for Head and neck cancer, malignant melanoma, cervical cancer and sickle cell disease
- Major contraindication: depressed bone marrow reserve, except in blast crisis of acute leukemia
- Most common adverse effects: gastrointestinal effects manifested by anorexia, nausea and vomiting, stomatitis, and diarrhea or constipation
- Most serious adverse effects: depression of bone marrow function, including leukopenia, anemia, and thrombocytopenia. Rapid decrease in white blood cell counts may occur within a short period, which is the desired effect for leukemia patients.
- Minimizing adverse effects: Monitor the patient's blood count before, during, and after treatment. If anemia occurs, the patient may receive blood transfusion without interrupting treatment cycles. Premedicate the patient with the appropriate antiemetic regimen.
- Most important patient education: Hydroxyurea is administered orally, take with or without food. If unable to vomiting occurs after taking hydroxyurea notify prescriber immediately. Advise the patient on careful handling of a cytotoxic agent, particularly to avoid contact with the skin or mucous membrane.

Drug Significantly Different From P Hydroxyurea

L-Asparaginase (Elspar) belongs to the group of miscellaneous drugs that are cell cycle–specific. The inhibitory action of this drug occurs in the postmitotic (G_1) phase of the cell cycle. L-Asparaginase is indicated in patients with ALL. In this condition, the tumor cells depend on exogenous asparagine for survival. When L-asparaginase is administered to the leukemic patient, the serum asparagine is hydrolyzed to nonfunctional aspartic acid and ammonia, depriving malignant cells of the required amino acid. Absence of asparagine causes rapid inhibition of DNA and RNA synthesis. Normal cells are able to synthesize asparagines and therefore are less affected than tumor cells by depletion of this enzyme.

L-Asparaginase does not appear to cross the blood–brain barrier and is not excreted in the urine. It is administered by the intramuscular or IV routes. Patients receiving this drug should be treated in the hospital because anaphylactic reactions can occur. There is no predictable or reliable way to test for hypersensitivity; therefore, treat each dose as if it had the possibility of causing a serious reaction. Toxicity is more common in adults than in children. A modified version of L-asparaginase, PEG-L-asparaginase (Oncaspar), is given to patients who are hypersensitive to the native form. In addition to anaphylaxis, other common side effects are hepatotoxicity, which occurs in most patients, hyperglycemia, pancreatitis, and decreased clotting factors, which may lead to bleeding problems such as intracranial hemorrhage and fatal bleeding associated with low fibrinogen. Depression of bone marrow function is rare and transient. Mild to severe CNS effects, manifested by somnolence, lethargy, drowsiness, and malaise, have been noted. These effects are usually reversible with discontinuation of L-asparaginase.

CHAPTER SUMMARY

- All cells, normal and malignant, progress through the different phases of the cell life cycle.
- In general, antineoplastic drugs are most effective on cells in the proliferative phases.
- Cell cycle–specific drugs exert their cytotoxicity at a particular phase or phases of the cell cycle and cause no substantial harm during the remaining phases.
- The major toxicities of antineoplastic drugs act on rapidly dividing cells, such as the bone marrow, GI mucosa, hair follicles, and gonadal cells.
- Hypersensitivity, anaphylactic reactions, and extravasations are the most common immediate reactions associated with chemotherapy administration.
- Health care workers can be exposed to chemotherapy through the following routes: skin and mucus membrane absorption, inhalation, and ingestion.
- The major teaching points to emphasize with a patient receiving chemotherapy are to (1) practice good body and oral hygiene; (2) eat a nutritious diet and drink plenty of fluids; (3) avoid injury, especially cuts to the skin;

(4) avoid possible sources of infection, such as animal excrement or people with colds, chickenpox, and herpes; and (5) pace activities of daily living to provide adequate rest and exercise.

QUESTIONS FOR STUDY AND REVIEW

1. What are the goals of chemotherapy?
2. What are the different strategies undertaken in the use of chemotherapeutic agents?
3. What are the basic features of a malignant cell?
4. What is the procedure for cleaning up a chemotherapy spill?
5. How are health care workers exposed to chemotherapy?
6. What are the nursing measures to take when an extravasation occurs?
7. What causes hypotension during an etoposide infusion?
8. What are the signs and symptoms of a hypersensitivity reaction?
9. Before starting a paclitaxel infusion, what must the person administering the drug check for?

NEED MORE HELP?

Chapter 56 of the Study Guide to Accompany *Drug Therapy in Nursing*, 4th Edition, contains NCLEX-style questions and other learning activities to reinforce your understanding of the concepts presented in this chapter. For additional information or to purchase the study guide, visit the**Point**.

REFERENCES

American Cancer Society. (2007). *Cancer facts & figures 2009*. Retrieved from *http://www. cancer.org*

Bedell, C. H. (2003). A changing paradigm for cancer treatment: The advent of new oral chemotherapy agents. *Clinical Journal of Oncology Nursing,* 7(Suppl 6):5–9.

DeVita, V. T., Hellman, S., & Rosenberg, S. A. (2008). Cancer: Principles and practice of oncology (8th ed.). Philadelphia, PA: Lippincott Williams & Wilkins.

National Institute of Occupational Safety and Health Standards. (2004). *Hazardous drug exposures in healthcare*. Publication no. 2004–165. Retrieved from *http://www.cdc.gov/ niosh/ topics/hazdrug/*

Mosteller, R. D. (1987). Simplified calculation of body-surface area. *New England Journal of Medicine,* 317:1098.

Polovich, M., Whitford, J., Olsen, M. (2009) *Chemotherapy and biotherapy: Guidelines and recommendations for practice.* Oncology Nursing Society. Pittsburgh, PA: Oncology Nursing Press.

Polovich, M., Blecher, C. S., Glynn-Tucker, E. M., McDiarmid, M., & Newton, S. A. (2003). *Safe handling of hazardous drugs*. Pittsburgh, PA: Oncology Nursing Society.

Yarbro, C. H., Frogge, M. H., Goodman, M., et al. (Eds.) (2011). *Cancer nursing: Principles and practice (7th ed)*. Boston, MA: Jones and Bartlett.

57

Drugs That Are Cell Cycle–Nonspecific

Learning Objectives

At the completion of this chapter the student will:

1. Differentiate a cell cycle–specific from a cell cycle–nonspecific agent.
2. Identify core drug knowledge about cell cycle–nonspecific drugs.
3. Identify core patient variables relevant to cell cycle–nonspecific drugs.
4. Relate the interaction of core drug knowledge to core patient variables for cell cycle–nonspecific drugs.
5. Generate a nursing plan of care based on the above interactions between core drug knowledge and core patient variables for cell cycle–nonspecific drugs.
6. Describe the nursing interventions to maximize therapeutic and minimize adverse effects of cell cycle–nonspecific drugs.
7. Determine key points for patient and family education for cell cycle–nonspecific drugs.
8. Discuss the treatment options for chemotherapy-induced nausea and vomiting.
9. State the rationale for using a combination of drugs in chemotherapy.
10. Identify the characteristics of drugs that are useful for combination chemotherapy.

Key Terms

acute emesis
alkylating agent
antitumor antibiotics
cell cycle–nonspecific
combination chemotherapy

delayed emesis
disease flare
emetogenics
hormones
hormone antagonists

liposomes
nitrosoureas
radiomimetic
tumor burden

Drugs That Are Cell Cycle–Nonspecific

C Alkylating Agents

P **cyclophosphamide**
busulfan
chlorambucil
melphalan
carboplatin
cisplatin
oxaliplatin

C Nitrosureas

P **carmustine**
lomustine
streptozocin

C Antitumor Antibiotics

P **doxorubicin**
doxorubicin HCl liposome
mitoxantrone
bleomycin

C Hormones and Hormone Antagonists

C Antiestrogens

P **tamoxifen**
adrenocorticosteroids (see also Chapter 35)
androgens (see also Chapter 54)
estrogens (see also Chapter 55)
progestins (see also Chapter 55)
antiandrogens (see also Chapter 54)
gonadotropin-releasing hormone analogues
goserelin acetate
leuprolide
aromatase inhibitor
anastrozole

The symbol C indicates the drug class.
Drugs in **bold type** marked with the symbol P are prototypes.
Drugs in blue type are closely related to the prototype.
Drugs in red type are significantly different from the prototype.
Drugs in black type with no symbol are also used in drug therapy; no prototype.

Cancer chemotherapy agents that are effective at specific phases in the cell's life cycle are classified as cell cycle–specific. Drugs that are effective through all phases of the cell cycle and are not limited to a specific phase are classified as **cell cycle–nonspecific.** This chapter focuses on the cell cycle– nonspecific antineoplastic drugs and the various management strategies used to ameliorate toxicities and maximize optimal therapeutic efficacy. Cell cycle–nonspecific drugs act on cells in both the proliferative and the nonproliferative phases of the cell cycle. They directly affect the deoxyribonucleic acid (DNA) molecule and do not display any specificity for cells that are dividing. They are considered more toxic than the cell cycle–specific drugs because their destructive action does not differentiate between normal and malignant cycling cells. Additionally, their toxicities occur throughout the cell cycle. This chapter also discusses the role of cytoprotectants and antiemetic agents, which have advanced the use of chemotherapeutic agents. Included in the cell cycle–nonspecific class of drugs are the alkylating agents, antitumor antibiotics, and hormonal drugs (hormones and hormone antagonists). Nonspecific agents are given in bolus doses because they cause cell death independently of the proliferative state of the cell. These agents also reduce the number of cells that make up a patient's tumor(s), which is known as the **tumor burden.**

This chapter also focuses on the important role of combination therapy: cell cycle–specific or cell cycle–nonspecific drugs, or both, used together to combat malignant neoplasms. The combination of a cell cycle–nonspecific and a cell cycle–specific drug can kill cells that are slowly dividing and those that are actively dividing. Cell cycle–nonspecific drugs also can help recruit cells into a more actively dividing state, which then makes them more sensitive to cell cycle–specific drugs. This chapter also discusses the rationale for implementing single-drug therapy and for designing effective combinations. Additionally, it includes some of the most common drug combinations in clinical use today. Finally, this chapter provides an overview of the newest type of chemotherapy, called targeted therapy.

The drug classes that are presented in this chapter include the alkylating agents, the antitumor antibiotics, and the hormone and hormone antagonists. Alkylating agents include nitrogen mustard and its derivatives, the nitrosoureas, and the platinum compounds. Prototypes for both the nitrogen mustard derivatives (cyclophosphamide [Cytoxan]) and the nitrosoureas (carmustine [BCNU]) are presented because they have significant differences. The prototype antitumor antibiotic is doxorubicin. The hormone and hormone antagonist group consists of adrenocorticosteroids, androgens, estrogens, progestins, antiestrogens, antiandrogens, gonadotropin inhibitors, and aromatase inhibitors. The prototype is the antiestrogen tamoxifen. Table 57.1 presents a summary of these antineoplastic drugs.

C ALKYLATING AGENTS

The **alkylating agents** attack cells in any phase of the cell cycle, including (for some agents) the resting phase. They exert their toxic effects by transferring their alkyl groups to various intracellular components, including nuclear DNA. Once the nucleotides have been alkylated, abnormal base pairing may occur, leading to DNA breakage (scission) and cross-linking. The damaged DNA molecule cannot replicate itself, and cell death results. The alkylating drugs are described as **radiomimetic,** so named because they mimic the actions of radiation therapy on the cells.

The alkylating drugs, the first modern chemotherapeutic agents, are a product of the secret wartime gas programs in the first and second World Wars. The exposure of seamen to mustard gas in World War II led to the discovery that alkylating drugs cause marrow hypoplasia, which led to their use in treating hematopoietic neoplasms such as Hodgkin's and non-Hodgkin's lymphoma.

Cyclophosphamide (Cytoxan), a nitrogen mustard derivative, is the prototype alkylating drug discussed here. Drugs closely related to cyclophosphamide include busulfan, chlorambucil, and melphalan.

Nursing Management of the Patient Receiving P Cyclophosphamide

Core Drug Knowledge

Pharmacotherapeutics

Cyclophosphamide is the most widely used alkylating agent. It has a broad spectrum of antitumor activity and plays a major role in the treatment of hematologic malignancies such as Hodgkin's and non-Hodgkin's lymphoma and multiple myeloma. It is the only alkylating agent that is effective against acute as well as chronic leukemias. Cyclophosphamide is an important component of regimens used in stem cell transplantation. It is also effective against solid tumors, such as breast cancer, small-cell lung cancer, endometrial cancer, and ovarian cancer. Cyclophosphamide is given intravenously or orally.

Pharmacokinetics

Cyclophosphamide and its active and inactive metabolites are well distributed throughout the body, including the brain and cerebrospinal fluid. The drug also distributes into breast milk and saliva. Most of the drug is metabolized in the liver, and about 60% of some metabolites bind extensively to plasma protein. It is exclusively excreted by the kidneys, primarily as metabolites; however, because of avid tubular reabsorption, only about 5% to 25% of the drug is excreted unchanged in the urine.

Pharmacodynamics

Cyclophosphamide exerts its toxic effects by transferring alkyl groups to nuclear DNA, leading to abnormal base pairing, DNA breakage and cross-linking, and cell death. During extensive first-pass hepatic metabolism, cyclophosphamide

TABLE 57.1	Summary of Selected Ⓒ Cell Cycle–Nonspecific Antineoplastic Drugs		
Drug (Trade) Name	**Selected Indications**	**Route and Dosage Range**	**Pharmacokinetics**
Ⓒ Alkylating Agents			
Ⓟ cyclophosphamide (Cytoxan)	Multiple approved indications: e.g. leukemia, lymphoma, **B**reast, genito-urinary, advanced ovarian, and cervical cancers	*Adult:* IV, single agent, 370 mg/m² on day 1, q4wk, depending on platelet count; in combination with cyclophosphamide, 300 mg/m² on day 1, q4wk. High dose therapy is used as a preparatory regimen for stem cell transplantation and for the decreasing tumor burden in patients with acute leukemia.	*Onset:* Rapid *Peak:* 1 h *Duration:* Unknown $t_{1/2}$: 4–6 h
cisplatin (Platinol, CDDP)	Testicular cancer and other genito-urinary tumors (bladder, prostate, metastatic ovarian, cervical, and endometrial)	*Adult:* IV, low level, 20–49 mg/mg²; moderate level, 50–75 mg/m²; and high level, 75–120 mg/m² or 3 mg/kg over 20–30 min or continuous 24-h infusion	*Onset:* 8–10 h *Peak:* 18–23 d *Duration:* 20–35 d $t_{1/2}$: 25–49 min; then 58–73 h
carboplatin (Paraplatin)	Ovarian cancer	*Adult:* IV, 300 mg/m² on day 1, q4wk, dose vary per protocol and AUC.	*Onset:* Rapid *Peak:* Unknown *Duration:* 48–96 h $t_{1/2}$: 1.1–2h, then 2.6–5.9 h
ifosfamide (Ifex)	Testicular cancer, sarcoma	*Adult:* 1–.2 g IV /day × 5 d repeat every 3 wk for testicular cancer. Dosing for other cancers such as sarcoma varies per protocol.	*Onset:* Rapid *Peak:* Unknown *Duration:* Unknown $t_{1/2}$: 3–10 h for low dose; 13.8 h for high dose
busulfan (Myleran)	Chronic myelogenous leukemia, used as high dose therapy for the preparatory regimen for stem cell transplantation.	*Adult:* PO, 4–8 mg/d until WBC decreases by half, then maintenance doses up to 4 mg/d. High dose therapies differ per protocol.	*Onset:* 0.5–2 h *Peak:* 2–3 h *Duration:* 4 h $t_{1/2}$: Unknown
chlorambucil (Leukeran)	Hodgkin's lymphoma, chronic lympho-cytic leukemia, non-Hodgkin's lym-phoma, breast and ovarian cancer	*Adult:* 0.1–0.2 mg/kg for 3–6 wk, then a maintenance dose not to exceed 0.1 mg/kg/d	*Onset:* Varies *Peak:* 1 h *Duration:* 15–20 h $t_{1/2}$: 1 h
mechlorethamine (nitrogen mustard, Mustargen)	Lung cancer, chronic lymphocytic leu-kemia, chronic myelogenous leukemia, Hodgkin's disease, lymphosarcoma, malignant effusions	*Adult:* IV, 0.4 mg/kg/course; intracavitary, 0.2–0.4 mg/kg	*Onset:* Immediate *Peak:* Seconds *Duration:* Minutes $t_{1/2}$: Minutes
melphalan (Alkeran)	Multiple myeloma, ovarian cancer	*Adult:* PO, 0.25 mg/kg/d × 7 d, followed by 3 wk drug free, then maintenance dose of 2 mg/d; IV, 16 mg/m² q3wk × 4 doses, then q4wk	*Onset:* Varies (PO), Rapid (IV) *Peak:* 2 h (PO), 1 h (IV)
Ⓒ Nitrosoureas			
Ⓟ carmustine (BCNU)	Palliative therapy of brain tumors, multiple myeloma, Hodgkin's lym-phoma, and non-Hodgkin's lymphoma as single-drug or combination therapy	*Adult:* IV, 150–200 mg/m² q6wk as a single dose or given over 2 d in divided doses as a slow infusion over 1–2 h, higher doses may be used in the setting of stem cell transplantation.	*Onset:* Immediate *Peak:* 15 min *Duration:* Unknown $t_{1/2}$: 15–30 min
streptozocin (Zanosar)	Pancreatic cancer, colon cancer, carcinoid tumors	*Adult:* IV, 500 mg/m² d for 5 d every 6 wk or 1 g/m²/wk for 2 wk; dosages not to exceed 1.5 g/m²/wk	*Onset:* Varies *Peak:* Unknown *Duration:* 24 h $t_{1/2}$: 35 min
lomustine (CCNU)	Hodgkin's disease, brain tumors	*Adult:* 130 mg/m² q6wk	*Onset:* 10 min *Peak:* 5 h *Duration:* 48 h $t_{1/2}$: 16–72 h

(Continued)

TABLE 57.1 **Summary of Selected** Ⓒ **Cell Cycle–Nonspecific Antineoplastic Drugs** *(continued)*

Drug (Trade) Name	Selected Indications	Route and Dosage Range	Pharmacokinetics
Ⓒ **Antitumor Antibiotics**			
P doxorubicin (Adriamycin)	Hematologic cancers (leukemias, Hodgkin's lymphoma, non-Hodgkin's lymphoma, multiple myeloma); solid tumors (breast, ovarian, prostate, stomach, thyroid, liver, small-cell lung, and head and neck cancers)	*Adult:* IV, 60–75 mg/m² as single injection every 21 d; alternate schedule, 30 mg/m² on each of 3 successive days for 4 wk; administered by slow IV push through a free-flowing IV line over 3–5 min or as a continuous 24 h infusion through a central venous access device	*Onset:* Rapid *Peak:* 2 h *Duration:* 24–37 h $t_{1/2}$: 12 min; then 3.3 h
doxorubicin HCl liposome (Doxil)	AIDS-related Kaposi sarcoma, ovarian cancer, multiple myeloma	*Adult:* IV, 20 mg/m² q3wk. doses up to 60 mg/m² is used in some indications.	*Onset:* Unknown *Peak:* Unknown *Duration:* Unknown $t_{1/2}$: 55 h
bleomycin (Blenoxane)	Lymphomas, squamous cell carcinoma, and testicular cancers	*Adult:* IV/IM/SC, 10–20 units/m² weekly or twice a week. Cumulative doses should not exceed 400 units.	*Onset:* Immediate *Peak:* IV, 10–20 min; IM/SC, 30–60 min *Duration:* Unknown $t_{1/2}$: 2 h
daunorubicin hydrochloride (Cerubidine, DNR)	Acute myelogenous leukemia, acute lymphocytic leukemia	*Adult:* IV, 30–60 mg/m²/d × 3d *Child:* IV, 25–45 mg/m²	*Onset:* Slow *Peak:* Unknown *Duration:* 8 d $t_{1/2}$: 20 h
daunorubicin citrate liposome (DaunoXome)	Advanced AIDS-related Kaposi sarcoma	*Adult:* IV, 40 mg/m² q2wk	*Onset:* Unknown *Peak:* Unknown *Duration:* Unknown $t_{1/2}$: 5.9–43.6 h
dactinomycin (Actinomycin, Cosmegen)	Testicular cancer, Ewing sarcoma, trophoblastic tumor, rhabdomyosarcoma, trophoblastic neoplasms	*Adult:* 500 mcg/d for a maximum 5 d *Child:* 15 mcg/d to a maximum of 500 mcg/d for 5 d	*Onset:* Rapid *Peak:* Unknown *Duration:* 9 d $t_{1/2}$: 37 h
idarubicin (Idamycin)	Acute myelogenous leukemia	*Adult:* 12 mcg/m²/d × 3 d in combination with cytarabine	*Onset:* Rapid *Peak:* Minutes *Duration:* Unknown $t_{1/2}$: 6–9.4 h
mitoxantrone (Novantrone)	Acute myelogenous leukemia, prostate cancer, multiple sclerosis	*Adult:* 12 mg/m² d × 2–3 d (used in combination with cytosine arabinoside in AML). Do not exceed 140 mg/ m²	*Onset:* Varies *Peak:* 10–14 d *Duration:* 28 d $t_{1/2}$: 5.8 d (median)
pentostatin (Nipent)	Alfa-interferon refractory hairy cell leukemia	*Adult:* IV, 4 mg/m² q other wk	*Onset:* Rapid *Peak:* 11 min *Duration:* Unknown $t_{1/2}$: 5.7 h
plicamycin (Mithramycin)	Testicular tumors, severe hypercalcemia	*Adult:* IV, 25–30 mcg/kg/d for 8–10 doses; severe hypercalcemia: 25 mcg/kg/d × 3–4 d	*Onset:* Rapid *Peak:* 4 h *Duration:* Unknown $t_{1/2}$: Unknown
Ⓒ **Hormones and Hormone Antagonists**			
Ⓒ *Antiestrogens*			
P tamoxifen (Nolvadex)	Breast cancers	*Adult:* PO, 20–40 mg/d	*Onset:* Varies *Peak:* 4–7 h *Duration:* Unknown $t_{1/2}$: 7–14 h

TABLE 57.1   Summary of Selected Ⓒ Cell Cycle–Nonspecific Antineoplastic Drugs   *(continued)*

Drug (Trade) Name	Selected Indications	Route and Dosage Range	Pharmacokinetics
Androgens			
fluoxymesterone (Halotestin)	Advanced breast cancer in premenopausal women	*Adult:* PO, 10–40 mg/d in divided doses	*Onset:* Rapid *Peak:* 2 h *Duration:* Unknown $t_{1/2}$: 9.5 h
testolactone (Teslac)	Advanced breast cancer	*Adult:* PO, 250 mg qid	*Onset:* Rapid *Peak:* Unknown *Duration:* Unknown $t_{1/2}$: Unknown
Estrogens			
estradiol (Estinyl)	Advanced breast cancer in postmenopausal women, prostate cancer	*Adult:* Breast cancer: PO, 0.5 mg/d initially, gradually increased to 3 mg/d in three divided doses; prostate cancer: PO, 0.15–2 mg/d. Also available as a vaginal cream and a transdermal patch.	*Onset:* Slow *Peak:* Days *Duration:* Unknown $t_{1/2}$: Unknown
Progestins			
medroxyprogesterone (Provera, Depo-Provera)	Advanced endometrial carcinoma	*Adult:* IM, 400–800 mg 2×/wk; PO, 200–300 mg/d	*Onset:* Slow, weeks *Peak:* Unknown *Duration:* Unknown $t_{1/2}$: Unknown
megestrol acetate (Megace)	Advanced endometrial carcinoma, breast cancer	*Adult:* PO, 40–320 mg/d	*Onset:* Slow *Peak:* Weeks *Duration:* Unknown $t_{1/2}$: Unknown
Antiandrogens			
bicalutamide (Casodex)	Advanced prostate cancer	*Adult:* PO, 500 mg once daily	*Onset:* Slow *Peak:* 31.3 h *Duration:* Days $t_{1/2}$: 5.8 d
flutamide (Eulexin)	Advanced prostate cancer	*Adult:* PO, 250 mg q8 h	*Onset:* Varies *Peak:* 2 h *Duration:* 72 h $t_{1/2}$: 6 h
nilutamide (Nilandron)	Advanced breast cancer in postmenopausal women with disease progression after tamoxifen	*Adult:* PO, 300 mg/d × 30 d, then 150 mg/d	*Onset:* Varies *Peak:* Unknown *Duration:* Unknown $t_{1/2}$: Unknown
Gonadotropin-Releasing Hormone (GnRH) Analogues			
goserelin (Zoladex)	Advanced prostatic cancer, advanced breast cancer, endometriosis	*Adult:* SC, 3.6 mg q28 d	*Onset:* Slow *Peak:* 12–15 d *Duration:* Unknown $t_{1/2}$: 4.2 h
leuprolide (Lupron, Lupron Depot)	Advanced prostatic cancer	*Adult:* SC, 1 mg/d *Depot:* IM, 7.5 mg monthly, q28–33 d	*Onset:* Slow *Peak:* Unknown *Duration:* Unknown $t_{1/2}$: Unknown
Aromatase Inhibitors			
anastrozole (Arimidex) Aromasin (Exemestane) Femara (Letrozole)	Indicated in breast cancer for adjuvant, first line or second line therapy.	*Adult:* PO, 1 mg daily 25 mg once daily after a meal 2.5 mg PO daily	*Onset:* Rapid *Peak:* Unknown *Duration:* Unknown $t_{1/2}$: 7 d

undergoes hydroxylation and is converted into a cytotoxic agent with wide clinical utility in the treatment of various tumors. It is particularly effective with leukemias because the abnormal leukocytes are very sensitive to this drug's effects.

Contraindications and Precautions

Patients with severely compromised bone marrow function and with known hypersensitivity to cyclophosphamide should not be treated with the drug. The drug is in pregnancy category D.

Adverse Effects

The dose-limiting toxicity associated with cyclophosphamide (at high dosage) is leukopenia. Leukocytes reach nadir within 2 weeks, with recovery after 3 to 4 weeks. At very high doses, cyclophosphamide has a propensity for inducing sterile hemorrhagic cystitis. This problem is manifested by hematuria, pain, and burning on urination caused by the irritation of the bladder wall by acrolein, a metabolic by-product of cyclophosphamide. Other adverse effects of high-dose therapy (120 to 270 mg/kg) include syndrome of inappropriate antidiuretic hormone. High doses can also cause cardiomyopathy in the form of chronic heart failure (CHF) and hemopericardium secondary to hemorrhagic myocarditis and myocardial necrosis. In addition, high-dose cyclophosphamide is associated with high levels of acute and delayed nausea and vomiting.

Hypersensitivity to cyclophosphamide has been observed in both unpretreated and pretreated patients. Reproductive effects such as amenorrhea, gonadal suppression, sterility, and ovarian fibrosis can occur. Secondary malignancies have been reported. Other adverse effects include alopecia and transverse ridging and hyperpigmentation of the nails. Nausea, vomiting, and anorexia also occur. Dizziness, nasal stuffiness, and rhinorrhea are less common.

Drug Interactions

Table 57.2 notes the effects of cyclophosphamide on other drugs. It is compatible with other common antineoplastic agents such as melphalan, paclitaxel, vinorelbine, idarubicin, cisplatin, and bleomycin. Interaction with some herbal medicines has been noted. Patients should report all medications, whether over-the-counter or prescribed, to the health care team.

Assessment of Relevant Core Patient Variables

Health Status

Assess any organ system that could be potentially compromised by cyclophosphamide therapy. Before initiating treatment, baseline tests to determine sufficient hematopoietic and renal function should be performed. Carefully assess patients with impaired renal function, myelosuppression, or a known hypersensitivity to cyclophosphamide; these conditions may preclude administration of the drug. Patients who have had prior radiation to the pelvis or bladder are at increased risk for hemorrhagic cystitis. BK virus has also been associated with higher risk of hemorrhagic cystitis in stem cell transplant patients who receive cyclophosphamide.

Life Span and Gender

Document the age and developmental status of the patient. Cyclophosphamide can cause secondary malignancies such as bladder cancer, acute myeloid leukemia, and non-Hodgkin lymphoma, which can occur up to 20 years after treatment. Long-term and high-dose therapy increases the risk of secondary malignancies. Patients should be counseled about this serious risk. Patients who develop bladder cancer usually have a history of hemorrhagic cystitis. Adolescent patients who received cyclophosphamide for cancer treatment as children seem to be at higher risk than other populations for secondary cancers. Because of possible reproductive adverse effects, discuss reproductive goals with patients of childbearing potential who are considering high-dose therapy. Also, assess the woman of childbearing age for pregnancy and explore contraceptive methods because cyclophosphamide is a pregnancy category D drug.

Lifestyle, Diet, and Habits

Assess the daily dietary habits and elimination patterns of patients taking the oral formulation of the drug.

TABLE 57.2	Agents That Interact with P Cyclophosphamide	
Interactants	**Effect and Significance**	**Nursing Management**
doxorubicin	Potentiates doxorubicin-induced cardiotoxicity	Dose modification is advised. Monitor cardiac function.
succinylcholine	Prolongs neuromuscular blocking activity	Administer with caution.
digoxin	Decreases pharmacologic effect	Digoxin dosage may need to be increased.
halothane and nitrous oxide	When used in conjunction, has produced mortality	Notify anesthesia department.
corticosteroids	Decreases conversion of cyclophosphamide to its active metabolites, decreasing activity	Notify health care provider for dose adjustment.

The metabolites of the drug should be excreted during the day. Instruct the patient to take all oral doses before 4 or 5 PM daily. If metabolite-rich urine stagnates, it can irritate and inflame the bladder wall. To promote diuresis and prevent this potential adverse effect of drug administration, the patient must drink at least 2 L of liquid a day. Assess activities of daily living, because the patient may have difficulty getting to the bathroom if he or she has impaired mobility.

Environment

Be aware of the environment in which the drug will be administered. High-dose intravenous (IV) cyclophosphamide therapy is usually given in an acute care facility, where patients can be adequately managed for potential major and acute toxicities, such as severe nausea and vomiting or hemorrhagic cystitis. For standard-dose IV and oral formulations, instruct the patient and caregiver about the necessity of retreatment hydration with vigorous oral intake, which can be accomplished in the home setting.

Nursing Diagnoses and Outcomes

- Risk for Infection related to suppression of bone marrow function
  Desired outcome: *The patient will be free from infection and exercise caution to avoid exposure to infection.*
- Risk for Injury associated with depression of bone marrow function and related bleeding and hypersensitivity reaction (anaphylaxis)
  Desired outcome: *The patient will attain pretreatment hematologic status, learn to monitor and prevent situations that may induce bleeding, and recognize and immediately report signs and symptoms associated with a hypersensitivity reaction.*
- Imbalanced Nutrition: Less than Body Requirements, related to nausea, vomiting, and taste alterations
  Desired outcome: *The patient will experience adequate emetic control, using pharmacologic and nonpharmacologic measures.*
- Impaired Urinary Elimination related to cyclophosphamide-induced urinary-bladder toxicity and nephrotoxicity.
  Desired outcome: *The patient will maintain fluid balance and be free from signs and symptoms of hemorrhagic cystitis as evidenced by adequate fluid intake and output with an absence of hematuria, pain, and dysuria. In addition, renal function will not be compromised, as shown by normal renal values.*
- Impaired Skin Integrity and Disturbed Body Image related to changes in skin pigmentation, nail conditions, and alopecia.
  Desired outcome: *The patient will be able to recognize and report any changes in the skin and integuments and will undertake measures to enhance appearance and body image.*

Planning and Intervention

Maximizing Therapeutic Effects

Before administering cyclophosphamide, ensure that the test results disclose adequate renal function and adequate hematopoietic reserves to achieve the intended therapeutic effects.

Minimizing Adverse Effects

The incidence of hemorrhagic cystitis can be reduced by a vigorous hydration regimen of at least 2 L of fluid a day and, in high-dose therapy, administering the uroprotectant agent mesna. Prehydrate the patient orally and intravenously with at least 2 L of normal saline solution. Potassium and magnesium additives may also be indicated. Monitor urine output vigilantly to ensure an output of at least half of the intake. Consider discontinuation of any medications that carry a high risk of renal toxicity to prevent compromising renal function. Assess for risk of nausea and vomiting and institute antiemetic therapy as appropriate.

Providing Patient and Family Education

- Emphasize methods of preventing the major toxicities of cyclophosphamide therapy.
- Encourage patients to drink large amounts of fluid, at least 2 L daily, to induce diuresis. Some of the pretreatment hydration can be accomplished at home; thus, if patients understand the reason for it, their adherence to the regimen the night before drug administration will be improved. Additional hydration will be given in the hospital to augment previous oral intake.
- Advise patients that temporary and reversible hair loss will occur. Refer patients to a wig specialist before treatment is initiated, and educate patients to refrain from using chemical treatments on the hair and from vigorous brushing. Teach patients to use mild shampoos and, if they have long hair, suggest that it be cut before

CRITICAL THINKING SCENARIO

DETERMINING THE MOST APPROPRIATE ANTIEMESIS REGIMEN TO PREVENT CHEMOTHERAPY-INDUCED NAUSEA AND VOMITING

Mrs. H., a 50-year-old patient with acute myelogenous leukemia, is being admitted to receive high-dose cyclophosphamide to induce stem cell mobilization in preparation for an autologous stem cell transplantation. She has been properly hydrated, and she needs to receive her antiemetic regimen prior to starting cyclophosphamide.

1. To determine the appropriate antiemesis regimen, it is necessary to assess Mrs. H. for which risk factors?
2. Explain the types of nausea and vomiting that this patient may develop and the appropriate class of medications to treat each type.
3. Name additional nonpharmacologic interventions that could be utilized for this patient.

chemotherapy starts. Each patient will have individual preferences that should be explored. Reassure patients that hair regrowth will occur; however, advise them that new hair may be a different color or texture.

- Review signs and symptoms of a hypersensitivity reaction with patients to alleviate their anxiety. Ask patients about other known sensitivity to drugs and determine whether patients have asthma.

- Instruct patients to notify the prescriber about other serious adverse effects. Signs and symptoms to report include lower volume of urine or less frequent urination than usual; blood in the urine, dysuria, or burning with urination; a temperature of 100.5°F or higher; excessive vomiting, diarrhea, or inability to keep food and fluids down that persists for more than 24 hours; and the presence of black stools, red rash, or unusual bruising, which are signs of bleeding.

- Reassure patients that nausea and vomiting can be relieved with antiemetic drug therapy and emphasize that they should request these agents when needed. Teach nonpharmacologic measures such as relaxation and always ask patients to initiate practices that have helped alleviate these symptoms in the past. Good emesis management is important because both acute and delayed emesis have distressing effects on physical and psychological functioning (see discussion below on the types of chemotherapy-induced emesis).

- Counsel patients about the long-term risks of secondary malignancies (e.g., leukemia, lymphoma, bladder and skin cancers) associated with cyclophosphamide therapy.

- If patients are taking an oral formulation of the drug, instruct them to ingest the drug early in the morning on an empty stomach, to drink at least 10 to 12 glasses of water daily, and to empty the bladder frequently. These practices ensure that the metabolites of the drug are excreted during the day and do not stagnate to erode the bladder wall.

- Discuss the need for sperm and egg banking with patients who are on high-dose therapy and are considering having children in the future.

Ongoing Assessment and Evaluation

When patients undergo subsequent courses of chemotherapy with cyclophosphamide, assess renal function and hematopoietic reserve. Assess the patient's hematologic status every week during the first months of therapy and until maintenance therapy is set, and then at intervals of 2 to 3 weeks. For high-dose regimens, also monitor cardiac function. Dose modification may be considered in patients with impaired renal, hematologic, or hepatic function.

Drugs Closely Related to
P Cyclophosphamide

Busulfan

Busulfan is used to treat chronic myelogenous leukemia. Both oral and IV formulations are also frequently used

MEMORY CHIP

P Cyclophosphamide

- Indicated for testicular, ovarian, and bladder cancers
- Major contraindications: severe depression of bone marrow function, serious infections, nursing mothers, and women and men with reproductive potential
- Most common adverse effect: hemorrhagic or nonhemorrhagic cystitis
- Dose-limiting effect: leukopenia
- **Life span alert: Patients on long-term therapy should be counseled about risks of secondary malignancy.**
- Maximizing therapeutic effects: Ensure that patient has adequate bone marrow reserve and good renal function.
- Minimizing adverse effects: Promote vigorous hydration and diuresis, and administer mesna, if indicated, to prevent hemorrhagic cystitis.
- Most important patient education: Instruct the patient to drink plenty of fluids and empty the bladder every 2 hours.
- **Patient safety alert: Obtain a current and accurate height and weight in order to calculate the body surface area. These numbers should be independently verified and not obtained from another provider's stated measurements to ensure that the proper dose of cyclophosphamide is administered. Death can result if inappropriate doses are administered.**

in high doses in the preparatory regimen for stem cell transplantations. The most notable toxicity of busulfan is myelosuppression, which can be severe and long lasting. Additionally, pulmonary fibrosis and seizures can occur with high-dose therapy. With high doses, prophylaxis with antiseizure medication is necessary. Prior to stem cell transplantation, hepatic venous occlusive disease is associated with doses greater than 16 mg/kg when combined with other chemotherapy agents.

Chlorambucil

Chlorambucil is indicated in the treatment of chronic lymphocytic leukemia and lymphomas. Pulmonary fibrosis and seizures can occur, just as with busulfan. Barbiturates may increase the toxicity of chlorambucil and should be avoided, or patients should be carefully monitored. Chlorambucil should be avoided within 4 weeks of radiation or cytotoxic therapy.

Melphalan

Melphalan is a bifunctional alkylating agent active against both active and dividing cells in the cell cycle. This drug is commonly used to treat multiple myeloma and in the preparatory regimen for stem cell transplantation in myeloma. In high doses, melphalan is notable for severe oral mucositis. Oral and IV formulations are available; the oral formulation must be administered on an empty stomach. Finally, melphalan is associated with a delayed nadir, which can last 4 to 6 weeks.

Drugs Significantly Different From P Cyclophosphamide

Cisplatin

Cisplatin (Cisplatinum, CDDP; Platinol-AQ) is a widely used heavy metal that acts as a bifunctional alkylating agent like cyclophosphamide. It also produces intrastrand and interstrand linking in DNA through covalent bonds with the platinum molecule, leading to breaking of DNA strands during cell replication. Cisplatin is clinically used to treat almost every solid tumor and lymphoma. The pharmacokinetics show rapid distribution of the drug to the tissues after IV infusion. Most cisplatin bonds to protein. It is believed to be metabolized in the liver and excreted in the urine.

Unlike cyclophosphamide, cisplatin has some unique features and adverse effects. Cisplatin belongs to a group of antineoplastic drugs called **emetogenics,** which have high potential for causing severe nausea and vomiting (Box 57.1). Approximately 75% of chemotherapy patients experience this distressing adverse effect, which can drastically affect physical functioning and quality of life. The risk factors that predispose the patient to this problem are listed in Box 57.2. The Black Box warning for cisplatin cites nausea and vomiting as dose-limiting effects.

Advances in understanding the pathophysiology of emesis have shifted attention from the roles of dopamine and serotonin in emesis to the potential role of substance P and the use of neurokinin-1 (NK-1) antagonists. The emetic center contains the chemoreceptor trigger zone and is stimulated through peripheral and central pathways. Peripheral stimulation occurs when chemotherapy causes damage to the gastrointestinal (GI) mucosa, activating afferent input through the vagus nerve. Serotonin is the neurotransmitter for peripheral stimulation. Substance P is found in vagal afferent neurons and binds to NK-1 receptors, causing vomiting. The study of this specific mechanism of vomiting has led to the development of a new class of antiemetics, NK-1 receptor antagonists.

Emesis associated with cytotoxic agents occurs in different patterns: acute, delayed, anticipatory, breakthrough, and refractory (Box 57.3). Cisplatin therapy can be associated with any of these patterns of nausea and vomiting, but it is primarily associated with **acute emesis** (vomiting within 24 hours after chemotherapy) and **delayed emesis** (nausea and vomiting 24 hours after chemotherapy). In cisplatin

---

Box 57.2 RISK FACTORS FOR NAUSEA AND VOMITING

Anxiety, expectations of severe side effects, and previous chemotherapy experience are predisposing factors to the adverse effects of nausea and vomiting. This type of nausea and vomiting is termed anticipatory. Certain patient characteristics and prognostic factors also affect the incidence of nausea and vomiting:

- Age: Younger patients experience nausea and vomiting more than older patients.
- Gender: A higher incidence of nausea and vomiting in women is thought to result from administration of more highly emetogenic drugs to women than to men and lower alcohol consumption among women.
- Alcohol and illicit drug intake: High alcohol consumption and use of illicit drugs are associated with a higher tolerance of nausea and vomiting.
- Performance status and motivation: Patients who have a better physical, emotional, and functional status have a better tolerance of emesis.
- History of motion sickness or severe emesis during pregnancy: These patients are more susceptible to chemotherapy-induced episodes of nausea and vomiting.

Box 57.1 RANKING CHEMOTHERAPEUTIC DRUGS ACCORDING TO EMETOGENIC POTENTIAL

The following antineoplastic drugs are listed according to their emetogenic potential. Highly emetogenic drugs begin the list; mildly emetogenic drugs complete it.

Cisplatin*	Procarbazine
Dacarbazine	Taxanes
Streptozocin	Mitomycin-C
Nitrogen mustard	Etoposide
Hexamethylmelamine	Methotrexate
Actinomycin D	Irinotecan
Cyclophosphamide*	Topotecan
Carboplatin*	Gemcitabine
Lomustine	Bleomycin
Carmustine	Vinca alkaloids
Anthracyclines	5-Fluorouracil
Ifosfamide*	Hormones
Cytosine arabinoside	Chlorambucil

*Associated with acute and delayed nausea and vomiting.

Box 57.3 TYPES OF EMESIS AND THEIR TREATMENTS

Acute: Occurs within 24 hours after chemotherapy
Delayed: Occurs more than 24 hours after chemotherapy; may severely affect a patient's food intake and prolong hospitalization. This type of nausea and vomiting is often underestimated by health care providers. Proactive treatment of delayed emesis is essential to decrease symptoms and increase quality of life in cancer patients receiving chemotherapy.
Anticipatory emesis: Learned response; occurs often if the patient has a negative experience with the first chemotherapy dose. Anticipatory nausea is difficult to treat; however, lorazepam and corticosteroids may be helpful. It can be minimized by effectively managing the first chemotherapy cycle and educating patients about adverse effects.
Breakthrough emesis: Occurs during a treatment cycle despite prophylaxis
Refractory emesis: Occurs after at least 1 cycle of chemotherapy; can persist despite attempts to prevent it

therapy, severe nausea and vomiting occur within 1 to 4 hours after treatment and usually last for 24 hours.

The drugs that are most effective in treating acute emesis from cisplatin therapy are the serotonin receptor antagonists. These first-line agents act by blocking serotonin from binding to receptors in the GI tract. The efficacy of these agents can be enhanced by using dexamethasone. For cisplatin-induced acute nausea, an NK-1 receptor antagonist is also indicated. Current clinical guidelines from the American Society of Clinical Oncology (Kris, Hesketh, Somerfield, et al., 2006) on antiemetics and the National Comprehensive Cancer Network guidelines (2009) recommend the use of all three drugs concurrently in managing the severe nausea that is related to cisplatin therapy. The National Comprehensive Cancer Network guidelines also state that lorazepam might also be added to this combination.

Delayed emesis from cisplatin therapy may persist for up to 5 days after treatment. The mechanism for delayed emesis is not as well understood. This type of emesis is usually treated with corticosteroids, NK-1 antagonists, lorazepam, and metoclopramide. Guidelines for treating various emetic patterns and adjunct nonpharmacologic treatments are found in Box 57.4 and Box 57.5. Antiemetics are discussed fully in Chapter 53; ondansetron is the prototype serotonin receptor antagonist drug presented.

The major dose-limiting adverse effect of cisplatin is nephrotoxicity, which is dose related and cumulative.

Box 57.4 GUIDELINES FOR MANAGING CHEMOTHERAPY-INDUCED EMESIS

1. Determine the emetogenic potential of the drug: high, intermediate, or low.
2. When combination agents are given, give the antiemetic appropriate for the chemotherapeutic agent with the highest risk.
3. For acute emesis, the agents with the highest therapeutic index are the serotonin antagonists. At equivalent doses, they have the same safety and efficacy profiles and can be used interchangeably.
4. The oral route is as effective and safe as the intravenous route.
5. For acute emesis with high-risk agents, the combination of a serotonin antagonist, an NK-1 antagonist, and a corticosteroid is recommended. A corticosteroid is suggested for patients treated with intermediate-risk agents, whereas for low-risk agents, no antiemetic is needed. Antiemetics should be given for each day of the chemotherapy. Lorazepam, a benzodiazepine, is sometimes added.
6. For delayed emesis, in patients receiving high-risk cisplatin, an NK-1 antagonist and a corticosteroid plus metoclopramide, lorazepam, or a serotonin antagonist is recommended. For intermediate- and low-risk agents, no preventive agent for delayed emesis is recommended.
7. Prevention of chemotherapy-induced emesis by using the most active antiemetic agents appropriate for the drug to prevent acute or delayed emesis is suggested. Such regimens should be used with all highly and moderately emetogenic chemotherapy treatment to avoid anticipatory nausea and vomiting with subsequent cycles. If anticipatory emesis occurs, behavioral therapy with systematic desensitization is effective and suggested.

Box 57.5 NONPHARMACOLOGIC TREATMENTS FOR CHEMOTHERAPY-INDUCED EMESIS

Nonpharmacologic methods for managing nausea and vomiting are adjuncts to antiemetic therapy, not substitutes for it. These include:

1. Music therapy
2. Moderate aerobic exercise
3. Acupressure wristbands
4. Behavioral interventions such as hypnosis, biofeedback, guided imagery, and cognitive distraction*

*Effectiveness believed to be from producing relaxation, giving the patient a sense of control, reducing feelings of helplessness, and diverting the patient's attention away from the acute situation to more neutral and relaxing images.

Pretreatment hydration and forced diuresis are required to prevent nephrotoxicity. Cisplatin differs from the prototype cyclophosphamide in that it carries a Black Box warning related to its possible nephrotoxic adverse effects. Amifostine, a Food and Drug Administration (FDA)–approved cytoprotectant, is indicated for minimizing the nephrotoxic effects of cisplatin in advanced ovarian cancer or non–small cell lung cancer as well as the peripheral neurotoxicities. Neurotoxicity and ototoxicity may also limit the dose or the length of therapy of cisplatin, because these adverse effects more commonly occur with larger doses or after repeated use. Peripheral neuropathy is common and can be debilitating. Neurotoxicity may also occur or worsen after cisplatin therapy has been discontinued, and some forms are irreversible. Ototoxicity, which may be bilateral or unilateral and possibly permanent, is more severe in children treated with cisplatin. Cumulative ototoxicity is common, although deafness has occurred rarely after an initial dose. Patients should be assessed for pre-existing hearing loss; assessment should continue concurrently during cisplatin therapy. Coadministration of cisplatin with other drugs that produce ototoxicity, such as loop diuretics, may produce additive ototoxicity and should be avoided. In addition, cisplatin can cause another serious adverse effect—an anaphylaxis-like reaction. Black Box warnings for cisplatin include both ototoxicity and anaphylaxis, and these warnings are not given for the prototype cyclophosphamide. Epinephrine, corticosteroids, and antihistamines are used to alleviate anaphylactic reactions. Also, the Black Box warning describes a risk of myelosuppression as a dose-limiting adverse effect.

Other potential adverse effects of cisplatin are electrolyte imbalances. Cisplatin therapy can cause hypomagnesemia, hypocalcemia, hyponatremia, hypokalemia, and hypophosphatemia; these electrolyte imbalances are believed to be related to renal tubular damage that occurs with cisplatin therapy. Hypomagnesemia may be severe in high-dose cisplatin therapy, and this effect appears to contribute to some of the vascular toxicities caused by cisplatin, such as Raynaud phenomenon. Patients with low magnesium levels may need a diet high in magnesium to help offset losses from cisplatin therapy. Examples of these foods are nuts, chocolate, whole-wheat breads and cereals, instant coffee and tea, oatmeal, beans, and peas. Calcium and magnesium compete to gain entrance into the intestines, so calcium-rich foods increase the body's requirements for magnesium. Calcium-rich foods, such as dairy products, should be limited when eating foods high in magnesium during cisplatin therapy.

When administering cisplatin, care should be taken not to use needles or administration sets containing aluminum because these devices result in precipitate formation or loss of drug potency; the drug reacts with aluminum.

Carboplatin

Carboplatin (Paraplatin; Paraplatin NovaPlus), another platinum compound, is very similar to cisplatin. It is used for a variety of malignancies, including many gynecologic cancers. Carboplatin exhibits less renal toxicity and neurotoxicity compared with cisplatin. However, the risk of myelosuppression appears greater, especially for anemia. Carboplatin carries a Black Box warning relating to anemia. Like cisplatin, carboplatin has a risk of anaphylaxis and nausea and vomiting. Unlike cisplatin, carboplatin causes thrombocytopenia, which can be dose limiting. Dosing is based on creatinine clearance, which seems to be the most reliable way of predicting toxicity and drug clearance. Health care providers must be knowledgeable in dose calculations and formulas that are unique to carboplatin to avoid accidental overdosing or underdosing.

Oxaliplatin

Oxaliplatin (Eloxatin) is another platinum compound similar to cisplatin. It is primarily used in combination with other chemotherapy agents for colorectal cancers. Oxaliplatin is well known for causing a rare but disturbing neuropathic side effect. The acute syndrome of pharyngolaryngeal dysesthesia, reported in 1% to 2% of patients, is exacerbated by cold. This neuropathic syndrome is characterized by feelings of dyspnea and/or difficulty swallowing without laryngospasm or bronchospasm. Although it can be frightening for patients, this condition is not life threatening. Proper instruction can prepare patients and help them avoid causative agents. They should be advised to avoid cold drinks, cold air, or cold food for up to one week after receiving the drug. Like cisplatin, oxaliplatin may cause anaphylaxis and carries a Black Box warning to that effect. Unlike cisplatin, oxaliplatin does not carry the risk of nephrotoxicity or ototoxicity.

© NITROSOUREAS

The **nitrosoureas** are alkylating drugs that are frequently classified separately from the others because they also have additional mechanisms of cytotoxicity. Like the alkylating agents, they cause breaks and cross-linking in DNA strands. They also inhibit DNA repair. Nitrosoureas are highly lipid-soluble drugs. As such, they cross the blood–brain barrier. They have broad clinical activity in treating lymphomas and certain solid tumors. Unlike most other chemotherapy agents, nitrosoureas are associated with a delayed nadir. Myelosuppression caused by these drugs can be severe, and the neutrophils (one type of white blood cell) reach nadir 4 to 6 weeks after therapy starts, rather than the typical 7 to 10 days. Examples of frequently used nitrosoureas are carmustine and streptozocin, which are discussed in this chapter. The prototype nitrosourea is carmustine (BCNU). Drugs closely related to the prototype are lomustine and streptozocin.

Nursing Management of the Patient Receiving [P] Carmustine
Core Drug Knowledge
Pharmacotherapeutics

Carmustine is a nitrosourea used in the palliative therapy of brain tumors, multiple myeloma, Hodgkin's and non-Hodgkin's lymphoma. It is also frequently used in high doses during the preparative regimen for stem cell transplantations in lymphoma patients. It may be administered as a single drug or in combination with other antineoplastic agents. It is given as a slow infusion to prevent severe pain and burning at the IV site.

Pharmacokinetics

After IV administration, carmustine is rapidly degraded. Most of the drug is excreted by the renal system in 96 hours, and about 10% is excreted by the respiratory system as carbon dioxide. This drug crosses the blood–brain barrier because of its high lipid solubility.

Pharmacodynamics

The mechanism of action of carmustine is similar to that of an alkylating drug. It alkylates DNA and ribonucleic acid (RNA), thereby blocking synthesis and repair. It also inhibits essential enzymes by carbamylation of the amino acids.

Contraindications and Precautions

Carmustine is contraindicated in patients who are hypersensitive to it. It should be used cautiously in those with impaired respiratory or bone marrow function. Accidental skin contamination can cause hyperpigmentation and brown discoloration of the affected area. The drug should be dispensed in glass; plastic containers should be avoided. Carmustine is a pregnancy category D drug.

Adverse Effects

The major toxic effect of carmustine is suppression of bone marrow function, which generally occurs 6 weeks after drug administration. This delayed suppression is cumulative and is manifested as thrombocytopenia and leukopenia. Pulmonary toxicity in the form of pulmonary inflammation and/or fibrosis is associated with prolonged therapy and cumulative doses of more than 1,400 mg/m². Pulmonary fibrosis can be irreversible. A Black Box warning relates to the risk of myelosuppression and pulmonary toxicity. As with alkylating agents, carmustine and the other nitrosoureas are associated with the development of secondary malignancies.

TABLE 57.3	Agents That Interact with ℗ Carmustine	
Interactants	Effect and Significance	Nursing Management
cimetidine	Increased toxicity and myelosuppression	Monitor blood counts.
digoxin, phenytoin	Decreased serum level	Measure serum level. Consult health care provider about dose modification if needed.

Nausea and vomiting also occur frequently with carmustine. In addition, the patient may complain of local reactions, such as intense pain and discomfort in the vein used for drug administration, flushing of the skin, and suffusion of the conjunctiva within 2 hours that can last for 4 hours after administration of the drug.

Drug Interactions
When given concomitantly with other drugs, carmustine exhibits certain effects, as shown in Table 57.3.

Assessment of Relevant Core Patient Variables
Health Status
Because the major carmustine-induced toxicities are related to bone marrow and pulmonary functions, assess patients for adequate bone marrow reserve and pulmonary function. Patients at risk are those with a history of lung disease, patients receiving a greater cumulative dose than 1,400 mg/m^2 of carmustine, and children treated with cumulative doses of 770 mg/m^2 to 1,800 mg/m^2 and cranial irradiation.

Life Span and Gender
If the patient is on prolonged therapy, regularly perform pulmonary assessments to monitor for pulmonary dysfunction and disease. The onset of pulmonary problems is usually delayed, and disease is chronic. Pulmonary fibrosis has been reported to occur up to 15 years later in patients who received cumulative doses of as much as 1,800 mg/m^2, concomitantly with irradiation, as adolescents. Among adults, the same outcome has been noted with prolonged therapy and large cumulative doses. Assess women of childbearing age for pregnancy and lactation because carmustine is a pregnancy category D drug. It is not known whether carmustine is excreted in breast milk; hence, breast-feeding women should be cautioned.

Lifestyle, Diet, and Habits
Forewarn patients about the acute onset of nausea and vomiting associated with carmustine therapy. Assess the effect that nausea and vomiting will have on the patient's diet and activities of daily living. Nausea and vomiting usually occur 2 to 4 hours after drug administration. Because the signs and symptoms of myelosuppression are delayed, explore whether the patient's activities of daily living might expose him or her to risks for infection and bleeding.

Environment
Be aware of the environment in which carmustine will be administered. It is usually given in an acute care setting so that medical and nursing support are easily available should a hypersensitivity reaction or anaphylaxis occur.

Nursing Diagnoses and Outcomes
- Pain related to discomfort of drug administration
  Desired outcome: The patient will be free from discomfort along the infusion route.
- Risk for Infection and Injury, especially bleeding related to suppression of bone marrow function
  Desired outcome: The patient will take steps to prevent exposure to potential sources of infection and bleeding, minimize risks for infection and bleeding, and comply with requirements for periodic blood counts.
- Impaired Gas Exchange related to drug-related pulmonary fibrosis
  Desired outcome: The patient will learn to recognize and report signs and symptoms of respiratory dysfunction. The patient will comply with the need to have pulmonary function tests during the course of treatment.
- Imbalanced Nutrition: Less than Body Requirements, because of drug-induced nausea and vomiting
  Desired outcome: The patient will expect emetic episodes and ask for antiemetics as needed. The patient will learn how to manage dietary intake and patterns to ensure adequate nutritional intake.
- Reproductive and Sexual Dysfunction resulting from drug therapy.
  Desired outcome: The patient will be aware of the physical changes in reproductive and sexual functions. The patient will accept these changes and explore ways to enhance sexual and reproductive health.

Planning and Intervention
Maximizing Therapeutic Effects
Be aware that after reconstitution, the carmustine solution is stable in a glass container for 24 hours at 4°C or for 8 hours at 25°C when protected from light.

Minimizing Adverse Effects
In patients undergoing therapy with carmustine, monitor hematologic indices regularly, especially because myelotoxicity is delayed. Also, monitor renal, hepatic, and pulmonary function tests to forestall any impending problems that might compromise the patient. If long-term therapy is planned, the prescriber should discuss the possible use of a central venous access device (e.g., an implanted port through which to deliver the drug). During drug administration, the patient

may experience intense discomfort. Exercise care to use a large vein for infusion if a central venous access device is not used. To minimize the pain, slow the infusion, and prolong the duration of administration. To minimize inflammation, flush the vein postinfusion with 125 mL of normal saline. Treat nausea and vomiting, which may occur within 2 hours of the treatment, with an adequate antiemetic regimen. Assess the patient for concurrent medication use because drug interactions can occur with phenytoin (Dilantin) or cimetidine. If the patient cannot be switched from these drug therapies, additional monitoring may be warranted.

Providing Patient and Family Education

Once the patient can be treated safely in an outpatient setting, develop an education plan that includes both the patient and significant caregivers.

- Teach patients about general adverse effects and adverse signs and symptoms specific to carmustine therapy, including infection and bleeding (which might have delayed onset) and pulmonary fibrosis if the patient will receive high-dose or long-term therapy.
- Inform patients about IV drug delivery and describe reportable signs and symptoms that might signal possible phlebitis or extravasation.
- Discuss the potential for nausea and vomiting and provide the appropriate antiemetic regimen.
- Identify reportable problems, such as inability to eat or drink for more than 24 hours or respiratory problems.
- Explain the need for regular blood counts and pulmonary testing. Advise patients to report any shortness of breath, dry cough, or temperature greater than 100.5°F, which may indicate the development of pulmonary toxicity.
- Advise patients to avoid taking aspirin or drugs that contain aspirin unless ordered by the prescriber and to report signs of bleeding, such as black stools, bloody gums, bruises, and red rash.
- Discuss patients' concerns and the impact of the adverse effects regarding reproductive and sexual functions and quality of life.
- Teach patients which problems are most important to report to the health care team. Make sure patients have phone numbers or beeper numbers to use when appropriate.

Ongoing Assessment and Evaluation

In patients undergoing therapy with carmustine, closely monitor complete blood counts every week for 6 weeks to ensure that they are adequate before retreatment. Monitor pulmonary function tests before and during the course of therapy so that patients at risk for pulmonary toxicity can be managed appropriately.

Drugs Closely Related to Carmustine

Streptozocin (Zanosar), another nitrosourea, is a product of the organism *Streptomyces achromogenes*. It is well known

---

MEMORY CHIP

P Carmustine

- Indicated for treating brain tumors, multiple myelomas, Hodgkin's and non-Hodgkin's lymphomas, and malignant melanoma
- Major contraindications: poor pulmonary function, which places the patient at risk of developing pulmonary toxicity, and known hypersensitivity to the drug
- Most common adverse effects: acute nausea and emesis
- Dose-limiting effect: delayed myelosuppression
- Most serious adverse effects: pain and burning at the site during drug infusion
- Maximizing therapeutic effects: After reconstitution, solution is stable in a glass container for 24 hours at 4°C or for 8 hours at 25°C when protected from light.
- Minimizing adverse effects: To decrease pain and burning during drug administration, infuse the IV slowly over 1 to 2 hours, increase the primary IV volume, and then infuse 125 mL of normal saline.
- Most important patient education: Instruct patient to comply with the prescribed hematologic monitoring.

---

for its efficacy in treating malignant islet cell tumors of the pancreas. Streptozocin is given intravenously. Patients may complain of pain and burning during the infusion. This discomfort can be minimized by slowing the infusion, increasing the volume used for dilution, and increasing the total volume of the primary IV infusion.

The most frequently reported adverse effect of streptozocin is severe nausea and vomiting. Another GI reaction is hepatotoxicity, manifested by an increase in liver enzyme and bilirubin levels, hypoalbuminemia, and jaundice. Streptozocin is infamous for its renal toxicity, which is dose limiting and may be fatal. The mechanism of nephrotoxicity is unclear. Early manifestations include hypophosphatemia, glycosuria, proteinuria, azotemia, and renal tubular acidosis. Patients with pre-existing renal disease are at risk. Closely monitor renal, hematopoietic, and hepatic functions at baseline and periodically during therapy so that the patient's organ systems are not severely compromised. Additionally, streptozocin has shown diabetogenic activity evidenced by altered glucose metabolism, a decrease in insulin levels, and elevated fasting blood glucose levels. This activity is thought to result from an increased uptake of the drug into the islets, which may occur in some patients.

Lomustine, another nitrosourea, is most commonly used in brain tumors and Hodgkin's lymphoma. In addition to the mechanisms of action of other nitrosureas, lomustine creates a by-product that prevents normal DNA function. It is an oral chemotherapy agent and should be administered on an empty stomach. The capsules come in different dosages and colors, and patients should be carefully instructed on proper administration to ensure safety. Lomustine is toxic to the liver. In addition, like the other nitrosoureas, it is highly emetogenic. Acute nausea usually occurs 3 to 6 hours after an oral dose and usually lasts about 24 hours.

C ANTITUMOR ANTIBIOTICS

Most **antitumor antibiotics** are isolated from fermented broths of various *Streptomyces* bacteria. Antitumor antibiotics interfere with DNA-directed RNA synthesis by inserting between the base pairs of DNA, binding to DNA, and changing the normal structure of the DNA and RNA chains. This action prevents the normal duplication and separation of these chains and inhibits further synthesis. The antitumor antibiotics are dactinomycin, bleomycin, doxorubicin, daunorubicin, mitomycin, idarubicin, pentostatin, epirubicin, plicamycin, and mitoxantrone. Liposomal versions of doxorubicin and daunorubicin are available (see Table 57.1). Several of these antibiotics, because they also induce double-stranded DNA breaks, are considered topoisomerase II inhibitors. These drugs include doxorubicin, daunorubicin, and idarubicin, which are anthracycline based (i.e., red pigmented), as well as mitoxantrone, a synthetic anthracenedione that is structurally similar to the anthracyclines. (Anthracyclines are a group of antitumor antibiotics that work similarly.) Their major dose-limiting toxicity is cardiotoxicity. Doxorubicin (Adriamycin) is currently the most useful and popular antitumor antibiotic. Therefore, it is described here as the prototype drug for this class. Drugs closely related to the prototype are doxorubicin HCl liposome and mitoxantrone. A drug significantly different from the prototype is bleomycin.

Nursing Management of the Patient Receiving P Doxorubicin HCl

Core Drug Knowledge

Pharmacotherapeutics

Doxorubicin was isolated from the soil fungus *Streptomyces peucetius var caesius*. Although doxorubicin is the most recently discovered anthracycline, it has gained the distinction of being the most commonly prescribed. It has wide clinical activity, particularly against hematologic cancers, such as the leukemias, Hodgkin's and non-Hodgkin's lymphoma, multiple myeloma, and solid tumors, such as carcinoma of the breast, ovary, prostate, stomach, thyroid, liver, and small-cell lung and head and neck cancers.

Doxorubicin may be used as a single drug or in combination with other drugs, such as vinblastine, cyclophosphamide, and paclitaxel. It is administered intravenously. Dose adjustments are necessary for patients who have poor bone marrow reserve because of age, prior therapy, or neoplastic marrow infiltration. Dose reductions are also recommended for patients with impaired liver function, as evidenced by elevated serum bilirubin levels and transaminases.

Pharmacokinetics

Doxorubicin is rapidly distributed in body tissues. It is metabolized in the liver and is primarily excreted in the bile. A small percentage is excreted in the renal system and may produce reddish discoloration of the urine. The pharmacokinetic profile of doxorubicin appears in Table 57.1. Recent advances in pharmaceutical technology led to the approval

by the FDA of two anthracycline antibiotics, daunorubicin and doxorubicin, in **liposomes.** Liposomes are microscopic spherical vesicles that encapsulate the drug molecules. This novel drug formulation enhances the therapeutic efficacy of the drug by increasing the concentration, delaying clearance, retarding metabolism, decreasing the volume of distribution of the drug, and shifting its distribution to the diseased tissues with increased capillary permeability.

Pharmacodynamics

Doxorubicin acts mainly by intercalation between specific base pairs within the cancer cell's DNA. This action results in blocking the synthesis of new RNA or DNA or preventing DNA strand scission. Normal proliferating cells are also affected by doxorubicin, which accounts for such adverse effects as myelosuppression, alopecia, and mucositis.

Contraindications and Precautions

Doxorubicin is contraindicated in severe CHF or any existing cardiomyopathy or marked myelosuppression from irradiation or chemotherapy. Precautions should be observed in patients with hepatic insufficiency because concentrations of active metabolites may be increased. A Black Box warning indicates that dosage should be reduced in patients with impaired hepatic function. Secondary acute myelogenous leukemia (AML) has been reported in patients treated with anthracyclines, including doxorubicin. The occurrence of refractory secondary leukemia is more common when such drugs are given in combination with DNA-damaging antineoplastic agents, when patients have been heavily pretreated with cytotoxic drugs, or when doses of anthracyclines have been escalated. A Black Box warning relates to this risk.

Doxorubicin is a pregnancy category D drug.

Adverse Effects

The adverse effects of doxorubicin may be grouped into acute, chronic, and local reactions. Acute toxicities include nausea, vomiting, suppression of bone marrow function, and mucositis. Alopecia is reversible; other cutaneous reactions are hyperpigmentation of the nail beds and dermal creases.

Cardiotoxicity is chronic and is the major toxicity that limits the use of doxorubicin; a Black Box warning relates to this severe adverse effect. This toxicity is cumulative and may manifest weeks or months after the initial treatment. Doxorubicin shows an affinity for myocytes, which are the cells of the heart muscle. The damaged myocytes are not easily replaced because they have a slow mitotic rate. The decreased number of myocytes and the ensuing interstitial edema weaken the pumping capacity of the heart muscle. Cardiac damage may range from insignificant electrocardiographic changes to more serious and potentially fatal complications, such as CHF.

Local adverse effects of doxorubicin include cutaneous effects, which can have devastating consequences for the patient. These include extravasation injury and radiation recall reaction. Anthracyclines such as doxorubicin are the most toxic vesicants. Extravasation is especially problematic with these drugs because anthracyclines bind to nucleic acids, causing destructive and prolonged tissue injuries. They form free radicals that are toxic to the tissues and especially impede wound healing. The DNA–doxorubicin complex is retained and recirculates in the tissues, setting up a pattern for continuous tissue damage (refer to Chapter 36 for extravasation management). Doxorubicin carries a Black Box warning relating to the risk of severe local tissue necrosis if extravasation occurs during administration.

Radiation recall is exhibited with doxorubicin as erythematous changes, which appear at a previously irradiated site. The phenomenon can occur weeks or months—even years—after radiation, but happens more frequently with short intervals between sessions and high-dose chemotherapy. These reactions are manifested by erythema (redness), blisters, hyperpigmentation, edema (swelling), vesicle formation, exfoliation (skin loss), and sometimes ulcer formation, which all may occur in the skin, lung, heart, and GI tract.

Drug Interactions

Drug interactions with doxorubicin are summarized in Table 57.4. Doxorubicin should not be mixed with the following drugs in solution because of incompatibility: aminophylline, cephalothin sodium, dexamethasone sodium phosphate, diazepam, hydrocortisone, furosemide, heparin, and fluorouracil.

Assessment of Relevant Core Patient Variables

Health Status

The risk for cardiotoxicity in patients receiving doxorubicin can be potentiated by concurrent therapy with cyclophosphamide and mediastinal irradiation. Ensure that initial cardiac evaluations, which might include an electrocardiogram (ECG) and a multigated radionuclide angiogram (MUGA), are made to establish a safe baseline for treatment. Before initiating treatment, obtain a careful history to ascertain that the patient does not have existing cardiomyopathy or hepatic insufficiency that might put him or her at risk during treatment.

Life Span and Gender

Document the age and gender of the patient. The risk of cardiac damage increases with age. Age influences cardiac

tolerance to anthracycline therapy. Children and the elderly are more susceptible than young adults to adverse cardiac effects at low cumulative doses. Children especially suffer more from the synergistic cardiotoxicities of mediastinal irradiation and doxorubicin. However, they have a better chance of recovering from CHF-related problems than adults do. Women, especially those younger than 50 years, are more likely to experience nausea and vomiting.

Assess the woman of childbearing age for pregnancy and explore her reproductive goals. Doxorubicin is a pregnancy category D drug and its potential effect on fertility is not known.

Lifestyle, Diet, and Habits

Assess the client for adequate nutritional intake. Malnutrition, particularly in children, potentiates cardiotoxicity. Also, assess the patient's anxiety about chemotherapy-related nausea and vomiting, which can substantially impair quality of life.

Environment

Be aware of the environment in which the drug will be administered. Doxorubicin is given in either an inpatient or outpatient setting because of the need to monitor adverse effects, especially the potential for extravasation, which requires prompt medical attention and necessitates patient education.

Nursing Diagnoses and Outcomes

- Risk for Infection related to suppressed bone marrow function
  Desired outcome: The patient will be free from infection and will exercise caution to avoid exposure to sources of infection.
- Risk for Injury related to cardiotoxicity, depressed bone marrow function, and associated bleeding
  Desired outcome: The patient will not suffer from any acute or chronic cardiotoxicity and will be able to recognize and promptly report any of its clinical manifestations. In addition, the patient will attain pretreatment hematologic status. The patient will learn to monitor and manage situations that may induce bleeding.
- Imbalanced Nutrition: Less than Body Requirements related to nausea, vomiting, and taste alterations
  Desired outcome: The patient will remain adequately nourished because emesis control will be achieved by pharmacologic and nonpharmacologic means.

TABLE 57.4	Agents That Interact with P Doxorubicin	
Interactants	**Effect and Significance**	**Nursing Management**
digoxin	Decreased serum levels and therapeutic effect of digoxin	Monitor serum digoxin levels.
heparin	Precipitate formation if mixed together	Administer doxorubicin and heparin separately.
barbiturates	Increased plasma clearance of doxorubicin	Notify health care provider for dosage considerations.

- Impaired Skin Integrity related to possible extravasation and radiation recall

  Desired outcome: *The patient will recognize and report signs and symptoms that suggest an extravasation or recall reaction. The patient will receive the doxorubicin dose without vascular or tissue damage.*

Planning and Intervention

Maximizing Therapeutic Effects

Recent advances in drug development have made possible the use of cardioprotectants in conjunction with anthracycline therapy. One such drug is dexrazoxane (Zinecard). Dexrazoxane is a potent intracellular chelating drug that interferes with iron-mediated free radical generation, thought to be responsible for anthracycline-induced cardiotoxicity. It is indicated to reduce the severity and incidence of cardiomyopathy associated with doxorubicin in women with metastatic breast cancer who have received a cumulative dose of 300 mg/m^2 and who, in their prescriber's opinion, would benefit from continuing treatment with doxorubicin. Dexrazoxane and doxorubicin may be used concurrently in children. The recommended dose of dexrazoxane to doxorubicin is at a ratio of 10:1 (e.g., dexrazoxane, 500 mg, to doxorubicin, 50 mg). If prescribed, give this by slow IV push or rapid IV infusion before administering doxorubicin. Do not allow the total elapsed time from the beginning of the dexrazoxane infusion to the initiation of doxorubicin to be more than 30 minutes. The adverse effects of dexrazoxane at the recommended dose are mild; however, dexrazoxane could add to the myelotoxic effects of doxorubicin.

Minimizing Adverse Effects

Before initiating doxorubicin therapy, carefully assess the patient's cardiac and hematopoietic functions, because of the extensive effect of the drug on the systems involved. Implement strategies using dose administration and scheduling to modify the risk for cardiotoxicity. The recommended maximum cumulative lifetime dose of doxorubicin is 550 mg/m^2. However, if the patient has previously had myocardial irradiation or cytotoxic drug therapy, the cumulative lifetime dose should be lowered to 400 mg/m^2. Modifying the dose and dosing schedule of the patient can ameliorate the cardiotoxic adverse effects. Multiple daily doses rather than large single boluses of the drug can also minimize cardiac damage.

Dose reduction to a cumulative dose of 400 mg/m^2 is advocated for patients who have had or who are receiving concurrent radiation therapy or cyclophosphamide. With regard to extravasation, prevention is the key. Prevention requires that medical and nursing personnel be skilled in venous access techniques, perform meticulous monitoring during drug administration, and know actions to undertake promptly in case extravasation occurs. Use large veins, with a new peripheral line for vesicant administration. Extravasation can occur even with a good venous return and without

the usual initial complaint of burning or pain at the injection site (see Chapter 36). Administer vesicants through the side port of a free-flowing IV set, allowing for dilution of drug and frequent blood return checks during administration. If the patient complains of any discomfort or if loss of blood return or swelling is noted, discontinue the vesicant administration immediately.

Providing Patient and Family Education

- Reassure patients that reddish urine after doxorubicin injection is a harmless and expected response to the drug. This reaction may happen within 1 to 2 days postinfusion.
- Explain that a substantial fraction of patients who receive this drug complain of acute nausea and vomiting. Reassure patients that proper antiemetics will be available, and tell them that they should ask for them if needed. Carefully review nonpharmacologic interventions, such as relaxation techniques, with patients and caregivers.
- Review signs and symptoms of extravasation. If a suspected extravasation occurs, provide and review a teaching card with directions for caring for an extravasation site, so that the patient can best participate in care. Reassure patients that adequate monitoring and follow-up, through telephone triage by the health care team, will be undertaken even in the home setting.
- Discuss with patients the signs and symptoms of other adverse effects, particularly cardiotoxicity and depressed bone marrow function, and encourage appropriate precautions. For example, encourage patients to keep appointments for cardiac function tests and caution against taking aspirin or drugs that contain aspirin, which may promote bleeding during suppression of bone marrow function.
- Remind patients who have had radiation therapy that recall reactions, manifested by redness, blistering, and hyperpigmentation, can have a delayed onset and should be reported promptly.

Ongoing Assessment and Evaluation

Advise the patient who continues taking doxorubicin to have periodic examinations of cardiac functions as ordered. Radionuclide ventriculography and echocardiography are useful methods to detect impending myocardial damage. Look for any significant changes in the ECG readings that might indicate potential problems, such as irreversible cardiac damage. Also assess the patient frequently for weight gain, presence of ankle edema, dyspnea, elevated blood pressure, and nonproductive cough, which are typical clinical signs of CHF.

Drugs Closely Related to P Doxorubicin

Doxorubicin HCl liposome (Doxil) is most commonly utilized for AIDS-related Kaposi sarcoma and ovarian cancer. The mechanism of action of doxorubicin HCl liposome

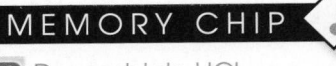

MEMORY CHIP

P Doxorubicin HCl

- Indicated for treating acute leukemias, soft-tissue and bone sarcoma, Hodgkin and non-Hodgkin lymphoma, breast and ovarian cancers, bronchogenic carcinoma
- Major contraindication: severe depression of bone marrow function
- Most common adverse effects: alopecia and nausea with vomiting
- Most serious adverse effects: cardiac damage, bone marrow depression, and extravasation
- Maximizing therapeutic effects: Administer dexrazoxane cardioprotectant therapy, if indicated.
- Minimizing adverse effects: Maintain maximum lifetime dose of 550 mg/m², if patient is receiving radiation or concurrent myelotoxic therapy, dose is 400 mg/m².
- Most important patient education: Warn patient of the appearance of red urine discoloration (harmless) after administration and of alopecia, which is reversible.

is described under Pharmacokinetics. Unlike the prototype, doxorubicin HCl liposome is not considered to be a vesicant because of the liposomal property of the drug. Instead, acute infusional hypersensitivity reactions have been reported in 10% of patients, necessitating slow administration over at least 30 minutes. Additionally, doxorubicin HCl liposome must be administered in D_5W instead of normal saline, and an in-line filter should not be used. A unique adverse effect of the drug that must be carefully assessed and managed is hand-and-foot syndrome. This condition is associated with erythema, edema, pain, and even desquamation. This condition can be dose limiting; however, once the drug is stopped, the condition resolves quickly.

Mitoxantrone, another antitumor antibiotic, is indicated for prostate cancer and AML. It works by causing cross-links and strand breaks in DNA, thus interfering with RNA and inhibiting topoisomerase II. Like doxorubicin, mitoxantrone is associated with cardiac toxicity and myelosuppression. Unlike doxorubicin, mitoxantrone is dark blue, and patients must be instructed that their urine and the sclera of the eyes can be colored blue-green for up to 72 hours after administration.

Drugs Significantly Different From
P Doxorubicin

Bleomycin (Blenoxane) is an antitumor antibiotic. Unlike doxorubicin, it is neither an anthracycline nor a cell cycle–nonspecific drug. Bleomycin is used to treat lymphomas, squamous cell carcinoma, and testicular cancers. It is given by IV, subcutaneous, or intramuscular routes. The recommended dosage is expressed in either units or milligrams (1 unit = 1 mg). Bleomycin is known for its pulmonary toxicity. For this reason, use of this drug has become limited. The early clinical features of bleomycin toxicity are dyspnea and rales, which can progress to pneumonitis and pulmonary fibrosis and may be fatal.

The treatment of bleomycin-induced toxicity consists of discontinuing the drug and administering corticosteroids. The practitioner should review pulmonary function tests and chest radiographs at baseline and periodically thereafter to monitor for adequate pulmonary reserve. Patients should be advised to notify health care providers—especially anesthesiologists—that they have received bleomycin therapy, because pulmonary toxicity is enhanced by a high intraoperative fraction of inspired oxygen.

Other adverse effects are cutaneous toxicity, which is often seen as urticaria or erythematous swelling and phlebitis at the injection site caused by the irritant properties of bleomycin. Following drug administration, patients may complain of fever and chills. Acetaminophen administered in appropriate doses around-the-clock can help alleviate the fever and chills in the first 24 hours after drug administration. Patients may also have nausea and vomiting, general weakness, and, sometimes, hypotension. These symptoms are considered to be an idiosyncratic reaction, similar to anaphylaxis, and are noted rarely and mostly in lymphoma patients. A test dose of 2 U of bleomycin may be administered before the first two treatments. Test doses are not always predictive of hypersensitivity and precautions should still be followed in the absence of a positive test dose reaction. Premedication with acetaminophen and diphenhydramine may be helpful.

C HORMONES AND HORMONE ANTAGONISTS

The **hormones** and **hormone antagonists** (antihormones) are a diverse group of drugs that are beneficial in treating neoplasms. Their use predates the first chemotherapeutic agent (nitrogen mustard) as the oldest form of cancer treatment. Hormones are hormonal or hormone-like drugs that inhibit tumor proliferation by blocking or antagonizing the naturally occurring substances that stimulate tumor growth.

Some hormones alter the cellular environment and affect the permeability of the cell membrane in ways that affect cell growth. This group (see Table 57.1) consists of adrenocorticosteroids, androgens, estrogens, progestins, antiestrogens, antiandrogens, gonadotropin inhibitors, and aromatase inhibitors. Hormonal therapy is recognized mostly for its efficacy in treating neoplasms that originate from tissues in which growth is hormonally mediated, notably prostate and breast cancers. The clinical responsiveness of breast tumors to hormonal manipulations was demonstrated more than 100 years ago. Over time, hormonal treatment of breast cancer has been accomplished by ablative surgery (oophorectomy, adrenalectomy, and hypophysectomy) or pharmacologically by using hormonal and antihormonal therapy.

C ANTIESTROGENS

Antiestrogens are first-line therapy for treating breast cancer in postmenopausal women. They act as agonists by binding to the estrogen receptors in the target cells, making the estrogen unavailable to the tumor. Tamoxifen is the most widely recognized antiestrogen. However, it is not a pure antiestrogen. Tamoxifen is a selective estrogen receptor modulator (SERM), one of a group of pharmacologic agents, often called "designer drugs," that produces estrogenic effects, alone or combined with antiestrogenic agents, at various sites in a woman's body. These sites include the breast, endometrium, cardiovascular system, brain, and bone. Two other SERM agents include Evista (Raloxifene) and Feresten (toremifene).

Tamoxifen possesses agonistic properties that stimulate endometrial proliferation, and it is known to induce estrogenic effects that are linked with thromboembolic events. These adverse effects have led to the search for pure antiestrogens, called selective estrogen receptor downregulators (SERDs). Fulvestrant (Faslodex), an SERD, is indicated as second-line therapy in postmenopausal women with metastatic breast disease. Because of its effectiveness and first-line use in treating advanced breast cancer, tamoxifen is the prototype antiestrogen drug.

Nursing Management of the Patient Receiving [P] Tamoxifen

Core Drug Knowledge

Pharmacotherapeutics

Tamoxifen (Nolvadex) is indicated as a first-line drug for treating advanced breast cancer in premenopausal and postmenopausal women. It is used in adjuvant therapy for the treatment of axillary node-negative breast cancer in women after mastectomy or segmental mastectomy, axillary dissection, and breast irradiation. In premenopausal women with metastatic breast cancer, tamoxifen is an alternative to oophorectomy and irradiation. It is the only drug approved to prevent breast cancer in high-risk women and to reduce the risk of contralateral breast cancer.

Pharmacokinetics

Tamoxifen is well absorbed, highly protein bound, and extensively metabolized in the liver after oral administration. It undergoes enterohepatic circulation, prolonging blood levels. It is taken up by tissues such as the lung, uterus, breast, brain, pancreas, and liver. It has a half-life of 7 to 14 days. Most tamoxifen is excreted in the bile and feces.

Pharmacodynamics

Tamoxifen, a potent nonsteroidal antiestrogenic drug, competes with estrogen for binding sites in tissues high in estrogen receptors, such as breast tissue. This mechanism deprives estrogen-sensitive tumors of estrogen. It may also stimulate the production of transforming growth factor-beta, which inhibits the growth of most breast cancer and other epithelioid cells.

Other favorable consequences of tamoxifen treatment have been reported; namely, increased bone mineral density in postmenopausal women and reduced cholesterol levels, which may account for a lower incidence of fatal myocardial infarction in women receiving adjuvant tamoxifen.

Contraindications and Precautions

Tamoxifen is contraindicated in patients with known hypersensitivity. Precautions should be observed when administering the drug to patients with myelosuppression and during pregnancy and lactation. Tamoxifen is a pregnancy category D drug. An increased incidence of endometrial changes, including hyperplasia, polyps, and endometrial cancer, has been reported with long-term tamoxifen therapy.

Adverse Effects

Short-term tamoxifen therapy is rarely associated with toxicity. Most patients taking this drug experience no toxicity whatsoever. These adverse effects, although they occur infrequently, are most common: hot flashes, particularly in premenopausal women, and mild nausea, which is transient and unaccompanied by vomiting. The severity of hot flashes diminishes with continued use of the drug. Other, less common adverse effects are headache, light-headedness, weight gain, vaginal bleeding and discharge, menstrual irregularities, fluid retention, visual side effects, and skin rash, all of which are reported in fewer than 1% to 2% of patients. Increased bone and tumor pain and a local **disease flare** (worsening of the disease) have been observed; they indicate that the tumor is responding to treatment. Hypercalcemia may occur but is infrequent. Data from long-term studies have clearly established the serious long-term effects of tamoxifen use, which include endometrial cancer, thromboembolic events (strokes and pulmonary embolism), and cataract formation requiring cataract surgery. Patients receiving long-term therapy should be monitored regularly. Adverse hematopoietic reactions are transient and uncommon, usually exhibited by thrombocytopenia.

Women at high risk for cancer or women with ductal carcinoma in situ who are receiving tamoxifen to prevent their risk of developing breast cancer are also at increased risk of cancer and thromboembolic events. Tamoxifen carries a Black Box warning that these women need special counseling to help them weigh the risks versus benefits of therapy.

Drug Interactions

Drug–laboratory test interactions have been reported with tamoxifen therapy, including elevated serum calcium and thyroxin levels. Other interactions are discussed in Table 57.5.

Assessment of Relevant Core Patient Variables

Health Status

Even though the adverse effects of tamoxifen are fairly mild, evaluate baseline hematopoietic test results, particularly platelet counts, to make sure that bone marrow function is adequate. Assess the tumor receptor status of the patient because the measurement of estrogen receptors provides important information for planning treatment. Also, screen the patient for a history of thrombophlebitis or endometrial cancer, which may modify the treatment plan. A baseline vision test may also be necessary.

TABLE 57.5	Agents That Interact with ℗ Tamoxifen	
Interactants	**Effect and Significance**	**Nursing Management**
oral anticoagulants	Increased risk of bleeding	Monitor prothrombin time. Notify health care provider for dose modifications. Monitor for signs of bleeding.
bromocriptine	Increased serum levels	Monitor tamoxifen serum levels.

Life Span and Gender

One of the most important issues confronting women receiving hormonal therapy is its effect on their sexual and reproductive health. Explore these concerns and discuss the various changes associated with tamoxifen therapy. Tamoxifen is the preferred adjuvant treatment for postmenopausal women who have breast cancer with nodal involvement and estrogen receptor–positive tumors. Assess the patient for pregnancy and explore the contraceptive practices of the patient because the drug can cause fetal harm.

Lifestyle, Diet, and Habits

Women taking tamoxifen experience no limitations in their functional capacities. Lifestyle is not normally affected, except possibly by physical changes, such as hot flashes, menstrual irregularities, weight gain, and vaginal bleeding. Explore with patients how these changes could affect their lifestyle. Although visual side effects are rare, caution patients about driving and performing tasks requiring visual acuity.

Environment

Be aware of the environment in which the drug will be administered. Tamoxifen is a fairly mild oral drug that does not usually require close monitoring. Patients take this drug at home and are instructed to have periodic checkups with their health care provider. Hematologic screenings can be done at an accredited laboratory that sends the findings to the prescriber for comparison with baseline values.

Nursing Diagnoses and Outcomes

- Pain related to discomfort produced by a flare reaction to drug therapy
  Desired outcome: *The patient will learn to recognize the signs and symptoms of a flare reaction and appreciate it as a positive response to tamoxifen therapy.*
- Reproductive and Sexual Dysfunction resulting from drug therapy
  Desired outcome: *The patient will be aware of the physical changes to reproductive and sexual functions. The patient will be accepting of these changes and will explore ways to enhance sexual and reproductive health.*
- Risk for Infection and Bleeding related to suppression of bone marrow function
  Desired outcome: *The patient will learn to recognize and report symptoms related to infection and bleeding and will implement measures to prevent unnecessary risks or injury that will compromise the hematopoietic and immune systems.*
- Risk for Impaired Skin Integrity related to skin rash and pedal edema
  Desired outcome: *The patient will report the appearance of skin rash and monitor peripheral edema from fluid retention. The patient will take steps to reduce edema from fluid retention, such as eating a low-salt diet.*
- Disturbed Sensory Perception (Vision and Balance) related to adverse effects of drug therapy
  Desired outcome: *The patient will recognize and report changes in visual acuity and other related symptoms, such as headache, dizziness, and light-headedness, to the caregiver. The patient will take the necessary precautions to avoid injury resulting from altered visual acuity.*
- Risk for Injury related to drug-induced hypercalcemia
  Desired outcome: *The patient will be knowledgeable about clinical manifestations of hypercalcemia, such as nausea, vomiting, constipation, decreased urine volume, malaise, and loss of muscle tone. The patient will also know to report these signs and symptoms immediately to the prescriber, who might consider the need for hospitalization. The patient's calcium level will normalize.*

Planning and Intervention
Maximizing Therapeutic Effects

Tamoxifen is very effective in treating metastatic breast tumors identified as estrogen receptor positive. This criterion is an important determinant in the patient's response to tamoxifen therapy. Ensure that the necessary testing is done to determine the patient's estrogen receptor status.

Minimizing Adverse Effects

Tamoxifen's adverse effects are generally mild and rare. To determine whether such effects occur, ensure monthly monitoring of blood counts, annual Papanicolaou smears, and regular visual function tests. The changes noted most often are those related to the menopausal symptoms and can be very bothersome, especially to premenopausal women. Teach these patients to implement comfort measures such as wearing absorbent cotton clothing, lowering the thermostat at home, avoiding caffeine and spicy foods, and exercising regularly. Discuss the patient's concerns and the effect of the adverse events on reproductive and sexual functions and quality of life. The occurrence of a disease flare is actually a positive sign of tumor response to the therapy. Advise the patient that she might experience initial bone and tumor pain and an increase in tumor size. If these symptoms are bothersome, assist the patient in obtaining a prescription for pain medication.

Providing Patient and Family Education

- Instruct patients to report signs and symptoms of a disease flare to the prescriber. If signs and symptoms are distressing, obtain the necessary supportive medications for her.
- Teach patients to recognize and report changes in visual acuity and other related symptoms, such as headache, dizziness, and light-headedness. If periodic vision checkups are ordered, emphasize their importance.
- Remind patients to report immediately any clinical manifestations of hypercalcemia, such as nausea, vomiting, constipation, decreased urine output, malaise, and loss of muscle tone. Hypercalcemia may require hospitalization.
- Teach patients to recognize and report the appearance of skin rash and peripheral edema.
- Educate patients regarding likely changes in reproductive or sexual function, such as irregular or missed menstrual periods or unscheduled vaginal bleeding.
- Reassure patients that all of the above symptoms are mild and rarely occurring adverse effects of tamoxifen therapy. These symptoms do not usually require discontinuing the drug.
- Counsel patients about contraception and warn that the drug can cause fetal harm.
- Advise patients taking long-term tamoxifen therapy to have annual pelvic examinations and Papanicolaou screening and to note and report any unusual vaginal bleeding.

Ongoing Assessment and Evaluation

Throughout tamoxifen treatment, monitor the patient's blood count regularly. Although hypercalcemia is uncommon, evaluate serum calcium levels during therapy to make sure that appropriate measures are initiated to correct this condition should it occur. Also assess the patient's vision, because of the possibility for corneal changes and decreased visual acuity.

Drugs Significantly Different From
P Tamoxifen

Adrenocorticosteroids

In addition to their cytotoxic effects, adrenocorticosteroids are used for their palliative benefits. For example, adrenocorticosteroids such as betamethasone, dexamethasone, and prednisone have anti-inflammatory properties and are useful in reducing the edema and associated symptoms in brain tumors. Adrenocortical steroids are effective in leukemias and lymphomas because of their suppressant effect on lymphocytes. Many of their adverse effects, such as increased appetite and a feeling of well-being, are an extension of their

MEMORY CHIP

P Tamoxifen

- Indicated for advanced breast cancer in postmenopausal women and cancers of tissues having specific hormone receptors, such as the prostate gland
- Major contraindications: allergy to the drug, pregnancy, and lactation
- Most common adverse effect: occurrence of hot flashes, especially among premenopausal women
- Most serious adverse effects: risk of endometrial cancer and thromboembolic events associated with long-term therapy
- Maximizing therapeutic effects: Instruct the patient to take his/her pills bid, in the morning and evening. Drug should not be discontinued without consulting the physician or nurse.
- Minimizing adverse effects: Teach the patient to regulate the home environment to a cooler temperature; to wear loose, cotton, layered clothing (for hot flashes); to eat small, frequent meals and to stay away from spicy foods (for nausea and vomiting); and to notify the physician immediately if symptoms of muscle weakness, pain and swelling of legs and ankles, mental confusion, and constipation are noted.
- Most important patient education: Counsel women about the possible risks of endometrial cancer and to have regular gynecologic checkups.

normal physiologic activity and are considered beneficial and palliative. Some of their adverse effects are glucose intolerance, peptic ulceration, manic psychosis, and suppression of cellular immunity, which predisposes patients to infection.

Androgens, Estrogens, and Progestins

Androgens, estrogens, and progestins are used to treat cancers of tissues that have specific hormone receptors—for example, mammary tissue and the prostate gland. Because these drugs have a greater degree of specificity for these tissues, their effects inhibit proliferation of the tumor.

Androgens control the growth and development of the male sex organs and maintain secondary sex characteristics. This group affects the release of various endogenous hormones, namely testosterone, follicle-stimulating hormone (FSH), and luteinizing hormone (LH). The two androgenic agents fluoxymesterone and testolactone are used palliatively for androgen-responsive recurrent breast cancer in postmenopausal women. These drugs are well tolerated, although they may exhibit adverse effects similar to those produced by the estrogens, including fluid retention, hypercalcemia, and liver impairment. Their most profound side effect is virilization in women, manifested by hirsutism, alopecia, acne, clitoral hypertrophy, and increased libido. Further discussion of testosterone is in Chapter 54, and luteinizing hormone is discussed again in Chapter 55.

Estrogens are necessary to develop and maintain secondary sexual characteristics, control the female menstrual cycle, and affect the maturation of long bones. They diffuse through the membrane of estrogen-responsive cells and bind to and activate receptors in the cell nucleus. They are believed to change the hormonal milieu of the cells, making them less conducive to growth. Estrogen-responsive cells (those that are sensitive to estrogen) are located in the reproductive system, breasts, pituitary, hypothalamus, liver, and bone. However, not all of the tumors that arise in these organs are estrogen sensitive. In many patients, after the initial hormonal manipulation, even as the estrogen-responsive cells are being destroyed, the cells that are not responsive to estrogen continue to proliferate. Therefore, the response is neither complete nor permanent. Estradiol is an estrogen given orally to treat advanced prostate cancer, adenocarcinoma, and metastatic breast cancer. Estradiol is also available as a vaginal cream that is well absorbed through the skin and mucous membranes. Additionally it is supplied as a transdermal patch. The adverse effects include gynecomastia, voice changes, hirsutism, change in libido, fluid retention, nausea, vomiting, and thrombophlebitis. Further discussion of estrogens is in Chapter 56.

Progestins are natural or synthetic substances that affect the actions of progesterone, a steroid that counteracts the actions of estrogens. Megestrol acetate (Megace) is a progestin indicated for treating carcinoma of the breast, endometrium, and kidney. It is also used for the treatment of anorexia and cachexia associated with cancer. Medroxyprogesterone is the other agent used in patients with advanced endometrial cancer. These agents are contraindicated during pregnancy because they have been found to cause fetal genital abnormalities. Progestins are also discussed in Chapter 56.

Antiandrogens

Antiandrogens compete with testosterone for androgen-receptor binding sites on target cells. The most frequently used antiandrogenic agents are bicalutamide (Casodex), flutamide (Eulexin), and nilutamide (Nilandron). These agents are used for advanced stages of prostate cancer. Adverse effects are gynecomastia, diarrhea, hot flashes, breast pain, impotence, loss of libido, and abnormal liver function test results. The patient's liver function should be monitored if the patient is on prolonged therapy.

Gonadotropin-Releasing Hormone Analogues

The gonadotropin-releasing hormone (GnRH) analogues are goserelin acetate (Zoladex) and leuprolide (Lupron). LH and FSH are gonadotropins that stimulate hormone secretion by the gonads. They play an important role in the maturation of the germ cell. GnRH regulates the release of these hormones from the pituitary gland. Goserelin inhibits the secretion of gonadotropin. When patients are on prolonged therapy with this drug, their serum testosterone level is decreased to a level equivalent to that associated with surgical castration. This drug is an alternative treatment for males with advanced prostate cancer who do not wish to undergo orchiectomy or estrogen therapy. It is also used in advanced breast cancer. Goserelin is well tolerated. In men, adverse effects are hot flashes, sexual dysfunction, and fewer erections. In women,

adverse effects are decreased bone mineral density, vaginal bleeding, and breast tenderness. Goserelin is available as a preloaded, disposable syringe with a 14-gauge needle that is injected subcutaneously into the upper abdominal wall. The other drug, leuprolide, has similar indications and also causes chemical orchiectomy in men who have metastatic prostate cancer. Leuprolide has fewer adverse effects than goserelin. It is available in three formulations: a subcutaneous injection, a depot suspension, and a suspension given intramuscularly. With both these medications, it is important to teach the patient the correct administration technique appropriate to the drug formulation and emphasize the importance of adhering to the dosage schedule. Two other drugs in this category indicated for the palliative treatment of advanced prostate cancer include; triptorelin (Trelstar), and histrelin (Vantas). Triptoerlin is available in a once monthly injection or a long acting injection given once every 84 days. Histrelin is inserted into the patient as a SQ implant that gives off continuous drug for 12 months. A drug similar but considered an antagonist is Degarelix (Firmagon). This drug is a new LHRH antagonist that was approved for use in 2008 to treat advanced prostate cancer. It is given monthly as an injection under the skin.

Aromatase Inhibitors

As tamoxifen became the mainstay for antiestrogen therapy in breast cancer, the role of aromatase was increasingly explored. Many breast cancers have estrogen receptors; the growth of these tumors is stimulated by estrogen. In postmenopausal women, the main source of estrogen is the conversion of precursors to estrogen (primarily estradiol); this conversion occurs through an enzyme called aromatase. Drugs in this class inhibit aromatase, thus decreasing the eventual levels of available estrogen. Anastrozole is a nonsteroidal aromatase inhibitor that is also considered an antiestrogen, similar to tamoxifen. It is indicated for the treatment of postmenopausal women who have locally advanced or advanced breast cancer that has and for those who have progressed after tamoxifen therapy. It is also approved for early breast cancer as adjuvant treatment. It is given orally and is well tolerated. It is important to discuss the patient's reproductive goals and warn patients that this drug can cause fetal harm. Anastrozole can interact with some herbal preparations. Two other aromatase inhibitors are Aromasin (exemestane) and Femara (Letrozole). The most common side effect of drugs in this category is joint pain. Aromatase inhibitors are often used first line or after treatment with tamoxifen to extend disease free survival. Aromasin is unique in that it inactivates aromatase.

MAXIMIZING CELL KILL: COMBINATION THERAPY

With rare exceptions, monotherapy in cancer is not curative because of drug resistance. Most cancers contain cells that are resistant to any single agent. In tumors that initially

BOX 57.6 FOCUS ON RESEARCH

Combination Therapy for Stage III Colon Cancer

Schmoll, H., Cartwright, T., et al. (2007). Phase III trial of capecitabine plus oxaliplatin as adjuvant therapy for stage III colon cancer: A planned safety analysis in 1,864 patients. *Journal of Clinical Oncology*, 25(1):102–109.

The Study

Researchers designed a study to compare the two adjuvant treatment options for stage III colon cancer in terms of toxicity and safety. Patients with the disease were randomly assigned to receive one of two regimens: either oral capecitabine plus intravenous oxaliplatin (XELOX) or a standard intravenous bolus of fluorouracil/leucovorin (FU/LV, as administered at the Mayo Clinic) on a 3-week cycle for eight cycles. The patient population consisted of 1,864 patients; of these, 938 received XELOX and 926 received FU/LV. Most treatment-related adverse events occurred at similar rates in both treatment arms. However, patients receiving XELOX experienced less diarrhea and alopecia, and more neurotoxicity, vomiting, and palmar planter syndrome than those patients receiving FU/LV. Compared with the FU/LV regimen, XELOX showed fewer grade 3/4 hematologic toxicities and more grade 3/4 gastrointestinal toxicities. Treatment-related mortality within 28 days from the last study dose was 0.6% in the XELOX group and 0.6% in the FU/LV group. In conclusion, this study proved that XELOX has a manageable tolerability profile in the adjuvant setting. Efficacy data will continue to be studied.

Nursing Implications

Nurses are challenged with understanding the toxicities of various regimens as well as the rationale for using one regimen over another. As more and more combination chemotherapy regimens are designed for various cancers, safety and toxicity data are extremely important when determining the most efficacious and tolerable regimen for the patient. Quality of life is an important consideration in the treatment of cancer. This study illustrates the importance of large randomized trials to answer questions of patient tolerability. Long-term survival data will also be an important next step in deciding the most appropriate regimen for this patient population. Nurses have a responsibility to assess carefully and to report any and all toxicities that patients experience so that these regimens can be fully understood and toxicities managed properly.

---

respond to an agent, further drug resistance may develop during treatment as a result of proliferation of pre-existing drug-resistant cells or because of increased mutations that lead to drug resistance. If a combination of drugs is used, cells that are resistant to one chemotherapy agent may be killed by another agent in the combination. Furthermore, many antineoplastic drugs are dose limited because of their cytotoxicity. The limits imposed by toxicities to the different organ systems are another rationale for using combination drugs to achieve better therapeutic outcomes.

Combination chemotherapy, first developed in the 1960s and 1970s, is one of the major advances in cancer therapy. It continues to guide the development of new treatment protocols for various malignancies. Combination therapy involves using two or more drugs proven effective against a tumor type (Box 57.6). It is considered superior to single-drug therapy because of higher tumor response rates and increased duration of remissions. The effectiveness of a particular antineoplastic drug is measured by objective criteria and tumor response (Box 57.7).

Many combination regimens in current use have proved to increase the response rate two to four times (Table 57.6). Two or more drugs can be administered simultaneously or in a preplanned sequence. In combination therapy, the response rates and survival are more dramatic because they accomplish the following objectives:

- Maximum cell kill within the range of toxicity tolerated by the patient
- A broader range of coverage against resistant cell lines in the heterogenous tumor population
- Minimal or slow development of new resistant cell groups

In designing successful drug combinations, the choice of drugs follows these principles:

- Selected drugs should be proven partially effective against the tumor when used alone.

- Ideally, the drugs used in combination are best if they do not have overlapping toxicities.
- The dosages and schedules for the various drugs should be maximized.
- Drugs should be administered at consistent intervals.
- Drugs should be selected to produce synergy.

Box 57.7 RATING TUMOR RESPONSE

How well a tumor responds to chemotherapy can be rated by the categories below.

Complete Response

All evidence of tumor (physical examination and radiologic studies) has disappeared and no new lesions have developed. Response must last for at least 4 weeks. The patient must have no cancer-related symptoms and all abnormal biochemical parameters must have returned to normal.

Partial Response

The sum of the product of the diameters of measured lesions decreases 50% or more for at least 4 weeks without cancer-related symptoms or weight or performance deteriorations. If there is no change in tumor size but the biochemical parameters decline by 80% or more, the patient is considered stable.

Stable Disease

Patients who do not meet the criteria for partial response but who are without signs and symptoms of progressive disease for at least 3 months comprise this category.

Progressive Disease

An increase exceeding 25% in the total area of the bidimensionally measured lesions, the appearance of new lesions, or greater or significant deterioration that cannot be attributed to treatment or medical conditions is considered disease progression.

TABLE 57.6	Common Combination Regimens	
Acronym	**Regimen**	**Indications**
ABVD	Doxorubicin, bleomycin, vinblastine with dacarbazine	Hodgkin lymphoma
AC	Doxorubicin, cyclophosphamide	Breast cancer
BEP	Bleomycin, etoposide, cisplatin	Testicular cancer
BIP	Bleomycin, ifosfamide, cisplatin, mesna	Cervical cancer
CAF	Cyclophosphamide, doxorubicin, fluorouracil	Breast cancer
CAP	Cyclophosphamide, doxorubicin, cisplatin	Non–small-cell lung cancer
RCHOP	Rituximab, cyclophosphamide, doxorubicin, vincristine	Non-Hodgkin lymphoma
CHOP-BLEO	Add bleomycin to CHOP	Non-Hodgkin lymphoma
CMF	Cyclophosphamide, methotrexate, fluorouracil	Breast cancer
CP	Cyclophosphamide, cisplatin	Ovarian cancer
DHAP	Cisplatin, cytarabine, dexamethasone	Hodgkin's lymphoma
EAP	Etoposide, doxorubicin, cisplatin	Gastric cancer
EC	Etoposide, carboplatin	Small-cell lung cancer
FAC	Fluorouracil, doxorubicin, cyclophosphamide	Breast cancer
FAM	Fluorouracil, doxorubicin, mitomycin	Gastric cancer
FAMTX	Fluorouracil, doxorubicin, methotrexate, leucovorin	Gastric cancer
ITP	Ifosfamide, Taxol, cisplatin	Genitourinary cancer
IVAC	Ifosfamide, vincristine, doxorubicin, cyclophosphamide	Multiple myeloma
ICE	Ifosfamide, carboplatin, etoposide	Lung cancer
MAID	Mesna, Adriamycin (doxorubicin), ifosfamide, dacarbazine (MAI is also commonly used and excludes dacarbazine).	Sarcoma
MOPP	Mechlorethamine, vincristine, procarbazine	Hodgkin lymphoma
MVAC	Vincristine, doxorubicin, cyclophosphamide	Lung cancer
MVP	Mitomycin, vinblastine, cisplatin	Lung cancer

CHAPTER SUMMARY

- Cell cycle–nonspecific drugs exert their cytotoxic activity irrespective of the phase of the cell life cycle.
- Cell cycle–nonspecific drugs are considered more toxic than cell cycle–specific drugs.
- Alkylating drugs are radiomimetic.
- The nitrosoureas are alkylating agents that are highly lipid soluble.
- The antitumor antibiotics that are considered both anthracyclines and topoisomerase II inhibitors are daunorubicin, doxorubicin, and idarubicin. Mitoxantrone is a synthetic anthracenedione.
- The most feared adverse effect of anthracycline therapy is cardiotoxicity.
- Some prognostic factors relating to a patient's tolerance to acute emesis are age, gender, and method of drug administration.
- The different groups of hormones used in cancer therapy are the adrenal corticosteroids, androgens, antiandrogens, estrogens, antiestrogens, gonadotropin-releasing hormone analogues, progestins, and aromatase inhibitors.
- Combination chemotherapy is superior to single-drug therapy because it kills a maximum number of cancer

cells within a toxicity range tolerated by the patient, it provides a broader range of coverage against resistant cells in the heterogenous tumor population, and it is characterized by minimal or slow development of new resistant cancer cells.
- Targeted therapies have been developed that work directly to prevent cancer cell development and growth. Because their primary effect is on cancer cells, these therapies are associated with fewer adverse effects than other chemotherapies.

QUESTIONS FOR STUDY AND REVIEW

1. What are anthracyclines, and which of the antitumor antibiotics are they?
2. Which cell cycle–nonspecific drugs are highly lipid soluble? What can they do?
3. What are the different groups of drugs used to control acute emesis?
4. What is the role of dexrazoxane in anthracycline therapy? How is it administered?
5. What are the characteristics of drugs that are useful for combination therapy?

NEED MORE HELP?

Chapter 57 of the Study Guide to Accompany *Drug Therapy in Nursing*, 4th Edition, contains NCLEX-style questions and other learning activities to reinforce your understanding of the concepts presented in this chapter. For additional information or to purchase the study guide, visit thePoint.

REFERENCES

American Society of Health-System Pharmacists. (2006). ASHP guidelines on handling hazardous drugs. *American Journal of Health-System Pharmacists*, 63:1172–1193.

Bremerkamp, M. (2000). Mechanism of action of 5-HT receptor antagonists: Clinical overview and nursing implications. *Clinical Journal of Oncology Nursing*, 4:201–207.

Camp-Sorrell, D. (2011). Chemotherapy: Toxicities and management. In C. H. Yarbro, M. H. Frogge, M. Goodman, & S. L. Groenwald (Eds.), *Cancer nursing: Principles and practice* (7th ed.). Boston, MA: Jones and Bartlett.

Campos, D., Pereira, J. R., & Reinhardt, R. R. (2001). Prevention of cisplatin-induced emesis by the oral neurokinin-1 antagonist, MK-869, in combination with granisetron and dexamethasone or with dexamethasone alone. *Journal of Clinical Oncology*, 19:1759–1767.

DeVita, V. T., Jr., Hellman, S., & Rosenberg, S. A., eds. (2008). *Cancer: Principles and practice of oncology* (8th ed.). Philadelphia, PA: Lippincott Williams & Wilkins.

Dibble, S. L., Isreal, J., Nussey, B., Casey, K., & Luce, J. (2003). Delayed chemotherapy-induced nausea in women treated for breast cancer. *Oncology Nursing Forum*, 30(2):40–47.

Fisher, B., Constantino, J. P., Redmond, C., et al. (1994). Endometrial cancer in tamoxifen-treated breast cancer patients: Findings from the National Surgical Adjuvant Breast and Bowel Project (NSABP) B-14. *Journal of the National Cancer Institute*, 86:527–537.

Kris, M. G., Hesketh, P. J., Somerfield, M. R., et al. (2006). American Society of Clinical Oncology guideline for antiemetics in oncology: Update 2006. *Journal of Clinical Oncology*, 24(18):2932–2947.

National Comprehensive Cancer Network. (2010). *Clinical practice guidelines in oncology: Antiemesis* (version 2, 2010). http://www.nccn.org/professionals/physician_gls/PDF/antiemesis

National Institute for Occupational Safety and Health. (2004). *Preventing occupational exposure to antineoplastic and other hazardous drugs in health care settings* (NIOSH publication no. 2004–165). Retrieved *from http://www.cdc.gov/niosh/docs/2004–165/*

National Study Commission on Cytotoxic Exposure. (1984). *Recommendations for handling cytotoxic agents.* Retrieved from *http://209.85.165.104/search?q=cache:hOiOOLc0pelJ:ctep.cancer.gov/handbook/append_13.html+National+Study+Commission+on+Cytotoxic+ Exposure&hl=en&ct=clnk&cd=1&gl=us*

Ozols, R. F., Herbst, R. S., Colson, Y. L., et al. (2007). Clinical cancer advances 2006: Major research advances in cancer treatment, prevention, and screening. A report from the American Society of Clinical Oncology. *Journal of Clinical Oncology*, 25(1):146–162.

Polovich, M., Whitford, J., Olsen, M. (2009) *Chemotherapy and biotherapy: Guidelines and recommendations for practice.* Oncology Nursing Society. Pittsburgh, PA: Oncology Nursing Press.

Pritchard, K. I. (2001). Selective estrogen receptor modulators in the prevention and treatment of breast cancer. *Clinical Oncology Updates*, 3(4):1–15.

Schuchter, L. M., Hensley, M. L., Meropol, N. J., et al., for the American Society of Clinical Oncology Chemotherapy and Radiotherapy Expert Panel. (2002). *2002 Update of recommendations for the use of chemotherapy and radiotherapy protectants: Clinical practice guidelines of The American Society of Clinical Oncology.* Retrieved from *http://www.asco. org/portal/site/ASCO/menuitem.c543a013502b2a89de912310320041a0/?vgnextoid=cda18c393c458010VgnVCM100000ed730ad1RCRD&vgnextfmt=default*

Answers to Questions for Study and Review

Unit 1: Foundations for Drug Therapy in Nursing

Chapter 1: Nursing Management of Drug Therapy

1.1. The nurse assesses core patient variables in several ways: the patient interview, the physical assessment, and the medical record. Data on some of the variables can be obtained from more than one source.

1.2. Core drug knowledge contains basic pharmacologic facts about the drug. The nurse needs to know this information to administer drugs safely, to determine interactions with core patient variables, to devise strategies, to maximize therapeutic effects and minimize adverse effects, and to educate patients and their families.

1.3. Learning about a prototype drug gives the nurse information about a group of drugs instead of just one drug, which simplifies learning and helps the nurse organize drug information logically.

1.4. Core patient variables may affect the form the patient education should take (i.e., written, visual with pictures, or spoken), who in the family should be included in the teaching, and what content is most important to include in the teaching.

Chapter 2: Pharmaceuticals: Development, Safeguards, and Delivery

2.1. The *United States Pharmacopeia* (USP) and the *National Formulary* (NF) are compendia of drugs available in the United States. The drugs are listed by their official names.

2.2. The "omics" technologies use knowledge of a person's DNA sequencing to predict which drugs would be most efficacious or undesirable for that particular patient. It is proposed that individualizing pharmacotherapy will maximize therapeutic effects and minimize adverse effects.

2.3. Drugs are classified according to chemical composition, physiologic effect, or therapeutic use. Organizing a multitude of drugs into family groups— drug classes—with similar characteristics facilitates learning about an individual drug within the group. A general characteristic of the drug class is likely to apply to a single drug within the class.

2.4. The 1938 Food, Drug, and Cosmetic Act prohibited the marketing of new drugs before they had been properly tested for safety. It further stipulated that pharmaceutical companies had to submit an investigational new drug application to the government for review of a drug's safety before it could sell the product. The Durham-Humphrey Amendment provided further safeguards. This amendment distinguished between legend drugs (requiring a prescription) and over-the-counter drugs (not requiring a prescription) and required that labels of legend drugs carry the legend: "Caution— Federal law prohibits dispensing without a prescription." It further specified certain drugs that could not be refilled without a new prescription from the health care provider. The Canadian Narcotics Control Act (1961) regulated possession, sale, manufacture, production, and distribution of narcotics.

2.5. Clinical trials proceed after extensive animal testing provides initial evidence of the safety and efficacy of a new drug. Clinical trials have four phases. Phase I establishes optimal dosage range and pharmacokinetics. Phase II closely monitors study participants for the drug's effectiveness and adverse effects. Phase III begins if no serious adverse effects have been identified in phase II. Beginning in this phase, double-blind studies (in which neither the investigator nor the study subject knows whether the drug being administered is a placebo or the new drug being studied) establish the drug's clinical effectiveness, safety, and dosage range. Phase IV consists of postmarketing studies. Some drugs make it through all phases of clinical trials without problems, only to have severe adverse effects show up after they are used more widely in the general population. Examples of this phenomenon are the links uncovered between felbamate and aplastic anemia and between troglitazone and hepatic failure.

2.6. Controlled substances are drugs defined and categorized according to their abuse potential and dependence-producing liability.

The 1970 Controlled Substance Act requires an accounting of all controlled drugs on a special record and an accounting of all discarded or wasted medication. Another licensed nurse must countersign the special record filled out by a first. Furthermore, all controlled substances must be kept under double lock. Only authorized people have access to the keys.

2.7. All patients should be taught not to share drugs with anyone else, to follow directions for use that appear on the drug label, to avoid drinking alcohol with any prescription or over-the-counter drug, and not to take a drug after its expiration date.

2.8. The patient teaching plan for drug therapy should include the drug name and reason for use; the dosage (amount, frequency, duration of therapy, what to do about a missed dose or a double dose); administration route; special directions or procedures (for drug administration, drug stability, storage, disposal); minor adverse effects and reportable serious adverse effects; drug interactions (among drugs and foods); effects of other disease states on drug therapy; and self-monitoring techniques.

Chapter 3: Drug Administration

3.1. The most frequently used drug administration route is the enteral route for oral drugs.

3.2. An enteric coating prevents the drug from breaking down in the stomach and thus prevents GI irritation and inactivation of the drug by stomach acid. Sustained release may also occur with enteric coating.

3.3. The parenteral route may be recommended for a patient who is unable to swallow, is confused and uncooperative with oral medications, is unconscious, or has a physiologic need to keep the GI tract empty (e.g., in

preparation for a diagnostic test or surgery, or to rest the tract). The parenteral route may be used when the drug has a high first-pass effect when administered orally, which eliminates most of the active drug, or when the drug will be inactivated by gastric acid.

3.4. The greatest risk for rapid drug toxicity is the intravenous route, especially in cases of continuous intravenous infusion.

Unit 2: Core Drug Knowledge

Chapter 4: Pharmacotherapeutics, Pharmacokinetics, and Pharmacodynamics

4.1. Pharmacokinetics is what happens to the drug as it moves through the body (i.e., the body's effect on the drug). Pharmacodynamics is the manner in which the drug produces its action in the body (i.e., the drug's effect on the body).

4.2. Lipophilic drugs are soluble in lipids, or fats. Because the cell membrane is composed primarily of lipids, being lipophilic allows a drug to pass through the cell membrane easily.

4.3. Hydrophilic drugs or particles are water soluble. Water solubility promotes excretion in the urine, which is water based.

4.4. Drugs attach to specialized receptors on the cell. Attachment to the receptor either turns on the receptor's specialized action or blocks other substances from attaching to the receptor.

4.5. One hundred percent of drugs that are given orally present to the liver first after absorption. If the drug is extensively metabolized, most of the drug dose will be lost before it enters the systemic circulation. Giving the drug by another route (such as the intravenous route or the sublingual route) bypasses the liver initially, allowing 100% of the drug dose to enter the systemic circulation.

4.6. In a person with renal insufficiency or hepatic dysfunction, the dose given may be lower than the typical dose given to other patients because improperly functioning kidneys cannot excrete drugs at the rate that is normally expected and a poorly functioning liver cannot metabolize drugs as rapidly. Both of these impairments increase the amount of circulating drug and prolong the effect from a drug dose. An increase in the amount of the circulating drug increases the therapeutic effects of the drug, but it also increases the risk for adverse effects.

4.7. A patient with decreased albumin levels who is receiving a drug that is known to be highly protein bound is at higher risk for adverse drug effects than a patient with normal albumin levels because drug that is bound to protein is not active. Only free drug is active and can create an effect. Because the protein albumin is low, there is no place for the drug to bind, and more drug than would normally be expected is free, active, and able to cause therapeutic and adverse effects.

Chapter 5: Adverse Effects and Drug Interactions

5.1. Rash, hives, redness, itching, swelling of the eyes or another body part, and difficulty swallowing or breathing (laryngeal edema) are all signs of allergic reactions to drug therapy. Complaints such as nausea or vomiting would more likely indicate adverse effects.

5.2. Changes in hearing and balance may naturally occur with aging, but they are also signs of ototoxicity. Thus, adverse effects could be misconstrued as age-related changes.

5.3. The circulating blood level of Drug A will be decreased. When Drug B stimulates the hepatic pathway, more of the isoenzyme

CYP3A4 will be active, leading to more metabolism of Drug A. As Drug A is metabolized at a faster than normal rate, the circulating level will decrease.

5.4. No, the circulating blood levels of the drug will differ. The effect of grapefruit juice on metabolism varies greatly among people because people have different amounts of CYP3A4 in their GI tract.

5.5. Owing to normal circulatory patterns, all the dose of the oral drug is presented initially to the liver, where damage may occur. When the drug is administered parenterally, the drug molecules first go to the heart, and then only about 25% of the molecules are sent to the liver. Because fewer drug molecules are present in the liver at any given time, less damage may occur.

5.6. The combination of these drugs will result in an additive CNS depressive effect, greatly increasing the risk for CNS toxicity.

5.7. As the nurse, you consider the possibility that Drug A and Drug B have had an interaction, producing decreased therapeutic response from Drug A. Look up both drugs and determine whether this is an accurate assessment.

Unit 3: Core Patient Variables
Chapter 6: Life Span: Children

6.1. In the infant and especially the neonate, immature liver function affects drug distribution. The neonate's immature liver produces fewer plasma proteins, especially albumin; many drugs bind strongly to albumin. The pharmacologic effects of drugs result from unbound, or free, drug. In the neonate and infant, more free drug is available because less drug is bound to plasma protein. This state results in increased blood levels of drugs and, in turn, more adverse effects and toxicity.

6.2. Body surface area is the external surface of the body expressed in square meters. The ratio of body surface area to weight is inversely proportional to length. Body surface area is determined to calculate the correct dose for many drugs given to pediatric patients.

6.3. An increased dose of some drugs may be given to the infant because the drug is diluted by the infant's higher body water content.

6.4. No. Some drugs have adverse effects only in children and are contraindicated in them. Most drugs are not supported by enough clinical study to determine what effects (therapeutic and adverse) they would have on a child. These drugs are used off-label in children. Caution and extra monitoring must be used when administering these drugs.

6.5. The correct dose is 250 mg every 12 hours. The dose is determined in the following manner:

25mg: 1kg:: x mg: 20kg (or can be

written $\dfrac{25mg}{1kg} = \dfrac{xmg}{20kg}$); solving for

x gives an answer of 500 mg per day.

As there are two doses in 24 hours (one dose every 12 hours), divide 500 mg by 2 to equal 250 mg per dose. The most common pediatric medication error is a misplaced decimal, resulting in a ten-fold error in the dose. In this case a misplaced decimal point could have resulted in a dose of 25 mg or 2500 mg being administered instead of 250 mg. To prevent administering the incorrect dose, double-check the dosage for each dose you administer, even though the physician and the pharmacist should have also calculated the dose. In some institutions, all doses are rechecked by two nurses; in others only certain medications are rechecked by two nurses, and the remaining drugs are double-checked by only one nurse.

6.6. Vastus lateralis or rectus femoris.

6.7. If past experiences were unpleasant, the child would more likely be fearful and anxious about this interaction or drug therapy. Because parents and sometimes other family members are normally responsible for seeing that the child receives the appropriate drug therapy at home, including family members in the planning and education relevant to drug therapy is crucial. Children also need to be involved, at an age-appropriate level, in their drug therapy.

Chapter 7: Life Span: Pregnant or Breast-Feeding Women

7.1. A drug assigned to FDA pregnancy category X should not be used because it is almost sure to harm the fetus. The benefits of drug therapy cannot compensate for the risk to the fetus.

7.2. Drugs that have low-molecular weight and are lipophilic and non-protein-bound will pass through the placenta's lipid membrane easily.

7.3. Gestational weeks 3 through 8 mark the period of organogenesis, which is when all major fetal organ systems are developing. Teratogenic exposure during this period may cause major malformations that are usually recognized at birth.

7.4. Physiologic changes in the renal system that increase drug excretion rates include an increase of 40% to 50% in blood flow. This increases filtration through the glomerulus about 50% and contributes to increased excretion rates.

7.5. Lipophilic or fat-soluble drugs will pass into breast milk due to the high fat content in breast milk.

Chapter 8: Life Span: Older Adults

8.1. Liver function and metabolism are impaired because of decreased mass of the liver, decreased hepatic blood flow and hepatic tissue perfusion, and changes in the phases of metabolism.

8.2. Normal renal function decreases with aging. Drugs that depend on renal elimination are not excreted as quickly in the older adult. This leads to elevated circulating active drug levels, which place the patient at risk for adverse effects or drug toxicity.

8.3. Polypharmacy is the simultaneous use of multiple prescription and over-the-counter drugs by one person, and it puts the patient at increased risk for drug interactions, adverse effects, and nonadherence with drug therapy. Polypharmacy occurs frequently in older adults because they often experience multiple health problems related to organ and body system deterioration with advanced age.

8.4. Adverse drug effects often mimic many changes which frequently occur naturally with advanced age.

8.5. Activity affects absorption and distribution of some drugs. Dietary habits indicate whether a patient is able to swallow oral tablets or pills. Quality of life may be impaired because of adverse effects of drug therapy. The patient may have strict habits about when the drug therapy is taken; following the patient's normal routine may be less stressful. The patient's economic status, including drug insurance coverage, may affect whether he or she obtains the prescribed drugs regularly.

Chapter 9: Lifestyle: Substance Abuse

9.1. Alcohol is a CNS depressant. In combination with other CNS depressants, alcohol can produce additive pharmacologic effects of CNS depression.

9.2. Drug abuse is the excessive self-administration of a drug (often dependence producing) for other than therapeutic purposes. Drug misuse is the inadvertent incorrect use of a drug, often because the individual lacks knowledge of the drug. Addiction is physical dependence on a drug, which leads to serious physical and behavioral problems. Without the drug, physical symptoms of withdrawal begin to occur. Withdrawal is marked by a variety of physical effects, including nausea, muscle cramping, dysphoria, and convulsions. Characteristics of addiction include compulsive drug use, drug craving, and drug seeking. Psychological dependence (habituation) is an intense desire or craving for the drug when it is not available.

9.3. Factors that place an individual at risk for substance abuse include chronic pain; struggles with self-esteem issues and peer pressure; poverty and illiteracy among the socioeconomically underprivileged; wealth and influence among the very privileged; profession (health care providers); history of child abuse or sexual assault; and family history of substance abuse, including alcoholism.

9.4. Methadone is an opioid with a dependence-producing liability. During therapy, patients develop a dependence on methadone. Oral methadone dosing suppresses opioid withdrawal symptoms, and the drug has a long duration of action (24 hours), which are advantages of methadone therapy.

9.5. Hallucinogenic drugs distort perceptions and reality. Nursing interventions for a "bad trip" rely on decreasing sensory stimuli and providing for safety and support.

9.6. Two major substances that are abused are alcohol and nicotine (cigarettes). Categories of additional drugs of abuse include CNS depressants (alcohol, marijuana, opioids, sedatives and hypnotics, antipsychotics, and antianxiety drugs), CNS stimulants (cocaine, amphetamines, caffeine), and mind-altering or psychedelic drugs (LSD, mescaline, MDMA). Some individuals use drugs to alter thoughts and feelings

Chapter 10: Lifestyle, Diet, and Habits: Nutrition and Complementary Medications

10.1. Adverse drug–nutrient interactions are most likely to occur if medications are taken over long periods, if several medications are taken, or if nutrition status is poor or deteriorating.

10.2. Drugs and nutrients can interact and alter metabolism by acting as structural analogues, competing with each other for metabolic enzyme systems, altering enzyme activity, and contributing pharmacologically active substances.

10.3. Foods can alter drug absorption by changing the acidity of the digestive tract, stimulating secretion of digestive enzymes, altering rate of absorption, binding to drugs, or competing for absorption sites in the intestines.

10.4. Patients may not consider these substances to be potentially harmful or capable of interacting with prescribed drug therapy and therefore may not volunteer this information unless directly questioned.

Chapter 11: Environment: Influences on Drug Therapy

11.1. The nurse assesses for exposure to chemicals in the workplace, home, and community. Exposure to these chemicals is thought to be responsible for alteration of the hepatic drug-metabolizing enzymes, resulting in decreased drug efficacy, prolonged pharmacologic effects, or increased toxicity.

11.2. Alcohol, tobacco, or exposure to chemicals (e.g., industrial chemicals, pesticides) may adversely affect the pharmacokinetics of certain drugs by altering hepatic drug-metabolizing enzymes and altering drug responses, which increases the patient's risk for drug reactions.

11.3. The nurse inquires about the patient's home and workplace environment because they may have a bearing on drug therapy. The nurse also obtains a complete patient history that also documents lifestyle habits (e.g., ethanol, tobacco), which may affect drug therapy, as well as exposure to workplace chemicals; these factors all influence the hepatic drug-metabolizing enzymes. This information is important and will help the nurse determine whether the desired effect of drug therapy is achieved.

11.4. The nurse collects the medical information, including medication history, from the patient or patient's family and then ensures that the dosages are appropriate for the patient. The nurse then compares the current orders of the health care provider to the medication history and communicates any discrepancies to the health care provider. Medication reconciliation is performed each time the patient moves from one environment to another.

Chapter 12: Culture: Considerations in Drug Therapy

12.1. A culture is a background of customs and traditions, values, institutions, art, history, and folklore that is shared by a people. An ethnic group has a common heritage linked by race, nationality, or language.

12.2. An awareness of cultural differences alerts the nurse to assess for factors that might have an effect on drug therapy, such as current health status, genetic variations in pharmacokinetics, self-medication (with traditional or alternative medicines), and dietary practices. This awareness also assists the nurse in forming a therapeutic relationship, in communicating effectively with the patient and family, and in providing appropriate and effective teaching.

12.3. Obtain an interpreter or translator. Speak to the patient. Speak slowly. Do not shout or exaggerate your mouth movements. Allow time for the patient to think and respond. Use as few words as possible. Use as many words in the patient's language as possible. Use nonverbal language.

12.4. If the patient is present oriented, explain problems that may occur now, if medicine is not taken as directed. If the patient is future oriented, she or he will be more receptive to learning that the medication will prevent future problems if taken as directed.

12.5. The genetic background of Mexican Americans is quite varied. Their bodies may not handle drugs in the same way as Hispanics. Drug information that is related to findings for Hispanic people can be generalized only tentatively to Mexican Americans.

12.6. This patient is at risk to have more adverse effects from the drug therapy than other patients. With less metabolism, more drug remains in the circulation to be active and to cause adverse effects (as well as more therapeutic effects). Serum levels of the drug can be monitored to determine if the patient is reaching toxic levels of the drug. A lower dose of the drug is warranted if the patient's serum level of the drug increases significantly.

Unit 4: Peripheral Nervous System Drugs

Chapter 13: Drugs Affecting Adrenergic Function

13.1. Drugs that stimulate the SNS attach to and stimulate the adrenergic receptors, creating the same effects as endogenous neurotransmitters (NE, Epi, DA) that stimulate those receptors.

13.2. Beta-1 blockade slows the speed of conduction in the heart, decreases the force of contraction, and slows down the pulse rate.

13.3. Epinephrine stimulates all beta and alpha receptors. It will initially stimulate beta receptors and cause vasodilation to organs and skeletal muscle. With larger doses, the effects of alpha stimulation are evident and there will be vasoconstriction. When the alpha effects become predominant, they will override the beta effects.

13.4. Dopamine is often dosed based on the clinical response it produces. When urinary output increases to a desired amount, it can be determined that there is enough dopamine to dilate the renal artery and provide adequate perfusion to the kidney. Dopamine also will increase blood pressure from stimulation of alpha receptors. An increase in blood pressure also will allow more perfusion to the organs.

13.5. Prazosin is an alpha-1 blocker and thus causes vasodilation. This decreases peripheral resistance and lowers blood pressure.

13.6. Phenylephrine stimulates alpha-1 receptors causing vasoconstriction, and thus increasing peripheral resistance. This is how it raises blood pressure. When used in cold preparations, the vasoconstriction decreases nasal congestion temporarily.

Chapter 14: Drugs Affecting Cholinergic Function

14.1. Cholinergic stimulation in the eye produces miosis (smaller pupils) and decreases intraocular pressure.

14.2. Cholinergic stimulation of the GI track increases gastric tone and motility to promote digestion and movement through the GI tract and defecation. Additionally, there is more saliva produced to help to break down food that is eaten. GU stimulation results in the relaxation of the deltrusor muscle of the bladder so that voiding can occur. (PSNS is the "rest and digest" system.)

14.3. Extra stimulation of cholinergic receptors may cause the following CV problems:

14.4. Neostigmine inhibits the breakdown of acetylcholinesterase, which is responsible for breaking down acetylcholine. Because it is not broken down as quickly, more acetylcholine is available in the synapse to activate the cholinergic receptors, indirectly increasing the cholinergic stimulation and effects.

14.5. Symptoms of cholinergic crisis include nausea and vomiting, diarrhea, salivation, sweating, peripheral vasodilation, bronchial constriction, and (if not recognized and attended to initially) respiratory arrest. The antidote is the anticholiergic drug atropine.

14.6. Cholinergic effects on the heart include slowing the rate, (decreased pulse), slowing the speed of conduction (decreasing pulse and ECG changes), decreasing the force of contraction (decreasing cardiac output, which will decrease blood pressure).

14.7. The action of atropine on the heart rate is dose dependent. In doses of 0.4 to 0.6 mg, atropine causes a slight sinus bradycardia through vagal stimulation. In larger doses (1 to 2 mg), it causes sinus tachycardia secondary to inhibition of vagal control of the sinoatrial node in the heart. Atropine is mostly given for its ability to increase the heart rate.

Unit 5: Central Nervous System Drugs

Chapter 15: Drugs Relieving Anxiety and Promoting Sleep

15.1. Lorazepam intensifies the effects of GABA, a neurotransmitter that inhibits the nervous system.

15.2. No, it would not continue to be effective. Lorazepam, like all benzodiazepines, allows tolerance to the dose to develop with chronic use. When tolerance develops, a larger dose is needed to achieve the same therapeutic effect. Stopping a benzodiazepine, such as lorazepam, suddenly causes the patient to experience withdrawal symptoms. Additionally, recurrent anxiety or rebound insomnia is likely.

15.3. Lorazepam is metabolized to an inactive metabolite, which can then be excreted renally. Other benzodiazepines are metabolized to active metabolites. With lorazepam, the liver does not have to do as much work to convert the drug to a form that can be eliminated.

15.4. Older adults are more at risk for sedation, ataxia, and confusion than younger adults. This combination places them at increased risk for falling in their homes.

15.5. Triazolam has a very quick onset but also a very short half-life. Because the effects of the drug wear off quickly, the patient may have problems with waking up early in the morning and not falling back asleep easily.

15.6. Eszopiclone is the only drug for insomnia that is approved for long-term use (up to 6 months of use). Unlike the benzodiazepines, eszopiclone does not seem to produce tolerance, even with long-term use. Withdrawal symptoms are possible after discontinuation, but they are mild in comparison to those experienced from benzodiazepine withdrawal.

Chapter 16: Drugs Treating Mood Disorders

16.1. Selective serotonin reuptake inhibitors (SSRIs), tricyclic antidepressants, and monoamine oxidase inhibitors (MAOIs) are the three main classifications of antidepressants.

16.2. When depressed, a patient often lacks the energy to carry out plans for suicide. However, after beginning antidepressant therapy, a patient may experience increased energy before mood improves. Therefore, you must assess the patient for thoughts of self-harm and reassure the patient that the full effects of therapy have not yet occurred. Suicide precautions may have to be implemented to maintain patient safety.

16.3. It is important to continue antidepressant therapy even after symptoms of depression improve; otherwise, the depressive symptoms will come back.

16.4. Gastrointestinal distress is sometimes reported with sertraline therapy. This distress frequently lessens early on, as the patient's body adapts to the drug. Giving the drug with meals may also decrease gastrointestinal distress.

16.5. Adverse effects such as blurred vision, dry mouth, and constipation are the anticholinergic effects frequently associated with nortriptyline therapy.

16.6. The patient taking phenelzine must adhere to a strict diet that excludes foods high in tyramine, such as aged cheeses (especially blue, Camembert, Swiss, and Stilton), tap beers, and some types of meats (pepperoni, salami).

16.7. Symptoms of an MAOI-induced hypertensive crisis are flushing of the face, occipital headache, sweating, suddenly elevated blood pressure, and fever.

16.8. Although lithium is still the first choice for treating bipolar disorder, antiepileptics such as carbamazepine (Tegretol), valproic acid (Depakote), and gabapentin (Neurontin) are increasingly used as well.

16.9. In general, the therapeutic range of lithium is a serum concentration between 0.6 and 1.2 mEq/L.

16.10. Lithium toxicity usually presents as diarrhea, vomiting, unsteady gait, weakness, and slurred speech. Symptoms of toxicities usually appear when the serum level of lithium is greater than 2 mEq/L.

Chapter 17: Drugs Treating Psychotic Disorders and Dementia

17.1. Low-potency typical antipsychotic drugs are more likely to produce these adverse effects: sedation and anticholinergic effects. High-potency typical antipsychotic drugs are more likely to produce extrapyramidal symptoms as an adverse effect.

17.2. EPS—extrapyramidal symptoms—come from the relative lack of dopamine stimulation and relative excess of cholinergic stimulation. There are four major presentations of EPS: (1) Parkinson-like effects (pseudoparkinsonism), which are symptoms that are typically seen with Parkinson disease (cog-wheeling muscle rigidity, fine tremor, slow motor responses, shuffling gait, and a flat affect [a mask-like facial expression]); (2) akathisia (a constant feeling of restlessness); (3) acute dystonia; and (4) tardive dyskinesia (involuntary lip-smacking, chewing, mouth movements, tongue protrusion, blinking, grimacing, and muscle twitching of the limbs). Tardive dyskinesia, unlike the other EPS adverse effects, is usually permanent once it occurs.

17.3. Typical antipsychotics treat the positive symptoms of psychotic illness (delusions and hallucinations). Atypical antipsychotics treat the positive symptoms as well as the negative symptoms (flat or blunted emotions, lack of pleasure or interest in things [anhedonia], and limited speech). Atypical antipsychotics also produce very few adverse effects.

17.4. Acute dystonia involves prolonged muscular contractions and spasms, especially in the neck (arching and twisting), the larynx and pharynx (contractions and spasms that may occlude the airway), back (arching), and eye (eye-rolling up toward the back of the head). Although all of the symptoms can be painful and require medical attention, airway occlusion can be life-threatening and constitutes a medical emergency.

17.5. Teach that the adverse effect is usually transient. Suggest that instead of giving two equal-sized doses daily to a patient, the larger dose or the entire daily dose could be taken at bedtime. Also, the patient can be encouraged to be as active as possible during the daytime hours to help ward off sedation.

17.6. Rivastigmine is an acetylcholinesterase inhibitor, which prevents the breakdown of acetylcholine. When acetylcholine is not broken down, its action is prolonged on cortical cholinergic receptors and in the synapse; there is also more effective neuronal transmission. This increase in acetylcholine activity decreases the dementia found in mild to moderate Alzheimer disease.

Chapter 18: Drugs Treating Seizure Disorders

18.1. A seizure is hyperexcitation of the neurons in the brain producing changes in level of consciousness and/or involuntary muscle activity. A convulsion is the jerky, involuntary muscle movement that can occur during a seizure.

18.2. Phenytoin slows the influx of sodium through the sodium channels into the cell. Sodium influx changes the negativity of the cell and produces an action potential. Slowing the influx of sodium lengthens the time between action potentials. Both seizures and some types of cardiac arrhythmias are caused by excessive firing of cells.

18.3. A benzodiazepine such as diazepam or lorazepam is the first-line drug of choice in treating status epilepticus.

18.4. The half-life of phenytoin lengthens considerably as the dose increases, so the drug dose should be titrated in small amounts to avoid making too big a change in the blood drug level.

18.5. Phenytoin is highly protein bound. When there is a lack of serum protein (albumin), as in a patient with low serum albumin levels, more drug is free and active than would usually be expected from the dose. Because more drug is active, it is more likely to cause adverse effects.

18.6. Ethosuximide reduces absence seizures by inhibiting the influx of calcium ions when they travel through a special set of channels, known as T-type calcium channels in the hypothalamus, the site of absence seizure formation.

18.7. Benzodiazepines suppress seizure activity by potentiating the effectiveness of the inhibitory neurotransmitter, GABA. Patients with seizures are believed to have a lack of GABA or an excess of glutamate, the opposing excitatory neurotransmitter.

Chapter 19: Drugs Producing Anesthesia and Neuromuscular Blocking

19.1. Producing general anesthesia with a single agent is not always desirable because too deep a level of unconsciousness may ensue. To overcome this limitation, a process called balanced anesthesia is used. Balanced anesthesia relies on a combination of drugs to produce loss of consciousness, analgesia, and muscle relaxation, while producing and maintaining a lighter stage of anesthesia. Drugs used in balanced anesthesia include inhaled or parenteral anesthetics, ultrashort-acting barbiturates, neuromuscular blocking agents, benzodiazepines, and opioid analgesics.

19.2. Patients need to be given anesthesia in a controlled environment, such as the operating suite or critical care unit. A cardiac monitor, blood pressure monitor, and ventilator must be available for immediate use. Full resuscitation capability is mandatory.

19.3. First, the emulsion is a great medium for bacterial growth. Be aware of how infusion time must be monitored as a safeguard against bacterial growth. Second, the emulsion vehicle contains soybean oil, glycerol, and egg phosphatide. Assess for hypersensitivity to any of

these elements before the drug is administered.

19.4. Local anesthetic agents are relatively free of adverse effects if they are administered at an appropriate dosage and in the correct anatomic location. However, systemic and localized toxic reactions may occur, usually because of accidental intravascular or intrathecal injection or the administration of an excessive dose of the local anesthetic agent. Systemic reactions to local anesthetics primarily involve the central nervous system and the cardiovascular system.

19.5. Nondepolarizing neuromuscular junction (NMJ) blockers induce muscle flaccidity, whereas depolarizing NMJ blockers excite the muscle, promoting contraction until it can no longer receive neurocommunication and becomes paralyzed.

19.6. In discussing Mrs. Smith's prognosis, you need to remember that the patient may be paralyzed but not deaf. Because you do not know the outcome of the charge nurse's conversation, you may suggest moving the discussion to an environment where the patient cannot overhear the conversation.

19.7. Education of a patient undergoing surgical anesthesia with succinylcholine as an adjunctive therapy may focus on the patient's inability to speak, move, or breathe unassisted while using this drug. Reassure the patient that he or she will be monitored constantly for safety. Also, explain that uncomfortable side effects such as muscle ache can be relieved with acetaminophen.

Chapter 20: Drugs Affecting Muscle Spasm and Spasticity

20.1. A muscle spasm is defined as a sudden, violent, involuntary

contraction of a muscle or group of muscles. Spasm is usually related to a localized skeletal muscle injury from acute trauma. Pain and interference with function attend muscle spasm, producing involuntary movement and distortion. Spasticity is a condition in which certain muscles are continuously contracted. This contraction causes stiffness or tightness of the muscles and may interfere with gait, movement, or speech. Damage to the portion of the brain or spinal cord that controls voluntary movement usually causes spasticity.

20.2. Cyclobenzaprine is chemically similar to amitriptyline. Combining these two drugs will increase anticholinergic effects. Monitor the patient for symptoms such as dry mouth, blurred vision, constipation, and urinary retention. Because cyclobenzaprine and diazepam are both CNS depressants, also monitor the patient for increased sedation. In the hospital, the bed should be in the lowest position with the side rails up. Caution the patient to call for help before attempting to ambulate. Assess the sedative effects before the patient drives a vehicle or performs tasks that require concentration.

20.3. Baclofen (Lioresal), diazepam (Valium), and dantrolene (Dantrium) can be used to manage spasm and spasticity. Dantrolene is generally reserved for patients with muscle spasticity.

20.4. Baclofen works at the spinal end of the upper motor neurons. Spasms caused by cerebrovascular accident (CVA) or Parkinson disease involve lesional or functional impairment of basal ganglia, which are above the spinal motor neurons.

20.5. Symptoms suggesting hepatitis in the patient on long-term dantrolene therapy include loss of appetite, nausea or vomiting, yellowed skin or eyes, and changes in stool or urine color.

20.6. No, botulinum toxin would be a poor choice for this patient with an acute injury. Botulinum toxin is used to manage chronic pain that has not responded well to other medical or physical treatment. This patient needs quick relief, but the onset of action for botulinum toxin may take up to 2 weeks. Similarly, the duration of effect is up to 3 months, which is much longer than most acute musculoskeletal injuries last.

Chapter 21: Drugs Treating Parkinson Disease and Other Movement Disorders

21.1. Dopaminergics increase the amount of dopamine in the brain. Anticholinergics decrease the amount of acetylcholine in the brain. Both effects restore the necessary balanced antagonism of these two neurotransmitters.

21.2. A substantial amount of carbidopa is destroyed in the periphery of the body before it reaches the brain. Carbidopa decreases the amount of levodopa that is destroyed and increases the amount of levodopa that reaches the brain. Because more levodopa can pass the blood–brain barrier, a lower dose is needed to induce effects.

21.3. Neuroleptic malignant syndrome is characterized by rapid onset of marked rigidity, akinesia, tremor, and hyperpyrexia. It may occur if carbidopa-levodopa therapy is stopped abruptly.

21.4. A bradykinetic episode is associated with the eventual ineffectiveness of carbidopa-levodopa therapy. The episode, also called the on–off effect, is characterized by akinesia followed by a return of drug effectiveness. The patient is at risk for injury during these

periods because hypotonia may occur.

21.5. Patients starting carbidopa-levodopa therapy should have a moderate amount of protein in divided portions throughout the day. They also should decrease their intake of pyridoxine, which is found in foods such as avocados, bananas, beef liver, oatmeal, halibut, chicken, pork, mashed potatoes, wheat germ, and sunflower seeds.

21.6. Throughout carbidopa-levodopa therapy, monitor patients for drug effectiveness, adverse effects, and the onset of new and progression of existing Parkinson symptoms.

21.7. Riluzole therapy aims to delay the need for tracheostomy or mechanical ventilation in the patient with amyotrophic lateral sclerosis (ALS).

21.8. Some of the most frequent adverse effects of riluzole are asthenia, dizziness, and vertigo. These are also signs of ALS progression.

21.9. Dietary restrictions associated with riluzole therapy include caffeine, food high in fat, and charcoal-broiled foods.

21.10. Glatiramer is a synthetic drug that modifies the immune system by acting as a decoy for autoimmune antigens that destroy the myelin sheath in the nervous system. Interferon beta is a drug developed by recombinant DNA technology. It works by decreasing levels of interferon gamma and other proinflammatory cytokines and increasing production of nerve growth factor.

21.11. All of the current drugs used to manage multiple sclerosis (MS) are administered parenterally. Some patients fear injections, and others do not have the manual dexterity or visual skill to self-administer parenteral drugs.

Chapter 22: Drugs Stimulating the Central Nervous System

22.1.

Short-Acting	Intermediate-Acting	Long-Acting
Ritalin	Ritalin SR	Metadate CD
Methylin	Methylin ER	Concerta
Methylin Chewable	Metadate ER	Ritalin LA
Focalin		Adderall XR
Dexedrine		
Dextrostat		
Adderall		

22.2. "Have you noticed any changes in behavior since your last visit?"

"Has your child complained of nervousness, insomnia, dizziness, or palpitations?"

"Has your child been eating meals regularly?"

"Have you noticed any changes in sleep since your last visit?"

"Tell me about your child's intake of caffeine-rich products."

"Has your child had any behavior problems at school?"

Observations should include height and weight measurements, blood pressure, and heart rate. Auscultate heart, lung, and bowel sounds. Palpate the thyroid. Coordinate periodic monitoring tests, including ECG, CBC, thyroid function tests, and blood glucose.

22.3. To adequately assess the effectiveness of dextroamphetamine, ask questions such as, "How many sleep attacks has your mother had today, yesterday, and on previous days?" "How many attacks per day was she having when you first brought her for treatment?" "Is your mother showing or complaining of any adverse effects, like hypertension, insomnia, irritability, hyperactivity, or psychosis?"

22.4. This patient describes caffeine withdrawal syndrome. Assess the difference between caffeine intake during the week and on weekends. Suggest that the patient decrease the amount of caffeine ingested during the week.

22.5. An important component of health promotion is encouraging and supporting the patient's commitment to weight loss. Remind the patient that sibutramine is only one component of weight loss strategy. Behavior modification and exercise are equally important to reach the patient's weight loss goal. It is also important to ensure that the patient understands that sibutramine may increase blood pressure and to make arrangements for serial checks of blood pressure.

22.6. Sibutramine works systemically by blocking the reuptake of norepinephrine, serotonin, and dopamine, resulting in a feeling of satiety. Orlistat works by inhibiting the absorption of fats from the GI tract. It does not have a systemic action.

Unit 6: Analgesic and Anti-inflammatory Drugs

Chapter 23: Drugs Treating Severe Pain

23.1. Because morphine is a CNS depressant, it suppresses the respiratory drive and decreases the respiratory rate. Acute pain indicates that the pain is of a severe, episodic type, and not a chronic condition. When morphine is being used to treat acute pain in an opioid-naive patient, the patient has not developed any tolerance to the effects of the drug. This includes tolerance to the respiratory depressive effects of morphine. Therefore, giving morphine to someone who has respiratory depression increases

respiratory depression and may cause respiratory arrest.

23.2. Patients who have been receiving morphine regularly every day for a long period (e.g., as for chronic pain) develop a tolerance to the respiratory depression that morphine may produce. They do not incur further respiratory depression from morphine. Patients with chronic pain who have a respiratory rate of 8 to 12 breaths/ minute may receive their next dose of morphine.

23. 3. Patients who abuse opioids or other CNS depressants may have cross-tolerance to the effects of morphine. For this reason, they may need a larger dose than other patients to achieve pain control.

23.4. A rescue dose is a dose of opioid used to treat breakthrough pain. It is ordered in addition to the baseline pharmacologic treatment for pain and is about 10% to 30% of the opioid dose the patient receives in 24 hours.

23.5. The half-life of naloxone is very short compared with the half-life of morphine and other opiates. Therefore, the effect of naloxone ends, and the respiratory depression from the opiates may recur. Multiple doses of naloxone may be necessary so that the patient does not revert to severe respiratory depression.

23.6. Codeine acts directly on the medullary cough center to depress the cough reflex. It also has a drying effect on the mucous membranes and can increase the viscosity of respiratory depression or arrest, because the patient is unable to independently clear his or her airway.

Chapter 24: Drugs Treating Mild to Moderate Pain, Fever, Inflammation, and Migraine Headache

24.1. Inhibition of certain prostaglandins interrupts the inflammatory cycle, thus decreasing pain and fever.

24.2. There are two isoforms of prostaglandins: COX-1 and COX-2. COX-1 maintains the functioning of many cells of the body. COX-2 is found mainly in areas of inflammation. Use of drugs that are nonselective, such as the NSAIDs, results in inhibition of both types of COX. When COX-1 is inhibited, the cytoprotective mechanism of the body is altered, and the patient is at a higher risk for adverse effects.

24.3. The most potentially serious adverse effects are bone marrow depression, blood dyscrasias, renal dysfunction, and hepatic dysfunction. These reactions can be decreased by careful assessment of medical problems and medications that contraindicate their use. Obtaining baseline laboratory tests and monitoring them throughout therapy will also decrease adverse effects. Teaching the patient the signs and symptoms of potential adverse effects and the importance of contacting the health care provider is another intervention to decrease the severity of adverse effects.

24.4. Aspirin is an irreversible inhibitor of cyclooxygenase; therefore, the antiplatelet action remains for the life of the platelet (8 days). NSAIDs are reversible inhibitors of cyclooxygenase, which means that the antiplatelet activity ceases when the blood levels decline. Aspirin is used in healthy people for protection from MI and stroke. NSAIDs do not offer protection from MI or stroke; they are actually associated with an increased risk of these disorders.

24.5. COX-2 inhibitors preferentially inhibit COX-2, decreasing inflammation. Because they do not affect COX-1 as much, their cytoprotective mechanism is not altered, which results in a decreased risk of GI bleeding. The second major difference is that COX-2 inhibitors do not alter platelet aggregation.

24.6. The triptans decrease migraine pain by stimulating the 5-HT$_{1B/1D}$ receptors located on cranial blood vessels and sensory nerves of the trigeminal vascular system. The resultant vasoconstriction decreases the throbbing sensation in the head. Stimulating the 5-HT$_{1B/1D}$ receptors also inhibits the release of proinflammatory neuropeptides, resulting in decreased vascular inflammation.

24.7. The pharmacodynamics of the triptans is limited to stimulating the 5-HT$_{1B/1D}$ receptors. Ergotamine and dihydroergotamine also affect serotonergic, dopaminergic, and alpha-adrenergic receptors as well as stimulating uterine contraction and inducing nausea and vomiting.

Chapter 25: Drugs Treating Rheumatoid Arthritis and Gout

25.1. Salicylates, NSAIDs, and acetaminophen control only the symptoms of the disease. Disease-modifying antirheumatic drugs (DMARDs) have the advantage of actually halting the progression of inflammatory diseases and the potential damage they may cause.

25.2. The major disadvantage of DMARDs is the frequency of potentially serious adverse effects, such as depressed bone marrow function, hepatotoxicity, and renal toxicity. Another disadvantage is that most of the common DMARDs have a long period before results of the therapy can be noticed by the patient.

25.3. Joint destruction begins in the early stages of the disease, even before some patients have physical symptoms. Using DMARDs within 3 months of diagnosis halts the progression of the damage and ultimately can decrease the extent of damage.

25.4. The autoimmune and inflammatory processes of the body have many substances that continue the cycle. Multiple classes of drugs may be used because they have different mechanisms of action that can affect the immune response, the inflammatory response, or both responses at different sites of the cycle or affect different substances within the cycle.

25.5. Tumor necrosis factor (TNF) is a cytokine produced by macrophages and activated T cells, which play an important role in rheumatoid arthritis (RA) by mediating cytokines that cause inflammation and joint destruction.

25.6. TNF inhibitors should not be given to any patient with an active infection, and they should be given very cautiously to an immunocompromised patient. The potential adverse effect common to all these drugs is an increased risk of serious infections. These drugs alter the immune and inflammatory responses; thus, the patient may acquire a life-threatening infection.

25.7. The biologic drugs have the same type of serious adverse effects: severe infections and malignancy. When given concurrently, they do **not** increase the efficacy of treatment but substantially increase the risk for serious adverse effects.

25.8. Colchicine decreases the inflammatory process induced by gout; therefore, it is used in acute gout. Allopurinol increases the excretion of uric acid. It is used as a prophylactic medication.

Unit 7: Hematopoietic, Cardiovascular, and Renal System Drugs

Chapter 26: Drugs Affecting Blood Pressure

26.1. Lifestyle changes of antihypertensive therapy include stopping smoking, controlling weight, limiting sodium intake, increasing potassium and calcium intake, restricting alcohol use, increasing aerobic exercise, and limiting cholesterol levels.

26.2. Thiazide diuretics are very effective in controlling hypertension and in preventing the sequelae that accompany uncontrolled hypertension. They are as effective as other drug classes, in some cases more effective, and less expensive. They should be the drug of first choice, unless there are other compelling reasons to use another drug class.

26.3. The angiotensin-converting enzyme (ACE) inhibitors prevent the conversion of angiotensin I to angiotensin II, which is a potent vasoconstrictor. By preventing vasoconstriction, ACE inhibitors decrease peripheral vascular resistance and therefore lower blood pressure. The effect of angiotensin II on aldosterone production is also blocked, preventing the sodium and fluid retention that aldosterone produces.

26.4. Aldosterone receptor blockers (ARBs) block the action of angiotensin II from all the different pathways where it is formed, not just the single substrate altered by ACE inhibitors. These drugs are effective in lowering blood pressure. In addition they seem to block deleterious effects from angiotensin II at the end-organ stage. ARBs do not cause the chronic cough that ACE inhibitors cause, and they are better tolerated by some patients.

26.5. The black box warning for these drug classes warn that the drug may cause serious fetal harm and potential death if used during the second or third trimester of a pregnancy.

26.6. Hyperkalemia (elevated potassium).

26.7. The following are safety measures used when administering nitroprusside: Always use an IV pump, preferably a volumetric pump, to infuse nitroprusside. Never allow the infusion solution to run by gravity. Monitor blood pressure constantly. Assess for signs of cyanide toxicity, thiocyanate toxicity, and methemoglobinemia. Do not infuse maximum dosage for longer than 10 minutes.

26.8. Dopamine increases renal perfusion. As the kidney becomes adequately perfused, it resumes its normal functioning and produces urine at a normal rate. Urinary output indicates if the dose of dopamine is sufficient to adequately perfuse the kidneys. The systolic blood pressure should rise from dopamine administration. If the diastolic pressure rises greatly, or disproportionately, it indicates that the alpha-2 effects of dopamine are overriding the beta-2 and dopaminergic effects. The drug rate needs to be decreased if this occurs.

Chapter 27: Drugs Affecting Urinary Output

27.1. Before thiazide therapy for hypertension is started, blood pressure, pulse, presence of edema, weight, and urinary output should be assessed.

27.2. Conditions treated by diuretic therapy include hypertension, chronic heart failure, pulmonary edema, peripheral edema (various causes), renal stones (thiazides), renal disease, increased intraocular pressure, and increased intracranial pressure.

27.3. Fluid and electrolyte problems that are likely to occur in patients receiving thiazide or loop diuretics are hypokalemia, hyponatremia, hypochloremia, hypomagnesemia, hypercalcemia (thiazides), hypocalcemia (loop), hyperglycemia, hyperuricemia, and elevated cholesterol and triglyceride levels.

27.4. Loop diuretics work in the loop of Henle, where more sodium is usually absorbed. Because loop diuretics promote more sodium loss than in the distal tubule, more potassium is lost.

27.5. Osmotic diuretics are different from thiazide or loop diuretics because they are composed of a sugar that passes through glomerular filtration but is not reabsorbed. The osmotic pressure that results pulls water into the vascular space and traps it until it is excreted in the urine.

27.6. Carbonic anhydrase inhibitors are used primarily to treat chronic open-angle glaucoma.

27.7. Blockade of the muscarinic receptors in the bladder restricts the bladder's ability to contract.

Chapter 28: Drugs Affecting Lipid Levels

28.1. High-density lipoprotein (HDL) cholesterol is believed to offer some protection against heart attack and is known as "good" cholesterol.

28.2. Elevated serum cholesterol levels lead to fatty deposits, or atherosclerosis, in the arteries. These deposits narrow the lumen of the vessel, increasing peripheral resistance and thus increasing blood pressure.

28.3. The patient is at risk of drug interactions because lovastatin is metabolized by the CYP3A4 hepatic pathway. If the patient is receiving other drugs that are also metabolized by CYP3A4, the metabolism of lovastatin is decreased, and increased drug levels result. If the other drug therapy inhibits the CYP3A4 enzyme, metabolism of lovastatin is also reduced.

28.4. Liver enzyme levels are frequently elevated from lipid-lowering drug therapy, regardless of the class of drug. If the levels rise more than three times the upper limit, evaluate the patient closely for liver impairment; unexplained and continued elevations indicate that a dose adjustment (smaller dose) is required, or the drug therapy should be stopped.

28.5. Transient, moderately elevated creatine kinase (CK) levels (i.e., 3 to 10 times above the upper limit of normal) do not indicate serious muscle damage from lovastatin. If CK levels reach greater than 10 times the upper limit of normal and the patient has symptoms, therapy should be stopped. This is to prevent serious myopathy and rhabdomyolysis, which can be fatal.

Chapter 29: Drugs Treating Heart Failure

29.1. Primary effects of digoxin include positive inotropic effect (increased force of contraction), negative chronotropic effect (decreased rate), and negative dromotropic effect (decreased speed of conduction).

29.2. Diuretics, ACE-inhibitors, and beta blockers all decrease mortality from CHF and form the basis of drug therapy. The cardiac glycoside digoxin does not decrease mortality from CHF, but it does decrease morbidity and therefore improves the quality of life for patients with CHF.

29.3. Digoxin is excreted renally. Therefore, serum drug levels will rise in the patient with decreased renal function above those normally expected for the dose administered. This makes the patient more at risk of having adverse effects. A smaller dose may be required.

29.4. Beta blockers block the effect of the sympathetic nervous system and cause vasodilation and decreased peripheral vascular resistance, which is helpful to patients with CHF. Beta blockers may also actually reverse the ventricular remodeling process that occurs in CHF by reducing left ventricular volumes and improving systolic function.

Chapter 30: Drugs Treating Angina

30.1. This prevents nitrate tolerance, which decreases the antianginal effects of the drug.

30.2. One every 5 minutes. Up to 3 tablets in 15 minutes may be given.

30.3. Nitroglycerin causes vasodilation, especially on the venous side. This allows blood to pool in the venous beds, decreasing blood pressure. The nurse should verify that the patient is not hypotensive prior to administering the drug.

30.4. Vasodilation of the vessels to the head has occurred in nurses from accidental exposure to nitroglycerin. Headache is a common adverse effect from this vasodilation.

30.5. Nitroglycerin decreases preload and afterload. This decreases the energy the heart must use to eject blood, thus decreasing the oxygen needs of the heart. Additionally, the coronary vessels are dilated, increasing blood flow to the heart. Circulation is also redirected to use the smaller vessels more, improving blood flow to the heart.

Chapter 31: Drugs Affecting Cardiac Rhythm

31.1. Ventricular arrhythmias (tachycardia and fibrillation) do not allow the ventricle to fill adequately with blood. The rapid contractions are also not effective at emptying the ventricle. Consequently, cardiac output decreases significantly. The body needs oxygenated blood to survive.

31.2. Proarrhythmia is the tendency of a drug to create a new arrhythmia or to exacerbate the arrhythmia it is supposed to be treating.

31.3. Antiarrhythmics alter the normal mechanisms that control heart rate and rhythm. Therefore, they can also cause an arrhythmia.

31.4. Class I antiarrhythmics depress phase 0. Class II antiarrhythmics depress phase 4 (depolarization). Class III antiarrhythmics produce a prolonged phase 3 (repolarization). Class IV antiarrhythmics depress phase 4 (depolarization) and lengthen phases 1 and 2 of repolarization.

31.5. Amiodarone is approved only for use in life-threatening arrhythmias such as recurrent ventricular fibrillation or recurrent, hemodynamically unstable ventricular tachycardia. It is also used as an unlabeled drug to treat atrial fibrillation.

31.6. Several electrophysiologic effects occur with the administration of amiodarone. An increased cardiac refractory period occurs, usually without influencing the resting membrane potential. Sinus rate decreases by 15% to 20%. The PR and QT intervals increase by about 10%. U waves appear and T waves are altered. These changes do not usually require discontinuation of amiodarone, although marked sinus bradycardia or sinus arrest and heart block can occur. QT prolongation can be associated with worsening of the arrhythmia, but this event is rare.

31.7. Amiodarone has a very long half-life. To quickly achieve a therapeutic level without waiting for steady state to occur, a loading dose is used. Because amiodarone is used for life-threatening arrhythmias, it is important to achieve a therapeutic effect as soon as possible so that the patient does not die.

31.8. Drink plenty of fluids and eat fresh fruits and vegetables. Include varied sources of fiber in the diet. Exercise if allowed by the physician. Discuss with physician the use of a stool softener (traps water in the stool).

Chapter 32: Drugs Affecting Coagulation

32.1. Heparin prevents fibrin formation. Warfarin interferes with the formation of prothrombin and factors VII, IX, and X.

32.2. An infusion control pump should be used to regulate the rate of heparin administration. Monitor activated partial thromboplastin time (aPTT) to prevent overdosage. Use general safety measures, such as placing the bed in a low position with the side rails up to prevent patient falls. Assess the patient regularly for signs of bleeding.

32.3. The aPTT should be monitored while the patient is receiving heparin. A therapeutic aPTT value is 1.5 to 2 times greater than the given control. The prothrombin time (PT) is monitored while the patient is taking warfarin. PT is considered therapeutic when it is approximately 1.5 times the given control or the INR value is between 2 and 3.

32.4. Warfarin interferes with the synthesis of vitamin K–derived clotting factors. Increases in vitamin K intake interfere with the action of warfarin if the increase occurs after the warfarin dosage has been titrated. Vitamin K does not affect the action of heparin.

32.5. Check for effectiveness of each therapy, as there may be a drug interaction via the P-450 system which may decrease the effectiveness of one or the other drug.

32.6. An anticoagulant lengthens clotting time and prevents future blood clots; thrombolytics break down a formed clot.

32.7. Antihemophilic factor (AHF) would be administered before and after surgery until the appropriate level of factor VIII is obtained, as determined by blood assays.

Chapter 33: Drugs Affecting Hematopoiesis

33.1. Erythropoietin, thrombopoietin, G-CSF, GM-CSF, and interleukin are the principal polypeptides and glycoproteins involved in hematopoiesis.

33.2. The kidneys produce erythropoietin, which is responsible for stimulating the production of red blood cells. When the kidneys are not functioning fully, they do not produce normal amounts of erythropoietin; thus, the patient becomes anemic.

33.3. The increased risk of infection can be fatal because the first line of defense against infection (the neutrophil) is decreased.

33.4. Platelets are fragments of large cells from the bone marrow called megakaryocytes. Thrombopoietin stimulates the production of megakaryocytes.

33.5. Fluid retention is the most common adverse effect from oprelvekin. Intake and output indicate if fluid retention is occurring. Additional fluid load can overburden the taxed heart and exacerbate the CHF, possibly causing pulmonary edema.

33.6. Thrombotic events can occur in patients with chronic renal failure receiving epoetin alfa; the risk increases when attempting to raise the hemoglobin and hematocrit to normal levels. The usual target range is 30% to 36% for hematocrit.

Unit 8: Respiratory System Drugs

Chapter 34: Drugs Affecting the Upper Respiratory System

34.1. Dextromethorphan and narcotic antitussive drugs have the same efficacy in alleviating cough. Narcotic antitussives are more sedating and have more potential adverse effects and more drug–drug interactions.

34.2. Antihistamines block the antigen–antibody reaction. In a viral syndrome, such as the common viral cold, there is no allergic reaction, only a viral infection.

34.3. Fexofenadine is a second-generation antihistamine that does not easily pass the blood–brain barrier. This results in less sedation than with first-generation antihistamines.

34.4. The advantage of inhaled antihistamines and steroids is that they act locally, are minimally absorbed, and thus induce few adverse effects.

34.5. Guaifenesin enhances the output of respiratory tract fluids by reducing the adhesiveness and surface tension of the respiratory fluids, allowing easier movement of the less viscous secretions. The result of this thinning of secretions is a more productive cough. With a more productive cough, the frequency of coughing should decrease.

Chapter 35: Drugs Affecting the Lower Respiratory System

35.1. Drugs can be grouped into mucolytic agents, such as acetylcysteine; bronchodilators, such as theophylline; and anti-inflammatory drugs, such as cromolyn sodium.

35.2. Theophylline acts by stimulating two prostaglandins, which results in smooth-muscle relaxation in both the bronchi and vasculature. Beta-adrenergic agonists are sympathomimetic agents. That means the drugs mimic the action of norepinephrine. In the lungs, norepinephrine stimulates bronchodilation. Anticholinergic agents block the action of acetylcysteine. When acetylcysteine stimulates the lungs, bronchoconstriction occurs; thus, when its action is blocked, the bronchi do not constrict.

35.3. Beta-adrenergic agonists, such as albuterol, have the quickest onset of action. They are referred to as "rescue drugs."

35.4. Glucocorticosteroids are the most powerful anti-inflammatory agents.

35.5. Both drugs are effective in reducing inflammation. Glucocorticoid steroids given orally have the potential to cause more adverse effects because they are systemic. Steroids given by inhalation have a local action; thus, they cause fewer adverse effects.

35.6. Cromolyn sodium works by stabilizing the mast cell. When the mast cell ruptures in response to an antigen, bronchoconstrictive substances such as histamine, bradykinin, serotonin, and leukotrienes are released. By stabilizing the mast cell, the drug prevents release of these substances. Glucocorticoid steroids have a multitude of actions. In the lungs, they decrease the effectiveness of inflammatory cells, thus keeping the bronchioles open. Leukotriene antagonists block the ability of leukotrienes to bind to their receptor sites. Because leukotriene binding to these sites is what causes bronchoconstriction, bronchoconstriction is blocked.

35.7. The beta-adrenergic agonist inhaler should be used first because it has the fastest onset. It will open the bronchial tree, so that the other drugs can be dispersed farther into the lungs to exert their action.

Unit 9: Gastrointestinal Tract Drugs

Chapter 36: Drugs Affecting the Upper Gastrointestinal Tract

36.1. The cause of peptic ulcers is the bacterium *Helicobacter pylori*. Without treatment to kill these bacteria, the ulcers almost always recur.

36.2. Highly acidic foods such as tomato juice and highly spiced foods may worsen gastroesophageal reflux disease (GERD) symptoms and may keep the patient from feeling relief from the pain and discomfort of GERD.

36.3. Omeprazole may interact with other drugs that also are metabolized through the cytochrome P-450 pathway (e.g., cyclosporine, disulfiram, and benzodiazepines). This interaction may produce elevated levels of these other drugs because their metabolism is decreased. Because omeprazole causes prolonged and substantial decreases in gastric acidity, drugs that depend on an acid environment for absorption may not be absorbed as well.

36.4. H_2 antagonists reduce gastric acid production by blocking histamine at the H_2-receptor site of parietal cells, resulting in a reduction in the hydrogen ion concentration and volume of gastric acid. H_1 antagonists are not effective at these sites and have no effect on gastric pH but are effective in relieving symptoms of allergic reactions. H_2 antagonists have no effect on the H_1 receptor sites.

36.5. Aluminum and magnesium are commonly combined in a preparation to balance the constipating effects of aluminum with the diarrheal effects of magnesium.

36.6. Patients with chronic renal failure tend to have elevated phosphate levels. Aluminum carbonate binds with the phosphate to return the patient's serum phosphate levels to normal.

36.7. The main adverse effects of orlistat are the GI symptoms of oily spotting, flatus with discharge of stool, fecal urgency, fatty or oily stool, oily evacuation, increased defecation, and fecal incontinence.

36.8. Serotonin receptors of the 5-HT$_3$ type are located peripherally on the vagal nerve terminal and centrally in the chemoreceptor trigger zone (CTZ). Stimulation of these receptors brings on nausea and vomiting. During chemotherapy, special mucosal cells in the small intestine release serotonin, which stimulates these receptors. Ondansetron blocks these receptor sites, thus preventing nausea and vomiting.

Chapter 37: Drugs Affecting the Lower Gastrointestinal Tract

37.1. Chew simethicone tablets thoroughly before swallowing. Shake suspension forms before measuring. Take after meals and at bedtime.

37.2. The unpleasant effects of atropine, such as dry mouth and tachycardia, discourage abuse of the drug for opioid effects.

37.3. Stool softeners should be used. Bearing down to defecate (Valsalva maneuver) increases the pressure in the eye. Stool softeners decrease the need to do this when defecating.

37.4. No. The kidney that is not functioning optimally does not excrete magnesium. Hypermagnesemia may develop from the additional magnesium provided by magnesium hydroxide.

37.5. Lactulose pulls ammonia from the bloodstream into the digestive tract. Patients with severe hepatic disease have excessive ammonia in their blood. Lactulose will therefore decrease ammonia levels.

37.6. Alosetron is limited to women because insufficient data exist to support its use in men. Alosetron is associated with the risk of severe constipation and ischemic colitis, which is why it is limited to patients with severe symptoms of IBS, in which diarrhea is the primary symptom.

37.7. Serotonin is a primary neurotransmitter affecting the enteric tract, and it plays a role in visceral sensation and the normal functioning of the tract, including secretion and motility. Abnormalities in motility and visceral sensation correspond to the pathology of many of the symptoms of IBS.

Unit 10: Antimicrobial Drugs

Chapter 38: Principles of Antimicrobial Therapy

38.1. For antimicrobial therapy to be effective, the guiding principle is to use "the right drug for the right bug."

38.2. Antimicrobials may be classified by the type of organism they affect or by their mechanism of action.

38.3. Antimicrobials work by inhibiting cell wall synthesis, inhibiting protein synthesis, inhibiting nucleic acid synthesis, disrupting the cell membrane permeability, inhibiting metabolic pathways, or inhibiting viral enzymes.

38.4. Selective toxicity means that the drug harms the pathogen but does not harm the host cell.

38.5. In the human host, many bacteria keep other microbes, such as fungus, in check. When the "good" bacteria are killed by antimicrobials, the nonsusceptible microbes can proliferate, causing an additional infection.

38.6. In the United States, the microbes that have developed substantial resistance include methicillin-resistant *Staphylococcus aureus* (MRSA), vancomycin-resistant *Enterococcus* (VRE), and multiple drug–resistant *Mycobacterium tuberculosis* (MDR-TB), as well as microbes that cause nosocomial infections.

38.7. Nurses can help meet the objectives of the CDC's campaign by consistently using aseptic technique for all procedures; obtaining culture specimens appropriately; contacting the physician or other health care providers with culture and sensitivity results; ensuring adherence to isolation procedures for themselves, visitors, and the physician; documenting improvement or worsening of symptoms of infection; and washing hands between contact with patients.

38.8. The best way to limit the risk of a nosocomial infection is handwashing before contact with each patient.

Chapter 39: Antibiotics Affecting the Bacterial Cell Wall

39.1. Penicillins bind with penicillin-binding proteins (PCPs) located inside the bacterial cell wall. Binding at these sites alters the way the bacteria are able to build their cell walls by affecting the development of cross-bridges that give the cell wall its strength. As the cell wall weakens, the internal osmotic pressure of the bacteria changes to allow the cell to absorb water, swell, and then burst. The body's immune system completes the process of fighting the infection and cleans up debris from ruptured bacteria. Penicillins also "turn on" autolysin, an enzyme

that actively promotes cell wall destruction.

39.2. Gram-negative bacteria have a cell wall envelope that actively keeps penicillin from entering the cell and binding to penicillin-binding proteins (PCPs). Penicillins cannot work if they cannot bind to these proteins.

39.3. Penicillins are classified by their spectrum of activity. The narrow-spectrum penicillins can eradicate a limited number of bacteria, the penicillinase-resistant penicillins are effective against bacteria that produce penicillinase, the aminopenicillins are effective against most gram-positive bacteria, and the extended-spectrum penicillins are specifically effective against *Pseudomonas* species.

39.4. Clavulanic acid, tazobactam, and sulbactam have very little antibacterial activity on their own. They fight beta-lactamase–producing bacteria by becoming "suicide agents." By binding to the active site of beta-lactamase, they enable penicillin to reach its target site within the bacterial cytoplasmic membrane and destroy the bacteria.

39.5. Imipenem, meropenem, and ertapenem are parenteral carbapenem beta-lactam antibiotics. They are all broad-spectrum, with imipenem having the broadest spectrum of the three. Meropenem (Merrem) and ertapenem (Invanz) are administered as single agents, whereas imipenem is combined with cilastatin (Primaxin) to reduce the potential for renal toxicity. Imipenem is indicated for severe resistant infections, especially nosocomial infections; meropenem is used for intra-abdominal infections and bacterial meningitis; and ertapenem is indicated to manage moderate to severe, complicated intra-abdominal infections,

skin and skin structure infections, pyelonephritis, acute pelvic infections, and community-acquired pneumonia. The drugs all have similar contraindications, precautions, and adverse effects. Of the three, imipenem is most likely to cause seizures, especially in patients with pre-existing seizure disorders or insults to the brain such as head trauma. Ertapenem is the only carbapenem not indicated for use in children.

39.6. Cephalosporins can be grouped into four generations. As the generations progress from first to fourth, the drugs have increasing activity against gram-negative bacteria, increasing resistance to destruction by beta-lactamases, and increasing ability to reach the cerebrospinal fluid (CSF).

39.7. Beta-lactam antibiotics include penicillins, cephalosporins, monobactams, and carbapenems. They are called beta-lactam antibiotics because they all contain a beta-lactam ring that is responsible for their antibacterial activity.

39.8. Vancomycin is reserved for serious infections because of its ability to cause serious adverse effects, especially ototoxicity and nephrotoxicity.

Chapter 40: Antibiotics Affecting Protein Synthesis

40.1. Tetracyclines have limited use because of emerging bacterial resistance. They are also associated with food interactions that decrease the absorption of the drug. They may not be used by pregnant or lactating women or children younger than 8 years because of their potential to damage primary teeth.

40.2. Aminoglycosides are used only in serious infections because of their potential to cause serious toxicities, including ototoxicity, nephrotoxicity, and neuromuscular blockade.

40.3. The most serious adverse effects of chloramphenicol therapy are irreversible bone marrow toxicity and life-threatening blood dyscrasias.

40.4. An antibiotic affects any bacterium within its spectrum. In the body, some bacteria are used to keep other organisms under control. When those bacteria are affected, organisms such as yeast can overgrow.

40.5. Patients receiving clindamycin therapy should be advised to stop the medication immediately if these symptoms occur and contact the provider. These symptoms may suggest antibiotic-associated colitis, also known as pseudomembranous colitis or *Clostridium difficile* colitis, which is associated with overgrowth of *C. difficile.*

40.6. Quinupristin/dalfopristin is a parenteral agent that is active against *E. faecium* but not *E. faecalis,* both of which may cause bacteremia. Linezolid is active against both *E. faecium* and *E. faecalis.* Additionally, linezolid is offered as both parenteral and oral preparations. Because linezolid induces monoamine oxidase (MAO) inhibition, however, it has many more potential drug interactions in addition to food and beverage interactions.

Chapter 41: Drugs That Are Miscellaneous Antibiotics

41.1. First-generation quinolones are used only to treat uncomplicated urinary tract infections (UTIs). Second-generation fluoroquinolones have better gram-negative and systemic activity. Third-generation fluoroquinolones have extended activity against gram-positive pathogens but are less active than second-generation drugs against *Pseudomonas* species. In addition to having the spectrum of activity of third-generation fluoroquinolones, the fourth-generation drugs are also active against *Pseudomonas* species and anaerobic bacteria.

41.2. Fluoroquinolones inhibit DNA gyrase. This enzyme, essential for the replication of bacteria, has a counterpart in human cells, but the human enzyme is not affected by fluoroquinolones.

41.3. Ciprofloxacin should not be given to children younger than 18 years or to women who are pregnant or breast-feeding. Fluoroquinolones have caused cartilage deterioration in immature animals and may induce arthropathies in infants and children.

41.4. Compounds that contain aluminum, calcium, iron, magnesium, or zinc bind with ciprofloxacin. This affinity results in decreased absorption and bioavailability of ciprofloxacin.

41.5. Daptomycin is the first of a new class of antibiotic that works in a totally different way than other antimicrobial drugs. At this time, no mechanism of resistance to daptomycin has been identified, there are no known transferable elements, or plasmids, that confer resistance, and cross-resistance has not been reported. To keep bacteria from becoming resistant to daptomycin, it should be used only after other antibiotics have been unsuccessful.

41.6. Parenteral polymyxin B is used only in clinical situations in which patients have not responded to other less toxic drugs, because of its potential to induce serious nephrotoxicity.

Chapter 42: Drugs Treating Urinary Tract Infections

42.1. One of the most common uses for sulfamethoxazole-trimethoprim (SMZ-TMP) is prophylaxis and treatment of *Pneumocystis carinii* pneumonia (PCP). SMZ-TMP is frequently used for respiratory infections caused by *Haemophilus influenzae* or *Streptococcus pneumoniae.* In the respiratory tract, these microbes may cause bronchitis, sinusitis, or pneumonia. It is also an alternative treatment for *Legionella pneumophila* pneumonia. GI infections treated with SMZ-TMP include shigellosis and salmonellosis. SMZ-TMP concentrates in prostate and vaginal fluids and thus is useful in prostatitis and some types of vaginitis. SMZ-TMP is also effective for sexually transmitted diseases, such as acute gonococcal urethritis and oropharyngeal gonorrhea.

42.2. Sulfonamides interrupt the formation of folate, which is necessary for the microorganism's biosynthesis of DNA, RNA, and protein. If the microorganism does not rely on folate for this action, the drug is ineffective.

42.3. Antibiotics used to manage UTIs reach high concentration in serum; thus, they can be used for infections other than those of the urinary tract. Urinary tract antiseptics have a direct local action on urine and achieve only very low serum concentrations. Therefore, they are systemically ineffective and useful only in UTI.

42.4. UTIs cause several uncomfortable symptoms, including lower abdominal pain, dysuria, and a feeling of urgency. Phenazopyridine is an analgesic that decreases these symptoms in the bladder. It is generally used for a few days, until the antibiotic is able to decrease the bacterial count enough to decrease these symptoms.

42.5. Use aseptic technique and follow these steps:

- Wash your hands
- Cleanse the wound completely and remove any remaining medication.
- Remove dead or burned skin and other debris.
- Wear sterile gloves to apply a thin layer (about 1/16 inch) to the wound.
- After application, cover the wound with a dressing or leave it uncovered, as ordered by the health care provider.

Chapter 43: Drugs Treating Mycobacterial Infections

43.1. Patients with pre-existing hepatic disorders, renal insufficiency, or malnutrition, those who abuse drugs or alcohol, and those older than 35 years are at greatest risk of hepatitis resulting from isoniazid therapy.

43.2. Chemoprophylaxis consists of single-drug therapy with isoniazid to prevent active TB. The patient is asymptomatic, and the therapy continues for 6 to 12 months. Active TB therapy requires a multidrug regimen (usually isoniazid, rifampin, and pyrazinamide) and is used in patients with signs and symptoms of TB. Therapy may last up to 18 months.

43.3. TB bacilli have the ability to become resistant to all of the anti-TB drugs. Additionally, resistance develops because of the duration of therapy. Finally, multidrug resistance, or MDR, occurs because adherence to the complete duration of therapy is difficult. Patients repeatedly start and stop their drug therapies, allowing the bacillus to become resistant.

43.4. There are three major obstacles to successful therapy with rifampin. The first obstacle is adherence. Rifampin is given for up to 18 months to treat TB and for 12 months to treat leprosy. The second obstacle is the potential for serious adverse effects. Close monitoring and serial laboratory testing are necessary to ensure the safety of the patient. The third obstacle is the drug–drug interactions induced by rifampin. The patient must understand the importance of contacting the prescriber before taking any new medications, especially prescription medications.

43.5. All mycobacterial infections require lengthy treatment. Patients have difficulty adhering to long-term therapies, especially when the drug therapy does not make the patient feel different.

Chapter 44: Drugs Treating Fungal Infections

44.1. Amphotericin B may produce nephrotoxicity; an infusion reaction marked by headache, chills, fever, rigors, hypotension, bronchospasm, and nausea and vomiting; electrolyte imbalances; and anemia.

44.2. Adverse effects of fluconazole therapy include elevated liver enzyme levels, hepatotoxicity, exfoliative skin disorders, and Stevens-Johnson syndrome.

44.3. Azole drugs that can be used to manage systemic fungal infections include fluconazole, itraconazole, ketoconazole, and voriconazole.

44.4. Griseofulvin therapy make take up to 12 months. Because it can cause blood dyscrasias and hepatic injury, the patient should have a CBC and liver function tests monitored during therapy.

44.5. Most azole drugs inhibit the metabolism of drugs that use the CYP3A4 enzyme system. When the metabolism of a drug is inhibited, the serum concentration of the drug increases, resulting in an increased risk for adverse effects and toxicity.

Chapter 45: Drugs Treating Viral Infections

45.1. Few effective antiviral drugs exist because a virus must replicate within the host cell. Drugs that affect the virus may also affect the host cell and do substantial harm.

45.2. Acyclovir is phosphorylated into its active form by the enzyme thymidine kinase. In its active form, acyclovir competes for a position in the DNA chain of the herpesvirus and terminates DNA synthesis.

45.3. Acyclovir should be given cautiously to patients with renal disease, seizures, and other neurologic disorders.

45.4. The interferons are used in managing hepatitis. The FDA approves each type of interferon for a specific subtype of virus; however, the interferons may also be used "off-label" for another subtype.

45.5. HIV drug resistance may occur in chronic HBV patients with unrecognized or untreated HIV infection.

45.6. Amantadine and rimantadine are effective for the prophylaxis or management of influenza A, whereas oseltamivir and zanamivir are effective for both influenza types A and B.

45.7. Although oseltamivir and zanamivir are useful to decrease the symptoms of influenza, they do not replace the need for a yearly influenza vaccination for patients who are immunocompromised.

45.8. Ribavirin is not generally used in adults because adult patients are usually not affected by respiratory syncytial virus (RSV). Moreover, ribavirin is a teratogen and may produce testicular lesions.

45.9. Ribavirin is used to treat RSV, whereas palivizumab and RSV-IG are prophylactic drugs given to infants at risk for RSV.

Chapter 46: Drugs Treating HIV Infection and AIDS

46.1. Blood testing is used to diagnose HIV. To detect antibodies to HIV, the patient may have an EIA, ELISA, rapid HIV test, or oral HIV test. If the patient tests positive with the EIA or ELISA, a WB test or other confirmatory test is performed to ensure accurate results. To test for presence of the virus itself, a PCR test may be done.

46.2. HIV has an affinity for CD4 cells. These cells are important for normal immune function. Destruction of these cells strips the person of protection against common organisms.

46.3. The CD4 cell count is an indication of the current immunologic status of the patient. The CD4 cell count indicates the amount of damage to the immune system. A viral load count reflects disease progression.

46.4. HIV, like other viruses, has the ability to mutate and thus become resistant to a drug. Use of HAART attacks the virus during multiple stages of the viral replication process. This approach prolongs the time before the virus becomes resistant to a specific antiretroviral drug.

46.5. Anemia, granulocytopenia, and thrombocytopenia are adverse effects that indicate a need to stop zidovudine therapy.

46.6. Tests recommended before zidovudine therapy begins include CBC, blood chemistry profile, CD4 cell count, and viral load. Renal and hepatic function tests should be considered if pre-existing damage is suspected.

46.7. Lifestyle, diet, and habit assessments and interventions that are important when initiating zidovudine therapy include highlighting the importance of adhering strictly to drug therapy; teaching that drug therapy does not affect the transmissibility of the disease; advising a high-carbohydrate, moderate-protein, and low-fat diet; taking zidovudine on an empty stomach; exploring the dangers of substance abuse during therapy and otherwise; and overcoming financial constraints to obtaining the prescribed drugs.

46.8. Protease inhibitors (PIs) work at the last stage of HIV replication. They prevent HIV from being successfully assembled and released from the infected CD4 cell.

46.9. Although nonnucleoside reverse transcriptase inhibitors (NNRTIs) work at the same site as nucleoside reverse transcriptase inhibitors (NRTIs), their mechanism of action is very different. NRTIs constrain HIV replication by incorporating into the elongating strand of viral DNA, which causes chain termination. NNRTIs do not incorporate into viral DNA; instead, they inhibit replication directly by binding noncompetitively to reverse transcriptase.

46.10. Entry inhibitors work by binding to gp41, thereby blocking its ability to bind to other cells. If HIV cannot bind to a cell, it cannot enter the cell; thus, it cannot replicate.

46.11. Many infections that generally do little harm to humans may cause great morbidity and mortality in immunocompromised patients. In a person with a competent immune system, the infections are kept under control. In a person with an immunocompromised system, these minor microbes can create serious illness, blindness, and even death.

46.12. Once inside the CD4 T cell, HIV viral RNA utilizes reverse transcriptase to convert it into DNA. A viral enzyme called integrase then helps to hide HIV's DNA inside the cell's DNA. When this occurs, the cell can begin producing genetic material for new viruses. Inhibiting integrase prevents HIV DNA from entering healthy cell DNA.

Chapter 47: Drugs Treating Parasitic Infections

47.1. Vision examinations are important for patients receiving chloroquine because the drug has potential adverse ophthalmologic effects, including retinopathy. Retinopathy, which can lead to blindness, can progress even after the drug is discontinued.

47.2. Chloroquine is used cautiously in children because they are extremely susceptible to chloroquine toxicity. Fatalities have occurred with relatively small doses.

47.3. Baseline evaluations that should precede long-term antimalarial therapy include CBC, liver function tests, kidney function tests, eye examination, gross hearing evaluation, and ECG.

47.4. A patient with alcoholism should be monitored during antiparasitic therapy to detect hepatotoxicity. Many of the antiparasitic drugs have the potential for causing hepatic toxicity. Alcohol is also hepatotoxic. Therefore, patients with alcoholism may have an increased risk of the hepatic toxicity associated with these drugs.

47.5. Nurses and other health care providers should protect themselves when administering pentamidine because pentamidine frequently causes cough and bronchospasm during inhalation. Patients with immunodeficiency diseases are at high risk for respiratory diseases, such as tuberculosis. During pentamidine therapy, these patients may cough and spread airborne pathogens.

47.6. Before administering pentamidine, evaluate the patient's baseline vital signs. Then with the patient supine, infuse pentamidine over 60 minutes. After the infusion, monitor the patient's blood pressure until it is stable.

47.7. Studies of mebendazole have demonstrated that it causes birth defects in animals and would probably cause similar birth defects in humans.

Unit 11: Endocrine Drugs
Chapter 48: Drugs Affecting Corticosteroid Levels

48.1. The effects of glucocorticoids on metabolism are potent and varied. They include increased blood glucose concentrations, increased breakdown of protein and use of fatty acids for energy, and increased loss of calcium from bones.

48.2. Untreated acute adrenal insufficiency is life threatening. Signs and symptoms include hypoglycemia; anorexia, nausea, and vomiting; hypotension; fluid and electrolyte imbalance—dehydration, hyponatremia, and hyperkalemia; dehydration; and fatigue, weakness, and malaise. Untreated chronic adrenal insufficiency is not immediately life threatening but impairs the person's ability to cope with stress.

48.3. Cushing syndrome is a disease of adrenal hyperfunction. Chronic pharmacologic dosing of corticosteroids can lead to the same physiologic effects as adrenal hyperfunction. These effects are known as cushingoid characteristics and include fat stores in the face (moon face), glaucoma and cataract formation, hirsutism and masculinization, cervicodorsal fat (buffalo hump), extremity thinning and atrophy, abdominal striae, protuberant abdomen, truncal obesity, edema caused by sodium and fluid retention, and brittle bones. Any excess of corticosteroids, whether from endogenous or exogenous causes, can result in cushingoid characteristics.

48.4. Three major actions of the adrenal steroids are (1) metabolic effects on carbohydrate, protein, and fat metabolism; (2) anti-inflammatory and immunosuppressant effects; and (3) sodium-retaining activity associated with potassium loss. The first two actions are classified as glucocorticoid actions, and the third is a mineralocorticoid action.

48.5. The two major clinical uses of adrenal steroids are replacement therapy in endocrine deficiency states and anti-inflammatory or immunosuppressive effects in nonendocrine states such as asthma or organ transplantation.

48.6. Exogenous administration of glucocorticoids suppresses the hypothalamic-pituitary-adrenal (HPA) axis, resulting in the adrenal glands losing their ability to synthesize cortisol and other glucocorticoids. Too abrupt cessation of glucocorticoid use may produce a withdrawal syndrome (i.e., hypotension, hypoglycemia, myalgia, arthralgia, and fatigue), leading to acute adrenal insufficiency (addisonian crisis), circulatory collapse, shock, and death.

48.7. Benefits of alternate-day therapy are reduced adrenal suppression, reduced risk of growth retardation, and reduced overall toxicity and cushingoid changes. The likelihood of adrenal insufficiency is decreased because over the long interval between glucocorticoid doses, plasma glucocorticoids decline to a level that is low enough to permit some production of ACTH and some synthesis of cortisol by the adrenals. The disadvantages related to alternate-day therapy include difficulty with patient adherence, potential for subtherapeutic plasma levels, and inconclusive data that adverse effects are substantially decreased.

48.8. Glucocorticoids interact with several types of drugs. Drugs that decrease the serum concentration of glucocorticoid drugs include barbiturates, hydantoins, and rifamycins. Monitor for therapeutic efficacy of glucocorticoid drugs if these other drugs are given concurrently. Glucocorticoid drugs may decrease the effects of anticholinesterase drugs, oral anticoagulants, and salicylates. Monitor the efficacy of those drugs when given concurrently with a glucocorticoid drug. When glucocorticoid drugs are given with oral contraceptives, monitor for possible steroid toxicity. Potassium-increasing diuretics enhance prednisone's potassium depletion.

48.9. Fludrocortisone is used in the treatment of primary (Addison disease) and secondary adrenocortical insufficiency. It also is used to treat salt-losing adrenogenital syndrome. An unlabeled use is the management of severe orthostatic hypotension. Fludrocortisone possesses both mineralocorticoid and glucocorticoid properties.

48.10. Patient teaching with fludrocortisone is just like patient teaching with the glucocorticoids because fludrocortisone has both mineralocorticoid and glucocorticoid properties. The patient receiving fludrocortisone is at risk for acute adrenal insufficiency when he or she experiences stressful situations during or after drug therapy. Moreover, the patient can develop adverse cardiovascular effects of hypertension, edema, chronic heart failure, and cardiomegaly from the mineralocorticoid actions of the drug. It is vital to stress the importance of regular follow-up visits with the prescriber and prompt reporting of adverse effects of dizziness, severe or continuing headaches, swelling of the lower extremities or feet, and unusual weight gain.

48.11. The major clinical indication for the adrenal steroid inhibitors is Cushing syndrome, which is a rare disorder of adrenal cortical hyperfunction. The prototype inhibitor is aminoglutethimide. Aminoglutethimide suppresses the function of the adrenal cortex and thus reduces the amount of endogenous cortisol.

Chapter 49: Drugs Affecting Blood Glucose Levels

49.1. Insulin lowers blood glucose levels by allowing glucose to leave the blood stream and enter the cells.

49.2. Glucagon helps regulate blood glucose levels. Falling blood glucose levels trigger the release of glucagon from the pancreas, as do sympathetic nerve impulses, exercise, infection, and trauma. In the liver, glucagon stimulates glycogenolysis and gluconeogenesis, resulting in a release of glucose into the blood. Glucagon helps to counterbalance the effect of insulin if insulin causes the blood glucose level to fall below normal.

49.3. A patient with type 1 diabetes mellitus has an absolute deficiency of endogenous insulin, and the disease can be controlled only by restoring insulin by injection. A patient with type 2 diabetes still has some natural insulin synthesis and secretion but the cells are resistant to insulin. This patient's diabetes can usually be controlled by diet, exercise, and oral antidiabetic

drug therapy, although insulin may be required in some patients.

49.4. Peptides in the digestive enzymes of the GI tract will destroy the insulin molecule so insulin cannot be given orally.

49.5. The effect of too much insulin would most likely be hypoglycemia and, in its most severe form, an insulin reaction. Early signs and symptoms are neurologic in nature and include irritability, tremors, headache, fatigue and malaise, diaphoresis, and tachycardia. A later symptom may be loss of consciousness.

49.6. Combining regular and a longer acting insulin provides an immediate onset of insulin (from the regular) to lower the current blood sugar level as well as a sustained effect (from the longer acting insulin) to maintain the glucose in a normal range throughout the day.

49.7. Regular, lispro, aspart, and glulisine insulins can be used as supplemental doses (correctional doses).

49.8. NPH is an intermediate-acting insulin. It is a suspension and is cloudy. Its pharmacokinetics include a definite peak and trough so glucose control can vary. It is often dosed twice a day to achieve glucose control. Glargine is a long-acting insulin. It is not a suspension and is clear in appearance. Its pharmacokinetics do not include a peak and trough, so glucose control is more constant throughout the day. It is dosed once daily at bedtime.

49.9. Hypoglycemia.

49.10. Arcabose reduces the rate of digestion of complex carbohydrates. Less absorption of glucose occurs, because the carbohydrates are not broken

down into glucose molecules. This decreases the blood glucose level.

49.11. Glucagon is used to increase the blood glucose level of patients experiencing severe hypoglycemia. In addition to knowing the symptoms of hypoglycemia the patient and family must be taught correct preparation and administration techniques as it is given SC or IM in the home setting. Furthermore, the family should be taught to provide supplemental carbohydrates as soon as possible after glucagons injection to restore liver glycogen and prevent secondary hypoglycemia.

Chapter 50: Drugs Affecting Pituitary, Thyroid, Parathyroid, and Hypothalamic Function

50.1. Calcium is used in many of the body's metabolic processes, including membrane transport processes, conduction of nerve impulses, muscle contraction, and blood clotting. Calcium levels are maintained within a narrow range by the interactions of parathyroid hormone, calcitonin, and vitamin D. These hormones alter calcium resorption from the intestine, affect osteoclast activity to alter the removal or deposit of calcium in bone, and affect the renal resorption of calcium.

50.2. A combination of neural and endocrine systems, originating in the hypothalamus, regulates central nervous system (CNS), autonomic nervous system (ANS), and endocrine functions. Major hypothalamic regulatory functions include somatic and visceral reactions, including temperature regulation, perspiration, GI activity, regulation of appetite and thirst, blood pressure, respiration, regulation of basic body rhythms (e.g., sleep and menstrual cycles), and complex behavioral and emotional reactions (e.g., sexual behavior and defensive reactions of fear and rage). To promote homeostasis, the hypothalamus transmits stimuli to the pituitary gland, causing hormonal release or hormonal inhibition. When stimulated by the hypothalamus, the pituitary gland releases vasopressin (ADH) to regulate water balance in the system or oxytocin to increase uterine contractions or stimulate milk let-down. The anterior pituitary releases various stimulating hormones that increase the activity of other endocrine glands in response to hypothalamic releasing factors. These other endocrine glands regulate growth, development, and metabolism. The activity of both the hypothalamus and pituitary is carefully balanced through a series of negative feedback signals that maintain the levels of hormone present within an effective range.

50.3. Patients receiving somatropin will require it over the long term. It is administered only by injection. The patient and family need to learn sterile technique and proper methods for reconstituting and storing the solution. In addition, they need to learn how to administer the injection and recognize the importance of rotating sites to prevent complications and ensure adequate absorption.

50.4. Signs and symptoms of hypothyroidism include lethargy, slowing of mental processes, neuropathies, decreased heart rate, decreased cardiac output, eyelid drooping, periorbital edema, enlarged tongue, decreased appetite, constipation, increased cholesterol levels, decreased deep tendon reflexes, decreased renal blood flow with decreased output, hypermenorrhea, decreased libido, pale and puffy skin, dry and brittle hair, brittle nails, and intolerance to cold.

50.5. Gallium can be extremely nephrotoxic. The patient will have to have renal function test results and serum electrolytes monitored closely. Renal failure can further complicate the patient's electrolyte disturbances. The patient needs to be well hydrated during the 5 days of treatment to flush the drug through the kidneys as quickly as possible.

50.6. Calcitonin, salmon is from an animal source, and there is a risk for allergic reaction, especially in patients with a known history of allergic reaction to animal products. A skin test should be administered before the drug is given. If no reaction is noted within 15 minutes of the skin test, the drug can be used. The patient should be evaluated periodically for any sign of the development of an allergic reaction and should be asked to report fever, rash, lethargy, or difficulty breathing.

Chapter 51: Drugs Affecting Men's Health and Sexuality

51.1. The primary effects of testosterone are normal growth and development of the male sex organs and development and maintenance of the male secondary sexual characteristics (e.g., male hair distribution, hair texture and color, laryngeal enlargement and vocal cord thickening [voice deepening], and alterations in body musculature and fat distribution). Secondary effects of testosterone are retention of sodium, potassium, and phosphorus; decreased urinary excretion of calcium; stimulation of the growth of skeletal muscle tissue and enhancement of the growth of long bones in prepubescent boys; ossification of the epiphyseal growth plates; and stimulation of the production of red blood cells by enhancement of the production of erythropoietic-stimulating factor.

51.2. The main risk is premature ossification of the epiphyseal growth plate, resulting in stunted growth.

51.3. cGMP (when activated by nitric oxide) stimulates smooth-muscle relaxation and allows the inflow of blood into the erectile tissue in the penis. Sildenafil inhibits the isoenzyme (phosphodiesterase [PDE] type 5) that metabolizes cGMP. The decrease in the metabolism of cGMP allows cGMP to remain active longer, promoting more smooth-muscle relaxation and inflow of blood. This creates an improved and more sustained erection.

51.4. Finasteride is a pregnancy category X drug. Absorption through the skin is increased if the drug is crushed or broken.

51.5. Poor systemic absorption decreases the risk of adverse effects. Therapeutic effect is achieved without systemic absorption with topical minoxidil.

Chapter 52: Drugs Affecting Women's Health and Sexuality

52.1. Progesterone is used to treat amenorrhea and abnormal uterine bleeding because after ovulation, the ovarian follicle is transformed into the corpus luteum, which secretes a great deal of progesterone (and estrogens). This rise in progesterone makes the endometrium ready for implantation. As progesterone levels (and estrogen levels) rise, production of FSH and LH lowers. This prevents further ovulation. When fertilization does not occur, the corpus luteum disintegrates, and progesterone levels fall. Menstruation occurs. Thus, depending on the timing and duration of therapy, either ovulation can be blocked or menses can be initiated.

52.2. The serious adverse effects from estrogen therapy are: increased risk of endometrial cancer, possibly increased risk of breast cancer, increased risk of thromboembolic disorders (including thrombophlebitis, MI, and pulmonary embolus PE), gallbladder disease, and hypertension.

52.3. Raloxifene can achieve the same effects as estrogen on increasing bone mineral density, and decreasing lipids. Raloxifene does not however have the same effects on uterine or breast tissue that estrogen does. Thus, the risk for endometrial and breast cancer is reduced. This is especially important for women who have high-risk factors for these cancers but also are at risk, or currently have, osteoporosis.

52.4. If a dose of an oral contraceptive is missed, it should be taken as quickly as possible; two tablets may be taken on the same day. Two missed pills should be made up over 2 days. If three consecutive pills are missed, the patient should begin a new cycle the day after the last pill was missed or 7 days after the last pill was taken. Another form of birth control should be used as a backup for at least 7 consecutive days of the new cycle and preferably for the rest of the cycle.

52.5. Instruct the patient to take alendronate at least 30 minutes before eating, drinking any beverage other than plain water, or taking any other medication. Swallow the medicine with 6 to 8 oz (180 to 240 mL) of plain water. Do not take with coffee, juice, or mineral water. The nurse should instruct the patient not to lie down for at least 30 minutes after swallowing the medication.

Chapter 53: Drugs Affecting Uterine Mobility

53.1. Slow upward titration of oxytocin more closely resembles oxytocin excretion, which naturally induces labor. Additionally, doing so minimizes adverse fetal and maternal effects.

53.2. The three phases of oxytocin response are 1) incremental phase (uterine activity increases evenly as the dose of oxytocin increases); 2) stable phase (uterine activity remains constant even if the oxytocin dose increases because the myometrial receptor sites are already full); and 3) hyperstimulation (the dose continually increases, the frequency of contractions increases, but the uterine pressure decreases so that the contractions are less effective).

53.3. Water intoxication can be fatal.

53.4. Nursing assessment that may help to minimize adverse oxytocin effects include maternal pulse rate, blood pressure, and fluid status; duration of contractions; time between contractions; fetal heart rate, and character of fetal movement.

53.5. Terbutaline is a beta agonist that selectively stimulates uterine receptors and stops uterine contractions.

53.6. If tachycardia, palpitations, and nervousness develop during terbutaline infusion, the nurse should slow the infusion, or possibly stop it, and notify the physician or nurse midwife.

53.7. Magnesium sulfate is the drug of choice to treat or prevent seizures associated with preeclampsia, eclampsia, and pregnancy-induced hypertension. It is also used off label to treat preterm labor.

53.8. Calcium gluconate.

53.9. The most common maternal adverse effects are: headache, hyporeflexia, weakness, thirst, flushing, and burning at infusion site. The most common fetal/neonatal adverse effects are: heart rate changes, neonatal hypotonia, and neonatal respiratory depression (possibly serious).

Unit 12: Immune System and Cancer Chemotherapy Drugs
Chapter 54: Drugs Affecting the Immune Response

54.1. Cytokines have the ability to activate and enhance host specific immune responses that are important for recognition of mutations (e.g., cancer cells) and transplanted tissue.

54.2. Interferons and interleukins are both naturally occurring biologic substances called cytokines or lymphokines because they are secreted by activated lymphocytes to create a cell-specific cytotoxic effect.

54.3. Interferons activate normal immunosurveillance properties, aiding in recognition of mutations evidenced as malignant cells. Also, their antiviral properties enhance their ability to destroy tumors that are viral in origin. In addition, their antiproliferative properties help them target rapidly proliferating cells, of which tumor cells are the most likely to demonstrate this property.

54.4. Interleukin-2 is a more potent cytokine that has greater proinflammatory activation, producing more infection and sepsis-like adverse effects. Use of interleukin-2 is also more limited than the interferons, because it does not have the same antiviral or antiproliferative properties.

54.5. Cyclosporine, a common macrolide polypeptide antibiotic agent with potent T lymphocyte–suppressing properties, is used to prevent and treat acute rejection in both solid organ and blood and marrow transplantation. It has also been used successfully to treat severe autoimmune disorders such as rheumatoid arthritis.

54.6. The three most common dose-limiting toxicities of cyclosporine are nephrotoxicity, neurotoxicity, and diabetes generation. Although hypertension may frequently occur, it only sometimes necessitates changing to another agent.

54.7. The most common toxicity limiting therapeutic use of thalidomide is its teratogenic effects, necessitating careful candidate selection and monitoring while proactively providing contraception.

54.8. All patients prescribed thalidomide must enter the S.T.E.P.S. program and consent to therapy while agreeing to not get pregnant or impregnate another. They must also consent to frequent monitoring of their pills, health practices and education reinforcement.

Chapter 55: Targeted Therapies

55.1. Epidermal growth factor receptor (EGFR), vascular endothelial grown factor (VEGF-1, 2, and 3), platelet-derived growth factor beta (PDGF-beta), and transforming growth factor alfa (TGF-Alfa). Intracellular tumor targets that have been identified include: platelet-derived growth factor (PGDF-alfa), hypoxia-inducible factor (HIF), c-Raf, b-raf, and transforming growth factor (TGF).

55.2. Cost and patient adherence.

55.3. Targeted therapies interfere with specific extracellular and intracellular molecules and receptor sites involved with carcinogenesis and tumor growth or proliferation. Chemotherapy is toxic to the cell cycle phases of all cells in the body, therefore causing damage to non-cancerous cells, which leads to a number of toxicities.

55.4. CYP-enzymes play an important role in the metabolism of many of the kinase inhibitors, which can lead to drug interactions. Patients on kinase inhibitors should have a full review of all medications to ensure a maximum benefit and decreased toxicities.

Chapter 56: Drugs That Are Cell Cycle-Specific

56.1. The goals of chemotherapy are cure, control, and palliation.

56.2. The different strategies include adjuvant, induction, consolidation, neoadjuvant, palliative, salvage, and intensification therapy.

56.3. Malignant cells are characterized by the following features:

- Uncontrolled cell proliferation
- Decreased cellular differentiation
- Inappropriate ability to invade surrounding tissue
- Ability to establish new growth at ectopic sites

56.4. To expedite the handling of a spill and to minimize undue patient and employee exposure, well-equipped chemotherapy spill kits should be readily available. To manage spills of chemotherapeutic agents, it is necessary to adhere to the following recommended sequence:

- Post a sign immediately to warn people away from the exposed area.
- Don two pairs of powder-free latex gloves, a disposable gown, and a face shield.
- Wear a NIOSH-approved respirator.
- Place an absorbent pad over the spill to contain it.
- Pick up glass fragments with a scoop and dispose of in a puncture-proof container.
- Clean the area with a detergent three times, from the least contaminated to the most contaminated areas.
- Rinse the absorbed spill area with clean water. Repeat the washing and rinsing.
- Dispose of all cleanup equipment according to institutional policy for chemotherapy waste.
- Document the spill according to institutional policy; usually,

spills of 5 mL or more are reportable. The following data should be included in the documentation: name of chemotherapy agent and approximate volume spilled, how spill occurred, procedures followed to contain and clean up spill, names of people who were exposed, and names of those who were notified of spill.

56.5. Exposure to chemotherapy can occur through the following routes: skin and mucous membrane absorption, inhalation, injection by needlestick, and ingestion.

56.6. The following steps should be taken:

- Stop the infusion immediately and restart the infusion at a new site.
- Apply warm or cold compresses as indicated to the extravasation site, and if prescribed, administer a local antidote, such as hyaluronidase, to minimize any tissue damage.
- Notify the health care provider.
- Rest and elevate the affected extremity for 48 hours.
- Apply a sterile dressing that allows the extravasation area to remain visible. Avoid any pressure to the site.
- Obtain a photograph of the site for baseline comparisons
- Document the following in the patient's medical record per institutional guidelines: date and time of extravasation, name of drug, approximate volume of infiltrate, needle gauge, site of extravasation, symptoms reported by the patient and assessed by the nurse, nursing measures implemented, name of health care provider notified, patient education provided, and nurse's signature.
- Consult the physician regarding need for referral to plastic surgeon, if appropriate.

56.7. The drug should never be administered by IV push or rapid IV infusion because doing so can cause hypotension.

56.8. Hypersensitivity or anaphylaxis-like reactions are manifested by hypotension, chills, fever, facial flushing, bronchospasm, dyspnea, and tachycardia.

56.9. Before administration of paclitaxel, check for premedication orders. To prevent severe reactions, premedication is necessary. Premedication usually consists of corticosteroids (dexamethasone), diphenhydramine, and an H_2-antagonist (e.g., cimetidine), which are given intravenously 30 minutes before the paclitaxel infusion.

Chapter 57: Drugs That Are Cell Cycle-Nonspecific

57.1. Anthracyclines are a group of antitumor antibiotics, which include doxorubicin, daunorubicin, their liposomal counterparts, epirubicin, and idarubicin.

57.2. The highly lipid-soluble nitrosoureas can cross the blood–brain barrier, which is critical in the treatment of central nervous system diseases.

57.3. The drugs used to control acute emesis are the serotonin antagonists (such as odansetron), the NK-1 antagonists (aprepitant), and the corticosteroids (dexamethasone). The anxiolytic lorazepam is an adjunct that may be added to combination therapy to treat emesis.

57.4. Dexrazoxane is a potent intracellular chelating drug that interferes with iron-mediated free radical generation, which is thought to be responsible for anthracycline-induced cardiotoxicity. It is used to decrease the incidence of cardiomyopathy in women with metastatic breast cancer who have received the maximum suggested dose of doxorubicin but would benefit from continuing treatment with doxorubicin. The recommended dose of dexrazoxane to doxorubicin is at a ratio of 10:1 (e.g., dexrazoxane, 500 mg, to doxorubicin, 50 mg). It should be given by slow IV push or rapid IV infusion before administering doxorubicin. The total elapsed time from the beginning of the dexrazoxane infusion to the initiation of doxorubicin should not be more than 30 minutes.

57.5. Drugs used in combination should have the following characteristics:

- Maximum cell kill within the range of toxicity tolerated by the patient
- A broader range of coverage against resistant cell lines in the heterogenous tumor population
- Minimal or slow development of new resistant cell groups

In designing successful drug combinations, the choice of drugs follows these principles:

- Selected drugs should be proven partially effective against the tumor when used alone.
- Ideally, the drugs used in combination are best if they do not have overlapping toxicities.
- The dosages and schedules for the various drugs should be maximized.
- Drugs should be administered at consistent intervals.
- Drugs should be selected to produce synergy.

Index

Note: Page numbers followed by b indicate boxed material; those followed by f indicate figures; those followed by t indicate tables. Drugs are listed in **boldface** type under their generic names; trade names are listed in CAPITAL LETTERS.

in pediatric patients, 71
in pregnancy, 85
Pharmacogenetics, 16, 149–153, 149f, 152b
Pharmacogenomics, 16, 149–153, 149f, 152b
Pharmacokinetics, 42–52. *See also specific drugs*
  absorption in, 42, 43, 44b
  of alcohol, 118
  in breast-feeding, 85
  clearance in, 52
  definition of, 42
  distribution in. *See* Drug distribution, in body
  environmental influences on, 143
  excretion in, 42, 49–50, 49b, 50f
  half-life and, 51
  malnutrition and, 132–133, 132b
  metabolism in, 42, 46–49, 47b, 47t
  in older adults, 97–99, 97b
  in pediatric patients, 71–73, 72t
  phases of, 42
  in pregnancy, 84–85, 85b, 86t
  steady state in, 51–52, 51f
Pharmacology, history of, 15
Pharmacotherapeutics, 42
  definition of, 2
  for older adults, 97
  for pediatric patients, 70–71, 70b, 71f
  in pregnancy, 84
Pharyngitis
  drug therapy for, 692, 694–697, 695t, 696t, 828t, 847t
  pathophysiology of, 694
Pharyngolaryngeal dysthesia, 1255
PHAZYME (**simethicone**), 786–787, 786t
Pheasant's eye, drug interactions of, 582t
PHENAZO (**phenazopyridine**), 883t, 888
Phenazopyridine, 883t, 888
Phencyclidine (PCP), 122, 125t
  bad trip from, 128b
  central nervous system effects of, 116
  street names for, 125t
Phendimetrazine, 394t, 396, 770t, 772
Phenelzine, 245t, 260–265
  adverse effects of, 246t, 261
  contraindications and precautions with, 261
  core drug knowledge for, 260–261, 262t, 263t
  core patient variable assessment for, 261–262
  drug interactions of, 261, 262t, 263t, 370
  drugs related to, 264–265
  food interactions of, 261, 263
  nursing diagnoses and outcomes for, 263
  ongoing assessment and evaluation for, 264
  pharmacodynamics of, 261
  pharmacokinetics of, 261
  pharmacotherapeutics of, 260–261
  planning and intervention for, 263–264
PHENERGAN (**promethazine**), 103t, 775t, 777
Phenobarbital, 235, 299t
  in breast milk, 89t
  drug interactions of
    calcitriol, 1103
    drug interactions of, 1181t
    imatinib, 1206t
    oxcarbazepine, 308
    primidone, 314
    tiagabine, 315
  metabolism of, in pediatric patients, 72–73
  for seizures, 314
Phenothiazines
  drug interactions of
    antacids, 761t
    atropine, 214, 215t
    bromocriptine, 369
    captopril, 502t
    carbidopa-levodopa, 366t
    codeine, 424t

dantrolene, 355t
dextroamphetamine, 390t
epinephrine, 173t
insulin, 1044t
metoprolol, 191t
nortriptyline, 257t
pentamidine, 1000t
phenytoin, 301t
propofol, 327t
propranolol, 191t
SIADH related to, 1074t
Phenotype variations, 149–151, 149f, 152b
Phenoxybenzamine, 185t, 188–189, 518–519
Phensuximide, 311
Phentermine, 394t, 395–397, 770t, 772
  adverse effects of, 395, 396
  contraindications and precautions with, 395
  core drug knowledge for, 395
  core patient variable assessment for, 395
  drug interactions of, 395, 395t
  drugs different from, 396–397
  nursing diagnoses and outcomes of, 396
  ongoing assessment and evaluation of, 396
  pharmacodynamics of, 395
  pharmacokinetics of, 395
  pharmacotherapeutics of, 395
  planning and intervention for, 396
Phentolamine, 185t, 188, 515t, 518–519
Phenylbutazone
  drug interactions of glyburide, 1054t
  gold salts, 469
  insulin, 1044t
  warfarin, 650t
Phenylephrine, 171t, 176–178, 521–522, 699t, 701t
  adverse effects of, 176, 177
  contraindications and precautions with, 176
  core drug knowledge for, 176, 177t
  core patient variable assessment for, 176–177
  drug interactions of, 176, 177t
  drugs related to, 178
  nursing diagnoses and outcome for, 177
  ongoing assessment and evaluation of, 178
  pharmacodynamics of, 176
  pharmacokinetics of, 176
  pharmacotherapeutics of, 176
  planning and intervention for, 177–178
1-[2-Phenylethyl]-4-acetyloxypiperidine, 117
Phenylpropanolamine
  drug interactions of
    caffeine, 399t
    phenelzine, 261
    selegiline, 265
Phenytoin, 297–309, 299t
  adverse effects of, 300–301, 303–304
  for arrhythmias, 618
  contraindications and precautions with, 298, 300, 300b
  core drug knowledge for, 297–301, 300b, 301t
  core patient variable assessment for, 301–302, 302b
  for digoxin toxicity, 585b
  drug interactions of, 301, 301t, 1181t
    calcitriol, 1102t
    carmustine, 1256t
    caspofungin, 655t
    dopamine, 180t
    ethosuximide, 310t
    furosemide, 540t
    imatinib, 1206t
    insulin, 1044t
    isoflurane, 323t
    levamisole, 1184–1185
    lorazepam, 229t
    omeprazole, 752t

oxcarbazepine, 308t
ranitidine, 756t
sertraline, 249t
tiagabine, 315t
  drugs different from, 306–309
  drugs related to, 305–306
  food interactions of, 133
  nursing diagnoses and outcomes for, 302
  off-label uses of, 298
  ongoing assessment and evaluation of, 304
  patient and family education on, 304, 305b
  pharmacodynamics of, 298
  pharmacokinetics of, 298
  pharmacotherapeutics of, 297–298
  planning and interventions for, 302–304
Philadelphia chromosome, 150
Phobias, 223
PHOSPHOLINE IODIDE (**demecarium**), 200t, 211
PHOSPHO-SODA (**sodium phosphate**), 792t, 795
Photosensitivity, 143
Physical dependence, 112
Physical examination, 7
Physical incompatibilities, 64–65
Physicians Desk Reference, 18t
Physiologic classification, 17
Physostigmine, 201t, 211
Phytomedicinals, 136
Phytonadione (**vitamin K**), 650t
Piggybacking, for intravenous drug administration, 36
Pills (tablets), 30–31
  boxes for, 106
  for older adults, 106
Pilocarpine, 199–204, 200t
  adverse effects of, 201–203
  contraindications and precautions with, 201
  core drug knowledge for, 199, 201–202, 202t
  core patient variable assessment for, 202
  drug interactions of, 202, 202t
  drugs closely related to, 203
  drugs different from, 203–204
  nursing diagnoses and outcomes for, 202
  ongoing assessment and evaluation of, 203
  pharmacodynamics of, 199, 201
  pharmacokinetics of, 199
  pharmacotherapeutics of, 199
  planning and interventions for, 202–203
PILOPINE HS. *See* **Pilocarpine**
Pimozide, 275t, 284, 379
  drug interactions of
    aprepitant, 777
    darunavir, 969
    erythromycin, 849t, 850
    itraconazole, 920
    saquinavir, 967t
    somatropin, 967t
    tipranavir, 970–971
Pindolol, 186t, 192-193
PINK BISMUTH (**bismuth subsalicylate**), 788t, 791
Pinworm infections
  drug therapy for, 1002t
  pathophysiology of, 985
Pioglitazone, 1043t, 1059–1060
Piper methysticum, drug interactions of, 347t, 355t
Piperacillin, 819t, 821t, 824–825
Piperacillin-tazobactam, 821t
Piperazine, drug interactions of, 1004
Piperonyl butoxide, pyrethrins with, 1007–1008
PIPRACIL (**piperacillin**), 819t, 821t, 824–825
Pirbuterol, 721t, 725